Workbook for

Surgical Technology: Principles and Practice

Workbook for

Surgical Technology: Principles and Practice

Eighth Edition

Prepared by

Elizabeth Ness, CST, BA
Program Coordinator
Surgical Technology
Macomb Community College
Clinton Township, Michigan

ELSEVIER

Elsevier
3251 Riverport Lane
St. Louis, Missouri 63043

WORKBOOK FOR SURGICAL TECHNOLOGY, EIGHTH EDITION ISBN: 9780323935333

International Standard Book Number: 9780323935333

Senior Content Strategist: Nancy O'Brien
Content Development Specialist: Elizabeth McCormac
Publishing Services Manager: Shereen Jameel
Project Manager: Aparna Venkatachalam

Printed in India

Last digit is the print number: 9 8 7 6 5 4 3 2

Preface

This new edition of the Workbook has been written to solidify a student's awareness of his or her grasp of the topics presented in *Surgical Technology: Principles and Practice*, eighth edition. The questions have been specifically designed to challenge students' strategic thinking skills and to get them to think creatively about scenarios that are commonplace in the modern operating room. The following exercises have been used to meet these goals:

- **Key Terms**. The most important key terms are presented to enhance clarification. Students are asked to differentiate between two terms that are commonly confused and whose precise definitions are key to understanding important concepts.
- **Short Answer** questions apply knowledge learned from the text to a variety of situations.
- **Matching:** These exercises allow students to define and categorize words within a specific area of surgical technology practice. This in turn enhances memorization of each term's meaning and significance.
- **Multiple choice** questions provide a way to differentiate and define information.
- **Labeling** exercises reinforce important anatomy concepts that a surgical technologist should be familiar with.
- **Case Studies** have been carefully written to improve students' critical thinking skills and challenge them to look at clinical situations from various points of view. The case studies also provide a basis for group discussion and knowledge sharing.
- **Skills Checklists** provide clear guidelines on how skills should be performed and help students self-evaluate the performance of core functions by practicing skills.

Contents

Contents

Workbook for

Surgical Technology: Principles and Practice

1 Surgical Technology: The Profession and the Professional

Student's Name ______________________________

KEY TERMS

Write the definition for each term.

1. ABHES: ______________________________
2. ACS: ______________________________
3. Allied health profession: ______________________________
4. AHA: ______________________________
5. AMA: ______________________________
6. ANSI: ______________________________
7. ARC/STSA: ______________________________
8. ASA: ______________________________
9. AST: ______________________________
10. Certification: ______________________________
11. Continuing education: ______________________________
12. CST: ______________________________
13. CST-CFA: ______________________________
14. Nonsterile team members: ______________________________
15. ORT: ______________________________
16. Professional characteristics: ______________________________
17. Proprietary school: ______________________________
18. Scrub: ______________________________
19. Sterile personnel: ______________________________
20. Surgical conscience: ______________________________
21. STSR: ______________________________

COMPUTER ASSIGNMENT

Research what the abbreviations for following organizations stand for and what each of them is responsible for.

1. AORN:

2. ARC/STSA:

3. CAAHEP:

4. NBSTSA:

SHORT ANSWERS

Provide a short answer for each question or statement.

1. What is an ethical dilemma?

2. What are the educational options for students who want to be surgical technologists?

3. Why is it important for a practicing surgical technologist to engage in continued education?

4. Name areas of potential employment for a graduate surgical technologist.

5. List career opportunities for surgical technologists.

6. Surgical conscience is a specific set of professional attributes that are associated with surgery; define:

   Accountability ______________________________

   ____

   Confidentiality ______________________________

   ____

7. List professional ethics for health care workers.

   ____

   ____

   ____

8. What are the characteristics of a professional?

   ____

   ____

9. What types of support and services are provided by AST?

   ____

   ____

   ____

MATCHING

Match the following individuals with a description of their roles. Individuals may have multiple roles, and each question may have more than one answer.

_____ 1. Maintain retraction of tissue

_____ 2. Scrub, gown, and glove self and team members

_____ 3. Communicate effectively with surgeon to prevent errors

_____ 4. Nonsterile team member who acts as an advocate for the patient and provides assistance to the sterile surgical team

_____ 5. Performs surgical maneuvers such as cutting tissue, maintaining hemostasis, and suturing under the direction of the primary surgeon

_____ 6. Specialist in the preparation, handling, and use of instruments

_____ 7. Prepares medications and solutions for use in the surgical wound

_____ 8. Teaches new employees and surgical technology students in surgery

_____ 9. Pursues an advanced degree in hospital administration and management

_____ 10. Trained in the processes of disinfection, inspection, assembly, and sterilization of instrument trays

_____ 11. Maintains a "dry" surgical site by operating suction devices and appropriate use of surgical sponge

_____ 12. Ensures patient chart, including results of diagnostic procedures, permits, and preoperative checklist, accompany the patient in surgery

_____ 13. Prepares instruments and supplies on the sterile field

_____ 14. Nonsterile person who completes documentation, performs skin prep, urinary catheterization, and assists in positioning the patient on the operating table

_____ 15. Assists in hemostatis by clamping blood vessels and securing them with suture

_____ 16. Assists surgeon in specific, well-defined tasks as needed during a procedure

a. Surgical technologist

b. Circulator

c. CST-CFA First Assistant

d. Preceptor

e. Second assistant

f. Leadership and management

MULTIPLE CHOICE

1. The surgical technologist working in a hospital or other facility that provides 24-hour care is usually required to:
   a. Work a double shift
   b. Work a 24 hour shift
   c. Work over time
   d. Be on "call"

2. All of the following are areas for graduate surgical technologists to work except:
   a. Hospitals
   b. Ambulatory surgery center
   c. RN OR educator
   d. Specialty practice

3. Reliability, trustworthiness, responsibility and honesty are all examples of which of the following?
   a. Self-regulation
   b. Integrity
   c. Tactfulness
   d. Respect for rules, regulations, and laws

4. Which of the following is one of the best known ethical standards in medicine?
   a. Ethical dilemma
   b. Empathy
   c. Practice equal rights
   d. Do no harm

5. Which of the following refers to a professional's accountability by admitting any mistakes immediately to prevent harm to the patient.
   a. Surgical conscience
   b. Commitment
   c. Tact and discression
   d. Self-regulation

CASE STUDIES

1. *Read the following case study and answer the questions based on your knowledge of the scope of practice for a surgical technologist:*

   You are a new student in the operating room. Halfway through the procedure you think you notice a tear in the sleeve of your gown. It is a very small tear and not very visible, and you are not sure what to do because you will be embarrassed and do not want to get in trouble. You do not think anyone will notice the tear.

   a. What should you do in this situation?

   b. Will you get in trouble?

2 Communication and Teamwork

Student's Name ____________________

KEY TERMS

1. Assertiveness: ____________________
2. Body language: ____________________
3. Consensus: ____________________
4. Facilitator: ____________________
5. Feedback: ____________________
6. Gossip: ____________________
7. Groupthink: ____________________
8. Message: ____________________
9. Norms: ____________________
10. Receiver: ____________________
11. Rumor: ____________________
12. Sender: ____________________
13. Therapeutic touch: ____________________
14. Win-lose solution: ____________________
15. Win-win solution: ____________________

SHORT ANSWERS

Provide a short answer for each question or statement.

1. What are the elements of positive listening skills?

____

____

2. What environmental barriers to good communication are common in the operating room?

____

____

3. When is communication considered successful?

____

____

MATCHING

Match each term with the correct definition regarding successful communication. Some terms may be used more than once.

______	1. Expressing one's own needs and rights while respecting the needs and rights of others.	a. Conciseness
______	2. Polite concise language without sany rudeness directed respectfully towards the other person.	b. Assertiveness
______	3. Reporting a problem or situation to appropriate personnel, not to someone who does not have any control of the situation.	c. Neutrality
______	4. The message delivered is concise and to the point.	d. Clarity
______	5. Taking consideration the person, time and place when communicating a need in reporting an event or situation.	e. Right person, right time, right place
______	6. Shifting gaze on the other person from one eye to the other.	f. Civility
______	7. A message that carries no emotion.	g. Follow chain of command
______	8. The message is delivered in simple, straight forward language that is understood by those receiving it.	h. Maintain eye contact

MATCHING

Choose from the terms of methods of communication failure listed and match them with their most correct description. You may use an answer more than once.

______	1. Personal views may not coincide with others, making assumptions of what is seen heard and understood based on our views.	a. Cultural competence
______	2. How we perceive a problem, situation, or action sometimes depends on our social and cultural background as much as our knowledge.	b. Emotions
______	3. A preexisting opinion about people based on affiliations, culture, economic status and disease.	c. Environmental barriers
______	4. How we feel at the time of communication, can effect the ability to send and receive messages.	d. Lack of a desire to communicate
______	5. Receiver does not have sufficient knowledge to understand exactly what the sender is trying to communicate.	e. Perception of the situation
______	6. Hearing is a particular problem in the operating room, background noises and muffled speech are all examples of:	f. Bias
______	7. To be successful in sending and receiving information, a person must want to communicate.	g. Lack of understanding
______	8. Skill and knowledge to communicate and integrate well with people from diverse backgrounds.	h. Social and cultural influences

MULTIPLE CHOICE

Choose the most correct answer to complete the question or statement.

1. Communication should take place with the:
   a. Right person, time, and place
   b. Right time, person, and situation
   c. Right situation, person, and place
   d. Right person, place, and things

2. Who is the "right person" to communicate a problem within the workplace?
   a. Top management in all situations so that you are sure the message reaches the most authoritative person
   b. Someone who seems to have the right answers most of the time
   c. One who can sympathize with the problem
   d. One who has the authority to help solve the problem

3. _______ maintains appropriate social boundaries when speaking to patients in the health care environment.
   a. A professional
   b. A department manager
   c. An instructor
   d. Someone who is mature in age

4. The professional understands that most patients _______.
   a. Are naturally concerned and worried
   b. Do not understand the surgery or its risks
   c. Have a high respect for health care workers
   d. Are well informed about the surgery, since they must sign the surgical consent

5. The operating room requires its personnel to work at a high level of mental, physical, and emotional strength. Because of this environment, the work is:
   a. Necessary
   b. Good
   c. Stressful
   d. Rehearsed

6. When working with people with problem behaviors, one must remember to focus on the behavior and not the _______.
   a. Person
   b. Attitude
   c. Team
   d. Task

7. A _______ is a group of people who come together to reach a common goal or set of goals.
   a. Gang
   b. Team
   c. Professional
   d. None of the above

8. Most role confusion is a result of poor:
   a. Teamwork
   b. Groupthink
   c. Attitude
   d. Communication

9. The goal of conflict resolution is to attempt to find a solution that is acceptable to all parties; this is called a _______-_______ solution.
   a. Win lose
   b. Win win
   c. Conflict resolution
   d. Open minded

10. In the role of _______, the surgical technologist tutors the student and shares the duties of a scrubbed technologist.
   a. Team leader
   b. Preceptor
   c. Manager
   d. Instructor

CASE STUDIES

1. *Read the following scenario and then answer the questions that follow:*

You are in the operating room and scrubbed in for an exploratory laparotomy. The anesthesiologist and your circulator are chatting about a movie they both recently saw. The surgeon remains focused on the field. At this point there is increased hemorrhage and the surgery becomes more intense. You interrupt the circulator in her conversation to alert her to the sudden hemorrhage, and ask for more sponges.

After the patient has been taken to the postanesthesia care unit (PACU) and is stable, your circulator comes to you and states that you made her look "stupid" in front of the surgeon and the anesthesiologist.

a. Is the circulator's evaluation of the situation valid?

b. How do you respond to her?

c. What is the real issue here, and does it matter who is right?

3 Medicolegal Aspects of Surgical Technology

Student's Name ______________________________

KEY TERMS

Write the definition for each term.

1. Abandonment: ______________________________
2. Accountability: ______________________________
3. Administrative law: ______________________________
4. Advance directive: ______________________________
5. Adverse event: ______________________________
6. Certification: ______________________________
7. Damages: ______________________________
8. Defamation: ______________________________
9. Delegation: ______________________________
10. Evidenced-based practice: ______________________________
11. Hospital policy: ______________________________
12. Incident report: ______________________________
13. Informed consent: ______________________________
14. Lateral abuse: ______________________________
15. Laws: ______________________________
16. Libel: ______________________________
17. Licensure: ______________________________
18. Malpractice: ______________________________
19. Medical power of attorney: ______________________________
20. Negligence: ______________________________
21. Perjury: ______________________________
22. Practice acts: ______________________________
23. Registration: ______________________________

24. Regulations:

25. Retained foreign object:

26. Sentinel event:

27. Sexual harassment:

28. Slander:

29. Standard of conduct:

30. Statutes:

31. Subpoena:

32. TIMEOUT:

33. Tort:

34. Unretrieved device fragment:

35. Vertical abuse:

SHORT ANSWERS

Provide a short answer for each question or statement.

1. Describe a sentinel event and what categorizes something as a sentinel event.

2. What are the requirements for the delegation of a task?

3. What is accountability, and how does it apply to the surgical technologist's role in the health care facility?

4. What does the Latin phrase *respondeat superior* mean?

5. Who is responsible when a delegated task results in patient harm or injury?

6. In legal terms, what does it mean for a person to "do no harm"? Contrast that with what it means to the operating room team to "do no harm." Are they the same?

7. Can an approved hospital policy contradict the law of the state?

8. What is negligence?

9. What are the four elements of negligence that must be proven in a lawsuit?

10. Why is documentation so important? Explain the medical consequences of poor documentation.

11. How does lateral abuse affect the work environment?

12. How can the receiver of verbal abuse approach the abuser?

13. How do you deal with problem behaviors in the operating room?

14. What is sexual harassment, and how does one deal with it in the operating room?

15. Bullying is the most common abusive behavior in health care. It is defined by The Joint Commission as:

____

____

____

16. List The Joint Commission five categories of work place violence.

1. ____
2. ____
3. ____
4. ____
5. ____

MATCHING

Choose from the terms listed and match them with their most correct description. You may use the same answer more than once.

_____ 1. Legal principles or rules established through legal precedents

_____ 2. Create standards that meet or exceed Joint Commission requirements.

_____ 3. State laws.

_____ 4. Violation may result in disciplinary action by the facility.

_____ 5. Regulations passed by agencies and departments of the government such as the FDA and OSHA.

_____ 6. Practice acts.

_____ 7. Created by specialists within the organization in consultation with The Joint Commission to create best practices.

_____ 8. State and federal laws that make specific behaviors illegal.

_____ 9. Laws that protect the right of individuals.

_____ 10. Rules established by the Environmental Protection Agency (EPA) for the handling of medical waste.

_____ 11. Branch of law that applies previous legal decisions to a case currently being judged.

_____ 12. Types of government law responsible for many agencies that administer laws having to do with health care including Health Insurance Portability and Accountability Act (HIPPA) and Medicare insurance.

a. Hospital policy
b. Statutes
c. Administrative law
d. Legal doctrines
e. Common law
f. Criminal law
g. Federal law
h. Civil law

MULTIPLE CHOICE

Choose the correct answer for the question or statement.

1. You are scrubbed on a case in which the surgeons are discussing the patient's personal affairs that have no bearing on the surgical procedure or medical condition. These comments make you feel uncomfortable; you would consider this:
   a. Not your concern
   b. Lateral abuse
   c. Sexual harassment
   d. Slander

2. Tammy is a program director who frequently talks about her supervisor. Tammy informs the class that her supervisor is uneducated and does not know the standards and guidelines. These comments are:
   a. Defamation
   b. Negligent
   c. Assault
   d. Slander

3. ____________ means deliberate efforts to erode the reputation of another person.
   a. Defamation
   b. Assault
   c. Battery
   d. Slander

4. __________ is the threat or attempt to harm another person.
   a. Battery
   b. False imprisonment
   c. Assault
   d. Slander

5. __________ involves contact with intent to injure and applies even if no injury occurred.
   a. Battery
   b. False imprisonment
   c. Assault
   d. Slander

6. Restraints become a method of managing a group of patients all in one place, possibly against their will. This type of case might be considered as:
   a. Battery
   b. False imprisonment
   c. Assault
   d. Slander

7. HIPAA protects a patient's ___________ and other health information through its privacy rule.
   a. Medical records
   b. Opinions
   c. Legal record including past convictions
   d. Constitutional rights

8. ____________ represent a permanent legal record of the patient's interaction with health care providers and services.
   a. Laboratory results
   b. Surgical consent
   c. Documentation
   d. Forms

9. The ___________ is the process in which the attending practitioner explains the risks, benefits, and alternatives of the surgery to the patient.
   a. Health literacy
   b. Signed consent
   c. Informed consent
   d. Discharge criteria

10. The surgical consent is signed by the ______.
    a. Nurse and anesthesiologist
    b. Surgeon and surgical technologist
    c. Patient, surgeon, and witness
    d. Patient, PCA, and surgeon

11. If a patient is mentally incompetent or incapacitated, who may sign the informed consent on behalf of the patient?
    a. A responsible guardian
    b. An agency representative
    c. A court representative
    d. All of the above

12. Which of the following legal doctrines represents *Res ipsa loquitor*?
    a. "Let the master respond"
    b. "The thing speaks for itself"
    c. "First do no harm"
    d. Doctrine of foreseeability

13. In an effort to prevent harm to the patient, the health professional should be able to predict specific risks associated with their duties that could injure the patient. Which of the following legal doctrines is this?
    a. *Primum non nocere*
    b. *Res ipsa loquitor*
    c. *Respondeat superior*
    d. Doctrine of forseeability

14. What is the most frequent cause of injury in the operating room?
    a. Burns
    b. Falls
    c. Incorrect patient positioning
    d. Wrong site surgery

15. While transporting a patient to the OR, the circulator realized she left the patient's oxygen tank in pre-op holding. She leaves the patient on the gurney in the hallway outside the door to the OR while she runs to get the O_2 tank; meanwhile the patient needed to use the restroom and tried to get off the gurney and fell on the floor. Which of the following is the circulator charged with?
    a. Assault
    b. Battery
    c. Abandonment
    d. Slander

16. Verbal abuse is a significant problem in the ______.
    a. Professional environment
    b. Operating room
    c. Family and work
    d. Work environment

17. What is verbal abuse?
    a. Vulgar remarks
    b. Violent public criticism demeaning another person
    c. Loud and abrasive comments or demands
    d. All of the ablve

18. Verbal abuse sometimes is built into the operating room ______.
    a. Culture
    b. Environment
    c. Management
    d. Surgeons

19. Most people are reluctant to report abuse in the workplace for fear of:
    a. Retaliation
    b. Losing their job
    c. More abuse
    d. Embarassment

20. ______ abuse takes place among staff members of equal rank and position.
    a. Lateral
    b. Verbal
    c. Vertical
    d. Physical

21. Sexual harassment is an extreme abuse of power in which a person engages in the following types of behavior:
    a. Expects sexual favors in exchange for personal or professional gain
    b. Directs sexually explicit comments toward another
    c. Directs vulgar of sexual innuendoes at another
    d. All of the above

22. Victims of sexual harassment should confront the perpetrator when sexual harassment occurs and afterward submit:
    a. A written report
    b. An oral report
    c. Nothing
    d. A warning to everyone in the department

23. Which of the following intentional torts would involve publicly discussing or depicting patients outside the health care environment?
    a. Defamation
    b. Assault
    c. Libel
    d. Invasion of privacy

24. Which of the following is a deliberate effort to erode the reputation of another person in a written form?
    a. Incident form
    b. Slander
    c. Libel
    d. Hospital policy

25. When handling the surgical specimen careful handling and documentation are essential; which of the following could happen if an error occured with improper labeling or loss of specimen?
    a. Disastrous consequences for the patient
    b. Delay in treatment
    c. Misdiagnosis
    d. All of the above

CASE STUDIES

1. *Read the following case study and answer the questions based on your knowledge of unintentional torts or civil wrongs.*

   You have just been served with legal documents that suggest that you were scrubbed in on a procedure in which your patient was burned. You are charged with negligence. For what reasons could you be charged with negligence in this situation?

2. You are a student who is about to graduate and is offered a job at your extern site. The surgeon you are working with is making sexual comments that make you uncomfortable.

   a. What should you do?

   b. Why is documentation so important in issues involving sexual harassment?

   c. Is this sexual harassment?

   d. How do you know it is sexual harassment/

3. *Read the following case study and answer the questions based on your knowledge of the scope and practice for a surgical technologist:*

You are a surgical technologist who has been hired as a new graduate in the local surgery center. You have worked there for about a month, and a seasoned certified surgical technologist is still acting as your preceptor. You have been assigned to work with Dr. Smith, who will be performing an open inguinal hernia procedure. You have never worked with this surgeon before. Once the procedure begins, the surgeon asks you to administer the local anesthetic. You know that as a surgical technologist, you are not allowed to administer medications.

a. Are you performing tasks delegated by the surgeon?

b. Is administration of a local anesthetic within your scope of practice?

c. Can you perform this task if the surgeon states that he will take the responsibility?

d. What should you do in this situation?

4 Health Care Facility Structure and Environment

Student's Name ______________________

KEY TERMS

Write the definition for each term.

1. Accreditation (of a health care facility): ______________________
2. Administration: ______________________
3. AHRQ: ______________________
4. AIA: ______________________
5. APIC: ______________________
6. Back table: ______________________
7. Biomedical engineering technician: ______________________
8. Case cart system: ______________________
9. Central core: ______________________
10. Chain of command: ______________________
11. Decontamination area: ______________________
12. Efficiency: ______________________
13. EPA: ______________________
14. Integrated operating room: ______________________
15. Job description: ______________________
16. Job title: ______________________
17. OSHA: ______________________
18. Personnel policy: ______________________
19. Postanesthesia care unit (PACU): ______________________
20. Risk management: ______________________
21. Semirestricted area: ______________________
22. The Joint Commission: ______________________
23. Traffic patterns: ______________________

24. Transitional area: ______

25. Unrestricted area: ______

SHORT ANSWERS

Provide a short answer for each question or statement.

1. The surgical department is structured and engineered with three objectives in mind. List the three objectives.

   a. ______

   b. ______

   c. ______

2. Traffic patterns in the operating room are restricted. Describe the typical traffic pattern for an operating room, and explain why the movement is restricted.

3. Name two basic principles of infection control used in the physical design of the operating room.

4. List departments that support the operating room.

5. Who is the operating room educator, and what are the job duties of this person in the operating room?

6. Describe the chain of command and give an example of why the chain of command is important for communicating within the department.

7. Design an operating room suite to include all ancillary areas and locations the following areas may be located. Include the following areas:
   Surgical waiting area, urgical offices, locker room, employee lounge, pre-op patient care holding area, scrub sinks, sterile instrument storage room, central core, equipment storage, decontamination, clean processing area, anesthesia department, and PACU

MATCHING

Match each term with the correct definition. Some terms may be used more than once.

_____ 1. Answers phone, relays messages within the surgical department. During emergency, assists management with rescheduling procedures and notifying all personnel of changes.

_____ 2. The patients primary physician in the operating room.

_____ 3. Provides direct patient care of daily living, including assisting with mobility, dressing, eating and toileting.

_____ 4. Specialist in performing procedures and tests measuring brain activity.

_____ 5. Prepares the sterile field, assists surgeon with draping, passing instruments, and accountability for all items in the sterile field used in surgery.

_____ 6. Performs diagnostic imaging procedures of patients, including x-ray, CT, and MRI.

_____ 7. Maintain meticulous assessment, monitoring, and adjustments of the patient's physiological status during surgery.

_____ 8. Performs circulating duties.

_____ 9. Provides extracorporeal (outside the body) oxygenation of the blood during cardiac bypass procedures.

_____ 10. Disinfection, decontamination, inspection, assembly, and sterilization of instruments and supplies.

_____ 11. Provides exposure, hemostasis, suturing, suctioning, and other tasks assigned by the surgeon.

a. Certified Surgical Technologist (CST)

b. Perfusionist

c. Anesthesia Provider

d. Perioperative Registered Nurse

e. Unit Clerk

f. Certified Surgical Technologist - Certified Surgical First Assistant (CST-CFA)

g. Surgeon

h. Patient Care Technician

i. Central Processing Technician

j. Radiology Technician

k. Electroencephalogram (EEG) Technician

MATCHING

Choose from the terms listed and match them with their most correct description. You may use the same answer more than once.

______ 1. Adjustable for height, degree of tilt in all directions used for positioning the patient.

______ 2. Large, stainless steel table on which all instruments and supplies except those in immediate use are placed.

______ 3. Small tables used for skin prep kits, power equipment, and extra sterile supplies that may be too heavy or bulky to place or open on to the back table.

______ 4. Smaller table with one open end that can be raised and lowered.

______ 5. The surface is covered with a firm removable pad.

______ 6. Holds wrapped basin sets.

______ 7. Designated for soiled surgical sponges.

______ 8. Is covered with a sterile drape and used for instruments and supplies that are needed immediately during surgery.

______ 9. Before surgery a sterile pack is opened on this table containing table covers, drapes, towels and gowns.

______ 10. Is designed to support the lip of the basin.

a. Back table
b. Mayo stand
c. Ring stand
d. Kick bucket
e. Prep tables
f. Operating room table

MULTIPLE CHOICE

Choose the most correct answer to complete the question or statement.

1. ____________ is the economic use of time and energy to save unnecessary work, material resources, and time.
   a. Efficiency
   b. Engineering
   c. Environment
   d. Operations

2. ____________ are physical routes for people and equipment in the health care facility, which are designed to prevent the transmission of disease.
   a. Airflow
   b. Traffic patterns
   c. Clean area
   d. Certain areas

3. The department is separated into three distinct areas:
   a. Restricted, semirestricted, and clean
   b. Unrestricted, clean, and dirty
   c. Unrestricted, clean, and restricted
   d. Unrestricted, semirestricted, and restricted

4. The locker room is a/an ____________ area.
   a. Restricted
   b. Transitional
   c. Semirestricted
   d. None of the above

5. Only personnel in complete scrub attire, including hair cap, mask, and facial hair covering, are permitted in the ____________ area.
   a. Restricted
   b. Unrestricted
   c. Semirestricted
   d. None of the above

6. The ____________ core contains clean and sterile equipment and supplies.
   a. Clean
   b. Sterile
   c. Central
   d. Equipment

7. The primary design goal of the floor plan is to create a clear separation between ____________ and ____________ equipment.
   a. Sterile, clean
   b. Soiled, contaminated
   c. Soiled, clean
   d. Dirty, soiled

8. ____________ in the surgical suite are stored in closed cabinets to keep them clean.
   a. Sterile supplies
   b. The computer and accessories
   c. Anesthesia drugs
   d. Anesthesia hoses and masks

9. The operating room table is adjustable for height, degree of tilt in all directions, orientation in the room, articular breaks, and ____________.
   a. Patient weight capacity
   b. Ability to be used for transport
   c. Safety features
   d. Length

10. The back table is a large, stainless steel table on which all instruments, supplies, and equipment needed for surgery are arranged, except for those needed for:
   a. Immediate use
   b. Delivery of anesthesia
   c. Later in the case
   d. Suturing

CASE STUDIES

1. *Read the following case study and, using the information given, create a line chain of command for the facility.*

   You have been recently hired at your local hospital. Mr. Hall is the Chief Operations Officer (COO). He has just been hired. He asks you if you could show him the chain of command for your area of surgical services. Because you work in a very small hospital, there are only two certified surgical technologists, you and one other scrub (Arlinda). Two nurses (Paul and Lydia) work in the OR.

   The charge nurse for your area is Mrs. Jones. She has worked at the hospital in this position for 25 years. The operating room staff educator's name is Abby. Mrs. Markus is the operating room nurse manager, and she reports to the director of perioperative services. His name is Mr. Smith. Mr. Smith reports to the vice president of patient care services, Mr. Zander.

   a. Design a linear chain of command including the name and titles of the individuals with the information provided.

2. *Your hospital has been bought out. They are looking for a new design for the operating room, and you have been chosen to be on the design team. They ask you to do the following:*

   a. Design an operating room.

b. Include all ancillary departments.

c. Include any other items you feel will enhance the department.

5 Supporting the Psychosocial Needs of the Patient

Student's Name ______________________

KEY TERMS

Write the definition for each term.

1. Anesthesia awareness: ______________________
2. Body image: ______________________
3. Maslow's hierarchy of human needs: ______________________
4. Patient-centered care: ______________________
5. Physiological: ______________________
6. Self-actualization: ______________________

SHORT ANSWERS

Provide a short answer for each question or statement.

1. What is the philosophy of Roger's patient-centered care?

____

____

2. What does Maslow's chart teach us about the needs of individuals?

____

____

3. Why would a patient feel a loss of security if he or she were about to undergo a surgical procedure?

____

____

4. Therapeutic supportive patient communication includes:

____

____

5. List effective ways of communicating with the elderly patient.

____

____

6. Explain developmental disability and how it affects communication.

____

____

7. What are some common fears of patients prior to surgery?

____

____

MATCHING

Define Maslow's triangular hierarchy with the correct definition and give an example of each.

1. ______ Sleep	a. Physiological
2. ______ Temperature	b. Protection
3. ______ Mobility	c. Relational
4. ______ Safety	d. Self-actualization
5. ______ Security	
6. ______ Belonging	
7. ______ Altered body image	
8. ______ Achieving personal goals	
9. ______ Elimination	
10. ______ Respiration	
11. ______ Love	
12. ______ Nutrition	

MATCHING

Match the appropriate developmental age groups to the following descriptions.

1. _______ Curious about their bodies, often insist on "helping" with their own care.
2. _______ The operating room is terrifying, there is a strong fear of the unknown, commonly view the hospital and OR as punishment.
3. _______ Very sensitive about body image, resistant to intrusion of privacy and physical exposure.
4. _______ Becomes extremely anxious and frustrated when separated from their primary care provider.
5. _______ Needs to be physically close to their caregivers, often accompanied to the OR by the primary care provider.

a. Infant	birth to 18 months
b. Toddler	19 months to 3 years
c. Preschool	3 to 6 years
d. School age	7 to 12 years
e. Adolescent	13 to 18 years

MULTIPLE CHOICE

Choose the most correct answer for each question or statement.

1. According to Maslow's hierarchy of needs, the most basic of human needs are:
   a. Psychological
   b. Physiological
   c. Metabolic
   d. Pathological

2. Maslow's hierarchy of human needs is depicted as a triangular hierarchy in which the critical needs to preserve life are at the base levels, and other needs that create the rest of the hierarchy are:
   a. Emotional
   b. Social
   c. Spiritual fulfillment
   d. All the above

3. A patient's fear that he or she will not awaken from the anesthetic, or will feel pain while remaining paralyzed, is called:
   a. Anesthesia
   b. Anesthesia awareness
   c. Anesthesia provider
   d. Anesthetic agents

4. Fear of ______ during or after surgery is common among patients who are about to receive a general anesthetic or undergo radical cancer surgery.
   a. Pain
   b. Physical exposure
   c. Loss of control
   d. Death

5. Fear of ______ is a normal protective mechanism.
   a. Pain
   b. Disfigurement
   c. Loss of control
   d. Death

6. Patients undergoing radical or reconstructive surgery have realistic fears about:
   a. Pain
   b. Disfigurement
   c. Loss of control
   d. Death

7. When patients enter the health care system, they often feel a loss of personal rights and ______.
   a. Pain
   b. Disfigurement
   c. Control
   d. Death

8. The fear of ___________ of the body is quite strong in many patients, especially adolescents.
   a. Pain exposure
   b. Physical exposure
   c. Control
   d. Death

9. __________ are powerful needs that determine sense of well-being through the acceptance and nurturing of others.
   a. Esteem
   b. Self-actualization
   c. Love and belonging
   d. Spiritual needs

10. Many patients are afraid that information about their health may not be held in confidence. This is a fear of:
    a. Loss of privacy
    b. Physical exposure
    c. Control
    d. Death

11. Patients often express their religious _________ while in the health care setting. _______ can be a major force for many patients and may even play an equal role in their well-being along with the surgical procedures they undergo.
    a. Love
    b. Belonging
    c. Self-actualization
    d. Faith

12. Maslow's model includes _______ and self-image because the perception we have of ourselves influences motivation and relationships, both social and personal.
    a. Self-esteem
    b. Feelings of acceptance
    c. Family needs
    d. Self-doubt

13. ______ is dependent not only on physical appearance but also on people's normal roles within their family and community.
    a. Self-esteem
    b. Feelings of acceptance
    c. Family needs
    d. Self-image

CASE STUDIES

1. *Read the following case study and answer the questions based on your knowledge of therapeutic communication and geriatric patients:*

You have been asked by the operating room (OR) supervisor to help transport an elderly patient to the pre-op holding area from her patient room. The patient was recently diagnosed with breast cancer. You enter the patient's room and introduce yourself. The following conversation ensues:

You: "Hello, sweetie. My name is Jane Smith, and I'm here to transport you to surgery today. Can you please tell me the name of your surgeon and the type of procedure you will be having today?"

Mrs. Smith: "Dr. Woods is my surgeon, and he is going to remove my cancer today."

You: "Could you be more specific, Mrs. Smith? Where is your cancer?"

Mrs. Smith: "The cancer is in my left breast. (pause) I'm worried about the surgery. My friend said that the procedure is very disfiguring."

You: "Many patients are afraid of surgery, Mrs. Smith."

Mrs. Smith: "I'm worried that I might die from the cancer if the doctor doesn't get it all out."

You: "Would you like to talk to someone about this before we go to surgery?"

Mrs. Smith: "No, I guess not. I'm ready to go."

You: "Okay, can I get you to scoot over to the OR stretcher for me?"

Now answer the following questions about this conversation:

a. Are you comfortable with the way this conversation has gone?

b. Was the conversation helpful in alleviating the patient's fear before you brought her to surgery?

c. Is the conversation you are having with the patient helpful or therapeutic?

d. Modify the conversation so that it becomes therapeutic for the patient. Change your responses above.

2. *Design a Maslow's hierarchy needs chart.*

a. Give an example of each area and how it pertains to the surgical patient.

b. How does the hierarchy relate to the CST during care of the surgical patient?

c. What happens if one area is not given the right attention at the right time?

6 Diagnostic and Assessment Procedures

Student's Name ______________________________

KEY TERMS

Write the definition for each term.

1. ABO blood group ______________________________
2. Acute illness ______________________________
3. Benign ______________________________
4. Chronic illness ______________________________
5. Complete blood count (CBC) ______________________________
6. Computed tomography (CT) ______________________________
7. Contrast medium ______________________________
8. Diastolic pressure ______________________________
9. Differential count ______________________________
10. Digital radiography ______________________________
11. Doppler studies ______________________________
12. Electrocardiography ______________________________
13. Endoscopic procedures ______________________________
14. Fluoroscopy ______________________________
15. Hematocrit (Hct) ______________________________
16. Hemoglobin (Hgb) ______________________________
17. Imaging studies ______________________________
18. Invasive procedure ______________________________
19. Magnetic resonance imaging ______________________________
20. Malignant ______________________________
21. Mean arterial pressure (MAP) ______________________________
22. Metastasis ______________________________
23. Neoplasm ______________________________

24. Nuclear medicine ____________________

25. Orthostatic (postural) blood pressure ____________________

26. Palpating ____________________

27. Partial thromboplastin time (PTT) ____________________

28. Positron emission tomography (PET) ____________________

29. Prothrombin time (PT) ____________________

30. Pulse pressure ____________________

31. Radioactive seed ____________________

32. Radionuclide or isotopes ____________________

33. Radiopaque ____________________

34. Sphygmomanometer ____________________

35. Staging ____________________

36. Systolic pressure ____________________

37. TNM classification system ____________________

38. Transcutaneous ____________________

39. Tumor marker ____________________

40. Vital signs ____________________

SHORT ANSWERS

Provide a short answer for each question or statement.

1. The vital signs include:

____

____

2. During surgery, why is it important to monitor vital signs?

____

____

3. What is the difference between acute and chronic illness? Give an example of each.

____

____

4. Name six different ways a patient's temperature might be taken?

 a. ______
 b. ______
 c. ______
 d. ______
 e. ______
 f. ______

5. Explain the three- or four-point scale used to report the strength of the pulse, as well as the terminology used to describe the pulse.

6. Describe the technique for measuring the respiratory rate.

7. Describe the technique of evaluating the pulse using the associated terms and definitions.

8. List the areas for measuring the pulse.

9. What can alter the respiratory rate?

10. What problems are associated with evaluation of a patient's blood pressure using a simple digital (automatic) sphygmomanometer?

11. Blood pressure varies by age and is affected by various other normal physiological conditions including:

____

____

12. Important normal physiological factors that influence blood pressure include:

____

____

13. List the technique for taking the blood pressure.

____

____

14. List the common errors associated with blood pressure measurement.

____

____

15. The CBC is a basic test used to evaluate the type and percentage of normal components in the blood. What five components are tested?

____

____

____

____

____

16. Positively charged electrolytes are called *cations*. Which cations are routinely tested during a routine blood workup?

____

____

MATCHING

Match each term with the correct definition.

1. ______ A combination of x-ray and digital technology in which images are captured and translated to a flat panel screen that is visible in normal lighting.
2. ______ Is generated by high-frequency sound waves.
3. ______ Uses radiofrequency signals and multiple magnetic fields to produce a high-definition image.
4. ______ Uses the combined technologies of computed tomography and radioactive scanning.
5. ______ X-ray and computer technologies are combined to produce high-contrast cross-sectional images.

a. Computed tomography (CT)
b. Magnetic resource imaging (MRI)
c. Fluoroscopy
d. Positron emission tomography (PET)
e. Ultrasound

MATCHING

1. ______ A person's blood type.
2. ______ Is a basic test used to evaluate the type and percentage of normal components in the blood.
3. ______ The mechanism of blood clotting.
4. ______ Cations and anions.
5. ______ Includes blood glucose, carbon dioxide, creatinine, urea nitrogen, bicarbonate, and several important electrolytes.

a. Complete blood count
b. Metabolic panel
c. Coagulation test
d. Arterial blood gases
e. ABO groups
f. Electrolytes

MATCHING

Match the blood pressure technique with its error. You may use the same answer more than once.

1. ______ Pressing the stethoscope too hard on the artery.
2. ______ Cuff is too loose for the patient.
3. ______ Cuff is too small for the patient.
4. ______ Failure to wait longer than 2 minutes before retaking the blood pressure.
5. ______ Cuff is deflated too quickly.
6. ______ Cuff is deflated too slowly.
7. ______ Air escapes from the cuff even when the valve is closed.
8. ______ Stopping deflation and reinflating the cuff.

a. Faulty equipment
b. False high diastolic
c. False low diastolic
d. False low systolic
e. False high systolic and diastolic

MULTIPLE CHOICE

Choose the most correct answer to complete the question or statement.

1. The most basic form of clinical assessment is (a/an):
   a. CT scan
   b. Chest radiograph
   c. ECG
   d. Vital signs

2. The body requires a core (internal) temperature of approximately 99° F, or
   a. 37.2° C
   b. 38.2° C
   c. 40° C
   d. 42° C

3. Axillary temperature readings are ______ than oral measurements.
   a. 0.3° to 0.6° C higher
   b. 0.5° to 1° F lower
   c. 0.5° C and 1.5° C lower
   d. 0.6° C and 1.6° C higher

4. Which statement about the use of thermometers is true?
   a. Rectal thermometers are the preferred method for measuring temperature.
   b. You do not need to wash your hands after taking a patient's temperature with a forehead or skin thermometer because it is not an invasive procedure.
   c. The rectal method is preferred over the tympanic method.
   d. Tympanic thermometers have a single-use probe cover that is used to prevent cross-contamination of patients.

5. The normal pulse rate for an adult is ______.
   a. 40 to 60 beats per minute
   b. 60 to 100 beats per minute
   c. 75 to 110 beats per minute
   d. 80 to 120 beats per minute

6. The pulse range for an athlete is:
   a. 50 to 100 beats per minute
   b. 60 to 100 beats per minute
   c. 75 to 110 beats per minute
   d. 80 to 120 beats per minute

7. ______ provides detailed information about heart conduction.
   a. ECG
   b. EEG
   c. Blood pressure
   d. Oximetry

8. The basic metabolic panel includes all of the following, *except:*
   a. Blood glucose
   b. Carbon dioxide
   c. Creatinine
   d. Oxygen

9. ______ is performed to assess the functional ability of the coagulation sequence.
   a. Electrolyte testing
   b. ABO group testing
   c. PTT
   d. Measurement of ABG levels

10. Electrolytes include all the following, *except:*
    a. Sodium
    b. Carbonic acid
    c. Potassium
    d. Calcium

11. Hypocalcemia is caused from a deficiency of what electrolyte?
    a. Calcium
    b. Potassium
    c. Sodium
    d. None of the above

12. Hyponatremia is caused from a deficiency of what electrolyte?
    a. Calcium
    b. Potassium
    c. Sodium
    d. None of the above

13. Hypokalemia is caused from a deficiency of what electrolyte?
    a. Calcium
    b. Potassium
    c. Sodium
    d. None of the above

14. Urinalysis is performed to assess the body's overall health, with particular focus on the urinary tract; a simple screening is performed to check for different substances to include all, *except:*
    a. Albumin
    b. Glucose
    c. Magnesium
    d. Leukocytes

15. One of the tests used to detect the type of infection is the:
    a. Biopsy and aspiration
    b. Sensitivity and aspiration
    c. Culture and biopsy
    d. Culture and sensitivity

16. The surgical removal of a small portion of tissue is a(n):
    a. Needle or trocar biopsy
    b. Brush biopsy
    c. Excision
    d. Smear

17. Biopsy obtained by passing a small cylandrical brush is used to sweep a hollow lumen or cavity for cells?
    a. Needle or trocar biopsy
    b. Brush biopsy
    c. Excision
    d. Core biopsy

18. What is used to sweep a hollow lumen or cavity for cells?
    a. Needle or trocar biopsy
    b. Brush
    c. Excision
    d. Smear

19. A procedure in which a core sample of tissue is removed with a hollow needle or trocar in one or more locations of the suspected area is called:
    a. Needle or trocar biopsy
    b. Brush biopsy
    c. Excision
    d. Smear

20. Fluid for pathological examination may be removed and placed on a microscopic slide sprayed with a cell fixative.
    a. Needle or trocar biopsy
    b. Brush biopsy
    c. Aspiration biopsy
    d. Smear

21. A procedure in which tissue is removed and immediately placed in liquid nitrogen is called:
    a. Frozen section
    b. Brush biopsy
    c. Excision
    d. Smear

22. An abnormal growth of tissue that can be benign or malignant
    a. Malignant tumor
    b. Benign tumor
    c. Metastasis
    d. Neoplasm

23. What is composed of cells belonging to a single tissue type and does not spread to distant regions of the body?
    a. Malignant tumor
    b. Benign tumor
    c. Metastasis
    d. Neoplasm

24. New tumors may develop from these "seed" cells.
    a. Malignant tumor
    b. Benign tumor
    c. Metastasis
    d. Neoplasm

25. What is composed of disorganized tissue that exhibits uncontrolled growth?
    a. Malignant tumor
    b. Benign tumor
    c. Metastasis
    d. Neoplasm

26. The culture and sensitivity test is used to:
    a. Determine the presence of a foreign body in tissue
    b. Identify the exact microorganism and appropriate antibiotic to treat the infection.
    c. Detect an infectious agent
    d. Detect the presence of pus in a wound

27. A neoplasm:
    a. Is usually malignant
    b. Does not undergo histological change
    c. Is always benign
    d. Is any abnormal growth

28. Malignant tumors:
    a. Closely resemble the tissue or origin
    b. Release toxins that kill normal cells
    c. Capture nutrients from normal cells
    d. Are single tissue type

29. Metastasis is:
    a. The spread of a benign tumor into other tissues
    b. A tumor that is confined and does not infiltrate the tissue bed
    c. A tumor that exhibits organized growth patterns
    d. Often propagated by seed cells that break away from the tumor, which spreads to distant locations of the body

30. Magnetic resonance imaging (MRI) uses magnetic energy to detect structural tissue abnormalities. Which of the following can cause distortion of MRI imaging?
    a. Biomedical devices
    b. Tattoos containing metal-based dye
    c. Vascular clips
    d. All of the above

31. Which of the following is used during surgery to provide moving images to be seen in real-time?
    a. MRI
    b. PET scan
    c. Fluoroscopy
    d. X-ray

32. Which of the following WBC levels indicate infection?
    a. 5000
    b. 12,000
    c. 8000
    d. 10,000

CASE STUDIES

1. *You are asked to take the patient's vital signs. You can only find one blood pressure cuff. It is intended for normal adults. Your patient's BMI is 40 (morbidly obese).*

    a. How will this cuff affect the blood pressure reading?

b. Can you use this cuff as long as you document which size you used?

c. While the cuff is being inflated, it suddenly pops off the patient's arm. How should you proceed?

7 Environmental Hazards

Student's Name ____

KEY TERMS

Write the definition for each term.

1. Airborne transmission precautions: ____
2. Blood-borne pathogens: ____
3. Electrocution: ____
4. Electrosurgical unit: ____
5. Eschar: ____
6. Flammable: ____
7. Grounding: ____
8. Hypersensitivity: ____
9. Impedance (resistance): ____
10. Latex: ____
11. Neutral zone (no hands) technique: ____
12. Occupational exposure: ____
13. Oxiders: ____
14. Oxygen-enriched atmosphere (OEA): ____
15. Personal protective equipment: ____
16. Postexposure prophylaxis: ____
17. Risk: ____
18. Sharps: ____
19. Smoke plume: ____
20. Standard Precautions: ____
21. Transmission-based precautions: ____
22. Underwriters laboratories: ____
23. Volatile: ____

SHORT ANSWERS

Provide a short answer for each question or statement.

1. What is the fire triangle? How do the components relate to each other?

2. What is a "source of ignition"?

3. What is a patient fire? What are the percentages of the most common locations where patient fires occur? What needs to be done to stop the profression of the fire?

4. List several fuels that are capable of causing surgical site fires and explain how to prevent them.

5. Name the common sources of ignition found in the operating room.

6. If a fire breaks out in the operating room, what three steps should be taken immediately to protect the patient and put out the fire?

7. What parts of a compressed gas cylinder should you inspect for safe operation?

8. Describe the recommended procedure for transporting compressed gas cylinders in the health care facility.

9. List the guidelines for storage of gas cylinders.

10. What is a Material Safety Data Sheet?

11. Why are Standard Precautions used in health care?

12. What diseases require airborne transmission precautions? Droplet precautions?

13. In the operating room, musculoskeletal injuries most often occur as a result of:

LABELING

Using the following triangle, draw in the three components required for fire. Under each of the three components, make a directory of the items specific to the operating room that fall into that section.

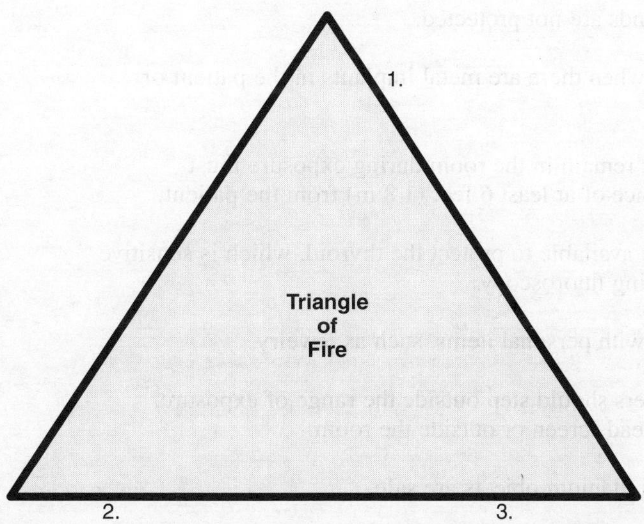

1.

2. ____

____

____

3. ____

____

____

MATCHING

Determine whether each statement refers to ionizing radiation (a) or magnetic resonance imaging (b).

a. Ionizing radiation

b. Magnetic resonance imaging

1. _______ A lead apron must be worn during fluoroscopy to prevent exposure to scatter radiation.
2. _______ Lead aprons must be stored flat or hung in a manner that prevents bending of the material.
3. _______ Remember that a lead apron protects only the areas of the body that are covered by the apron.
4. _______ The primary risk is the presence of metal, which can be drawn from its source and into the path of the powerful magnetic field. For this reason, absolutely no metal objects are permitted in the environment during this process.
5. _______ The eyes and hands are not protected.
6. _______ Cannot be used when there are metal implants in the patient or staff members.
7. _______ Those who must remain in the room during exposure must maintain a distance of at least 6 feet (1.8 m) from the patient.
8. _______ Neck shields are available to protect the thyroid, which is sensitive to radiation, during fluoroscopy.
9. _______ Cannot be used with personal items, such as jewelry.
10. _______ Nonsterile workers should step outside the range of exposure, either behind a lead screen or outside the room.
11. _______ Only plastic and titanium objects are safe.
12. _______ Lead glasses should be worn during exposure to a fluoroscope.
13. _______ The safest place to stand is at a right angle to the beam on the side of the radiograph machine or origin of the radiation beam.

MATCHING

1. _______ ECRI
2. _______ CDC
3. _______ APIC
4. _______ EPA
5. _______ FDA
6. _______ TJC
7. _______ OSHA
8. _______ NIOSH

a. National Institute for Occupational Safety and Health
b. The Joint Commission
c. Occupational Safety and Health Administration
d. Centers for Disease Control and Prevention
e. Association for Professionals in Infection Control and Epidemiology
f. Agency for Healthcare Research and Quality
g. U.S. Environmental Protection Agency
h. U.S. Food and Drug Administration

MULTIPLE CHOICE

Choose the most correct answer to complete the question or statement.

1. Materials and substances that burn are called:
   a. Flammable
   b. Flame resistant
   c. Flame retardant
   d. High alert

2. Which of the following statements is true regarding the high fire risk in the operating room?
   a. Oxygen is heavier than air and settles on the floor.
   b. Oxygen is lighter than air and tends to float above the anesthesia machine.
   c. Oxygen may become confined in areas such as the groin and the axilla.
   d. When nitrous oxide decomposes in the presence of heat, oxygen molecules are produced, creating an oxygen-rich environment.

3. An environment that has a concentration of oxygen greater than 21% is called an:
   a. Oxygen-poor atmosphere
   b. Oxygen-enriched atmosphere
   c. Operating room oxygen
   d. Oxidizer

4. Which of the following are/is considered flammable?
   a. Endotracheal tubes
   b. Surgical drapes
   c. Fibrin glue
   d. All of the above

5. Which of the following are/is considered source(s) of ignition?
   a. Surgical drapes
   b. Laser
   c. Chlorhexidine
   d. Alcohol prepping solution

6. Which of the following acronyms should you remember if you are trying to put out a fire?
   a. PASS
   b. RACE
   c. RICE
   d. PAST

7. Compressed _____________ is used as a power source for instruments, such as drills, saws, and other high-speed tools.
   a. Oxygen
   b. Argon
   c. Nitrogen
   d. Nitrous oxide

8. Which of the following compressed medical gases is used as an anesthetic gas?
   a. Oxygen
   b. Nitrous oxide
   c. Argon
   d. Carbon dioxide

9. Chemicals that are transferred from larger containers to smaller containers must be labeled with the exact information found on the ___________.
   a. MSDS sheets
   b. Original container
   c. OSHA regulation sheets
   d. Manufacturer's directions

10. With regard to toxic chemicals in the operating room, which of the following statements is true?
    a. The cumulative effects can be much greater than the effects of any single exposure.
    b. Many of the chemicals are hazardous, but they usually produce only short-term effects.
    c. Guidelines for handling chemicals are designed to help in the development of risk strategies.
    d. Only the emergency department is required to maintain MSDS for chemicals.

11. Nonresistant materials include:
    a. Metal
    b. Water
    c. Human body
    d. All of the above
    e. None of the above

12. TB is a type of ___________ transmission.
    a. Bloodborne
    b. Airborne
    c. Contact
    d. Standard

13. Rubella is a type of ___________ transmission.
    a. Bloodborne
    b. Airborne
    c. Contact
    d. Standard

14. Influenza is a type of ___________ transmission.
    a. Droplet
    b. Bloodborne
    c. Contact
    d. Standard

15. ___________ is a naturally occurring sap obtained from rubber trees.
    a. OPA
    b. Radiation
    c. Latex
    d. None of the above

16. Scaling, drying, and cracks in skin are symptoms of what type of allergic skin reaction?
    a. Contact dermatitis (nonallergic)
    b. Allergic contact dermatitis
    c. Natural rubber latex allergy
    d. Hypersensitivity

17. ___________ causes dermatitis on contact with the object.
    a. Contact dermatitis (nonallergic)
    b. Allergic contact dermatitis
    c. Natural rubber latex allergy
    d. Hypersensitivity

18. ___________ is the amount of physical effort needed to perform a task, such as moving an object.
    a. Posture
    b. Repetitive motion
    c. Exertion
    d. Contact stress

19. ___________ is a critical component of musculoskeletal stress.
    a. Posture
    b. Repetitive motion
    c. Exertion
    d. Contact stress

20. ___________ places stress on tendons and muscles.
    a. Posture
    b. Repetitive motion
    c. Exertion
    d. Contact stress

21. When ___________, keep the object close to your body.
    a. Lifting
    b. Pushing and pulling
    c. Bending
    d. Standing

22. When ___________, place one foot behind the other, with back foot braced comfortably.
    a. Lifting
    b. Pushing and pulling
    c. Bending
    d. Standing

CASE STUDIES

1. *Read the following case study and answer the questions based on your knowledge of fire in the operating room:*

   You are scrubbed in for an endoscopic procedure. The surgeon has disconnected the light cord from the endoscope and placed it on the surgical drapes without turning it off.

   a. What can you say to the surgeon about safety related to this?

   b. What is your own role here?

2. *Read the following case study and answer the questions based on your knowledge of fire in the operating room:*

   You are searching the OR suite for something that smells as if it is overheating. You see that a C-arm fluoroscopy machine is plugged into the wall. While you are calling the radiology department to come and check out the machine, it bursts into flames.

   a. Using the acronym RACE, describe the actions you will take.

      R ______

      A ______

      C ______

      E ______

8 Microbes and the Process of Infection

Student's Name ______________________________

KEY TERMS

Write the definition for each term.

1. Aerobes: ______________________________
2. Aerosol droplets: ______________________________
3. Anaerobes: ______________________________
4. Bioburden: ______________________________
5. Contaminated: ______________________________
6. Cross-contamination: ______________________________
7. Culture: ______________________________
8. Diffusion: ______________________________
9. Direct transmission: ______________________________
10. Droplet nuclei: ______________________________
11. Endospore: ______________________________
12. Entry site: ______________________________
13. Fomite: ______________________________
14. Infection: ______________________________
15. Inflammation: ______________________________
16. Necrosis: ______________________________
17. Nosocomial infection: ______________________________
18. Opportunistic infection: ______________________________
19. Pathogen: ______________________________
20. Prion: ______________________________
21. Resident microorganism: ______________________________
22. Sterile: ______________________________

23. Suppurative: ______________________________

24. Vector: ______________________________

25. Virion: ______________________________

26. Virulence: ______________________________

SHORT ANSWERS

Provide a short answer for each question or statement.

1. List the tools for identifying microbes and give an example of each.

____

____

2. A surgical site infection may start as an abscess. What exactly is an abscess?

____

____

3. Bacteria that cause infection are called pathogenic. List common pathogenic microbes.

____

____

4. List the most important methods of disease prevention in the health care facility.

____

____

5. List physiological risks for surgical site infection.

____

____

6. Describe and provide examples of nosocomial infection.

____

____

MATCHING

Match the microbe with the correct definition and example.

1. _______ an organism lives on or within another organism (the host) and gains an advantage at the expense of that organism.
2. _______ one organism uses another to meet its physiological needs but causes no harm to the host. For example, the normal human intestinal tract contains many different types of bacteria, such as *Escherichia coli,* that are essential for metabolism.
3. _______ only about 3% to 5% of all microbes are pathogenic. However, nonpathogenic microbes (those that do not usually cause disease) that live in and on the body can become pathogenic under certain conditions.
4. _______ each of the organisms benefits from their relationship in the environment. For example, *Staphylococcus aureus* inhabits normal, healthy skin.

a. Commensalism

b. Mutualism

c. Parasitism

d. Opportunistic organisms

MATCHING

Match the disease transmission with the proper term.

1. _______ *Staphylococcus aureus*
2. _______ Talking, coughing, or sneezing
3. _______ Food
4. _______ Blood-borne pathogens
5. _______ Vector

a. Direct contact

b. Airborne transmission

c. Transmission by body fluids

d. Oral transmission (ingestion)

e. Fly

MATCHING

1. _______ Straight or curved rod shaped bacteria, which can occur singly or in pairs, chains or filaments.
2. _______ Comma-shaped bacteria.
3. _______ Single spherical-shaped bacteria.
4. _______ Curved or spiral-shaped bacteria that may be coiled or loosely curved.
5. _______ Spherical-shaped bacteria.
6. _______ Spherical-shaped bacteria in groups of four or in clusters.
7. _______ A pair of spherical-shaped bacteria.
8. _______ A chain of spherical-shaped bacteria.

a. *Vibrio*

b. *Cocci*

c. *Spirochetes*

d. *Staphylococci*

e. *Streptococci*

f. *Bacilli*

g. *Diplococci*

h. *Micrococci*

MULTIPLE CHOICE

Choose the most correct answer to complete the question or statement.

1. Virology is the study of:
   a. Disease mechanisms, diagnosis, and treatment
   b. Bacteria
   c. Microbes
   d. Viruses
2. Which of the following is *not* a characteristic of eukaryotic cells?
   a. Multicellular
   b. Double-layer membrane
   c. Cell membrane
   d. Include bacteria and Archaea
3. The primary structural difference between the prokaryote and eukaryote is:
   a. Prokaryotes are more like human cells.
   b. Prokaryotes have a semipermeable cell membrane.
   c. Prokaryotes have no distinct nucleus.
   d. Eukaryotes are not pathogenic.
4. The __________ protects the cell from drying and provides resistance to chemicals and invasion by viruses.
   a. Cell wall
   b. Capsule
   c. Cell membrane
   d. Spores
5. The __________ is also called the slime layer.
   a. Cell wall
   b. Cell membrane
   c. Outside layer of the nucleus
   d. Capsule
6. __________ is a process in which particles are engulfed.
   a. Phagocytosis
   b. Pinocytosis
   c. Active transport
   d. Endocytosis
7. The human intestinal tract contains many different types of bacteria, such as *Escherichia coli,* which are essential for digestion. This is an example of:
   a. Mutualism
   b. Parasitism
   c. Symbiosis
   d. Commensalism
8. What is the most effective way of controlling cross-contamination in the health facility environment?
   a. Handwashing
   b. Sterilization of instruments before surgery
   c. Keeping patient rooms clean
   d. Providing lockers for each employee
9. In the __________ phase, symptoms begin to appear.
   a. Incubation
   b. Prodromal phase
   c. Acute phase
   d. Convalescence
10. In the __________ phase, the organism is at its most potent.
    a. Incubation
    b. Prodromal phase
    c. Acute phase
    d. Convalescence
11. In the __________ phase, the pathogens actively replicate.
    a. Incubation
    b. Prodromal phase
    c. Acute phase
    d. Convalescence
12. During the __________ phase, proliferation of the infectious organism slows and symptoms subside.
    a. Incubation
    b. Prodromal phase
    c. Acute phase
    d. Convalescence
13. The prion diseases are very significant in the surgical setting because:
    a. They spread rapidly
    b. All surgical patients are at risk
    c. It is impossible to know who is a carrier
    d. They are resistant to all usual methods of destruction
14. Skin and mucous membrane are considered the first line of defense against disease because:
    a. Skin can be sterilized using disinfectants
    b. Once the skin is broken, infection can develop
    c. Skin contains many blood vessels
    d. Skin is very strong
15. Which surgical wound is associated with a higher risk of infection in the postoperative patient?
    a. Clean
    b. Clean-contaminated
    c. Contaminated
    d. All the above
16. The cardinal signs of inflammation are:
    a. Heat, redness, pain, swelling
    b. Pus, pain, redness, swelling
    c. Heat, pus, fever, pain
    d. Both A and C

17. Surgical site infection begins when a pathogenic or nonpathogenic microorganism colonizes sterile tissues. This can be caused by:
    a. Contamination of the tissues, such as a ruptured bowel or a traumatic wound caused by a foreign object
    b. External contamination of the wound during convalescence
    c. Poor surgical technique
    d. All of the above

18. Bacteria that causes infection is called:
    a. Contagious
    b. Toxic
    c. Pyogenic
    d. None of the above

19. Surgical site infection represents:
    a. The greatest cause of hospital-acquired infection
    b. The second most common cause of hospital-acquired infection
    c. The most avoidable cause of hospital-acquired infection
    d. The main reason for a hospital to lose accreditation

20. Bacteria require basic elemental nutrients, *except:*
    a. Oxygen
    b. Sulfur
    c. Water
    d. Carbon

21. All of the following are Gram-positive bacteria, *except:*
    a. *Staphylococcus epidermidis*
    b. *Streptococcus Pyogenes*
    c. Gonorrhea
    d. *Streptococcus Pneumoniae*

22. A ___________ is a nonliving infectious agent that ranges in size from 10 to 300 nm.
    a. Bacterium
    b. Virus
    c. Fungi
    d. Prion

23. The ___________ is a unique pathogenic substance.
    a. Bacteria
    b. Virus
    c. Fungi
    d. Prion

24. ___________ are found worldwide on living organic substances, in water, and in soil.
    a. Bacteria
    b. Viruses
    c. Fungi
    d. Prions

25. ___________ are a group of single-cell eukaryotic organisms.
    a. Protozoa
    b. Virus
    c. Fungi
    d. Algae

26. ___________ are eukaryotes that belong to the plant kingdom; they include sponges and seaweed.
    a. Protozoa
    b. Virus
    c. Fungi
    d. Algae

27. ___________ exists from the time of birth.
    a. Innate immunity
    b. Adaptive immunity

28. ___________ conferred through exposure to a specific substance or microbe called an *antigen.*
    a. Innate immunity
    b. Adaptive immunity

29. ___________ develops when the body receives the specific disease antibodies from an outside source.
    a. Active immunity
    b. Passive immunity
    c. Vaccination
    d. Hypersensitivity

30. Immune response to a substance is referred to as:
    a. Active
    b. Passive
    c. Vaccines
    d. Hypersensitivity

31. ___________ is a process mediated by the immune system.
    a. True allergy
    b. Passive
    c. Vaccines
    d. Hypersensitivity

32. In certain diseases, the body does not recognize "self." This is known as ___________
    a. True allergy
    b. Autoimmunity
    c. Vaccines
    d. Hypersensitivity

33. There are two types of true allergic reactions:
    a. Immediate and reaction
    b. Reaction and delayed
    c. Delayed and immediate
    d. Immediate and true

34. The most widespread cause of surgical site infection is:
   a. *Streptococcus pyogens*
   b. *Staphylococcus epidermidis*
   c. *Staphylococcus aureus*
   d. *Pseudomonas aeruginosa*

35. The resident bacteria of the GI tract that are the most common cause of urinary tract infections are:
   a. *Staphylococcus epidermis*
   b. *Escherichia coli*
   c. *Neisseria gonorrhoeae*
   d. *Pseudomonas aeruginosa*

36. Spore-forming anaerobic bacterium that causes rapid tissue death in deep sounds deprived of oxygen causing gas gangrene is:
   a. *Salmonella typhi*
   b. *Escherichia coli*
   c. *Clostridium tetani*
   d. *Clostridium perfringens*

37. Spore-forming bacteria that cause severe diarrhea are:
   a. *Clostridium difficile*
   b. *Clostridium perfringens*
   c. *Salmonella typhi*
   d. *Salmonella enterica*

38. A virulent form of *staphylococcus* that is mainly transmitted by direct contact with hands, equipment, and supplies is:
   a. *Escherichia coli*
   b. *Clostridium difficele*
   c. *Pseudomonas aeruginosa*
   d. Methicillin-resistant *staphylococcus aureus and epidermis*

CASE STUDIES

1. *Read the following case study and answer the questions based on your knowledge of microbiology.*

   You are a new surgical technologist setting up for a craniotomy. You are opening your supplies to get ready to set up for the procedure. You have just been informed that the patient is undergoing a brain biopsy for suspected Creutzfeldt-Jakob disease. You recall learning about prions in your microbiology class. What should you do?

9 Sterile Technique and Infection Control

Student's Name ______________________________

KEY TERMS

Write the definition for each term.

1. Antiseptic: ______________________________
2. Chemical barrier: ______________________________
3. Containment and confinement: ______________________________
4. Contaminated: ______________________________
5. Contamination: ______________________________
6. Double gloving: ______________________________
7. Disinfection: ______________________________
8. Gross contamination: ______________________________
9. Hand hygiene: ______________________________
10. Handwashing: ______________________________
11. Hands-free technique: ______________________________
12. Instructions for use (IFU): ______________________________
13. Laminar air flow: ______________________________
14. Neutral zone: ______________________________
15. No-touch technique: ______________________________
16. Nonsterile: ______________________________
17. Nonsterile team members: ______________________________
18. Physical barrier: ______________________________
19. Postexposure prophylaxis (PEP): ______________________________
20. PPE: ______________________________
21. Sharps: ______________________________
22. Squames: ______________________________
23. Sterile field: ______________________________

24. Sterile item: ____________________

25. Sterility: ____________________

26. Strike-through contamination: ____________________

27. Surgical conscience: ____________________

28. Surgical hand antisepsis: ____________________

29. Surgical scrub: ____________________

30. Surgical site infection (SSI): ____________________

31. Surgical wound: ____________________

SHORT ANSWERS

Provide a short answer for each question or statement.

1. List examples of hazardous medical waste materials.

____

____

____

____

2. Where is the sterile field? What is the center of the sterile field?

____

____

3. Sterile objects are contained or confined to create barriers to avoid contact with __________ areas or objects.

4. What should be done before opening any sterile packages?

____

____

____

5. The primary purpose of shoe covers is to ____________________.

6. ______________, ______________, and ______________ are the three types of hand hygiene practiced in the operating room.

7. Masks must be worn in all restricted areas of the operating room. They should not be worn around the neck *at any time* because ____________________

____

____

8. Home-laundered head caps are not sanctioned by any infection control agency because ______

9. What are the two methods for performing surgical hand antisepsis? ______

10. Sterile gowning and gloving takes place immediately after ______

11. The sterile towel, gown, and gloves should be opened on a clean surface away from where sterile instruments and other equipment have been opened to prevent ______

12. Describe the purpose of good hand hygiene and why it is essential for health care professionals. ______

13. Double gloving is perferred over single gloving because ______

14. Closed gloving technique is used when ______

15. Open gloving technique is used for ______

16. When gloving another person, you should open the glove, grasp the upper edges, and offer it with the palm of the glove facing ______

17. If a surgical team member contaminates their glove during surgery, the circulator will remove it. This is done by offering the contaminated hand with the palm facing ______

MATCHING

Match each term with the correct definition.

1. ______ are made of a lint-free synthetic material that is woven loosely enough to allow the breath to pass through effectively but tightly enough to filter 99% of particles of 5 micrograms or larger.
2. ______ are often worn by nonsterile perioperative personnel, for comfort and to prevent contamination of the surgical field through bacterial shedding from the arms.
3. ______ of any kind is a potential source of pathogens.
4. ______ are worn to reduce contamination of the surgical field by loose hair and dandruff from the scalp.
5. Perioperative personnel should wear ______ that are comfortable and easy to keep clean and that protect the wearer against foot injury.
6. ______ are worn any time surgical staff leave the department temporarily.
7. OSHA mandates the use of ______ as part of its blood-borne pathogen standard to protect workers exposed to splashing and splatter of blood and other body fluids.
8. The ______ is designed to prevent the shedding of skin particles and hair into the environment and to protect the wearer from contact with soil and body fluids.

a. Protective eyewear/face shield
b. Head coverings
c. Jewelry
d. Scrub suit
e. Cover gowns/Lab coats
f. Nonsterile cover jacket
g. Masks
h. Shoes and covers

MATCHING

Match each term with the correct transmission precautions.

______ 1. C-Difficile
______ 2. Measles
______ 3. Haemophilius influenzae type B
______ 4. Herpes
______ 5. HIV
______ 6. Varicella
______ 7. Impetigo
______ 8. Nisseria meningitidis
______ 9. MRSA
______ 10. Streptococcal pharyngitis
______ 11. Abscess
______ 12. Rubella
______ 13. HBV

a. Airborne transmission precautions
b. Blood-borne transmission precautions
c. Droplet transmission precautions
d. Contact transmission precautions

MATCHING

Match each area with the required air pressure that is required in the following areas.

______ 1. Clean work room	a. Positive
______ 2. Soiled work room	b. Negative
______ 3. Sterile processing clean work room	
______ 4. Sterile processing decontamination	
______ 5. Operating room	
______ 6. Sterile storage rom	

MULTIPLE CHOICE

Choose the most correct answer to the question or statement.

1. Which of the following is contamination occuring when fluid from a nonsterile surface penetrates the protective wrapper of a sterile item?
   a. tear in kimguard wrapper
   b. safety seal missing
   c. tear in plastic outerwrap
   d. strike-through

2. After an item has been sterilized, its sterility is maintained by:
   a. Surgical technologists
   b. Asepsis
   c. Decontamination
   d. Aseptic technique

3. The ethical and professional motivation that regulates a professional's behavior regarding disease transmission is known as:
   a. Tort
   b. Surgical law
   c. Surgical conscience
   d. Asepsis

4. A scrub suit must be changed if it:
   a. Is contaminated by blood or body fluid
   b. Comes in contact with the patient
   c. Comes in contact with any nonsterile item

5. Long-sleeved cover jackets are worn in the OR by the:
   a. Surgeon
   b. Scrub
   c. Circulator
   d. All of the above

6. At the end of the shift, the surgical technologist may place the scrub suit in his or her locker if:
   a. It is unsoiled
   b. It does not have gross contaminants on it
   c. The surgical technologist has worked less than 8 hours in it
   d. The surgical technologist must never place the scrub suit in their locker at the end of a shift

7. When changing from street clothes to a scrub suit for entering the operating room, the surgical technologist puts on which of the following items first?
   a. Scrub suit
   b. Shoe covers
   c. Cover jacket
   d. Mask

8. The term for the area under the fingernails is:
   a. Sublingual
   b. Subungual
   c. Buccal
   d. Ungal

9. In the surgical scrub, which of the following comes first?
   a. Scrubbing the forearms
   b. Scrubbing the fingers
   c. Remove debris from under the nail beds
   d. Applying the soap from fingers to elbows to "wash" the hands and arms

10. The surgical scrub extends to:
    a. 2 inches above the elbows
    b. The elbows
    c. Just below the elbows

11. When sterile supplies have been opened, the sterile setup is vulnerable to contamination. Once the sterile supplies have been opened, (select all that apply):
    a. They remain sterile for one hour
    b. You must tape the OR door closed
    c. They remain sterile for two hours
    d. They must be continuously monitored to ensure sterility

12. ______ is a way of making decisions and acting on proven methods.
    a. Evidence-based practice
    b. Surgical conscience
    c. Asepsis
    d. Aseptic technique

13. ______ is based on surgical conscience: that is, the ethical and professional motivation that regulates a professional's behaviors regarding disease transmission.
    a. Evidence-based practice
    b. Law
    c. Asepsis
    d. Aseptic technique

14. ______ occurs when the surgeon's gloved hand accidentally touches the nonsterile edge of the surgical drape.
    a. Contamination
    b. A surgical error
    c. Antisepsis
    d. Aseptic technique

15. The ______ is worn by both sterile and nonsterile surgical personnel in the perioperative environment.
    a. Scrub suit
    b. Body lotion
    c. Leather shoes
    d. Lab coat

16. At the close of the case, gown and gloves are removed:
    a. By pulling gloves off first
    b. By removing the gown first and then gloves
    c. By breaking all the ties with gloved hands after removing gloves
    d. By pulling from the back

17. Before opening a sterile pack, the scrub should also check the outside package for the:
    a. Right size
    b. Integrity
    c. Right wrap
    d. Colored tape

18. What operating room furniture should the large pack be placed on before opening?
    a. Ring stand
    b. Mayo stand
    c. Back table
    d. Prep stand

19. What operating room furniture should the instrument tray be placed on prior to opening?
    a. Ring stand
    b. Mayo stand
    c. Back table
    d. Prep stand

20. What operating room furniture should the basin set be placed on before opening?
    a. Ring stand
    b. Mayo stand
    c. Back table
    d. Prep stand

21. Items wrapped in ______ are delivered directly to the scrub by grasping the top edges of the wrapper and peeling the wrapper apart to reveal the sterile item.
    a. Sterile wrap
    b. Sealed pouches
    c. Sealed wrap
    d. Original package

22. What color is a biohazard bag?
    a. Clear
    b. Blue
    c. Red
    d. Yellow

23. The relative humidity of the operating room is within what range?
    a. 25%–65%
    b. 30%–70%
    c. 20%–60%
    d. 20%–70%

24. The recommended air exchanges per hour in the operating room is:
    a. 20–25
    b. 25–30
    c. 30–35
    d. 35–40

25. The range of temperature in the operating room is:
    a. 60–70 degrees F
    b. 65–70 degrees F
    c. 60–65 degrees F
    d. 68–75 degrees F

26. Unidirectional ultra-clean delivery system directing air away from the sterile field creating a "curtain" of air around the sterile field is called:
    a. Negative pressure
    b. Positive pressure
    c. Laminar air flow
    d. Scavenging system

27. Which of the following would require use of ethyl or isopropyl alcohol combined with skin emollients?
    a. Hand hygiene
    b. Surgical scrub
    c. Surgical rub

28. Which of the following would require use of a sterile brush?
    a. Hand hygiene
    b. Surgical scrub
    c. Surgical rub

CASE STUDIES

1. *You are about to begin clinicals and your instructor informed you one of the new students from another program accidently went to a restricted area of the department where she works. Your instructor has now asked you to name all of the zones of the operating room and their associated areas by function as well as describe the required attire for each of the zones.*

10 Decontamination, Sterilization, and Disinfection

Student's Name ______________________________

KEY TERMS

Write the definition for each term.

1. Antiseptic ______________________________
2. Antisepsis ______________________________
3. Bactericidal ______________________________
4. Bacteriostatic ______________________________
5. Bioburden: ______________________________
6. Biofilm ______________________________
7. Biological indicators ______________________________
8. Bowie Dick test ______________________________
9. Case cart system ______________________________
10. Cavitation ______________________________
11. Central processing technician ______________________________
12. Chemical indicator ______________________________
13. Chemial sterilization ______________________________
14. –cidal ______________________________
15. Clean ______________________________
16. Cleaning ______________________________
17. Contaminated ______________________________
18. Decontamination ______________________________
19. Detergent ______________________________
20. Disinfection ______________________________
21. Enzymatic cleaner ______________________________
22. Ethylene oxide (EO) ______________________________
23. Event-related sterility ______________________________

24. Exposure time

25. Fungicidal

26. Gas plasma sterilization

27. Germicidal

28. Gravity displacement sterilizer

29. High-level disinfection (HLD)

30. High-vacuum sterilizer

31. Cobalt-60 radiation

32. Inanimate

33. Implant

34. Immediate-use sterilization

35. Material Safety Data Sheets

36. Medical device

37. Noncritical items

38. Nonwoven

39. Peracetic acid

40. Personal protective equipment (PPE)

41. Physical monitor

42. Prion

43. Reposable

44. Reprocessing

45. Reusable

46. Sanitation

47. Sharps

48. Single-use items

49. Spaulding system

50. Sporicidal

51. Sterile processing department

52. Sterilization

53. Terminal cleaning

54. Turnover ____________________

55. Ultrasonic cleaner ____________________

56. Viricidal ____________________

57. Washer-sterilizer/decontaminator ____________________

58. Woven wrappers ____________________

SHORT ANSWERS

Provide a short answer for each question or statement.

1. Before the washer-sanitizer cycle is finished, the instruments are considered __________. What is the purpose of the washer-sterilizer?

____

____

2. After the instruments are taken to the clean assembly area, what are the next steps for?

____

____

3. Items with a lumen should have a small amount of __________ flushed through them immediately before sterilization.

____

____

MATCHING

Match each term with the correct definition. Some terms may be used more than once.

1. _______ Provides recommended practices and technical information for U.S. medical professions.
2. _______ Accreditation agency for all health care organizations in the United States.
3. _______ Professional association for perioperative nurses.
4. _______ An organization for which standards are developed with the support of the U.S. Food and Drug Administration.
5. _______ Agency of the federal government that provides research and protocols in all areas of public health.
6. _______ Organization that oversees compliance with environmental and patient safety regulations.

a. AAMI

b. AORN

c. CDC

d. TJC

MULTIPLE CHOICE

Choose the most correct answer to complete the question.

1. ________ is a chemical used to remove microorganisms on tissue.
   a. An antiseptic
   b. A disinfectant
   c. Sterilization
   d. All of the above

2. The system that assigns a patient care device a risk category for reprocessing on the specific regions of the body where the device is used is the ________ system.
   a. Spaulding
   b. Sterilization
   c. Dewey
   d. Maslow

3. Which of the following body tissues presents a high risk in the Spaulding system?
   a. Hands
   b. Intact skin
   c. Vascular system
   d. Mucosal membranes

4. ________ is a skilled, certified profession requiring expertise in the science and practice of materials management, decontamination, and sterilization.
   a. Perioperative nursing
   b. Anesthesiology
   c. Central processing technician
   d. Certified nurse's aides

5. The ________ is used to transport sterile and nonsterile instruments and equipment to and from the main operating room area.
   a. Crash cart
   b. Elevator
   c. Case cart

6. The washer-sterilizer or washer-disinfector is used to process all instruments that can tolerate
   a. Heat
   b. Water turbulence and high-pressure steam
   c. Strong disinfectant
   d. Cold solutions

7. After cleaning and disinfection, instruments are ________ to ensure smooth mechanical action.
   a. Unratcheted
   b. Lubricated
   c. Disinfected
   d. Wiped down with alcohol

8. Instruments that have ________ must be disassembled before cleaning and sterilization.
   a. Removable parts
   b. Ratchets
   c. Sharp edges
   d. Blades

9. Instrument trays have a perforated bottom so that:
   a. Steam can circulate up through the tray and adequately cover all surfaces of the instruments.
   b. They are easier for the surgical team to handle.
   c. The instruments are easily put into sets by central processing.
   d. The towels in the instrument sets cannot be damaged by the steam.

10. Which of the following statements is *not* true regarding the use of peel pouches?
    a. Items wrapped in peel pouches must not be placed inside an instrument tray.
    b. Double pouches are unnecessary and may prevent sterilization of the item.
    c. The item in the pouch should clear the seal by at least 1 inch.
    d. Peel pouches are intended for items such as bone rongeurs, rasps, and multiple instruments.

11. Which type of sterilization method requires an aeration?
    a. Steam
    b. Steam under pressure
    c. Ethylene oxide
    d. Gas plasma

12. Which of the following sterlization methods cloth or cellulose cannot be used and it requires items that are going to be sterilized to be clean and dry?
    a. Vaporized hydrogen peroxide
    b. Flash
    c. Ethylene oxide
    d. Steam

13. Which of the following high-level disinfectants could also be used as a sterilizing agent?
    a. Gas plasma
    b. Peracetic acid
    c. Glutaraldehyde
    d. Steam

14. The following are high-level disinfection semi-critical items, except:
    a. Operating room table and accessories
    b. Respiratory therapy equipment
    c. Bronchoscopes
    d. Anesthesia equipment

15. The following are low-level disinfection noncritical items, *except:*
    a. Stethoscopes
    b. Furniture in the surgical suite
    c. Bronchoscopes
    d. Blood pressure cuffs

16. Which is the cleaning process that removes debris from instruments in a process called cavitation?
    a. Cobalt-60
    b. Peracetic acid
    c. Ultrasonic
    d. Hydrogen peroxide

17. What is the exposure time for a wrapped tray of instruments at 250 degrees F?
    a. 15 minutes
    b. 20 minutes
    c. 30 minutes
    d. 45 minutes

18. What is the minimum exposure time for a wrapped tray of instruments at 270 degrees F?
    a. 15
    b. 20
    c. 30
    d. 45

19. Which is used to monitor air in the chamber of high-vacuum sterilizers?
    a. Bowie Dick
    b. Chemical indicator
    c. Mechanical indicator
    d. External chemical indicator

20. Which is the bacteria used to monitor steam sterilization effectiveness?
    a. *Bacillus subtilis*
    b. *Geobacillus stearothermophilis*
    c. *Stearothermophilius bacillus*
    d. *Geobacillus subtilis*

21. During surgery, if there is blood spilled on the floor in the operating room, what should the circulator do?
    a. Wipe and clean the area with a hospital-grade disinfectant
    b. Call housekeeping
    c. Cover it
    d. Do nothing

22. Routine cleaning of the operating room at the close of surgery each day is:
    a. Environmental
    b. Decontamination
    c. Damp dusting
    d. Terminal

CASE STUDIES

1. *Read the following case study and answer the following questions.*

   You are working in an ambulatory ophthalmic surgery center. You have a dual role at the facility—you scrub in surgery and also process and sterilize the instruments. Some of Dr. Smith's patients have developed some postoperative complications after cataract surgery recently.

   a. What is the most probable condition that has occured?

b. What are the causative factors that can contribute to this condition?

c. List AAMI guidelines for processing of ophthalmic instruments to prevent TASS.

11 Surgical Instruments

Student's Name ______________________________

KEY TERMS

Write the definition for each term.

1. Alloy: ______________________________
2. Anastomosis: ______________________________
3. Box lock: ______________________________
4. Chisel: ______________________________
5. Curettage: ______________________________
6. Dilator: ______________________________
7. Double-action rongeur: ______________________________
8. Elevator: ______________________________
9. Gouge: ______________________________
10. Hemostat: ______________________________
11. Rongeur: ______________________________
12. Resection: ______________________________
13. Serosa: ______________________________
14. Shank: ______________________________
15. Single-action rongeur: ______________________________
16. Tenaculum: ______________________________

LABELING

Label the following diagram of a locking clamp.

1. ______________________________
2. ______________________________
3. ______________________________
4. ______________________________
5. ______________________________

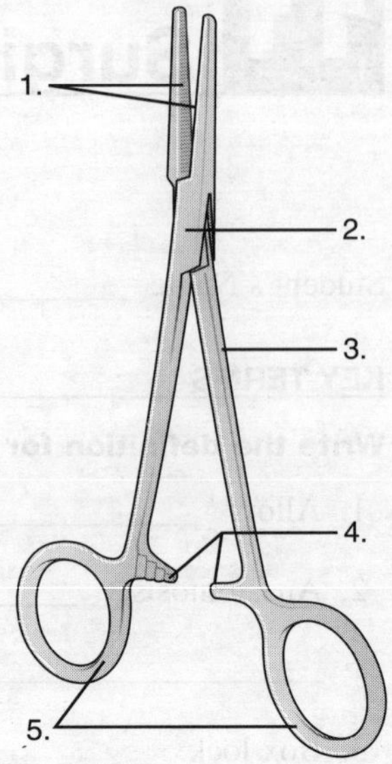

MATCHING

Match each instrument with its classification or function.

1. ______ Crile
2. ______ Allis
3. ______ Babcock
4. ______ Adson
5. ______ Poole
6. ______ Chisel
7. ______ Baumgartner
8. ______ Key
9. ______ Curved Mayo
10. ______ Sarot
11. ______ Kelly
12. ______ Gelpi
13. ______ Leksell
14. ______ Cobb
15. ______ Senn
16. ______ Weitlaner
17. ______ Pituitary
18. ______ Harrington

a. Cutting
b. Clamping/grasping
c. Hemostatic clamp
d. Suturing/needle holder
e. Dilator
f. Handheld retractor
g. Stapling
h. Hemostatic clip
i. Rongeur
j. Self-retaining retractor
k. Probing
l. Periosteal elevator
m. Tissue forcep
n. Atraumatic clamp
o. Filing bone
p. Suction
q. Scraping tissue or bone

19. ______ GIA

20. ______ Russian

21. ______ Osteotome

22. ______ Israel

23. ______ Yankauer

24. ______ Mayo-Hegar

25. ______ Metzenbaum

26. ______ Curette

27. ______ Kerrison

28. ______ Duval

29. ______ Mosquito

30. ______ Debakey

31. ______ Richardson

32. ______ Kocher Oschner

33. ______ Clip applier

34. ______ Balfour

35. ______ Frazier

36. ______ Deaver

37. ______ LDS

38. ______ Rasp

39. ______ Gigli

40. ______ Rake

MATCHING

Match each stapler with the name and function.

1. ______ Performs end-to-end intestinal resection and anastomosis.
2. ______ Right angle used to fit around deep structures for resection and anastomosis.
3. ______ Used for linear side-to-side and end-to-side anastomosis.
4. ______ Suture line is placed around the full circumference of a tubular structure.
5. ______ Places a single line of staples across skin edges.
6. ______ V-shaped staples used to occlude vessels or ducts.

a. Skin stapler
b. GIA Gastrointestinal anastomosis stapler
c. EEA End-to-end anastomosis stapler
d. TA Transverse anastomosis stapler
e. Purse-string stapler
f. Hemostatic clips

MATCHING

Match the correct knife handle with the correct blade.

1. ______ Microblade
2. ______ # 10
3. ______ # 11
4. ______ # 12
5. ______ # 15
6. ______ # 20
7. ______ #21
8. ______ #22

a. # 3 Short
b. # 3 Long
c. # 7
d. #. 4 Short
e. #. 4 Long
f. # 9
g. Beaver

SHORT ANSWERS

Provide a short answer for each question or statement.

1. Explain the difference in a self-retaining retractor and a handheld retractor. Also, give an example of each and the surgical procedure for which you would use the retractor.

2. You are the scrub for an exploratory laparotomy, where the surgeon is irrigating the abdomen. What suction tip would you use and why?

3. You are the second circulator in the room and the circulator asks you to get an EEA stapler. What type of surgical procedure would you use the stapler for?

4. You are scrubbed on an open reduction internal fixation (ORIF) of the ankle, and the surgeon asks for an elevator. What type of elevator would you use and why?

5. During a transurethral resection of the prostate (TURP), the surgeon asks for an instrument to relieve a stricture of the urethra. What type of instrument would you give the surgeon?

6. You are scrubbed on a thyroidectomy and the surgeon asks for a vessel clip. What type would you give the surgeon and why?

7. You are scrubbed on a total knee arthroplasty, and the surgeon asks for an instrument to scrape out a portion of diseased bone. What type of instrument would you give the surgeon?

MULTIPLE CHOICE

Choose the correct answer for each question.

1. An example of an angled instrument is a(n):
   a. Schnidt
   b. Mixter
   c. Osteotome
   d. Deaver

2. Which instrument penetrates the tissue rather than just holding it?
   a. Tenaculum
   b. Babcock
   c. Kelly
   d. Lowman

3. Which instrument is used to grasp the fallopian tube or intestinal tissue?
   a. Allen
   b. Babcock
   c. Kocher
   d. Adson

4. All of the following are types of elevators, *except:*
   a. Penfield
   b. Curette
   c. Cobb
   d. Key

5. Which instrument is used to remove bone using a biting action?
   a. Rongeur
   b. Osteotome
   c. Curette
   d. Chisel

6. Which instrument is used to remove excess fluid from the throat?
   a. Poole
   b. Yankauer
   c. Frazier
   d. Joseph

7. Choose the self-retaining retractor that is used during abdominal surgery.
   a. Finochietto
   b. Balfour
   c. Gelpi
   d. Weitlaner

8. Which instrument is used to clamp small blood vessels?
   a. Babcock clamp
   b. Duval lung clamp
   c. Mosquito hemostat
   d. Crile hemostat

9. What classification is a Kocher?
   a. Clamping
   b. Grasping
   c. Retracting
   d. Cutting

10. What classification is a Babcock?
    a. Clamping
    b. Grasping
    c. Retracting
    d. Cutting

11. What classification is a hemostat?
    a. Clamping
    b. Grasping
    c. Retracting
    d. Cutting

12. What classification is a Richardson Eastman?
    a. Clamping
    b. Grasping
    c. Retracting
    d. Cutting

13. Which needle holder has a curved tip?
    a. Baumgartner
    b. Mayo-Hegar
    c. Sarot
    d. Heaney

14. __________ reduces glare but is also prone to staining.
    a. Highly polished or mirror finish
    b. Satin finish
    c. Black chromium
    d. Titanium anodizing

15. __________ instruments resist staining.
    a. Highly polished or mirror finish
    b. Satin finish
    c. Black chromium
    d. Titanium anodizing

16. __________ is a finishing method that imparts color and hardness to the surface of titanium.
    a. Highly polished or mirror
    b. Satin
    c. Black chromium
    d. Titanium anodizing

17. __________ finish is used on laser surgery instruments.
a. Highly polished or mirror finish
b. Satin
c. Black chromium
d. Titanium anodizing

18. The __________ is a small cup with a sharpened, serrated, or smooth rim at the end of the handle.
a. Rongeur
b. Osteotome
c. Curette
d. Shears

19. A __________ is used to remodel bone.
a. Rasp
b. Curette
c. Chisel
d. Osteotome

20. If an instrument has a gold finish on the ring fingers or handle indicates the working tip or edge of the instrument has:
a. Stainless steel
b. Tungsten carbide
c. Chromium
d. Nickle

21. Supercut scissors have serrations in the cutting edge of the blade. If the surgeon requests a supercut scissor what color handle will you look for on the scissors you have on the back table?
a. Gold
b. Anodized
c. Black
d. Satin

CASE STUDIES

1. *Briefly describe the following surgical instrument grades and finishes. Be sure to include the materials of which they are made and the purposes for which they are used.*

a. Surgical-grade instruments

b. Floor-grade instruments

c. Bright (or mirror) finish instruments

d. Satin finish instruments

e. Ebony finish instruments

f. Disposable instruments

12 Perioperative Pharmacology

Student's Name ______________________________

KEY TERMS

Write the definition for each term.

1. Adverse reaction: ______________________________.
2. Agonist: ______________________________.
3. Allergy: ______________________________.
4. Antagonist: ______________________________.
5. Antibiotics: ______________________________.
6. Bioavailability: ______________________________.
7. Chemical name: ______________________________.
8. Concentration: ______________________________.
9. Contraindication: ______________________________.
10. Contrast media: ______________________________.
11. Controlled substances: ______________________________.
12. Diluent: ______________________________.
13. Dosage: ______________________________.
14. Dose: ______________________________.
15. Drug: ______________________________.
16. Drug administration: ______________________________.
17. Generation: ______________________________.
18. Generic name: ______________________________.
19. Half-life: ______________________________.
20. Hypersensitivity: ______________________________.
21. Intraosseous: ______________________________.
22. Intrathecal: ______________________________.
23. Parenteral: ______________________________.
24. Peak effect: ______________________________.

25. Pharmacodynamics: ______.

26. Pharmacokinetics: ______.

27. Pharmacology: ______.

28. Prescription: ______.

29. Proprietary name: ______.

30. Side effects: ______.

31. Therapeutic window: ______.

32. Topical: ______.

33. Trade name: ______.

34. Transdermal: ______.

35. U.S. Pharmacopeia (USP): ______.

SHORT ANSWERS

Provide a short answer for each question or statement.

1. Drugs used in modern medicine are derived from a number of synthetic and natural sources. Name the sources, and give an example of each.

2. The Joint Commission (TJC) requires health care organizations develop policies that agree with state laws regulating who may handle drugs and in what circumstances. What activities must be regulated?

3. Describe the medication process.

4. The FDA maintains strict regulatory control on devices and substances used on or in the body, which includes:

5. List the four types of allergic reactions, and explain the differences between them.

   a. ______

   b. ______

   c. ______

   d. ______

6. Who or what indicates or recommends a route for drug administration to a patient?

7. If you are scrubbed and you are about to label the medication on your table, what information must be on the label?

8. List the 10 elements that have the most influence on drug errors.

a.

b.

c.

d.

e.

f.

g.

h.

i.

j.

9. What are the three commonly used staining solutions and what are they used for during the intraoperative period?

a.

b.

c.

10. Name a topical antibiotic commonly used for wound irrigation?

11. What is the difference between a staining agent, a dye, and a contrast medium?

12. What is the difference between colloids and crystalloids? Give an example of each.

a. Example of a colloid: ______________________

b. Example of a crystal: ______________________

13. List the seven drug rights and define.

a. ______________________

b. ______________________

c. ______________________

d. ______________________

e. ______________________

f. ______________________

g. ______________________

14. List the protocol for receiving and dispensing drugs on the sterile field.

____

____

15. Using the drug label in Fig. 12.1 in the text, answer these questions:

a. What is the generic name?

____

b. What is the *proprietary* name?

____

c. What is the dosage form?

____

d. What is the dosage and route of administration?

____

e. What are the contraindications?

____

MATCHING

Match each term with the correct definition.

_____ 1. A sterile solution intended to bathe or flush open wounds or body cavities; used topically, never parenterally.

_____ 2. A drug delivery system that often contains an adhesive backing that is applied to an external site on the body.

_____ 3. A solution for the preparation of an iced saline slush, which is administered by irrigation and used to induce regional hypothermia (in conditions such as certain open heart and kidney procedures) by its direct application.

_____ 4. A semisolid dosage form that contains a gelling agent to provide stiffness to a solution or colloidal solution or dispersion.

_____ 5. A product that is packaged under pressure and contains therapeutically active ingredients that are released on activation of an appropriate valve system; it is intended for topical application to the skin as well as local application into the nose (nasal aerosols), mouth (lingual aerosols), or lungs (inhalation aerosols).

_____ 6. An alcoholic or hydroalcoholic solution.

_____ 7. An emulsion, semisolid dosage form used for external application to the skin or mucous membranes.

_____ 8. A mixture of dry drugs or chemicals that on addition of suitable vehicles yields a solution.

_____ 9. A solid dosage form containing medicinal substances.

_____ 10. A material containing drug intended to be inserted securely or deeply in tissue for growth, slow release, or formation of an organic union.

_____ 11. A clear homogeneous liquid that contains one or more chemical substances dissolved in a solvent.

_____ 12. A solid oral dosage form consisting of a shell and filling.

_____ 13. A small piece of flat absorbent material that contains a drug.

_____ 14. Substance intended for external application of consistency to adhere to the skin and attach to a dressing; intended to afford protection and support.

_____ 15. A liquid minutely divided as by a jet or stream of air.

_____ 16. A liquid preparation of increased strength and reduced volume that is usually diluted before administration.

_____ 17. A small, round, solid dosage form containing a medicinal agent intended for oral administration.

_____ 18. A porous, interlacing, absorbent material that contains a drug.

_____ 19. A material usually covered by or impregnated with a drug that is inserted into a body cavity.

a. Aerosol
b. Capsule
c. Cement
d. Concentrate
e. Cream
f. Emulsion
g. Film
h. Gel
i. Graft
j. Implant
k. Inhalant
l. Injection
m. Irrigant
n. Packing
o. Patch
p. Pellet
q. Pill
r. Plaster
s. Powder for solution
t. Solution
u. Solution for slush
v. Sponge
w. Spray
x. Swab
y. Tablet
z. Tincture

______ 20. A dosage form consisting of at least two immiscible liquids, one of which is dispersed as droplets within the other liquid.

______ 21. A class of inhalations consisting of a drug or combination of drugs that are carried into the nasal passage, where they exert their effect.

______ 22. A small sterile solid mass consisting of a highly purified drug intended for implantation in the body.

______ 23. A sterile preparation intended for parenteral use. Five classes of injections are defined by the USP.

______ 24. A thin layer or coating.

______ 25. A slip of skin or other tissue for implantation.

______ 26. A substance that produces a solid union between two surfaces.

MATCHING

Match the route of administration with the dosage form.

1. ______ Sublingual
2. ______ Intravenous
3. ______ Vaginal
4. ______ Intraosseous (IO)
5. ______ Subcutaneous (SQ)
6. ______ Intradermal (ID)
7. ______ Transdermal
8. ______ Intraperitoneal
9. ______ Ingestion
10. ______ Inhalant
11. ______ Intramuscular (IM)
12. ______ Instillation
13. ______ Rectal
14. ______ Buccal
15. ______ Nasal
16. ______ Intraspinal

a. Parenteral

b. Oral

c. Topical

MATCHING

Match the following blood and blood products.

______	1. Concentration of several hemostatic proteins that have been prepared from whole blood.	a. Whole blood
		b. Granulocytes
______	2. Essential for blood coagulation containing coagulation factors, RBCs, and white blood cells administered to patients with bleeding disorders.	c. Packed red blood cells
______	3. Extracted from whole blood and contains normal amounts of coagulation factors.	d. Leukoreduced red blood cells
______	4. Used in patients with hemophilia who require invasive procedures.	e. Factor concentrates
______	5. Contains serum and blood cells, plus anticoagulants and preservatives.	f. Washed red blood cells
______	6. Administered to patients who demonstrate repeated hypersensitivity to blood or blood components.	g. Cryoprecipitate
		h. Platelets
______	7. Administered to patients with a history of non-hemolytic febrile transfusion reactions.	i. Fresh frozen plasma
______	8. Administered to increase the oxygen-carrying capacity of blood.	
______	9. Obtained from an AO Rh-compatible donor used in treatment of severe neutropenia.	

MATCHING

Match the following hemostatic agents and tissue sealants; there may be more than one answer for each item, match all that apply.

1. ______ Fibrant sealant applied to the surface of tissues to bind them together.
2. ______ Collagen absorbable hemostat manufactured from bovine collagen supplied in dry form as powder, sheets, and sponges.
3. ______ Oral anticoagulant using vitamin K antagonist in treatment of venous thromboembolism, pulmonary embolism, and cardiac abnormalities that increase the risk of embolism.
4. ______ Used for the immediate breakdown of systemic blood clots in myocardial infarction, ischemic stroke, and pulmonary embolism.
5. ______ Topical powder applied dry or mixed with isotonic saline for use as a spray, by drop, or soaking sponges.
6. ______ Inhibits blood clot formation but does not dissolve clots.
7. ______ Mesh, granular, or fluff topical mechanical hemostatic agent.
8. ______ Induces blood coagulation.
9. ______ Absorbable dry sponge applied to develop clot formation.
10. ______ Hemostatic material applied to the surface of bleeding bone.
11. ______ Hemostatic material available in mesh, fluff, or powder form.
12. ______ Injectable anticoagulant used in treatment of venous thromboembolism, pulmonary embolism, and cardiac abnormalities that increase the risk of embolism.

a. Coagulant
b. Anticoagulant
c. Thrombolytic drug
d. Warfarin
e. Heparin
f. Floseal
g. Surgiflo
h. Topical thrombin
i. Gelatin
j. Collagen
k. Cellulose
l. Gelfoam
m. Gelfilm
n. Surgifoam
o. Surgical
p. Avitene
q. Bone wax (Ostene)

MATCHING

Match the agents to the conditions they are used for.

1. ______ Used in PACU to prevent or reduce vomiting.	a. Corticosteroid
2. ______ Used to treat certain types of cancers.	b. Antidiabetic
3. ______ Group of drugs for the body's response in autoimmune disease manifestations.	c. Oxytocin
4. ______ Osmotic diuretic used to reduce cerebral edema and intraocular pressure.	d. Antibiotic
5. ______ Used to treat bacterial infections.	e. Antifungal
6. ______ Used to manage insulin.	f. Antineoplastic
7. ______ Used to stimulate production of urine by the kidneys.	g. Anticholinergics
8. ______ Used to treat superficial and systemic fungal infections.	h. Adrenergic
9. ______ Used to augment contractions during labor.	i. Diuretic
10. ______ Used in the treatment of asthma and during anesthesia emergencies such as anaphylactic shock.	j. Mannitol
	k. Antiemetic
11. ______ Used to control airway secretions and to regulate heart rate in selected patients.	

MATCHING

Match the anesthetic agents to their function.

______ 1. Natural or synthetic opiates used for moderate to severe pain control.	a. Benzodiazepine
______ 2. Inhalation anesthetic safely used for both adults and pediatric patients, with a rapid emergence causing it to be useful for outpatient surgery.	b. Barbiturate
	c. Ketamine
______ 3. Reduces anxiety and provides muscle relaxation.	d. Propofol
______ 4. Used in conjunction with general anesthesia to paralyze skeletal muscles, as an essential component to anesthesia.	e. Narcotic
______ 5. Commonly used for the induction of anesthesia, additionally for treatment of seizure disorders.	f. Neuromuscular blocking agent
______ 6. Used for induction and maintenance used in low doses on short procedures for short surgical procedures that do not require unconsciousness.	g. Nitrous oxide
	h. Isoflurane
______ 7. Short rapid-acting dissociative anesthesia that can cause delirium in adults.	i. Sevoflurane
______ 8. Widely used inhalation anesthetic with systemic effects superior to other inhalation agents.	j. Desflurane
______ 9. The most common intravenous sedative used for induction and maintenance of general anesthesia.	k. Enflurane (Ethrane)
______ 10. Colorless, odorless inhalation anesthetic delivered in a gaseous form.	
______ 11. Inhalation anesthetic ideal for outpatient surgery providing rapid emergence used on adults but not used with pediatric patients due to a high incidence of bronchospasm and laryngospasm.	

MULTIPLE CHOICE

1. Which of the following osmotic diuretics is used to reduce intraocular pressure and cerebral edema?
   a. Rantidine
   b. Mannitol
   c. Prednisol
   d. Ergometrine

2. Shich of the following medications can be administered intravenously?
   a. Gelfoam
   b. Thrombin
   c. Ostene
   d. Heparin

3. Using the federal drug schedules of controlled substances, which schedule of drug has a high potential for abuse and has an accepted medical use with restrictions in the United States in which the abuse can lead to severe psychological of physical dependence?
   a. Schedule I
   b. Schedule II
   c. Schedule III
   d. Schedule IV

4. Drugs used to reduce the bodys immune response are ____________.
   a. Diuretics
   b. Anticholinergics
   c. Antiinfective
   d. Corticosteroids

5. Which type of drugs administered in the PACU to prevent or reduce nausea and vomiting postoperatively?
   a. Antiemetic agent
   b. Histamine receptor
   c. Anticholinergic
   d. Adrenegic

CASE STUDY

Read the following case study and answer the questions at the end of the case study.

1. You are assigned to relieve on a lunch break in room 2. The surgical technologist you are relieving reports off to you counts and medications in the field. You notice none of the medications, syringes, or irrigation solutions are labeled. What should you do?

13 Anesthesia, Physiological Monitoring, and Post Anesthesia Recovery

Student's Name ______________________________

KEY TERMS

Write the definition for each term.

1. Airway: ______________________________
2. Amnesia: ______________________________
3. Analgesia: ______________________________
4. Anesthesia: ______________________________
5. Anesthesia care provider (ACP)(AP): ______________________________
6. Anesthesia machine: ______________________________
7. Anesthesia technician: ______________________________
8. Anesthesiologist: ______________________________
9. Anesthetic: ______________________________
10. Amnesia: ______________________________
11. Anxiolytic: ______________________________
12. Apnea: ______________________________
13. Auscultation: ______________________________
14. Aspiration: ______________________________
15. Bier block: ______________________________
16. Breathing bag: ______________________________
17. Bronchospasm: ______________________________
18. Central nervous system depression: ______________________________
19. Coma: ______________________________
20. Consciousness: ______________________________
21. Delirium: ______________________________
22. Discharge against medical advice: ______________________________
23. Emergence: ______________________________

24. Endotracheal tube: ______________________

25. Esmarch bandage: ______________________

26. Extubation: ______________________

27. Gas scavenging: ______________________

28. General anesthesia: ______________________

29. Glasgow coma scale: ______________________

30. Handover: ______________________

31. Homeostasis: ______________________

32. Hypothermia: ______________________

33. Induction: ______________________

34. Intraoperative awareness (IOA): ______________________

35. Intravascular volume: ______________________

36. Intubation: ______________________

37. Laryngeal mask airway (LMA): ______________________

38. Laryngoscope: ______________________

39. Laryngospasm: ______________________

40. Malignant hyperthermia (MH): ______________________

41. Moderate sedation: ______________________

42. Monitored anesthesia care (MAC): ______________________

43. Nasopharyngeal airway: ______________________

44. Neuromuscular blocking agent: ______________________

45. Oropharyngeal airway (OPA): ______________________

46. Perfusion: ______________________

47. Physiological monitoring: ______________________

48. Pneumatic tourniquet: ______________________

49. Postanesthesia care unit (PACU): ______________________

50. Preoperative medication: ______________________

51. Protective reflexes: ______________________

52. Pulmonary embolism (PE): ______________________

53. Pulse oximeter: ______________________

54. Regional block: ____________________

55. Sedation: ____________________

56. Sedative: ____________________

57. Sensation: ____________________

58. Topical anesthesia: ____________________

59. Unconsciousness: ____________________

LABELING

Label the laryngeal mask.

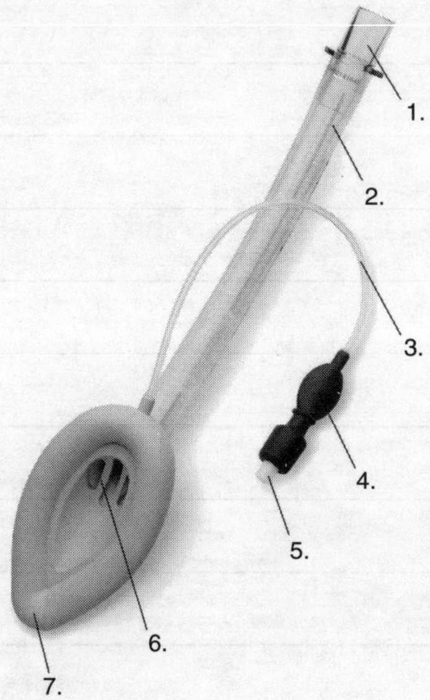

Courtesy LMA North America.

1. ____________________
2. ____________________
3. ____________________
4. ____________________
5. ____________________
6. ____________________
7. ____________________

SHORT ANSWERS

Provide a short answer for each question or statement.

1. Anesthesia means "without sensation." What is the goal of surgical anesthesia?

2. List the primary goal of the ACP.

3. What seven things help the surgeon, the ACP, and the patient decide which type of anesthetic will be best for the individual during the procedure?

   a.

   b.

   c.

   d.

   e.

   f.

   g.

4. Hospitals and other surgical facilities have individual check-in protocols. Which specific details are always verified?

   a.

   a.

   c.

   d.

   e.

   f.

   g.

   h.

   i.

5. What are the four phases/stages of anesthesia?

a. ______________________________

b. ______________________________

c. ______________________________

d. ______________________________

MATCHING

Match each term with the correct definition.

______ 1. Diminished mental, sensory, and physical capacity. It is another way of expressing sedation.

______ 2. The loss of recall (memory) of events.

______ 3. Loss of pain sensation. Specialized nerves transmit signals from the source of pain to the brain. Particular drugs interrupt these pain nerve pathways.

______ 4. The awareness of stimuli, including hearing, sight, smell, taste, touch, temperature (heat and cold), pressure, and pain.

______ 5. The deepest state of unconsciousness, in which most brain activity ceases.

______ 6. A state of awareness in which a person is able to *sense the environment and respond to it*.

______ 7. Severe depression of the central nervous system (CNS) resulting in the *inability to respond to external stimuli*. Deep unconsciousness, such as that achieved during general anesthesia, results in the absence of protective mechanisms, such as swallowing, coughing, blinking, and shivering.

______ 8. A *state of consciousness* described along a continuum. At one end, a person is fully aware of the surroundings and able to respond to stimuli. At the other end is unconsciousness, in which the patient is not aware of the environment and cannot respond to external stimuli including those that are noxious (e.g., pain, cold, heat).

a. Sensation

b. Analgesia

c. Consciousness

d. Sedation

e. Central nervous system depression

f. Unconsciousness

g. Coma

h. Amnesia

MATCHING

Match each parameter measured with the physiological monitoring device.

Parameters measured:

______ 1. Core body temperature

______ 2. Rapid administration of fluids and bloods

______ 3. Myocardial ischemia

______ 4. Detects air embolism

______ 5. Assess valve function

______ 6. Assessment of cardiac preload

______ 7. Auscultation of breathing and heart sounds

______ 8. Measures central venous pressure

______ 9. Ventilator disconnection during general anesthesia

______ 10. Blood oxygen saturation

______ 11. Heart rate

______ 12. Measurement of arterial blood pressure

______ 13. Evaluates myocardium

______ 14. Cardiac preload

______ 15. Heart rate

______ 16. Heart rhythm

______ 17. Adequacy of ventilation

______ 18. Delivered oxygen concentration

______ 19. Gross indication of renal perfusion and intravascular volume

______ 20. Assessment of descending aortic flow

______ 21. Monitor airway pressure

______ 22. Blood pressure

______ 23. Obtain samples of arterial blood for analysis

______ 24. Detection of air embolism

______ 25. Airway pressure

______ 26. Assess intravascular volume

______ 27. Cardiac output

______ 28. Drug administration

a. Pulse oximetry

b. Automatic blood pressure cuff

c. Electrocardiography

d. Capnography

e. Oxygen analyzer

f. Ventilator pressure monitor

g. Temperature-monitoring probe (Foley type)

h. Urine output using Foley catheter

i. Central venous catheter

j. Arterial catheter

k. Precordial doppler

l. Transesophageal echocardiography

m. Esophageal doppler

n. Transpulmonary indicator dilution

o. Esophageal and precordial stethoscope

MATCHING

Match the type of regional anesthesia to method of anesthesia delivery

______ 1. Intravenous block where blood is temporarily displaced from a limb and replaced by a local anesthetic with use of a pneumatic tourniquet.

______ 2. Injection of an anesthetic into superficial tissues to produce a small area of anesthesia.

______ 3. Anesthesia applied on skin, mucous membranes, and superficial eye tissues.

______ 4. Anesthesia agent injected into tissue to anesthetize a group of fine superficial nerves in a small area.

______ 5. Anesthesia injected into the epidural space often used for OB GYN.

______ 6. Injection of anesthesia into the subarachnoid space.

a. Topical anesthesia
b. Local infiltration
c. Nerve block
d. Bier block
e. Spinal anesthesia
f. Epidural

MULTIPLE CHOICE

Choose the most correct answer to complete the question or statement.

1. ________________ is an invasive airway that extends from the mouth to the trachea.
   a. OPA (Oropharyngeal airway)
   b. LMA (Laryngeal mask airway)
   c. NPA (Nasopharyngeal airway)
   d. ET tube (Endotracheal tube)

2. ________________ provides passage between the nostril and the nasopharynx.
   a. OPA (Oropharyngeal airway)
   b. LMA (Laryngeal mask airway)
   c. NPA (Nasopharyngeal airway)
   d. ET tube (Endotracheal tube)

3. ________________ is inserted over the tongue to prevent the tongue or epiglottis from falling back against the pharynx.
   a. OPA (Oropharyngeal airway)
   b. LMA (Laryngeal mask airway)
   c. NPA (Nasopharyngeal airway)
   d. ET tube (Endotracheal tube)

4. ________________ is inserted without the aid of a laryngoscope and fits snugly over the larynx.
   a. OPA (Oropharyngeal airway)
   b. LMA (Laryngeal mask airway)
   c. NPA (Nasopharyngeal airway)
   d. ET tube (Endotracheal tube)

5. The ________________ phase involves continuation of the anesthetic agent.
   a. Induction
   b. Maintenance
   c. Emergence
   d. Recovery

6. Post-anesthesia care is provided in the ________________ phase.
   a. Induction
   b. Maintenance
   c. Emergence
   d. Recovery

7. During the ________________ phase, general anesthesia begins with the administration of the drug ending with loss of consciousness.
   a. Induction
   b. Maintenance
   c. Emergence
   d. Recovery

8. The ________________ phase is the withdrawing of the anesthetic.
   a. Induction
   b. Maintenance
   c. Emergence
   d. Recovery

9. During ________________ the patient is relaxed, and protective reflexes are lost.
   a. Stage 1
   b. Stage 2
   c. Stage 3
   d. Stage 4

10. ________________ begins with the administration of induction drugs and ends with loss of consciousness.
    a. Stage 1
    b. Stage 2
    c. Stage 3
    d. Stage 4

11. During what stage can anesthesia overdose resulting in severe respiratory and circulatory collapse occur?
a. Stage 1
b. Stage 2
c. Stage 3
d. Stage 4

12. During ____________________, delirium ensues, marked by unconsciousness and exaggerated reflexes.
a. Stage 1
b. Stage 2
c. Stage 3
d. Stage 4

13. ____________________ is induced with the drug ketamine.
a. Dissociative anesthesia
b. Regional anesthesia
c. Conscious sedation
d. Nonreceptive sedation

14. ____________________ provides reversible loss of sensation in a specific area of the body without affecting consciousness.
a. Dissociative anesthesia
b. Regional anesthesia
c. Conscious sedation
d. Nonreceptive sedation

15. MAC stands for:
a. Monitored anesthesia consciousness
b. Monitored anesthetic care
c. Monitored anesthesia care
d. None of the above

16. A ____________________ anesthetic is an injection into superficial tissue to produce a small area of anesthesia.
a. Topical
b. Local
c. Spinal
d. Nerve

17. A ____________________ anesthetic provides anesthesia to a specific area of the body supplied by a major nerve or nerve plexus.
a. Topical
b. Local
c. Spinal
d. Nerve

18. A ____________________ anesthetic is used on mucous membranes and on superficial eye tissue during ophthalmic surgery.
a. Topical
b. Local
c. Spinal
d. Nerve

19. A(n) ____________________ is injection of anesthetic into the intrathecal space.
a. Intravenous block
b. Nerve block
c. Epidural
d. Spinal block

20. A ____________________ is a also known as Bier block.
a. Intravenous block
b. Nerve
c. Epidural
d. Spinal

21. A ____________________ is produced when the anesthetic agent is injected into the epidural space.
a. Intravenous block
b. Nerve block
c. Epidural
d. Spinal block

22. When the body is in a balanced physiological state, it is in:
a. Hemostasis
b. Balanced anesthesia
c. Homeostasis
d. Topical anesthesia

23. Electrocardiography (ECG) measures the:
a. Heart rate per minute
b. Electrical activity of the brain
c. Electrical activity of the heart
d. Respiratory rate per minute

24. Which of the following would *not* be needed for a Bier block procedure?
a. Enflurane
b. Esmarch bandage
c. IV
d. Pneumatic tourniquet

25. Type of shock caused by severe bacterial infection resulting in hypovolemia is called:
a. Hypovolemic
b. Cardiogenic
c. Anaphylaxis
d. Septic

26. Type of shock is the depletion of the total intravascular volume caused by redistribution of body fluids from trauma or burn, or external fluid loss from vomiting, diarrhea, polyuria, or blood lost is called:
a. Hypovolemic
b. Cardiogenic
c. Anaphylaxis
d. Septic

27. Rare physiological response to all volatile anesthetic agents and succinylcholine, symptoms including high core temperature, tachycardia, tachypnea, and increased muscle rigidity is called:
    a. Hemorrhage
    b. Shock
    c. Malignant hyperthermia
    d. Laryngospasm

28. Dantrolene (Dantrium) is an emergency drug used to treat:
    a. Cardiopulmonary arrest
    b. Malignant hyperthermia
    c. Septic shock
    d. Hypovolemic shock

29. ______________ complications can be managed by an anelgesic.
    a. Respiratory
    b. Pain
    c. Cardiovascular
    d. Metabolic

30. The patient history includes all of the following, *except*:
    a. Age
    b. Allergies
    c. Current medications
    d. Future pathology

31. After receiving the handover, the PACU nurse performs a patient:
    a. Head-to-toe assessment
    b. Pain assessment
    c. Social assessment
    d. Wound assessment

32. Bowel sounds are assessed by:
    a. Observation
    b. Palpation
    c. X-ray
    d. Auscultation

33. Assessment for dehydration includes:
    a. Cardiac dysrhythmia
    b. Alteration in consciousness
    c. Physical signs and symptoms
    d. Blood tests

34. Patients are discharged from the PACU only when they:
    a. Meet discharge criteria
    b. Meet the respiratory standards
    c. Achieve PACU standards
    d. Become normotensive

35. Your male surgical patient is about to be discharged from PACU. Which of the following does *not* meet the criteria for discharge?
    a. The patient arranged for transportation before being admitted for the procedure.
    b. The PACU has called a cab to deliver the patient to his apartment.
    c. The patient has asked his friend to assist him to his home.
    d. The patient's mother has arrived to drive him home and stay with him for the day.

36. It is the responsibility of ______________ to educate the patient before the individual is discharged from the hospital to go home.
    a. The surgical technologist
    b. The surgeon
    c. The anesthesia care provider
    d. Nursing personnel trained in discharge planning

CASE STUDY

1. *You are about to scrub in on a case and the anesthesia care provider informs you and the circulator that the patient has a family member who has experienced malignant hyperthermia in the past.*

    a. What should you do prior to surgery in preparation for the case?

b. What items are available on the malignant hyperthermia cart?

c. The procedure has begun and the ACP alerts the team the patient is exhibiting an extremely high core temperature, tachycardia, tachypnea and increased muscle rigidity. What should you do?

14 Death and Dying

Student's Name ______________________________

KEY TERMS

Write the definition for each term.

1. Advance health care directive: ______________________________
2. Coroner's case: ______________________________
3. Cultural competence: ______________________________
4. Determination of death: ______________________________
5. DNAR: ______________________________
6. DNR: ______________________________
7. End of life: ______________________________
8. Heart beating cadaver: ______________________________
9. Kübler-Ross, Elisabeth: ______________________________
10. Living will: ______________________________
11. Non–heart beating cadaver: ______________________________
12. Postmortem care: ______________________________
13. Required request law: ______________________________
14. Rigor mortis: ______________________________

SHORT ANSWER

Provide a short answer for each question or statement.

1. From a medical point of view, the *end of life* is:

____

____

2. The term *brain* dead refers to:

____

____

3. ________________ is the right of every individual to make decisions about how he or she lives and dies.

4. ________________ issues arise when decisions about end-of-life care fall to the family when the patient is unable to communicate his or her wishes.

5. ________________ or ________________ expresses the patient decision to decline lifesaving efforts.

6. ________________ care is the medical and supportive care provided to the dying patient.

7. Describe briefly the difference between a living will and a DNR order.

____

____

8. The surgical technologist should refrain from providing information to family or friends about ________________ of the patient.

MATCHING

Match the term with the description.

1. _______ It may occur during the dying process, but treated clinically.
2. _______ A natural first response, a defense mechanism.
3. _______ The idea that death is no longer a source of psychological conflict.
4. _______ Refusing nutrition or treatment.
5. _______ "I just want to experience one pain-free day with my family."

a. Denial
b. Bargaining
c. Anger
d. Acceptance
e. Depression

MULTIPLE CHOICE

Choose the most correct answer to complete the question or statement.

1. Which of the following is a famous physiatrist who constructed the death and dying model that is most frequently recognized today?
   a. Maslow
   b. Freud
   c. Piaget
   d. Elisabeth Kübler-Ross

2. During the dying process, ________________ is a defense mechanism that forestalls the full impact of the fact of death until the mind is ready to accept it.
   a. Denial
   b. Acceptance
   c. Bargaining
   d. Anger

3. A dying patient may express anger to:
   a. Gain control over the environment
   b. Get even with the physician
   c. Pass through the stages of dying even if the person is not angry
   d. Keep from becoming depressed

4. It is the responsibility of the ________________ to convey information about the patient's medical condition to the family and/or friends.
   a. Operating room scheduler or secretary
   b. Surgeon only
   c. Physician and nurses
   d. Operating room staff

5. The order to ________________ is made official by signing a DNR order, which is charted in the patient's medical record.
   a. Not resuscitate
   b. Call the doctor
   c. Add additional medications
   d. Sign a surgical consent form

6. Examples of palliative care include all of the following, *except*:
   a. Debulking of a tumor
   b. X-ray films
   c. Debridement of a pressure wound
   d. Insertion of a gastric feeding tube

7. If there is a sudden death in the operating room, it is appropriate for the technologist only to:
   a. Provide details about the cause of death
   b. Provide details about what occurred in the operating room
   c. Offer an acknowledgment of loss
   d. Discuss the laboratory test values

8. For surgical technologists to recognize and acknowledge the fact of death and what this means to the patient in that moment and time, they should:
   a. Focus on what the patient is experiencing in the operating room or holding area
   b. Observe facial expressions and gestures
   c. Be alert to any changes in mood or signs of anxiety and fear related to death and isolation
   d. All of the above

9. Medical interventions for a dying patient include all of the following, *except:*
   a. Respiratory support (artificial respiration)
   b. Intravenous feeding
   c. Dialysis
   d. Pain medications

10. The ______________ of death is considered by some to be too constricting and does not allow for individualism in the experience of death.
   a. Stage theory
   b. End-of-life theory
   c. Spiritual theory
   d. Psychological theory
   e. Examination

11. ______________ is the right of every individual to make decisions about how he or she lives and dies.
   a. DNR
   b. Advance directive
   c. Self-determination
   d. Living will

12. A ______________ specifies the exact nature of palliative care that a patient accepts.
   a. Living will
   b. Advance directive
   c. DNR
   d. Assisted suicide

13. When no verifiable permission has been granted for organ donation by the patient, the ______________ may act as a surrogate for the patient.
   a. Surgeon
   b. Family
   c. Chaplain
   d. Nurses

14. In the operating room, death is a(n) ______________ event.
   a. Rare
   b. Occasional
   c. Weekly
   d. Daily

15. For a coroner's case, all of the following are mandatory for an autopsy, *except:*
   a. Death of an incarcerated individual
   b. Unwitnessed death
   c. Death from a diagnosed terminal illness in which the patient was being treated for
   d. Suicide

16. Donors are registered in different ______________ of the country and the data are exchanged with recovery organizations.
   a. Parts
   b. States
   c. Regions
   d. Counties

17. Reactions and coping skills available to health care professionals are influenced by the following factors, *except:*
   a. Lack of support
   b. The health care professional's beliefs and values
   c. Previous experience with death
   d. Emotional well-being

18. A ______________ cadaver is maintained on cardiopulmonary support to provide tissue perfusion.
   a. Non-heart-beating
   b. Heart-beating

19. The cornea, bone and skin can be harvested from a ______________ cadaver.
   a. Non–heart-beating
   b. Heart-beating

20. Organ and tissue donation arises as a(n) ______________ issue when the patient has not left a clear directive before death.
   a. Moral
   b. Ethical

21. ______________ prepares the body for viewing by the family and assists in further handling procedures carried out by the morgue and mortuary.
   a. Rigor mortis
   b. Operating room
   c. Postmortem care
   d. All the above

22. The process of recovery is administered through:
   a. Donors
   b. Tissue banks
   c. Recipients
   d. Organized recovery
   e. All the above

CASE STUDIES

1. *Read the following case study and answer the questions based on your knowledge of death and dying.*

   You are called in for an exploratory laparotomy. Upon arrival to the hospital, you learn your patient has a ruptured aneurysm. You prepare the operating room and scrub, then notice the patient is brought in and is not breathing. The surgeon makes the incision and the abdomen is filled with blood and your patient crashes. After a very brief silence, you patient dies on the table.

   a. What is your role as a surgical technologist at this point?

   b. The patient's family wants to see their family member. Who stays with the family while they say goodbye?

   c. What is the ethical thing to do with this patient?

   d. Do you remove all the cords, clean the patient up before the family visit? Why?

15 Energy Sources in Surgery

Student's Name ______________________________

KEY TERMS

Write the definition for each term.

1. Ablation: ______________________________
2. Active electrode: ______________________________
3. Argon: ______________________________
4. Bipolar circuit: ______________________________
5. Capacitive coupling: ______________________________
6. Carbon dioxide: ______________________________
7. Cavitron ultrasonic surgical aspirator (CUSA): ______________________________
8. Coagulum: ______________________________
9. Cryoablation: ______________________________
10. Cryosurgery: ______________________________
11. Cutting mode: ______________________________
12. Direct coupling: ______________________________
13. Dispersive electrode: ______________________________
14. Electrosurgery: ______________________________
15. Electrosurgical unit (ESU): ______________________________
16. Electrosurgical vessel sealing: ______________________________
17. Eschar: ______________________________
18. Excimer: ______________________________
19. Fulguration: ______________________________
20. Holmium: YAG: ______________________________
21. Impedance: ______________________________
22. Implanted electronic device (IED): ______________________________
23. Insulate: ______________________________

24. Laser: ______

25. Laser classifications: ______

26. Laser head: ______

27. Laser medium: ______

28. Monopolar circuit: ______

29. Nonconductive: ______

30. Optical resonant cavity: ______

31. Patient return electrode (PRE): ______

32. Phacoemulsification: ______

33. Potassium-titanyl-phosphate (KTP): ______

34. Pulsed wave lasers: ______

35. Q-switched lasers: ______

36. Radiant exposure: ______

37. Radiofrequency: ______

38. Return electrode monitoring (REM): ______

39. Selective absorption: ______

40. Smoke plume: ______

41. Ultrasonic energy: ______

LABELING

Name the bovie tip and description of use.

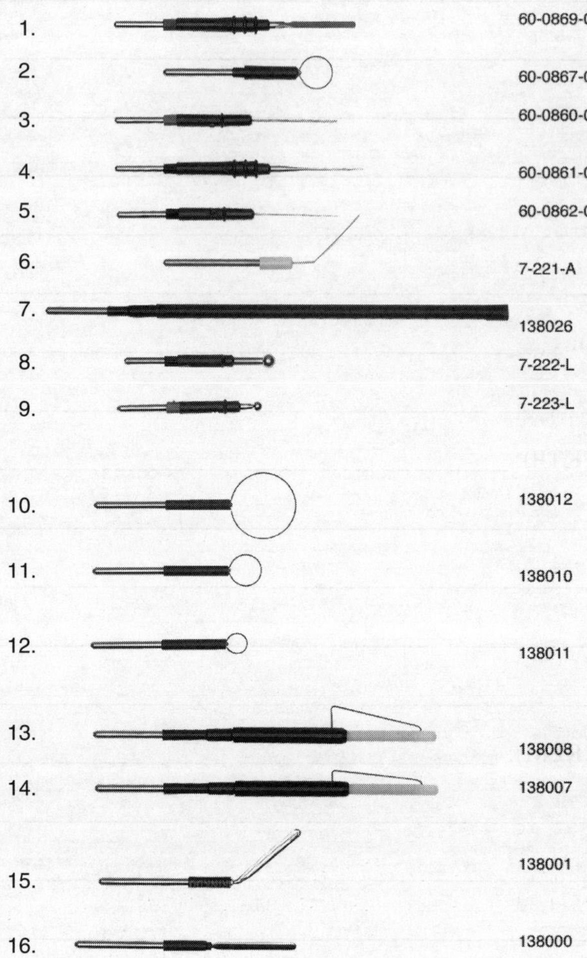

Courtesy Conmed, Inc.

1. ______________________________

2. ______________________________

3. ______________________________

4. ______________________________

5. ______________________________

6. ______________________________

7. ______________________________

8. ______________________________

9. ______________________________

10. ______________________________

11. ______________________________

12. ______________________________

13. ______________________________

14. ______________________________

15. ______________________________

16. ______________________________

SHORT ANSWERS

Provide a short answer for each question or statement.

1. Which variables cause tissue to react to electrosurgery?

2. Describe the difference between electrosurgery and ultrasonic energy.

3. What is the difference between monopolar and bipolar delivery of ESU?

4. What is capacitive coupling and why would it occur in endoscopic procedures more often than in open procedures?

5. How do lasers work?

6. How are lasers classified?

7. Lasers are grouped into two categories according to the duration of the output waves. What are the two groups?

   a. ______________________________

   b. ______________________________

MATCHING

Match each laser classification with the correct definition.

1. ______ Laser printers.
2. ______ Can cause severe eye injury when viewed directly or by reflection. These lasers do not cause injury when the laser beam is diffused and do not normally present a fire hazard.
3. ______ Can cause permanent eye damage if viewed directly or if viewed indirectly by reflection, may also ignite materials and cause skin burns. Most surgical lasers are in this category.
4. ______ Laser pointers and bar code scanners.
5. ______ Normally does not cause eye injury if viewed momentarily but presents a hazard if viewed with collecting optics (e.g., fiberoptic cable, magnification loupe, or microscope.)

a. Class 4
b. Class 3b
c. Class 3a
d. Class 2
e. Class 1

MATCHING

Match the laser with the correct description.

1. ______ Invisible to the human eye, and the beam has a high affinity for water, and functions at a superficial depth.
2. ______ Has a high affinity for tissue protein but little for water. Of all the laser types, has the greatest ability to coagulate blood vessels.
3. ______ A laser that offers two wavelengths, which allows two separate sets of laser characteristics to be selected at any time.
4. ______ This laser beam is outside the visible light range, penetrates all types of tissue, and is extremely versatile, able to cut, shave, contour, ablate, and coagulate tissue.
5. ______ This laser produces a cool beam by stripping electrons from the atoms of the medium in the chambers stimulating short bursts of laser light delivered to target tissue through fiberoptic bundles.
6. ______ Solid lasing material used to remove superficial skin defects and tattoos.
7. ______ A visible blue-green beam that is absorbed by red-brown pigmented tissue, such as hemoglobin.
8. ______ This pulsed dye laser beam is formed when fluorescent liquid or other dyes are exposed to argon laser light.

a. Argon gas laser
b. Carbon dioxide laser
c. Holmium:YAG laser
d. Nd:YAG laser
e. KTP laser
f. Excimer laser
g. Tunable dye laser
h. Ruby and alexandrite

MULTIPLE CHOICE

Choose the most correct answer to complete the question or statement.

1. Resistance to the flow of electricity:
   a. Impedance
   b. Frequency
   c. Circuit
   d. Current

2. The cutting mode causes tissue burning with the loss of water content is:
   a. Blended mode
   b. Cryoablation
   c. Desiccation
   d. Electrosurgical waveforms

3. The ______ provides radio frequency powers and controls for all types of ESU.
   a. Generator
   b. Duty cycle
   c. Desiccation
   d. Electrosurgical waveforms

4. Electrosurgical vessel sealing uses high-frequency, bipolar electrosurgery, low voltage, and physical pressure to create a weld in tissue. All of the follow are true statements, *except:*
   a. The vessel-sealing system is used during resection procedures that traditionally do not require clamping, suturing, and cutting.
   b. Electrosurgical vessel sealing uses a microprocessor that controls and programs the system.
   c. The vessel sealing system provides tissue impedance monitoring.
   d. Electrosurgical vessel sealing system has an alarm that automatically stops the current when the tissue seal is achieved.

5. ______ is a specific burn hazard of monopolar endoscopic surgery, occurring when current passes unintentionally through instrument insulation.
   a. Direct coupling
   b. Capacitive coupling

6. The safety system used in ESU monitoring impedance in the electrode stopping the current if is too high:
   a. PAE
   b. REM

7. ______ is the flow of electricity from one conductive substance to another.
   a. Direct coupling
   b. Capacitive coupling

8. The active electrode is the actual contact point at the tissue and is contained at the:
   a. Tip of the electrosurgical unit (ESU) handpiece or "pencil"
   b. Grounding plate
   c. Generator's plug in
   d. Foot pedal

9. The function of the ______ is to capture electrical current from the active electrode and transmit it back to the power unit.
   a. Bipolar circuit
   b. Bayonet
   c. Return electrode
   d. Pencil type of handpiece

10. In the ______ mode, the electrode is held above the tissue, without contact, and the air between the electrode and tissue acts as a conductor, allowing the high-voltage current to flow between the tissue and the electrode.
    a. Blended
    b. Cutting
    c. Desiccation
    d. Microbipolar cutting

11. Procedure in which a probe is inserted into a tumor or tissue mass. High-pressure argon gas is injected into the probe causing the tissues to freeze destroying the tissue.
    a. Ultrasound
    b. Phacoemulsification
    c. Cryoablation
    d. Laser

12. When laser light is directed at a surface, which of the following would *not* occur?
    a. Absorption
    b. Coagulation
    c. Reflection
    d. Scattering

13. ______ is the use of an extremely cold probe or substance to destroy tissue.
    a. Ultrasound
    b. Phacoemulsification
    c. Cryoablation
    d. Cryosurgery

14. ______ is created when electricity is transformed into mechanical energy generated by high-frequency vibrations and the focus on friction.
    a. Ultrasound
    b. Phacoemulsification
    c. Cryoablation
    d. Ultrasonic energy

15. ______ is performed by inserting a series of needle probes directly into the tumor under direct fluoroscopic imaging.
    a. Ultrasound
    b. Phacoemulsification
    c. Ablation
    d. Cryosurgery

16. Placement of the patient return electrode is extremely important when placing the grounding pad. Which of the following is incorrect related to placement of the pad?
    a. Place on a large muscle
    b. Place over a bony prominence
    c. Have complete contact with the skin surface
    d. Inspect the patients skin before applying the grounding pad

17. Where should the ESU pencil placed during surgery?
    a. On top of the patient
    b. On top of the drapes
    c. Tucked under the neck of the patient
    d. In a nonconductive safety holder

18. Forcep style ESU that the circuit flows from the generator through the cable to the tips of the forcep.
    a. Monopolar
    b. Bipolar
    c. Cryosurgery
    d. Ultrasound

19. Protective eyewear for laser procedures must:
    a. Have a clear lens
    b. Bear an inscription on the lens detailing the optical density and label of the specific laser type
    c. Have an opening on the sides of the eyes
    d. Have a clear amber lens

20. When a smoke evacuator is used to suction the smoke plume from the surgical site the tip of the nozzle must be within __________ of the site to be effective.
    a. 2 inches
    b. 4 inches
    c. 6 inches
    d. 1 foot

21. Both laser and ESU plumes contain:
    a. Dead and living cells
    b. Hydrogen cyanide
    c. Formaldehyde and acrolein
    d. Biological particles, such as cancer cells
    e. All of the above

CASE STUDIES

1. Your patient is coming to surgery today, and your surgeon would like to use the laser in the procedure. What safety precautions will the operating room team have to understand and undertake before the laser is used for the patient's procedure?

16 Moving, Handling, and Positioning the Surgical Patient

Student's Name ______________________________

KEY TERMS

Write the definition for each term.

1. Abduction: ______________________________
2. Compression injury: ______________________________
3. Dependent area of the body: ______________________________
4. Embolism: ______________________________
5. Fowler position ______________________________
6. Gurney: ______________________________
7. Hyperextension: ______________________________
8. Hyperflexion: ______________________________
9. Ischemia: ______________________________
10. Kraske position: ______________________________
11. Lateral transfer: ______________________________
12. Lateral position: ______________________________
13. Lithotomy position: ______________________________
14. Range of motion: ______________________________
15. Reverse Trendelenburg: ______________________________
16. Roller board: ______________________________
17. Shearing injury: ______________________________
18. Transfer board: ______________________________
19. Trendelenburg position: ______________________________

LABELING

Label the operating room table in the following figure.

1. ______________________________
2. ______________________________
3. ______________________________
4. ______________________________
5. ______________________________
6. ______________________________
7. ______________________________
8. ______________________________
9. ______________________________
10. ______________________________
11. ______________________________

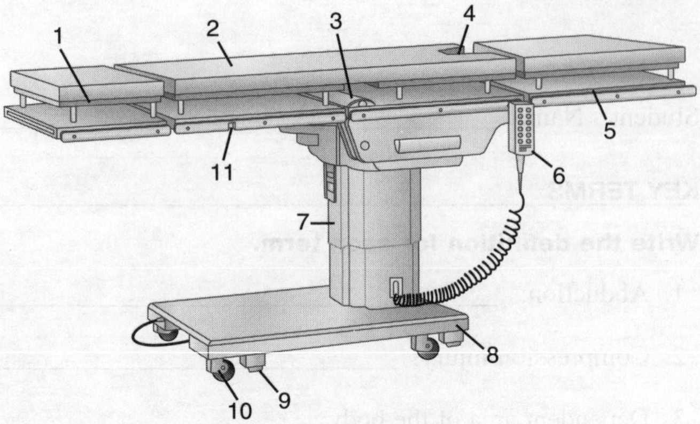

Modified from Martin JT, Warner MA: *Positioning in anesthesia and surgery*, ed 3, Philadelphia, 1997, WB Saunders.

SHORT ANSWERS

Provide a short answer for each question or statement.

1. What type of activity would or could cause a shearing injury?

2. Health care workers are at risk for skeletal injury while moving and transferring patients. List guidelines for preventing injuries to themselves when moving and handling patients.

3. Accident and injury to patients can be reduced when individuals take responsibility for the possible risks. List causes of injury to the patient when moving and handling the patient during transport and transfer.

4. What are the guidelines that all health care workers should use to identify and validate the patient's identity?

5. List the steps used to perform the log roll and assisted lateral transfer for the patient from a gurney to the operating room table.

____

____

MATCHING

Match each term with the correct definition. Some terms may be used more than once.

1. _______ Position in which the patient's head is tilted down.
2. _______ Position in which the patient is lying on the back.
3. _______ Sitting position.
4. _______ Position in which the patient's feet are tilted down.
5. _______ Position in which the patient is lying with the front of the body (the abdomen) on the operating room table.
6. _______ Position used for gynecological, urology, and some rectal procedures.
7. _______ Position used for head, neck, eye, ear, breast, abdominal, and vascular procedures.
8. _______ A type of prone position in which the patient's hips are flexed.
9. _______ Sitting position used for cranial, facial, and reconstructive breast procedures.
10. _______ Side-lying position.
11. _______ Position used for access to the perianal region, buttocks, posterior spine, and posterior lower legs.
12. _______ Position used for anorectal procedures.
13. _______ Position used to provide exposure to the lateral flank and lateral thorax.
14. _______ Position to access the lower abdominal and pelvic organs.
15. _______ Position used for procedures of the upper abdomen and neck.

a. Reverse Trendelenburg position
b. Prone position
c. Lithotomy position
d. Trendelenburg position
e. Supine position
f. Jackknife (Kraske) position
g. Lateral position
h. Fowler position
i. Modified Fowler
j. Lateral decubitis

MATCHING

Match the potential sources of injury with the correct term.

1. _______ Flexion of a joint beyond its normal anatomical range.
2. _______ Tissue injury caused by continuous pressure over an area.
3. _______ Loss of skin and deep tissue related to continuous pressure over an area of the body.
4. _______ Loss of blood supply to a body part either by compression or blockage of the blood vessels, can cause tissue death from lack of oxygen to the tissue.
5. _______ Skin inflammation that can occur when a patient is pulled over a high friction of surface such as a bed sheet or blanker.
6. _______ Extension of a joint beyond its normal anatomical range.

a. Decubitus ulcer
b. Shearing injury
c. Compression injury
d. Hyperextension
e. Hyperflexion
f. Ischemia

MULTIPLE CHOICE

Choose the most correct answer to complete the question or statement.

1. Which of the following terms means movement of a joint or body part away from the body?
   a. Abduction
   b. Adduction
   c. Hyperextension
   d. Ischemia

2. Health care workers are at high risk for injury while caring for, moving, and transferring patients because:
   a. They do not use proper body mechanics when moving a patient.
   b. The tasks are unpredictable.
   c. A sudden shift of the patient's weight may put the worker off balance.
   d. All of the above.

3. Transport and transfer injuries occur more often when:
   a. There is sufficient help.
   b. Personnel assisting in the transfer or transport have a plan.
   c. Personnel are rushed.
   d. The patient is cooperative.

4. Which of the following statements is true regarding patient transfers?
   a. One person should be in charge of the move and guide the others.
   b. It is best to make a plan as you move the patient so that the move is individualized.
   c. The patient's right to modesty is forfeited at admission.
   d. It is best to move the patient without blankets so that the patient does not get tangled up in them.

5. The most important part of transporting patients is:
   a. Proper identification before you transport them
   b. Proper positioning on the cart
   c. Keeping the patient warm while in the hallways
   d. Greeting the patient in a friendly manner and introducing yourself

6. The first step in transferring a mobile patient to a stretcher is to:
   a. Lower the bed rails and align the patient's bed and the stretcher
   b. Make sure the locks are engaged on both the patient's bed and the stretcher
   c. Identify the patient
   d. Let the surgeon know that the patient is about to be transferred

7. _______________ people should be present during the transfer of a mobile and alert patient.
   a. Two or three
   b. Three or four
   c. Four or five
   d. Five or six

8. The transfer of a conscious patient from a stretcher to an operating table starts with aligning the head of the stretcher with the head of the operating table and then:
   a. Opening up the back of the patient's gown
   b. Identifying the patient
   c. Freeing up the IV tubing
   d. Locking the wheels of the stretcher and the operating room table

9. During the transfer of a conscious patient to the operating room table, the duties of the STSR include:
   a. Protecting the patient's neck and airway
   b. Holding the IV tubing
   c. Controlling the slide board
   d. Nothing, the STSR is preparing the sterile field for surgery and is not needed for assistance during the transfer of a conscious patient to the OR table

10. Position a morbidly obese patient on a ________________ surgical table.
    a. Standard
    b. Double
    c. Jackson frame
    d. Bariatric

11. When a patient is placed in the supine position, where is the safety strap placed?
    a. 2 inches below the knees
    b. On the lower abdomen
    c. 2 inches above the knees
    d. On the knees

12. When the patient is positioned in the prone position, the arms should be extended no greater than:
    a. 30 degrees
    b. 60 degrees
    c. 90 degrees
    d. 120 degrees

13. These are used on the patient during surgery to prevent blood pooling and embolism (clot formation):
    a. Bear hugger
    b. Sequential compression device
    c. Hypothermia blanket
    d. Warming blanket

14. The minimum number of people required to perform a lateral transfer of a patient from the stretcher to the operating room table is:
    a. 4
    b. 2
    c. 3
    d. 6

15. Movement of an extremity toward the body is called:
    a. Abduction
    b. Adduction
    c. Circumflexion
    d. Rotation

16. When positioning a pregnant patient, a wedge pad should be placed under the ________________ flank to prevent uterine compression on the vena cava, which can cause hypotension and compromise fetal circulation.
    a. Upper thoracic
    b. Left upper thoracic
    c. Right flank
    d. Left buttock

CASE STUDIES

1. *Read the following case study and answer the questions based on your knowledge of patient positioning and use of the operating room table.*

   You have been asked to set up the operating room for a procedure. Today your surgeon will perform a right nephrectomy in operating room 2. The surgeon has told the team that he will be making a flank incision.

   a. In what position will the patient be placed?

b. What position will the patient be in for administration of the general anesthetic?

c. What positioning devices will be needed for this patient?

2. *Read the following case study and answer the questions based on your knowledge of the pregnant patient.*

You are called in for an emergency appendectomy. You are told upon arrival that your patient is pregnant.

a. What position will the patient be placed in?

b. What position devices should you have available?

c. What additional positioning device should be available for positioning your pregnant patient for her appendectomy and why?

17 Surgical Skin Preparation and Draping

Student's Name ______________________________

KEY TERMS

Write the definition for each term.

1. Antiseptic: ______________________________
2. Debridement: ______________________________
3. Fenestrated drape: ______________________________
4. Impervious: ______________________________
5. Incise drape: ______________________________
6. Residual activity: ______________________________
7. Retention catheter: ______________________________
8. Single-stage prep: ______________________________
9. Solution: ______________________________
10. Squaring the incision: ______________________________
11. Straight catheter: ______________________________
12. Two-stage prep: ______________________________

LABELING

In the drawings below, use a colored pen or pencil to indicate the prep for the procedure listed.

1. Anterior head and neck

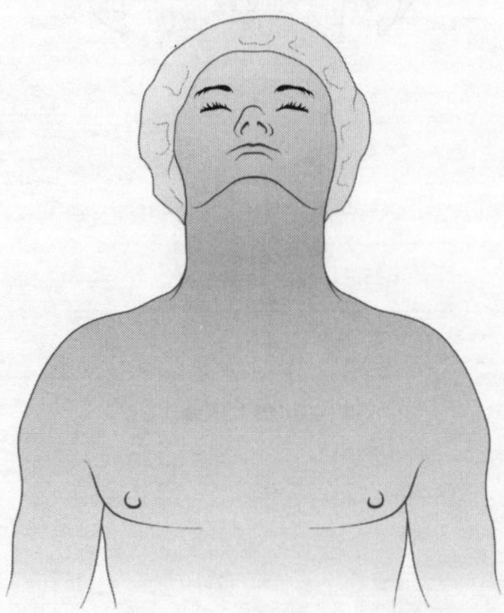

2. Shoulder

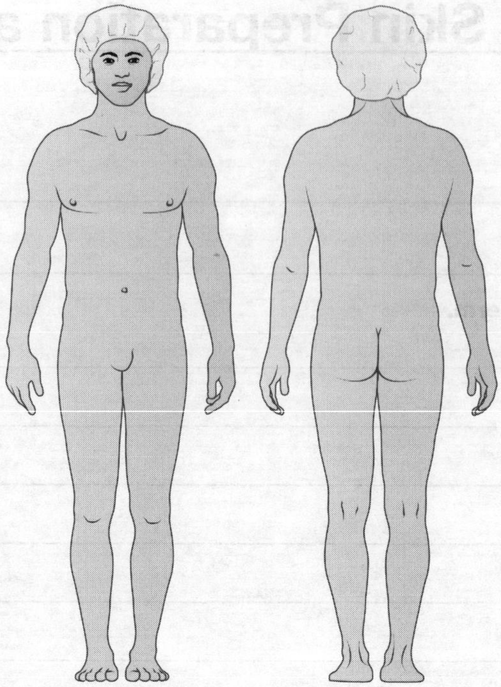

3. Abdomen

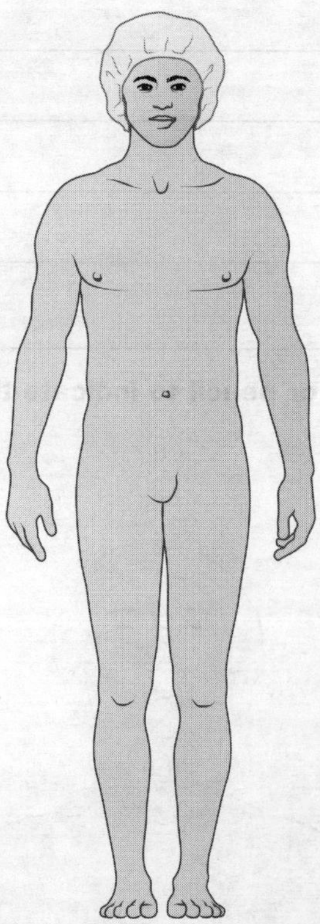

SHORT ANSWERS

Provide a short answer for each question or statement.

1. List the supplies needed for urinary catheterization.

2. List the steps of urinary catheterization.

3. List the two types of catheterizations and define. List the types of catheters necessary to perform these types of catheterizations.

4. What are the CDC guidelines for indications in the operating room for the use of indwelling urethral catheters?

5. Antiseptics used for surgical skin prep are mainly evaluated according to what primary criterias?

6. Why is iodine a risk of thermal burn when it is heated (warmed)?

7. Hair removal requires a verbal or written order by the surgeon. What guidelines should be followed for hair removal?

8. The flank and back areas are prepped in the same manner as the abdomen; describe the technique.

9. What are the principles of surgical draping?

10. List the technique on how to drape equipment such as the operating room microscope.

____

____

11. List the sequencing and order of the layers of draping materials used during draping the patient for an abdominal procedure.

____

____

12. List the technique in removing drapes.

____

____

MATCHING

Match each term with the correct definition. Some terms may be used more than once.

1. _______ destroys microorganisms by *desiccation* (drying) of the cell proteins.
2. _______ has not been approved as a first-choice skin prep by The Joint Commission or CDC.
3. _______ Although it normally is nonirritating to tissue, first-degree and second-degree chemical burns can result from improper prep technique or if the patient is sensitive to iodine.
4. _______ A solution that was removed as a safe skin prep agent. This agent was found to be absorbed through damaged skin of all ages, it was also found to cause damage to the central nervous system in infants.
5. _______ is extremely flammable and volatile.
6. _______ has been linked to hearing loss when accidently introduced in the inner ear.
7. _______ should never be used on mucous membranes or the eyes or in any open wound.
8. _______ should never be used during prep of the eye, ear, or face. Not recommended for use on large open wounds, burns, or infants younger than 2 months of age.

a. Hexachlorophene
b. Iodophors
c. Alcohol 70%
d. Chlorhexidine gluconate (CHG)

MULTIPLE CHOICE

Choose the most correct answer to complete the question or statement.

1. Prewarming a prep solution in a microwave or uncontrolled or unmonitored systems create a risk of:
   a. Allergies
   b. Chemical burn
   c. Fire
   d. Thermal burn

2. Surgical prep agents can cause skin irritation, rash, or other conditions except:
   a. Sterilization of the skin
   b. Chemical and thermal burns
   c. Fire
   d. Allergy

3. Alcohol and alcohol-based prep solutions are volatile and flammable. When alcohol solution or volatile fumes come in contact with heat sources, they can easily cause:
   a. Allergies
   b. Chemical burn
   c. Fire
   d. Thermal burn

4. Serious ____________ can occur when prep solutions are allowed to pool under the patient during surgery.
   a. Allergies
   b. Chemical burns
   c. Fires
   d. Thermal burns

5. During the cleansing process, the surgeon removes all foreign material and trims away devitalized tissue called:
   a. Trauma
   b. Cardiac/vascular
   c. Autograft
   d. Debridement

6. ____________ is a type of tissue that is removed from one site on the patient and grafted to another site.
   a. Trauma
   b. Cardiac/vascular
   c. Autograft
   d. Debridement

7. ____________ wounds are almost always contaminated because they are caused by external forces and often occur in environments that are mildly or grossly contaminated.
   a. Trauma
   b. Cardiac/vascular
   c. Autograft
   d. Debridement

8. ____________ require(s) a large area of exposure.
   a. Trauma wounds
   b. Cardiac/vascular inscisions
   c. Autografts
   d. Debridement

9. ____________ are folded in a specific way before sterilization so that they can be positioned over the operative site and unfolded in a way that prevents contamination.
   a. Towels
   b. Gowns
   c. Drapes
   d. All the above

10. A retention catheter with a small, inflatable balloon at the tip is called a ____________ catheter.
    a. Robinson
    b. Malecot
    c. Fogarty
    d. Foley

11. Catheterization of a female surgical patient requires the ____________ position.
    a. Supine
    b. Prone
    c. Lithotomy
    d. Knees slightly flexed

12. Which of the following statements is true regarding the technique for placing a Foley catheter?
    a. The assisting hand does not contact sterile supplies, including the catheter itself.
    b. Both hands must remain sterile for the procedure.
    c. If the catheter is placed before the prep has been done, it is not done using aseptic technique.
    d. The insertion hand does not contact sterile supplies.

13. Healthy skin contains colonies of:
    a. Infection
    b. Bacteria
    c. Grease
    d. Water

14. When is hair removed from the surgical site?
    a. Always
    b. When it will interfere with the procedure, and when the surgeon orders it
    c. When the patient has excess hair
    d. When the patient is a high risk for surgical site infection

15. Which of the following is not true related to performing the surgical prep?
    a. Antiseptic soap solution may be used, followed by a coating of antiseptic solution
    b. Antiseptic solution may be used alone
    c. The prepping agent is selected by the surgeon based on the area to be prepped and any sensitivities the patient may have to prep solutions
    d. The prep used is based on the preferences of the hospital infection control nurse

16. The basic principles of the skin prep:
    a. Is a method to prevent surgical site infection
    b. Is performed prior to draping
    c. Is a method to reduce the number of transient and normal microorganisms to an absolute minimum
    d. All of the above

17. Surgeons apply the surgical drapes in a prescribed order based on:
    a. Aseptic technique
    b. Surgical practice
    c. The patient's risk of infection
    d. Hospital policy

18. To ensure a moisture barrier between the patient and the sterile field, surgical drapes are made of woven and ________ materials.
    a. Polypropylene
    b. Linen
    c. Synthetic
    d. Polyester

19. A draping routine usually begins with:
    a. A plain sheet
    b. A stockinette
    c. A fenestrated drape
    d. A towel or sticky drape

20. The sterile drape that is coated with adhesive on one side and may be impregnated with antiseptic is called a(n):
    a. Three-quarter drape
    b. Fenestrated drape
    c. Half-sheet
    d. Incise drape

21. The procedure drape, or specialty drape, is placed on the patient:
    a. Before the half-sheet
    b. Before the incise drape
    c. First
    d. Last

22. Which of the following rules of asepsis apply to placement of the surgical drapes?
    a. Handle drapes with as much movement as you need to ensure proper placement.
    b. When placing a drape, do not touch the patient's body.
    c. After a drape has been placed, shift or move the drape to make a good fit for the patient and the procedure.
    d. Use perforating towel clips to secure drapes

23. The sterile technique required for catheterization entails application of sterile gloves using open gloving technique and keeping:
    a. Both hands and arms sterile
    b. Both hands unsterile, because this is not a sterile procedure
    c. One hand sterile for insertion of the catheter and using the other gloved hand for exposure of the meatus
    d. Both hands sterile

24. ____________ is the most common hospital acquired infection.
    a. Surgical site
    b. Urinary catheterization
    c. Improper prep
    d. All the above

25. Which of the following is recommended to mark the surgical site?
    a. Sharpie
    b. Pen with a ball point
    c. Gentian violet
    d. All of the above

26. Which of the following drapes has a fenestration?
    a. U-drape
    b. Perineal
    c. Utility
    d. Laparotomy

27. How many milliliters of sterile water are required to inflate the 5cc balloon on a Foley catheter?
    a. 5
    b. 10
    c. 7
    d. 6

CASE STUDIES

1. *Read the following case study and answer the questions based on your knowledge of surgical drapes.*

   You are about to scrub for a knee arthroscopy. Your patient is asleep under general anesthesia. He has been prepped, and you are about to drape him. What will you need to have ready for the surgeon so that you can drape the patient? List your supplies in the order you will use them.

18 Surgical Skills I: Planning a Case, Opening, and Start of Surgery

Student's Name ____________________

KEY TERMS

Write the definition for each term.

1. Blunt dissection: ____________________
2. Case planning: ____________________
3. Count: ____________________
4. Dissecting sponge: ____________________
5. Event related: ____________________
6. Graft: ____________________
7. Implant: ____________________
8. Radiopaque: ____________________
9. Raytec: ____________________
10. Sterile setup: ____________________
11. Surgeon's preference card: ____________________
12. TIMEOUT: ____________________
13. Universal Protocol: ____________________

SHORT ANSWERS

Provide a short answer for each question or statement.

1. What are the four categories of surgery by objectives?

   a. ____________________

   b. ____________________

   c. ____________________

   d. ____________________

2. What items are typically found on the surgeon's preference card?

3. What items are included in a surgical count?

4. Who is responsible for ensuring that no item is left in a patient?

5. When are surgical counts performed?

6. Items are usually counted in a specific order; what is that order?

7. Why is a TIMEOUT performed?

8. List synthetic implant materials.

MATCHING

Match each term with the correct description.

1. _______ Means to remove a large portion but not all of a tumor.
2. _______ Separation of one tissue plane from another with use of scissors to increase the space between the layers.
3. _______ Separation of tissue without using sharp instruments.
4. _______ This term means to carefully separate anatomical structures by cutting with instruments, small firm sponges, or the fingers.
5. _______ Enable precise reviewing of an anatomical area.
6. _______ This term usually refers to the removal of a limb or digit.
7. _______ To constrict a vessel or duct using a suture tie.
8. _______ This refers to the joining of two hollow anatomical structures (vessels, ducts, tubes, or hollow organs) using sutures or surgical staples.
9. _______ The use of sharp surgical instruments such as a scalpel and scissors to cut away dead tissue.
10. _______ The spaces and tissues that are accessed through the surgical incision.
11. _______ To bring a tissue structure partially outside the body.
12. _______ To raise or lift an anatomical structure, sometimes without removing it.
13. _______ A large portion or segment of tissue is removed.
14. _______ The removal of tissue, usually a mole or small lesion using cutting instruments or electrosurgery.
15. _______ The sterile area immediately around or in the surgical incision.
16. _______ This refers to an undesirable pucker in skin as a result of poor suture placement.
17. _______ In surgical terms, this means to “bring together” tissues by suturing or other means.

a. Amputate
b. Anastomose
c. Approximate
d. Blunt dissection
e. Debridement
f. Dog ear
g. Debulk
h. Dissect
i. Elevate
j. Excise
k. Exposure
l. Exteriorize
m. Ligate
n. Resection
o. Surgical field
p. Surgical wound
q. Undermine

MATCHING

Match each term with the correct definition as it applies to implants and grafts.

1. ______ Tissue used to cover large defects in the skin.
2. ______ Graft made from nonliving cadaver bone.
3. ______ Grafts made from a combination of cadaver bone, morcellated allograft bone and marrow.
4. ______ Used as a biological dressing for burns, skin ulcers, and infected wounds.
5. ______ Any type of tissue replacement or device placed in the body.
6. ______ Tissue graft derived from human tissue.
7. ______ Graft taken from pig tissue.
8. ______ Tissue obtained from the patient's body and implanted in another site.
9. ______ Graft taken from a species different from that of the patient.
10. ______ Migration of epithelial cells into the wound during healing.
11. ______ Graft taken from beef origin.

a. Allogeneic graft
b. Allograft
c. Amniotic membrane and unbilical cord
d. Autograft
e. Bovine graft
f. Composite graft
g. Epithelialization
h. Implant
i. Porcine graft
j. Xenograft
k. Wound cover

MULTIPLE CHOICE

Choose the most correct answer to complete the question or statement.

1. Case planning combines knowledge of:
   a. Surgical procedure and surgical techniques
   b. Anatomy and pathology
   c. The patient's diagnosis
   d. The patient's prognosis

2. When opening packages sealed with tape, why should you break the tape rather than peel the tape off?
   a. To prevent the outer wrapper from ripping, causing contamination
   b. So that you have to look at the tape to see whether it is sterile
   c. To prevent strike-through
   d. To prevent the inner wrapper from ripping

3. Which of the following is *not* a recommendation for opening a case?
   a. Open the scrubbed surgical technologist's gown and gloves on a small table or Mayo stand.
   b. Never unwrap a heavy item by holding it in midair.
   c. Do not open small sterile items into the genesis instrument tray.
   d. Open extra sutures, special equipment, and implants so that the surgeon does not have to wait for them during the procedure.

4. After the case has been opened, the surgical technologist's next immediate task is to:
   a. Load the knife blade
   b. Dress the Mayo stand
   c. Perform a surgical hand scrub
   d. Organize the instruments

5. Using a methodical method for all sterile set-ups in the learning stages:
   a. Makes the instruments easy for the surgeon to reach
   b. Contaminates the back table
   c. Improves efficiency and decreases great stress and errors
   d. Is against the Association of Perioperative Registered Nurses (AORN) standards

6. After finishing the surgical scrub, which task is done next?
   a. Arrange towels, gowns, and gloves in order of use
   b. Gown and glove self
   c. Organize the knife and the instruments
   d. Put all sponges in one location so you are ready to count

7. The selection of suture material is almost always prescriptive, or:
   a. Written on the surgeon's case plan ahead of time
   b. Delayed until the surgeon can prescribe the type she wants
   c. Determined only after the surgeon has taken a look at the surgical wound
   d. Delayed until the surgeon has discussed surgical wound closure with the patient.

8. If the count is incorrect:
   a. A radiograph should be taken immediately.
   b. The surgeon should not be bothered.
   c. The surgeon is notified and the count repeated.
   d. The circulator should call the house supervisor for an incident report.

9. A retained item can cause patient injury from all of the following, *except*:
   a. X-ray exposure sickness
   b. Infection
   c. Organ perforation
   d. Obstruction

10. Immediately after gowning and gloving, the technologist must complete:
    a. Scattering the case
    b. The sterile setup or setting up a case
    c. Preparation of the operating room
    d. The surgical count

11. After you scrub and as you first approach the pile of sterile equipment, do not move anything until:
    a. You have a plan
    b. You count the instruments
    c. You load the blade on the knife handle
    d. You move the drapes and put them in order

12. Tissue derived from human tissue acquired from a tissue bank is called:
    a. Allograft
    b. Synthetic implant
    c. Autologous autograft
    d. Silicone

13. Tissue obtained from the patient's own body, implanted into another site, is called:
    a. Allograft
    b. Silicone
    c. Synthetic implant
    d. Autologous autograft

CASE STUDIES

1. *Read the following case study and answer the questions based on your knowledge of case preparation.*

   It is 6:30 AM, and you are assigned to operating room 6 with your preceptor, who has called and said that she will be late because she has a flat tire. She has asked that you go ahead and get the room ready for the day, "pick the case," and then place the sterile unopened packs onto the furniture where they will be opened soon. She does not want you to "open the case" until she gets there to assist you. How should you proceed?

19 Surgical Skills II: Intraoperative and Immediate Postoperative Period

Student's Name ____________________

KEY TERMS

Write the definition for each term.

1. Absorbable suture: ____________________
2. Adhesion: ____________________
3. Anastomosis: ____________________
4. Approximate: ____________________
5. Biopsy: ____________________
6. Capillary action: ____________________
7. Dehiscence: ____________________
8. Detachable suture: ____________________
9. Evisceration: ____________________
10. Frozen section: ____________________
11. Hematoma: ____________________
12. Hemostasis: ____________________
13. Inert: ____________________
14. Interrupted sutures: ____________________
15. Nonabsorbable suture: ____________________
16. Primary intention: ____________________
17. Reverse cutting needle: ____________________
18. Swage: ____________________
19. Tensile strength: ____________________
20. Tie on a passer: ____________________

SHORT ANSWERS

Provide a short answer for each question or statement.

1. List types of surgical sponges and their uses that are commonly used in the operating room.

2. List Halstead's principles of surgery and define.

   1.
   2.
   3.
   4.
   5.
   6.
   7.

3. What are the primary techniques of hemostasis used in surgery?

   a.
   b.
   c.
   d.

4. What are the three categories of physical structures of sutures?

   1.
   2.
      2a.
      2b.
   3.

5. List classifications of wounds and provice characteristics and examples of each.

 1. ______________________________

 2. ______________________________

 3. ______________________________

 4. ______________________________

6. All substances, including suture products, that bear the USP label must meet minimum standards. What are the standards for sutures?

____

____

7. List the physical characteristics of sutures that influence a surgeon's decision in choosing a suture.

 1. ______________________________

 2. ______________________________

 3. ______________________________

 4. ______________________________

 5. ______________________________

 6. ______________________________

 7. ______________________________

 8. ______________________________

 9. ______________________________

 10. ______________________________

8. List materials that are the most inert in tissue.

____

____

9. Describe the types of suture needles.

____

____

10. List important considerations that may determine which type of suture is selected to be used in particular tissues.

____

____

____

____

____

____

11. What are the purposes of wound dressings?

____

____

LABELING

Label the following pictures with the type of suture technique shown.

1. ____

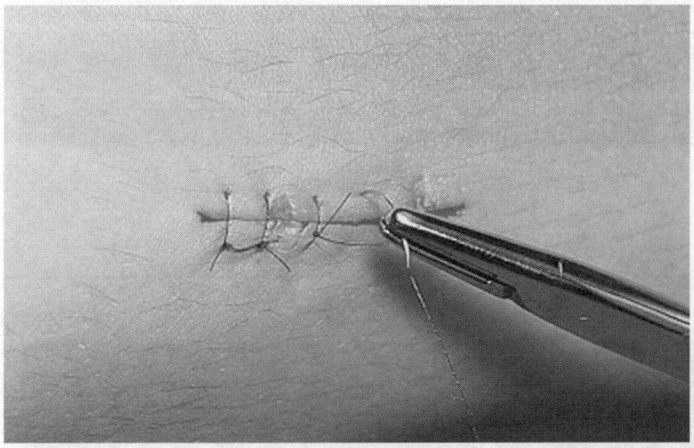

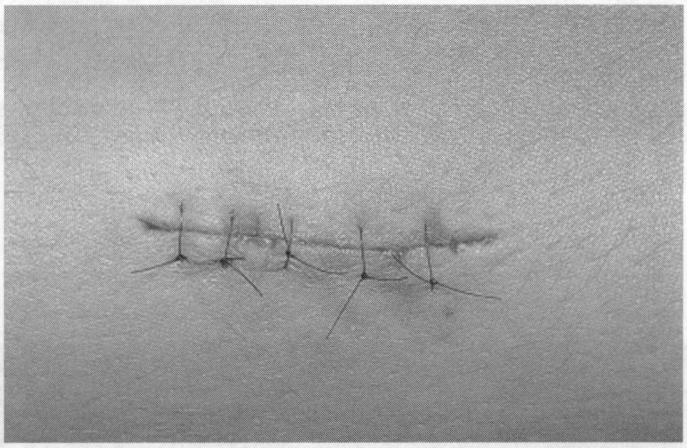

2. ____

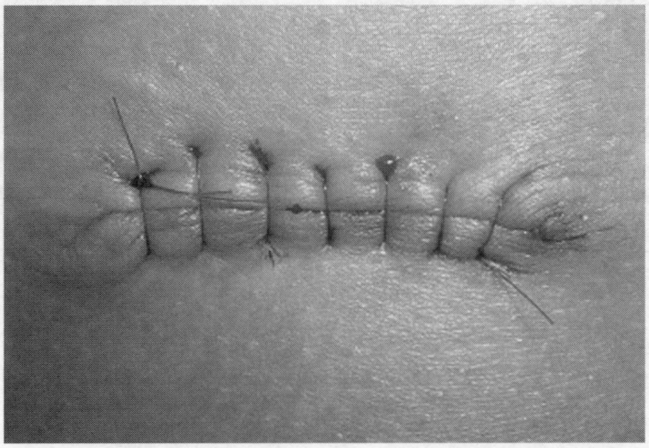

3. ____

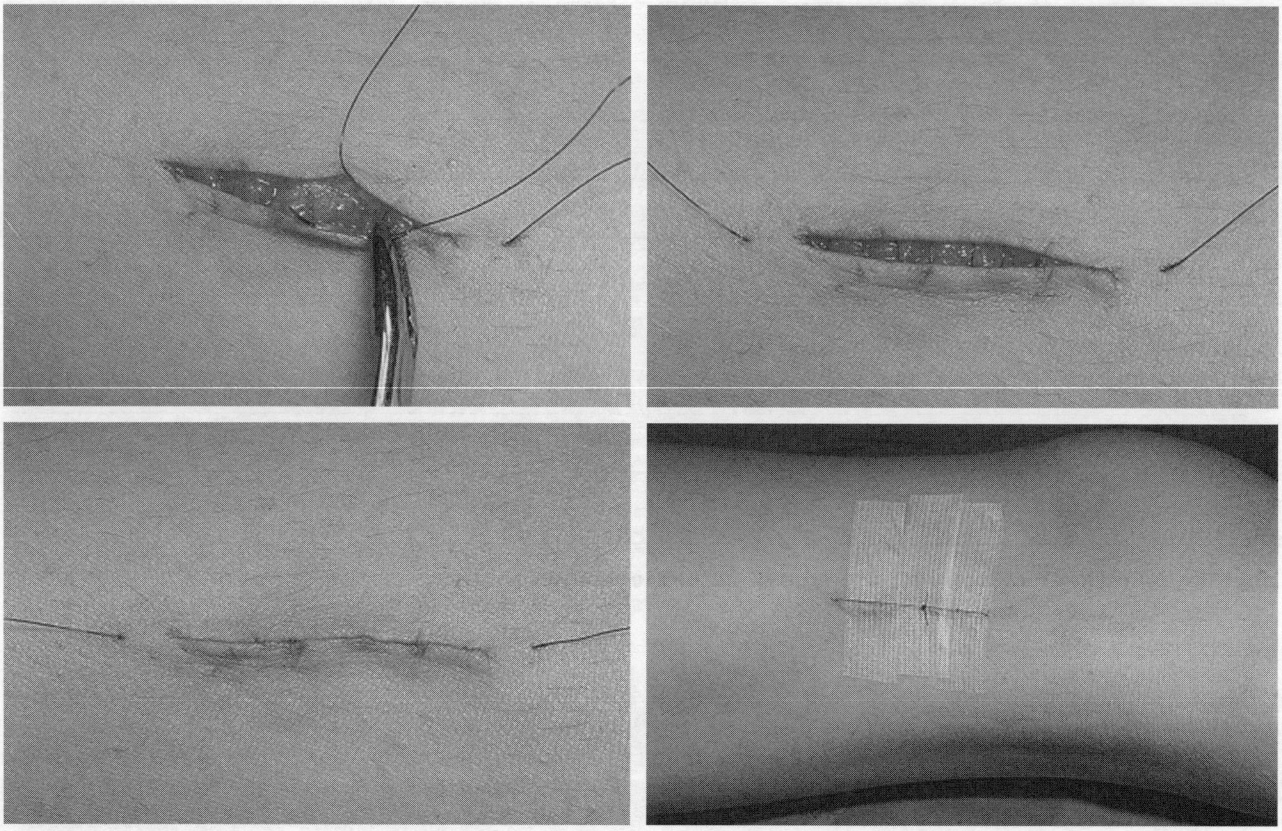

4. ____

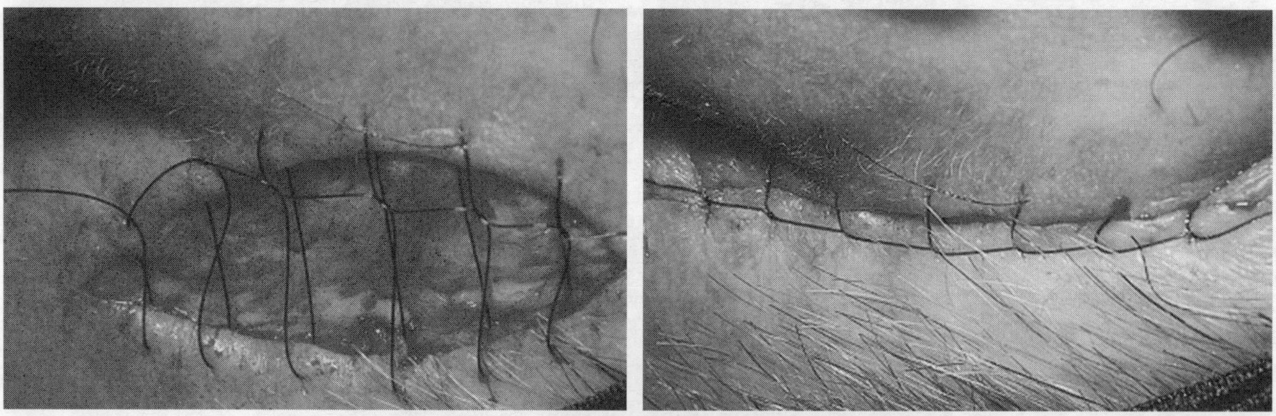

5. ______________________________

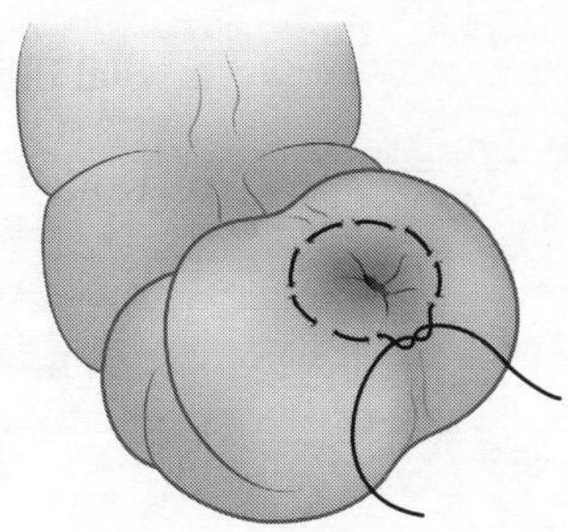

6. ______________________________

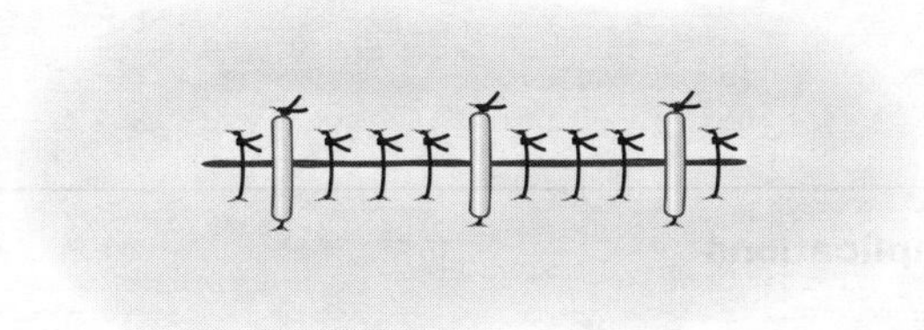

MATCHING I

Match the wound drains to the category of wound drainage system

1. _____ Jackson Pratt
2. _____ Malecot
3. _____ Penrose
4. _____ Stoma pouch
5. _____ Pezzar
6. _____ Chest drainage tubes
7. _____ Hemovac

a. Passive drain

b. Suction drain

c. Water-sealed drainage system

d. Collection of body fluids from an artificial orifice

MATCHING II

Match the following dressings

1. _____ ABD pad
2. _____ Tube stockinet
3. _____ Telfa
4. _____ Coban
5. _____ Adaptic - petroleum based agent
6. _____ Elastoplast
7. _____ 4 x 4 gauze sponges
8. _____ Kling gauze

a. Flat dressing
b. Rolled dressing

MATCHING III

Match the following wound complications

1. _____ Tissue breakdown at the edges of the wound causing the wound edges to open up
2. _____ Bands of scar tissue in the abdominal area, pelvic organs, and peritoneum
3. _____ Usually occurs during the first week post op beginning with an excess of inflammation and serious discharge from the wound
4. _____ collection of blood that forms in a wound due to incomplete hemostasis or capillary bleeding
5. _____ tissue breakdown of the wound with protrusion of the abdominal contents outside of the wound, can involve the omentum and or bowel
6. _____ Collection of fluid that develops in the wound during healing caused by tissue trauma incurred during the procedure, acting as a physical barrier between the wound edges preventing healing

a. Surgical site infection
b. Seroma
c. Hematoma
d. Dehiscence
e. Evisceration
f. Adhesions

MULTIPLE CHOICE

Choose the most correct answer to complete the question or statement.

1. Which of the following specimens might be sent to the pathologist on a Telfa sponge?
   a. Adenoid tissue
   b. Prostate from a transurethral resection of the prostate (TURP)
   c. Uterus and fallopian tubes
   d. Breast tissue for frozen section

2. Which of the following specimens must be sent to the pathologist dry?
   a. Colon polyps
   b. Bronchial washings
   c. Kidney stones
   d. Tonsils

3. Which sponge is used to make a sponge stick?
   a. Laparotomy
   b. Raytec
   c. Kittner
   d. Tonsil

4. Which type of sponge is packaged in groups of 10?
   a. Kittner
   b. Cherry
   c. Raytec
   d. Laparotomy

5. Which type of sponge would be appropriate for "packing" the abdominal cavity?
   a. Kittner
   b. Raytec
   c. Laparotomy
   d. Neuro patties

6. Uncontrolled oozing or insecure hemostasis can lead to a:
   a. Hematoma
   b. Contusion
   c. Seroma
   d. Compartment syndrome

7. Tissue breakdown at the wound margins which causes the wound to open up is called:
   a. Evisceration
   b. Adhesions
   c. Dehiscence
   d. Hematoma

8. Suture materials are used for all of the following, *except:*
   a. Approximation
   b. Ligation of tubular structures
   c. Hemostasis
   d. Coagulation

9. Which of the following is the *largest* suture?
   a. # 1 Ethibond
   b. # 0 silk
   c. 3-0 Vicryl
   d. 11-0 chromic

10. The physical characteristics of a suture include which of the following?
    a. Size
    b. Elasticity
    c. Memory
    d. Effect of the suture on the tissue

11. A bridal suture used in ophthalmic surgery is also called a(an):
    a. Retention suture
    b. Subcutaneous suture
    c. Traction suture
    d. Vertical mattress suture

12. The _______ of suture refers to the amount of force needed to break the suture.
    a. Knot strength
    b. Tensile strength
    c. Tissue drag
    d. Biological environment

13. Sutures made of multifilament strands can hold body fluids which can retain and carry infections by the sutures by:
    a. Osmosis
    b. Wicking or capillary action
    c. Monofilament
    d. Inert

14. A wound that is not sutured and must heal from the base is healing by: __________
    a. Delayed union
    b. First intention
    c. Secondary intention
    d. Third intention

15. Which of the following is the first phase of wound healing?
    a. Healing phase
    b. Remodeling phase
    c. Proliferative phase
    d. Inflammatory phase

16. Which of the following is *not* considered a risk factor in wound healing?
    a. Nutritional status
    b. Chronic disease
    c. Obesity
    d. Healthy 20-year-old athlete

17. Which type of sponge is used in neurosurgical procedures?
    a. Pusher
    b. Kitner
    c. Laparotomy
    d. Cottonoid

18. Which type of sponge is used for blunt dissection?
    a. Cottonoid
    b. Peanut
    c. Tonsil
    d. Patty

19. Removal of an entire mass of suspicious area of tissue:
    a. Core needle biopsy
    b. Fine needle aspiration
    c. Excisional biopsy
    d. Incisional biopsy

20. Tissue biopsy with use of a long fine needle to aspirate small pieces of tissue:
    a. Core needle biopsy
    b. Fine needle aspiration
    c. Excisional biopsy
    d. Incisional biopsy

21. Tissue biopsy with use of a large bore hollow trocar or needle:
 a. Core needle biopsy
 b. Fine needle aspiration
 c. Excisional biopsy
 d. Incisional biopsy

22. Partial removal of a tissue mass:
 a. Core needle biopsy
 b. Fine needle aspiration
 c. Excisional biopsy
 d. Incisional biopsy

23. Immediate analysis of tissue for malignancy is called a frozen section, the tissue is sent to the pathology department:
 a. In Normal Saline solution
 b. Fresh with no fixative
 c. In Formalin
 d. In sterile water

24. When handling forensic evidence such as bullets how should you handle the item?
 a. Handle item with hemostatic forceps
 b. Handle item with tooth forceps
 c. Handle item carefully to avoid scratching or distorting
 d. Send the item to pathology

25. Which type of needle is used on the liver?
 a. Cutting
 b. Blunt
 c. Taper
 d. Taper cut

26. Which type of needle would be used on soft tissues such as the gastrointestinal tissue?
 a. Cutting
 b. Blunt
 c. Taper
 d. Reverse cutting

27. Which type of needle would be used on tendons or skin?
 a. Cutting
 b. Blunt
 c. Taper
 d. Spatula

28. Which type of suture is used to provide additional support to wound edges?
 a. Retention
 b. Vertical mattress
 c. Horizontal mattress
 d. Purse-string

29. Commonly called a stick tie:
 a. Tie on a passer
 b. Free tie
 c. Suture ligature
 d. Reel

CASE STUDIES

1. *You have been precepting new students in the operating room and know how challenging it is to learn sutures. You want to create something to simplify the process of learning sutures. You decide you are going to make a suture square:*

Using the squares below, categorize the sutures from the text. After you have finished that, use a colored pencil to make the suture name in the same color as the suture package.

	Synthetic Sutures	Natural Sutures
Absorbable sutures		
Nonabsorbable sutures		

20 Minimally Invasive Surgery

Student's Name ______________________

KEY TERMS

Write the definition for each term.

1. Active electrode monitoring (AEM): ______________________
2. Arthroscopy: ______________________
3. Auxiliary water channel: ______________________
4. Biopsy channel: ______________________
5. Camera control unit (CCU): ______________________
6. Cannula: ______________________
7. Capacitative coupling: ______________________
8. Control head: ______________________
9. Direct coupling: ______________________
10. Elevator channel: ______________________
11. Endocoupler: ______________________
12. Gain: ______________________
13. High definition (HD): ______________________
14. Imaging system: ______________________
15. Insertion tube: ______________________
16. Instrument channel: ______________________
17. Insufflation: ______________________
18. Intravasation: ______________________
19. Light cable: ______________________
20. Light source: ______________________
21. Optical angle: ______________________
22. Pixel: ______________________
23. Pneumoperitoneum: ______________________

24. Port: ______________________________

25. Resectoscope: ______________________________

26. Standard definition (SD): ______________________________

27. White balance: ______________________________

SHORT ANSWER

Provide a short answer for each question or statement.

1. Describe the difference between rigid endoscopy and flexible endoscopy.

____

____

2. What are the special considerations when prepping and draping for MIS procedures?

____

____

3. What are the components of the surgical imaging system?

____

____

4. The guidelines for taking care of the fiberoptic cables include:

   a. ______________________________

   b. ______________________________

   c. ______________________________

   d. ______________________________

   e. ______________________________

   f. ______________________________

   g. ______________________________

5. What is the procedure for white balancing?

____

____

6. Describe the process of insufflation.

____

____

7. What is the procedure for insertion of a Veress needle?

____

____

8. What is the purpose of continuous irrigation and fluid distension? Which types of procedures is it commonly used during?

____

____

MATCHING

Match each term with the correct definition. You may use the same answer more than once.

1. _______ In minimally invasive surgery, the inflation of the abdominal or thoracic cavity with carbon dioxide gas.
2. _______ Refers to the abdomen when it is distended with carbon dioxide gas.
3. _______ A trocar that is rounded at the tip.
4. _______ In MIS suturing and knot tying, technique performed "inside the body."
5. _______ A device that controls and emits light for delivery in endoscopic procedures.
6. _______ A sharp, rod-shaped instrument used to puncture the body wall.
7. _______ Connects the camera to the telescope.
8. _______ Long, narrow instruments with an optical lens used during endoscopic surgery.
9. _______ A hollow tube that holds the trocar.
10. _______ A spring-loaded needle used to deliver carbon dioxide gas during insufflation.
11. _______ The suture or pre-tied loop used when a tissue structure requires ligation rather than suturing.
12. _______ The fiberoptic light cable that transmits light from the source to the endoscopic instrument.
13. _______ Refers to the rigid lensed instrument used in minimally invasive surgery.
14. _______ Instrument passed through a natural orifice for assessment or surgery of a hollow organ, duct, or vessel performed with a flexible, semi-rigid or rigid endoscope.

a. Light source
b. Light cable
c. Endoscope
d. Cannula
e. Blunt trocar
f. Telescopic instruments
g. Intracorporeal
h. Veress needle
i. Insufflation
j. Pneumoperitoneum
k. Trocar
l. Ligation loop
m. Endocoupler

MATCHING II

Title Match the parts of a flexible endoscope

____1. Receives the biopsy forceps, brushes, and other instruments used to obtain specimens

____2. Connects with the digital camera, optical system control handles, suction and irrigation

____3. Used to insufflate the lumen of the gastrointestinal tract to create space in the same way as a pneumoperitoneum

____4. Port located near the junction of the control head and insertion tube

____5. Channel used to clear blood and tissue debris from the lens

____6. Component of the endoscope that enters the patient's body

a. Air channel

b. Auxillary water channel

c. Biopsy channel

d. Instrument channel

e. Insertion tube

f. Control head

MULTIPLE CHOICE

1. Patient position for laparoscopic procedures of the upper abdomen and lower esophagus is:
   a. Reverse Trendelenburg
   b. Beach chair
   c. Semi fowlers
   d. Trendelenburg

2. Patient position for laparoscopic procedures of the lower abdomen and pelvis is:
   a. Jack knife
   b. Trendelenburg
   c. Reverse Trendelenburg
   d. Kraske

3. Patient position for laparoscopic procedures of the shoulder is:
   a. Trendelenburg
   b. Beach chair
   c. Decubitis
   d. Lateral decubitis

4. Patient position for video-assisted thoracoscopic procedures is:
   a. Supine
   b. Prone
   c. Beach chair
   d. Lateral decubitis

CASE STUDIES

1. *You are scrubbed in on a laparoscopic procedure that is about to finish. Your responsibility as a surgical technologist is to properly handle and care for the laparoscope in a manner that prevents damage. What does that include?*

   a. ____________________

   b. ____________________

c. ____

d. ____

e. ____

2. *During a laparoscopic procedure an emergency situation occurs, and the surgeon needs to convert to an open procedure. What will the process be while you are converting to an open case?*

a. ____

b. ____

c. ____

d. ____

e. ____

f. ____

21 Robotic-Assisted Surgery

Student's Name ______________________________

KEY TERMS

Write the definition for each term.

1. Bedside unit: ______________________________

2. Docking: ______________________________

3. Hand controllers: ______________________________

4. Haptic feedback (force pressure): ______________________________

5. Modular robotic system: ______________________________

6. Near-infrared imaging: ______________________________

7. Port: ______________________________

8. Registration (of a digital image): ______________________________

9. Remote data display: ______________________________

10. Reposable: ______________________________

11. Robotic-assisted surgical system (RAS): ______________________________

12. Scaled movement: ______

13. Surgeon console: ______

14. Surgical access: ______

15. Wristed instruments: ______

SHORT ANSWER

Provide a short answer for each question or statement.

1. Robotic-assisted surgery evolved from the technology of minimally invasive surgery. Describe the similarities.

2. What does the U.S Food and Drug Administration define robotic-assisted surgical device as a subtype of?

3. Differentiate between the Veress needle technique and Hasson techniques for creation of pneumoperitoneum.

MATCHING I

Match each term with the correct definition.

1. _______ Accessory equipment tower in which equipment such as energy modalities, system electronics, video controller, and touch screen are placed where signals relayed by fiber optic cables to the surgeon console can be controlled.
2. _______ Refers to providing sense of touch.
3. _______ Freely moveable unit system that features a single instrument and its arm that is attached to a dedicated base.
4. _______ Nonsterile control station where the surgeon sits or stands while operating.
5. _______ CT or MRI scans can be displayed on the screen monitor at any time.
6. _______ Describes instruments that feature a long shaft, working tip, and head that attaches to the robotic arm.
7. _______ Used to move the surgical instruments during the procedure.
8. _______ Provides three-dimensional images, as well as an endoscopic field of vision that can be panned or out without loss of image, quality, or light.
9. _______ Refers to the tips of the robotic instruments in a nose-up and nose-down position.
10. _______ Surgeon console system referred to as immersive featuring a cockpit-style viewer.
11. _______ Used on some systems to activate the energy instruments.
12. _______ Surgeon console system that has no cockpit or hood.
13. _______ Refers to the tips of the robotic instruments making right and left turns in a space.
14. _______ Receptacle for the surgical instruments and endoscope that are inserted into designated arms.

a. Surgeon console
b. Open console design
c. Closed console design
d. Remote data display
e. Hand controllers
f. Foot controls
g. Bedside unit
h. Modular robotic system
i. Optics
j. Vision tower
k. Wristed
l. *Pitch*
m. *Yaw*
n. Haptic

MATCHING II

Match each type or robotic system with the correct definition.

_______ 1. Robotically controlled bronchoscope with a high degree of flexibility and high-definition 3-D vision used during bronchoscopy for taking biopsies and some therapeutic procedures.

_______ 2. A modular system with freely moveable bedside carts for each instrument and the endoscope. It is a robotic-assisted digital system featuring an open surgeon console and uses standard, reusable, minimally invasive instruments and trocar-cannula systems.

_______ 3. System features modular, freely moveable bedside carts for wristed instruments and the robotic endoscope providing 3-D viewing and motionless endoscopic field of vision. The surgical non-haptic instruments are reposable, and the system uses compatible energy devices.

_______ 4. Semi-robotic platform that features a flexible endoscope and robotically controlled instruments commonly used in transoral and transanal surgical procedures.

_______ 5. System has a closed surgeon console, single bedside cart with multiple instrument arms mounted on a central column, robotic endoscope, and 3-D viewing. Instrumentation is reposable, the system does not have haptic feedback.

_______ 6. Orthopedic robotic-assistive system used to enable accurate bone preparation and tissue balancing for total or partial joint replacement.

a. Versius (CMR Surgical)
b. daVinci
c. Senhance
d. Joint arthroplasty system
e. Flex Robotic (Medrobotics, Inc.)
f. Monarch Platform (Auris Health)

MULTIPLE CHOICE

1. Cause of conversion from a robotic case to an open case is:
   a. Loss of vision
   b. Instrument failure
   c. Hemorrhage
   d. All of the above

2. After placing the Veress needle, why is a small amount of saline lightly injected or dropped into the needle hub?
   a. To create negative pressure
   b. To create pneumoperitoneum
   c. If the saline flows, the Veress needle is in proper placement
   d. If the saline does not flow, it means the Veress needle is in proper placement

3. Robotic team member responsible for direct patient care, protecting the sterile field, assisting the anesthesia provider, and assisting in setting up the robotic equipment and driving the base unit or patient cart into place:
   a. Assistant surgeon
   b. Circulating nurse
   c. Surgical technologist
   d. Robotics coordinator

4. What type of serious complications can pneumoperitoneum cause related to anesthesia during the procedure?
   a. Decreased lung capacity
   b. Increased body temperature
   c. Increased lung capacity
   d. Decreased body temperature

CASE STUDIES

1. *You are assigned to scrub in the robotics room. What are the steps in preoperative preparation as well as the initial setup of the sterile field and start of surgery?*

22 General Surgery

Student's Name ______________________

KEY TERMS

Write the definition for each term associated with the abdomen.

1. Abdominal peritoneum: ______________________
2. Adhesions: ______________________
3. Direct inguinal repair: ______________________
4. Fistula: ______________________
5. Hernia: ______________________
6. Incarcerated hernia: ______________________
7. Incisional hernia: ______________________
8. Indirect inguinal hernia: ______________________
9. Linea alba: ______________________
10. McBurney incision: ______________________
11. Resection: ______________________
12. Ventral hernia: ______________________
13. Viscera: ______________________

Write the definition for each term associated with the bowel.

1. Anastomosis: ______________________
2. Billroth I procedure: ______________________
3. Billroth II procedure: ______________________
4. Exploratory laparotomy: ______________________
5. Gastrostomy: ______________________
6. Isolation technique: ______________________
7. Laparotomy: ______________________
8. Morbid obesity: ______________________
9. -ostomy: ______________________

10. Stoma: ______________________________

11. Stoma appliance: ______________________________

Write the definition for each term associated with the liver and spleen.

1. Cirrhosis: ______________________________

2. Lobectomy: ______________________________

3. Segmental resection: ______________________________

Write the definition for each term associated with the breast.

1. Body image: ______________________________

2. Needle wire localization: ______________________________

3. Mastectomy: ______________________________

4. Modified radical mastectomy: ______________________________

5. Sentinel lymph node biopsy (SLNB): ______________________________

6. Skin flap: ______________________________

7. Subcutaneous mastectomy: ______________________________

8. Technetium-99: ______________________________

LABELING

Label the axillary anatomy of the breast.

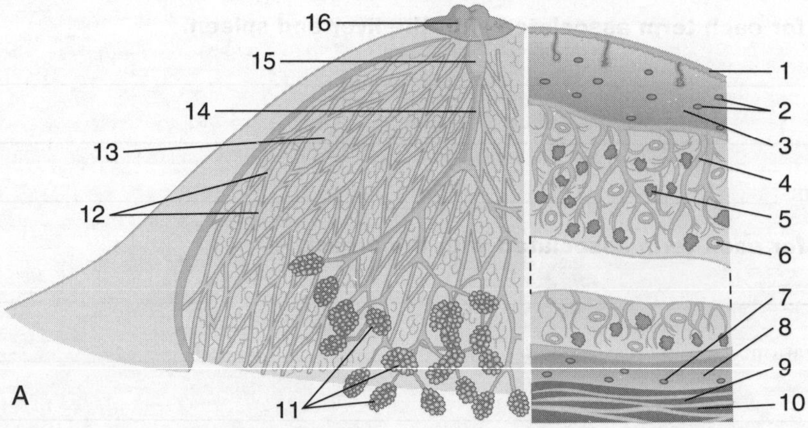

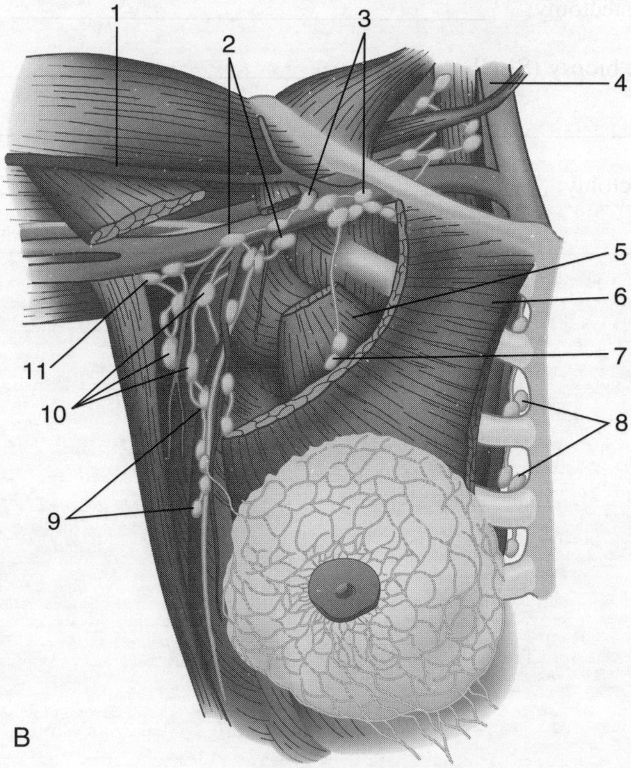

A. 1. ______________________________

2. ______________________________

3. ______________________________

4. ______________________________

5. ______________________________

6. ______________________________

7. ______

8. ______

9. ______

10. ______

11. ______

12. ______

13. ______

14. ______

15. ______

16. ______

B. 1. ______

2. ______

3. ______

4. ______

5. ______

6. ______

7. ______

8. ______

9. ______

10. ______

11. ______

LABELING

Label the biliary and hepatic anatomy.

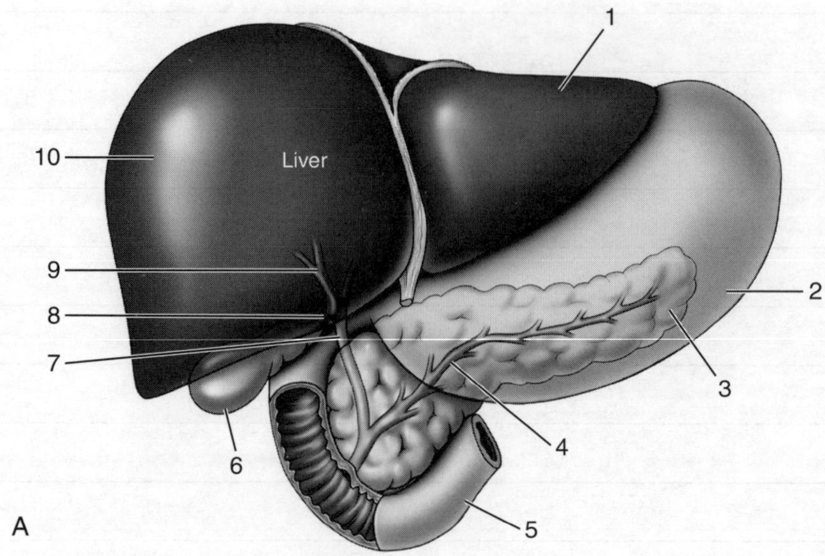

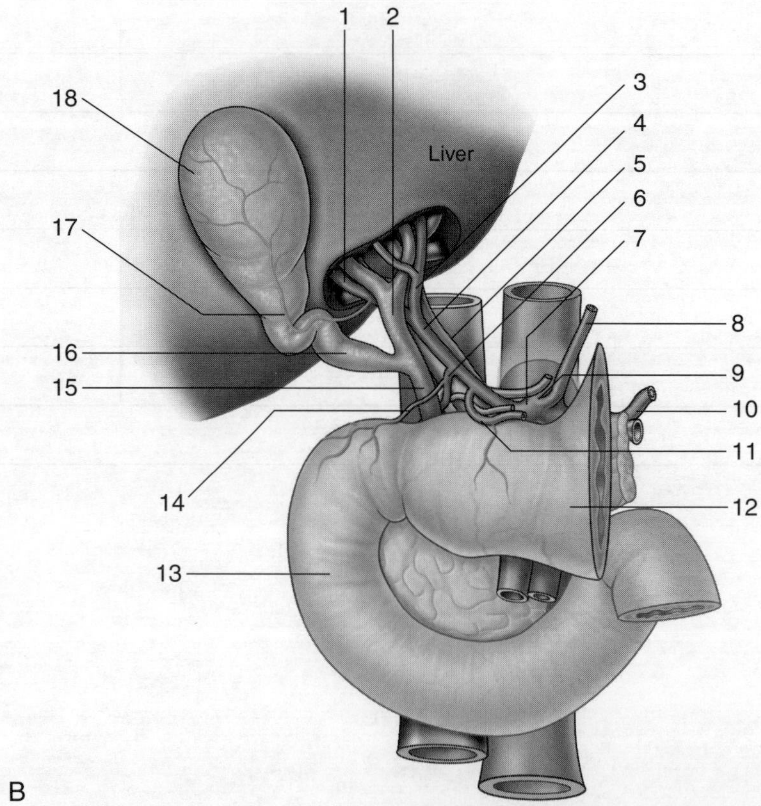

A. 1. ______

2. ______

3. ______

4. ______

5. ______

6. ______

7. ______

8. ______

9. ______

10. ______

B. 1. ______

2. ______

3. ______

4. ______

5. ______

6. ______

7. ______

8. ______

9. ______

10. ______

11. ______

12. ______

13. ______

14. ______

15. ______

16. ______

17. ______

18. ______

LABELING

Draw in the following types of abdominal incisions.

1. Subcostal

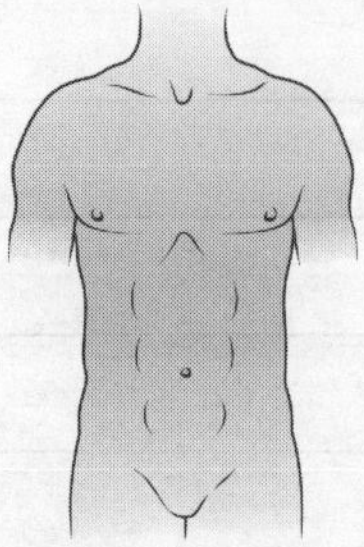

2. Paramedian

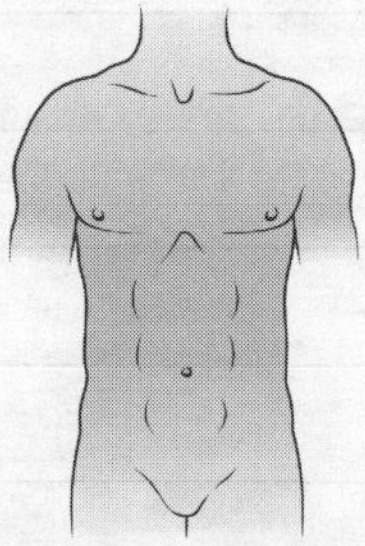

3. McBurney

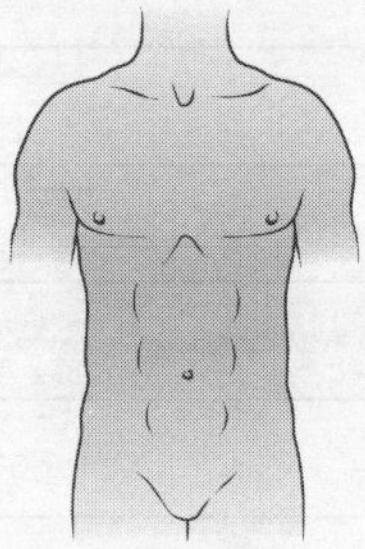

4. Pfannenstiel

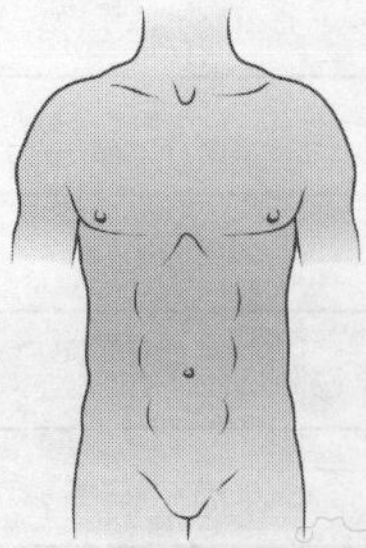

5. Upper midline

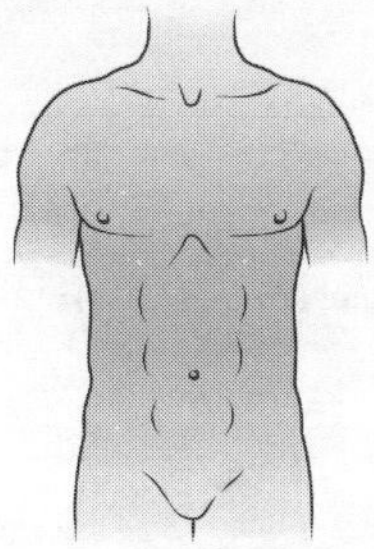

6. Upper abdominal transverse

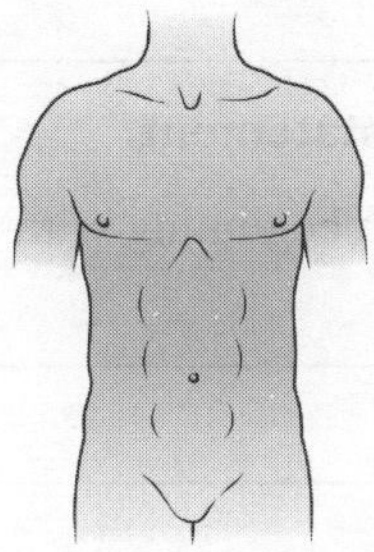

7. Oblique

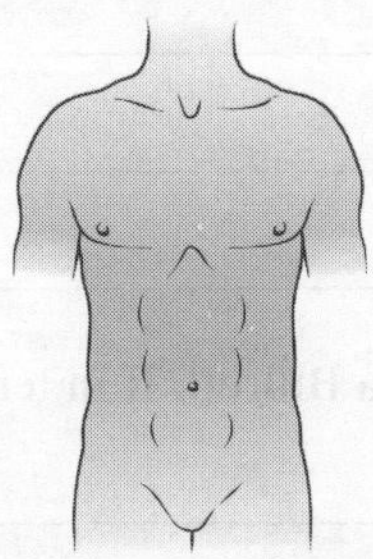

8. Lower midline

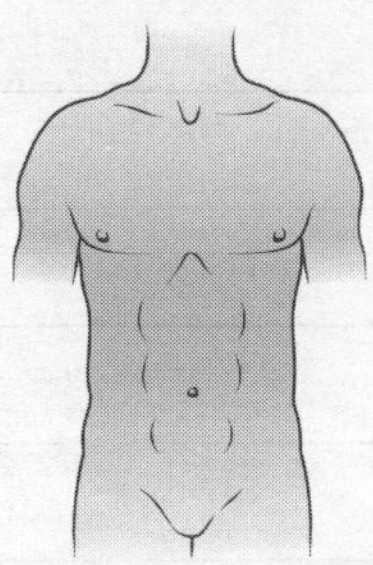

9. Draw the four quadrants of the abdomen and label them.

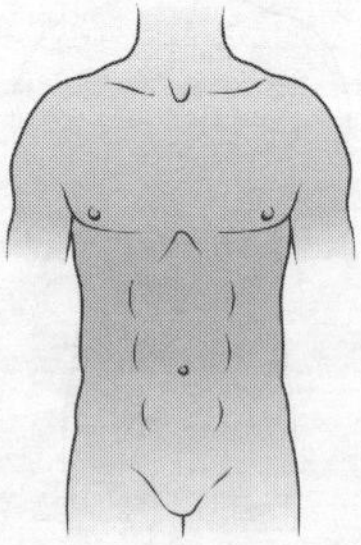

SHORT ANSWER

Provide a short answer for each question or statement.

1. List the three anatomical sections of the stomach beginning with the upper portion.

   a. ______________________________

   b. ______________________________

   c. ______________________________

2. What are the components of the Hesselbach triangle?

   a. ______________________________

   b. ______________________________

   c. ______________________________

3. What is the difference between a Billroth I and a Billroth II in terms of resection and anastomosis?

   ____

   ____

4. What are the tissue layers of the abdominal wall from outer to inner?

   a. ______________________________

   b. ______________________________

   c. ______________________________

   d. ______________________________

   e. ______________________________

5. What are the layers of the intestine from inner to outer?

   a. ______________________________

   b. ______________________________

   c. ______________________________

6. Define the following intestinal conditions.

   a. Volvulus: ______________________________

   b. Intussusception: ______________________________

   c. Paralytic ileus: ______________________________

   d. Peptic ulcer: ______________________________

7. Define the following endoscopic procedures, and what organs are being viewed for diagnosis.

   1. EGD: ______________________________

   2. Colonoscopy: ______________________________

   3. Sigmoidoscopy: ______________________________

   4. ERCP: ______________________________

   5. Choledochoscopy: ______________________________

MATCHING I

Match each term with the correct definition.

1. _______ Hernia that results from a defect in the inguinal floor. The defect is located in the Hesselbach triangle.
2. _______ Herniated tissue that is trapped in an abdominal wall defect causing loss of blood supply.
3. _______ A tract or tunnel through the tissue developing an epithelial lining preventing the wound from healing in an incisional hernia.
4. _______ Abdominal wall defect occurring in the linea alba at the umbilical ring.
5. _______ Postoperative herniation of tissue into the tissue layers of an abdominal incision.
6. _______ Hernia protrusion of the abdominal viscera into the inguinal canal from the deep inguinal ring.
7. _______ Hernia in which abdominal tissue has become trapped or strangulated by surrounding tissue between the layers of an abdominal wall defect.
8. _______ A type of incisional hernia.
9. _______ Rare hernia that occurs between the transverse abdominis and rectus muscles.

a. Ventral hernia

b. Direct inguinal hernia

c. Incisional hernia

d. Incarcerated hernia

e. Umbilical

f. Fistula

g. Indirect inguinal hernia

h. Strangulated hernia

i. Spigelian

MATCHING II

Match each type of breast procedure with the correct definition.

1. _______ Removal of a wire localized tissue mass for pathologic examination.
2. _______ The entire breast is removed and sentinel node biopsy or axillary dissection is performed.
3. _______ Removal of a breast mass ensuring margins are completely free of cancer cells. Axillary node dissection may be performed at the same time.
4. _______ Procedure in which a hook wire device is inserted into a breast mass using guided imagery.
5. _______ Procedure that removes the breast while leaving the skin, nipple, and areola intact.
6. _______ Skin sparing procedure in which one or more lymph nodes are removed to determine whether a tumor has metastasized; nodes are identified by isosulfan blue dye or technetium-99.
7. _______ Procedure that removes breast tissue, including the skin, areola, and nipple. The axillary lymph nodes are not removed.
8. _______ The entire breast, all axillary nodes, and chest wall muscles are removed.

a. Wire localization
b. Excisional biopsy
c. Lumpectomy
d. Radical mastectomy
e. Modified radical mastectomy
f. Sentinel lymph node biopsy
g. Simple mastectomy
h. Subcutaneous mastectomy

MATCHING III

Match the portions of the gastrointestinal tract.

1. _______ 10-inch tubular structure extending from the pharynx to the stomach entering the abdominal cavity at the diaphragm.
2. _______ The first portion of the large intestine.
3. _______ The distal 4 to 5 inches of the intestine.
4. _______ Extends from the distal ileum to the rectum and is divided into five sections.
5. _______ Area where muscular sphincters control the release of feces.
6. _______ Slender worm-shaped tube at the terminal end of the cecum that has no function.
7. _______ The first portion of the small intestine.
8. _______ The second portion of the small intestine.
9. _______ Sphincter that communicates the stomach with the esophagus.
10. _______ Connects to the esophagus containing the fundus, body, and antrum.
11. _______ The area where the rectum terminates.
12. _______ The distal portion of the small intestine connecting to the large intestine.

a. Jejunum
b. Pylorus
c. Rectum
d. Anal canal
e. Esophagus
f. Stomach
g. Cecum
h. Veriform appendix
i. Large intestine
j. Ileum
k. Cardia
l. Anal canal

MULTIPLE CHOICE

1. Removal of the entire breast, all axillary nodes, and chest wall muscles is called:
   a. Lumpectomy
   b. Sentinel lymph node biopsy
   c. Modified radical mastectomy
   d. Radical mastectomy

2. Injection of dye or radioactive material to provide visibility of nodes for removal is called:
   a. Lumpectomy
   b. Sentinel lymph node biopsy
   c. Modified radical mastectomy
   d. Radical mastectomy

3. Removal of a breast mass to confirm a diagnosis or to treat malignancy is called:
   a. Radical mastectomy
   b. Modified radical mastectomy
   c. Lumpectomy
   d. Sentinel lymph node biopsy

4. Removal of the entire breast and sentinel node biopsy or performing axillary dissection is called:
   a. Radical mastectomy
   b. Modified radical mastectomy
   c. Lumpectomy
   d. Sentinel lymph node biopsy

5. During a cholecystectomy, what is ligated?
   a. Common bile duct and cystic artery
   b. Common bile duct and cystic duct
   c. Cystic duct and cystic artery
   d. Common bile duct and common bile artery

6. During a cholecystectomy, which is preserved?
   a. Cystic duct
   b. Common bile duct
   c. Cystic artery
   d. Common bile artery

7. Which of the following is the procedure to treat gastroesophageal reflux disease (GERD)?
   a. Lap band gastroplasty
   b. Roux-en-y gastric bypass
   c. Nissen fundoplication
   d. Laparotomy

8. Which of the following procedures is performed to treat cancer of the head of the pancreas?
   a. Billroth I
   b. LeFort I
   c. Billroth II
   d. Whipple

9. Insulin and glucagon are synthesized in the region of the pancreas called:
   a. Islets of Langerhans
   b. Pancreatic duct
   c. Sphincter of Wirsung
   d. Ampulla of Vater

10. Bile enters the duodenum through an opening called:
    a. Islets of Langerhans
    b. Pancreatic duct
    c. Duct of Wirsung
    d. Ampulla of Vater

11. The release of bile and pancreatic enzymes is controlled by a sphincter in the ampulla called the sphincter of:
    a. Wirsung
    b. Odi
    c. Vater
    d. Langerhans

CASE STUDIES

1. *You are scrubbed in on an emergency endoscopic appendectomy. What are the steps (in order) for performing an appendectomy?*

____

23 Gynecological and Obstetrical Surgery

Student's Name ______________________

KEY TERMS

Write the definition for each term associated with gynecology and reproduction.

1. Ablate: ______________________
2. Adnexa: ______________________
3. Coitus: ______________________
4. Colposcopy: ______________________
5. Cystocele: ______________________
6. Dermoid cyst: ______________________
7. Electrolytic fluid: ______________________
8. Episiotomy: ______________________
9. Fibroid: ______________________
10. Hyperplasia: ______________________
11. Incomplete abortion: ______________________
12. LEEP: ______________________
13. Leiomyoma: ______________________
14. Menarche: ______________________
15. Menorrhagia: ______________________
16. Missed abortion: ______________________
17. Obturator: ______________________
18. Papanicolaou (Pap) test: ______________________
19. Parturition: ______________________
20. Perineum: ______________________
21. PID: ______________________
22. Transcervical: ______________________

Write the definition for each term associated with obstetrics.

23. Amniotic fluid: ____

24. Amniotic membranes: ____

25. Apgar score: ____

26. Birth canal: ____

27. Breech presentation: ____

28. Cerclage: ____

29. Cord prolapse: ____

30. Eclampsia: ____

31. Ectopic pregnancy: ____

32. Epidural: ____

33. Fetal demise: ____

34. Gestational age: ____

35. Incompetent cervix: ____

36. Labor: ____

37. Meconium: ____

38. Normal spontaneous vaginal delivery: ____

39. Nuchal cord: ____

40. Placenta: ____

41. Placental abruption: ____

42. Placenta previa: ____

43. Prenatal: ____

44. Presentation: ____

45. STD: ____

46. Suprapubic pressure: ____

47. Uterus: ____

LABELING

Label the structures of the vulva.

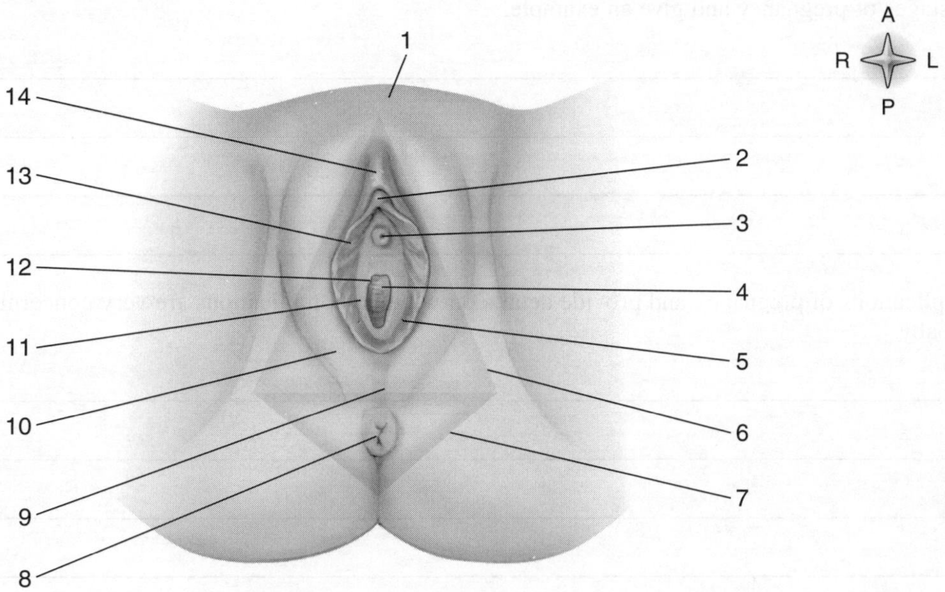

From Thibodeau G, Patton K: *Anatomy and physiology*, ed 6, St Louis, 2007, Mosby.

1. ______________________________

2. ______________________________

3. ______________________________

4. ______________________________

5. ______________________________

6. ______________________________

7. ______________________________

8. ______________________________

9. ______________________________

10. ______________________________

11. ______________________________

12. ______________________________

13. ______________________________

14. ______________________________

SHORT ANSWER

Provide a short answer for each question or statement.

1. Explain the stages of pregnancy and give an example.

2. List the complications of pregnancy and provide details on why the complications are very concerning for the mother and baby.

3. List the gynecologic diagnostic tests performed on pregnant women.

4. What is an Apgar score? List the assessment parameters.

5. Define a cesarean delivery and list conditions that would indicate a reason for a cesarean delivery.

MATCHING I

Match each term with the correct definition.

1. __________ Herniation of the bladder into the vaginal wall.
2. __________ Mass that arises from the germ layers of the embryo that contains tissue remnants, including hair and teeth.
3. __________ Endometrial tissue growth outside of the uterine cavity.
4. __________ Fibrous, benign tumor of the uterus that usually arises from the myometrium.
5. __________ Excessive proliferation of tissue.
6. __________ Sexually transmitted disease or other disease arising from an infection that causes scarring of the fallopian tubes and adhesions in the abdominal and pelvic cavities.
7. __________ Bulging of intestinal tissue into a weakened posterior vaginal wall.
8. __________ Excessive menstrual bleeding.
9. __________ Persistent or bleeding ovarian follicle that fails to regress after ovulation.
10. __________ Diagnosed in women with persistent multiple cystic follicles.
11. __________ Weakness and stretching of the cardinal ligaments can result in this condition.
12. __________ Implantation of the embryo outside the intrauterine cavity.

a. Ovarian cyst
b. Hyperplasia
c. Polycystic ovary syndrome
d. Uterine prolapse
e. Cystocele
f. PID
g. Rectocele
h. Ectopic pregnancy
i. Dermoid cyst
j. Leiomyoma
k. Menorrhagia
l. Endometriosis

MATCHING II

Match the surgical procedure with the correct definition.

1. __________ Removal of a circumferential core of tissue around the cervix.
2. __________ Ligation is performed to block the passage of ova through the tube and prevent implantation in the uterus.
3. __________ The removal of the uterus by a combined laparoscopic and vaginal approach.
4. __________ Surgical removal of the uterus and cervix through a transpelvic incision.
5. __________ Involves the dissection and wide removal of the uterus, fallopian tubes, ovaries, supporting ligaments, upper vagina, and pelvic lymph node chains.
6. __________ Complete removal of rectum, the distal sigmoid colon, the urinary bladder and distal ureters, and the internal iliac vessels and their lateral branches. All pelvic reproductive organs and lymph nodes, as well as the entire pelvic floor, pelvic peritoneum, levator muscle, and perineum, are removed.
7. __________ A fiber optic scope is inserted through the cervix and into the uterus.
8. __________ Removal of a benign leiomyoma of the myometrium to control bleeding and prevent pressure on other structures in the pelvis.
9. __________ Sharp and smooth curettes are used to remove the surface of the endometrium through a transvaginal approach.
10. __________ A transcervical approach is used to remove the uterus.
11. __________ Herniated tissue of the anterior and posterior vagina is reduced, and the vaginal walls are reconstructed.
12. __________ To create a functional vagina to facilitate sexual intercourse.
13. __________ A small, hollow tract that connects the bladder to the vagina.
14. __________ Shirodkar procedure performed on the cervical os to prevent spontaneous abortion of pregnancy.
15. __________ Wall may be everted and sutured to the skin to prevent recurrence.
16. __________ Surgical removal of the labia, as well as other structures of the vulva according to the extent of the pathology.

a. LAVH
b. TAH
c. Simple vulvectomy
d. Pelvic exenteration
e. Hysteroscopy
f. Cone biopsy of the cervix
g. Vesicovaginal fistula
h. Radical hysterectomy (Wertheim procedure)
i. Myomectomy
j. Bartholin gland cyst
k. Dilation and Curettage
l. Laparoscopic tubal ligation
m. Cerclage
n. Vaginal hysterectomy
o. Repair of a cystocele and rectocele
p. Vaginoplasty

MULTIPLE CHOICE

1. The first closing count of a cesarean section begins during closure of the:
   a. Uterus
   b. Peritoneum
   c. Fascia
   d. Subcutaneous

2. Which of the following is a hysterectomy clamp?
   a. Allen
   b. Heaney
   c. Harrington
   d. Pennington

3. Which of the following is a bladder retractor used during a cesarean section?
   a. DeLee
   b. O'Connor O'Sullivan
   c. Heaney
   d. Jackson

4. During a cesarean section, which of the following is a suction catheter used to suction the baby's mouth and nose?
   a. Asepto
   b. Yankauer
   c. Toomey
   d. DeLee

5. During a cesarean section, the incision in the uterus is extended with which of the following?
   a. Jorgensen scissors
   b. Heaney scissors
   c. Bandage scissors
   d. Jameson scissors

6. When a patient is positioned for a cesarean section, to prevent hypotension from pressure on the vena cava by the fetus, how is the patient positioned?
   a. Low lithotomy
   b. Modified left lateral with a wedge support under the patient's left hip
   c. Modified right lateral with a wedge support under the patient's right hip
   d. Supine

CASE STUDIES

1. *Many gynecology procedures are performed with the patient in the lithotomy position. What are the critical safety considerations for the lithotomy position?*

   1. ______________________________

   2. ______________________________

3. ______________________________

4. ______________________________

5. ______________________________

6. ______________________________

7. ______________________________

8. ______________________________

9. ____

10. ____

2. *You are scrubbed on a laparoscopic tubal ligation. Please answer the following.*

a. Define laparoscopic tubal ligation.

b. What position will the patient be in?

c. What instrument trays will you use?

d. What type of prep will be used?

e. How will you drape?

f. What type of setup will you use?

g. What anatomy do you need to be aware of?

24 Genitourinary Surgery

Student's Name ______________________

KEY TERMS

Write the definition for each term.

1. Arteriovenous fistula (or AV shunt): ______________________
2. Calculi: ______________________
3. Extracorporeal shockwave lithotripsy (ESWL): ______________________
4. Foley catheter: ______________________
5. Glomerular filtration rate (GFR): ______________________
6. Indwelling catheter: ______________________
7. Meatotomy: ______________________
8. Percutaneous: ______________________
9. Reflux: ______________________
10. Resectoscope: ______________________
11. Retrograde pyelography: ______________________
12. Specific gravity: ______________________
13. Staghorn stone: ______________________
14. Stent: ______________________
15. Tamponade: ______________________
16. Torsion: ______________________
17. Transurethral: ______________________

LABELING I

Identify the urinary catheters in the following figure, starting left to right.

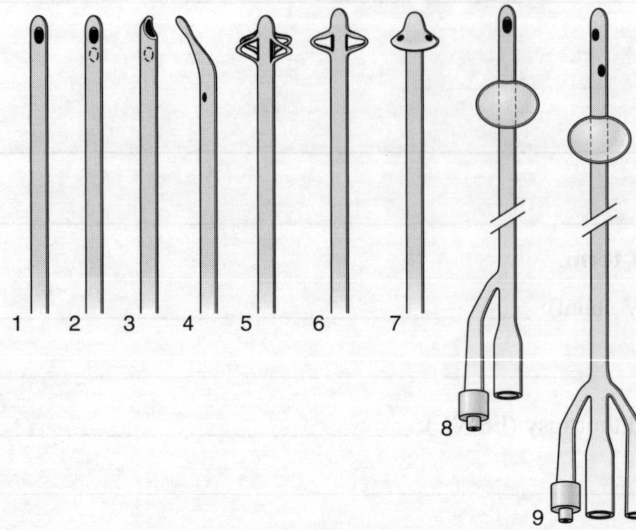

Modified from Walsh PC, Retik AB, Vaughan Ed, et al: *Campbell's urology*, ed 8, Philadelphia, 2002, WB Saunders.

1. ________________________

2. ________________________

3. ________________________

4. ________________________

5. ________________________

6. ________________________

7. ________________________

8. ________________________

9. ________________________

LABELING II

Identify the components of the male reproductive system.

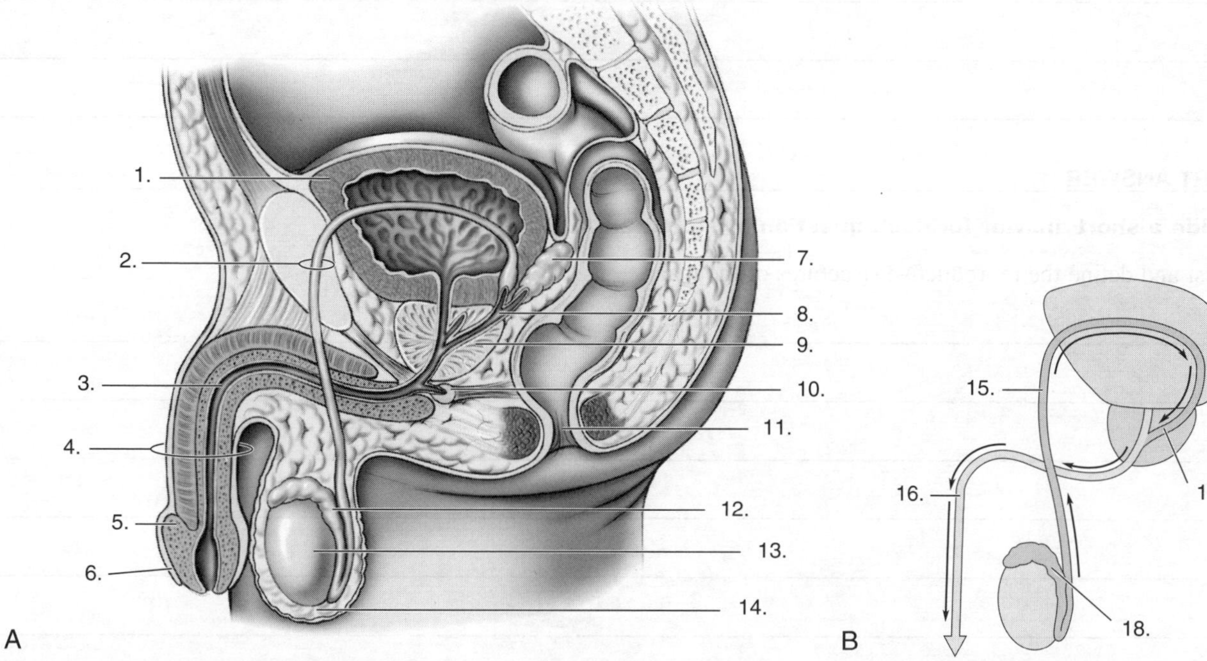

From Herlihy B, Maebius NK: *The human body in health and disease*, ed 2, Philadelphia, 2003, WB Saunders.

1. ______________________
2. ______________________
3. ______________________
4. ______________________
5. ______________________
6. ______________________
7. ______________________
8. ______________________
9. ______________________
10. ______________________
11. ______________________
12. ______________________
13. ______________________

14. ______

15. ______

16. ______

17. ______

18. ______

SHORT ANSWER

Provide a short answer for each question or statement.

1. List and define the reproductive structures of the male.

______

______

______

______

______

______

2. What is dialysis and how does it work?

______

______

______

______

______

______

MATCHING I

Match each term with the correct definition.

1. _______ A small incision made in the urethra to reduce scarring or relieve a stricture.
2. _______ Fluid-filled cyst at the spermatic cord.
3. _______ Congenital defect in which the external urethral meatus is located on the bottom side of the penis.
4. _______ Fluid-filled sac arising in the layers of the tunica vaginalis of the testicle.
5. _______ Process by which urine is secreted from the bladder.
6. _______ A procedure in which ultrasonic sound waves are delivered from outside the body and used to pulverize kidney stones.
7. _______ Congenital condition in which the external urethral meatus is located on the top of the penis rather than the tip.
8. _______ Removal of all or part of the prepuce (foreskin) of the penis.
9. _______ Condition in which the foreskin cannot be retracted from the glans.
10. _______ Surgical creation of vascular access for patients undergoing hemodialysis.

a. Hypospadias
b. Hydrocele
c. Spermatocele
d. ESWL
e. Phimosis
f. Micturition
g. Epispadias
h. Urethrotomy
i. AV shunt
j. Circumcision

MATCHING II

Match the term with the correct definition pertaining to the diagnostic test.

1. _______ Is performed to detect specific substances, both normal and abnormal, in urine.
2. _______ The presence or absence of specific substances in the blood reveals kidney function.
3. _______ Measures the rate of creatinine clearance from the blood.
4. _______ A test that assesses the elimination of urea from the liver.
5. _______ Tissue removed from the genitourinary (GU) tract for microscopic pathological testing.
6. _______ Is the preferred method for imaging tumors of the kidney.
7. _______ C-Arm real-time radiography.
8. _______ Radiographic studies using a contrast media to obtain radiographs of the renal pelvis and calyces.
9. _______ Radiograph of the kidney, ureters, and bladder used to outline structures of the urinary system.
10. _______ This study provides images of the bladder while it is emptying with use of contrast medium.
11. _______ Provides an extremely detailed assessment and is commonly used in the diagnosis of tumors.
12. _______ Radioisotope scanning in GU studies to detect metastasis arising from a primary tumor of the prostate.
13. _______ Retrograde injections are made using a catheter inserted into the ureter with contrast medium instilled in the catheter.
14. _______ One of the first-line imaging techniques used in GU medicine.

a. Tissue biopsy
b. Blood test
c. Computed tomography (CT)
d. Urinalysis
e. Blood urea nitrogen
f. Ultrasonography
g. Kidney, ureter, and bladder x-ray (KUB)
h. Glomular filtration rate (GFR)
i. Fluoroscopy
j. Magnetic resonance imaging (MRI)
k. IV urography
l. Micturating cystourethrogram (MCU)
m. Nuclear imaging
n. Retrograde ureteropyelogram

MULTIPLE CHOICE

1. Which procedure is removal of an enlarged prostate through an incision in the lower abdominal wall through the bladder?
   a. Transurethral resection of the prostate
   b. Open perineal prostatectomy
   c. Robot-assisted laparoscopic prostatectomy
   d. Suprapubic prostatectomy

2. The cortex of the kidney is covered with a strong fibrous tissue is called which of the following?
   a. Renal calyces
   b. Hilium
   c. Gerota's capsule
   d. Renal pyramids

3. Which of the following surgical procedures is removal of one or both testicles performed in cases of torsion or cancer?
   a. Phimosis
   b. Orchiectomy
   c. Hydrocelectomy
   d. Circumcision

4. Drainage and removal of a benign fluid-filled sac that develops in the anterior testis is which of the following?
   a. TURP
   b. Penectomy
   c. Orchiectomy
   d. Hydrocelectomy

5. Which of the following is a specimen evacuator collection device used to remove pieces of tumor during a TURP?
   a. Asepto
   b. Ellik
   c. Bulb
   d. Van Buren

6. Which of the following urethral catheters is used to traverse the urethra through an enlarged prostate?
   a. Coude
   b. Whistle tip
   c. Robinson
   d. Foley

CASE STUDIES

1. *You are about to scrub for a cystoscopy when the operating room supervisor delivers a surgical technology student to you and asks you to serve as her preceptor for the case. Your student has never seen a cystoscopy before, and you decide to describe the procedure to her before you start. What steps would you describe to her to explain the procedure?*

   a. ______________________________

   b. ______________________________

   c. ______________________________

   d. ______________________________

   e. ______________________________

   f. ______________________________

   g. ______________________________

   h. ______________________________

   i. ______________________________

   j. ______________________________

25 Ophthalmic Surgery

Student's Name ______________________________

KEY TERMS

Write the definition for each term.

1. Accommodation: ______________________________
2. Cataract: ______________________________
3. Cryotherapy: ______________________________
4. Diathermy: ______________________________
5. Enucleation: ______________________________
6. Evisceration: ______________________________
7. Exenteration: ______________________________
8. Focal point: ______________________________
9. Glaucoma: ______________________________
10. Keratoplasty: ______________________________
11. Muscle recession: ______________________________
12. Muscle resection: ______________________________
13. Phacoemulsification: ______________________________
14. Pterygium: ______________________________
15. Refraction: ______________________________
16. Spatula needle: ______________________________
17. Strabismus: ______________________________

SHORT ANSWER

Provide a short answer for each question or statement.

1. Explain the concept of refraction.

____

____

2. List and define the different types of diagnostic testing for the eye.

   a. _______________

   b. _______________

   c. _______________

   d. _______________

3. List the supplies needed for the sterile prep setup.

   a. _______________

   b. _______________

   c. _______________

   d. _______________

   e. _______________

   f. _______________

   g. _______________

   h. _______________

4. How should the instruments be cared for before, during, and after surgery?

5. What challenges does microsurgery present?

a.

b.

c.

6. List the guidelines for handling the microscope.

1.
2.
3.
4.
5.
6.
7.
8.
9.
10.

7. What is the protocol for the care of the microscope?

1. ______________________________

2. ______________________________

3. ______________________________

8. What is the role of the surgical technologist during eye surgery?

a. ______________________________

b. ______________________________

c. ______________________________

d. ______________________________

e. ______________________________

f. ______________________________

g. ______________________________

h. ______________________________

i. ______________________________

MATCHING I

Match each term with the correct definition. You may use the same answer more than once or not at all.

1. _______ Performed for treatment of glaucoma to create a channel for the aqueous humor to drain from the anterior chamber.
2. _______ Procedure performed for detached retina.
3. _______ A process in which high-frequency sound waves are used to fragment tissue, such as a cataract.
4. _______ The procedure performed for a corneal transplant.
5. _______ Surgery in which the eye muscle is moved back to release the globe.
6. _______ Surgical shortening of an eye muscle to pull the globe into correct position.
7. _______ Creation of a permanent opening in the tear duct for drainage of tears.
8. _______ Surgical removal of the eyeball (globe) but eye muscles are left intact.
9. _______ Removal of nodal tissue arising from a sebaceous gland excised from the tarsal plate.
10. _______ Surgical removal of the contents of the eyeball, with the sclera and muscle attachments left intact.
11. _______ Removal of the entire contents of the eye socket, including the globe, muscles, fat, and eyelids.
12. _______ A technique in which a cold probe is used to freeze tissue, such as the sclera, ciliary body (for glaucoma), or retinal layers, after detachment.
13. _______ Low-power cautery used to mark the sclera over the area of retinal detachment.

a. Dacryocystorhinostomy
b. Trabeculectomy
c. Exenteration
d. Diathermy
e. Cryotherapy
f. Enucleation
g. Phacoemulsification
h. Muscle recession
i. Evisceration
j. Muscle resection
k. Chalazion
l. Scleral buckling
m. Keratoplasty

MATCHING II

Match the drug with the brand name. You may use the same answer more than once or not at all.

1. _______ Constricts the pupil, used in intraocularly during anterior segment surgery.
2. _______ Stains the cornea yellow-green when used as a topical stain. When administered through an IV in angiography to diagnose retinal disorders
3. _______ Is a cholinergic, constricts the pupil, and is used topically to lower intraocular pressure in glaucoma.
4. _______ Injected subconjunctively for prophylaxis after eye procedures.
5. _______ Constricts the pupil.
6. _______ Mydriatic used to dilate the pupil but permit focusing for examination of the retina, testing refraction, and easier removal of the lens.
7. _______ Used to irrigate the eye to keep the cornea moist during surgery.
8. _______ Topical anesthetic applied directly to the eye providing loss of corneal sensation.
9. _______ Viscoadherent maintains a deep chamber for procedures of the anterior segment.
10. _______ Viscoelastic used to maintain separation between tissue and maintain pressure in the anterior chamber.
11. _______ Injectable anesthetic often used as a nerve block. Provides anesthesia of deep tissues.
12. _______ Osmotic diuretic administered intravenously to reduce intraocular pressure.
13. _______ Anticholinergic used for dilation of the pupil and for examination of the fundus and refraction.
14. _______ Adrenocorticosteroid anti-inflammatory agent injected subconjunctivally after surgery for prophylaxis.

a. Ancef, Kefzol

b. Occucoat

c. Miostat

d. Neo-Synephrine

e. Healon

f. Xylocaine

g. Tetracaine hydrochloride

h. BSS

i. Mydriacyl

j. Mannitol (osmitrol)

k. Decadron

l. Miotics

m. Pilocarpine hydrochloride

n. Fluorescein

MULTIPLE CHOICE

1. Ophthalmic sutures range in size from:
   a. 2-0 to 8-0
   b. 4-0 to 12-0
   c. 1-0 to 8-0
   d. 4-0 to 7-0

2. Which instrument is used to measure intraocular pressure?
   a. Sound
   b. Caliper
   c. Tonometer
   d. Depth gauge

3. Ophthalmic sponges are made from what type of material?
   a. Lint-free cellulose
   b. Oxidized cellulose
   c. Gelfoam
   d. Dry sponge sheets

4. During a lateral rectus resection, which suture is placed through the sclera as a traction suture?
   a. 7-0 nylon
   b. 3-0 nylon
   c. 6-0 vicryl
   d. 4-0 silk

5. An abnormal inversion of the lower eyelid, which causes the eyelashes to rub on the cornea.
   a. Strabismus
   b. Ectropion
   c. Entropion
   d. Chalazion

6. Which of the following is a circular cutting instrument that produces a tissue button during a corneal transplant?
   a. Spatula needle
   b. Vannas
   c. Westcott
   d. Trephine

7. Which of the following is a muscle hook?
   a. Jameson
   b. Vannas
   c. Westcott
   d. Trephine

8. An outwardly turned eyelid that creates an overflow of tears and exposes the conjunctiva, which becomes dry and irritated.
   a. Ectropion
   b. Enucleation
   c. Entropion
   d. Strabismus

CASE STUDIES

1. *You are a student assigned at a children's hospital and have been assigned to scrub in eye surgery with a preceptor who quizzes you frequently when you are ssigned to her. All of your cases in the room that day are to correct strabismus.*

   a. What is strabismus?

   b. What are the two common surgical procedures to correct strabismus? Provide a description of each procedure.

26 Surgery of the Ear, Nose, Pharynx, and Larynx

Student's Name ______________________________

KEY TERMS

Write the definition for each term.

1. Cerumen: ______________________________
2. Cholesteatoma: ______________________________
3. Effusion: ______________________________
4. Epistaxis: ______________________________
5. Evert: ______________________________
6. Hypertrophy: ______________________________
7. Ossicles: ______________________________
8. Ototoxic: ______________________________
9. Packing: ______________________________
10. Papilloma: ______________________________
11. Paranasal sinus: ______________________________
12. Paresis: ______________________________
13. Perforation: ______________________________
14. Phonation: ______________________________
15. Polyp: ______________________________
16. Sensorineural hearing loss: ______________________________
17. Transcanal: ______________________________
18. TM: ______________________________
19. Transsphenoidal: ______________________________
20. Tympanostomy tube: ______________________________

SHORT ANSWER

Provide a short answer to each question or statement.

1. List methods of external examination of the ear and diagnostic procedures performed to evaluate the ear.

2. List functions and names of instruments used for nasal procedures.

   a. Retractors

   b. Knives

   c. Elevators

   d. Forceps

   e. Rongeur

   f. Gouge/chisel/osteotome

   g. Rasp/saw

   h. Scissors

3. List instruments needed for a tonsillectomy.

____

____

MATCHING I

Match each term with the correct definition.

1. _______ A benign tumor of the middle ear caused by shedding of keratin in chronic otitis media.
2. _______ Defect in the the tympanic membrane that can be caused by trauma or infection.
3. _______ Enlargement of the tonsils that can cause airway obstruction or sleep apnea.
4. _______ A benign epithelial tumor characterized by a branching or lobular shape.
5. _______ Fluid in the middle ear.
6. _______ Bleeding arising from the nasal cavity.
7. _______ Vibration of the vocal cords during speaking or vocalization.
8. _______ The most common cause of a break in the ossicle chain, which erodes the ossicles.
9. _______ Paralysis of a structure, such as vocal cord paresis.
10. _______ Excessive proliferation of mucosal epithelium.
11. _______ Hearing impairment arising from the cochlea, auditory nerve, or central nervous system.
12. _______ Can cause infection, otorrhea, bone destruction, hearing loss, and paralysis of the facial nerve.

a. Cholesteatoma
b. Papilloma
c. Polyp
d. Perforation
e. Epistaxis
f. Effusion
g. Hypertrophy
h. Paresis
i. Sensorineural hearing loss
j. Phonation
k. Cholesteatoma

MATCHING II

Match each term with the correct definition.

1. _______ A surgical opening is made in the tympanic membrane to release fluid.
2. _______ Close a small, nonhealing hole in the tympanic membrane.
3. _______ Surgical removal of a cholesteatoma and mastoid bone, with or without reconstruction.
4. _______ Removal of diseased bone, the mastoid air cells, and the soft tissue lining the air cell of the mastoid.
5. _______ The reconstruction of the ossicles to restore conduction to the oval window, performed to treat profound hearing loss related to sclerosis of the stapes.
6. _______ Is used to transmit external sound directly to the VIII cranial nerve, to treat sensineural hearing loss.

a. Mastoidectomy/tympanomastoidectomy
b. Cochlear implant
c. Myringotomy
d. Tympanoplasty
e. Stapedectomy/ossicular reconstruction
f. Myringoplasty

MATCHING III

Match each term with the correct definition.

1. _______ Is performed to treat disease of the paranasal sinus, nasal cavity, and skull base and to improve nasal airflow.
2. _______ Maxillary sinus is exposed by making an incision in the gingival-buccal sulcus (the junction of the gum and upper lip).
3. _______ Removal of any bony obstruction at the frontal sinus to increase airflow through the nose.
4. _______ Surgical manipulation of the septum to return it to the correct anatomical position or to gain access to the sphenoid sinus for removal of a pituitary tumor.
5. _______ Is performed to reshape the external nose for aesthetic or functional purposes.
6. _______ Is performed to reduce ear, nose, and throat infection, and improve the airway.
7. _______ Surgical removal of the adenoids.
8. _______ Performed to reduce and tighten oropharyngeal tissue to improve obstructive sleep apnea.
9. _______ Endoscopic assessment of the larynx.
10. _______ Is performed in the emergency department, ICU, or operating room to create an airway for the patient.

a. Septoplasty
b. Endoscopic sinus surgery (ESS)
c. Tracheostomy/tracheostomy
d. Tonsillectomy
e. Caldwell-Luc
f. Laryngoscopy
g. Adenoidectomy
h. Turbinectomy/turbinate reduction
i. Rhinoplasty
j. UPP

MULTIPLE CHOICE

1. Which of the following is performed that involves removal of the larynx often including wide excision and tissue grafting as a part of the procedure?
   a. Total glossectomy
   b. Temporomandibular joint arthroplasty
   c. Radical neck dissection
   d. Laryngectomy

2. Procedure performed to treat malignant tumors; removal of all cervical lymph nodes and surrounding structures including the spinal accessory nerve, jugular vein, and sternocleidomastoid muscle.
   a. Radical neck dissection
   b. Laryngectomy
   c. Modified neck dissection
   d. Glossectomy

3. Which of the following is a type of salivary gland?
   a. Thyroid
   b. Parotid
   c. Cervical
   d. Adenexa

4. Which of the following is surgical removal of the entire tongue?
   a. Uvulopalatoplasty
   b. Tonsillectomy and adenoidectomy
   c. Modified radical neck dissection
   d. Glossectomy

5. Which of the following is an ear dressing consisting of several gauze sponges held in place with a molded plastic shield secured with Velcro straps?
   a. Colloid
   b. Fiberglass
   c. Glasscock
   d. Fluffs

CASE STUDIES

1. *If you are about to scrub for a radical neck dissection, you will have to know the extent of the dissection or the degree of pathology. What are the three types of neck dissection? What is involved in each?*

   a.

   b.

   c.

27 Oral and Maxillofacial Surgery

Student's Name ______________________________

KEY TERMS

Write the definition for each term.

1. Arch bars: ______________________________
2. Bicortical screw: ______________________________
3. Blowout fracture: ______________________________
4. Dentition: ______________________________
5. LeFort I fracture: ______________________________
6. LeFort II fracture: ______________________________
7. LeFort III fracture: ______________________________
8. Mastication: ______________________________
9. Maxillomandibular fixation (MMF): ______________________________
10. Occlusion: ______________________________
11. Odontectomy: ______________________________
12. Oromaxillofacial surgery: ______________________________
13. Subciliary incision: ______________________________
14. Transconjunctival incision: ______________________________

LABELING

Facial trauma may involve the many bones of the face and frontal sinus. To increase your knowledge of the anatomy of the bones of the face, label the following diagram.

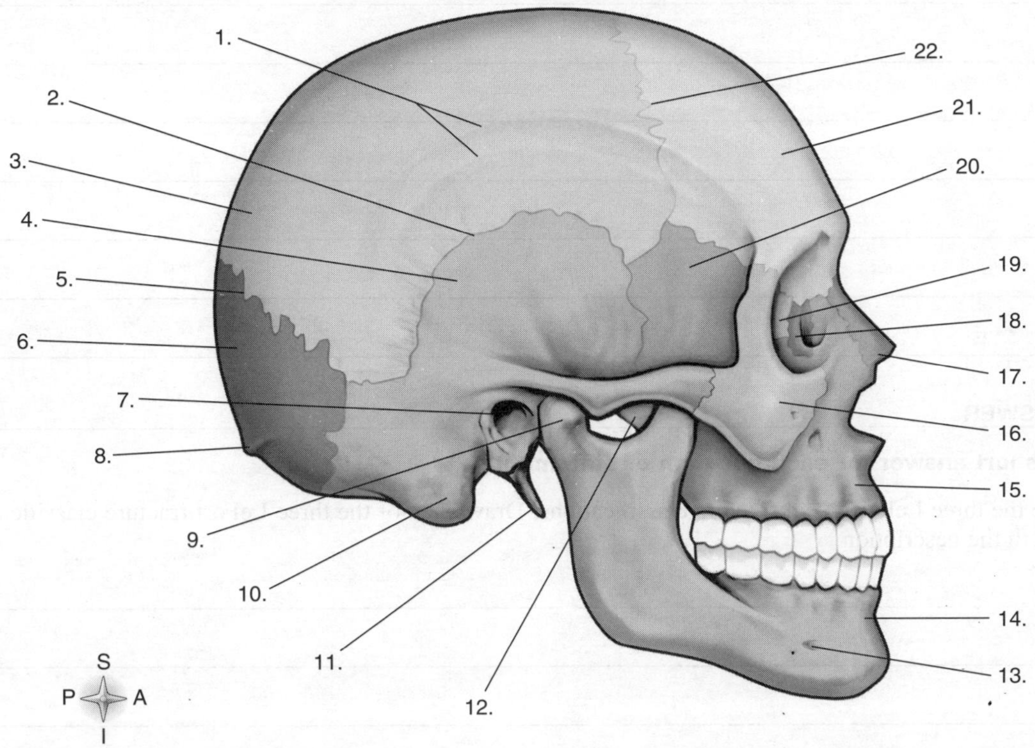

Modified from Thibodeau GA, Patt KT: *Anthony's textbook of anatomy and physiology*, ed 17, St Louis, 2003, Mosby.

1. ______________________________

2. ______________________________

3. ______________________________

4. ______________________________

5. ______________________________

6. ______________________________

7. ______________________________

8. ______________________________

9. ______________________________

10. ______________________________

11. ______________________________

12. ______________________________

13. ______________________________

14. ____________________

15. ____________________

16. ____________________

17. ____________________

18. ____________________

19. ____________________

20. ____________________

21. ____________________

22. ____________________

SHORT ANSWER

Provide a short answer for each question or statement.

1. Describe the three LeFort facial fracture classifications. Draw each of the three LeFort fracture classifications underneath the description.

   1. ____________________

   2. ____________________

   3. ____________________

MATCHING

Match each term with the correct definition. You may use the same answer more than once or not at all.

1. _______ Procedure to wire the jaws in a closed position with arch bars.
2. _______ Chewing
3. _______ Involved in "blowout" fractures.
4. _______ Mandible
5. _______ Maxilla
6. _______ Open reduction and internal fixation of a fracture.
7. _______ Procedure performed to remove teeth.

a. Maxillomandibular fixation
b. ORIF
c. Mastication
d. Upper jaw bone
e. Orbital floor
f. Frontal sinus
g. Lower jaw bone
h. Odontectomy

MULTIPLE CHOICE

1. Which of the following is a transverse fracture of the maxilla?
   a. LeFort I
   b. LeFort II
   c. LeFort III
   d. Odontectomy

2. Which gauge stainless steel wire is used for application of arch bars?
   a. 30–32 gauge
   b. 16–18 gauge
   c. 24–26 gauge
   d. 34–36 gauge

3. Which of the following is a pyramidal fracture of the maxilla?
   a. LeFort I
   b. LeFort II
   c. LeFort III
   d. Mandibular osteotomy

4. What must remain with the patient at all times postoperatively after arch bar application?
   a. Wire twisters
   b. Needle nose pliers
   c. Wire scissors
   d. Utility scissors

5. Which of the following fractures of the mid-face is the entire facial bone separated from the frontal bone through the zygoma?
   a. ORIF mandible
   b. ORIF maxilla
   c. LeFort I
   d. LeFort III

CASE STUDIES

1. *You are assigned to an ORIF repair of a mandible. Describe the purpose and steps of an open reduction and internal fixation of a mandibular fracture. What needs to be at the patient's bedside postoperatively?*

28 Plastic and Reconstructive Surgery

Student's Name ______________________

KEY TERMS

Write the definition for each term.

1. Aesthetic surgery: ______________________
2. Allograft: ______________________
3. Autograft: ______________________
4. Biological graft: ______________________
5. Biosynthetic graft: ______________________
6. Composite graft: ______________________
7. Debridement: ______________________
8. Dermatome: ______________________
9. Eschar: ______________________
10. Fasciotomy: ______________________
11. Full-thickness skin graft (FTSG): ______________________
12. Hypertrophic scar: ______________________
13. Keloid: ______________________
14. Mohs micrographic surgery: ______________________
15. Plication: ______________________
16. Porcine: ______________________
17. Ptosis: ______________________
18. Rule of nines: ______________________
19. Split-thickness (or partial-thickness) skin graft (STSG): ______________________
20. Synthetic grafts: ______________________
21. Undermine: ______________________
22. Xenograft: ______________________

LABELING

Label the following diagram. Name the type of skin graft in diagram A, then name the tissue layers. What type of skin graft is diagram B? Label the components of a hair follicle in diagram C.

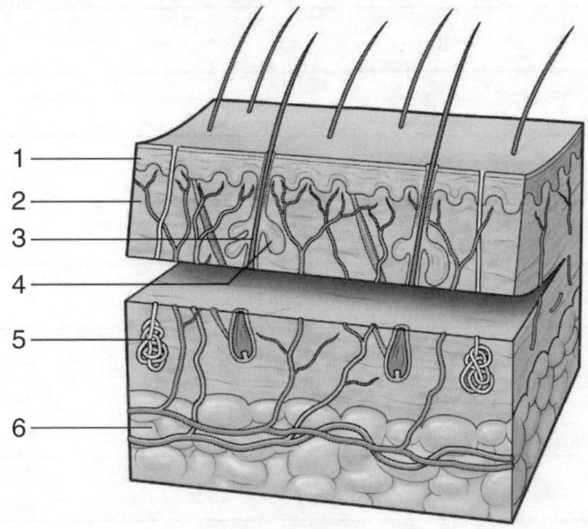

A

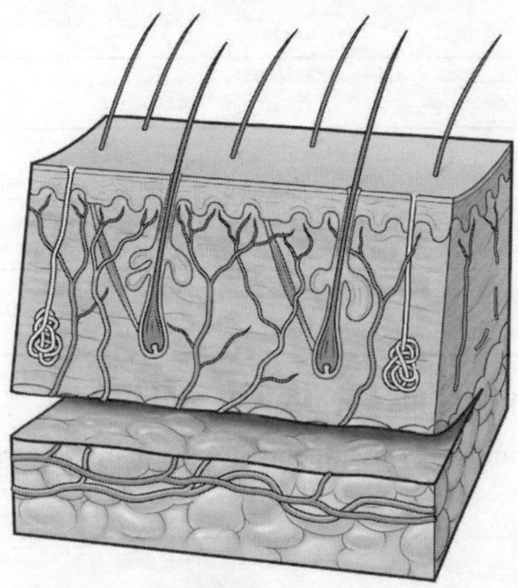

B

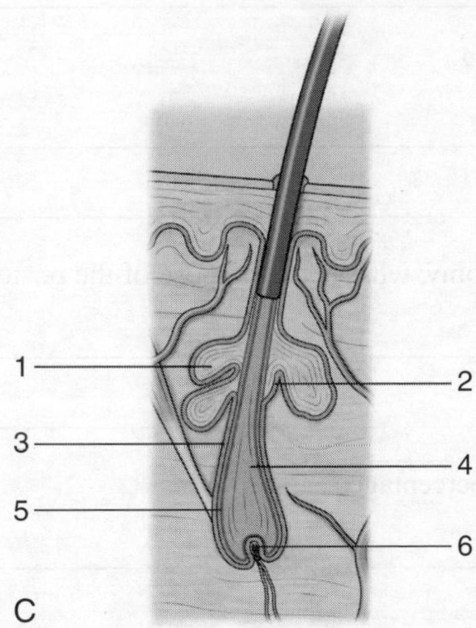

C

From Velasco J. Ballo R, Hood K, Jolley J, Rinewalt D, Veenstra B, *Essential Surgical Procedures*, Philadelphia 2016 Elsevier

A. Type of skin graft: ______

1. ______
2. ______
3. ______
4. ______
5. ______
6. ______

B. Type of skin graft: ______

C. Label the structures of a hair follicle.

1. ______
2. ______
3. ______
4. ______
5. ______
6. ______

SHORT ANSWER

Provide a short answer to complete each question or statement.

1. What advances the aging process and what treatments are available to arrest the process?

______

______

2. What are the specific goals of plastic surgery?

______

______

3. Following an abdominoplasty or panniculectomy, what is the purpose of the postoperative position?

______

______

4. Describe the Rule of Nines and identify the percentages.

______

______

5. List types of dermatomes.

____

____

6. List the different types of skin graft materials.

____

____

7. List different types of implant materials or injectable fillers used for a mentoplasty.

____

____

8. Describe a debridement of a burn.

____

____

____

____

MATCHING I

Match each term with the correct description.

1. _______ An unsevered graft raised from the donor site to provide coverage and vascularization to a soft tissue defect.
2. _______ A graft transferred from one individual (human) to another.
3. _______ A biological graft taken from one area of the body and transplanted to another area in the same patient.
4. _______ A biological graft consisting of more than one tissue type.
5. _______ A graft that contains only the dermis used to replace skin that has been lost as a result of trauma or disease.
6. _______ A graft derived from manufactured materials.
7. _______ A graft containing the dermis and epidermis used to cover a deep defect.
8. _______ Tissue taken from one species and grafted to another.
9. _______ Graft in which the entire graft is raised, excised, and transferred to another recipient site of the body.
10. _______ A graft derived from live tissue.

a. Allograft
b. Full-thickness skin graft
c. Biological graft
d. Xenograft
e. Split-thickness skin graft
f. Composite graft
g. Autograft
h. Synthetic graft
i. Pedicle graft
j. Free flap graft

MATCHING II

Match each term with the correct description.

1. _______ Is performed to remodel a previous scar or to remove a keloid.
2. _______ Is the removal of nonviable tissue from a burn or a nonhealing or traumatic wound.
3. _______ Reduction and removal of the loose apron of adipose tissue that arises from the lower abdomen.
4. _______ Resection of the eyelid to improve vision of the upper visual fields.
5. _______ Is performed to lift the supportive structures of the brow and alleviate drooping of skin, muscle, and fascia.
6. _______ Redundant and sagging supportive tissue of the face is reduced or modified to provide a more aesthetic appearance.
7. _______ Surgical modification of the external ear.
8. _______ Is performed to increase the size and improve the shape of the breast or create a new breast after mastectomy.
9. _______ Is performed to reduce excess breast tissue.
10. _______ Transverse rectus abdominis myocutaneous flap performed to reconstruct the breast without the use of implants.
11. _______ Is performed to remove excess deep fat with a cannula.
12. _______ Is performed to remove excess skin and adipose tissue from the abdominal wall.
13. _______ Performed to increase the height of the cheekbone for aesthetic purposes.
14. _______ Placement of a synthetic implant in the chin.

a. Malar augmentation
b. Liposuction
c. Abdominoplasty
d. Augmentation mammoplasty
e. Scar revision
f. Otoplasty
g. Panniculectomy
h. Brow lift
i. Debridement
j. TRAM
k. Blepharoplasty
l. Reduction mammoplasty
m. Rhytidectomy
n. Mentoplasty

MULTIPLE CHOICE

1. When performing a split-thickness skin graft, what is applied to the skin graft site to reduce friction?
   a. Vaseline
   b. Mineral oil
   c. Surgilube
   d. Lidocaine gel

2. During a split-thickness skin grafting procedure what is the graft mesher used for?
   a. Aerating the graft
   b. Increasing the surface area of the graft
   c. Improving contact between the graft and recipient site
   d. All of the above

3. Which of the following is treatment for a condition in which there is a pointed appearance of the ear at the top of the ear where it is normally rounded?
   a. Otoplasty
   b. Mentoplasty
   c. Correction of Stahl's ear
   d. Correction of syndactaly

4. Which is the technique of excising a malignant skin lesion by systematic removal of the margins and immediate microscopic examination, and additional tissue is removed until the margins of tissue are free of cancer cells?
   a. MOHS
   b. STSG
   c. FTSG
   d. DIEP

5. Which type of dressing is used after an STSG is placed to maintain contact between the skin graft and the tissue bed below it with a bolster that is secured over the graft with sutures?
   a. Glasscock
   b. Cast
   c. Stent
   d. Flat

CASE STUDIES

1. *Your patient is coming to surgery for debridement of a burn. Describe the different types of burns listed below using the American Burn Association classification system so you are familiar with the severity of the burn you will be treating.*

   a. Superficial partial-thickness, first-degree

   b. Partial-thickness, second-degree

   c. Full-thickness, second-degree

   d. Full-thickness, third-degree

29 Orthopedic Surgery

Student's Name ______________________

KEY TERMS

Write the definition for each term.

1. Alloy: ______________________
2. Aponeurosis: ______________________
3. Arthrodesis: ______________________
4. Bioactive implant: ______________________
5. Biocompatibility: ______________________
6. Biomechanics: ______________________
7. Broaches: ______________________
8. Cannulated: ______________________
9. Casting: ______________________
10. Closed reduction: ______________________
11. Comminuted: ______________________
12. Compartment syndrome: ______________________
13. Compression: ______________________
14. Cruciate: ______________________
15. Dislocation: ______________________
16. Distraction: ______________________
17. External fixation: ______________________
18. Internal fixation: ______________________
19. Open reduction: ______________________
20. Orthopedic system: ______________________
21. Press-fit: ______________________
22. Ream: ______________________
23. Reduction: ______________________

24. Replantation: ____________________

25. Tap: ____________________

26. Traction: ____________________

SHORT ANSWER

Provide a short answer for each question or statement.

1. What are the three stages of bone healing, and what occurs during each phase?

   a. ____________________

   b. ____________________

   c. ____________________

2. How are joints classified?

   a. ____________________

   b. ____________________

   c. ____________________

   d. ____________________

3. List the types of saws used in orthopedic surgery, including the movement/direction of the blade.

4. List the different types of instruments used in orthopedic surgery and give an example.

5. List the different types of fracture patterns and give an example of each.

6. Describe reduction and fixation of fractures.

7. List the parts of a screw and define.

8. List and define the different types of screws.

9. List the functions of a plating system.

10. List and define the different types of plates.

11. Define and give an example of the following: IM rod, wires and cables, K-wires, and Steinmann pins.

12. Traction is used for:

    Describe two types of traction.

13. List and define the different types of arthroplasty materials used for joint replacement.

14. Describe the following drill attachments and accessories.

a. Burr: ______________________________

b. Chuck: ______________________________

c. Depth gauge: ______________________________

d. Drill bit: ______________________________

e. Drill guide: ______________________________

f. Reamer: ______________________________

g. Shaver: ______________________________

h. Tap: ______________________________

15. List hemostatic agents used on bone.

____

16. Describe laminar air flow.

____

17. List various dressing materials and uses applied in the operating room at the end of the case.

____

MATCHING I

Match each of the following types of joint.

1. ______ The fluid located in joints.
2. ______ Composed of a bony protuberance and an open collar component allowing rotation (first and second vertebrae of the neck).
3. ______ Has limited movement or a fixed articular surface such as between the bones of the cranium
4. ______ Has a rocker-and-cradle component, allowing extension and flexion only (elbow).
5. ______ The most freely movable type of joint allowing flexion, extension, abduction, adduction, rotation, and circumduction (hip).
6. ______ Freely movable synovial joint (shoulder).
7. ______ Joint in which the two components have a complimentary convex-concave shape in which the bones slide over each other. The body only has one, which is the thumb.
8. ______ Joint in which a small protrusion slides within a slightly elliptical component allowing flexion, extension, abduction, and adduction. (carpal bones of the wrist).
9. ______ Joint in which relatively flat surfaces of bone slide over each other (vertebrae).
10. ______ Joint in which bones are connected by cartilage and only slightly movable (symphasis pubis).

a. Hinge joint
b. Saddle joint
c. Gliding joint
d. Ball and socket joint
e. Pivot joint
f. Condyloid joint
g. Synovial
h. Diathrosis (synovial joint)
i. Amphiarthrosis (cartilaginous joint)
j. Synarthrosis (suture joint)

MATCHING II

Match the parts of the bone and different orthopedic pathology.

______ 1. Compact bone found in the shaft of long bones, at the ends of joints, and in vertebrae where it is surrounds the softer cancellous bone.

______ 2. Torn or detached tendon, ligament, or muscle often occurring as a sudden event or trauma.

______ 3. Membrane covering the bones.

______ 4. Partial or complete tearing away of tissue such as bone, tendon, muscle, or ligaments from the normal point of attachment.

______ 5. Damage and disease of soft connective tissues caused by repetitive motion or repeated stress.

______ 6. Found in the ends of long bone, containing red and yellow marrow, is also called spongy bone.

______ 7. The ends of the long bones.

______ 8. A break of the continuity of bone due to trauma or disease.

______ 9. The middle shaft of the bone.

a. Avulsion
b. Fracture
c. Cortical bone
d. Cancellous bone
e. Periosteum
f. Diaphysis
g. Epiphysis
h. Overuse injury
i. Rupture

MATCHING III

Match the procedure.

______	1. Performed to restore mobility to the hand and fingers by releasing constricted palmar fascia.	a. Triple arthrodesis
______	2. Fusion of the talocalcaneal, talonavicular, and calcaneocuboid joint.	b. Bankart procedure
______	3. Performed to treat a tear in the ACL to provide stability to the knee.	c. Bunionectomy
______	4. Reduction or removal of an enlarged hallux valgus.	d. Dupuytren contracture
______	5. Performed to reattach the labrum to the glenoid rim to correct recurrent glenohumeral dislocation.	e. Cruciate ligament repair

MULTIPLE CHOICE

1. Which is the longest bone in the body?
   a. Tibia
   b. Fibula
   c. Femur
   d. Phalanges
2. Application without an incision of an external fixator is which of the following?
   a. ORIF
   b. CREF
   c. CRIF
   d. OREF
3. Which of the following is a bone holding clamp?
   a. Cobb
   b. Langenbeck
   c. Hibbs
   d. Lowman
4. The single largest patient risk associated with casting is?
   a. Dupetryns
   b. Compartment syndrome
   c. Carpel tunnel
   d. Cardiac arrest
5. Which of the following is the most common site for bone graft harvesting?
   a. Ischium
   b. Femur
   c. Iliac crest
   d. Sacrum

CASE STUDIES

1. *Your patient has arrived for an arthroplasty. Describe patient risks associated with polymethylmethacrylate (PMMA), which is also called bone cement, and the technique used to reduce the hazards of PMMA.*

2. *You have just been called in for orthopedic trauma. Knowing the types of bone fractures helps you choose the type of instrumentation needed for the repair. Working from left to right, label the fractures pictured in the following figure.*

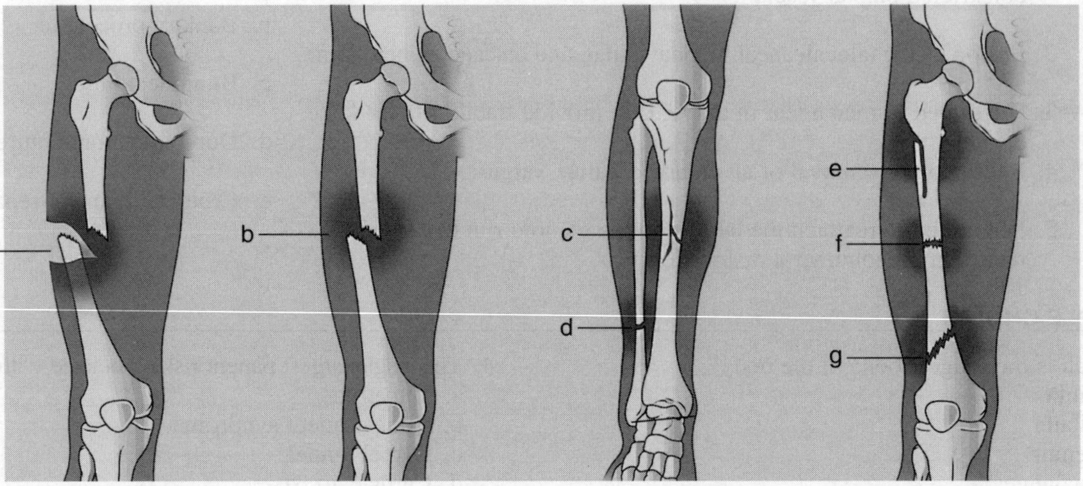

a. ______________________________

b. ______________________________

c. ______________________________

d. ______________________________

e. ______________________________

f. ______________________________

g. ______________________________

30 Vascular and Microvascular Surgery

Student's Name ______

KEY TERMS

Write the definition for each term.

1. Aneurysm: ______
2. Angioplasty: ______
3. Arteriosclerosis: ______
4. Arteriotomy: ______
5. Atherosclerosis: ______
6. Bifurcation: ______
7. Doppler duplex ultrasonography: ______
8. Embolus: ______
9. Endarterectomy: ______
10. Endovascular: ______
11. Hemodialysis: ______
12. Hemodynamic: ______
13. Hybrid operating room: ______
14. In situ: ______
15. Infarction: ______
16. Intimal hyperplasia: ______
17. Intravascular ultrasound: ______
18. Ischemia: ______
19. Lumen: ______
20. Microsurgery: ______
21. Percutaneous: ______
22. Stent: ______
23. Thrombus: ______

24. Umbilical tape: ______

25. Venous stasis: ______

26. Vessel loop: ______

SHORT ANSWER

Provide a short answer for each question or statement.

1. List the structures of the blood vessel and define.

______

______

2. Define blood pressure and list factors that affect normal blood pressure.

______

______

3. List the major arteries of the body in their designated locations provided below.

   a. Thoracic cavity: ______

   b. Head: ______

   c. Upper extremeties: ______

   d. Abdomen: ______

   e. Lower limbs: ______

4. List the diagnostic procedures associated with peripheral vascular surgery.

   a. ______

   b. ______

   c. ______

   d. ______

5. List and give an example of instruments used in peripheral vascular surgery.

   a. ______

   b. ______

   c. ______

d.

e.

f.

6. List the sutures, accessories, vascular graft materials, and medications used for peripheral vascular surgery.

a.

b.

c.

d.

7. Define the following surgical procedures.

a. Endarterectomy

b. Intraoperative angiography

c. Angioplasty

d. Insertion of a vena cava filter

e. Vascular access for renal hemodialysis

f. Arteriovenous shunt

g. Arteriovenous fistula

h. Thrombectomy

i. Carotid endarterectomy

j. Abdominal aortic aneurysm

k. Aortobifemoral bypass

l. Axillofemoral bypass

m. Femorofemoral bypass

n. In situ saphenous femoropopliteal bypass

o. Femoropopliteal bypass

MATCHING I

Match the following.

1. ______ Carries blood back to the heart from the peripheral tissues.	a. Arteries
2. ______ Carries oxygenated blood from the heart to the rest of the body.	b. Pulmonary arteries
3. ______ Moves blood to the lungs and back to the heart.	c. Veins
4. ______ Carries blood to all organs and tissues of the body except the lungs and then returns it to the heart.	d. Systemic circulation
	e. Pulmonary circulation
5. ______ Carries deoxygenated blood from the heart to the lungs.	

MATCHING II

Match each disease process with the correct definition.

1. ______ Ballooning of an artery as a result of weakening of the arterial wall caused by atherosclerosis, infection, or anatomical defect.	a. Aneurysm
	b. Arteriosclerosis
2. ______ Clot of blood, air, or atherosclerotic plaque or fat that moves freely in the vascular system.	c. Atherosclerosis
3. ______ Drop in blood pressure related to reduced blood or fluid volume.	d. Embolus
4. ______ Abnormally high blood pressure.	e. Hypotension
5. ______ Blockage in an artery, leading to ischemia and tissue death.	f. Hypovolemia
6. ______ A stationary clot in the arterial or venous system.	g. Hypertension
7. ______ The most common form of arteriosclerosis, which causes plaque to form on the inner surface of an artery.	h. Infarction
	i. Ischemia
8. ______ Decrease or absence of blood supply to a localized area.	
	j. Thrombus
9. ______ Abnormal decrease in blood pressure.	
10. ______ Disease characterized by thickening, hardening, and loss of elasticity of the artery walls.	

MATCHING III

Match the following agents.

1. ______ Heparin	a. Vasodilator
2. ______ Gelfoam	b. Topical hemostatic
3. ______ Avitene	c. Anticoagulant
4. ______ Papaverine	
5. ______ Surgicel	
6. ______ Thrombin	

MATCHING IV

Match the following; items may have more than one answer.

1. _______ Used to create a tubular space through tissue in which a graft can be threaded.
2. _______ Used for retraction of blood vessels.
3. _______ Glasses with mounted oculars used to magnify the surgical field.
4. _______ Used to prevent suture material from cutting through the arterial wall.
5. _______ Placed on tips of mosquito forceps to prevent damage to the suture on a double-ended suture.

a. Loupes
b. Shods/paws/boots
c. Loop
d. Umbilical tape
e. Pledget
f. Tunneler

MULTIPLE CHOICE

1. Which type of aneurysm is characterized by a hematoma that arises from a blood vessel?
   a. Fusiform
   b. Saccular
   c. Pseudo
   d. Dissecting

2. Which type of aneurysm is characterized by a bulging that is symmetrical?
   a. Fusiform
   b. Saccular
   c. Pseudo
   d. Dissecting

3. Which type of catheter is used to perform an embolectomy?
   a. Foley
   b. Filiform
   c. Coude
   d. Fogarty

4. Which type of aneurysm is characterized by its protrusion from one wall only?
   a. Fusiform
   b. Saccular
   c. Pseudo
   d. Dissecting

5. Which type of aneurysm results from a tear in the intima of the vessel that gives rise to splitting of the arterial wall?
   a. Fusiform
   b. Saccular
   c. Pseudo
   d. Dissecting

CASE STUDIES

1. *You are relieving the surgical technologist on a bilateral femoropopliteal bypass.*

   a. What is the first thing you should do when you scrub in?

b. What types of medication should you have on the field?

c. What types of sponges should you have on the field?

d. What extra sterile equipment should you have on the field?

e. What is the technique used in a femoropopliteal bypass?

f. After the case, what should you do?

31 Thoracic and Pulmonary Surgery

Student's Name ____________________

KEY TERMS

Write the definition for each term.

1. Apnea: ____________________
2. Arterial blood gases (ABGs): ____________________
3. Bleb: ____________________
4. Closed chest drainage: ____________________
5. Diffusion (oxygen): ____________________
6. Dyspnea: ____________________
7. Empyema: ____________________
8. Expiration: ____________________
9. Hemothorax: ____________________
10. Hypoxia: ____________________
11. Inspiration: ____________________
12. Perfusion (oxygen): ____________________
13. Pneumothorax: ____________________
14. Pulmonary function tests (PFTs): ____________________
15. Ventilation: ____________________

LABELING I

Draw a diagram of the bilateral lungs. Be sure to label your drawing. Include the tollowing structures in your drawing.

Cartilaginous rings

Trachea

Apex

Primary bronchi

Superior lobe

Secondary bronchi

Tertiary bronchi

Bronchiole

Inferior lobe

Hilus

Base

Inferior lobe

Middle lobe

Superior lobe

SHORT ANSWER

Provide a short answer for each question or statement.

1. What organs and structures are located in the mediastinal space?

2. Explain the pleural cavity. Include in your explanation the pleural sac, pleural space, and negative pressure.

3. What diagnostic tests would be done on a patient who will undergo lung and respiratory surgical procedures?

4. What position and incisions would most likely be used for patients undergoing pulmonary procedures?

5. List the equipment, supplies, and medication associated with thoracic and pulmonary surgery.

6. List the different types of instruments associated with thoracic and pulmonary surgery.

7. Define the following surgical procedures associated with thoracic and pulmonary surgery.

   a. Insertion of chest tube

   b. Rigid bronchoscopy

   c. Flexible bronchoscopy

   d. Mediastinoscopy

   e. VATS

f. Endobronchial ultrasound

g. VATS lung biopsy

h. Lung volume reduction surgery

i. Thoracotomy

j. Lobectomy

k. Pneumonectomy

l. Decortication of the lung

m. Lung transplantation

____

____

____

MATCHING

Match the medical diagnosis with the correct surgical intervention. You may use the same answer more than once or not at all.

1. ________ Decortication of the lung
2. ________ Mediastinoscopy
3. ________ VATS
4. ________ Lung transplantation
5. ________ Lung volume reduction
6. ________ Lobectomy
7. ________ Chest tube insertion for bleeding
8. ________ Chest tube insertion for spontaneous collapse lung
9. ________ Thoracotomy
10. ________ Pneumonectomy
11. ________ Bronchoscopy

a. Dyspnea and hypoxia caused by pulmonary emphysema
b. Bronchitis
c. Removal of a small portion of lung tissue for pathological assessment with use of a thoracoscope
d. Thymus and lymph node biopsy to establish a diagnosis or determine cancer
e. End-stage pulmonary disease
f. Removal of a portion of the lung for treatment of cancer, cysts, localized infection, or trauma to a portion of the lung to prevent the spread of cancer
g. Hemothorax
h. Thoracic emergency such as an open or penetrating wound
i. Bronchiectasis, pulmonary obstruction, extensive or chronic abscess, or a palliative measure to slow the progression of cancer
j. Pneumothorax
k. Aspiration of a foreign body
l. Empyema

MULTIPLE CHOICE

1. Excessively deep respiration:
   a. Apnea
   b. Hyperventilation
   c. Hyperpnea
   d. Dyspnea

2. Cessation of breathing:
   a. Dyspnea
   b. Apnea
   c. Cyanosis
   d. Hypoventilation

3. Bluish tint to the skin seen in patients with poor oxygenation:
   a. Apnea
   b. Dyspnea
   c. Dysphasia
   d. Cyanosis

4. Difficulty or painful respiration:
   a. Dyspnea
   b. Dysphasia
   c. Diaphoresis
   d. Apnea

5. Which of the following is used during bronchoscopy to collect sputum of fluid samples?
   a. Ellik
   b. Toomey
   c. Lukens
   d. Chest drainage tube

CASE STUDIES

1. *Your patient has a lung disease and will have to undergo lung transplantation. Answer the following questions about your patient and the procedure to better understand the operation.*

   a. What disease processes might precipitate the patient's need for a transplant?

   b. In what position will your surgical patient be placed for the procedure?

   c. Will your patient need to go on bypass for the procedure?

32 Cardiac Surgery

Student's Name ______________________

KEY TERMS

Write the definition for each term.

1. Aneurysm: ______________________
2. Aortotomy: ______________________
3. Apex: ______________________
4. Arrhythmia: ______________________
5. Arteriosclerosis: ______________________
6. Atherosclerosis: ______________________
7. Bicaval cannulation: ______________________
8. Bradycardia: ______________________
9. Cardiac cycle: ______________________
10. Cardioplegia: ______________________
11. Coarctation: ______________________
12. Conduit: ______________________
13. Congenital: ______________________
14. Cross-clamp: ______________________
15. Diastole: ______________________
16. Endovascular repair: ______________________
17. Femoral cannula: ______________________
18. Fibrillation: ______________________
19. Infarction: ______________________
20. Ischemia: ______________________
21. Off-pump procedure: ______________________
22. Pacemaker: ______________________
23. Shunt: ______________________

24. Stenosis: ____________________

25. Sternotomy: ____________________

26. Systole: ____________________

27. Tachycardia: ____________________

28. Thoracoabdominal aortic aneurysm: ____________________

29. Thoracotomy: ____________________

30. Type A aortic dissection: ____________________

SHORT ANSWER

Provide a short answer for each question or statement.

1. What structures are in the thoracic cavity?

____

____

2. List the diagnostic tests associated with cardiac surgery.

____

____

3. List the equipment, supplies, and medication associated with cardiac surgery.

____

____

4. Describe the following items and equipment associated with cardiac surgery.

   a. Cardiac catheterization

   ____

   ____

   b. Vessel and patch grafts

   ____

   ____

   c. Prosthetic valves

   ____

   ____

d. Pacemaker

e. Cardiopulmonary bypass machine

5. Define the following surgical procedures.

a. Median sternotomy

b. CABG

c. Resection of a left ventricular aneurysm

d. Aortic valve replacement

e. Mitral valve repair and replacement

f. Resection of an aneurysm of the ascending aorta

g. Resection of an aneurysm of the ascending arch

h. Resection of an aneurysm of the descending thoracic aorta

____

____

i. Endovascular repair of a thoracic aneurysm

____

____

j. Insertion of an artificial cardiac pacemaker

____

____

k. Temporary pacemaker

____

____

l. Insertion and removal of an intraaortic balloon catheter

____

____

m. Left ventricular assist device

____

____

n. Heart transplantation

____

____

MATCHING

Match each term with the correct definition.

1. ______ Weakening of the heart muscle caused by obstruction of coronary arteries.
2. ______ Buildup of plaque or cholesterol deposits in the lining of the arteries.
3. ______ Chaotic disorganized stimulation of one or both atria that prevents atrial contraction.
4. ______ Disease of the arteries characterized by loss of elasticity and hardening of arterial walls.
5. ______ Weakening of the wall of an artery or the heart chamber, leading to thinning and ballooning.
6. ______ Cause for this would include valve disease, coronary artery disease, and congenital heart disease.
7. ______ Heart rate below 60 beats/min.
8. ______ Possible narrowing of aortic and mitral valve or valves.
9. ______ Cardiac muscle that beats abnormally fast.

a. Aneurysm
b. Arteriosclerosis
c. Atrial fibrillation
d. Bradycardia
e. Heart transplantation
f. Atherosclerosis
g. Myocardial infarction
h. Valve stenosis
i. Tachycardia

MULTIPLE CHOICE

1. Heart rate over 120 beats per minute:
   a. Atrial flutter
   b. Atrial fibrillation
   c. Ventricular fibrillation
   d. Ventricular tachycardia

2. Heart rate of 240 - 350 beats per minute:
   a. Ventricular tachycardia
   b. Atrial flutter
   c. Atrial fibrillation
   d. Ventricular fibrillation

3. Chaotic disorganized stimulation of one or both ventricles that does not pump the blood:
   a. Ventricular tachycardia
   b. Atrial fibrillation
   c. Ventricular fibrillation
   d. Bradycardia

4. Which of the following is a combination of congenital defects including pulmonary stenosis, ventricular septal defect, right ventricular hypertrophy, and displacement of the aorta?
   a. Tetralogy of Fallot
   b. Circle of Willis
   c. Wilm's
   d. Hirschsprung's

5. Which incision is used for incision for placement of a permanent pacemaker?
   a. Median sternotomy
   b. Thoracoabdominal
   c. Subxiphoid
   d. Subclavian

CASE STUDIES

1. *You are assigned to scrub for the surgeon who is performing grafting of the saphenous vein during a CABG. What supplies should you have available, and what are the steps of the procedure?*

33 Pediatric Surgery

Student's Name ______________________________

KEY TERMS

Write the definition for each term.

1. Acquired abnormality: ______________________________
2. Bolus: ______________________________
3. Child life specialist: ______________________________
4. Choana: ______________________________
5. Coarctation: ______________________________
6. Congenital: ______________________________
7. Ductus arteriosus: ______________________________
8. Embryonic life: ______________________________
9. Exstrophy: ______________________________
10. Fetus: ______________________________
11. Genetic abnormality: ______________________________
12. Homeostasis: ______________________________
13. Isolette: ______________________________
14. Magical thinking: ______________________________
15. Mutagenic substance: ______________________________
16. Nephroblastoma: ______________________________
17. Neutral tube defect: ______________________________
18. Omphalocele: ______________________________
19. Pyloric stenosis: ______________________________
20. Teratogen: ______________________________

SHORT ANSWER

Provide a short answer for each question or statement.

1. Name three perioperative interventions used to maintain normothermia.

   a. ______

   b. ______

   c. ______

2. What is the surgical technologist's responsibility in reporting and calculating blood loss in pediatric patients?

3. Babies with esophageal atresia or a transesophageal fistula usually are low-birth-weight babies. Why?

4. What is Hirschsprung disease?

5. What is epispadias?

6. What is the primary differences regarding electrosurgery in the pediatric patient versus the adult patient?

7. List important considerations in pediatric anesthesia that differ physiologically and anatomically from adults.

8. List the specialty instrumentation related to pediatric surgery.

9. Thermoregulation is important during pediatric surgery. List and define the two risks that pediatric patients are particularly vulnerable to.

____

____

10. List the developmental stages of the child, and list a psychological characteristic.

____

____

____

____

11. Define the following surgical procedures.

 a. Repair of a cleft lip

 ____

 ____

 b. Repair of a cleft palate

 ____

 ____

 c. Orchiopexy

 ____

 ____

 d. Pyloromyotomy

 ____

 ____

 e. Correction of choanal atresia

 ____

 ____

 f. Repair of pectus excavatum

 ____

 ____

 g. Nephrectomy in Wilms tumor

 ____

 ____

h. Repair of myelomeningocele

______

______

i. Correction of syndactyly

______

______

MATCHING

Match each medical diagnosis with the correct definition.

1. ______ Congenital blockage of an orafice or tubular structure.
2. ______ Chest wall deformity in which the sternum protrudes outward.
3. ______ Complex set of congenital anomalies involving the lower genitourinary tract and skeletal system.
4. ______ Congenital narrowing of the thoracic aorta that restricts blood flow to the lower body.
5. ______ Congenital anomaly in which abdominal viscera develops outside the body in which there is no membrane or peritoneal sac covering the contents.
6. ______ Wilms tumor.
7. ______ Congenital abnormality resulting from lack of folic acid in the mother's diet causing specific spinal cord defects such as spina bifida or anencephaly.
8. ______ Congenital anomaly in which the abdominal viscera develops outside the body contained within a peritoneal sac.
9. ______ A thickening of the pylorus that results in stricture at the gastric outlet.
10. ______ The opening of the urethra is fully exposed on the dorsum of the penis.
11. ______ Chemical change in the genetic structure that can cause skeletal deformity, microcephaly, and delayed development.
12. ______ Environmental agent (chemical or drug) that injures an embryo or a fetus.

a. Pyloric stenosis
b. Bladder exstrophy
c. Pectus carinatum
d. Atresia
e. Omphalocele
f. Neural tube defect
g. Coarctation of the aorta
h. Nephroblastoma
i. Gastroschisis
j. Epispadias
k. Teratogen
l. Mutagenic substance

CASE STUDIES

1. *There are items both in the environment and the diet of a pregnant woman that can cause developmental defects to the fetus. What are they, and what types of defects do they contribute to?*

34 Neurosurgery

Student's Name ______________________

KEY TERMS

Write the definition for each term.

1. Aneurysm: ______________________
2. Arteriovenous malformation (AVM): ______________________
3. Astrocytes: ______________________
4. Bone flap: ______________________
5. Craniectomy: ______________________
6. Cranioplasty: ______________________
7. Craniotomy: ______________________
8. Embolization: ______________________
9. Intracranial pressure (ICP): ______________________
10. Spondylosis: ______________________
11. Stereotactic: ______________________

SHORT ANSWER

Provide a short answer for each question or statement.

1. The brain is divided into three main sections. What are they?

   a. ______________________

   b. ______________________

   c. ______________________

2. Describe the three protective layers of membranes known as the meninges that protect the brain and spinal cord.

   a. ______________________

   b. ______________________

   c. ______________________

3. What are the lobes of the cerebrum, and what is each lobe responsible for controlling?

   a. ______________________________

   b. ______________________________

   c. ______________________________

   d. ______________________________

4. What are the major structures of the midbrain?

5. If it is necessary for a patient's hair to be removed for a cranial procedure, what is the protocol?

6. Why would your patient undergo a rhizotomy?

7. What is a disc herniation and why does it occur?

8. List the spinal vertebrae and how many vertebrae are in each section.

9. Hemostasis of the wound edge of an incision into the scalp for a craniotomy is achieved and maintained with the use of what?

10. What is CJD?

11. What are common diagnostic procedures that might be performed during the perioperative phase?

12. List the instruments associated with neurosurgery.

13. List two types of head stabilizers used for cranial surgery.

14. List two types of operating room tables used for neurosurgery.

15. Name a frame used for a posterior lumbar laminectomy.

16. Define the surgical procedure.

a. Craniectomy

b. Cerebral aneurysm

c. Arteriovenous malformation resection

d. Correction of craniosynostosis

e. Cranioplasty

f. Ventriculoperitoneal shunt

g. Transsphenoidal hypophysectomy

h. Stereotactic

i. Endoscopic ventriculoscopy

j. Anterior cervical discectomy with fusion – Open

k. Posterior cervical laminectomy

l. Lumbar laminectomy with discectomy

m. Microdiscectomy

n. Posterior lumbar interbody fusion

o. Rhizotomy

p. Ulnar nerve transposition

q. Carpal tunnel release

r. Thoracic corpectomy

MATCHING I

Match each term with the correct definition. You may use the same answer more than once or not at all.

1. ______ Narrow path that leads directly into the fourth ventricle.
2. ______ Outer tissue layer of the cerebrum.
3. ______ Continuous connection between the spinal cord and the pons.
4. ______ Layer of meninges that is closest to the brain.
5. ______ Ligament that connects one spinous process of a vertebra to another vertebra.
6. ______ Small bulges that occur throughout the surface of the cerebrum.
7. ______ Large, deep furrows in the cerebrum.
8. ______ Covers and protects the brain.
9. ______ Area of brainstem responsible for vital functions of the circulatory system, respiration, and heart rate.
10. ______ The outermost layer of the meninges.

a. Skull
b. Cerebral aqueduct
c. Medulla oblongata
d. Cerebral cortex
e. Medulla
f. Gyri
g. Fissures
h. Ligamentum flavum
i. Pia mater
j. Dura mater

MATCHING II

Match the following cranial nerves.

1. ______ Controls lateral movement of the eye.
2. ______ Controls muscles of the tongue.
3. ______ Has two parts: a cranial portion and a spinal portion.
4. ______ Sense of smell.
5. ______ Sensations of the face, forehead, mouth, nose, and top of the head.
6. ______ Sense of taste and pharyngeal movement.
7. ______ Conveys impulses for sight.
8. ______ Controls hearing and equilibrium.
9. ______ Controls muscles that move the eye and iris.
10. ______ Controls muscles of the face and scalp, tears, and salivation.
11. ______ Innovates pharyngeal and laryngeal muscles, heart, pancreas, lungs, and digestive systems.
12. ______ Controls oblique muscles of the eye.

a. I (Olfactory)
b. II (Optic)
c. III (Oculomotor)
d. IV (Trochlear)
e. V (Trigeminal)
f. VI (Abducens)
g. VII (Facial)
h. VIII (Vestibulocochlear)
i. IX (Glossopharyngeal)
j. X (Vagus)
k. XI (Accessory)
l. XII (Hypoglossal)

MULTIPLE CHOICE

1. Which of the following is a cerebral aneurysm clip?
   a. Filshie
   b. Falope
   c. Yasargil
   d. Hulka

2. Which of the following are small square felted sponges used to control bleeding on neural and vascular tissue?
   a. Tonsil
   b. Cottonoid
   c. Peanut
   d. Pusher

3. Which of the following is a spinal retractor?
   a. Taylor
   b. Charnley
   c. Lowman
   d. Lewin

4. When closing for a craniotomy, which is the first layer that is closed?
   a. Galea
   b. Skin
   c. Subcutaneous
   d. Dura

CASE STUDIES

1. *Your patient's illness has been recently diagnosed as an endocrine-dependent malignant tumor of the pituitary gland.*

   a. What signs or symptoms did your patient most likely have when she arrived at the physician's office?

   b. What procedure will the surgeon suggest to the patient as a potential cure?

   c. How will the surgeon describe to the patient the potential postoperative complications for this procedure?

   d. Where will the incision be?

e. Once the tumor is resected, what will be used to pack the floor of the sella to prevent or manage a CSF leak?

2. *Your surgical case today is an open craniotomy for removal of a tumor. The surgeon is going to create and remove a bone flap for access to the tumor. As the scrub, what is your responsibility with regard to the bone if it is removed from the patient?*

35 Emergency Trauma Surgery

Student's Name ______________________________

KEY TERMS

Write the definition for each term.

1. Advance Trauma Life Support (ATLS): ______________________________
2. Algorithms: ______________________________
3. Autotransfusion: ______________________________
4. Blunt injury: ______________________________
5. Cardiac rupture: ______________________________
6. Cardiac tamponade: ______________________________
7. Coagulopathy: ______________________________
8. Compartment syndrome: ______________________________
9. Contusions: ______________________________
10. Damage control surgery: ______________________________
11. Definitive diagnosis: ______________________________
12. Definitive procedure: ______________________________
13. Exsanguinating: ______________________________
14. Flail chest: ______________________________
15. Focused assessment with ultrasound for trauma (FAST): ______________________________
16. Hemorrhagic shock: ______________________________
17. Hemothorax: ______________________________
18. Metabolic acidosis: ______________________________
19. Occult injury: ______________________________
20. Penetrating injury: ______________________________
21. Pneumothorax: ______________________________
22. Resuscitation: ______________________________

SHORT ANSWER

Provide a short answer for each question or statement.

1. Describe damage control surgery and the goals of damage control surgery.

2. List the trauma system and define.

3. List and define the lethal triad.

4. List the ATLS principles of trauma management.

5. List and define the A, B, C, D, E primary patient assessment performed by first responders.

6. List and give an example of the preoperative care of the patient.

7. List the proper way to manage the sterile field in an emergency trauma.

8. Describe disseminated intravascular coagulation (DIC).

9. How should forensic evidence be handled?

10. List and give an example of the following surgical procedures related to trauma.

a. Laparotomy with staged closure

b. List steps of damage control techniques for abdominal trauma.

c. Abdominal compartment syndrome

d. Orthopedic trauma

e. Emergency treatment of orthopedic fractures

f. Thoracic injury

g. Blunt cardiac rupture

h. Penetrating cardiac wound

i. Flail chest

j. Aortic injury

k. Hemothorax

____

____

l. Laceration of the lung

____

____

m. Trauma of the brain and spinal cord

____

____

n. Trauma related to major peripheral vascular trauma

____

____

MULTIPLE CHOICE

1. Prehospital care of the trauma patient morbidity and mortality are partially related to the time elapsed between the first critical hour of care after injury is referred to as the:
   a. ABCDE
   b. Resuscitation
   c. Secondary survey
   d. Golden hour

2. Which of the following is a hematoma between the dura and the brain?
   a. Intracerebral hematoma
   b. Subdural hematoma
   c. Subarachnoid hematoma
   d. Arteriovenous hematoma

3. Which of the following is the most common cause of penetrating brain injury?
   a. Knife wounds
   b. Motor vehicle accident
   c. Gunshot wounds
   d. Traumatic subarachnoid hemorrhage

4. Which of the following would most likely cause thoracic injuries, sternal and rib fractures, flail chest, cardiac contusion, aortic injuries, and hemo- or pneumothorax during a motor vehicle accident?
   a. Windshield
   b. Ejection from the vehicle
   c. Rollover
   d. Steering wheel

5. Which of the following is vascular failure caused by severe blood loss and the most common cause of mortality in trauma?
   a. Hemorrhagic shock
   b. Hypothermia
   c. Metabolic acidosis
   d. Hypokalemia

CHART COMPLETION

Complete the following chart.

Techniques for Temporary Abdominal Closure

Technique	Description	Mechanism
1. ________________	A perforated plastic sheet covers the viscera, and a sponge is placed between the fascial edges. The wound is covered by an airtight seal, which is pierced by a suction drain connected to a suction pump and fluid collection system.	The (active and adjustable) negative pressure supplied by the pump keeps constant tension on the fascial edges while it collects excess abdominal fluid and helps resolve edema.
2. ________________	A perforated plastic sheet covers the viscera, damp surgical towels are placed in the wound, and a surgical drain is placed on the towels. An airtight seal covers the wound, and negative pressure is applied through the drain.	The negative pressure keeps constant tension on the fascial edges, and excess fluid is collected.
3. ________________	Two opposite Velcro sheets (hooks and loops, one on each side) are sutured to the fascial edges. The Velcro sheets connect in the middle.	This technique allows for easy access and stepwise reapproximation of the fascial edges.
4. ________________	The viscera are covered with a sheet (e.g., ISODrape, Microtek [Microban], Huntersville, NC). Horizontal sutures are placed through a large-diameter catheter and through the entire abdominal wall on both sides.	The sutures keep tension on the fascia and may be tightened to allow staged reapproximation of the fascial edges. This may be combined with a vacuum system.
5. ________________	A sterile x-ray film cassette bag or sterile 3-L urology irrigation bag is sutured between the fascial edges or the skin and opened in the middle.	This is an easy technique that allows for easy access. The bag may be reduced in size to approximate the fascial edges.
6. ________________	An absorbable or nonabsorbable mesh or sheet is sutured between the fascial edges. Examples are Dexon, Marlex, or Vicryl mesh. Examples of sheets are Silastic or silicone sheets.	The mesh or sheet may be reduced in size to allow for reapproximation. Nonresorbable meshes may be removed or left in place at the end of the open abdominal period.

Modified from Diaz J, Duton W, Miller R: The difficult abdominal wall. In Townsend CM Jr, Beauchamp RD, Evers BM, Matto x KL, editors: *Sabiston textbook of surgery*, ed 19, Philadelphia, 2012, WB Saunders.

36 Disaster Preparedness and Response

Student's Name ______________________________

KEY TERMS

Write the definition for each term.

1. Agency for Healthcare Research and Quality (AHRQ): ______________________
2. All-hazards approach: ______________________
3. American Red Cross: ______________________
4. Bioterrorism: ______________________
5. Declared state of emergency: ______________________
6. Disaster: ______________________
7. Disaster recovery: ______________________
8. Emergency: ______________________
9. Federal Emergency Management Agency (FEMA): ______________________
10. Logistics supply chain: ______________________
11. Mass casualty event: ______________________
12. Mitigation: ______________________
13. National Fire Protection Agency (NFPA): ______________________
14. Natural disaster: ______________________
15. Pandemic: ______________________
16. Shelter-in-place: ______________________
17. Surge capacity: ______________________
18. Vulnerability: ______________________

SHORT ANSWER

Provide a short answer for each question or statement.

1. What is the difference between a disaster and an emergency?

2. List types of natural disasters.

3. List types of intentional violence/terrorism disasters.

4. What is bioterrorism?

5. Define the three levels of disasters.

6. What role does the community play in disaster preparation?

7. List the primary objectives of a local disaster plan.

MATCHING

Match each term with the correct definition.

______ 1. An important activity in infection control during a disaster.

______ 2. Ensures that a disaster response is consistent with the doctrines and laws of the country.

______ 3. Way of moving people away from a disaster to protect them from catastrophic morbidity and mortality.

______ 4. A process of putting family members in contact with each other during or after a disaster.

______ 5. Social and psychological assistance needed in every disaster.

______ 6. Protects people from extreme weather, including environmental conditions.

______ 7. Form the process of transport and distribution of materials, goods, food, and other necessary supplies.

______ 8. A designated area for placing the dead, far from the emergency department outside the building to avoid patients and the public.

a. Shelter
b. Evacuation
c. Temporary morgue
d. Logistics
e. Mental health needs
f. Health messages in the community
g. Department of Homeland Security
h. Reunification

MULTIPLE CHOICE

Choose the most correct answer for each question or statement.

1. ______ is a process in which casualties are given emergency medical treatment according to the probability of their survival.
   a. Surge capacity
   b. Communication
   c. Triage
   d. Medical facility evacuation

2. A major health facility has the ability to ______ using satellite or high frequency radio.
   a. Analyze surge capacity
   b. Communicate
   c. Perform triage
   d. Evacuate injured people

3. ______ of a medical facility may sometimes be necessary because of structural hazards or immediate threat from fire, chemical, or bioterrorism.
   a. Surge capacity
   b. Communication
   c. Triage
   d. Evacuation

4. ______ is the ability of a health care facility to quickly increase its capability to receive and treat patients.
   a. Surge capacity
   b. Communication
   c. Triage
   d. Medical facility evacuation

5. Roles are assigned using a *job action sheet* (JAS). This is a tool used to define:
   a. Surge capacity
   b. Staff assignments
   c. Triage
   d. Medical facility management team

6. During a disaster, individual health care workers may be asked to:
   a. Perform tasks outside their scope of practice
   b. Perform tasks outside their usual role
   c. Perform management tasks even though they have no experience
   d. Be a spokesperson for the hospital

7. During a disaster, the press and other media require:
   a. Food and water from the health facility
   b. The ability to examine patients
   c. Lists of the dead
   d. A designated media representative to work in the communication area to control accuracy in reporting

CASE STUDIES

1. *Read the following case study and answer the question based on your knowledge of the health care disaster plan.*

   A mass casuality event has occurred in the community. The hospital has activated its emergency plan, including the deployment of all staff, and you have been informed to report to the hospital.

   What would you imagine your role as a surgical technologist to be during a mass casuality event?

NOTES

NOTES

NOTES

NOTES

SURGICAL TECHNOLOGY

PRINCIPLES AND PRACTICE

SURGICAL TECHNOLOGY

PRINCIPLES AND PRACTICE

Eighth Edition

Joanna Kotcher Fuller, BA, BSN, RN, RGN, MPH
Emergency Medical Coordinator, Medical Emergency Relief International, UK-Global

CONSULTING EDITOR
Elizabeth Ness, CST, BA
Program Coordinator
Macomb Community College
Clinton Township, Michigan

ELSEVIER

Elsevier
3251 Riverport Lane
St. Louis, Missouri 63043

SURGICAL TECHNOLOGY: PRINCIPLES AND PRACTICE, EIGHTH EDITION ISBN: 978-0-323-68018-9

Notice

Practitioners and researchers must always rely on their own experience and knowledge in evaluating and using any information, methods, compounds or experiments described herein. Because of rapid advances in the medical sciences, in particular, independent verification of diagnoses and drug dosages should be made. To the fullest extent of the law, no responsibility is assumed by Elsevier, authors, editors or contributors for any injury and/or damage to persons or property as a matter of products liability, negligence or otherwise, or from any use or operation of any methods, products, instructions, or ideas contained in the material herein.

Previous editions copyrighted 2018, 2013, 2010, 2005, 1994, 1986, 1981

International Standard Book Number: 978-0-323-68018-9

Senior Content Strategist: Nancy O'Brien
Content Development Director: Laurie Gower
Content Development Specialist: Betsy McCormac
Publishing Services Manager: Julie Eddy
Senior Project Manager: Richard Barber
Book Designer: Renee Duenow

Printed in Canada

Last digit is the print number: 9 8 7 6 5 4 3

CONTRIBUTORS AND REVIEWERS

CONTRIBUTORS

BROCK HOLTZCLAW, BAS, ASST, CST/CSFA
Robotic Specialists
Main Operating Room
Our Lady of the Lake
Department of Surgery
Baton Rouge, Louisiana

INSTRUCTOR AND STUDENT RESOURCES

Test Bank, Review Questions

RACHAEL WILKERSON, CST
Adjunct Assistant Professor and
Clinical Instructor
Santa Fe College Surgical Technology
Program
Gainesville, Florida

REVIEWERS

SUSAN M. ASSAF, RN, MSA
Retired, Surgical Technologist Program
Macomb Community College
Macomb, Michigan

KELSEY BEMUS, CST, CRCST
Certified Surgical Technologist
Neurosurgery
Beaumont Hospital
Royal Oak, Michigan

JESSICA DENYS, CST
Certified Surgical Technologist
Operating Room
Troy Beaumont, Macomb Community College
Troy, Michigan

REBECCA ANN DUCLO, BSN, RN
Clinical Coordinator/Educator
Operating Room
Children's Hospital of Michigan
Detroit, Michigan

JOSHUA HARVILLE, RN
Orthopedic, Neuro, and Spine Coordinator
Operating room/Surgery
Ascension Providence Rochester
Rochester Hills, Michigan

KRISTY KAUFMAN, BS, CST
Certified Surgical Technologist
William Beaumont Hospital
Troy, Michigan

JESSICA MINARD, BSN, RN
Nurse Manager
Operating Room and Sterile Processing Department
Ascension Macomb Oakland Hospital - Madison Heights
Campus
Madison Height, Michigan

CATERINA ONWELLER, CST
Certified Surgical Technologist
Main Operating Room
Beaumont Healthcare
Troy, Michigan

JANE E. SERRA, BSN, CNOR
Retired, RN, Perioperative Nurse Educator
Surgical Services
Detroit Medical Center
Detroit, Michigan

CATHRYN S. SMYTH
Surgical Technologist,
Specialty Coordinator, Colorectal and bariatric surgery
William Beaumont Hospital
Troy, Michigan

KAY STEELE, CST
Certified Surgical Technologist
Surgical Services Area D
Beaumont Hospital
Troy, Michigan

TINA STOPCZYNSKI, CST
Certified Surgical Technologist
Children's Center for Surgery
Beaumont Health Royal Oak Campus
Royal Oak, Michigan, Adjunct Faculty
Surgical Technology Program
Macomb Community College
Macomb, Michigan

DANUTA TYLECKA, CST
Certified Surgical Technologist
Surgery, Beaumont Hospital
Troy, Michigan

DANIELLE COOK, MS, CST
Program Director/Instructor
Surgical Technology Program
Moraine Park Technical College
Fond du Lac, Wisconsin

DEBRA M. CREWS, RN, CNOR, KCSA, CST/CSFA, FAST
Assistant Professor, Program Director/Coordinator
Surgical Technology
Southcentral Kentucky Community & Technical College
Bowling Green, Kentucky

CARRIE DELINE, CST, AA
Program Director
Surgical Technology
Columbia Public Schools
Columbia, Missouri

DENISE D. DURAN, CST, AAS
Clinical Coordinator
Surgical Technology
Eastern Iowa Community College
Bettendorf, Iowa

JAMES BRYAN HIGH, MA, CST
Surgical Technology Instructor
Huntsville Hospital
Huntsville, Alabama

SHAWN JEUNE, MS, APRN-ACNS, RN, CST, CNOR
Program Director, Surgical Technology
Adult Health Clinical Nurse Specialist
Hudson Valley Community College
Troy, New York
Albany Medical Center
Albany, New York

APRIL NICHOLE KESLER, CST, AAS
Program Coordinator
Surgical Technology
Northwestern Michigan College
Traverse City, Michigan

REBECCA LYNN LAWSON, CST, AAS, BA
Associate Professor, Program Coordinator
Surgical Technology
Southeast Kentucky Community & Technical College
Pineville, Kentucky

ELIZABETH NESS, CST, BA
Program Coordinator
Surgical Technology
Macomb Community College
Clinton Township, Michigan

KATHY PATNAUDE, CST, BS, FAST
Program Director
Surgical Technology
Midlands Technical College
Columbia, South Carolina

TINA K. PUTNAM, CST, CRCST
Assistant Professor
Surgical Technology
Lord Fairfax Community College
Middletown, Virginia

ELIZABETH A. ROMEO, ST
Surgical Technologist
McLaren Macomb
Mt. Clemens, Michigan

SHANNON E. SMITH, MHSC, CSFA, CDEI
Program Chair
Surgical Technology
Vincennes University
Vincennes, Indiana

MATTHEW WAKEEN, CST, BS
Program Director
Surgical Technology
Eastern Iowa Community College
Bettendorf, Iowa

DOUGLAS F. WYSE, BS, AS, CST
Clinical Instructor
Surgical Technology
Keiser University
Tampa, Florida

ROBERT YOUNG, BS, MBA, CST
Department Chair/Program Director
Surgical Technology
Keiser University
Tampa, Florida

PREFACE

This eighth edition of *Surgical Technology: Principles and Practice* contains new material that advances the surgical technologist's knowledge and practice to keep up with a quickly changing profession. Today's surgical technologists are required to practice more advanced skills based on advanced technologies in the areas of robotic and computer guided procedures, digital and optical innovations that provide greater precision, and new man-made and natural materials, which have advanced the safety of surgical practices in nearly every medical specialty. Along with these advances comes greater responsibility and the need for more advanced problem-solving skills. This edition initiates students into what is now a highly technical field of practice.

A new chapter on robotic surgery and introductory robotic and image-guided procedures along with advanced guidelines and skills are presented in straightforward language. Terminology used in this edition has been harmonized with the common language of surgical technique, infection control, and sterile technique (previously called "aseptic technique"). The *guidelines* for sterile technique and infection control have been completely harmonized with those of the American College of Surgeons, the Centers for Disease Control and Prevention, and the Association of Perioperative Registered Nurses. A common language among these organizations has already been established and adopted by accredited health care facilities in the United States. The addition of these guidelines in the 8th edition provides both the language and the practices for surgical technology students to learn and use on the job.

Another new feature in this edition is greater exposure to self-learning resources. These occur throughout the book. They are intended to enhance certain topics by offering new insights, expanded technical facts, and interesting background material about a topic.

Essential surgical skills are now presented in two consecutive chapters: *Surgical Skills I* and *Surgical Skills II.* These chapters follow a time-based progression of surgical technology skills as they are actually performed from the time a procedure is scheduled to the time the patient leaves the operating room. The focus is on the surgical technologist as strategic thinker (planning and executing tasks), skilled surgical assistant, infection control agent, and patient advocate.

New illustrations and photos occur throughout the book and include updated images that clarify the role of the modern surgical technologist.

I would like to thank all the students and their dedicated instructors who have learned or taught from this textbook through its many editions. The greatest gift we can offer a student is to respect each one and offer the chance and opportunity to fulfill their professional and personal goals. I hope I have contributed to this worthy goal.

ACKNOWLEDGMENTS

I first want to thank Nancy O'Brien, Senior Content Strategist, for her professional wisdom and continued guidance during the writing and production of this 8th edition of *Surgical Technology: Principles and Practice*. She has contributed to my professional and personal development in many ways, and I am truly grateful for all I have learned from her.

Elizabeth McCormac, Content Development Specialist, and Richard Barber, Project Manager, have provided important support during manuscript preparation. Both have taken care to ensure continuity of the work with regular and timely communication.

New to this edition is a chapter dedicated to robotic surgery. A special thanks to consultant, Brock Holtzclaw, Assistant Robotics Program Coordinator, Our Lady of the Lake Regional Medical Center, Baton Rouge, Louisiana. His expertise as a surgical technologist and staff trainer in robotic surgery have been invaluable in providing the most up-to-date entry-level skills for the da Vinci Robotic Systems (Intuitive, Inc.).

Curriculum Consultant Elizabeth Ness, Program Coordinator, Macomb Community College, Clinton Township, Michigan has provided chapter reviews to ensure compliance with the Core Curriculum of the Association of Surgical Technologists and reflections as a long-time instructor who is very familiar with the Curriculum and the educational and certifying bodies that support it. Her contributions have been valuable and much appreciated.

As always, I am very grateful for the support of a number of manufacturers who have supplied photos and technical information about their products. We received continuous, timely support to the Robotics chapter from CMR Surgical. CMR also provided high-quality photos and technical information of their products. Intuitive, Inc. provided photos of their most updated daVinci systems. Medtronic has continued to provide high quality photos of their latest products to provide students insight into cutting-edge surgical technology. Scanlan provided a large number of high-resolution images in the area of video assisted thoracic surgery (VATS). Finally, I would like to thank Aesculap, Inc for their continued support with images of surgical instruments.

CONTENTS

PART I: SURGICAL TECHNOLOGY PRINCIPLES

PART II: SURGICAL TECHNOLOGY PRACTICE

SURGICAL TECHNOLOGY: THE PROFESSION AND THE PROFESSIONAL

1

LEARNING OBJECTIVES

After studying this chapter, the reader will be able to:

1. Describe how the profession of surgical technology originated
2. Describe the process of training the surgical technologist
3. Discuss the services provided by the Association of Surgical Technologists and its support agencies
4. Discuss the role of the surgical technologist
5. Discuss career opportunities available to the surgical technologist
6. Discuss professional ethics and behaviors that define it

TERMINOLOGY

Allied health profession: A branch of health care personnel that includes primary care workers; health promotion advocates and administrative and rehabilitative workers; and diagnostic professionals.

Assistant circulator: The surgical technologist in the nonsterile role of the surgical team responsible for monitoring the conditions in the operating room that are related to patient care, safety, documentation, distribution of sterile supplies, and counts.

Certification: Acknowledgment by a private agency that a person has achieved a stated level of knowledge and skill. Certification is usually established by graduation from an accredited institution and passing a written examination.

Continuing education: More formally called professional development. It is education undertaken after one has achieved professional status. Continuing education (CE) credits are provided by a professional organization.

CST: Certified surgical technologist. A surgical technologist who has successfully passed the certification examination required to achieve this status.

CST–CFA: Certified surgical technologist–certified first assistant. A surgical technologist with advanced training who has successfully passed the certification examination for surgical first assistants.

Ethical dilemma: A situation in which one must make a decision and none of the options are acceptable.

Nonsterile team members: Surgical team members who handle only nonsterile equipment, supplies, and instruments. The circulator is the primary nonsterile team member.

Proprietary school: Private, for-profit school.

Scrub: Role and name commonly applied to the surgical technologist or licensed nurse in the sterile scrub role during surgery.

Sterile team member: Members of the surgical team who have performed a hand and arm hygiene procedure. They don sterile gown and gloves and either perform the surgery or assist as a team member.

Surgical conscience: Accountability and admission of errors for actions carried out by the surgical team.

Surgical technology is part of a larger health sector called **allied health professions.** This family of professions includes medical technologists, nuclear medicine technologists, bioengineers, respiratory therapists, laboratory technologists, anesthesia technicians, cardiac perfusionists, and many others. Allied health professionals contribute to the well-being and health of the patient through technical expertise and patient care in line with the standards, guidelines, and ethics of their profession. This chapter explores the role of the surgical technologist, history of the profession, education, professionalism, and professional ethics.

SHORT HISTORY OF THE PROFESSION

Surgeons have always needed skilled assistants, including those whose specific role was centered around surgical instrumentation. The role of the surgical nurse has been well documented since the late 19th century. In the late 1800s she prepared instruments for surgery, and in the early 1900s she assisted in surgical procedures and in the administration of ether, called "etherizing." Her duties from about the 1920s to the 1940s were similar to those of today's circulating nurse (described later). She also instructed student nurses. Often, the operating room supervisor was the only graduate nurse in surgery, and it was her duty to oversee the student nurses as they completed their rotation.

The need for other types of surgical assistants became critical during World War II. During World War I, Army corpsmen worked on the battlefield to offer aid and comfort to the wounded, but they had no role in surgery. World War II dramatically changed that. The development of antibiotics, such as penicillin and sulfa, allowed war surgeons to operate on and save the lives of many more patients than was previously possible. Technological advances created a need for more trained personnel who could assist the surgeon.

The increase in battlefield survivors created a dramatic shortage of nurses. In addition to the nurses needed to staff the field hospitals, many more were needed at base hospitals. At home, extra nurses were trained to attend to the wounded who returned from battle. To supply the field hospitals in the Pacific and European theaters, the Army began training corpsmen to assist in surgery, a role that previously had been filled only by nurses. By this time, however, corpsmen were expected to administer anesthesia or perform segments of the surgery.

When nurses were not available, such as on combat ships, corpsmen worked under the direct supervision of the surgeons. The Army referred to these corpsmen as operating room technicians (ORTs). Thereafter, the military played a significant role in defining the role of the ORT. Each branch of the military provided specific training for the ORT.

After World War II, the Korean War caused a continued shortage of highly trained nurses, who were needed in many other areas of combat medicine. At this time operating room supervisors began to recruit former corpsmen to work in civilian surgery. Registered nurses continued to fill the role of "instrument nurse" until about 1965, when the role changed to "circulating" or nonsterile nurse. At this point hospitals began training civilian ORTs.

In the early 1960s the first steam sterilizer was introduced along with the concept and standards of aseptic technique to prevent postoperative infection. In 1967, prompted by the need for guidelines and standards in the training of paramedical surgical personnel, the Association of Operating Room Nurses (AORN) published a training manual called *Teaching the Operating Room Technician*. In 1968 the AORN board of directors created the Association of Operating Room Technicians (AORT), which led to formal training for the civilian ORT in **proprietary schools** across the United States.

Along with organizational independence came steps toward formalizing the technologist's education. The AORT created two new committees, the Liaison Council on Certification for the Surgical Technologist (LCC-ST) and the Joint Review Committee on Education. In 1970 the first certifying examination for ORTs was administered, and those who passed were given the title Certified Operating Room Technician (CORT). In 1973 the AORT became independent from the AORN, and the AORT changed its name to the Association of Surgical Technologists (**AST**). The certified technician became known as the certified surgical technologist (**CST**).

SURGICAL TECHNOLOGIST'S ROLE

The exact job description of today's surgical technologist varies by the type of surgical facility and the individual surgical technologist's (ST's) specialization. An overview of the surgical technologist's role in surgery is presented here. Chapter 18 describes the duties and roles of the ST in greater detail. A formal job description written by the AST is on the association's website (http://www.ast.org).

TASK INTEGRATION

An important concept for surgical technology students and experienced professionals alike is task integration. The ST does not work in isolation. His or her tasks and responsibilities fit into a more complex order involving many other professionals. Health care professionals understand that individuals achieve success as part of a team. Becoming a "team player" is extremely important in modern complex medical-surgical care.

SCRUB ROLE

As a member of the sterile team, the ST performs hand and arm antisepsis, dons sterile gown and gloves, and is an active participant in surgery. In very simple terms, the sterile team, which includes the surgeon and assistant(s), delivers direct surgical care by performing the surgery. The ST supports the surgeon's and assistant surgeon's work. In this position the ST is often referred to as the **scrub**. The scrub also assists the surgeon in specific, well-defined tasks as needed during the procedure. The term *scrub* has been used to describe this role for many years and predates the current title *surgical technologist*. Even though the role has evolved, the name remains as part of a tradition. The scrub role can be fulfilled by various professionals, including registered nurses (RNs), licensed vocational nurses (LVNs), and licensed practical nurses (LPNs). The ST in the scrubbed role may also be referred to as STSR (surgical technologist scrub role), scrubbed ST, or simply ST. In this text the term *scrub* is used interchangeably with *scrubbed ST*.

Surgical procedures require many different instruments, supplies, and equipment specific to the type of surgery being performed. These range from a relatively small number of basic instruments to very large instrument "sets" of specialty instruments for a specific body system such as orthopedics or ear-nose-throat (ENT) surgery. Complex operations require hundreds of items to be immediately available for the surgeon's use. Some instruments require assembly "on the field" (the immediate sterile work area of the team); sutures must be prepared; and supplies such as sponges, medications, solutions, and electronic devices must be carefully handed to the surgeon throughout the procedure. These are presented as needed at the precise moment they will be used. This is accomplished by learning each step of a particular surgery and the specific preferences of the surgeon.

The scrub protects the sterile field from contamination and communicates effectively with the surgeon to prevent errors, such as passing the wrong instrument or passing it in the wrong orientation. Errors consume valuable time and cause disruptions that are distracting to the surgeon and are not conducive to safe surgery. This means that the scrub must always keep the instrument tables neat and orderly. The scrub communicates with the circulator to receive other items needed during a surgical procedure. The knowledge and skills required to be a surgical technologist are learned step by step through study and practical experience in surgery.

ASSISTANT CIRCULATOR

The surgical technologist in the circulator role is identified as an **assistant circulator,** ST circulator, or STCR—surgical technologist circulating role. A registered nurse is required to be immediately available (present) in surgical cases. He or she is the primary circulator. In this text the term *ST circulator* refers to the assistant circulator position.

Whereas the scrub is a **"sterile" team member** who remains at the sterile field throughout the surgery, the circulator is a **"nonsterile" team member** who is responsible for many different tasks, including direct patient care. Traditionally, this role was fulfilled exclusively by a registered perioperative nurse. In the past decade the surgical technologist's role has expanded to include some of the circulator's responsibilities. The exact duties vary somewhat by state, region, and health facility.

The circulator's role is quite different from that of the scrub. The circulator does not directly contact (touch) any sterile instruments, supplies, or equipment. Instead, he or she obtains, delivers, and prepares the nonsterile equipment. The circulator also distributes and opens sterile instruments and other supplies for the sterile team members using a method that protects the sterile items from contamination. The circulator is also responsible for positioning the patient before surgery, assisting the anesthesia care provider, and receiving tissue and other types of specimens from the sterile field and preparing them correctly for the pathologist. He or she ensures that the patient chart, including results of diagnostic procedures, permits, and preoperative checklist, is available at the time of surgery and makes preparations for the next surgery on the schedule. Other duties of the circulator include performing the surgical skin prep and urinary catheterization. The circulator is the main communicator between the surgical team and personnel outside the operating room and is also responsible for case documentation and many other tasks. The role is described fully in later chapters. The AST website also provides a basic description of the ST assistant circulator role, which can be adapted to state and regional practice.

SECOND ASSISTANT

Most surgical procedures require one or more assistants to the surgeon. The *first assistant* may incise or remove tissue, insert sutures, clamp and manipulate tissues, remove fluids from the incision site, and many other tasks. When two assistants are needed, the surgical technologist may step into the *second assistant* position. The second assistant performs tasks that do not involve cutting into or removing tissue. The tasks of the second assistant include but are not limited to the following:

- Tissue retraction
- Uses suction and surgical sponges to maintain a "dry" surgical wound (incision)
- Assists with hemostasis as directed by the surgeon
- Assembles and attaches wound suction devices at the close of surgery
- Applies wound dressings at the close of surgery
- Steadies and maintains the position of the insertion tube during endoscopic surgery
- Irrigates the surgical wound when required

The scope of practice for an allied health professionals is defined in each state's Practice Acts. These are discussed in detail in Chapter 3.

OTHER PERIOPERATIVE RESPONSIBILITIES

Emergency Duty

The surgical technologist working in a hospital or other facility that provides 24-hour care is usually required to be on "call." This means that the surgical technologist is available outside normal working hours to respond to emergency cases. It is a normal requirement for surgical technologists to rotate through a "call" schedule.

Preparation of Surgical Instruments and Equipment

Preparing surgical instruments and equipment includes cleaning, disinfection, sterilization, assembly, and storage. More complex tasks require advanced training, especially for robotic, fiber-optic, and endoscopic equipment. Information can be found at https://www.iahcsmm.org/.

Patient Care

The surgical patient is exposed to numerous risks. Some are directly related to the technology used to perform surgery; other risks are related to the hospital and operating room environment. The direct care that the surgical technologist, nursing, and medical team provide helps mitigate or eliminate these risks. In the last decade, the AST has expanded the role of the surgical technologist to include direct patient care, including psychosocial support. This expanded role is defined in the Association's guidelines, position statements, and surgical technologist responsibilities (refer to the AST website).

Leadership and Management

Unique opportunities in leadership and management are available to experienced surgical technologists. Specialty services such as orthopedics, ophthalmology, and neurosurgery need team leaders to facilitate and coordinate teams and to manage equipment in specialty departments.

Surgical technologists may choose to pursue an advanced degree in hospital administration and management. At advanced levels, the integrated experience of both technology and patient care is an excellent springboard for a broader managerial career.

Preceptor

Surgical technologists may be asked to act as preceptors, teaching students or recently graduated STs in the sterile and nonsterile role. Some people enjoy this role and are natural teachers. Others are uncomfortable with the responsibility or simply prefer to remain in their traditional role. Serving as a preceptor requires patience and a willingness to share knowledge and experience.

SURGICAL TECHNOLOGY EDUCATION AND CERTIFICATION

Surgical technologists may be trained in a short certificate program (9 to 12 months) or a 2-year associate degree course. The AST recognizes the associate degree as the *educational model that must be offered to prepare graduates to fulfill the entry-level duties of the surgical technologist.* The current surgical technology program model includes classroom studies ("tabletop" learning) and skills development in a lab setting. Students are required to complete clinical training in a health facility where they are able to participate directly in surgery under the supervision of a skilled mentor and clinical instructor. More detailed information on the surgical technology curriculum and surgical cases required for graduation can be found on the AST website.

CERTIFICATION

All health care professionals are required to demonstrate competence in their area of practice before they are allowed to serve the public. Competency is usually measured by accreditation of the schools they attend, graduation, and a passing score on an examination. When all the requirements have been met, they are granted the right to practice. Some professions use a licensing procedure, whereas others prefer **certification** as a public record of their achievements. Surgical technologists may take the profession's national certification exam after meeting the educational requirements. If they are successful on the exam, they are granted certification.

IMPORTANT TO KNOW *Students who graduate from an accredited program are required to take the certification exam as a means of maintaining the school's accreditation status.*

The comprehensive certification exam covers the principles and basic practices of surgical technology, including basic sciences and patient care in the operating room. To maintain certification, practicing STs must earn **continuing education** (CE) credits. A list of activities that qualify for CE credit and the current regulations for maintaining certification can be found on the AST website. The National Board of Surgical Technology and Surgical Assisting (NBSTSA), which provides credentialing services for surgical technology, provides a Candidate Handbook for students. The handbook covers eligibility to take the certification exam and other topics important to the process. The Handbook can be accessed at https://www.nbstsa.org/sites/nbstsa/files/pdf/2019_CSTrev2.pdf.

REQUIRED SKILLS

Many professions, including the allied health professions, require specific skills. The manual skills required of the surgical technologist are acquired first in the lab setting. These are refined in clinical practice. Other skills such as adaptability, decision making, and communication take more time. However, these "soft" skills are highly valued and worth the effort to master.

ORGANIZATIONAL SKILLS

The ST is required to have excellent organizational skills. This is the ability to prioritize tasks and equipment in a logical and efficient manner. For example, the surgical technologist is required to prepare, assemble, and physically arrange instruments and equipment in the order in which they will be needed. This requires the surgical technologist to be familiar with all the steps of the surgery. A single procedure may require hundreds of items. Instruments, sutures, sponges, needles, electrosurgical devices, solutions, and medications must all be immediately available at the time they are needed. Materials must be organized in a logical and methodical way so that they can be quickly passed to the surgeon at the correct time. Additional items needed during the course of the surgery require interaction between the ST and the circulator. Timing is very important. The needed items must be obtained in advance of their actual use on the surgical field. However, it is not practical to obtain every item at the start of surgery. The ST must request the items at the ideal time. This allows the circulator time to obtain and distribute the item while avoiding clutter on the surgical tables. Some items (certain drugs and chemicals) must only be distributed immediately before use.

It is also important to keep the instrument tables free of clutter with equipment arranged *precisely and logically.* A disorganized table results in wasted time and increases the chance that an item is miscounted or lost during surgery.

MANUAL DEXTERITY

The surgical technologist must work with precision, sometimes quickly and deliberately. Equipment must be assembled and handled efficiently without confusion. This requires manual skills and keen observation. Excellent hand-eye coordination is required to master the skills needed to prepare for and assist during surgery. Speed is not always the most important skill; in fact, if the scrub tries to work too fast, organization can break down, instruments can be dropped, and injuries can occur.

PROBLEM SOLVING

Problem-solving skills refers to the methods we use to overcome difficulties in carrying out tasks. For example, let's suppose that you are moving into a new house. The sum of your belongings fills many boxes. How will you pack your boxes to increase efficiency as you move in? How do you avoid a situation in which everything is disorganized? Will you list every item in every box? Maybe you prefer to pack the boxes according to which room the contents were kept before the move. How will you find items that will be needed as soon as you move, such as cleaning supplies and simple hardware tools?

Problem solving requires strategic thinking: you must look at all the possibilities, prioritize the most important facts or steps, and develop a strategy to accomplish the task or reach a conclusion.

The surgical technologist must be adept at problem solving because a large part of the job requires it.

IMPORTANT TO KNOW *Just like math or reading skills, problem-solving skills can be developed during your program and on the job.*

TIME MANAGEMENT

Time management is a skill required by all professionals and others who lead busy lives. We all need to balance our private lives with the demands of work. The surgical technologist usually has an event-filled workday and is required to be available for emergencies while on call. It is important to start developing time management skills before you start your career, when time pressures become even greater. There are many websites that present time management methods. Some are directed at health care professionals and others focus on business. Two excellent resources are https://www.thebalancecareers.com/ and https://www.mindtools.com/Apps. Enter "time management" in the search boxes for links to the topic.

PEOPLE SKILLS

People skills are sometimes called "soft skills." They include how we communicate, relationship building, conflict management, and generally getting along with others. They are the basis of our relationships with others and often determine how others interact with us. Health professionals have a duty to develop their people skills. They must gain the trust of their patients and colleagues and the public. In different situations they must demonstrate respect, empathy, interest in their surroundings, responsiveness, and trust in others.

AST: THE ASSOCIATION OF SURGICAL TECHNOLOGISTS

The AST is the professional organization in surgical technology. The association supports students and graduate surgical technologists through its many services and publications. The association leadership includes a board of directors and three national standing committees, including a Bylaws and Parliamentary Procedure Committee, an Education and Professional Standards Committee, and a State Assembly Leadership Committee. Each of these committees has specific roles and responsibilities, which are described in the AST website at http://www.ast.org/AboutUs/Leadership/. State assemblies, local chapters of AST, link surgical technologists to their national association and provide forums for learning, discussion, and advocacy. The association is actively involved in training and curriculum development. At the national level, AST supports student and graduate surgical technologists, the public, and teaching institutions. Support services provided by AST are shown in Box 1.1.

It is important for surgical technology students to become active members of AST and to promote the standards of the profession. Participation in conferences and educational seminars allows the ST exposure to new ideas and technology and the chance to meet others in the profession.

BOX 1.1 Support and Services Provided by AST

1. Maintains the Practice Standards, Code of Ethics, and Code of Conduct for surgical technologists
2. Publishes a professional journal, *The Surgical Technologist*, which provides news, legislative updates, and articles for professional development
3. Holds annual conferences for surgical technologists, assistants, and educators
4. Maintains a membership registry
5. Provides opportunities for continuing education (professional development)
6. Provides leadership, standards, and direction for the profession through its Standing Committees
7. Represents surgical technologists and advocates for standards in patient care through state and federal legislative bodies and the general public
8. Maintains regional and local chapters of the Association of Surgical Technologists
9. Provides academic scholarships through its foundation

The website of the Association of Surgical Technologists can be accessed at http://www.ast.org.

AFFILIATED ORGANIZATIONS

As a body of professionals, surgical technologists are supported by a number of key organizations. Each has a designated role in promotion, certification, accreditation, and continuing education. These are shown in Box 1.2. Details about the organizations and their collaborative roles can be found on the AST website and on the websites of each organization.

Other organizations that are not directly involved in surgical technology but commonly referred to in health care delivery are shown in Box 1.3.

CAREERS FOR CERTIFIED SURGICAL TECHNOLOGISTS

FACILITY-BASED SURGICAL TECHNOLOGIST

The combination of health care and technological expertise provides a wide range of roles and responsibilities for the surgical technologists. Most graduates work in hospitals and ambulatory surgery centers; this is the role that entry-level STs are trained to perform.

STs may also work as contracted agency personnel. In this position they are not permanent employees of a particular medical facility, but rather work under short-term contracts in different hospitals. This provides a variety of experiences in different locations.

MILITARY SERVICE

The military offers a surgical technology program for a specific setting through its operating room specialist course. The educational program parallels civilian requirements, with additional

BOX 1.2 Affiliated Organizations

ARC/STSA Accreditation Review Council on Education in Surgical Technology and Surgical Assisting https://www.arcstsa.org/

ABHES Accrediting Bureau of Health Education Schools http://www.arcstsa.org

ASA Association of Surgical Assistants https://www.surgicalassistant.org/

CAAHEP Commission on Accreditation of Allied Health Education Programs https://www.caahep.org/

FFST Foundation for Surgical Technology ffst.org

NBSTSA National Board of Surgical Technology and Surgical Assisting https://www.nbstsa.org/

JC The Joint Commission https://www.jointcommission.org/

BOX 1.3 Professional Health Care Organizations

American College of Surgeons (ACS)
American Medical Association (AMA)
American National Standards Institute (ANSI)
American Society of Anesthesiologists (ASA)
Association for Professionals in Infection Control and Epidemiology (APIC)
Association for the Advancement of Medical Instrumentation (AAMI)
Association of periOperative Registered Nurses (AORN)
Centers for Disease Control and Prevention (CDC)
Emergency System for Advance Registration of Volunteer Health Professionals (ESAR-VHP)
Environmental Protection Agency (EPA)
Food and Drug Administration (FDA)
International Association of Healthcare Central Service Materiel Management (IAHCSMM)
Medical Reserve Corps (MRC)
National Disaster Life Support Education Consortium (NDLSEC)
National Fire Protection Association (NFPA)
National Institute for Occupational Safety and Health (NIOSH)
Occupational Safety and Health Administration (OSHA)
World Health Organization (WHO)

training in combat and war surgery. The military program was the prototype for surgical technologists and remains dedicated to high standards, offering care to the war wounded and other military personnel and civilians in combat areas where the armed forces are deployed. Opportunities in military surgery extend to more complex tasks associated with emergency settings.

SPECIALTY PRACTICE

The facility-based surgical technologist may be employed in one or more surgical specialties, such as orthopedics, neurosurgery, cardiac surgery, obstetrics, or plastic surgery. Qualified STs at the mid-level and advanced stages of their career can provide expert assistance in these specialties, and their work is in high demand.

Many surgical technologists work as private scrub assistants in a surgical specialty. Examples include orthopedics, plastic, ENT, and ophthalmic surgery. These positions require advanced-level experience and management and leadership skills. Private scrubs are often required to provide preoperative education to patients in the office practice, schedule cases, manage the surgical equipment, and help patients and their families with administrative tasks associated with insurance and compensation. Educational requirements for the role of specialist begin with certification in basic surgical technology. More advanced education in patient care and management may also be required to provide care in the medical office.

CERTIFIED SURGICAL TECHNOLOGIST–CERTIFIED FIRST ASSISTANT

The Certified Surgical Technologist–Certified First Assistant (**CST-CFA**) assists the surgeon directly. The primary tasks are listed here. There are many other skills and duties required of the surgical assistant:

- Provides wound exposure by tissue retraction
- Assists in hemostasis (preventing excess blood loss) by clamping blood vessels and securing them with suture, and sponging the incision
- Safe use of electrosurgical equipment
- Tissue retraction
- Suturing tissue planes or applying surgical staples
- Applying complex dressings and fluid collection devices

The ST surgical assistant works under the direction of the surgeon at all times. State Practice Acts determine the scope of the role and responsibilities of the assistant. Surgical technologists represent one among several professions that can attain professional status as a surgical assistant. Others include the registered nurse first assistant, the physician assistant first assistant, and the surgical assistant nurse practitioner. Expanded professional roles of the RN and physician's assistant usually involve greater responsibility because these individuals provide complex perioperative care to the surgical patient.

Preparation for the CST-CFA role includes certification in entry-level surgical technology and graduation from an NBSTSA-recognized first assistant program. Refer to the NBSTSA for further information on eligibility (https://www.nbstsa.org/policies.html).

The Association of Surgical Assistants (ASA) website can be accessed at http://www.surgicalassistant.org.

EDUCATOR AND CLINICAL INSTRUCTOR

Certified surgical technologists may become formal instructors in the classroom or clinical setting. They may also move into administrative or management roles such as department head or program director of a surgical technology program. In these roles they implement the required curriculum for their institutions and may also manage the department. The need for qualified instructors has increased with the demand for more graduates in the profession.

MEDICAL INDUSTRY REPRESENTATIVE

A surgical technologist with advanced training and experience may work as a representative in the medical services and equipment industry. Service representatives are responsible for advising and training hospital and private clinical staff in the use of a company's products. They often travel to clinical sites and are available on call to answer questions and provide immediate technical assistance during surgery that involves their company's equipment. In this role they ensure safe use of the equipment, train operating room personnel in its use, and provide technical expertise to manage equipment problems.

The educational requirements for the role of medical services representative include entry-level certification plus experience and additional training in management and service provision, which is provided by the company. More advanced positions in medical industry management may require a degree in business administration.

MATERIALS PROCESSING MANAGEMENT

Materials management or central sterile processing is a specialty that focuses on the preparation and care of medical instruments and equipment used in surgery. This field is growing in complexity and scope. It requires expertise in instrument technology and a thorough training in health and safety standards. The scope of duties and responsibilities includes disinfection and sterilization processes, assembly of surgical instrument sets, and management of complex instrument systems. It may also include managing and ordering other supplies used in surgery and maintaining accurate records of processing, use, and distribution. The surgical technologist may manage a materials processing department or function under the supervision of others.

The educational requirements for the role of materials management and processing are basic entry-level certification and at least 1 year of experience in operating room technology. Some hospitals may require separate training and certification as a central processing technician. Refer to the International Association of Healthcare Central Service Materiel Management for more information (https://www.iahcsmm.org/).

OTHER CAREER OPPORTUNITIES

The surgical technologist has many opportunities in a variety of settings. Many positions may require further education and certification. These are listed in Box 1.4.

Watch Chapter 1: Overview of the Surgical Technologist on the Evolve website: http://evolve.elsevier.com/Fuller/surgical.

BECOMING A HEALTH CARE PROFESSIONAL

The journey from student to health care professional is a process that includes learning new skills and acquiring knowledge. You will have "hands-on" practice for many of the technical skills and the opportunity to connect classroom knowledge directly to your work. In addition to the practice and theory, you will begin to develop **professional behaviors.** This is just as important as all the other knowledge and skills you acquire as a surgical technologist.

BOX 1.4 Career Opportunities for Surgical Technologists

- Anesthesia technician
- Central supply manager
- Educator
- Assistant in obstetrics
- Materials manager
- Medical sales
- Organ and tissue procurement or preservation
- Surgical first assistant
- Research assistant
- Office manager
- Surgery scheduler

IMPORTANT TO KNOW *Employers, instructors, colleagues, and patients can recognize professionalism in the health care worker before observing their skill and knowledge.*

WHAT IS A PROFESSIONAL?

Most people think of a professional as someone who is highly trained and uses his or her skills in the public sector. But the term *professional* means much more than being good at one's vocation. A true professional exhibits specific behavior that others recognize and respect. All health care providers go through the process of becoming a professional. It is a normal part of learning and maturing in a chosen vocation. Failure to develop professionalism often results in failure to maintain employment or even to become employed.

Many students are more concerned about demonstrating hands-on skills than professional attributes. However, lack of professionalism, difficulty with patient interaction, communication problems, and team integration are often more significant problems in the clinical area.[1]

Some believe that professionalism cannot be taught but only acquired by observation and interaction with others. The process of developing professionalism is enhanced when colleagues, instructors, and our mentors give us feedback on our behavior and attitudes.

CHARACTERISTICS OF A PROFESSIONAL

Integrity

A person with integrity is reliable, trustworthy, responsible, and honest. Professionals who have a high level of integrity are respected by others both in and out of the workplace.

Self-Regulation

This term relates to a person's ability to adjust their behavior regardless of mood and emotions. People who effectively regulate their emotions in the workplace demonstrate an ability to remain calm and reasonable even under stress. Professionals are expected to manage their personal affairs so that they don't interfere with professional responsibilities.

Truthfulness

A truthful person does not lie to others and does not attempt to cover up mistakes. This is extremely important in medicine and allied health professions. Mistakes can result in patient harm. Admitting a mistake opens the door for concrete actions to correct it. The phrase **surgical conscience** refers to a professional's accountability in surgery. It means admitting a mistake in the perioperative environment. Mistakes that are not reported immediately may have devastating implications for patient safety.

Commitment

Professionals honor their commitments to others. In other words, professionals are serious about their responsibilities (stated and unstated). When taking on a task, the professional knows what is involved and completes it on time. Professionals are committed to their profession and the responsibilities that go with it. They do not quit when situations or tasks are difficult or uncomfortable; they persevere until the job is done or the situation is resolved.

Politeness

The professional is polite and respectful of others in speech and action. In modern culture, it may seem that being polite and even *civil* is somehow outdated or no longer required. Regardless of what we hear or see in popular culture, politeness demonstrates respect and must never be taken for granted. Respect is critical in all social interaction. Lack of respect for others and for institutions, laws, and standards leads inevitably to the breakdown of civility. In the health care setting, lack of respect to colleagues often leads to poor communication and poor patient care.

Tact and Discretion

Professionals are tactful in their speech. Being tactful means to consider the impact of what you are saying *before* you say it. For the person who is not accustomed to speaking tactfully, this requires some restraint. Tactful speech patterns take some time to develop, but with time, they become part of one's personal "vocabulary." Discretion is knowing what *not to say* in certain environments. Professionals do not discuss the private affairs of others. They do not say things that startle or offend others. This includes vulgar language and sexual innuendos. Students who are new to surgery learn that not everyone outside the profession wants to hear the details of their work, especially when it includes graphic descriptions of the surgery or of a patient's disease.

Attention to Personal Hygiene and Appearance

As a professional you deliver personal care to your patients. This requires strict attention to personal hygiene and appearance. Good personal hygiene includes care of the hair, nails, skin, feet, genitals, and teeth (dental hygiene). The body must be kept clean to prevent the spread of infection and to eliminate offensive body odors associated with poor hygiene. Perfumes and scented toiletries (e.g., deodorants, after-shave lotion, skin creams) must not be used because they can be offensive and may trigger an allergic reaction in others.

The professional guidelines for hygiene and infection control are discussed in Chapter 9.

Respect for Rules, Regulations, and Laws

The nature of health care requires professionals to comply with many types of regulations and standards—including those of their professional association and workplace. Professionals may disagree with regulations and rules but must never challenge them during the course of work. Disagreements should be aired away from the public and only with the appropriate people in the workplace—*never with patients*.

Perspective

The ability to put events in perspective and enjoy the lighter side of work and life is a great asset. Humor, when expressed appropriately, can ease tension and relax the social atmosphere. However, not all humor is appropriate. Humor that is sarcastic, mean-spirited, prejudicial, or crude may create tension and disdain among team members.

PROFESSIONAL ETHICS FOR HEALTH CARE WORKERS

Professional ethics is the standard of behavior that society expects of those who provide services. Medical ethics defines the conduct of those in the health professions.

Ethical behavior in health care is based on a few very powerful directives.

Respect Human Individuality and Uniqueness

Each individual has needs that are specific to his or her personality, medical condition, psychological state, emotions, social life, and culture. Respect is demonstrated when health professionals treat the patient as a person with a name, a history, and a lifetime of experiences. Health workers must show respect for the individual's uniqueness at all times.

When we encounter a patient who acts or looks very different from what we consider "normal" or "mainstream," we sometimes are caught off guard or even feel offended. Health professionals learn to curb these feelings and transform them into therapeutic action. A person may behave outside the norm, but he or she is human, with all the needs and pain of any human being. It is these characteristics to which health professionals must respond, not the patient's lifestyle, appearance, or mannerisms.

Practice Your Profession With Empathy

Empathy is understanding what the other person feels. It requires health professionals to move beyond aspects of the patient's condition that offend their senses or make them emotionally uncomfortable and instead focus on the use of their professional and personal skills. Empathy allows us to respond humanely but without pity.

Practice Equal Rights

All patients have the right to equal treatment regardless of age, gender identification, physical attributes, mental capacity, ethnicity, or socioeconomic status. Advocating for justice may mean speaking out in the workplace when equal rights are violated. It also means monitoring and challenging our own beliefs and perhaps even our prejudices. Health professionals must be culturally and socially sensitive. To act without sensitivity is to act without justice.

Respect All Confidences Entrusted to You

Confidential information about the patient must not be shared with others outside the therapeutic environment. Confidence among coworkers is also an expected ethical behavior. Gossip is an insidious but common breach of confidentiality. It results in enormous cost in emotional hurt and can affect the professional and personal lives of people in profound ways that we may never realize.

Respect the Free Will of the Patient

All patients have the right to refuse care and to participate in their care. They have the right to receive information about their condition from their physicians and nurses and to ask for advocacy. Health care workers are expected to respect and respond to patients' freedom to make choices and express needs and concerns.

Do No Harm

One of the best-known ethical standards in medicine is *"Do no harm."* It makes a promise to every patient that no matter what treatment or advice is given, the patient will not be injured *as a result* of the treatment. It is an implied contract between the patient and the health care professional and the basis of trust in this relationship. Surgical technologists work with complex instruments and equipment. Used incorrectly or without regard to safety can result in patient injury and even death. This is only one example in which the ST is responsible for preventing patient harm. Throughout this text, safety of the patient is emphasized with explanations, diagrams, and illustrations. It cannot be overstated how important this concept is. Every health care worker is directly responsible for his or her actions in promoting and practicing patient safety.

Surgical Conscience

Surgical conscience is taking responsibility for one's actions. This includes errors that may result in serious injury even when the error is not witnessed by others. Examples are contamination of the sterile field, preparing or administering the wrong drug, or forgetting to implement a safety measure resulting in injury.

Impairment in the Workplace

An impaired team member is a major threat to the safety of the patient and others in the environment. Health care professionals have both a legal and an ethical responsibility to report suspected impairment of a coworker or, if needed, to seek treatment for themselves. Self-destructive behavior, such as substance abuse, is not a weakness; it is an illness. In reporting these behaviors, team members protect not only everyone in the environment but also the abuser.

Refusal to Perform an Assigned Task

The surgical technologist has the right to opt out of participation in certain types of cases that violate his or her ethical or religious values. The facility must be informed of this when the surgical technologist is hired. It is not ethical to suddenly refuse to follow a directive unless the case is one that could never have been anticipated by the staff member. When offered a position, the surgical technologist should discuss the matter with human resources, which may require a written list of cases in which he or she declines to participate on the basis of ethical or religious beliefs.

Refusal to Work With a Specific Individual

To suddenly refuse to scrub a case, or worse, to walk out in the middle of a case, could be interpreted as abandonment of the patient and grounds for probation or immediate dismissal. If the reason for refusal is a personality clash, steps must be taken to resolve the problem, because it can ultimately lead to poor patient care.

Ethical Dilemmas

An **ethical dilemma** is a *personal conflict* that arises from the need to make a decision based on choices that are not completely acceptable. A common example is the overloaded lifeboat. If everyone remains on the lifeboat, it will probably sink. To remove individuals and prevent the boat from sinking will result in the immediate death of those thrown overboard. Neither option is satisfactory from an ethical viewpoint. Society tries to resolve dilemmas in many areas of medical ethics through ethics committees, public debate, and even laws.

Professional Codes of Ethics

Professional organizations, such as the AST, the American Nurses Association, the American Hospital Association (AHA), and the American Medical Association (AMA), have created codes of ethics that reflect expectations of those professionals as they make decisions involving ethical issues. By acting in accordance with these ethics, professional health care workers demonstrate their advocacy for human rights, patient protection, and the laws of society. In all situations, the health care worker is the patient's advocate; the health care worker is doing what the patient would do if he or she were able. The AST code of ethics can be found on the association's website.

PREPARING FOR EMPLOYMENT

Students can improve their chance for successful employment by exploring the job market and how to achieve their goals while still learning the profession. Beyond academic accomplishments, which are necessary to employability, there are important behaviors that can tip an employer's decision to hire someone else with greater professionalism or "soft" skills. The following guidance can help students grow professionally and increase their chances of being hired into a rewarding job.

Think of yourself as a professional from the first day of school. Would you consider yourself prepared to enter a highly professional environment? If not, what changes should you start to make in your attitudes and behavior?

Never pass up an opportunity to expand your skills and knowledge. Challenge yourself to learn as much as you possibly can as a student. Even the least interesting subjects deserve your attention and effort.

Develop and refine your time management skills. Find ways to manage your time by observing others who have achieved this goal. Speak to other professionals about how to prioritize activities.

Explore your career possibilities as a graduate surgical technologist. Picture yourself in the career that you want. Make a detailed plan to achieve that goal. If you are unable to map out the way to achieve your goal, it is unlikely you will achieve it. Seek information from many sources—not only online, but by talking with people who have already achieved the goal. Never hesitate to ask questions. People are usually happy to talk to students about their goals.

Develop an awareness of your teamwork skills. Evaluate your ability to get along with others on a team. Watch others who have good teamwork skills. Practice identifying what those skills are.

Getting Hired

To be successful, you must become familiar with the hiring process. This includes the application, cover letter, the interview itself, a thank-you note to the person who interviewed you, and, if you are successful, your acceptance note or letter.

There are many good websites that provide assistance and coaching on preparation for employment. Some of the most important points about the process are the following:

1. **Prepare your resume.** Start building your resume skills while you are still a student. There are many different models available in books and on the Internet. Remember that the resume is the first thing a prospective employer sees concerning your abilities and professionalism. Important elements are the contact information, participation in professional groups or associations, work history, and academic history. You should also cite at least two references from people who can vouch for your abilities and skills. Be sure to spell-check your resume before sending it out. Never lie or "push the truth" on an application or resume. References will be validated and dates checked for accuracy.
2. **Research various employers.** The first step in seeking employment is correspondence with the health facility. Visiting or writing to the human resources department is a good place to start. Find out what qualifications are necessary at a specific health care facility. When it is time to send in your resume and request for interview, you will have the essential information you need to approach the employer.
3. **Develop your list of references.** References are professionals who are familiar with you or your work and can provide a letter of recommendation.
4. **Practice filling out job applications.** Use these practice applications to learn what to say and how to say it. Seek out individuals who can help with this.
5. **Prepare for an interview.** As you approach the last few months of your course, research the type of questions you may be asked on an interview. Know ahead of time how you would answer. Do not try to rehearse a speech, but instead think clearly about how and what you want to communicate. It is helpful to speak with someone else in the profession who can help with interview preparation.

KEY CONCEPTS

- The profession of surgical technologist developed out of a need for qualified personnel who were familiar with the technical aspects of surgery and could assist in intraoperative patient care.
- The US military has trained surgical technologists since World War II and continues to do so today.
- The Association of Surgical Technologists is the professional organization for surgical technologists. It provides its members with opportunities for career planning, training materials, national conferences, and professional and legislative support.
- Surgical technologists may be employed in a health care facility, hospital, or private clinic. Many develop expertise in specialty areas such as orthopedics, cardiac surgery, eye surgery, and ENT surgery.
- Surgical technologists are required to have the same qualities as any other health professional. Honesty, professionalism, respect for others, empathy for patients and other staff members, and the ability to work on a team are necessary.

REVIEW QUESTIONS

1. In what ways does certification affect the quality of practice in surgical technology?
2. What is meant by professionalism?
3. Why should surgical technologists develop professional behavior?
4. What is meant by "Do no harm"?

CASE STUDIES

CASE 1

Intensive student experiences, such as those in allied health, often change an individual's general outlook and reflection on one's accomplishments. In a group setting, discuss what changes you hope will occur (in addition to achieving technical expertise and acquiring knowledge in the profession) and those that seem highly challenging. What strategies can you adopt to overcome the more difficult challenges?

REFERENCE

1. Freeman J, Rogers J. A comparison of rank ordered professional attributes by clinical supervisors and allied health students. *Inet J Allied Human Sci Prac.* 2010;8(3). Article 5 http://ijahsp.nova.edu/articles/Vol8Num3/Freeman.htm. Accessed July 23, 2015.

BIBLIOGRAPHY

Accreditation Review Council on Education in Surgical Technology and Surgical Assisting (ARC/STSA): http://www.arcst.org.

Army-Portal MOS 68D – Operating Room Specialist: http://www.army-portal.com/jobs/medical-service/68d.html. Accessed July 24, 2015.

Association of periOperative Registered Nurses (AORN). *Standards, Recommended Practices and Guidelines*. 2014 edition. Denver: AORN; 2014.

Association of Surgical Technologists (AST): Standards of practice. http://www.ast.org. Accessed July 23, 2015.

Association of Surgical Technologists: *Surgical technology: a growing career*. Accessed October 12, 2011.

National Board of Surgical Technology and Surgical Assisting (NBSTSA): http://www.nbstsa.org.

US Army Medical Department Center and School; U.S. Army Health Readiness Center of Excellence: http://www.cs.amedd.army.mil/ahs.aspx. Accessed July 24, 2015.

US Department of Labor Bureau of Labor Statistics: Occupational outlook: surgical technologists. http://www.bls.gov/ooh/healthcare/surgical-technologists.htm. Accessed July 24, 2015.

2 COMMUNICATION AND TEAMWORK

LEARNING OBJECTIVES

After studying this chapter, the reader will be able to:

1. Describe the elements of good communication
2. Demonstrate body language and describe its meaning
3. List the qualities of good communication
4. Discuss barriers to communication
5. Discuss different types of verbal abuse and why it is so destructive
6. Discuss problem behavior in the workplace
7. Define sexual harassment and discuss how to manage it in the workplace
8. Describe the characteristics of good teamwork
9. Explain how poor teamwork results in poor patient care
10. Discuss how computers are used in the perioperative environment
11. Identify the physical components of the computer
12. Discuss how computer networks and the Internet are used in a professional medical setting

TERMINOLOGY

Assertiveness: Communicating one's personal and professional needs to others; protecting one's own rights while respecting those of others.

Body language: Communication through facial expressions, posture, and gestures.

Consensus: Agreement among members of a group.

Facilitator: A group leader who coordinates the direction and flow of a group meeting without influencing the content of people's contributions. It is similar to an enabling position, in which people are encouraged to express ideas without fear of judgment.

Feedback: The response to a message; a component of effective communication.

Groupthink: In sociology and group behavior theory, the conformity of a group to one way of thinking and behaving. Groupthink creates two factions: those who agree (in-group) and those who disagree (out-group). This generates resentment and conflict in the workplace.

Message: The idea, concept, thought, or feeling expressed during communication.

Norms: Behaviors that are accepted as part of the environment and culture of a group. Norms are usually established by custom and popular acceptance rather than by law, although the two may not be mutually exclusive.

Receiver: The person to whom a message is communicated by a sender.

Sender: The person who communicates a message to another.

Rumor: A rumor is information with questionable validity.

Therapeutic touch: The purposeful touching of another person to convey empathy, care, and tenderness.

Win-lose solution: In conflict resolution, a solution that leaves one party satisfied but the other party dissatisfied.

Win-win solution: In conflict resolution, a solution that allows both parties in a conflict to gain.

Communication skills are among the most important tools for health care professionals to acquire. Technical information must be relayed accurately and precisely in terms that are understood by others. Communication in the workplace requires tact, respect for others, and discretion. Communication can reassure an anxious patient and demonstrate sensitivity. Individuals who develop these qualities are respected by others and sought after for career advancement.

Surgery is performed by *teams* of health professionals. Within the team, each person has a role and tasks. The ability to form a cohesive group quickly and efficiently—even among those who do not know each other—is one of the challenges of teamwork. *Communication skills or lack of them can make or break team relationships and productivity.* Some teams in the perioperative setting are more or less permanent. Department committees, policy groups, and surgical specialty teams meet regularly to communicate policy for scheduling, for training, or for social functions. Hundreds of models are available to help people form teams, get along, be productive, and enjoy the process. No matter what model (if any) is used, the process requires active participation, good communication skills, and willingness to work toward common goals.

PART I: COMMUNICATION

WHY STUDY COMMUNICATION?

Good communication is not accidental—it requires skill and practice. Even under the best of circumstances, communication can be difficult. Many health care workers are surprised to find that the greatest challenge in their work is not the work itself, but the interactions and social climate of the workplace. In the health care setting, the exchange of information is everyone's responsibility. In patient care, effective communication is essential to understand the patient's physical and psychosocial needs. Clear communication among coworkers is important because it contributes to safety and efficiency in the workplace. It gives personnel the information needed to establish priorities and act on them. Good communication clarifies relationships, solves problems, and helps establish professional and social boundaries. It increases teamwork and reinforces team goals. Poor communication can result in serious errors, conflict, and stress.

IMPORTANT TO KNOW *A 2013 study reported in the* Journal of Patient Safety *found that 440,000 patients die each year from* preventable *medical errors. The Joint Commission's analysis of the data from 2012, 2013, and first 6 months of 2014 found that 80% of the errors involved miscommunication.*

ELEMENTS OF COMMUNICATION

The primary **message** is the actual information being exchanged. The message also carries a tone, which is determined by *how* the message is expressed. Most people have experienced communication that is neutral in substance but delivered in a way that conveys an emotion or attitude, for example. Examples include a tone that is negative, positive, angry, respectful, or derisive. Tone can be conveyed in all types of communication (e.g., spoken, written). The message **sender** is the one conveying the information that is directed toward the **receiver.**

For communication to be considered effective in the workplace, one additional element is required. **Feedback** is a response by the receiver who acknowledges receipt of the message and its content. The feedback should demonstrate that the receiver understands the information and knows how to act on it. **Clarification** of a message is needed when the receiver understands some, but not all, of the message. In this case he or she should ask for more information. Communication is successful when the message is understood in content and tone the way it was intended by the sender.

VERBAL COMMUNICATION

SUCCESSFUL SPOKEN COMMUNICATION

When developing any skill, including communication, the professional should set objectives, or goals, as a way of measuring success.

The objectives of spoken communication in the health care environment are the following:

1. **Clarity.** The message is delivered in simple, straightforward language that is well understood by those receiving it.
2. **Neutrality.** The message carries no emotion. This is achieved by avoiding "charged" words because these interfere with the meaning and are a distraction to the receiver. Tone of voice can also set undesirable tones of impatience, lack of confidence, and even unprofessionalism.
3. **Conciseness.** The message is brief and to the point. The message should be delivered avoiding unnecessary words and sentences. If clarification or additional information is needed, the receiver should indicate this as feedback.
4. **Civility.** Concise language does not have to be sharp to the point of rudeness. Polite communication is based on respect for the other person.
5. **Assertive not aggressive. Assertiveness** is the ability to express one's own needs and rights while respecting the needs and rights of others. It demonstrates confidence without being confrontational. An assertive person communicates self-worth without showing arrogance or dominance.
6. **Right person, right time, right place.** In a busy workplace people often feel pressed to communicate to their managers and colleagues with urgency, even when the subject at hand is not critical. It is important to consider person, time, and place when communicating a need or reporting an event or situation. The person to whom you are reporting *should be one who needs to know the information. If an action is required, the person should have the ability to solve the problem and the authority to do so.* If the person receiving the message cannot immediately respond, they should know to whom it should be referred. Timing is very important. Pick a time when the other person is not distracted with other tasks or is in the middle of a conversation with someone

else. This is common courtesy. The person you have sought out will be much more receptive to your communication when he or she is not unnecessarily interrupted. Finally, pick the right place. This depends on whether the information is confidential or might cause distraction to others in the vicinity. Be alert to cues that the other person is not listening or wants to terminate the conversation. Such cues include looking away or from side to side, fidgeting, and backing up.

7. **Follows chain of command.** This is a further detail concerning authority to act in a specific situation. Before going to a staff member with a problem, use the "need to know" test. Ask yourself whether this person needs to know the information you have. If the message is urgent, do not delay. However, do not rush to someone with a problem that is not under that person's control.
8. **Maintain eye contact.** In maintaining relaxed eye contact, shift your gaze on the other person from one eye to the other. A fixed stare can convey emotional intensity.

IMPORTANT TO KNOW *In some cultures, direct eye contact with another person carries specific meaning. It is considered impolite for an Arab woman to make casual eye contact with a male, outside those of her family. In Chinese culture, one who makes eye contact with another person shows dominance and authority over that person. In many different cultures, children are taught not to make eye contact with their elders because it shows defiance or disobedience.*

9. **Avoid background conversation.** On the telephone, do not carry on a secondary conversation with others in the vicinity. It is disruptive to the person at the other end of the line and prolongs the conversation unnecessarily.

LISTENING SKILLS

People find it easy to talk with those who have good listening skills. Good listeners are often placed in key positions because of their ability to communicate ideas in a concise, accurate, and nonjudgmental way. People seek them out for advice because they know they will be heard fairly and with respect.

Listening requires active participation. Passive listening frequently leads to inaccurate interpretation or an inappropriate response. Parts of the message may be lost because the listener is distracted or impatient to speak.

Many people begin to formulate a response before they have heard everything the sender has to say. Their thoughts are focused on what they want to say, and they fail to receive the message. Box 2.1 presents positive listening skills.

HANDWRITTEN COMMUNICATION

Handwritten communication in health care is reserved for specific uses. These usually relate to patient safety or legal issues. Therefore great care must be taken to ensure that the words are clearly written or printed using the appropriate type of pen or marker. Handwriting or hand printing is used routinely in the following circumstances and many others not listed here:

- Signatures used to indicate the staff member has completed a task or is attesting to the validity of an action. These include signing off the surgical count (discussed in Chapter 19), preoperative checklist, self-identification on lab requisitions, and more.
- Signatures of witnesses to specific events such as the patient informed consent documents
- Any patient progress notes that are not routinely completed electronically
- Information required for tissue specimens obtained during surgery or other invasive procedure

Except for a signature, which is distinctive by its style, all handwritten and hand-printed information should be easy to read. Illegible notes waste time and can cause serious medical errors.

IMPORTANT TO KNOW *Special rules apply to handwritten notes containing the names and dosages of medications. These are discussed in Chapter 12.*

NONVERBAL COMMUNICATION

BODY LANGUAGE

The way we use posture, gestures, and expressions to convey ideas and messages is called **body language**. These cues can emphasize the message or convey a meaning that differs significantly from what was intended. Table 2.1 provides some common examples of body language observed in Western culture. When acquiring good communication skills, we should examine our own body language during conversation. Does your body language convey what you mean? Or is it a barrier to your communication? Be careful about using gestures. Those that are used in one culture may have a completely different meaning in another.

Gestures to Avoid in Our Multicultural Community

- Thumbs up is used liberally in America and in social media. However in Australia, Greece, and the Middle East it is a vulgar sign similar to the American middle finger.
- The "OK sign" is a vulgarity in Brazil, Germany, and Russia. It refers to a body orifice.
- Pointing at someone while speaking to them is a loud expression of your negative opinion of them. This is especially true in Asian and Latin American cultures.
- Placing the palm up in someone's face is an extreme insult in Greece.
- Eye contact is a sensitive issue. In Latin America and all African countries, eye contact is interpreted as a challenge to the other person. Between the sexes in the Middle East, eye contact is not allowed. Likewise, eye contact between a child and adult is a challenge of authority.
- Sitting posture can also be misinterpreted. Crossing the legs is considered rude in many cultures, including the Middle East, South Africa, and Japan.

BOX 2.1 Positive Listening Skills

1. Focus on the sender. Avoid listening to background noise or other conversations.
2. Avoid listening for what you want to hear; you may misinterpret the message.
3. Do not judge the sender. If you are preoccupied with personal details about the sender, you cannot interpret the message accurately.
4. Watch for nonverbal cues, such as facial expressions and body position.
5. Ask for clarification!
6. Rephrase the sender's content so that both of you know the message is understood—for example, "You mean that..."
7. If the sender begins to get sidetracked from the topic, redirect the conversation. Ask questions about the original issue or ask the sender to return to the topic.
8. If you find that your attention has drifted, ask the sender to repeat what was just said.
9. Do not assume background information unless you know it. If the message seems unreasonable, there may be circumstances of which you are unaware. Be open to the possibility that a much bigger picture is involved than the one you see.
10. When asking another to change his or her tone or language, be sure to state your own feelings about it—for example, "I wish you wouldn't criticize me in front of everyone, it's really humiliating."

TABLE 2.1 Examples of Body Language in Western Culture

Element of Body Language	What It Might Mean
Hands on hips	Authority or anger
Arms folded across the chest	Resentment or guarding
Eye contact	Attention and respect for the speaker, confidence
Lack of eye contact	Lack of social comfort (note that people of different cultural backgrounds may not hold eye contact with the speaker because of their culture or faith)
Eyes cast downward	Contemplation, embarrassment, or contrition
Backing up	Social distance that is too close or a desire to leave
Rigid posture	Restrained emotions or tension
Upright posture	Confidence or a sense of well-being
One eyebrow raised	Doubt or mistrust
Mouth covered by hand	Shock or sudden grief; embarrassment

- Displaying the bottom of one's feet is an extreme insult in Asian culture.

Does it mean that a colleague at your work will take offense at misguided gestures? Probably not. However, patients should not be exposed to these gestures. Whether we respect others who exist within boundaries of their culture depends on whether we want them to respect us.

Therapeutic Touch

Therapeutic touch is a method of conveying care and empathy to others. Comforting others by touch is universal. Training in therapeutic touch is becoming more popular as part of a holistic approach to disease and wellness. However, it must be used with care in the professional environment. Touch can be misinterpreted and even have a negative impact on the patient. However, touch remains a powerful source of comfort to many patients. Experienced health care workers learn to observe the patient's body language before offering a soothing hand. The patient has a right to decline to be touched, even when it might be comforting.

COMPUTERS IN THE PERIOPERATIVE ENVIRONMENT

Information technology is the use of computers and other electronic equipment to create, store, transmit, and retrieve information. Computer technology is incorporated into many different types of equipment and biomedical devices used in the perioperative environment. Some of these include the following:

- Secure computer systems for recording patient information (patient charts) and other medical records
- Preference cards for surgeons (indicates the surgeon's choice of equipment, supplies, positioning, and other important information)
- Diagnostic imaging equipment (e.g., radiography, magnetic resonance imaging [MRI], computed tomography [CT], fluoroscopy)
- Digital cameras and image output on monitors (screens) during surgical procedures
- Robotic surgical systems
- Surgical navigation (computer-guided surgery)
- Computer tracking of hospital supplies, instruments, and equipment during reprocessing (e.g., disinfection, sterilization)

Hardware (Physical Components)

The physical parts of a computer are the central core unit and peripherals. The core unit contains the wiring and complex circuits that run the computer and store data. The peripherals are other types of equipment that *interface* with (work with) the computer and are part of its operation, such as the computer screen, keyboard, and mouse. The basic hardware components are described in Table 2.2.

Computer Software

The term *software* is used to describe programs that control the tasks a computer can perform. Software is stored in the

TABLE 2.2 Basic Computer Hardware

Component	Description
Central processing unit (CPU)	The computer memory (internal) and electronic components that enable programming and output
Memory	Also called RAM or random access memory, this connects with the main electrical circuits to perform all the tasks needed to operate the computer. Data placed in RAM must be saved on other hardware called the *drive*
Motherboard	The primary circuits that run the computer
Drive	Internal or external device that stores the computer's data. External data drives such as flash drives are portable and can be moved from one computer to another for reading. Internal drives are identified by a letter on some types of computers
Monitor	The computer's screen where data are viewed by the user. The screen is also called the *display* or *output display*. Two types are commonly used—the liquid crystal display (LCD) and the cathode ray tube (CRT)
Modem/wireless card	An electronic device that makes the transmission to or from a computer via a communication line
Keyboard	Alphanumeric device for inputting data into the computer
Mouse	The user's steering component for inputting data on the monitor. It provides a visual cue on the monitor and signals the computer to perform a task associated with that cue
Speakers	Like other types of speakers, these provide sound output from the computer
Hard copy	Data computer output that has been reproduced in the form of a CD, DVD, or paper printout
Printer/scanner/fax	Output and input devices that produce paper and electronic documentation
USB port	A type of serial port for connecting peripheral devices to a computer system

electronic components of a computer. The computer needs instructions from the software to perform the tasks that individuals require it to do. Unlike a mechanical device, which performs physical work, the computer sorts and computes information electronically. These tasks are made possible through the computer software.

To further define what software actually is, we need to know that the computer operates by reading a set of instructions that tell it what to do and how to do it. These instructions are contained in a code (called *machine code*), which is a series of billions of on-off switches. Combinations of on-off codes create endless possibilities for storing and manipulating information (data) based on the on-off switch codes.

Data in the memory of the computer are organized into blocks of eight switches. Each switch is called a *bit*, and each block is called a *byte*. Computer programs (software) are described as having a certain number of bytes that operate in an exact way, giving the computer instructions to perform different tasks associated with that program.

Computer Networks

The term *computer network* refers to two or more computers that are connected electronically. Networks allow the transfer of information from one computer to another.

The Internet is a vast computer network; the World Wide Web is part of the Internet. The Web is a method of exchanging files, documents, graphics, and other discrete packets of information through the Internet. The method used to exchange and transfer the data is complex and beyond the scope of this discussion. However, it is important to understand that the Web is only one of many types of information systems that use computer networking.

An intranet is a system of multiple computers within a facility or organization that allows communication only within that system. Medical facilities often have their own intranet, which transmits useful information such as medical references, articles, and announcements about upcoming events. More important, hospital intranets publish the facility's policies and safety protocols so that everyone on the staff can continually update information about safety issues and patient care. Email is also part of the intranet system in most organizations. To access the intranet, you must use a password (Box 2.2). When you log onto your employer's intranet server, always remember to log off before you quit the session. This prevents others from accessing information that you have entered.

Navigating the Internet

Research on the Internet is performed through a search engine. This is a computer program that is available as a free download or to purchase. The search engine allows the user to type in a topic or phrase, which is sent out through the network. The program then returns information in data blocks called *links*, which are listed by their Internet title and address. The user can open these links and access the material within. An example of a reliable search engine is Google.

A vast amount of information is available on the Internet and World Wide Web. Traditional research sources (e.g., databases, periodicals, books, CD-ROMs, videos, DVDs) have largely moved to the Internet. When these tools are used appropriately, research can be done quickly and efficiently. However, so much information is available that it sometimes is difficult to determine whether the source is reliable and the information is correct. Remember that anyone can post almost anything on the Internet, regardless of whether it is valid. It is up to the user to select information carefully and review the copyright restrictions. Always scan your choices before you start opening files on the Internet. If you are doing professional research, use professional sites. If you want to buy

BOX 2.2 Passwords

A password is a code that each user types on the keyboard to start a computer session. Passwords are also used to gain access to programs or request data from a public or institutional computer. Health care providers may access an institution's computers through their individual password, given to them at the time of employment. The password must never be given to anyone else. It connects a specific user to data entry and retrieval. Access to patient information is privileged and belongs only to the person given the password. Remember that when you use an institution's computer, you must also log off (remove the password from the computer memory) so that others will not use your access after you leave the computer.

a product or research products for sale (e.g., surgical equipment), use the commercial sites.

For academic research, it is wise first to locate an academic institution or professional association most appropriate to the topic and then search for the desired topic. For example, if you want to research a disease, instead of simply typing the name of the disease in the search box, try locating a medical or academic link first. Use websites from organizations such as the Centers for Disease Control and Prevention (CDC), the American Medical Association (AMA), or the Mayo Clinic. These organizations' websites have extensive search engines that will give you accurate and authoritative information. If you do not know any professional organizations, use an Internet search engine to find one. Searching key terms such as *surgical organizations, infectious diseases,* or *medical reference* will also give you authoritative links. Look at the Internet address of the link before you randomly click on any of the choices. Educational institutions have "edu" in the address. Professional organizations have "org" in the address. If the address ends in "com," the site is a commercial one, with a focus on products to sell.

Email

Most people are familiar with email, even if they do not use it regularly. This process allows individuals or groups to contact each other through electronic mail programs on a network or the Internet and to send and receive messages, documents, and graphics electronically.

Health care institutions often set up email systems for their employees as a means of communicating messages and sending documents. New employees are instructed in how to access their mail and send messages within the system.

Professional electronic communication follows guidelines that are standard within professional communities. They apply to formal emails written to professional colleagues and managers.

- Professional emails should be as concise and short as possible. Use single line points whenever possible.
- Always include a subject heading. The heading should be short, clearly defining the purpose of the message. Avoid using an old string for a new email subject. If the message does not relate to the string, create a new subject heading.
- It is appropriate in professional transmissions to begin the email with a greeting, as in a letter (e.g., *Dear Dr. X…*). Even if you are communicating by a first name, include a greeting (e.g., *Dear Sandra*).
- Avoid emotional language and emotionally charged words in all professional communications.
- Emojis and SMA text abbreviations are *not appropriate* in professional communications.
- Do not forward an email or attachment to someone else without the author's permission. This demonstrates your respect for the author's privacy.
- When a message is sent to more than four people, the names should first be formatted as a group and the email sent to the name of the group. This protects the confidentiality of the group members.
- Never "reply to all" unless the message applies to everyone in the group.
- Compress heavy attachments before sending them as a courtesy to the receiver.
- Avoid sending attachments that contain information already stated in the body of the email.
- Remember that any email can be used as a legal document. What you say in an email can be stored and retrieved later. Use words carefully and professionally.
- Observe patient confidentiality requirements in all communication. Refer to Chapter 3 for an expanded discussion on confidentiality.
- Always include your name and contact information at the end of the email, even if the other person has this information already. This demonstrates that you want to be contacted and makes it easier for the other person.

An example of a well-written professional email is shown in Box 2.3.

BOX 2.3 Example of a Professional Email

Subject: Orthopedics hardware meeting
Dear Elliot,
It was great talking to you about the new orthopedic equipment. I am particularly interested in the titanium plates.
Can we set up a meeting to talk further about this?
I am available most afternoons. You can reach me by phone or at this email address.
I look forward to talking with you, and thanks again for your support to our department.
Sincerely,
John Douglas, CST
Orthopedics Coordinator
St. Mary's Hospital
123 5th St.
Newtown, CA
Mobile 555-666-6666

CULTURAL COMPETENCE

Cultural competence (sometimes called *cultural intelligence*) is the skill and knowledge to communicate and integrate well with people from diverse backgrounds and cultures. In health care it includes the ability to care for people across many different cultures and belief systems; it is also necessary to work with others of different backgrounds and cultures. To communicate successfully with patients and colleagues, health care workers need to understand different cultures and identify the ways communication can be improved for everyone's benefit.

Cultural competence requires is a set of skills, behaviors, and attitudes that enables people to interact effectively with others of different cultures and subcultures. It means putting aside personal bias or stereotyping (positive or negative) and actively seeking ways to understand the other person's needs and understanding. Patients from different cultures may have different beliefs about the origin of sickness and disease, and their coping mechanisms may be completely different from our own experience or understanding. In health care, cultural competence has a strong influence on patient care. Knowing some important beliefs and values of the patient improves the quality of communication with both the patient and his or her family. Poor understanding of the patients' values and beliefs can cause fear and mistrust of the health care providers and systems, noncompliance with medical advice, or avoidance of health care altogether.

The process of building cultural competence starts with self-assessment of our own beliefs that shape our behavior and attitudes toward others. Many people are surprised to discover their own bias for or against different cultures and subcultures. Self-awareness about bias helps health professionals move toward equal care and respect for all. We have all heard negative comments about newcomers' language, beliefs, and traditions. Whatever bias or prejudice is felt in parts of our society, health care workers have a professional ethical responsibility to demonstrate respect and equality of care to everyone in their care.

Equality of care does not mean we should try to change someone's beliefs or traditions to match our own. Social and interpersonal **norms** are imbued in people from the time they are born. Cultural beliefs and value systems cannot be switched off and on. If we accept the responsibility to provide equal care to all, then we must actively acquire knowledge and understanding about the values and health care beliefs of other cultures. This is best done through self-study and programs that teach health workers about the importance of cultural communication and prominent belief systems among different cultural groups. Excellent resources for learning are shown in Box 2.4.

BOX 2.4 Self-Guided Learning—Cultural Competence

The National Center for Cultural Competence provides a free, excellent self-guided course in four modules: https://nccc.georgetown.edu/bias/

The Nebraska Action Coalition has produced the following slide presentation and other resources for cultural competency. Although intended for nurses, they are applicable for all health care professionals: https://neactioncoalition.org/cultural-intelligence-for-the-nursing-profession/

The United States Department of Health and Human Services offers this website with online training links for health care professionals: https://www.thinkculturalhealth.hhs.gov/education/

COMMUNICATION WITH PATIENTS

Surgical technologists play a part in communication with patients and their caregivers—the family or friends of the patient. Communication with the patient combines clinical knowledge with care for the patient as an individual. Communication with the patient's family and friends requires specific qualities that require different skills.

PROFESSIONAL RELATIONSHIP

The relationship among the health professional, the patient, and his or her family has particular characteristics based on the professional relationship:

- The professional relationship requires a level of formality during communication between the health care professional and the patient or caregivers. Some formality is required to maintain the emotional distance required of professionals.
- When the patient is removed from the company of family, *it is a significant separation.* The family is naturally concerned and often worried. The health professional may be the only "emotionally neutral" person in the setting, and the family needs this neutrality for reassurance.
- The family may believe that the health professional has privileged or undisclosed information that is hidden from them. This is not the same as mistrust in the professional. It is simply part of the relationship and must be considered during communication.
- Family members may be self-conscious or embarrassed to show their emotions in front of the health professional. When a health professional steps into an emotional setting, he or she does not need to be drawn into the emotion of the context. Setting these boundaries is very important.
- The health professional may feel awkward about dealing with the family's emotions and relationship with the patient. Health professionals, especially those who are starting their career, may feel inadequate or out of place in the company of the patient and his or her family. This uncomfortable feeling may result in poor or inappropriate comments during communication.

All students in health care go through a period of discomfort when first introduced to patient and family communication. However, with experience, increased understanding of difficult situations usually results in increased skills in this area. Instructors and other mentors can be very helpful during the learning period.

COMMUNICATION FAILURE

Communication can fail for many reasons. The following are some of the most common:

- **Perception of the situation.** Our perceptions of the environment may not coincide with those of others. We make assumptions about what we see, hear, and understand based on our perception of the situation.
- **Bias.** *Personal bias* is our preexisting opinions about people based on affiliations, culture, economic status, and even their diseases. Bias is an effective communication stopper

because it does not allow new ideas or opinions to develop or to be revealed. The biased receiver already "knows" all he or she wants to know and is firmly rooted in a point of view.

- **Environmental barriers.** Communication sometimes fails simply because the environment prevents reception. Hearing is a problem in the operating room. Masks can muffle our speech; background noises such as suction, irrigation, power equipment, or loud music can distort communication.
- **Lack of understanding.** Sometimes the receiver does not have enough knowledge to understand exactly what the sender is trying to communicate. This is why *clarification* is so important in communication.
- **Social and cultural influences.** How we perceive a problem, situation, or action sometimes depends on our social and cultural background as much as our knowledge. These affect the way we evaluate and comprehend what is being communicated. Communication in any form is integrated into what we already know and believe. In a sense, there is no "pure" communication; each of us has a unique point of view of ourselves and the environment.
- **Emotions.** How we feel at the time of communication can have a powerful effect on our ability to receive and send messages. Communication is extremely difficult when people are overcome by emotions such as anger, resentment, fear, and anxiety.
- **Lack of a desire to communicate.** To be successful in sending and receiving information, a person must *want* to communicate. The desire to communicate creates greater attention, focus, and concentration, which are necessary for clarity and understanding.

VERBAL BLOCKING

Sometimes health care workers block communication with patients and each other. The most common causes are the following:

- Fear of escalating emotions
- Fear of being unable to handle a difficult topic
- Lack of confidence in managing sensitive discussions
- Lack of privacy to discuss the topic
- Environment is unsuitable for the discussion (too loud, too distracting, too many people)
- Mistrust in colleagues, ability to maintain confidentiality

Examples of Blocking Others' Need to Communicate

Blocking communication can be related to the examples above, or it can be due to insensitivity.

Minimizing the importance of the topic and needs of the sender:

A: "I want to talk to you about the mistake I made in surgery this morning."

B: "Oh, I'm sure no one noticed it."

Blocking the other's emotion:

A: "It was so upsetting."

B: "But you're OK now, right?"

Normalizing violent behavior:

A: "I'm so upset. Dr. X shoved me against the lockers when we were in the dressing room."

B: "Oh, you aren't the only one. He's done that before when he was really angry."

Defending or justifying behavior in others:

A: "The nurse told me that my surgery would take a long time."

B: "Don't worry, she says that to all the patients. It's just so the family doesn't worry when the case takes too long."

A: "Sometimes I wish my pregnancy didn't show. Dr. X put his hand right on my belly in the break room."

B: "Well he was just patting the *baby.* There's nothing wrong with that!"

PART II: TEAMWORK AND PROBLEM BEHAVIORS

A team is a group of people who come together to achieve common goals. The surgical team is only one type of team that plans and implements patient care in the operating room. In this type of structure, surgical technologists work with their peers to design instrument sets, order equipment, and update the surgeons' procedural changes. The team may or may not have a team leader.

The surgical technologist may also participate in other types of interdepartmental teams to improve care or produce information for surveillance and monitoring. Within a team, different personalities, work styles, values, and cultures are brought together. In spite of these different views and ways of working, the individuals on a team must identify and prioritize the steps of the process to reach the desired objectives.

The surgical team includes the surgeons, anesthesia provider, assistants, surgical technologist, and registered nurse. They all work together on a single procedure. Communication usually is focused and task oriented.

A *group* does not necessarily have a common goal, but the people in the group can share a common profession, interest, or other identifier. Group work and teamwork are very similar. Interpersonal relationships and the ability to resolve differences are equally important in a team and in a group. When people work on the same shift in the operating room, they form a group. An understanding is formed among them that they will help each other with certain tasks and try to resolve work-related obstacles.

CHARACTERISTICS OF GOOD TEAMWORK

Good teamwork is the result of good communication and healthy relationships within the team. This doesn't mean there are no conflicts. Conflict in groups is normal because people have different ideas, problem-solving skills, values, and beliefs. The qualities of a good team reflect how conflict is managed. Individuals can retain valued traits, such as genuineness, self-assertion, and empathy, yet at the same time be willing to discuss, yield, and accept change.

Many different social and professional models of team building and collaboration have been devised. There is no "best" model for every situation. People work in teams for immediate (emergency) results, long-term project goals, creative output, and many other reasons. The dynamics of team interaction always include common social and psychological behavior.

Conflict cannot be managed unless people communicate about their problems. Discussion means that the group must admit that a problem exists. Identifying the problem requires sharing of experiences and interpretations of events without judgment. Members of successful groups do not accuse others of wrongdoing. They focus on the problem, not the person. They simply state the facts and relate the effect.

Ability to Yield

Yielding in teamwork does not mean giving up one's values or beliefs. It means accepting the fact that others have valid points of view. People who are able to yield are open minded and retain a sense of fairness during team interaction. A team member who tries to gain control of all decisions and conversations is unable to accept that others also have valid ideas. Such individuals cannot imagine any way but their way and make little or no attempt to broaden their thinking.

Flexibility

The ability to accept change is crucial to good teamwork. Many people experience change as a positive event, but others are very uncomfortable with it. One of the purposes of a team is to adjust to a changing environment, such as unfolding events during a surgical procedure, a change in instrumentation, or new responsibilities. *When teams are confronted with change, they must adjust their ways of working to accommodate the change.* Team members must identify new tasks or procedures and implement them with as little disruption as possible. This requires personal flexibility and acceptance, which are positive character traits found in the successful professional.

Civility

Civility concerns the manner in which people speak to and behave toward each other. The attributes of acceptable behavior include respect, gratitude, and acceptance. The operating room culture does not always promote these attributes. This does not mean that they are unimportant. On the contrary, teams that honor and practice these qualities maintain a pleasant work atmosphere, are efficient, and show a high level of professionalism. They experience fewer conflicts, and team members show high self-esteem. Unfortunately, groupthink and aggressive behavior often overcome civility in the operating room. The most powerful way to instill civility in a group is to model it.

Polite behavior is not complicated or difficult. Saying "thank you" or "please" makes people feel appreciated and respected. Offering to help another person even if you have not been asked and responding to requests for help without resentment create an atmosphere of cohesion among coworkers. Speaking with others in a calm manner without sarcasm promotes evenness and reduces stress.

Ability to Collaborate

Collaboration is working together for a common purpose. In the operating room, individuals contribute their skills, time, and energy to the care of the surgical patient. Even though individuals have different skills, knowledge, and training, they do not exert authority; they simply contribute what is required and is within their ability. Successful patient outcomes can improve when each team member recognizes the relationship between his or her role and the roles of others. Each person understands that his or her contribution is one of many and that problems or strengths in one area affect the entire collaborative effort.

Setting team priorities requires cooperation, which is agreement on what the goals are and how they will be reached. Everyone may understand the goal, but people may disagree on how to reach it. For example, during surgery, the surgeon's goal is to work quickly without pauses in the flow of the procedure. The ST's goal is to remain ahead of the surgeon, anticipating what will happen next and what instruments and supplies will be needed, at the same time providing what is needed in the present. To do this, the ST must use every moment to prepare, as well as work in the present.

Consider a scenario in which the surgeon places used instruments out of the ST's reach. Suction, hemostats, and needle holders soon pile up out of reach of the ST. The surgeon has created a situation in which the surgical technologist cannot do his or her work. (Normally the ST must continually retrieve instruments from the field, wipe them down, and replace them on the Mayo stand.) The ST reminds the surgeon of the need to return instruments. The surgeon is frustrated because he or she must periodically collect the instruments and return them to the ST. The ST must spend time requesting the instruments and sorting them. Cooperation is lacking. The solution, of course, is for the surgeon to place the used instruments within the ST's reach immediately after using them. In this case, it would be helpful for the ST to point out that the procedure would go more quickly and more smoothly if the used instruments were placed within reach. The surgeon may be unaware of this need or may not have thought about the effect of his or her work habits on the achievement of the overall goal. Resolving this type of situation need not cause stress or tension. Each person must simply state their needs, and together they reach a consensus (agreement) on the matter.

TEAM CONFLICT

Conflict on teams can take several forms. No matter what form it takes, conflict on a team creates stress, lack of motivation, and reduced productivity across the entire team.

INTERPERSONAL CONFLICTS

Personality clashes, attempts to gain control of the group, and power plays are some causes of team conflict. All teams experience interpersonal conflicts from time to time. However, chronic conflict is intolerable for most teams. Those not in the conflict are frustrated because they cannot solve the problem and often resent the people involved for creating the tension. Team cohesion disintegrates, and members worry about productivity, safety, and accountability. Resolving the conflict may require mediation if the individuals involved cannot resolve

BOX 2.5 Guidelines for Serving as a Preceptor

1. If you are a student now, notice the problems you encounter. Think of the preceptors from whom you have learned the most and consider why you learned from them.
2. Develop a plan with the person for whom you are serving as preceptor. Discuss with the learner what each of you will do and how it will be done. For example, as the preceptor, you might start the case and then allow the learner to step in and complete it. You might also have the student perform certain tasks while you do others.
3. Never try to perform the same task at the same time as your student. For example, if the learner is passing instruments, allow your student time to think and act. Silently point to the correct instrument, but do not reach for it; this would result in hand collisions on the Mayo stand and frustration for everyone.
4. If the learner is struggling, try to help by coaching quietly in the background. If this is insufficient, ask the learner whether you should take over for a while. This allows the student to regain composure.
5. Never make a learner feel inadequate or foolish; this will only intensify the person's lack of confidence. Encouragement is much more productive than criticism. If you cannot contain negativity, ask to be excused from preceptor duties.
6. Always introduce the learner to the surgical team before beginning the procedure. This allows the learner to feel like part of the team and encourages confidence.
7. Respect the learner as a person. Remember that the learning phase is only one aspect of this person's life. You have a privileged job in helping the student achieve goals. You are also in a position to hurt the student's confidence. This is especially true of adult learners, who may not be accustomed to steep learning curves.
8. If the surgeon becomes irritated or anxious because of the learner's lack of experience, support the learner. If the situation becomes critical, ask the learner to wait until the critical situation has passed. Then, invite the student back into the case after assessing whether the surgeon is tolerant.

their differences. Particularly in health care, the overall goal (patient care) must not suffer because of individuals' inability to get along. In case of interpersonal conflict, the team leader must step up to help solve the conflict or refer the people involved to a human resources manager.

CONFLICT BETWEEN TEAM GOALS AND PERSONAL GOALS

Sometimes, personal or professional goals of individuals on a team interfere with the team goals. For example, a student ST is assigned to scrub with a staff ST. The overall goal is to complete the surgery in a safe and efficient manner. The role of the staff ST is to teach. The goals of the student, however, are to learn about the procedure and practice skills that will allow him or her to work independently without a preceptor. The student is eager to learn and apply hands-on skills during the procedure. The staff ST may not want to give up control of the case out of concern that the surgeon will become tense or angry when the pace and rhythm of the procedure is interrupted or the student makes an error. The goals of the student and the staff ST do not match and are likely to cause tension. By discussing each other's goals, the student and staff ST can acknowledge the conflict and find a solution that works for both. Box 2.5 provides guidelines for preceptors.

ROLE CONFUSION

Role confusion in the context of team conflict occurs when individuals are uncertain of what is expected of them in the workplace. This is a common problem among teams and groups of people, especially those in complex work situations. The following comments are common expressions of role confusion:

"That's not *my* job."

"I thought *you* were supposed to do that."

"What am *I* supposed to do about that?"

"No one told *me* that was part of my job description."

Most role confusion is a result of poor communication and lack of a defined job description. Every new employee must be given a detailed job description. A change in tasks or roles must be clarified by the team leader or manager to avoid problems.

As a student, you may be asked to carry out tasks that you are not confident doing. In this case, ask for support from the person who has delegated the task. When working on a team, ask for clarification of what is expected of each person. *Do not give up responsibility for a task after you have accepted it.* If you cannot complete it, you must report back to the person who assigned the task.

CONFLICT RESOLUTION

The goal of conflict resolution is to attempt to find a solution that is acceptable to all parties. This is called a **win-win solution.** Another type of resolution is a **win-lose solution,** in which one party is satisfied but the other is not. In extreme cases, a lose-lose situation will occur, where neither party has a satisfactory resolution.

The goal of conflict resolution is to find a win-win solution. This requires behaviors such as flexibility, willingness to yield, and the ability to focus on the problem, not the people. The following are some steps for resolving conflicts:

- When discussing the problem, recognize that you might have a personal opinion or bias about the situation. Consider the problem as objectively as possible.
- Remain open-minded about solutions. Do not get stuck on a single fact or solution.
- Gather information about the problem before discussing it. Discuss the available information with the team before looking for a solution.
- View the problem as a team problem, not as *your* problem. Brainstorm for solutions. Offer suggestions without deep analysis. Brainstorming allows people to suggest creative or different solutions without fear of judgment.

- Address any interpersonal conflicts in the team before other problems are solved. Tension in the team competes for energy needed for other types of problem solving.
- Formulate a plan for improvement that includes necessary behaviors and the rationale for changes.
- Try to reach a win-win solution. If such a solution is not reached, go back over the plan and evaluate whether concessions can be made to achieve a more satisfactory resolution.
- Seek outside help if the conflict cannot be resolved.

TEAM MANAGEMENT

Surgical technologists are increasingly required to be team managers. They may manage other technologists on a specialty team or serve as managers for projects. Few technologists just coming out of school have previous management training; therefore they must learn how to develop those skills on the job and by further education. Management practices have changed significantly in the past decade. Professional teams are more participatory in decision making, and a completely top-down approach is reserved for emergency situations in which the team leader must make decisions that have immediate consequences.

Management styles were first popularized in the 1970s, when businesses began to seek methods of training managers for increased production. Early texts identified these styles based on the behavior of the manager and the context. The modern team leader is a **facilitator** or enabler. Managers are trained to develop the ideas of individual team members, clarify their common goals, and help set a course that will accomplish the objectives. An effective team leader will follow these guidelines:

- Listen to everyone with equal attention and respect.
- Set realistic goals.
- Keep the team focused and interested in the goals.
- Be alert for friction among team members.
- Remain unemotional in team interactions.
- Enable every team member to participate in discussion and input.
- Recognize that new ideas can be brought to the team in many ways; integrate them into the objectives.
- Allow team members to make mistakes.
- Remember to encourage team members frequently; point out accomplishments.
- Meetings should be short, well planned, and focused.
- Allow others to speak more frequently than you do.
- Do not become involved in department politics, and do not criticize management.
- ***Be generous with your knowledge and humble about your opinions.***

OVERCOMING TEAM NEGATIVITY

Teams and groups can lose their ability to work well together for many reasons. Some of the most common reasons involve poor team leadership and demoralization by individuals who spread negativity.

Chronic Complainers

Legitimate complaints about conditions in the workplace are important and should be addressed because they can lead to creative solutions that produce a safer and more efficient workplace. However, when people complain without the intention of seeking solutions, they erode morale and sometimes create conflict. Chronic complaining can be contagious. When it becomes part of the workplace culture, it spreads discontent. Habitual complaining is usually not about occasional incidents. Habitual complainers are usually unhappy about many aspects of their lives. They do not look for solutions; they simply want everyone to know how they feel and seek out others to hear and validate their many complaints. Although it is helpful for people to share problems, chronic complaining is not usually directed at these goals. The following guidelines can be used when dealing with chronic complainers:

- Do not become a complainer yourself. The complainer seeks out others to agree with him or her to validate their unhappiness. This only perpetuates the problem. Offer a solution or suggest how the person might solve the problem. If the complainer rejects the solution immediately or gives more examples of how bad things are, you know that the individual is not interested in seeking solutions but simply wants to state and restate the negative aspects of work or of his or her personal life.
- Just listen. Sometimes silence has a powerful effect on the complainer. Listen without emotion and then simply exit the conversation politely. This is not a satisfying response to the complainer, and the person may stop.
- Confront the complainer. Complainers often dominate locker room conversation or complain in front of patients. If you are in the presence of a patient and the complainer begins complaining, simply say, "Not now" or "This isn't the time." Speak to the complainer in private and tell the person the effect that complaining has on patients and the team. If necessary, remove yourself from the situation.

Overly Critical People

Criticism is a helpful tool in correcting work habits or raising awareness about harmful or unsafe situations. When offered appropriately, criticism is specific, nonjudgmental, and *focused on the problem, not on the person.* When criticism is used to exercise power over others or boost one's own self-confidence, however, it can be very destructive. People who habitually criticize are usually insecure in their own lives. They use criticism as a way to soothe the anxiety they experience as a result of self-dissatisfaction. Nevertheless, this does not give them the right to demoralize or demean others. Some critics are expert at finding vulnerabilities in their coworkers and using these to demonstrate their superiority or authority.

Habitually critical people are often defensive and may become resentful when confronted with their behavior. However, it is important to point out when their criticism is causing conflict.

- State that you find the person's behavior distressing rather than helpful.
- Tell the person that if he or she wishes to discuss your work, you will do so in private. This formalizes the critical process and removes its ability to cause embarrassment in front of others.

Gossip and Rumors

Gossip is the telling and retelling of events about another's personal life, professional life, or physical condition. It is insidious behavior that hurts people, erodes teamwork, and damages group cohesion. Gossip is not the same as the normal sharing of news or events that occur in people's lives. It is communication about another person or event that is confidential or personal. The goal of gossip is to shock or evoke intrigue. As gossip spreads, the story may change slightly and facts may become blurred so that the only importance of the story is its ability to entertain at the expense of someone else.

A rumor is information with questionable validity. The damaging effect of a rumor is that, after the story begins to circulate, people assume that it is true and react as if the rumor were fact. If the **rumor** is unpleasant news, conflicts arise, and people may become resentful, angry, or even fearful. Ironically, people who spread rumors are often unable to validate the rumor. As with gossip, the value of the rumor lies in its effect on others during the telling and retelling, not in whether it is based on reality.

Adopt the following rules in coping with gossip and rumors:

- Do not perpetuate rumors or gossip about others. If you find yourself participating in spreading rumors or gossip, some self-reflection is necessary to explore why you find it necessary to behave in this way.
- Call attention to the behavior. One very effective way to do this is to make a remark such as, "We shouldn't be talking about Dr. X. That's his personal business." (Note that it is important not to accuse the other person; that is, do not say, "*You* shouldn't…") You might also say, "It's not fair to talk about someone when he can't defend himself." The point is to reinforce to the gossiper that you do not want to perpetuate gossip.

Groupthink

Groupthink is collective behavior and thinking. It is based on peer pressure and occurs when members of a group are polarized in their opinions, ways of doing things, and means of expression. It produces two categories of people: those who are "in" and those who are "out." People avoid becoming isolated and strive to become part of the "in" group, so they alter their own values to avoid being shut out. In this way, group culture is created and maintained.

Groupthink establishes unwritten, unspoken rules. Those who do not follow the rules may be criticized or ostracized by their peers. Standards of practice are deeply affected by groupthink.

Groupthink is usually a negative force because it does not allow freedom of speech or action without the implied threat of isolation. A surgical technologist should be an independent and critical thinker, uphold high standards, and act in a professional manner in every situation.

KEY CONCEPTS

- *Effective communication skills are extremely important in the health care professions. Patient safety and teamwork are based on the ability to deliver and receive information in all forms.*
- *The elements of communication are a sender, a receiver, the message, the means of communication, and feedback about the message.*
- *Verbal communication is written and spoken. Our choice of words and tone of voice can often alter the meaning of a message, resulting in positive or negative reactions in those with whom we are communicating.*
- *Communication is influenced by culture, attitude, point of view, emotions, and the desire (or lack of desire) to communicate.*
- *The qualities of good communication include focused listening, assertiveness, respect, and clarity.*
- *Stressors in the environment can block good communication and teamwork.*
- *Characteristics of good teamwork include yielding, the ability to change, civility, and collaboration.*
- *Team conflict often arises when the goals of the team conflict with the priorities of individuals.*
- *Role confusion is an important source of team conflict. Clarification of everyone's role on the team is of utmost importance.*
- *Conflict resolution is a learned skill that can benefit all health care professionals.*
- *Computer technology is now an integral part of many medical devices and is also a common method of documentation and communication in health care facilities. The surgical technologist is required to have fundamental computer skills needed to fulfill documentation requirements and, in many operating rooms, access to the surgeon's preference cards necessary to prepare for a case.*
- *The most basic physical components of the computer include the central processing unit, keyboard, mouse, and monitor. Entry-level computing and digital communication require the use of these devices to access data stored in the computer.*
- *Health facilities use a computer network system or intranet to allow communication and access to important data by employees. The network, which requires a password to enter (log on), is a group of internally connected computers located throughout the health care facility. In many modern operating rooms, computer stations are located inside or near each suite for convenient access. The Internet is an internationally connected network that is separate from an intranet. The Internet is accessible by the public, whereas use of an intranet is restricted to facility employees.*

REVIEW QUESTIONS

1. Give three examples of groupthink that you have observed.
2. What is the purpose of having teams?
3. What are the characteristics of good communication?
4. Why does communication sometimes fail?
5. What does it mean to withhold information deliberately?
6. What are some constructive ways to work with chronic complainers?
7. What would you do if you believed a coworker was spreading rumors about you?
8. What are the causes of cultural discrimination?
9. Why is it important to develop and keep public trust for a health care worker?

CASE STUDIES

CASE 1

You are among six surgical technologists on an orthopedics team in a large hospital. The team leader is aggressive and rude to you. You feel that his technical expertise is lacking and that he was made team leader because of his relationships with the sales representatives. How will you handle your working relationship with this person? How can you reduce your own stress?

CASE 2

You are a new employee in a large hospital operating room. You have been assigned a preceptor with whom you have difficulty working. You are not learning much because she won't let you do anything except observe. When you tell her you would like to do more, she declares, "You're not ready to do anything; just watch." After several weeks, the situation has not changed. What will you do?

BIBLIOGRAPHY

Costello J, Clarke C, Gravely G, D'Agostino-Rose D, Puopolo R. Working together to build a respectful workplace: transforming or culture. *AORN J*. 2011;93(1):115–126.

Develop Cultural Intelligence - Online Course. FutureLearn. https://www.futurelearn.com/courses/develop-cultural-intelligence. Published 2019. Accessed March 25, 2019.

Hu Y, Parker S, Lipsitz S, et al. Surgeon leadership style and team behavior in the operating room. *J Am Coll Surg*. 2015;221(4):S133.

Workplace Violence Prevention in Health Care - Rulemaking. Dir.ca.gov. http://www.dir.ca.gov/OSHSB/Workplace-Violence-Prevention-in-Health-Care.html. Published 2019. Accessed March 25, 2019.

MEDICOLEGAL ASPECTS OF SURGICAL TECHNOLOGY

3

LEARNING OBJECTIVES

After studying this chapter, the reader will be able to:

1. Differentiate among law, standards of practice, and codes of conduct
2. Define risk management
3. Explain the difference between licensure, certification, and registration
4. Identify and discuss abuse and violence in the perioperative environment
5. Define sentinel event
6. Identify common areas of negligence in perioperative practice
7. Discuss the importance of documentation in the perioperative setting
8. Explain informed consent
9. Discuss adverse events in the perioperative environment
10. Discuss different examples of negligence that occur in the perioperative environment
11. Describe what a legal document is
12. Differentiate between a law and a standard
13. Discuss the reasons why sexual harassment, bullying, and extreme forms of verbal abuse exist in the perioperative environment
14. Define and give examples of advance care directives

TERMINOLOGY

Abandonment: A health professional's failure to stay with a patient and provide care, especially when there is an implied contract to do so.

Accountability: Accepting responsibility for one's actions. In a professional context, this means that roles and actions accepted by an individual within the context of their occupation require the person to accept responsibility for the consequences of carrying them out.

Administrative laws: Laws created by an agency or a department of the US government.

Advance directive: A document in which a person gives instructions about his or her medical care in the event that the individual cannot speak for himself or herself. Examples are a living will and a medical power of attorney.

Adverse event: An unanticipated, undesirable, or potentially dangerous occurrence in a health care organization.

Code of conduct: A set of rules or guidelines an organization writes for its members. The rules pertain to how people behave and are based on the principles that the organization values, such as professionalism and personal integrity.

Damages: Compensation (money) for an injury caused by negligence.

Delegation: The assignment of one's duties to another person. In medicine, the person who delegates a duty retains accountability for the action of the person to whom it is delegated.

Evidence-based practice: Professional practices and their standards based on established scientific research rather than opinion or tradition.

Horizontal abuse: Verbal abuse or sabotage of people of equal job or professional ranking.

Hospital policy: Rules or regulations that hospital employees are required to follow. They are created to protect patients and employees from harm and to ensure smooth operation of the hospital.

Informed consent: A process or legal document that describes the patient's surgical procedure and the risks, consequences, and benefits of that procedure.

Libel: A deliberate attempt to discredit another person in writing.

Negligence: Negligence as it applies to health professionals can occur in two ways: it can be a failure to do something that a reasonable person, guided by the ordinary professional considerations, would do; or it can be the act of doing something that a reasonable and prudent person would not do.

Perjury: The crime of intentionally lying or falsifying information during court testimony after a person has sworn to tell the truth.

Practice Acts: State laws that establish and regulate the conditions under which professionals may practice, including licensure, registration, educational requirements, scope of duties, and functions.

Regulations: Laws that are enforced by state and federal agencies.

Retained foreign object: An item that is inadvertently left inside the patient during surgery.

Sentinel event: A patient safety event that is not related to the patient's illness or underlying condition, resulting in death, permanent harm, or severe temporary harm requiring intervention to sustain life.

Sexual harassment: An extreme abuse of power in which an individual uses sexualized language, gestures, or unwanted touch to coerce or intimidate another person.

Slander: A deliberate attempt to discredit another person through speech.

Statutes: Laws passed by federal or state legislative bodies.

Subpoena: A court order requiring its recipient to appear and testify at a trial or deposition. Medical records can also be the subject of subpoenas.

Tort: Legal wrongdoing that results in injury to a person or property.

TERMINOLOGY (Cont.)

Universal protocol: A procedure in which the surgical team affirms the identity of the patient, correct procedure and location (side), verification of informed consent, and other documents necessary to proceed with the surgery. The procedure is mandated by The joint commission.

Unretrieved device fragment: A portion of a medical device that has broken off or come apart in the body and is not detected or removed. Examples are fragments of a broken surgical needle and a hinge pin of a surgical instrument.

Vertical abuse: Bullying, attempts to devalue, intimidate, or embarrass an individual. This occurs between two people of different levels of hierarchy in an organization.

Health professionals in all settings are guided in their practice by standards, laws, regulations, and policies. They also follow an ethical code, which is expected of people who are highly accountable to the public. Laws reflect society's rules, which have been created by the people and enforced by their government. Law in most societies is intended to protect individuals from harm and promote a peaceful society. Violation of the law has legal consequences.

TYPES OF LAW

There are many different types of laws, sources of laws, and legal specialties. The surgical technologist is mainly concerned with **statutes** and liability. These will be the focus of this chapter. However, other forms of law will also be defined.

FEDERAL LAW

The federal government is responsible for many agencies that administer laws having to do with health care. Examples are the Health Insurance Portability and Accountability Act of 1996 (HIPAA) Privacy Rule (see later) and the laws concerning Medicare insurance.

STATE LAW

State laws are enacted by state and federal governments. The statutes that most concern the surgical technologist are the state Practice Acts that define the *scope of practice.*

State Practice Acts

Under the US Constitution, each state has the power to pass laws that define and regulate its health professions. These state laws are called **Practice Acts.** They are enacted by state legislature and may be modified by further legal proceedings. The purpose of a Practice Act is to "protect and benefit the public" by defining the type and level of education and experience required for the profession. The Practice Acts also define the scope of practice for health care professionals. This is a description of what health care professionals are allowed and not allowed to do in their practice.

The current laws are more detailed than in the past. In many states, surgical technologists are specifically named in the statutes, whereas they were not in the past.

Surgical technologist Practice Acts vary from state to state. For this reason, graduates and students should access their state laws to study the statutes. Surgical technologists can research their state Practice Acts online by searching *state legislature* plus [the state] plus *surgical technologist.* Other key words to replace *legislature* are *state register* and *statute.* Because of the varied roles of the surgical technologist, there is active debate about surgical technologists' range of allowable duties. Legislators (those who make the laws) must ensure a balance between reimbursement for state and federal medical services and the realities of an available workforce. Lobbyists (those who propose change in the law) are concerned with advocacy and protection of the profession and appropriate advancement, leading to greater esteem and financial reward. Both groups are motivated to protect the public and provide a high standard of care. Surgical technologists can become involved in their state legislative activities by contacting their state assembly.

ADMINISTRATIVE LAW AND REGULATIONS

The branch of law that deals with federal and state agencies is called **administrative law.** The laws that are enforced by the agencies are called **regulations.** Government agencies are established to oversee large programs affecting the environment, commerce, housing, health care, and many other areas of public concern. They issue regulations to enforce the standards each agency develops to meet its objectives. For example, the Occupational Safety and Health Administration (OSHA) issues and enforces regulations that reduce employee injury in the workplace. Another agency involved in health care is the US Food and Drug Administration (FDA), which establishes laws that govern the safety of medicines and medical devices.

Hospitals and other health care facilities are required to follow government regulations that concern patient and employee safety, management of medicines and medical devices, and other areas. Violation of a regulation is punished by a fine and can affect an organization's accreditation. Health professionals are required to adhere to the regulations. These are available to new employees and are kept on file for employee reference. Individual employees are not fined, only the institution. Employees are expected to follow the regulations that affect the overall compliance of their facility.

CIVIL LAW

Civil laws are those that protect the *rights* of individuals. Civil law is implicated when one person or organization violates the rights of another. This area of the law includes important categories that apply to all health care workers.

Tort Law

Tort law is a branch of civil law. Actions that result in physical or psychological harm or injury to another is called a **tort.** A tort is classified as intentional (done on purpose with intent to harm) or as a result of negligence (see the next section). Tort cases are handled in the civil court.

NEGLIGENCE TORT **Negligence** is the most common cause of injury in the health care setting. It is defined by The Joint Commission (TJC) as "the failure to use such care as a reasonably prudent and careful person would use under similar circumstances." In other words, the negligent person fails to act in a situation that he or she *should have known about* or acted in a way that he or she *should have known* might result in harm. Negligent acts are unintentional.

> The Joint Commission. Sentinel event glossary of terms. n.d. http://www.jointcommission.org/sentinelevents/se_glossary.htm.

That is, the negligent person did not intend to cause injury.

Refer to Common Acts of Negligence in the Perioperative Setting later in this chapter for a complete description of common actions of negligence (negligence torts).

INTENTIONAL TORT Intentional tort is intentional wrongdoing that results in injury or harm to another person. Examples are as follows:

- Battery: Harmful contact with another person with intention to harm, such as a physical attack on another person
- Assault: The threat or attempt to harm another person, regardless of whether the threat is carried out
- Invasion of privacy: This refers to publicly discussing or depicting patients outside the health care environment. It also includes any mention or photos of patients on public media unless the patient has provided specific permission to do so.
- False imprisonment: A person is restrained against their will by another who has no legal authority to do so, such as when a person is prevented from leaving their car or house by physical restraint or threats of violence
- Defamation: Deliberate efforts to erode the reputation of another person. If the actions are verbal, it is **slander.** If the statement is written, it is **libel.**

MEDICAL MALPRACTICE Malpractice is also part of civil law. It is defined by TJC as "improper or unethical conduct or unreasonable lack of skill by a holder of a professional or official position." Cases of malpractice are brought about against professionals who do not practice their professional skills when these skills are required or expected. Examples of medical malpractice are the following:

- The surgeon allows an untrained assistant to complete the surgical procedure while the surgeon takes a break
- A missed diagnosis by a physician
- Operating on the wrong patient or wrong side

CRIMINAL LAW

Criminal laws are state and federal laws that make specific behaviors illegal. The punishments for violation of criminal laws are imprisonment and fines. An important difference between criminal law and civil law is that the state is the accuser of a crime, whereas in civil law the accuser is the individual that was harmed. Examples of criminal law are homicide (murder), theft, robbery, and sex crimes.

COMMON LAW

Common law is a branch of law that applies previous legal decisions to a case currently being judged. Legal *doctrines* are the legal principles or rules that have been established through legal precedents. Examples of legal doctrines that may apply to health care are listed in Box 3.1.

CORPORATE LAW

A registered corporation is treated as a person under the law. This means that it can be liable in a lawsuit. Health care institutions that are also corporations are accountable for the protection and safety of their patients.

FACILITY STANDARDS AND POLICIES

Hospitals and other health care facilities are accredited by TJC through a rigorous process of performance evaluation in key areas of patient care. To achieve and maintain accreditation, facilities must establish standards and policies that meet or exceed those expected by TJC. Accredited hospitals and other health care facilities are also required to provide orientation training for their employees and to supply documents that detail their policies. New employees and students must be familiar with the policies that affect their professional role and duties. Violation of **hospital policy** may result in disciplinary action by the facility (which may jeopardize one's job in the future). Forgetting a policy or not knowing a policy is not considered an acceptable reason for failure to comply. Policies are usually logical and are beneficial for a smooth-running workplace. They are created by specialists within the organization, in consultation with TJC, who advises on best practices based on risk analysis and specific research in the areas of safety that are affected by those practices.

The operating room *procedure manual* is distinct from the hospital policy. It describes the operating room protocols for specific practices such as disinfection and sterilization methods, room turnover procedures, and chemical and laser safety precautions. Separate policy manuals may be used to detail the safe and careful use of particular equipment, protocols for

BOX 3.1 Examples of Legal Doctrines

- *Respondeat superior:* "Let the master respond." Historically, the surgeon or health care facility was held responsible for the acts of others on the surgical team through a doctrine called "borrowed servant." However, individual professionals on the surgical team are now held accountable for their own acts whether they are unintentional, negligent, or delegated.
- *Res ipsa loquitur:* "The thing speaks for itself." The defendant is judged to be guilty of an act of negligence even though there is no direct evidence of harm. This is based on the fact that the act is so obvious that "the thing speaks for itself." An example is leaving an instrument or sponge in the patient, which is an obvious source of harm and needs no other evidence that it is harmful.
- *Primum non nocere:* "First, do no harm." Many medical organizations use this slogan to emphasize that professionals have a legal and ethical responsibility to ensure that their care does not cause injury or harm.
- *Doctrine of foreseeability:* This concept is embodied in the laws regarding negligence in which a health professional should be able to predict specific risks associated with their duties that could injure a patient and take the appropriate precautions to prevent that harm. Areas included are electrosurgery, laser use, patient positioning, and other usual activities with inherent risk.

moving and handling patients, preparation of the patient for surgery, and other specific areas of care.

STANDARDS OF PRACTICE, POSITION STATEMENTS, AND CODES OF CONDUCT

STANDARDS OF PRACTICE

Laws protecting society from harm are supported by professional standards of practice (also called *practice standards*). These are not laws. They are technical guidelines that detail the methods and techniques for specific procedures. Examples are the method to use during the surgical hand and arm scrub or the required technique for the surgical count. Medical, allied health, and professional nursing organizations such as the American Academy of Surgeons, the Association of Surgical Technologists (AST), and the Association of periOperative Registered Nurses each publish standards of practice. Professional standards should be based on evidence derived from recent peer-reviewed scientific data. This demonstrates their scientific validity. Health care workers are required by their professional organizations to follow its standards. This is known as **evidence-based practice,** because it relies on science rather than opinion or tradition.

Perioperative practice covers a wide range of topics and subspecialties. This means that some procedures are common to several different professions that provide standards of practice for the same or similar procedures. Sometimes there are discrepancies in practice standards among professional organizations, and questions arise as to which is correct. In this case, the *sources* of the technical information used to validate the standard must be cited.

New technology and research can cause standards to become quickly outdated or obsolete. Therefore professional organizations normally review the scientific literature frequently (at least yearly) so that practices keep pace with current medical science. However, professional institutions do not rush to change a standard based on a single new study, especially if the study itself does not follow appropriate research techniques or if there was a conflict of interest on the part of the researcher.

POSITION STATEMENT

In addition to technical and professional standards, organizations publish *position statements.* These are public declarations of the organization's *opinion* on issues related to professional practice and policy. A position statement may not be used to bypass law, Practice Acts, or hospital policy. Instead, position statements are used to publicly state the organization's point of view.

AST publishes position statements on its website: http://www.ast.org.

CODE OF CONDUCT

A code of conduct is an organization's rules or guidelines for the *behavior* of its members. The purpose of a code of conduct is to ensure that the actions of individuals in that profession or organization are consistent with its core values. These are not laws, and there is no legal consequence for violating the code of conduct unless a standard coincides with an existing law. However, violation of the professional code of conduct may result in disciplinary action by the organization. This may include revoking membership in the organization or privileges to practice in a particular institution. The AST code of conduct is shown in Box 3.2.

BOX 3.2 Code of Ethics of the Association of Surgical Technologists

1. To maintain the highest standards of professional conduct and patient care.
2. To hold in confidence, with respect to the patient's beliefs, all personal matters.
3. To respect and protect the patient's legal and moral rights to quality patient care.
4. To not knowingly cause injury or any injustice to those entrusted to our care.
5. To work with fellow technologists and other professional health groups to promote harmony and unity for better patient care.
6. To follow principles of asepsis.
7. To maintain a high degree of efficiency through continuing education.
8. To maintain and practice surgical technology willingly, with pride and dignity.
9. To report any unethical conduct or practice to the proper authority.
10. To adhere to the Code of Ethics at all times with all members of the health care team.

Association of Surgical Technologists https://www.ast.org.

RIGHT TO PRACTICE

The right to practice a health profession is granted when the individual completes all the requirements of the profession, including education, demonstration of skills, and education, number of clinical or contact hours, and a successful written examination. In health care and some other professions there are three types of documentation that demonstrate that someone has met all the requirements to practice their profession. These are certification, licensure, and registration.

CERTIFICATION

Certification is validation that an individual has met the requirements needed to practice a particular profession. Certification to practice a profession may or may not be required by law (refer to Chapter 1 for details on certification for surgical technologists).

LICENSURE

Licensure is a legal requirement for certain professions. Professional licenses are issued by the state in which a professional intends to work. Examples of licensed health professionals are medical doctors, registered nurses, respiratory therapists, and radiology technologists. Licensure allows states to monitor and regulate professionals to protect the public. Most states allow *reciprocity*, which means that a person licensed in one state may apply for licensure in a different state. If the conditions of licensure are different from those in which the person is licensed, additional testing, study, or internship can be undertaken to meet the new requirements.

REGISTRATION

Registration of health professionals is an administrative process carried out for public protection. The state government maintains an official record of the health professional's vital statistics, address, and place of employment. Registration allows the state to accurately identify health professionals to monitor the person's whereabouts and to carry out criminal background checks. Some states require surgical technologists to register to practice.

COMMON ACTS OF NEGLIGENCE IN THE PERIOPERATIVE SETTING

When a civil lawsuit is brought into action because of negligence, the plaintiff (the person bringing the suit) seeks money (called **damages**) to compensate for the injury caused by the negligence. Examples of negligent actions common in health care are discussed in detail later in this chapter.

It is important for the surgical technologist to be aware of common forms of negligence and intentional wrongdoing in the perioperative environment.

UNINTENDED RETAINED FOREIGN OBJECTS

A **retained foreign object** is an instrument, sponge, needle, or instrument fragment **(unretrieved device fragment)** unintentionally left in the patient as a result of surgery or other invasive procedure. A retained object can result in infection, tissue destruction, and hemorrhage. Delayed healing and unresolved pain are additional consequences. Accountability for a retained object lies with the entire surgical team. The standard for preventing retained objects is the sponge, sharps, and instrument count (commonly called the *count*). The scrub and the circulator are responsible for the surgical counts, which must be performed in an exact way at prescribed times during the surgery. This protocol is fully described in Chapter 18. Surgical counts are documented according to hospital policy, and extra precautions may be taken under specific circumstances.

BURNS

Burns are the most frequent cause of injury in the operating room. Injuries are the result of misuse or negligent operation of electrosurgical equipment, heating blankets, hot solutions, hot instruments, lasers, and chemicals. Every person who works with these devices and agents is responsible for learning about the risks and must be able to demonstrate their safe use. The following are examples of actual cases of burn injuries caused by negligence:

- During laser surgery of the upper respiratory tract, special precautions for a laser-safe endotracheal tube are neglected. The endotracheal tube bursts into flames, causing third-degree burns of the patient's face and throat.
- Sparking from the electrosurgical device ignites a wet alcohol prep solution and surgical drapes, resulting in third-degree burns of the peritoneal cavity and thorax.
- A warm air blanket that covers the patient's body is connected improperly. The warm air hose accidentally disconnects from the blanket but is undetected by the surgical team. The patient suffers extensive burns that are not discovered until the end of surgery when the drapes are removed.
- An improperly placed dispersive electrosurgical pad allows current to flow to the electrocardiographic leads, resulting in serious burns under the leads.
- A stainless steel retractor is removed from the steam sterilizer and immediately placed in the patient. The abdominal contents are burned by the hot instrument.
- Skin prep solutions are allowed to pool under the patient. After the procedure, the drapes are removed to reveal blistering of the skin.
- Irrigation solutions are kept in warmers at excessively high temperatures. The lining of the body cavity in which the irrigation solution is used is burned by the hot solution.
- A hot ultrasound coagulation/dissecting instrument is inadvertently placed on the patient's skin, causing a second-degree burn.

FALLS

Patient falls are the *leading* cause of death in hospitalized people older than 65 years. Hospital employees are also at risk for falls, which contribute to injury, lost workdays, reduced patient care, and expense in worker compensation claims. The following are examples of common circumstances in which falls occur in the perioperative environment:

- The side rails on a stretcher are not kept raised, or a safety strap is not secured on the operating room table.
- A sedated or disoriented patient climbs over the side rails or becomes entangled between the rails.
- Unsafe transfer techniques are used to move a patient to and from a wheelchair, resulting in a fall.

INCORRECT PATIENT POSITIONING

The patient can be seriously and permanently injured as a result of improper positioning for the surgical procedure. Overextension of limbs, pressure on bony prominences, loss of circulation as a result of poor or improperly placed padding, and restricted ventilation are some consequences of improper positioning. The surgeon, anesthesiologist, nurse anesthetist, surgical assistant, and circulator work collaboratively while positioning the patient to ensure safety.

OPERATING ON THE WRONG PATIENT OR WRONG SITE

No excuse is acceptable for operating on the wrong patient or the wrong site or doing the wrong procedure. The consequences of these errors are so grave that TJC requires surgical teams to comply with a specific protocol in which the entire team participates. The **Universal Protocol** or **TIMEOUT** is a verification procedure in which the team pauses just before surgery and verbally recites essential information about the operative site and side, patient identity, position, and other crucial information about the patient and procedure. Surgery may not proceed until the protocol is completed. A record of the TIMEOUT is included in the operative record or other permanent form in the patient's chart. The Universal Protocol is fully described in Chapter 18.

INCORRECT IDENTIFICATION OR LOSS OF A SPECIMEN

Any tissue or foreign object removed from the patient during surgery requires careful handling and documentation. If the specimen is removed to confirm or rule out malignancy, improper labeling or loss of the tissue can have disastrous consequences for the patient, including misdiagnosis or a delay in appropriate treatment. All foreign bodies and tissue specimens must be examined by the hospital pathology department. A key responsibility of the surgical technologist is to handle and maintain specimens properly. The surgical team must identify, label, and ensure delivery of specimens to the pathology department or other area specified by hospital policy. This procedure is described in Chapter 19.

MEDICATION ERRORS

Surgical technologists are required to transfer medicines to the surgical field, to mix solutions, and to prepare medicines for administration. They are also required to label medicines received on the sterile field, which is necessary when drugs are transferred from their original container into another container or delivery system for use in surgery.

Studies in the past decade have shown that labeling errors are among the most prevalent and serious errors occurring during surgery. These can result in the wrong drug being transferred or administered, or the wrong strength mixed at the sterile field as a result of miscalculation or some other error. The complete procedure for handling medicines in the operating room can be found in Chapter 12.

ABANDONMENT

Abandonment is neglect of a patient or leaving a patient unattended while under the direct care of a health care professional. An abandoned patient can suffer a fall or other injury such as aspiration (breathing in fluid), choking, cardiac arrest, or other life-threatening events. These can happen very quickly and may be irreversible by the time help arrives. Examples of abandonment follow:

- A patient is left unattended in the operating room suite.
- A staff member leaves the operating room at the change of shift once the patient is on the operating table, and no relief is available.
- A patient is being transported to the operating room by stretcher and is left unattended in a hallway.
- A staff member leaves the workplace without notifying anyone.
- A health professional delegates care of the patient to a colleague who is unqualified to provide safe care.

FAILURE TO COMMUNICATE AND MISCOMMUNICATION

Failures in communication can occur when a member of the team neglects to pass on vital information that requires action. The information can be about the condition of the patient or some important aspect of a procedure. Communication is often difficult in the operating room environment because staff are required to carry out multiple tasks and to continually anticipate new ones. Distraction is a major cause of neglecting to carry out a task. Recent studies have also shown that the noise level related to devices and loud music played during surgery can contribute significantly to poor communication and decreased safety for patients.

LOSS OF OR DAMAGE TO THE PATIENT'S PROPERTY

Patients sometimes arrive in surgery with dentures, jewelry, hearing aids, glasses, and other personal items. Loss or damage of these can be very stressful for the patient. Any personal property removed from the patient must be properly labeled with the patient's name and hospital number. Their property is then transferred to a designated area for safekeeping according to hospital policy.

NEGLIGENT DELEGATION

Delegation is the transfer of duty to perform a task from one person to another. Delegation of tasks to the surgical technologist is sometimes but not always defined by state Practice Acts. Surgical technologists are routinely delegated tasks by the surgeon and sometimes by nurses, so it is best to check the Practice Acts and professional standards for the medical profession as well as for surgical technologists. Some surgical technologists and surgical first assistants are eager to accept responsibilities, whereas others feel uncomfortable with some of the tasks they are asked to do. In either case, it is wise to learn the statutes that apply to surgical technologists ahead of time.

The basic guidelines for accepting a delegated task can be summarized in the following points:

- The delegee (the person to whom the task is delegated) must be *legally allowed to* perform the task. The legality of a task may be determined by the state's Practice Acts and by hospital policy standards of practice. Legal accountability may rest with both the delegee and the person delegating the task. This is because it is assumed that both professionals know their scopes of tasks or practice. The legality of the delegated action may depend on whether the task is being directly supervised or not.
- The delegee must have received the appropriate training to perform the task safely.
- The delegee must be competent and able at the time of delegation to perform the task.

Accountability is taking responsibility for one's actions, including professional duties. As surgical technologists now take on a wider scope of tasks than in the past, they are obliged to accept the personal responsibility that goes along with it.

IMPORTANT TO KNOW *When a surgical technologist accepts a delegated task, he or she must agree to be identified as having carried out the task in the formal documentation* *process, including signing off on the task. Otherwise, the technologist should not agree to perform the task.*

This is for the protection of both the delegee and the delegator. It is an ethical and legal consideration, because taking the responsibility for an act also includes accepting the consequences of one's actions. If any form of coercion is routinely used in the delegation of tasks for which the delegee feels uncomfortable, for any reason, this should be documented and taken to the supervisory level, all the way through the chain of command, if necessary. This helps protect and promote everyone's rights to act legally and safely.

ABUSE AND DISRUPTIVE BEHAVIOR IN THE OPERATING ROOM

It has been well established by health care professionals that abuse or disruptive and violent behavior is an extensive problem in the perioperative environment. The operating room (OR) is a unique environment that has traditionally embraced hierarchy and authoritarian practices that normalize abuse. Professionals sometimes train in an environment of aggressive and even violent behavior such as bullying and throwing objects at team members. There is no evidence that the problem is worsening, but professional associations are recognizing and speaking out about the extent and consequences of these behaviors.

TJC has issued a zero-tolerance policy for any form of abuse or violence and requires health care institutions to take specific measures to address it. Organizations such as the American College of Surgeons, American Medical Association, American Nurses Association, and Association of periOperative Nurses have developed strict codes of conduct that discourage abusive behavior and punish those who violate it. It is important that students coming into a health care profession and even experienced professionals understand how to recognize abuse and what recourse is available to the victim.

DEFINING THE BEHAVIORS

A vocabulary for communication about workplace abuse, violence, and disruptive behavior has developed in professional journals and codes of conduct.

Bullying

Bullying is the most common abusive and potentially destructive behavior in health care. It is defined by TJC as:

- Verbal abuse
- Threatening, intimidating, or humiliating behaviors (including nonverbal actions)
- Work interference—sabotage—which prevents the individual from performing required tasks

TJC also recognizes five categories of violence occurring in the workplace:

- Threat to professional status (public humiliation)
- Threat to personal standing (name called, insults, teasing)
- Isolation (withholding information)
- Overwork (impossible deadlines)
- Destabilization (failing to give credit where credit is due)

Cases that have been reported in peer-reviewed literature include instances in which surgical staff were physically injured by surgical instruments and equipment, which were thrown or dropped on them by an abusive team member.

Bullying may be focused on individuals by whom the bully (or bullies) feel threatened. The target may be better educated or have other enviable qualities. Sometimes the bully will pick someone who has little ability to fight back or is otherwise vulnerable. The target may also be in a minority cultural or ethnic group.

Hazing is a specific type of bullying that is inflicted on student doctors, nurses, and surgical technologists who are new in the profession. Hazing includes actions intended to humiliate and embarrass the victim. In severe cases hazing may even result in physical injury.

Abuse is often described as **horizontal** (lateral) or **vertical. Horizontal abuse** takes place among staff members of equal rank and position. Vertical abuse occurs when a person of authority abuses one in a lower rank (chief surgeon to surgical intern; head nurse to nursing assistant; surgeon to surgical technologist). Vertical abuse can also occur when the person of lower rank abuses the one of higher rank, but this occurs more rarely.

Sexual Harassment

Sexual harassment is defined legally by the US Equal Employment and Opportunities Commission (EEOC). Sexual harassment and other forms of abuse are *illegal.* Over the past 20 years, sexual harassment has increasingly been condemned in the workplace. Incidents that used to be accepted as the norm in team relationships are no longer tolerated by institutions or health care workers themselves. No one in any profession is obliged to tolerate implied or actual physical or verbal sexual aggression. Employees who feel they are the target of sexual harassment should document and report each instance of harassment as it occurs. The person who is alleging harassment should retain an exact duplicate of the report. If the perpetrator is a superior, the report should be made above his or her administrative level or up the chain of command. Sometimes victims of sexual harassment do not report the abuse because they are afraid of losing their job. Talking about the abuse to peers often reveals others with the same experience, and the collective documentation can force institutions to act.

Disruptive Behavior

The American Medical Association, in its Code of Medical Ethics, defines disruptive behavior as "any abusive conduct, including sexual or other forms of harassment, or others forms of verbal or nonverbal conduct that harms or intimidates others to the extent that quality of care of patient safety could be compromised."

The following are listed in the code:

- Physically threatening anyone (in the hospital)
- Making threatening or intimidating physical contact with another person
- Throwing things

- Threatening violence or retribution
- Sexual and other harassment
- Persistent inappropriate behavior rising to the level of harassment

EFFECTS OF WORKPLACE ABUSE

Abusive behaviors in the health care environment have serious consequences. Victims suffer physiological and psychological effects. Bullying in particular can result in depression, anxiety, hypertension, headaches, and emotional exhaustion. Victims lose their motivation to work and may even leave their profession. Suicide has been traced back to cases of severe and persistent bullying.

The impact on patients is also severe. Abuse has been reported to result in poor patient care, increased medical errors, reduced productivity, and a threat to patient safety. For this reason, sexual harassment and bullying are considered sentinel events.

PREVENTION

Professional organizations, psychologists, and others have suggested that workplace bullying and other types of abuse are a reporting, identification, and management problem.

The victims of abuse often do not report the abuse or identify the abuser for fear of retaliation from the abuser. In the past it was standard practice for administrators to ignore reports of abuse to keep high-profile (and highly profitable) doctors on staff. Whistleblowers (those who report abuse) may be considered disruptive to the organization and at risk for losing their own job. This has changed in recent years. Now, professional health care organizations encourage staff to report all violations of professional codes and provide a means to do so.

Sometimes staff do not know if they are being bullied or sexually harassed. They know how they are affected but are uncertain if what they experience is actual abuse. This uncertainty and the fear they will not be taken seriously contribute to the lack of reporting. When there is no reporting, there can be no action to address it. This is a problem in workplaces that have tolerated bullying and other types of abuse for a long time so that even severe behavior becomes normalized. Now, specific behaviors are published in policy manuals and codes of conduct, making it easier for victims to clearly identify abuse.

An administration that does not address a problem as soon as it occurs gives implied permission for it to continue. TJC has placed health facility managers and administrators in control of programs to stop abuse and disruptive behavior in the workplace. In 2009 TJC released a mandatory Leadership Standard that requires action by the health care facility and its managers. Additional guidelines are now in place for the development of strict policies, processes, training, and reporting violence in the workplace.

A zero-tolerance culture that has the necessary tools and procedures in place to address abuse are key to stopping it. Prompt reporting when an incident occurs is crucial to address the problem. TJC has identified workplace intimidation and abuse as a sentinel event that requires reporting as a condition of accreditation.

BOX 3.3 Resources for Legal Information on Forms of Workplace Abuse

Equal Employment Opportunity Commission https://www.eeoc.gov/laws/types/sexual_harassment.cfm

The Joint Commission Workplace Violence Prevention—Bullying https://www.jointcommission.org/workplace_violence_prevention_-_bullying/

EEOC extended definition of sexual harassment https://www.un.org/womenwatch/osagi/pdf/whatissh.pdf

American College of Surgeons Statement on Harassment, Bullying, and Discrimination https://www.facs.org/about-acs/statements/117-harassment

MORE INFORMATION

Box 3.3 provides resources for more information about forms of abuse and extensive definitions for legal purposes.

INCIDENTS IN THE HEALTH CARE SETTING

The day-to-day activities in the health care environment are always subject to unexpected events that must be managed. Incidents are also called **adverse events.** A **sentinel event** is a specific category (see later). How an event or incident is handled depends on the type of incident, especially if patients or staff have been harmed or injured. Aside from the possible need for a medical or surgical response, there may be legal consequences. This discussion provides guidance in the reporting procedures for legal purposes. All health care facilities are required to have detailed guidelines and standards to follow in response to unexpected events. These include a wide spectrum of emergency events and non-emergency situations. It is likely that at some time the ST will need to report or be interviewed after an incident that he or she was involved in or witnessed.

HOW TO REPORT AN INCIDENT

The first step in reporting an incident is to notify the operating room supervisor of the event, who will determine the type of report to make, on which form, and to whom it will be directed. Examples of outside agency reporting requirements are shown in Table 3.1. *Internal* reporting is required for all incidents that involve injury and many other events that may result in harm or injury. Incidents may also be reported for cases of internal conflict on the team during surgery, bullying, sexual harassment, and other forms of coercion.

Following an incident or "near miss," in which an event almost occurred but was averted, the risk management department is notified, and an investigation is initiated to assess the causes of the event, the injuries (if applicable), and the outcome. If the event involves an injury to a patient or staff member, the injury is treated immediately to prevent complications. A report of the event is made as soon as possible,

TABLE 3.1 Examples of Agency Reporting Requirements Following an Incident*

Adverse Event	Agency
Severe injury related to the malfunction of a medical device	Food and Drug Administration (FDA)
Needlestick or other sharps injury	Occupational Safety and Health Administration (OSHA)
Severe injury of an employee while at work	Occupational Safety and Health Administration (OSHA)
Sentinel event	The Joint Commission (TJC)

*Additional internal reporting is required.

which will lead to an investigation. Remember that the purpose of the report is only to report it, not to make a judgment about an event.

The reports are never placed in the patient's chart, but a description of the event and any injury is reported in the progress notes. An annual review of policies and procedures helps to determine whether these must be modified to further manage risk.

The report lists the date and time that the incident occurred, who was there, and what happened, exactly as it occurred without emotion or embellishment. The main reasons for the report are for quality assurance or risk reduction and to provide details in case legal action is taken by any of the individuals involved.

SENTINEL EVENTS

A sentinel event is a specific type of adverse event. It is defined by TJC as a *Patient Safety Event.* It is defined as an event that was "not related to the natural course of the patient's illness or underlying condition" and results in

- Death
- Permanent harm
- Severe temporary harm and intervention required to sustain life

To see a complete description of sentinel events go to the following The Joint Commission website: https://www.jointcommission.org/-/media/tjc/documents/resources/patient-safety-topics/sentinel-event/20200101_23_camac_22_se.pdf.

Sentinel events require specific documentation by the health care facility who submits the report to TJC. TJC then begins a process of review and analysis of the event to determine how and why the event happened so that appropriate measures can be implemented to prevent future events. An important resource on patient safety for surgical technologists and other perioperative professionals is the institution originally formed as the ECRI. The institute is a leading authority on patient safety used by many different professional organizations. The Patient Safety Authority collects and analyzes national data on sentinel and other safety-related events and publishes reports and case studies.

The specific ECRI website on patient safety is https://www.ecri.org/search-results?phrase=patient%20safety.

IMPORTANT TO KNOW *Sentinel event reporting is only one type of reporting required for events relating to harm and safety. Refer to your health facility policy manual for other types of reports required by your institution.*

HOW TO WRITE AN INCIDENT REPORT

A report is required whenever an event occurs that has resulted or may result in death, injury, or harm. *Harm* includes psychological as well as physical injury.

Incident reports are completed using the hospital's designated form. The forms include the date, location, and time of the incident and a description of the incident written in his or her own words by an individual involved. The statement must include *who* was involved, *where* the incident occurred, *when* it took place, and *how* it happened. Any number of people involved in the incident may submit their own reports.

These guidelines can be followed in writing the narrative part of the report:

1. **Write and submit the form as soon as possible after the event.** If you are uncertain whether an incident report is needed, check with the operating room supervisor.
2. **State only the facts, and do not give your opinion about the incident.** An example of a proper statement is, "Dr. X smelled strongly of alcohol. His speech was slurred." or "The needle count was incorrect at the close of surgery. An x-ray was taken but did not reveal the needle, and the needle was not found outside the patient."
3. **Use professional and precise language whenever possible.** It is *more proper* to state, "Dr. X looked agitated and angry. He refused to let us time take a sponge count and proceeded to throw surgical scissors off the sterile field onto the floor." Language such as the following should be *avoided*: "Dr. X was acting horrible. He wouldn't even take a sponge count, and he smashed the Metz across the room."
4. **Write in the first person.** For example, "When I arrived in operating room 4, I saw the patient lying on the floor" is better than "The patient was seen by the surgical tech (me) on the floor in room 4."
5. **Do not be intimidated by others who want to protect individuals.** In some circumstances, employees may wish to protect others who were involved. Always use good ethical judgment; keep the safety of the patient in mind.
6. **Take your time in writing the report.** Try to write the report in a location where you are undisturbed by others. Fill out the form carefully and thoughtfully.
7. **Submit the incident report directly to the operating room supervisor or other designated personnel.** Do not leave the report where others can find it. Do not place it in the patient's chart.
8. **After an incident report is submitted to the risk management or legal department, an informal investigation may be conducted, or the hospital's insurance company will be notified.** Further action is then taken if needed.

WHISTLEBLOWING

Whistleblowing refers to a policy in which institutions encourage their employees to report acts of misconduct or suspected negligence. The policy has gained momentum in the past few years as equal rights in the workplace have increased. Health care workers no longer take the blame for wrongdoing by those in a position of authority. Historically, it was common for a nurse or technologist to remain silent to "protect" the surgeon or institution. However, more and more professionals are finding out that this may not be the best action, and it certainly is no longer expected of professionals working in the health care system.

RISK MANAGEMENT

Risk management is a process used to prevent adverse events in the perioperative environment and other health care settings. Safety in the environment is a chief concern of all hospital administrators, and risk management is taken very seriously. Throughout this textbook, you will find many discussions about safety for patients and staff. These are intended to alert the student to potential risks and actions needed to reduce or mitigate them. Because of the complex nature of medical and surgical technology, specific measures required to ensure safety are discussed in the context of the activity or device.

The primary goal of risk management programs is to prevent harm and injury to patients, staff, and visitors to the health facility.

> Further information is available at TJC website on patient safety: https://www.jointcommission.org/topics/patient_safety.aspx.

The most basic steps taken to prevent harm and injury are the following:

- Increase awareness of the problem through education for all staff
- Promotion of safety measures through training and visual cues such as signs and posters
- Compliance with safety measures such as the Universal Protocol
- Coordination with TJC for follow-up after an adverse event
- Frequent opportunities for staff training
- Stringent policies for reporting unsafe conditions or equipment
- Coordination and cooperation with risk management managers for timely data reports and implementation of new policies

LEGAL DOCUMENTS

Standards in health care require all patient encounters with the system be documented in a specific way. TJC has specific rules that apply to documentation. Individual health care facilities develop their own documents based on the rules. Learning how to document correctly is an important part of becoming a health care provider.

Medical records are protected by law. Losing or misplacing a record or part of a record is a serious event. The use of electronic documentation is now common in most facilities and requires all personnel to become familiar with specific operating systems. General documents that the surgical technologists are likely to encounter are discussed later in this section. Specific documents are described within their subject in the text—for example, specimen and pathology documentation is detailed in Chapter 19.

HEALTH INSURANCE PORTABILITY AND PRIVACY ACT (HIPPA)

The federal Health Insurance Portability and Privacy Act (HIPAA) was passed by Congress in 1996. Within the act is a Privacy Rule that protects the confidentiality of an individual's health information (called *protected health information*). This includes identifiable health information relating to the individual's past, present, or future physical or mental health or condition and information about payments for health care. The Privacy Rule applies to all of information through any medium, including electronic, paper, or oral means. Box 3.4 specifies information that cannot be shared. All employees of the health care facility must sign a confidentiality statement in which they agree to abide by the HIPAA Privacy Rule.

> The complete HIPAA document can be accessed at http://www.hhs.gov/ocr/privacy/hipaa/understanding/srsummary.html.

Taking photographs of the patient is ***never*** permitted without the patient's or guardian's specific written permission beforehand. This includes photos and videos that are necessary to the medical or surgical care of the patient and those used for educational purposes. Likewise, photographs of the medical or surgical facility may not be made without express written permission by the facility administration.

GUIDELINES FOR DOCUMENTATION

Documentation is the means of making a permanent legal record of the patient's interaction with health care providers

BOX 3.4 Health Privacy Act Identifiers That May Not Be Shared

Individual identifiers include but are not limited to the following:

- Name and address
- Birth date
- Social Security number
- Photographs
- Medical record numbers
- Fax numbers
- Email addresses
- Health plan beneficiary numbers
- Account numbers
- Certificate/license numbers
- Vehicle identifiers and serial numbers, including license plate numbers

and services. It is a way for health professionals to communicate patient procedures, diagnoses, treatments, conditions, and recommendations for care. Many health professionals will consult the patient's medical record, so it is done in a standardized manner. Separate forms are required for many different types of documentation, but the method of documentation is consistent among health care facilities. The importance of correct documentation cannot be overstated. A mistake in documentation can lead to serious medical errors.

The following general guidelines should be followed for health care documentation:

1. Every document must contain the patient's unique identifiers, including patient name, hospital or Social Security number, and other information required specifically for that health facility.
2. The date must be accurate. Never predate or postdate a document. Always document the correct time.
3. If you make an error in handwritten documentation, make a single line through the part that is incorrect and write in the correct information. Initial the change. Never use opaque liquids or tapes to blank out the error—only a strikethrough of the error is acceptable.
4. If the documentation is performed in writing, make sure it is legible, using *black* ink only. Documents must be kept clean and dry to prevent smearing. It is good practice to document away from areas where spills or splashes can occur.
5. Use brief, exact wording when documenting. Documentation is a record of facts only.
6. Remember that your documentation will be read by many professionals. Use correct spelling, and do not use SMS language.
7. Avoid abbreviations.
8. When performing computer-based documentation, remember to log off when finished. Do not allow someone else to use your password, and do not give your password to anyone else.
9. The person performing the documentation must be identified by a signature. Never sign another person's document or allow someone else to sign for you.

IMPORTANT TO KNOW *The Joint Commission has developed a list of abbreviations that must not be used in documentation because they can be misread or misinterpreted. These are mainly related to drug administration and are shown in Table 3.2. The list also appears in Chapter 12 for emphasis.*

MEDICAL RECORDS AND DOCUMENTS

PATIENT MEDICAL RECORD

The patient's medical record is the sum of all encounters with the health care system, including reports, assessments and investigations, surgical procedure records, nursing notes, anesthesia records, counts records (sponge, needles, instruments), and dates of admission and discharge.

Medical records may be stored electronically or in paper form. If the record is in paper form, the record may contain more than one file; these files are usually dated by year. The patient medical record "travels" with the patient whenever he or she is admitted to the health care facility. Although the patient may not physically carry it, it is present during all health care encounters so that records can be kept in real time. All records are kept in the medical records department of the hospital.

IMPORTANT TO KNOW *Every item in the patient's medical record is a legal document. This means that all or part of the record can be demanded by court order. The medical record is subject to state and federal confidentiality and privacy laws.*

TABLE 3.2 The Joint Commission List of Do Not Use Abbreviations

Do Not Use	Potential Problem	Use Instead
U (unit)	Mistaken for "0" (zero), the number "4" (four) or "cc"	Write "unit"
IU (International Unit)	Mistaken for IV (intravenous) or the number 10 (ten)	Write "International Unit"
Q.D., QD, q.d., qd (daily) Q.E.D., QOD, q.o.d., qod (every other day)	Mistaken for each other Period after the Q Mistaken for "I" and the "O"mistaken for "I"	Write "daily" Write "every other day"
Trailing zero (X.0 mg)* Lack of leading zero (.X mg)	Decimal point is missed	Write X mg Write 0.X mg
MS MSO_4 and $MgSO_4$	Can mean morphine sulfate or magnesium sulfate Confused for one another	Write "morphine sulfate" Write "magnesium sulfate"

Applies to all orders and all medication-related documentation that are handwritten (including free-text computer entry) or on preprinted forms.
*Exception: A "trailing zero" may be used only where required to demonstrate the level of precision of the value being reported, such as for laboratory results, imaging studies that report the size of lesions, or catheter/tube sizes. It may not be used in medication orders or other medication-related documentation.

BOX 3.5 Information Included in the Patient Consent Form

1. A detailed description of the procedure
2. The disease or medical conditions that can require this surgery
3. Treatment options—an explanation of alternative treatment for the patient's condition
4. A detailed explanation of all the possible risks associated with the procedure
5. The benefits of the procedure
6. The site and side of the procedure
7. How the patient should prepare for the procedure (includes eating and drinking restrictions, personal hygiene, medications to take)
8. What to expect during recovery and home care after the surgery including follow-up care, wound management, diet, and activity
9. The statement of consent. This includes admission of having read and understood the verbal and written consent and admission of "no guarantee" that the procedure will be effective. The consent also authorizes the surgeon to perform any emergency procedures that are required.
10. The patient must state that he or she was offered a translator or interpreter during the discussion.

INFORMED CONSENT

All patients have the legal and ethical right to be thoroughly informed about the details of any invasive procedure before the procedure begins. The process must include an opportunity for the patient or responsible person to ask questions about the procedure. A patient's operative consent form, or **informed consent,** is a process in which the risks, benefits, and alternatives of the surgery or treatment are communicated to the patient, who must sign the form.

All invasive procedures require informed consent, including blood transfusion and administration of anesthesia. Anesthesia consent is required as a process separate from the surgical consent. Some facilities have specific consent forms for elective procedures that result in sterilization and for implantation of medical devices.

If the procedure is elective, the surgical consent may be prepared in the surgeon's office and signed several days before the scheduled date of the surgery. In emergency situations, the consent is prepared as close to the time of surgery as possible. The responsibility for obtaining the consent lies with the patient's treatment team. The consent is legal only when all elements are included (Box 3.5).

If the patient is unable to understand or sign the process and has a legal guardian or representative (called a "surrogate decision maker"), this person is responsible for understanding and signing the document. Patients who are not native speakers of English may need an interpreter to ensure comprehension. Those with hearing impairment must have a qualified interpreter present. The surgeon or surgeon's representative may make a note in the patient's chart verifying that the patient appeared to understand the consent and that it was not signed under coercion or pressure.

BOX 3.6 Special Considerations in Obtaining Informed Consent

- If the patient is a minor, the parent or legal guardian may sign.
- If the patient is illiterate, he or she makes an X, which is followed by the witness's signature and the words "patient's mark."
- If the patient is mentally incompetent or incapacitated, a responsible guardian, agency representative, or court representative may sign.
- In the case of an emancipated minor,* a responsible relative or a spouse may sign.
- In an emergency, consent for immediate lifesaving treatment is not necessary. Verbal consent by telephone is permitted, but only if two registered nurses obtain the verbal permission. Written consent must then be obtained later.

*The definition of an emancipated minor varies among states.

The consent is then signed by the patient or person authorized to give the consent and the surgeon.

In an emergency situation, when the patient is incompetent or unconscious and has no representative, the decision to act in beneficence may override other considerations. This is a decision made by the attending physician. In some cases, a court order may be required for medical or surgical intervention. The laws concerning this vary by state. Special cases determine who can provide consent (Box 3.6).

Patients who agree to participate as subjects in experimental surgery or other types of research must be fully informed of the risks and possible outcomes. These are contained in a special informed consent document designed by the Institutional Review Board according to FDA regulations.

Witness to the Consent

A witness signature to the consent is required in all cases. By law, any adult, such as a legal guardian, spouse, or agency representative, can witness the patient's signature. The witness is only attesting to the fact that *he or she observed the signing* by the physician and patient, not that the patient understood the information. However, hospital policy may state who may or may not act as a witness in the perioperative environment. The attending surgeon may not act as a witness to the consent because of conflict of interest. Many health care facilities do not allow other members of the surgical team who will be performing the surgery, such as the surgical technologist, to witness the consent for the same ethical reasons.

INTRAOPERATIVE RECORD

The *intraoperative record* is specific documentation about the surgical procedure and includes information on patient assessment, as well as technical information about the equipment and devices, drains, and implants used during the procedure. Implants require registration of the type, manufacturer, identification number, size, and other identifiers. The patient position and prep site must be indicated, along with details about specimens and medications. The names of all perioperative personnel who participated in the procedure, including those who filled in during breaks, are listed, and those who participated in the counts must sign at the close of surgery.

ANESTHESIA RECORD

The anesthesia record is a document of the intraoperative anesthesia process including the type, drugs and solutions used, methods, and any complications that occurred during the surgery. It is also used to document physiological monitoring, any unexpected interventions performed, and the outcome of the procedure. There is a section on the record for drains, for fluid loss during surgery, and for replacement fluids or blood products given during the procedure.

PATIENT CHARGES

Patient charges are documented in a variety of locations in the chart. Usually, there is a dedicated form in the patient chart for stating the service or equipment and appropriate charge. The process for documenting charges is part of the operating room policy and is easily accessed through the department.

BIRTH AND DEATH CERTIFICATES

Birth certificates (also called a certificate of live birth) and death certificates (also called a registration of death) are legal records issued by the county or state where the event occurred. The information required is obtained by the health facility and then submitted to the vital records office of the county or state. Information required for a death certificate is provided by the attending physician or the coroner.

SPECIMEN AND PATHOLOGY RECORDS

Documentation must accompany all tissue or other specimens obtained during surgery. A description of the tissue, its origin, time of recovery, and any special identifiers must be included. Specimen identification is critical in the prevention of medical errors. Incorrect or lost documentation may result in delays or even failure to assess the tissue. All health care facilities publish a manual that specifically states how to submit a specimen and what information is required. A complete discussion of the care of specimens and their documentation is included in Chapter 19.

ADVANCE HEALTH CARE DIRECTIVE

An **advance directive** is a document in which a patient gives instructions about his or her medical care in the event that the individual cannot speak for himself or herself because of incapacity.

In recent years the advance directive has become complex and detailed. Along with increased longevity in Western countries, people are concerned about their ability to manage end-of-life choices. In the past the order DO NOT RESUSCITATE simply meant that the patient wanted no medical intervention in the near-death situation. People are now able to select specific interventions that they wish to decline such as intubation, tube feeding, and mechanical respiration.

If the patient is incompetent or a minor, a guardian or family member may sign the advance directive. Various forms of advance directives can be used, and states have different regulations and standards for the implementation of directives. For example, an individual may refuse mechanical ventilation but accept medication. If the patient is considered to be in a persistent vegetative state, the guardian may request withdrawal from mechanical support systems. In most institutions, the advance directive must be reactivated with each separate hospital admission. The following sections explain the different types of advance directives.

Organ Donation

Patients have the right to refuse the removal of their organs for transplantation after their death. Several religions and cultures forbid or limit certain types of organ transfers. Others may not provide consent for organ donation based on fears that the organs may be removed before death is pronounced. Regardless of the reason, documentation of this directive should be included in the patient's chart. Organ transplantation itself requires extensive documentation consistent with the complex nature of the procedure. Organ transplant is discussed in Chapter 14.

Refusal of Blood or Tissue Products

Patients may refuse blood or tissue products because of their faith or personal beliefs. Simply stating that one belongs to a certain faith does not automatically restrict medical intervention. If the patient is unable to communicate his or her wishes, lifesaving measures may be initiated. An advance directive is needed if the normal process of patient care, including transfusion, is unwanted. Patients who decline medical intervention including blood transfusion may accept alternative therapies such as autotransfusion or transfusion of specific blood products. Permits and informed consent remain necessary even in emergency cases.

Medical Power of Attorney

The patient may assign a specific person to act as his or her proxy with regard to medical treatment. After the medical power of attorney is prepared and signed, the proxy thereafter can speak on behalf of the patient regarding his or her medical treatment. The medical power of attorney does not give up legal authority in any area except medical treatment.

CIVIL LAWSUITS

In a civil lawsuit the plaintiff (the one bringing charges against another) must prove that a tort was committed, and, if the plaintiff is successful, they may be awarded monetary compensation, also called *damages*.

In this case, legal representation is required for both the plaintiff and the defendant (the one being sued). Certain terms are important to understand the basic process of a lawsuit. If negligence is suspected and a lawsuit is to be filed, the medical professional will receive a summons or **subpoena,** which is an order to appear as a witness to an incident. A meeting then takes place in which testimony is given, called the deposition.

The deposition is recorded by a court reporter, and all lawyers involved in the case are allowed to question the witness. If a surgical technologist is required to testify about an incident at the hospital, the individual should check with the hospital administration before doing so. In some cases, the hospital (or its insurance carrier) may provide a lawyer to be present during the testimony. The person giving a deposition who is directly involved in the lawsuit will have an attorney present. Unless a settlement is made early in the case, a jury is called to hear the evidence and produce a verdict. Testimony given during a court trial is given under oath. Lying under oath is **perjury,** which is punishable by law. Once the verdict is given, the judge decides on the amount and type of damages awarded to the plaintiff.

LIABILITY INSURANCE

Health professionals can protect themselves against liability for acts of negligence by purchasing liability insurance. In the past, it was very rare for a surgical technologist to be named in a lawsuit; however, the trend is changing. This may be due to the higher profile of the profession, the fact that surgical technologists are assuming more high-risk roles, or because of shifts in accountability within the legal system. Certainly, there is an increasing trend to shift responsibility from the surgeon to other members of the surgical team. Nevertheless, any individual on the surgical team and the health facility itself can be held liable.

There are two schools of thought regarding whether an individual should take out malpractice insurance. One is that if one does take malpractice insurance, one is more likely to be named in a lawsuit. The other is that it is wiser to prepare oneself in the event a lawsuit is brought and won. Both are valid arguments. It is wise to review the options and the liability protection available.

PATIENTS' RIGHTS

Government agencies and established laws are created to protect patients. Professional organizations for health care workers establish and publish codes of ethics. These codes outline the behaviors expected of any member of the health profession. A health professional is thus expected to act in a certain way and within the ethical standards of the profession and the laws of the state. Health professionals have an unspoken contract to maintain a particular kind of relationship with their patients. The American Hospital Association (AHA) has developed guidelines to help patients understand their rights in the hospital setting.

These can be found on the AHA website at. http://www.aha.org/advocacy-issues/communicatingpts/pt-care-partnership.shtml

KEY CONCEPTS

- Laws concerning the practice of medicine, nursing, and allied health have been established to protect the public.
- The surgical technologist's scope of tasks is defined by state law.
- The medical and nurse Practice Acts of each state provide information about the roles and responsibilities of health care workers.
- Health care policies are established by professional organizations and by health care facilities.
- Delegation is an important legal and professional concept in medicine. It is the transfer of responsibility for a task from one person to another. The conditions of delegation must be determined to protect the patient from harm.
- Civil liability derives from an act committed against a person or property. Acts of negligence in health care are causes of civil liability.
- Negligence is the most common cause of patient injury and death in health care.
- Examples of negligence include patient burns, falls, medication errors, improper patient positioning, abandonment of a patient, and retained surgical items. Failure to care for a surgical specimen correctly and failure to communicate about a potentially dangerous situation are also considered negligence.
- The patient's record is a legal document. Laws regarding the use of patient information are strictly enforced.
- Documentation in the perioperative environment is necessary to protect the patient.
- A sentinel event is one in which there is potential or actual injury or death in the work environment. A report must be completed for any sentinel event.
- A legal action may be brought against any health professional when a negligent act results in harm.
- Standards, policies, and guidelines are not laws, but noncompliance of them can result in serious consequences.
- Forgetting a policy or claims that the policy was unknown to a professional are not acceptable as reasons to not comply.
- Regulations are created by government agencies to protect the public from harm by medical devices, medicines, and chemicals.
- The patient's record is a legal document. Laws regarding the use of patient information are strictly enforced.
- The HIPAA protects the patient's right to privacy concerning their medical care, past, present, and future.
- Informed consent is a process in which a planned invasive procedure is explained in detail to the patient and signed by a witness and the patient or their representative.
- A legal action (lawsuit) may be brought against any health professional when a negligent act results in harm.
- Documents that make up the patient's medical record are legal documents that can be used in a legal action.
- Negligence occurs when a health care professional fails to act in a way that prevents injury or acts in a way that causes injury or death.
- A leading cause of patient injury in surgery is a retained foreign object. This occurs when a sponge, instrument, or device fragment is unintentionally left in the incision.
- Abuse in the perioperative environment is a persistent problem that affects patient safety.
- Bullying is the most common abusive and potentially destructive behavior in health care. It involves threatening,

intimidating, or humiliating behaviors, interference with another's work, and verbal abuse.

- Sexual harassment is illegal under the EEOC as a form of sex discrimination.

REVIEW QUESTIONS

1. Define the relationship between accountability and delegation.
2. Who may delegate a task? Under what circumstances can a task be delegated?
3. What is sexual harassment? Why do you think people tolerate it in the workplace?
4. Negligence is the most common cause of lawsuits in medical practice. Define negligence and give three examples of negligent acts or behavior.
5. What are state Practice Acts?
6. What are the causes of negligence in the operating room?
7. What is informed consent? Why is it necessary? Why do you think it is called "informed" consent? Why not just "consent"?

CASE STUDIES

CASE 1

You are assigned to scrub on a case, and you have just finished setting up the back table and instruments. The surgeons are gowned and gloved. The circulator is completing the skin prep using an alcohol-based antiseptic. As soon as she finishes, the surgeons ask for drapes. You see that the patient's skin is still quite wet with the prep solution, and you hesitate in starting the draping, knowing that the prep solution has not dried. You remark on this to the surgeon, and he replies, "Come on—come on, let's get going on this." A few minutes later, the edge of the drape catches fire. The fire is quickly extinguished, revealing a second-degree burn of the patient's skin. Who do you believe is responsible? What documentation is needed? Who should be notified?

CASE 2

Your patient is a 70-year-old man scheduled for a hernia repair. Your role is assistant circulator. The registered nurse circulator asks you to go to the holding area to see whether the patient has arrived. When you arrive at the holding area, the patient is there with the surgeon. The patient's speech is slurred, and he appears to have difficulty hearing the surgeon. As the surgeon looks over the chart, he notices that the patient has not signed the operative permit. He asks you to witness the patient's signing. What will you do?

CASE 3

While scrubbed on a case involving surgical treatment of carpal tunnel syndrome, you complete the instrument, sponge, and needle count. You are missing a needle. You tell the surgeon that the count is incorrect. He replies, "Oh, don't worry. The needle can't be in the wound, it's too small. I would be able to see it. Let's close." What will you do?

CASE 4

While in the locker room, you notice that one of your coworkers is emptying the pockets of her scrub suit. There are two vials of injectable medications. You cannot see what they are. She puts them in her purse and leaves. What do you do?

CASE 5

You have been called into the office of the hospital's attorney to answer questions about a case 2 months earlier in which you scrubbed. The case involves the retained needle in the patient undergoing carpal tunnel surgery (see case 3), who is suing the hospital and staff. Based on how you answered the question in case 3, what are your thoughts as you wait to see the hospital's attorney?

CASE 6

You have been asked to help position an 80-year-old man for hip surgery. He is under general anesthesia and is intubated. After the surgery, the anesthesiologist discovers that the patient's right ulna is fractured. The surgeon says, "We'd better fix this ulna now." Think about the events in this procedure. Who is responsible for the fracture? Can the surgeon repair the ulna without a permit? What (if anything) is the appropriate action for you as a surgical technologist at this point?

BIBLIOGRAPHY

Agency for Healthcare Research and Quality. *Patient Safety Network Reporting Patient Safety Events*; 2019. Available at, Retrieved https://psnet.ahrq.gov/primers/primer/13/Reporting-Patient-Safety-Events. Accessed June 13, 2019.

Association of Surgical Technologists (AST): *Standards of practice.* http://www.ast.org.Accessed June 13, 2019.

Association of Surgical Technologists (AST): *Code of ethics.* http://www.ast.org.Accessed June 13, 2019.

Pham JC, Girard T, Pronovost PJ. What to do with healthcare incident reporting systems. *J Public Health Res.* 2013;2(3):e27. https://doi.org/10.4081/jphr.2013.e27.

The Joint Commission. *Sentinel Event Policy and Procedures*; 2017. Available at https://www.jointcommission.org/sentinel_event_policy_and_procedures/. Accessed June 9, 2019.

United States Department of Health and Human Services, Office for Civil Rights: *Summary of the HIPAA privacy rule.* http://www.hhs.gov/ocr/privacy/hipaa/understanding/summary/privacysummary.pdf. Accessed July 19, 2011.

University of Washington School of Medicine: Informed consent: ethics in medicine. http://depts.washington.edu/bioethx. Accessed July 18, 2011.

Virginia Board of Health Professions, Virginia Department of Health Professions. Study into the need to regulate surgical assistants & surgical technologists in the Commonwealth of Virginia. Accessed http://www.dhp.virginia.gov/bhp/studies/SurgicalAssistant_Technologist ReportFinal.doc; 2010. Accessed January 23, 2012.

Workplace Violence Prevention in Health Care - Rulemaking. Dir.ca.gov. http://www.dir.ca.gov/OSHSB/Workplace-Violence-Prevention-in-Health-Care.html. Published 2019. Accessed March 25, 2019.

4 HEALTH CARE FACILITY STRUCTURE AND ENVIRONMENT

LEARNING OBJECTIVES

After studying this chapter, the reader will be able to:

1. Describe the principles of operating room design
2. Identify common items found in the surgical suite
3. Discuss the functions of various work areas in the surgical suite
4. List common hospital ancillary services and describe their functions
5. Describe three types of ambulatory surgery facilities discussed in this chapter
6. Discuss the advantages and disadvantages of ambulatory surgical facilities
7. Define *health care insurance* and discuss the ways patients pay for care
8. Define *chain of command*
9. Identify perioperative professionals and their roles

TERMINOLOGY

Accreditation (of a health care facility): The process by which a hospital or other health care facility is evaluated by an independent organization. Accredited facilities are those that meet the standards of the accreditation agency.

Administration: Individuals who manage an institution, plan its activities, and provide oversight for day-to-day operations and employees. The administration is also a liaison between the facility and the community, government, and media.

Back table: A large stainless steel table on which most of the sterile surgical supplies and instruments are placed for use during surgery. Before surgery, the back table is covered with a sterile drape, and sterile instruments and other equipment are opened onto its surface.

Biomedical engineering technician (also called biomedical engineers): Professional who specializes in the maintenance, repair, and safe operation of devices used in patient care.

Case cart system: A method of preparing equipment and instruments for a surgical case. Equipment is prepared and assembled by the central services or supply department and sent to the operating room in a closed stainless steel cart.

Chain of command: A hierarchy of personnel positions that establishes both vertical and horizontal relationships between positions.

Decontamination area: A room or department in which soiled instruments and equipment are cleaned of gross matter and decontaminated to remove microorganisms.

Efficiency: The economic use of time and energy to prevent unnecessary expenditure of work, materials, and time.

Integrated operating room: A type of structural and engineering design in which digital and computerized components such as cameras, monitors, and environmental controls can be controlled from a central location in the room. Components such as endoscopic control units and monitors are built into the room structure rather than as separate portable units.

Job description: A document that specifies the duties, responsibilities, location, pay, and management structure of a job.

Job title: The name of a job, such as "certified surgical technologist" or "chief of surgery."

The Joint Commission (TJC): The accrediting organization for hospitals and other health care facilities in the United States.

Kick bucket: A stainless steel bucket mounted in a frame on wheels used for soiled surgical sponges during the procedure.

Mayo stand: A small open-ended adjustable table used during surgery. Instruments and supplies to be required immediately are placed on the Mayo stand.

Personnel policy: A policy that sets forth the health care facility's job descriptions, role delineations, requirements for employment, and rules of conduct for personnel.

Postanesthesia care unit (PACU): The critical care area where patients are taken after surgery for monitoring and evaluation as they emerge from anesthesia.

Ring stand: A stainless steel frame designed to hold sterile fluid basins during surgery.

Risk management: The process of tracking, evaluating, and studying accidents and incidents to protect patients and employees. Risk management results in changes in policy or enforcement of policy if the risk reaches an unacceptable level.

Transitional area: An area in which surgical personnel or visitors prepare to enter the semi-restricted areas. Transitional areas include the locker rooms and changing rooms.

Unrestricted area: An area where people dressed in street clothes may enter.

The services provided in the health care setting require specific facilities and staff capable of delivering those services. Neither of these elements of health care can exist without the other. The facility itself must provide a safe environment for patients, staff members, and visitors. It must also *enable* the work of health care personnel in a way that encourages efficiency of time, movement, and space. This is done through the administrative and management process.

This chapter is an introduction to the perioperative environment and to the health care facility as a whole. It explains the rationale for operating room design and standards. It also provides important information about the professionals who work in the facility—specifically, what their roles are and how those roles fit into the larger organizational structure. Environmental safety for patients and perioperative personnel includes the methods, guidelines, and standards related to operating room technology. This topic is crucial for patient care and the occupational safety of everyone who works in the surgical environment.

STANDARDS AND RECOMMENDATIONS

Technical standards and recommendations for the physical perioperative environment are set by several different agencies and regulatory bodies that are concerned with safety, including infection control, structural engineering, and safety in the workplace. Some of the agencies listed here will be seen in later chapters covering additional focal areas, especially in the area of environmental safety, which is covered in Chapter 7:

- **Association for Professionals in Infection Control and Epidemiology** (APIC) conducts research and establishes guidelines for infection control measures (http://www.apic.org).
- **Agency for Healthcare Research and Quality** (AHRQ) National Guideline Clearinghouse (searchable database) (http://www.guideline.gov/browse/by-topic.aspx).
- **American Institute of Architects** (AIA) sets standards for health care facility engineering (http://www.aia.org).
- **Environmental Protection Agency** (EPA) sets and enforces regulations related to safety in the environment, including hazardous chemicals and radiation (http://www.epa.gov).
- **Facility Guidelines Institute** (FGI) is a nonprofit organization that publishes guidelines for health care facility design (http://www.fgiguidelines.org/about-fgi).
- **Occupational Safety and Health Administration** (OSHA) regulates occupational hazards and safety https://www.osha.gov/index.html).

ACCREDITATION

Accreditation, as it pertains to health care institutions and facilities, is the process by which a team of professionals evaluates a health care institution's practices and policies and the outcomes of patient care.

THE JOINT COMMISSION *is the primary accreditation organization for all health care facilities (http://www.jointcommission.org).*

The facility is awarded accreditation when these standards are met. Accreditation is a voluntary process, but government agencies and insurers use accreditation to determine whether an institution qualifies for patient care reimbursement. Accreditation implies a high standard of care and a commitment to public safety and welfare.

To earn accreditation by The Joint Commission, the institution must meet or exceed the high standards set by the commission. The Joint Commission bases its own standards on those of professional and governmental agencies. The Joint Commission is governed by a board of commissioners composed of members of the American College of Physicians, American Society of Internal Medicine, American College of Surgeons, American Dental Association, American Hospital Association, American Medical Association, and selected professionals. The Joint Commission standards apply to every area of the health care facility and focus on patient safety, protection, and quality care.

ALIGNMENT OF TERMINOLOGY

This chapter, like all those of this edition of *Surgical Technology: Principles and Practice,* introduces and uses technical terminology that is in line with major health care organizations and written policies such as the Association of perioperative Registered Nurses, the American College of Surgeons, the Centers for Disease Control and Prevention, and The Joint Commission. Alignment of terms ensures accurate and precise communication among health care professionals, associations, policies, and guidelines, which are reviewed yearly to assess them for currency (Do they reflect updated studies and research?), accuracy, and clarity of meaning.

SECTION I: THE PERIOPERATIVE ENVIRONMENT

PRINCIPLES OF OPERATING ROOM DESIGN

The surgical department (operating room) is structured and engineered to provide a safe and efficient environment for patients and staff members (Fig. 4.1). Many different designs can be used, but all must achieve the following objectives:

1. Infection control
2. Environmental safety
3. Efficient use of personnel, time, space, and material resources

INFECTION CONTROL

Infection control is a multidisciplinary process that involves many different areas of expertise and practice. The physical design of the operating room is one focal area. It is based on two basic principles:

- Physical separation between the surgical environment and any source of contamination
- Containment of sources of infection

Clean and *contaminated* areas (those with the greatest potential sources of infection) are physically separated

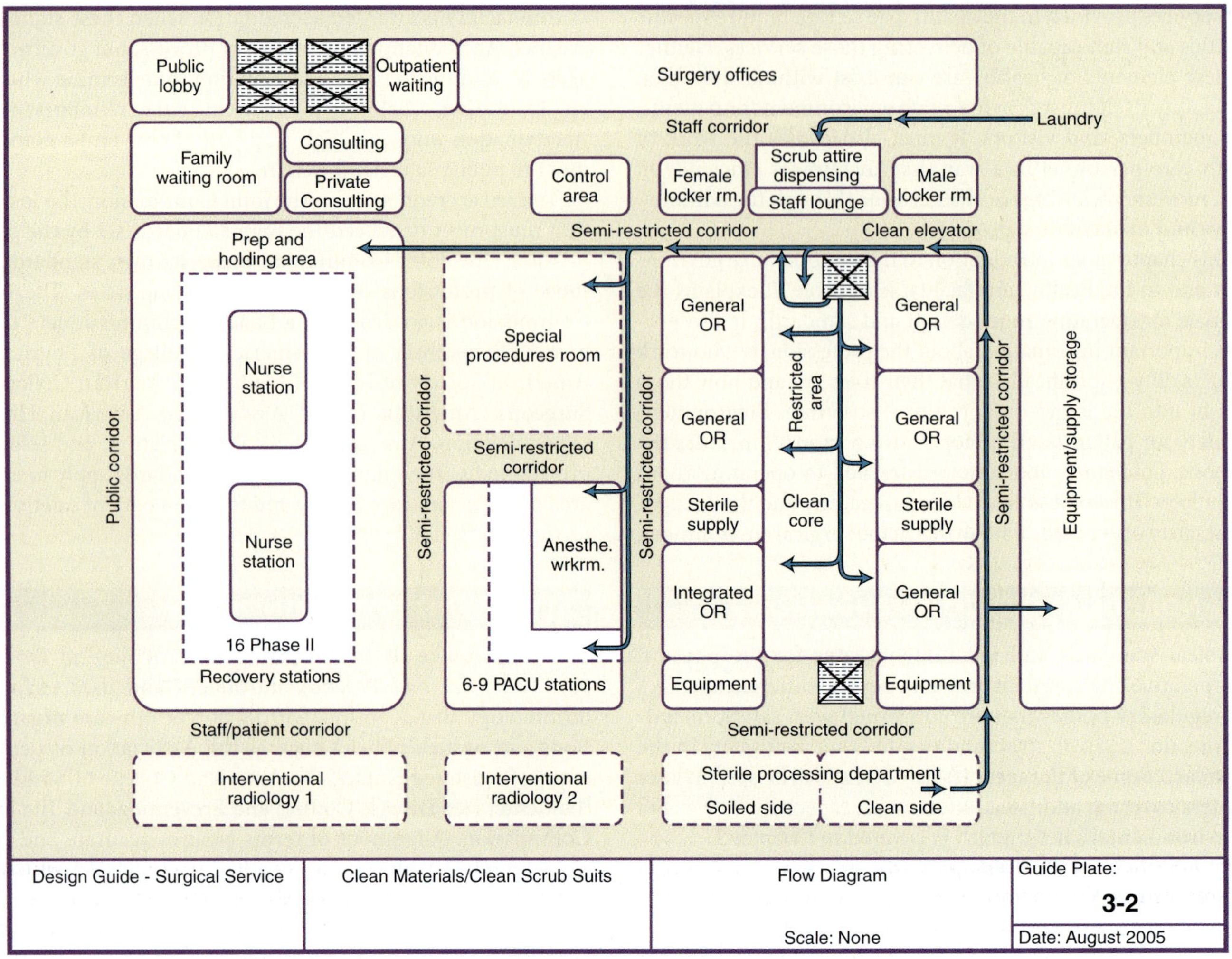

FIG. 4.1 Example of operating room design.

when possible. For example, the cleaning and decontamination area is separated from the procedure rooms (individual rooms where surgery is performed) by walls and corridors. The **decontamination** area is where surgical instruments and equipment are disinfected after use. The surgical department (operating room) itself is separated from hospital corridors and units by doors that remain closed at all times.

When complete physical separation is impossible, contaminated objects are *contained* or confined within a prescribed area or barrier. For example, the air in the surgical suite cannot be completely separated from the air directly outside the suite; therefore, it is contained by keeping the doors closed and by maintaining air pressure in the suite higher than it is outside. Nonporous materials are used for floors so that soil, debris, and body fluids remain on the surface, from which they can be easily removed with disinfectant.

ENVIRONMENTAL SAFETY

The surgical environment contains many potential hazards. Some of these are obvious, but others are not. For example, although explosive anesthetic gases are no longer permitted, high-level energy sources such as laser and electrosurgical devices are used routinely. Strong chemicals including sterilizing agents are used to prepare surgical instruments and clean environmental surfaces. Extremely hot temperatures are used in the decontamination of equipment. High-pressure gas canisters are used to contain medical gases and oxygen, which support combustion and fire. Environmental engineering in the operating room follows national medical engineering standards for electrical circuits, inline gases, lighting, and other utilities. Strict safety standards ensure that patients and staff members are protected from extreme hazards and accidents such as fire, explosion, and electrocution. These are discussed in Chapter 7.

EFFICIENCY

Efficiency is the economical use of time and energy to save unnecessary work, material resources, and time. Efficient use of space contributes to safety. Work in the operating room is strenuous, and intelligent design can reduce physical stress by reducing movement and creating work systems that minimize strain. Time-saving practices are implemented not only to increase the number of patients served but also to make the best use of people's skills and abilities. In an emergency, time

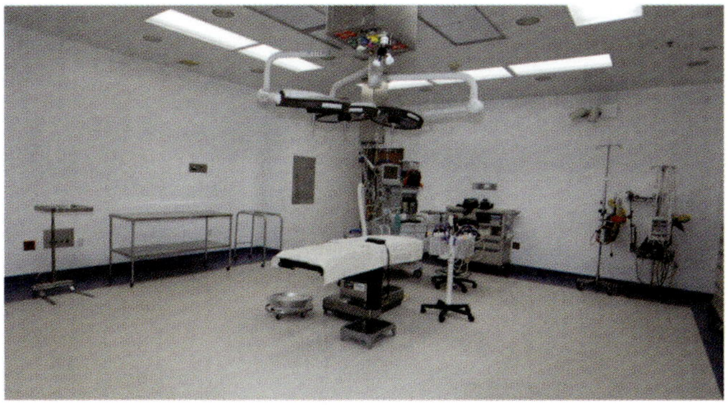

FIG. 4.2 Operating room suite.

is sometimes the most important factor in achieving a good outcome. Proper storage of sterile supplies and efficient use of space protect the sterility of the items and enable staff members to find what they need quickly and retrieve it safely. For example, equipment that is stacked too high for safe retrieval or equipment that obstructs hallways results in the risk of injury for patients and employees.

OPERATING ROOM DESIGN

The design of the operating room is purposely created to establish zones to prevent the transmission of infectious microorganisms. Specific guidelines are enforced for the movement of staff and equipment from one zone to another. These are often called *traffic patterns.* When traffic patterns are enforced in the operating room, they include entry *into* the operating room and movement of people and equipment *within* the department. Traffic patterns create boundaries between areas that carry the highest potential sources of infection and those that are the cleanest (most *aseptic*).

Each zone is also defined by the activities that are carried out there. These are also strictly defined along with the correct operating room apparel for that zone.

NOTE *Since the definition and guidelines are closely associated with infection control, these are discussed in detail in Chapter 9.*

SURGICAL SUITE

EQUIPMENT AND FURNITURE

Equipment, furniture, and supplies in the surgical suite are stored in a standardized way that is familiar to all personnel. This facilitates efficient setup and the ability to locate stored supplies rapidly. Every piece of equipment has a designated location. Basic components are standard to most surgical suites. Equipment needed during surgery includes the operating table, instrument tables, ring stands for solutions, computer station, digital imaging equipment, and electrosurgical unit. All rooms contain an anesthesia machine and physiological monitoring equipment. Sterile supplies are stored in recessed cabinets or in substerile rooms immediately outside the suite. Fig. 4.2 shows a standard operating room with furniture and equipment in place.

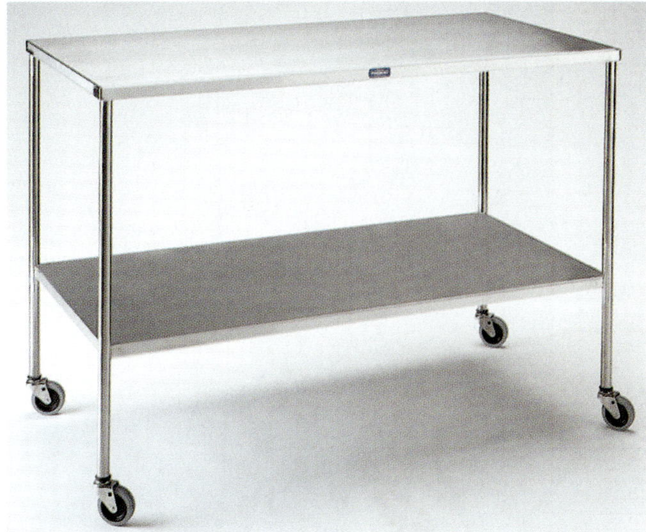

FIG. 4.3 Back table. (Courtesy Pedigo Products, Vancouver, WA.)

The operating table is adjustable for height, degree of tilt in all directions, orientation in the room, articular breaks ("table breaks"), and length. This allows the patient to be positioned in any anatomical position to expose the surgical site fully and maintain safety. The table surface is covered with a firm, removable pad. (The operating table is discussed in detail in Chapter 16.)

The **back table** is a large, stainless steel table on which all instruments and supplies except those in immediate use are placed (Fig. 4.3). For some procedures, more than one back table may be needed. Just before surgery, a sterile pack (table cover with towels and drapes enclosed) is opened onto the table. This provides a sterile surface on which instruments and sterile supplies are distributed. After gowning and gloving, the scrubbed surgical technologist arranges all the equipment in an orderly manner.

Other small tables are used for skin prep kits, power equipment, and extra sterile supplies that may be too heavy or bulky to place on the back table during surgery.

The **Mayo stand** (also called *the Mayo)* is a smaller table with one open end. Its height is adjustable (Fig. 4.4). It is also covered with a sterile drape and is used for instruments and supplies that are needed immediately during surgery. The Mayo stand is placed over or alongside the patient for quick access to instruments. As the case progresses, new instruments or supplies are added to the Mayo stand, and others are placed in reserve on the back table.

The **kick bucket** is constructed of stainless steel and fitted into a wheeled frame (Fig. 4.5). It has a specific use and is not a trash receptacle. The kick bucket is designated for soiled surgical sponges. During surgery, it is placed in a strategic location near the surgical field so that the scrub can drop sponges directly into it.

The **ring stand** is used to contain one or two basins (Fig. 4.6) and is designed to support the lip of the basin, which has been previously wrapped and sterilized. Before surgery, the wrapped basin is placed in the ring stand and the wrapper

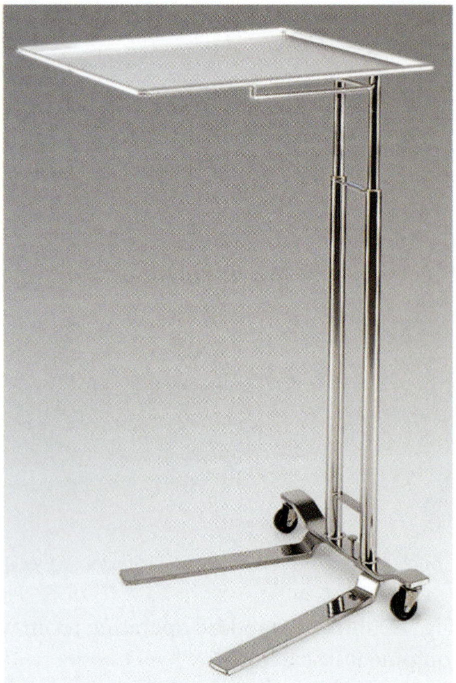

FIG. 4.4 **Mayo stand.** (Courtesy Pedigo Products, Vancouver, WA.)

opened up to expose the basin. Sterile water or saline is poured into the basin for use during surgery.

SPECIAL PROCEDURE ROOM

Some types of surgical procedures require specialized rooms that contain the equipment and technology of that specialty. For example, transurethral (through the urethra) procedures of the genitourinary tract require continuous irrigation and a specialty operating table. Most health care facilities have a separate procedure for endoscopy procedures, which can be located in the operating room or a separate department. A cystoscopy room may also be located in the operating room or a special department. Other procedures, such as fluoroscopy-assisted cryosurgery, are performed in the interventional radiology or nuclear medicine department or the emergency department.

AIRFLOW AND VENTILATION

The airflow and ventilation in the operating room are strictly regulated to reduce airborne particles that may carry infectious microorganisms. The surgical technologist should be aware of the environmental regulations and guidelines. These are discussed in detail in Chapter 9.

LIGHTING

Many different light sources are used in the operating room. Overhead surgical lighting illuminates the surgical field, whereas room lighting is recessed into the ceiling fixtures. Light that is used for endoscopic surgery is derived from fiber-optic cables that are integrated into the instruments. Many modern light systems provide direct visualization on high-definition screens using the same technology as television and computer monitors. Modern surgical lighting is usually derived from LED (light-emitting diode) sources and halogen. LEDs are the newest generation of high-intensity light and are replacing halogen lamps because of their relatively cool temperature and the energy-saving features of LEDs. Halogen lamps provide extremely intense light that is less fatiguing to the eyes than other types of light of equal intensity. Energy emitted by both halogen and LED lighting is given off as light rather than as heat, making it safe to use in surgery.

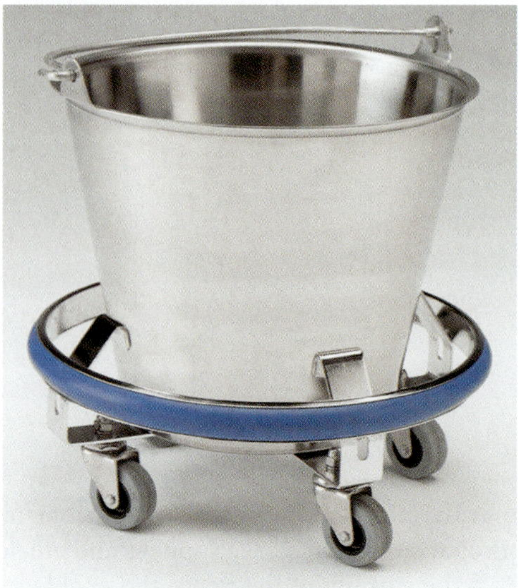

FIG. 4.5 **Kick bucket.** (Courtesy Pedigo Products, Vancouver, WA.)

GASES

A number of different types of compressed gases are used as adjuncts to anesthesia and as power sources for pneumatic devices used during the surgical procedure. Oxygen, compressed air, nitrous oxide, and nitrogen are available through inline systems in most hospitals and outpatient surgical centers. Gas lines terminate at hoses that drop from an overhead panel in each surgical suite. Each hose is fitted with a safety valve to provide direct connections with anesthesia or surgical equipment. Facilities that do not have an inline supply of gases such as nitrogen and compressed air must use compressed gas cylinders that are stored in a designated room within the surgery department. Safety laws and procedures related to the storage and use of compressed gases are strictly monitored by The Joint Commission. A complete discussion on the use of compressed gas, including gauges, fittings, storage, and safety precautions, is found in Chapter 7.

Suction is needed during surgery to evacuate fluids, including blood from the surgical incision (wound), and to remove any fluids from the patient's airway during anesthesia. Like inline gas supply, suction is supplied through line systems that terminate at outlets or hoses fitted with safety valves. Suction tubing is fitted between collection units and safety valves. The strength of the vacuum is measured in pounds per square inch and is adjustable.

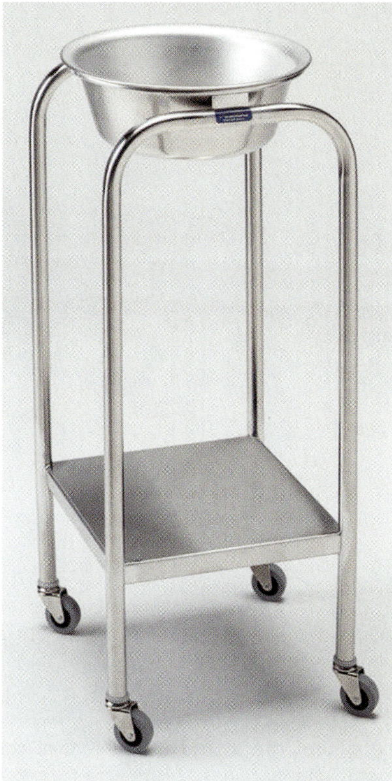

FIG. 4.6 Single ring stand. (Courtesy Pedigo Products, Vancouver, WA.)

ELECTRICITY

Electrical outlets in the operating room are necessary for a wide variety of equipment and medical devices. Because of the high risk associated with electrosurgical devices and electricity in general, there are numerous codes and standards related to electrical equipment and the types of outlets used. Perioperative personnel have many opportunities to learn about the safe use of electricity and other forms of energy in surgery. Chapter 15, Energy Sources in Surgery, discusses the actual use of electricity and other energies, how they are used in medical devices, and safety guidelines to protect patients and staff.

WORK AREAS

Surgical departments can vary widely in size, the use of space, and the types of work areas that they contain. Regardless of the exact appropriation of space, every department strives to maintain the principles of asepsis—separating and confining contaminated areas to keep them apart from clean and sterile areas. The following are some examples of units in the surgical department.

SURGICAL OFFICES

A front office situated near the main entry doors serves as a reception and central communication area for the department. General incoming calls may be received in and referred from this office. Because of its location, the office is also a monitoring point for personnel entering the department. Other offices include those of the operating room supervisor, head nurse, anesthesia director, and other department heads. Dictation rooms are set up for surgeons to make postsurgical reports and for general communication needs.

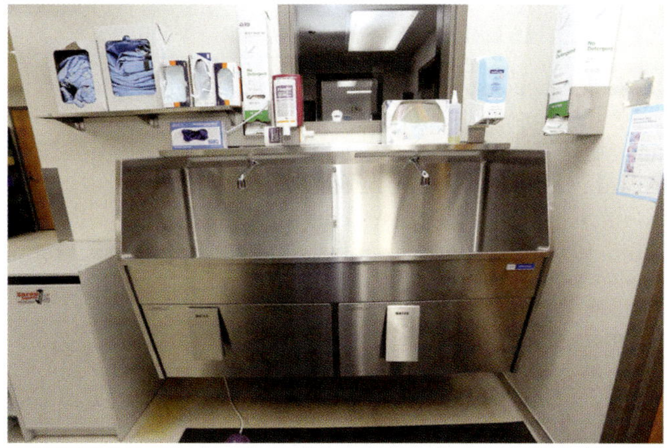

FIG. 4.7 Scrub sink area.

LOCKER ROOM/LOUNGE AREA

The locker room is a **transitional area** for those who need to change from street clothes to surgical attire. Clean scrub attire is located outside the locker room to protect it from contamination by fluids or soil inside the locker room. Locker and changing rooms for staff may be entered directly from outside the department using a key card or coded lock. A separate door leads into the semi-restricted area, allowing staff to transition into the next level of environmental asepsis. Locker room facilities include showers and lavatories. Because the locker room itself is a transitional area, operating room attire must not be kept inside lockers along with street clothes, bags, and other personal items.

If the locker room leads directly into the lounge area, it is separated from the nonrestricted area. The areas are clearly delineated so that personnel dressed in street clothes do not frequent the lounge, offices, or other locations used by those who work in restricted zones. The lounge area often presents a problem for infection control, because personnel in street clothes may have easy access, and traffic control may be limited or even absent.

PREOPERATIVE PATIENT CARE AREA

Surgical patients are transported to the preoperative care area before being taken into the operating room. Outpatients (i.e., those coming from outside the hospital) may be escorted to a changing area and then to the preoperative care area. Patients arrive via gurney or wheelchair and await surgery. This may also be referred to as the holding area and is a check-in point where the surgeon, anesthesiologist, and circulating nurse can confirm that all laboratory and preoperative documentation are in order; the information on the preoperative checklist can also be verified here. In some health care facilities, emergency patients may be brought directly from the emergency department or other facility departments to the operating room suite without passing through the preoperative area.

SCRUB SINKS

Scrub sinks are located outside the operating rooms so that personnel can proceed directly to surgery immediately after hand antisepsis (Fig. 4.7). Scrub sink areas contain antiseptic hand rub, masks, face shields, protective eyewear, brushes, and surgical soap. The area around the scrub sink is kept clean and free of surface water.

STERILE INSTRUMENT ROOM

Sterile wrapped supplies are stored in designated restricted areas adjacent to the operating rooms nearby. Specialty rooms, such as those used for orthopedics, genitourinary procedures, or cardiothoracic surgery, often have their own sterile supply rooms close by. Case cart systems are used in nearly all health facilities to decrease the number of instrument sets stored in the operating room.

CENTRAL CORE

Most operating rooms are designed so that the suites are positioned around one or more central atriums. The core of the atrium is referred to as the *central core*. This area is commonly used to store sterile supplies. Separate doors connect the central core to individual surgical suites. Fig. 4.8 shows a suture supply area in the central core connected to an adjacent operating suite.

EQUIPMENT STORAGE

Large equipment, such as the operating microscope, operating table attachments, and other heavy equipment, is kept in clean designated storerooms. Equipment must be arranged in a way that prevents damage during movement into and out of the room. Thousands of dollars of the operating room's yearly budget are spent on equipment repair as a result of poor storage systems in the operating room department. Many of these accidents occur when equipment is poorly stored in a space that is too small or in a manner that makes the equipment difficult to remove.

UTILITY WORKROOM AND DECONTAMINATION AREA

Soiled instruments and equipment are decontaminated and washed in a utility workroom or central processing area. Some operating rooms use a combination of systems, holding back certain specialty instruments for decontamination and sterilization in the utility workroom and sending the remainder to central processing. The workroom is located in an area convenient to the staff but well contained and away from all restricted areas to prevent cross-contamination of sterile and clean equipment and supplies.

When a **case cart system** is used, sterile supplies (e.g., wrapped instrument sets, single-use items, and drapes) are placed on a closed or open stainless steel cart by personnel in the central processing department. The case carts are usually prepared ahead of time (in many facilities, they are prepared the night before) and are sent to the operating room by central service personnel. As new cases are added to the schedule over the workday, new case carts are assembled. After surgery, soiled instruments and equipment are placed on a cart and returned to the utility workroom and/or the central processing decontamination area, where the cart and instruments are decontaminated. The equipment can then be assembled on trays, wrapped, and resterilized. Designated elevator systems are used to transport carts into and out of the operating room to the central service.

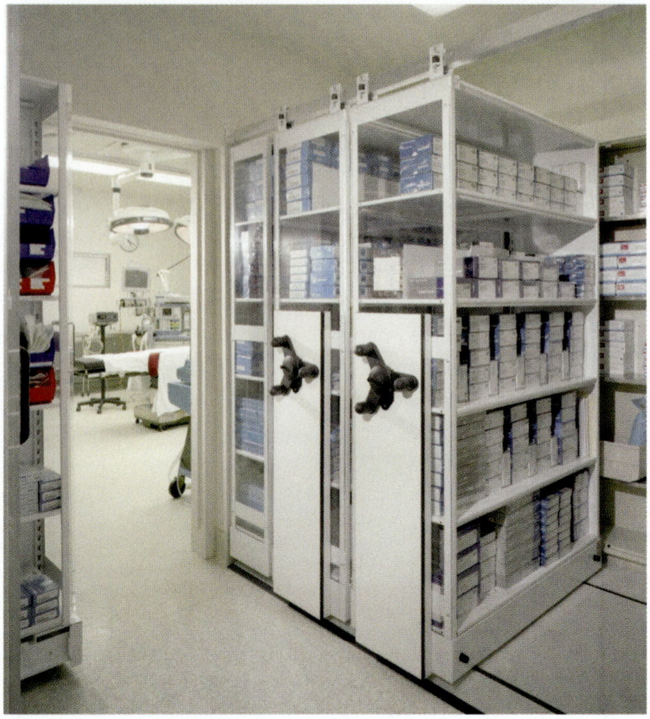

FIG. 4.8 Sterile sutures are stored in the central core adjacent to the operating room suite. (Courtesy Spacesaver Corp., Fort Atkinson, Wis.)

CLEAN PROCESSING AREA

Any instruments that are not sent out of the department for decontamination and sterilization are brought to a clean processing area for assembly after decontamination in the department. This area usually contains at least one sterilizer. Items that are particularly delicate or that are used infrequently may be handled in this way. Likewise, if an item must be reused in a later case and there is not enough time to send it to the central processing department, it may be cleaned and prepared in the operating room decontamination area and wrapped for sterilization in the clean processing area. In the past, high-speed steam sterilizers ("flash sterilizers") were located in small ("substerile") rooms between the operating suites. In this location the sterilizers were used to sterilize items needed quickly during surgery. Current guidelines require that sterilizers are installed in satellite processing areas in a separate location within the operating room but not in substerile rooms. Some surgical facilities may still access high-speed sterilizers in the substerile room but against current guidelines.

ANESTHESIA DEPARTMENT

The anesthesia workroom contains clean respiratory equipment, anesthetic agents, and adjunctive drugs. Tubes, hoses, valves, airways, and other equipment are stored in the workroom and organized neatly to avoid damage and to enable personnel to locate the items quickly. This semi-restricted area may also have its own separate office. Furthermore, the anesthesia workroom may be used to store clean physiological monitoring equipment. Sterile supplies and equipment used for intravenous access and for local and regional anesthesia are usually maintained in a separate sterile room in the anesthesia department.

POSTANESTHESIA CARE UNIT

A patient emerging from anesthesia faces many physiological risks. These include airway obstruction, cardiac arrest, hemorrhage, neurological dysfunction, hypothermia, and pain. Therefore, patients are taken directly from surgery to the **postanesthesia care unit (PACU)**. Critical care nurses in the PACU assist the patient in recovery from conscious sedation or general anesthesia. They assess, monitor, and document the patient's recovery from the time of arrival until the patient is discharged back to the hospital unit, other health care facility, or home. (Refer to Chapter 13 for a complete discussion of the postanesthesia recovery unit.)

SURGERY WAITING AREA

The surgery waiting area for the patient's family is located outside traffic areas leading into the operating room but near the department. This waiting area allows families to be close to the operating room in a quiet environment. This is an area where the surgeon and other surgical staff may communicate directly with family members. Some facilities also have side rooms where the surgeon may consult with the family in a secluded area.

INTEGRATED OPERATING ROOM SYSTEMS

The **integrated (hybrid) operating room** provides centralized control of surgical devices and equipment through a sterile remote- or voice-activated system. This enables the surgeon to activate endoscopic controls, imaging components, operating lights, table adjustments, insufflators, environmental controls, and many other devices that previously were managed individually. Integrated systems allow the surgical team to view patient monitoring output, as well as diagnostic imaging, on the central monitor or "inside" the image seen by the endoscopic camera. A nonsterile workstation in the system provides secondary control of equipment and a standard computer for intraoperative documentation and access to patient records. Integrated operating room systems allow for advances in technology through software design that can be updated periodically.

SECTION II: AMBULATORY AND OUTPATIENT SURGERY

The development of short-acting, fast-emergence anesthetics and minimally invasive surgical technology has led to an increasing trend in the use of free-standing, office-based, and outpatient ambulatory surgical facilities. Approximately 60% of surgeries are currently performed as ambulatory cases.

Ambulatory and outpatient surgical facilities are self-contained to include the same basic perioperative services and functions as the hospital-based operating room. They tend to be fast paced with rapid patient turnover throughout the surgical day. They accommodate surgeons and their patients in specific specialties such as general surgery, cosmetic plastic, reconstructive, orthopedic, bariatric, and ophthalmic surgery or a combination of specialties according to the surgeons who practice in the facility.

TYPES OF AMBULATORY FACILITIES

By definition and regulation, ambulatory patients should be discharged the same day as surgery, or in special cases, observed in the facility for 24 hours postoperatively. The ambulatory facility design and administration is determined by the type and proposed use of the facility as follows.

FREESTANDING FACILITY

The freestanding ambulatory surgery center (ASC) must provide a clear delineation between perioperative care and emergency or inpatient services. This enhances the focus on ambulatory care and contributes to a design and patient flow specific to the needs of the "day case" patient. However, the freestanding clinic is mandated to have a practical plan in the event of perioperative emergencies, including the transfer of patients requiring urgent care.

INTEGRATED HOSPITAL-BASED OUTPATIENT SERVICES

Integrated hospital-based outpatient clinics are those that share surgery facilities with inpatient care areas. Although they share the basic premises and some services, the outpatient clinic must have dedicated areas for preoperative and postoperative (recovery) care that are separate from the inpatient facilities.

SELF-CONTAINED HOSPITAL OUTPATIENT FACILITY

This type of outpatient facility is independent of the inpatient services and areas. They operate and manage separate reception and admission areas and have operating rooms and PACUs that are completely separate from the hospital's services. This separation allows sharing of some resources with the hospital while focusing on non-emergent care.

OFFICE-BASED OUTPATIENT SURGERY

Office-based surgical care has a number of advantages and disadvantages for patient and surgeon. The advantages are mainly convenience for the patient and the surgeon and lower cost per surgery. The disadvantages are limitations in resources, including staff and equipment, and capacity to handle emergencies.

OUTPATIENT FACILITY DESIGN

Outpatient surgical facilities contain departments and work areas similar to the acute care setting with some differences. The workflow and traffic pattern follow the same rules of sterile technique as the acute care setting. The traffic patterns and workflow must conform to the standards and regulations (see later).

BOX 4.1 Designated Areas of the Ambulatory Surgery Facility

- Public access areas:
  - Waiting room(s)
  - Reception area
  - Private space for interviews
  - Medical records area
  - Patient preparation
  - Dressing rooms
  - Preoperative unit for administering medications, starting intravenous lines, checking patient documents
- Staff areas
  - Changing areas with lockers
  - Lounge
- Individual operating rooms
- Separate instrument processing areas—clean and soiled
- Postoperative care area
  - Phase 1 acute care
  - Phase 2 recovery lounge
- Clean storage areas for instruments, medical devices, and supplies
- Designated environmental services areas
- Medical gas storage
- Chemical storage
- Housekeeping supply storage

FUNCTIONAL AREAS OF AN AMBULATORY SURGERY FACILITY

The functional areas of the ambulatory surgery facility are very similar to those of the hospital-based operating room, but some may lack the support services found in acute care hospitals. However, increased regulations and stricter qualifications for facility accreditation have resulted in an increase in support services in the ambulatory surgery facility. The main areas of the ambulatory facility are listed in Box 4.1.

Fig. 4.9 illustrates the flow of activities between areas of the ambulatory facility.

REGULATION AND ACCREDITATION OF AMBULATORY SURGICAL FACILITIES

The increased utilization of these facilities has brought about needed regulatory changes to ensure patient and staff safety. Accreditation of facilities not only is a measure of quality patient care but also is linked to government funding.

ASCs are regulated at the federal level by the Centers for Medicare and Medicaid Services, which is a federal agency within the Department of Health and Human Services. At the state level they are regulated by the state's department of health. Locally only the zoning and building departments are involved with ASCs. Accreditation of ASCs is achieved by meeting the guidelines and quality standards of The Joint Commission.

NOTE *Requirements for certification of ASCs by the Centers for Medicare and Medicaid Services can be found at https://www.cms.gov/Medicare/Provider-Enrollment-and-Certification/CertificationandComplianc/ASCs.*

Guidelines for specific specialties within the ambulatory care environment are regulated through the professional associations of the specialty.

COMPARISON OF THE AMBULATORY SURGERY CENTER AND HOSPITAL-BASED OPERATING ROOMS

It is important that health care personnel working in the ambulatory surgery environment understand that the standard of care, guidelines for safety, and perioperative procedures are no different than those at a hospital-based facility, as long as those standards are met. There are advantages and disadvantages to ambulatory surgery. The advantages have created the rapid growth of all types of ambulatory care. The challenges and disadvantages have motivated professional organizations and agencies to create and enforce guidelines for greater safety and protection of patients and staff.

DISADVANTAGES OF AMBULATORY SURGERY

1. Ambulatory facilities may lack sufficient physical space or staff to carry out perioperative activities related to disinfection and sterilization of instruments and equipment (Bringhurst, 2019).
2. Staff may be assigned to areas they are not usually assigned to, such as stock management, risk management, and environmental safety (Davidson, 2014).
3. Staff are responsible for ensuring that equipment and instruments are processed according to the same high standards as those for any health care facility. This may require special staff training or retraining.
4. Medical-legal responsibilities are increased among ambulatory staff. This is inherent in the facility's ability to handle acute emergencies. In any case the facility must be able to transfer emergency patients quickly and efficiently.
5. Unlike the acute care facility, the ambulatory facility does not usually have centralized support staff and services for infection control, patient safety, pharmacy, and environmental safety. These roles are either absent or delegated to existing clinical personnel who may not have the qualifications or resources to take on the additional activities.
6. Because patients are discharged the same day as surgery, there is usually no skilled care available after discharge. This may affect the patient's compliance with postoperative orders.

ADVANTAGES OF AMBULATORY SURGERY

As ambulatory surgery becomes increasingly common, even for complex cases, the advantages have been well documented.

Patient Acceptance

The experience of having ambulatory surgery is usually comforting, with personable staff who demonstrate care at all levels. This may be related to the size of the facility, which creates a sense of security in patients in spite of the fast pace.

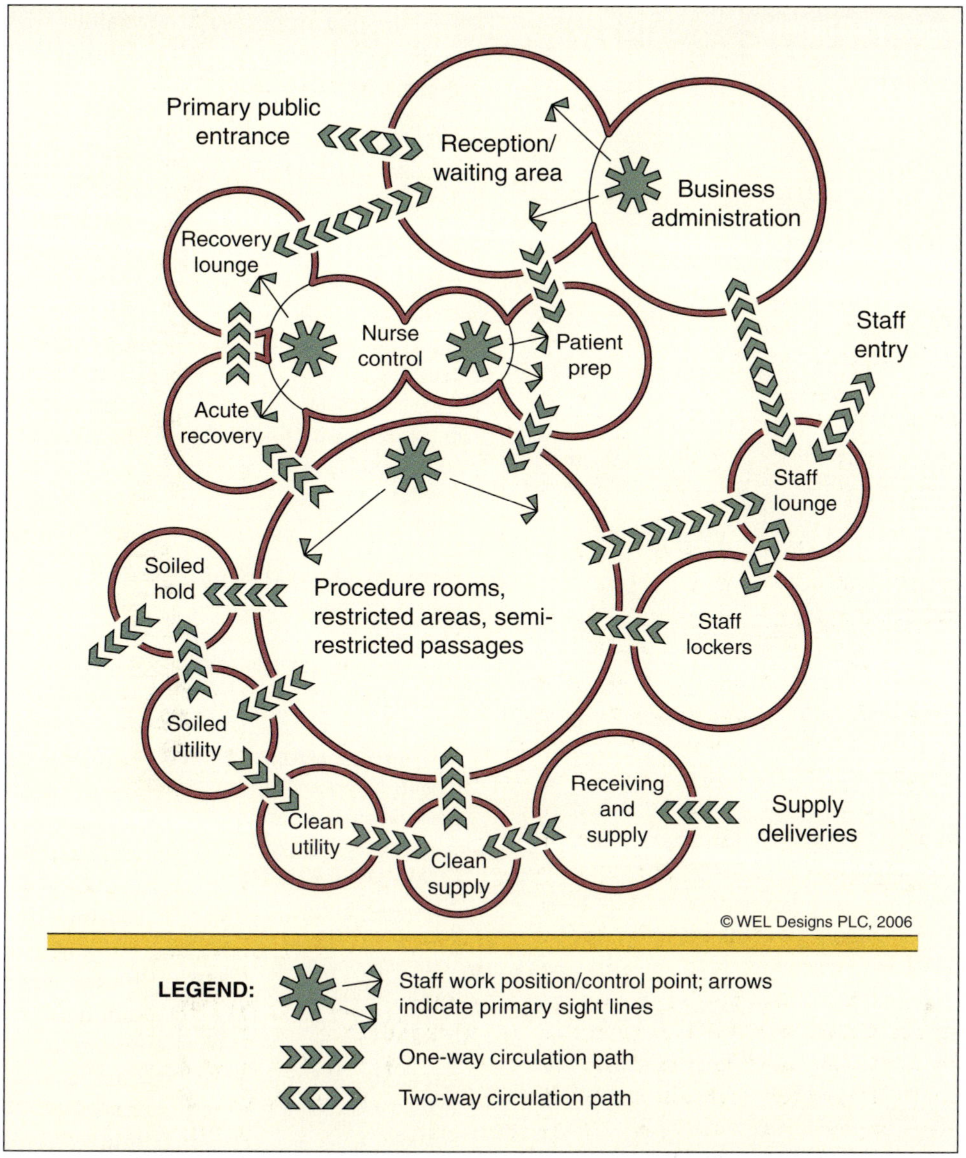

FIG. 4.9 Ambulatory surgery center design. (From Lindeman WE. Design and construction of an ambulatory surgery center. *AORN J.* 2008;88[3]:369–389. doi:10.1016/j.aorn.2008.04.016.)

Cost Effectiveness

Patients are able to take advantage of the lower price of ambulatory surgery as compared to inpatient acute care. Reimbursement from the government and insurance companies means that more patients have access to surgical interventions than in the past.

Ease of Scheduling Cases

Surgeons generally have greater control over scheduling ambulatory cases. Because emergencies are not performed in the setting, and most procedures are routine according to the specialty, there is little chance of a procedure getting "bumped" or postponed. Patients also have more control over the date and time of their procedures.

Control Over the Surgical Environment and Supplies

It has been observed and documented that staff working in ambulatory facilities have more control of the physical resources such as equipment, instruments, and supplies as compared with the large acute care facility. Staff have greater opportunities to develop supportive relationships with patients. This may be related to the amount of time spent on preparing the patient for surgery and ensuring that the patient is "discharge ready." Because patients return home or to the home of others after the procedure, they often require more detailed explanations for surgical aftercare. This creates a closer relationship between patients and professionals.

Efficiency

Ambulatory surgical facilities can be extremely efficient in time—for the surgeon and the patient. Preoperative preparation takes place in the surgeon's office, where required documents can be explained and signed. Surgeons can operate in a number of facilities close to their practice, which can save time in travel. The same is true for patients who are often able to select a surgery center close to their home. Waiting times between surgical procedures is also reduced because there are few "unknown factors," such as emergency cases that can contribute to delays.

BOX 4.2 Hospital Departments

PATIENT MEDICAL SERVICES

Diagnostic Services
- Radiology
- Clinical Laboratory/Pathology
- Diagnostic Imaging (e.g., computed tomography, magnetic resonance imaging)

Patient Care Units (wards)
- Cardiovascular
- Labor and Delivery
- Medical/Surgical
- Neonatal
- Neurological
- Orthopedic
- Pediatric
- Trauma
- Psychiatric
- Renal Dialysis

Intensive and Critical Care Units (ICUs)
- Cardiac Telemetry
- Cardiac (CICU)
- Medical (MICU)
- Neonatal (NICU)
- Neurocritical Care Unit (NCCU)
- Operating Room
- Postanesthesia Care (PACU)
- Trauma (TICU)
- Pediatric (PICU)

Anesthesia and Pain Management
Blood Bank
Outpatient or Ambulatory Surgery
Emergency Department (ED or ER)
Rehabilitation
Physical Therapy
Outpatient Medical Clinics
Nuclear Medicine
Food and Nutrition Services
- Dietitian
- Outpatient Nutrition Services

PSYCHOSOCIAL AND OUTREACH SERVICES

Patient Education
Community Health Services
Home Health Services
Hospice
Adult Day Care Services
Hospital Chaplaincy
Occupational Therapy

EMPLOYEE AND ADMINISTRATIVE SERVICES

Human Resources
- Employee Education

Employee Health Services and Insurance
Accounting
Patient Accounts
Reimbursement
Managed Care
Auditor
Payroll

ENVIRONMENTAL SERVICES

Infection Control
Maintenance
Bioengineering (Clinical Engineering)
Housekeeping

MATERIALS MANAGEMENT

Central Supply
Distribution

COMMUNICATIONS

Switchboard
Paging System
Telecommunications
Mobile Radio Communications
Electronic Communications

SAFETY

Risk Management
Security

RECORDS AND CLERICAL SERVICES

Medical Records
Admissions

SECTION II: HEALTH CARE FACILITY DEPARTMENTS AND FUNCTIONS

TEAM APPROACH TO PATIENT CARE

Perioperative staff members work in coordination with many different professionals and departments in the health care facility. The operating room often seems isolated and independent from other departments of the hospital. Physical barriers and procedures necessary to maintain strict asepsis seem to foster an atmosphere of independence. In fact, the operating room could not function without the collaborative efforts of the departments outside the operating room. The efforts of many departments and caring staff members contribute to safe surgery and uneventful recovery. Perioperative staff members must communicate effectively with those outside the operating room and help facilitate a cohesive team approach. Knowledge about the roles of other departments and the activities they perform contributes to this team approach.

Sometimes, departments face multiple demands that may exceed their limits of available personnel and time. Patience, respect, and professionalism build good interdepartmental relationships, help reduce stress, and improve patient care.

Departments in the health care facility are distinguished by function (what they do) or by **administration** (the sector in which they are managed, such as nursing administrator or medical director). Box 4.2 lists the hospital departments found in most facilities.

PATHOLOGY

The pathology department receives all tissue samples and other specimens from surgery. A *pathologist* is a specialist medical doctor (MD) who examines specimens to determine the type of tissue or other material, to identify disease within the tissue, and to create a permanent legal record. If the surgeon requires an immediate tissue evaluation, as in the case of a suspected malignancy, the pathologist is available to perform immediate analysis. The specimen is frozen with liquid nitrogen and sliced into sections for microscopic examination. Immediate tissue analysis provides the information needed to make decisions about the need for more extensive surgery during the same procedure.

NUCLEAR MEDICINE AND INTERVENTIONAL RADIOLOGY

Nuclear medicine involves the use of radioactive materials or radiopharmaceuticals to diagnose and treat disease. These special procedures are performed in a designated nuclear medicine department that has the technical capacity to handle a variety of different procedures following the strict regulations needed to ensure patient and staff safety.

Interventional radiology uses radiography, magnetic resonance imaging (MRI), computed tomography (CT), ultrasound, and other imaging techniques to guide instruments into vessels and organs. Surgical technologists may be required to assist in interventional radiology because sterile technique is required. Examples of interventional radiology procedures are angiography, angioplasty, insertion of a gastrostomy tube, needle biopsy, and stereotactic procedures.

INFECTION CONTROL

Infection control personnel are specialists in the prevention and control of hospital-acquired infection. The health care environment is a potential source for the spread of many types of infection. Whenever people are in close proximity, especially people who are already ill or are debilitated by surgery, nutritional problems, stress, or trauma, the potential for infection is high. The infection control department develops policies on the basis of the standards and recommendations of The Joint Commission, the Centers for Disease Control and Prevention, APIC, OSHA, and the National Institute for Occupational Safety and Health.

The objectives of infection control are to reduce the number of infections by prevention and to study the causes of infection within the facility. Infection prevention policies affect every department of the hospital. Important goals in infection control include educating staff members and patients, tracking policy compliance, and investigating the sources of infection.

BIOMEDICAL ENGINEERING

Biomedical engineering technicians (also called *biological engineers*) maintain the safety and operating condition of many of the hospital's medical devices, including those used in surgery. The complexity of sophisticated devices requires technicians who are specially trained in biomedical engineering. The biomedical engineering department is usually a separate department, but there may be an office dedicated to surgical equipment near the surgery department. Technicians may be called to the operating room in the event of equipment failure during surgery.

MATERIALS MANAGEMENT

The materials management department of a health care facility is the purchasing and logistics center for goods and supplies needed for the delivery of health care. It is also responsible for ordering new supplies and for implementing tracking systems to maintain the supply chain.

CENTRAL SUPPLY

Disposable items, linens, and equipment are distributed to hospital departments by the central supply department. Items are usually tracked by computer, and distribution is carefully managed to control hospital costs. In some health care facilities, this department may be responsible for receiving soiled equipment used in surgery. In this case, wrapping and sterilization are performed in separate areas of the department.

PHARMACY

The pharmacy distributes medications to patient care units in the hospital. Medications and anesthetic agents used in the operating room are received from the pharmacy, either by regular delivery or by special requisition. Many modern surgical departments have their own pharmacy, which is stocked from the central pharmacy or directly from the vendors. Anesthetic agents are usually stored in the anesthesia department or pharmacy located in the surgical department.

LABORATORY

Diagnostic tests are performed in the hospital laboratory, where clinical laboratory personnel examine and analyze body fluids, tissues, and cells. Laboratory personnel perform chemical, biological, hematological, immunological, microscopic, and bacteriological tests. They also perform blood-typing procedures. The data and results obtained in the laboratory are returned to the physician to aid in the evaluation and treatment of the patient.

BLOOD BANK

The blood bank provides blood products for transfusion in the surgical, postanesthesia care, and medical units of the hospital. Because of the stringent protocols regulating blood product transfusion, strict methods are followed for their handling, storage, transport, and identification. The surgical technologist may interact with blood bank personnel and should be familiar with the institution's policy regarding ordering and transporting blood products.

RISK MANAGEMENT DEPARTMENT

Because of the many environmental risks and the possibility for errors and omissions by personnel, surveillance is required to track the number and exact nature of adverse or sentinel events in a given time period. The cause of each event is studied, and policies are enacted to prevent future incidents of the same type. For example, if the incidence of chemical burns among staff members was increasing, the **risk management** team would investigate the circumstances, time of day, personnel involved (e.g., housekeeping, nursing), and other important aspects to identify the cause. The team would then develop a plan to reduce the number of incidents. The team may change existing policies regulating the use of chemicals or give personnel intensive training. After the plan is implemented, an evaluation is performed to determine whether the measures taken actually did reduce the number of chemical burns. Incident reports (see Chapter 3) are very important to risk management because they contain the information needed to analyze incidents and develop a plan of intervention.

COMMUNICATION SYSTEMS

The central communication point of a health care facility is designed to redirect calls to specific individuals or departments. With new voice and communication technology, staff can receive and transmit information through many different types of systems that reduce the need for hospital-wide intercom paging. Wireless, voice-controlled communication using smartphones and voice badges allows facility staff to communicate instantly with each other without the delay common in older pager systems. Modern intercom systems are designed for hands-off use and can be integrated for use inside and outside the health care facility. The operating room intercom system can be set up for voice control communication so that the surgeon can communicate directly with other departments such as pathology without stepping away from the surgical field. Messaging systems can now use smartphones to provide pages, text messages, and alerts sent through a web-based console. Web-based and satellite-based systems also allow teaching and telemedicine during surgical procedures.

MEDICAL RECORDS

The medical records department is responsible for receiving, maintaining, and transferring all patient records. Because patient records are legal documents, strict protocols determine when signatures are required, who may make entries, what must be included, and where the patient's documents are stored. Many, but not all, health care facilities use electronic record systems. When an electronic system is in use, patient records are accessed through a strictly monitored password system.

FACILITIES MAINTENANCE

The facilities maintenance department is responsible for environmental systems in the hospital. These systems include the hospital's power source (regular and emergency), ventilation, inline gases, suction, electricity, water, light, heat, cooling, and humidity control. Standards for environmental control and safety are established by The Joint Commission and government agencies. Perioperative personnel should never ignore or try to repair a system that malfunctions. Maintenance personnel are available at all times to respond to environmental emergencies.

ENVIRONMENTAL SERVICES

Environmental services personnel perform essential cleaning and decontamination services for all departments of the hospital. In the operating room, they maintain a clean environment and decontaminate the floors, furniture, and other surfaces between cases (called *room turnover*). They work with other team members to ensure rapid turnover from one case to the next.

SECURITY

Security services are provided in large- and medium-sized health care facilities. Security officers are responsible for monitoring public activities in the facility, including traffic and staff identity. They respond to public disorder within the boundaries of the facility and are in direct communication with local enforcement authorities. Security personnel are not members of the police department. Their role is to reduce the level of security incidents and to implement training programs for security personnel.

NUTRITIONAL SERVICES

Nutritionists are licensed health care professionals who advise and perform care related to the nutritional status of patients. Nutritionists consult with medical and nursing personnel to provide a plan of care for a patient whose medical condition either contributes to or is caused by a diet that is harmful. They are also consulted for patients with particular dietary needs such as those with kidney disease or patients who have undergone gastric procedures for obesity control. In addition to advising in special cases, they may also coordinate with dietary services in planning meals for the general patient population.

SECTION III: HEALTH CARE ADMINISTRATION

HEALTH CARE PROVIDERS

Most large health care organizations provide primary health care, inpatient and outpatient, diagnosis, and outpatient rehabilitation services. Primary or secondary (preventive) medical care is provided in a fixed location, such as the community hospital. The community hospital, whether privately or publicly owned, brings together people with different professional skills to provide coordinated services. Larger hospitals or medical centers also operate satellite facilities in rural or urban areas away from the central facility. Satellite facilities deliver various types of care or treatments. Services may include but are not limited to ambulatory surgery centers, clinics, urgent care centers, laboratory and radiology centers, physicians' offices, extended care, and rehabilitation facilities.

Surgery is performed in many different settings, including hospitals, community health centers, and freestanding clinics that may be privately owned or operated by nonprofit organizations.

Ambulatory surgical centers perform minor surgery that does not require postoperative hospital recovery. Ambulatory surgery and outpatient surgery departments in hospitals are also becoming increasingly popular. In addition, some types of surgery are being performed in surgeons' offices.

Surgery that requires general anesthesia, conscious sedation, or complex local anesthesia is performed in a hospital facility, where perioperative services are coordinated with the services of other departments. This setting provides continuity of care and ensures that emergency services are immediately available. This chapter focuses on the hospital-based surgical department. However, the principles of administration, organization, and physical layout are similar for all settings.

HEALTH CARE FINANCING

Health care financing in the United States is mainly divided among government structures, employer contributions, and private insurance.

GOVERNMENT ASSISTANCE

Government-assisted health care systems are managed by state and federal agencies. The *Medicaid system* assists in medical care for specific low-income families and individuals with special needs, including disability. The program is jointly funded by the state and federal government. Eligibility is dependent on both economic and health qualifications.

The *Medicare system* operates like an insurance plan in which individuals pay into a fund through their employment taxes and can later draw on the fund after the age of 65 years for certain medical costs. The plan includes hospital and medical insurance and is administered to people with specific types of permanent disability. Individuals or their spouses who pay into the Medicare system through their taxes generally do not pay for hospital insurance. Certain medical and prescription drug insurance is partly covered under a monthly premium paid by the individual through Social Security taxes.

PRIVATE INSURANCE

Private medical insurance programs require regular payments by an individual or group of individuals, who in turn receive partial or total payment for specific types of medical care. Insurance companies may contract specific health organizations to provide services at a reduced rate for their beneficiaries. These organizations are referred to as *preferred provider organizations* or PPOs. The *health maintenance organization* (HMO) is another system of health care delivery used by insurance companies. The HMO contracts specific health care providers to deliver services using techniques and standards that are designed to be economical and efficient. The HMO sets guidelines for care that must be followed by the contracted health care providers.

PAYMENT SYSTEMS

The specific payment systems in the insurance industry use standardized codes for diagnoses and treatment modalities. The *diagnosis-related group* (DRG) is a list of services or "products" that hospitals deliver. For example, a surgical procedure is one type of product. The system of DRGs is used by Medicare and insurance companies to determine the amount of money the system pays out for its beneficiaries.

The International Classification of Diseases (ICD) code is an assigned number for specific medical conditions. The ICD code is used in combination with the DRG to determine the amount of money that the insurance company or Medicare provides for its beneficiaries. Another system used by medical providers is the Current Procedural Terminology (CPT) code, which is created and maintained by the American Medical Association to provide consistent terminology for medical procedures.

MANAGEMENT STRUCTURE

Hospital management and operational staff members are usually organized into separate bodies or groups of people whose joint functions and roles enable patient and community services. The board of directors or trustees is responsible for hiring the chief executive officer (CEO). It determines the hospital's administrative and development policies and mission statement, and it reviews the procedures for safe, ethical patient care.

The administrative sector designs and implements personnel procedures, policies, and financial systems. It communicates with the public and handles overall institutional issues, such as public relations and quality assurance.

The medical and other professional staff delivers services according to the privileges granted to them by license and state codes. Management within these sectors is usually organized by departments and professions. Medical staff members are usually managed by the chief or head physician of the department. Professional nurses are managed by the nursing department. Allied health staff members are managed by their own department heads, or they may be administered by the nursing department. The management structure can be horizontal (many people sharing the same level of management) or vertical (fewer people at the management level).

CHAIN OF COMMAND

The **chain of command** defines the relationship between management and staff members. An employee reports (is responsible) to his or her immediate line manager.

The chain of command is important for several reasons. Management systems rely on the flow of information *from* specific people in particular positions *to* people in other specific positions. Certain information is critical to the outcome of the work. For example, a safety warning about equipment is directed to all staff members who use that equipment. The direct link between the staff members and their immediate manager may be the most important source of that information. In another example, an incident in surgery must be reported to the individual positioned to act on the consequences of that incident. This includes not only immediate action on health and safety but also the process of analysis and risk management. Certain people in the chain of command are responsible for these tasks. Following the chain of command puts the person (or position) previously designated as the most appropriate in charge of the response.

The types and volume of responsibility required of managers in today's hospitals are much greater than ever before. The chain of command defines the domains and specific areas of focus for each manager. It allows managers to focus their attention where it is intended. This creates a more smoothly running department and better patient outcomes.

The chain of command is important for the resolution of questions regarding policy and protocol. Each staff member has a line manager whose tasks include resolving issues or directing them to another appropriate source. For example, if a staff member experiences abusive treatment in the operating room, that staff member must present the situation to his or her line manager. The line manager must be made aware of staff relations in the department and is best placed to counsel the individual and refer the situation to another authority if necessary. Except in unusual circumstances, it is almost always unwise to skip the chain of command when reporting incidents or seeking information, as this may be interpreted as a lack of respect for one's direct line manager or a lack of faith in that person's ability to manage. This reflects badly on the manager to his or her own manager and peers.

STAFF ROLES

PERSONNEL POLICY

The responsibilities and functions of all employees in the surgical department are clearly defined in writing in the hospital manual covering its **personnel policy.** These policies are written to clarify job descriptions and to establish the accountability of each employee. They include topics such as employee safety, how to respond in emergency situations, insurance issues, and ethical conduct. These policies comply with state and federal laws and ensure that the hospital meets the minimum standards set by The Joint Commission. Policies must be strictly followed, because they define the practices necessary for the safe and efficient operation of the department. Employees are required to read these policies and often must sign a form stating that they understand the policies for the hospital to enforce compliance.

Each member of the hospital staff has defined duties and responsibilities. These are often referred to as a **job description.** A job description for each position is necessary to ensure that every person knows what is expected of him or her. The job description is a management tool to ensure that all tasks have been assigned appropriately. It is equally important for the individual to know exactly what his or her role is. The job description includes a **job title,** which identifies the position by name. This is another method of clarifying roles and responsibilities.

Many different professional personnel make up the modern perioperative team. Some roles overlap, whereas others are specific to a particular job according to professional standards, policy, training, and individual capability.

PERIOPERATIVE PROFESSIONALS

Surgeon

The surgeon is the patient's primary physician in the operating room and is responsible for guiding the surgical procedure. The surgeon operates under the prescribed policies of the hospital in which he or she works and is licensed under the medical Practice Acts in his or her state. The surgeon may be qualified as an MD, doctor of dental surgery, doctor of dental medicine, doctor of osteopathic medicine (DO), or doctor of podiatry.

Assistant Surgeon

The assistant surgeon is an MD licensed to perform and assist in surgery. The assistant provides direct care to the patient according to the delegation of the surgeon and the needs of the patient. The assistant surgeon is qualified to deliver emergency care during a procedure and must be able to take charge of the surgical case in the event that the primary surgeon is unable.

Anesthesia Provider

The anesthesia provider is an MD, DO, or certified registered nurse anesthetist and is a specialist in anesthesia and pain management. The anesthesia provider is responsible for the meticulous assessment, monitoring, and adjustment of the patient's physiological status during surgery. He or she consults with the surgeon on the patient's specific physiological and medical condition before surgery and follows this care through the postsurgical recovery period.

Perioperative Registered Nurse

The perioperative registered nurse (RN) holds a current license in nursing and may also have advanced certification in perioperative nursing (certified nurse–operating room). The perioperative nurse functions as a circulating nurse (circulator) or as a scrub. Additional training permits a registered nurse to become a registered nurse–first assistant.

Physician Assistant

A physician assistant (PA) is a medical professional who practices medicine under the supervision of a physician. A PA is required to pass a national certification examination and earn the title of physician assistant–certified. A PA in the operating room has received additional training in surgery. The PA may perform first-assistant tasks under the direct supervision of the surgeon and according to hospital policy.

Licensed Practical Nurse

The licensed practical nurse (LPN) (or licensed vocational nurse [LVN] in some states) has completed a 1- to 2-year program in a college or vocational or technical school. After completing a state-approved practical nursing program, an LPN or LVN becomes licensed after passing the National Council Licensure Examination for Licensed Practical Nurses, which is the national qualifying examination for LPNs. In the operating room, the LPN or LVN usually functions in the role of scrub.

Certified Surgical Technologist

The role of the certified surgical technologist (CST) is discussed throughout this text. The CST prepares equipment and instruments before surgery, ensuring that all devices are safe and operative. Surgical technologists also assist in preparation of the patient immediately before surgery. They help position the patient, perform the antiseptic skin prep, and assist the surgeon in applying sterile drapes to protect the surgical site from contamination. They arrange the equipment, maintain it during surgery, and pass instruments to the surgeons. They are also responsible for setting up and maintaining instruments during the procedure and for safely handling and transporting soiled instruments for reprocessing. In addition, the CST may also function as the assistant circulator, which is described in detail in Chapter 19.

Certified Surgical Technologist–Certified Surgical First Assistant

The certified surgical technologist–certified surgical first assistant (CST-CSFA) is a CST who has completed an educational program in surgical assisting. For the purposes of patient reimbursement through Medicare, he or she is a "nonphysician surgical assistant." Certification requirements are established by the National Board of Surgical Technology and Surgical Assisting. The CST-CSFA provides exposure (retraction), hemostasis (controlling bleeding in the surgical wound), suturing, suctioning fluids from the wound, and other tasks as directed by the surgeon. The CST-CSFA may be hired by a specialist surgeon or health care facility to perform in a role specific to that specialty, such as ophthalmic surgery, ear, nose, and throat surgery, or orthopedic surgery.

Certified Surgical Assistant or Nonphysician Surgical Assistant

The certified surgical assistant or nonphysician surgical assistant is an allied health qualification achieved by certification through the National Surgical Assistant Association. Qualifications for certification include graduation from an accredited surgical assistance school, military training, or a foreign medical degree. Physician assistants and registered nurses may also apply for qualification, which is recognized by the Accreditation Review Council on Education in Surgical Technology and Surgical Assisting and approved by the Commission on Accreditation of Allied Health Education Programs. There are also other credentialed surgical assistants (i.e., Surgical Assistant-Certified (SA-C)).

Certified Anesthesia Technologist

The certified anesthesia technologist is a member of the anesthesia patient care team and department. Anesthesia technologists directly assist the anesthesiologist, residents, and nurse anesthetist. They prepare and maintain equipment and supplies needed for the administration of anesthetics and calibrate monitoring devices used during surgery. They assist with laboratory tests and obtain blood products and pharmaceuticals. Depending on their expertise, they may also perform technical and support roles in procedures involving anesthesia.

Operating Room Educator

The operating room nurse educator may be a registered nurse or CST with extensive operating room experience. This individual develops and implements educational programs, seminars, and in-services (informational training on new products or techniques) within the department. Not all surgical departments have a designated educator; some provide training on a more informal basis. The surgical technologist instructor is designated by the health care facility to orient and teach newly recruited surgical technologists or those in a specialty.

Independent surgical technology instructors are affiliated with their educational institution, not with the health care institution in which students have internships. The instructor upholds the policies of the health care institution and supervises students in compliance with these standards. The students also interact with health care facility staff members who may delegate individual tasks in accordance with the goals and objectives of the educational program. Cooperation and good communication between the surgical technology instructor and operating room staff ensure that students complete their educational requirements while following the policies of the health care institution in which they are learning.

Surgical Orderly or Aide

The surgical orderly participates in many types of patient care services, including transportation of the patient to and from the surgical department. The orderly may also participate in "turnover" (preparation of the surgical suite for the next patient). Orderlies often assist in the preparation of supplies and instruments for decontamination and sterilization. The work is demanding, because many members of the surgery department make many requests for their attention.

Central Sterile Processing Technician

The central processing or sterile processing technician is responsible for the safe management and sterilization of equipment in preparation for and after its use in surgery and other care units. These technicians are knowledgeable about the process of sterilization and decontamination, asepsis, and standard precautions. They assemble instruments and safely process them according to hospital standards. They also keep hospital and operating room inventories of instruments and equipment and may be responsible for ordering supplies.

PATIENT CARE TECHNICIAN

The patient care technician (PCT) is a multidisciplinary nursing assistant. He or she provides direct patient care in activities of daily living. These include patient mobility, dressing, eating, and toileting. The certified PCT may also perform phlebotomy (venipuncture), electrocardiography, and other technical roles.

Radiology Technician
Medical and technical radiology professionals may be involved in the perioperative setting before, during, and after surgery. The radiologist MD is responsible for the medical interpretation of diagnostic images produced by CT, fluoroscopy, MRI, and other complex imaging. Radiology technicians perform imaging procedures in the interventional radiology department or as on-call personnel who perform imaging in other departments of the health care facility, including surgery.

Electroencephalogram Technician
The electroencephalogram (EEG) technician is a specialist in measuring the brain's activities through a variety of procedures and tests, usually in a special department of the health care facility. The EEG technician may also perform brain activity monitoring duties during specific surgical procedures.

Medical Industry Representative
The medical industry representative is employed by surgical equipment and instrument companies to provide guidance and training on the company's products. The industry representative may be present in the operating room during procedures in which their products, such as orthopedic implants, are being used. Their role is to train members of the surgical team on the proper use of the products.

Cardiovascular Perfusionist
The role of the cardiovascular perfusionist is to provide extracorporeal (outside the body) oxygenation of the blood during cardiac bypass procedures in which the heart is placed in standstill. The perfusionist is responsible for setting up all equipment and for its safe operation during surgery.

Health Care Facility Management
The CEO of the health care facility is responsible for the overall operational planning and implementation of the facility's strategic plan. This role may be shared with the chief operational officer (COO), who is expected to assume the role of CEO in that individual's absence. Additional roles of the CEO are ensuring that the facility complies with regulatory requirements and developing good communication among departments within the facility. The executive officer provides leadership within the facility and in the community.

Chief Operational Officer
The COO is responsible for oversight of the health care facility with a particular focus on the functioning of the medical services, personnel, and fiscal areas. This individual works with all levels of operations, developing strategic plans for operation and implementing them. The operational department covers a broad range of areas, including workforce recruitment and safety, information technology, communications, liaison with educational institutions, and research. The COO is a manager who troubleshoots problems in the actual day-to-day operations from a global perspective.

Director of Surgical Services/Operating Room Supervisor
The director of surgical services (also known in some areas as the operating room supervisor) is responsible for overseeing all clinical and professional activities in the department. Using evidence-based standards, he or she creates and implements policies about clinical and professional practices in the operating room. The operating room supervisor may represent the department at supervisory meetings, where he or she helps coordinate activities in other departments with those of the operating room.

Perioperative Nurse Manager
A perioperative nurse manager may assist the operating room director with his or her duties or may have separate responsibilities. If the director is absent from the department, the nurse manager may assume the role of supervisor if necessary. The nurse manager is responsible for the day-to-day activities of the operating room, although the individual may or may not participate in surgical procedures. The nurse manager is usually an RN with a bachelor of science in nursing and a master's degree in management. Responsibilities may include ordering and management of devices and materials, environmental safety, education, infection control, staff scheduling, and resolving staffing problems. The nurse manager is often responsible for organizing triage and emergency responses in the operating room.

Unit Clerk/Secretary
The surgical unit clerk or secretary receives scheduling requests from the surgeons or their representatives. The secretary must also answer the telephone and relay messages within and out of the surgical department. In the event of emergency, the secretary must assist the manager in rescheduling any cases that have been canceled and notify all personnel involved in these cases. The unit clerk maintains an orderly schedule and coordinates the scheduling needs of many different surgeons. The individual is knowledgeable about medical and surgical terminology, has excellent communication skills, and is able to cope with a variety of stressful situations.

KEY CONCEPTS

- *The operating room is designed and engineered to provide infection control; environmental safety; and efficient use of personnel, time, space, and resources.*
- *The layout of the surgical department is based primarily on the principles of infection control—confining and containing areas and sources of contamination.*
- *Traffic patterns in the surgical department contribute to infection control and are strictly enforced.*
- *Operating room equipment and furniture are managed in a way that promotes safety and efficiency.*
- *The physical environment of the operating room, such as lighting, air exchange, temperature, and humidity, is strictly controlled. Standards for these elements are enforced by accreditation and safety organizations.*
- *Basic equipment and furniture needed for surgery are kept in each surgical suite. Special procedure rooms contain supplies and equipment for surgical specialties such as*

genitourinary surgery, orthopedics, and plastic surgery.
- *Designated areas of the surgical department include the individual operating (procedure) rooms, instrument storage areas, anesthesia workroom, and scrub sink areas.*
- *The health care facility has many different departments that interact with each other to provide patient care. Coordination among departments is essential for smooth teamwork.*
- *Perioperative personnel rely on departments such as interventional radiology, materials management, pharmacy, and the blood bank for day-to-day activities in surgery.*
- *All health care facilities have a mission statement and community goals on which they base their policies, procedures, and activities.*
- *Hospital policies are established in consultation with accreditation and safety organizations. All employees must be familiar with personnel, health, and safety policies. They are also required to understand the policies of the department in which they work.*
- *An organizational chart establishes the relationships between management and staff. These are ranked by chain of command.*
- *All personnel are required to have a job description so that they know what is expected of them.*
- *The surgical department employs many different types of professional and nonprofessional staff. Everyone has a responsibility to coordinate their work with others and to become familiar with each other's roles in the workplace.*

REVIEW QUESTIONS

1. How is the floor plan of the operating room related to patient safety?
2. What is a restricted area in the operating room?
3. What is an integrated operating room?
4. What is the purpose of hospital accreditation?
5. What types of problems might employees experience if they are not familiar with the policies of their employer?
6. What is the purpose of a chain of command?

CASE STUDIES

CASE 1

The floor plan of the surgical department is one of the main strategies for infection control. Working in a group, design a floor plan that meets the criteria discussed in this chapter without duplicating the designs already shown.

CASE 2

The concept of *chain of command* was introduced in this chapter. The importance of this concept is often overlooked as simply a paper exercise that only concerns management. However, in actual practice, it is extremely important. Analyze the following situation and discuss how chain of command affects the outcome:

A single mother employee is experiencing difficulty in the workplace because of difficulties balancing care of her children with the work schedule. If she could change her work schedule to coincide with the hours she is needed at home, it will solve the problem. She sends an email to someone in human resources who she believes may be more sympathetic than her line manager—after all, it is a human resources problem. What effect will this have on resolution of the problem? What reaction do you feel the line manager may have? What about the person in human resources?

CASE 3

An employee's job description is an important document for clarification of roles, responsibility, and accountability. What is the effect of a job description that is extremely vague? What is the relationship between a job description and chain of command?

REFERENCE

Bringhurst J. Special problems associated with reprocessing instruments in outpatient care facilities: physical spaces, education, infection preventionists, industry, reflections. *Am J Infect*. 2019;47. https://doi.org/10.1016/j.ajic.2019.03.006.

Davidson J. Why a column on ambulatory best practices? AORN Journal. 2014;99(5):612–615. https://doi.org/10.1016/j.aorn.2014.01.018.

BIBLIOGRAPHY

ASHRAE Standing Standard Project Committee 170 (SSPC 170): ANSI/ASHRAE/ASHE Standard 170, Ventilation of Health Care Facilities. http://sspc170.ashraepcs.org. Accessed July 11, 2011.

Association of Surgical Technologists. Job description: surgical assistant. http://www.ast.org. Accessed February 20, 2020.

Association of Surgical Technologists. Job description: surgical technologist. http://www.ast.org. Accessed February 20, 2020.

Lindeman, William E. "Design and construction of an ambulatory surgery center". AORN Journal. 2008; 88(3):369–389. https://doi.org/10.1016/j.aorn.2008.04.016.

US Department of Labor, Occupational Safety and Health Administration: surgical suite module. http://www.osha.gov/SLTC/etools/hospital/surgical/surgical.html. Accessed February 20, 2020.

Recommended practices for environmental cleaning: In *Perioperative Standards and Recommended Practices*, Denver, CO, 2019, AORN, Inc.

5 SUPPORTING THE PSYCHOSOCIAL NEEDS OF THE PATIENT

LEARNING OBJECTIVES

After studying this chapter, the reader will be able to:

1. Define patient-centered and outcome-oriented care
2. Discuss the basis of human needs as described in Maslow's hierarchy and Roger's humanistic theory
3. Discuss a person's needs for safety, belonging, esteem, and actualization
4. Discuss preoperative patient fears and their basis
5. Define spirituality as it applies to patient care
6. Discuss special needs patients and their psychosocial care in the perioperative environment

TERMINOLOGY

Anesthesia awareness: A rare phenomenon in which a fully unconscious patient under general anesthesia retains the sense of hearing and pain during the surgery and is able to recall the experience.

Anxiolytic: A medication that prevents anxiety—often administered preoperatively for patients who are highly anxious.

Body image: The way an individual perceives himself or herself physically in the eyes of others.

Maslow's hierarchy of human needs: A model of human needs developed by psychologist Abraham Maslow.

Patient-centered care: Therapeutic care, communication, and intervention provided according to the unique needs of the patient and centered on those needs.

Self-actualization: A person's ability to plan for and achieve their life goals.

Supportive communication: A purposeful method of communication in which the caregiver responds to the explicit or implicit needs of the patient. Listening is emphasized.

As a member of the patient care team in the operating room, the surgical technologist directly contributes to the patient's physical and psychological well-being. Patients undergoing surgery are often fearful and worried about the outcome of the surgery but also the processes that they cannot control. Surgical technologists in different health care settings have varying levels of social and professional contact with patients. In some settings, the ST may have only brief encounters with patients, whereas in others, contact is extensive. For example, the ambulatory surgical center usually involves more contact. Regardless of how brief or extended the professional relationship is, the ST can anticipate the patient's immediate needs through verbal and nonverbal cues.

Empathy for the patient evolves from recognizing the patient's physical and psychosocial needs. Every patient is unique, and a positive surgical outcome depends on holistic **patient-centered care**—which is based on many different dimensions of care according to the patient *as an individual.* These unique needs are revealed through information from others, the patient's records, accurate observation, and good communication with the patients.

BASIC HUMAN NEEDS

Health care workers are often required to study the importance of basic human needs in patient care.

MASLOW'S HIERARCHY OF NEEDS

In the 1970s psychologist Abraham Maslow developed a theory about human needs. His model, known as **Maslow's hierarchy of human needs,** is depicted as a triangular hierarchy of needs (Fig. 5.1). This model, along with more contemporary ones, is still used to describe fundamental human needs. This model is taught as a way of understanding and

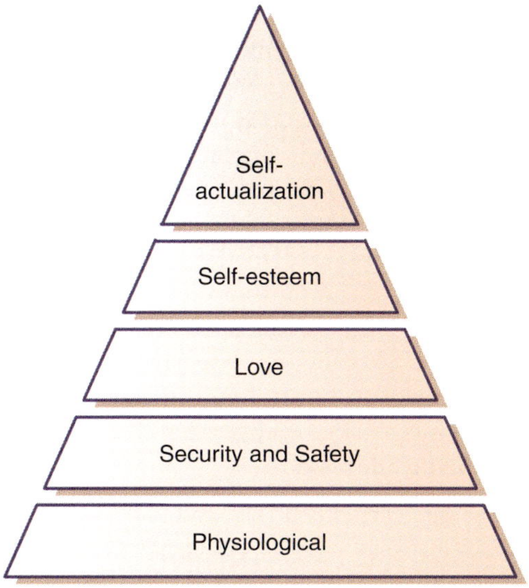

FIG. 5.1 Maslow's hierarchy of human needs. (Redrawn from Maslow AH, Frager RD [Editor], Fadiman J [Editor]: *Motivation and personality*, ed 3. Copyright 1987. Reprinted with permission of Ann Kaplan.))

helping patients cope with the health care process. According to Maslow's model, the most basic requirements for life must be fulfilled for the higher levels to be achieved. In other words, a level of need cannot be met until the one below it has been fulfilled. Maslow's model provides a useful guide for patient care and a method of prioritizing the patient's needs.

ROGERS' PATIENT-CENTERED CARE

Another prominent psychologist, Carl Rogers, worked with Maslow and developed his own theories of personal growth and development. This is called the *person-centered approach.* Rogers believed that every person has the potential for well-being and that, provided with the right environment and humanistic experiences, people will gravitate toward good psychological and physical health. He believed that each person lives a unique experience of life and that individuals "know" or sense what is best for their own emotional and social fulfillment. Among the most important determinants are love, empathy, unconditional acceptance, and "genuineness." According to Rogers' theory, these qualities of human interaction provide the highest level of freedom for self-fulfillment.

LEVEL 1: PHYSIOLOGICAL NEEDS

The most basic of human needs are physiological. These involve the biochemical, mechanical, and physical processes necessary to preserve life (Table 5.1).

LEVEL 2: THE NEED FOR SAFETY AND SECURITY

Safety and security are closely associated with each other. These needs can apply to our health, the ability to care for one's self, to have shelter, and freedom from real or perceived physical or psychological harm.

In the physical realm, people need to be safe from any threat to their well-being. When people are unable to create safety in their lives, it often leads to anxiety and even fear. These fears can diminish the ability to make decisions, have relationships with others, and care for oneself. Most surgical patients experience anxiety. There are many causes directly related to the surgery. But more subtle causes can be related to their concerns about the association of illness and surgery to their independence and the ability to make a living and support their family. Severe anxiety in the presurgical period contributes to alterations in physiological processes, which in turn affect the response to anesthesia. Anxious patients are more likely to have problems such as delirium as they emerge from general anesthesia. Anxiety is also linked to increased requirements for postoperative analgesia and contributes to poor communication between the patient and nursing or medical staff.

Fear of surgery can be complex, involving previous social and emotional experiences. Even though patients may understand the process and objectives of the surgery, their emotions can be overwhelming.

Common Patient Fears

The following are fears that are common to many patients.

ANESTHESIA Many patients fear that they will not awaken from the anesthetic or that they will feel pain while remaining paralyzed (called **anesthesia awareness**). Although this condition is real, it has been given a great deal of attention by the media and depicted in fictional movies. This has created a public fear that is unwarranted. The anesthesia care provider normally explains the process to the patient ahead of the surgery. An empathetic anesthetist or anesthesiologist can relieve many of the patient's anxieties related to the anesthetic agents, physiological care during anesthesia, and the experience of emergence from general anesthesia. Patients who are at high risk for anesthesia awareness can be monitored during surgery for electrical activity, which can be managed with anesthetic agents.

DEATH Fear of death during or after surgery is often greater in a patient who is about to receive a general anesthetic or radical cancer surgery. The concept of being held unconscious and in another's control increases feelings of impending death.

PAIN Fear of pain is a normal protective mechanism. However, surgical patients sometimes have extreme fear of postoperative pain. Perhaps they have unanswered questions about their postoperative care, or they may have experienced severe pain follow surgery in the past.

DISFIGUREMENT Patients undergoing radical or reconstructive surgery have realistic fears about disfigurement. Body image is very important to psychological and social well-being. People identify themselves with physical self-image,

TABLE 5.1 Basic Physiological Needs of the Patient

Need	Management in the Perioperative Environment
Nutrition, water	Administration of intravenous replacement fluids and nutritive or electrolyte fluids
Shelter	Control of temperature through cloth blankets, air heating, or cooling blankets
Air and oxygen	Maintenance of an open airway Provision of the proper mix of oxygen with anesthetic or room air Attention to signs of oxygen deficit
Rest and sleep	Protection from environmental stress such as noise, light, or cold
Elimination	Catheterization or opportunity to void as needed
Movement	Freedom from restraint and assistance with movement when the patient is unable to move on his or her own Protecting the patient from harm
Freedom from pain	Observation of the patient for signs of pain Administration of pain medication Exercise care when moving the patient

which often influences their ability to relate to others. Disfigurement is attached to social stigma and rejection, which are powerful triggers for fear and anxiety. Patients undergoing radical cosmetic surgery or reconstructive procedures can be particularly fearful.

LOSS OF CONTROL When patients enter the health care system, they often feel a loss of personal rights and control. For the surgical patient, these feelings are intensified with the anesthesia experience. The patient may also anticipate immobilization as a result of pain or loss of function. Whereas some patients are stoic about their surgery, others may act regressive, exhibiting childlike behaviors including helplessness.

PHYSICAL EXPOSURE The fear of physical exposure of the body and loss of self-dignity is strong in many patients, especially adolescents. It is very important to cover the patient's body at all times unless absolutely necessary for a procedure.

LOSS OF PRIVACY Many patients are afraid that information about their health may not be held in confidence. They fear that the information may result in loss of employment or that it will injure their relationships with others. The ethical responsibility to hold all patient information in strict confidence cannot be overemphasized. (Refer to Chapter 3 for a more complete discussion of patient privacy.)

Supporting the Fearful Patient

Surgical patients need to trust in those who care for them, not only for comfort and a sense of well-being but also for reduction of stress that can prolong recovery after surgery. Acknowledgment of the patient's fears and showing empathy can ease the patient's anxiety. The patient feels greater security when team members explain, honestly and professionally, what is occurring and why, in a way that is not overly technical. Never dismiss or make light of the patient's feelings. For example, the patient safety strap is secured as soon as the patient is transferred to the operating table. Rather than saying jokingly, "I'm putting this strap over you so that you don't get away," it is better to use reassuring statements such as, "The operating bed is very narrow. I'm putting this strap over your legs to remind you to stay centered on the bed." This statement acknowledges that there is a safety issue but that it is being addressed.

LEVEL 3: LOVE AND BELONGING

Love and belonging are powerful needs. They determine our sense of well-being through the acceptance and nurturing of others. Love and belonging affirm our humanity and provide emotional fulfillment.

People identify with groups that give them a sense of belonging and of being needed. Sports activities, clubs, and family life are important to many people's sense of belonging. If these suddenly become unavailable because of illness or a disability, it can be very disturbing. Social and medical science research have demonstrated that a sense of belonging has a dramatic effect on physical and emotional health. People who are actively involved in their community and family experience a sense of connectedness that is related to good health and even longevity. Social and personal support seem to have positive effects on the immune system and seem to decrease stress, which is a determinant of many diseases.

Family and Community Support

Family support of the patient is extremely important during illness. The surgical patient is often accompanied in the preoperative period by family members and partners, who wait for them during the procedure and postoperative recovery period. The support and care of family and friends is reassuring and healing. Family members may accompany the patient as he or she is taken to the operating room. The moment of separation can be very emotional. A professional, caring attitude toward patients and family is important for all.

LEVEL 4: ESTEEM

Esteem is a measure of respect and admiration for a person. How others perceive us as a person is critical to how we see and care for ourselves. When others judge a person to be *unworthy* as a human, that person reflects these judgments on him- or herself. Think about specific populations in the community who are disrespected for their culture, economic status, faith, or other characteristics. The person who experiences disrespect in the community develops low self-esteem, which often leads to lack of motivation, self-neglect, and poor health.

Body image is closely related to self-esteem. Body image is the way we perceive ourselves physically in the eyes of others. When we are comfortable with our body image, we feel good about ourselves. When a person's body image is altered suddenly or is perceived to be altered, feelings of embarrassment, rejection, and isolation can arise. Patients who need counseling to adjust to sudden changes in their appearance can be guided to support groups or trained specialists.

LEVEL 5: SELF-ACTUALIZATION

Self-actualization features prominently in both humanistic theories presented by Maslow and Rogers. Self-actualization is an individual's ability to plan and achieve his or her life goals based on the physical, social, and psychological freedom (the lower levels of the pyramid) to pursue those achievements. Personal goals are whatever that person defines as a goal or an achievement. The frustration and grief many patients feel during illness can be related to their actual or perceived inability to achieve important life goals, which contribute to their identity. Surgical patients are vulnerable to this risk because of the added psychological burden of altered body image or loss of function. Perioperative caregivers can help their patients through this difficult situation by acknowledging the patient's feelings of loss.

SUPPORTIVE PATIENT CARE

When learning how and when to provide supportive patient care, health care workers must first explore their own attitudes and beliefs because these can interfere with their ability to provide honest, meaningful communication. Professional development in this area can be transforming for the health professional. Some of the more important attitudes that must be explored are the following:

- What are my own beliefs about how to cope with stress?
- Do I hold prejudice against any particular faiths?
- What are my beliefs about psychological disability?
- How do I act around people with severe physical disability?
- How do I normally respond to older adults in the community?
- What are my personal opinions about morbidly obese individuals?
- Do I like children? Do I like being around them?
- What are my assumptions about blind people? Do I assume they need my help in the community?
- What do I know about people who are traumatized? How much of this knowledge is based on what I've seen in the popular media (e.g., TV, movies)?
- Do I know how I would cope if faced with a life-threatening illness?
- What is my attitude toward immigrants, illegal or otherwise?
- What are my core beliefs about faith and spirituality?

It is difficult for anyone to step outside their own beliefs and attitudes to see from another's perspective; however, in health care, this is required. Professionals must explore their own attitudes, which may be stereotypic or prejudicial and ultimately interfere with their care of others. It is a process that requires continual reflection if we truly want to be health professionals.

IMPORTANT TO KNOW *Students are encouraged to assess their personal biases confidentially by using an online tool developed by the Harvard University program* Project Implicit. *The online tool is located at https://implicit.harvard.edu/implicit/takeatouchtest.html.*

SUPPORTIVE PATIENT COMMUNICATION

Today's health care system is fast paced and demanding. The surgical patient is in the center of a storm of activity, in a very busy environment that is unfamiliar and authoritative. Patients have little or no control over what is happening and are handed from one person to the next, often with no knowledge about the roles of the people involved in their care.

Perioperative personnel can alleviate some of the patient's fears and concerns by using **supportive communication techniques**. This is a specific way of communicating that encourages the patient to express concerns. The health care provider then responds to those concerns first by *acknowledging them* and then showing empathy and support.

Supportive Listening

Make eye contact (as appropriate within the patient's culture) and listen attentively. Do not allow yourself to be distracted while communicating with the patient. If your attention is split, you may convey a lack of concern. When people seek comfort from others, whether in the health care setting or in social relationships, they need time to express themselves. Listening—not talking—becomes a valuable means of support, as long as the support person listens attentively and shows that they are listening carefully.

Provide Information

Although some patients do not want to know the details of their surgery, most are eager to understand what is occurring around them. Look and listen for cues that the patient needs information. Be honest about what you do not know. Patients are often unaware of the professional roles of different staff members caring for them. If you are asked a medical question or one that requires assessment or other specialized skills, refer the question. It is better to delay an answer than to mislead the patient or worse, give inaccurate information. The patient may not ask specific questions but instead show concern or worry about some aspect of the environment.

Example question: "I heard that I'll need at least four more surgeries before I can use my arm again. But I have two young kids at home . . ."

Possible response: "Well it all depends on how quickly you are able to recover from this first procedure. It would be best to talk it over with Dr. X after the surgery. If you like, I can tell him you are concerned."

Give Reassurance

The caregiver can provide reassurance while anticipating the patient's concerns.

Example: "Are you wearing dentures? You will need to remove them just before you receive the anesthesia. I will make sure they are in the recovery room for you."

Provide Clarification

Clarification demonstrates that you are listening carefully and supportively.

Example: "Let me understand better. When you say that *you have no one to help you*, do you mean that no one has made arrangements for your home care after the surgery?"

Example: "Does your aunt plan to wait for you here, or should I show her where the surgical waiting area is?"

Example: "Are you cold? We keep the temperature a bit low for safety reasons. I'll get you a warm blanket."

PATIENTS WITH SPECIAL NEEDS

All patients should be supported as they go through the surgical process. However, patients with special needs are likely to require specific types of support. This is especially true of those who are unable to understand or cope with their environment. Patient groups with special needs include children, some older adults, and people with disabilities, especially those that affect their ability to cope in the perioperative environment.

IMPORTANT TO KNOW *Many patients with special needs require specific care related to their medical and physiological requirements. These are discussed in the appropriate chapters such as patient positioning, moving and handling, and anesthesia.*

FEAR IN THE DISORIENTED PATIENT

Fear and anxiety can be overwhelming in patients who do not understand their environment, do not have coping mechanisms for the situation, or are unable to express their emotions or needs. Patients known to have special needs will usually be managed by the anesthesia team and circulating nurse, who have training and experience in psychology. An **anxiolytic** drug is usually administered to patients at risk for severe anxiety.

Specific techniques can be used to support the patient. Remember that the patient may not be oriented or able to respond. Calming techniques are meant to provide an atmosphere that is quiet, comforting, and attentive.

1. Maintain quiet in the room.
2. Soft music may be used to increase a sense of calm in the room, according to facility policy.
3. When speaking to the patient use short, direct sentences. Long explanations or chatter are usually counterproductive. Even if the patient cannot fully understand, a calm but direct way of speaking can sometimes decrease anxiety.
4. Keep your voice calm when speaking to the patient and others in the room.
5. When touching the patient, such as placing the safety strap or ECG leads, use movements that express confidence rather than hesitancy.
6. Watch the patient for any signs of increased agitation, which should be reported to the anesthesia team.
7. Cover the patient with a warm blanket unless there is a risk of hyperthermia. This can provide a feeling of security.

PEDIATRIC PATIENTS

Children need particular support according to their age. Pediatric patient groups are defined according to approximate chronological age ranges. The age group reflects the developmental stage, as shown in Table 5.2.

Developmental Stages of Children

Children of different developmental stages have predictable fears, responses, and reactions to unfamiliar environments such as the operating room. Knowledge of these stages can help the surgical technologist understand the behaviors exhibited by children in the operating room.

Infants need to be physically close to their caretakers. They should be held as much as possible until the procedure begins. When infants are separated from the familiar sight, feel, and smell of their primary caregiver, they are difficult to comfort and may cry continually. For this reason, they are often brought into the operating room and undergo anesthesia while being held by the family member with whom they are most comfortable.

Toddlers become frustrated and anxious when separated from their primary caretaker. The operating room environment can be terrifying to a toddler. Toddlers are especially difficult to comfort; they require patience and understanding from their caregivers. Stronger restraint (or more restrainers) usually causes increased resistance and fear. Taking the time to instill calm is the humane way to provide medical intervention. When this is unsuccessful, rapid sedation may be required. Many hospitals and surgical centers provide opportunities for a child to visit the facility before the scheduled surgery day. This provides an opportunity for the child to experience the environment before the procedure.

Preschoolers have a strong fear of the unknown. These patients commonly view the hospital and surgical experience as a type of punishment and may believe that their family has abandoned them. Prone to fantasy, they may imagine that they

TABLE 5.2 Pediatric Age Groups

Development Stage	Age Range
Infant	Birth to 18 months
Toddler	19 months to 3 years
Preschool	3 to 6 years
School age	7 to 12
Adolescent	13 to 18 years

will be mutilated by surgery. They are concrete thinkers and understand words literally, often in exaggerated terms. Presurgical visits to the facility can also provide reassurance for this age group.

School-age children are more compliant and cooperative with health care personnel, but many tend to withdraw from their caregivers. They are curious about their bodies and often insist on "helping" with their own care. They are very sensitive about body exposure, which can be particularly stressful. This age group uses information-seeking as a coping strategy for fear. Their curiosity can overcome fear, and they welcome simple explanations about their environment.

Adolescents are very sensitive about body image and physical changes. They resist any intrusion on their privacy and physical exposure. They also fear loss of control. At times stoic and curious, they are grateful for concrete information about the surgical environment and the procedure itself. Among their many concerns, potential isolation from their peers and fear of being "left out" because of illness are very important. A more extensive discussion on the needs of the pediatric patient can be found in Chapter 33.

OLDER PATIENTS

Elderly patients are disproportionately affected by stereotyping. The older patient is often spoken to as one may talk to a very young person. This is called *infantilizing* the person—"treating the elderly patient as a small child." This includes speech patterns that use short sentences with simple grammatical structures spoken in a high-pitched voice by the care provider. Another example is using the plural "we" instead of "you."

Example: "And how are we doing today? Did we remember to take our medicine last night?"

Better: "Hello Mrs. X, how are you doing? I need to check that you *did take* the medication that was prescribed to help you sleep last night."

Research in this area has shown poor medical outcomes for patients who are exposed to this type of condescending communication. Instead, speak to the older patient as you would to any adult and provide clarification as necessary.

The following guidelines can be helpful when offering support to the older patient:

- Do not use clichés. Do not reach for the first available, easiest response. For example, if the patient says that she is a burden to others in her illness, do not respond with, "Oh, I'm sure you're no bother." Instead, support the patient in her feelings by active listening. Acknowledge her worries. Instead of negating her concern, acknowledge it. It is not necessary to find a solution, but it is important to listen and provide an opportunity for her to speak more about the problem.
- Do not refer to the patient by diminutives such as "sweetie" or "honey." These names are offensive to many patients and can be interpreted as a lack of respect. Always address the patient by his or her proper name.

IMPORTANT TO KNOW *In some regions of the United States, health care workers refer to themselves, others in the clinical area, and their patients by their first name. Use discretion when adapting this practice. Do not assume that the older patient is cognitively impaired. The normal aging process does not include dementia. Some patients are slightly disoriented in the hospital. This is often related to poor eyesight or hearing. Perioperative caregivers should support patients by orienting them to the physical environment and by providing information about their surroundings.*

- The patient's chart should alert caregivers to any sensory deficits and this should be managed appropriately. Specific care of the patient with sight and hearing deficits are discussed in Chapters 25 and 26.

PATIENTS WITH A DEVELOPMENTAL DISABILITY

Developmental disabilities refer to a large group of diseases or conditions that affect movement, posture, cognitive ability, and behavior. The following conditions are included in but not limited to this category:

- Cognitive disability
- Learning disabilities
- Asperger disorder
- Autism spectrum disorders

There is a very large spectrum of diseases that can be regarded as developmental and learning disabilities. For the purposes of this discussion, it is important to understand that the syndromes are complex. Although many exhibit common features, each patient expresses the condition according to his or her personality, environment, previous experience in the health care system, and complex emotional factors.

The Person Is Not the Disease

In caring for patients with developmental delay, it is important to use terms that respect the individual and that apply to that patient. For example, Down syndrome is only one of many chromosomal defects resulting in development and learning disability. When speaking about a patient with family members, and colleagues, use "people-first" language. A person with a disability *has* the disability. He or she is not a "victim" of Down syndrome or "afflicted by cerebral palsy." These phrases define the patient as a disease. Some guidelines for people-first language are as follows:

- Name the person first, not the disability:
  A person with a disability, *not a disabled person*
  An adult with autism, *not an autistic adult*
- Use neutral expressions:
  An individual who had a stroke, *not a stroke victim*
- Use preferred language:
  Use cognitive disability, *not mentally retarded*

The perioperative experience for patients with learning or developmental disability may not require special techniques outside of empathetic, safety-conscious care. In cases in which patients are difficult to provide care to because of agitation, the anesthesia team provides guidance to prevent patient injury related to uncoordinated or erratic movement

SPIRITUAL NEEDS OF THE PATIENT

Spirituality is a sense or understanding of something more profound than humanity that is not perceived by the physical senses. Spirituality is not necessarily the same as religion, although they are often expressed as a single entity. It is an awareness or belief in an energy or power greater than humankind. This power may be referred to as creator, spirit, or God(s), or the patient may have no name for it. In the religious setting, spiritual life is integrated into rituals (practices that have special meaning) and ceremonies common to those who practice a particular faith.

Patients often express their religious faith while in the health care setting. The expression may be through prayer or other sacred rituals. Ritual defines life-changing events and is important to physical and mental healing. For many it *is* the healing force. Health professionals may avoid becoming involved in the spiritual needs of the patient because they are uncomfortable or perhaps have not faced this dimension of care in the past. With today's short-stay practices, patients can come into the health care facility and leave the same day, even after complex procedures. Caregivers in this environment do not have the opportunity to witness spiritual practices as they apply to sickness and healing. However, it is important for all health care professionals to learn at least the basic beliefs of the people in their community. These faith groups are likely to be the most common encountered in a health care facility. Faith can be a major force for many patients and may even play an equal role in their well-being along with the medical or surgical procedures they undergo.

SELF LEARNING: Box 5.1 shows links to resources for learning about different practices and beliefs of various faiths.

Patients may bring religious items into the health care setting that reinforce their faith and provide a source of strength. These may be items that assist in prayer such as icons, religious jewelry, and prayer books. It is very important to safeguard these items to prevent their loss. Jewelry may not be worn during surgery. If a patient is reluctant to remove an item, the caregiver needs to carefully explain what the risks are. Whenever possible, a family member can take care of the item until the patient returns from surgery.

All operating room staff should learn where the prayer areas are in their facility and how to contact the facility's chaplain. The health facility's chaplaincy staff are highly trained in providing spiritual support to patients and their families. If a chaplain of a particular faith is not on staff, one can be found through the chaplaincy's resources.

Many faiths have specific religious laws that relate to or are frequently encountered in health care. These are contained in the rules or canons. Some practices that are often subject to ruling are the following:

- Abortion
- Alternative medicines or substances for healing
- Amputation
- Artificial insemination
- Autopsy
- Bathing restrictions
- Birth control
- Burial of an amputated limb
- Complex diet restrictions
- Cremation (may be forbidden)
- Cutting of any body hair (e.g., forbidden in Sikhism)
- Disposition of the placenta
- Donation of organs
- Donation of the deceased's body
- Embalming (may be forbidden)
- Euthanasia
- Medicines derived from blood products
- Opioids or stimulants
- Spiritual objects attached to the body (see Sikhism)
- The use of blood or blood products
- Unction during sickness and death (anointing with sacred oil)

Note that cultural practices may be strictly practiced but not required by religious law.

BOX 5.1 Resources for Self-Learning About Faiths and Cultures

An excellent resource for learning about spiritual, religious, and cultural beliefs is The Cultural Sensitivity Handbook published online by the Healthcare Chaplaincy at http://www.healthcarechaplaincy.org/docs/publications/landing_page/cultural_sensitivity_handbook_from_healthcare_chaplaincy_network.pdf.

Another comprehensive source is Rosewell Park Cancer Institute, "Caring Across Cultures and Belief Systems in an Interfaith World": https://www.roswellpark.org/sites/default/files/node-files/page/nid940-21946-caring-across-cultures-web.pdf.

Both sources include the most recent information about faiths that have sanctions for receiving blood and blood products, medications, and other practices encountered in the health care system. Note that Jehovah Witnesses are not the only faith that is concerned about these practices.

IMPORTANT TO KNOW *All health facilities maintain directives and requirements for the disposition of body parts, including the placenta.*

KEY CONCEPTS

- The needs of humans have been summarized in a theory known as Maslow's hierarchy of human needs. This theory, which is commonly used to identify areas of focus for patient care, includes physiological needs, protection, and relational and personal needs.
- Communication with the patient establishes the basis of all care.
- In patient-centered care, the surgical team bases its assessments, planning, and interventions on the patient *as an individual.*
- Supportive communication is a learned skill that all health care professionals can develop.

- Special patient populations have particular psychosocial support.
- Patients use different types of coping strategies for dealing with preoperative anxiety.
- Patients with a severe hearing deficit or language barrier require an interpreter to ensure their understanding of the surgical procedure and its consequences.
- Patients who are fearful or anxious about their surgery may exhibit regressive behavior.
- Pediatric patients, especially adolescents, are particularly sensitive about body exposure and self-image.
- Developmental disabilities are a large group of diseases or conditions that affect movement, posture, cognitive ability, behavior, and learning processes.
- Patients often seek comfort through their faith and religious rituals.
- Most religions have specific rules or practices that are encountered in their health care. These are regarded as sacred to their faith, and all efforts are made to accommodate them in the health care setting.
- Some faith communities advocate specific disposition of body parts that have been surgically removed. Efforts are made to accommodate the beliefs within the boundaries of public health considerations.

All surgical staff are encouraged to find out where the health facility's chaplaincy services and chapels are located to support the patient's and their families' spiritual needs.

REVIEW QUESTIONS

1. Define patient-centered care.
2. Discuss the domains of Maslow's hierarchy.
3. What is body image? In what ways does body image influence a patient's anxiety about surgery?
4. What methods would you use in supportive communication?
5. Why should health care workers examine their values concerning special needs populations?
6. What is developmental disability?
7. Why is body image a source of anxiety for adolescents?
8. Why might the patient with a sensory deficit be particularly anxious in surgery?

SCASE STUDIES

CASE 1

A patient has arrived for a scheduled C-section. When you arrive at the patient holding area to check her chart, she informs you that she wants to take the placenta home to bury it. What should you do with this information?

CASE 2

There is debate among health care professionals, including allied health, whether spirituality should be included in their curricula. Briefly provide your arguments on both sides of this issue.

CASE 3

A patient has expressed that he worries that after his surgery he will no longer be able to play with his grandchildren. What specific needs is he expressing? How would you respond to him?

CASE 4

Today you are working in the outpatient clinic. Your patient is a 38-year-old mother of two. She is scheduled to have a hernia repair under general anesthetic. You are escorting her to the operating room when she tells you that she saw a program on television about a woman who underwent surgery and felt everything that was done to her, even though she had general anesthesia. She appears quite anxious as she tells the story.

To what is this patient referring? How can you provide support and reassurance?

BIBLIOGRAPHY

Aust H, Rüsch D, Schuster M, Sturm T, Brehm F, Nestoriuc Y. Coping strategies in anxious surgical patients. *BMC Health Serv Res.* 2016;16:250.

Collier R. Person-first language: noble intent but to what effect. *CMAJ: Can Med Assoc J.* 2012;184(18):1977–1978.

Dreger V, Tremback T. Management of preoperative anxiety in children. *AORN J.* 2006;84(5).

Kourkouta L, Papathanasiou IV. Communication in nursing practice. *Materia Socio-Medica.* 2014;26(1):65–67.

Park Cancer Institute Rosewell. Caring across cultures and belief systems in an interfaith world. Retrieved at https://www.roswellpark.org/sites/default/files/node-files/page/nid940-21946-caring-across-cultures-web.pdf. Accessed on June 16, 2019.

Thompson DG. Tielsch-Goddard A Improving management of patients with autism spectrum disorder having scheduled surgery: optimizing practice. *J Pediatr Health Care.* 2014;28(5):394–403. https://doi.org/10.1016/j.pedhc.2013.09.007. Epub 2013 Nov 25.

6 DIAGNOSTIC AND ASSESSMENT PROCEDURES

LEARNING OBJECTIVES

After studying this chapter, the reader will be able to:

1. Describe the proper procedure for taking the patient's vital signs
2. Accurately document vital sign measurements
3. Describe the use of an electrocardiograph
4. List and define commonly used imaging studies
5. Discuss basic blood and urine chemistry tests
6. Describe different methods of tissue biopsy
7. Describe the effects of malignancy on the body
8. Discuss cancer screening

TERMINOLOGY

ABO blood group: Inherited antigens are found on the surface of an individual's red blood cells. These antigens identify the blood group (i.e., type A blood has type A antigens). Also known as blood type.

Acute illness: Sudden onset of disease or trauma or disease of short duration, usually 3 weeks or less.

Benign: A term used to characterize a tumor that does not have the capability to spread to other parts of the body and is usually composed of tissue similar to its tissue of origin.

Chronic illness: An illness that has continued for months, weeks, or years.

Complete blood count (CBC): A blood test that measures specific components, including the hemoglobin, hematocrit, red blood cells, and white blood cells.

Computed tomography (CT): An imaging technique that allows physicians to obtain cross-sectional x-ray views of the patient. The result is a CT scan.

Contrast medium: A fluid that is not penetrable by x-rays, used to determine the contours of a part of the body.

Diastolic pressure: The pressure exerted on the walls of the blood vessels during the resting phase of cardiac contraction.

Differential count: A test that determines the number of each type of white blood cell in a specimen of blood.

Digital radiography (DR): An imaging system that uses flat panel detectors to capture images, which are then immediately translated into digital data.

Doppler studies: A technique that uses ultrasonic waves to measure blood flow in a vessel.

Electrocardiography: A noninvasive assessment of the heart's electrical activity displayed on a graph, the electrocardiogram. In the United States, electrocardiogram is abbreviated correctly as ECG. EKG is the European abbreviation.

Endoscopic procedures: Medical assessment of body cavities using a fiber-optic instrument (endoscope).

Fluoroscopy: A radiological technique that provides real-time images of an anatomical region.

Gantry: The circumferential opening in the O-ring fluoroscopy machine. The gantry is positioned within the long axis of the operating table enabling it to produce 3-D images.

Hematocrit (Hct): The ratio of red blood cells to plasma, measured as a percentage.

Hemoglobin (Hgb): The oxygen-carrying molecule found in red blood cells. The amount of hemoglobin in the patient's blood is measured in grams per deciliter (g/dL).

Imaging studies: Diagnostic tests that produce a picture or image.

Invasive procedure: A medical or nursing procedure in which the skin is penetrated, or a body cavity is entered.

Magnetic resonance imaging (MRI): A diagnostic technique that uses radiofrequency signals and magnetic energy to produce images.

Malignant: A term used to characterize tissue that shows disorganized, uncontrolled growth (cancer). Malignant tissue has the potential to spread to distant areas of the body. It is then termed metastatic.

Mean arterial pressure (MAP): The average amount of pressure exerted throughout the cardiac cycle.

Metastasis: The spread of cancerous cells to a local or distant area of the body.

Neoplasm: A tumor, which may be benign or malignant.

Nuclear medicine: Medical procedures that use radioactive particles to track target tissues in the body.

Orthostatic (postural) blood pressure: Refers to a technique used to check the patient's blood pressure in the upright and recumbent positions.

Palpating: Assessing a part of the body by feeling the outline, density, movement, or other attributes.

Partial thromboplastin time (PTT): A test of blood coagulation used in patients receiving heparin to determine the correct level of anticoagulation.

Positron emission tomography (PET): A type of medical imaging that measures specific metabolic activity in the target tissue.

Prothrombin time (PT): A measurement of the time required for blood to clot.

Pulse pressure: A measurement of the difference between the systolic pressure and diastolic pressure. This can be a significant sign of metabolic disturbance.

Radioactive seeds: Small particles of radioactive material implanted in tissue for cancer treatment.

Radionuclides or isotopes: In nuclear medicine, radioactive particles are directed at the nucleus of a selected element to create energy. These special elements are referred to as radionuclides or isotopes.

Radiopaque: A substance that is impenetrable by x-rays.

Sphygmomanometer: An instrument used to measure blood pressure.

Staging: An international method of classifying tissue to determine the level of metastasis in cancer.

Systolic pressure: The pressure exerted by blood on the walls of vessels during the contraction phase of the cardiac cycle.

TNM classification system: An international system for determining the extent of metastasis and the level of cell differentiation, two important factors in the treatment and prognosis of cancer.

Transcutaneous: Literally "through the skin"; it refers to a procedure in which a needle or other medical device is inserted through the skin.

Tumor marker: An antigen present on the tumor cell, or a substance (protein, hormone, or other chemical) released by cancer cells into the blood.

Vital signs Cardinal signs of well-being: Cardinal signs of well-beingpain, temperature, pulse, respiration, and blood pressure. These are measured to assess a patient's basic metabolic status.

The first step in medical and surgical decision making is assessment, which provides clues and information about the nature of the patient's illness and the possible causes. In this process, a general assessment is followed by more complex investigations.

Diagnostic procedures and tests are often performed to confirm or rule out a diagnosis. In some cases, invasive tests are required. An **invasive procedure** involves penetrating intact skin or mucous membrane or inserting a medical device into a body cavity. Noninvasive procedures are limited to skin contact or no direct contact with the body. Interventional radiology procedures combine technologies such as x-ray or other imaging tools with invasive techniques.

This chapter is an orientation to commonly performed tests and diagnostic procedures. Surgical technologists participate in a variety of invasive diagnostic procedures described in this chapter and throughout the book. **Endoscopic procedures,** in which a fiber-optic instrument is passed through a body cavity for examination and biopsy, are described in Chapters 20 and 22 and in each procedural chapter according to specialty. Bacteriological and other tests required for the investigation of infectious diseases are described in Chapter 8. Diagnostic tests associated with a particular medical specialty are described in the chapter associated with that specialty.

CONCEPTS RELATED TO PATHOLOGY

Pathology is the study of disease and can also refer to a specific illness. Illness can be caused by a number of different environmental and physiological conditions, or one single factor. The term *etiology* means *cause*. For example, you might see "etiology unknown" written in the patient's chart. This means that the cause of the disease or condition was unknown at the time of examination. Primary health care providers use the word *idiopathic* to mean that the condition arose suddenly or spontaneously without apparent cause, such as "idiopathic hypertension," meaning the patient developed high blood pressure without an apparent cause. The terms *morbidity* (rate of illness in the population) and *mortality* (rate of death in the population) are used in the field of epidemiology, which focuses on population health. For example, syncytial rhinovirus (a common cold virus) is associated with high morbidity and low mortality in most populations.

When a patient is being assessed, specific terms are used to describe the disease process and outcome. When discussing the disease itself, we usually refer to its *course*. For example, "the patient experienced abdominal pain throughout the course of the infection." A more formal term referring to the origin and development of the disease is *pathogenesis*. *Signs* of a condition are the measurable evidence (e.g., rash, fever, injury, loss of function). For example, signs of disease may include "There is marked swelling of the lower lid, with serosanguinous drainage at the medial punctum." *Symptoms* are what the patient reports: for example, "The patient reports gradual loss of vision in the left eye over 5 days."

Events related to the disease state are also qualified using specific terms. A *complication* of disease is separate from the primary problem but occurs at the same time or as a consequence of the main problem. A complication usually causes the main problem to be more serious or complex. For example, "The nonunion fracture was caused by postoperative infection, complicated by poor nutritional intake." Sometimes, the term *exacerbation* is used to mean worsen or become more serious. A *syndrome* is a unique group of signs associated with a specific disease.

The course of the disease is defined by specific terms. The *prognosis* is a prediction of the outcome of a condition or medical intervention. This is usually expressed with general terms such as excellent, good, or poor. If the disease subsides (goes into *remission*) and then returns again, it is called a *relapse*. An illness that will result in death is said to be *terminal. A condition can be acute (came on suddenly) or chronic (long term).*

The treatment of disease also uses special vocabulary. *Curative* refers to treatment that is meant to resolve the medical problem. However, *palliative* care is intended to make the condition more tolerable, without actually curing it.

VITAL SIGNS

Taking a patient's **vital signs** allows an overall evaluation of the person's well-being. This is the most basic form of clinical assessment. In some facilities, the surgical technologist may be required to measure the patient's vital signs. These are documented and reported to the registered nurse or surgeon. The surgical technologist is not expected to interpret the measurements or make a diagnosis on the basis of the results. However, *accurate measurement* is always required. The vital signs include the following:

- Temperature
- Pulse
- Respiration
- Blood pressure

During general anesthesia or deep sedation, vital signs are measured almost continuously with complex biomedical devices. In simple procedures performed with a local anesthetic, noninvasive techniques are used.

Baseline values (i.e., those taken at the beginning of an assessment period) may vary from "normal" limits.

TEMPERATURE

Normal body temperature is 98.6°F (37.2°C) with normal variations of 1°F (0.6°C). The body requires a core (internal) temperature of approximately 99°F (37.2°C) to maintain physiological functions. The core temperature is regulated by the hypothalamus through a complex feedback system that balances the core temperature with environmental factors. However, when environmental factors or disease exceed the body's ability to adjust, vital functions deteriorate, and this can result in serious tissue injury or death.

Temperature is recorded and documented in degrees Celsius. The formula for conversion from the two systems is as follows:

$$\text{Fahrenheit} \rightarrow \text{Celsius}^{\circ}\text{ C} = {}^{5}\!/_{9}\ ({}^{\circ}\text{F} - 32)$$

$$\text{Celsius} \rightarrow \text{Fahrenheit }{}^{\circ}\text{F} = {}^{\circ}\text{C} \times {}^{9}\!/_{5} + 32$$

Methods of Measuring Temperature

The site where the temperature is measured affects the reading.

- The oral temperature is measured under the tongue *(sublingually)*. The tongue is highly vascular and accurately reflects the core temperature. The normal oral temperature in a person at rest is 98.6°F (37°C). The normal range is 96.4° to 99.1°F (35.8° to 37.3°C).
- Temporal artery temperature measured with a temporal artery thermometer (TAT) is approximately 0.8°F (0.4°C) higher than the oral temperature.
- The *tympanic* temperature accurately assesses core temperature through the external auditory canal.
- The *rectal* temperature varies from 0.7° to 1°F (0.4° to 0.5°C) higher than the oral value.
- The *axillary* temperature is measured at the axilla. Readings are 0.5° to 1°F (0.3° to 0.6°C) lower than the oral value.
- The forehead, or skin, temperature varies with environmental changes.

Use of Thermometers

Always wear gloves when taking the patient's temperature. Probe and tympanic thermometers can harbor an infectious biofilm that may not be visible. Even though only the probe cover comes in contact with patient tissue, the units are often heavily laden with bacteria.

The TAT has replaced many other types of patient thermometers in the clinic setting. The thermometer probe is noninvasive and accurate when used properly. It can be used on patients of all ages. After disinfection with an alcohol wipe, the probe is gently swiped in a straight line from the center of the forehead laterally to cross the temporal artery, lifted from the skin, and placed briefly behind the ear lobe. It is not placed at the temple, which is a common user error.

The *electronic probe thermometer* consists of a sensing probe connected to a handheld reader with a light-emitting diode (LED) or liquid crystal display (LCD) format. This type of thermometer is used primarily for oral and axillary measurements. A clean probe cover must be used on each patient to prevent the spread of infection. The measurement is displayed after about 30 seconds.

To use the electronic thermometer, make sure the batteries are charged and the unit is clean. Insert the tip into a new disposable probe cover and press gently. This attaches the cover to the probe. Then, proceed as follows:

- *Oral temperature:* Gently insert the probe under the patient's tongue.
- *Axillary temperature:* When the thermometer is used in the axilla, make sure the tip of the probe does not extend outside the body. In children, it is best to hold the upper arm in contact with the body to ensure an accurate reading. Stabilize the probe until the reading is obtained.
- *Rectal temperature:* Rectal temperature readings are seldom performed or required except in critical care and during general anesthesia because safer and more accurate technologies have been developed. Have the patient lie on his or her side with the uppermost knee flexed. The probe tip should be lubricated after the probe cover is applied. Spread the buttocks with one hand and gently insert the probe approximately 1½ inches (3.75 cm). If stool is encountered during insertion, remove the probe, replace the cover, and begin again. Stabilize the probe until the reading is completed. The risk of puncturing the rectal mucosa and musculature exists when a rectal probe is used. This method is used only when *no other method is available.* The tympanic or temporal methods are preferred over the rectal method. Remove the probe and dispose of the cover in a hazardous waste container. Wash your hands thoroughly and record the measurement.
- *Tympanic membrane thermometer:* This may be used on conscious or unconscious patients. It is the preferred method of temperature assessment in the clinical setting. The tympanic thermometer receives infrared signals from the eardrum. It provides an accurate reading of core temperature, because the tympanic membrane shares its

TABLE 6.1 Normal Pulse and Respiratory Rates by Age*

Age (Years)	Normal Pulse Rate (Range) (Beats per Minute)	Normal Respiration (Breaths per Minute)
0	120 (70–190)	30–40
1	120 (80–190)	21–40
2	110 (80–130)	25–32
4	110 (80–120)	23–30
6	100 (75–115)	21–26
8	100 (70–110)	21–26
10	90 (70–110)	21–26
12	90 (70–110)	18–22
14	85 (65–105)	18–22
16	85 (60–100)	16–20
18	75 (55–95)	12–20
Adult	75 (60–100)	10–20
Athlete	50-60 (50–100)	10–20

*Male children may have slightly lower values.

blood supply with the carotid artery. The instrument is shaped like an otoscope, and single-use probe covers are used to prevent cross-contamination among patients. To use the thermometer, clean the probe using a soft alcohol wipe. Place a disposable probe cover over the tip. Direct the tip into the external ear canal. Rotate the thermometer slightly to seat it into the ear canal and retract the skin in front of the ear to seat the tip. Release the skin before taking the reading. Remember that the infrared beam must "see" the tympanic membrane for an accurate reading. Press the activate button and wait for an audible beep from the thermometer. Remove the earpiece gently and dispose of the cover. Record the measurement.

Glass thermometers, which contain a colored solution, have been replaced by electronic or digital instruments. Mercury is no longer used in the manufacture of glass thermometers because of concerns with environmental safety. Health care workers may occasionally be required to use a glass thermometer, which first must be briskly shaken to lower the liquid column.

MEASURING THE PULSE

The pulse is a reflection of the stroke volume (amount of blood pumped through the heart) of each beat. The pulse is felt in the artery as it expands with each heartbeat. The normal heart rate varies according to age, condition, and metabolic level. Disease or injury alters the metabolic level and affects the heart rate, rhythm, and strength. Table 6.1 lists normal resting pulse rates by age. The normal pulse rate for an adult is 60 to 100 beats per minute.

The *strength* of the peripheral pulse can vary with changes in metabolism, disease, or injury. A normal pulse feels elastic

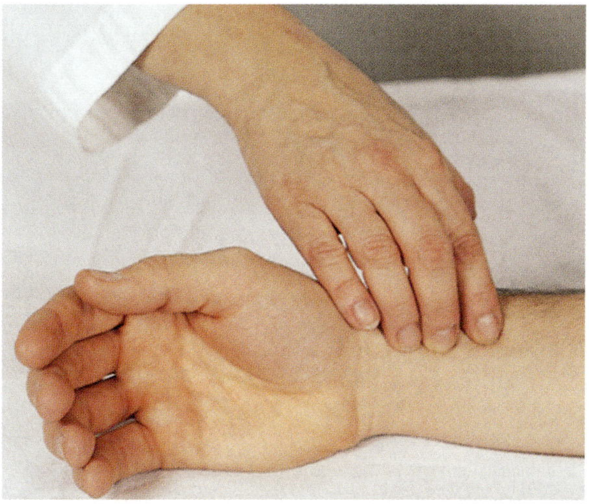

FIG. 6.1 Measuring the radial pulse. (From Jarvis C, ed. *Physical Examination and Health Assessment.* 5th ed. Philadelphia: Saunders; 2008.)

and has moderate strength. A "bounding" pulse is one that feels exceptionally strong, whereas a weak pulse may be barely palpable or "thready." A three-point or four-point scale is used to report the strength of the pulse:

- Bounding: 3+
- Normal: 2+
- Weak 1+
- Absent: 0

The pulse is measured by **palpating** (feeling) an artery. The radial artery located on the inner side of the wrist (Fig. 6.1) is commonly used to measure pulse, but any other artery can be used. Box 6.1 describes the location and method of palpating major arteries.

Always use the pads of your first three fingers to measure the pulse, because the thumb has its own pulse, which may be confused with the patient's pulse. Also, applying excessive pressure depresses the artery and stops circulation.

When you have located the pulse, count the number of beats in 30 seconds and multiply this number by 2 to get the beats per minute. The baseline reading (the first taken) should be counted for a full minute. Further, if at any time the pulse is irregular, you must count for 60 full seconds. Keep in mind that an irregular pulse or a missed beat may result in a difference of 4 or 5 beats per minute in the measurement.

RESPIRATION

The respiratory rate is an objective assessment of the number of breaths per minute. It is altered by exertion, metabolic stress, strong emotion, and the effect of specific drugs, which can depress or stimulate the autonomic nervous system.

The respiratory rate is measured by observing the patient's thorax and abdomen and recording the breaths per minute. It is measured when the patient is unaware, because people often alter their breathing pattern when under observation. To measure the respiratory rate, count the number of breaths in 30 seconds and multiply this number by 2. Normal respiratory rates are listed in Table 6.1.

BOX 6.1 Location and Method of Palpating Major Arteries

- The temporal artery is located between the ear and outer eye in the depression above the cheek bone.
- The carotid artery is located in the depression between the sternocleidomastoid muscle and the trachea, at the side of the neck midway between the clavicle and the jaw.
- The brachial artery can be felt in the groove that runs along the side of the biceps muscle on the inside (medial aspect) of the upper arm. To locate this artery, flex the biceps to locate the groove and then relax the muscle to palpate. This pulse can also be felt in the antecubital fossa behind the elbow. This is the artery used to measure the patient's blood pressure.
- The radial artery is most often used to assess a patient's pulse in the clinical setting because it is easily accessible. Palpate this artery by placing the fingers on the radial bone and sliding them slightly toward the inner wrist so that they rest in the groove next to the bone.
- The femoral artery is very important in surgery. This artery is most often used to cannulate the larger vessels of the trunk for an angiogram (arteriography) and in the placement of stents. To palpate the artery, place your fingers in the deepest furrow of the groin where the upper leg joins the pelvis. You may have to press firmly, because the femoral artery lies deep in the fascia and muscle.
- The popliteal artery is an extension of the femoral artery. It can be felt at the back of the knee in the depression at the top of the tibia, behind the patella.
- The dorsalis pedis branches from the popliteal artery and is located over the front of the foot in the depression between the great and second toes.
- The posterior tibial artery lies in the furrow between the Achilles tendon and the tibial process (ankle bone).

NOTE *Medical assessment of breath sounds, such as tone, pitch, pattern, and rhythm, is required for complex assessment of respiratory disease.*

BLOOD PRESSURE

Blood pressure is the force exerted on the vessel walls by the blood as it is pumped through the body. Vascular pressure changes during the cardiac cycle (filling of the heart chambers and shunting of blood through the heart). When the blood is forcefully pumped through the left ventricle, the pressure is at its greatest. This is called the **systolic pressure.** As the heart muscle relaxes between contractions, the blood pressure is lowered. This is called the **diastolic pressure.** The **mean arterial pressure (MAP)** is the average amount of pressure exerted throughout the cardiac cycle. When blood pressure is assessed, the difference between the diastolic and systolic pressures can be a significant sign. This is called the **pulse pressure.** Fig. 6.2 shows changes in pressure that occur throughout the cardiac cycle. Many diseases cause changes in blood pressure. It is also important to understand how normal physiological processes can affect blood pressure.

Factors That Affect Blood Pressure

Normal blood pressure for an adult is 120/80 mm Hg. Blood pressure varies by age and is affected by various other normal physiological conditions, including the following:

- Weight
- Exertion
- Stress
- Strong emotion

Gender is another factor; blood pressure tends to be lower in adult women than in men. Important normal physiological factors that influence blood pressure include the following:

- *Cardiac output:* The total amount of blood pumped through the heart in 1 minute.
- *Stroke volume:* The amount of blood pumped during ventricular contraction. The total blood volume alters the cardiac output.
- *Peripheral vascular resistance:* The static pressure of the blood vessels against the flow of blood. As the blood vessels contract and relax, peripheral vascular resistance changes. Vessel obstruction also increases vascular resistance.
- *Resilience of the cardiac and vascular systems:* The elasticity of the vessels and heart muscle directly affects vascular pressure.

Procedure for Taking Blood Pressure

A simple blood pressure assessment requires both the diastolic and systolic measurements.

Blood pressure is measured with an electronic (digital) or manual **sphygmomanometer,** which requires the use of a stethoscope. The stethoscope method provides a more thorough assessment.

The method used to take the blood pressure is critical to obtaining a correct reading. Table 6.2 lists common errors in blood pressure measurement. A sphygmomanometer has three components: the cuff, the pump, and the gauge. A manual blood pressure apparatus has a round gauge with numerical values and a pointer. Electronic blood pressure devices display the measurement on an LED or LCD panel attached to the control unit. The blood pressure cuff is an inflatable bladder covered with fabric that is secured to the patient's limb with Velcro.

Blood pressure can be measured in several locations on an arm or a leg. For adults, the most common location is the upper arm (i.e., the brachial artery). The cuff should be no larger than 40% of the circumference of the person's upper arm. Cuffs are available in many sizes, from pediatric to extra large. An incorrectly sized cuff is a common error in blood pressure measurement (see Table 6.2). This can lead to a falsely high or low reading.

The patient should be sitting or lying in a relaxed position. The arm must be at the level of the heart, and it should be supported on a surface. The person taking the reading may also support the arm, but it must be at heart level. Wrap the cuff around the patient's upper arm so that the air tubes are in line with the inner arm and brachial artery (Fig. 6.3).

HOW TO USE A MANUAL SPHYGMOMANOMETER

1. Before taking a reading, you must locate the general systolic pressure. Palpate the brachial artery, which is

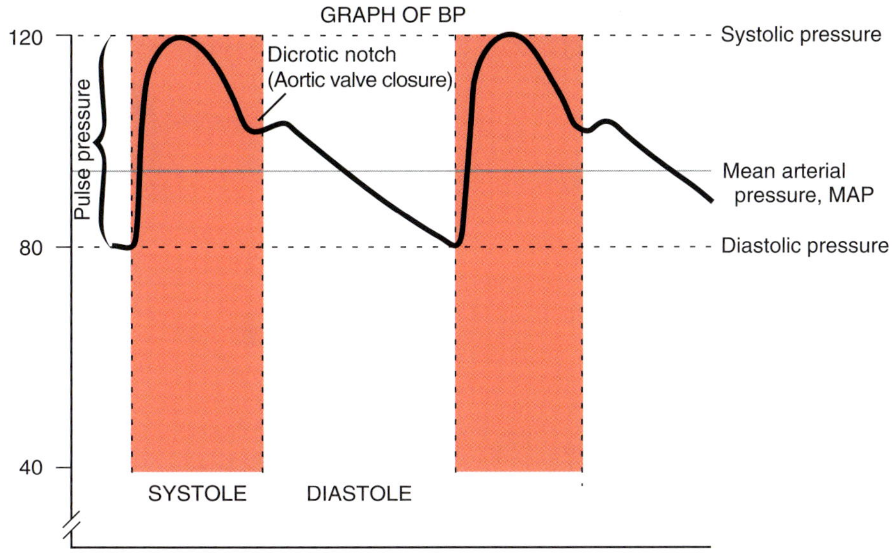

FIG. 6.2 Graph of the cardiac cycle. (From Jarvis C, ed. *Physical Examination and Health Assessment.* 5th ed. Philadelphia: Saunders; 2008.)

TABLE 6.2 Common Errors in Blood Pressure Measurement

Result of Measurement	Cause of Inaccuracy
• False high systolic and diastolic pressures	• Blood pressure taken when patient is upset or anxious • Measurement taken after exertion • Wrong size cuff (too narrow) • Cuff too loose or unevenly wrapped • Arm below heart level
• False low systolic and diastolic pressures	• Arm above heart level • Failure to inflate cuff sufficiently
• False low systolic pressure	• Failure to inflate cuff sufficiently • Cuff deflated too quickly
• False low diastolic pressure	• Stethoscope pressed too hard on artery
• False high diastolic pressure	• Cuff deflated too slowly • Stopping deflation and reinflating • Failing to wait longer than 2 minutes between readings
• Any type of error	• Working too fast • Faulty technique • Defective equipment

just above the antecubital fossa. Center the cuff above the fossa. Do not allow the cuff to slide down, because this obscures the measurement.

2. With your fingers over the brachial artery, inflate the cuff until the arterial pulse is no longer palpable. Continue to inflate another 25 to 30 mm above this point.

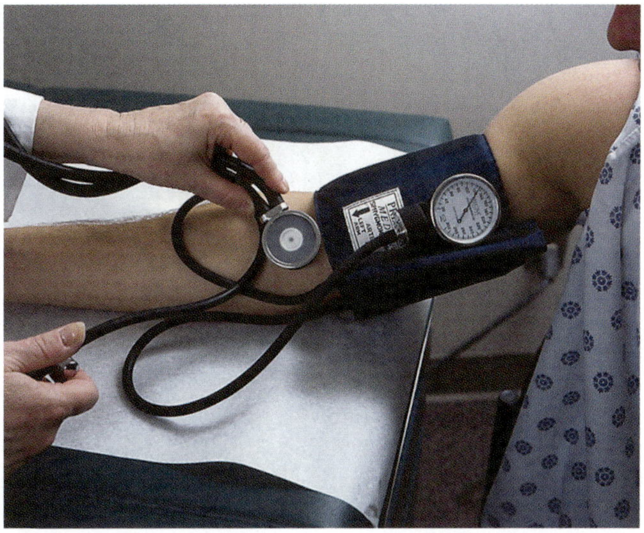

FIG. 6.3 Correct positioning of the blood pressure cuff. (From Jarvis C, ed. *Physical Examination and Health Assessment.* 5th ed. Philadelphia: Saunders; 2008.)

3. Release the cuff and wait 10 to 15 seconds. This allows blood to return to the artery.
4. Place the bell end of the stethoscope over the artery and inflate the cuff to the level you previously measured.
5. Slowly deflate the cuff and listen for the first sound of the pulse. Observe the correct level on the gauge or liquid column. *This is the systolic reading.*
6. Continue to deflate until you hear a muffled pulse and then the disappearance of the pulse. The diastolic measurement is the point where the pulse was no longer audible.
7. If the difference between the muffled sound and no sound is greater than 10 mm Hg, you must document all three measurements. In some facilities, the middle sound is always documented.
8. To document the blood pressure, write the systolic pressure over the diastolic pressure (e.g., 140/70). If you document the middle sound, it is written between

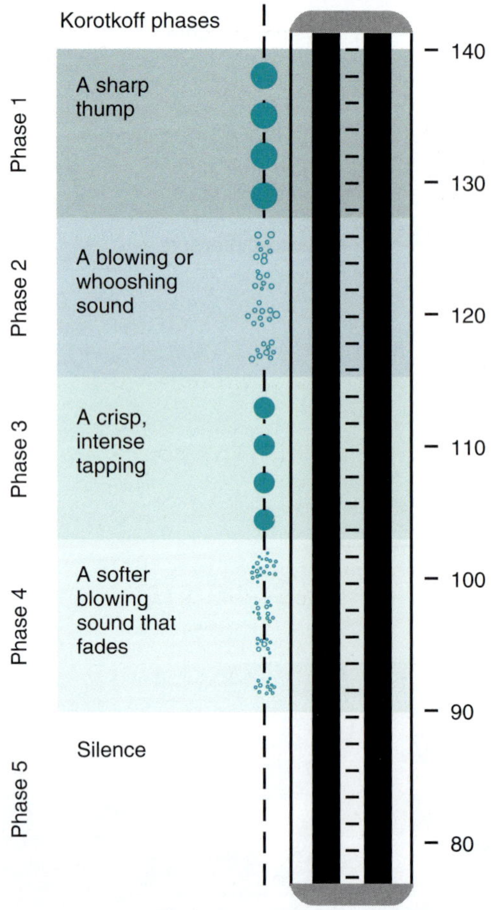

FIG. 6.4 Korotkoff sounds and blood pressure. Taking the blood pressure with a sphygmomanometer and stethoscope provides a detailed assessment of the sounds. (From Perry AG, Potter P, eds. *Basic Nursing*. 11th ed. St Louis: Mosby; 2012.)

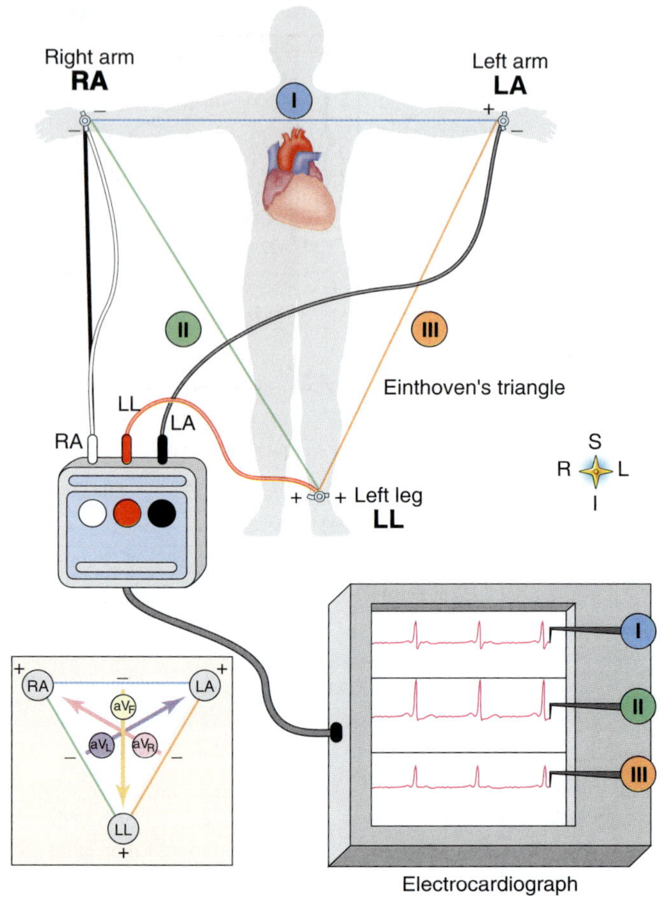

FIG. 6.5 Three-lead electrocardiogram (ECG). (From Thibodeau G, Patton K, eds. *Anatomy and Physiology*. 6th ed. St Louis: Mosby; 2007.)

the diastolic and systolic pressures (e.g., 140/97/70). Documentation also includes identification of the artery used for measurement, and the side. Fig. 6.4 shows the relationship between auscultatory sounds and pressure.

If the patient is to be assessed for **orthostatic (postural) blood pressure,** the pulse and blood pressure are measured with the patient in the recumbent position and again while the individual is sitting or standing. The patient's posture for each reading must be indicated in the documentation.

NOTE *A simple digital (automatic) sphygmomanometer provides the pulse rate, systolic pressure, diastolic pressure, and MAP. However, it does not measure important anomalies in the auscultatory sounds, and readings may be inaccurate, depending on the quality of the instrument and its maintenance.*

OXYGEN SATURATION

Oxygen saturation is often measured along with the other vital signs. This is performed with a pulse oximeter that attaches to the finger. The device measures the level of oxygen in the blood using spectrometry.

ELECTROCARDIOGRAPHY

Electrocardiography measures the electrical activity of the heart and displays it on a graph, known as an **electrocardiogram (ECG),** for evaluation. To obtain the readings, electrodes are placed at strategic locations on the chest wall and extremities. These coincide with the heart's conductivity pattern. A 12-lead ECG is used for a complete assessment; a simple assessment can be made with a three-lead ECG (Fig. 6.5). ECG monitoring is a routine procedure for any patient undergoing general anesthesia or sedation, in the postoperative period, and for selected high-risk patients.

The ECG machine has a console with a roll of paper that feeds automatically when the leads are in place and the machine is activated. Electrical activity through the heart is graphed by time and strength of impulse. This produces characteristic patterns indicating normal or abnormal conduction, which are recognizable to trained personnel.

As a diagnostic tool, an ECG provides detailed information about heart conduction. Each phase of the cardiac conduction system is represented on the graph. The waveforms correspond to the impulses that stimulate heart action, which pushes the blood through the chambers and valves. One complete heart cycle is represented by a series of waves, which

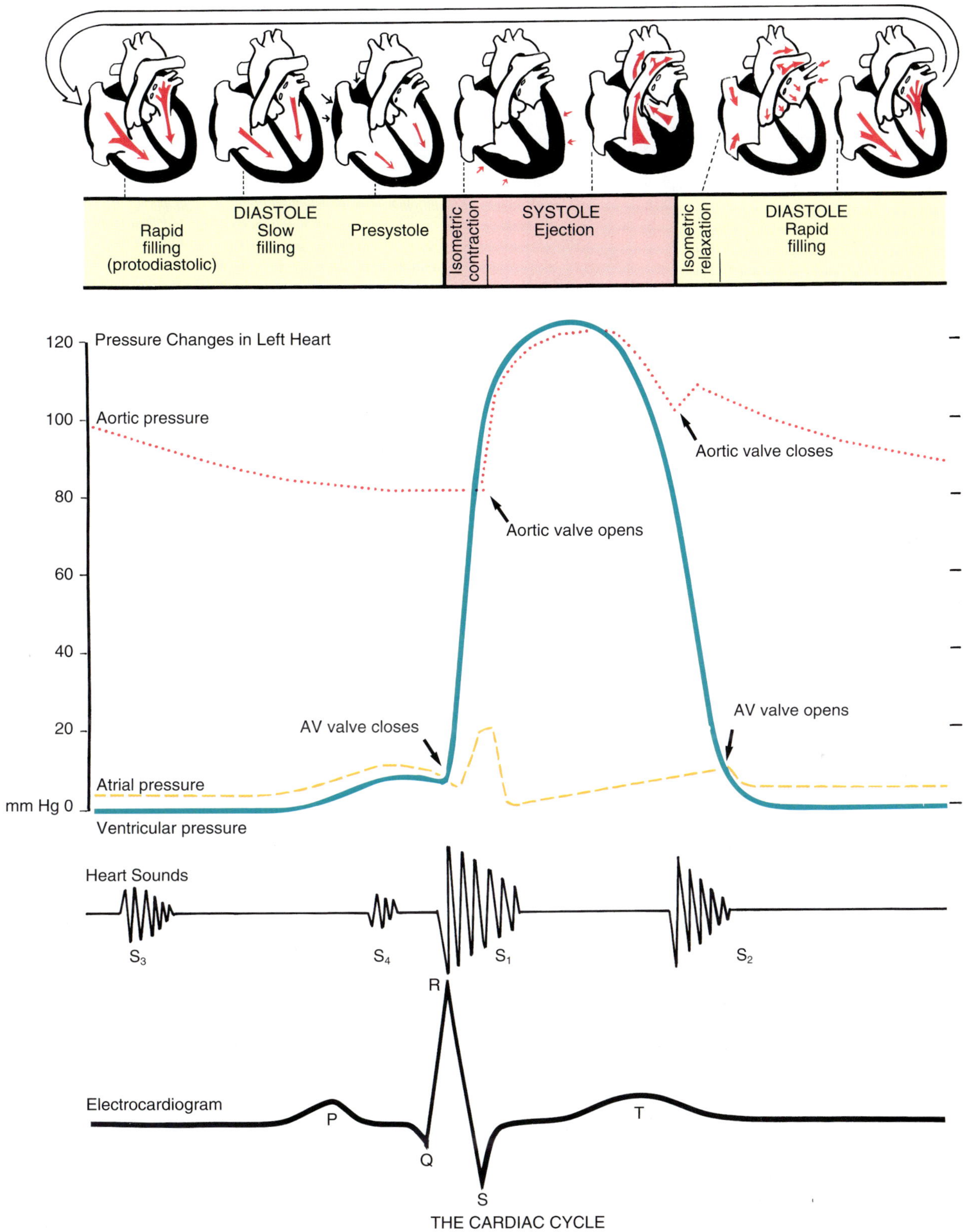

FIG. 6.6 Cardiac cycle QRS wave. *AV,* Atrioventricular. (From Jarvis C, ed. *Physical Examination and Health Assessment.* 5th ed. Philadelphia: Saunders; 2008.)

have characteristic peaks, troughs, and duration. This is called a *QRS wave.* A normal QRS wave form is shown in Fig. 6.6. Certain kinds of patterns and variations indicate disturbances in the conduction system that may be caused by disease, physiological disorder, and certain drugs.

IMAGING PROCEDURES

As the name implies, **imaging studies** involve a "picture" of the patient's anatomy. Imaging studies provide information about the function and shape of regional anatomy. Selected

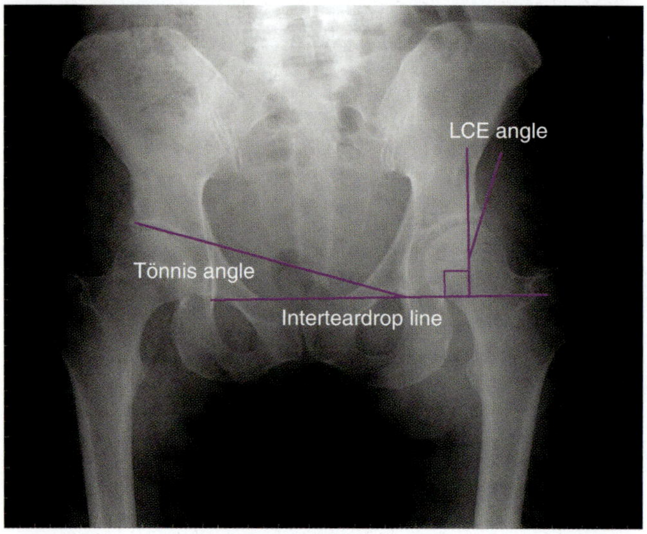

FIG. 6.7 Flat radiograph of the pelvis showing dislocation of the left hip. (From Canale S, Beaty J. *Campbell's Operative Orthopaedics.* 12th ed. Philadelphia: Elsevier Mosby; 2013.)

studies are performed in the perioperative environment during surgery or in a separate department of the facility.

RADIOLOGY

X-rays are electromagnetic particles with a relatively short wavelength. A radiographic (x-ray) image is created when radiation passes through structures and strikes a medium positioned in line with the penetrating rays. X-rays penetrate body tissue at different rates according to density. Some materials and tissue do not allow full penetration of the x-rays (Fig. 6.7). X-ray images are recorded, and the output is available as electronic data. Historically, all radiographs were recorded onto film. This method has been replaced in most facilities by **digital radiography** (**DR**), in which the image is immediately transferred electronically to a computer system. The images produced by DR are far superior to those using flat film.

NOTE *Because radiographs use gamma radiation, all personnel must wear protective attire that prevents the penetration of radiation. (Safety precautions and protection against gamma radiation in the perioperative environment are discussed in detail in Chapter 7.)*

The images formed by x-rays display contrasts in density. An extremely dense substance produces a white image, whereas air produces a black image. Contours and outlines of organs, systems, and tissue are displayed as a combination of white, black, and grays. Color 3-D images are also possible. Diagnostic x-rays are often used to confirm a condition or to provide baseline studies for comparison following a surgical procedure. Baseline x-rays are taken in the radiology department as part of the preoperative preparation of the patient. Many different forms of x-ray imaging are used in modern diagnostic medicine. Radiography is also used in combination with other imaging techniques such as computed tomography (CT) and fluoroscopy.

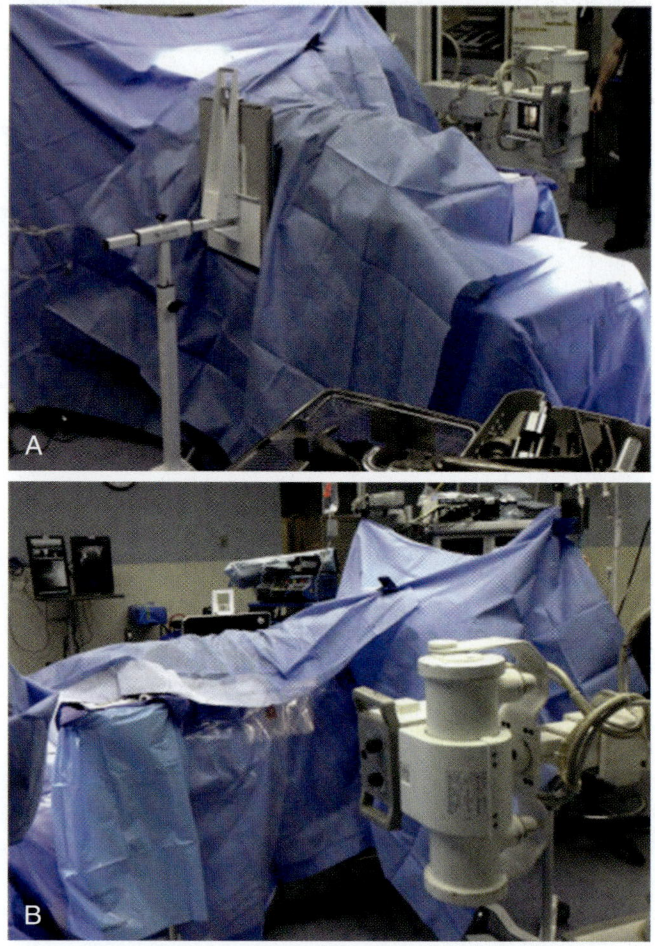

FIG. 6.8 (A and B) Example of intraoperative room setup during AP pelvic radiograph. The patient is in a lateral decubitus position. A temporary sterile drape is over the patient. The x-ray cassette is held on a portable stand with the longer side of the cassette vertical and the short-side horizontal. The x-ray is shot cross-table. (From Ezzet KA, Mccauley JC. Use of intraoperative x-rays to optimize component position and leg length during total hip arthroplasty. *J Arthroplasty.* 2014;29[3]:580–585. doi:10.1016/j.arth.2013.08.003.)

Standard Radiography

The standard x-ray film is obtained with a fixed or portable x-ray machine. Both types are used in operating rooms. The portable machine is transported to the operating room on an on-call basis so that images can be obtained during surgery as needed. Many types of x-ray procedures can be performed intraoperatively. They are most commonly used during orthopedic surgery, biliary procedures, and vascular surgery. An x-ray film might also be taken when a surgical count cannot be resolved and the risk exists that an item was left in the patient.

Intraoperative anteroposterior x-ray films are obtained with the use of a Bucky platform. This is a Plexiglas or carbon platform mounted on the operating bed frame. The technician slides the film into the platform from the head or foot of the table. When done properly, this does not risk contamination of the sterile field. However, the target of the radiograph must be protected from contamination by the overhead tube. The machine is brought into position at the sterile field only after the area is protected with sterile drapes (Fig. 6.8). A draped, portable radiographic film stand is used when other

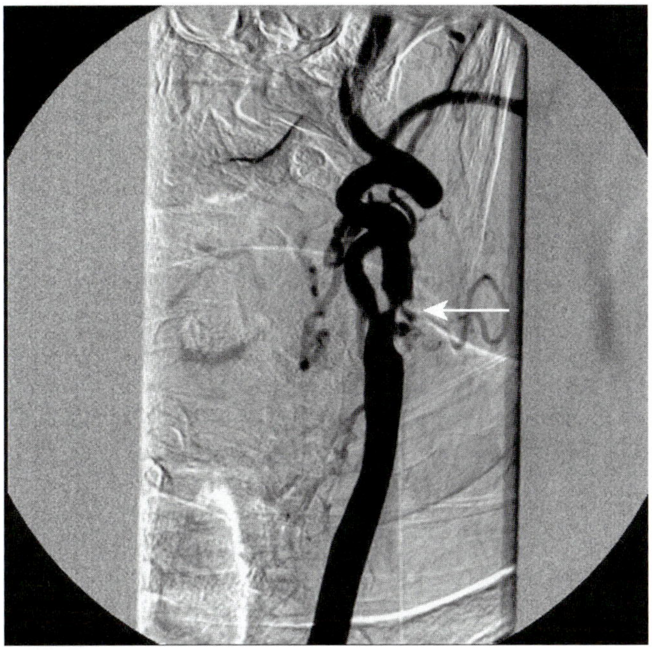

FIG. 6.9 Carotid angiography using a contrast medium injected intravenously. (From Cameron J, Cameron A. *Current Surgical Therapy.* 11th ed. Philadelphia: Saunders; 2014.)

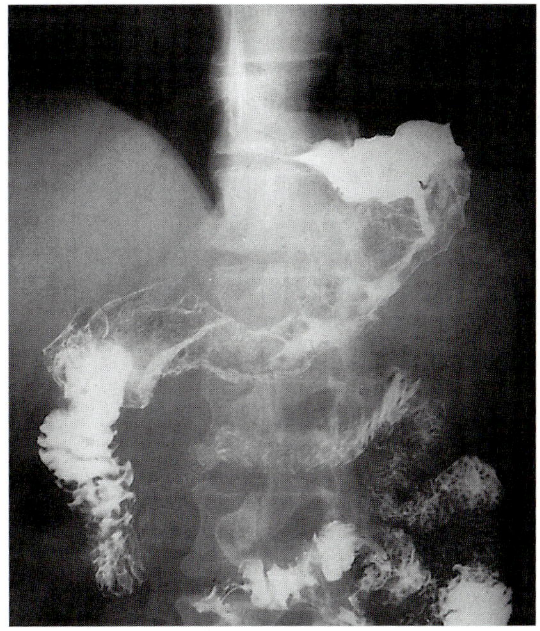

FIG. 6.10 Barium study of the stomach showing extensive gastric carcinoma. (From Garden O, Bradbury A, Forsythe J, Parks R. Principles and Practice of Surgery. 6th ed. Edinburgh: Churchill Livingstone; 2012.)

views are required. In these cases, the scrub protects the sterile field, including instrument tables and other draped equipment, from contamination by the overhead radiograph machine.

Contrast Radiography

The term **radiopaque** refers to substances that x-rays cannot penetrate. In diagnostic medicine, a drug called a **contrast medium** is injected, instilled, or ingested to outline hollow organs or vessels before x-ray films are taken. The liquid contrast medium produces a solid, white field in the area of the medium. Crevices, deviations, and the shape of a hollow structure can be clearly viewed on x-ray or by fluoroscopy. (Contrast media are discussed in Chapters 6 and 12.)

Contrast radiography carries a risk of allergy to the radiopaque medium, especially when the agent is injected. A careful patient history is used to determine whether the patient has had any previous reaction to contrast media. Allergy to iodine or agents containing iodophor may indicate sensitivity to contrast media. There is no evidence that allergy to shellfish indicates sensitivity or allergy to contrast media.

Specific details for intraoperative contrast studies are described in the surgical procedure chapter for that specialty. Contrast studies are used in nearly every medical specialty. The most commonly performed are the following:

- *Cholangiography:* A contrast medium is injected into the biliary tree. This outlines the ducts of the biliary system for suspected stones, tumor, or dilation.
- *Angiography:* A contrast medium is injected into the cardiovascular system to determine areas of stricture or other anomalies of blood flow in vessels (Fig. 6.9).
- *Myelography:* A contrast medium is injected into the subarachnoid space for visualization of the spinal cord and nerve roots.
- *Retrograde pyelography:* A contrast medium is instilled into the urinary tract for visualization of the bladder, ureter, and kidney. This procedure is used to identify stones, strictures, tumor, or other anomalies of the urinary system.
- *Gastrointestinal studies:* In studies of the gastrointestinal system, barium, a radiopaque element, is used to fill and outline the structures. An upper gastrointestinal study is used to identify problems in the esophagus, stomach, and small intestine. For a study of the large intestine, barium is instilled into the distal colon and rectum (Fig. 6.10).

Digital and Computed Radiography

DR is performed using flat panel x-ray detectors, which capture the x-rays. The panel plate is then removed and the data transformed into digital displays. DR requires a much lower dose of radiation than the older flat film method. However, radiation precautions must still be observed. DR data can be read almost immediately.

Computed radiography uses a photo-stimulated luminescent screen, which detects the x-rays. The internal cassette is transferred to a reader, which transforms the data into digital images. Although the reader is fast, it does require an extra step to download and read the cassette.

FLUOROSCOPY

Fluoroscopy uses x-ray and digital technology. Images are captured and translated to a flat panel screen that is visible in normal lighting. A digital monitor allows the moving images to be seen in real time. Fluoroscopy is used diagnostically and intraoperatively during procedures using contrast media or during implantation of a biomedical device.

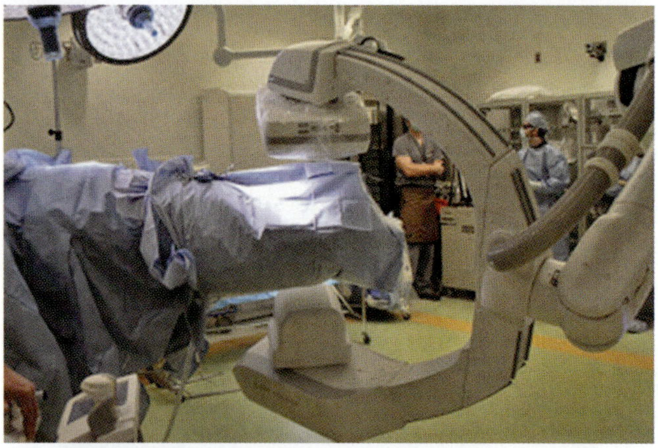

FIG. 6.11 Robotic C-arm in place for acquisition of 3-D imaging. Sterile three-quarter drapes were placed over the operative extremity before positioning the C-arm. (From Cancienne JM, et al. Use of a hybrid operating room to improve reduction of syndesmotic injuries in ankle fractures: a case report. *J Foot Ankle Surg*. 2016;55[5]:1052–1056. doi:10.1053/j.jfas.2015.10.003.)

Mobile C-Arm

The mobile C-arm fluoroscope is used in surgery for real-time imaging (Fig. 6.11). The head of the fluoroscope is directed through the body onto an image intensifier on the underside of the C-arm. The C-arm can be moved into place so that the operating bed is centered between the tube and the intensifier. Multiple images can be taken by moving the machine along the axis of the operating table. The C-arm is draped before positioning to allow freedom of movement along the sterile field and has replaced portable x-ray machines in many hospitals.

O-Arm

The O-arm has become the standard image-guided system for use in spinal surgery (Fig. 6.12). The device is an open tube, referred to as the **gantry.** This is the housing for the x-ray tube. The patient is positioned within the gantry, which can be moved along the long axis of the operating table. Images are created in multiple locations along the diameter of the tube and projected to a flat panel screen. The O-arm has the capacity to project up to 391 images within the 360-degree gantry. Moving images in two dimensions, 3-D images are produced in real time, and these can be frozen and stored individually (Fig. 6.13). The O-arm provides superior images over those produced by conventional or 3-D C-arm. The result is more accurate placement of surgical screws during spinal column surgery. Also, the O-arm reduces the patient's exposure to x-rays, which is an important consideration in pediatric surgery.

COMPUTED TOMOGRAPHY

Computed tomography (CT) combines x-ray and computer technologies to produce high-contrast cross-sectional images. This technique allows precise tissue differentiation and determination of the dimensions of anatomical structures. CT is enhanced with contrast media to assess structures such as ducts, blood vessels, and the gastrointestinal system.

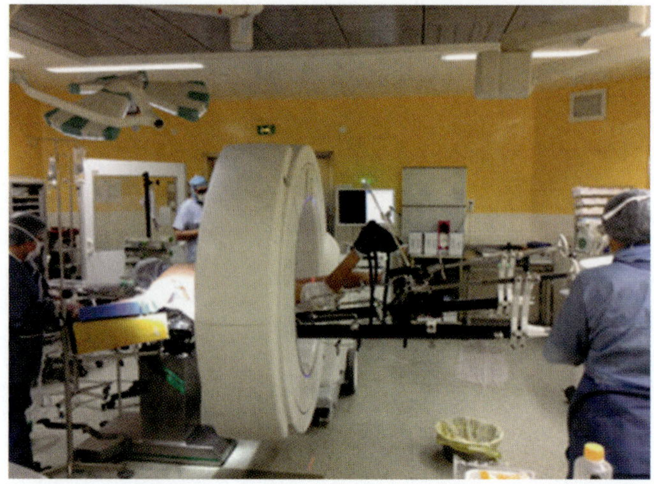

FIG. 6.12 The O-ARM device (Medtronic, Sofamor, Broomfield, CO) is introduced to check for possible conflict with the operating table and then removed for preparing of the operative site. (From Sebaaly A, et al. The added value of intraoperative CT scanner and screw navigation in displaced posterior wall acetabular fracture with articular impaction. *Orthop Traumatol Surg Res*. 102[7]:947–950, 2016. doi:10.1016/j.otsr.2016.07.005.)

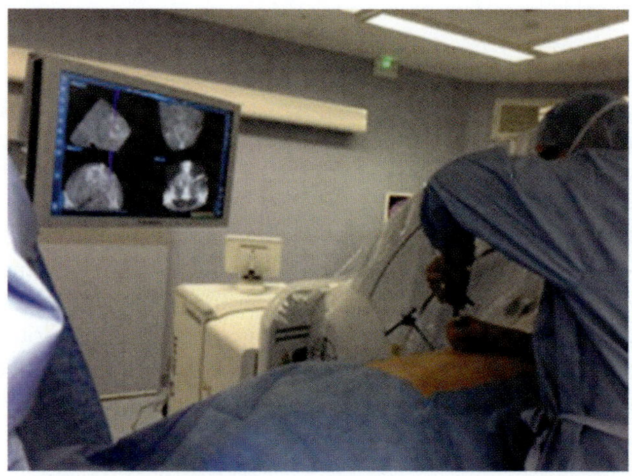

FIG. 6.13 Access to the surgical field with an O-type system (O-Arm, Medtronic). (From Tonetti J, et al. Role of 3D intraoperative imaging in orthopedic and trauma surgery. *Orthop Traumatol Surg Res*. 2019. doi:10.1016/j.otsr.2019.05.021.)

MAGNETIC RESONANCE IMAGING

Magnetic resonance imaging (MRI) uses radiofrequency signals and multiple magnetic fields to produce a high-definition image (Fig. 6.14). In this process, the patient is exposed to electromagnetic energy, which is emitted inside a closed body tube or an open platform. MRI produces 2-D or 3-D digital images in cross section and is mainly used to detect structural abnormalities, including tumors. Because the process involves a high level of electromagnetic energy, any metal in range of the device may be drawn toward the source of emission. This poses a genuine risk for injury to the patient and personnel working in the area. Images can also be distorted by the presence of metallic substances in the tissue. These include biomedical devices such as a pacemaker, vascular clips, and certain kinds of tattoos containing metal-based dye. MRI is performed in the interventional medicine or radiology

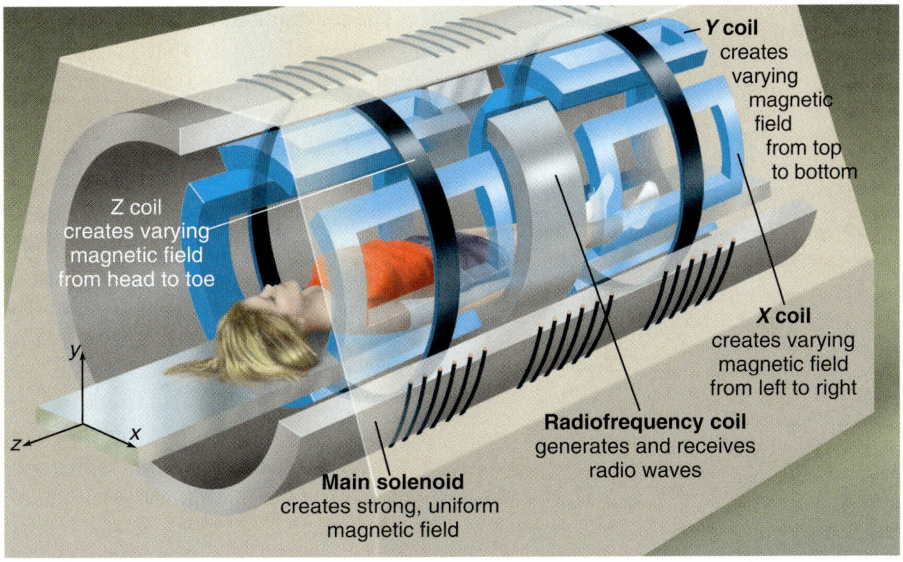

FIG. 6.14 Magnetic resonance imaging (MRI) apparatus. (From Giambattista A, Richardson R, Richardson BM, eds. *College Physics*. 2nd ed. New York: McGraw-Hill; 2007. Reproduced with the permission of the McGraw-Hill Companies.)

department and, occasionally, intraoperatively in facilities that have a dedicated surgical suite.

POSITRON EMISSION TOMOGRAPHY

Positron emission tomography (PET) uses the combined technologies of CT and radioactive scanning. PET is performed to produce an image not of a structure but rather of a metabolic process. In this technique, a biological substance to be followed in the body is "labeled" with radioactive atoms. The labeling is performed by injection. During PET, the radioactive particles emitted by the atoms are traced and computed to provide an image of the physiology and biochemical properties of the tissue. These are displayed in 3-D color representations of the structure, such as the brain or heart.

ULTRASOUND

Ultrasound energy is generated by high-frequency sound waves. As a diagnostic tool, the sound waves are directed at tissue, which reflects the waves back to produce a real-time image. The images are digitalized for viewing, storage, and reproduction. Ultrasonic waves can be clearly traced through liquid or semiliquid substances. When the ultrasound probe is applied to skin or mucous membrane for deep tissue assessment, a gel coating is used as an interface because the high-frequency waves cannot be precisely tracked through air.

Ultrasound has many applications, both intraoperatively and outside surgery. It is commonly used to obtain images of abdominal viscera and for pregnancy assessment. The images represent tissue density. The outline and internal density are identified by shades of black, white, and gray. When combined with the Doppler technique, ultrasound is used in vascular surgery to track the movement of blood and provide a screen image of velocity and viscosity. An intraoperative ultrasound probe is used to assess vascular structures and tissue density. Echocardiography is used in the same way to demonstrate motion of the heart.

Doppler studies use ultrasound for specific measurement of vascular flow. The Doppler probe, or transducer, provides **transcutaneous** (through the skin) measurement of vascular obstruction. The sounds reproduced by the Doppler technique differ in pitch and quality and correspond to the movement of blood through a vessel. Doppler sounds can be directly interpreted, or they may be transmitted as wave signals and digitally displayed on a screen for interpretation.

BLOOD TESTS

Blood tests are routinely performed to assess the blood's chemistry, function, structure, and composition. The structure and type of blood cells present are also important assessment findings. Many hundreds of blood tests can be done and are routinely performed in the health care setting. The most basic tests are the **complete blood count (CBC),** tests for coagulation, overall blood chemistry, and verification of blood type. The arterial blood gas (ABG) test is performed in critical care situations, including during surgery.

COMPLETE BLOOD COUNT

The CBC is a basic test used to evaluate the type and percentage of normal components in the blood (Table 6.3). A blood sample is drawn from the vein and centrifuged. This separates it into cellular and liquid components for evaluation. The CBC is a basic blood test used for screening medical, infectious, and other types of diseases. When formulating a diagnosis, physicians always consider variations in normal blood values along with other signs and symptoms; they are never considered in isolation.

The blood components measured are the following:

- ***Hemoglobin (Hgb):*** The oxygen-carrying protein attached to red blood cells (erythrocytes) is measured in grams per deciliter (g/dL).

TABLE 6.3 Components of the Complete Blood Count

Component	Normal Values
Hematocrit (Hct)	Men 45% (38%–51%) Women 40% (36%–47%)
Hemoglobin (Hgb)	Men 14–17 g/dL Women 12–16 g/dL Children 12–14 g/dL
Erythrocytes	Men 5.0 (4.5–6.0) million Women 4.5–5.5 million
Reticulocytes	1.0%
Leukocytes, total (WBC)	5,000–10,000 (100%)
DIFFERENTIAL WHITE BLOOD CELLS	
Segmented neutrophils	2,500–6,000 (7%–40%)
Band neutrophils	0–500 (0–5%)
Eosinophils	50–300 (1%–3%)
Basophils	0–100 (0–1%)
Monocytes	200–800 (4%–8%)
Lymphocytes	1,000–4,000 (7%–40%)
Platelets	200,000–500,000

- *Red blood cell count:* Erythrocytes make up most of the volume in the peripheral blood. They are produced in red bone marrow and live for about 120 days. Their main function is to deliver oxygen to cells.
- ***Hematocrit (Hct):*** The percentage of red blood cells in the blood (by volume).
- *Platelet count:* Platelets have important functions in the blood clotting mechanism, including clot retraction and activation of coagulation factors.
- *Differential leukocyte count:* White blood cells (leukocytes) are essential to the immune process. The **differential count** measures the number of each type of leukocyte by volume of blood. These are *monocytes, macrophages, band neutrophils, eosinophils, basophils, and lymphocytes.*

METABOLIC PANEL

The metabolic panel includes a number of tests to determine the serum levels of substances that are crucial for metabolism. Many types of metabolic panels can be done. The *basic metabolic panel* includes blood glucose, carbon dioxide, creatinine, urea nitrogen, bicarbonate, and several important electrolytes. The exact tests included in any metabolic panel are determined by health care regulatory agencies and may change with reimbursement regulations.

COAGULATION TESTS

A number of blood studies may be performed to determine coagulation, which is a critical factor for the surgical patient. The tests are used to assess disease states and to monitor patients who are receiving antiplatelet drugs for a clotting disorder.

The mechanism of blood clotting is an extremely complex physiological activity that is divided into two processes, the *intrinsic pathway* and the *extrinsic pathway*. The extrinsic pathway occurs at the tissue level, and the intrinsic pathway occurs in the vascular system. Both systems activate a chemical called *factor X* and the formation of *fibrin* for clotting. The chain reaction of physiological events in the coagulation process is controlled by many chemicals, called *factors,* which are identified by Roman numerals. These are released in specific order, and if one is missing, the clotting mechanism is altered.

The **prothrombin time (PT)** and **partial thromboplastin time (PTT)** are determined to evaluate the extrinsic coagulation system. They are also used for screening congenital deficiencies of factors II, V, VII, and X.

The PT is a measurement of coagulation time. The PT is generally used to monitor the patient on long-term anticoagulant therapy.

The PTT or activated partial thromboplastin time (APTT) is commonly performed to assess the functional ability of the coagulation sequence. In this test, partial prothrombin is added to coagulated blood. The test is most commonly used to determine the effects of heparin therapy or to screen for clotting disorders.

ARTERIAL BLOOD GASES

ABG analysis measures the pH of the blood and also the levels of oxygen and carbon dioxide. The values provided must then be interpreted to formulate a diagnosis.

Blood gas analysis is often performed in critical care situations but may also be required urgently during surgery. Blood drawn for ABG testing is usually taken from the radial artery and must be kept cold during transport, because temperature affects the accuracy of the results.

ABO GROUPS

A person's blood type, or **ABO blood group,** is based on inherited antigens found on the surface of an individual's red blood cells. The *Rh type* refers to whether a specific antigen called *Rh* is present. An individual is typed as Rh positive or Rh negative according to whether this antigen is present.

The four significant ABO antigens are A, B, O, and AB. Individuals who lack A and B antigens are typed as *O*. Those who have type A antigens are typed as *A*. Those with B antigens are typed as *B*, and those with both A and B are typed as *AB*.

An individual develops antibodies to the antigen he or she does not have. For example, a person with type A antigens develops antibodies to type B antigens. In the case of a transfusion, the antigen reaction is predictable when the ABO group is known.

The significance of the ABO grouping is that a transfusion of blood containing antibodies to the specific antigens of the blood group can cause a transfusion reaction. This can be a mild allergic reaction or a life-threatening condition. Blood incompatibility can lead to a hemolytic reaction in which the recipient's blood cells are destroyed. For this reason, any

TABLE 6.4 Electrolytes

Cations	Anions
Sodium ($Na+$)	Chloride ($Cl-$)
Potassium ($K+$)	Phosphate ($PO_4{}^{3-}$)
Magnesium (Mg^{2+})	Bicarbonate ($HCO_3{}^{-}$)
Calcium (Ca^{2+})	Sulfate ($SO_4{}^{2-}$)

patient receiving blood products must be tested for blood grouping before a transfusion is performed.

ELECTROLYTES

Body fluids contain both organic and inorganic substances. These substances are essential for homeostasis. Molecules of inorganic substances are capable of splitting to yield a charged particle or substance, called an *electrolyte.* Positively charged electrolytes are called *cations,* and those that are negatively charged are called *anions* (Table 6.4). Cations function mainly in the transmission of nerve impulses to muscles. The highest percentage of positive ions is found in the blood, cells, intercellular spaces, and the gastrointestinal tract. Electrolyte imbalance can result in severe physiological disturbances. The cations potassium, sodium, calcium, and magnesium are routinely measured in blood. Several anions are measured directly (e.g., ion gap). For more complex information on this topic, a blood chemistry or pathophysiology text should be consulted.

Potassium

Potassium is mainly found in cells. It is necessary for the transmission of nerve impulses to skeletal, smooth, and cardiac muscle. It also functions in the conversion of carbohydrates for cellular energy and is critical in maintaining osmolality in cells. *Hypokalemia* (decreased serum potassium) can result from persistent and severe vomiting and diarrhea, extensive tissue trauma, or shock. Certain drugs can also cause a decrease in potassium.

Sodium

Sodium is the most plentiful electrolyte found outside the cell. It is responsible for regulation of body and cellular fluids and plays a critical role in the transport of substances into and out of the cell. It binds with specific negatively charged electrolytes to maintain the blood pH. *Hyponatremia* (low sodium) is caused by prolonged vomiting and diarrhea, the use of certain diuretics, and surgery.

Calcium

Calcium is found in cells and in the extracellular fluid. It is most important in promoting myocardial contraction and in the conversion of thrombin to prothrombin, which is part of the blood-clotting mechanism. Calcium contributes to cell permeability and is necessary for the development and maintenance of bone tissue. *Hypocalcemia* can result from parathyroid disease, vitamin D deficiency, and specific drugs such as corticosteroids and some diuretics.

Magnesium

Magnesium is important in the neurotransmission of all muscles but especially the myocardium. Like calcium, it contributes to cell permeability and also protein and carbohydrate metabolism. Magnesium is necessary for the transport of sodium and potassium through the cell membrane. Hypomagnesemia can be caused by drugs such as corticosteroids, laxatives, and some diuretics.

URINALYSIS

Standard urinalysis is performed to assess the body's overall health, with particular focus on the urinary tract. Simple screening is performed with a dipstick coated with reagents that register the levels of different substances in the urine. These substances are as follows:

- Albumin
- Bilirubin
- Glucose
- Ketones
- Leukocytes
- Blood nitrite
- Urobilinogen

The pH and specific gravity are also assessed. The color, clarity, and odor of the urine are interpreted in the overall assessment. The sample is centrifuged to create sediment, which is examined for microorganisms, crystals, cells, and casts. Urine culture is performed to determine the exact organism associated with a urinary tract infection.

MICROBIOLOGICAL STUDIES

Tissue specimens and fluid suspected of being infected are analyzed to determine the presence and type of microorganisms. Samples that are suspected or known to be contaminated are taken intraoperatively in selected procedures, usually using sterile culture swabs. This is based on evidence of pus, inflammation, or devitalized tissue. A sample confirms the diagnosis and aids treatment decisions. One of the tests used to detect infection is the culture and sensitivity (C&S) test. In this test, a sample is allowed to incubate on a culture medium. After colonization, a number of tests are performed on the colonies to identify the exact microorganism. The sensitivity test exposes the cultured microorganisms to a variety of antibiotic substances during incubation. This determines which of the antibiotics interferes with growth.

PATHOLOGICAL EXAMINATION OF TISSUE

Pathology is the study of diseases. Tissue pathology is the examination of tissue for the presence of disease. In surgery, pathology specimens are routinely obtained and sent to the pathology department for analysis. Each type of tissue requires special care to ensure that the cells are not damaged.

TISSUE BIOPSY

Biopsy is the removal of tissue for analysis and diagnosis. Protocols for tissue preservation vary according to the type of tissue, whether it will be examined immediately, and how it is to be analyzed. The protocol for handling specimens is developed by the facility's pathology department and is available to all perioperative personnel for study. (Chapter 21 presents information on the handling of specimens.) Biopsy specimens can be obtained in a number of ways:

- *Excision:* Surgical removal of tissue to check for disease. Please refer to Chapter 19 for specific biopsy procedures.
- *Needle* or *trocar biopsy:* The removal of tissue with a hollow needle or trocar, which is inserted into the tissue. A core sample of the tissue is removed in one or more locations of the suspected area. The needle can be inserted through the skin (percutaneously) or into tissue exposed during surgery. A hollow trocar may be used to remove a large core of tissue such as bone marrow.
- *Brush biopsy:* A biopsy brush, a very small cylindrical brush, is used to sweep a hollow lumen or cavity for cells. This technique is commonly used in diagnostic procedures of the throat structures and bronchi. The procedure removes only superficial cells and does not cut into the tissue. After biopsy, the brush is withdrawn and immediately swished in liquid preservative or saline to prevent drying.
- *Aspiration biopsy:* A microscope slide, which is sprayed with a cell fixative. The specimen can then be examined microscopically by the pathologist.
- *Frozen section:* Immediate microscopic and gross (without aid of a microscope) examination of suspect tissue is performed by *frozen section.* In this procedure, the tissue is removed and placed in liquid nitrogen. This freezes the sample. It is then sliced into single-cell sections and analyzed microscopically. A surgical procedure is purposefully scheduled with a frozen section to determine the need for radical or more extensive excision of a tumor. A permanent section fixes the tissue slices on slides for preservation.

CANCER TERMS AND CONCEPTS

Surgery is commonly performed to diagnose or treat cancer. Terms related to cancer treatment, classification, and diagnosis are used in the perioperative setting. A basic understanding of these terms and their origin is an important aspect of surgical practice.

DEFINITIONS

A **neoplasm,** or tumor, is an abnormal growth. A tumor is classified as malignant or benign. A **malignant** tumor is composed of disorganized tissue that exhibits uncontrolled growth. Malignant tissue has the potential to spread from the original site (called the *primary tumor*) to other parts of the body. A **benign** growth is composed of cells belonging to a single tissue type and does not spread to distant regions of the body. Any word with the ending *-oma* refers to a tumor (e.g., osteoma, leiomyoma, and lymphoma).

COMPARISON OF MALIGNANT AND BENIGN TUMORS

A benign tumor often resembles the tissue in which it originates. It does not undergo histological change (changes in the tissue type) but remains consistent during growth. These tumors are usually encapsulated or confined and do not infiltrate the tissue bed. A benign tumor may continue to grow but does not take over the functions of the original tissue. In contrast, a malignant tumor develops a disorganized vascular system and usually contains different types of cells or tissue. It invades the tissue of origin and captures its nutrients and often its blood flow. Malignant cells release toxins that kill normal cells, and the tumor grows quickly and invasively. Cells from the malignancy break off and enter the lymph system, where they are transported to other areas of the body. New tumors may develop from these seed cells; this is called **metastasis.** Eventually, the tumor disrupts or halts the normal function of vital organs. Malignancy usually results in death unless it is treated early.

A benign tumor may impinge on nearby tissue or organs. This can interrupt blood supply, cause pain, or alter the function of healthy tissue. However, the tumor grows slowly compared to malignant tissue, and the benign tissue does not invade the healthy tissue or deplete its nutrients.

EFFECTS OF MALIGNANCY ON THE BODY

Malignancy causes specific injury to the body:

- The risk of thrombosis (blood clot) is increased as a result of inappropriate production of clotting factors by the tumor itself. The tumor may also block blood vessels, resulting in clotting.
- Pain is caused by direct injury to tissue or by pain mediators released by the tumor. As the tumor impinges on healthy tissue, the tissue dies, resulting in severe pain.
- Cachexia (tissue and body wasting) is characteristic of malignancy. As the tumor destroys tissue, the patient's metabolism is altered. Nutrients normally received by healthy tissue for growth and repair are captured by the malignant tissue, which continues to grow and spread.
- Anemia occurs as a result of internal bleeding and the body's inability to replace red blood cells.
- As the malignancy spreads, changes occur in the function of the target tissue. This results in many different disease conditions, depending on the organ or tissue function.

DIAGNOSTIC METHODS

Several tests are commonly performed to screen for suspected cancer. The exact type of test depends on the affected tissue.

Tumor Markers

A **tumor marker** is an antigen present on the tumor cell or other substance (protein, hormone, or other chemical) released by the cells into the blood. Some markers are specific for certain types of cancer cells. Markers are not always reliable for diagnosing malignancy, because some benign tumors can also release markers. Tests for tumor markers are most useful in patients undergoing treatment when a comparison provides information over the course of therapy. An assessment tool for the detection of prostate cancer is measurement of the tumor marker prostate-specific antigen. Another common assessment marker is CA-125, which is present in some types of ovarian cancer.

Biopsy

A tissue biopsy is a sample of tissue, cells, or fluid that is removed from the body and examined for suspected disease. A tissue biopsy can be a small segment of the suspected tissue, a cell washing, a smear, or a blood sample. The Pap smear (Papanicolaou test) is a familiar type of routine biopsy for cervical cancer. The frozen section specimen described previously is another type of biopsy.

Tumor Staging

Two methods are used to classify malignant tumors; this is called **staging.** One is by analysis of the cellular characteristics, and the other is by the spread of cancer (i.e., the metastatic pattern). Staging provides a basis on which to select the most beneficial treatment. It also indicates the progress of treatment and the outcome, or *prognosis.* The staging process is an internationally used system called the **TNM classification system** (Box 6.2). *T* refers to the extent of the tumor, *N* refers to the lymph node involvement, and *M* is the extent of metastasis. Tumors are also graded according to the level of cellular differentiation. Grades I through IV indicate decreasing levels of differentiation. Grade I cells show the most differentiation. Decreased differentiation indicates more serious disease; thus grade IV has greater risk of lethality than grade I.

BOX 6.2 Tumor-Node-Metastasis (TNM) Classification System

TUMOR	
Tx	Tumor cannot be assessed
T0	No evidence of a primary tumor
Tis	Carcinoma in situ
T1–T4	Increasing tumor size or involvement of healthy tissue
NODES	
Nx	Lymph nodes cannot be assessed
N0	No evidence of lymph node involvement
N1–3	Increasing involvement of regional lymph nodes
METASTASIS	
Mx	Metastasis not assessed
M10	No evidence of distant metastasis
M1	Distant metastasis confirmed and site indicated

CANCER PREVENTION AND SCREENING

Many forms of cancer can be treated in the early stages of the disease. Public health promotion and screening procedures enable people to learn about cancer and protect themselves against some cancers.

An updated review of screening recommendations can be found on the National Cancer Institute's website at http://www.cancer.gov.

NUCLEAR MEDICINE

Nuclear medicine involves the use of radioactive particles, which are directed at the nucleus of a selected element to create energy. These special elements are referred to as **radionuclides** or **isotopes.** Radionuclides emit gamma radiation and can be used for diagnosis and treatment. Administered intravenously, orally, or by direct deposition, they can be traced to reveal the structure and function of an organ, system, cavity, or tissue.

RADIATION THERAPY

Tissue destruction by ionizing radiation is used in the treatment of a neoplasm. The delivery and implantation systems for radiation therapy include needles, seeds, and capsulated implants. Radiation therapy procedures are carried out in designated areas of the hospital or health care facility by specially trained personnel. In addition to implantation procedures, intraoperative radiation therapy is used to deliver a single dose of radiation to a specific area of the body.

In needle delivery systems, cesium-137, a radioactive isotope, is enclosed in dose units and contained in special hollow needles for insertion into tissue. The needles are placed around the borders of the tumor. These are connected by heavy sutures and secured to the patient's skin. The needles remain in place for up to 7 days.

Radioactive seeds can be implanted directly into the tumor mass and may be left in the patient indefinitely. Cesium-137, iodine-125, and iridium-192 are used in this procedure. Seeds are generally used in tumors that cannot be removed by surgical resection because of precarious location or size. The procedure may be performed intraoperatively or in the interventional radiology department.

Short-acting radiotherapy in high doses can be delivered through *brachytherapy.* In this procedure, a capsule containing high-dose radiation is implanted using a special catheter. Radioactive pellets are inserted into the implanted catheter for several days and then removed. This treatment is used in breast and prostate cancer.

Historical Highlights

For many years, it was thought that an allergy to shellfish meant that a patient was also allergic to injectable iodinated contrast media. There were never any clinical data to support this, but the misinformation continued to be widespread. The theory was formally debunked in the early 2000s. Allergic reactions to injectable contrast media do occur in about 3% of cases, but these are entirely *unrelated to shellfish*.

For more information, see the U.S. Department of Health and Human Services, Agency for Healthcare Research and Quality website, Reaction to Dye, available at https://psnet.ahrq.gov/webmm/case/75/reaction-to-dye, or search for "AHRQ dye."

KEY CONCEPTS

- The first step in medical and surgical decision making is assessment of the problem.
- An invasive procedure involves breaking intact skin or mucous membrane or inserting a medical device into a body cavity. Noninvasive procedures are limited to skin contact or no direct contact with the body.
- The vital signs include temperature, pulse, respiratory rate, and blood pressure, and in the health care setting, measurement of the patient's level of pain.
- Filling of the heart chambers and shunting of blood through the heart is called the *systolic pressure*. As the heart relaxes between contractions, the pressure decreases. This is called the *diastolic pressure*.
- An ECG machine measures the electrical activity of the heart.
- The images formed by x-rays display contrasts in density. An extremely dense substance produces a white image, whereas air produces a black image.
- The term *radiopaque* refers to substances that x-rays cannot penetrate.
- In surgery, the mobile C-arm fluoroscope is used for real-time imaging.
- The O-arm uses fluoroscopy to produce high-resolution 3-D images and is used primarily during spinal surgery.
- In computed tomography, x-ray and computer technologies are combined to produce high-contrast cross-sectional images.
- Magnetic resonance imaging uses radiofrequency signals and magnetic energy to produce images.
- Positron emission tomography uses the combined technologies of CT and radioactive scanning.
- During ultrasound imaging, high-frequency sound waves are directed at tissue. These are reflected back to produce an image of the tissue.
- Doppler studies use ultrasound to measure vascular flow. The reflected sound waves can be interpreted directly or transmitted as waveforms on a digital output monitor.
- The complete blood count is a basic test used to evaluate the type and percentage of normal components in the blood.
- The prothrombin time is a measurement of coagulation time.
- The ABO blood groups, also known as blood types, are categorizations based on inherited antigens found on the surface of an individual's red blood cells.
- Electrolytes are vital for homeostasis and are responsible for nerve impulses, fluid balance, the transport of substances into and out of the cell and for maintaining the blood pH.
- Biopsy is the removal of tissue for analysis and diagnosis.
- Excision is the surgical removal of a small portion of tissue. Excision usually refers to removal by cutting (also called excisional biopsy).
- Brush biopsy is performed with a very small cylindrical brush used to sweep a hollow lumen or cavity for cells.
- In an aspiration biopsy, fluid for pathological examination is removed from semisolid tissue by aspirating fluid (removal with a syringe).
- A smear is obtained by passing a swab or small brush over superficial tissue. The swab is then passed over a glass microscope slide and sprayed with a cell fixative.
- A frozen section is removal of tissue for immediate pathological assessment. The tissue specimen is frozen and passed through a device that produces single-cell sections for examination.
- A neoplasm, or tumor, is excessive, disorganized growth of tissue.
- A malignant neoplasm consists of nondifferentiated cells that have the potential to break loose from the original site and spread to other parts of the body.
- Tissue destruction by ionizing radiation is used in the treatment of a neoplasm. The delivery and implantation systems for radiation therapy include needles, seeds, and capsulated implants.

REVIEW QUESTIONS

1. Describe the factors that can increase core temperature in the clinical setting.
2. Which methods of temperature assessment accurately reflect core temperature?
3. How do you correctly document the patient's vital signs? Give examples and explain what they mean.
4. What are the causes of a falsely high blood pressure reading?
5. What is "postural" blood pressure?
6. To what do the peaks and troughs on the ECG reading correspond?
7. What is the purpose of a contrast medium?
8. What is the differential leukocyte count?
9. Compare the main differences between a malignant and a benign tumor.
10. What is a tumor marker?

11. Why do you think people do not take advantage of screening procedures for cancer?

CASE STUDIES

CASE 1

While assisting the circulator during outpatient surgery under local anesthesia, you are asked to take the patient's vital signs for the duration of the case. Explain the following:

1. You do not know what the patient's normal vital signs are. Do you need to know this to carry out this role?
2. You cannot find an available digital blood pressure apparatus, so you must use a stethoscope and manual sphygmomanometer. Is this important to document?
3. The circulator asks you to record all three elements of blood pressure. What does he mean, and how do you measure it?
4. You are required to take vital signs every 15 minutes. You have missed one blood pressure reading. The next diastolic reading you get is elevated by 20 points. The pulse rate is elevated by 15. Should you report this immediately or repeat the measurement?

CASE 2

During emergency surgery, you are assisting the circulator. You are asked to rush to the laboratory and pick up 2 units of blood for the patient. You arrive at the lab and are handed 2 bags of blood. When you return to the operating room, you discover that the patient's name as documented with the blood is incorrect. How should this have been prevented?

CASE 3

According to your knowledge of arterial blood gases, why would getting blood gases be an emergency procedure? Why do you think the blood must be arterial rather than venous blood?

BIBLIOGRAPHY

Chernecky C, Berger B. *Laboratory Tests and Diagnostic Procedures*. 2nd ed. St Louis: Mosby; 2008.

McPhee S, Papadakis M, Tierney L. *Current Medical Diagnosis and Treatment*. 46th ed. New York: McGraw-Hill; 2007.

Porth C. *Pathophysiology Concepts of Altered Health States*. 6th ed. Philadelphia: Lippincott Williams & Wilkins; 2007.

7 ENVIRONMENTAL HAZARDS

LEARNING OBJECTIVES

After studying this chapter, the reader will be able to:

1. Identify the risks that are present in the operating room
2. Explain the importance of the fire triangle
3. Discuss fuels and sources of ignition commonly found in the operating room
4. Describe how to respond appropriately to a patient fire
5. Identify methods associated with preventing fires in the operating room
6. Describe measures to safely store, transport, and use compressed gas cylinders
7. Identify precautions to prevent exposure to ionizing radiation
8. Describe methods to avoid chemical injury
9. Describe toxic substances in smoke plume
10. Define Standard Precautions
11. Discuss techniques to prevent sharps injuries
12. Identify the practice for transmission-based precautions
13. Identify methods of properly handling and disposing of hazardous waste in the operating room
14. Describe the symptoms of true latex allergy
15. Identify necessary precautions to prevent latex reaction in allergic patients
16. Describe correct body mechanics for lifting, pulling, and pushing heavy equipment

TERMINOLOGY

Airborne transmission precautions: Precautions that prevent airborne transfer of disease organisms in the environment.

Blood-borne pathogens: Harmful microorganisms that may be present in and transmitted through human blood and body fluids.

Electrocution: Severe burns, cardiac disturbances, or death as a result of electrical current discharged into the body.

Electrosurgical unit (ESU): Medical device commonly used in surgery to coagulate blood vessels and cut tissue.

Eschar: Burned tissue fragments that can accumulate on the electrosurgical tip during use; eschar can cause sparking and become a source of ignition.

Flammable: Capable of burning.

Grounding: A path for electrical current to flow unimpeded through a material and disperse back to the source or disperse into the ground.

Hypersensitivity: A cell-mediated immune response to a substance in the body.

Impedance (resistance): The ability of a substance to stop or alter the flow of electrons through a conductive material.

Latex: A naturally occurring sap obtained from rubber trees that is used in the manufacture of medical devices, supplies, and patient care items.

No-hands technique: A method of transferring sharp instruments on the surgical field without hand-to-hand contact. A neutral zone is identified, and sharps are exchanged in this zone.

Occupational exposure: Exposure to hazards in the workplace; for example, exposure to hazardous chemicals or contact with potentially infected blood and body fluids.

Oxidizers: Agents or substances capable of supporting fire.

Oxygen-enriched atmosphere (OEA): An environment that contains a high percentage of oxygen and therefore presents a high risk for fire.

Personal protective equipment (PPE): Clothing or equipment that protects the wearer from direct contact with hazardous chemicals or potentially infectious body fluids.

Postexposure prophylaxis (PEP): Recommended procedures to help prevent the development of blood-borne diseases after an exposure incident such as a needlestick injury.

Risk: The statistical probability of a given event on the basis of the number of such events that have already occurred in a defined population.

Sharps: Any object that can penetrate the skin and has the potential to cause injury and infection. Sharps include but are not limited to needles, scalpels, broken glass, broken capillary tubes, and exposed ends of dental wires.

Smoke plume: Smoke created during the use of an electrosurgical unit (ESU) or laser. This smoke contains toxic chemicals, vapors, blood fragments, and viruses.

Standard Precautions: Guidelines issued by the Centers for Disease Control and Prevention (CDC) to reduce the risk of transmission of blood-borne and other pathogens.

Transmission-based precautions: Guidelines to prevent the spread of infectious disease by patients known to be infected.

Underwriters Laboratories (UL): A nonprofit agency that tests and certifies electrical equipment in the United States.

Volatile: A substance such as alcohol with a low boiling point and that converts to a vapor at low temperature.

The potential for accidents and injury in the operating room is one of the highest in the health care setting. High-voltage equipment, chemicals, exposure to blood and body fluids, and stress injury are some of the risks that perioperative personnel encounter daily.

Management of environmental risks requires knowledge of the risk, a plan of action, and continuous monitoring. A successful injury reduction plan considers both the human factor and the technological aspects. Education, awareness, and compliance with recommendations and safety protocols are equally important. This chapter discusses hazards in the operating room environment and provides a basis for knowledge and understanding of the hazards for patients and personnel.

RISK AND SAFETY

Risk is the statistical probability of a harmful event; it is defined as the number of harmful events that occur in a given population over a stated period. In other words, risk represents the number of times an event actually occurs under specified conditions in a specific environment. For example, the risk of contracting human immunodeficiency virus (HIV) as a result of working in the health care environment is based on the number of people who have contracted HIV through **occupational exposure** in the past (based on yearly statistics). Risk and probability are not difficult to measure when sentinel event reporting is performed each time there is an accident or injury in the workplace. Statistics are collected and analyzed so that risk can be measured and policies put in place to prevent future accidents. People often ignore risk factors because they believe themselves to be immune from harm or they believe that they will somehow escape the danger. They know that risk exists, but not for themselves. Taking risks means trying to beat the odds, but it does not change the probability that a given event will occur.

In the health care setting, taking a risk for oneself often means risking the safety of the patient and staff members.

HUMAN AND TECHNICAL FACTORS THAT CONTRIBUTE TO RISK

Most of the discussions in this chapter focus on the technical aspects of accident and injury. However, human factors also contribute to risk. Some of the human causes of injury include the following:

- Fatigue in the workplace
- A work culture focused on the completion of tasks rather than the methods used to complete the tasks safely
- Rushing through tasks to get the work done
- Lack of knowledge about the risks involved
- Emotional strain and stress, which may influence work habits

A culture of safety is crucial to injury reduction in the workplace. This means that staff members must have *awareness* of the risk, *accept* the responsibility for harm reduction, and *act* on prevention measures.

The risks discussed in this chapter focus on the three types of potential injury that represent the most common sources of accidents:

- *Technical risk factors:* Hazards related to medical devices and energy sources
- *Chemical risk factors:* Hazards related primarily to liquid, gas, and solid chemicals in the perioperative environment
- *Biological risk factors:* Hazards related to the transmission of infectious diseases

SAFETY STANDARDS AND RECOMMENDATIONS

A number of private, professional, and government organizations create standards and recommendations aimed at reducing injury in the health care setting:

- *ECRI Institute:* A nonprofit research organization designated as an evidence-based practice center by the U.S. Agency for Healthcare Research and Quality and a collaborating agency of the World Health Organization. Note that ECRI is not an acronym. The initials ECRI have a historical origin. http://www.ecri.org
- *Association for Professionals in Infection Control and Epidemiology (APIC):* http://www.apic.org
- *Centers for Disease Control and Prevention (CDC):* An agency of the federal government and the central authority on infectious diseases. http://www.cdc.gov
- *U.S. Environmental Protection Agency:* http://www.epa.gov
- *U.S. Food and Drug Administration (FDA):* http://www.fda.gov
- *The Joint Commission:* http://www.jointcommission.org
- *Occupational Safety and Health Administration (OSHA):* http://www.osha.gov

These organizations can be contacted for further information on patient and occupational risks in surgery. Standards are periodically updated and renewed. The surgical technologist should remain current because hazards and risks change as new technologies develop.

FIRE

Historically, fire in the operating room has been a great risk. In the past, many fires were associated with flammable anesthetics and unregulated combustible materials. Although these are no longer used, fire is still a real risk. All accredited health care facilities have a responsibility and mandate to orient employees and students to fire safety practices, including the use of fire extinguishers and facility evacuation procedures.

Fire requires three components:

- *Oxygen* (available in the air or as a pure gas)
- *Fuel* (a combustible material)
- *Source of ignition* (usually in the form of heat)

These components are commonly present in the operating room (Fig. 7.1).

OXYGEN

Oxygen is a medical gas. Normal air contains about 21% oxygen. An environment that contains a greater concentration

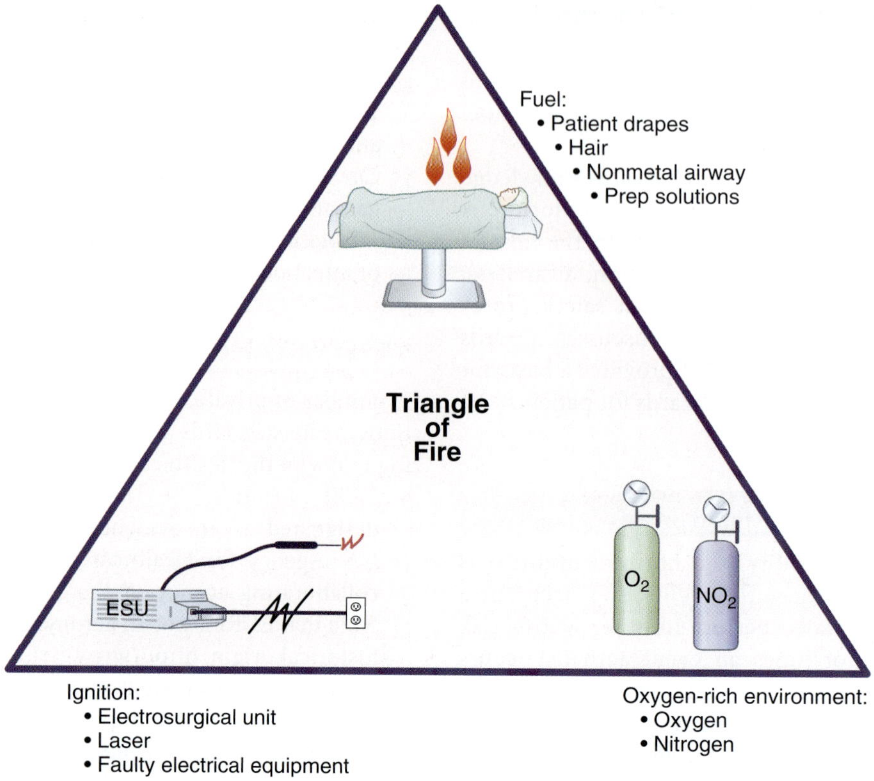

FIG. 7.1 The triangle of fire.

of oxygen is called an **oxygen-enriched atmosphere (OEA).** The operating room is an OEA because oxygen is used in conjunction with general anesthetics and in patient care. Consequently, the risk of fire is high. Oxygen is heavier than air, so it settles under drapes and in confined areas, such as body cavities, where it remains trapped. Further, oxygen molecules are produced when nitrous oxide, used in anesthesia, decomposes in the presence of heat, and this adds to the accumulated level of oxygen.

As the concentration of oxygen increases in the environment, so does the *speed* of ignition, *duration* of the fire, and the *temperature* of the flames. Items that would not normally burn in atmospheric air are highly flammable in the presence of oxygen. Oxygen and nitrous oxide are called **oxidizers** because they are capable of supporting fire.

FUELS

Any material capable of burning is potential fuel for a fire. Materials and substances that burn are described as **flammable.** Note that the words *flammable* and *inflammable* have the same meaning; both indicate combustibility. Sources of fuel commonly found at the surgical site are listed in Table 7.1. Although many items used in the surgical setting are considered "flame resistant" or "flame retardant," they may easily catch fire and continue to burn when ignition occurs in an OEA.

Alcohol

Alcohol is now commonly used in skin prep solutions and is a high-risk source of fuel in surgical fires. An alcohol concentration greater than 20% is flammable and highly **volatile** (i.e., vaporizes at a low temperature). Most skin prep solutions contain 70% alcohol. Vapor from alcohol can be trapped under drapes. When the vapor is ignited, the fire is hidden from view. Second- or third-degree burns can occur within moments of ignition. Most fires arising from alcohol prep solutions occur in combination with an electrosurgical spark (ignition). Although alcohol is highly volatile, it is widely used because it is inexpensive, readily available, and effective. Chemicals such as cyanoacrylates (fibrin glue), which are used as tissue glue and for taking tissue grafts, and methyl methacrylate (bone cement) are volatile and flammable. Petroleum products, such as ointments, can also ignite.

Rubber and Plastics

Rubber, plastic, Silastic, and vinyl materials are flammable. Medical devices made of these materials are common in surgery. Disposable anesthesia equipment, such as endotracheal tubes, airways, masks, cannulas, and corrugated tubing, are a hazardous source of fuel. Endotracheal tubes, except those made especially for laser surgery, are frequently the cause of patient fires during laser surgery of the head, neck, and face. An endotracheal fire can begin as an explosion, causing extensive burns within seconds. The fire moves quickly along the oxygen path and spreads to the lungs, face, hair, and drapes. Surgical drapes and gowns are flame resistant; however, they can ignite easily in an OEA. The operating table mattress and positioning devices made of foam and liquid gels are also potential fuel. As these items burn, they release toxic gases that are an additional source of injury.

TABLE 7.1 Fuel Sources at the Surgical Site

Fuel Source	Fire Prevention
Oxygen-rich environment (OEA)	Tent drapes away from the patient's head during surgery.
Dry sponges and drapes	Place the tip of the electrosurgical unit (ESU) in a holder. Use wet towels, wet sponges, or nonflammable drapes at the operative site.
Endotracheal tube and other flammable anesthesia equipment	Use only laser-approved airways and endotracheal tubes. Use a reflective shield between the patient's head and the surgical field.
Volatile prep solutions	Drape the patient only after all prepping solutions are dry. Tent drapes to allow the escape of vapors when an alcohol-based prep is used. Always check for solutions pooling under the patient before draping.
Lanugo (fine body hair on the patient)	Use a water-based gel on lanugo near laser or ESU sites.
Petroleum-based products	Do not use around laser or ESU sites.
Suction catheter and other peripheral venous catheter (PVC) devices	Do not use around laser or ESU sites.
Smoke plume evacuator tip	Use a noncombustible evacuator tip. Use moist sponges around the laser area.
Gastrointestinal gas	Use suction to remove gases at the operative site.

Intestinal Gas

The intestine normally produces hydrogen, oxygen, nitrogen, carbon dioxide, and methane. Some gases are produced by normal bacteria in the gastrointestinal tract, and others are ingested with food. Forty percent of these gases are contained in the large bowel. Hydrogen and methane are present in sufficient quantities and concentration to be important risks. Methane is explosive at concentrations of 5% to 15%.

SOURCES OF IGNITION

Any heat-producing device has the potential to cause a fire. The more intense the heat, the more rapidly oxidation and ignition are likely to occur. Many potential sources of ignition can be found in the operating room.

Approximately 13% of surgical fires involve lasers (ECRI Institute, 2015). Laser surgery of the trachea and adjacent structures is performed in an OEA close to flammable material. During laser surgery of the neck and throat, a nonflammable endotracheal tube and aluminum-coated drapes are used. Despite these precautions, laser energy remains a potent source of ignition in an OEA during surgery.

The **electrosurgical unit (ESU)** uses electrical energy to coagulate and cut tissue. The active electrode can reach 1292°F (700°C), which is hot enough to ignite surgical drapes and other supplies. The tip of the active electrode can become coated with **eschar** (oxidized tissue residue), which holds heat in much the same way as charcoal. Eschar causes sparking and ignition. Small bits of eschar can be released into the wound as burning embers (e.g., into the throat during neck surgery).

Sparking can occur when the active electrode comes in contact with metal. Sparks can ignite volatile gases, liquids, drapes, and sponges, especially in an OEA. (Chapter 15 presents a complete discussion of the hazards associated with the ESU.)

Other, less obvious devices can ignite combustible materials in surgery. These include power instruments, burrs, drill bits, saws, and the harmonic scalpel, which uses high-frequency sound waves to cut and coagulate tissue. When high-speed drills are used, the active tip is irrigated to prevent the buildup of heat created by friction between the metal tip and the bone. Hot drill bits, saw blades, and other metal tips should never be placed in contact with drapes or other combustible materials.

Light sources used in surgery are intense and bright. Although modern surgical lights are cooler than in the past, these light sources are still a risk. Fiber-optic light, which is used in endoscopic instruments, is particularly intense. The light source is delivered through a fiber-optic cable. When the cable is detached from the endoscope, light emitted from the cable can easily ignite drapes, cloth, or other materials. (The safe use of fiber-optic light is fully described in Chapter 22.)

An electrical short or other malfunction can cause sparking (electrical arcing), which can ignite combustible materials on the surgical field. If an electrical device malfunctions during surgery, it must be removed from service immediately and sent out of the department for repair by the bioengineering department or manufacturer. Perioperative staff should never attempt to repair malfunctioning electrical equipment.

PATIENT FIRE IN THE OPERATING ROOM

Patient fire is a devastating event. Approximately 21% of patient fires occur in the airway, 44% on the face, 8% inside the patient, and 26% on the skin (Eagan, 2012). It takes only moments for a flash fire to engulf the patient. To stop the progression of the fire, *the triangle of fire must be broken.* This means that one or more components (fuel, oxygen, or source of ignition) must be removed from the fire.

WHAT TO DO IN A FIRE

During a patient fire, time is critical. Three steps are immediately taken to protect the patient and stop the fire:

1. Shut off the flow of all gases to the patient's airway.
2. Remove any burning objects from the surgical site.
3. Assess the patient for injury and respond appropriately.

The anesthesia provider reduces the flow of oxygen in the event of fire around the airway. At the same time, burning objects are removed from the field as safely as possible. The surgical technologist must stand by for direction from the surgeon and other staff members in the room. He or she should always have sterile saline or water immediately available on the back table. These may be needed to extinguish a patient fire. Patient fires can usually be contained when one of the elements of the fire has been removed. The next phase of the emergency focuses on the patient's injuries.

RACE

If the fire extends beyond the immediate patient area, the surgical team must activate the hospital fire plan. This plan is based on four immediate actions, which are easily remembered by the acronym *RACE:*

Rescue patients in the immediate area of the fire.

Alert other people to the fire so that they can assist in patient removal and response. Activate the fire alert system.

Contain the fire. Shut all doors to slow the spread of smoke and flame. Always shut off the zone valves controlling inline gases to the room.

Evacuate personnel in the areas around the fire.

If the fire is limited to a small area, appropriate extinguishing agents may be used to put it out. Personnel should never let a fire get between them and the exit.

EXTINGUISHERS

Fire drills are held regularly in all health care facilities. Staff training on fire includes emergency response, the location of fire extinguishers and fire escape routes, and procedure to activate the fire alert system. Most fire extinguishers used in the operating room are water based, carbon dioxide, or dry powder. Carbon dioxide is the preferred type for operating room fires.

During fire extinguisher training, employees and students are asked to remember the acronym PASS:

Pull the ring from the handle.

Aim the nozzle at the base of the fire.

Squeeze the handle.

Sweep the fire with tank contents.

FIRE PREVENTION

Fire prevention is the responsibility of everyone working in the operating room. Risk reduction strategies have been developed by the Joint Commission, ECRI, Association of periOperative Registered Nurses (AORN), and other professional organizations concerned with the protection of patients and staff members. The following strategies are the focus of risk management:

- Participation in fire drills
- Demonstration of the use of firefighting equipment
- Developing methods for rescue operations
- Gas shutoff procedures
- Location of ventilation and electrical systems
- Review of code "red" (fire alert) policies
- Review of fire department procedures
- Developing a safety culture

ECRI and AORN have established fire risk management strategies on the basis of current recommendations for perioperative personnel. These are shown in Tables 7.2 and 7.3.

COMPRESSED GAS CYLINDERS

Although most surgical facilities use inline gases, gas cylinders are still commonly used. Gases such as oxygen, nitrous oxide, argon, and nitrogen are often available as backup or as the primary source of gas.

- *Oxygen* is contained in portable tanks and is used when inline systems are not available or when patients are transported.
- *Compressed* nitrogen and air are used as power sources for instruments such as drills, saws, and other high-speed power tools.
- *Argon* is used during laser surgery.
- *Nitrous oxide* is an anesthetic gas.
- *Carbon dioxide* is used for insufflation of the abdominal cavity, most commonly during laparoscopy.

Compressed gas cylinders are made of heavy steel and are able to withstand the high pressure of the gas and resist puncture or breakage. The wall of a large cylinder is approximately ¼ inch (0.63 cm) thick, and the gas is pressurized to 2200 pounds per square inch (psi). A regulator is fitted into the cylinder stem valve by a threaded connection. The regulator contains two gauges; one displays the flow of gas from the regulator to the equipment being used, and the other shows the amount of gas in the tank (in psi). The regulator is activated by a valve handle. A valve stem or hand wheel is fitted into the top of the tank. Gas flows through the regulator when the tank valve is opened.

The contents of gas cylinders are identified by a stamp or stencil on the tank itself or by a cylinder tag.

IMPORTANT TO KNOW *All safety organizations publish warnings against using a tank's color to identify the gas contained inside. Tank colors vary from vendor to vendor, and there is no international standard for tank color. Safety guidelines mandated by OSHA and the Compressed Gas Association (CGA) advise that only the cylinder tag or stamp/stencil located on the cylinder itself should be used to identify the gas.*

GAS CYLINDER HAZARDS

Two types of hazards are associated with compressed gas cylinders: physical hazards, which are related to the high pressure in the cylinder, and chemical hazards, which are related to the flammability and oxidative qualities, toxicity, or other properties of the gas.

Any compressed gas cylinder can explode or rupture, because the gas is under extremely high pressure. If the gas is also flammable or supports combustion (e.g., oxygen and

TABLE 7.2 Fire Management Strategies: Ignition

Risk	Management
Electrosurgical unit (ESU)	• Use the lowest possible power setting. • Place the patient return electrode on a large muscle mass close to the surgical site. • Large reusable return electrodes should be used according to the manufacturer's instructions. • Always use a safety holster. • Do not coil active electrode cords. • Inspect the active electrode to ensure its integrity. • Do not use the ESU in the presence of flammable solutions. • Ensure that electrical cords and plugs are not frayed or broken. • Do not place fluids on top of the ESU control unit. • Do not use the ESU near oxygen or nitrous oxide. • Ensure that the ESU active electrode tip fits securely into the active electrode handpiece. • Ensure that any connections and adaptors used are intended to connect to the ESU and fit securely. • Do not bypass ESU safety features. • Ensure that the alarm tone is always audible. • Remove any contaminated or unused active accessories from the sterile field. • Keep the active electrode tip clean. • Use wet sponges or towels to help retard fire potential. • Never alter a medical device. • Do not use rubber catheters or protective covers as insulators on the active electrode tip. • Use *Cut* or *Blend* instead of *Coagulation* when possible. • Do not open the circuit to activate the ESU. • Make sure the active electrode is not activated near another metal object that could conduct heat or cause arcing. • After prepping, allow the prep solution to dry and the fumes to dissipate. Wet prep and fumes trapped beneath drapes can ignite. • Provide multidisciplinary in-service programs on the safe use of ESUs based on the manufacturer's instructions.
Argon beam coagulator	• Argon beam coagulators combine the ESU spark with argon gas to concentrate and focus the ESU spark. Argon gas is inert and nonflammable, but because it is used with an ESU, the same precautions as with an ESU should be taken. • Always use a safety holster. • Make sure the active electrode is not activated near another metal object that could conduct heat or cause arcing.
Laser	• Use a laser-specific endotracheal tube (i.e., a tube that has laser-resistant coating or contains no material that will ignite) if head, neck, lung, or airway surgery is anticipated. • Wet sponges around the tube cuffs may provide extra protection to help retard fire potential. Moist towels around the surgical site may also retard fires. • Keep towels moist and away from the edge of the surgical site to retard fires. • Do not use liquids or ointments that may be combustible. • Inflate cuffed tube bladders with tinted saline so that inadvertent rupture may be detected during chest or upper airway surgery. • Do not use uncuffed, standard endotracheal tubes in the presence of a laser or the ESU. • If an endotracheal tube fire occurs, oxygen administration should be stopped, and all burning or melted tubes should be removed from the patient immediately. • Prevent pooling of skin prep solutions. • Have water and the correct type of fire extinguisher available in case of a laser fire. • Ensure that the alarm tone is always audible.
Fiber-optic light sources and cables	• Ensure that the light source is in good working order. • Place the light source on standby or turn it off when the cable is not connected. • Place the light source away from items that are flammable. • Do not place a light cable that is connected to a light source on drapes, sponges, or anything else that is flammable. • Do not allow cables that are connected to hang over the side of the sterile field if the light source is on. • Make sure light cables are in good working order and do not have broken light fibers.
Power tools, drills, and burrs	• Instruments and equipment that move rapidly during use generate heat. Always make sure they are in good working order. • A slow drip of saline on a moving drill or burr helps reduce heat buildup. • Do not place drills, burrs, or saws on the patient when they are not in use. • Remove instruments and equipment from the sterile field when not in use.

Continued

TABLE 7.2 Fire Management Strategies: Ignition—cont'd

Risk	Management
Defibrillator paddles	• Select paddles that are the correct size for the patient (e.g., pediatric paddles on a child). • Ensure that the gel recommended by the paddle manufacturer is used. • Adhere to appropriate site selection for paddle placement. • Contact between the paddles and the patient should be optimal, and no gaps should be present before the defibrillator is activated.
Electrical equipment	• Ensure that all equipment is inspected periodically by biomedical personnel for proper function. • Check the biomedical inspection stickers on the equipment; they should be current. • Do not use equipment with frayed or damaged cords or plugs. • Remove any equipment that emits smoke during use.

Modified from the Association of periOperative Registered Nurses (AORN). Fire prevention in the operating room. In *Standards, Recommendations, Practices and Guidelines*. Denver: AORN; 2007.

TABLE 7.3 Management Strategies: Fuel and Oxidizers

	FIRE RISK—FUEL
Fuel Sources	**Management Strategies**
Bed linens Caps, hats Drapes Dressings Gowns Lap pads Shoe covers Sponges Tapes Towels	• Assess the flammability of all materials used in, on, or around the patient. Linens and drapes are made of synthetic or natural fibers. They may burn or melt, depending on the fiber content. • Do not allow drapes or linens to come in contact with activated ignition sources (e.g., laser, electrosurgical unit [ESU], light sources). • Do not trap volatile chemicals or chemical fumes beneath drapes. • Moisten drapes, towels, and sponges that will be near ignition sources. • Ensure that oxygen does not accumulate beneath drapes. • If drapes or linens ignite, smother small fires with a wet sponge or towel. Remove burning material from the patient. • Extinguish any burning material with the appropriate fire extinguisher or with water, if appropriate.
• Prep solutions	• Use flammable prep solutions with extreme caution. • Do not allow prep solutions to pool on, around, or beneath the patient. • After prepping, allow the prep solution to dry and the fumes to dissipate. • Do not activate ignition sources in the presence of flammable prep solutions. • Do not allow drapes that will remain in contact with the patient to absorb flammable prep solutions.
Skin degreasers	• Skin degreasers may be used before skin prep to degrease or clean the skin or as part of the dressing. These products may contain chemicals that are flammable. Allow all fumes to dissipate before beginning surgery. The laser or ESU should not be used after the dressing is in place.
• Body tissue and patient hair	• The patient's own body can be a fuel source. Coat any body hair that is near an ignition source with a water-based jelly to retard ignition. • Ensure that surgical smoke from burning patient tissue is properly evacuated. Surgical smoke can support combustion if allowed to accumulate in a small or enclosed space (e.g., the back of the throat).
• Intestinal gases	• The patient's intestinal gases are flammable. The ESU or laser should be used with caution whenever intestinal gases are present. Do not open the bowel with the laser or ESU when gas appears to be present. • Use suction during rectal surgery to remove any intestinal gases that may be present.
Oxygen	• Oxygen should be used with caution in the presence of ignition sources. Oxygen is an oxidizer and is capable of supporting combustion. • Ensure that anesthesia circuits are free of leaks. • Pack wet sponges around the back of the throat to help retard oxygen leaks. • Inflate cuffed tube bladders with tinted saline so that inadvertent ruptures can be detected. • Use suction to help evacuate any accumulation of oxygen in body cavities such as the mouth or chest. • Do not use the laser or ESU near sites where oxygen is flowing. • Use a pulse oximeter to determine the patient's oxygenation level and the need for oxygen. • Allow oxygen fumes to dissipate before using the laser or ESU. • Oxygen should not be directed at the surgical site.

Continued

TABLE 7.3 Management Strategies: Fuel and Oxidizers—cont'd

	FIRE RISK—FUEL
	• Ensure that drapes are configured to help prevent oxygen accumulation when mask or nasal oxygen is used. • With a large fire, turn off the gases; with an airway or tracheal fire, disconnect the breathing circuit and remove the endotracheal tube. • Stop supplemental oxygen for 1 min before using electrocautery or laser for head, neck, or upper chest procedures.
Nitrous oxide	• The strategies to manage oxygen should also be used to manage risks associated with nitrous oxide.

From the Association of periOperative Registered Nurses (AORN). Fire prevention in the operating room. In *Standards, Recommendations, Practices and Guidelines*. Denver: AORN; 2007.

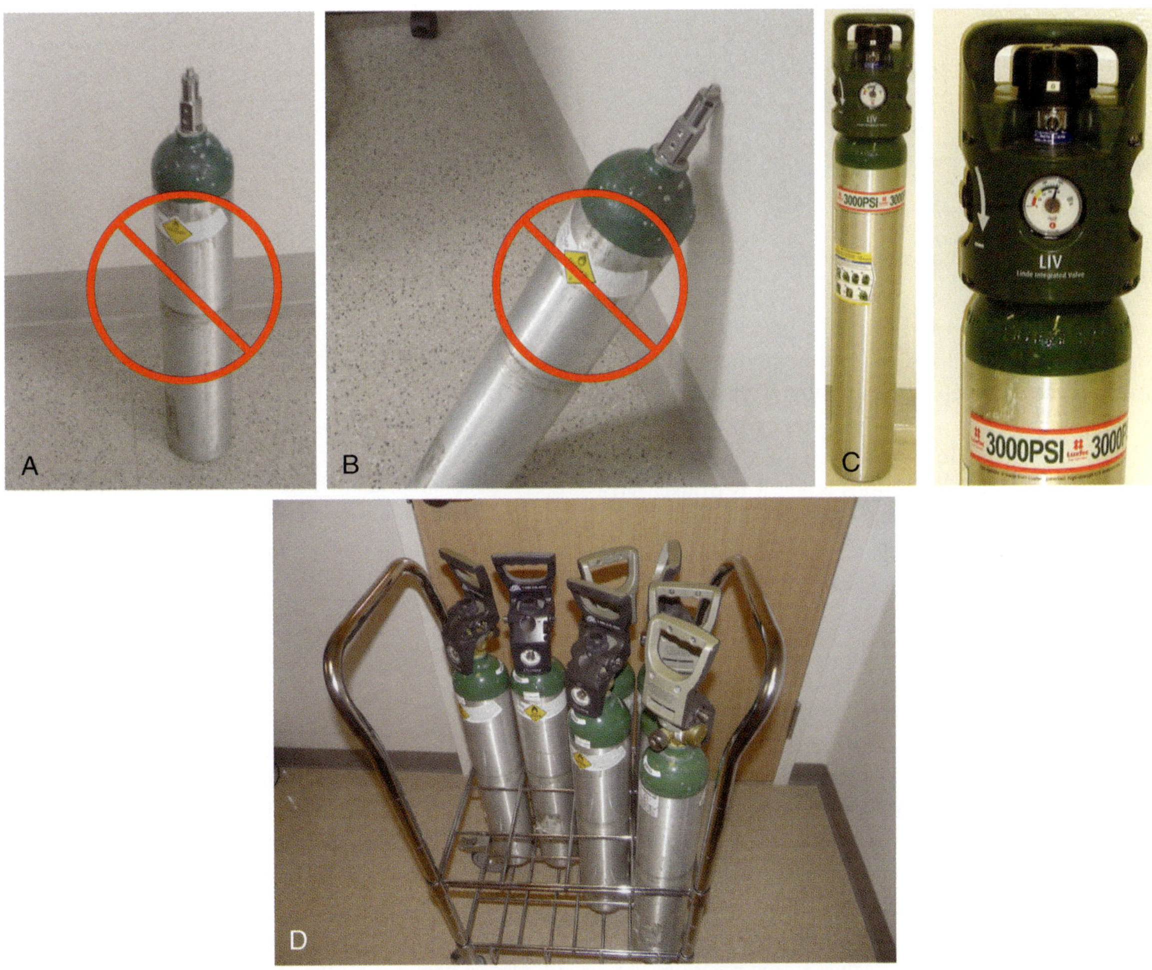

FIG. 7.2 Handling of compressed gas cylinders. (A, B, and C) Never stand gas cylinders unless they are secured in a storage rack. (D) Storage rack for oxygen cylinders. (From Ehrenwerth J, Eisendraft J, Berry J. *Anesthesia Equipment: Principles and Applications.* 2nd ed. Philadelphia: Saunders; 2013.)

nitrous oxide), the risk increases significantly. Cylinders must be handled with care. A leak in a tank or separation of the valve from the tank can propel the tank with the force of a missile, sending it through walls and into objects and people. A cylinder explosion sends high-speed metal particles from the fragmented cylinder into the environment in the same way that a bomb causes injury from shrapnel. Cylinder storage is therefore very important. Gas cylinders must be stored in an upright position in a storage container or rack with chains to hold the cylinders in place. Cylinders must never be left standing upright without the appropriate supports. Oxygen cylinders are now available at extremely high pressures, thus increasing the risk of accidents. Fig. 7.2 demonstrates the correct and incorrect methods of storing cylinders.

PREVENTING CYLINDER ACCIDENTS

Many modern operating rooms have inline gas outlets that dispense oxygen, nitrogen, and air. Even so, gas cylinders, especially oxygen and nitrogen, are common in the hospital environment. The surgical technologist should be familiar with the following procedures for opening, adjusting, and connecting the cylinder to a hose for use in pneumatic-powered surgical instruments:

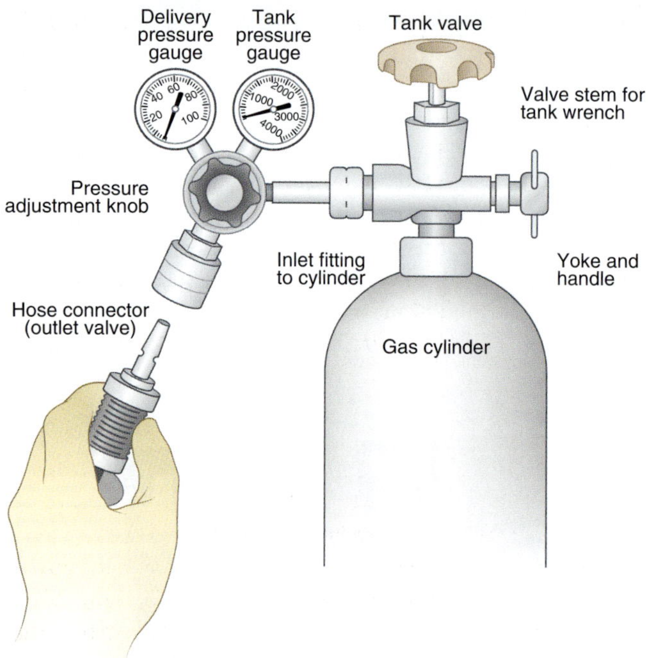

FIG. 7.3 Gas regulator and valve.

1. The gas cylinder has two valves, as shown in Fig. 7.3. One opens the cylinder and allows gas to flow to the regulator. This valve is located on top of the cylinder. Cylinders have either a hand wheel or stem valve with no turn wheel. The stem valve is operated using a valve *spindle key,* which remains with the cylinder at all times while it is in use. Do not use a wrench or other tool to operate the stem valve, because this can result in damage to the valve stem. Only tools that are provided with the cylinder should be used to operate the valve.
2. The second valve is located on the regulator. This valve controls the flow from the regulator to the tubing connected to the user end. It must be adjusted according to the specific requirements of the instrument or device that uses the gas.
3. The right-hand gauge displays the pressure in the cylinder. The left-hand gauge displays the pressure in the power hose connected to the instrument.
4. If the regulator is already attached to the cylinder, *slowly* turn the valve to "crack" it open and then turn the valve to the fully open position. With the valve in this position, the tank pressure is displayed on the right-hand pressure gauge.
5. Do not use the tank if the pressure is less than 500 psi because this means that there is insufficient gas remaining in the tank. A small amount of residual gas (and pressure) in the tank prevents debris (e.g., rust, dust) from entering the hose. Particles entering the hose can damage the equipment or cause injury. Therefore, it is unsafe to run the tank dry.
6. Attach the connector hose securely to the regulator outlet. Most connectors can be attached by pushing and turning firmly.
7. Turn the regulator wheel handle to set the pressure at the correct level. The required pressure level depends on the instrument manufacturer's specifications. Some instruments must be running to set the correct pressure. Make sure that the correct pressure is maintained throughout use.

BOX 7.1 Guidelines for the Storage and Transport of Gas Cylinders

1. Label storage areas with the names of the gases stored there.
2. Never use a gas cylinder that is not labeled properly.
3. A gas cylinder must be secured at a point approximately two thirds of its height at all times. Each cylinder should be secured individually with a chain, wire cable, or cylinder strap.
4. Store cylinders so that the valve is accessible at all times.
5. Never store oxygen cylinders in the same area as flammable gases.
6. Cylinders must never be stored in public hallways or other unprotected areas.
7. Never use grease or oily materials on oxygen cylinders or store them near these cylinders.
8. Always secure a gas cylinder before transporting it. Use a caged rack, chain, or other secure device designed to prevent the cylinder from falling or tipping over.
9. Do not store cylinders of different gases together or allow one to strike another.
10. Never store gas tanks near heat or where they may come in contact with sources of electricity.
11. Never roll, drag, or slide a gas cylinder. Always use a hand cart to transport a tank.
12. Do not tamper with tank safety devices.
13. Always read the identification label of any gas cylinder. Do not rely on the color for identification.
14. Do not attempt to repair a cylinder or valve yourself. The tank must be returned to the bioengineering department or regulator supplier for repair.
15. Never use pliers to open a cylinder valve. Cylinders are equipped with a wheel or stem valve to initiate the flow. Operation of stem valves requires a key, which must remain with the cylinder at all times.
16. Make sure all compressed gas storage areas have adequate ventilation.

8. After use, turn off the tank pressure valve and then bleed the gas remaining in the air hose by activating the instrument.
9. Close the regulator valve by rotating the regulator dial. The pressure should now read zero.
10. Do not return a tank to storage if the pressure is below 500 psi. The tank must be replaced.
11. *Regulators are gas specific and are not interchangeable.* Do not attempt to modify a regulator gauge to fit the gas you are using.

All personnel should be familiar with the safety precautions used for the storage and transport of gas cylinders. These are described in Box 7.1.

ELECTRICAL HAZARDS

Electrical malfunctions are a leading cause of hospital fires in the United States. Accredited hospitals are required to install explosion-proof outlets and to comply with building and environmental codes enacted to prevent electrical fires. However, electrical equipment must also be maintained. The probability of malfunction increases as devices become technologically more sophisticated and have greater requirements for repair and maintenance.

The nature and mechanics of electrical energy are described in Chapter 15. A few points are extracted here for the sake of discussion. The characteristics of electricity (the flow of electrons) are current, voltage, impedance (resistance), and grounding.

- *Current* is the rate of electrical (electron) flow. Direct current (DC) is low voltage and originates from a battery. Alternating current (AC) is transmitted by a 220 V or 110 V line, such as that normally found in wall outlets. The available power is much higher with AC than with DC.
- *Voltage* is the driving force behind the moving electrons.
- **Impedance (resistance)** describes the ability of a substance to stop the flow of electrons (electricity). Electricity follows the path of least resistance. Nonresistant materials include metal, water, and the human body. When electricity enters the body and is not directed back to the source, severe burns and cardiac arrest can result. This is commonly referred to as **electrocution.**
- **Grounding** is the discharge of electrical current from the source to the ground, where it is dispersed and rendered harmless. As long as electrical current can travel unhindered through the body and is directed back to its source, electrocution does not occur. An improperly grounded electrical device can send electricity through the patient but does not control its dispersal to the ground. Normal grounding is established by the use of a three-prong plug. Two of the prongs send the current through the device. The ground wire, or third prong, connects the device to the ground. If no ground wire is used, current can leak into other conductors and will follow a nonresistant path.

HOW TO PREVENT ELECTRICAL ACCIDENTS

- Equipment with frayed cords or devices with exposed wires must never be used.
- Cords must not be spliced or threaded through solid obstacles.
- All switches must be protected from moisture.
- Only devices intended for use around fluids should be used.
- All equipment must be properly grounded.
- Any instrument or device must be switched to the off position before the power plug is removed.
- All equipment used in the operating room must be inspected and must be approved by **Underwriters Laboratories (UL).** This agency develops and maintains standards of safety for consumer electrical products. Electrical items that do not have a UL approval rating must not be used.

The most common source of electrical injury to the surgical patient is the ESU. (Chapter 18 presents a complete discussion of the risks and proper use of the ESU and other power equipment.)

IONIZING RADIATION

X-ray machines, fluoroscopes, and unshielded radioactive implants produce ionizing radiation in amounts high enough to damage tissue. Exposure occurs when workers are not protected during procedures that use radiography or fluoroscopy. Hazard warnings should be posted whenever radiographic or fluoroscopic studies are in progress. The extent of tissue damage depends on the duration of exposure, the distance from the source of radiation, and the tissue exposed. Repeated exposures have cumulative effects. Among the risks of overexposure to radiation are genetic mutation, cancer, cataract, burns, and spontaneous abortion. Certain areas of the body are more vulnerable than others. These are the areas in which cell reproduction is the most rapid, including the ovaries, testes, lymphatic tissue, thyroid, and bone marrow.

X-ray and fluoroscopy are frequently used in diagnostic areas and in the operating room. Lead shields are the most effective method of blocking radiation. The distance from the radiation source, the duration of exposure, and the quality of the shielding are the most important parameters determining risk and protection.

SAFETY PRECAUTIONS DURING THE USE OF IONIZING RADIATION

- Although lead aprons are uncomfortable and heavy, team members should wear them under their sterile gowns during any procedure that requires radiation. Many lead aprons shield only the front of the body; personnel should face the radiation source during exposure.
- A lead apron must be worn during fluoroscopy to prevent exposure to scatter radiation.
- Lead aprons must be stored flat or hung in a manner that prevents bending of the material.
- Remember that a lead apron protects only the areas of the body that are covered by the apron. The eyes and hands are not protected.
- Lead glasses should be worn during exposure to a fluoroscope.
- Neck shields are available to protect the thyroid, which is sensitive to radiation.
- Nonsterile workers should step outside the range of exposure, either behind a lead screen or outside the room. Those who must remain in the room during exposure must maintain a distance of at least 6 feet (1.8 m) from the patient. The safest place to stand is at a right angle to the beam on the side of the radiograph machine or origin of the radiation beam.
- In the radiology department, the walls are lined with lead to protect workers when diagnostic studies are performed. In this circumstance, personnel may be able to step behind the lead wall while the equipment is in operation.
- Whenever possible, a mechanical holding device should be used to support radiograph cassettes to prevent exposure to the hands.
- Lead-impregnated gloves must be worn any time the hands are directly exposed to the radiation beam, or when radioactive implants or dyes are handled.
- Dosimeters are available to measure the cumulative radiation dose for those who are often exposed to radiation.
- Perioperative staff members should rotate through cases involving ionizing radiation. This prevents overexposure of the same staff members.

IMPORTANT TO KNOW *Scrubbed members of the surgical team must don a lead apron before performing hand antisepsis, gowning, and gloving (Fig. 7.4).*

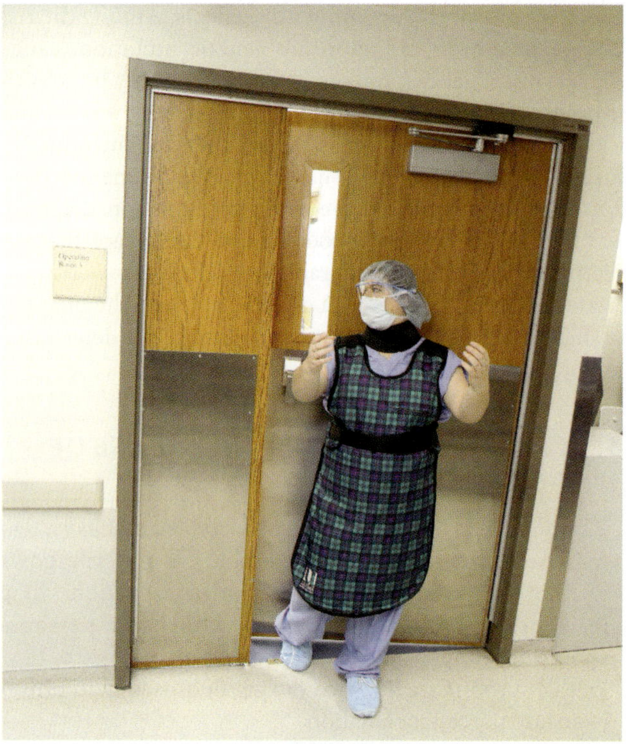

FIG. 7.4 Scrubbed team members must don a lead apron before performing hand antisepsis, gowning, and gloving. Here, the scrub is entering the operating room following hand antisepsis.

MAGNETIC RESONANCE IMAGING

Magnetic resonance imaging (MRI) is a technique used to identify and analyze body tissues. Although similar to other types of imaging, MRI does not use any type of radiation such as that found in x-ray or fluoroscopy. Unlike conventional radiation, MRI produces a 3-D picture of the body. The important component in the MRI machine is a set of very powerful magnets that cause the protons of water molecules in the body to align in one direction and then in the opposite direction. Rapid sequence imaging captures the tissues as they are realigned in the second phase.

Perioperative staff members may assist during MRI procedures. MRI provides a 3-D view of the patient's anatomy using radiofrequency. Whenever MRI is used, the primary risk is the presence of metal in the environment, which can be forcibly drawn from its source and into the path of the powerful magnetic field. The magnetic field of the MRI machine is strong enough to forcefully pull objects into the central tube as large as a hospital bed. For this reason, absolutely no metal objects are permitted in the MRI environment and fringe areas. A substantial risk of injury exists from certain types of metal implants in the patient or staff members and personal items, such as scissors or jewelry. Only plastic and titanium objects are safe to use during MRI procedures.

TOXIC CHEMICALS

Perioperative staff are exposed to many different types of chemicals. The majority of these are hazardous and can produce serious effects, such as respiratory or skin problems, genetic changes, and fetal injury. It is important to remember that, although exposure to a particular chemical may be brief, constant exposure to chemicals in a variety of work situations has a cumulative effect. For example, in a given day, a surgical technologist might be exposed to glutaraldehyde disinfectant, vapor from methyl methacrylate cement, formaldehyde used as a specimen preserver, a phenolic agent used during environmental cleaning, and peracetic acid used as a sterilizing agent. Although the effects of any single exposure may be limited, the cumulative and synergistic effects can be much greater.

BOX 7.2 Reading a Chemical Label

The National Fire Protection Association (NFPA) uses a diamond-shaped diagram of symbols and numbers to indicate the hazards associated with a particular chemical.
Blue: Health hazard
Red: Flammability
Yellow: Reactivity
White: Other hazards

Each category is given a score that corresponds to the hazard level:
4 Extreme
3 Serious
2 Moderate
1 Slight
0 Minimal

Standards and guidelines for handling chemicals are designed to reduce the risk of occupational exposure and associated injuries. All hazardous chemicals approved for use in the United States are issued a *Material Safety Data Sheet* (MSDS). The MSDS describes the chemical, precautions for handling the chemical, hazards associated with the chemical, and firefighting techniques and first aid for exposure. Each department in the health facility is required to maintain an MSDS for chemicals used in that department, and employees must have access to these.

EXPOSURE

Toxic chemicals can enter the body through the respiratory tract, by direct skin contact, by splash contact, or by ingestion. **Personal protective equipment (PPE)** protects personnel against high concentrations of chemicals. Exposure to an airborne chemical (vapor) is measured by concentration, in parts per million (ppm) or milligrams of substance per cubic meter of air (mg/m^3). Every chemical used in the health care setting has a safe limit of exposure, which is determined by government agencies.

PREVENTION

Chemicals used in the health care setting must carry a label containing information about the chemical, including its intended safe use, toxicity, and postexposure measures. All personnel must be familiar with chemical labels and know how to interpret them (Box 7.2). When working with any chemical, know and use the appropriate concentration and the correct procedure for using it safely (e.g., glutaraldehyde must be used under a hood to prevent respiratory irritation). Hazard warning labels are posted on the

TABLE 7.4 Hazardous Chemicals Commonly Used in the Operating Room Environment

Substance	Use	Precaution
Anesthetic gases	General anesthesia	Must be scavenged by anesthesia machine. Be wary of possible fetal injury.
Ethylene oxide	Sterilization	Objects must be aerated in the chamber. Personnel should wear a dosimeter to measure exposure. Do not handle objects until aeration is complete.
Peracetic acid	Sterilization	Use goggles, a face shield, and gloves when operating sterilizer.
Glutaraldehyde	Disinfection	Use only under a hood. Wear gloves, a mask, and goggles.
Phenolic compounds	Decontamination (environmental)	Use correct dilution. Wear gloves and goggles.
Sodium hypochlorite (1 ppm)	Decontamination (environmental)	Use correct dilution. Wear gloves and goggles.
Formaldehyde	Tissue preservative	Wear a mask, gloves, and goggles.
Methyl methacrylate	Bone cement	Do not wear soft contact lenses while using this substance; it causes corneal burns and melts contact lenses. Wear a mask, gloves, and goggles.
Fibrin glue	Tissue glue	Wear goggles, gloves, and a mask.

container and in storage areas. Chemicals transferred from larger containers to smaller ones must be labeled with the exact information found on the original container. Table 7.4 lists the chemicals commonly found in the operating room environment.

SMOKE PLUME

A **smoke plume** is created during laser surgery and electrosurgery. Smoke plumes contain harmful toxins that must be removed from the immediate surgical environment, because they are known to contain benzene, hydrogen cyanide, formaldehyde, blood fragments, and viruses and are potentially harmful when inhaled. All safety organizations, including the National Institute for Occupational Safety and Health (NIOSH), recommend an efficient evacuation and filtering system. A suction tip at the exact site where smoke is generated filters the smoke and absorbs minute toxic particles. This equipment must be used according to the manufacturer's instructions. Filters are considered to be toxic waste and are handled according to institutional and government policy. (The details of smoke plume control and risks are discussed in Chapter 15.)

STANDARD PRECAUTIONS

Sources of infection and the ways diseases are spread from one person to another are discussed in Chapters 8 and 9. This section is an overview of guidelines that have been established to prevent the disease transmission in the health care facility, especially diseases caused by direct contact with blood and body fluids.

NOTE *The practices and standards to prevent the spread of infection are discussed in Chapter 9, Aseptic Technique and Transmission-Based Precautions.*

STANDARD PRECAUTIONS

Standard Precautions are used in all patient care settings–necessary for the protection of patients and staff. They are the minimum practices required of health workers to prevent disease transmission. Box 7.3 lists the basic guidelines. An extended discussion of Standard Precautions can be found in Chapter 9 *Sterile Technique and Infection Control*.

IMPORTANT TO KNOW *The principle on which Standard Precautions are based is that any person may harbor potentially infectious microorganisms. Therefore, the practices of the standard apply to all patients and all actual or possible contact with blood and body fluids.*

LATEX ALLERGY

Sensitivity and true allergy to latex rubber are risks to both patients and personnel. True allergy is differentiated from other types of immune responses. True allergic response, which is mediated by the immune system, is described in Chapter 8. Box 7.4 lists sources of latex found in the health care setting.

Latex is a naturally occurring sap obtained from rubber trees. It is used commercially in the manufacture of many products, including medical devices, supplies, and patient care items. True allergy is an abnormal immune response to a substance.

BOX 7.3 Recommended Practices for Preventing Transmissible Infections in the Perioperative Setting

1. Health care workers should use Standard Precautions when caring for all patients in the perioperative setting.
2. Hand hygiene should be performed before and after each patient contact.
3. Protective barriers must be used to reduce the risk of skin and mucous membrane exposure to potentially infectious material.
4. Health care practitioners should double-glove during invasive procedures.
5. Contact precautions should be used in providing care for patients who are known or suspected to be infected or colonized with microorganisms that are transmitted by direct or indirect contact with patients or items and surfaces in the patients' environments.
6. Droplet precautions should be used when caring for patients who are known or suspected to be infected with microorganisms that can be transmitted by infectious large-particle droplets that generally travel short distances [i.e., 3 feet (0.9 m) or less]; diseases caused by such microorganisms include diphtheria, pertussis, influenza, mumps, and pneumonic plague.
7. Airborne precautions should be used when caring for patients who are known or suspected to be infected with microorganisms that can be transmitted by the airborne route; diseases caused by such microorganisms include rubella, varicella, and tuberculosis.
8. Health care workers should be immunized against epidemiologically important agents according to the regulations of the CDC.
9. Work practices must be designed to minimize the risk of exposure to pathogens.
10. Personnel must take precautions to prevent injuries caused by needles, scalpels, and other sharp instruments.
11. The activities of personnel with infections, exudative lesions, nonintact skin, and/or blood-borne diseases should be restricted when these activities pose a risk of transmission of infection to patients and other health care workers.
12. Policies and procedures that address responses to threats of intentionally released pathogens should be written, reviewed periodically, and readily available within the practice setting.
13. Policies and procedures that address responses to epidemic or pandemic pathogens should be written, reviewed periodically, and readily available within the practice setting.
14. Personnel should demonstrate competence in the prevention of transmissible infections.

Previous exposure and sensitization are required for the body to initiate the formation of antibodies against the allergen.

Latex allergy is a local or systemic reaction mediated by the body's immune system. The reaction causes the release of histamines, which occur normally in the body. This causes edema (swelling) and redness. When histamines are released in massive amounts, the reaction can be life-threatening. The extent of the reaction depends on the exact location and nature of the contact. Allergies are a response to proteins within a substance.

Hypersensitivity is a cell-mediated response. It is a type of delayed reaction that causes dermatitis on contact with the object. In the case of latex gloves, supplies, and medical devices, this reaction is generally related to chemicals in the latex product rather than the latex itself.

Nonallergic dermatitis (skin inflammation) is caused by many irritants found in the operating room environment. Chemicals, antiseptic residue from surgical scrub or hand washing, and glove powder are known to cause irritation in some sensitive individuals.

The operating room environment has many potential sources of latex. The most common concern among surgical personnel is latex gloves. Most surgical and examination gloves contain latex because of its strength and resilience. However, non-latex gloves are available. Box 7.4 lists common sources of latex.

All health facilities have a latex-safe cart available for patients known to be allergic to latex. The cart contains supplies needed for the management of patients with latex sensitivity. Latex cannot be eliminated from the medical environment completely, but risk reduction is an important factor in preventing injury.

Patients and perioperative personnel can be exposed to latex through the skin, circulatory system, respiratory system, and mucous membranes. Gloves and glove powder containing latex molecules are a major concern, but many other medical devices contain latex as well.

Latex can cause skin reactions, including sores, skin cracks, lumps, and itching. Latex can come in contact with the circulatory system through intravenous catheters, tubing, and other intravascular devices. If the latex reaches the bloodstream, large amounts of chemical mediators are released. These can cause severe bronchial obstruction, pulmonary edema, and death.

Individuals who are at the greatest risk of latex allergy are the following:

- People who have had repeated surgeries or frequent contact with medical devices, especially in early childhood
- Individuals who have a positive reaction to a serum latex antibody test
- Anyone with a history of asthma or allergies to particular foods

PREVENTION AND RISK REDUCTION

Prevention of latex injury requires identification of those at risk and avoidance of contact with devices that contain latex. A supply area containing latex-free devices should be maintained for patients known to be allergic to latex. If the patient is known to be latex sensitive, a warning sticker is placed on the person's chart. The information is also included in the patient surgical checklist.

TABLE 7.5 Allergic and Nonallergic Skin Reactions

Type of Reaction	Symptoms/Signs	Cause	Prevention/Management
Contact dermatitis (nonallergic)	Scaling, drying, and cracks in the skin. Bumps and sores, especially on the dorsal side of the hand, caused by gloves.	Skin irritation caused by gloves, powder, soaps, and detergents. Incomplete rinsing after hand washing and surgical scrub. Incomplete hand drying.	Use alternative products. Rinse hands thoroughly after exposure to detergents and antiseptics. Dry hands completely before donning gloves.
Allergic contact dermatitis (delayed hypersensitivity or allergic contact sensitivity)	Blistering, itching, and crusts, similar to a poison ivy reaction. Cracks that occur on the hands or arms after skin exposure, caused by gloves.	Chemicals used in latex processing, including accelerators (thiurams, carbamates, benzothiazoles).	Correctly identify cause. Use gloves that do not contain these chemicals.
Natural rubber latex (NRL) allergy (IgE/histamine mediated) (type I immediate hypersensitivity)	Hives in the area of contact with NRL. Generalized redness, nasal irritation, wheezing, swelling of the mouth, and shortness of breath. Can progress to anaphylactic shock.	Direct contact with or breathing in natural latex proteins, including those contained in glove powder or found in the environment.	Eliminate or drastically reduce exposure to NRL protein. Use non-latex, powder-free gloves.

BOX 7.4 Common Sources of Latex

- Blood pressure cuffs
- Blood pressure tubing
- Bulb syringe
- Catheters, internal and external
- Esmarch bandages (used with pneumatic tourniquet)
- Gloves, sterile and nonsterile
- Intravenous catheters
- Medical tape
- Needles
- Oxygen delivery systems
- Pneumatic tourniquet
- Rebreathing bag for anesthesia machine
- Respiratory tubing and all connectors
- Stethoscope
- Syringes
- Tubing
- Urinary drainage systems
- Wound drains

Workers who believe they are sensitive or allergic to latex should be tested. The use of low-allergen latex and powder-free gloves is recommended by NIOSH and other organizations concerned with the health risks of latex in the health care setting.

MUSCULOSKELETAL RISKS

Musculoskeletal injury is a risk to all personnel working in the operating room. The lumbosacral area, wrist, shoulder, and neck are particularly vulnerable. The causes of musculoskeletal injury are classified according to the types of movement and the workload involved.

Exertion is the amount of physical effort needed to perform a task, such as moving an object. The amount of exertion required for a task varies with the duration and nature of the task; it can also be modified by changing one's posture or grip.

Posture is a critical component of musculoskeletal stress. Twisting or turning the body disrupts normal balance. Other high-risk positions include bending, kneeling, reaching overhead, and holding a fixed position for a long time.

Repetitive motion places stress on tendons and muscles. Factors that affect the risk are the speed of the movement, the required exertion, and the number of muscles needed to complete the action.

Contact stress is excessive direct pressure against a sharp edge or hard surface. Increasing the pressure increases the risk of damage to nerves, tendons, and blood vessels.

RISK PREVENTION

In the operating room, musculoskeletal injuries most often occur as a result of the following:

- Lifting, positioning, transporting, and transferring the patient (see Chapter 16)
- Retrieving and shelving heavy instrument trays overhead or near the floor
- Moving heavy equipment (e.g., the operating table, operating microscope, imaging equipment)
- Catching items that are falling
- Tripping over tubing or electrical cords
- Balancing a heavy instrument tray in the hand while distributing it onto the sterile field
- Attaching cords to wall sockets or overhead inline connectors
- Climbing over operating room clutter or trying to retrieve a heavy item from a cluttered environment

Prevention of musculoskeletal injuries involves creating a safe work environment and using good body mechanics. Fatigue and stress affect muscle control, which can lead to injury. Standing and walking for long periods put extra stress on muscles, tendons, and joints. Perioperative personnel can reduce muscle fatigue while standing by placing the feet shoulder width apart. If a lift (raised platform) is used, it should accommodate a wide stance. Two lifts may be needed so that the scrubbed technologist is not required to step up and down while working between the instrument table and the patient.

Shifting the body weight back and forth on a level surface can reduce muscle strain. Standing on one foot for long periods, however, increases stress and puts the body off balance. Elevating the feet during breaks helps increase circulation to the legs.

Support stockings and leggings significantly reduce muscle ache. These can be purchased in medical supply stores. Supportive shoes distribute pressure on the foot to prevent heel spurs and arch problems.

Heavy items such as large instrument trays must be stored at elbow height, never above the head or at floor level. If they must be stored at floor level, attention to good body mechanics in retrieving these items helps prevent lower back injury. The appropriate way to shelve equipment is to place the heaviest items even with the elbows and smaller items on the shelves above and below this height.

Reducing clutter is another way to prevent musculoskeletal injury. When the surgical suite is crowded with equipment, workers are inclined to shift their weight off balance to move around. Tubing and power cords are added risks. Reducing clutter usually requires planning. Extra space may not be available for the equipment needed, but clutter can be consolidated. Bring in only what is needed for immediate use. Avoid draping cords over furniture and equipment. Consolidate extra supplies on a designated cart, which can be placed away from traffic areas.

The use of mechanical and hydraulic lifting equipment is the best way to prevent injury related to patient handling. The Occupational and Safety Administration now recommends that health care workers avoid lifting patients in all circumstances. Refer to Chapter 16 for further description of patient handling and transfer.

BODY MECHANICS

Developing good body mechanics is a conscious activity. Students and new employees should learn these methods before entering the clinical area for work. If you are injured on the job, obtain medical care as soon as possible.

When *lifting an object,* keep it close to your body. This reduces the force of exertion. Fig. 7.5 demonstrates force exerted on the back in various lifting positions. Fig. 7.6 illustrates safe and unsafe lifting techniques.

- Always bend at the knees when raising or lowering a heavy object. This takes pressure off the lower back and uses the body's heaviest muscles to do the work. Remember to keep your back straight and legs wide apart with both feet flat on the floor for balance.
- Never lock the knees and bend over to pick up an object (Fig. 7.7). This puts stress on the lower back and does not permit use of the thigh muscles to help lift the body.

When *pushing a cart* ahead of you from a standstill, place one foot behind the other. The back foot should be braced comfortably. Use the back foot to push off while transferring your weight to the front foot. Pushing is the preferred method of transporting objects rather than pulling. Make sure you can see any obstacles in your path.

- When *pulling a cart* toward you, use the same stance as in pushing. Use your front leg to exert backward pull while the back foot maintains balance and support.
- When *performing a horizontal transfer* (straight across from one surface to another), use abdominal and arm muscles actively. Do not simply lean back and pull.
- When it is necessary to *bend or reach upward* to connect an electrical outlet or inline gas connection, never twist your body or balance on one foot (Fig. 7.8). This combination not only places the body off balance but it also increases the risk of back injury, because the standing leg is locked in position.
- To lift an object, use your abdominal muscles to hold the weight of your upper body. When the abdominal muscles are not engaged in exertion, the back muscles, especially those in the sacral and lumbar region, must support the entire trunk; this is a common cause of back injury. Tighten your abdominal muscles as you lift and notice that your back feels much more supported.

KEY CONCEPTS

- The risk of accident and injury in the operating room is one of the highest in the health care setting.
- Management of environmental risks requires a knowledge of the risks, a plan of action, and monitoring.
- Risk is the statistical probability of a harmful event and is defined as the number of harmful events that occur in a given population over a stated period.
- A work culture of safety is critical to injury reduction.
- Fire requires three components: oxygen, fuel, and a source of ignition.
- The operating room is an oxygen-enriched environment that supports combustion and fire.
- As the concentration of oxygen increases in the environment, so do the speed of ignition, duration, and temperature of a fire.
- Medical devices made of flammable materials are common in surgery.
- Any heat-producing device has the potential to cause a fire.
- Sparking can occur when an active electrode comes in contact with metal. Sparks can ignite volatile gases, liquids, drapes, and sponges, especially in the presence of oxygen.
- During a fire, the most important priority is protecting the patient.

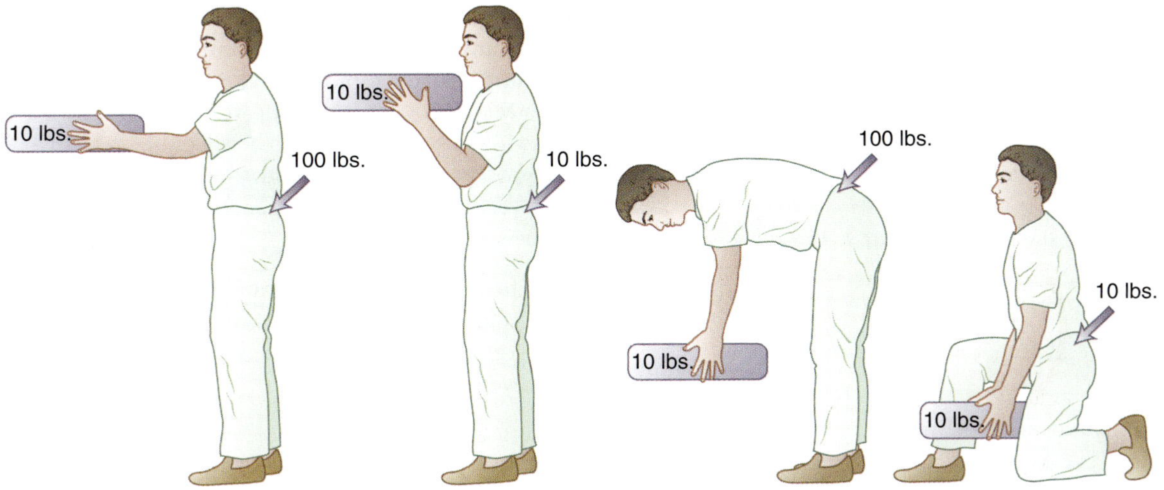

FIG. 7.5 Weight on the back in various lifting positions. (Redrawn from Saunders DH, Saunders R. *Evaluation, Treatment, and Prevention of Musculoskeletal Disorders*. 1st vol, 3rd ed. Chaska, MN: Saunders Group; 1995.)

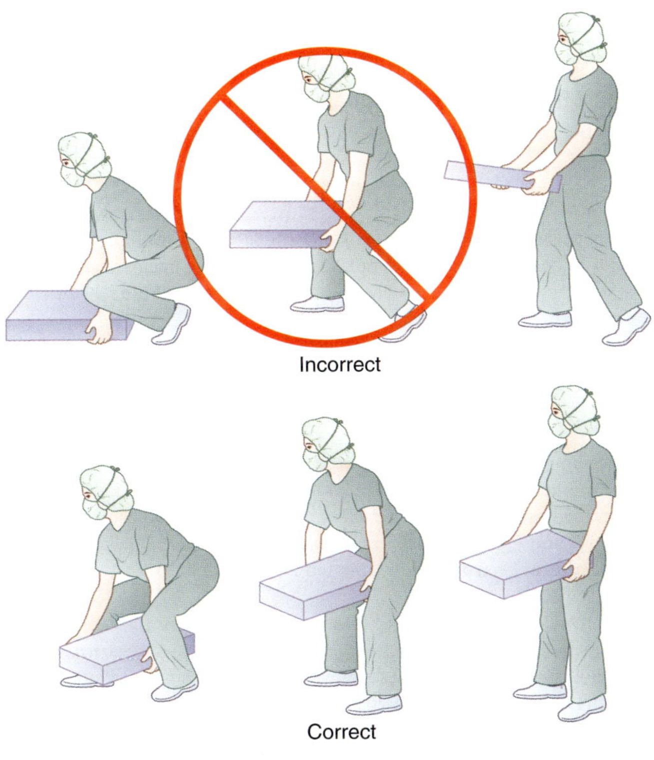

FIG. 7.6 Correct and incorrect mechanics of lifting.

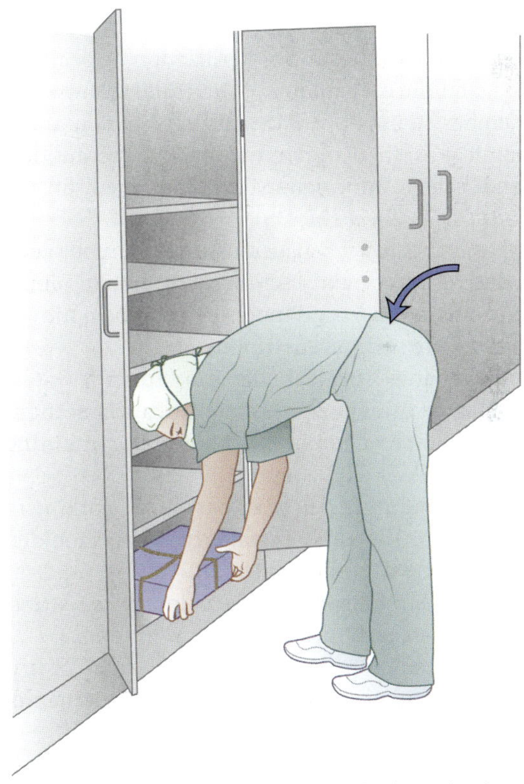

FIG. 7.7 Unsafe body mechanics: locking the knees creates the potential for back injury.

- Immediate action during a fire is described by the acronym RACE: **r**escue patients in the immediate area of the fire; **a**lert other people to the fire so that they can assist in patient removal and response; **c**ontain the fire; and **e**vacuate personnel in the areas around the fire.
- Compressed gases in steel cylinders are associated with serious accidents and fatalities related to the explosion or rupture of the tank.
- A ruptured gas cylinder can become a projectile capable of penetrating walls. Safe handling techniques can prevent rupture.
- The most common source of electrical injury to the surgical patient is the electrosurgical unit (ESU).
- Ionizing radiation used in the operating room and interventional radiology departments can cause tissue damage. The most important method of reducing risk is to prevent exposure by using lead shields, aprons, and other protective devices.
- Magnetic resonance imaging uses radiofrequencies to provide a three-dimensional view of the patient's anatomy. Metal can be drawn into the magnetic field, causing severe injury or death.

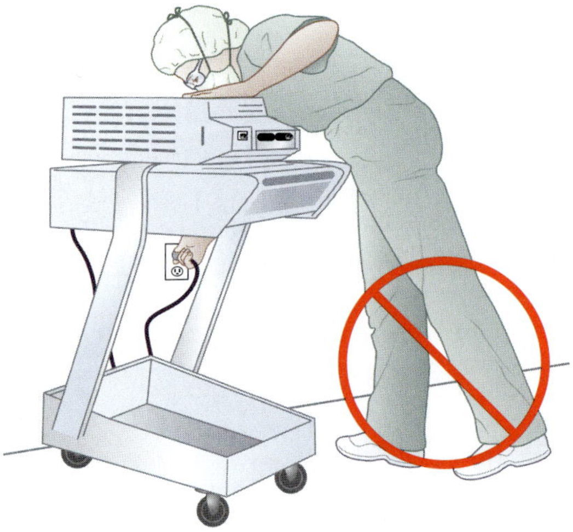

FIG. 7.8 Bending and twisting at the same time creates the risk of back injury. Avoid putting weight on one foot, which decreases balance.

- Dangerous chemicals are used in the perioperative environment for disinfection, sterilization, specimen preservation, and the preparation of surgical implants.
- All staff members must have access to information about specific chemicals in their work environment. Precautions, hazards, and safety information are contained in the Material Safety Data Sheet (MSDS).
- Smoke plume is created whenever tissue is burned, such as during electrosurgery and laser surgery. Smoke plume is known to contain toxins and therefore must be removed from the immediate surgical environment.
- Many medical and surgical devices contain latex. Prevention of latex injury requires identification of those at risk and avoidance of contact with devices containing latex.
- Musculoskeletal injury is a risk to all personnel working in the operating room. The lumbosacral area, wrist, shoulder, and neck are particularly vulnerable.
- The primary causes of musculoskeletal injury are stress, lack of balance, overexertion, and repetitive motion.
- Good body mechanics prevents musculoskeletal injury. However, staff members often neglect good mechanics because of personnel shortages, rushing, or fatigue.

REVIEW QUESTIONS

1. What is the definition of risk? What is meant by risk management?
2. Under what circumstances might perioperative personnel bypass safety precautions?
3. Describe the elements of the fire triangle.
4. What characteristics of oxygen make it particularly dangerous in the perioperative environment?
5. What is an endotracheal fire?
6. Define the RACE procedure during a fire.
7. What are the elements of the PASS procedure for the use of fire extinguishers?
8. What is the rationale behind Standard Precautions?
9. What is the minimum safe distance from a source of ionizing radiation during radiography?
10. What is a Material Safety Data Sheet?

CASE STUDIES

CASE 1

You have finished a busy day at work and are passing through one of the hospital wards to see a friend. As you walk past a utility room, you see that a small fire has started near the linen cart. What do you do?

CASE 2

After a case in outpatient surgery, you are hurrying to clean up so that you can scrub on the next case. You suddenly cut your hand on a sharp retractor that has been soaking in an instrument basin. You decide not to tell anyone because you are sure there won't be any consequences, and you don't have time to fill out an incident report or go to the emergency department. Two weeks later, you regret your decision and are worried about the incident. You may face disciplinary action for not reporting the injury, but you are extremely worried. What would you do?

REFERENCES

ECRI Institute. Surgical fire prevention: Educational resources and custom consulting services. https://www.ecri.org/Accident_Investigation/Pages/Surgical-Fire-Prevention.aspx. Accessed June 23, 2019 Copyright 2016 ECRI Institute.

Council on Surgical and Perioperative Safety. Preventing surgical fires. http://www.cspsteam.org/7-fire-safety. Accessed June 23, 2019.

BIBLIOGRAPHY

Association of periOperative Registered Nurses. Fire safety in perioperative settings. *AORN J*. 2007;86(suppl 1):S141.

Centers for Disease Control and Prevention, Centers for Disease Control and Prevention: *Sharps safety for healthcare settings*. http://www.cdc.gov/sharpssafety/. Updated February 11, 2015. Accessed June 23, 2019.

Centers for Disease Control and Prevention, Centers for Disease Control and Prevention: *Workplace safety and health topics — Electrical and magnetic fields*. http://www.cdc.gov/niosh/topics/emf/. Updated April 21, 2014. Accessed June 23, 2019.

Healthcare Environmental Resource Center. Sterilants and Disinfectants in Healthcare Facilities. http://www.hercenter.org/hazmat/steril.php Copyright 2015 Healthcare Environmental Resource Center. Accessed June 23, 2019.

Occupational Safety and Health Administration. Bloodborne Pathogens—OSHA's Bloodborne Pathogens Standard and Needlestick Prevention. https://www.osha.gov/SLTC/bloodbornepathogens/gen_guidance.html. Accessed June 23, 2019.

Occupational Safety and Health Administration. Safety and Health Topics: Compressed Gas and Equipment. https://www.osha.gov/SLTC/compressedgasequipment/ June 23, 2019.

Occupational Safety and Health Administration. Safety and Health Topics: Laser Hazards. https://www.osha.gov/SLTC/etools/hospital/surgical/lasers.html. Accessed June 23, 2019.

MICROBES AND THE PROCESS OF INFECTION

8

LEARNING OBJECTIVES

After studying this chapter, the reader will be able to:

1. Explain different classifications of organisms and the binomial system
2. Describe components of the cell and cell transport
3. Discuss methods of identifying microbes
4. Identify the basic components of a biological microscope and describe their functions
5. Relate the study of microbiology and the process of infection to surgical practice
6. Describe blood-borne pathogens
7. Describe the phases of types of infections
8. List and describe types of bacteria and the diseases they cause
9. Explain the significance of multidrug-resistant organisms
10. List and describe types of viruses and the diseases they cause
11. List and describe types of fungi and the diseases they cause
12. List and describe types of protozoa and the diseases they cause
13. Describe the body's defense mechanisms against infection
14. List the ways a person acquires immunity to pathogenic organisms
15. Relate a good surgical outcome to the patient's immune response

TERMINOLOGY

Aerobes: Organisms that favor an environment with oxygen. Strict aerobes cannot live without oxygen.

Aerosol droplets: Droplets of moisture small enough to remain suspended in the air; such a droplet can carry microorganisms within it.

Anaerobes: Organisms that prefer an oxygen-poor environment. Strict anaerobes cannot survive in the presence of oxygen.

Bioburden: A measure of the number of bacterial colonies on a surface.

Contaminated: A surface, substance, or tissue that is not completely free of microorganisms.

Culture: The process of growing a microbe in a laboratory setting so that it can be studied and tested.

Diffusion: Uniform dispersal of particles in a solution or across a membrane.

Direct transmission: The transfer of microbes to an item or tissue by direct physical contact with the microbes.

Droplet nuclei: Dried remnants of previously moist secretions containing microorganisms. Droplet nuclei are an important source of disease transmission.

Endospore: The dormant stage of some bacteria that allows them to survive in extreme environmental conditions, including heat, cold, and exposure to many chemicals. Endospores are commonly referred to as spores.

Entry site: In microbial transmission, the sites where microorganisms enter the body.

Fomite: An intermediate inanimate source of infection in the process of disease transmission. An object, such as a contaminated surgical instrument or medical device, can become a fomite in disease transmission.

Infection: The invasion and proliferation of pathogenic microorganisms in the body.

Inflammation: The body's nonspecific reaction to injury or infection that results in redness, heat, swelling, and pain.

Necrosis: Tissue death.

Nosocomial infection: Another term for hospital-acquired infection (HAI) or health care–acquired infection; an infection acquired as a result of being in a health care facility.

Opportunistic infection: Infection in a weakened individual; the host may be debilitated by another disease or their immune system may be compromised.

Pathogen: A disease-causing (pathogenic) microorganism.

Prion: An infectious protein substance that is resistant to common sterilization methods.

Resident microorganisms: The microorganisms that normally colonize certain tissues of the body, usually without harm to the host.

Sterile: Completely free of all microorganisms.

Suppurative: Having developed pus and fluid.

Vector: A living intermediate carrier of microorganisms from one host to another.

Virion: A complete virus particle.

Virulence: The degree to which a microorganism is capable of causing disease.

Microbiology is the study of microscopic organisms called microbes or microorganisms. In the operating room, we are particularly concerned with preventing infections caused by bacteria and viruses transmitted by instruments, equipment, and personnel. To understand how disease is transmitted and prevented, we first need to study the organisms themselves and the diseases they cause. This chapter in particular explains the relationship between microbes and infection. Box 8.1 presents a short summary of important events in the history of microbiology.

Microbiology is a highly complex field with many subspecialties. *Medical microbiology* is the study of infectious diseases caused by microorganisms. Subspecialties of medical microbiology are concerned with specific species (e.g., virology, bacteriology, parasitology).

Pathology is the study of disease mechanisms, diagnosis, and treatment. Nonmedical microbiology includes the study of microbes in the environment or those used in commercial products. Plant microbiology is an important field of study for understanding habitats in the environment and the preservation of species. The study of microbial diseases in plants often focuses on the development and protection of food crops.

Epidemiology is the study of disease or event (e.g., trauma) patterns. Epidemiology specifically focuses on the incidence (number of *new* cases or events in a given time period), affected populations, and the existing burden of the disease (total number of cases per population at a given time).

A new field of study related to infectious disease is called *emerging diseases*. This is related to new diseases or known diseases that have not previously been a public health problem but are becoming a threat.

BOX 8.1 Important Events in the History of Microbiology

1677: Anton van Leeuwenhoek develops the light microscope and observes "little animals" under magnification.
1796: Edward Jenner develops the first smallpox vaccination.
1850: Ignaz Semmelweis discovers the association between hand washing and a decrease in puerperal infection.
1861: Louis Pasteur disproves the theory of spontaneous generation and develops the germ theory of infection.
1867: Joseph Lister first practices surgery using antiseptic practices.
1876: Robert Koch offers the first proof of the germ theory using *Bacillus anthracis*.
1882: Robert Koch develops the Koch postulates. Paul Ehrlich develops the acid-fast stain.
1884: Christian Gram develops the Gram stain.
1885: Louis Pasteur develops the first rabies vaccine.
1892: Dmitri Iosifovich Ivanovski discovers the virus.
1900: Walter Reed proves that mosquitoes carry yellow fever.
1910: Paul Ehrlich discovers a cure for syphilis.
1928: Alexander Fleming discovers penicillin.
1995: The first microbe genome sequence (for *Haemophilus influenzae*) is published.

CLASSIFICATION OF ORGANISMS

A simple definition of an organism is a living thing or system capable of reproduction, reaction to stimuli, growth, and maintenance or metabolism. There are many different types of organisms. A mammal is an organism and so are one-celled bacteria.

Science uses several different methods to classify organisms. The oldest method was developed 300 years ago by Carolus Linnaeus, and his system is called the *Linnaean system*. The Linnaean system classifies living things as either plant or animal according to evolutionary descent. Of course, since Linnaeus's work, classification (taxonomy) has become much more sophisticated and complex. A commonly used system in biology has eight categories or classifications, listed here from smallest to largest:

- Species
- Genus
- Family
- Order
- Class
- Phylum
- Kingdom
- Domain

BINOMIAL SYSTEM

The *binomial system* is a method of naming organisms. Each organism is named specifically according to its genus and species, which are Latin or Greek words. For example, human beings are classified as genus *Homo* and species *sapiens*. The disease typhoid is caused by the bacterium *Salmonella typhi*. When the scientific name of an organism is typed, the genus is capitalized *(Salmonella)*, and both the genus and species are italicized *(Salmonella enterica)*; when the scientific name is handwritten, the capitalization stays the same, and the name (both parts) is underlined.

CELL AND ITS COMPONENTS

Cell theory was developed in the 1600s, shortly after the invention of the microscope. This theory is the basis of modern biology and states that

1. The cell is the fundamental unit of all living things.
2. All living things are composed of cells.
3. All cells are derived from other cells.

The cell is the basic unit of a living organism. Cellular organisms are divided into two types, prokaryotes and eukaryotes, each descended from different groups. Fig. 8.1 shows both types of cells.

CELLS OF EUKARYOTES (COMPLEX ORGANISMS)

Plants, animals, and single-celled organisms are composed of many types of cells. This basic type of cell in a complex organism such as a mammal is called a *eukaryotic cell*. All cells that make up the human body are eukaryotic. Different tissues are composed of variations of the eukaryotic cell. For example, a muscle cell has features that distinguish it from a nerve cell

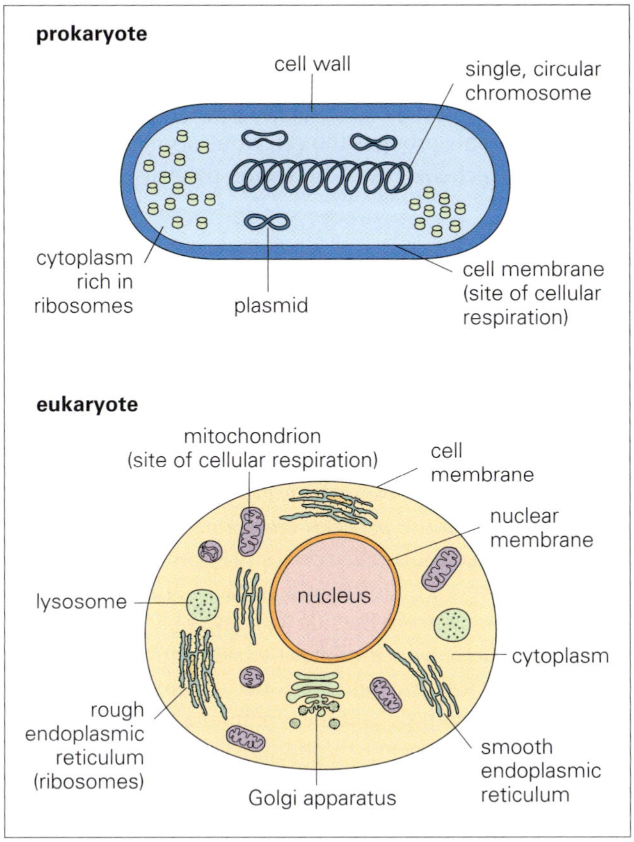

FIG. 8.1 Eukaryotic and prokaryotic cells. Only bacteria and the Archaea groups are prokaryotes. (From VanMeter K, Hubert R, eds. *Microbiology for the Healthcare Professional.* 2nd ed. St Louis: Elsevier; 2016.)

(neuron). However, both are eukaryotic. The cells of a fish or a fungus are also eukaryotic cells.

The eukaryotic cell is the basic cell that makes up multicellular organisms and some types of single-celled organisms. There are many different kinds of eukaryotic cells, but all have the same basic structure, which includes a cell membrane and many specialized structures inside the cell.

Eukaryotic cells are surrounded by a double-layered membrane. The inside of the cell contains a semi-clear liquid, called *cytosol,* and small bodies called *organelles,* which perform the cell's metabolic functions.

Organelles

Eukaryotic cells have many types of smaller interior organs called organelles (Fig. 8.2):

- *Nucleus, chromatin, chromosomes:* The *nucleus* is the largest organelle. It is surrounded by a complex membrane that forms interconnected folds called the *endoplasmic reticulum.* The nucleus contains a protein substance called *chromatin* that contains the cell's deoxyribonucleic acid (DNA). This enables the cell to replicate. During reproduction, the chromatin forms double strands called *chromosomes.*
- *Nucleolus:* The nucleus also contains a *nucleolus,* which has proteins and ribonucleic acid (RNA), which is also necessary for cell reproduction. RNA transfers the cell's genetic information from the DNA in the nucleus to the ribosomes along the folds of the endoplasmic reticulum. These small organelles are the site of protein synthesis for cell reproduction.

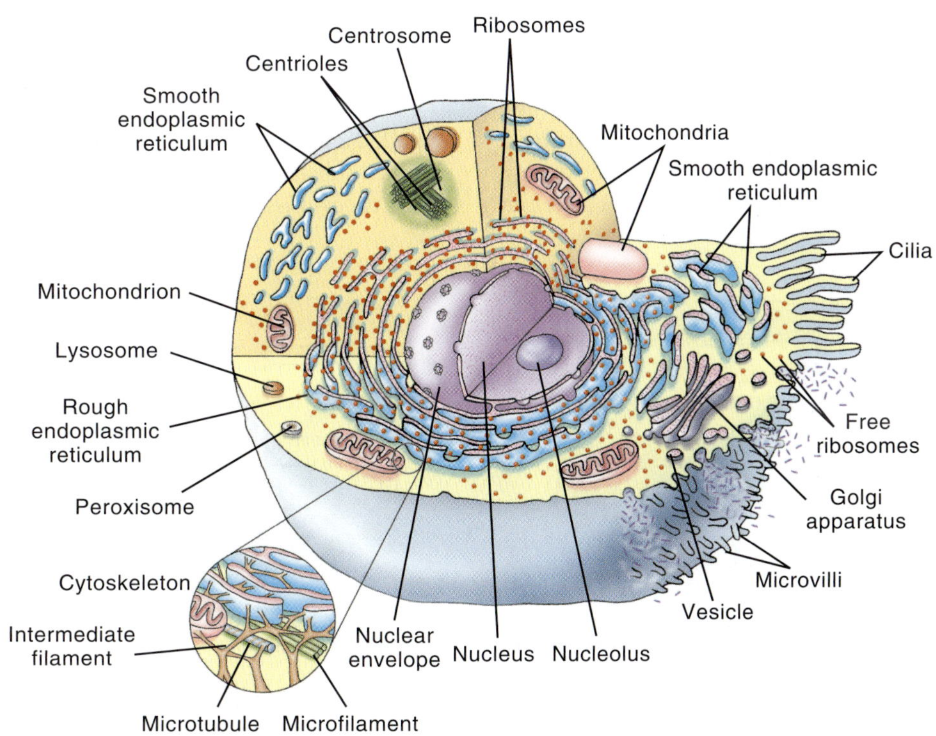

FIG. 8.2 Eukaryotic cell demonstrating organelles, which are units of metabolic function within the cell. (From Thibodeau G, Patton K, eds. *Anatomy and Physiology.* 6th ed. St Louis: Mosby; 2007.)

- *Inner membranes and their vacuoles and Golgi apparatus:* The cell has a complex network of membranes that form compartments for the organelles. This system is called the *endomembrane system.* The endomembrane can "pinch off" to form new closed compartments as needed; these are called *vacuoles,* which may store molecules or transfer waste out of the cell. They also wall off any harmful substances inside the cell. Smaller sacs, called vesicles, store substances and transport waste. The *Golgi apparatus* is another extension of the endomembrane. This organelle stores and modifies large molecules and transports them inside the cell.
- *Mitochondria:* The *mitochondria* are composed of an outer membrane and many inner compartments. Mitochondria synthesize *adenosine triphosphate (ATP),* which provides energy for cell metabolism.

CELLS OF PROKARYOTES (MICROBES)

A *prokaryote* is one of a group of single-celled microbes that includes only bacteria and a smaller, primitive group of single-celled organisms called *Archaea.* In medicine, we are mainly concerned with bacteria, because they cause disease.

- *Genetic material:* A prokaryotic cell (bacterium) does not develop into a complex organism with tissue differentiation. It remains as a single cell, but it multiplies into colonies. One of the main differences between prokaryotes and eukaryotes is that prokaryotes have no nucleus. The genetic material for prokaryotic cells is coiled in an area called the nucleoid. This structure contains chromosomes, but DNA may also lie outside this region in a small circular molecule called a plasmid. The only true organelle of the prokaryote is the ribosome, which synthesizes protein.
- *Cell membrane:* All prokaryotes are surrounded by a cell membrane, and some have a rigid *cell wall.* The cell wall is very important in the classification of bacteria.
- *Flagellum and pili:* A long filament extends from the surface of the cell. This structure may occur as a single strand *(flagellum)* or in small "tufts" *(flagella).* The flagella are used for movement. *Pili* are another type of surface extension on bacterial cells. A single *pilus* attaches to another bacterium as a means of infusing its cytoplasm and genetic material. Some bacteria can attach their pili to human tissue and alter the body's immune response to the bacteria.
- *Capsule or slime layer:* Some bacteria have a *capsule,* or *slime layer.* This protects the cell from drying and provides resistance to chemicals and invasion by viruses.

CELL TRANSPORT AND ABSORPTION

Cells absorb molecules and other substances across their outside membranes and synthesize others from substances inside the cell. The movement of substances occurs by two different methods, namely *passive transport* and *active transport.* Passive transport is the simple movement of particles in a solution. An example of passive transport is **diffusion.** When salt is added to water, the salt crystals simply disperse in the water. No energy is needed for this to occur. When the particles cross a permeable membrane, such as that of a cell, it is called *osmosis* (Fig. 8.3). The cell membrane is selective and allows only certain substances to cross. Water tends to move from the side with fewer particles to the side with more particles, which dilutes the side with more particles. Water continues to move until the concentration and water pressure are equal on both sides of the membrane (Fig. 8.4).

To function, cells require some substances to be unequal in their distribution between the outside and inside of the cell. The cell does this by "pumping" the substance across the membrane rather than simply allowing it to disperse as in passive transport. The pumping is accomplished by chemical or electrochemical action that requires cellular energy. This type of transport is called *active transport.*

Endocytosis is a type of active transport in which the cell *carries a substance into the interior* by engulfing it. In pinocytosis, the cell takes in water and small particles by surrounding them with a membrane-covered blister or vesicle. The material is completely enclosed by the membrane and moved to the interior of the cell, where it is transported to the needed location or outside the cell.

In *phagocytosis,* large particles such as microbes are engulfed and digested by a cell structure called a *lysosome.* The digested substances are then released from the cell by a process called *exocytosis* (Fig. 8.5).

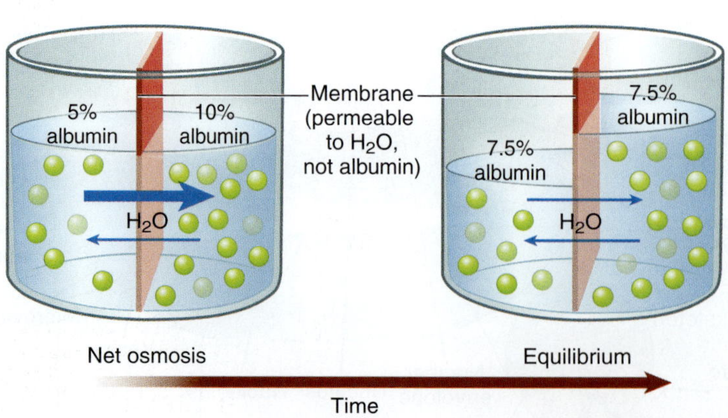

FIG. 8.3 The process of osmosis, which is the passage of water through a selectively permeable membrane. On the *left,* the container holds two concentrations of albumin. On the *right,* the membrane has allowed water, but not albumin, to pass through, creating equilibrium. (From Patton KT, Thibodeau GA. *The Human Body in Health & Disease.* 6th ed. St Louis: Elsevier; 2014.)

TOOLS FOR IDENTIFYING MICROBES

The study of microbes in medicine includes identifying them and testing their sensitivity to antimicrobial agents. This requires special laboratory procedures and tools. Most basic laboratory procedures focus on the bacteria, because this group of microbes causes most infectious diseases, and accurate identification is often critical for treatment and prevention.

Culture

To identify a specific type of bacteria, a sample must be allowed to grow (colonize) outside the body. This is called a bacterial **culture.** After a sample of tissue or fluid is obtained, a very small amount of the sample is applied to a special plate or test tube that contains a semisolid or liquid medium conducive to microbial growth. There are many different types of culture media, which are composed of various substances that support bacterial growth. The most common types are shown in Box 8.2. After the bacteria are inoculated into the culture medium, the plate or test tube is placed in a warm culturing oven for several days to a week to allow the bacteria to proliferate. Samples of the newly cultured microbes are then ready for testing and identification. Bacteria are routinely tested for their sensitivity to antimicrobials (antibiotics). This is performed by inoculating a culture plate with the microbe and placing small paper discs impregnated with various antibiotic agents on the

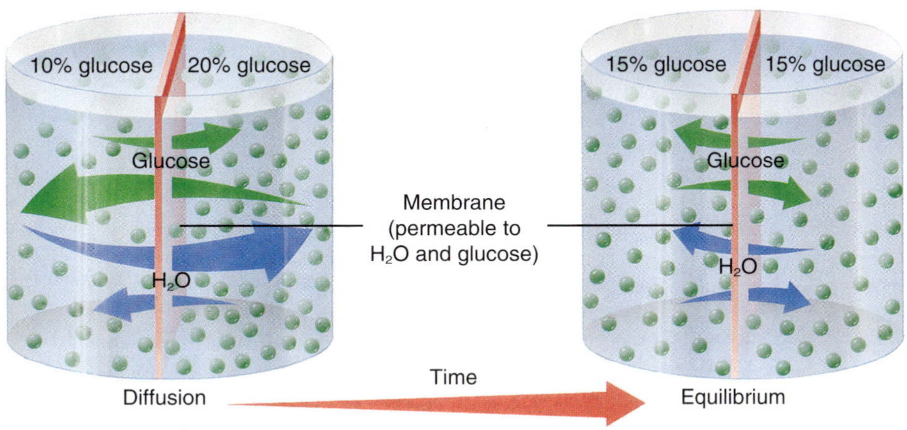

FIG. 8.4 Diffusion across a membrane. The container on the *left* shows two separate concentrations of glucose. The membrane allows glucose to pass through until the two sides are equal in concentration. (From Thibodeau G, Patton K, eds. *Anatomy and Physiology*. 6th ed. St Louis: Mosby; 2007.)

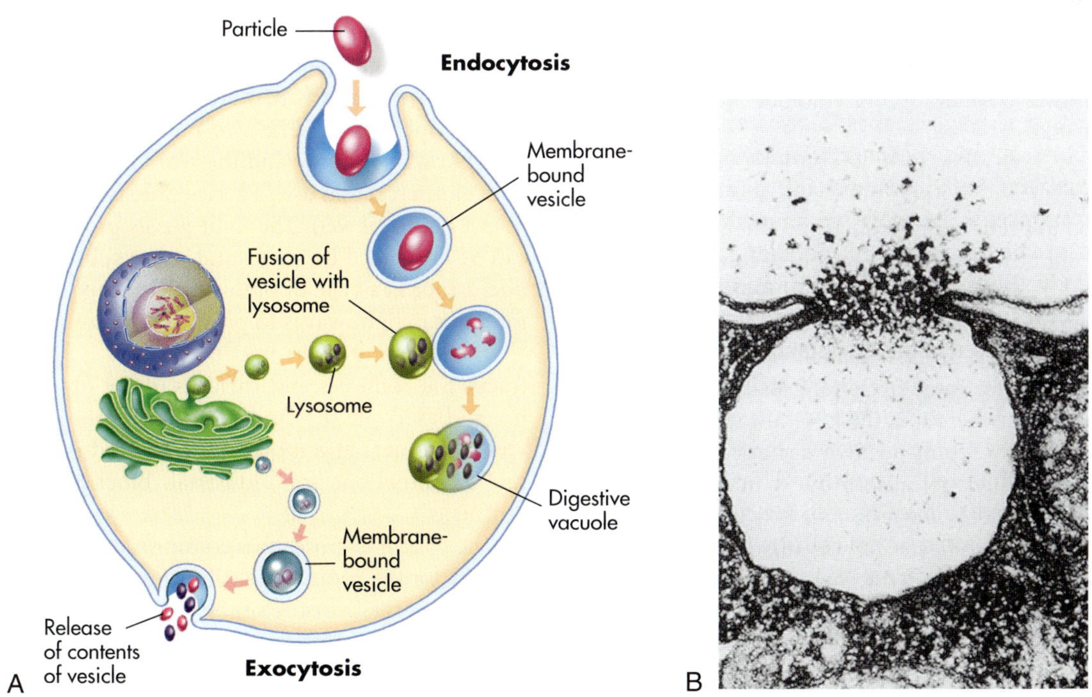

FIG. 8.5 Endocytosis and exocytosis. Materials are transported into and out of a cell by means of a vesicle. Fusion of the vesicle with the lysosome causes the material to break down. The contents of the vesicle are released by exocytosis. (From McCance KL, Huether S. *Pathophysiology: The Biologic Basis for Disease in Adults*. 7th ed. St Louis: Elsevier; 2015.)

BOX 8.2 Types of Culture Media

Defined: Consists of specific substances or recipes.
Complex: Does not contain specific measured substances. These are made of different proteins known to promote bacterial growth.
Selective: Are made of specific substances that support the growth of individual types of bacteria.
Anaerobic: These support only anaerobic bacteria.
Transport: These media are used only for transporting specimens that will be cultured at a later time.

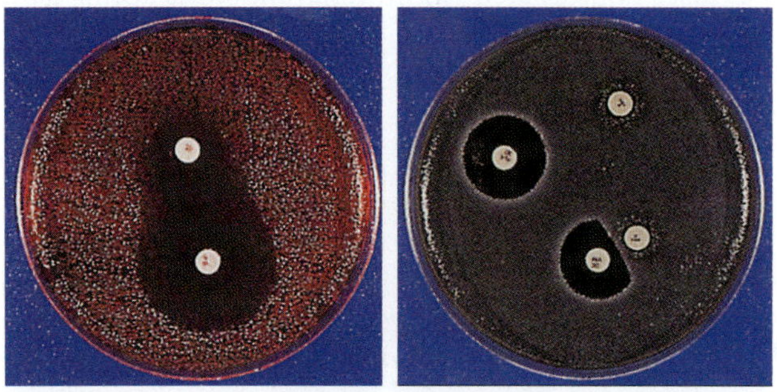

FIG. 8.6 Testing for culture and sensitivity. This is a common method of determining which antibiotics are effective against a specific bacterium or fungus. Various types of antibiotic agents impregnated on paper are positioned in the culture medium, which has been inoculated with the microorganism. Note the areas of no colonization around some of the squares. (From Goering R et al. *Mims' Medical Microbiology*. 4th ed. St Louis: Mosby; 2008.)

sample. This procedure is called *culture and sensitivity testing.* The antimicrobial agents that prevent microbial growth of the particular bacteria show no cultures in that region of the culture plate. The microbe is said to be *sensitive* to that chemical. The antimicrobial discs that are *not* effective at halting microbial growth show a proliferation of colonies in the region of that agent (Fig. 8.6).

Staining

Staining is used to prepare a microbial specimen for examination under the microscope. A large variety of colored stains are available to perform specific tests in the laboratory.

Gram staining is routinely performed to differentiate bacteria into two primary groups, namely gram-positive and gram-negative bacteria. Some bacterial cells have a very thin cell wall, whereas in others it is thick. Gram staining reveals the thicker wall of the gram-positive bacteria. The bacteria with the thinner wall do not absorb the stain and are gram-negative. The *acid-fast staining technique* is used primarily for the identification of *Mycobacterium* organisms, especially *M. tuberculosis.* In this procedure, the bacteria are exposed to an acidic stain that is taken up by the cell wall and is visible under microscopy.

See the tables on the Evolve website that review staining techniques and culturing techniques: http://evolve.elsevier.com/Fuller/surgical.

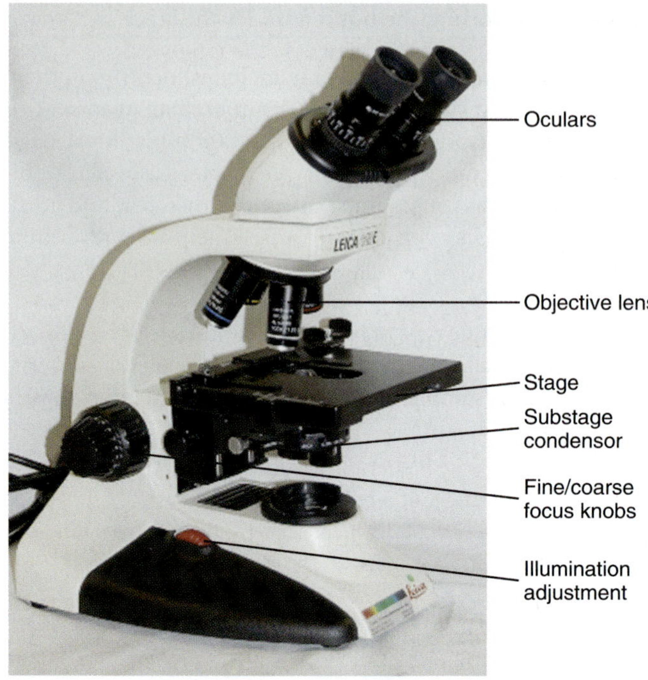

FIG. 8.7 Light microscope showing the lens system and parts. (From VanMeter K, Hubert R, eds. *Microbiology for the Healthcare Professional.* 2nd ed. St Louis; Elsevier; 2016.)

Another staining technique is that used for observing bacterial endospores, which are present in some bacilli. This test uses the stain malachite green. *Capsule staining* is used to detect the outer gelatin layer of the bacterial spore. This test differentiates spores with a thin outer slime layer.

Microscopy

The laboratory microscope is one of the most important tools used to identify and study microbes. The microscope magnifies specimens to identify their shape, size, staining properties, and other important attributes. A discussion of the use of the microscope follows. The two main types of microscopes are the *optical microscope* and the *scanning probe microscope.* The optical microscope uses a series of lenses to focus light on the object being viewed. The light waves provide contrast, which can be enhanced by stains and other substances. The *electron microscope* is a type of optical microscope that uses electrons rather than light waves to provide contrast.

The *scanning probe microscope* uses a physical probe that tracks the contours and surfaces of the object and creates an image based on the findings. This type of microscope can view the object at a molecular level and is used in extremely fine examinations for industrial, biochemical, and medical purposes.

The *optical microscope* is commonly used in medical microbiology for the routine identification and study of tissue, cells, and microorganisms. A simple optical microscope is pictured in Fig. 8.7. Many different types of optical microscopes use an exterior or interior light source to illuminate the subject.

PARTS OF A MICROSCOPE A biological microscope has one or two eyepieces, a series of lenses, a light source, focus adjustment, and a strong base that stabilizes the microscope. Modern microscopes use an electric light source contained inside the body or located at the bottom under the stage, where the specimen slide is placed for viewing. The following parts make up the microscope:

1. *Ocular (eyepiece):* One or two oculars are located at the top of the microscope. The viewer looks into the eyepieces, through which the image of the object is viewed. The eyepieces are directly in line with the series of lenses that focus the light and bring the image into clear view.
2. *Tube:* The tube, or viewing tube, connects the eyepiece to the objective lens, which is located directly over the stage.
3. *Arm:* The arm connects the viewing tube to the base and balances the microscope. It is also used for carrying the microscope; one hand is placed on the base and the other around the arm.
4. *Objective lens:* This set of lenses is located at the bottom of the tube. The lens powers, or magnification, differ among microscopes. The common laboratory microscope has 10×, 40×, and 100× lenses. These are in line with the eyepiece lens, which is usually 10×. Thus the collective magnification is 10 times the power of the objective lens.
5. *Focus adjustment knobs:* Two focus adjustment knobs are located near the arm. These provide fine and coarse focus by moving the serial lenses vertically. Because the focus adjustment moves the objective lenses directly over the subject, the danger exists of direct contact (and damage) to the objective lens. Some microscopes have a rack stop to prevent this.
6. *Rack stop:* This is a vertical adjustment that prevents direct contact between the objective lens and the specimen. The rack stop is common on student microscopes to prevent damage to the objective lens (and slide).
7. *Nosepiece:* This is a round fitting for the objective lenses. The nosepiece revolves to place one of the objective lenses directly over the subject being viewed.
8. *Stage:* This is the flat area just under the objective lenses where the specimen slide is placed. The stage can be moved with knobs so that the specimen can be scanned from side to side or up and down. The slide is secured on the stage by a clip mechanism.
9. *Illuminator (light source):* Intense, evenly distributed light is needed to view the specimen. This is provided by the light source, which is located under the base of the microscope directly under the condenser. Tungsten or quartz halogen light bulbs are commonly used in laboratory microscopes.
10. *Condenser:* This mechanism is located under the stage and contains two sets of lenses that focus light on the subject. The condenser has a diaphragm, or iris, that can be adjusted to allow more or less light into the viewing area. The condenser is operated with a diaphragm lever located just under the stage.

USE OF THE MICROSCOPE Using a microscope properly requires "hands-on" instruction and practice. The microscope itself is a delicate and expensive instrument with numerous components. In addition, the specimen itself requires preparation. If the slide is prepared improperly, the specimen will be damaged or obscured.

Guidelines for caring for the microscope include the following:

1. Always carry the microscope by the arm and the base, using both hands.
2. Use only laboratory-grade, lint-free lens paper to clean the objective lenses. The lenses are very delicate and can be easily scratched with coarse paper. Lint from cleaning materials can obscure the lenses.
3. Provide a clutter-free surface for the microscope during use.
4. Always store the microscope with the objective lenses in their highest position to prevent damage.
5. Never attempt to insert a slide with the objective lenses lowered.
6. Store the microscope in a dust-free environment with a cover.

The microscope requires some setting up and adjustments in the illumination system before use. Once these are accomplished, a simple specimen can be used to practice with the microscope. Follow these steps to prepare a simple specimen for viewing under the microscope:

1. Prepare the specimen using a glass slide and cover slip. (Slides that have been commercially prepared beforehand are best for learning in the beginning.)
2. Make sure the lowest power objective is in position over the stage. It should be placed in its closest position over the specimen.
3. Position the slide specimen on the stage and secure the spring clip. The stage should be centered under the objective.
4. Observe the specimen through the eyepiece. Slowly raise the objective using the coarse adjustment knob. Use the fine focus adjustment to clarify the image.
5. Use the condenser diaphragm to adjust the amount of light, which is critical for a clear view.
6. View the specimen on the next highest power by turning the nosepiece. Do not move the specimen.
7. Use the fine focus adjustment to clarify the image.

Immersion oil is required to view images with the red-coded objective lens. This further focuses the light.

MICROBES IN THE ENVIRONMENT

Many microbes inhabit the environment in numerous habitats. Humans and other species are in constant contact with microbes in the environment. We can describe the relationship between the microbe and the body in three ways. These are commensalism, mutualism, and parasitism. In these relationships, the *host* is the organism that is occupied by the microbe.

In *commensalism,* one organism uses another to meet its physiological needs but causes no harm to the host. For example, the normal human intestinal tract contains many different types of bacteria, such as *Escherichia coli.* The bacteria survive in balance with the body as long as they remain in the intestine. However, if *E. coli* escape the intestine and enter the **sterile** tissues of the body, such as when the bowel is perforated by trauma or disease, the result can be fatal.

In *mutualism,* each of the organisms benefits from their relationship in the environment. For example, *Staphylococcus aureus* inhabits normal, healthy skin. These bacteria proliferate in this environment, and they protect the skin from other invading organisms. However, the stress of disease, a break in the skin, and other conditions cause the bacteria to multiply rapidly and create infection. Bacteria that reside in a healthy individual are called *normal flora,* whereas those that we encounter briefly are referred to as *transient flora.*

A *parasite* is an organism that lives within another organism and gains an advantage at the expense of that organism. Infectious disease is the result of a parasitic relationship between the host and the invading organism. **Infection** is the proliferation of a harmful microbe in the host.

Organisms that cause infectious disease are called *pathogenic* organisms. However, not every contact with a **pathogen** results in infection. Certain conditions must be favorable for the pathogen to gain entry into the body and proliferate:

1. *The microbe must have an entry site and an exit site.* Microbes are often environmentally suited to a specific body system, and their **entry site** and exit site are often the same.
2. *Microbes must be present in sufficient numbers.* An infection or disease can be established only if a sufficient number of disease organisms are present. The number of microbe colonies on a surface is referred to as the **bioburden.**
3. *The environment must be well suited to the pathogen.* Once the pathogen gains entry into the body, the conditions for nutrition, oxygen requirements, pH, and temperature must be conducive to bacterial colonization and proliferation.
4. *The host is unable to overcome the harmful mechanisms of the pathogen.* Infection develops only if the host's natural or artificial immunity cannot prevent the microbes from multiplying.

Chain of Infection

Disease transmission can be understood by looking at the chain of events or conditions necessary for an infection to be carried from one individual to another. This process is often called the *chain of infection* (Fig. 8.8), because if any link in the chain is broken, disease transmission cannot occur.

PRESENCE OF AN INFECTIOUS AGENT For microbes to cause an infection, the agent must be present in the host environment.

The following groups of organisms are responsible for specific infections:

- Bacteria
- Virus
- Fungus
- Prion
- Protozoa

Bacteria are responsible for most infections in humans. However, only about 3% of all bacterial species are pathogenic.

RESERVOIR The reservoir for a microbe is its normal habitat where it lives and proliferates. For example, the human body is a reservoir for *Staphylococcus aureus,* which normally resides on our skin without causing harm. On the other hand, the bacterium that causes tetanus normally inhabits soil and animal feces. Examples of reservoirs are people, food, water, animals, and soil.

EXIT PORTAL The exit portal refers to the way in which an organism leaves the body. For microbes to infect more than one individual, they must have a means to leave the host organism and enter another. For example, infectious gastrointestinal microbes leave the body of an infected individual through its feces. Human immunodeficiency virus (HIV) leaves the body through blood and other body fluids. The virus that causes the common cold exits the body through the respiratory system—through nasal and other secretions produced by that system.

METHOD OF TRANSMISSION Once an infectious microbe leaves one host, it must have a means of transmission. The following are methods of transmission that are important in the study of infectious disease:

Direct contact (touching) with the organism may result in an infection. This is a common means of transmission in the health care setting. For example, patient care equipment such as stethoscopes and blood pressure cuffs can carry a very large bioburden of *S. aureus* bacteria. Unless these are disinfected between patients, they can be a cause of infection for each patient they are used on. Contaminated instruments can carry infection to the surgical patient. This concept is the basis of aseptic technique. Contact transmission can occur through an intermediary source. The source can be nonliving **(fomite)** or living **(vector).** A nonsterile

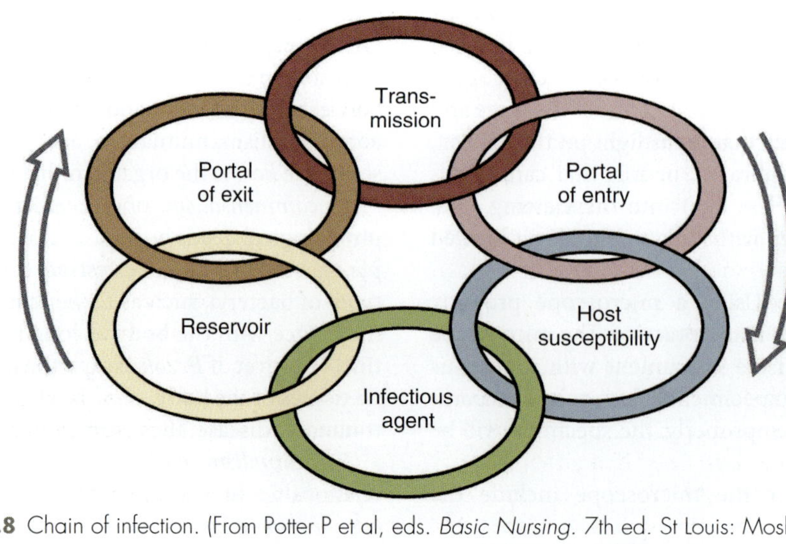

FIG. 8.8 Chain of infection. (From Potter P et al, eds. *Basic Nursing.* 7th ed. St Louis: Mosby; 2011.)

(contaminated) surgical instrument can become a fomite by transmitting microorganisms into sterile tissue. Instruments and medical devices can harbor pathogenic bacteria encased in dried blood and body tissue that was not removed during the cleaning process. Other common fomites in the hospital are bed linens, wound dressings, and contaminated urinary catheters. Insects or rodent vectors carry pathogens from one surface to another or between hosts. Certain bacteria are capable of sticking together by forming a slime layer. This layer can exist on the surfaces of inanimate things as well as those that are alive. The sticky layer that contains these bacteria is called a *biofilm* and is an important concept in surgery. Biofilm may form on surgical instruments and resist normal cleaning methods. Biofilm can then infect the patient by direct contact.

Droplet transmission is the spread of microorganisms by water droplets in the air. Water droplets are released in the environment during talking, coughing, or sneezing. Infectious microbes inhabiting the respiratory system of an individual are rapidly spread to others through droplet transmission. Water droplets are relatively heavy and do not remain suspended in the air. We wear masks that cover the nose and mouth in surgery to prevent the shedding of bacteria from our breath into the sterile tissues of the patient and other surfaces in the perioperative environment. Water droplets can also be transmitted to other individuals who breathe them in. Another example of contamination by water droplets occurs during surgery when potentially infectious blood splatter or other aerosolized body fluids are released into the air.

Airborne transmission also occurs via **droplet nuclei.** These are the dried remnants of previously moist particles containing living microorganisms. Unlike droplet transmission described above, droplet nuclei or **aerosol droplets** can remain suspended in the air because of their small size (usually 1 to 5 μm). They are infective for long periods of time and transmit disease when individuals breathe in the particles. Aerosol droplets can also settle on surfaces and transmit disease by direct contact.

Oral transmission occurs when a pathogen is ingested in food or water or through fecal-oral transmission. Poor hygiene among patients and hospital staff contributes to the spread of pathogens in this way. Frequent hand washing in the health care setting is very important in the prevention of oral disease transmission.

PORTAL OF ENTRY For a microbe to cause disease, it must first enter the body. The entry site is called the portal of entry. Examples of portals of entry are the skin, respiratory tract, mucous membranes, and gastrointestinal tract.

SUSCEPTIBLE HOST The final link in the chain of infection is a susceptible host. The infectious microbe cannot continue to proliferate without another host. Although some microbes can enter a dormant stage for long periods of time, proliferation and growth requires a host body. For example, an unvaccinated child with the measles virus can transmit the disease through respiratory secretions but only if another unvaccinated individual comes in contact with it. The vaccinated child is protected and therefore not susceptible. A susceptible host can also be an individual who is weakened by other circumstances such as poor nutrition, injury, advanced age, or another disease.

PHASES OF INFECTION

The course of an infection follows a pattern of distinct phases.

1. *Incubation:* In this phase, the pathogens actively replicate, but the host shows no symptoms. This may be a short period (hours), or it may continue for days or even months. The incubation period is affected by the physical status of the host, the port of entry, and the number of infectious organisms present in the body.
2. *Prodromal phase:* In this phase, symptoms begin to appear. They may be very mild or vague at the start of the infection or may include certain clinically important signs of the disease.
3. *Acute phase:* In this phase, the organism is at its most potent, and the symptoms are very apparent. Cellular damage and destruction of tissue are characteristic of many diseases at this stage.
4. *Convalescence:* During this phase, proliferation of the infectious organism slows and symptoms subside. Tissue begins to heal, and the body starts to regain strength and normal function.

These stages apply to diseases that resolve with treatment or by natural course. However, not all diseases resolve. A *chronic infection* may develop in some individuals. Weeks or months may be required for resolution, when all the disease organisms are eliminated from the body. Further, a person may harbor disease organisms but show no signs or symptoms; this person is referred to as a *carrier.*

HOSPITAL-ACQUIRED INFECTION

A hospital-acquired infection (HAI), also called a **nosocomial infection,** is an infection acquired while the patient is in a health care institution. The most common HAI is urinary tract infection in patients who have been catheterized. In the United States, about 2 million patients a year develop infections, including surgical site infections, as a result of hospitalization. Seventy percent of the bacteria that cause these infections are resistant to at least one of the drugs commonly used to treat that infection. The spread of an HAI from person to person is called *cross-contamination.* Introduction of an infection from one part of the body to another is called *self-infection* or autoinfection.

SURGICAL SITE INFECTION

Surgical site infection begins when a pathogenic or nonpathogenic microorganism colonizes the sterile wound (incision tissues). This can be caused by contamination:

- Of the tissues before surgery, such as a ruptured bowel or a traumatic wound caused by a foreign object
- During surgery because of poor sterile technique (discussed in Chapter 9)
- Of the incision after surgery

Some wound infections are minor, involving only the skin, whereas others occur in deep tissue or body cavities. The infection may remain localized or spread throughout the body. The patient's general condition at the time of surgery is a predictor of risk. Certain surgical patients have a high physiological risk of infection (Box 8.3).

The severity of the infection is influenced by the type, **virulence,** and number of invading bacteria, as well as the organism's sensitivity to antibiotic treatment.

Infections are usually treated at the first signs. A culture specimen is taken if there is exudate present, and antibiotic treatment may be initiated immediately. The wound is observed for further signs of infection and the patient monitored closely.

A small, localized area of infection sometimes develops at the wound site. This type of *abscess* is easily treated. However, a surgical site infection that spreads and becomes systemic can cause serious disease or death. In moderate-to-severe infection, the patient's temperature becomes elevated soon after surgery. The patient may experience pain at the incisional site or deep within the wound.

BOX 8.3 Physiological Risks for Surgical Site Infection

- Age: The immune system of an older patient is less responsive than that of a younger patient. Tissues heal more slowly, and innate body defenses are less effective. Older patients are often undernourished.
- Undernourishment or malnourishment: Essential proteins required for tissue healing and body defenses against infection are often missing in the diet of these patients. Low body fat predisposes the patient to lowered body temperature, which increases physiological stress.
- Diabetes mellitus: The diabetic patient is at extremely high risk of infection because of problems with the circulatory system, which must be properly functioning to support a healthy immune system. Poor peripheral and visceral circulation prevents the flow of nutrients and oxygen to traumatized tissue, which increases the overgrowth of both resident and disease-producing microorganisms.
- Substance or alcohol abuse: These patients are often malnourished. Liver damage related to substance abuse and alcohol abuse leads to poor conversion of glycogen to glucose, which is necessary for cellular metabolism. Immune function is often depressed.
- Immune suppression: Patients with acquired immunodeficiency syndrome (AIDS) or other immune diseases, those undergoing cancer therapy, and those who have been prescribed high doses of corticosteroids have impaired immune function.
- Long preoperative stay in the hospital: A prolonged preoperative stay allows the body to incubate and colonize bacteria and other microorganisms commonly found in the hospital environment, especially antibiotic-resistant forms.
- Surgical wound classification: Contaminated wounds are associated with a higher risk of infection in the postoperative patient.
- Long operative procedure: Long procedures put the patient at higher risk for exposure to airborne pathogens and direct contact with contaminated medical devices and instruments.

Exudate (an accumulation of pus, drainage, dead cells, and serum) may appear around the incision. The wound then is described as **suppurative.** The site becomes extremely tender or painful. If the infection is localized, antimicrobial therapy may be initiated and the infection eradicated. Deep infections, however, may lead to widespread areas of tissue death, accumulation of pus, and breakdown of the sutured tissue layers.

Infection occurring at the surgical site can cause other problems such as breakdown of the incision layers. As suture materials degrade in the presence of bacteria, the wound may split open, a condition known as *dehiscence.*

A large accumulation of pus leads to the spread of infection into adjacent tissues. An uncontrolled infection in a body cavity results in inflammation of the lining of that cavity (e.g., peritonitis in the abdomen). This can be rapidly fatal as vital organs are infected.

Treatment

A superficial surgical site infection is usually treated at the first signs. A culture specimen is taken; this is a sample of the wound exudate, which is incubated and allowed to proliferate for testing. The wound is observed for further signs of infection and the patient monitored closely. Deep infection may not be diagnosed until days after the surgery and is often accompanied by pain and fever. Antibiotic treatment is started immediately. If the symptoms do not resolve, the wound may be incised again so that pus, necrotic tissue, and devitalized tissue can be removed. This procedure is called an *incision and drainage* (I & D). Advanced treatment includes intravenous (IV) antibiotic therapy and continuous wound drainage. If the infection remains localized, the prognosis for resolution is good. However, systemic infection can result when bacteria migrate into the vascular system, causing septicemia and widespread organ damage.

When infection is present, the wound cannot be sutured, because infected tissues cannot withstand the tension of sutures and bacterial toxins rapidly break most suture materials. Instead, the wound is packed with gauze dressings and allowed to heal from the bottom to the exterior.

Isolation

Certain diseases and infections require the patient to be isolated from others in the environment. Patients with highly resistant bacterial infections are treated in the hospital using isolation procedures in which equipment and supplies needed for patient care are contained in the patient's room. Nurses and other care providers must put on gowns, face masks, and gloves while handling any contaminated medical supplies and must discard protective equipment in the patient's room before leaving. The procedures used when caring for an isolation patient are called *transmission-based precautions.*

Patients with highly contagious infections that are transmitted primarily through droplet transmission are almost never brought into the operating room for treatment.

DISEASE PREVENTION

The most important reason for studying certain aspects of microbiology is *disease prevention.* No other area of health care has a greater impact on populations, including patients undergoing surgery. Important methods of disease prevention in the health care facility include the following:

- Hand washing
- Learning and practicing Standard Precautions and isolation precautions
- Learning and practicing aseptic technique
- Good personal hygiene practices
- Strict disinfection and environmental cleaning in the facility
- Proper use of antiseptics and chemical disinfectants
- Isolation of infected patients according to standard guidelines

Note that hand washing is the most important and effective method of disease prevention in the health care facility and in the community.

Standard Precautions and transmission-based precautions are standards established by the Centers for Disease Control and Prevention (CDC) that establish special techniques to stop the spread of infection in the health facility environment. Standard Precautions are discussed thoroughly in Chapter 7.

The most recent version of the standards is available in the following CDC document: 2007 Guideline for Isolation Precautions: Preventing Transmission of Infectious Agents in Healthcare Settings, available at http://www.cdc.gov/hicpac/2007IP/2007isolationPrecautions.html.

MICROORGANISMS AND THE DISEASES THEY CAUSE

BACTERIA

Bacteria are prokaryotic organisms. They represent a very large population of microbes in the environment and affect animals, humans, and plants. Most live without causing harm to other organisms; however, a few species cause serious disease. Bacteria that cause infection are called *pathogenic.* This group includes streptococcal, staphylococcal, meningococcal, pneumococcal, and gonococcal organisms and the coliform (intestinal) bacilli. These organisms typically cause suppuration (pus) and tissue destruction that can lead to systemic involvement and ultimately may be fatal.

Structure

Bacteria represent the largest variety of infectious microorganisms and cause the greatest number of postoperative infections and other HAIs. Bacteria exist in a variety of shapes, sizes, and forms, which are created by the cell wall. Bacteria can exist singly or in groups, called colonies. Fig. 8.9 shows a generalized bacterium.

Identification of specific bacteria is an important goal in the diagnosis of infectious diseases. Many tests can be performed on bacterial cells to identify their exact classification and disease potential. Other tests are performed to determine the organism's susceptibility to antibacterial drugs.

Bacteria are partially classified according to their shape (Fig. 8.10). This can be determined by staining the bacteria and observing them under a microscope. Bacteria take the following basic shapes:

- Rod-shaped bacteria are *bacilli,* which occur singly or in pairs, chains, or filaments. Rods can be slightly curved or straight.
- Curved or spiral-shaped bacteria are *spirochetes,* which may be coiled or loosely curved.
- Spherical bacteria are *cocci,* which occur singly (micrococci), in chains (streptococci), in pairs (diplococci), in groups of four, or in clusters (staphylococci).
- *Vibrio* are comma shaped.
- Other shapes that are sometimes seen are square and tetrahedral, but these are less common.

Motility

Bacteria move using a number of different mechanisms. The flagella and pili described earlier are the most common methods. The flagella rotate and propel the cell in different directions. Pili also create motility by anchoring to a surface and retracting, which allows the pili to move the cell along. Some

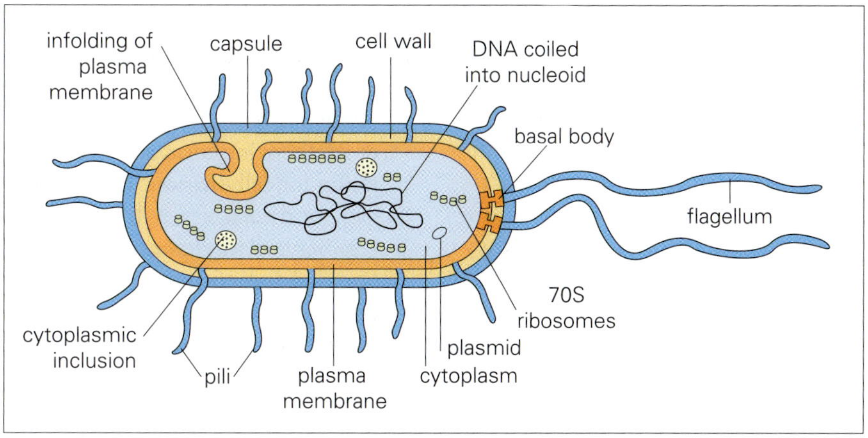

FIG. 8.9 Generalized bacterial cell. Note both the cell wall and the plasma membrane, which differentiate the prokaryote from most eukaryotic cells. A wide variation in morphology is seen among bacteria types. (From Goering R, Dockrell H, Wakelin D, et al, eds. *Mims' Medical Microbiology.* 4th ed. St Louis: Mosby; 2008.)

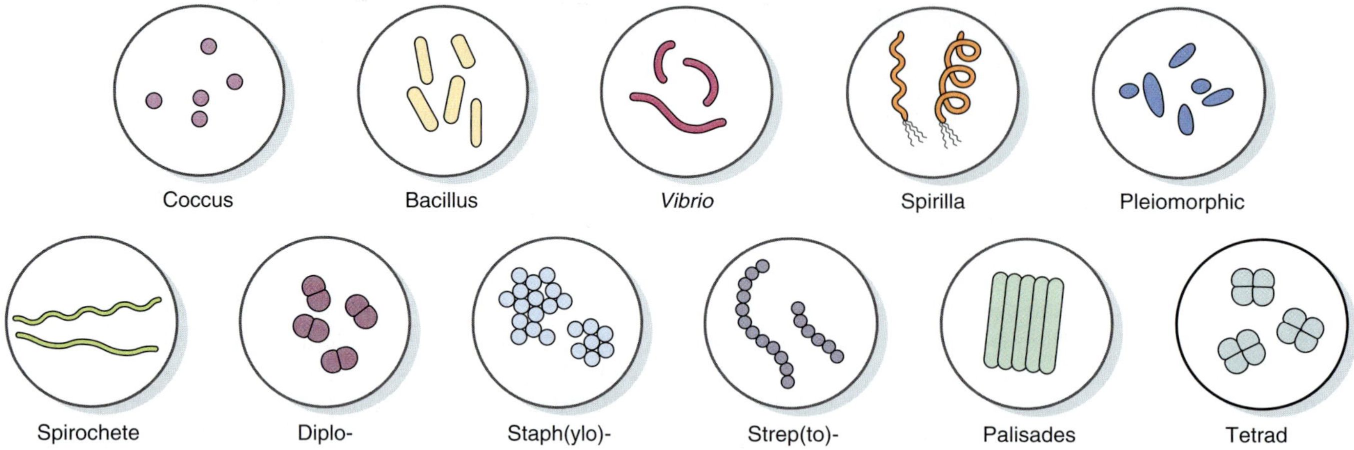

FIG. 8.10 Bacteria morphology. (From VanMeter K, Hubert R, eds. *Microbiology for the Healthcare Professional*. 2nd ed. St Louis: Elsevier; 2016.)

bacteria move by using the host's cytoskeleton, a network of filaments within the cytoplasm.

Environmental and Nutrient Requirements

Important environmental parameters for all microorganisms include temperature, oxygen, pH, moisture, and atmospheric pressure. Bacteria are found everywhere in the natural world, living under a wide variety of conditions. Those that infect humans require moderate conditions.

Bacteria that produce spores can live in temperature ranges of −4° to 194°F (−20° to 90°C). Oxygen requirements for bacteria vary widely. Some require oxygen to live and grow (strict **aerobes**). Others cannot live in the presence of oxygen; these are called strict **anaerobes.** Anaerobes are important in the process of infection, because they can proliferate in deep traumatic or surgical wounds. *Facultative* bacteria can live with or without oxygen.

Bacteria have evolved to withstand extremes of the pH spectrum. For example, the normal pH of blood is 7.35 to 7.45. *Helicobacter pylori* can invade the gastric mucosa and reproduce at a pH of 2. The normal pH in the body prevents most pathogenic organisms from proliferating, but a change in pH can destroy the normal "resident" bacteria and allow pathogens to invade the body.

Bacteria that are significant in infectious disease prefer a moist environment. One method of destroying bacteria is *desiccation* (drying). Resistance to drying makes bacteria such as mycobacteria, which cause tuberculosis (TB), a public health problem, because the bacteria can spread through dried sputum.

Bacteria obtain nutrient substances from their immediate environment. Some bacteria can synthesize many nutrients from substances available within the cell. Others require a more complex variety of organic compounds, which they take in from their environment. Most bacteria require basic elemental nutrients:

- Carbon
- Oxygen
- Nitrogen
- Hydrogen
- Phosphorus
- Sulfur
- Potassium

Reproduction

Bacterial cells reproduce by asexual fission into two new cells. In this process, the genetic material is replicated and moves to separate areas of the cell. A septal membrane develops, splitting the mother cell into two halves, which separate into daughter cells.

Some bacteria are capable of producing a vegetative reproductive form called an **endospore** (commonly referred to as a *spore*). This is a dormant phase in the reproductive cycle in which the bacteria form a thick, multilayered protein wall around their genetic material. The wall resists extreme environmental conditions such as boiling, drying, chemical destruction, and high pressure. When environmental conditions are favorable, the spore becomes active, and reproduction (colonization) begins. Two spore-forming bacteria are *Clostridium tetani* (tetanus) and *Bacillus anthracis* (anthrax).

Bacterial Growth

Bacteria grow at a rate that corresponds to their environment and nutritional status. A favorable environment that meets the bacteria's essential requirements results in more rapid colonization than an environment in which the bacteria must compete for resources. In the laboratory, bacteria can be provided with essential environmental and nutritive requirements. In this way, their growth patterns can be studied.

Bacteria show four characteristic phases of growth:

1. *Lag phase:* This period occurs immediately after the growth medium is inoculated with the sample bacteria. During this phase, the bacteria do not divide, but they may be processing or synthesizing components of the growth medium in preparation for cell division. This is a period of increased metabolism for the bacteria as they adjust to the environment.
2. *Exponential (log) phase:* This phase is characterized by active and sometimes rapid cell division. The rate is usually constant and depends on the growth medium. This rate is often referred to as the *doubling time* or *generation time* of the bacteria.
3. *Stationary phase:* In this phase, the bacteria have used up their available nutrition in the growth medium and the amount of space available for growth. The byproducts of reproduction have accumulated, and these inhibit further growth. During this phase, cell division stops.

TABLE 8.1 Bacterial Toxins and Diseases

Bacteria	Exotoxin	Tissue Damaged	Mechanism	Disease
Clostridium tetani	Tetanospasmin	Neurons	Spastic paralysis	Tetanus
Clostridium perfringens	Alpha toxin	Erythrocytes, platelets, leukocytes, endothelium	Cell lysis	Gas gangrene
Clostridium botulinum	Neurotoxin	Nerve–muscle junction	Flaccid paralysis	Botulism
Corynebacterium diphtheriae	Diphtheria toxin	Throat, heart, peripheral nerve	Inhibits protein synthesis	Diphtheria
Shigella dysenteriae	Enterotoxin	Intestinal mucosa	Fluid loss from intestinal cells	Dysentery
Escherichia coli	Enterotoxin	Intestinal epithelium	Fluid loss from intestinal cells	Gastroenteritis
Vibrio cholerae	Enterotoxin	Intestinal epithelium	Fluid loss from intestinal cells	Cholera
Staphylococcus aureus	Alpha toxin	Red and white cells (via cytokines)	Hemolysis	Abscesses
	Hemolysin	Red and white cells (via cytokines)	Hemolysis	Abscesses
	Leukocidin	Leukocytes	Destroys leukocytes	Abscesses
	Enterotoxin	Intestinal cells	Induces vomiting, diarrhea	Food poisoning
	Toxic shock syndrome toxin (TSST) 1	—	Release of cytotoxins	Toxic shock syndrome
	Epidermolytic	Epidermis	Cell lysis	Scalded skin syndrome
Streptococcus pyogenes	Streptolysin O and S	Red and white cells	Hemolysis	Hemolysis, pyogenic lesion
	Erythrogenic	Skin capillaries	Inflammation	Scarlet fever
Bacillus anthracis	Cytotoxin	Lung	Pulmonary edema	Anthrax
Bordetella pertussis	Pertussis toxin	Trachea	Destruction of epithelium	Whooping cough
Legionella pneumophila	Numerous	Neutrophils	Cell lysis	Legionnaires' disease
Listeria monocytogenes	Hemolysin	Leukocytes, monocytes	Cell lysis	Listeriosis
Pseudomonas aeruginosa	Exotoxin A	Cell lysis	Cell lysis	Various infections

4. *Death phase:* In the restricted culture medium, the death phase follows the stationary phase. The bacteria can no longer survive, and the colony dies out, usually at the same rate as the growth phase.

Pathogenicity

Bacteria cause disease by gaining entry into the host and colonizing tissue. Bacteria have many different mechanisms for adhering to host cells and evading the immune system. They can overcome and destroy the body's defensive white blood cells. Some are capable of hemolysis, the destruction of red blood cells. One of the most potent pathogenic mechanisms of bacteria is the release of toxins by the bacterial cell.

Endotoxins are chemicals contained within the cell wall of bacteria. When the bacterial cell ruptures, endotoxins are released into the bloodstream and spread to different organ systems. The toxic effects of these substances include fever, diarrhea, shock, extreme weakness, and sometimes death.

Exotoxins are proteins produced as a result of bacterial metabolism. Exotoxins break down the surrounding tissue, which allows the pathogen to spread and colonize freely. Exotoxins enter specific body cells and disrupt the cell's chemical and physical structure. For example, *Clostridium botulinum* produces a highly concentrated toxin that damages the nerve–muscle mechanism and causes paralysis in the host. Exotoxins released by bacteria and other microbes are listed in Table 8.1.

Important Bacterial Pathogens

GRAM-POSITIVE COCCI Gram-positive cocci are responsible for about one-third of all bacterial infections in humans. Many are responsible for surgical site infections. They cause suppurative infection, and some are resistant to antibiotic therapy.

The streptococci are further classified by their ability to reduce the levels of iron in hemoglobin through hemolysis. Two groups of hemolytic streptococci are the *alpha-hemolytic* streptococci and the *beta-hemolytic* streptococci.

STAPHYLOCOCCUS AUREUS *S. aureus* is the most widespread cause of surgical site infections. It normally resides on healthy skin, but when transmitted to the surgical wound by direct or indirect contact, it can cause an infection. Between 30% and 70% of people are skin carriers of *S. aureus*. When confined to the surgical wound itself, it produces copious amounts of pus; the organism also causes endocarditis (infection of the lining of the heart) when it colonizes heart valves. Invasion of the bone causes osteomyelitis.

STAPHYLOCOCCUS EPIDERMIDIS *S. epidermidis* is a normal resident of the skin. However, it can cause infection in other parts of the body when spread by medical devices such as catheters, prosthetic valves, and orthopedic implants.

STREPTOCOCCUS PYOGENES Many HAIs are caused by *S. pyogenes* (a group A beta-hemolytic streptococcus). This potentially lethal pathogen causes surgical site infection; it spreads via the lymphatic system to other sites in the body, causing anaerobic infection and tissue death. Burn patients are particularly vulnerable to streptococcal infection. Surgical site infection is most commonly caused by **direct transmission** from a contaminated surface.

STREPTOCOCCUS PNEUMONIAE *S. pneumoniae* is the primary cause of pneumonia and otitis media (middle ear infection). This pathogen is spread mainly through the respiratory tract. It colonizes the nose and nasopharynx and then spreads to the lungs and middle ear. The bacteria are coated with a thick capsule and cell wall, which prevent its destruction by the body's white blood cells. Because of this resistance mechanism, respiratory disease caused by *S. pneumoniae* can be fatal in children and older adults.

Gram-Negative Rods and Cocci (Aerobic)

PSEUDOMONAS AERUGINOSA *P. aeruginosa* is found in the normal gastrointestinal tract and in sewage, dirt, and water. It has emerged as an increasingly important pathogen in hospitalized patients. It can infect nearly all body systems. *P. aeruginosa* infection is especially prevalent in burn patients who lack healthy skin as a barrier against airborne bacteria. *P. aeruginosa* can cause septicemia (systemic vascular infection), osteomyelitis, urinary tract infection, and endocarditis. It is highly resistant to antimicrobial agents.

NEISSERIA GONORRHOEAE Gonorrhea is a sexually transmitted disease spread from person to person by direct contact with *N. gonorrhoeae*. The infection usually remains localized in the reproductive tract, but it may become systemic. The bacteria can cause blindness in the newborn of an infected mother; however, this can be prevented by instilling antibiotic drops into the newborn's eyes. If the disease is not treated, it may lead to sterility and endocarditis.

NEISSERIA MENINGITIDIS Bacterial meningitis is a highly contagious infection of the meninges, which cover the brain and spinal cord. Two forms of the disease are caused by *N. meningitidis*, one that is transient and resolves spontaneously and a more serious form that can result in seizures, respiratory arrest, and coma.

BORDETELLA PERTUSSIS *B. pertussis* is a bacterium that causes whooping cough, a life-threatening disease in children. Vaccination against *B. pertussis* has reduced the mortality rate significantly. Before the vaccine was developed, whooping cough was a major killer of children.

ENTERIC BACTERIA The enteric bacteria are also gram-negative rods; however, they are facultative anaerobes and can grow in an oxygen-poor environment. This group of pathogens inhabits the intestinal tracts of humans both in a disease state and as resident (normal) bacteria.

ESCHERICHIA COLI *E. coli* are resident bacteria of the gastrointestinal tract. Postoperative infection caused by this bacterium occurs when the organisms are transmitted via a contaminated object such as an endoscope or catheter. Direct transmission occurs when the gastrointestinal tract is perforated and the bowel contents spill into the sterile peritoneal cavity. *E. coli* is the most common cause of urinary tract infections. In the bloodstream, *E. coli* can spread to other organs and cause severe tissue destruction or death.

SALMONELLA ENTERICA *S. enterica* is a common cause of food poisoning (acute gastroenteritis). The bacterial infection is spread from person to person by contaminated food and fecal contact. The disease causes diarrhea, vomiting, and fever, which usually resolve without treatment.

SALMONELLA TYPHI As mentioned previously, the bacteria *S. typhi* causes the disease typhoid. The infection is spread via contaminated water and food. In communities where sewage treatment is lacking, the bacteria can contaminate local drinking water and cause widespread infection. Bacterial colonies can persist in the intestine long after antibiotic treatment, and a disease carrier may continue to infect others while showing no symptoms.

When ingested, the bacteria penetrate the intestinal wall and enter the mesenteric lymph nodes. They release a powerful endotoxin that enters the bloodstream and causes septicemia, cardiovascular infection, and death. Several types of typhoid vaccine are available, but the vaccine is usually given only to individuals at risk, such as those traveling or working in an area where sanitation is poor.

Spore-Forming Bacteria

The spore-forming bacteria are significant because of their ability to resist destruction. They are extremely important in the health care setting. In the perioperative environment, any process of sterilization is defined by its ability to destroy not only all microbes but also bacterial spores.

CLOSTRIDIUM PERFRINGENS *C. perfringens* is an anaerobic bacterium that causes rapid tissue death in deep wounds deprived of oxygen. This is a relatively rare infection, but it does occur in health care settings. Historically, it has been a common infection of deep, penetrating combat wounds. In true gas gangrene, the tissue is destroyed by the toxins of the *C. perfringens* bacilli. *C. novyi* bacilli, another type of clostridia, invade the necrotic tissue and release toxic gases. Systemic absorption of these gases is fatal. The disease is transmitted directly from a contaminated source to an open or penetrating wound.

CLOSTRIDIUM TETANI *C. tetani* is the causative bacteria of tetanus, a disease of the nervous system. *C. tetani* bacterium is an anaerobic organism commonly found in soil and the intestinal tracts of humans and other mammals. The toxins released by the bacilli travel along the peripheral nerve pathways, eventually reaching the central nervous system (CNS). Severe muscle spasms, convulsions, and eventual paralysis of the respiratory system lead to death from asphyxia. Transmission is through direct contact with the bacilli, usually through an open or penetrating wound.

CLOSTRIDIUM DIFFICILE *C. difficile* is a spore-forming bacterium that causes severe diarrhea. It is easily spread among patients who are immunocompromised, and the infection can be rapidly fatal. Strict attention to asepsis, especially hand washing, is needed to control its spread in the health care setting.

Mycobacterial Infections

As mentioned previously, the bacillus *Mycobacterium tuberculosis* causes the disease TB. The human strain of the bacterium causes dense nodules or tubercles to form in localized areas of the body, including the lungs, liver, spleen, and bone marrow.

TB is a serious concern in areas where people live or work in crowded conditions. Multidrug-resistant strains of *M. tuberculosis* are increasingly common throughout the world. TB kills about 3 million people and infects about 9 million every year worldwide. The organism primarily causes respiratory disease, but it can also infect other areas of the body, including vital organs. The infection is spread by inhalation of the bacteria in droplets or dust containing dried mycobacteria. The infection can be introduced into the body via medical equipment such as respiratory, diagnostic, or anesthesia equipment.

After the bacteria have entered the respiratory system, they are engulfed by white blood cell components. The mycobacteria that are not destroyed by the body become encased in granular "tubercles," which remain in the lungs. These become calcified and fibrotic. If the infected person's immune system becomes weakened, the bacteria can again become proliferative.

RICKETTSIAE Rickettsiae are a type of bacteria carried by specific species of ticks, mites, and fleas. The insect transmits the bacteria to its host through a skin bite. Once the bacteria enter the host's body, they move through the bloodstream and attach to the inner lining of the blood vessels (endothelium). The cell then ingests the bacteria, which continue to multiply and enter other host cells. Rickettsiae are identified by staining, using the same techniques as those for bacteria in general.

Diseases caused by rickettsiae include typhus, Q fever, and Rocky Mountain spotted fever. Rickettsial disease can persist in the body for long periods of time. Prevention of disease involves avoiding exposure to ticks, fleas, and mites that carry the bacteria.

Important bacterial diseases are listed in Table 8.2.

Multidrug-Resistant Pathogenic Bacteria

Certain strains of bacterial pathogens have evolved to be partly or completely resistant to the most powerful antimicrobial agents available. Certain strains of bacteria are of grave concern, because they are easily transmitted, colonize rapidly, and can be lethal. The symptoms of these infections are the same as with the original nonresistant strains. However, treatment becomes problematic, because resistance leads to the spread of the infection and severe debilitation and/or death.

Treatment with antimicrobial agents destroys some pathogens, but the more resistant microbes survive and are transmitted to other hosts. The resistance is passed to succeeding generations of microbes through simple replication or via plasmid exchange, which carries the genes of the resistant strain to other microbes. Resistance occurs when the antibiotic used only partly destroys the pathogen or when antibiotic treatment is stopped before the microbes are destroyed.

Natural selection of resistant strains has been hastened by a combination of microbe strength and the indiscriminate and improper use of antibiotics. *Antibiotic-resistant* bacterial infection is a primary focus of public and clinical health researchers. Unfortunately, as new and more powerful drugs are developed, resistant strains also develop. The incidence of multidrug-resistant organisms (MDROs) in the United States has increased steadily over the past few decades.

Strict isolation protocols are used for patients with an MDRO. The surgical technologist must be knowledgeable about these protocols, which are established by the health institution in which the technologist works. In addition to following all protocols, all health care workers must carefully practice hand-washing procedures. These are discussed in detail in the next chapter.

METHICILLIN-RESISTANT *STAPHYLOCOCCUS AUREUS* AND *EPIDERMIS* Methicillin-resistant *S. aureus* (MRSA) is a virulent form of *Staphylococcus* that is transmitted primarily by direct contact with the hands, equipment, and supplies. Health care workers who carry the bacteria in their respiratory systems may become carriers of the disease. They do not become ill but can transmit the pathogens to others in their environment. MRSA can occur in surgical incisions and burns and on urinary catheters, chest tubes, and other common devices used in the health care setting.

Recently, MRSA has been discovered in the community, outside the health care setting. The infection can be fatal and is particularly serious in debilitated patients. Vancomycin has traditionally been used to treat MRSA. However, a new strain has developed—vancomycin-resistant *S. aureus* (VRSA). Methicillin-resistant *S. epidermis* is another MDRO found in the clinical setting and is implicated as a source of wound infection.

VANCOMYCIN-RESISTANT AND VANCOMYCIN-INTERMEDIATE-RESISTANT Staphylococcus Aureus Infection with VRSA was first diagnosed in the United States in 1997. Since then, the incidence of the infection has increased steadily, and a new strain has also emerged, vancomycin-intermediate-resistant *S. aureus* (VISA). These strains can be treated with other antibiotics. However, the infection can be fatal in severely debilitated patients.

VANCOMYCIN-RESISTANT ENTEROCOCCI Vancomycin-resistant enterococci (VRE) infection is transmitted by direct contact or through intermediate sources, including furniture, equipment, and the hands of health care workers. Enterococci inhabit the intestines and female genital tracts of healthy individuals. However, patients previously treated with vancomycin, surgical patients, and those who are debilitated or have a suppressed immune system are at particular risk for VRE infection. The bacteria are transmitted through contact with stool, urine, or blood and by the hands of health care workers. The bacteria cause urinary tract infections, septicemia (blood infection), and wound infection.

MULTIDRUG-RESISTANT TUBERCULOSIS Multidrug-resistant tuberculosis (MDR TB) has emerged in the past few decades as

TABLE 8.2 Important Bacterial Infections

Organism	Major Infection	Less Common Infection	Vaccine Preventable
GRAM-POSITIVE COCCI			
Staphylococci			
S. epidermidis	Bacteremia in immunocompromised individuals	Most often associated with indwelling devices	No
S. saprophyticus	Urinary tract infections	—	No
S. aureus	Boils, impetigo, wound infections, osteomyelitis, septicemia	Pneumonia, endocarditis, toxic shock syndrome, food poisoning	No
Streptococci			
Beta-Hemolytic			
S. pyogenes (group A)	Tonsillitis, impetigo, cellulitis, scarlet fever (rheumatic fever, glomerulonephritis)	Puerperal sepsis, erysipelas, septicemia	No
Alpha-Hemolytic			
S. pneumoniae	Pneumonia, otitis media	Meningitis, septicemia	Yes (some serotypes)
S. viridans	Dental caries	Subacute bacterial endocarditis	No
Group D Streptococci			
S. faecalis (enterococci) (Enterococcus faecalis)	Urinary tract infections, wound infections, intra-abdominal abscess	Bacteremia, endocarditis	No
GRAM-NEGATIVE COCCI AND COCCOBACILLI			
Neisseria			
N. meningitidis	Meningitis, septicemia	Arthritis	Yes (serogroups A/C)
N. gonorrhoeae	Gonorrhea, pelvic inflammatory disease	Arthritis, conjunctivitis	No
AEROBIC GRAM-POSITIVE BACILLI			
Spore-Forming			
Bacillus			
B. anthracis	Anthrax	—	Yes
Non–Spore-Forming			
Listeria			
L. monocytogenes	Neonatal sepsis, meningitis	Septicemia in immunocompromised individuals	No
Corynebacterium			
C. diphtheriae	Diphtheria	Skin infections	Yes
C. urealyticum	Cystitis	—	No
C. jeikeium	Infection associated with prosthetic devices and intravenous or cerebrospinal fluid (CSF) catheters		No

Modified from Hart T, Shears P, eds. *Color Atlas of Medical Microbiology.* London: Mosby; 2000.

a serious public health risk worldwide, including in the United States. It is also a risk for all health care workers. Transmission is the same as for nonresistant TB. However, MDR TB continues to increase in virulence and is fatal without treatment. A newer strain, called extensively drug-resistant TB (XDR TB), is rare but has a greater risk of mortality. This strain is resistant to both the first- and second-line drugs normally used to treat TB. All strains of TB are transmitted by airborne particles and droplets, direct contact with inanimate objects, and direct contact with an infected individual.

MISCELLANEOUS BACTERIAL PATHOGENS

Haemophilus influenzae—Meningitis
Klebsiella pneumoniae—Pneumonia
Porphyromonas gingivalis—Periodontal disease and intestinal infection
Streptococcus mutans—Dental caries
Moraxella catarrhalis—Upper respiratory infection
Acinetobacter—Wound and systemic infection, especially in immunocompromised patients
Treponema pallidum—Syphilis
Streptococcus agalactiae—One of the group B streptococcal bacteria found normally in the vagina but may infect the newborn during birth
Mycobacterium leprae—Hansen's disease (leprosy)

Chlamydia trachomatis—Genital and reproductive system infection
Gardnerella vaginalis—Genital infection
Mycoplasma hominis—May be related to pelvic infection
Proteus mirabilis—Urinary tract infection
Bartonella—Opportunistic bacterial infection

VIRUSES

A virus is a nonliving infectious agent that ranges in size from 10 to 300 nm. A virus is not a cell. It is referred to as a *virus particle.* A complete virus particle is called a **virion.** These agents cause some of the most lethal infections known. Although they can be extremely pathogenic, they are unable to metabolize outside the host cell. While inside the host's cells, they are unable to infect another individual. Viruses are transmitted by inhalation, in food or water, and by direct transmission from an infected host via blood or body fluids. Some viruses may also be transmitted by insects. Viruses are found throughout the living environment and cause disease in many different organisms.

Classification

Viruses are classified by a number of complex systems and categories, such as by morphology (shape and structure), chemical composition, and method of replication.

Morphology

A virion consists of a double or single strand of either DNA or RNA. This genetic material is surrounded by a protein coating (capsid). The total structure is called a nucleocapsid. Depending on the type of virus, the nucleocapsid can take on many different complex geometric shapes. Some virions are enclosed in a membrane, or envelope, derived from the host cell (Fig. 8.11). A virion has no organelles.

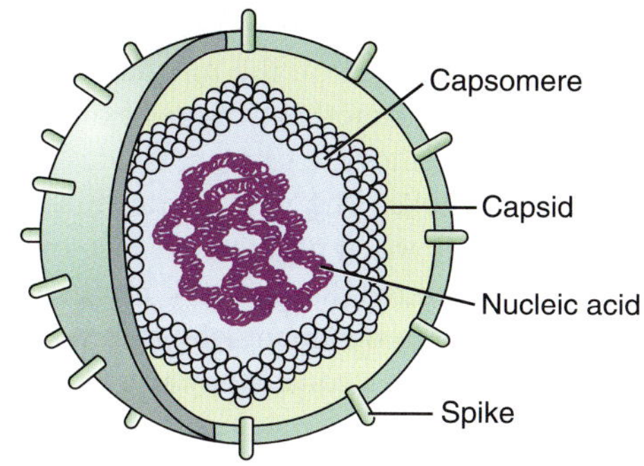

FIG. 8.11 Virus morphology. (From VanMeter K, Hubert R, eds. *Microbiology for the Healthcare Professional.* 2nd ed. St Louis: Elsevier; 2016.)

Replication and Transmission

Although viruses contain genetic material, they cannot replicate without a host cell. To replicate, they inject their DNA or RNA into another cell and dissolve its genetic material. The virus uses the host cell's physiological mechanisms to replicate its own genetic material. The virus then synthesizes new capsids, assembles new virions, and ruptures the cell to release them. The cycle of replication and lysis (bursting) of the host cell is called *lysogenesis.*

Some types of viruses remain inside the host cell in latent form. In this state, the virus is not infective, but it continues to replicate. Under certain favorable conditions, the virus begins to replicate more actively and produces disease symptoms, perhaps years later. Examples of viruses that follow this cycle are the herpes simplex virus and the poliovirus.

A virus that invades bacterial cells is called a *bacteriophage.* Bacteriophages are widely dispersed throughout living organisms and may display a parasitic, commensal, or symbiotic relationship with their bacterial host. Bacteriophages can replicate and spread or remain inside the bacterial cell. Bacteriophages are currently being tested for use in medicine and food production as a way to destroy harmful bacteria.

Viruses are also capable of transforming normal cells into cancerous cells, which lose their original functional and metabolic characteristics through genetic changes. These cells divide rapidly and develop into tumor tissue. Specific cancer-inducing viruses include the hepatitis A virus (HAV) and certain types of human papillomavirus (HPV).

Pathogenicity

Pathogenicity is defined less clearly in viruses than in bacteria. We know some of the mechanisms that create and sustain viral disease in certain strains. These include the following:

- *Ability to enter a healthy cell:* The virus enters the host cell by attaching to its membrane or wall, where it is absorbed by phagocytosis.
- *Ability to develop:* The virus is able to redirect the cell's genetic material to viral replication rather than cell reproduction.
- *Ability to resist the host's defense mechanisms:* The virus may be recognized by the body's immune system, which attacks its own cell, killing it.
- *Cell transformation:* The virus's ability to mutate the cell can result in the formation of cancer growth in some cells.
- *Ability to synthesize substances not normally produced by the host cell.*
- *Ability to initiate structural changes in the host cell:* These changes lead to cell death or to abnormalities that alter the cell's functions.

Pathogenic Viruses

HUMAN IMMUNODEFICIENCY VIRUS/ACQUIRED IMMUNODEFICIENCY SYNDROME Infection with HIV is pandemic (a worldwide epidemic). Approximately 33.4 million cases of HIV have been reported worldwide (UNAIDS, 2015). The global effect of AIDS has changed practices and procedures in health care dramatically.

HIV is transmitted via blood-to-blood contact, sexual contact, and contact with certain body fluids. The body fluids known to transmit HIV are the following:

- Blood
- Semen
- Vaginal secretions
- Breast milk
- Cerebrospinal fluid
- Synovial fluid
- Amniotic fluid
- Any body fluid containing blood

HIV may be transmitted when the body fluids of an infected person are deposited on the mucous membranes or into the vascular system of another person. Sexual contact and use of contaminated needles are primary modes of transmission in the general public. The risk of transmission during sexual contact increases when partners are also infected with another sexually transmitted disease. HIV can be transmitted to the fetus in utero and to the infant who receives breast milk from an infected mother. A neonate may also be infected during delivery.

Casual contact with an infected person does not transmit the virus. Although HIV has been found in saliva, tears, and sweat, the number of pathogens found in these body fluids has been very small. Contact with these fluids has not been shown to result in the transmission of HIV. Occupational risk to health care workers is highest in needle stick and other sharps injuries. There is little evidence of a risk of transmission from an infected health care worker to a patient.

A person infected with HIV may show no symptoms yet still transmit the disease to others. This is because early in the disease process, the body's immune system is able to attack the virus. As long as such individuals are not tested, they may continue to transmit the disease to others without realizing that they are infected. Weeks after the initial infection, mild illness occurs, followed by increasingly serious disease manifestations. Years may pass before symptoms of AIDS begin to appear. The conversion from HIV infection to AIDS-related complex to AIDS is poorly understood. HIV infection is confirmed by the presence of specific antibodies.

AIDS is not a separate disease organism but a syndrome that results from infection with HIV. Patients with AIDS lack normal immune response, and certain diseases are common in these individuals. A true diagnosis of AIDS is made when the presence of one or more of these diseases is confirmed (Box 8.4). Currently, AIDS has no cure. However, the disease can now be controlled with drug therapy.

Extensive information about AIDS and its treatment can be found on the websites for the CDC and the United Nations Committee on HIV/AIDS.

BOX 8.4 Opportunistic Infections and Tumors in Acquired Immunodeficiency Syndrome (AIDS)

VIRUSES

Disseminated cytomegalovirus (lungs, retina, brain)
Herpes simplex virus (HSV-1 and HSV-2) (lungs, gastrointestinal tract, central nervous system [CNS], skin)
JC papovavirus (brain: progressive multifocal leukoencephalopathy)
Epstein–Barr virus (EBV)

BACTERIA

Mycobacteria (e.g., *Mycoplasma avium, Mycobacterium tuberculosis*: disseminated, extrapulmonary)
Salmonella (recurrent, disseminated; septicemia)

PROTOZOA

Toxoplasma gondii (disseminated, including the CNS)
Cryptosporidium (gastrointestinal tract: chronic diarrhea)
Isospora (gastrointestinal tract: diarrhea persisting longer than 1 month)

FUNGI

Pneumocystis jiroveci (lungs: pneumonia)
Candida albicans (esophagus, lung)
Cryptococcus neoformans (CNS)
Histoplasma capsulatum (disseminated, extrapulmonary)
Coccidioides (disseminated, extrapulmonary)

TUMORS

Kaposi sarcoma
B cell lymphoma (e.g., brain; some are EBV induced)

OTHER

Human immunodeficiency virus (HIV) encephalopathy (AIDS dementia complex)

*Also pyogenic bacteria (e.g., *Haemophilus, Streptococcus, Pneumococcus* spp.), which cause septicemia, pneumonia, meningitis, osteomyelitis, arthritis, abscesses, and other diseases; multiple or recurrent infections, especially in children.
†Associated with human herpesvirus 8, an independently transmitted agent; 300 times more common in AIDS than in other immunodeficiency conditions.

VIRAL HEPATITIS Viral hepatitis is a disease of the liver that is caused by one of five significant viruses. The hepatitis B, C, and D viruses are blood-borne pathogens, which are transmitted when blood from an infected person enters the body of another person (a transmission similar to that for HIV). Hepatitis A and hepatitis E are transmitted through contaminated food or water.

HAV is transmitted by ingestion and by close contact with an infected person. Fecal and oral routes are the common modes of transmission. This virus cannot be cultured, but hepatitis can be diagnosed through a serological test that shows the presence of antibodies to HAV. Hepatitis A is rarely fatal, and one infection results in permanent immunity to the disease.

Infection with the hepatitis B virus (HBV) can cause chronic hepatitis, cirrhosis, massive liver **necrosis,** and death. Like HIV, HBV is transmitted through blood and body fluids. The virus is 100 times more infective than HIV. It can be spread through sexual contact and is found in most body secretions. Infected mothers also pass it to infants in 70% to 90% of births. Infected infants have a 90% chance of becoming chronic (long-term) carriers.

The incubation period of HBV is 10 to 12 weeks, during which time the virus can be detected through serological testing. The disease causes general weakness, arthralgia, myalgia, and severe anorexia. Fever and upper abdominal pain may also be present. Some patients develop cirrhosis and liver cancer as a complication of the disease. There is no cure for the disease, so only the symptoms are treated. However, a safe, effective vaccine is available, and all health care workers and those coming in contact with blood products or body fluids should be vaccinated.

Hepatitis C virus (HCV) is transmitted by blood transfusions and blood products. The virus is also found in saliva, urine, and semen. Health care workers, those who receive blood transfusions, IV drug abusers, organ transplant recipients, and hemodialysis patients are at high risk for the disease. The symptoms are similar to but milder than those of hepatitis B. About 50% of patients develop chronic hepatitis and cirrhosis and may require liver transplantation. The highest rates of infection are found in transfusion recipients and IV drug abusers. HCV is a causal agent of liver cancer.

Hepatitis D virus (HDV) is associated with HBV as a coinfection. It is a blood-borne virus that is acquired as a secondary infection with HBV or as a result of HBV. When the two infections occur together, they result in more rapid liver destruction and more severe clinical manifestations than HBV alone.

Hepatitis E is caused by the hepatitis E virus. It causes serious acute liver disease and is transmitted by contaminated water. The disease does not develop into a chronic form.

HUMAN PAPILLOMAVIRUS HPV is a potentially cancer-producing virus that occurs in about 15% of the population. Approximately 40 types of HPV exist, although only a few of them are oncogenic. The virus is found throughout the animal population but is species specific. It is transmitted through sexual contact and therefore is a significant public health concern. Both men and women can be affected. Chronic HPV infection may develop into cervical cancer in women and noninvasive penile and anal cancer in men. The virus types are divided into two groups: high risk and low risk (for cancer association). Some of the low-risk types cause genital warts (condylomata), which can be removed. However, the virus may persist in the body after removal of the lesions.

HPV may cause no symptoms and can lie dormant for many years. Predictors for HPV in women include the following:

- Women younger than 25 years of age
- Multiple sex partners
- Early onset of sexual activity (younger than 16 years old)
- Male partner with a history of multiple partners

Predictors in men include multiple partners. Disease rates are higher in the males having sex with males (MSM) population.

A vaccine for HPV is available for girls and young women. No evidence supports the effectiveness of the vaccine in men. A routine Papanicolaou (Pap) test is one of the best methods of detecting cervical cancer in women. The Pap test detects changes in the cervical endothelium caused by HPV.

MISCELLANEOUS PATHOGENIC VIRUSES This group of viruses and the diseases they cause are of public health concern but are not necessarily related to surgery:

- Rubella
- Varicella zoster—chicken pox
- Variola—German measles
- Morbillivirus—measles
- Enterovirus—polio
- Lyssavirus—rabies

Information on HPV from the CDC can be found at https://www.cdc.gov/hpv/.

PRIONS The **prion** (a proteinaceous, infectious particle) is a unique pathogenic substance. It is a protein particle that contains no nucleic acid. It is believed to be a modified form of normal cellular protein that arises through mutation. It is then transmitted by ingestion or direct contact, especially during medical or surgical procedures. Prions are resistant to all forms of disinfection and sterilization that are normally used in the medical setting. They cannot be cultured in the laboratory, and the immune system does not react to them. Only a few prion diseases affect human beings. The most important is Creutzfeldt–Jakob disease (CJD) and the newly emergent variant of CJD.

CJD is a rare, transmissible disease of the nervous system that is progressive and always fatal. The disease may have an incubation period of up to 20 years. Although CJD is not contagious, it is transmissible. The mechanism of transmission is currently unknown. CJD represents a threat in the health care setting because it is known to be transmitted by contaminated electrodes during neurosurgical stereotactic surgery, corneal grafts, and direct contact with neurosurgical instruments that have been used on patients with CJD. For these reasons, current infection control standards require the use of disposable instruments for these types of surgical procedures or specialized decontamination procedures. Protocols for CJD have been established to help prevent transmission.

FUNGI

Fungi are found worldwide on living organic substances, in water, and in soil. More than 70,000 species of fungi exist, but only 300 are pathogenic. They are composed of eukaryotes classified into two groups, molds and yeasts.

Characteristics

Yeasts are unicellular, and molds are multicellular. Like the bacterial endospore, fungal spores are resistant to heat, cold, and drying. They have a cell wall and obtain their nutrients through absorption. Fungi are distinct from plants and animals. They occur as a single cell or as filaments called *hyphae.* These occur as a complex mass called a *mycelium.* The mycelium is divided into compartments, each containing a nucleus. Many fungi are visible without a microscope, and colonies may be grown in the laboratory for identification and drug sensitivity testing.

Identification

Fungi can be identified in the laboratory by direct observation of their form after culture. A specimen of the fungus is allowed to grow in a suitable medium and then observed for the shape, pattern, and color of the fungal colony. Further testing can be performed by staining the cells and observing them under the microscope.

Reproduction

Fungi are capable of sexual or asexual reproduction, depending on the species and environment. Sexual reproduction takes place in the mycelium, which contains the sex cells needed for meiosis (reproductive cell division). Spores are released through sexual reproduction, and these may go on to produce a new colony. Fragmentation of the mycelium may also initiate the growth of a new colony.

Transmission to Humans

Fungal diseases occur as superficial or deep mycoses. Superficial fungi, which affect the skin, hair, nails, mouth, and vagina, are transmitted by direct contact with the source and cause mild disease symptoms. The yeast *Candida albicans* is normally established in the oral cavity of the newborn and persists as a commensal organism throughout life. At times of immune stress or disease, oral *Candida* can proliferate. Deep fungi enter the body through the respiratory tract or through breaks in the skin or mucous membranes. Medical devices, such as catheters and IV cannulas, can also infect a healthy individual. In the health care setting, fungi can survive in the heating and cooling ducts of the ventilation system, releasing spores into the environment from which patients and workers can become infected.

Pathogenicity

Deep or disseminated fungal infections can be fatal. Patients who are immunosuppressed or who are weakened by metabolic disorders, infectious diseases, or trauma are at high risk for serious *mycotic* (fungal) disease. Healthy individuals are rarely infected with deep mycosis. Pathogenic fungi are described in Table 8.3.

Pathogenic Fungi

ASPERGILLUS FUMIGATUS *A. fumigatus* is a significant fungal pathogen. It is an **opportunistic infection** in immunosuppressed patients. This fungus invades the body through the lungs and blood vessels and can cause vascular thrombosis and partial blockage of the airways. In a severely compromised patient, invasive *Aspergillus* infection is often fatal.

CANDIDA ALBICANS *C. albicans* is a common opportunistic infection. It is a normal resident of the mouth, vagina, and intestine. However, it can proliferate in individuals who are immunosuppressed or weakened by disease and in patients taking antibiotics. When localized in the oral cavity or vagina, the infection can usually be treated successfully with antifungal drugs. Systemic or disseminated infection can spread to any location in the body, including the heart, kidneys, and other vital organs.

PNEUMOCYSTIS JIROVECI Infection with *P. jiroveci* (formerly known as *P. carinii*) is widespread in the general population but usually produces only mild symptoms. Pneumocystis pneumonia (PCP) is a common respiratory disease among patients with AIDS. Patients who are immunosuppressed, including those receiving immunosuppressive drugs for organ transplantation, are at high risk for the disease. The infection is difficult to diagnose, because the symptoms are nonspecific and the fungus cannot be isolated from the patient's sputum through normal methods.

CUTANEOUS MYCOSES Superficial fungal infections invade the superficial layers of the skin. The filaments of the fungus spread into dead (keratinized) skin, hair, and nails. These cause irritation and oozing and may encourage the development of a superficial bacterial infection.

PROTOZOA

Characteristics

Protozoa are a group of single-celled eukaryotic organisms. Protozoa are free-living in a variety of freshwater and marine habitats. Approximately 65,000 different species have been identified (compared to 4500 species of bacteria). A large number of protozoa are parasitic in animals, including human beings. Most have complex life cycles with intermediate hosts that facilitate their transmission and reproduction. Single-celled protozoa reproduce by binary fission, and they can infect any tissue or organ of the body. The organisms usually enter through an insect bite or by ingestion. Once in the body, they selectively reproduce in particular anatomical structures, such as the intestine, skin, blood, liver, or CNS. Protozoa feed on a wide variety of substances in the environment, including algae and bacteria. These are absorbed through the cell membrane.

The structure of protozoa varies widely by species, which allows identification by microscopic examination. Most protozoa have a well-defined shape and cell membrane, or envelope. They range in size from 1 to 300 micrometers. Many have an outer layer, called an *ectoplasm,* which contains the organelles used for feeding, locomotion, and defense. The cytoplasm contains organelles usually found in eukaryotic cells (described previously).

Mobility

Protozoa move through their watery environment by a variety of mechanisms. These are used to classify the protozoa. *Ciliates*

TABLE 8.3 Medically Important Fungal Infections

Type of Fungus	Location	Disease	Causative Organism
Superficial	Keratin layer of skin, hair shaft	Tinea nigra, pityriasis versicolor	*Trichosporon*
			Malassezia
			Eosinophilia
Cutaneous	Epidermis, hair, nails	Tinea (ringworm)	*Microsporum*
			Trichophyton
			Epidermophyton
Systemic	Internal organs	Coccidiomycosis	*Cryptococcus*
		Histoplasmosis	*Candida*
		Blastomycosis	*Aspergillus*
		Paracoccidioidomycosis	*Pneumocystis*

Modified from Goering R, Dockrell H, Zuckerman M, et al, eds. *Mims' Medical Microbiology.* 4th ed. St Louis: Mosby; 2008.

are protozoa that move by multiple projections (cilia), which extend as hair-like fibers around the periphery of the ectoplasm. The cilia move in waves, providing locomotion. *Flagellates* have a single flagellum ("tail") or multiple flagella that propel them in different directions. *Amoebae* move by using a pseudopod (false foot), which extends and pulls the cell along. Amoebae are attracted or repelled by concentration gradients in their environment, and they feed by absorption through the pseudopod.

Pathogenicity

Protozoa cause a wide variety of diseases in animals and human beings. These diseases are often characterized by destruction of the host cells by ingestion. Protozoa are able to resist or avoid many of the body's defenses by changing the antigens on their surface or by ingesting the immune complement of the cell, thereby disabling it. Widespread cell destruction results in the disease characteristics of different protozoan species and of the tissue they invade.

Gastrointestinal disease is characterized by simple diarrhea or dysentery. Protozoa feed on the mucosa and red blood cells of the host. This can result in severe dehydration, anemia, perforation of the intestine, and proliferation in other organs.

Protozoan diseases of the CNS can result in severe destruction of nerve cell tissue or blood vessels, leading to encephalitis and death. Malaria is the most significant protozoan disease of the CNS and a major killer of children in Africa and Asia. Protozoa that infect blood and organs destroy blood cells and tissue, including the liver, kidneys, heart, and lymph system. Important pathogenic protozoa are described in Table 8.4.

ALGAE

Algae are eukaryotes that belong to the plant kingdom; they include sponges and seaweed. They are classified as microbes but have no pathogenic effect on human beings. Structurally, they vary widely, from single-celled organisms to colonies and large plants that can reach several hundred feet in length. They occur in freshwater and saltwater sources globally. Widespread commercial harvesting of algae for food products, manufacturing, and agriculture threatens these species, which are important in the food chain and in the ecology of wetlands and waterborne animals.

IMMUNITY

The immune system defends the body against harmful substances, including disease microorganisms. *Immunity* is the body's ability to accept substances that are part of the body ("self") and eliminate those that are not ("nonself"). The study of immunity and the immune system is often difficult, because it involves many terms and complex concepts.

The body has two general types of immunity, innate and adaptive:

- *Innate immunity* (also called *nonspecific immunity*) exists from the time of birth. This type of protection is not targeted at a specific substance but occurs as a physiological reaction whenever an injury occurs or foreign substances are present in the body.
- *Adaptive immunity* is conferred through exposure to a specific substance or microbe called an *antigen*. When exposure occurs, the immune system develops *antibodies*, which are specific proteins that can stay in the system and trigger it to launch its defenses during subsequent exposure to the microbe or substance.

INNATE IMMUNITY

Chemical and Mechanical Body Defenses

The body has many different chemical and mechanical defenses against infection. These are sometimes called "first-line" defenses against infection.

TABLE 8.4 Important Protozoan Parasites

Anatomical Location	Species	Disease	Method of Transmission
Intestine	*Entamoeba histolytica*	Amebiasis	Ingestion of parasite cysts in water or food
	Giardia intestinalis	Giardiasis	
	Cryptosporidium spp.	Cryptosporidiosis	
	Microsporidia	Microsporidiosis	
Urogenital tract	*Trichomonas vaginalis*	Trichomoniasis	Sexual contact
Blood and tissue	*Trypanosoma* spp.	Trypanosomiasis Sleeping sickness Chagas' disease	Reduviid bug Tsetse fly
	Leishmania spp.	Visceral leishmaniasis (kala-azar) Cutaneous leishmaniasis	Sand fly
	Plasmodium spp. (*P. vivax*, *P. ovale*, *P. malariae*)	Malaria	*Anopheles* mosquito
	Toxoplasma gondii	Toxoplasmosis	Ingestion of cysts in raw meat; contact with infected cat feces

Modified from Goering R et al, eds. Mims' Medical Microbiology. 4th ed. St Louis: Mosby; 2008.

- Intact skin, including the mucous membranes, serves as an excellent barrier against the transmission and spread of infection. The normal flora of the skin, fatty acids derived from perspiration, excretions of sebaceous glands, and the rapid growth of keratin prevent bacterial entry into deeper tissues. Specific skin tissues are specialized in their ability to defend the body against infection. For example, skin appendages such as the eyelashes and nasal and ear hair prevent contamination by dust and droplets.
- The respiratory system has many different defense mechanisms. Microscopic cilia that line the respiratory tract continually sweep particles from the surface of the tract. The action of the cilia moves material toward the mouth and nose and prevents it from settling in the lower respiratory tract. Mucus in the respiratory system traps particles and bacteria, which are forced out through the cough reflex.
- Bacteriostatic chemicals in saliva, low pH in the stomach, and resident flora in the intestine prevent infection. Gastrointestinal transmission occurs by ingestion (eating or drinking food or water contaminated with infectious microorganisms). We ingest many different types of foreign material and bacteria each day. Despite the body's defenses, virulent disease organisms can quickly invade the tissues of the intestine and proliferate.
- **Resident microorganisms** compete with invading microbes for the environment. Shortly after birth, an infant's body begins to acquire a wide variety of bacterial colonies in certain tissues of the body. Resident microorganisms are found in areas of the body that communicate with or are exposed to the outside environment. The gastrointestinal system has a complex environment that includes different resident bacteria that can be harmful outside of the gastrointestinal system. All other tissues in the body are normally sterile. The resident microbes help prevent invading, potentially disease-causing microorganisms from colonizing in tissue.
- The inflammatory response is the body's innate immune response to injury. The four classic signs of **inflammation** are heat, redness, swelling (edema), and pain.
- Almost immediately after tissue injury, blood vessels temporarily constrict at the site of injury. Constriction of capillaries helps reduce bleeding and restricts the movement of any microbial toxins present. This is rapidly followed by localized arterial and venous dilation. As a result, the injured area becomes red and warm. Local capillaries become more permeable, which allows plasma to escape into the surrounding tissue. The plasma dilutes any toxins in these tissues; it also increases the thickness (viscosity) of the local blood supply and encourages clotting. These processes result in swelling, pain, and impaired function of the affected part.
- When microorganisms invade the body, a cellular response is initiated. Specialized white blood cells (leukocytes) rush to the site and surround and engulf them. This process, called phagocytosis, is an immune response triggered by the process of inflammation. Once the microorganism is inside the leukocyte, the leukocyte's lysosomes fuse with the microorganism and digest it. Nonliving remnants of the microorganism are then released from the leukocyte. Two types of "digesting cells," called *phagocytes*, are involved in this process. *Neutrophils* are carried to the site of infection within 90 minutes. Within about 5 to 48 hours, *macrophages* arrive and continue to engulf and digest large amounts of bacteria. Regional lymph nodes collect cellular debris and act as centers for more intensive phagocytic activity. Pus at the site of an infection is composed of dead cells, lymphocytes, and living and dead pathogens.

ADAPTIVE IMMUNE SYSTEM

The *adaptive immune system* is triggered by exposure to a specific potentially harmful substance, such as a disease microorganism in the environment or through a vaccination. This protein substance is referred to as an *antigen*. When exposed to an antigen, the body forms antibodies, which attach to the cells and remain there temporarily or throughout life.

- Antigens are *nonself* substances that trigger the immune system to launch a defense.
- Antibodies are self-substances that provide protection to the body.

ACTIVE IMMUNITY

Active immunity develops when the body is stimulated to form its own antibodies against specific disease antigens. This type of immunity is usually permanent. The best immunity is formed from a live antigen.

Active immunity can occur after vaccination or exposure to the disease. In this process, T and B lymphocytes are activated to bring about the production of antibodies (proteins that remain in the immune system memory). When the body is exposed to the disease pathogen again, the antibodies are activated and quickly destroy the organisms. Immunity can last for years or a lifetime.

A person can develop active immunity in two ways:

1. By getting the disease
2. By vaccination, which is an injection containing a small amount of disease antigen. The antigen is modified to prevent the recipient from developing the disease, but it is effective in stimulating the formation of antibodies.

PASSIVE IMMUNITY

Passive immunity develops when the body receives the specific disease antibodies from an outside source. This eliminates the need for the body to synthesize them. Passive immunity, which is temporary, occurs when:

1. The fetus receives antibodies in utero from the mother's immune system or breast milk (natural immunity).
2. A person receives a specific antibody for a specific antigen, created in equine or human tissue. The antibody is usually given by injection. Tetanus antitoxin is an example of an injectable antibody.

VACCINES

Vaccination provides a form of adaptive immunity. Vaccines are modified forms of disease organisms that create immunological memory in the body. They produce the same immunological response as the disease itself, without the risks involved in the disease process. Vaccination provides artificial immunity against specific organisms.

Vaccines are classified into two main types and their subtypes:

1. Live attenuated vaccines
   - Viruses
   - Bacteria
2. Inactivated vaccines
   - Whole
   - Fractional

Live attenuated vaccines contain modified disease organisms, either viruses or bacteria. Modification of the organism prevents the recipient of the vaccine from experiencing the effects of the disease, but immunity is still conferred. Examples of attenuated vaccines licensed in the United States are polio, measles, mumps, varicella, and rubella.

Inactivated vaccines contain whole viruses or bacteria, or fractional components of the organisms. Protein-based fractional vaccines are called toxoids; these are inactivated bacterial toxins.

HYPERSENSITIVITY

Immune response to a substance is referred to as hypersensitivity. Hypersensitivity only occurs in individuals who have previous exposure and sensitivity to the substance. A hypersensitivity reaction may be mild, producing a rash, mild respiratory distress leading to asthma, or gastrointestinal symptoms. The reaction can be immediate or delayed for up to 12 hours after exposure. A severe immediate reaction is referred to as *anaphylactic shock,* which can be quickly fatal.

ALLERGY

True allergy is a process mediated by the immune system. A substance that causes a hypersensitivity reaction is called an *allergen.* Allergens gain entry into the body by many routes. In the perioperative environment, it is very important to know the patient's allergies. These may include medications and latex rubber, which is contained in many medical devices, including surgical gloves.

Immediate and Delayed Reaction

The two types of true allergic reactions are immediate and delayed. Delayed reactions are mediated by T lymphocytes, whereas immediate reactions are mediated by antibodies. Allergic reactions are divided into four categories:

- *Type I:* These reactions are characterized by inflammation of tissues, which is caused by the release of *histamine* in the body. This causes increased permeability of blood vessels and constriction of bronchioles, leading to difficulty breathing. The most extreme form of sensitivity is anaphylactic shock, which can lead to death.
- *Type II:* A type II reaction is called a *cytotoxic reaction.* It causes the onset of powerful immune defense mechanisms, which can result in injury or death. Mismatched blood transfusion and hemolytic disease in newborns are type II reactions.
- *Type III:* Type III reactions are caused by antigen–antibody complexes, which produce tissue damage when they trigger an immune response. An example of a type III reaction is allergy to antibiotics. Symptoms include itching, rash, severe tissue swelling, and fever. This usually resolves in several days.
- *Type IV:* Type IV reactions are cell-mediated reactions (not related to antibodies) that occur 24 to 72 hours after exposure to the agent. An example of this delayed hypersensitivity is a positive reaction to the tuberculin skin test, in which a small amount of killed *Mycobacterium tuberculosis* is injected into the skin.

Autoimmunity

In certain diseases, the body does not recognize "self." Consequently, it mounts a mild-to-severe immune response to its own tissues, causing fever, swelling, and tissue destruction. Examples of autoimmune diseases are rheumatoid arthritis, systemic lupus erythematosus, and ulcerative colitis (single organ autoimmune disease).

KEY CONCEPTS

- Microbiology is the study of microorganisms and their relationship with the environment.
- The Linnaean system of classification is used in biology to distinguish specific groups of organisms.
- Living cellular organisms are divided into two groups: eukaryotes and prokaryotes.
- Eukaryotic cells are the cells of complex organisms such as mammals.
- Bacteria belong to the prokaryote class of cells.
- Microbes are identified by their morphology, staining tendencies, and reactions to biochemical tests. Gram staining is a basic test performed for differentiation.
- Chemical tests can be performed on bacteria only if they are grown in a laboratory environment (culturing). After culturing, the bacteria are tested for sensitivity to antimicrobial drugs (culture and sensitivity).
- Microbes are classified by types according to the Linnaean system. The major groups are bacteria, viruses, fungi, protozoa, rickettsiae, and prions.
- Cells contain various types of organelles, which aid in the cell's metabolism.
- Substances move into the cell mainly by diffusion, osmosis, active transport, and pinocytosis.
- The relationship between a microbe and its host depends on the environment, the condition of the host, and the condition of the microbe.
- The biological relationship between organisms living together is called *symbiosis.* If neither organism is harmed, the association is called *commensalism;* if the association benefits both, it is *mutualism,* and if one is harmed and the other benefits, it is *parasitism.*
- Bacteria are the most important group of microbes in medicine, because they cause most diseases.

- Bacteria vary in their environmental and physiological needs. These include nutrition, oxygen requirements, pH, and temperature.
- Oxygen requirements are particularly important in wound management. Aerobic bacteria require oxygen, and anaerobic bacteria do not. Anaerobic bacteria produce powerful toxins that can be fatal in the host.
- Bacterial toxins are produced by living bacteria as products of metabolism (exotoxin), or the toxins are released after the bacteria die (endotoxin).
- Specific types of bacteria live normally in human tissues. These are called resident flora, and they aid in digestion and defense against disease.
- Prions and viruses are nonliving but able to cause disease.
- Creutzfeldt–Jakob disease and variant CJD are fatal, transmissible diseases of the nervous system. They are important in surgery, because although rare, the prion responsible for the diseases cannot be destroyed by normal sterilization methods.
- Hepatitis and HIV/AIDS are the most important infectious diseases caused by viruses. The hepatitis B virus and HIV are blood-borne microbes transmitted through contact with body fluids.
- Disease transmission occurs only when certain conditions are met. These include a method of transmission, a portal of entry into the body, a sufficient dose of microbes, a suitable environment for microbe reproduction, and insufficient resistance in the host.
- Infectious disease is transmitted by direct contact, airborne droplets, oral transmission, and ingestion of microbes.
- Urinary catheterization causes the greatest number of hospital-acquired infections (HAIs) in the United States. Surgical site infection is the second most frequent HAI.
- Multidrug-resistant organisms have evolved because of the overuse and misuse of antimicrobial agents worldwide.
- The immune system defends the body against infection by innate immunity and adaptive immunity. Innate immunity is present at birth, and adaptive immunity is conferred by previous exposure to the disease-causing organism, either naturally or by immunization.
- Hypersensitivity to a substance in the environment is also mediated by the immune system and can result in serious illness or death.

REVIEW QUESTIONS

1. In what ways are viral and bacterial diseases transmitted?
2. What particular protection does the bacterial spore provide in prolonging the life of bacteria?
3. Why are antibiotics not effective against viral infections?
4. What is resident flora? What protection does it provide?
5. How do viruses replicate?
6. How is hepatitis B transmitted?
7. What characteristics make CJD such a risk?
8. Define these terms: antibody, antigen, passive immunity, and active immunity.
9. What is the most important method of preventing disease transmission in the health care setting?

CASE STUDIES

CASE 1

Direct contact with pathogenic microorganisms is the most common cause of hospital-acquired infection. How might a dermal (skin) *Staphylococcus* infection of a staff member result in a urinary traction infection of a patient? Describe a possible pathway of contamination during a normal workday.

BIBLIOGRAPHY

Atkinson W, Hamborsky J, McIntyre L, Wolfe S, eds. *Epidemiology and Prevention of Vaccine-Preventable Diseases*. 12th ed. Washington, DC: Public Health Foundation; 2011. Accessed June 20, 2019. http://www.cdc.gov/vaccines/pubs/pinkbook/index.html. September 21, 2015.

Centers for Disease Control and Prevention. Prion diseases: about prion diseases. February 5, 2016. http://www.cdc.gov/prions/index.html. Accessed June 20, 2019.

Centers for Disease Control and Prevention. Healthcare-associated infections (HAIs). http://www.cdc.gov/hai/. May 27, 2016. Accessed January 11, 2016.

Centers for Disease Control and Prevention. *HIV/AIDS*. HIV Basics. http://www.cdc.gov/hiv/basics/index.html. Accessed June 20, 2019.

Control Practices Advisory Committee. *2007 Guidelines for Isolation Precautions: Preventing Transmission of Infectious Agents in Healthcare Settings*. https://www.cdc.gov/anthrax/pdf/infection-control-guidelines-for-healtcare-setting-2007.pdf. Accessed June 20, 2019.

World Health Organization. *WHO Guidelines on Hand Hygiene in Health Care*. WHO; 2009. https://www.who.int/gpsc/5may/tools/978 9241597906/en/. Accessed June 20, 2019.

STERILE TECHNIQUE AND INFECTION CONTROL

9

LEARNING OBJECTIVES

After studying this chapter, the reader will be able to:

1. Review guidelines related to sterile technique
2. Clearly define terms related to sterile technique
3. Explain the concepts of barriers and containment
4. Demonstrate sterile techniques
5. Describe surgical attire
6. Demonstrate methods of hand hygiene using the correct technique
7. Demonstrate correct gowning and gloving techniques
8. Demonstrate how to introduce sterile items onto the sterile field
9. Demonstrate and describe methods used to maintain the sterile field
10. Demonstrate the principles of Standard Precautions
11. Describe important components of OSHA's bloodborne pathogens standard
12. Discuss the purpose and procedures used in transmission-based precautions

TERMINOLOGY

Antiseptic: A chemical agent used on the skin to inhibit the proliferation of microorganisms.

Blood-borne pathogen: Infectious microorganisms in blood that can be transmitted by direct contact with blood or other body fluids of an infected person.

Chemical barrier: The residual action of a disinfectant or antiseptic that prevents recolonization (regrowth) for a limited period of time.

Containment and confinement: A foundation concept of sterile technique in which sterile and nonsterile surfaces are separated by physical barriers or space.

Contamination: The potential or actual transfer of microorganisms to a previously sterile surface.

Contaminated: Describes a sterile surface which has come in contact with a nonsterile surface.

Double gloving: Wearing two pairs of gloves, one over the other, to reduce the risk of contamination as a result of glove failure or puncture.

Disinfection: A process that results in the destruction of microorganisms on an inanimate (nonliving) object or surface.

Gross contamination: Contamination of a large area of tissue or the environment by an actual or potentially infective material.

Hand hygiene: Procedures related to hand care and cleansing.

Hand washing: A specific technique used to remove soil, debris, and dead cells from the hands. Hand washing with an antiseptic also reduces the number of microorganisms on the skin.

Hands free technique (HFT):: A method of passing sharp instruments within the sterile field to a team member so as to prevent injury. See text for complete description.

Instructions for Use (IFU): A manufacturer's instructions for the use of a medical device by skilled professionals.

Laminar air flow: An unidirectional ultraclean air delivery system that creates a "curtain" of super clean air around the sterile field.

Neutral zone: An area of the sterile field designated for the exchange of sharps. A magnetic pad or basin can be used for sharps so that hand-to-hand exchange can be avoided.

No-touch technique: All sharp items used in surgery are handled with an instrument, not the hand to prevent injury and transmission of blood-borne disease.

Nonsterile: An area or device that is not sterile is described as nonsterile or contaminated.

Nonsterile (unscrubbed) team members: In surgery, team members who remain outside the boundary of the sterile field and do not come in direct contact with sterile equipment, sterile areas, or the surgical wound.

Physical barrier: In surgery, a barrier that separates a sterile surface from a nonsterile surface. Examples are sterile surgical gloves, gowns, and drapes.

Post-exposure prophylaxis (PEP): Voluntary procedures a person may undertake following potential exposure to blood-borne pathogens.

Protective personal equipment (PPE): Equipment worn to minimize exposure to hazards that cause serious workplace injuries and illnesses. (Occupational Safety and Health Administration, https://www.osha.gov/SLTC/personalprotectiveequipment/)

Restricted zone: An area of the operating room with the most stringent methods to reduce the presence of infectious microorganisms in the environment. The main difference between semi-restricted and restricted is the requirement for surgical masks in restricted zones.

Semi-restricted zone: An area of the operating room that has specific requirements for the use of surgical attire and access to other areas of the department.

Sharps: Any objects that can penetrate the skin and can cause

TERMINOLOGY (CONT.)

injury and infection, including but not limited to needles, scalpels, broken glass, and exposed ends of wire sutures.

Squames: Dead skin cells that are normally shed from the epidermis as new skin cells emerge. Squames may potentially transmit pathogenic bacteria.

Sterile field: An area that includes the draped patient, draped tables, and sterile equipment in the immediate area of the patient. The surgical incision is the center of the sterile field.

Sterile item: Any item that has been exposed to a process that destroys all microbes, including spores.

Sterility: A state in which an inanimate or animate surface harbors absolutely no viable microorganisms.

Strikethrough contamination: An event in which fluid from a nonsterile surface penetrates the protective wrapper of a sterile item, causing it to become contaminated.

Surgical conscience: In surgery, the ethical motivation to immediately report surgical errors including contamination of the sterile field.

Surgical hand antisepsis: The application of a specific antiseptic to all surfaces of the hands and arms prior to donning gown and gloves before a surgical procedure.

Surgical scrub: A specific method used to wash the hands and arms using detergent-based antiseptic before donning sterile surgical gown and gloves just before surgery.

Surgical site infection (SSI): Postoperative infection of the surgical wound.

Surgical wound: All the tissue layers of the surgical incision. This is the center of the surgical field.

Unrestricted zone: An area of the operating room that is maintained at a high level of environmental cleanliness without restrictions on attire.

Sterile technique involves *specific practices* that are carried out to prevent contamination and infection of the surgical wound. The development of sound sterile technique takes time and practice. When students first begin to learn aseptic technique, with its many rules and procedures, they often feel awkward and worry about making errors. This is a normal reaction to a completely new way of performing tasks, such as pouring liquid from a bottle or gowning and gloving. The learning process always feels uncomfortable, especially when others are watching. However, the learning environment is where mistakes can be corrected as soon as they occur. There is no easy way to assimilate new ways of doing things except by practice. Repeated practice develops competence and confidence.

Sterile technique is employed routinely during preparations for surgery and in the intraoperative period. This chapter covers the preoperative and intraoperative techniques and recommendations required to prevent contamination of the surgical site. Other topics such as sterilization, disinfection, and surgical skin antisepsis of the patient's skin before surgery are covered in other chapters that are devoted to these topics.

This chapter also introduces the surgical technologist to infection control guidelines and regulations. This is a broad area of theory and practice that includes measures that reduce the risk of infectious disease transmission in patients and perioperative personnel.

The detailed version of Standard Precautions and transmission-based precautions can be accessed at https://www.cdc.gov/infectioncontrol/basics/standard-precautions.html.
OSHA's bloodborne pathogens standard can be accessed at https://www.osha.gov/SLTC/bloodbornepathogens/worker_protections.html.

PART I: FOUNDATION CONCEPTS IN STERILE TECHNIQUE

PRACTICE GUIDELINES

The guidelines provided in this textbook are evidence-based, thorough, rigorous, *up-to-date* research and review. Agencies that are widely accepted as *primary sources* for conducting research and/or establishing guidelines in perioperative patient care and safety are shown in Box 9.1. The organizations' mission statements are also included.

It is important to note that as new research is performed, accrediting agencies update their guidelines and recommendations. This means that practice guidelines are subject to change, which can occur at any time. Health care professionals and facilities are required to keep up with changes to maintain currency in their practices.

As surgical personnel gain experience, they clarify their own practices and compare them with those of the people around them. Even after acquiring excellent technique, people may consciously (or unconsciously) disregard certain practices because of lack of peer or administrative support, lack of professional motivation, or simple apathy. Some professionals become very discouraged when others in the department do not support efforts to maintain high standards. Despite evidence-based guidelines, actual practice can vary slightly according to the setting and the policies of individual institutions.

Surgical personnel can and should discuss the sterile technique practices of their team, department, or institution as long as they have evidence to demonstrate that these practices should be changed. Always remember, however, that as a student, criticism of those in your internship facility will probably not be welcomed. All individuals must try to practice the highest standards possible, even if their colleagues are not supportive.

TERMS USED IN THE GUIDELINES

Terms used in this chapter to describe the guidelines have been adopted from the Association of periOperative Registered Nurses (AORN) *Guidelines for Perioperative Practice*, 2019. The AORN guidelines have been compiled from a variety of sources and reflect rigorous research and review. Many of the guidelines are mandated by federal agencies. Others have been researched and reviewed by agencies listed in Box 9.1. This chapter contains the 2019 guidelines that are most applicable to surgical technologists. The full guidelines and references can be obtained from AORN and specific government agencies cited in this chapter.

BOX 9.1 *Primary Sources* of Research and Establishment of Guidelines and Standards for Perioperative Practice

1. **Agency for Healthcare Research and Quality (AHRQ):** http://www.ahrq.gov/
"The Agency for Healthcare Research and Quality's (AHRQ) mission is to produce evidence to make health care safer, higher quality, more accessible, equitable, and affordable, and to work within the U.S. Department of Health and Human Services and with other partners to make sure that the evidence is understood and used." (AHRQ statement, 2020)
2. **American College of Surgeons:** https://www.facs.org/
"The American College of Surgeons is dedicated to improving the care of the surgical patient and to safeguarding standards of care in an optimal and ethical practice environment."
3. **Association for the Advancement of Medical Instrumentation (AAMI):** http://www.aami.org/standards/
"AAMI is the primary source of consensus standards, both national and international, for the medical device industry, as well as practical information, support, and guidance for healthcare technology and sterilization professionals."
4. **Association of periOperative Registered Nurses:** http://www.aorn.org
"The mission of the Association of periOperative Registered Nurses (AORN) is to promote safety and optimal outcomes for patients undergoing operative and other invasive procedures by providing practice support and professional development opportunities to perioperative nurses. AORN will collaborate with professional and regulatory organizations, industry leaders, and other health care partners who support the mission."
5. **Centers for Disease Control and Prevention (CDC) Healthcare Infection Control Practices Advisory Committee (HICPAC):** https://www.cdc.gov/infectioncontrol/guidelines/index.html
"HICPAC is a federal advisory committee appointed to provide advice and guidance to DHHS and CDC regarding the practice of infection control and strategies for surveillance, prevention, and control of healthcare-associated infections, antimicrobial resistance and related events in United States healthcare settings."
6. **Occupational Safety and Health Administration (OSHA):** http://www.osha.gov/index.html
"To ensure safe and healthful working conditions for working men and women by setting and enforcing standards and by providing training, outreach, education and assistance."

Recommendation: The guideline uses the word "should," and the guideline is backed up by evidence.
Regulatory Requirement: The guideline uses the word "must" and is mandated by government regulation.
Permissible: An action is possible. There is no evidence against the use of an action. The guideline uses the word "may."

IMPORTANT TERMS RELATED TO STERILE TECHNIQUE

The terms and concepts defined here are key to learning and practical application of sterile technique. A review of Chapter 8 on the process of infection will clarify the following concepts.

STERILITY

When a surface is sterile, it is completely free *of all living microorganisms, including bacterial spores.* A sterile surface is known to be sterile only after it has been proven to have been processed with a prescribed method of sterilization. After sterilization, the object must be maintained in an environment known to prevent contamination. The sterilization method must also have been tested to determine the efficiency of the process used for sterilization (discussed in Chapter 10). **Sterility** is absolute. Something is either sterile or not sterile—there is no "partial sterility." An area or device that is not sterile is described as **nonsterile** or **contaminated.**

Surgery is performed under sterile conditions. All instruments, medical devices, supplies, and materials used in a surgical procedure are sterile. Sterile drapes are placed around the surgical incision site extending over the patient's body, on all instrument tables, and on equipment that is required to be sterile. Members of the sterile team wear sterile gowns and gloves.

STERILE FIELD

The **sterile field** is the physical space occupied by the draped patient, draped instrument tables and equipment, and the scrubbed, gowned, and gloved sterile team members. The superficial and deep tissues of the surgical incision are collectively called the **surgical wound.** This is the center of the sterile field. During surgery, the sterile field is tightly controlled and has defined boundaries, which the entire team monitors during a procedure. This is to ensure that sterile surfaces and items remain within the sterile field and **nonsterile team members** remain outside the boundaries of the sterile field. Sterile team members—those who have performed hand antisepsis and donned a sterile gown and gloves—move within the sterile field to perform surgery. Specific rules of sterile technique are used to create and maintain the surgical field.

CONTAMINATION

Surgical **contamination** occurs when potentially pathogenic microorganisms are introduced into the surgical wound, or any sterile area of the sterile field, including surgical instruments, devices, supplies, and drugs used during surgery.

Recall from the previous chapter that the process of contamination occurs by any of the following:

- *Direct physical contact* by between a sterile surface and one that is nonsterile
- *Droplet contact* such as that which occurs when microorganisms are released in coughing, sneezing, and talking
- *Airborne particles* such as dust and lint, which can carry potentially pathogenic microorganisms
- *Vectors* (pathogen-carrying vermin such as insects), which gain entry into wrapped sterile supplies

The term *contaminate,* as it applies to the perioperative environment, is defined as follows:

- An area or item that was previously sterile but comes in contact with a contaminant. For example, a sterile instrument falls to the floor. The instrument is contaminated. The surgeon's gloved hand accidentally touches the nonsterile edge of the surgical drape. His glove is contaminated. The scrubbed surgical technologist accidentally punctures her glove with a suture needle. The needle is contaminated (remember that skin is not sterile).
- An event in which a **sterile item** or surface has come in contact with a nonsterile item or surface. For example, an infected appendix has ruptured, spilling infectious materials into the abdominal cavity. **Gross contamination** of the peritoneal cavity has occurred.

Strikethrough is a specific type of contamination of a sterile surface by penetration of a nonsterile fluid through its sterile covering.

DISINFECTION

Disinfection is a process that results in the destruction of microorganisms on an inanimate (nonliving) object or surface. Disinfectants vary in their ability to destroy certain types of microorganisms. This is discussed in detail in Chapter 10.

ANTISEPSIS

Antisepsis is the destruction of microorganisms on living tissue–mainly the skin. **Antiseptics** are used in hand hygiene, including surgical hand antisepsis and for the perioperative preparation of the patient's surgical site. Refer to Section V for a complete description of surgical hand antisepsis.

BARRIERS

One of the foundation principles of sterile technique is the concept of a barrier between sources of contamination and a sterile surface. To better understand and practice sterile technique, consider the concept of **containment and confinement.** A **physical barrier** can be used to separate a nonsterile surface from one that is sterile. For example, sterile gloves prevent direct contact between the sterile surgical instruments with the nonsterile hand.

Head covers (discussed later) are barriers that *contain* hair and dander. A **chemical barrier** is produced by the residual effect of the antiseptic used during the patient skin prep surgical hand antisepsis or hand rub.

Space is another type of barrier. As you study sterile technique, you will learn the accepted distances between a sterile and nonsterile surface so that you can maintain that distance in practice. This space is perceived, first consciously and then unconsciously. Over time, surgical personnel develop a sense of when nonsterile objects are too close to the field. A specific guideline for the distance required between a sterile and nonsterile surface is defined later.

PART II: OPERATING ROOM DESIGN AND ENVIRONMENT

FUNCTIONAL ZONES OF THE OPERATING ROOM

In Chapter 4 the concepts of specific zones or areas of the operating room (OR) were introduced. In this section these concepts are expanded and integrated into the practice of sterile technique. The functional areas of the operating room are separated into zones, which are assigned using the following criteria:

- The function and activities carried out in that zone
- Surgical attire required for that zone
- Access into and out of the zone
- Heating, ventilation, and air conditioning (HVAC) requirements
- Surface cleaning requirements

The operating room is divided into three zones: *unrestricted, semi-restricted,* and *unrestricted.* Table 9.1 lists each zone and the functional areas within it. The restrictions for each zone increase so that a fully restricted zone has the highest level of environmental **asepsis.**

IMPORTANT TO KNOW *There may be disagreement among professional organizations with regard to assigning levels of asepsis to specific zones.*

TABLE 9.1 Zones of the Operating Room and Their Associated Areas by Functions*

Unrestricted	Semi-restricted	Restricted
Staff locker room/changing areas	Preoperative patient care area*	Operating room
Loaner instrument drop off area	Postoperative patient care area*	Sterile core
Any room accessible to the public	Corridor from unrestricted to restricted area	Scrub sink area
Administrative offices	Satellite sterile processing area	
Medical records storage	Sterile processing clean and decontamination room†	
Meeting and lecture rooms	Procedure rooms†	
Soiled linen storage area		

*Note that an unrestricted area becomes semi-restricted when located within a semi-restricted zone.
†Association for the Advancement of Medical Instrumentation (AAMI) considers these as restricted areas.
Modified from Wood A. *Guidelines for Perioperative Practice.* Denver: Association of PeriOperative Registered Nurses (AORN); 2019.

The **unrestricted zone** is maintained at the lowest level of asepsis. The unrestricted zones are those in which there are no guidelines with regard to levels of asepsis. There are, however, safety guidelines, such as the use of protective footwear, which are set by regulatory agencies such as OSHA or the facility itself.

The **semi-restricted zone** has specific requirements for the use of surgical attire and access to other areas of the department. The primary difference in surgical attire between semi-restricted and restricted zones is the use of a surgical mask.

The **restricted zone** carries the highest standards for asepsis and most stringent guidelines for attire and access. Table 9.2 shows the requirements for attire and access for each zone. Specific HVAC requirements are discussed in the following section.

OPERATING ROOM ENVIRONMENT: HVAC

The specific design and parameters for heating, ventilation, and air conditioning are crucial for infection control in the health care facility in general, and the operating room specifically. The specific parameters for the operating room are shown in Table 9.3.

IMPORTANT TO KNOW *Air conditioning, in the context of HVAC systems, refers to physically conditioning the air. This includes regulation of temperature and humidity, air movement, air exchange, and air filtration.*

The parameters for HVAC are established according to the activities and functions carried out in a specific area or zone. Guidelines may be regulated at the state or local level and are necessary to obtain facility accreditation.

The surgical technologist is not usually involved in the planning or maintenance of environmental conditions. However, it is important to understand how and why HVAC contributes to a clean environment.

TEMPERATURE AND HUMIDITY

Temperature and humidity influence the proliferation of microbial colonies and contribute to the comfort of those in the area. The operating room environment is kept cool deliberately. However, the temperature inside individual operating and procedure

TABLE 9.2 Recommendations for Attire and Access for Each Zone

	Attire	Access	Other
Unrestricted	None Street clothes permitted	Access from outside the building, semi-restricted, or other restricted area	
Semi-Restricted	Surgical attire required: scrub clothes and head/beard covering, clean shoes. Mask is required whenever open sterile supplies are present.	Access from unrestricted, other semi-restricted, or restricted area	Area must be protected against contamination by personal items (e.g., backpacks, briefcases, mobile phones).
Restricted	Surgical attire required: clean scrub clothes, head/beard covering, mask, clean shoes.	Accessible only from a semi-restricted area	Area must be protected against contamination by personal items (e.g., backpacks, briefcases, mobile phones).
	Visitors are required to wear clean surgical attire or single-use jumpsuit that covers street clothes.		Facility may require masks where wrapped sterile goods are stored.

TABLE 9.3 Recommended Environmental Parameters for Specific Areas in the Operating Room Department

Area	Minimum Total Air Changes per Hour	Temperature °F (°C)	Relative Humidity	Pressure Relative to Adjacent Areas
Operating room	20	68°–75° (20°–24°)	20%–60%	Positive
Sterile processing clean workroom	4	68°–73° (20°–23°)	Maximum 60%	Positive
Sterile processing decontamination room	6	60°–73° (16°–23°)	NR	Negative
Clean workroom	4	NR	NR	Positive
Soiled workroom	10	NR	MR	Negative
Sterile storage room	4	Maximum 75° (24°)	Maximum 60%	Positive

NR, No recommendation.
From Wood A. *Guidelines for Perioperative Practice*. Denver: Association of PeriOperative Registered Nurses (AORN); 2019.

rooms may be adjusted to prevent patient hypothermia or to deliberately induce patient hypothermia as required.

Humidity is controlled to prevent the growth and spread of fungi and water-borne bacteria. This is achieved by humidification and dehumidification systems.

AIR CHANGES AND FILTERING

To maintain clean air in a closed space, fresh air from outside or air that is highly filtered must be changed at a constant rate. The changes are expressed as the number of air changes per hour (ACH). Fresh air is needed to remove particles and other contaminants from the air, without causing air turbulence. The fresh air may be obtained from outside, or by conditioning the air using a filtration system. High-efficiency particulate air (HEPA) filters are commonly used to remove particles, including bacteria, mold ranging from 1 to 5 microns in size, and virus particles, which are much smaller.

AIR PRESSURE AND FLOW

Air pressure in a closed space can be increased (positive pressure) or decreased (negative pressure) relative to the pressure adjacent to that space. The air pressure in the operating room is higher than the adjacent spaces. This prevents air from the adjoining space from flowing into the operating room. This is especially important when the doors are opened. Air can also be directed away from the sterile field during surgery by the installation of a unidirectional ultraclean delivery system called **laminar air flow.** This system creates a "curtain" of super clean air around the sterile field. When laminar air flow is used, the sterile field, including instrument tables, must be positioned inside the curtain.

IMPORTANT TO KNOW *Personnel must not walk or stand between the air flow curtain and the sterile field.*

PART III: PERSONAL CLEANLINESS AND HAND HYGIENE

PERSONAL CLEANLINESS

Personnel working in the operating room must be particularly meticulous about personal hygiene to maintain good health, prevent cross-infection to others, and minimize the spread of microbes in the surgical environment. Individuals with acute or chronic skin conditions resulting in inflammation and infection may be a significant source of microbial transmission to patients, equipment, and other staff members. Sebum, produced normally by the skin glands, protects and maintains suppleness. However, sebum is also a medium for bacterial colonization. Daily bathing and shampooing are necessary to reduce sebum and bacteria.

Bacteria shed from the nasopharynx and skin are a particular risk to patients and other staff members. Individuals with a respiratory infection can contaminate the environment, including sterile surfaces. Droplets containing pathogenic microorganisms are forcefully spread by coughing and sneezing. These microbes can spread from the hands of the infected person to surfaces in the environment, where they are transferred to others who contact those surfaces.

ROUTINE HAND WASHING

All perioperative personnel must perform routine **hand washing** according to current guidelines. This is an *event-related* practice—performed before or after a specific task or event. *It the most important tool for preventing infection in the health care setting.* Organic debris, soil, and microorganisms can exist on the hands without any visible evidence. As staff move from one task to another, touching patients and equipment, they can easily transmit pathogens by direct or indirect contact. Antiseptic liquid soap and hand rub gel, dispensed from wall-mounted containers, are used in the health care setting for routine hand hygiene. Dispensers are refilled with individual vacuum-sealed bags to prevent microbial colonization inside the dispenser. Paper towels are available for drying after hand washing.

Hand hygiene should be performed using a systematic method. Refer to Fig. 9.1, which demonstrates the recommended technique.

Fingernails

Perioperative personnel are required to maintain their nails in a manner that enables them to carry out tasks safely, prevent infection, avoid injuring patients, and increase manual dexterity. Nails should be trimmed often and maintained no longer than 2 mm. The cuticle should be trimmed carefully to prevent tearing and infection. The subungual area (under the nails) should be cleaned routinely. A nail cleaner is preferred over a nail brush, which can cause small abrasions that can harbor pathogens.

Long nails, nail extenders, and wraps must not be worn by surgical personnel. Long nails, whether natural or artificial, increase microbial colonization. Long nails can also injure a patient and prevent personnel from performing their duties safely and efficiently.

The current recommendations on nail polish state that a multidisciplinary team in the clinical setting determines whether fingernail polish, including UV-cured gels, can be worn in the perioperative environment. In the absence of an infection control team, the decision is made by the health care facility. There is a potential risk that bacteria may colonize in chipped old nail polish and that chips may be transferred to the sterile field. UV-cured nail polishes can soften and damage the nails, allowing their penetration by pathogenic microorganisms.

Perioperative personnel must remove all hand jewelry before starting work. This includes bracelets, rings, and watches, which increase the bacterial load on the hands and prevent effective hand antisepsis.

HAND HYGIENE

Hand hygiene for surgical personnel is the specific care and cleansing of the hands. The skin carries both resident and transient flora (bacteria) as discussed in Chapter 8. The purpose of rigorous hand hygiene in health care is to reduce the number of bacteria to an absolute minimum and prevent cross-infection. The surgical environment is a critical care area in which hand hygiene is crucial for patient safety.

All health care professionals are required to wash their hands frequently in the course of their duties. Perioperative personnel expand these duties to include surgical preparation of the hands and arms. Frequent use of antiseptic products, especially antiseptic soaps, can cause skin dryness and temporary loss of natural oils that protect the skin and keep it supple. Dry skin is vulnerable to increased sloughing of surface skin cells and the development of skin cracks, where bacteria can colonize. Perioperative personnel must take extra care of their hands to prevent these problems.

Hand Lotions and Creams

Commercially prepared liquid antiseptic soaps and gels contain emollient additives to maintain skin softness and prevent its breakdown. However, accumulation of skin emollients contained in hand-rub products can create a sticky residue on the skin. This is uncomfortable and makes gloving more difficult. Skin residue can be removed by a thorough wash or hand scrub with no decrease in the efficacy of subsequent uses of the product. Additional application of creams or lotions may be necessary to provide increased protection. It is important to select a lotion that is water soluble and does not contain petroleum products, which can interfere with the barrier properties of latex gloves.

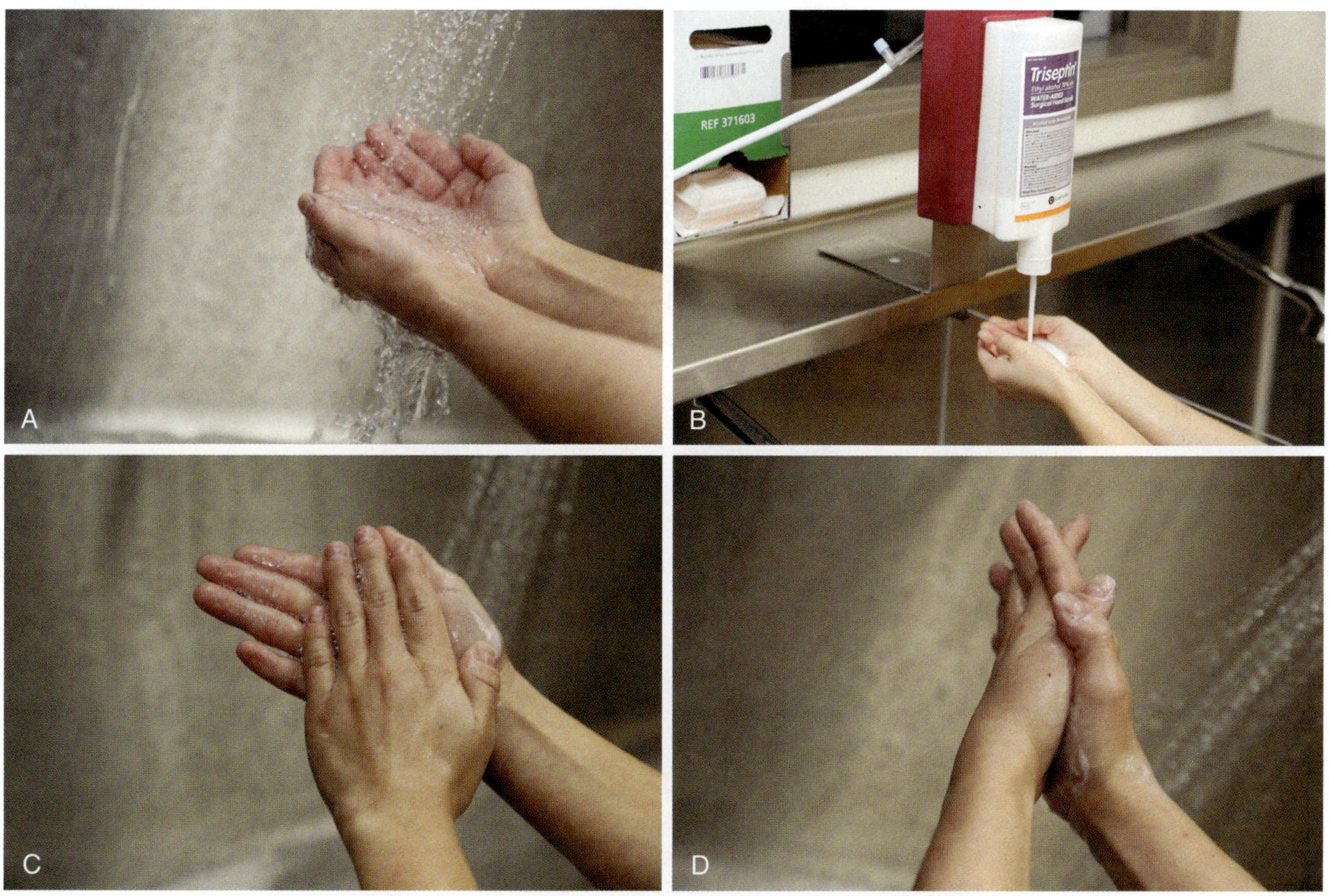

FIG. 9.1 Procedure for routine hand hygiene. (A) Remove *all* jewelry from hands and forearms and wet the hands to 2 inches above the wrists under running water. (B) Apply liquid antiseptic soap according to manufacturer's instructions. Cover all surfaces of the hands up to 2 inches above the wrists. (C) Rub hands together, palm to palm in a circular motion. (D) Spread the fingers and weave the two hands together, rubbing continuously.

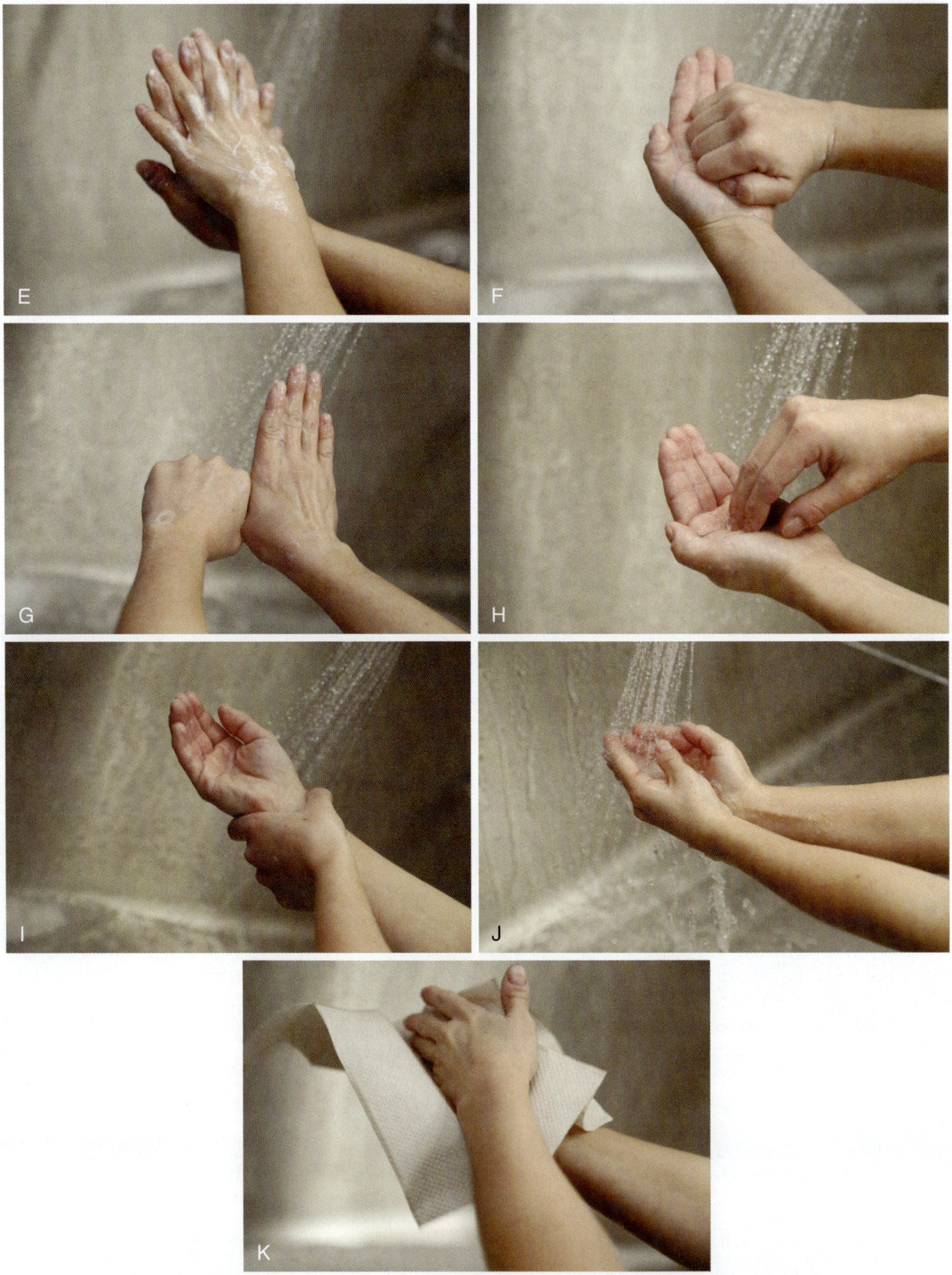

FIG. 9.1, cont'd (E) With the right palm over the back of the left hand, interlace the fingers and rub vigorously. Repeat with the opposite hand. (F) While clasping the fingers of one hand into the cupped fingers of the opposite hand, wash the backs of all the fingers by running them in a horizontal direction back and forth. (G) Clean the web space between the thumb and first finger by clasping the thumb of one hand into the opposite palm. Reverse for the opposite hand. (H) Rub the fingertips of one hand into the opposite palm using a circular motion. Repeat on the opposite hand. (I) In a back-and-forth motion, rub soap to 2 inches above the wrists. (J) Rinse hands under running water, keeping fingers pointed downward, hands lower than elbows, making sure that all traces of soap are removed. (K) Dry the hands using paper towels. A fresh towel should be used to turn the tap off as necessary.

IMPORTANT TO KNOW *Current recommendations are to use a facility-approved hand care product that is compatible with the use of latex gloves. Perfumed lotions must not be used, because they can increase or cause nausea in patients and may increase skin irritation.*

Dermatitis and Other Skin Conditions

Perioperative staff such as surgical technologists who perform hand hygiene and surgical hand antisepsis many times a week are at risk of developing dermatitis. This may take the form of irritation, general skin breakdown, or infection. Dermatitis can be prevented by using alcohol gel instead of soap and by reducing the temperature of the water used for hand hygiene. Water should be maintained between 70°F and 80°F. Any employee who develops a skin condition should seek advice from a qualified dermatologist. Causes can be eliminated and solutions developed, which may involve simply changing the type of gloves worn or changing the methods and materials used in hand hygiene.

IMPORTANT TO KNOW *Preventing dermatitis is much easier than treating it after it develops, and it may have consequences for infection control. People with dermatitis may not use effective hand hygiene methods, which can lead to cross-infection to patients.*

PART IV: SURGICAL ATTIRE

PURPOSE

Perioperative staff are required to wear specific surgical attire and to adhere to the recommendations and guidelines associated with it. The purpose of surgical attire is to maintain the high level of asepsis required in the surgical environment. Surgical attire, when worn properly, can help prevent disease transmission. Specific attire such as protective eyewear, nonpermeable gowns, and footwear are required to prevent the wearer from exposure to potentially infectious blood and body fluids. Specific guidelines on the density and composition of cloth used in manufacturing are available at http://www.cdc.gov/niosh/npptl/pce.html. Recent changes in the guidelines for surgical attire have been made in response to new research in this area.

SCRUB SUIT

The scrub suit includes pants, and shirt or tunic worn over the pants (Fig. 9.2). Cloth scrubs are manufactured from fabrics that shed little or no lint to prevent microbial transmission by airborne particles. The scrub suit prevents the shedding of skin particles and hair into the environment and helps protect the wearer from contact with soil and body fluids. Perspiration and normal exudate from sebaceous glands in the skin contain large colonies of bacteria, which are shed with friction and movement. The scrub suit helps prevent the release of these substances but is not a barrier against contamination by blood and other contaminants, which may soak through the material and contaminate the wearer.

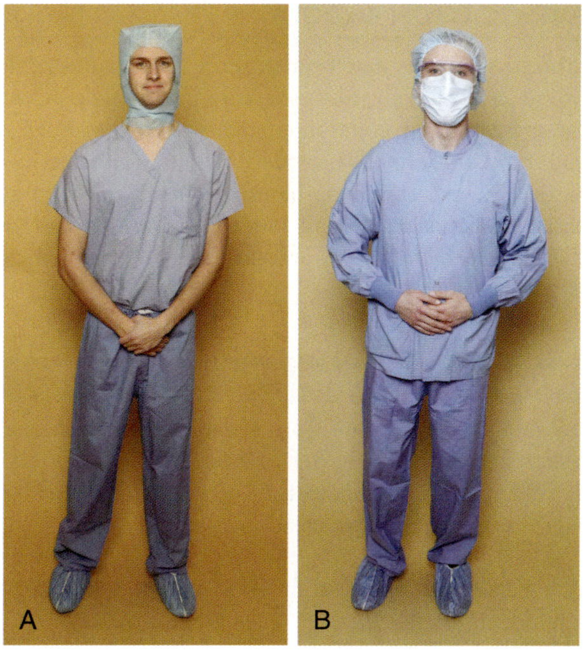

FIG. 9.2 Surgical attire. (A) Basic scrub suit: top and pants. The head cover is designed to enclose the entire hairline, including the nape of the neck. (B) Nonsterile attire for use in restricted areas including **nonsterile team members** during surgery, wherever sterile instruments and supplies are exposed, and whenever working in areas where surgical instruments are being wrapped and prepared for sterilization.

PERSONAL CLOTHING WORN UNDER THE SCRUB SUIT

Personal clothing such as T-shirts and thermal tights are sometimes worn by surgical personnel for warmth. Antiembolism stockings and tights may also be worn to support healthy venous circulation and prevent varicose veins—a hazard for all health facility staff, especially surgical personnel.

There are no current (2020) guidelines *restricting* the use of personal clothing under the scrub suit. Personnel should, however, select materials that are close fitting and low-linting. The clothing must be freshly laundered.

NOTE *The length of the sleeves and neckline style may be determined by facility policy.*

PERSONAL HANDHELD ELECTRONIC EQUIPMENT

Personal electronic devices such as mobile phones and tablets can carry a large burden of microbes. Any outside equipment should be cleansed according to the manufacturers' instructions before bringing it into the OR.

IDENTIFICATION BADGES

Identification badges may be attached to the scrub suit using a lanyard or clip. Lanyards, especially those made of woven fabric or nylon, may come in contact with the wearer's skin. Perspiration and skin oils provide a medium for bacterial colonization. These items must be cleaned regularly to prevent bacterial transmission. Many surgical facilities now require staff to wear a name tag to prevent the problems associated with lanyards.

HEAD COVERING

Disposable head covers are worn to reduce contamination by loose hair, dandruff, and bacteria. The scalp and hair are a rich source of *Staphylococcus aureus* and other bacteria, which proliferate under surgical caps. Head coverings confine the hair to prevent it from being shed in the perioperative environment. Head covers are available in different styles, including bouffant, hood, and skull cap.

Cloth head covers have become popular in recent years. However, they can present a problem when not laundered according to guidelines. All surgical attire, including cloth head covers, must be laundered according to guidelines by the health care facility or accredited laundry service (see the following section).

Current guidelines (2020) do not recommend one style of head covering over another except to emphasize that the cap must contain all hair and cover the scalp line, nape of the neck, and sideburns. Beards require a beard mask. Female Muslim team members may require head coverings that also cover their necks to be aligned with the beliefs of their faith and culture. Employers are required by the U.S. Equal Employment Opportunity Commission to comply with these needs as long as they do not compromise other standards for hygiene or safety. A disposable head and neck cover is illustrated in Fig. 9.3.

Guidelines • Head Covering

(Association of periOperative Registered Nurses. Guidelines for perioperative practice. 2020. Surgical attire. *Head covering.* Standard No. 5.)

1. Wear clean surgical attire and a surgical head covering when entering an operating room or invasive procedure room for any reason (e.g., stocking supplies, delivering equipment, transporting specimens). [Recommendation]
2. Cover the scalp and hair when entering the semi-restricted and restricted areas. [Recommendation]
3. Cover a beard when entering the restricted areas and while preparing and packaging items in the clean assembly section of the sterile processing area. [Recommendation]
4. No recommendation can be made for the type of head covers worn in the semi-restricted and restricted areas. [No Recommendation]
5. No recommendation can be made for covering the ears in the semi-restricted and restricted areas. [No Recommendation]
6. Remove head coverings at the end of the shift or when they are contaminated. [Recommendation]

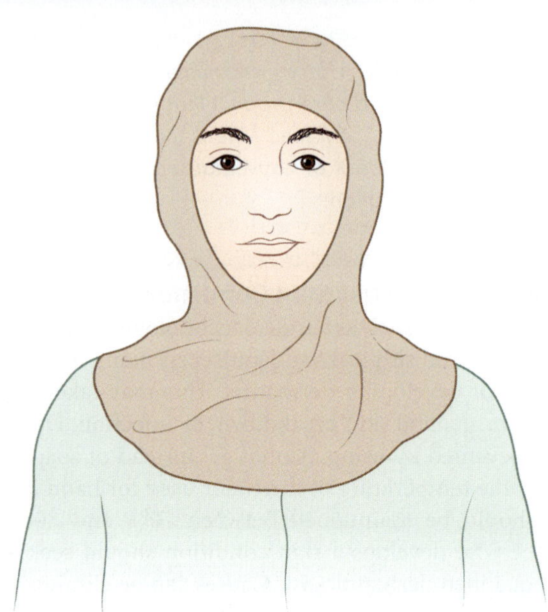

FIG. 9.3 Extended head covering for personnel who require the head and neck to be covered. See text for explanation.

SHOES, SHOE COVERS, AND BOOTS

Shoes worn in the operating room provide several levels of protection to the wearer. When made of solid nonfabric material, closed in front and back, they protect against direct contact with blood and body fluids. They can also prevent injury from objects, including sharp instruments that fall from the surgical field. Shoes are integral to foot, leg, and back health. A well-fitting, quality shoe is well worth the investment in preventing back problems and cushioning the feet during many hours of standing and walking. This may not be apparent in the first few years of employment but can become a significant source of pain and discomfort later in a career. It is also important to consider grip. During an emergency, staff must be able to move quickly. Backless shoes may become a particular hazard.

Fluid-resistant **shoe covers** are used whenever gross contamination by blood or other body fluids is anticipated. Protective shoe and leg covers or boots are worn for specific procedures in which a large amount of blood or body fluid spillage is anticipated, such as obstetrical, cystoscopy procedures, and major orthopedic cases.

Guidelines • Shoes

(Association of periOperative Registered Nurses. Guidelines for perioperative practice. 2020. Surgical attire. *Shoes.* Standard No. 6.)

1. Clean shoes should be worn entering the semi-restricted or restricted areas. [Recommendation]
2. Protective footwear that meets the health care organization's safety requirements should be worn. [Recommendation]
3. Fluid-resistant shoe covers or boots must be worn in instances when gross contamination can reasonably be anticipated. [Regulatory Requirement]
4. Shoe covers worn as PPE must be removed immediately after use. After removal, discard the shoe covers and perform hand hygiene. [Regulatory Requirement]

PROTECTIVE EYEWEAR AND FACE SHIELDS

Protective eyewear or face shields are required by OSHA as part of the bloodborne pathogens standard to protect workers exposed to splashing and splatter of blood and body fluids. They also provide physical protection during procedures in which bone is drilled or cut with power instruments. To be effective, protective eyewear must have side shields (Fig. 9.4). Ordinary eyeglasses do not provide sufficient protection.

Guidelines • Protective Eyewear and Face Shields

(Association of periOperative Registered Nurses. Guidelines for perioperative practice. 2020. Transmission-based precautions. *Personal protective equipment.* Standard No. 2.)

Perioperative personnel must wear eye protection when splashes, spray, spatter, or droplets of blood or other potentially infectious materials may be generated and eye contamination can be reasonably anticipated. [Regulatory Requirement]

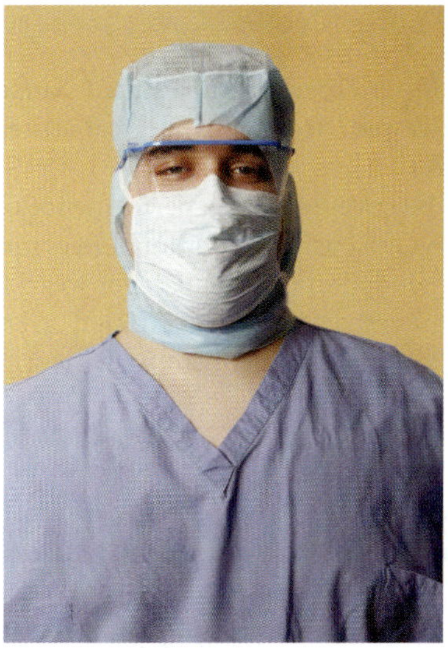

FIG. 9.4 Protective eyewear. Surgical team members are required to wear eye protection or full face shields during any procedure in which there is a danger of exposure to splashing by blood and body fluids. Eyewear must cover the entire eye, brows, and temples.

SURGICAL MASK

A surgical mask is worn to *protect the intraoperative environment* from possible contamination by aerosol droplets generated by the mouth, oropharynx, nose, and nasopharynx. A mask is also worn to *protect the wearer* from contamination by potentially infectious material by splashes, spray, spatter, or blood.

Masks are worn in the restricted areas of the operating room, including locations where sterile instruments and supplies are open and in the scrub sink area, where staff are in the process of or have completed surgical hand antisepsis. In some facilities, masks may also be required in semi-restricted areas.

The most important factor that contributes to the efficiency of a mask is its fit. Face masks are meant to filter the exhaled breath of the wearer. Masks that are secured by elastic ear loops may not provide protection. When securing a face mask, do not cross the ties. This causes the mask to tent at the sides, allowing exhaled breath to escape. The top ties should maintain the top portion of the mask. The bottom ties should be comfortable but not loose because this allows exhaled breath to escape at the bottom of the mask.

Masks must never be worn around the neck because pathogens on the mask can be transferred to the scrub top. A clean mask should be used for every surgical or invasive procedure and whenever it becomes moist. When removing the mask, untie it and discard it in the appropriate receptacle, handling only the ties. Always perform hand hygiene after handling a used mask.

Guidelines • Surgical Mask

(Association of Perioperative Registered Nurses. Guidelines for perioperative practice. 2020. Transmission-based precautions. *Personal protective equipment.* Standard No. 2.)

1. Perioperative personnel must wear masks when splashes, spray, spatter, or droplets of blood or other potentially infectious materials may be generated and nose or mouth contamination can be reasonably anticipated. [Regulatory Requirement]
2. Perioperative personnel should wear clean surgical attire and a surgical head covering when entering an operating room or invasive procedure room for any reason (e.g., stocking supplies, delivering equipment, transporting specimens). [Recommendation]
3. When open sterile supplies are present, perioperative personnel should wear a clean surgical mask that covers the mouth and nose and is secured in a manner that prevents venting at the sides of the mask. [Recommendation]
4. The Centers for Disease Control and Infection (2017) recommends that a surgical mask that fully covers the mouth and nose be worn when a surgical procedure is beginning or in progress or when sterile surgical instruments are open. [Recommendation]

NONSTERILE COVER JACKET

Long-sleeved cover jackets (also called warm-up jackets) made of the same material as other scrub attire are worn by nonsterile perioperative personnel to contain skin **squames** and prevent them from contaminating the surrounding environment. Jackets may be worn by the circulator during a surgical procedure. A nonsterile cover jacket is considered surgical apparel. Like all other cloth surgical apparel, guidelines for laundering the cover jacket are the same as those for the scrub suit. This means that cover jackets must not be stored in lockers, which are a potential source of bacterial proliferation. Nonsterile jackets should be worn in a way that prevents contamination of the sterile field—closed at the front.

Guidelines • Long-Sleeved Cover Jackets

(Association of periOperative Registered Nurses. Guidelines for perioperative practice. 2020. Surgical attire. *Long sleeves.* Standard No. 3.)

1. Arms may be covered during performance of preoperative patient skin antisepsis. [Conditional Recommendation]
2. No recommendation can be made for wearing long sleeves in the semi-restricted and restricted areas other than during performance of preoperative patient skin antisepsis. [No Recommendation]

LAB COATS AND COVER GOWNS

Lab coats and reusable cover gowns are often seen in conjunction with scrub attire both outside and within the surgical department. Some facilities require a lab coat or disposable cover gown to be worn over scrub attire when surgical staff leave the operating room. This may be for identification or other reasons. There is no evidence that a cover gown or lab coat protects the scrub attire from contamination. However, research has also demonstrated that personnel tend to wear cover apparel laden with bacteria for days and even weeks before laundering. Reusable cover attire may be worn within the health facility provided it is clean.

Guidelines • Lab Coats and Cover Gowns

(Association of periOperative Registered Nurses. Guidelines for perioperative practice. 2020. Surgical attire. *Cover apparel.* Standard No. 4.)

If worn, cover apparel (e.g., lab coats) should be clean. [Recommendation]

LAUNDERING SURGICAL ATTIRE

Laundering of scrub attire according to state and federal regulations for infection control is required in accredited health care facilities. The purpose of knowing about these guidelines is to understand why surgical attire must be laundered by the facility or other service provider that is certified to handle medical laundry. The regulations include standards for water temperature and the use of detergents capable of removing body fluids. Scrub attire is laundered daily by a health care–accredited laundry facility or at the health care organization according to state regulatory requirements or according to the Centers for Disease Control and Prevention (CDC) recommendations. Scrub attire must not be stored in lockers, which are a potential source of infectious microbes.

Guidelines • Laundering Scrub Attire

(Association of periOperative Registered Nurses. Guidelines for perioperative practice. 2020. Surgical attire. *Laundering.* Standard No. 1.)

1. Clean surgical attire should be worn when entering the semi-restricted and restricted areas. [Recommendation]
2. After each daily use, scrub attire should be laundered at
   a. A health care–accredited laundry facility,
   b. The health care organization according to state regulatory requirements, or
   c. The health care organization according to Centers for Disease Control and Prevention recommendations for laundering in the absence of state requirements [Recommendation]
3. Laundered surgical attire should be stored in enclosed carts, cabinets, or dispensing machines that are cleaned and disinfected regularly. [Recommendation]
4. Scrub attire that has been penetrated by blood, body fluids, or other potentially infectious materials must be removed immediately or as soon as possible, and replaced with clean attire. [Regulatory Requirement]
5. Surgical attire should be removed before leaving the health care facility. [Recommendation]
6. No recommendation can be made regarding personal clothing worn under scrub attire. [No Recommendation]

PART V: SURGICAL HAND ANTISEPSIS

INTRODUCTION TO SURGICAL HAND ANTISEPSIS

Surgical hand antisepsis is performed immediately before donning sterile gown and gloves for a surgical or other invasive procedure. Before performing the surgical hand antisepsis, the ST should open his or her gown and gloves in the assigned operating room. Gown and gloves must be opened onto a surface that is separate from other sterile supplies to prevent their contamination during gowning and gloving.

The surgical technologist should perform surgical hand antisepsis ahead of the surgeons in order to have time to perform the sterile setup.

There are two methods for performing surgical hand antisepsis:

1. The surgical *hand rub*
2. The surgical *hand scrub*

All supplies needed for the surgical hand antisepsis are available near the scrub sink area. These include masks, face shields, and protective eyewear, nail cleaners, and sterile scrub sponges. Defogger should also be available for eyewear. Antiseptic soap and alcohol-based hand rub are available in wall dispensers. Water taps are foot, knee, or motion activated. Before performing surgical hand antisepsis, the surgical technologist should don safety eye protection or face shield and mask. A face shield is worn as necessary for the planned surgical procedure. The scrub top should be tucked in to prevent it from becoming wet and prevent it from contaminating the hands and arms once the surgical hand antisepsis has been performed.

SURGICAL HAND SCRUB

The traditional surgical hand scrub, which has been used for many years, has been modified by infection control agencies and professional associations. New guidelines have been established after thorough research and peer review. Important revisions in the technique include the following:

- The scrub *brush* has been replaced with a *sponge* to prevent microabrasions in the skin, which can induce bacterial colonization.
- Instead of prescribing the same amount of scrub time for all antiseptic agents (5 to 10 minutes), the scrub time is determined by the manufacturer of the scrub antiseptic (usually 2 to 5 minutes). This ensures that most effective antisepsis with the least amount of chemical exposure.
- The counted stroke method, which prescribed the number of strokes for each surface of the hands and arms, has been replaced by the timed method.

Antiseptic preparations which reduce the number of microbes and provide *continuous antimicrobial action are preferred.* This is important, because bacteria can proliferate quickly in the moist environment between the gloves and skin. The surgical hand scrub is illustrated in Fig. 9.5.

Two sets of guidelines are presented here. They do not contradict each other but simply provide two acceptable methods.

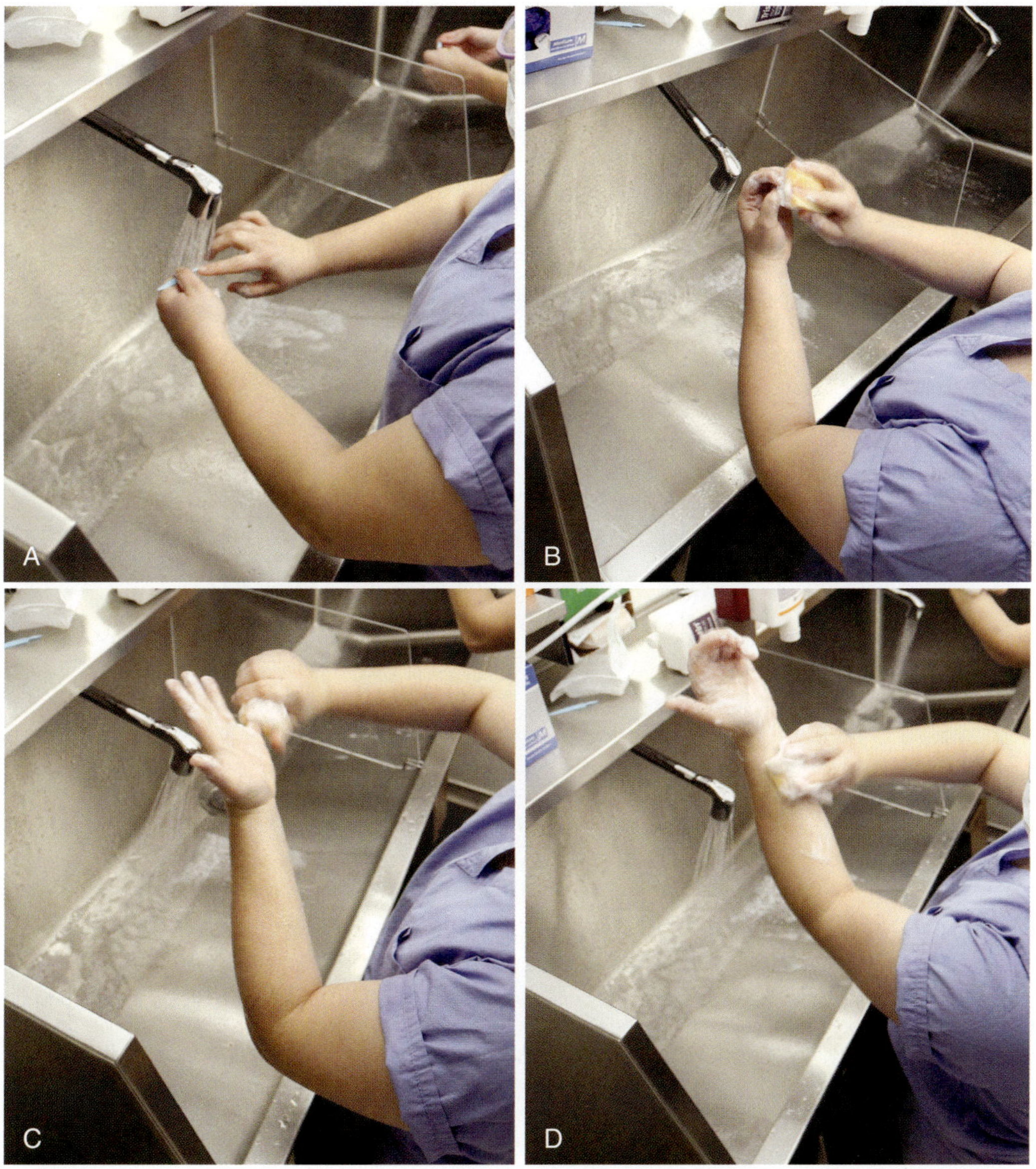

FIG. 9.5 Procedure for surgical hand scrub. (A) Turn on water. Using a nail cleaner, carefully clean the subungual areas of both hands while holding the hands under the running water. Discard the nail cleaner in the proper receptacle. (B) Surgical hand scrub. Unwrap the scrub sponge and dispense soap unless the sponge is impregnated with antiseptic soap. Begin timing the scrub. Begin with the nails. Pass the nails back and forth across the sponge. (C) Surgical hand scrub. Each finger has four sides. Scrub each side of each finger individually, between the fingers in the web spaces. (D) Surgical hand scrub. The dorsal and palm side of the hand are scrubbed.

Continued

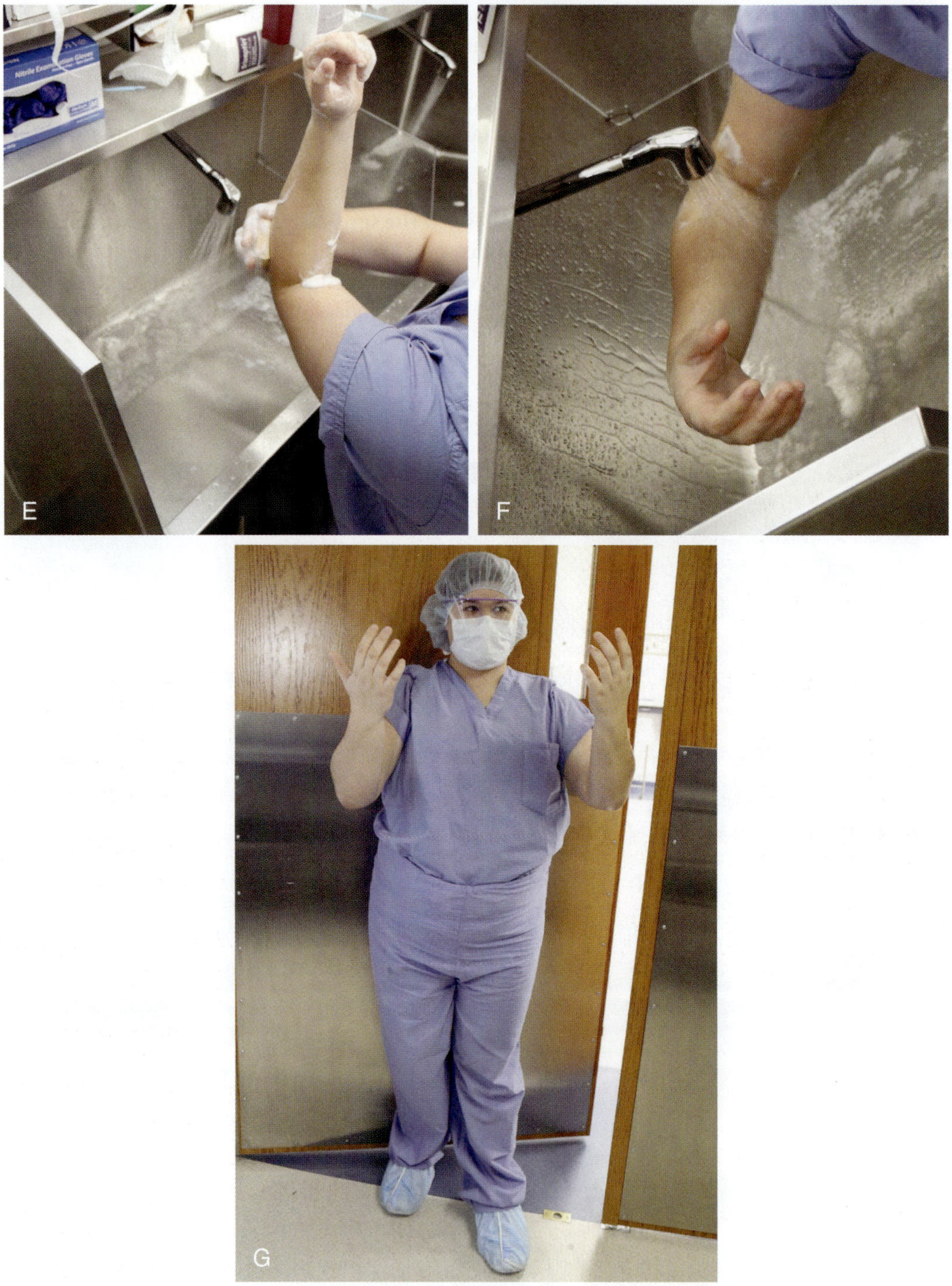

FIG. 9.5, cont'd (E) Surgical hand scrub. The forearm has four planes. Scrub each plane separately in a circular motion to 2 inches above the elbow. (F) Surgical hand scrub. Keep the hands higher than the elbows at all times, with upper arms well away from the body. Rinse by passing the fingers, then hands, then arms under the water, keeping them above the elbow. (G) Surgical hand scrub. Proceed to the operating room, continuing to hold arms above the elbows away from the scrub suit. Push the door open with your back. Proceed with drying, gowning, and gloving.

Guidelines • Performing Surgical Hand Scrub

(Association of PeriOperative Registered Nurses. Guidelines for perioperative practice. 2020. Hand hygiene. *Surgical hand antisepsis.* Guideline No. 4.3.1.)

1. Perform a standardized surgical hand antisepsis protocol using a surgical hand scrub in the following order:
   a. Remove jewelry from hands and wrists (e.g., rings, watches, bracelets).
   b. Don a surgical mask.
   c. If hands are visibly soiled, wash hands with soap and water.
   d. Remove debris from underneath fingernails using a disposable nail cleaner under running water.
   e. Apply the amount of surgical hand scrub product recommended by the manufacturer to the hands and forearms using a soft, nonabrasive sponge.
2. Visualize each finger, hand, and arm as having four sides. Wash all four sides effectively, keeping the hands elevated.
3. Scrub for length of time recommended by the manufacturer. The scrub should be timed to allow adequate product contact with skin.
4. For water conservation, turn off water when it is not in use, if possible.
5. Avoid splashing surgical attire.
6. Discard sponges, if used.
7. Rinse hands and arms under running water in one direction from fingertips to elbows.
8. Hold hands higher than elbows and away from surgical attire.
9. In the OR procedure room, dry hands and arms with a sterile towel using sterile technique before donning a surgical gown and gloves. [1 through 9 Recommendation]

Guidelines • Performing the Surgical Hand Scrub (CDC)

(Centers for Disease Control and Prevention, National Center for Emerging and Zoonotic Infectious Diseases [NCEZID], Division of Healthcare Quality Promotion [DHQP]. Jan 31 2020. Available at https://www.cdc.gov/handhygiene/providers/index.html.)

1. Remove rings, watches, and bracelets before beginning the surgical hand scrub.
2. Remove debris from underneath fingernails using a nail cleaner under running water.
3. Performing surgical hand antisepsis using either an antimicrobial soap or an alcohol-based hand sanitizer with persistent activity is recommended before donning sterile gloves when performing surgical procedures.
4. When performing surgical hand antisepsis using an antimicrobial soap, scrub hands and forearms for the length of time recommended by the manufacturer, usually 2–6 minutes.
5. Long scrub times (e.g., 10 minutes) are not necessary.

SURGICAL HAND RUB

The surgical hand rub can be used to prepare the hands and arms before gowning and gloving. Because the application of hand rub products does not remove debris, the hands—including the subungual area—and arms must be thoroughly washed and dried before the product is applied.

Many studies have demonstrated that, when performed properly, the antiseptic hand and arm rub is as effective as the surgical scrub unless the hands or arms are grossly soiled.

To be completely effective, all surfaces of the hands and arms must be wet with the antiseptic product. The effectiveness of the product depends on the amount of time it has contact with the skin as stated by the manufacturer's guidelines. A period of 2 to 3 minutes is standard. Alcohol rub products are not dried off with a towel but are allowed to air dry. Surgical hand antisepsis using an antiseptic rub is illustrated in Fig. 9.6.

Guidelines • Performing the Surgical Hand Rub

(Association of PeriOperative Registered Nurses. Guidelines for perioperative practice. 2020. Hand hygiene. *Surgical hand antisepsis.* Guideline No. 4.3.1.)

1. Perform surgical hand antisepsis using a surgical hand rub according to the manufacturer's instructions for use. [Recommendation]
   a. Perform a standardized surgical hand antisepsis protocol using a surgical hand rub in the following order:
   b. Remove jewelry from hands and wrists (e.g., rings, watches, bracelets).
   c. Don a surgical mask.
   d. If hands are visibly soiled, wash hands with soap and water.
   e. 4. Remove debris from underneath fingernails using a disposable nail cleaner under running water.
   f. 5. Dry hands and arms thoroughly with a disposable paper towel.
   g. Apply the surgical hand rub product to the hands and arms according to the manufacturer's instructions for use (e.g., amount, method, time).
   h. Allow hands and arms to dry completely before using sterile technique to don a surgical gown and gloves.

PART VI: DRYING THE HANDS, GOWNING, AND GLOVING

The sterile gown and gloves provide a barrier between the wearer's skin and scrub suit and the sterile field. There are many different types of sterile gowns and gloves available on the market. Surgical facilities select those that fit the needs of their patients and types of surgical procedures performed.

DRYING THE HANDS

After the *surgical antiseptic scrub,* personnel should proceed to the designated operating room with the elbows and keep hands up as shown in Figure 9.5. This prevents water dripping from the arms to the hands (after a wet scrub). This position also ensures that the hands and arms do not brush against the scrub suit, which would contaminate them. The towel is grasped without hesitation, ensuring that it does not unfold until clear of the table.

The method used to dry the hands and arms is the most efficient. The most common error in surgical technique during the process is contamination of the towel as it brushes the scrub suit. This is avoided by holding the towel away from the body and bending slightly at the waist. The technique for drying is illustrated in Fig. 9.7. When the process is completed, the towel should be handed off to the circulator or dropped into the kick bucket.

UNASSISTED GOWNING

Surgical gowns are worn by all sterile personnel. The gown is donned immediately before the start of surgery and may be changed during surgery if it is contaminated or penetrated by blood or other fluids. Most single-use gowns, particularly those used in procedures in which a high level of liquids are anticipated, have a moisture-proof barrier that is laminated to the gown from the axillary line to the hips. The gown is a wraparound type, which covers the front and back of the wearer. However, the back is still considered nonsterile because it cannot be viewed by the wearer.

The surgical technologist or scrub nurse dons a sterile gown immediately after drying the hands.

When gowning, consider the gown as having two surfaces: an inside surface that will contact the nonsterile scrub suit and bare skin of the hands and arms and an outside surface that will be considered sterile only from the waist to the axillary line and from the hands to the elbows.

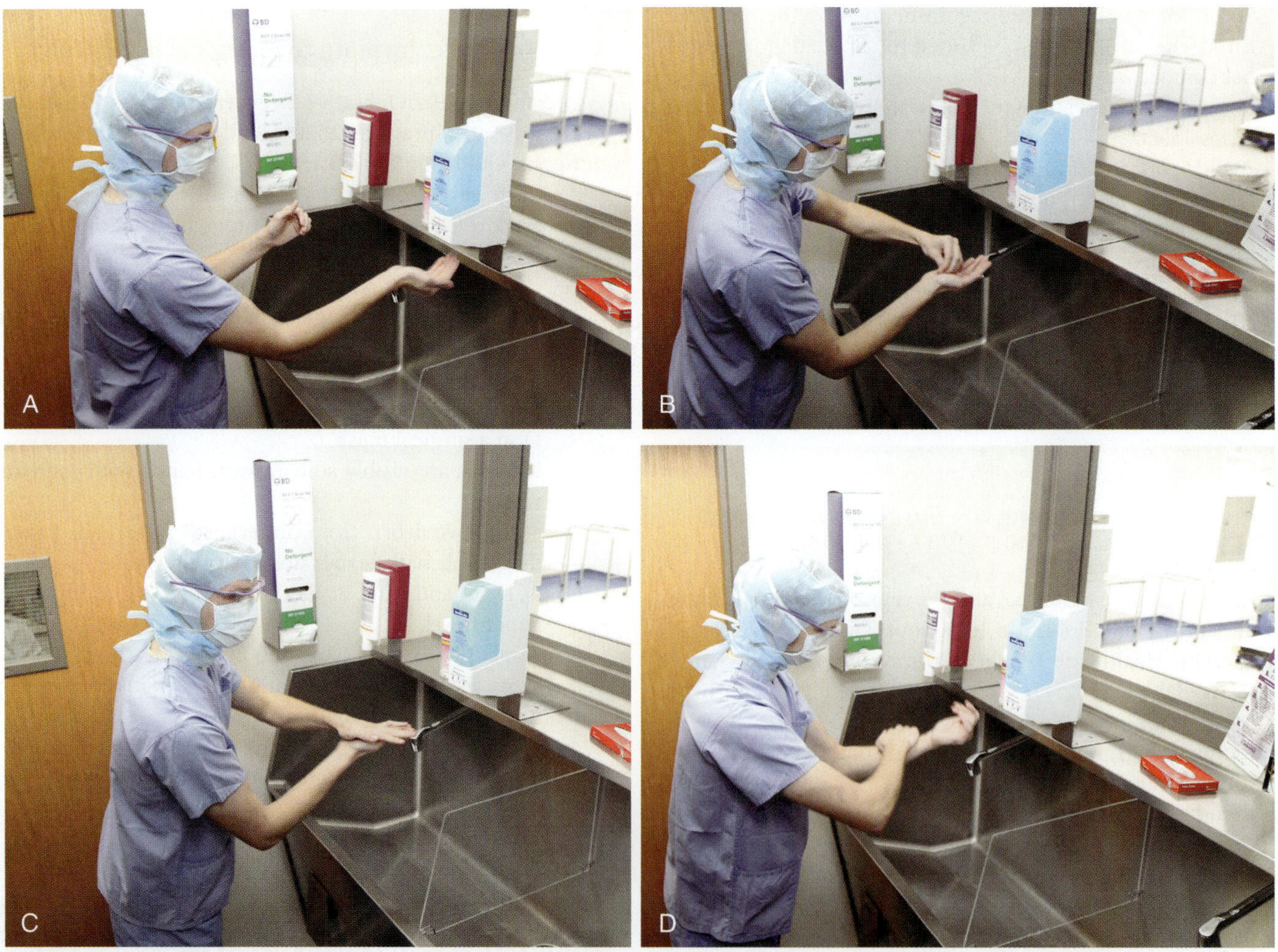

FIG. 9.6 Surgical hand antisepsis using a hand rub. (A) If hands are visibly soiled, clean nails and perform hand hygiene. Dry hands thoroughly before starting surgical hand antisepsis. Following the manufacturer's guidelines, dispense the correct amount of antiseptic into the palm of one hand. (B) Using the other hand, dip fingers into the antiseptic. Use circular motion to expose the fingernails and tips to antiseptic. (C, D) Spread antiseptic to the entire hand, including the individual fingers, wrist, forearm, and elbow, covering all surfaces. (E) Repeat steps on the other hand and arm.

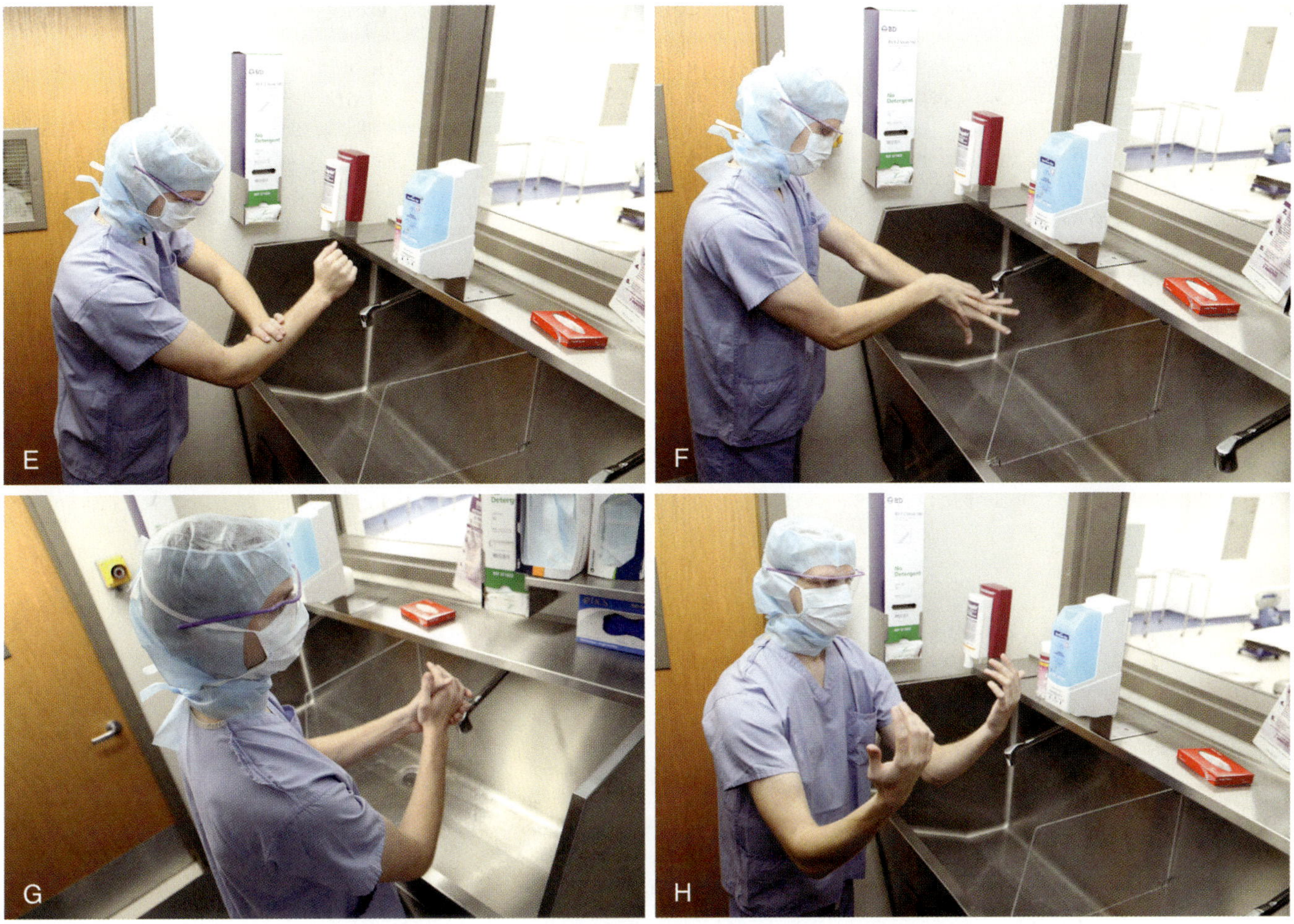

FIG. 9.6, cont'd (F) Dispense 2 to 5 mL of antiseptic into the palm of one hand to thoroughly cleanse the hands again. Cover all surfaces. The backs of the fingers are covered by interlocking cupped hands together and applying antiseptic with a back-and-forth movement. (G) Apply antiseptic to the web of the thumb and palm by interlocking them. (H) Proceed to the OR with forearms flexed above the elbows. Allow hands and arms to air dry before gowning and gloving.

Surgical gowns are folded inside-out before packaging. This allows scrubbed personnel to grasp the presenting surface of the gown with bare hands to put it on, because that surface will be the nonsterile side. Care must be taken not to grasp the gown at the neckline, because the sterile (outer) section of the gown may become contaminated.

Before gowning it is important to step away from any nonsterile surfaces. The circulator should stand by to assist in the final steps of gowning by securing the ties at the neck and inner flap in back. The most common error made in unassisted gowning is advancing the arms and hands too far into the cuff. Do not advance the hands beyond the seam between the sleeve and cuff.

The final step in gowning is securing the gown back flap that wraps around to the front. This is sometimes referred to as "turning the gown." This is done after gloving (see the following section on closed gloving).

The technique for unassisted gowning is illustrated in Fig. 9.8.

CLOSED (UNASSISTED) GLOVING

Many types of surgical gloves are commercially available. The common considerations in choosing gloves are the glove material, strength, thickness, economy, and comfort. Tactile sensation is important, especially in surgical specialties that require the use of fine instruments and in which delicate tissues are encountered. Thicker gloves are more appropriate for repeated contact with heavy instruments or if copious bleeding is likely.

Double gloving (wearing two pairs of surgical gloves) has been demonstrated to reduce the risk of glove failure, which increases with surgical time and prolonged handling of tissues and supplies. Glove punctures are associated with the transmission of blood-borne pathogens to health care workers and microbial contamination of the surgical site. The CDC recommends double gloving for all invasive procedures. No set rule governs glove sizes when double gloving. The outer glove can be one size larger or smaller or the same size. Using colored gloves

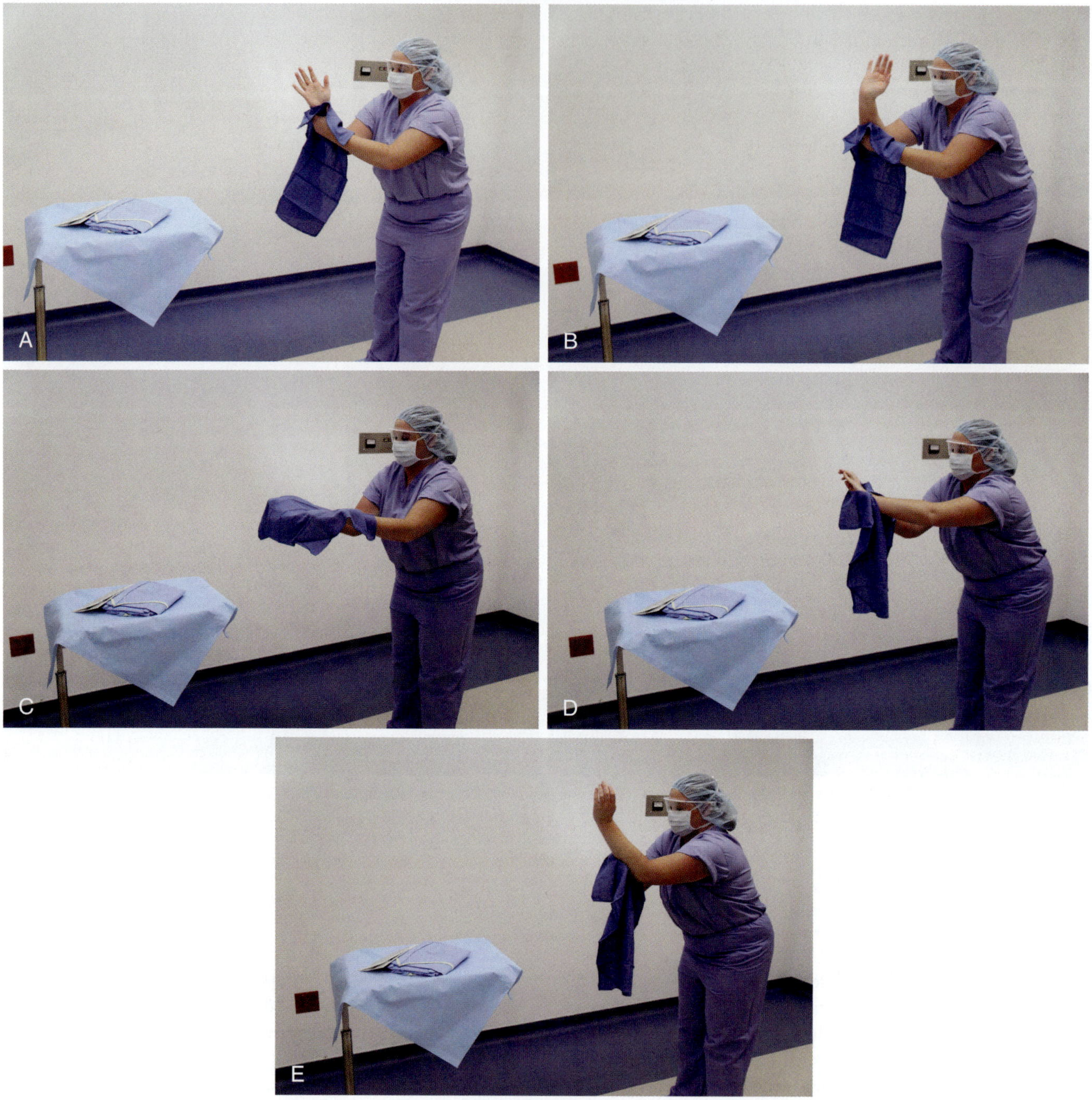

FIG. 9.7 Procedure for drying the hands and arms after the surgical scrub. (A) Grasp the towel and remove it from the table by lifting it up and away. (B) Allow the towel to unfold so that the long edge hangs between your hands. Bend forward slightly to prevent the towel from touching the scrub suit. Use one end of the towel for one hand and arm and the other end for the opposite hand and arm. (C). Blot the skin working from hand to wrist to arm without moving back over a previously dried area. (D) Keep the towel in front of you where you can see it. After drying one hand and arm, place the opposite hand under the towel at the other end as shown. (E) Allow the used end of the towel to drop down. Repeat the first three steps on the other hand.

as the first pair makes it easier to detect a puncture in the top glove. However, if there is any doubt, gloves must be changed.

Current guidelines recommend the use of gloves that feature a perforation indicator system. This consists of gloves that, when punctured, release a small amount of sterile dye, which is visible to the wearer. The system increases the detection of glove perforation significantly.

HISTORICAL HIGHLIGHT

Before the development of the surgical glove, surgeons operated bare handed and disinfected the hands by dipping them into 5% hypochlorite solution (household bleach). Early surgical gloves were made of thick rubber and were washed and disinfected after each case by the instrument nurses.

Closed gloving is performed immediately after gowning. It is the most effective method for preventing contact between the skin and the outside of the sterile glove. When you are learning the closed gloving technique, think of the glove as having two surfaces or planes: the inside and the outside. Before the gloves are touched, the entire glove is sterile, inside and outside. As soon as gloving is initiated, however, the *inside* surface is considered nonsterile.

One of the best ways to acquire the technique for closed gloving is to have an experienced person glove while you are also gloving in a practice session or dry run. Follow each step as the other person gloves. The experienced person must move slowly so that the student can follow these actions. The actions will have to be repeated to firmly establish the correct technique.

Always stand next to (not across) from the demonstrator to avoid confusion about which way the hand and glove are oriented. Take your time when learning to glove. It is better to be methodical and slow at first. Speed and efficiency will follow with practice. Students are often nervous when learning to glove. In practice sessions without a patient, the hands

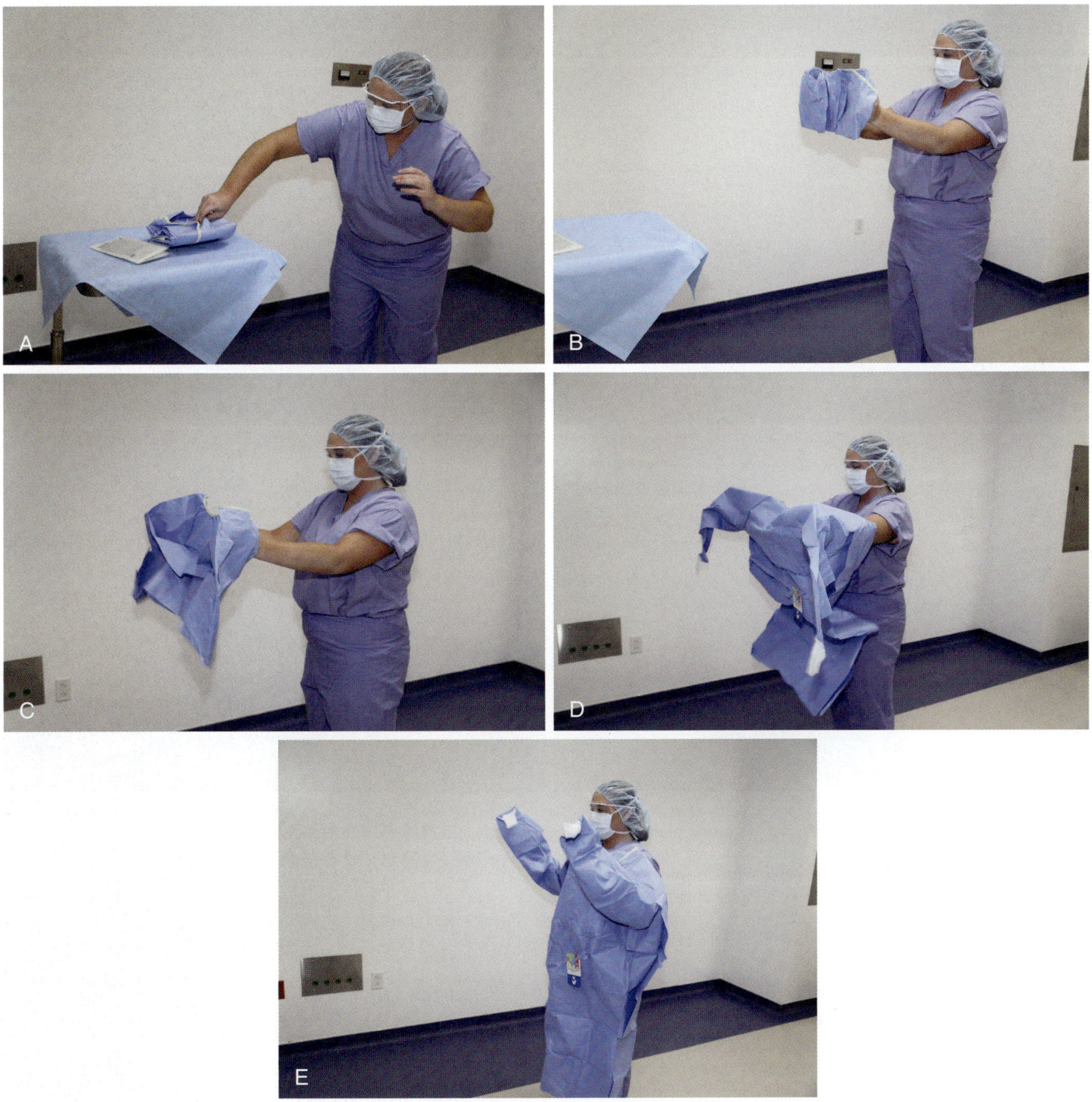

FIG. 9.8 Procedure for gowning oneself. (A) Grasp the gown just below the neckline and lift it up and away from table. (B) Step back from the table. Place each hand at the sleeve entry. (C) When hands are securely in place, allow the gown to unfold. Advance the hands slightly into the sleeves. (D) As the gown drops, slowly advance arms into the sleeves. (E) Do not allow the hands to pass the sleeve-cuff seam. Proceed with gloving.

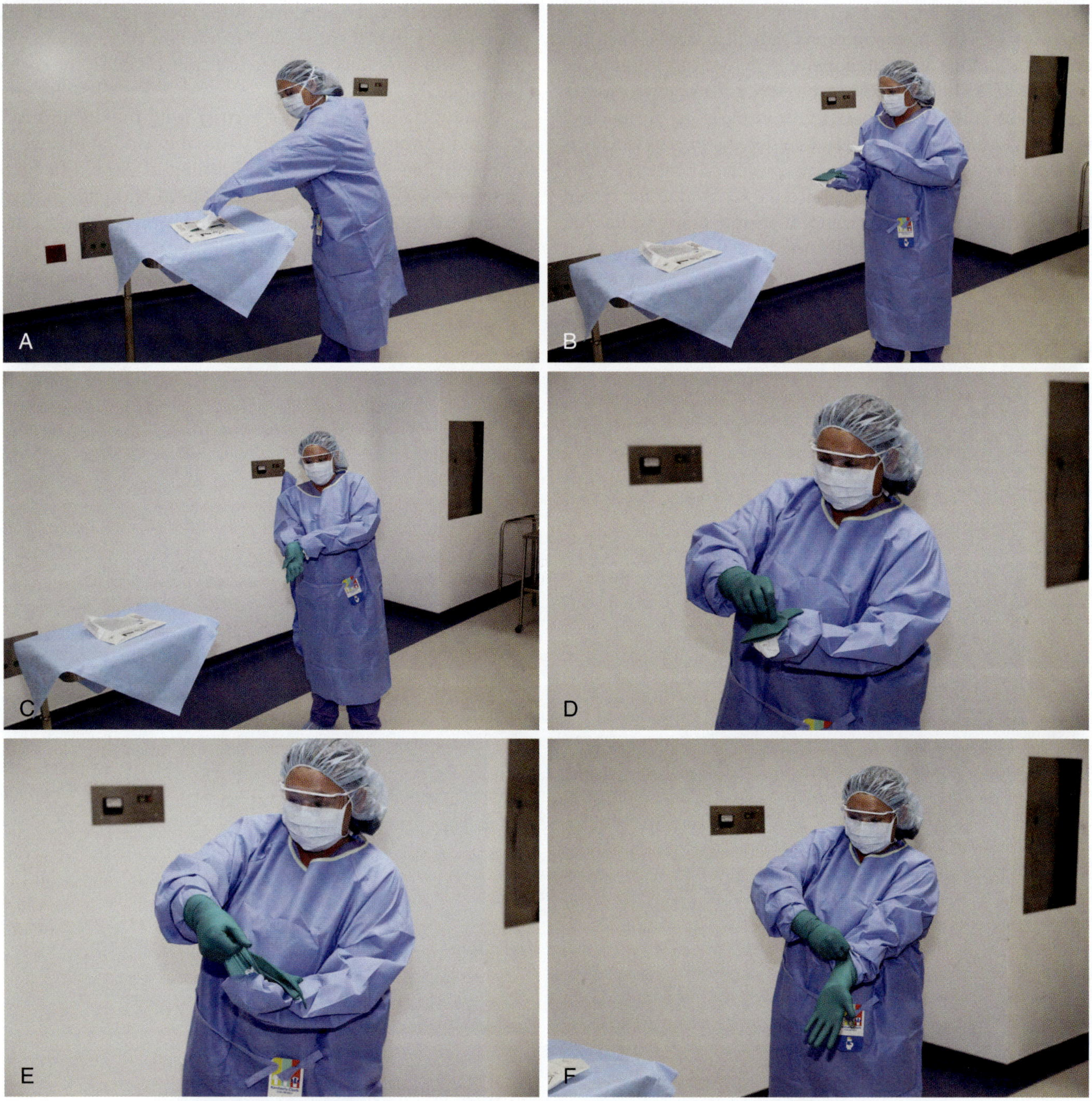

FIG. 9.9 Closed gloving technique. (A) With hands protected by the gown sleeve, open the glove wrapper. (B) Remove the first glove and place it with the glove's cuff fold in line with the open end of the gown cuff. The glove must be positioned with its palm down. The hand being gloved is facing palm up. (C) In this step the glove's cuff is pulled down and over the open gown cuff. This is done by grasping only the top layer of the glove. (D) Repeat steps A through C on the other hand. (E) Closing the gown flap. Pass the pull tab to the circulator using sterile technique. As the circulator holds the tab, turn so that the flap closes the back of the gown. Grasp the sterile tie. The circulator pulls the tab free. (F) Tie the gown as shown.

can be dusted with cornstarch, which dries the skin and helps gloves slide onto the hand more easily.

The technique for closed gloving is illustrated in Fig. 9.9.

Guidelines • Unassisted Gowning and Gloving

(Association of PeriOperative Registered Nurses. Guidelines for perioperative practice. 2020. Sterile technique. *Donning gown and gloves*. Standard No. 2.)

1. Select the surgical gown by task and anticipated degree of exposure to blood, body fluids, or other potentially infectious materials, as determined by the following factors:
   a. Team member's role
   b. Type of procedure (e.g., minimally invasive versus open, superficial incision versus deep body cavity incision)
   c. Procedure duration

   d. Anticipated blood loss
   e. Anticipated volume of irrigation fluid
   f. Possibility of handling hazardous medications
   g. Anticipated patient contact (e.g., splash, soaking, leaning)

[Recommendation]

2. Perform surgical hand antisepsis before donning a sterile gown and gloves. [Recommendation]
3. Use sterile technique when donning and wearing a sterile gown. [Recommendation]
4. When donning the sterile gown without assistance, prevent contamination of the sterile field by:
   a. Following the manufacturer's instructions for donning, if available
   b. Opening and donning the sterile gown and gloves away from the sterile field
   c. Not opening sterile gloves directly on top of the open sterile gown
   d. Completely drying hands and arms prior to donning the gown
   e. Only touching the inside of the sterile gown when picking it up for donning
   f. Not touching the sterile glove wrapper or gloves until the sterile gown has been donned [Recommendation]
5. Consider the following parts of the gown to be **sterile:**
   a. The front of a sterile gown from the chest to the level of the sterile field
   b. The gowns sleeves from the cuff to 2 inches above the elbow, circumferentially [Recommendation]
6. Consider the following parts of the surgical gown to be **contaminated** or **nonsterile:**
   a. The neckline, shoulders, and axillary regions
   b. The gown back
   c. The sleeve cuffs after the scrubbed team member's hands pass through and beyond the cuff

[Recommendation]

7. Scrubbed team members should wear two pairs of sterile surgical gloves (i.e., double glove), and use a **perforation indicator system.** [Recommendation]
8. Use sterile technique when donning, wearing, and changing sterile gloves. [Recommendation]
9. Perform gloving without assistance by touching only the inside of the glove. [Recommendation]

Perform initial gowning and gloving with assistance in the following order:

1. The team member being gloved should don a surgical gown with the gown cuffs remaining at or beyond the fingertips.
2. A scrubbed team member should hold open the glove to be donned.
3. The person donning the glove should insert his or her hand into the glove with the gown cuff touching only the inside of the glove. [Recommendation]

OPEN GLOVING

Open gloving is used during sterile procedures that do not require a sterile gown, such as preoperative skin preparation of the patient, assisting in minor skin procedures, catheterization.

When gloving, consider the two surfaces of the glove, the outside and the inside. The glove has a cuff that exposes the *inside* of the glove. This inner surface is considered the nonsterile surface, even though it is sterile until touched with the bare hand. The outside remains sterile. The wrapper is considered sterile to within 1 inch (2.5 cm) of the edges. The technique for open gloving is illustrated in Fig. 9.10.

When learning to glove, students sometimes experience difficulty removing the glove from the open sterile wrapper. Very thin or short-cuffed gloves are difficult to put on without contaminating the sterile side of the glove or the glove wrapper. Remember that as long as you do not touch the sterile surface with your nonsterile fingers, you have not contaminated either one.

ASSISTED GOWNING AND GLOVING

The surgical technologist usually assists the surgeons and surgical assistants in gowning and gloving. The surgical technologist may also require assisted gowning and gloving in case of contamination during surgery. Gowning and gloving of the other team members precede all other activities and are as much a social tradition as a necessary part of the surgical routine. During gowning and gloving, the surgeon greets the scrub, circulator, and anesthesiologist and may introduce other members of the team. This time allows formal acknowledgment of the team members and what is to be done before the actual start of surgery. The surgeon also may clarify the need for special instruments or equipment at this time. Interaction among the team members during the process of gowning and gloving often sets the tone for the entire surgery.

When the sterile team members enter the operating room, the scrub hands an unfolded towel to the surgical team leader (lead surgeon) and then to the other members of the team.

GOWNING OTHER TEAM MEMBERS

Before gowning another team member who has just performed surgical hand antisepsis, pass a towel (if a surgical scrub was performed). When passing the towel, drape one end over the other person's extended hand so that the long end extends from the palm. Gowning follows immediately as shown in Fig. 9.11.

IMPORTANT TO KNOW *The correct method for gowning another person is to ensure that the gown cuff remains at or beyond the fingertips.*

Watch Chapter 9: Scrubbing, Gowning, and Gloving on the Evolve website. http://evolve.elsevier.com/Fuller/surgical.

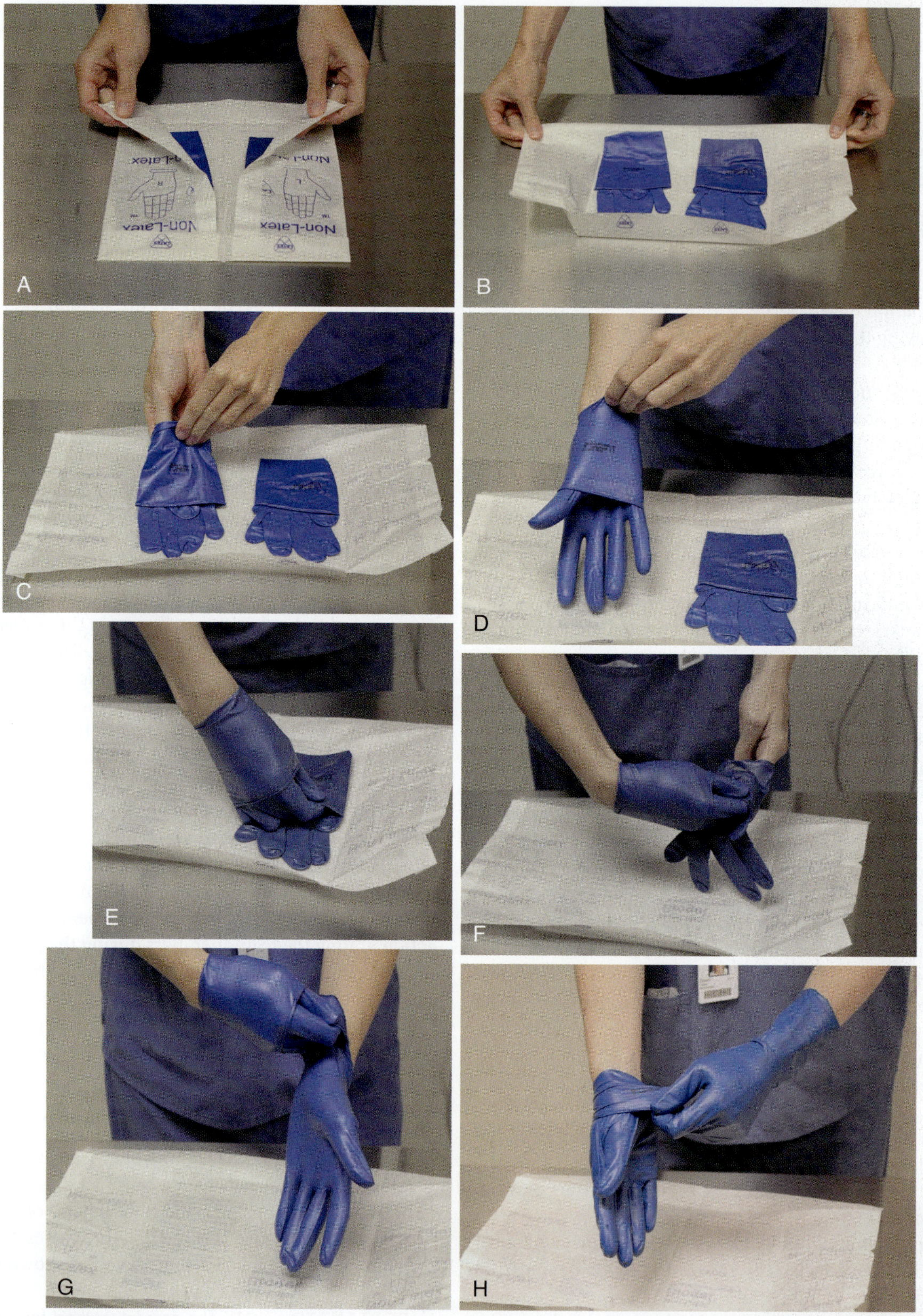

FIG. 9.10 Open gloving. (A) Perform hand hygiene before gloving. Open the glove wrapper by grasping the edges only. (B) Expose the gloves and give a slight tug on the wrapper to release the folds and keep it open. (C) Without touching the wrapper, slide one hand into either glove. (D) Pull the glove over the wrist but *do not unfold the cuff.* (E) Grasp the other glove by its cuff as shown. (F) Slide the hand into the glove without allowing it to contact the outer surface of the glove. (G) Pull the glove up without touching bare skin. (H) Unfold the cuff of the opposite hand without touching bare skin. (From Ehrlich RA, Coakes DM. *Patient Care in Radiography With an Introduction to Medical Imaging.* 9th ed. St Louis: Elsevier; 2017.)

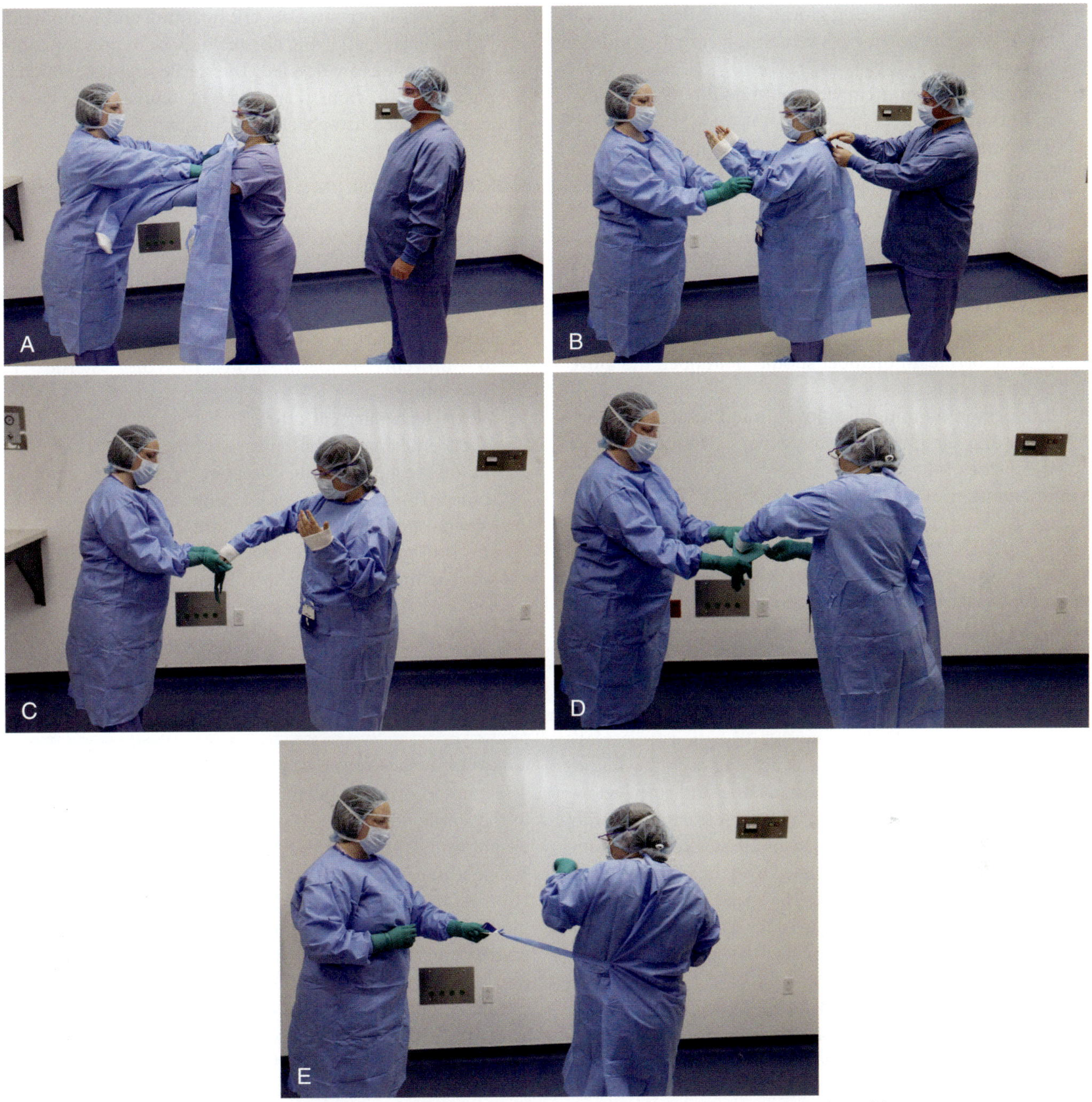

FIG. 9.11 Assisted gowning and gloving. (A) Make a wide cuff at the neck and shoulders of the gown to protect your gloved hands. As the other team member steps forward, maintain a hold on the gown. The other person will insert his or her arms into the sleeves. The circulator stands by to pull the gown back and up. (B) As the circulator ties the gown, gently pull the sleeves back to expose the fingers only. (C) Grasp the first glove (by convention this is the right hand) at the cuff. Grasp the glove under the cuff and spread the opening with your thumbs held well away from the glove or tucked securely under the cuff. Orient it so that the palm is facing toward the other person who inserts his or her hand into the glove. Allow the cuff to recoil *without snapping*. (D) Assisted gowning and gloving. Repeat the process with the other glove. (E) Turn the gown and pass the tie.

GLOVING OTHER TEAM MEMBERS

The scrubbed surgical technologist gloves other sterile team members as soon as they have been gowned.

Note that gloving another person following contamination of the glove, the cuff of the gown may remain at wrist level.

Guidelines • Gowning and Gloving Others

(Association of PeriOperative Registered Nurses. Guidelines for perioperative practice. 2020. Sterile technique. *Donning and gowns and gloves*. Guideline No. 2)

1. Perform initial gowning and gloving with assistance in the following order:

a. The team member being gloved should don a surgical gown with the gown cuffs remaining at or beyond the fingertips.
b. A scrubbed team member should hold open the glove to be donned.
c. The person donning the glove should insert his or her hand into the glove with the gown cuff touching only the inside of the glove.

[Recommendation]

2. When the gown cuff is at the wrist level, perform gloving with assistance in the following order:
   a. The team member being gloved should leave the gown cuff at wrist level, leaving the fingers and hand exposed.
   b. A scrubbed team member should hold open the glove to be donned.
   c. The person donning the glove should insert his or her hand into the glove with the gown cuff touching only the inside of the glove.

[Recommendation]

SURGICAL HELMET SYSTEM

The surgical helmet system (SHS) was developed to reduce the risk of **surgical site infection** in selected high-risk surgical procedures, especially total joint arthroplasty. The SHS works by isolating the scrubbed surgical team member's environment. A surgical helmet system consists of a nonsterile plastic head frame and a sterile hood, which fits over the frame. A sterile "toga" is a sterile face shield, head cover, and gown extension that is fitted into the head frame. The frame is equipped with a filtered ventilation system. Some systems are also equipped with an LED head lamp. The system is donned over the standard scrub suit, surgical mask, and head cover. The mask can be removed from the back of the helmet hood by the circulator once the helmet is in place. The sterile gown is donned after the helmet and hood.

NOTE *The effectiveness of surgical helmet systems in lowering the postoperative infection rate has been the subject of many research studies. At this time there is no consensus on their capacity to reduce postoperative infections.*

PART VII: PREPARING THE STERILE FIELD

OPENING A SURGICAL CASE

Preparing sterile equipment and supplies for a surgical case involves two distinct steps: (1) opening the case, which is performed by nonsterile staff, and (2) the case setup, performed by a scrubbed team member (e.g., the scrubbed surgical technologist). The surgical technologist and circulating nurse often open their case together in nonsterile roles until it is necessary for the ST to perform surgical hand antisepsis. She or he then returns to the designated operating room to don a sterile gown and gloves to perform the case setup. This section covers the creation of the sterile field. The case setup is discussed in detail in Chapter 19.

To begin case preparation, OR furniture and equipment are moved into place, allowing adequate space to prevent contamination as supplies are opened. The sterile supplies, which have been gathered previously, are brought in on a closed case cart. These are opened using sterile technique.

Guidelines • Opening a Surgical Case or Invasive Procedure

(Association of periOperative Registered Nurses. Guidelines for perioperative practice. 2020. Sterile technique. *Before preparing the sterile field.* Guidelines No. 1.)

1. Before preparing a sterile field, implement practices to prevent contamination of the sterile field. [Recommendation]
2. Wear clean surgical attire and a surgical head covering when entering an OR invasive procedure room for any reason (e.g., stocking supplies, delivering equipment, transporting specimens). [Recommendation]
3. When open sterile supplies are present, wear a clean surgical mask that covers the mouth and nose and is secured in a manner that prevents venting at the sides of the mask. [Recommendation]
4. Perform hand hygiene before opening sterile supplies. [Recommendation]

CREATING THE STERILE FIELD

The method used for opening a sterile item and distributing it to the sterile field depends on what it is, how it is wrapped, its weight, and its size. There are many different kinds of packaging systems used in commercial manufacturing of sterile supplies. However, all are designed to be distributed using sterile technique. High-quality packaging tends to open cleanly and easily, whereas inferior packaging may tear or delaminate during opening, resulting in contamination of the contents of the package.

Heavy sterile equipment and supplies are opened in place. This means that the *wrapped* sterile item is positioned on an instrument table, ring stand (for large basins), or small side table. The item's wrapper is then opened using sterile technique. Lighter items can be passed directly to the scrubbed surgical technologist or other scrubbed team member. They may also be placed securely on the sterile field.

Before opening any sterile package, always check the integrity of the outside of the package and the external chemical indicators that validate exposure to the sterilization process. Any packages with tears, holes, or water marks are contaminated and should be removed from the room for reprocessing. Wrapped packages stored in plastic or wire bins may be subject to frequent handling. Fraying of the wrapper may indicate a hole that is too small to see. Packages that show areas of fraying should be removed from the stock and reprocessed.

When opening a case, discard clean wrappers into designated receptacles (for clean trash and clean linen). Do not place wrappers on the operating table or other surfaces in the OR.

DRAPING THE BACK TABLE

It is necessary to drape at least one table or surface when opening a case. The back table is usually the first surface to be draped. A *basic pack,* also called a *procedure pack,* is opened in place on the back table. The pack may include surgical gowns, towels, and drapes. Preassembled case packs can be custom designed by the institution to include surgical supplies routinely used in specific types of surgery. Some commonly preassembled packs include abdominal, orthopedic, and minor surgery packs. The technique used to open the basic pack is illustrated in Fig. 9.12.

IMPORTANT TO KNOW *Remember that sterile drapes, including table covers, must never be adjusted after they have been placed. When draped, tables are only sterile at table height. Adjusting a drape brings a nonsterile surface into a sterile one. This rule also applies to the draped patient. Items that fall below the surface of the drape are considered contaminated.*

OPENING ENVELOPE-WRAPPED PACKS

The envelope technique for wrapping supplies and instruments is very common. The technique is illustrated in the following chapter (Chapter 10). Reading this section will be helpful in learning how to unwrap an item that has been packaged in this way.

Packages wrapped envelope style feature four flaps, each one covering a side of the item. To unwrap the pack using sterile technique, the flaps must be opened in a specific order regardless of the pack's size. The flap farthest away is opened first, then the side flaps, and finally the near flap. This technique is shown in Fig. 9.13.

INSTRUMENT TRAYS

Instruments are prepared as full sets either in trays that are wrapped with textile wrappers, or prepared in closed systems

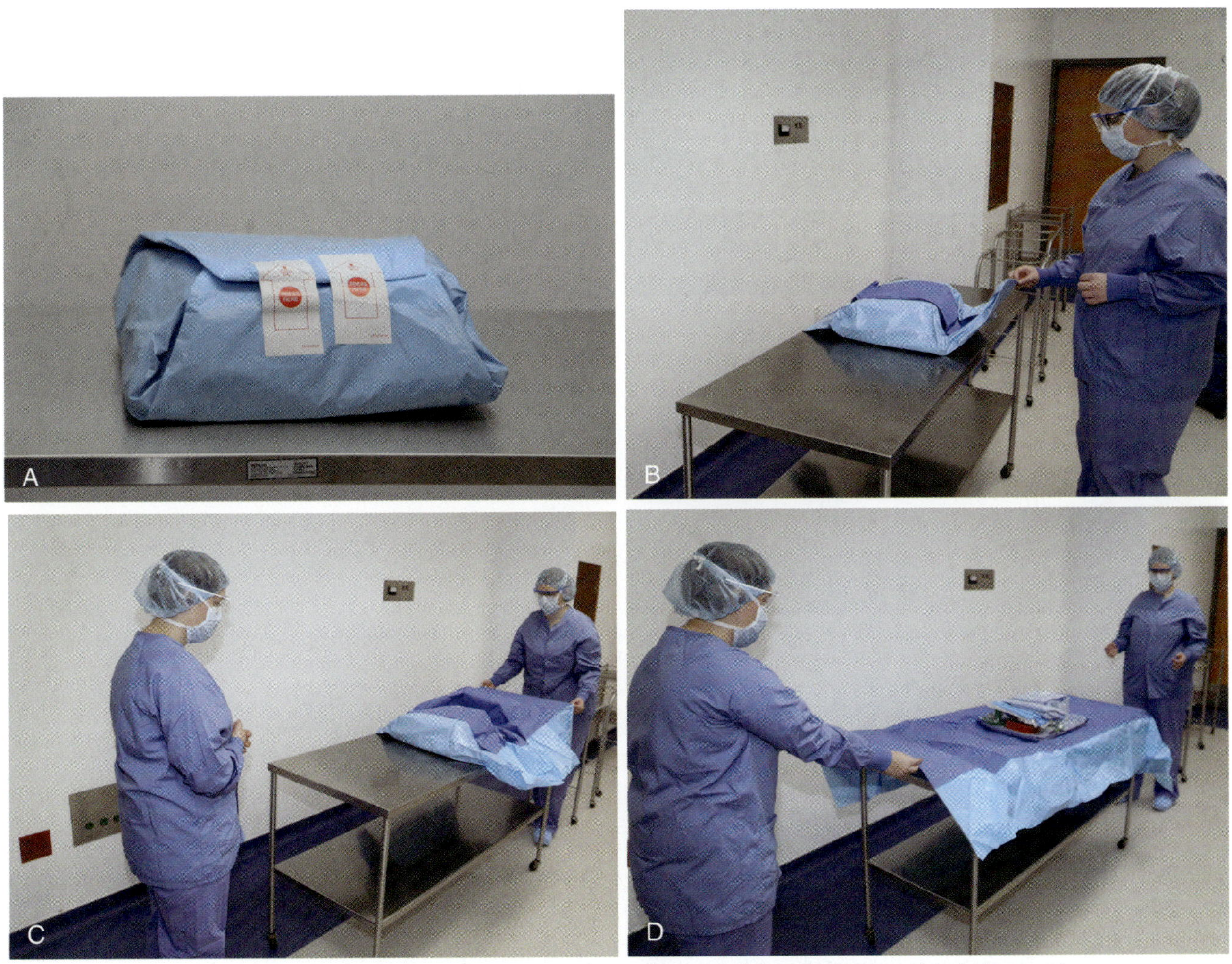

FIG. 9.12 Opening a basic pack. (A) Center the pack on the table and orient it so that the long ends of the outside drape line up with the long end of the table. Note: Packs differ in the way they have been folded. Commercially prepared packs and drapes have printed diagrams on the drape showing how to open correctly. (B) Grasp the folded edge closest to you with both hands and peel the edges back from the center. (C) Move to the other side of the table and repeat this process on the opposite top fold. Allow 1 inch (2.5 cm) of margin between the edge of the drape and your nonsterile hand. Note: Two people may open the pack as shown. (D) As the sides of the wrapper are opened, do not adjust its position on the table.

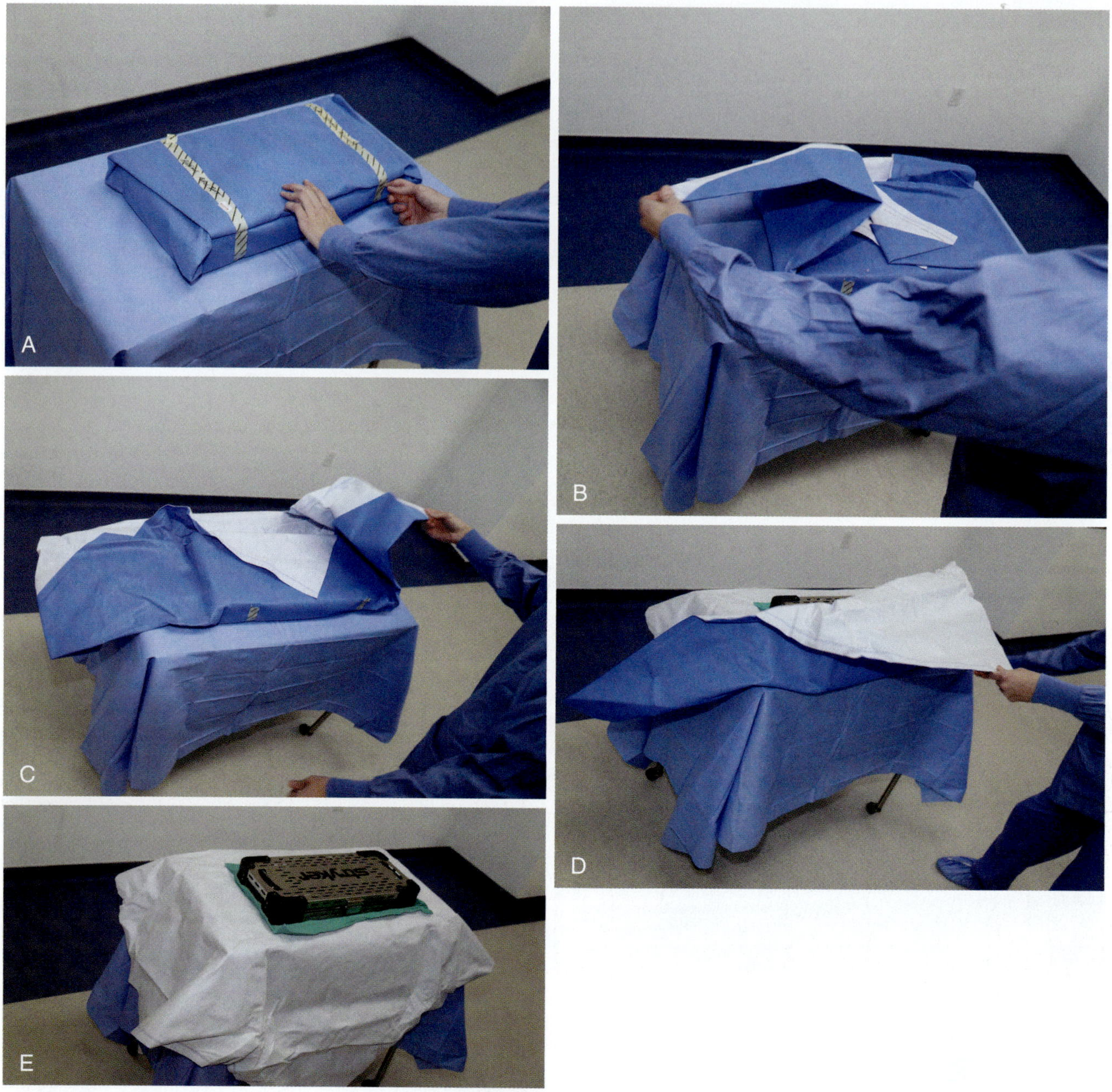

FIG. 9.13 Open large packs wrapped envelope style as follows. (A) After checking exterior sterilization monitors, break the wrapping tape. (B) Open the first flap by placing yourself in front of it first and pulling it toward you. (C) Open the side flaps. (D) Open the final flap by positioning yourself in front of it and pulling it toward you. Never reach across the pack to peel back a section. (E) The sterile tray is exposed on the inner sterile surfaces of the drape.

(sterile barrier system). Separate techniques to open them using sterile technique are required. It is important to follow the manufacturer's instructions for use when using a closed barrier system. A barrier system is illustrated in Chapters 10 and 18. Heavy instrument trays that are not contained in a sterile barrier system must be opened on a small table. The wrapped tray is placed on the table and the wrapper opened to create a small sterile field. The scrubbed surgical technologist may move the tray onto the back table or leave it in place as part of the sterile field.

BASINS

Basins are used to hold large quantities of sterile water, or saline may opened in place. Do not reach over the basin to open it. It is better technique to move around the sterile package and pull the flaps toward you.

PEEL POUCHES

Items wrapped in sealed pouches are delivered to the sterile field by grasping the top edges of the wrapper and peeling the

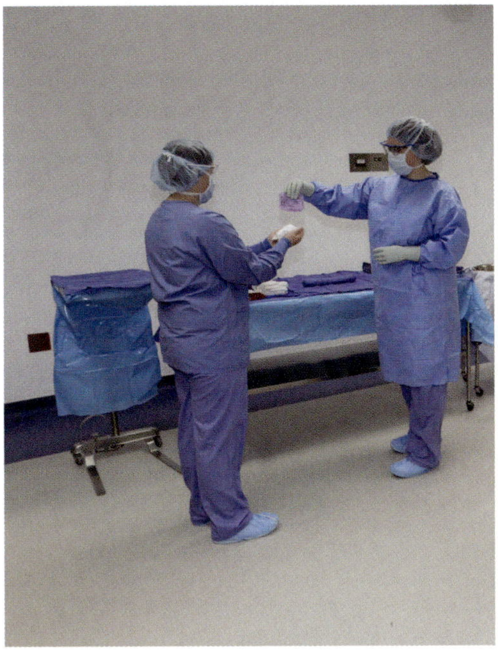

FIG. 9.14 Opening a small peel pouch. Grasp each side of the wrapper using both hands. Peel the sides apart to expose the contents so that it can be removed.

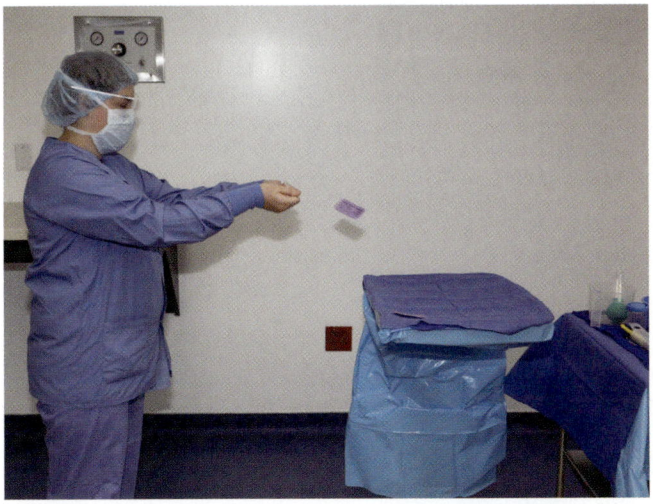

FIG. 9.15 Popping or flipping a suture packet. Grasp each side of the wrapper using both hands. Peel the sides down carefully about halfway. Peel the remaining portions down forcefully. This causes the packet to eject. Note that this technique takes some practice to refine. Used suture packets and wrappers can be used for practice.

wrapper apart to reveal the sterile item (Fig. 9.14). Suture packets can also be flipped onto the field (Fig. 9.15). This is done by opening the peel pouch halfway and then quickly popping the wrapper open the rest of the way to propel the contents out of the package and onto the sterile field. Do not reach over the sterile surface when flipping items onto the field. Take care to avoid flipping the item past the sterile field and onto the floor.

When opening a peel pouch wrapper, do not allow the item to slide out of the package; this contaminates it, because *the edge of the sterile package is never considered sterile.* The safest way to deliver items is to present them to a sterile team member directly.

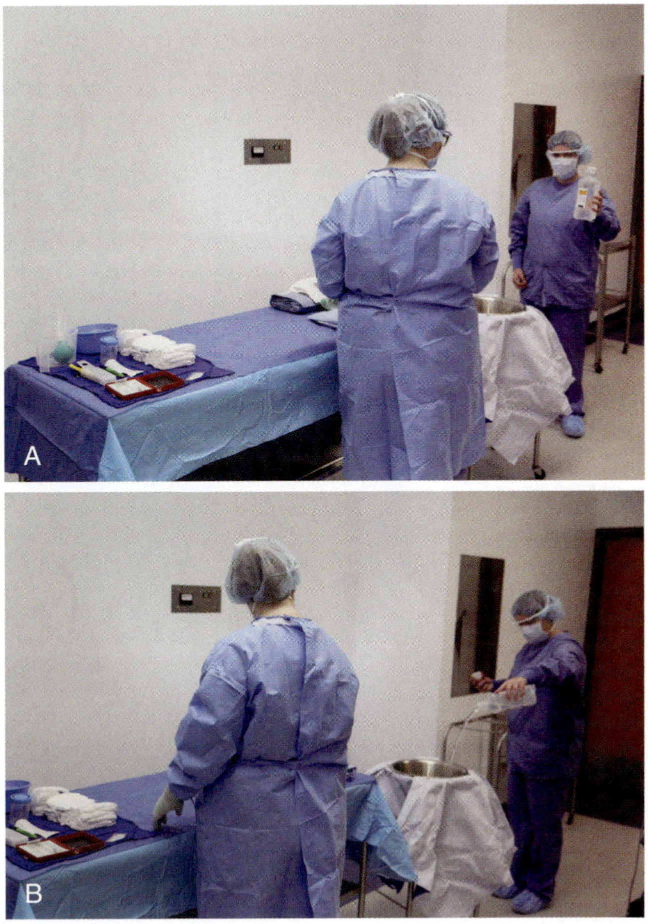

FIG. 9.16 Pouring sterile solutions in a basin. The entire contents of the bottle must be distributed at one time. Distribution of water and saline solution follows the same guidelines as for the distribution of any drug.

SHARPS

Scalpel blades and other **sharps** should be passed directly to the sterile surgical technologist or unwrapped in an open area where they are in plain view. Blades, trocars, and other sharps should not be opened onto instrument trays, because the sharps can be hidden by other instruments. If a sharp item is accidentally covered during opening, warn the scrubbed team of its location to prevent injury during the setup.

FLUIDS

Fluids are distributed on the sterile field so that the fluid does not come in contact with the side of the bottle or any area below the sterile lip. Fluid containers are manufactured so that the cap can be removed while preserving the sterility of the inner lip. When large quantities of fluids are poured, such as those used for irrigation, the bottle is held away from the edge of the basin (Fig. 9.16). Refer to Chapter 12 for required procedures for receiving medications on the sterile field.

SMALL WRAPPED PACKAGES

Small packages may be wrapped envelope style or in blister packs. Small packages in envelope wraps are opened in the same way as large packs (Fig. 9.17). When opening and

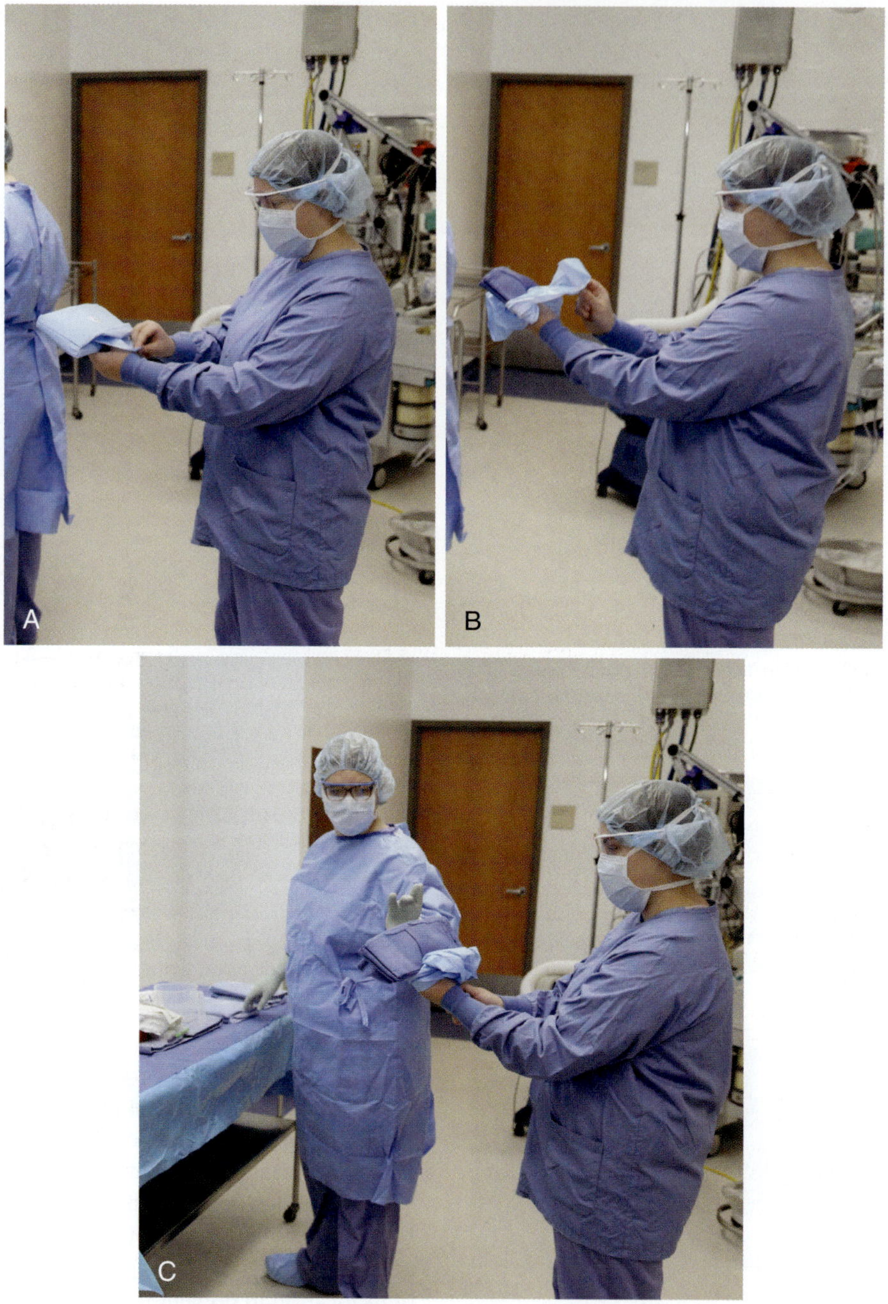

FIG. 9.17 Opening and distributing small packs.

distributing blister packs, peel the top away from the blister portion without contaminating the contents or the edge of the blister portion. The contents must be offered directly to the scrubbed team member or the blister portion turned over so that the contents fall on the sterile table. This must be done carefully to prevent the sterile contents from coming in contact with the nonsterile edge of the package.

Guidelines • Opening Sterile Items

(Association of periOperative Registered Nurses. Guidelines for perioperative practice. 2020. Sterile technique. *Opening sterile items.* Guidelines No. 4 and 5.)

1. Open, dispense, and transfer sterile items to the sterile field by methods that maintain the sterility and integrity of the item and the sterile field. [Recommendation]
2. Introduce sterile items to the sterile field as close as possible to the time of use. [Recommendation]
3. Immediately before presenting items to the sterile field, inspect sterile items for the following:
   a. Sterility of the contents, as noted on the packaging
   b. The expiration date, when applicable
   c. Package integrity
   d. Product integrity (e.g., discoloration or particulate formation in medications and solutions)
   e. Verification that the external chemical indicators have changed to the correct color, indicating that the parameters for sterilization have been met [Recommendation]
4. Deliver items to the sterile field in a manner that prevents unsterile objects or unscrubbed team members from leaning or reaching over the sterile field. [Recommendation]

5. Present sterile items directly to the scrubbed team member or placed securely on the sterile field. [Recommendation]
   a. Present heavy or sharp items directly to a scrubbed team member or opened them on a separate clean, dry surface. [Recommendation]
6. Open items packaged in sterile barrier systems according to the manufacturers' IFU [instructions for use], if available. [Recommendation]
   a. Inspect rigid sterilization containers for intact external locks, secured latch filters, valves, and tamper-evident devices, and for the correct color change to external chemical indicators before they are opened onto a clean, flat, and dry surface.
   b. An unscrubbed person should lift the lid up and toward himself or herself while moving the lid away from the container.
   c. The nonsterile person should inspect the integrity of the lid filter or valve and consider the contents to be contaminated if the filter is dislodged, damp, or not intact (e.g., holes, tears, punctures).
   d. A scrubbed team member should lift the inner basket(s) out of and above the container without contacting the unsterile surfaces of the table or container. Before the instruments are placed on the sterile field, the scrubbed surgical technologist should examine the internal chemical indicator for the correct color change and inspect the inside surface of the container for debris, moisture, contamination, or damage.
   e. If there are any filters in the bottom of the container, an unscrubbed person should inspect the integrity of the filters. [Recommendation]
7. When transferring medications and sterile solutions (e.g., normal saline) to the sterile field, transfer as close to the time of use as possible.
   a. Transfer in a slow, controlled manner using a sterile transfer device (e.g., sterile vial spike, filter straw, plastic catheter) unless the item is packaged for sterile delivery to the sterile field.
   b. Transfer into a receptacle that is placed near the sterile table's edge or is held by a scrubbed team member.
   c. Verify and label the medication or solution immediately after transfer.
   d. Do not remove medication vial stoppers from vials for the purpose of pouring medications unless they are specifically designed for removal and pouring by the manufacturer.
   e. Pour medications or sterile solutions from the container only once, and do not replace the cap. Discard any remaining fluids in the opened container at the end of the procedure. [Recommendation]

PART VIII: MAINTAINING THE STERILE FIELD

One of the most important duties of the surgical technologist is the shared responsibility with other members of the surgical team to maintain the sterile field. This includes preventing contamination, knowing when it occurs, and responding as quickly as possible to avoid extending the contamination.

BREAKS IN STERILE TECHNIQUE

A break in sterile technique is an event that results, or may have resulted, in contamination of a sterile surface within the sterile field. Breaks in sterile technique can be divided into four types that help to define the action required to mitigate the potential harm. Although there are a variety of ways in which a sterile break can occur, the most common are described in this section.

In terms of response to breaks, four types have been identified:

- Type 1: The break is recognized immediately.
- Type 2: The break is recognized shortly after it occurs.
- Type 3: The break is recognized much later after it occurs.
- Type 4: The break is never recognized.

The nature of contamination is that the longer it remains unnoticed, the greater the chance that the area of contamination will spread. For example, when the gloved hand of a team member is contaminated, further contact with sterile areas extends the contamination. This means that contamination must be reported to the team *as soon as it occurs or is suspected to have occurred.*

Management of breaks in technique requires a clinical decision. Simple breaks such as contaminating the glove when it is immediately recognized may be handled by changing the glove. Breaks that are more serious require a team decision based on the extent and nature of the break, when it was discovered, and patient risk. The lead surgeon has the final decision, but the team should provide input.

REMOVING GOWN AND GLOVES

To remove only the glove, the sterile team member presents the contaminated gloved hand to the circulator, palm upward. The circulator, wearing nonsterile gloves, grasps the contaminated glove below the wrist and removes it (see Fig. 9.19).

The technique for removing both gown and gloves is shown in Figs. 9.18 and 9.19.

CONTAMINATED INSTRUMENTS AND EQUIPMENT

Breaks in sterile technique should be treated on a case-by-case basis. Ideally, the contaminated item or equipment is removed from the sterile field. If this is not possible, the contaminated area must be contained. Instruments and other small items can be passed off to the circulator.

When draped equipment or the sterile field becomes contaminated, all items that have potentially become contaminated must be removed from the sterile field. In extreme cases, this may mean that the entire setup must be removed.

One area of contamination that is of particular risk is instruments that have not been thoroughly cleaned before sterilization. This includes stainless steel instruments and endoscopic systems. This topic is discussed in Chapters 10 and 11. Organic material,

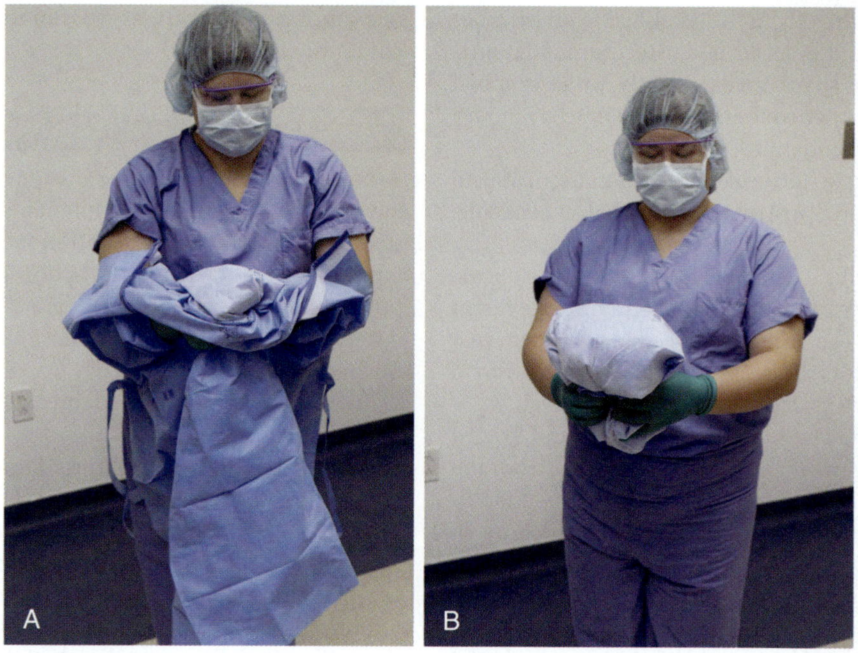

FIG. 9.18 Removing the gown without making skin contact with the outside surfaces.

including blood, tissue debris, hair, and bone particles present on an instrument, may prevent the sterilizing agent from making contact with all surfaces of the instrument. This means that there is no way to ensure that sterilization was achieved. If the instrument was part of a set, the entire set must be removed from the sterile field. Likewise, anyone who handled the instrument itself or the set must change gloves. Any other surface that came into contact with the instrument or set must also be removed.

Guidelines • Contamination of the Sterile Field

(Association of periOperative Registered Nurses. Guidelines for perioperative practice. 2020. Sterile technique. *Maintaining the sterile field*. Standard No. 6.)

1. Continually maintain the sterile field. [Recommendation]
2. Monitor for contamination of the sterile field and potential breaks in sterile technique and correct them immediately. [Recommendation]
   a. When a break in sterile technique occurs, take corrective action immediately unless the patient's safety is at risk. When a break in technique cannot be corrected immediately, take corrective action as soon as it is safe for the patient. [Recommendation]
3. Consider instruments contaminated when they are found:
   a. Assembled or clamped closed
   b. With organic material (e.g., blood, hair, tissue, bone fragments) on or in the instrument
   c. With other debris (e.g., bone cement, grease, mineral deposits) on or in the instrument [Recommendation]
4. When an item or items are found to be contaminated, take the following corrective actions, at a minimum:
   a. Remove the contaminated item(s).
   b. Remove any other items that may have come in contact with the contaminated item(s).
   c. Remove the gloves of any team member who may have touched the contaminated item(s).
   d. Take any additional corrective actions required after thoughtful assessment and informed decision making based on the specific factors associated with the individual event. [Recommendation]

COVERING THE STERILE SETUP

The Association of periOperative Registered Nurses (AORN) have published new guidelines for maintaining the sterile field. One of these recommends that the sterile setup or portions of it can be covered during times of increased activity in the room when there is a higher-than-normal likelihood of contamination by airborne particles. Fig. 9.20 demonstrates how to cover and uncover the sterile setup without contaminating it.

Technique for Covering a Sterile Setup

1. To safely cover the sterile setup, two cuffed, sterile drapes are required. The first drape is placed by the sterile surgical technologist so that the cuffed edge is just past the halfway point of the setup. It is carefully unfolded, allowing the fan folds to open up. The cover drape must not be adjusted once it is placed.
2. A second drape is applied so that the cuffed edge overlaps the first drape. This drape is then unfolded in the same manner as the first, observing all rules of sterile technique.
3. To remove the drape, the circulator places his or her hands under the cuff of the uppermost drape. The drape is lifted straight up while the person steps back away from the table. Do not allow the drape to slide or come back in contact with the sterile setup.
4. The second drape is removed using the same technique. Done properly, this maneuver ensures that the sterile setup is not contaminated. This practice is not used to bypass the requirement to monitor the setup at all times. Individual facilities may or may not adapt this practice.

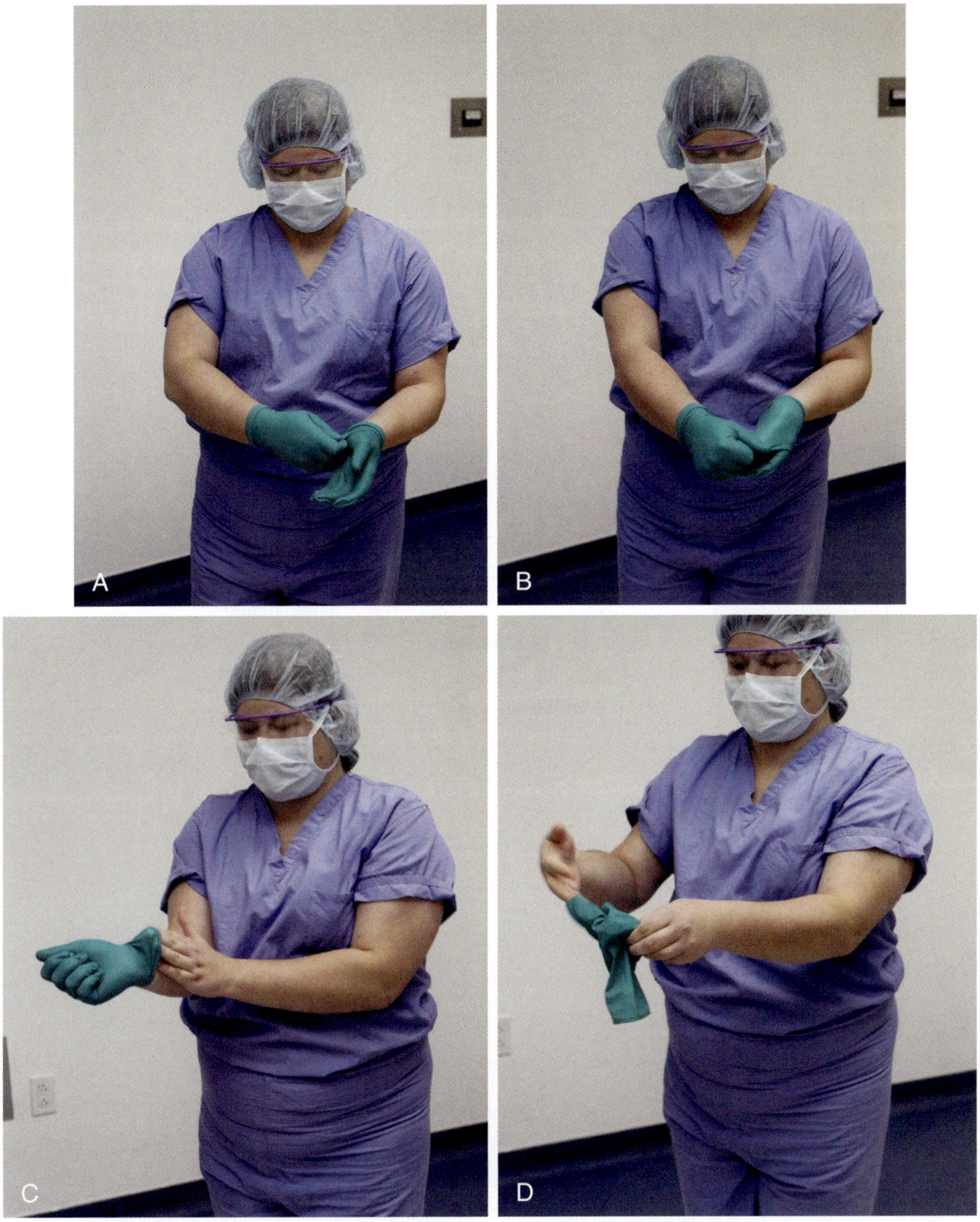

FIG. 9.19 Removing soiled gloves without making skin contact with the outside surfaces.

An alternative method of covering the sterile setup is using a commercially made system (CFI Medical). This can be viewed at http://cfimedical.com/sterile-z-back-table-cover/.

Guidelines • Covering the Sterile Field

(Association of periOperative Registered Nurses. Guidelines for perioperative practice. 2020. Sterile technique. *Maintaining the sterile field*. Standard No. 6.)

1. Cover the sterile field if it will not be used immediately (e.g., procedural delay, sterile field for closure, multiple tables) or during periods of increased activity (e.g., preincision, repositioning). [Recommendation] If the sterile field is in use, the portion of the sterile field that will not be immediately used (e.g., implants, instruments not in use) may be covered. [Conditional Recommendation]
   a. Cover the sterile field with a sterile drape in a manner that allows the cover to be removed without compromising the sterility of the table (e.g., bringing a portion of the table cover up and over the field from below the level of the table surface, cutting the drape down the middle). The sterile field may be covered with a sterile drape designed for this purpose or by the sterile two-"cuffed"-drape method.

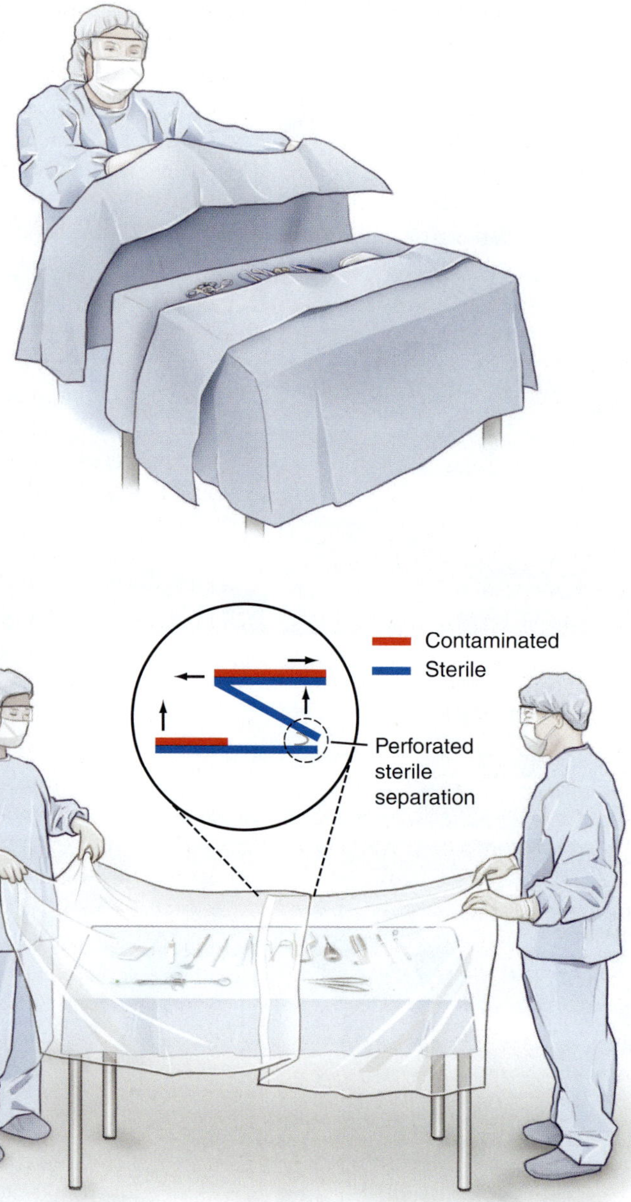

FIG. 9.20 Covering and uncovering the sterile field. (Top) Sterile drapes are cuffed and directly applied to the sterile set-up. These can be removed by the nonsterile circulator by reversing the process. (Bottom) A sterile commercial "Z" drape is applied to the sterile set-up using standard surgical technique. To remove the drape, the short ends are grasped and pulled apart by nonsterile personnel. The drape separates at the perforation, allowing each end to be removed aseptically.

MOVEMENT WITHIN AND AROUND THE STERILE FIELD

The movement of staff and equipment around the sterile field results in an increase in air movement with the potential for airborne contamination. It also increases the risk of contamination by team members and equipment.

When the sterile field is raised or lowered, such as during procedures in which one or all of the team members are seated, the level of the sterile field must be maintained throughout the procedure and team members must not shift their positions. Changing position, such as from sitting to standing, brings nonsterile surface, into direct contact with sterile ones.

Guidelines • Movement Around the Sterile Field

(Association of periOperative Registered Nurses. Guidelines for perioperative practice. 2020. Sterile technique. *Movement around the sterile field.* Standard No. 7.)

1. Move within or around a sterile field in a manner that prevents contamination of the sterile field. [Recommendation]
2. Scrubbed team members should
   a. Remain close to the sterile field and touch only sterile areas or items
   b. Keep their hands and arms above waist level at all times
   c. Not fold their arms with their hands positioned in the axillary area

  d. Avoid changing levels, and be seated only when the entire procedure will be performed at that level
  e. Not turn their backs on the sterile field
  f. Turn back to back or face to face while maintaining distance from each other, the sterile field, and unsterile areas during position changes
  g. Not be positioned between the horizontal unidirectional ultraclean air delivery system air curtain and the surgical site
  h. Not leave the sterile field to retrieve items from the sterilizer
  i. Use shielding devices (e.g., lead aprons, mobile shields) that reduce radiological exposure in order to stay near the sterile field when radiology equipment is used [Recommendation]
3. Unscrubbed team members should:
  a. Face the sterile field on approach
  b. Not walk between sterile fields or scrubbed persons
  c. Not reach over an uncovered sterile field
  d. Stay as far back from the sterile field and scrubbed persons as possible
  e. Remain outside of a vertical unidirectional ultraclean air delivery system air curtain
  f. Not walk between the horizontal unidirectional ultraclean air delivery system air curtain and the sterile field [Recommendation]
4. Limit nonessential conversations in the presence of a sterile field. [Recommendation]
5. Keep doors to the operative or invasive procedure room closed as much as possible except during the entry and exit of patients, required personnel, and necessary equipment. [Recommendation]
6. Keep the number and movement of individuals in an operative or invasive procedure room to a minimum. [Recommendation]

PART IX: INFECTION CONTROL IN THE PERIOPERATIVE ENVIRONMENT

The practice of sterile technique is a powerful tool in preventing postoperative infection in surgical patients. Health care professionals must also understand and carry out standards that are equally important in preventing the spread of infection in the health care environment. All health care providers have a duty to protect their patients and themselves against infectious disease.

Sources of infection and the ways diseases are spread from one person to another are discussed in Chapter 8. In this section, transmission precautions and recommendations are linked with activities in the perioperative environment. Note that many of the guidelines in this section are regulated by government mandate. This means that they are *required by government agencies.*

STANDARD PRECAUTIONS

Standard Precautions are fundamental to preventing the transmission of infectious disease in the health care setting. Standard precautions are used by all personnel in all health care settings. The assumption is that *any person* may harbor potentially infectious microorganisms. Therefore, Standard Precautions apply to all patients in all types of patient care environments. The guidelines focus on the handling of tissues, blood, body fluids, and any other potential infectious material.

Guidelines • Standard Precautions

(Association of periOperative Registered Nurses. Guidelines for perioperative practice. 2020. Transmission-based precautions. *Standard Precautions*. Standard No. 1.)

1. Use Standard Precautions when caring for all patients.[1,2] [Recommendation]
2. All personnel in the health care organization should follow established hand hygiene practices. [Recommendation]
3. Provide the patient with a clean, safe environment. [Recommendation]
4. Perioperative personnel must wear PPE whenever the possibility exists for exposure to blood, body fluids, or other potentially infectious materials. [Regulatory Requirement]
5. All people who enter the health care facility should practice respiratory hygiene and cough etiquette. [Recommendation]
6. Clean reusable medical equipment (e.g., blood glucose meters, blood pressure cuffs, pulse oximeter probes, surgical instruments, endoscopes) that has been used for one patient and disinfect or sterilize equipment in accordance with the manufacturer's written instructions for use (IFU) before use for another patient and when soiled. [Recommendation]

PERSONAL PROTECTIVE EQUIPMENT

Personal protective equipment (PPE) must be used by perioperative personnel whenever there is a risk of coming into direct contact with blood, body fluids, or other potentially infectious material. It must protect the skin, mucous membranes, eyes, and respiratory tract. It must be designed according to the type of transmission anticipated. For example, protective eyewear and face shields must cover the front and sides to prevent blood and tissue splatter from entering the eyes and mouth. A surgical mask is not sufficient to provide protection. Personnel who work in the decontamination area, hand washing soiled instruments and transferring them to mechanical washers, must wear nonpermeable high-cuffed gloves, face protection, gowns, and aprons while carrying out their duties. Simply wearing a cloth surgical gown and single-use patient care gloves does not provide sufficient protection.

Guidelines • Personal Protective Equipment

(Association of periOperative Registered Nurses. Guidelines for perioperative practice. 2020. Transmission-based precautions. *Personal protective equipment*. Standard No. 2.)

1. Perioperative personnel must wear PPE when exposure to blood, body fluids, or other potentially infectious materials is anticipated. [Regulatory Requirement]
2. The health care organization must provide PPE to personnel at no cost. [Regulatory Requirement]
3. Perioperative personnel must wear gloves when contact of the hands with blood, body fluids, or other potentially infectious materials can be reasonably anticipated,. [Regulatory Requirement] including when
4. Perioperative personnel must wear gowns when contact of the arms or clothing with blood, body fluids, or other potentially infectious materials can be reasonably anticipated. [Regulatory Requirement]
5. Perioperative personnel must wear eye protection when splashes, spray, spatter, or droplets of blood or other potentially infectious materials may be generated and eye contamination can be reasonably anticipated. [Regulatory Requirement]
6. Perioperative personnel must wear masks when splashes, spray, spatter, or droplets of blood or other potentially infectious materials may be generated and nose or mouth contamination can be reasonably anticipated. [Regulatory Requirement]
7. When respiratory protection is needed, wear a National Institute for Occupational Safety and Health (NIOSH)-approved, fit-tested, surgical N95 respirator or higher level respirator in accordance with the facility's respiratory protection program. [Recommendation]
8. Perioperative personnel must wear fluid-resistant surgical hoods when gross contamination can reasonably be anticipated (e.g., during orthopedic surgery). [Regulatory Requirement]
9. Perioperative personnel must wear fluid-resistant shoe covers or boots when gross contamination can reasonably be anticipated (e.g., during orthopedic surgery). [Regulatory Requirement]
10. Perioperative personnel must remove PPE and clothing as soon as possible after exposure to blood, body fluids, or other potentially infectious materials. [Regulatory Requirement]
11. Perioperative personnel must remove all PPE before leaving the work area and must place used PPE in a designated area or closed container for storage, washing, decontamination, or disposal. [Regulatory Requirement]

OSHA BLOODBORNE PATHOGENS STANDARD

The OSHA bloodborne pathogens standard reduces health care worker *exposure* to blood, body fluids, and other potentially infectious disease materials through multifaceted controls, plans, and practices.

PATIENT CARE EQUIPMENT AND LINENS

- Patient care equipment and linens must be handled in a way that prevents contact with skin and clothing.
- Handle soiled linens with gloved hands only.
- Hold soiled linen away from your body and place it in a biohazard laundry bag for disposal. Always wear gloves when handling patient care items.
- All contaminated single-use (disposable) items must be placed in biohazard bags for disposal.
- Sharps for disposal are contained in a special puncture-proof container and disposed of as contaminated waste.
- Multiple-use items must be decontaminated between patients.

More information on the OSHA standards is available at https://www.osha.gov/OshDoc/data_BloodborneFacts/bbfact01.pdf.

SHARPS INJURY

The most common means of transmission of **blood-borne pathogens** to health care workers is through sharps injuries. **Sharps** are such a threat to health care personnel that OSHA has issued the Bloodborne Pathogen Standard, a special set of regulations (rules) for handling and disposing of sharps.

Common sources of injury include the following:

- Hypodermic needles
- Suture needles
- Scalpel blades
- Needle-point electrosurgical tips
- Trocars, such as those used to perform endoscopic surgery or to place wound drains
- Sharp instruments, such as skin hooks, rakes, and scissors
- Metal guide wires and stylets
- Orthopedic drill bits, screws, pins, wires, and cutting tips, such as saw blades and burrs

Certain tasks are associated with a high risk of sharps injury:

- Passing and receiving a scalpel
- Preparing and passing sutures
- Collision of two individuals' hands when they reach for the same sharp instrument
- Mounting or removing a scalpel blade from the handle
- Manually retracting tissue
- Suturing

The risk of sharps injury can be reduced by following recommended guidelines and standards. This means performing tasks in a specific way. All health care workers are responsible for their own safety and the safety of others on the team. Therefore, compliance with guidelines is a combined ethical and safety issue.

RISK REDUCTION

- Whenever possible, retractable or self-sheathing needles and scalpels should be used.
- Blunt suture needles are now recommended over sharp needles.
- If hollow-bore hypodermic needles are used, they must never be recapped by hand. The cap is replaced by grasping it with an instrument. Removable needles must be handled

only with an instrument, never by hand. Self-sheathing needles have nonremovable parts.

- Scalpel blades must be mounted and removed with an instrument.
- Used disposable syringes and needles, scalpel blades, and other sharp items should be placed in appropriate puncture-resistant containers located as close as practical to the area where the items were used. The container must be removed and replaced at frequent intervals to prevent overflow, another common source of sharps injury.
- During surgery, sharps are contained on a magnetic board or in a special holder that can be contained and disposed of properly.
- All health care employees should be immunized against the hepatitis B virus (HBV).

NEUTRAL ZONE AND NO-TOUCH TECHNIQUE

Use of a **neutral zone** during surgery was developed because the evidence shows that most sharps injuries in surgery occur when instruments are passed and received. The technique uses a designated space on the sterile field where sharps can be placed and picked up so that the surgical technologist and surgeon do not hand sharps to each other directly. These guidelines are regulated. The **no-touch technique** is used for handling sharps.

Guidelines • Sharps Safety

(Association of periOperative Registered Nurses. Guidelines for perioperative practice. 2020. Work Practice Controls Standard No. 4, 7.)

1. Work practice controls must be used during handling of sharp devices (e.g., scalpels, hypodermic needles, suture needles, bone fragments, K-wires, burrs, saw blades, drill bits, trocars, bone cutters, towel clips, scissors, electrosurgical tips, skin hooks, retractors). [Regulatory Requirement]
2. Use a neutral zone or **hands-free technique** (HFT) for passing sharp instruments, blades, needles, and devices. [Recommendation]
3. When using a neutral zone,
   a. Identify and designate the neutral zone in the preoperative briefing
   b. Use an instrument mat, magnetic pad, basin, or designated area on the Mayo stand as the neutral zone
   c. Give verbal notification when a sharp is in the neutral zone
   d. Place one sharp at a time in the neutral zone
   e. Orient the sharp for easy retrieval by the surgeon or first assistant
   f. Ensure the sharp is handled by only one team member at a time
4. Place sharp items in the neutral zone after use.

[Recommendation]

5. The perioperative team may use a no-touch technique when handling sharps (e.g., loading, manipulating, removing). [Conditional Recommendation]
6. The perioperative team may use a blunt instrument (e.g., forceps or the suture packet to load and position the suture needle on the needle holder without touching the needle. [Conditional Recommendation]
7. The perioperative team may use a blunt instrument (e.g., forceps) to manipulate and guide the suture needle through tissue. Do not manipulate suture needles with gloved hands. [Conditional Recommendation]
8. If a neutral zone is not being used, a blunt instrument (e.g., forceps) may be used to turn the suture needle 90 degrees toward the box lock of the needle holder before returning the loaded needle holder. [Conditional Recommendation]
9. An instrument for loading or removing a scalpel blade on a knife handle or a single-handed scalpel blade remover should be used when a safety-engineered device is not available. [Recommendation]
10. Sharp devices must be contained, transported, and disposed of safely. [Regulatory Requirement]
11. Select sharps containers using functionality, accessibility, accommodation, and visibility criteria. [Recommendation]
12. Keep sharps disposal receptacles in an upright position when in use. [Recommendation]
13. Replace sharps containers before overfilling occurs. [Recommendation]
14. Use container devices with enhanced engineering features (e.g., counterbalanced tray, one-hand sharp deposit, hand-entry restriction, tamper-proof locks). [Recommendation]
15. Contain and isolate sharps on the sterile field (e.g., back table, Mayo stand) with a sharps containment device such as a magnetic sharps box or tray.
    a. The scrub person should account for and confine all sharps on the sterile field. [Recommendation]
    b. Segregate contaminated, reusable sharps (e.g., skin hooks, trocars) from non-sharp instruments after use, for transport to the decontamination area. [Recommendation]

HUMAN FACTOR

Although the nature of blood-borne disease, its transmission, and prevention methods are known, the human factor must be included in the planning and implementation of any risk reduction program. The following are some reasons people have difficulty with risk reduction:

- Working too quickly
- Distraction from the task at hand
- Failure to comply with precautions and standards ("It can't happen to me")
- Extreme fatigue
- Distraction related to environmental noise, including loud music and conversation. Recent studies have shown that loud music playing during surgery contributes to medical errors because it prevents clear communication.
- Lack of support in designing and maintaining a prevention program
- Difficulty abandoning old and valued methods of working
- Difficulty adapting to newer, safer medical devices

POSTEXPOSURE PROPHYLAXIS

Postexposure prophylaxis (PEP) is a risk-reduction strategy that is used following direct contact with blood or other body fluids. It involves the administration of drugs and testing. PEP is voluntary; no health care worker should be coerced into receiving it. However, the decision must be made quickly, because the preventive drugs are most effective when given within 24 hours after exposure.

Components of Postexposure Prophylaxis

Individuals exposed to HBV should be tested for HBV surface antigen, and an immunization series should be initiated. Health care workers who have not been previously vaccinated should be given hepatitis B immune globulin (HBIG) if the incident involved mucous membrane exposure or penetrating exposure to a patient's blood or other body fluids.

PEP for HIV consists of a regimen of antiviral drugs followed by regular testing. PEP must be initiated soon after exposure and has a limited effect, and additional health risks are associated with the medications used. Because PEP must be initiated within a brief period after exposure, it is vital that health care workers be evaluated rapidly and that the patient be screened for HIV before leaving the health care setting.

Antibodies generally take 25 days to 3 months to appear on standard HIV tests. The attending physician assesses the patient's HIV exposure risks. PEP includes the use of two or three antiretroviral agents to prevent the virus from attacking the immune system. These drugs are administered orally, and the regimen usually lasts for 1 month. These antiretroviral agents have a number of side effects that must be considered before PEP is initiated.

Guidelines • OSHA Bloodborne Pathogens Standard

(Association of periOperative Registered Nurses. Guidelines for perioperative practice. 2020. Transmission-based precautions. *OSHA bloodborne pathogens standard.* Standard No. 6.)

1. Perioperative personnel must follow the OSHA Bloodborne Pathogens standard when there is a risk of exposure to blood, body fluids, and other potentially infectious materials. [Regulatory Requirement]
2. Perioperative personnel must use engineering controls (e.g., safety-engineered devices) and work practice controls (e.g., neutral zone, hands-free technique). [Regulatory Requirement]
3. Perioperative personnel must wash their hands and skin with soap and water or flush their mucous membranes with water immediately or as soon as possible after coming into direct contact with blood, body fluids, or other potentially infectious materials. [Regulatory Requirement]
4. Food and drink must not be taken into the semi-restricted or restricted areas of the perioperative suite. Food and drink must not be kept in refrigerators, freezers, or cabinets or on shelves, countertops, or workspaces where blood or other potentially infectious materials are present. [Regulatory Requirement]

TRANSMISSION-BASED PRECAUTIONS

Transmission-based precautions are implemented when a patient is known or suspected to have a highly infectious disease and Standard Precautions are insufficient to prevent transmission to others. These guidelines are used in addition to Standard Precautions.

Airborne transmission precautions reduce the risk of transmission of airborne agents by droplet nuclei up to 5 micrometers in size (see Chapter 8). Because of their small size, such droplets remain suspended in the air and disperse widely in the environment.

A patient with a disease that can be spread by airborne transmission must wear a surgical mask during transport. Health care personnel must wear respiratory protection when within 3 feet (0.9 m) of such a patient. Masks must pass NIOSH-approved high-efficiency particulate air (HEPA) standards to be completely effective.

Airborne transmission precautions must be taken for the following diseases:

- Measles
- Varicella (including disseminated herpes zoster)
- Tuberculosis

NOTE *More detailed information on tuberculosis can be obtained from the CDC publication* Guidelines for Preventing the Transmission of Tuberculosis in Health Care Facilities.

Droplet precautions are implemented to reduce the risk of infectious disease transmission by large, moist aerosol droplets. These are spread from the mouth, nose, oropharynx, and trachea to a susceptible host. The traveling distance of droplets is 3 feet (0.9 m) or less, and they do not remain suspended in the air. Patients with any of the diseases that can be transmitted in this way must be separated from other patients by at least 3 feet (0.9 m), and health care workers must wear a mask when within 3 feet (0.9 m) of the patient.

A partial list of the infections for which droplet precautions should be implemented includes the following:

- Invasive infection with *Haemophilus influenzae* type B
- Invasive infection with *Neisseria meningitidis*
- Streptococcal pharyngitis
- Rubella

Contact precautions are used with patients known or suspected to harbor an infection transmitted by direct contact. In addition to Standard Precautions, the following steps are required:

- Gloves must be worn and hands must be washed before and after contact with the patient.
- Health care personnel must wear protective gowns.
- All items that come in contact with the patient must be disinfected or sterilized.

Contagious conditions for which implementation of contact precautions is required include the following:

- Infection with the herpes simplex virus
- Impetigo
- Uncontained abscesses, cellulitis, or decubitus ulcers
- Disseminated herpes zoster
- Infection with *Clostridium difficile*
- Infection with any multidrug-resistant bacterium

HAZARDOUS WASTE

The EPA defines medical waste as any solid waste generated in the diagnosis, treatment, or immunization of humans or animals, in research that involves people or animals, or in the production or testing of biologicals. For example, this includes the following:

- Soiled or blood-soaked bandages
- Culture dishes and other glassware
- Discarded surgical gloves after surgery
- Discarded surgical instruments and scalpels
- Needles used to give injections or draw blood
- Cultures, stocks, and swabs used to inoculate cultures
- Removed body organs (e.g., tonsils, appendices, limbs)

Besides the EPA, the federal agencies associated with the regulation of various aspects of medical waste include the FDA, OSHA, and the Nuclear Regulatory Commission (NRC). Medical waste disposal also is regulated at the state level, and each state has laws that apply specifically to medical waste.

Infectious waste must be separated from all other waste and placed in red biohazard disposal bags. (The common term for medical waste is *red bag waste*.) The biohazard symbol may or may not appear on the bag. The bag color and biohazard symbol are a form of hazard communication to anyone who later handles the waste material. Any person handling infectious waste, from the point of generation until its destruction, must wear PPE. Gloves must be worn at all times. Face shields and protective gowns protect the handler from splash hazards.

Guidelines for the handling and disposal of waste in the operating room environment include the following:

- Always wear gloves when handling any object contaminated with blood or body fluids.
- Red waste bags for infectious material must be available during case cleanup.
- Do not place noninfectious waste in red waste bags. The cost of processing is 10 times higher for infectious waste than for noninfectious waste.
- Place all sharps in an impenetrable sharps container.
- Do not overload sharps containers. Container overflow is one of the major causes of blood-borne disease transmission among health care workers.
- If it is necessary to examine items in a refuse bag, separate the items carefully by spreading them on an impermeable sheet or drape. Never handle waste material unless you can see what is contained in the refuse bag. Sharps may be present among trash and cause serious injury.
- Handle suction canisters and other blood containers with extreme caution. The practice of opening suction canisters used during surgery and pouring the contents into an open hopper puts workers at extremely high risk for disease transmission. Blood and fluid solidifiers are available. After fluids are solidified, they can be placed in tear-resistant plastic bags.
- Bags must not be loaded beyond their tensile strength. Double bagging may be necessary.
- Separate soiled reusable linen from disposable paper products and unsoiled items at the point of use.
- Keep all contaminated (soiled) or potentially contaminated waste separate from uncontaminated goods.
- Do not compact waste contained in plastic bags. Pack loosely and secure the open end.
- When transporting medical waste, do not use trash chutes or dumbwaiters. Use a transport cart.

A designated area of the operating room is reserved for the disposal of infectious waste. This must be completely separated from restricted and semi-restricted areas of the department. Biohazard signs should be posted in areas of waste disposal.

KEY CONCEPTS

- Evidence-based practice is a way of making decisions and acting on proven methods. It uses rational decision making rather than opinion or past practice. Methods derived through evidence-based practice can be traced to accepted authority (peer review) and the highest level of professional inquiry.
- Professional surgical technologists are engaged in health care practices that use evidence-based knowledge and methods. The modern surgical technologist must be familiar with evidence-based thinking and acting.
- Sterile technique is a method of preventing the contamination of instruments, supplies, and equipment used in critical and semi-critical areas of the body.
- Sterile technique is based on a set of principles that must be learned and practiced until they are intuitive.
- The basis of sterile technique is the concept of barriers between contaminated and sterile surfaces. Sterile objects or surfaces are contained or confined to prevent their contact with nonsterile objects.
- A contaminated surface is one that has been suspected of or has actually come in contact with a nonsterile surface.
- The domains of sterile technique include surgical attire, hand hygiene, gowning and gloving, surgical drapes, and techniques for handling sterile equipment.
- Perioperative personnel are required to wear scrub suit attire that has been freshly laundered and not previously worn.
- A surgical head cover is worn to cover all hair, the scalp, and hairline. During surgery, a sterile gown and gloves are worn as barriers between nonsterile skin and scrub attire and the surgical field.
- The sterile field is the area covered by sterile drapes. It includes scrubbed personnel who are gowned and gloved. The draped patient is the center of the sterile field.
- Surgical conscience is the practice of sterile technique, reporting when sterility has been broken, and taking measures to reestablish sterility. In cases of gross contamination of the surgical wound, medical therapy may be initiated to prevent infection.

REVIEW QUESTIONS

1. What is the purpose of sterile technique?
2. How do standards agencies decide on rules of sterile technique?
3. What strategy would you advise for another student who is extremely nervous about gowning and gloving?

4. As a student, would you let the surgeon know if he contaminated his glove during surgery?
5. How would you go about researching a question related to sterile technique? Would you use Wikipedia?
6. While putting on sterile gloves, you touch the glove wrapper with your finger. Is the wrapper still sterile?
7. What is the sterile field?
8. Why do we need to practice Standard Precautions?
9. What is hazardous waste?
10. What does PPE protect us from?
11. What is the bloodborne pathogens standard? Why is it important to your profession?

CASE STUDY

There are an infinite number of ways that sterile technique can be broken before and during surgery. However, some are very common. Provide an example of how sterile technique can be broken for each of the following scenarios.

1. During steam sterilization
2. While opening a case
3. While delivering solutions
4. During hand antisepsis or scrub
5. During surgery

REFERENCE

1. Association of periOperative Registered Nurses (AORN). *Guidelines for Perioperative Practice*. 2020 ed. Denver: AORN; 2019.

BIBLIOGRAPHY

Berrios-Torres SI, Umscheid CA, Bratzler DW, et al. Centers for disease control and prevention guideline for the prevention of surgical site infection, 2017. *JAMA Surg*. 2017;152(8):784–791. [IVA].

Hopper WR, Moss R. Common breaks in sterile technique: clinical perspectives and perioperative implications. *AORN J*. 2010;91(3):350–367. https://doi.org/10.1016/j.aorn.2009.09.027.

Occupational Safety and Health Administration (OSHA): Bloodborne pathogens. Available at https://www.osha.gov/bloodborne-pathogens/general. Accessed Nov. 11, 2020.

World Health Organization (WHO). *WHO Guidelines on Hand Hygiene in Health Care*. Geneva: World Health Organization; 2009. http://apps.who.int/iris/bitstream/10665/44102/1/9789241597906_eng.pdf. Accessed October 21, 2015

DECONTAMINATION, STERILIZATION, AND DISINFECTION

10

LEARNING OBJECTIVES

After studying this chapter, the reader will be able to:

1. Correctly use terms related to disinfection and sterilization
2. Explain the Spaulding system of classification
3. Describe the steps of reprocessing surgical instruments from the point of use to sterilization
4. Discuss the principles and processes of decontamination
5. Explain the rationale for specific methods of wrapping of instruments and loading of the steam sterilizer
6. Explain the principles of gas sterilization
7. Describe special processing required for instruments exposed to Creutzfeldt–Jakob disease
8. Distinguish between disinfection and sterilization
9. Recognize the hazards associated with the use of chemical disinfectants
10. Describe terminal cleaning of the operating room environment

TERMINOLOGY

Antiseptic: A chemical used to remove microbes from the skin.

-cidal: A suffix indicating death. For example, bactericidal means "able to kill bacteria."

Bactericidal: A bactericidal is a chemical that kills bacteria.

Bacteriostatic: Chemical agent capable of inhibiting the growth of bacteria.

Bioburden: The number of contaminating microbes on an object.

Biofilm: Dense colonies of bacteria that adhere tightly to surfaces.

Biological indicator (BI): A quality control mechanism used in the process of sterilization. It consists of a closed system containing harmless, spore-forming bacteria that can be rapidly cultured after the sterilization process.

Bowie-Dick test: A test that identifies air leaks and ineffective air removal in the steam sterilization process.

Case cart system: A method of transporting surgical supplies and equipment to and from the instrument processing and supply areas.

Cavitation: A process during ultrasonic cleaning in which air bubbles implode (burst inward), releasing particles of soil or tissue debris.

Chemical indicator (CI): A method of testing a sterilization parameter. Chemical strips sensitive to physical conditions, such as temperature, are placed with the item being sterilized and change color when the parameter is reached; sometimes called a chemical monitor.

Chemical sterilization: A process that uses chemical agents to achieve sterilization.

Clean: The absence of soil on a surface.

Cleaning: A process that removes organic or inorganic soil or debris using friction, detergent, and water.

Contaminated: Rendered nonsterile and unacceptable for use in critical areas of the body.

Decontamination: A process in which soiled medical devices, including instruments, are made safe for personnel to handle.

Detergent: A chemical that breaks down organic debris by emulsification (separation into small particles) to aid in cleaning.

Disinfection: Destruction of microorganisms by heat or chemical means. Disinfection does not produce sterility because not all microbial forms are destroyed in the process.

Environmental cleaning: The process of cleaning the surfaces in patient care areas, including the operating room. This includes floors, cabinets, equipment, lights, and furniture.

Enzymatic cleaner: A specific chemical used in detergents and cleaners to penetrate and break down biological debris, such as blood.

Ethylene oxide (EO): A highly flammable gas that is capable of sterilizing an object.

Event-related sterility: A wrapped sterile item may become contaminated by environmental conditions or events, such as a puncture in the wrapper. Event-related sterility refers to sterility based on the absence of such events. The shelf life of a sterilized pack is event related, not time related.

Exposure time: This is the amount of time goods are held in specific conditions during disinfection or the sterilization process. Exposure time varies with the size of the load, type of materials being sterilized, and the type of agent used. Exposure time is sometimes called the hold time.

Gas plasma sterilization: A process that uses the form of matter known as plasma during the sterilization process.

Gravity-displacement sterilizer: A type of steam sterilizer that removes air by gravity.

TERMINOLOGY (CONT.)

High-level disinfection (HLD): A process that reduces the bioburden to an absolute minimum.

High-vacuum sterilizer: A type of steam sterilizer that removes air in the chamber by vacuum and refills it with pressurized steam. Also known as a pre-vacuum sterilizer.

Immediate-use steam sterilization (IUSS): Rapid sterilization of instruments to be used immediately. This process was previously called flash sterilization.

Implant: Defined by the U.S. Food and Drug Administration (FDA) as "a device that is placed into a surgically or naturally formed cavity of the human body if it is intended to remain there for a period of 30 days or more."

Ionizing radiation: A method of bulk sterilization used by manufacturers to sterilize prepackaged equipment using cobalt-60 radiation.

Low-level disinfection: A method used to disinfect patient care items that contact only the skin.

Material Safety Data Sheet (MSDS): A government-mandated requirement for all chemicals used in the workplace. The MSDS describes the formulation, safe use, precautions, and emergency response.

Medical device: Any equipment, instrument, implant, material, or apparatus used in the diagnosis, treatment, or monitoring of patients.

Nonwoven: A fabric or material that is bonded together as opposed to a process of interweaving individual threads.

Peracetic acid: A chemical used in the sterilization of critical items.

Personal protective equipment (PPE): Approved attire that acts as a complete barrier between the wearer and the environment.

Physical monitor: A device that automatically provides output on the physical parameters of the sterilization process. Output includes printouts, gauges, and a digital display.

Prion: An infectious protein particle that is a unique pathogenic substance containing no nucleic acid. The prion is resistant to most forms of disinfection and sterilization normally used in the health care setting.

Reposable: An instrument that may be reprocessed a limited number of times. After the specific number of reprocessing events, the instrument must be withdrawn from use.

Reprocessing: Activities or tasks that prepare used medical devices for patient use.

Reusable: A designation used by manufacturers to indicate that a medical device can be reprocessed for use on more than one patient.

Sharps: Any objects used in health care that are capable of penetrating the skin, causing injury.

Single-use items: Instruments and devices intended for one-time use on one patient only.

Spaulding system: A system used to determine the level of microbial destruction required for medical devices and supplies. Each level is based on the risk of infection associated with the area of the body where the device is used.

Sporicidal: Able to kill spores.

Sterile Processing Department (SPD): The hospital department where medical devices and equipment are reprocessed; this process may also take place in a Central Processing (CP) department.

Sterilization: A process by which all microorganisms, including bacterial spores, are destroyed.

Terminal cleaning: A daily process in which exposed surfaces of the operating room are cleaned and disinfected.

Turnover: Cleaning, disinfection, and preparation of the operating room between patients.

Washer–sterilizer/disinfector: Equipment that washes and decontaminates instruments so that they can be safely handled by personnel.

Woven wrappers: Also called linen or cloth wrappers, these are fabric cloths used to wrap clean, disinfected supplies in preparation for a sterilization process.

In the community, people avoid infection through hygiene practices, public health measures such as vaccination, and healthy lifestyle behaviors. In the perioperative setting, patients are vulnerable to infection by instruments, equipment, surgical drapes, and medical supplies used during a surgical procedure. The environment, including the operating room furniture (e.g., instrument tables, operating table), floors, and even the air, is also a potential source of infection. This chapter describes the principles and methods required to prevent disease transmission by instruments, medical devices, supplies, and the surgical environment. The concepts and practices presented in this chapter bring together the science of microbiology and aseptic technique. The health care facility is a congested setting in which pathogens have ample opportunity to thrive. All procedures for decontamination of equipment and the surgical environment are performed to prevent disease transmission and apply to patients and staff.

All instruments used in a surgical procedure must be sterile—completely free of microbes. The procedures required to prepare instruments are called the reprocessing cycle. All of the activities in the cycle are performed according to standards that have been validated by research and are required by professional organizations.

STANDARDS IN SURGICAL DECONTAMINATION, DISINFECTION, AND STERILIZATION

Standards for the reprocessing of instruments, devices, and equipment in the perioperative environment are based on evidence established only after research has been conducted to prove the validity of a practice. The following organizations are responsible for performing this research or validating standards based on the evidence. The organizations are listed in alphabetical order:

- *Association for the Advancement of Medical Instrumentation (AAMI):* The AAMI provides recommended practices and technical information for the US medical professions. Standards are developed with the support of the U.S. Food and Drug Administration (FDA). http://www.aami.org
- *Association of periOperative Registered Nurses (AORN):* AORN is the professional association for perioperative nurses that performs research and publishes standards and guidelines of practice for all areas of perioperative care. http://www.aorn.org
- *Association of Surgical Technologists (AST):* The AST is the professional organization of surgical technologists that

publishes guidelines for many practices in the perioperative setting. http://www.ast.org

- *Centers for Disease Control and Prevention (CDC):* The federal agency that provides research and protocols in all areas of public health. http://www.cdc.gov
- *Centers for Disease Control and Prevention–Healthcare Infection Control Practices Advisory Committee (CDC-HICPAC):* Joint federal agencies that provide research and protocols in all areas of public health and infection control, including those in the professional environment. http://www.cdc.gov/hicpac/pubs.html
- *ECRI Institute:* Research and consulting organization that applies scientific research to determine which medical procedures, devices, drugs, and processes are best for patient care. http://www.ecri.org
- *The Joint Commission (TJC):* The accreditation agency for all health care organizations in the United States. It oversees compliance with environmental and patient safety regulations and enforces compliance with standards. http://www.jointcommission.org/
- *U.S. Food and Drug Administration (FDA):* The federal agency responsible for the regulation of medical devices, drugs, food, and cosmetics. http://www.fda.gov/

Standards and regulations are implemented through the policies of the health care provider. Management teams in infection control and in the **Sterile Processing Department (SPD)** or Central Processing Department (CPD) develop ways to implement the standards and monitor the outcomes, whereas the actual tasks are performed by perioperative and SPD staff. These areas are discussed below. Surgical technologists have a very important role in implementing standards related to infection control. It is important for students and working technologists to keep up with changing standards and help others become aware of new standards.

PRINCIPLES OF DECONTAMINATION, STERILIZATION, AND DISINFECTION

IMPORTANT TERMS

Before studying the material in this chapter, the reader should become familiar with basic terminology related to the processes discussed. Ongoing research and new technology often produce new terms. It is important to learn updated terms, because they accurately describe current technology that has been validated by standards agencies. The following are basic definitions used throughout the chapter.

- An **antiseptic** is a chemical used to remove microorganisms *on skin* or other tissue. This process is referred to as *antisepsis.* Surgical hand rubs and soaps contain an antiseptic. The patient's skin is cleaned with an antiseptic just before surgery to reduce the number of microorganisms. Some chemicals have dual-purpose qualities (i.e., they may be used on tissue and objects). However, if a chemical is labeled a *disinfectant,* it is intended for inanimate (nonliving) surfaces only.
- **Bacteriostatic** refers to a process or chemical that inhibits bacterial colonization (growth) but does not destroy bacteria.
- As discussed in Chapter 8, the **bioburden** is the number of live *bacterial colonies* on a surface before it is sterilized. For example, endoscopes used in gastrointestinal procedures contain a high level of bioburden and require meticulous cleaning and **high-level disinfection (HLD)** after use. A **biofilm** is composed of dense colonies of microbes that are attached to surfaces. These films are extremely resistant to physical cleaning and chemical removal. Biofilms can be a source of infection. **Contaminated** refers to any surface or tissue that has come in contact with a *potential* or actual source of microorganisms.
- **Cleaning** is the process of removing surface soil, blood, body fluids, and other kinds of organic debris with detergents and mechanical action (scrubbing or washing).
- **Disinfection** is a process that removes most but not all microbes on inanimate surfaces. Most disinfectants are not safe for use on tissues. Some disinfectants are formulated for use on surgical equipment, whereas others are used for environmental cleaning.
- **Reprocessing** refers to all the steps necessary to render soiled **medical devices,** including surgical instruments, safe for use on the patient.
- **Sterilization** is a process that results in the complete destruction of all forms of life on an object. An object is either sterile or not sterile. There are no "levels" of sterility.
- **Terminal cleaning** of the operating room environment takes place daily. The process includes removal of organic soil from all exposed surfaces of the critical and semi-critical areas of the operating room.
- Terminal **decontamination** is a process in which instruments and supplies are processed so that they are safe for staff to handle during subsequent stages of reprocessing.

SPAULDING CLASSIFICATION SYSTEM

The **Spaulding system** provides health care professionals a way to determine if a patient care device requires sterilization, disinfection (reduction of microbes but not complete eradication), or only surface cleaning to remove traces of organic soil. The system allows health care workers to select the exact method of reprocessing according to where in the body the item will be used. The system is based on *the level of risk for infection associated with that part of the body.*

These classifications do not specify the method used to reprocess the equipment. The method is determined by what the instrument or equipment is made of and by the manufacturer's recommended method.

- HIGH RISK is assigned to CRITICAL ITEMS. Critical items are those that come in contact with *sterile body tissues* such as internal organ systems and the vascular system. Examples are surgical instruments, vascular cannulas, and hypodermic needles. All medical devices in this category must be sterile.
- INTERMEDIATE RISK is assigned to SEMI-CRITICAL ITEMS. Semi-critical devices are those used on *nonintact skin* or mucous membranes. Any device in this category requires HLD. Examples are endotracheal tubes and airways, rectal instruments, and vaginal instruments.

- LOW RISK is assigned to NON-CRITICAL ITEMS. These are items that only come in contact with *intact skin.* Examples are a blood pressure cuff and stethoscope. These require cleaning with a low-level disinfectant.

STERILE PROCESSING DEPARTMENT

In most large health care facilities, high volume reprocessing takes place in the health facility's Sterile Processing Department (SPD). The personnel responsible for this are the *sterile processing technicians.* This is a skilled, certifiable profession that requires expertise in the science and practice of materials management, decontamination, and sterilization. In smaller facilities, surgical technologists may fill the role and perform tasks required for processing surgical equipment.

All instruments and equipment used in surgery are transferred to the SPD or other stand-alone area of the hospital for reprocessing. A high level of coordination is required between perioperative personnel and the CP staff to ensure a smooth **turnover** of supplies. Sterile processing personnel must ensure that equipment is safe and ready for scheduled surgery and that thousands of instruments are organized and processed according to standards. Perioperative staff members are under pressure to deliver equipment that is fully intact, with no missing parts, and ready for immediate use in the surgical field. This collaboration works when staff members from the departments understand and respect each other's roles. A bond of trust exists as well. The CP staff must handle extremely sharp and potentially dangerous equipment that arrives directly from the operating room. The surgical technologist has a responsibility to prepare equipment for processing in a way that protects CP personnel from injury. CP staff members must appreciate the need for instrument trays to be complete and ready for use in time for a scheduled procedure.

Personnel in both departments also must understand the critical nature of their work—disease prevention and safety for patients and staff.

QUALITY CONTROL MONITORING

Procedures and methods for reprocessing medical devices must be monitored to ensure patient safety. Monitoring means *checking, recording,* and *reporting.* Quality control includes monitoring the *technologies* (such as the steam sterilizer or instrument washer) used in reprocessing, as well as the *human* factor. (Is the person following the correct procedure? Do they understand the process? Are they protecting themselves from injury during the process?) The human and technical aspects are equally important.

REPROCESSING SINGLE-USE DEVICES

Single-use, or disposable, medical devices and products have come into widespread use in the past two decades. The debate over environmental damage, use of shrinking natural resources, and waste is a separate issue and should be an ongoing discussion. The trend favoring disposables is unlikely to change as long as patients and medical professionals create a demand for such products even though they are environmentally unsound.

The increased acceptance of single-use products has created a need for regulations and recommendations covering reprocessing of these items. **Single-use items** are those meant to be used on one patient, only once. These are manufactured under FDA approval for their intended use on one patient. However, many items opened for surgery are never used and eventually discarded as waste. To cut costs and retrieve the high cost of these items, some institutions reprocess the items. Commercial reprocessing services are available for instruments and equipment *approved for reprocessing* by the manufacturer. However, unless the manufacturer states specifically that the item can be reprocessed by the health care facility, the safety of a single-use device may be compromised. The health care facility is liable for any patient injury that occurs as a result of malfunction of a reprocessed single-use item that is not approved for multiple use.

REPOSABLE INSTRUMENTS

Reposable instruments or components are those that may only be reprocessed a specific number of times. The exact number and method of reprocessing is established by the manufacturer. Examples of reposable instruments are some robotic instruments and detachable endoscopic cutting instruments such as scissors whose tips do not retain their sharpness. The reposable scissor tips are fitted to a nondisposable handle. Tracking the number of times a device is reprocessed is sometimes problematic. Therefore some manufacturers have made the decision to retire their reposable instruments in favor of a disposable-only format.

IMPORTANT TO KNOW *The surgical technologist must ensure that reposable instruments and instrument components are not discarded inadvertently.*

LOANER INSTRUMENTS

Specialty instruments and surgical implant sets used on loan from sources outside the health care facility may arrive through health care industry representatives or other sources. Sometimes instruments are wrapped and have undergone a sterilization process. *The sterility of these items must not be assumed.* This is because there is no way to track the conditions under which the instruments were stored or transported. Therefore all loaner instruments should be processed first by decontamination and then by a sterilization method approved for those particular instruments by the manufacturer. In most cases, the health care facility will have a contractual agreement with the industry representative covering how the instruments are transported and cared for while on loan, including decontamination and sterilization before and after use.

REPROCESSING CYCLE

Reprocessing is a step-by-step procedure that follows an exact protocol. It starts at the point of use in surgery and ends with

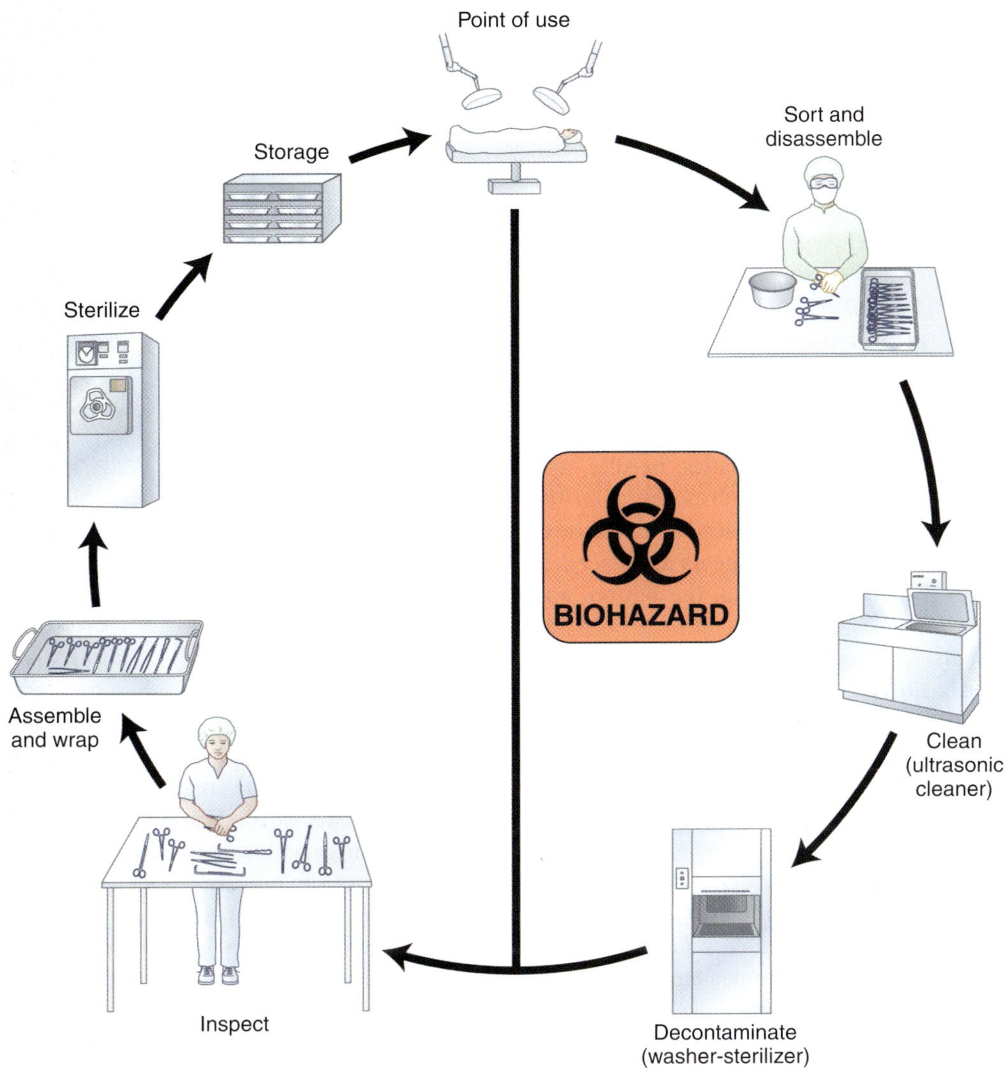

FIG. 10.1 Cycle of reprocessing, starting at the point of use.

equipment that is ready and safe for the surgical patient (Fig. 10.1). The correct order of the stages of the cycle are as follows:

1. *Point-of-use cleaning:* The ST prevents the buildup of blood and tissue debris on instruments during the surgical procedure.
2. *Sorting and disassembly:* At the end of the procedure, the ST prepares the soiled instruments for the next stage by sorting the instruments and disassembling those with multiple parts.
3. *Cleaning the instruments:* Instruments are cleaned to remove tissue and other debris in preparation for the next phase.
4. *Decontamination:* Instruments are put through a rigorous process of washing and decontamination to make them safe for handling.
5. *Sorting and inspection:* Instruments and other devices that have been decontaminated are separated by type and inspected for damage, malfunction, or incomplete cleaning.
6. *Assembly:* Instruments are assembled in standardized sets according to a specific type of surgery.
7. *Wrapping:* Instrument sets and single items to be sterilized by steam or gas are wrapped in a prescribed way to protect their sterility after reprocessing.
8. *Storage:* Wrapped sterile instruments are stored in a specific way and place to prevent their contamination during storage.

CLEANING AT THE POINT OF USE

The preparation of equipment and instruments for patient use begins at the point of use in surgery. In the perioperative environment, this means during surgery and immediately afterward. During surgery, instruments and equipment exposed to blood and body tissue are kept free of blood and debris to prevent caking and drying. Dried blood and tissue debris make instruments difficult to operate and should not be re-introduced into the surgical wound. Frequently wiping instruments helps to reduce biofilm that adheres to instruments and can prevent sterilization. A sponge moistened with water can be used for this purpose, or instruments can be placed in a basin of water. Suction tips and other cannulated (hollow tube) instruments should be periodically flushed with water. Saline is not used on instruments at any stage, because it causes pitting, rusting, and corrosion.

Non-immersible sterile equipment exposed to blood and body fluids should also be wiped down periodically during surgery. This includes digital cameras, light cables, and power equipment.

CLOSE OF SURGERY

At the close of surgery, the ST separates the equipment by category:

- Sharp
- Delicate
- Heavy
- Non-immersible
- Immersible

Disposable **"sharps"** such as scalpel blades, needles, and other disposable cutting instruments are disposed of in the proper container. Sharp instruments are placed in a puncture-proof container to prevent injury. Instruments are placed in a separate basin, with the heaviest ones on the bottom and lighter ones on top.

Delicate instruments that require hand washing are placed in a separate tray or basin. Water that was used to soak the instruments during surgery is suctioned off before the equipment is transported out of the room; this prevents spills and contamination of the environment. The equipment is placed on a covered or closed transportation cart for transfer to the decontamination area.

NOTE *All instruments opened on the sterile field must be processed regardless of whether they were used in the surgical procedure. Instruments may have been contaminated by air droplets or by direct contact. These events would not have been observed by the ST or other members of the team. These items should be separated from grossly soiled instruments for transport.*

TRANSPORT OF SOILED INSTRUMENTS TO DECONTAMINATION AREA

After surgery, all instruments and soiled equipment must be transported to the decontamination area in closed containers or a closed *case cart* (Fig. 10.2). Using the **case cart system,** sterile instruments and supplies are loaded onto a **clean** cart before surgery for transport to the surgical suite. The ST is responsible for loading the cart and transferring it to the decontamination area for processing. If a case cart system is not used, all soiled items must be contained in leak-proof bags for transportation to the decontamination area. An alternative method of containing contaminated instruments is by using a *biohazard transport container*. This is a heavy plastic tray fitted with safety locks that prevent leakage and allow contaminated instruments to be safely transported to the decontamination area. The composition of the container allows it to be exposed to high temperature and chemicals, and some models are red with the biohazard symbol clearly stamped into the container. Current vendors are Healthmark and Instrusafe.

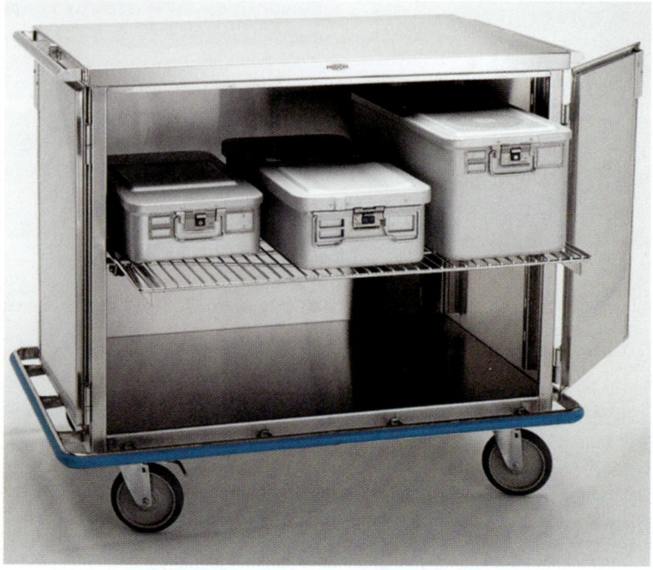

FIG. 10.2 Case cart used to transport sterile packs to the surgical suite and return them to the decontamination area after surgery. (Courtesy Pedigo Products, Vancouver, WA.)

Regardless of the system used, it must be completely closed and leak-proof and carry an orange or red biohazard label. This is an occupational regulation. The ST should transport the instruments as soon as possible to the decontamination area after surgery. Ideally, they should be washed within 20 minutes. This is to prevent blood, tissue, and biofilm from drying on the surfaces, where it can be difficult to remove and can impede sterilization. Upon arrival in the decontamination area, the case cart is unloaded for washing. The cart itself is then decontaminated in a designated washer for that purpose. Clean carts are then ready for preparation of another surgical procedure.

NOTE *Fiber-optic endoscopes are often processed by perioperative staff and stored in a location near the point of use, separate from the decontamination area. Cleaning, disinfection, and sterilization require special techniques that are closely associated with the instrument design. Chapter 20 presents a complete discussion on the processing of fiber-optic equipment.*

INSTRUMENT CLEANING AND DECONTAMINATION

To prevent cross-contamination the decontamination area is completely separated from areas where clean equipment is being processed. Sinks for washing soiled instruments are designated for that purpose only. Equipment and tools needed to clean instruments, such as brushes and stylets, are available in the decontamination area. The ultrasonic cleaner and washer–sterilizer are also located here. A source of deionized or distilled water is necessary for rinsing instruments and compressed air for drying tubular instruments. Chemicals such as detergents, disinfectants, and enzymatic cleaners are available. Eye wash stations are located throughout the department so that they can be accessed within 10 seconds of a chemical eye injury.

DECONTAMINATION ATTIRE (PPE)

All staff members who work in the decontamination area must wear **personal protective equipment (PPE)** in compliance with the Occupational Safety and Health Administration (OSHA) regulations. This is necessary to protect staff from potential infection from splashes and skin contact with contaminated instruments.

PPE includes the following:

- Protective eyewear (i.e., goggles with side shields) or a full face shield
- Mask
- Cuffed gloves approved for contact with chemicals
- Full protective body suit or gown with a waterproof apron and sleeves
- Waterproof shoes and covers

NOTE *PPE, by definition, must be impenetrable by liquids. Routine surgical attire, except for face shields and goggles, does not qualify as PPE.*

SORTING INSTRUMENTS

After arriving in the decontamination area from a surgical procedure, the instruments are sorted. Although some sorting takes place at the point of use, all instruments must be broken down into parts and separated by weight and complexity before decontamination. This is done to prevent damage to delicate items and prevent injury during reprocessing. It is also important to gather the small parts of instruments (pins, gaskets, screws) and keep them together to prevent their loss during reprocessing.

Items are removed from the transport cart and grouped together by category:

- Non-immersible equipment or instruments
- Instruments with sharp edges or points
- Gaskets, screws, pins, and other small parts
- Heavy instruments
- Delicate instruments
- Heat- and pressure-sensitive instruments
- Instrument containers
- Basins and cups
- Tubing, suction tips, or other hollow instruments
- Instruments or equipment requiring repair or replacement

After sorting, instruments and equipment must be cleaned before they are disinfected. Dried blood, body fluids, and tissue debris remaining on instruments can trap microorganisms and become contaminants. This debris can also cause instrument damage and malfunction.

Cleaning is performed by hand, ultrasonic cleaner, followed by the automated washer/disinfector/sterilizer.

HAND CLEANING THE INSTRUMENTS

After the instruments have been sorted, delicate instruments that could be damaged in an automated washer–sterilizer are soaked in enzymatic **detergent.** While immersed in the soaking solution, instruments can be hand cleaned using warm water and enzymatic cleaner. The temperature of the water bath should be determined according to directions from the detergent manufacturer. Some enzymatic detergents are deactivated at temperatures over 140°F (90°C). During hand cleaning, the instruments should be held under the water line to prevent the release of contaminated airborne droplets.

Areas that are difficult to clean are scrubbed with a small brush. Particular attention is paid to hemostats and other clamps, orthopedic rasps, and other instruments that trap bits of soft tissue or bone. Items with a lumen such as suction devices and tubing are cleaned with a soft, narrow brush. The correct-size brush must be used to be effective. Brushes that are bent or have sections of missing bristles are not efficient for removing tissue and biofilm. Suction tips are cleared with a stylet, a fine wire that is passed through the instrument to push out debris. Instruments with channels and valves require disassembly for complete cleaning. Small parts should be kept together in one location to prevent loss.

Equipment and specialty instruments that are not immersible are cleaned according to the manufacturer's specifications. After cleaning, instruments must be completely rinsed in distilled or deionized water to remove all traces of detergent and debris.

ULTRASONIC CLEANING

The ultrasonic cleaner removes debris from instruments by a process called **cavitation.** High-frequency sound waves are generated through a water bath, causing tiny air bubbles trapped within the debris to implode (explode inwardly); this releases the debris from the instrument.

The ultrasonic cleaner has one or more recessed sinks that are filled with water and **enzymatic cleaner** intended for use in the system. Many instruments are damaged by ultrasonic energy, and manufacturers of medical devices are careful to state whether the item can be exposed to ultrasonic energy.

To be effective, all instruments must be fully opened before placing them in the ultrasonic bath. Valves, stopcocks, and channels must be opened to allow the water bath to contact all surfaces of the instrument, including the inside channels.

The ultrasonic water bath can become heavily soiled with tissue debris and other organic soil after repeated use. Water that is visibly soiled should not be used, because the water can become a source of bacterial contamination. Certain bacteria can colonize in soiled water, leaving heat-resistant biofilm on the surface of the equipment's recessed sinks. Some manufacturers of the equipment specify that fresh water and cleaner should be used on each batch of equipment. Each day, the sinks must be emptied and dried. The chambers are then wiped down with 70% alcohol.

NOTE *Ultrasonic cleaning alone does not decontaminate or sterilize instruments.*

WASHER-STERILIZER/DISINFECTOR

After hand washing or a cycle in the ultrasonic cleaner, instruments are subjected to a cycle in the washer-disinfector, also called a **washer-sterilizer/disinfector.** This equipment has a single front-loaded chamber or operates using a tunnel system where a large quantity of instruments can be run at one time. In both systems, instruments are loaded into the washer's trays securely to prevent damage during processing. Only detergent that is recommended by the equipment manufacturer is used. This ensures that the detergent is compatible with the system and complies with safety standards.

The full cycle includes immersion in a water bath and forceful water spray. Some washer-sterilizer systems have an ultrasonic phase as part of the cycle. Finally, the load is rinsed and dried. Most instrument washers have an optional sterilization cycle.

To process equipment in the washer-sterilizer/disinfector, the instruments are opened and the hinges extended to their widest adjustment. The instruments are then placed in metal baskets and loaded into the washer chamber. Steel basins, bowls, and containers are also processed in an automatic washer. These are not placed in with the instruments but processed separately to prevent damage to the instruments and ensure their complete contact with water and steam.

At the conclusion of this process, the instruments can be handled by personnel.

After cleaning and disinfection, instruments are lubricated to ensure smooth mechanical action. This process is used on stainless steel instruments and other selected equipment according to the manufacturer's recommendations. Only lubricants approved for use on specific medical devices are used; a variety of lubricants are available. Although oils may be needed for the internal mechanisms of power equipment, these must not be used for surface lubrication. This is because the sterilization process may not penetrate the oil. Steel instruments may be dipped in a combined lubricating and protective "instrument milk" as the final stage in cleaning and decontamination. Instrument milk can also be added to the rinse cycle of some washer-sterilizers/disinfectors.

SPECIAL HANDLING OF OPHTHALMIC INSTRUMENTS

Ophthalmic instruments require special reprocessing to prevent toxic anterior segment syndrome (TASS). This is an acute inflammatory condition in which the anterior segment of the eye becomes damaged, with possible injury to the intraocular tissue and loss of vision. This condition occurs postoperatively and is most often seen after cataract surgery. The condition has been associated mainly with instrument reprocessing. The causative factors may be contaminated ultrasonic cleaners, contaminated instruments, detergent and enzymatic cleaner residue on instruments, and the use of glutaraldehyde during sterilization. Other factors include incomplete instrument cleaning resulting in residue from viscoelastic material (used during cataract surgery) and steam impurities occurring during sterilization.

Special reprocessing methods used on ophthalmic instruments to prevent TASS must be used. These are described in Box 10.1.

BOX 10.1 General Guidelines for Processing of Ophthalmic Instruments to Prevent Toxic Anterior Segment Syndrome (TASS)

- During surgery, instruments should be wiped clean with a lint-free sponge and water.
- At the end of the procedure, the instruments must be immediately submersed in sterile water.
- Single-use cannulas (fine suction tubing) should be used if possible. If these are not available, the lumens of the cannulas must be flushed with sterile water immediately after the procedure.
- All phacoemulsification tips, tubing, handpieces, and other components must be flushed before they are disconnected at the close of surgery according to the manufacturer's instructions.
- Only single-use brushes and syringes are used to clean ophthalmic instruments. These should be discarded after use.
- Items that have been manually or ultrasonically cleaned should be wiped with alcohol before sterilization and according to the manufacturer's instructions.
- All instruments should be inspected thoroughly for residue before sterilization.

For detailed guidelines on reprocessing ophthalmic equipment to prevent TASS, refer to the AAMI standard, AAMI ST79, and the American Society of Cataract and Refractive Surgery (ASCRS).

INSTRUMENTS EXPOSED TO PRION DISEASE

A **prion** is a protein particle that is not a cell and is not related to bacteria or viruses. Creutzfeldt–Jakob disease (CJD) and *variant* CJD are fatal diseases caused by prions. These are highly infective in central nervous system tissue, and they are of special concern in the processing of instruments and equipment used on patients with known or suspected prion disease. Prions are not destroyed by normal means of mechanical or **chemical sterilization**. Because of this, disposable supplies and instruments are used whenever practical in cases in which patients present with a high or known risk for having CJD or other spongiform infection. During surgery on patients with known or suspected disease, instruments must be kept moist throughout the surgical procedure, preparation, and transport of equipment to the decontamination area. This is because the prion is rapidly adherent to dry stainless steel but less viable in the presence of moisture. The current guideline for disinfection and sterilization of instruments that have been or are suspected to have been in contact with prions is that published by the Society for Healthcare Epidemiology of America (SHEA).

SORTING AND INSPECTION

After the decontamination process, all instruments are safe for handling. They are taken to the clean assembly area for sorting and inspection. The clean processing area is separated from the decontamination area to prevent cross-contamination. The area includes a workroom with ample table space for sorting and assembling instrument sets (Fig. 10.3A). Attire in the

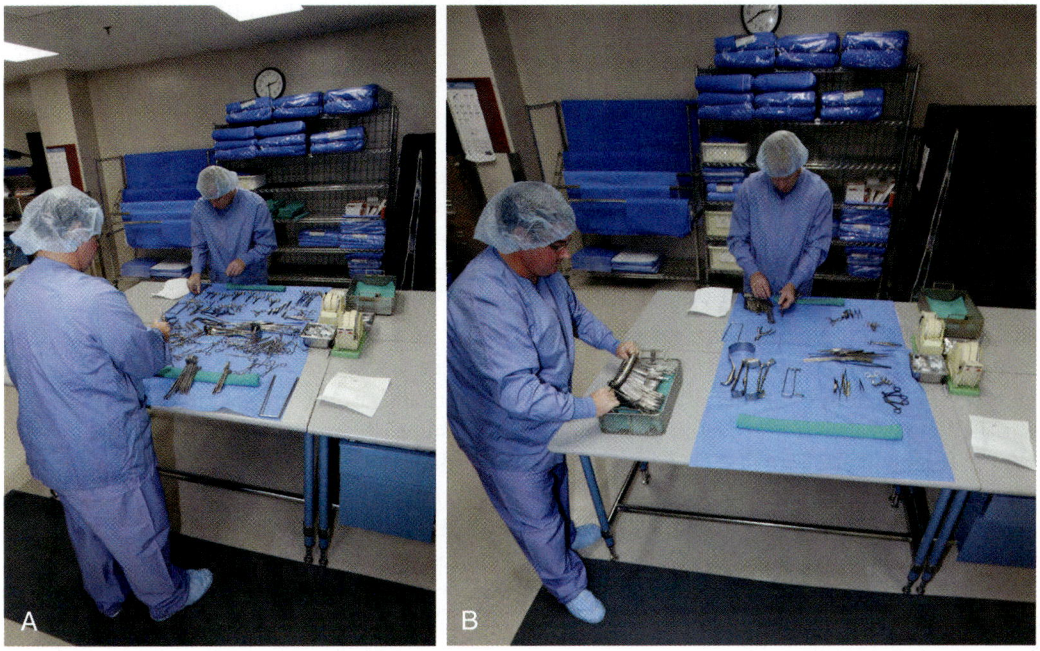

FIG. 10.3 (A) Sorting and inspecting instruments in a clean processing area following washing and decontamination. (B) Instrument sets are put together and placed correctly in sterilization trays.

clean assembly area includes a clean scrub suit, long-sleeved jacket, and head covering.

Large-volume sterilizers are located adjacent to the clean work area for easy transfer of instruments once they have been arranged in sets and wrapped for a specific sterilization process.

ASSEMBLING INSTRUMENT SETS

Before instruments are assembled and wrapped for sterilization, they must be inspected for soil, stains, corrosion, function, and structural soundness. This is a specific skill that is fully described in Chapter 11.

Instrument sets are groups of instruments that are needed for specific types of surgical procedures. Sets may contain a few or hundreds of separate instruments. After inspection, instruments are stored in the reprocessing areas as single instruments or wrapped in sets ready for sterilization. Lists of all instrument and equipment sets are maintained in a computer database or hard copy. These are kept in the clean processing area where the sets are assembled (Fig. 10.3B). Instrument lists are consulted to be sure that all needed instruments are included in the set and for counting purposes.

NOTE *Surgeons may request additions to a standard instrument set. It is important to communicate this information to those responsible for maintaining and updating the instrument lists.*

Guidelines • Instrument Set Assembly

Instruments are assembled in a way that protects them and facilitates sterilization.

1. Hinged instruments are opened (unlocked) and strung together with an instrument stringer or in racks designed to hold the instruments in an open position during the sterilization process.
2. Sharp or pointed items are turned downward to prevent injury and damage to the sterile wrapper.
3. Sharp and pointed instrument tips may be covered with plastic tip protectors to protect them from damage and prevent injury to the ST.
4. Some instruments must be disassembled for reprocessing. Any instrument that was not disassembled before disinfection may not be clean and should be returned for disassembly and repeat disinfection.
5. Instrument trays have a perforated bottom that allows the sterilant to circulate up through the tray and adequately cover all surfaces of the instruments. Make sure no instrument tips are caught in the perforations, where they could be damaged. A cloth towel may be placed on the bottom of the tray to prevent damage to the instrument tips during the sterilization process. Paper should not be used for this unless it is formulated without cellulose.
6. Heavy instruments are placed on the bottom of the tray, and the others are packed or nested so that they cannot shift and damage each other during processing.
7. For items with a lumen, a small amount of sterile, deionized (distilled) water should be flushed through the item immediately before steam sterilization only. This water vaporizes during sterilization and forces air out of the lumen. Any air that is left in the lumen may prevent sterilization of its inner surface. Remove stylets from suction tips for assembly so that the sterilant can freely circulate inside the lumen.
8. Instrument trays should not contain separate items wrapped in peel pouch packages. Air can become trapped inside the pouches and prevent steam from reaching all the surfaces of the items inside.

9. Elastic bands must not be used to group instruments, because these cannot be sterilized effectively except by ethylene oxide.
10. Synthetic wrapping material should not be used inside instrument trays to separate instruments or for lining the tray bottom. The material may prevent penetration of the sterilant to the instruments.
11. Power-driven surgical instruments (e.g., drills, reamers, and saws) should be disassembled before steam sterilization. Hoses can be coiled loosely during packaging, and all delicate switches and parts should be protected during preparation. Before sterilization, power-driven instruments should be lubricated according to the manufacturer's specifications. They should also be tested before wrapping. Finally, before processing, make sure that all switches and control devices are in the safety position.

Containers that allow systematic organization and separation of specialty instruments such as ophthalmic and microsurgery sets are used to protect the instruments during reprocessing and for use on the sterile field.

PACKAGING SYSTEMS USED IN STERILIZATION

All items to be sterilized by pressurized steam, ethylene oxide, ozone, or gas plasma methods must be wrapped using approved methods and materials. The primary purpose of a wrapping system is to protect the item from contamination after sterilization.

There are several systems commonly used to package surgical instruments and supplies at the health care facility.

QUALITIES AND TYPES OF WRAPPING SYSTEMS

A quality wrapping system accomplishes the following:

- Allows the sterilant to penetrate the wrapper and reach all parts of the device
- Allows complete dissipation of the sterilant when the process is finished
- Contains no toxic ingredients or non-fast dyes
- Does not create lint
- Resists destruction by the sterilizing process (e.g., melting, delamination, blistering, and alteration of the chemical structure of an item)
- Permits complete enclosure of the package contents
- Produces a package strong enough to withstand storage and handling
- Is convenient to work with (i.e., pliable and easy to handle)
- Facilitates a method of opening and distributing the device that prevents contamination at the point of use
- Is cost-effective
- Matches the method of sterilization to be used

Cloth Wrappers

Reusable cloth wrappers are woven from high-quality cotton or a combination of cotton and polyester. **Woven wrappers** are sufficiently dense to protect goods from contamination, yet porous enough to allow penetration of steam or gas. The thread count (number of threads per square inch) must be at least 140 for an effective wrapper. Two double-thickness cloth wrappers or the equivalent (one double-thickness wrapper of 280-count cloth) are used to wrap items. Before use, all cloth wrappers must be laundered. This ensures a minimum level of moisture in the cloth, which prevents superheating during sterilization. Before use, cloth wrappers must be inspected on a light table to detect any pinholes or tears in the cloth, which must be repaired before use for sterilization processes. This is usually done in the SPD. Defective materials are referred for repair.

Single-Use Nonwoven Materials

Disposable **nonwoven** wrappers are intended for one-time use only. These materials are manufactured from spun, heat-bonded fibers such as polypropylene. They are available in light and heavy weight and various sizes. Lightweight fabrics require the same treatment as cloth wrappers (i.e., four thicknesses for complete protection). Heavier fabrics may be used according to the manufacturer's specifications. These are valuable for wrapping heavy instruments and flat-surfaced items such as basins and trays or heavy linen packs.

Paper derived from cellulose is *not* used for wrapping items for sterilization because the sterilization process may break down the material. Further, paper recoils when the package is opened, making it difficult to distribute the goods inside aseptically.

Peel Pouch

Combination synthetic and paper wrappers, commonly called *sterilization pouches* or *peel pouches*, are available in various compositions and styles. These are double-sided bags made from medical-grade paper and transparent polypropylene–polymethylene. This material is available in many different sizes and comes from the manufacturer as a roll of continuous wrap, or as single-item pouches. The item is placed inside the pouch, and the opening is closed using a heat seal device. Self-seal pouches are also available.

- Items wrapped in peel pouches must not be placed inside an instrument tray. The sterilant might not penetrate the pouch.
- Double pouches are unnecessary and may prevent sterilization of the item.
- The item in the pouch should clear the seal on all four sides by at least 1 inch (2.5 cm).
- Peel pouches are intended only for lightweight instruments and devices. Using this system for heavy items (e.g., bone rongeurs, rasps, and multiple instruments) usually leads to tearing, loss of integrity of the pouch, and contamination of the item.
- Air should be evacuated from the pouch before it is sealed. Otherwise, the package can rupture during sterilization.
- When a mechanical heat-sealing device is used, the seal should be checked very carefully to ensure that no air pockets have formed along the seal.

Closed Sterilization Containers

Manufactured closed containers are used to hold equipment for sterilization (Fig. 10.4). These are convenient and safe for vapor,

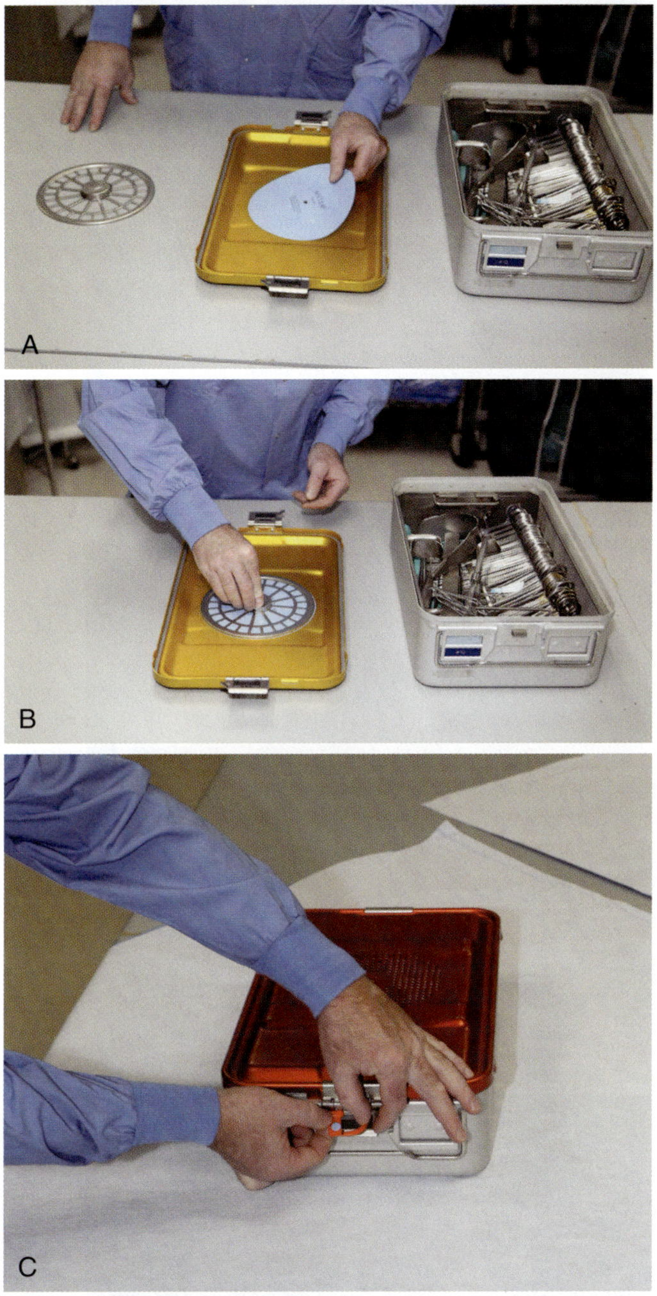

FIG. 10.4 Closed sterilization tray. (A and B) This system consists of a lightweight metal container fitted with a filter. Instrument trays are placed inside the container, which can then be sterilized without a wrapper. (C) Each container is fitted with a lightweight plastic cable lock that must be broken before the container is opened.

gas, and conventional steam sterilization. Sterilization containers incorporate disposable filters into the construction of the container, and a tamper-proof seal is used to verify that the cover of the container was not removed before use. When sterilization containers are used, the manufacturer's recommendations must be followed. Some containers are suitable only for a single method, whereas others are suitable for a number of different sterilization methods. Rigid sterilization containers are not meant to be used for nonsterile instrument storage.

Before preparing instruments in a closed container, make sure that the filter has not expired. Filters are changed after a designated number of cycles have been used on the container. It is also necessary to match the container with the method of sterilization to ensure compatibility. Fig. 10.5 demonstrates the preparation of instruments in a closed sterilization container. A clean filter is loaded into the container lid. Note that plastic locks are fastened to each side of the tray. After sterilization, these plastic locks remain in place until the ST removes them on the sterile field.

WRAPPING METHODS USING CLOTH AND SYNTHETIC MATERIALS

Goods are wrapped in sheets of cloth or bonded synthetic material, and the most common methods are the envelope technique (see Fig. 10.5) and the square wrap. Items may be single wrapped or double wrapped according to the specifications of the *wrapper* and in accordance with standard protocols for wrapping. Basins are also wrapped using the envelope method (Fig. 10.6). Note that a surgical towel can be placed between the basin and nested containers. However, do not placed items wrapped in pouches in the pack, because these can trap air and prevent thorough sterilization.

EQUIPMENT TRACKING

Regardless of the type of packaging or wrapping system used, each package must be properly labeled. The date of processing, name of the item, a lot control number, batch number, employee initials, and the department to receive the package must be included on the label. The lot control number is used to identify items that have been included in a sterilization load that may have yielded a positive biological or mechanical control test result. Any information written by hand on the outside of a wrapped package is usually placed on the sealing tape, the main purpose of which is to verify the parameters of the sterilization process (discussed in following sections).

A variety of computer-based technologies allow for the accurate management and tracking of surgical supplies and equipment. Bar code scanning allows the Central Supply and Surgical Processing Departments to track specific instrument sets and identify their location at any given time. These programs identify instrument sets that have been used a certain number of times and automatically advise sterile processing personnel to take a routine action, such as holding an instrument set for the sharpening of scissors or replacing certain reusable items.

To improve the management of single-use items, special cabinets and carts have been designed to allow personnel to obtain items through a computerized system. Items are stored in the cabinet and retrieved by pushing the button associated with that item. A computer printout in a central inventory office tells the supply or stock personnel to replace that item. These systems may be connected to the hospital billing system. In this way, equipment charges are automatically assigned to individual patients.

STERILIZATION

Instruments and equipment used in critical areas of the body must be sterile—completely free of all forms of microorganisms.

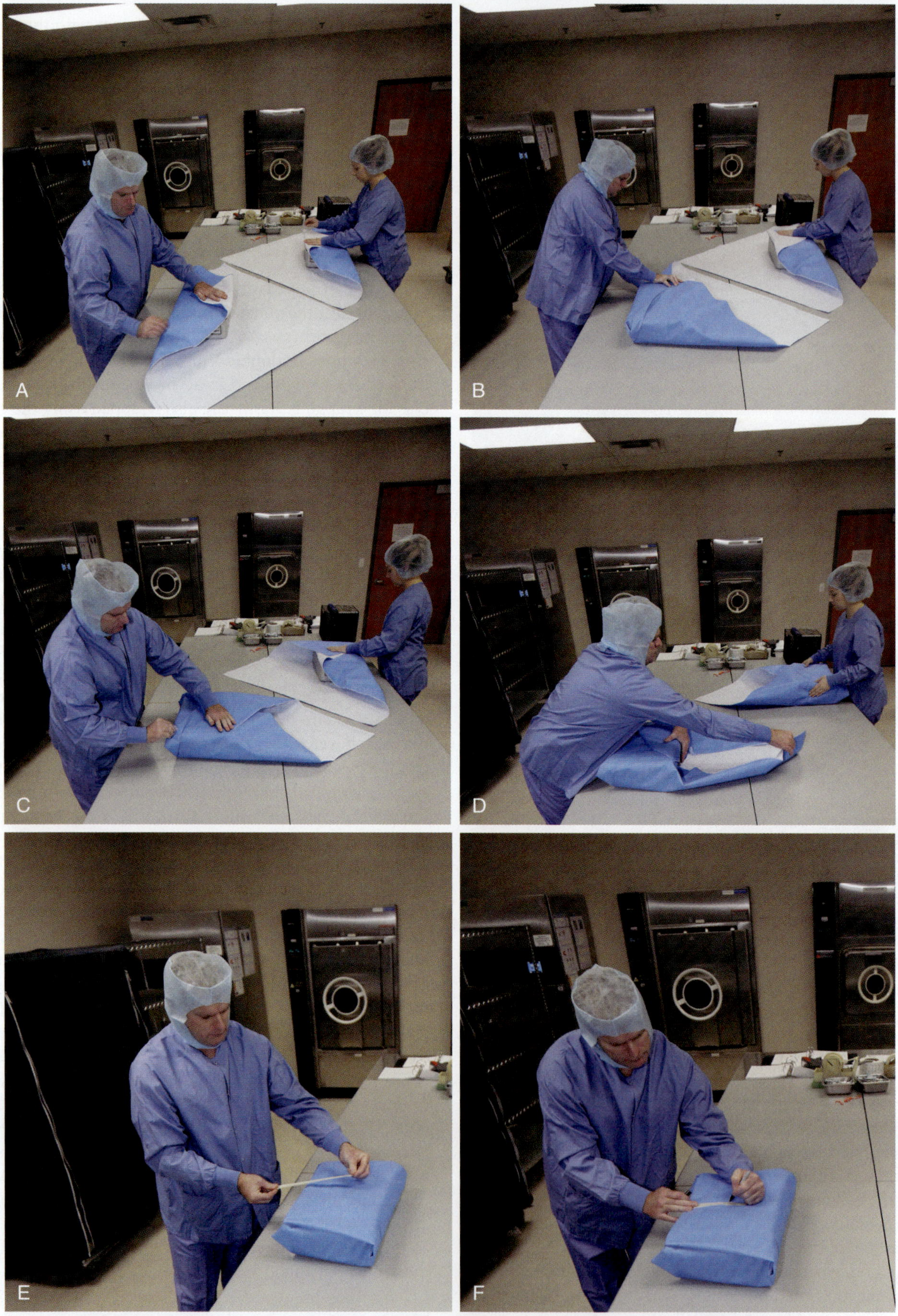

FIG. 10.5 Method of wrapping items in woven or synthetic sheets. (A) The tray is set on the wrapper diagonally. (B) The first wrap is taken from the near side. (C) Then, the side wraps are folded over. (D) The last fold is taken from the side opposite the first wrap. The tail of the last wrap can be folded over and tucked inside. (E) Chemical indicator tape is placed over the last flap. (F) The date of processing is written on the tape. A batch indicator may also be applied to the outside of the wrapper.

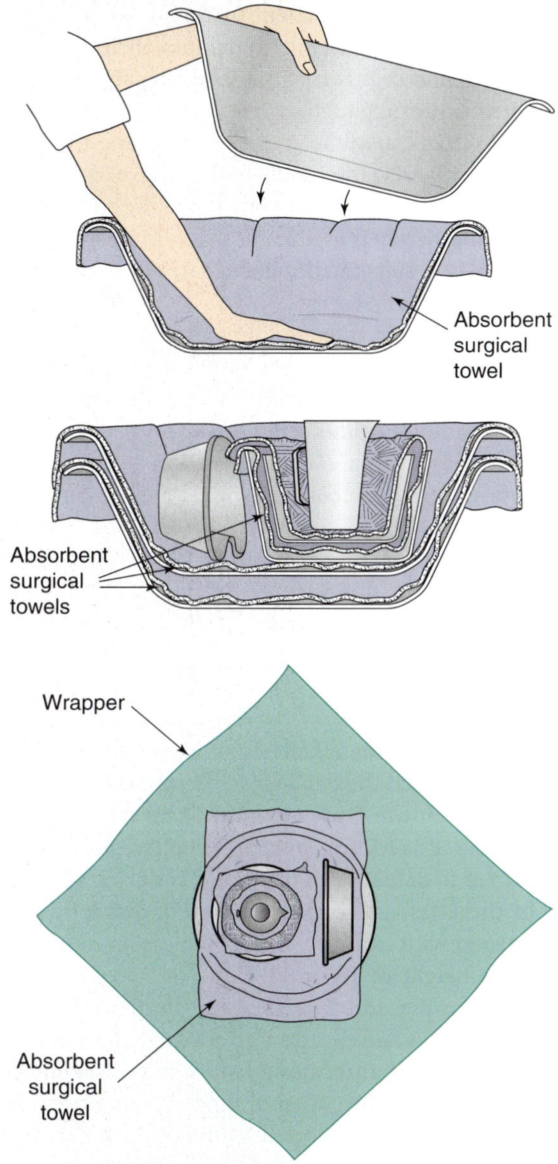

FIG. 10.6 Correct method of wrapping basins and other containers. A surgical towel can be placed between the basins. Small cups and pitchers should be placed on their sides.

Current methods of sterilization in the health care setting include the following:

- High-temperature steam under pressure
- Ethylene oxide (EO) gas
- Hydrogen peroxide gas plasma
- Hydrogen peroxide vapor
- Peracetic acid vapor
- Ozone
- Dry heat
- **Ionizing radiation**

The enormous variety of instruments and equipment used in surgery does not fit easily into a generalized protocol for selecting a sterilization method. The basic criteria are the safety of the process, its efficiency, and the economy of the product. Safety for the patient and for staff using the sterilization method is the most important criterion. Efficiency must be considered because a busy surgical facility must have rapid turnover between cases. This includes the sterilization time of instruments that are used in consecutive cases. Economy is also important because health care facilities must operate within a prescribed budget.

All devices used in the health care setting, including surgery, are sold or leased by manufacturers with instructions and guidelines for their care, including methods of reprocessing. Modern medical instruments and devices include a wide range of digital, electronic, electric, pneumatic, and lensed instruments and equipment. The complexity of methods and materials means that *the instrument manufacturer's recommendations for a sterilization process should be followed exactly.* Patient safety cannot be ensured unless devices are handled according to the manufacturer's recommendations. Manufacturers are liable for any injury caused by their products as long as the products are used and reprocessed according to their specifications. The selection criteria used by manufacturers are validated by research institutions so that they can be safely adopted by professional organizations and health care facilities. The student or newly hired technologist should become familiar with the approved reprocessing methods used for specific equipment in his or her facility.

MONITORING THE STERILIZATION PROCESS

The consequences of a sterilization failure can be extremely serious in human terms. Reprocessing instruments and equipment depends on human and technical factors. On the human side, knowledge and skills are applied at each stage of the reprocessing cycle. The technical aspects of sterilization must be monitored to ensure that the conditions required for sterilization have been met. To prevent surgical site infection (SSI), specific parameters are tested on every load of goods being sterilized, *regardless of the sterilization method*. By monitoring the parameters, we know that the conditions for sterilization have been reached.

NOTE *Monitors do not guarantee or ensure sterility. They are intended only to verify that the conditions required for sterilization have been achieved.*

Process monitoring is divided into categories according to the mechanism of the system. These are *physical, chemical,* and *biological* monitoring. These are also referred to as indicators, for example, **chemical indicators (CIs)** and biological indicators (BIs). The terms *monitoring* and *indicator* are synonymous.

NOTE *The category of the indicator refers to the indicator, not the parameter being tested.*

MECHANICAL MONITORING

All modern sterilizers provide immediate feedback on parameters such as time (duration of the cycle), temperature, and moisture. The monitoring output is recorded and displayed by printouts, gauges, and digital readings on the front panel of the equipment (Fig. 10.7). These provide valuable information and the means to detect a mechanical or digital malfunction. This type of monitoring is called mechanical monitoring

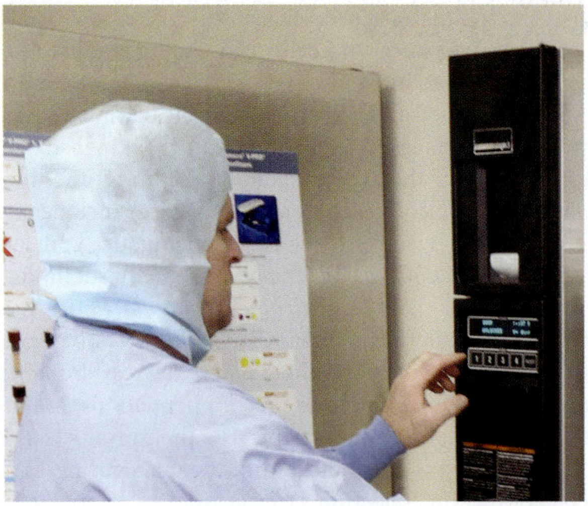

FIG. 10.7 All sterilizing systems perform digital monitoring, which is displayed on the front panel and should be printed out at the conclusion of each load.

or digital monitoring. To recognize when there is a technical fault in the sterilizer, the system's operator must know what the baseline or normal readings should be. Surgical technologists who operate sterilizer systems must be familiar with the baseline readings, which are on file in the workroom. The system printouts are kept and recorded by the department because they may be needed for validation at the time of the sterilizer operation or a later time.

CHEMICAL INDICATORS

In this test, commercially prepared paper strips or tape are chemically treated to change color when exposed to specific parameters of the sterilization process such as temperature and concentration of chemical sterilant (Fig. 10.8A). Chemical monitoring strips are routinely placed inside and on the outside of all packs to be sterilized (Fig. 10.8B). When sterile goods are distributed, the monitor must be checked to ensure it has changed color. Indicators inside packs are retrieved once the pack is opened on the sterile field. The ST must verify that the monitor has changed before proceeding with the setup.

BIOLOGICAL INDICATORS

A **biological indicator (BI)** is a harmless bacterium encased in a self-contained unit. The BI is placed in selected loads to be sterilized. After sterilization, the vial is retrieved and the bacteria rapidly cultured in an incubator. Only biological testing can determine whether the parameters were effective in the destruction of microbes in the load. If the bacteria are viable and grow, the load is most likely not sterile.

Biological controls should be administered at least once weekly in all sterilizers. Biological monitors are always used when an artificial **implant** or prosthesis is sterilized. If any indicator shows a positive result, all items included in that load are withdrawn from use. The infection control department will be notified and the event documented. If the items have already been used in patient treatment, additional safety precautions are immediately implemented, including notification of the surgeon or other primary health care provider who used the items during patient care.

Rapid biological monitoring uses an enzyme that binds to spores. After the sterilization process, the level of enzyme is measured. This corresponds with destruction of the bacterial spores. The monitoring system is used for both high-pressure steam and EO sterilization. Results can be obtained in 1 to 4 hours, depending on the sterilization process.

The bacteria used during biological monitoring differ according to the sterilization process.

- Steam sterilization: *Geobacillus stearothermophilus*
- EO sterilization: *Bacillus atrophaeus*
- Vaporized gas plasma: *Bacillus subtilis*
- Peracetic acid: According to the manufacturer's specifications
- Immediate-use steam sterilization: *Geobacillus stearothermophilus* enzyme (fluorescence testing)
- Ozone sterilization: *Geobacillus stearothermophilus*

AIR DETECTION

To test and monitor the efficiency of the *high-vacuum steam sterilizer*, a test called the daily air removal test (DART) is performed using a Bowie-Dick monitor. There are also commercially available tests for this purpose. High-vacuum sterilizers are monitored to detect air in the chamber during the exposure phase. In these tests, a special package of correctly wrapped towels is taped with heat-sensitive chemical monitor tape and stacked to a height of 10 or 11 inches (25 to 27.5 cm). The package is then placed by itself in the sterilization chamber, and the sterilizer is run for the appropriate length of time. An unsatisfactory DART indicates a failure in the vacuum pump system or a defect in the gasket of the sterilizer door. Unsatisfactory results must be reported to the biomedical engineering staff so that they can inspect the sterilizer, especially the vacuum system and door seals.

STEAM STERILIZATION

Steam sterilization is the most widely used, effective, and efficient method of sterilization in the health care setting. Normal atmospheric steam is not hot enough to completely destroy microbes and spores. However, steam under pressure reaches the extremely high temperatures necessary for sterilization. Steam under pressure coagulates the nucleic acids and protein that make up the cell's genetic and enzymatic material. Pressurized steam also destroys the cell's resilient outer wall and bacterial spores.

Modern steam sterilizers are classified as **high-vacuum sterilizers.** The high-vacuum system quickly and forcefully evacuates air from the chamber and replaces it with bursts or pulses of steam. Stainless steel instruments, other items made of stainless steel, and woven (cloth) materials are routinely sterilized with steam. However, many items used in surgery cannot tolerate high pressure, high temperature, or exposure to steam. The appropriate processing method

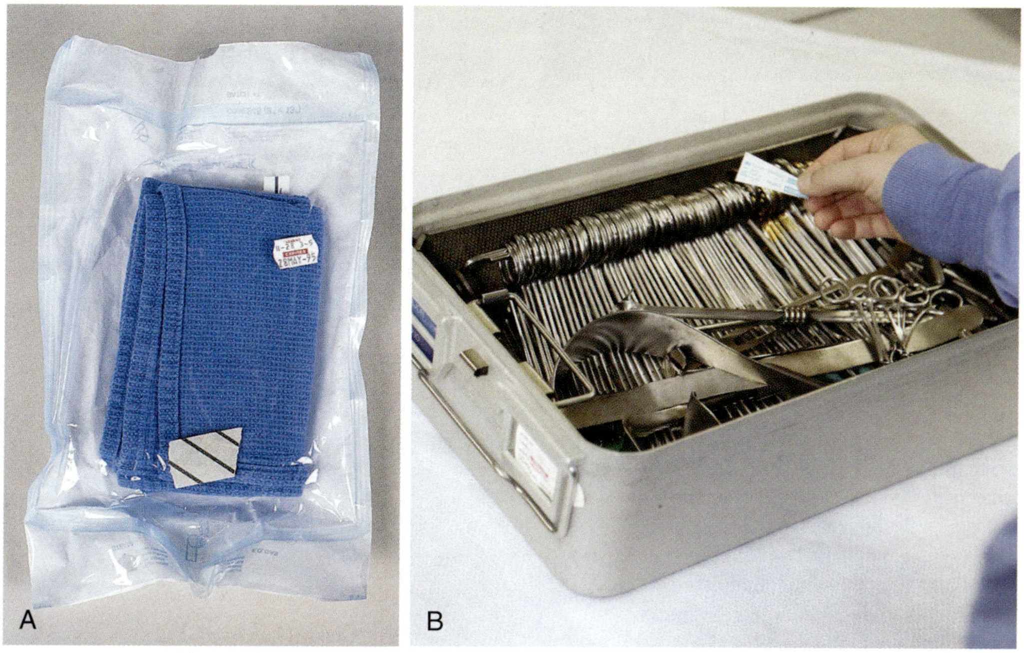

FIG. 10.8 (A) Chemical monitor. Sterilization tape becomes striped when exposed to specific parameters used in the sterilization process. (B) Paper monitors impregnated with a heat-sensitive chemical must be placed inside every item to be sterilized. (A, From Elkin MK, Perry AG, Potter PA. *Nursing Interventions and Clinical Skills*. 3rd ed. St Louis: Mosby; 2004.)

should always be verified directly with the manufacturer's manuals or company representative. Many power-driven instruments and those that contain an optical system or microprocessor cannot be steam sterilized. Some synthetic materials, such as Silastic, Teflon, polyethylene, polypropylene, and other complex polymers, may also be altered during steam sterilization.

The entire process of heating, pressurizing, and timing the load is called a *cycle*. Modern steam sterilizers have preprogrammed cycles for these parameters. A steam sterilizer has a central chamber where goods are placed and a mechanism for creating extremely high pressure. Steam enters the chamber, air is removed, and the internal pressure increased. This process heats the steam to the very high temperatures required for sterilization.

PARAMETERS FOR STEAM STERILIZATION

Steam sterilization is achieved according to the temperature, pressure, and **exposure time** of the items in the chamber. These depend on the type of steam sterilizer, the size of the load, the temperature, whether items are wrapped, and the type of materials or supplies being processed.

Effective steam sterilization requires a specific concentration of moisture. If too little moisture is present, items become superheated and eventually can be burned. Too much moisture leaves items wet after removal from the chamber; this can result in contamination of the item. The amount of moisture in the steam is referred to as the *steam quality*. Water is converted to steam at 212°F (100°C). At this temperature, steam is ineffective for sterilization. Steam that contains more than 97% water is necessary for sterilization to be achieved. As pressure is decreased with the evacuation of air from the chamber, the temperature of the steam rises to extremely high temperatures capable of destroying all forms of microbial life.

Box 10.2 shows a system of six classes of indicators used with steam sterilization.

WATER QUALITY

Manufacturers of high-pressure steam sterilizers recommend that water used during steam sterilization is treated to remove minerals. If unfiltered contaminants remain in the system, this can result in instrument stains and corrosion. The presence of orange, white, brown, or black spots on sterilized items may indicate the presence of excess minerals in the water supply. As these minerals become deposited in the box locks of surgical instruments, they can impair instrument function.

CORRECT LOADING OF A LARGE-CAPACITY STEAM STERILIZER

Large steam sterilizers are used for bulk processing of hospital equipment, including surgical instruments, basins, linen, drapes, and towels. They are usually located in the Sterile Processing Department. The loading technique used for any sterilizer influences the outcome. Large sterilizers used for bulk linens, basins, and complex instruments multiply the problems of air pockets, overheating, and proper steam drainage. Careful loading of items in the steam sterilizer is critical, because if the load is too dense or improperly positioned, air may become trapped in pockets. Items in these air pockets will not be sterilized.

BOX 10.2 Classes of Indicators for Steam Sterilization

A system of six classes of indicators is used for quality assurance with steam sterilization. Although the different classes are numbered, there is no associated ranking of the indicators. Each type produces different information about the performance of the sterilizer, and each type has a specific use.

- Class 1 (single parameter): These are process indicators. This can be tape or a label indicating only that an individual item or unit was directly exposed to the sterilization process. An example is tape that changes color when exposed to the critical temperature required in steam sterilization.
- Class 2 (specialty indicators): These are used for specific tests that measure parameters. Examples include the **Bowie-Dick** and daily air removal tests for the presence of pure air (no steam) in the sterilization chamber.
- Class 3 (single parameter): This class includes indicators that respond to only one critical parameter with an exact value. An example is a heat-sensitive pellet (encased in a glass tube) that melts only at a certain temperature that is consistent with the sterilization method. The pellet is placed in specific areas of the sterilization chamber.
- Class 4 (multiparameter): These are represented by multivariable indicators that react to two or more parameters. An example is internal chemical indicators printed on a paper strip.
- Class 5 (integrating parameters): This class includes indicators that react to all critical values over a specified range in the sterilization process. These are the most exacting and accurate of all indicators.
- Class 6 (emulating indicators): Class 6 indicators are used for internal pack control of each cycle run, not for the overall performance of the sterilizer for all cycles.

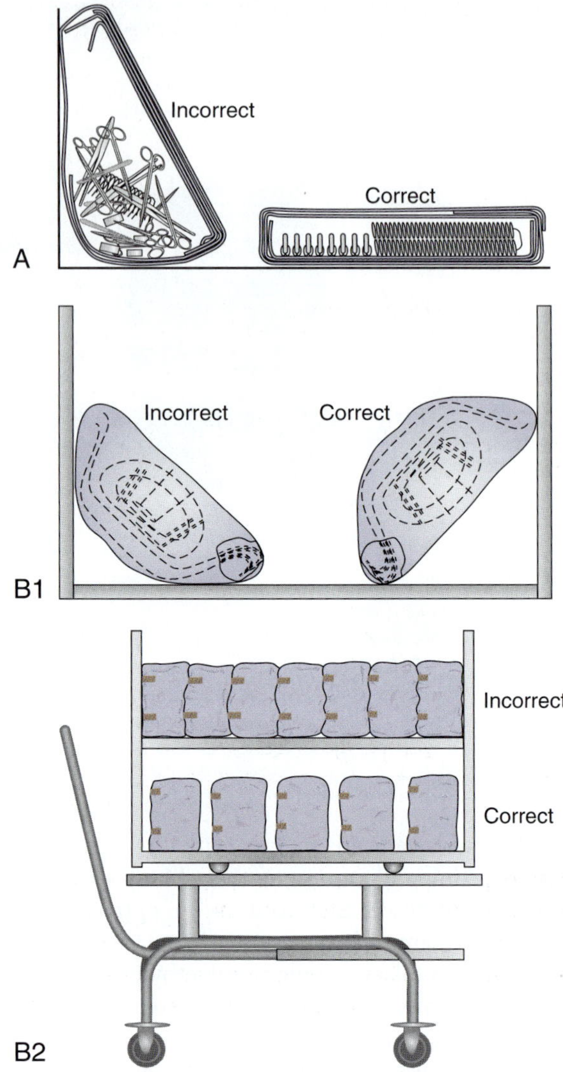

FIG. 10.9

- Instrument pans with mesh or wire bottoms are placed flat on the sterilizer shelf.
- Linen packs, because of their density, require special attention. Linen packs are best sterilized by placing the packs on their sides.
- Packs and instrument trays should be placed so that they do not touch, or touch only loosely, and small items should be placed crosswise over each other.
- Heavy packs should be placed at the periphery of the load, where steam enters the chamber.
- Basins, jars, cups, or other containers should be placed on their sides. Any item with a smooth surface on which water can collect and drip during the cooling phase of the sterilization cycle should be placed at the bottom of the load. Fig. 10.9 shows correct methods of loading a gravity-displacement sterilizer.

PHASES OF STEAM STERILIZATION

There are three distinct phases in all types of steam sterilizers:

1. *Conditioning (sometimes called preconditioning):* Air is removed from the chamber and replaced with steam.
2. *Exposure or holding time:* Goods in the chamber are exposed to superheated steam at a precise temperature and duration. This duration depends on the size of the load, complexity of materials being sterilized, and whether the items were wrapped before sterilization.
3. *Exhaust and drying:* Pressure in the chamber is reduced and the load is exposed to cool air.

Tables 10.1 and 10.2 show total cycle times for gravity-displacement and dynamic (high-vacuum) sterilizers. These exposure times and temperatures do not reflect the entire time needed to include all phases of the sterilization process. These minimum standards ***apply only to the exposure time.*** The total time includes all phases, including the preconditioning phase, the exposure phase (sometimes called the *kill time*), a factor of safety time, and an exhaust phase. Most sterilizers also include a drying phase. These times may vary from load to load, depending on the items to be sterilized.

IMPORTANT TO KNOW *When operating the sterilizer, always check the parameters required for the item being sterilized. The exact time, temperature, pressure, and type of sterilization to use are available from the manufacturer of the item being sterilized.*

TABLE 10.1 Cycle Times for Gravity-Displacement Steam Sterilization

Item	Exposure Time at 250°F (121°C)	Minimum Drying Time	Exposure Time at 270°F (132°C)	Minimum Drying Time	Exposure Time at 275°F (135°C)*	Minimum Drying Time*
Wrapped instruments	30 min	15 to 30 min	15 min	15 to 30 min	10 min	30 min
Textile packs	30 min	25 min	25 min	15 min	10 min	30 min
Wrapped utensils	30 min	30 min	15 min	15 to 30 min	10 min	10 min

*From AORN. *Guidelines for Perioperative Practice*, 2015. Denver: AORN; 2015.
From Rutala W, Weber D, Healthcare Infection Control Practices Advisory Committee (HICPAC). Atlanta: Centers for Disease Control and Prevention; 2008.

TABLE 10.2 Cycle Times for Dynamic Air Removal (Pre-vacuum) Steam Sterilization

Items	Exposure Time at 250°F (121°C)	Minimum Drying Time	Exposure Time at 270°F (132°C)	Minimum Drying Time	Exposure Time at 275°F (135°C)*	Minimum Drying Time*
Wrapped instruments	NA		4 min	15 to 30 min	3 min	16 min
Textile packs	NA		4 min	5 to 20 min	3 min	3 min
Wrapped utensils	NA		4 min	20 min	3 min	16 min

Note: Exposure and drying times for enclosed rigid sterilization containers are specified by the manufacturer and vary according to design. Always check the manufacturer's specifications for sterilization.
*From AORN. *Guidelines for Perioperative Practice*, 2015. Denver: AORN; 2015.
From Rutala W, Weber D, Healthcare Infection Control Practices Advisory Committee (HICPAC). Atlanta: Centers for Disease Control and Prevention; 2008.

To assist in the removal of moisture and to prevent wet packs, the sterilizer operator may use a dry cycle as part of the steam sterilization process. Regardless of whether a dry cycle is used, items that have been steam sterilized should be allowed to remain in the sterilizer chamber for 15 to 30 minutes after the cycle to prevent the formation of condensate. Do not crack the door of the sterilizer during the drying phase unless the manufacturer recommends it, as this can result in inefficient cooling and drying of the load.

After the packs have passed through the final phase (drying), they must remain on the sterilizer racks for cooling. Never place warm packs on a cool surface, as this will result in condensation and wet packs (Fig. 10.10).

NOTE *Packages that are discovered to be wet after removal from the steam sterilizer, even though they have passed through a drying and cooling phase, are considered contaminated. This is because moisture wicks bacteria from a nonsterile surface onto a sterile surface.*

IMMEDIATE-USE (FLASH) STEAM STERILIZER

A high-speed pre-vacuum sterilizer is used in the operating room and in other areas of the hospital to sterilize items for immediate use. The immediate-use steam sterilizer uses extremely high temperatures to achieve a short cycle.

In the past, the term *flash sterilization* was used to describe this process. In 2010 standards agencies agreed that the term *flash sterilization* does not reflect the complexity of sterilization for immediate use. Therefore the term has been replaced with **immediate-use steam sterilization (IUSS).** Standards for IUSS have been adapted by professional organizations, including AST.

Sterilizers employed for immediate use are usually located in the restricted substerile room just outside the operating room where surgery is performed. This type of sterilizer is used *only when no alternative is available.* Ideally, items to be sterilized for immediate use should be in a covered metal tray. However, some immediate-use sterilizers can be used with a drying cycle that is suitable for items wrapped in a single layer of woven material. Unwrapped items coming from the immediate-use sterilizer are wet, as there is no drying cycle for unwrapped goods.

AAMI RECOMMENDED PRACTICES FOR IMMEDIATE-USE STEAM STERILIZATION

1. Implants (items that remain inside the body such as bone plates and replacement joint components) must never be sterilized immediately before use except in a documented emergency situation when no other option is available. If an implant must be sterilized in an emergency, a rapid readout biological indicator must be used.
2. The manufacturer's specifications for exposure time and temperature must be followed.
3. If a covered sterilization container is used to sterilize instruments immediately before use, parameter values specified by the manufacturers of the container and the instrument must be followed.
4. Some instruments and equipment cannot be sterilized using IUSS. Always verify an instrument's status before processing it using IUSS.

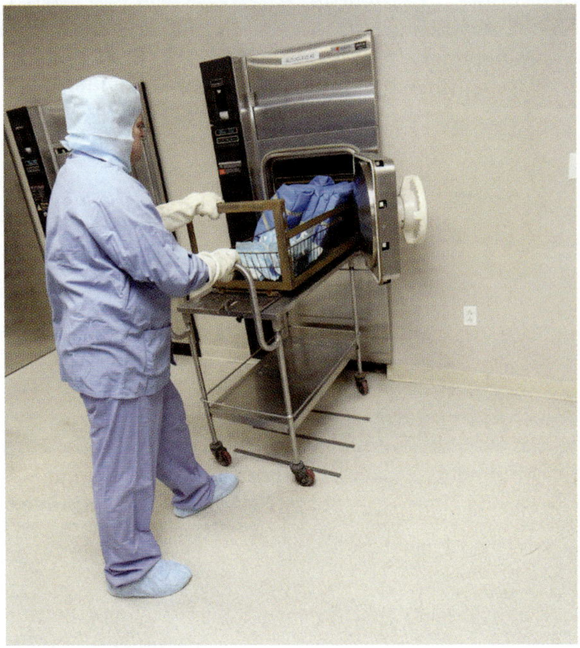

FIG. 10.10 Items that have been steam sterilized and allowed to dry in the chamber must be removed on their racks and remain on them until cool. They should not be placed on a cool surface, as this causes condensation of moist air, leading to wet packs and contamination.

5. Immediate-use sterilizers must be located in an area where unwrapped sterile items can be transported directly from the sterilizer to the sterile field.
6. Items for IUSS are not wrapped unless this is permitted by the manufacturer's specifications.
7. Sterilization monitors for temperature must be used with every load.
8. Items that are sold by the manufacturer as sterile devices intended for single use only must never be sterilized for immediate use.
9. Sterilization containers with tamper-proof seals may be used for IUSS. Always follow the manufacturer's instructions for use.
10. Items to be processed using IUSS must first be cleaned and decontaminated following the same procedures required for terminal decontamination of all instruments.
11. Do not use wrappers or pouches for IUSS loads unless the manufacturer guidelines specifically approve it.

Table 10.3 shows the parameters for immediate-use steam sterilization.

REMOVING ITEMS FROM THE IMMEDIATE-USE STERILIZER

Current standards for removing items from IUSS specify doing it in a way that prevents contamination of the items and injury to staff. To remove items from the sterilizer chamber, the circulator puts on sterile gloves and grasps the handles of the sterilization tray using sterile transfer handles. The tray is offered to the ST at the sterile field, who removes the items from the tray with care to prevent contamination. The tray should not be transferred to the sterile field, and the ST should not leave the sterile field or the room to retrieve the item from the sterilizer, as this is poor aseptic technique. Items that have just been sterilized by IUSS will be very hot. The ST should allow them to cool before use on the sterile field. If a closed sterilization tray has been used during sterilization, the circulator uses transfer forceps to deliver the sterilization tray containing the IUSS container.

ETHYLENE OXIDE STERILIZATION

Ethylene oxide (EO) is a highly flammable liquid that, when blended with inert gas, produces effective sterilization by destroying the deoxyribonucleic acid (DNA) and protein structure of microorganisms. EO is used in a 100% pure form, blended with carbon dioxide gas, or mixed with hydrochlorofluorocarbons (HCFCs). In 2016 the Environmental Protection Agency (EPA) began regulating the use of HCFCs, which are no longer available for use in the United States. This is related to the known effect of HCFCs on ozone depletion. However, 100% EO is still available and can be used with other inert gases such as carbon dioxide.

EO is used to sterilize items that are heat and moisture sensitive. It can be used for delicate instruments, including microsurgical instruments and those with optical systems. It is highly penetrating, which makes it ideal for complex instruments with delicate inner components.

The EO sterilizer operates at a low temperature. The temperature of the gas directly affects the penetration of items in the chamber. Operating temperatures range from 85°F to 100°F (29°C to 37.7°C) for a "cold" cycle and 130°F to 145°F (54°C to 63°C) for a "warm" cycle.

Humidity is required to make spores less resistant to the EO gas. The preferred moisture content for EO sterilization is 25% to 80%. The length of exposure depends on the type and density of material to be sterilized, temperature, humidity, and the concentration of the gas.

ETHYLENE OXIDE STERILIZATION SAFETY PRECAUTIONS

Environmental and safety hazards are associated with EO. Exposure to the gas can cause burns to skin and mucous membranes. Prolonged occupational exposure to EO gas is known to cause respiratory damage. EO is a stable compound with a long half-life. Its advantage as a penetrating sterilant also poses hazards. It is difficult to remove, and the level of EO residue is not the same in all materials. In addition, it reacts with many different substances, causing them to disintegrate or create other toxic compounds, such as ethylene glycol and ethylene chlorohydrin. These chemicals are also difficult to remove from the environment.

To prevent injury from EO exposure, OSHA requires air sampling in areas likely to contain high concentrations of EO. Personnel who routinely work in the presence of EO sterilizers and loads should wear a dosimeter badge that measures EO exposure. Goods that have been sterilized with EO must

TABLE 10.3 Immediate-Use Steam Sterilizer Parameters

Type of Sterilizer	Load	Temperature	Exposure Time
Gravity displacement	Metal instruments (nonporous, without lumens) only	270° to 275°F (132° to 135°C)	3 min
	Porous items with lumens; complex power instruments (always consult the manufacturer)	270° to 275°F (132° to 135°C)	10 min
Dynamic (pre-vacuum)	Metal instruments (nonporous without lumens)	270° to 275°F (132° to 135°C)	4 min
Pressure pulse/steam flush	Nonporous/mixed porous and nonporous	270° to 275°F (132° to 135°C)	4 min

Note: The exposure and for enclosed rigid sterilization containers are specified by the manufacturer and vary according to design. Always check the manufacturer's specifications for sterilization using these systems.
From Rutala W, Weber D, Healthcare Infection Control Practices Advisory Committee (HICPAC). Atlanta: Centers for Disease Control and Prevention; 2008.

undergo an aeration cycle. This allows all traces of EO to dissipate. Aeration takes place *in the same chamber as the sterilization process.* This is necessary to prevent EO exposure to staff while transporting goods from the EO sterilizer to the aeration chamber. The manufacturer's recommendations for aeration are critical to the safety of both the patient and the hospital personnel handling equipment that has been gas sterilized.

NOTE *Aeration of items sterilized in EO is a critical step in processing. Cutting the aeration time short may result in serious injury. Never rinse items that contain residual traces of EO. When mixed with water, EO forms byproducts that can be harmful.*

PREPARATION OF ITEMS FOR GAS STERILIZATION

All items to be gas sterilized must be *clean* and *dry*. Any water left on equipment bonds with EO gas and produces a toxic residue that can cause burns or a toxic reaction in those who come in contact with it. Any organic material or soil exposed to EO may also produce toxic residues. Therefore all items processed for EO gas must be completely clean. Items are loaded in the sterilizer loosely so that the gas is free to circulate over every surface.

Every attempt should be made to load items that have similar aeration requirements. Some items must not be gas sterilized. These include acrylics and some pharmaceutical items.

Any instruments with fittings or parts should be disassembled before EO sterilization to facilitate exposure to the gas.

Wrapping techniques for EO sterilization are the same as for high-pressure steam sterilization. However, some materials are not suitable for EO processing. These include wrappers made of natural fiber combined with nylon and rayon, polyester, and polyvinyl chloride (PVC). Double-wrapped peel pouches are not suitable for some EO sterilizers. Always follow the manufacturer's recommendations before processing.

ETHYLENE OXIDE LOADING AND STERILIZATION

The EO sterilizer is loaded in such a way that gas can penetrate all surfaces of the packages. Packages must not touch the bottom or top of the chamber and must be placed loosely on their sides. The EO sterilizer is preprogrammed for exposure time, temperature, and aeration parameters. The sterilizer is operated from the control panel by trained CP technologists.

VAPORIZED HYDROGEN PEROXIDE STERILIZATION

Hydrogen peroxide gas is used with or without a plasma cycle on items that are heat and moisture sensitive. During the sterilization process, hydrogen peroxide is exposed to a vacuum. This creates a vapor that is forced into the central chamber where the goods have been loaded. When a gas plasma cycle is included, radiofrequency energy in the form of gas plasma is transmitted through the vapor, which excites the hydrogen peroxide molecules. This action destroys microorganisms by interfering with the cell membrane, genetic material, and cell enzymes.

Items for vaporized hydrogen peroxide (VHP) must be clean and completely dry. They are packaged in trays, pouches, and wraps specifically recommended by the manufacturer. Cloth and cellulose products cannot be processed by **gas plasma sterilization.** Only specific nonwoven wrapping materials can be used (e.g., Tyvek or Mylar wrappers). Materials compatible with VHP sterilization are listed in Box 10.3.

Preparation of materials for VHP is the same as for EO sterilization. Items are decontaminated as usual, dried, assembled, and wrapped according to the manufacturer's specifications. Quality control indicators to verify sterilization parameters are used just as with other sterilization procedures. This technology has instrument lumen restrictions that must be correlated with the manufacturer's instruments.

The sterilization cycle has four phases:

1. *Vacuum phase:* Air is evacuated from the chamber to reduce the pressure.

BOX 10.3 Materials Compatible With Gas Plasma Sterilization

METALS
- Stainless steel 300 series
- Aluminum 6000 series
- Titanium

NONMETALS
- Glass
- Silica
- Ceramic

PLASTICS AND ELASTOMERS
- Acrylonitrile butadiene styrene (ABS)
- Chlorinated polyvinyl chloride (CPVC)
- Ethylene propylene diene monomer rubber (EPDM)
- Polycarbonate (PC)
- Polyether ketone (PEEK)
- Polyetherimide (Ultem)
- Polyethersulfone (PES)
- Polyethylene
- Polymethyl methacrylate (PMMA)
- Polymethylpentene (PMP)
- Polyphenylene oxide (Noryl, PPO)
- Polypropylene (LDPP, HDPP)
- Polypropylene copolymer (PPCO)
- Polysulfone (PSF)
- Polyvinyl chloride (PVC)
- Polyvinylidene fluoride (PVDF)
- Teflon (PTFE, PFA, FEP)
- Tefzel (ETFE)
- Most silicones and fluorinated silicones

2. *Injection phase:* Liquid hydrogen peroxide is injected into the central chamber, where it is vaporized.
3. *Diffusion phase:* Hydrogen peroxide vapor disperses throughout the load.
4. *Plasma phase:* Radiofrequency energy breaks apart the hydrogen peroxide vapor, creating a plasma cloud containing free radicals and ultraviolet light. The compounds recombine into oxygen and water and are dissipated from the chamber. This completes the cycle.

The exposure time depends on the type and size of the load but ranges from 30 to 60 minutes. No toxic chemicals are created by this process, and aeration time is not necessary. At the end of the sterilization cycle, hydrogen peroxide gas is converted to its molecular components, water and oxygen.

LIQUID PERACETIC ACID STERILIZATION

Peracetic acid solution is a liquid chemical made up of 35% peracetic acid, hydrogen peroxide, acetic acid, sulfuric acid, and water. This system is an alternative to cold sterilization processing, which is commonly performed with a glutaraldehyde solution. **Peracetic acid** is used in a closed commercial processing system that is frequently used for fiber-optic endoscopes. During the sterilization process, peracetic acid inactivates many cell systems through a chemical process called *oxidation*. As the peracetic acid decomposes after the sterilization process, it converts to acetic acid (vinegar) and oxygen. Peracetic acid does not leave a chemical residue, but it must be rinsed thoroughly from instruments.

OZONE STERILIZATION

Ozone sterilization uses a molecular form of oxygen (three oxygen atoms) at low heat for sterilization of moisture- and heat-sensitive instruments and equipment through a process of oxidation. The process has four separate phases that are repeated in the sterilization process. Following the cycle, ozone is converted back to oxygen and water. This method is environmentally friendly and safer than EO, but as yet has not been approved for many materials and instruments. The process can be used for rigid diagnostic instruments, stainless steel, and synthetic substances such as PVC, silicone, and polytetrafluoroethylene (PTFE [Teflon]). It is not approved for implants. The sterilization time exceeds 4 hours. This method is used only on equipment for which the manufacturer has approved ozone sterilization, usually in closed containers or nonwoven pouches approved for exposure to ozone.

COBALT-60 RADIATION

Most equipment available prepackaged from a manufacturer has been sterilized by cobalt-60 radiation, which destroys all microorganisms through destruction of the DNA. Items such as sharps, sutures, sponges, and disposable drapes are just a few of the many types of presterilized products available.

Also included are anhydrous materials such as powders and petroleum goods. These products have traditionally been sterilized by dry heat in the hospital setting. However, the current trend is moving away from dry heat sterilization because of its inconvenience and because these substances now are available as single-use items that are packaged in one-dose containers to prevent cross-contamination. Items intended for single use, whether supplies for use in the surgical field or other substances meant to be used only once, must never be re-sterilized by conventional methods (steam sterilization, EO, or chemical sterilization) without the manufacturer's express recommendation to do so. The item might change in composition or deteriorate and could become a hazard to the patient or personnel.

STORAGE OF WRAPPED STERILE GOODS

After an item has been decontaminated, sorted, wrapped, and sterilized, consideration must be given to how the item can be kept sterile. **Event-related sterility** is the accepted standard.

Event-related sterility is based on the principle that sterilized items are assumed to be sterile while wrapped unless environmental conditions or events interfere with the integrity of the package. Historically, a wrapped, sterilized item was assigned a time limit after which the item could no longer be considered sterile. However, this standard has changed, with research showing that sterility is based on events that cause a sterile pack to lose its ability to remain sterile. A pack is considered no longer sterile when the following are true:

- It shows sign of exposure to liquid (e.g., water stain, discoloration in the wrapper).
- The wrap is torn, punctured, or otherwise damaged.
- The pack has been stored in a location that has no environmental controls, including those for vermin.
- The packs have been transported using a soiled or open system.

NOTE *Sterile packs that have been dropped on the floor are considered contaminated if only one wrapper was used to contain the item or if the pack appears damaged.*

Guidelines • Storage

Items should be stored according to the following guidelines:

- Sterile items should be stored in areas that are separate from those used to store clean nonsterile items.
- Sterile items must never be stored near sinks or other areas where they can be exposed to water.
- Packages should be placed loosely on shelves to prevent crushing, tearing, or damage to items and wrappers. Fig. 10.11 illustrates an acceptable method of storing sterile goods in bins. The items are loosely packed to allow easy access and prevent overhandling of packages, which can lead to contamination.
- Sterile items should be stored in critical areas or in the sterile core when possible. They should be placed in a draft-free area away from vents and windows. The area must be dust and lint free. Fig. 10.12 shows a system of movable storage racks for storing sterile instrument sets and other equipment. Movable cabinets allow personnel to access equipment easily.
- If items are stored in open bins, the bins or drawers should be shallow to prevent excess handling of the items. Mesh or basket containers are preferable to those with a solid surface where dust and bacteria can collect.
- Heavy items must never be stacked on top of lighter ones. Stacking heavy instrument trays poses a risk that wrappers will be torn as the top tray is removed.
- Seldom-used items can be wrapped in protective dust covers.
- Wrappers should be inspected for damage and expiration before they are opened for use.
- Items commercially prepared and sterilized by manufacturers may be considered sterile indefinitely as long as the wrapper is intact. An expiration date printed on the package shows the maximum length of time for which the manufacturer can guarantee product stability and sterility.

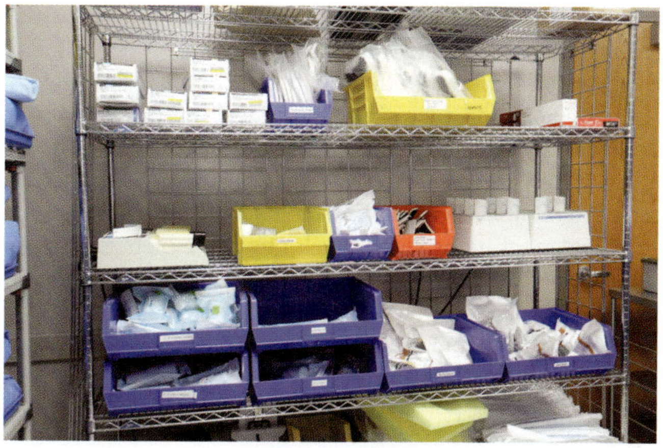

FIG. 10.11 Correct method of storing small sterile items. They are placed loosely in bins and trays to prevent overhandling of the packages, which can lead to weak areas in the wrapper and contamination.

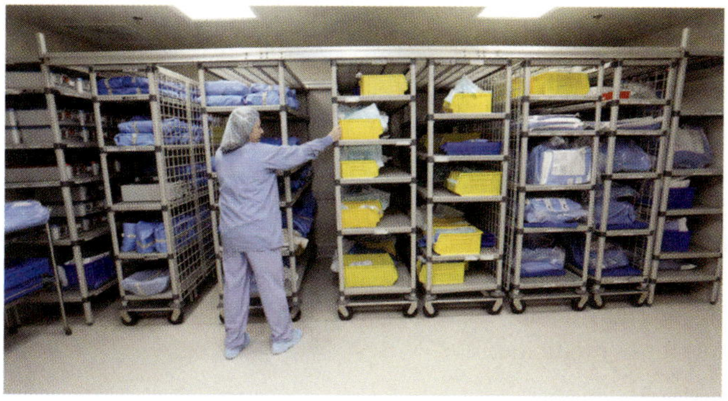

FIG. 10.12 Storage system for sterile goods. This system uses sliding racks, which allow staff to access equipment easily while maintaining correct storage parameters for wrapped goods.

DISINFECTION

Disinfection is the destruction of some but not all types and forms of microorganisms on an inanimate object. By definition, disinfection is not sterilization, because the disinfection process does not result in the complete destruction of all microorganisms. The Spaulding system provides two disinfection levels—high level and low level.

HLD is the most effective process for destroying microbes on a surface. HLD does not destroy bacterial spores; therefore it is used only for instruments that will be used in semi-critical areas of the body (e.g., nonintact skin and mucous membranes). Instruments and other items that are semi-critical include the following:

- Anesthesia equipment
- Gastrointestinal endoscopes
- Bronchoscopes
- Respiratory therapy equipment

HLD is used for flexible and rigid endoscopes that are used in noncritical areas of the body. Processing takes place in a special area of the operating room adjacent to or near the point of use, such as the endoscopy department or cystoscopy suite.

The process uses a commercial reprocessing unit with specific chemical disinfectants approved for HLD. Before any instrument is disinfected, it must be thoroughly cleaned to remove all traces of blood, tissue, and body fluids. Cleaning is carried out systematically so that no areas are overlooked.

A complete discussion of the techniques used in the reprocessing of endoscopes can be found in Chapter 20.

Low-level disinfection is performed on equipment that comes in contact with intact skin but not mucous membranes or tissue deeper than skin. Low-level disinfectant is used as a cleaning agent in environmental decontamination and includes health care devices such as blood pressure cuffs, stethoscopes, intravenous stands, and patient furniture. It is also used on items brought into the operating room from outside. Personnel items such as cell phones, tablets, and briefcases must be wiped clean with low-level disinfectant before they can be carried into the semi-restricted and restricted areas of the department.

ENVIRONMENTAL DISINFECTANTS

Environmental disinfectants are used for routine low-level disinfection and environmental decontamination. These disinfectants contain enzymes and other chemicals that destroy or inhibit microbes by changing cell proteins (denaturation) or by drying (desiccation) them.

Common terms used to describe chemicals and the process of disinfection help distinguish chemicals and also clarify their action.

The suffix **-cidal** means to kill. A **bactericidal** chemical is one that kills bacteria, and a viricidal chemical kills viruses. A **sporicidal** chemical destroys bacterial spores, and a fungicidal agent is one that kills fungi. The term *germicide* ("germ killing," or germicidal) is commonly used by the general public but not in medicine.

USE OF CHEMICAL DISINFECTANTS

Disinfectants commonly used in patient care are categorized by chemical type (Table 10.4). The selection of a disinfectant is based on the result required. Some disinfectants are effective at destroying a limited number of microorganisms; others destroy all organisms, including bacterial spores. Some are extremely corrosive, whereas others are relatively harmless to common materials found in the hospital.

Factors that affect a disinfectant's activity (or "-cidal" ability) include the following:

1. *Concentration of the solution:* Every chemical disinfectant is used at a prescribed dilution. Chemicals may require premixing with water. This must be done with a measuring device.
2. *The bioburden on the object:* As the bioburden increases, the effectiveness of the disinfectant may decrease.
3. *Water hardness and pH:* The mineral content and pH of the water used for dilution may alter the action of the chemical.
4. *Presence or absence of organic matter on the item:* Nearly all disinfectants are weakened in the presence of organic material such as blood, sputum, or tissue residue. Therefore items to be disinfected must undergo cleaning (removal of organic debris and soil) and thorough drying before the disinfection process.

DISINFECTANT SAFETY

Many disinfectants are unsafe for use on human tissue, including skin. This means that employees must be extremely cautious when handling them. Warnings and instructions for use must be strictly followed. Do not be misled by the mild odor of some disinfectants. Many chemicals do not emit noxious fumes but are still toxic.

Every health care facility is required by law to provide employees with information about hazards in their work environment. This includes specific training and information about the chemicals they handle. Every chemical used in the workplace has a corresponding **Material Safety Data Sheet (MSDS)**, as mandated by OSHA. The MSDS describes the chemical, potential hazards, and what to do if the chemical comes in contact with the skin or is splashed into the eyes. The MSDS for each chemical is easily accessed and should be read by all who work in the perioperative environment. (A more complete discussion of chemical safety is presented in Chapter 7.)

Safety Guidelines • Disinfectants

1. All disinfectants should be stored in well-ventilated rooms, and their containers should be kept covered.
2. All personnel handling disinfectants must wear PPE.
3. The dilution ratio of a liquid chemical should never be changed except by hospital protocol.
4. A measuring device designated for mixing liquid disinfectants with water should always be used. Personnel should not rely on haphazard techniques or guesswork when preparing solutions.
5. Two disinfectants should never be mixed; this could create toxic fumes or unstable and dangerous compounds.
6. Liquid chemicals should be disposed of as directed by hospital policy and the chemical's label instructions. Some chemicals are unsafe for disposal through standard sewage systems.
7. An unlabeled bottle or container should never be used and should be discarded. Personnel should always be aware of what chemical is being used and its specific purpose.

CHEMICAL DISINFECTANTS FOR MEDICAL DEVICES

The chemicals most commonly used in HLD are glutaraldehyde and ortho-phthalaldehyde (commercially prepared as Cidex and Cidex OPA). Cidex OPA is quickly replacing glutaraldehyde.

GLUTARALDEHYDE

Glutaraldehyde is a high-level disinfectant that is sporicidal, bactericidal, and viricidal. It is tuberculocidal in 20 minutes. This disinfectant is weakened considerably by unintentional dilution, which occurs if instruments are wet when placed in the immersion tank. Glutaraldehyde is also weakened by the presence of organic matter (tissue debris or body fluids). When glutaraldehyde solutions are mixed and kept for repetitive use, the solution must be completely renewed after 14 days because it is ineffective after that time. In addition, during its time in use, the solution must be evaluated often with test

TABLE 10.4 Properties of Disinfectants

Chemical	Level of Disinfection	Kills Spores	Kills HIV	Kills Mycobacterium Tuberculosis	Kills HBV	Uses	Risk
Isopropyl alcohol (70% to 90%)	Intermediate (some semi-critical and noncritical items)	No	Yes	Yes	Yes	Limited; no longer used as a general disinfectant	Flammable; can damage lensed instruments
Phenolic detergent compounds	Low	No	Yes	Yes	No	Environmental cleaning only	Highly toxic
Glutaraldehyde (2%)	High (critical items)	Yes	Yes	Yes	Yes	Endoscopes, respiratory equipment, anesthesia equipment, immersible items. Long shelf life. Disinfectant active for long periods when used properly.	Vapor causes eye, skin, and nasal irritation. Improperly rinsed endoscopes can cause tissue damage.
Stabilized hydrogen peroxide (6%)	High (critical items)	Yes	Yes	Yes	Yes	Must contact all surfaces when used as a sterilant	Can cause tissue irritation
Formalin (37% formaldehyde)	High	Yes	Yes	Yes	Yes	Currently used for specimen preservation	Highly noxious fumes; carcinogenic
Iodophor (free iodine in a detergent–disinfectant solution)	Intermediate to low, depending on concentration	No	Yes	Yes	Yes	As a disinfectant, limited to use in cleaning hydrotherapy tanks and thermometers, environmental cleaning	May cause reactions in sensitive individuals
Quaternary ammonium detergent	Low (noncritical items)	No	Yes	No	No	Limited effectiveness; used for low-level environmental disinfection	May cause reactions in sensitive individuals
Sodium hypochlorite (5%, 500 ppm)	Low (noncritical items)	No	Yes	No	Yes	1:100 ppm for spot disinfection and blood spills; environmental cleaning	Fumes can irritate skin and mucous membranes

HBV, Hepatitis B virus; *HIV*, human immunodeficiency virus.

strips to ensure that the proper concentration is maintained (2% glutaraldehyde).

Occupational hazards of glutaraldehyde most commonly arise when the solution is kept in open immersion baths in a poorly ventilated work area. The safe levels of formaldehyde or glutaraldehyde in the air are under 0.2 ppm. Any amount over that causes irritation of the eyes and nasal passages. Glutaraldehyde is toxic to tissue; items that have been disinfected or sterilized in glutaraldehyde must be completely rinsed with sterile distilled water before they are used on a patient.

ORTHO-PHTHALALDEHYDE

Ortho-phthalaldehyde 0.55% (Cidex OPA) is a non-glutaraldehyde-based, high-level disinfectant that can be used on immersible medical devices. Instruments and equipment are thoroughly cleaned, dried, and placed in the solution for 12 minutes at 20°C. An automatic endoscope reprocessor can achieve HLD in 5 minutes. The items must be thoroughly rinsed with water three times.

PHENOLICS

Phenol (carbolic acid) is formulated as a detergent for hospital cleaning. It is not sporicidal, but it is tuberculocidal, fungicidal, viricidal, and bactericidal. Because scant information is available on the specific effects of phenol on microorganisms, its use is restricted to disinfection of *noncritical items*. It is extremely important to follow the manufacturer's instructions for dilution and mixing, because phenolic mixtures can be toxic. Phenol has a very noxious odor and causes skin lesions and respiratory irritation in some individuals.

QUATERNARY AMMONIUM COMPOUNDS

Quaternary ammonium compounds, or *quats*, are fungicidal and bactericidal, but are not effective at killing spores. This group of disinfectants is less effective in hard water, which can limit their use in some regions. Benzalkonium chloride and dimethyl benzyl ammonium chloride are common quaternary ammonium compounds that are widely used as disinfectants. Quats are mainly used for low-level disinfection.

HYPOCHLORITE

Hypochlorite is sporicidal and tuberculocidal and effective against the human immunodeficiency virus (HIV). The CDC recommends this product for use in spot cleaning of blood spills, because it is fast acting. However, it is deactivated in the presence of organic material; therefore the area must be cleaned before hypochlorite is applied. The chemicals in the hypochlorite family are not used on instruments, because they are corrosive. However, they are widely used for **environmental cleaning,** because they are effective and inexpensive. Sodium hypochlorite, for example, is common household bleach. Hypochlorite must be diluted properly to prevent respiratory irritation and skin burns.

ALCOHOL

Alcohol is a commonly used disinfectant that is composed of two components: ethyl alcohol and isopropyl alcohol. Both are water soluble (mix easily in water). Alcohol is not sporicidal, but it is bactericidal, tuberculocidal, and viricidal. It is effective against cytomegalovirus and HIV. Alcohol's optimum disinfection ability occurs at 60% to 70% dilution. Alcohol must never be used on surgical instruments, because it is not sporicidal and is very corrosive to stainless steel.

Alcohol greatly reduces the number of bacteria on skin when used as a surgical hand rub. However, it also removes fatty acids from the skin and has a drying effect when used routinely.

Because it is highly flammable and volatile, alcohol must never be used around electrosurgery instruments or lasers. It must be stored in a cool, well-ventilated area. Skin preparation solutions that contain alcohol must be allowed to dry completely before draping.

ENVIRONMENTAL CLEANING

The perioperative environment carries a high risk for infection transmission. This is related to the number of patient contacts, surface contact ("high-touch areas"), and the level of contamination on these surfaces. Maintaining a clean environment is everyone's responsibility, with specific duties assigned to housekeeping personnel who carry out cleaning processes required to meet infection control standards.

Disinfection or sanitation is the process by which surfaces, materials, and equipment are cleaned with specific substances (disinfectants) that render them safe for their intended use. Any item that is exposed to or soiled with organic matter such as blood, tissue, or body fluid is considered contaminated. *Cleaning* refers to the process by which any type of soil, including organic material, is removed. This is accomplished with detergent, water, and mechanical action. Cleaning precedes all disinfection processes. The purpose of sanitation and disinfection is to prevent cross-contamination between patients and personnel.

ROUTINE DECONTAMINATION OF THE SURGICAL SUITE

Before the Workday

The recommended practice before the first case of the day is damp dusting of surgical lights, furniture, and fixed equipment in the operating suite. A clean, lint-free cloth and a hospital-grade chemical disinfectant are used.

During Surgery

The principles of Standard Precautions apply to all surgical procedures, and all cases are considered potentially contaminated and treated accordingly. The role of the ST in maintaining a clean environment has been discussed earlier. There should be increased emphasis on the handling of contaminated sharps. These include needles, scalpel blades, drill bits, and broken glass. Sharps must be segregated from all other equipment on the sterile field and off.

The following activities, which are part of the Standard Precautions, must be performed to prevent cross-contamination with blood-borne pathogens. The following duties are performed by the circulator or other nonsterile personnel:

- Any blood spills or contamination by other organic material should be removed promptly with a hospital-grade disinfectant. All articles used and discarded in the course of surgery must be placed in leak-proof containers. This prevents spilling of contaminated liquid onto other surfaces.
- Any contaminated or suspect item must be handled in a manner that protects personnel from contamination. An instrument can be used to transfer contaminated articles to a waste or other receptacle *(no-touch method)*.
- Tissue specimens, blood, and all other body fluids must be placed in a leak-proof container for transport out of the department. The outside of any specimen container that is passed off the surgical field to the circulator must be cleaned with a hospital-grade disinfectant.
- Because paper products are difficult or impossible to decontaminate, every effort should be made to keep patients' charts, laboratory slips, radiograph reports and radiographs, and any paper documentation free of contamination.
- Contaminated sponges must be collected in a kick bucket in which a plastic bag or liner has been previously placed. Sponges must not be lined up on the floor for counting. Sponges should be counted and immediately placed in plastic bags representing increment numbers such as five or ten sponges.
- Instruments that fall off the surgical field must be retrieved by the circulator (with gloves protecting the hands) and placed in a basin containing a noncorrosive disinfectant. In this way, organic debris on the instrument is prevented from drying and becoming airborne.

Environmental Cleaning After Surgery

After instruments, supplies, and contaminated equipment have been removed from the surgical suite, the walls, floors, furniture, and fixtures are cleaned.

- Floors are cleaned with disinfectant and may be wet-vacuumed. A 3- to 4-foot area (about 1 to 1.2 m) around the sterile field is considered efficient for routine decontamination between cases.
- The pads of the operating table are removed to expose the undersurface of the table. All surfaces of the table and pads are cleaned, with particular attention to the hinges, pivotal points, and casters.
- The operating table is moved aside for cleaning underneath and to check for any items that may have dropped to the floor during surgery.
- All soiled operating room equipment is cleaned with disinfectant.
- Walls, doors, surgical lights, and ceilings are spot cleaned if they are soiled with blood, tissue, or body fluids. Additional attention is given to supply cabinet doors, especially the latches and handles.
- All contaminated items used during the cleaning process are removed from the room.

After decontamination, all furniture is repositioned, and clean linen is placed on the operating table. Clean liner bags are then placed in kick buckets and linen frames.

Terminal Cleaning

Terminal cleaning takes place at the close of each workday. All perioperative areas are terminally cleaned with special attention to the operating and procedure rooms themselves. All exposed surfaces are cleaned and disinfected using an approved hospital disinfectant designated for use as an environmental cleaning/disinfecting agent.

The following areas are targeted:

- Operating room table, including the mattress, extensions, safety straps, and positioning equipment
- Patient transfer devices such as roller boards and transfer boards
- All furniture, including instrument tables, prep stands, chairs, stools, and desks
- Overhead procedure lights
- Storage equipment such as storage cabinets and supply carts
- High-touch areas such as door and cabinet handles, latches, and door edges
- Anesthesia equipment including carts, heavy equipment, and the anesthesia machine
- Patient monitors
- Communication and computer equipment, including computer accessories
- Light switches, cords, and cables
- Fixed equipment such as the suction regulator, suction holders, viewing monitors, electrosurgical equipment, gas regulators, microscope, etc.

Terminal cleaning also includes the postoperative care unit, preoperative holding areas, sterile processing areas, and instrument storage areas.

KEY CONCEPTS

- The practice of aseptic technique is based on the separation between sterile and nonsterile surfaces. The purpose of practicing aseptic technique is to prevent infection.
- Correct use of terms related to sterility and disinfection demonstrates understanding of the concepts and their importance in preventing infection.
- The Spaulding system separates medical devices and instruments according to the location of their use in the body, and thus the level of asepsis required—sterilization, disinfection, or cleaning.
- Systematic methods are used in the sterilization and disinfection of surgical devices and instruments so that no step is missed in the process. All surgical technologists are required to know what method to use and how to perform that method.
- Decontamination of instruments and devices is critical to prevent the transmission of infection from one individual to another.
- Surgical instruments and devices are made of many different types of materials whose physical properties require specific

methods of cleaning, disinfection, and sterilization. One of the primary goals in reprocessing is to use the most effective means while also considering safety and economics.

- Correct wrapping of surgical equipment and loading in the steam sterilizer are essential to achieve and maintain the sterility of an item. If this phase of the process is incorrect, the whole process may be invalid.
- Biological monitoring during sterilization is performed by exposing the load to harmless bacterial spores, which are then recovered and cultured.
- Steam under pressure is the most common and economical method of sterilizing surgical equipment.
- The IUS sterilizer is used to rapidly sterilize clean decontaminated equipment for immediate use. This method is used only when no other method is available. Implants are not sterilized in an IUS sterilizer except in an emergency and must be monitored with a biological control system.
- Other methods of sterilization include ethylene oxide gas, gas plasma, liquid peracetic acid, and ionizing radiation (commercial use only).
- All equipment used on a patient must be cleaned and decontaminated before sterilization.
- Disinfection is performed on equipment used in semi-critical areas of the body. High-level disinfectants are capable of destroying bacteria and their spores.
- Low-level disinfection is used for environmental cleaning.

REVIEW QUESTIONS

1. What is bioburden?
2. Why are instruments processed in the washer–decontaminator sterilizer?
3. What is the purpose of wrapping instruments for sterilization?
4. What disinfectant is approved for cleaning blood spills in the surgical suite?
5. Why doesn't a control monitor determine that sterilized goods are sterile?
6. What is DART?
7. Describe each of the three levels of the Spaulding classification system.
8. What is immediate-use processing?
9. What is terminal disinfection?
10. Why are sterile packages given a lot number?

CASE STUDY

As a student ST you are assigned to assist in the clean processing area of the operating room. Your health facility also has a Central Supply Department that has decontamination and sterilization services for the rest of the facility. In your assigned area, you will be asked to assist in assembling instrument trays correctly, ensuring that monitoring systems are in place, and loading the steam sterilizer. Your mentor will run the loads, but you are expected to retrieve and interpret the output data from the system. You will start your work by receiving instruments that have come out of the washer-sterilizer/disinfector. The instruments are in wash trays. They are decontaminated and dry, and your mentor for the day has removed them from the system and placed them in the clean workroom. Your workroom has files containing the contents of all instrument sets, logs to identify the sterilization loads by their number, the date of the run, and additional space to record which type(s) sterilization monitors were used for the run.

1. List the tasks you must complete up to the point but not including putting the instrument sets together. List small and large details of your tasks.
2. After completing these tasks, you will prepare the instruments and assemble them in perforated sterilization trays. How will you do this? Thinking strategically, how do you know which sets must be assembled? What monitors should you use? Consider documentation and instrument tracking. How should you prepare the instruments for sterilization before wrapping? Your final output is the prepared instrument tray that is not yet wrapped.
3. Now you will wrap the instrument sets and load the sterilizer. List the steps and any details regarding documentation. You also have a number of single instruments that must be wrapped separately. Explain how you might handle these.
4. Your mentor has selected the correct settings for your load, which has now completed its cycle. You will remove the instruments following the dry cycle. How will you unload the sterilizer? What documentation might be necessary at this stage?
5. What questions do you have for your mentor? Was anything unclear? What did you learn?

BIBLIOGRAPHY

American Society of Cataract and Refractive Surgery and the American Society of Ophthalmic Registered Nurses: *Recommended practices for cleaning and sterilizing intraocular surgical instruments.* https://www.aao.org/clinical-statement/guidelines-cleaning-sterilization-intraocular. Accessed July 20, 2019.

Association for the Advancement of Medical Instrumentation. Comprehensive guide to steam sterilization and sterility assurance in health care facilities. *ANSI/AAMI ST79*. 2006.

Association of periOperative Registered Nurses. *Guidelines for Perioperative Practice*. Denver: AORN; 2015.

Centers for Disease Control and Prevention. *Infection Control. Sterilizing Practices. Guideline for Disinfection and Sterilization in Healthcare Facilities*; 2008. https://www.cdc.gov/infectioncontrol/guidelines/disinfection/sterilization/sterilizing-practices.html. Accessed July 21, 2019.

Rutala WA, Weber DJ. Disinfection, sterilization, and antisepsis: an overview. *Am J Infect Control*. 2016;44(suppl 5):e1–6.

Rutala WA, Weber DJ. Guideline for disinfection and sterilization of prion-contaminated medical instruments. *Infect Control Hosp Epidemiol*. 2010;31(2):107–117.

Rutala WA, Weber DJ. Selection of the ideal disinfectant. *Infect Control Hosp Epidemiol*. 2014;35(7):855–865. https://doi.org/10.1086/676877.

The Joint Commission: *Standards FAQs details: laryngoscope–blades and handles–how to clean, disinfect and store these devices.* https://www.jointcommission.org/mobile/standards_information/jcfaqdetails.aspx?StandardsFAQId¼508&StandardsFAQChapter%20Id¼69.%2046. Accessed February 4, 2015.

SURGICAL INSTRUMENTS 11

LEARNING OBJECTIVES

After studying this chapter, the reader will be able to:

1. Review information on instrument manufacturing
2. Identify the different types of finishes on surgical instruments
3. Differentiate types of instruments by their design
4. Differentiate types of instruments by their function
5. Classify instruments by tissue type
6. Demonstrate how to pass basic instruments to the surgeon
7. Describe how to inspect instruments for defects

TERMINOLOGY

Alloy: A combination of several different kinds of metals. Alloys are used in the manufacturing of stainless steel.

Anastomosis: A surgical procedure in which tubular or hollow structures such as blood vessels or segments of intestine are connected by sutures or staples.

Box lock: The hinge point of many surgical instruments

Chisel: An orthopedic instrument used to shave bone; one side is straight and the other is beveled.

Curettage: The removal of tissue by scraping with a surgical curette.

Dilator: Graduated, smooth instrument that is used to increase the circumference of an orifice.

Double-action rongeur: A bone-cutting instrument with two hinges in the middle. This increases the leverage and strength of the instrument.

Elevator: A straight instrument with a curved sharp or dull tip used to separate tissue layers such as periosteum from bone.

Gouge: A hollow chisel used to cut into and remove portions of bone, often used for bone grafting.

Hemostat: A surgical clamp most often used to occlude a blood vessel.

Resection: A surgical technique in which a section of an organ or tissue is usually removed because of disease or trauma. Resection requires closure or repair of the remaining tissue edges along the line of resection.

Rongeur: A single or double hinged instrument with sharp, cup shaped, or delicate angled tips that is used to extract pieces of bone or other connective tissue.

Serosa: The delicate outer tissue layer of most organs.

Shank: The area of a surgical instrument between the box lock and the ring fingers.

Single-action rongeur: A bone-cutting instrument that has one hinge used to cut and extract bone or tissue.

Tenaculum: A grasping instrument with sharp pointed tips, generally used to manipulate or grasp tissue such as the thyroid or cervix.

INTRODUCTION

Expertise in surgical instrumentation is among the most important roles of a surgical technologist. Familiarity with instruments and their names (sometimes different from one region to another and even among health facilities) is *also one of the most difficult* learning curves for students in surgery.

The purpose of this chapter to provide the basis for understanding how instruments are made and the relationship between design and function. It is not a catalog for the memorization of instruments.

Important to know: *The most effective way to learn the names and use of instruments is to study them in association with the surgeries they are used in rather than in isolation.*

This is because a relatively small number of instruments are used compared to the thousands contained in different catalogs. In this text, surgical instruments are illustrated within their specialty chapter to reinforce the association and aid in memorization. Classification of instruments in groups according to function and association with tissue types encourages critical thinking during surgery. Finally, surgical technologists should know how to evaluate surgical instruments for soundness. This is an important role that has implications for patient safety and a technically smooth surgical procedure. Even if the facility's instruments are processed in a separate area such as the central processing department, the responsibility for providing safe instruments *lies with everyone involved in their use and processing.*

Note: Specific instruments pictured in the chapter are meant to be *examples* of different types of instruments. Note also that there are several ways to pass each type of instrument. The figures shown here are commonly used but other techniques are used according to the surgical procedure and specific anatomical considerations. Variations may also occur depending on whether the scrubbed ST stands next to the surgeon or across from her or him. In all instances, safety takes precedence over all else.

INSTRUMENT MANUFACTURING

The instrument manufacturing process, the origin of the materials, and the quality control on the finished product determine the quality and safety of surgical instruments. High-quality surgical instruments are constructed using specific types of metals. An **alloy** is any metal that contains two or more types of metallic elements. Stainless steel, which is the preferred alloy for surgical instruments, contains copper, titanium, molybdenum, and nickel and other metal combinations. In general, high-quality stainless steel contains a greater percentage of chromium, which resists corrosion and increases the strength of the stainless steel.

Poor-quality stainless steel has a low percentage of chromium and tends to develop hairline fractures that are sometimes not visible without magnification. However, these fractures become deeper with repeated use, finally resulting in breakage. Poor-quality instruments contain soldering defects that contribute to breakage and create microscopic burrs and sharp points that puncture and cut tissue. This is especially critical for ophthalmic and microsurgery instruments. Microscopic ridges and troughs in the surface of the steel can slice through delicate tissue and collect tissue debris. Biofilm in these small defects may not be removed in the disinfection and sterilization process, increasing the risk for patient infection.

INSTRUMENT GRADES

Within the stainless steel and surgical instrument industry, grades are assigned according to the quality of the stainless steel used in the manufacturing process. In the current global market, surgical instruments can be assembled in one country, with steel obtained from another. Quality may not be consistent. Surgical instruments are used in a variety of settings besides surgery. These settings include biological science laboratories, classrooms, and goods manufacturing. There are five different grades of stainless steel. Three of these are commonly used in the manufacturing of surgical instruments. Note that there are no universal standards for the manufacturing of stainless steel. Each instrument company grades its own products:

1. Surgical grade—has the highest level of chromium. The highest quality of surgical grade is called *premium* surgical grade by the steel industry. There are two types of surgical grades. The highest grade is used for cutting instruments needed to hold their sharpness. Intermediate surgical grade is used for instruments that are not subjected to a high impact and are not used for cutting.
2. Floor grade—contains lower percentage of chromium and are generally reserved for use in laboratories and other biomedical settings. Floor-grade instruments are prone to bending and breaking. It is important that these are not mixed with higher-grade instruments during reprocessing because they can be further weakened by ion transfer between the two grades.
3. Disposable grade—cannot withstand repeated exposure to high temperatures and are prone to breakdown with repeated use. Disposable grade instruments are meant for one time use only.

INSTRUMENT FINISHES

High-quality stainless steel resists corrosion and staining. However, even high-quality instruments can become damaged when subjected to harsh chemicals, frequent ultrasonic cleaning, and repeated sterilization. Different types of finishes on instruments protect them from environmental damage and also have specific uses in surgery. The most common finishes are easy to recognize:

1. *Highly polished* or *mirror finish* instruments resist staining. However, they are highly reflective and produce glare under strong lighting.
2. *Satin finish* reduces glare but is also prone to staining.
3. *Black chromium finish* is used on laser surgery instruments. The black finish absorbs all light and prevents reflection of laser energy into adjacent tissues.
4. *Titanium anodizing* is a method that imparts color and hardness to the surface of titanium. Anodizing is performed by passing an electric current through the surface metal, resulting in oxidation. Different colors are achieved by adjusting the oxide level of the coating. This process is commonly used in the manufacture of orthopedic implants such as plates and screws. Color coding allows easy matching of implant components and specialized tools. Titanium is extremely hard and resistant to corrosion and pitting, a quality that is essential in orthopedics. However, it is also very expensive.
5. *Anodizing* is used in the manufacturing of lightweight aluminum instrument sterilization trays. Without the anodizing process, aluminum trays would easily scratch, which can result in the proliferation of biofilm within the defects. The process allows the manufacturing of large instrument trays without the added weight of stainless steel.
6. *Gold dip* finish on the handles of an instrument usually means that the working tip or edge of the instrument has tungsten carbide inserts that are highly resistant to scratching, pitting, and dulling. Tungsten carbide scissors hold their cutting edge much longer than other types of metals. The tungsten carbide inserts in needle holders prevent the needle from slipping or rotating and increases grip at the jaws.
7. Black handles on cutting instruments can indicate that one of the cutting edges is micro-serrated. Instrument companies promote these under different names such as supercut, tough cut etc. However, instruments with a black finish are used in laser surgery to reduce hazardous reflection of laser energy.

INSTRUMENT NAMES

Like surgical procedures which, in previous times were named after (or by) the surgeon who developed the technique, that tradition carries on today with surgical instruments. Unfortunately for students of surgery who labor to learn the correct name for each instrument, this creates confusion and even disputes about which name is correct. Below are some examples of surgeons who have invented and trademarked specific instruments in different surgical specialties. One of the problems students encounter in learning instrument names is the use of the inventor's name which is attached to a type of instrument without further clarification. For example, there are many different types of *Debakey* clamps, just as there are many different types of *Cloward* retractors. An internet *image search* for each of the following provides insight into numbers of different instruments whose names include their inventor's identity. These are just a few of the many surgeons who have contributed to the standard and specialty instruments in common use today.

- *Dr. Michael Debakey* was a renowned cardiovascular surgeon who invented many hundreds of surgical techniques, devices, and specialized instruments.
- *Dr. Victor Satinsky and Dr. Denton Cooley* invented many innovative vascular clamps which are standard instruments in modern surgery.
- *Dr. Ralph Cloward* developed modern techniques in spinal surgery and innovative instruments that are commonly used today. These include the self-retaining Cloward blade retractors, anterior fusion retractors, vertebral spreaders, depth gauges, and elevators.
- *Dr. Ramon Castroviejo* was a pioneer in eye surgery who developed or refined many techniques used today. He invented many different types microsurgical eye instruments including spring needle holders, forceps, spring scissors, and callipers.

It is important to keep in mind that instrument names are adapted *regionally* and by different *facilities.* This means that students do need to know the names and types of the most common instruments in a specialty, but be prepared for variations.

COMMON TYPES OF INSTRUMENTS BY FUNCTION

Learning surgical instrument names and uses can be facilitated by knowing the categories they belong to. The Association of Surgical Technologists uses the following nomenclature for the categorization of surgical instruments. Students should be aware that there are other common systems of nomenclature used by instrument manufacturers and others involved in education.

- Cutting/dissecting
- Clamping/occluding
- Grasping/holding
- Retracting/exposing
- Aspirating/suctioning
- Suturing
- Stapling
- Dilating
- Probing
- Accessory
- Microinstruments
- Viewing

CUTTING INSTRUMENTS

The common *surgical scalpel* (knife) is used for sharp cutting. A disposable scalpel blade is detachable from the knife handle, although one piece single-use scalpels are available. Surgical blade handles and blades are numbered according to their size and shape. There are two systems used to identify the blade type. The most common is the Bard-Parker system. Each specific number handle is designed for specific blades (Figs. 11.1 and 11.2). The number of the blade corresponds to a specific size and shape. This numbering system is consistent across

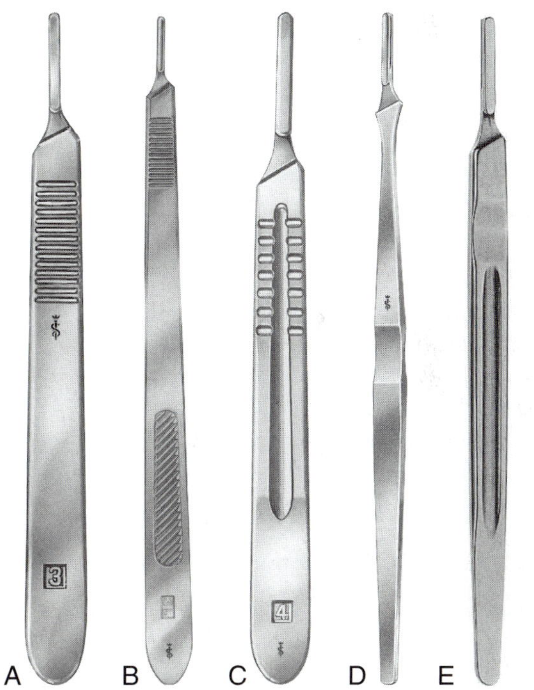

FIG 11.1 Bard-Parker knife handles. A, #3. B, #3 Long. C, #4. D, #7. E, #9 (Photo courtesy of Aesculap, Inc., Center Valley, PA.)

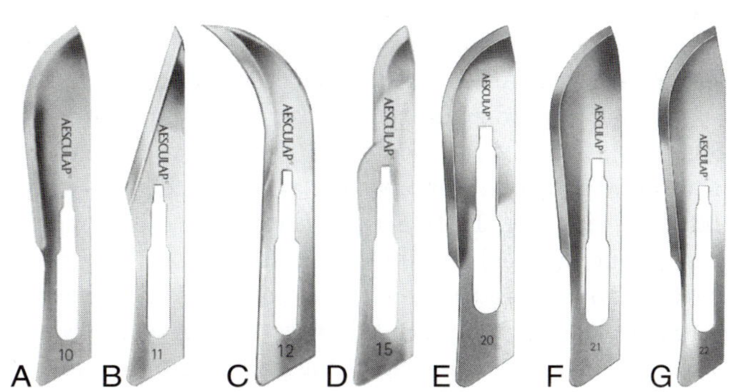

FIG 11.2 Bard-Parker knife blades. A, #10. B, #11. C, #12. D, #15. E, #20. F, #21. G, #22. (Photo courtesy of Aesculap, Inc., Center Valley, PA.)

TABLE 11.1 Commonly Used Surgical Blades and Handles

Handle Size	Fits Blade	Features
3, 3L (long), 7, 9	10	Curved edge, curved tip
	11	Straight edge, pointed tip
	12	Hook edge, pointed tip
	15	Narrow, curved edge, curved tip
4, 4L	20	Same as 10; larger one often used for skin incision
	23	Slightly curved edge, sharp tip

Note: Handles 4 and 4L are used with blade nos. 21 through 28.

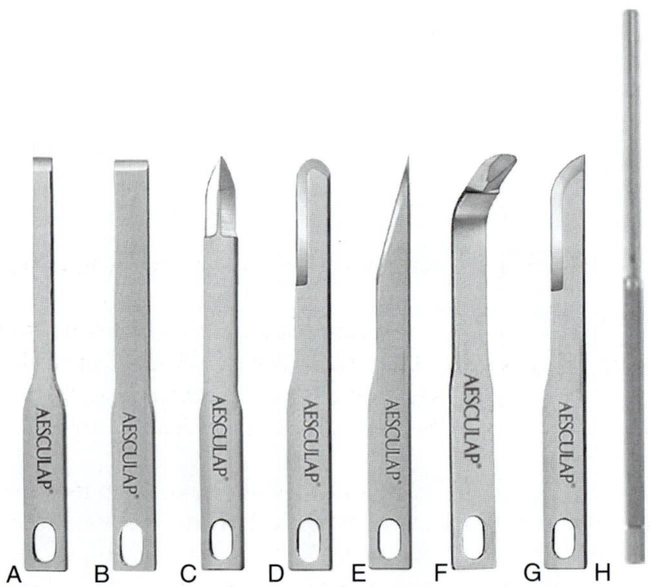

FIG 11.3 Micro Blades (also called Beaver Blades). A, #361. B, #362. C, #363. D, #364. E, #365. F, #366. G, #367. H, Handle for micro blades. (Photo courtesy of Aesculap, Inc., Center Valley, PA.)

all manufacturers. Table 11.1 shows which blades fit specific handles. Another common system of blades and handles, separate from the one just described, is the Beaver or *Micro blade* system. These blades are smaller and more delicate than the Bard-Parker system. These blades are designed for use in plastic, ophthalmic, and ear surgery and in general microsurgery (Fig. 11.3). Other types of knives are one piece instruments or are used in specializations such as orthopedic, ENT, and plastic surgery (Fig. 11.4). *Scissors* (Fig. 11.5) are among the most frequently used and important instruments in surgery. Careful handling and processing of scissors is necessary to maintain blade alignment and sharpness. High-quality surgical scissors are distinguished by the precision of the cutting edges, balance, and metal composition. Scissors are described according to the combination of round and sharp points.

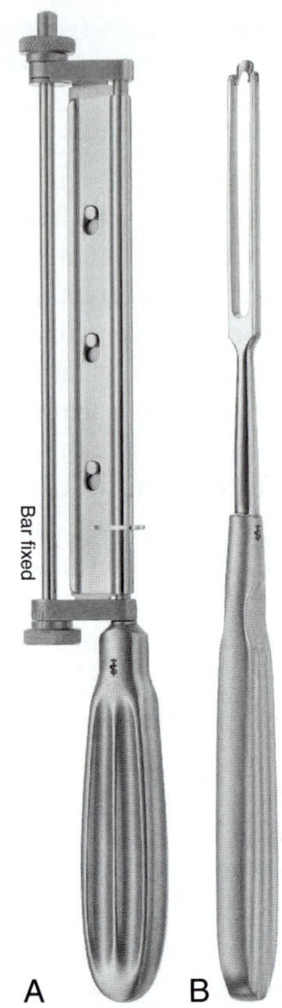

FIG 11.4 Specialty Knives. A, Watson skin graft knife. B, Ballenger swivel knife (ENT). (Photo courtesy of Aesculap, Inc., Center Valley, PA.)

These are sharp-sharp, sharp-round, and round-round. Scissors with extremely sharp points are used to sever very small areas of tissues during dissection. The blades of high-quality scissors are coated with tungsten or other hardened alloy to maintain sharpness. Surgical scissors are available in a wide variety of sizes and types. Small, sharp-tipped scissors, such as iris scissors, are used for extremely fine dissection in plastic surgery.

- Round-tipped, light dissecting scissors, such as Metzenbaum scissors, are extensively used on delicate tissue in many different surgical specialties. Fibrous connective tissue requires heavier scissors, such as the curved Mayo scissors.
- Straight Mayo scissors are used for cutting sutures and other materials, such as surgical mesh used to reinforce tissue, and hemostatic materials, such as oxidized cellulose. Note that tissue scissors such as the Metzenbaum must never be used to cut sutures as this leads to dulling of the blades.
- Wire-cutting scissors are used for stainless steel and other metal suture materials.
- Plastic surgery scissors are shorter than general surgery scissors and have very fine tips and blades.

A **rongeur** is used to cut and extract tissue and is distinguished by having a *spring-loaded* hinge (Fig. 11.6). The tips are cupped, and the edges are sharp. A rongeur may have a

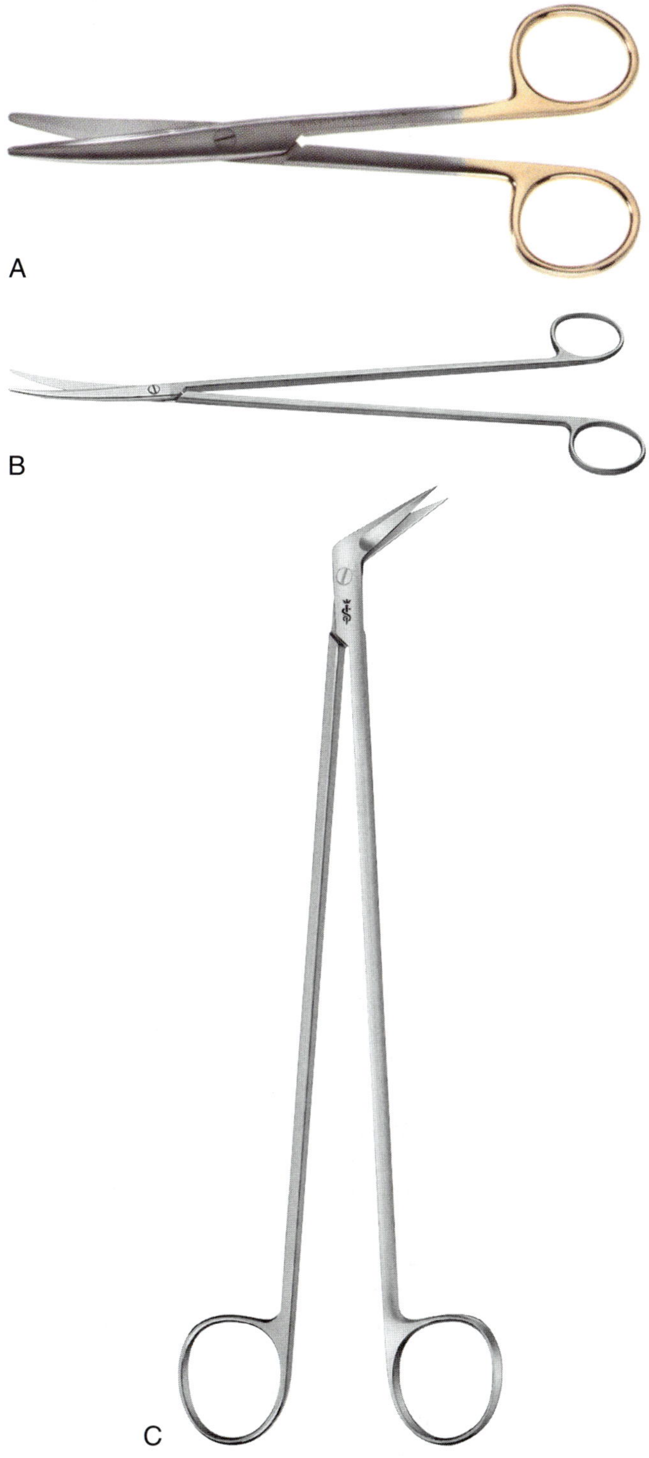

FIG 11.5 Tissue Scissors. A, Mayo. B, Metzenbaum. C, Potts. (A and B, Courtesy and © Becton, Dickinson and Company; C, Photo courtesy of Aesculap, Inc., Center Valley, PA.)

single hinge **(single-action rongeur)** or two hinges **(double-action rongeur).** A double-action rongeur creates twice the leverage of a single-action rongeur. Heavy rongeurs are used in orthopedic procedures. A long-handled delicate rongeur, such as the Kerrison rongeur, is used in spinal surgery. Fine-tipped rongeurs, such as the Kerrison, are categorized by the angle of their tips and described as either *up-biting* or *down-biting*. The angle of the rongeur tips allows the surgeon to cut

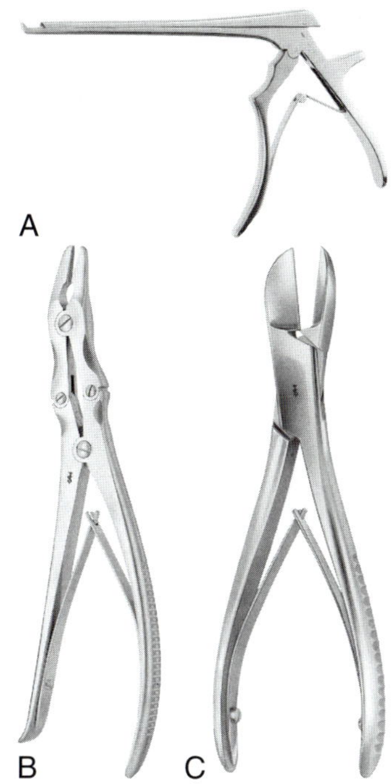

FIG 11.6 Rongeurs and Bone cutting forceps. A, Kerrison up bite (Neuro). B, Leksell double action (Ortho). C, Liston single action. (Photo courtesy of Aesculap, Inc., Center Valley, PA.)

and remove tissue from areas that are difficult to reach, such as around the spinous processes.

Shears (Fig. 11.7) are large cutting instruments used to sever bone. Their most common use is for cutting a rib needed to enter the chest cavity. Some shears are designed so that the cutting edge is to the left or right of the hinge. These are called *side-cutting* shears.

A *curette* (Fig. 11.8) is a small cup with a sharpened, serrated, or smooth rim at the end of the handle. Curettes are used in many specialties for scooping out tissue, including bone and soft tissue. Very fine curettes are used in ear, paranasal, and spinal surgery. Larger, heavier curettes are used in orthopedic procedures. Soft tissue curettes are used in gynecological surgery for endometrial **curettage.** These may be sharp or round-edged.

A **chisel** is an orthopedic cutting instrument that is used with a mallet (like chisels used in carpentry). Chisels are available in many widths and sizes that fit a particular specialty. For example, a chisel used in paranasal surgery is much more delicate than one designed for the large bones of the leg. The chisel and *osteotome* are often confused with one another. The osteotome is beveled on both sides, whereas a chisel blade is beveled on one side only (Fig. 11.9). The chisel produces a straight-sided cut. Both types of instruments are quite heavy and sharp. They are maintained in a metal rack where their blades cannot touch each other.

A **rasp** (Fig. 11.10) is used to remodel bone in the same way as its counterpart in carpentry. Many sizes, shapes, and surfaces are available. Fine rasps are used for delicate bones and surfaces such as the nasal sinuses. Heavy rasps are used to ream the medullary canal of long bones in preparation for an implant or smoothing heavy bone.

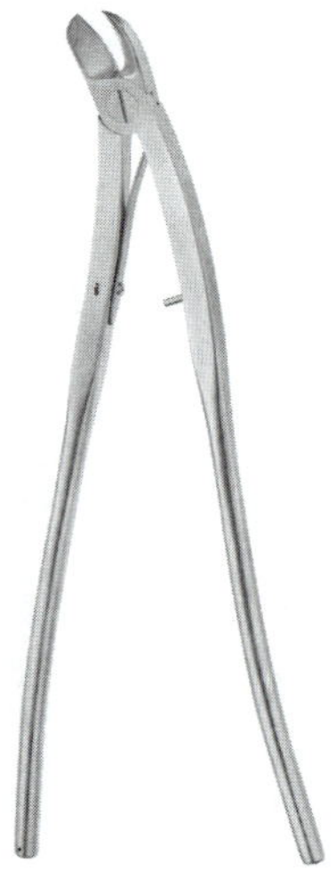

FIG 11.7 Shears. Bethune rib. (Photo courtesy of Aesculap, Inc., Center Valley, PA.)

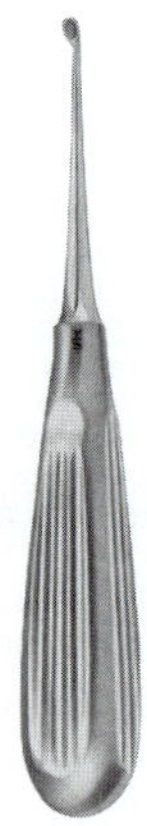

FIG 11.8 Bone curette (Photo courtesy of Aesculap, Inc., Center Valley, PA.)

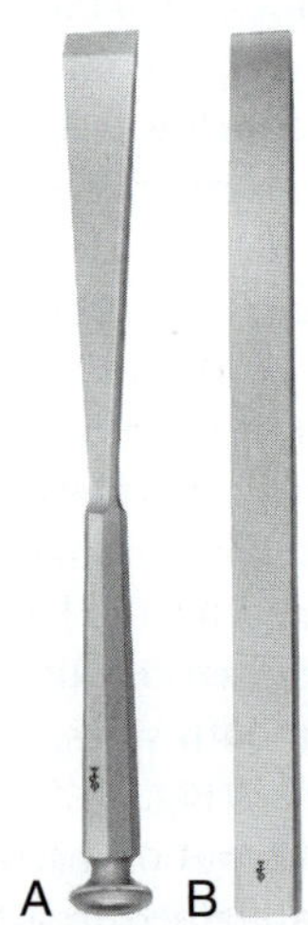

FIG 11.9 Chisel and Osteotome. A, Chisel. B, Osteotome. (Photo courtesy of Aesculap, Inc., Center Valley, PA.)

Drills are used very commonly in orthopedic surgery to create the holes needed for screws or wire or in craniotomy surgery to remove a section of bone in the cranium. Most drills are power driven, but hand drills are also available.

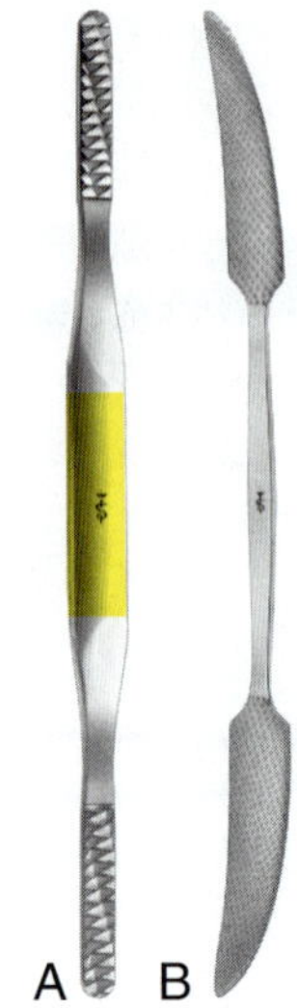

FIG 11.10 A. ENT Foman nasal rasp B. Orthopedic Putti bone rasp. (Photo courtesy of Aesculap, Inc., Center Valley, PA.)

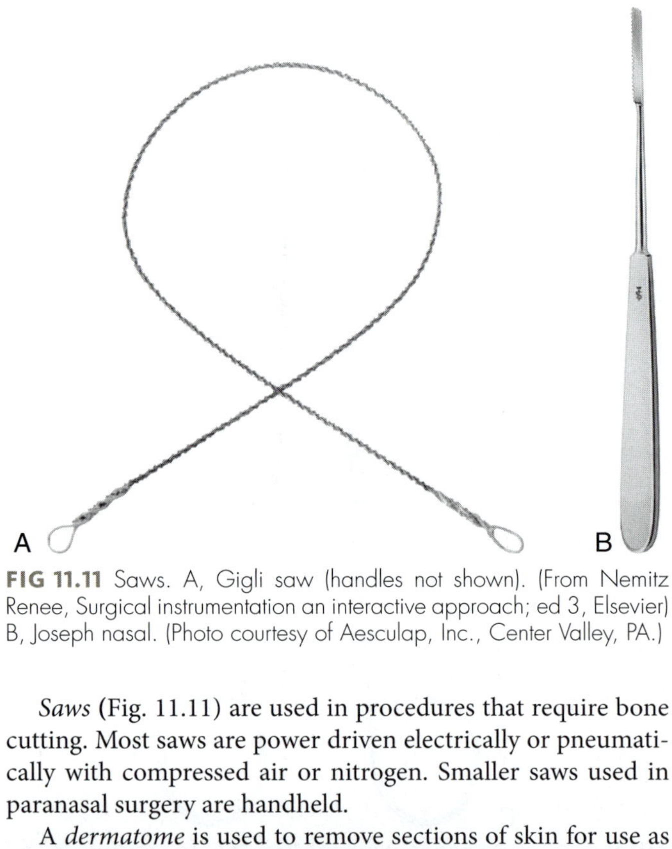

FIG 11.11 Saws. A, Gigli saw (handles not shown). (From Nemitz Renee, Surgical instrumentation an interactive approach; ed 3, Elsevier) B, Joseph nasal. (Photo courtesy of Aesculap, Inc., Center Valley, PA.)

Saws (Fig. 11.11) are used in procedures that require bone cutting. Most saws are power driven electrically or pneumatically with compressed air or nitrogen. Smaller saws used in paranasal surgery are handheld.

A *dermatome* is used to remove sections of skin for use as a skin graft. There are several different types of dermatomes. The most commonly used dermatomes, are discussed in detail in Chapter 28.

A **wire cutter** (Fig. 11.12) is another type of cutting instrument used to cut steel suture or small metal orthopedic pins.

An **elevator** (Fig. 11.13) is used to separate tissue layers. The most common uses are in orthopedic, nasal, vascular, and neuro surgery. The heavy, orthopedic elevator, such as the Lambotte elevator, slices bone tissue and is used with a mallet. The small, square-tipped Key elevator also has a sharp edge but is much more delicate. Very finely balanced elevators are used in soft tissue surgery such as in neuro and

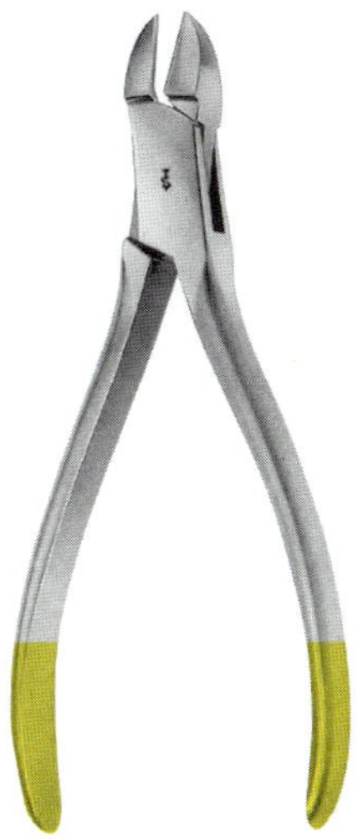
FIG 11.12 Wire cutter used to cut steel sutures and small orthopedic pins. (Photo courtesy of Aesculap, Inc., Center Valley, PA.)

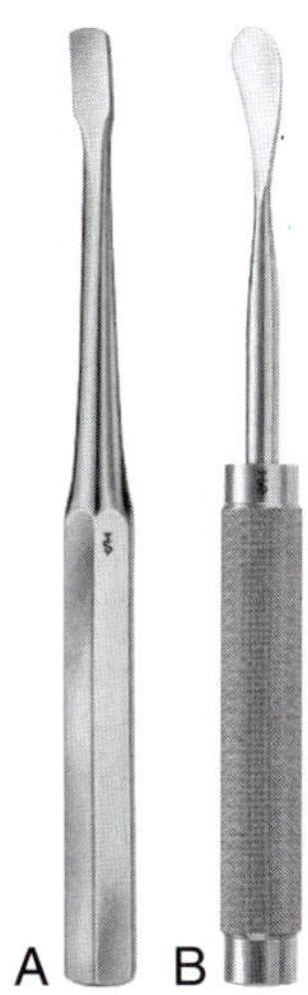

FIG 11.13 Elevator. A, Key. B, Cobb. (Photo courtesy of Aesculap, Inc., Center Valley, PA.)

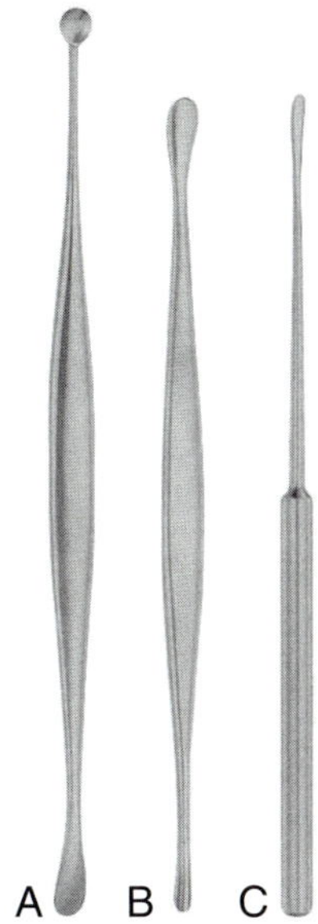

FIG 11.14 Dissector. A, Penfield #1. B, Penfield #2. C, Penfield #4. (Courtesy and © Becton, Dickinson and Company.)

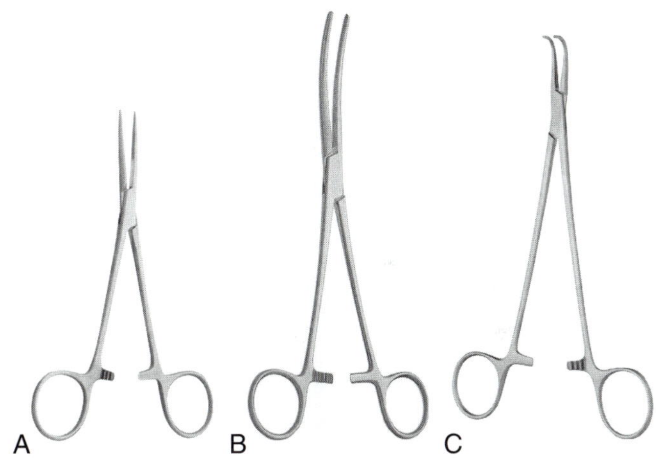

FIG 11.15 Hemostatic Clamp. A, Kelly. B, Mayo. C, Right angle (Mixter)19 A2228. (Courtesy and © Becton, Dickinson and Company.)

vascular procedures. In vascular surgery, elevators are used to separate atherosclerotic plaque from the inside of a blood vessel. These delicate elevators are well balanced and convey excellent tactile information from the working end to the surgeon's hand.

A **dissector** is used to lift and separate tissues similar to the elevator mentioned above. However, the dissector tends to have sharper edges. These are used in neurosurgery, plastic surgery, and in vascular procedures, where delicate tissue separation is required. A common dissector is the Penfield dissector, which is available in a number of different designs as shown in Fig. 11.14.

CLAMPING AND OCCLUDING

These instruments are used to grip tissues and organs, and in the case of occluding instruments, block the flow of body fluids including blood. The common *hemostatic clamp* provides a secure hold on tissue, sometimes to maintain pressure while the tissue is being ligated (tied or sewn with suture). There are many different types of **hemostats** of varying weights and lengths (Fig. 11.15). The tip of the instrument may be straight, curved, or right angled. These are also used to clamp tissue and to carry suture ties around deep structures.

A *partial occlusion* or atraumatic clamp has locking ratchets, but the tips and shanks do not fully lock down in a firm grip. An example is the intestinal clamp, which has longitudinal rather than horizontal serrations. During vascular surgery, blood flow must be temporarily stopped without damaging the vessel. *Vascular clamps* (Fig. 11.16) rather than hemostats are used in this case. These partially occluding clamps have enough pressure to slow or stop blood flow, but they do not bruise or crush the vessel. They are recognizable by their relatively light weight, delicate structure, and single or double ridges that run longitudinally along the jaws. The small bulldog and aneurysm clamp are spring-loaded and used mainly in neurovascular and cardiac surgery.

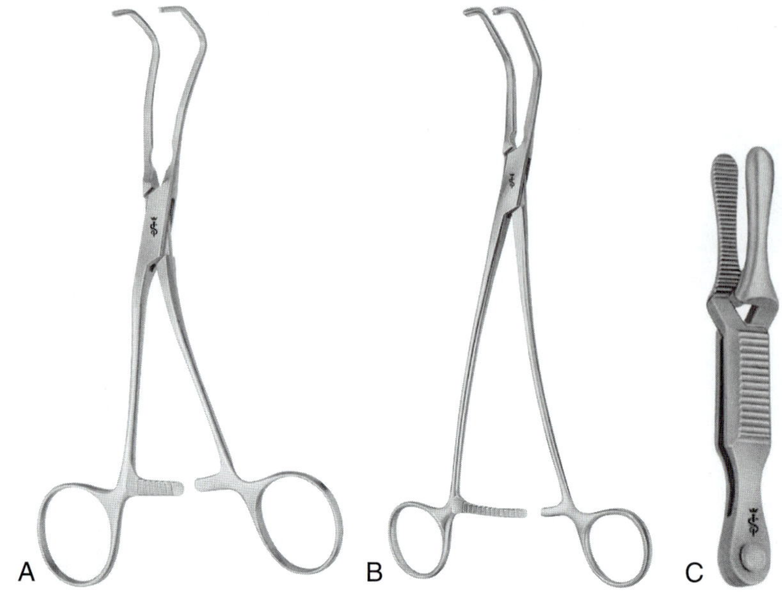

FIG 11.16 Vascular clamp. A, Cooley. B, Statinsky. C, Bulldog. (Photo courtesy of Aesculap, Inc., Center Valley, PA.)

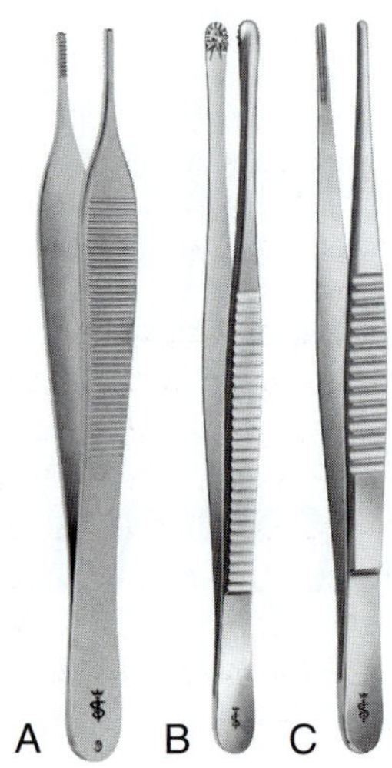

FIG 11.17 Thumb forceps. A, Adson serrated. B, Russian. C, DeBakey. (Photo courtesy of Aesculap, Inc., Center Valley, PA.)

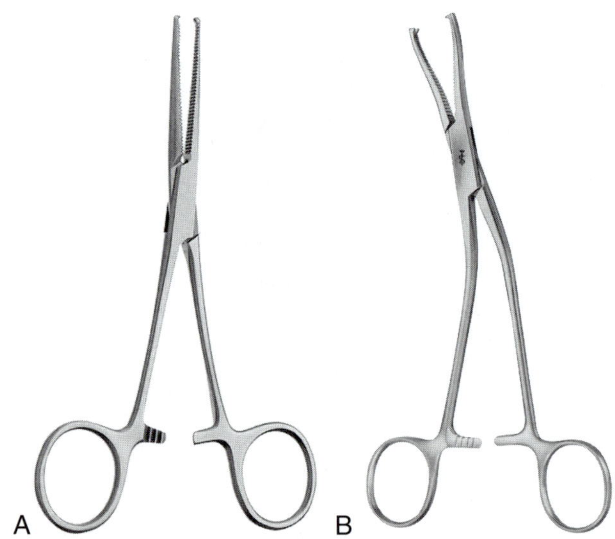

FIG 11.18 Connective tissue clamp. A, Kocher. B, Meniscus. (A, Courtesy and © Becton, Dickinson and Company; B, Photo courtesy of Aesculap, Inc., Center Valley, PA.)

GRASPING AND HOLDING

Grasping and holding instruments are necessary for both superficial and deep tissues of all types. Thumb forceps (also called "pick ups" (Fig. 11.17) are V-shaped instruments often used in the surgeon's nondominant hand during tissue dissection, manipulation, and suturing. Toothed forceps have one or more sharp teeth at the tips that mesh with slots on the opposite tine; 1 × 2 forceps have one tooth on one tine and two on the other. Smooth forceps have no teeth. Instead, the tines may be serrated to allow an atraumatic hold. Vascular forceps have the same fine rounded serrations as the vascular clamp.

Note: The term *forceps* is also used to describe a small number of hinged instruments which are used to grasp tissue.

Deep connective tissues such as ligament, tendon, and cartilage require grasping clamps with heavy teeth that bite into the tissue for a secure hold (Fig. 11.18). Bone holding instruments are designed to clamp around the bone's circumference or penetrate and hold the bone between sharp teeth.

The **tenaculum** is a specific type of holding clamp whose tips contain very sharp teeth that mesh together while penetrating the tissue in a pincer hold (Fig. 11.19). A tenaculum may have two or four separate teeth, which are extremely sharp. Examples are the cervical tenaculum used in gynecological procedures and the thyroid tenaculum.

Delicate tissues such as lung and intestine require grasping instruments that hold the tissue without causing bruising or any other injury. Examples include the Duval lung clamp and Babcock clamp commonly used to manipulate the fallopian tube or small intestine (Fig. 11.20).

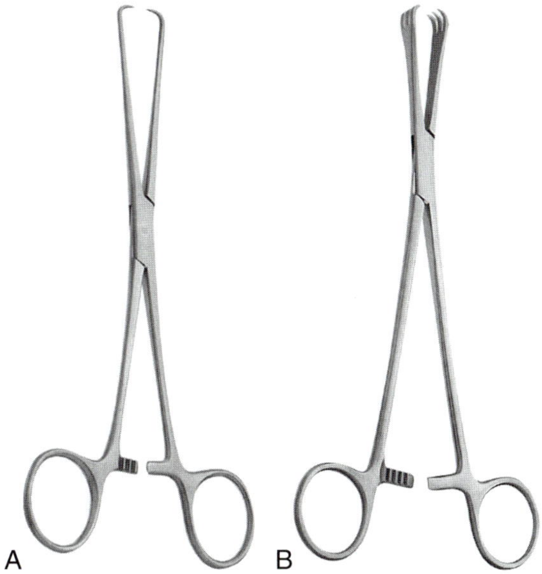

FIG 11.19 Tenaculum. A, Single toothed. B, Multiple tooth. (Courtesy and © Becton, Dickinson and Company.)

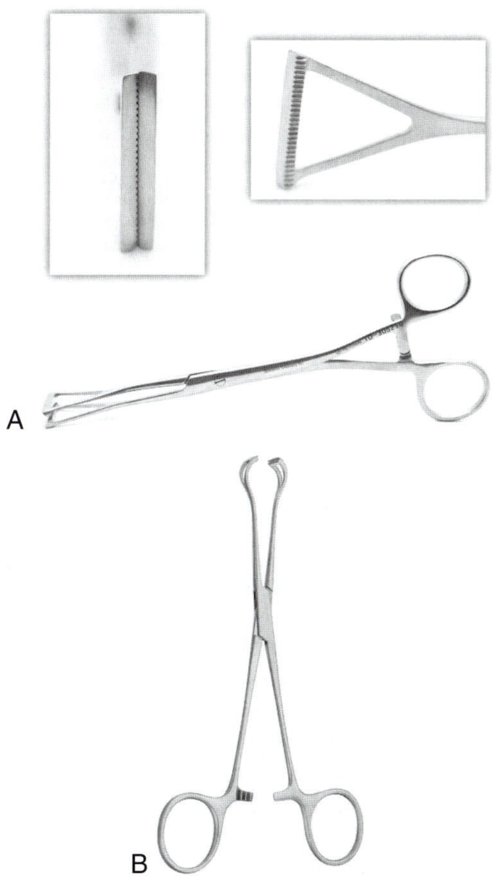

FIG 11.20 Atraumatic clamp. A, Duval lung. B, Babcock. (A, From Millennium Surgical Corp; B, Courtesy and © Becton, Dickinson and Company)

RETRACTION/VIEWING INSTRUMENTS

The body contains many complex tissue layers with individual structures occurring at different angles. Retractors are used to hold tissue structures away from other structures in order to expose deeper anatomy. Most retractors have a right angle or curved design. One end lies more or less flat and parallel to the body surface, whereas the other end curves inward or at a right angle to hold back the tissue within the surgical wound. The working end can be deep or shallow, depending on the type of retractor. The malleable or ribbon retractor is flat, spatula-shaped, and is designed to be bent into a curve according to the needs of the procedure. The overall size of the instrument can be very large, such as those used in abdominal or thoracic surgeries, or very small for use in eye and microsurgery.

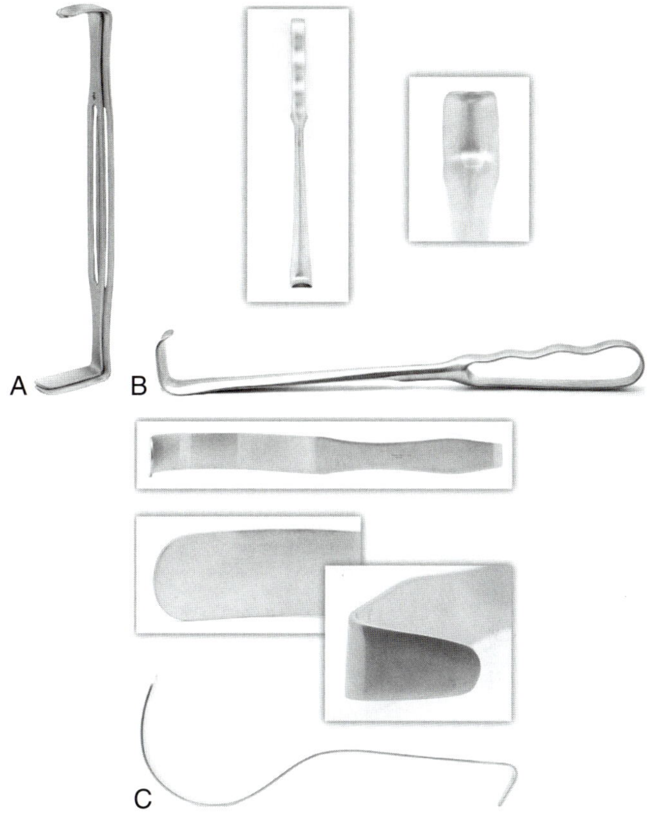

FIG 11.21 Handheld retractors. A, U.S. Army (also called Army-Navy). B, Richardson. C. Deaver. (A, Photo courtesy of Aesculap, Inc., Center Valley, PA.; B, C, From Millennium Surgical Corp.)

Handheld (Fig. 11.21) retractors range in size from the very fragile skin hook used in plastic surgery to the large, 4-inch (10-cm) wide Deaver retractor used in abdominal procedures.

The rake retractor, as its name implies, is shaped like a small claw or rake with sharp or dull points. The rake can be large, such as the Israel retractor, or very small, such as the double-ended Senn retractor. Blunt-tipped rakes are used near nerve tissue and large blood vessels, whereas sharp-tipped rakes are primarily used in connective tissue. The hook retractor is a type of a handheld retractor, which terminates in a sharp rounded hook. Small hooks are commonly used in delicate plastic surgery. The large bone hook is used to manipulate a bone.

Self-retaining retractors hold the tissue against the walls of the surgical wound by mechanical or spring action (Fig. 11.22). Large self-retaining retractors such as the Finochietto, Balfour, and Omni retractors have blade attachments, which are designed to retract specific organs or tissues during abdominal surgery. A number of self-retaining rake retractors have claw tips that grip the tissue. These tips can be sharp or dull. Examples are the Weitlaner and Gelpi retractors

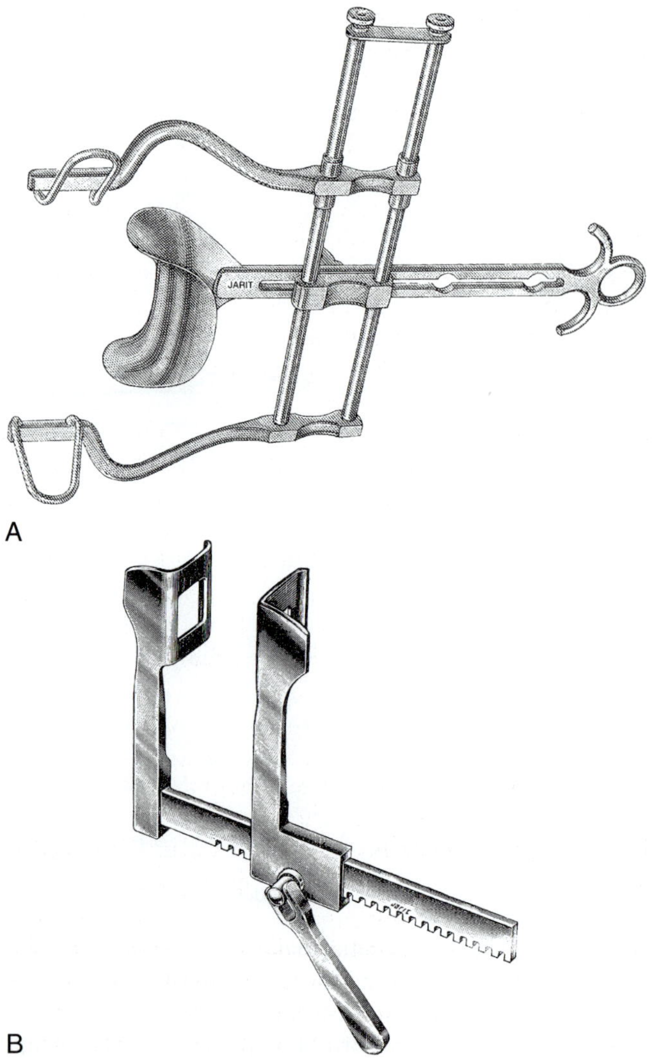

FIG 11.22 Self-retaining retractor, large. A, Balfour. B, Finochietto. (A, Courtesy Jarit Surgical Instruments, Hawthorne, NY; B, Courtesy and © Becton, Dickinson and Company)

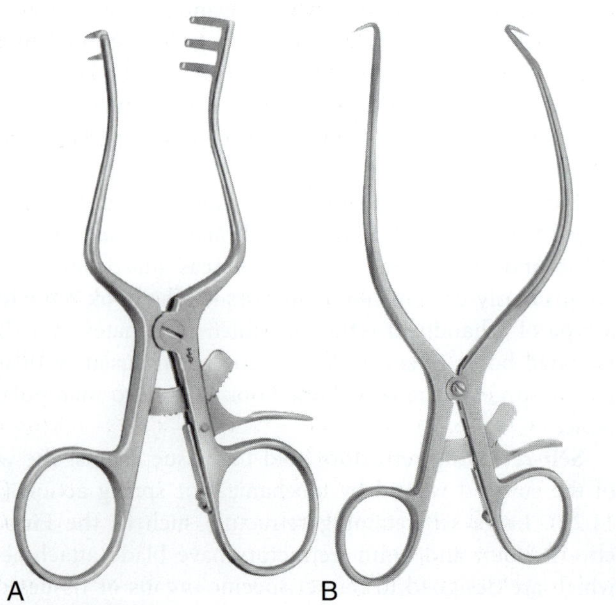

FIG 11.23 Self-retaining retractor, small. A, Weitlaner. B, Gelpi. (A, Photo courtesy of Aesculap, Inc., Center Valley, PA. B, Courtesy and © Becton, Dickinson and Company)

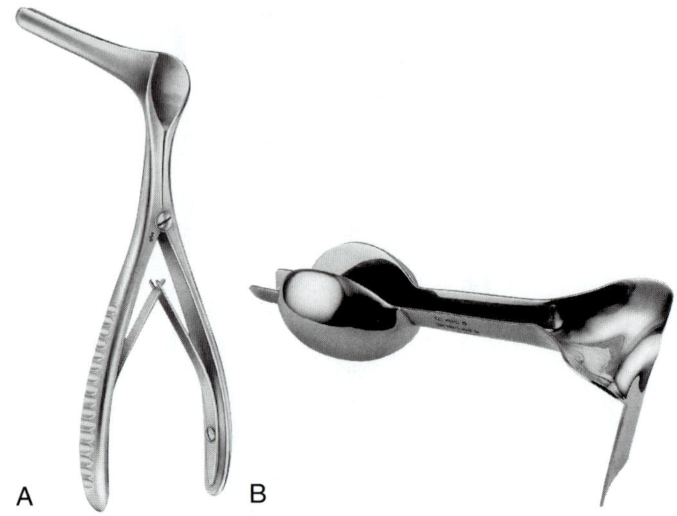

FIG 11.24 Speculum. A, Nasal. B, Vaginal. (A, Photo courtesy of Aesculap, Inc., Center Valley, PA. B, © 2016 Symmetry Surgical Inc.; Photo courtesy of Symmetry Surgical, Inc.)

(Fig. 11.23) used in general surgery and the Beckman retractor used in back and orthopedic surgery. Very delicate self-retaining retractors are spring loaded, similar to the action of a common safety pin. An example is the McPherson self-retaining lid speculum that is used to retract the eyelid. Lid retractors are shown in Chapter 26.

The **Speculum** (Fig. 11.24) is a specific type of retractor used to hold open a natural body opening such as the nose, ear canal, or vagina. The speculum can be handheld or self retaining. During ear surgery, the one piece speculum is handheld or positioned in a speculum holder. The nasal speculum is opened and closed by operating the handles.

A similar category of viewing instruments includes those that magnify, light, and project the surgical field onto a screen. This includes invasive cameras and lighted instruments such as telescopes used in minimally invasive surgery (MIS). These are discussed in detail in Chapter 20.

ASPIRATING/SUCTIONING INSTRUMENTS

Suction (aspiration) is needed during a surgical procedure to clear blood, fluids, and small bits of tissue debris from the surgical site and provide an unobstructed view of the anatomy. Suction is derived from a wall or ceiling boom attached to a disposable suction canister set below the level of the operating table. A pressure regulator is attached to the system to allow variable levels of suction pressure. A sterile suction tip is fitted with sterile tubing, which is passed off the sterile field and attached to the canister during surgery. Suction tips vary in length and diameter from very small (for eye surgery and microsurgery) to larger tips for general surgery and orthopedics. Tips are straight or angled and may have a removable shield or guard that reduces the suction pressure. For example, the Poole suction tip is designed for abdominal surgery and has a removable perforated guard that protects bowel and intestinal organs from injury by spreading the suction pressure over many small holes in the guard. The Yankauer or tonsil suction tip is unguarded to provide maximum suction pressure. The more delicate Frazier

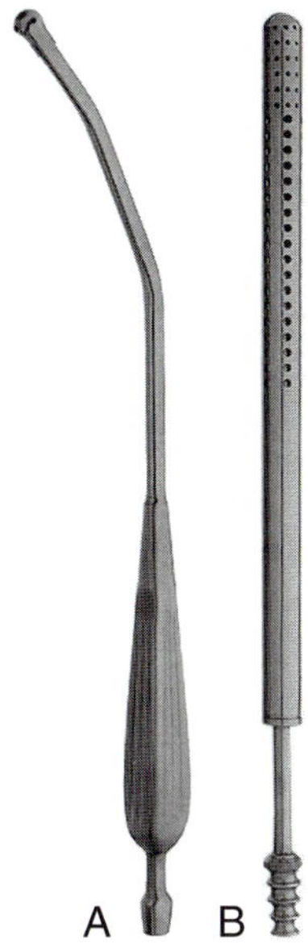

FIG 11.25 Suction tips. A, Yankauer. B, Poole. (Courtesy and © Becton, Dickinson and Company)

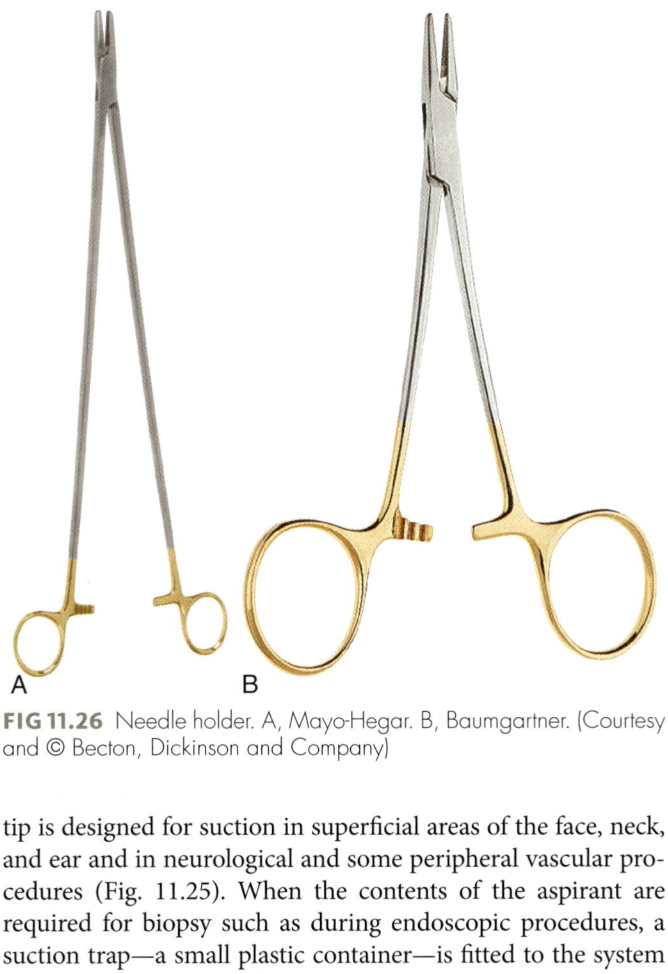

FIG 11.26 Needle holder. A, Mayo-Hegar. B, Baumgartner. (Courtesy and © Becton, Dickinson and Company)

tip is designed for suction in superficial areas of the face, neck, and ear and in neurological and some peripheral vascular procedures (Fig. 11.25). When the contents of the aspirant are required for biopsy such as during endoscopic procedures, a suction trap—a small plastic container—is fitted to the system to collect the tissue and fluid.

SUTURING INSTRUMENTS

A suturing instrument called a *needle holder* (Fig. 11.26) is used to grasp a needle/suture combination and advance it into tissues. Needle holders are designed for all types of tissues and surgical specialties. The tips or jaws of the instrument are used to grasp a needle and vary by shape and strength according to the size of suture needles. The heaviest needle holders have large blunt nose tips and strong shanks for use with larger needles and suture materials. Examples are the Heaney or Mayo-Hegar needle holder used for connective tissues such as ligaments. Smaller, more delicate needle holders are used in eye surgery as well as plastic and vascular procedures. Most high-quality needle holders have a tungsten carbon insert in the jaws for added durability and grip. These prevent the needle from rotating or slipping. Very fine sutures require fine needle holders. A sharp-tipped needle holder, such as the Sarot needle holder, is used for fine sutures (i.e., 4-0 and smaller). If the needle holder is too heavy, the surgeon will lose the feel of the needle. On the other hand, a lightweight or fine-tipped needle holder does not have enough surface area at the tip to grasp a heavy needle. A needle holder that is too delicate for the needle will cause the needle to twist during use and may damage the instrument tips. Needle holders are ratchet or spring-locked. The smallest needle holders, used in eye surgery are discussed later (see Microinstruments).

STAPLING INSTRUMENTS

Surgical staples have replaced many traditional suturing techniques for both open surgery and minimally invasive procedures. Surgical stapling instruments are used for **resection** and anastomosis of tissue and hollow organs such as the gastrointestinal and respiratory tracts. The instruments themselves are available as single-use medical devices or as reusable stainless steel instruments. Both types require manufactured cartridges of staples made of titanium, stainless steel, nylon, or absorbable polymer. The stapler is capable of firing a single or multiple rows of staples to approximate tissue in a linear or circular pattern. Cutting/stapling instruments divide a tissue plane and also fire one or more rows of staples to seal the division. The cutting assembly includes an anvil, which clamps the tissue against the staple cartridge. There are wide variations in assembly and component parts and the surgical technologist is urged to become familiar with the different types. Companies that manufacture the instruments have training available both online and in classroom settings with the opportunity to work with the instruments in the lab. The most common types of surgical staplers are known by their generic names as shown in Fig. 11.27.

- *Skin stapler:* Places a single line of staples across the incision edges.
- *Gastrointestinal anastomosis (GIA) stapler:* Used for linear *side-to-side* and *end-to-side* **anastomosis.**
- *EEA (End-to-end anastomosis) stapler:* Performs *end-to-end* intestinal resection and anastomosis.
- *TA (Transverse anastomosis) stapler:* Has a right-angled firing anvil that fits around deep structures for resection and anastomosis.
- *Purse-string stapler:* Performs the same function as a purse-string suture. In this technique, a suture is placed around the full circumference of a tubular structure such as the intestine. The ends of the suture are then tightly drawn to close down the opening in the structure.

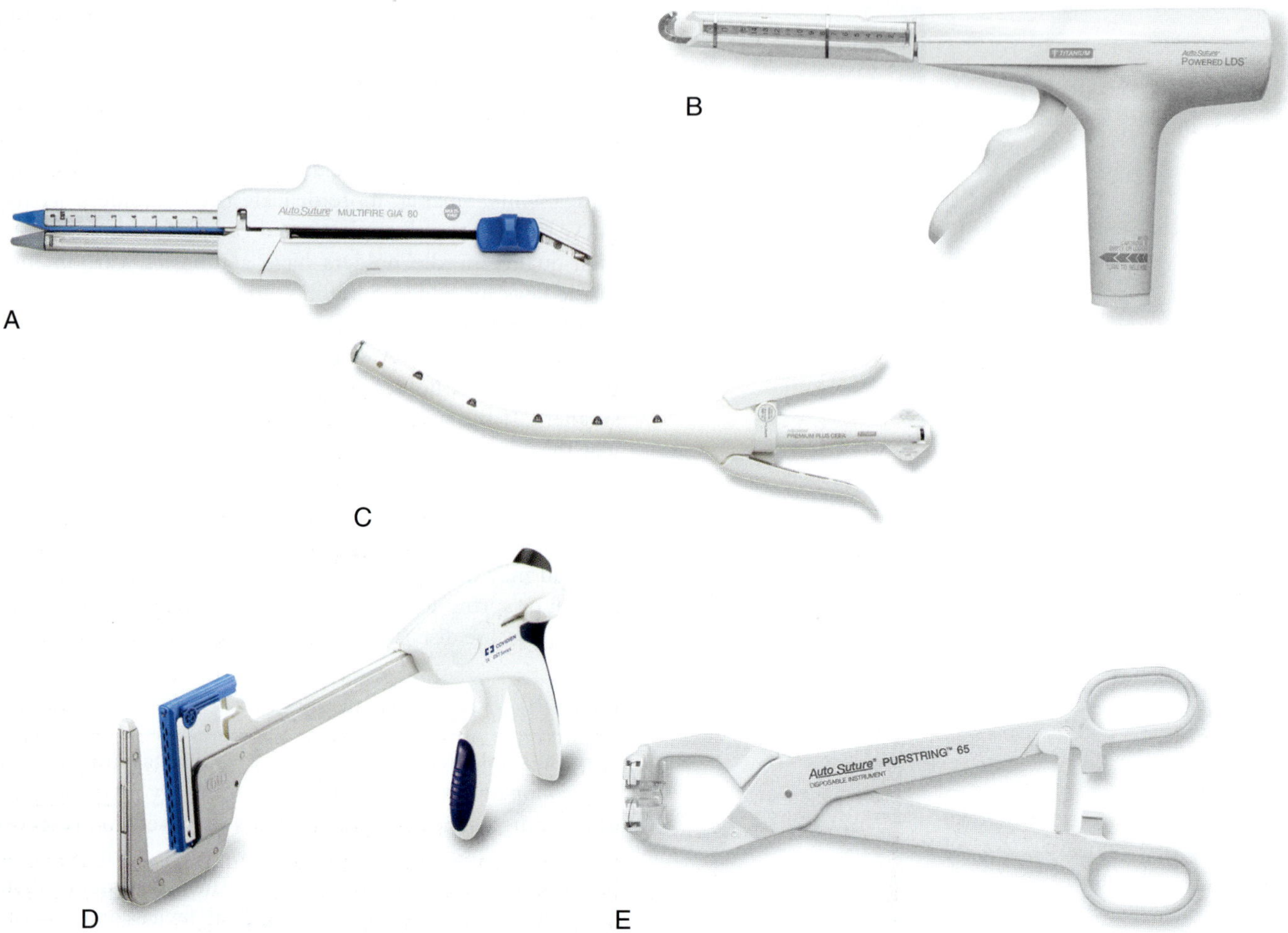

FIG 11.27 Stapling instruments. A, Gastrointestinal anastomosis GIA. B, Ligating dividing stapler LDS. C, End-to-end anastomosis EEA. D, Transverse anastomosis TA. E, Purse-string stapler. (A, C, and D, All rights reserved. Used with the permission of Medtronic; B and E, Copyright 2012 Covidien. All rights reserved. Used with the permission of Covidien.)

NOTE: *Endoscopic staplers used in minimally invasive surgery are discussed in Chapter 20.*

Hemostatic or *vessel clips* are small, V-shaped staples that close down and occlude a vessel or duct. These are applied by hand but require a clip applier matched to the size clip to be used. Clips are available in cartridges that are color coded by size (colors vary according to manufacturers). Clips may be made of stainless steel, titanium, tantalum, or absorbable polymer. Common surgical staplers and hemostatic clips are shown in Fig. 11.28.

DILATING INSTRUMENTS

A **dilator** (Fig. 11.29) is a slender, tube-like instrument with rounded ends. Dilating instruments are used to stretch or widen an existing lumen in the body. For example, urethral dilators are used to relieve a **stricture** in the urethra or to increase the circumference to allow the passage of surgical instruments. Cervical dilation is performed before curettage to allow the passage of curettes into the uterus. Surgical dilation is performed by increments using several different sizes starting with a very slender dilator and increasing the size as needed to widen the opening. Dilators are available as sets and may be made of stainless steel, aluminum, or malleable polyvinyl material.

PROBING INSTRUMENTS

A probing instrument is a slender rod with a blunt tip, used to explore and assess the consistency of tissue or to diagnose and treat a fistula (Fig. 11.30). The small diameter of the probe facilitates its use inside narrow tissue spaces. The lacrimal probe is used to locate a stricture or other type of blockage in the lacrimal (tear) duct. The laryngeal probe is used to gently explore the larynx tissues to identify a growth and to evaluate the consistency of the tissues. A fistula usually develops in conjunction with an infection. In this process, draining serous fluid and pus creates a hollow track in tissues. These tracks can penetrate the tissues in many different directions and may emerge on the surface of the body. Surgical treatment of the fistula involves probing the tracts and obliterating its walls so that the tissues can approximate and heal.

ACCESSORY INSTRUMENTS

This category includes instruments that do not easily fit into other existing categories. It includes instruments such as the

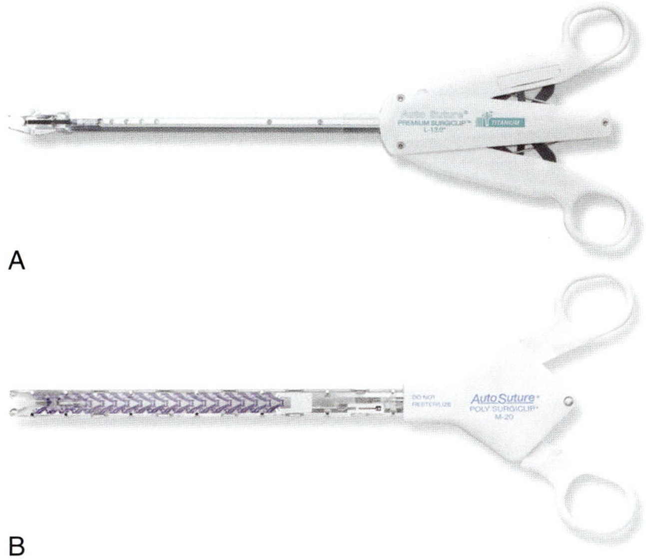

FIG 11.28 Hemostatic clip applier. A, Stainless steel clips. B, Synthetic absorbable clips. (All rights reserved. Used with the permission of Medtronic.)

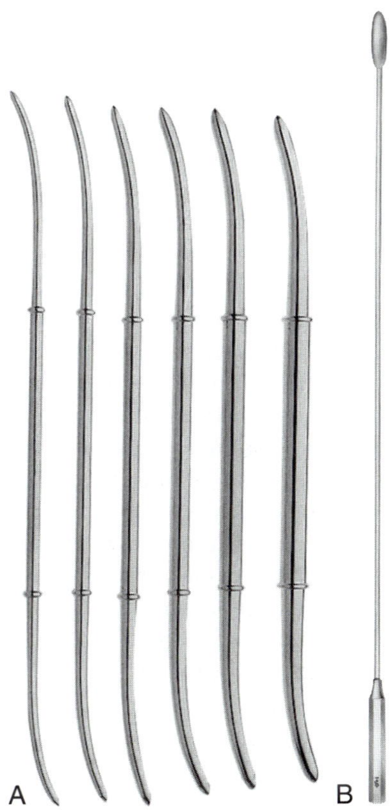

FIG 11.29 Dilating instruments. A, Hank uterine dilators. B, Bakes gall duct. (A, Courtesy and © Becton, Dickinson and Company; B, Photo courtesy of Aesculap, Inc., Center Valley, PA.)

towel clamp, which is used to grasp surgical towels in the draping process, and sponge forceps, which are used to grip a folded surgical sponge. Measuring instruments are also important groups of instruments in this category. Tissue and hollow structures are measured for many purposes. For example, the uterine sound is inserted into the cervix to measure the depth of the uterus from the cervix to the fundus. This is done to prevent uterine perforation during curettage. Orthopedic calipers are used to measure the bone for a joint implant. A depth gauge is used in orthopedic surgery to determine the depth of a drill hole so that the correct length of screw is implanted.

A *sizer* is a trial, reusable replica of an implantable prosthesis. Rather than opening and contaminating many expensive implants during surgery, the sizer allows the surgeon to test a replica first. For example, before a cardiac valve is inserted, a sizer is used to determine the correct size.

MICROINSTRUMENTS

Microinstruments are used during any surgery that is performed using an operating microscope or magnification loupes, which are worn like eyeglasses (Fig. 11.31). Specialties that require microinstruments include microvascular, eye, and ear surgeries; neuro- and tuboplasty; and vasectomy reversal. Microsurgical instruments have many of the same categories as their counterparts in other specialties but with distinctive differences in design and scale. Some microsurgical instruments are used in more than one specialty such as micro needle holders and tissue forceps, whereas others are designed for use in only one specialty, such as many ear instruments. Microinstruments are made of stainless steel and titanium and are finished to a dull sheen or black ceramic coating to reduce glare. The handles are often bayonet shaped. The sense of touch transmitted from the tissue, through the surgical instrument to the surgeon's hand, is extremely critical in microsurgery. The instruments are finely balanced, and the techniques of holding and operating the instruments are different from those of larger instruments. Instead of a ratchet lock, most instruments either have no locking mechanism or use a simple clip that is set between two leaf springs. The jaws of the instrument are opened or closed by applying gentle pressure on the leaf springs. The tissue forceps are extremely fine. A pin stop is set into the handle to prevent the two tips from crossing over each other (called *scissoring*) during use. Needle holders can accommodate suture as small as 11-0 and are locking or nonlocking. Microsurgical scissors are available as straight, curved, or angled from 45 to 125 degrees.

Scissor blades are available in many different styles within the normal configuration of sharp-sharp, sharp-curved, or curved-curved tips. Scissor and forceps handles are often bayonet shaped or have a leaf-spring design, which increases their sensitivity and precision.

Microsurgical instruments are managed on the surgical field with special racks with silicon padding to prevent damage to the instruments and to provide a means of segregating the types for easy identification. Commonly used specialty instruments and illustrated in the surgical procedure chapters. See also Chapter 30 for more in-depth information on microsurgery.

USE OF INSTRUMENTS BY TISSUE TYPE

The selection of a particular surgical instrument is based on the tissue type, depth of the surgical wound, technical requirements of the procedure, and surgeon's preference or experience. Tissues vary in texture, strength, elasticity, water and fat

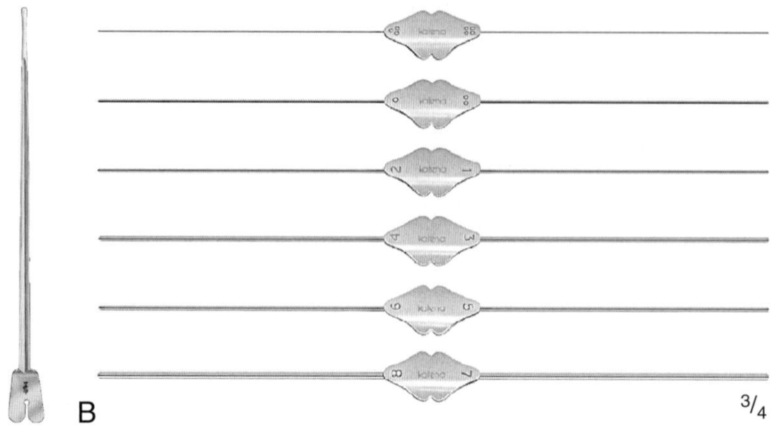

FIG 11.30 Probe. A, Grooved director tongue tie probe. B, Lacrimal. (A, Courtesy and © Becton, Dickinson and Company; B Katena Eye Instruments, Denville NJ.)

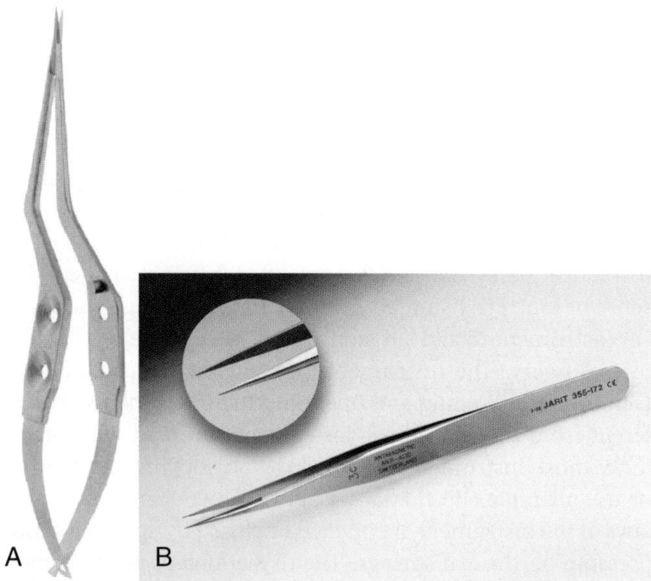

FIG 11.31 Microinstruments. A, Tindall micro scissors. B, Micro Jeweler's forceps. (A, Courtesy and © Becton, Dickinson and Company; B, From Nemitz. *Surgical Instrumentation: An Interactive Approach*. 3rd ed. St. Louis: Elsevier; 2019.)

content, and permeability. Table 11.2 shows a basic guideline for different types of tissues and the common types of instrument used on these tissues. Naturally, there will be exceptions, and the list is not exhaustive.

SKIN

Skin is elastic, relatively fibrous, and strong. In most surgical procedures, skin is incised rather than cut with scissors. This is because the elastic quality of skin makes it difficult to cut an even line with scissors. The scalpel is more precise and extremely sharp, which prevents the skin from dragging through the instrument as it cuts. As a general rule, only toothed, hooked, or serrated instruments are used to grasp the skin. This is because skin is relatively tough compared with other tissue types, and smooth jawed instruments do not have enough "bite" to hold the skin.

VISCERAL SEROSA

The viscera, or organs of the body, are each covered by a fine membrane called the **serosa**. This membrane is easily punctured, and the underlying tissue layers can bleed profusely. Therefore, atraumatic instruments are needed when handling this tissue. These include nonpenetrating forceps (smooth forceps), wide retractors that do not cut into the tissue, and suction tips that have a guard to decrease the suction pressure on the tissue. Babcock clamps are commonly used to grasp the viscera. Vascular forceps are often used during dissection and tissue mobilization of visceral serosa.

LUNG, SPLEEN, LIVER, AND THYROID

These highly vascular tissues are very delicate, bleed profusely, tear easily, and have little or no elasticity. A strong membrane covers and protects these organs. However, these tissues must be handled by hand or with atraumatic (round tipped) instruments. The liver and spleen can "break" or develop fissures when traumatized. Only partially occluding clamps and smooth tissue forceps are used on these tissues. However, during the dissection of adjacent tissues, very fine-toothed, vascular forceps and long curve-tipped clamps can be used. When the spleen, liver, and intestines are retracted, the retractor blade must be sufficiently wide to distribute the pressure. Edges must be protected with sponges to prevent the retractor edge from cutting into the tissue or bruising it. A wide Deaver, Richardson, or Harrington retractor is often used for the liver and spleen. Lung tissue is held with broad-tipped, partially occluding clamps such the Duval lung clamp.

PERITONEUM

The lining of the body cavities is smooth, elastic, and strong. Normal peritoneal tissue is dissected with the Metzenbaum scissors and may be grasped with toothed forceps, broad tipped hemostats, or Allis clamps.

ADIPOSE TISSUE

Loose connective tissue, such as the subcutaneous tissue of the abdomen, has a high fat content. It does not compress well and tends to fragment into small pieces when clamped. Adipose tissue has few blood vessels compared with other types of tissue. This allows the use of penetrating instruments, such as a handheld rake or Weitlaner self-retaining retractor. The Allis clamp, which has a T-shaped serrated tip, is often used

TABLE 11.2 Tissue Types and Appropriate Instruments				
TISSUE TYPE	**INSTRUMENT TYPE**			
Connective	**Thumb Forceps**	**Scissors**	**Tissue Clamp**	**Retraction**
Skin • Elastic • Resilient	Toothed, delicate, such as Adson Short to medium length, single-toothed	Use scalpel for incision Use fine-tipped short scissors, such as Westcott or tenotomy scissors for trimming and fine dissection	Not used on skin	Skin only, small rakes, sharp or rounded tips, such as Senn or double hook Plastic surgery skin hooks Self-retaining small spring, s 'such as Green Skin plus fat layer—use rake retractors, Army-Navy
Adipose (loose connective tissue) • Lobular • Sparse blood vessels • Oily • Tends to break apart when clamped	Toothed if used on body wall fat, medium length	Metzenbaum curved scissor electrosurgical unit (ESU)	For controlling bleeders use Mosquito, Kelly, Crile, or Mayo clamps	Handheld rake size depends on the depth of incision Shallow Weitlaner self-retaining or small rake Israel rake for deep adipose layers Large abdominal retractor for very deep layers: use Deaver or Richardson
Ligament • Strong • Fibrous • Elastic	Toothed Broad-tipped or heavy for large ligaments	Mayo scissor for broad ligaments May require incising with knife	Use strong ligament clamps, such as Heaney, for uterine ligaments For joint surgery, use Kocher clamp for grasping For hemostasis, use Mayo clamp	Fibrous sheath: use nonslip self-retaining retractor Single ligament: use vessel loop
Tendon • Tough • Stringy • Extremely strong • Avascular	Toothed forceps Heavy for large tendons, lighter for finer ones	Metzenbaum scissors for larger tendon Tenotomy scissors for delicate tendon	Use tendon clamp where available Avoid crimping tendon with hemostatic clamps	Tendon retractor when available Can use rubber loop to retract
Abdominal viscera • Delicate • Each encapsulated by thin, strong serous tissue	Use long, smooth tissue forceps or vascular forceps for suturing Babcock clamps for intestine, reproductive organs Allis clamps may be used on stomach borders	Always use fine Metzenbaum scissors for dissection, medium or long sometimes used for incising serosa of the spleen, liver, pancreas, uses ESU for dissecting	Non-occlusive clamps including Bainbridge, Babcock, Doyen, and Duval are used on fragile abdominal organs	Use broad, smooth, handheld retractors with adequate sponge packs to prevent injury to organ. Use Deaver, Richardson, Harrington, retractors.
Bone • Strong • Resilient • Springy or spongy • Covered with a tough periosteal layer	Forceps are not commonly used on bones Use broad-toothed forceps when needed	Bone rongeurs and single- and double-action cutters with various tips Saw, Gigli manual or power saws Drills Shaver Reamer Osteotome Chisel Elevator Knives, such as a Meniscus knife	Bone clamps, Lewin Bone hook	Handheld retractors for specific parts of the anatomy • Bennet—hip • Blount—knee • Meyerding—shoulder • Smillie—knee
Muscle • Fibrous • Vascular • Strong	Toothed forceps used for general manipulation	Heavy or lightweight dissection scissors (Mayo or Metzenbaum)	Striated muscle not normally clamped except to grasp bleeders	Handheld retractor for isolated muscle groups

to clamp or grasp adipose tissue. The high fat content of this tissue can cause instruments to become slippery and difficult to handle. In this case, they can be wiped down with a damp sponge during surgery. Toothed forceps are used for suturing adipose tissue.

MUSCLE

Striated muscle tissue is moved aside, or the muscle bundles are manually separated rather than cut whenever possible during surgery. This is because muscles are normally slow to regain function when severed and nearly all surgical incisions are oriented on the long axis of the muscle. Large muscles are elastic and fibrous, allowing for the use of toothed forceps and clamps. On rare occasions, when a muscle tissue must be severed, it is often grasped with Allis clamps and severed with heavy Mayo scissors or the electrosurgical unit.

BONE

Bone tissue is resilient and somewhat springy. Large bones are manipulated using traction or leverage rather than direct pulling. Bone retractors, such as the Bennett and Scoville retractors, have a toothed tip or a reverse curve that can be inserted under another bone for leverage. Other types of bone clamps, such as the Lewin clamp, wrap around the bone for manual traction. Bone tissue is usually cut or morcellated using power instruments including saws, drills, and rasps. Manual cutting instruments include the osteotome, chisel, and **gouge**. These are used with an orthopedic mallet.

CARTILAGE, TENDON, AND FASCIA

Cartilage, tendon, and fascia are extremely strong and resilient. The cartilaginous joint surfaces (those within a capsule) are naturally lubricated with synovial fluid, which has an oily consistency. These tissues can be quite slippery, requiring toothed clamps or those with ridges to maintain grip. Tendons are also covered by a sheath that is strong and smooth. These connective tissues are often handled using Kocher clamps, which have a single or double tooth at the tip increasing the instrument's grip. More specialized tendon clamps, such as the Martin clamp, have double rows of heavy teeth and are frequently used in knee surgery for grasping the medial and lateral tendons. Cartilage clamps, like tendon clamps, have heavy broad teeth. These tissues have little or no blood vessels, so toothed instruments can be safely used on them. Fascia can be grasped with Kocher clamps. Strong dissecting scissors, such as curved Mayo scissors, are used on fascia and large tendons.

PASSING SURGICAL INSTRUMENTS DURING SURGERY

One of the fundamental skills required of a surgical technologist is passing instruments to the surgeon during a procedure. The following techniques are provided as a guideline.

1. Instruments are passed to the surgeon in a way that prevents injury to the surgeon and scrubbed technologist. Many instruments have sharp edges or points. Accidents and injury can be prevented by following a standard technique.
2. While passing an instrument, it should be oriented in a way that facilitates its immediate use. Whenever possible, the surgeon should receive an instrument in the same position (spatial orientation) as that during its actual use in the body. This contributes to efficiency of motion. Note that the orientation of the instrument must be relative to the surgeon's operative hand.
3. Instruments should be passed purposefully and securely. This ensures that the surgeon knows that he or she has contact with the instrument without turning away from the surgical wound. The scrub should keep contact with the instrument until the surgeon grasps it. This prevents the instrument from dropping.
4. Instruments should be passed by grasping them in the midsection. This balances the instrument. Try to avoid handling the tip of an instrument as this can result in a tear in the glove or injury.
5. When passing a power driven instrument (drill, saw, etc.) or a stapling instrument, always place it in safety mode first to avoid inadvertent engagement and injury.
6. During surgical procedures in which the sterile field does not provide a flat surface, such as when the patient is in beach chair position or lateral decubitus, a magnetic mat should be available on the surgical field to prevent instruments from sliding to the floor during the procedure. A mat can also be used when the patient is positioned for long periods in Trendelenberg or reverse Trendelenberg position.

SPECIFIC INSTRUMENT TECHNIQUES

Specific instruments require handling techniques according to the type and design of the instrument. The following discussion and photos are provided as a guideline. Common hand signals used by some surgeons are also shown.

Knives and Scalpels

Single piece knives and scalpels with detachable blades must be passed with caution. Disposable knife blades are mounted on a handle and removed using a needle holder. This technique is shown in Fig. 11.32. Ideally, knives and scalpels should be passed on the sterile field in a basin using a "no-touch" technique. However, if the need arises to pass the scalpel by hand, it is important to grasp it in the middle, *blade down*. Do not lose contact with the scalpel until you feel the surgeon has grasped it. Fig. 11.33 illustrates this technique.

NOTE: *The preferred method is to place the scalpel in a shallow tray on the sterile field to avoid hand-to-hand contact with the instrument. If necessary, the scalpel can be carefully passed by hand. This is discussed fully in Chapters 9 and 18.*

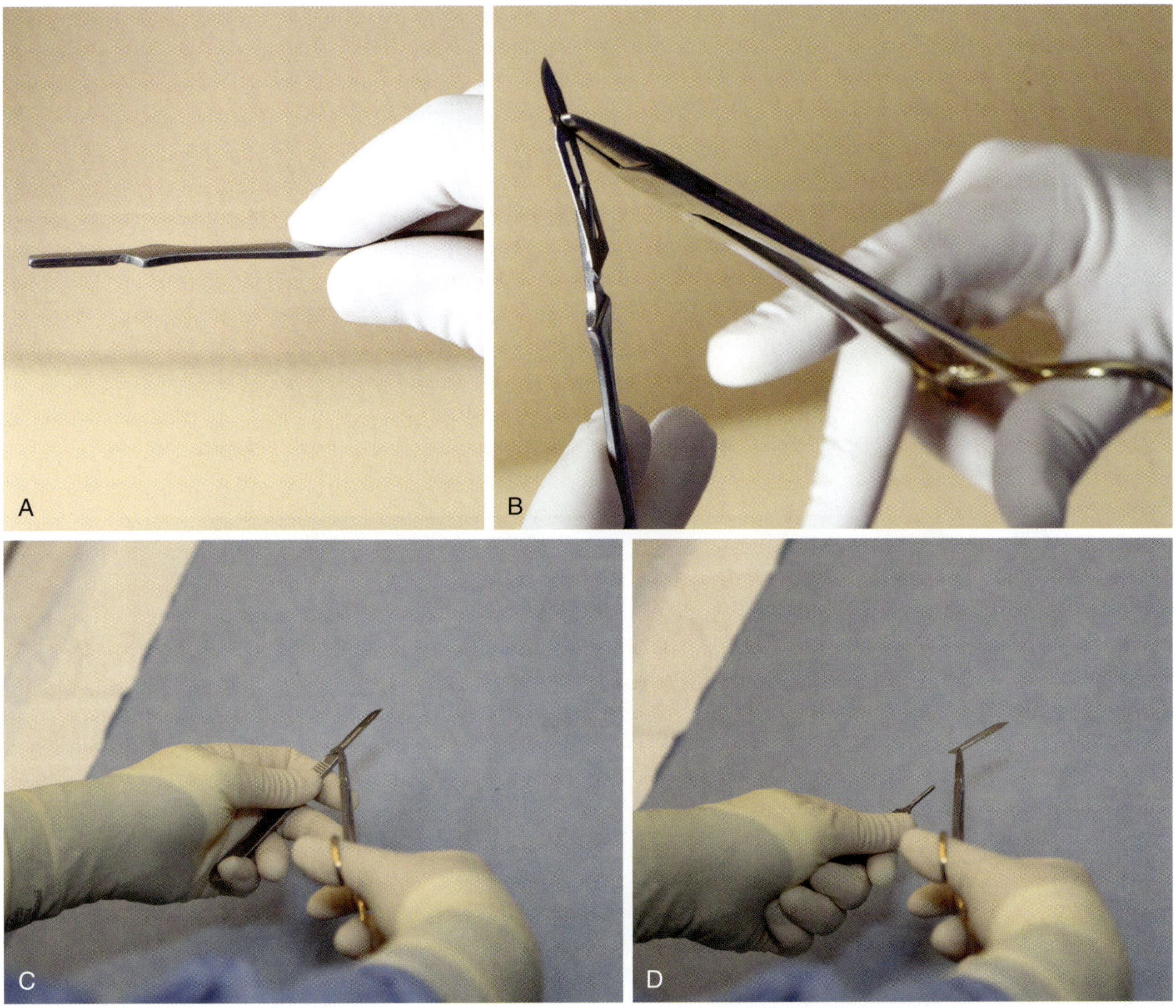

FIG 11.32 Loading and disarming a knife blade. A, Slot located on the sides of the Bard-Parker handles. B, The blade is fitted into the slots using a needle holder. C, To remove the blade, use a needle holder to lift the lower corner of the blade slightly. D, With the corner elevated, pull the blade out of the slot.

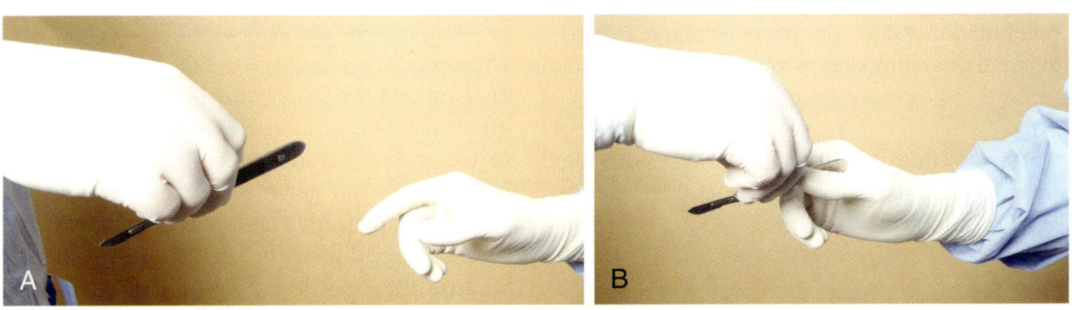

FIG 11.33 Passing the knife. A, The ST grasps the scalpel handle approximately 1/3 the distance from the blade. B, The knife handle is purposefully placed into the surgeon's hand. Do not release the handle until you feel the surgeon has grasped it.

Tissue Forceps

Tissue forceps should be passed with tips down. There are several ways to pass tissue forceps. They can be grasped at midsection or at the end opposite the tip and placed in the surgeon's hand as shown in Fig. 11.34.

Scissors

Scissors are usually passed in a way that the handles contact the surgeon's palm, with the points pointing toward the back of his or her hand (Fig. 11.35). This orientation places the curve of the scissor pointing upward during use in the body.

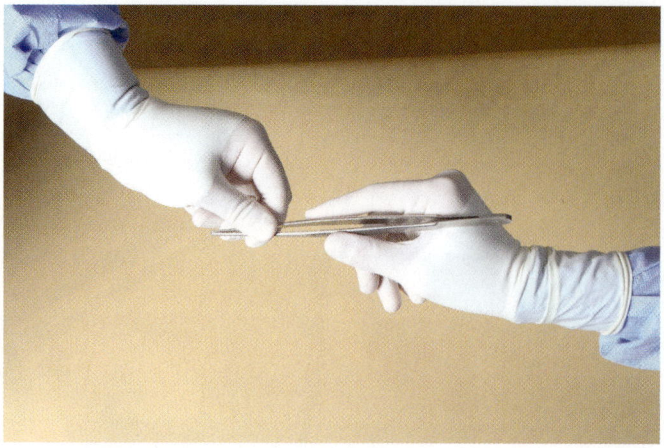

FIG 11.34 Passing tissue forceps. Grasp the forceps close to the tips and place the instrument in the web of the surgeons thumb and forefinger. Take care to not snag your glove on the tip of forceps with teeth.

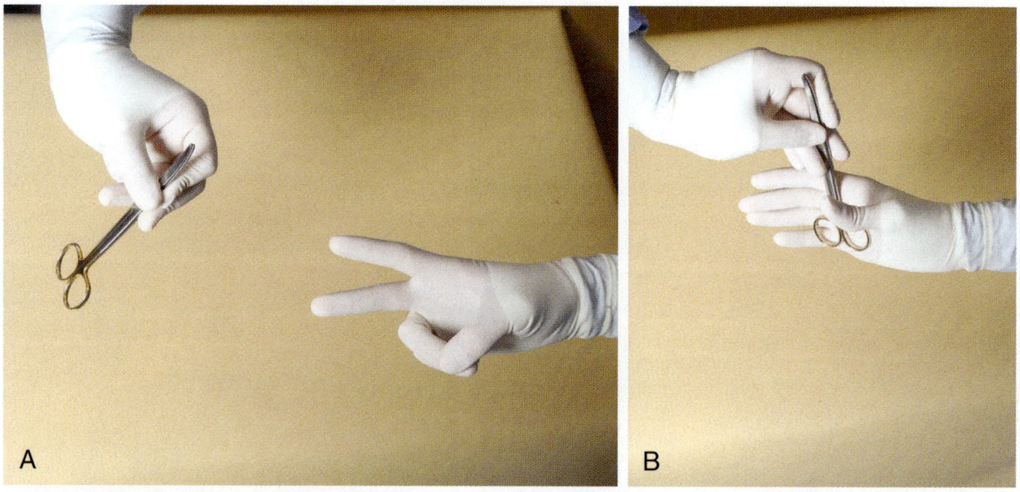

FIG 11.35 Passing scissors. A, The surgeon may signal for scissors. Hold the scissors at the fulcrum while passing the instrument. B, Place the scissors in the surgeon's palm as shown, blades pointing up.

Clamp

A hemostatic clamp is passed with the tips pointing upward and the finger rings in contact with the surgeon's palm. Angled clamps such as a right-angle or curved clamp are usually passed with the angled section pointing downward. The same technique is used for vascular clamps and dissecting clamps as shown in Fig. 11.36.

Retractor

The retractor is passed with the right angle blade(s) pointing down toward the wound. A self-retaining retractor should be passed in the *closed* position (Fig. 11.37).

Needle Holder

The needle holder and suture are passed so that the point of the needle is oriented upward, in ready position for use. Drape the long suture end over the back of the hand or grasp it lightly during passing to prevent it from being caught in the surgeon's palm as he or she receives the instrument (Fig. 11.38). Sutures are usually passed on a one to one basis. That means that the scrub should receive one suture needle back from the surgeon as the next one is passed. A microsurgical needle holder may have a spring lock or no lock at all. It must be passed gently to prevent the needle from dislodging from the tip. Pass the needle holder as shown in Fig. 11.39.

Refer to Chapter 19 for a complete discussion on handling sutures and needles.

TROUBLESHOOTING SURGICAL INSTRUMENTS

The surgical technologist takes a proactive role in checking instruments for safety and integrity. This can be done during processing or after the procedure when instruments are sorted and prepared for terminal disinfection. Stainless steel instruments can get mechanically or structurally damaged or there can be defects on the surface that lead to weakness. Damaged instruments must be withdrawn from service because they can lead to patient injury and lost operating time. The parts of a box-lock instrument are illustrated in Fig. 11.40.

The following discussion, along with Figs. 11.41 through 11.44, illustrate areas of potential damage and how to troubleshoot for defects.

SCISSORS

1. Look for pitting, chipping, and fractures along the blade edges. Vertical cracks in the blade can cause injury to

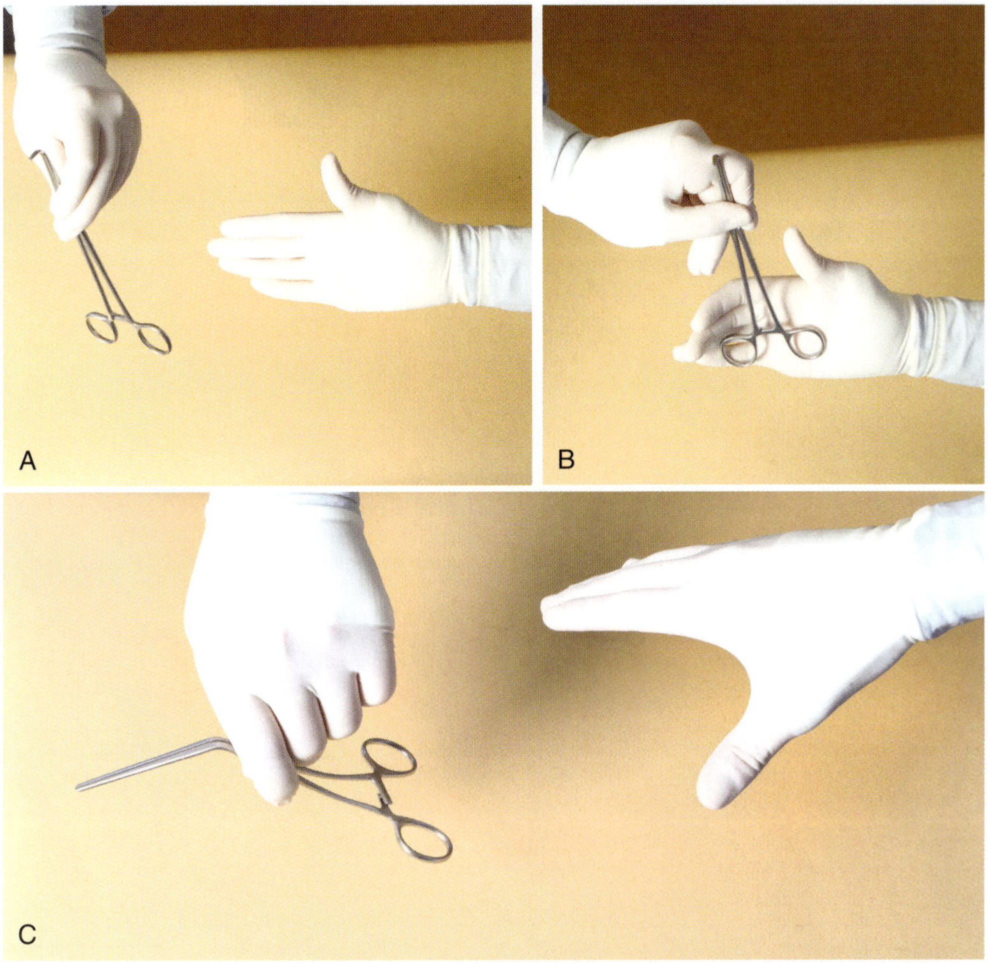

FIG 11.36 Passing a hemostatic clamp. A, The clamp is positioned for passing as shown. B, Place the clamp firmly against the surgeon's palm. C, Technique for the underhand passing of a vascular clamp.

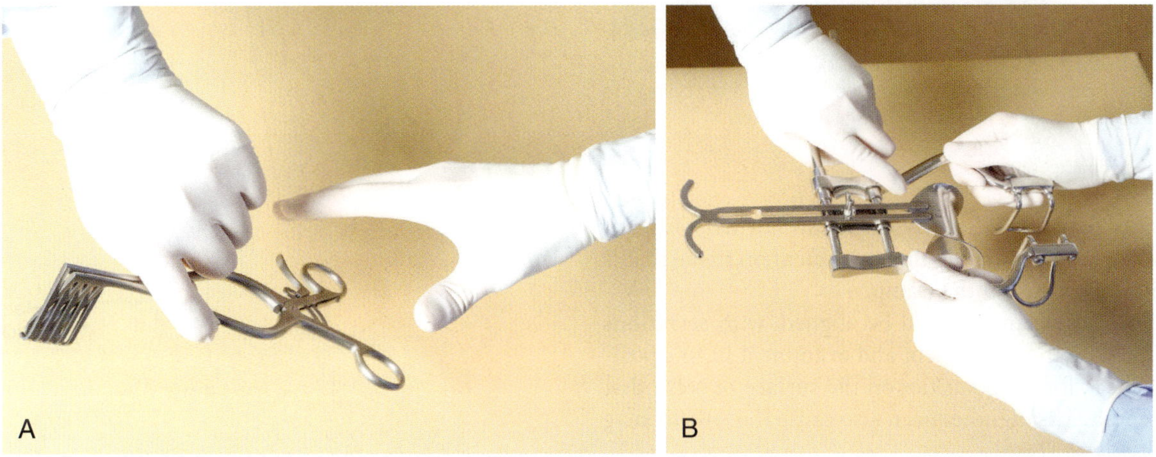

FIG 11.37 Passing a retractor. Retractors are placed in position for use with tips down. A, Passing a small self-retaining retractor. B, Passing a large abdominal retractor.

the tissue and may mean that the instrument cannot be repaired.

2. Check that the scissor tips precisely meet and are not bent or chipped. Sharp dissection scissors can develop burrs on the tips, usually from misuse or rough handling with heavier instruments. When the scissors are opened and closed, there should be no grinding of tips or shanks, which would indicate rough edges or bent tines.
3. The center hinge screw of the scissors can become worn with time. When the scissors are opened and closed, they should feel snug but not tight at the center screw.

HEMOSTATIC CLAMP

1. Examine the **box lock** closely for cracks, pitting, and tissue debris. Small cracks in the surface can lead to breakage

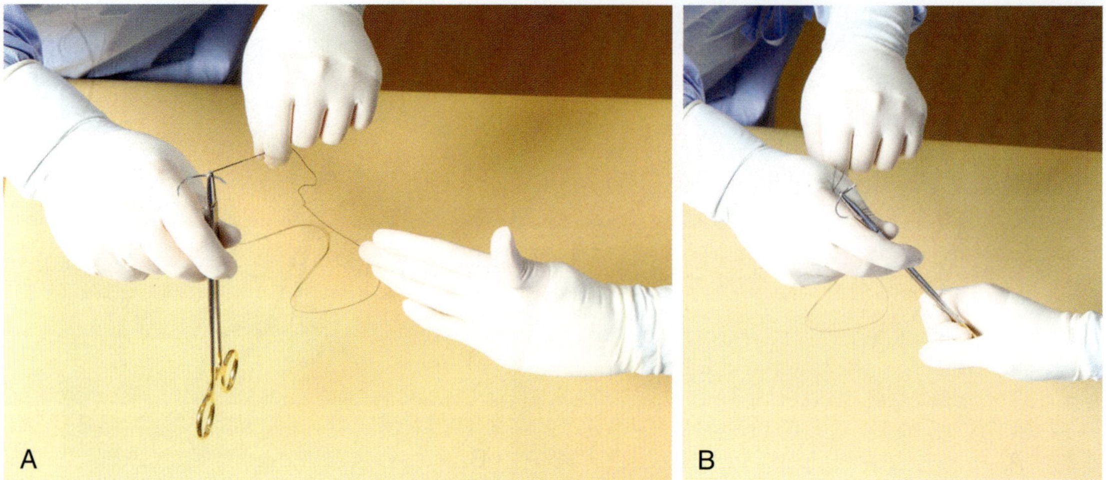

FIG 11.38 Passing the needle holder. A, The needle holder is passed so that the point of the needle is directed upward, in the position for suturing. B, To avoid placing the suture itself in the surgeon's palm, the end can be held back momentarily or draped over the back of the scrub's hand.

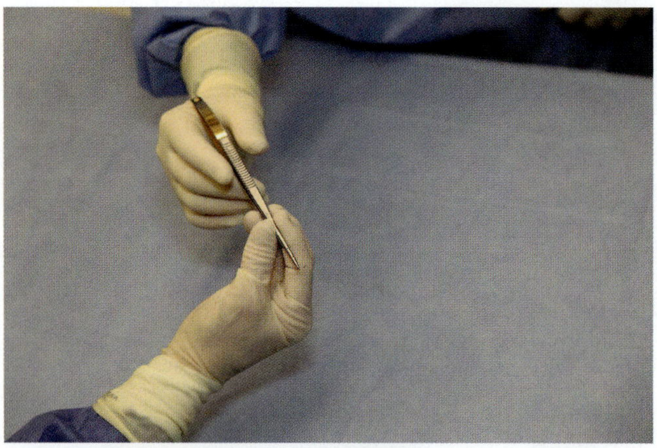

FIG 11.39 Passing the spring lock needle holder. A spring lock needle holder is passed gently to avoid opening the catch and dropping the suture. The needle holder is in position for immediate use.

with repeated use. These may be due to normal wear but can also be caused by using the instrument on tissue that is too thick or fibrous for the clamp.

2. The jaws of the clamp should be aligned, with serrations meshed. Close the instrument and examine it in this position to check for irregularities on the surface or teeth that do not mesh. Misalignment can also cause the jaws to snag on each other.
3. Check for a loose box lock. Open the instrument and examine for "play" in the box lock by gently pushing one handle up and the other down. A very small amount is normal, but if the box is loose, it needs repair.
4. Check that ratchets are aligned and that they do not spring open unexpectedly. The instrument should close easily and the ratchets click into place with moderate pressure. Loose or worn ratchets close too easily and do not hold the instrument closed. There should be 1/16 to 1/8 inch of space between the ratchets.

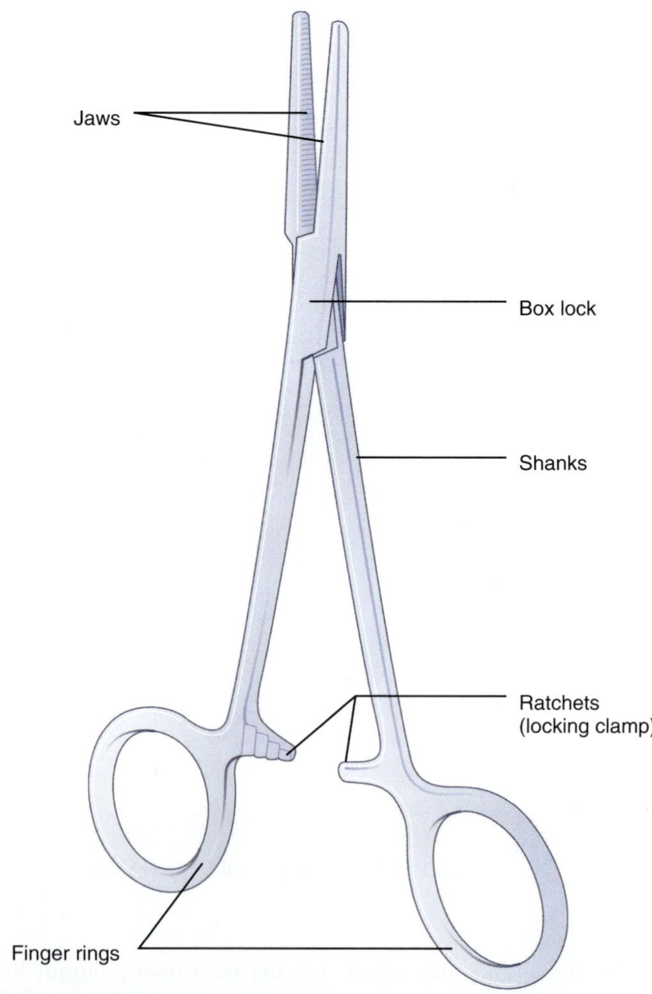

FIG 11.40 Parts of a box lock instrument. (Courtesy Teleflex, Research Triangle Park, NC.)

RONGEUR

1. Rongeurs such as the one shown are complex instruments with multiple pins, springs, and screws. If these are loose,

they can be lost in the surgical wound. Look for loose or missing screws and pins. Test the screw connecting the handle to the body by gently pushing the handles back and forth. The front handle should not rattle. The top shaft is secured to the body by a pin. A loose or faulty pin prevents the rongeur from opening and closing. Vibration in the front handle indicates a loose screw at the hinge shown.

2. The spring in the center of the handle allows the handle to snap back to the neutral position after closing. A worn spring causes the handle to lose tension.
3. The rongeur's cutting edge at the tip must be periodically sharpened. Ensure that there are no pits or cracks and that the tips do not stick or grind when opened and closed. Tissue not removed during reprocessing can easily build up in the tip, causing an infection hazard, as well as damage to the instrument. The tip should be visually inspected and should be able to cut through a thin strip of paper, approximately the same thickness as a business card.
4. The tip of the rongeur opens and closes by a sliding pin mechanism in the shaft. The central screw connects the handle to the body. All of these mechanisms must slide smoothly, without sticking.

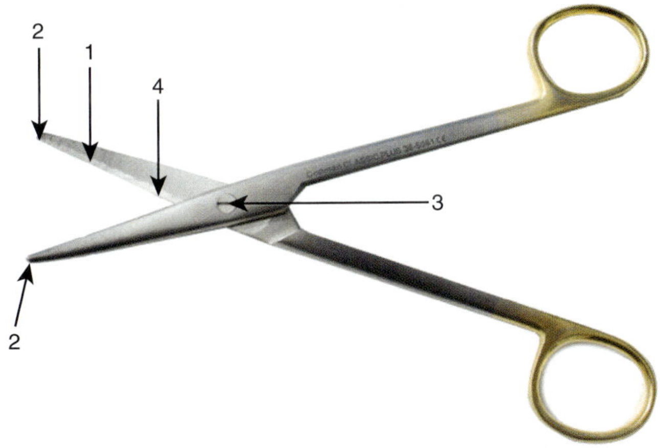

FIG 11.41 Inspecting scissors for damage or loss of function. (Courtesy Bramstedt Surgical Inc., Lino Lakes, Minn.)

NEEDLE HOLDER

1. Needle holders and dissection scissors are the most frequently used instruments. They must be frequently checked for mechanical breakdown and signs of wear that can lead to breakage. Look for cracks in the box lock and in the jaws of the instruments. Even small hairline fractures are enough to take an instrument out of service for repair.
2. The tungsten carbide inserts can wear down and require replacement. The insert should feel uniformly coarse all along their length. Test the inserts to see if they mesh together when the instrument is locked by holding the closed instrument up to the light and looking for gaps along the length of the inserts.
3. Like other instruments with a box lock, the needle holder can lose accuracy when the box lock is worn or loose. When the instrument is opened and closed, it should feel smooth and responsive but not tight or sticky.
4. Check the ratchets for alignment and fit. The closed instrument should have 1⁄16 to 1⁄8 inch of space between the ratchets in order to maintain the correct pressure. The needle holder should remain secure in the first ratchet position.

Watch Chapter 11: Basic Instrumentation on the Evolve website. http://evolve.elsevier.com/Fuller/surgical

KEY CONCEPTS

- Knowing the names of surgical instruments and how they are used is a fundamental skill in surgical technology. Instruments are generally named according to their type and shape and often include the name of the instrument's designer.
- Modern surgical instruments are manufactured in a global market where materials may be derived from one country, whereas assembly and distribution take place

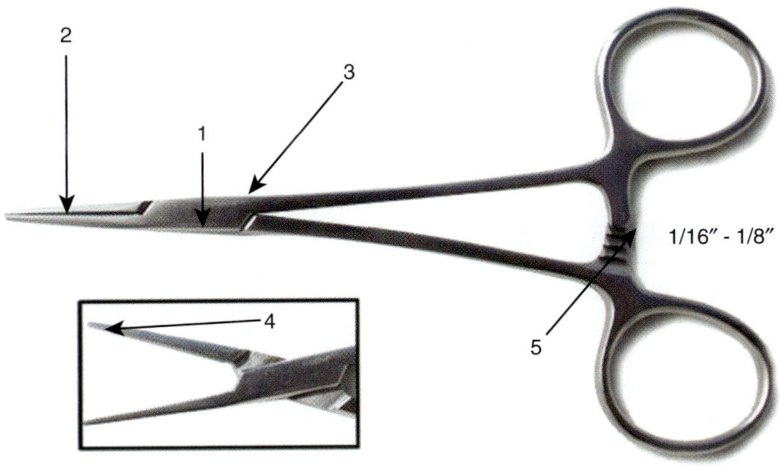

FIG 11.42 Inspecting a hemostat for damage or loss of function. (Courtesy Bramstedt Surgical Inc., Lino Lakes, Minn.)

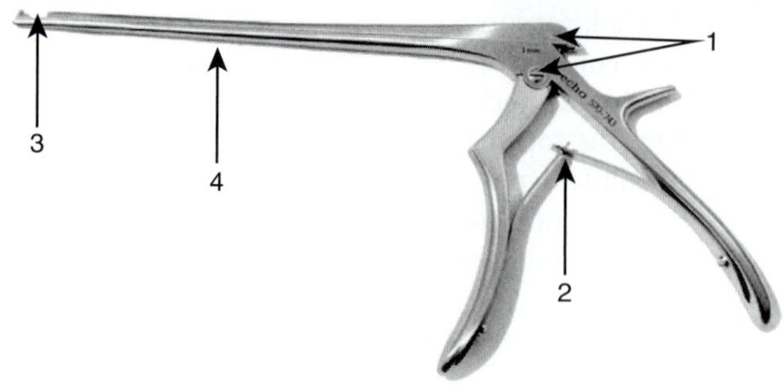

FIG 11.43 Inspecting a rongeur for damage or loss of function. (Courtesy Bramstedt Surgical Inc., Lino Lakes, Minn.)

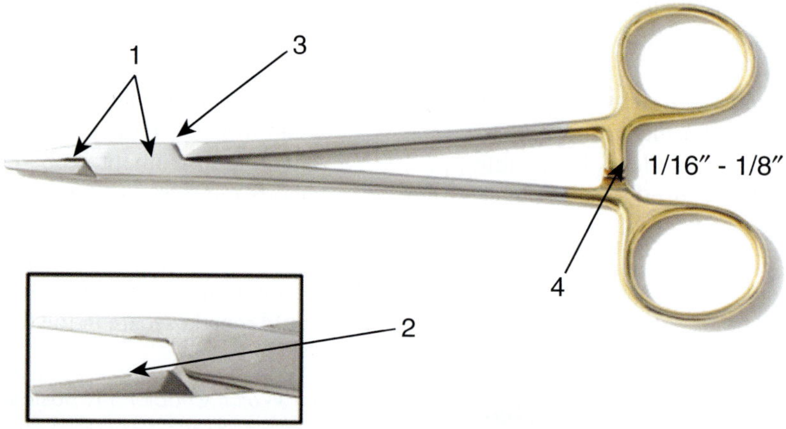

FIG 11.44 Inspecting a needle holder for damage or loss of function. (Courtesy Bramstedt Surgical Inc., Lino Lakes, Minn.)

elsewhere. Quality control varies and there is a wide variety of workmanship among instrument manufacturers worldwide.

- Metal finishes have significance in the quality of an instrument and in its function. Surgical technologists must be knowledgeable about the relationship between a particular metal finish and function of the instrument.
- One of the most important ways in which a surgical instrument is classified is by type, which also identifies its function or use in surgery. The ability to identify types of instruments is the first step in more complex differentiation.
- Structural, functional, and surface defects in a surgical instrument are associated with patient injury. The surgical technologist is responsible for identifying defects, including incomplete cleaning, cracks, chips, broken parts, and insulation failure before an instrument is used in surgery.

REVIEW QUESTIONS

1. What is the relationship between the characteristics of a particular type of tissue and the instruments that are used on that tissue?
2. On what types of tissues would you *not* use an instrument with teeth (one that punctures)?
3. What is the advantage of having a right-angled instrument?
4. List the correct scalpel blade numbers and their handles.
5. How would you protect the cutting edges of instruments from damage during surgery?
6. What is the function of a self-retaining retractor?
7. Describe your personal plan for learning the names and uses of instruments.

CASE STUDIES

CASE 1

You are scrubbed on a large case with your preceptor. Loud music is playing, and it is difficult to hear the surgeon's requests for instruments. You know the instruments but have not had much experience with them. You make many mistakes, and the surgeon becomes irritated. What is the best plan of action?

CASE 2

You have opened a case and are now scrubbed, preparing instruments for the start of surgery. Among the sterile goods is a complex instrument that you have not seen before. The instrument has been disassembled for sterilization, and you must now put it together. Little time is left, and you have 12 separate parts to assemble. What is the correct action? Consider the importance of not wasting operating time, the need for your attention at the sterile field, and prioritization of your time.

CASE 3

The surgeon asks for a particular instrument during a stressful procedure. You pass the instrument she requested. She states, "Don't give me what I ask for, give me what I need." What does this mean?

BIBLIOGRAPHY

Nilsen E. Managing equipment and instruments in the operating room. *AORN Journal*. 2005;81:349.

Spry C. Care and handling of basic surgical instruments. *AORN Journal*. 2007;86:S77.

12 PERIOPERATIVE PHARMACOLOGY

KNOWLEDGE AND SKILLS REVIEW

The following skills and knowledge should be reviewed before you start this chapter:
Aseptic technique
Law and documentation

LEARNING OBJECTIVES

After studying this chapter, the reader will be able to:

1. List the sources of drugs
2. Explain different drug resources available
3. Discuss the importance of drug regulation
4. Understand how drugs are named and formulated
5. Correctly identify and interpret the components of a drug label
6. Discuss ways to prevent drug errors
7. List and use the seven rights of the medication process
8. Recognize the elements of a prescription and how drugs are ordered drug
9. Apply the correct protocol for receiving drugs on the sterile field
10. Accurately convert values within and between measurement systems
11. List and describe different drug delivery devices
12. Describe the role of the surgical technologist in handling drugs
13. List drug administration routes
14. Describe the principles of pharmacokinetics
15. Describe the principles of pharmacodynamics
16. Explain the different drug categories and give examples of drugs in each category

TERMINOLOGY

Adverse reaction: An unexpected, harmful reaction to a drug.
Agonist: A drug that produces a response in the body by binding to a receptor.
Allergy: Hypersensitivity to a substance; a response produced by the immune system.
Antagonist: A drug or chemical that blocks a receptor-mediated response.
Antibiotics: Drugs that inhibit the growth of or kill bacteria.
Bioavailability: The extent and rate at which a drug or its metabolites (products of breakdown) enter the systemic circulation and reach the site of action.
Chemical name: The name of a drug that reflects its molecular structure.
Concentration: The quantity of a substance per unit of volume or weight.
Contraindications: Circumstances that make use of a protocol, drug, or procedure medically inadvisable because they increase the risk of injury or harm.
Contrast media: Radiopaque solutions (i.e., not penetrated by x-rays) that are introduced into body cavities and vessels to outline their shape.
Controlled substances: Drugs that have the potential for abuse. Controlled substances are rated according to their risk potential; these ratings are called schedules.
Diluent: The liquid component of a drug that must be mixed with a powder to form the required drug.
Dosage: The prescribed amount of a drug. Dosage is expressed as a quantity of drug per unit of time.
Dose: The quantity of a drug to be taken at one time or the stated amount of drug per unit of distribution (e.g., 0.5 mg per milliliter of solution).
Drug: A chemical substance that, when taken into the body, has a physiological effect.
Drug administration: The giving of a drug to a person by any route.
Generation: In pharmacology, refers to a drug group that was developed from a previous prototype (e.g., first-generation cephalosporin).
Generic drug: A drug that is manufactured and sold under its assigned name.
Generic name: The formulary name of a drug that is assigned by the U.S. Adopted Names Council.
Half-life: The time required for one-half of a drug to be cleared from the body.
Hypersensitivity: Allergic immune response to a substance causing a range of symptoms from mild inflammation to anaphylactic shock and death.
Intraosseous: Administration of a drug directly into the bone marrow.
Intrathecal: Administration of a drug into the spinal canal.
Luer-Lok syringe tip: Connection between the needle and syringe. This tip requires a twist and is the most secure type.
Onset: The point at which a drug begins to exert a physiological effect in the body.
Parenteral: Administration of a drug by injection.
Peak effect: The period of maximum effect of a drug.
Pharmacodynamics: The biochemical and physiological effects of drugs and their mechanisms of action in the body.

TERMINOLOGY (CONT.)

Pharmacokinetics: The movement of a drug through the tissues and cells of the body, including the processes of absorption, distribution, and localization in tissues; biotransformation; and excretion by mechanical and chemical means.

Pharmacology: The study of drugs and their action in the body.

Prescription: An order for a licensed drug written by an authorized health care provider.

Proprietary name: The patented name given to a drug by its manufacturer.

Side effects: Anticipated effects of a drug other than those intended. Side effects may be uncomfortable for the patient or may have a positive outcome.

Slip tip: Syringe-needle connection. The syringe tip is smooth and tapered making it easy to disconnect.

Therapeutic window: Range of drug doses that can treat disease effectively while staying within the safety range.

Topical: Refers to the application of a drug to the skin or mucous membranes.

Trade name: The name given to a drug by the company that produces and sells it.

Transdermal: Administration of a drug by absorption through the skin, such as with ointments or patches impregnated with the drug.

U.S. Pharmacopeia (USP): An organization that establishes standards for drugs approved by the U.S. Food and Drug Administration (FDA) for their labeled use.

The study of drugs is called **pharmacology.** The term **drug** is defined as a substance intended for use in the diagnosis, cure, relief, treatment, or prevention of disease or intended to affect the structure or function of the body.[1] This qualification is associated with regulations that protect the public from harm resulting from medical or pharmacological intervention.

This chapter describes basic principles of pharmacology, drug regulation, and the drug *process*—the steps required in ordering, preparing, and administering a drug, including the role of the surgical technologist. Drug errors and how to prevent them are presented as a vital part of the drug process. Finally, drug categories are introduced, along with examples of specific substances in selected categories. Anesthetic and adjunct drugs are also discussed in preparation for the study of anesthesia in the next chapter.

Pharmacological terms used in the chapter have been standardized to match the U.S. Food and Drug Administration (FDA) terminology so that students can research topics easily and accurately. The classification system and drug categories presented follow the American Hospital Formulary Service (AHFS), which is the current system used in the United States. Students are urged to become familiar with these classifications rather than relying on lay drug terminology and brand names of drugs.

A review of basic math is located in Appendix 2.

NOTE *Ophthalmic drugs are located in Chapter 25, Ophthalmic Surgery.*

SECTION I: PHARMACOLOGY BASICS

SOURCES OF DRUGS

Drugs used in modern medicine are derived from natural and synthetic sources:

- Animal and human proteins
- Minerals
- Elemental metals
- Plants
- Synthetic chemicals

Most drugs are derived from synthetic molecules. These might mimic, or act like, substances found in nature, but they have been modified during the manufacturing process to make them safer to use. Throughout history, healers of all cultures have used biological (natural) substances in the treatment of medical and psychological illness. Traditional healing with plants has guided the development of modern pharmaceuticals. Today, herbal medicines have returned to modern therapy as a component of healing. Other biological substances include proteins and hormones derived from animal or human sources. These are used in many different medicinal and immunological agents and also for tissue grafting.

Purified metals, salts, and other elements are used alone or as components of drugs. For example, barium is a naturally occurring metal used for diagnostic procedures, and electrolytes, which are necessary for life, are administered to balance cell function. The pharmaceutical industry also uses *biotechnology* to manufacture certain drugs, including those derived from human-made molecules and natural sources such as animal or plant substances. Biotechnology is not the source of the drug; it is the *process* used in manufacturing. In this process, genetically modified microorganisms are used for the production of chemicals, which are then purified to form the drug.

Drugs are manufactured in the United States as patented products. This means that the drug company that invented the drug owns a patent on it, and no other company can make the drug until the patent runs out.

DRUG INFORMATION RESOURCES

Drug information, including a drug's biochemical action, the correct **dosage**, and other technical data, is widely available in books and online. Reference books are used by clinicians to research technical information about a drug—its action, dose, and form, how the drug is metabolized, its interaction with other drugs, and other details important for the prescriber and other health care providers.

- *The Physicians' Desk Reference (PDR)* is used by many primary health care providers—especially prescribers and pharmacists. It contains detailed information about **prescription** and over-the-counter (OTC) drugs needed for safe administration. The PDR is updated yearly, and the entries are made by subscription.
- *The United States Pharmacopeia–National Formulary (USP-NF)* is the complete reference of all drugs, dietary supplements, and devices marketed for medical use in the United States. The reference is composed of many different standards sections, which describe packaging, storage, and labeling requirements for drugs.
- *The AHFS* has several publications. These include drug handbooks and references related to prescribing, consumer

BOX 12.1 Drug Information Resources Online

FDA Orange Book:
https://www.fda.gov/drugs/drug-approvals-and-databases/approved-drug-products-therapeutic-equivalence-evaluations-orange-book
U.S. Drug Enforcement Administration (DEA) List of Controlled Substances:
https://www.deadiversion.usdoj.gov/schedules/
Institute for Safe Medication Practices (ISMP):
http://www.ismp.org
National Coordinating Council for Medication Error Reporting and Prevention (NCCMERP):
http://www.nccmerp.org
The Joint Commission (TJC) National Patient Safety Goals:
http://www.jointcommission.org/standards_information/npsgs.aspx

drug resources, indexing and categories of drugs, and drug licensing.

Reputable *online drug resources* are often a good way to research drugs at all levels. A starter list of organizations and their websites useful for health care workers is given in Box 12.1.

Pharmacology textbooks are written for specific audiences. Texts may focus on specific areas of health care such as cancer medicine and pain management. There are many reference texts on pharmacology subspecialties such as pharmacokinetics and pharmacodynamics.

REGULATION OF DRUGS, SUBSTANCES, AND DEVICES

The laws appropriate to prescriptions, dispensing, and administration of drugs are defined by each state's *practice acts.* The Joint Commission requires health care organizations to develop policies that are in compliance with state laws, which regulate who may prescribe, dispense, and administer drugs. This means that health care institutions or organizations may not establish independent policies or guidelines that violate state practice acts. It is important for the surgical technologist to know both the health care institution's policy and the state's laws regarding drugs. To find out your state's laws, search "practice act," plus the state, plus the profession you are interested in researching. For example, to research the practice acts for surgical technologists in Utah, type "practice acts Utah surgical technologist." When researching practice acts, be sure to look for the current version of the law.

The following roles and who may perform them are regulated by law:

- Procurement and secure storage
- Prescription, ordering, and transcription of drug orders
- Preparation and dispensing of drugs
- Administration of drugs

Federal regulation of drugs is the responsibility of the FDA. This agency maintains strict regulatory control on devices and substances used on or in the body. These include the following:

- Prescription drugs
- Generic drugs
- Non-prescription drugs sold OTC
- Food supplements
- Cosmetics
- Medical devices, including implants and equipment used in the delivery of drugs
- Wound closure materials, such as suture
- Biologicals (materials made from live tissue)
- Devices that deliver potentially harmful levels of radiation

In the United States, drugs are approved for medical use only after rigid testing and application to the FDA. The FDA authorizes the sale and distribution of drugs and is responsible for ensuring that approved drugs meet consumer safety requirements. It approves drug literature and labeling so that health care providers and the public are informed about the nature and use of a drug and all the risks associated with it.

To protect the public from harm, prescription and OTC medicines must meet standards for quality, purity, identity, and strength. These standards are set by the **U.S. Pharmacopeia (USP).** All substances that meet these standards bear the initials *USP* after their generic name. Approved substances are published in the USP-NF. The World Health Organization (WHO) publishes an international formulary, the *International Pharmacopoeia.*

PRESCRIPTION AND OVER-THE-COUNTER DRUGS

A prescription drug is one that is regulated by the FDA. A prescription is authorization to obtain a licensed drug. Only certain state-licensed professionals (e.g., a doctor, dentist, osteopath, advanced practice nurse, or physician's assistant) may provide a prescription. Prescription drugs are differentiated from OTC drugs, which are available to the public without authorization. These groups of substances make up a large commercial market. Because these drugs require no authorization, the public may purchase them without medical supervision.

HERBAL REMEDIES AND FOOD SUPPLEMENTS

The FDA does not regulate herbal substances as drugs. Instead, it classifies them as food supplements. Companies within and outside the United States may market substances to the American public without the stringent testing and quality control required for prescriptions and OTC drugs. Many herbal drugs produce physiological changes in the body and may interfere with the action of regulated medicines.

The FDA regulates dietary substances such as vitamins and minerals less stringently than it does prescription and OTC drugs. Some supplements such as folic acid and vitamin A are known to be beneficial in the treatment or prevention of specific diseases. However, the manufacturer of dietary supplements does not have to *prove* efficacy of a supplement to market it. Manufacturers do have to prove that the products meet safe manufacturing standards.

CONTROLLED SUBSTANCES

Controlled substances are drugs that carry a high risk of abuse or addiction and are specifically designated and

BOX 12.2 Federal Drug Schedules of Controlled Substances

- Schedule I:
  The drug has a high potential for abuse.
  There is no accepted safety for use of the drug under medical supervision.
- Schedule II:
  The drug has a high potential for abuse.
  It has an accepted medical use with restrictions in the United States.
  Abuse may lead to severe psychological or physical dependence.
- Schedule III:
  The drug has less abuse potential than Schedules I and II.
  It has an accepted medical use in the United States.
  Abuse of the drug can lead to low or moderate physical dependence or high psychological dependence.
- Schedule IV:
  The drug or other substance has a low potential for abuse relative to the drugs or other substances in Schedule III.
  The drug has a currently accepted medical use in treatment in the United States.
  Abuse of the drug may lead to limited physical or psychological dependence relative to the drugs in Schedule III.
- Schedule V:
  The drug has low abuse potential compared with Schedule IV.
  It has an accepted medical use.
  Abuse can lead to limited physical or psychological dependence as compared with substances in Schedule IV.

regulated by state and federal law. The designation (called a *schedule*) is based on the risk of abuse or dependency. Controlled drugs include both prescription and illegal substances. The regulating body for controlled substances is the federal Drug Enforcement Administration (DEA) http://. Controlled drug schedules are shown in Box 12.2. Schedule I drugs carry the highest risk of abuse.

PREGNANCY CATEGORIES

Drugs are classified by pregnancy category (A, B, C, D, and X) to inform health care workers and patients of the potential risk to the fetus if a pregnant woman takes the drug. The categories are described as follows:

- A: No demonstrated risk to the fetus.
- B: Animal studies have not demonstrated risk and there are no adequate and well-controlled studies in pregnant women, or studies in animals show risk to the fetus but well-designed studies in people do not.
- C: Inadequate studies have been performed in animals and people; some studies show risk to the fetus in animals.
- D: There is a risk to the human fetus, but the benefits may outweigh the risks in certain situations.
- X: Drugs have been proven to pose a risk that outweighs the benefit of the drug.

Most drugs are listed as category D, because it is unknown whether they pose a risk, and testing would be unethical under any circumstances.

DRUG NOMENCLATURE

Drug *nomenclature* is a system of identifying drugs by name. Three methods are used in the international nomenclature system—generic name, trade name, and chemical formula.

GENERIC NAME

The **generic name** of a drug is assigned by the United States Adopted Names (USAN) Council at the time that the drug is invented and accepted for marketing. The USAN ensures that generic drug names do not sound or look alike to prevent drug errors. The manufacturer may market its drug under its own **trade name** (e.g., Lipitor), but the generic name must be assigned by the USAN. Examples of generic names are *acetaminophen* (trade name Tylenol) and *atenolol* (trade name Tenormin).

A **generic drug** is one that is manufactured and marketed without a trade name. Generics have the identical properties of their trade name counterparts. Generic drugs are substantially cheaper (sometimes up to 10 times less expensive) for the consumer because there are no advertising and few marketing costs associated with them. By law, drugs with the same generic name must have the same chemical composition as the identical drug with a trade name, regardless of how many companies produce it. Generic drugs are tested and regulated by the same standards as identical brand name drugs. By law, they are the same as branded drugs in dosage form, strength, safety, performance, and intended use. In general, generic drugs are much more widely available than branded equivalents. Using generic drugs can save consumers a considerable amount of money with no loss of quality or safety.

TRADE (PROPRIETARY) NAME

When a drug is developed, the company that produces the drug obtains a patent for it and gives it a trade name (known also as the brand name or **proprietary name**) under which the drug is marketed. Trade names apply to both prescription and OTC drugs. Drug patents and their names are currently granted for 20 years. After that time, the exclusive rights to the drug formula and name expire, allowing other companies to produce the same drug with their own trade names or as a generic drug. Surgical technologists may be familiar with prescription drug trade names that are used in the health care setting. It is important, however, for all professionals involved in the drug process to know and use the drug's generic name. This helps prevent ambiguity and may reduce drug errors in the clinical setting.

TABLE 12.1 Drug Nomenclature

Trade Name	Generic Name	Chemical Name
Zoloft	sertraline HCl	(1S-cis)-4-(3,4-dichlorophenyl)-1,2,3,4-tetrahydro-N-methyl-1-naphthalenamine hydrochloride
Cipro Ciproxin	ciprofloxacin	1-cyclopropyl-6-fluoro-4-oxo-7-piperazin-1-yl-quinoline-3-carboxylic acid
Lasix	furosemide	4-chloro-2-(furan-2-ylmethylamino)-5-sulfamoylbenzoic acid

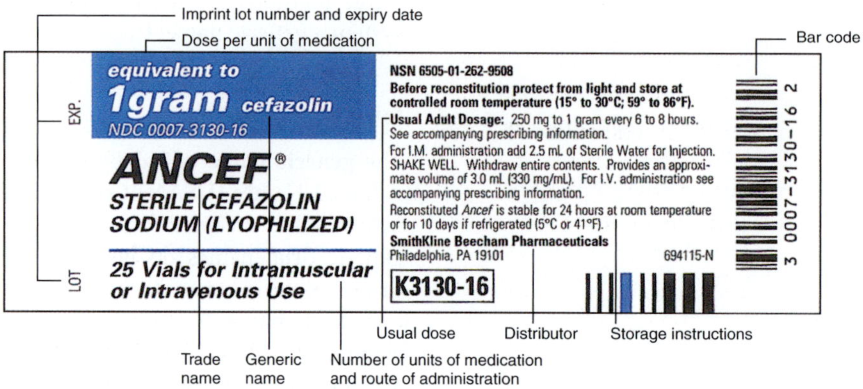

FIG. 12.1 Drug labels. Note dose, strength, bar code, and use. (From Kee J, Hayes E, McCuiston L. *Pharmacology*. 5th ed. Philadelphia: WB Saunders; 2006.)

CHEMICAL NAME

The **chemical name** of a drug is derived from its molecular formula. Some examples of drug nomenclature are shown in Table 12.1. The chemical formula is listed in the package insert and usually referred to for scientific purposes rather than during the medication process. The chemical is the *active ingredient*. This is the specific chemical or compound responsible for the drug's therapeutic action. Drugs also contain *inactive ingredients* that have no therapeutic effect. These are added for preservation, for color, or to bind the ingredients.

DRUG LABELS

All pharmaceutical products and implants are commercially labeled both inside and outside the package. The FDA regulates labeling to protect the public from harm resulting from misinformation or lack of information regarding the drug's use. A drug *insert* is a leaflet that accompanies prescription and some nonprescription drug packages. The insert is a detailed description of the drug's composition, intended use, action, adverse reactions, warnings, and dosage.

The package or container label is printed in ink and stamped on the container or carton. This information has specific importance to the health care providers who will dispense or administer the drug.

Critical information on the container label includes the following:

1. *Name of the drug including proprietary and generic name*
2. *Dosage form:* For example, solution, capsule, or dry powder for reconstitution
3. *Amount contained in the package:* For example, 1 gram, or 2 mg per mL
4. *Indications:* The labeled purpose of the drug—what it is used for
5. *Dosage:* The therapeutic amount to administer
6. *Route of administration:* How the drug is to be given (e.g., intravenous or intramuscular injection)
7. *Bar code:* This is a computer label that can be scanned and traced to ensure that the drug is not counterfeit and that the actual drug is the same as its label states it is. The label includes the product code, expiration date, manufacturing number, and quantity.
8. *Lot number:* When each drug batch is mixed in the drug laboratory, it is assigned a lot number in the event that a batch must be recalled from use for safety purposes.
9. *Expiration date:* The date beyond which the drug must not be used. The date is stamped onto the container in addition to that in the bar code.

Drugs must not be used beyond the specified expiration date. Over time, many drugs lose their efficacy or may become toxic. The expiration date indicates when the drug must be withdrawn from the market and destroyed.

Fig. 12.1 illustrates two different drug labels as seen on the outside of the drug package.

DRUG FORMATS

Drugs and other medical substances are manufactured so that they are compatible with how the drug is administered and how it reaches the target tissue. The format is not the same as the route of administration. This is an important point to remember. The format is also called the *dosage form* or therapeutic presentation (e.g., tablet, liquid, or cream). For example, drugs that are intended to reach the central nervous system (CNS) quickly are formulated as liquid intravenous injection or a tablet placed under the tongue, where it is rapidly absorbed through the mucous membrane. Tablets meant for oral administration must be resistant to breakdown until they reach the gastrointestinal (GI) system, where they will be absorbed through the stomach lining. Skin patches or films impregnated with medication keep the drug in contact with the skin, which slowly absorbs the drug at measured intervals.

The surgical technologist encounters many different drug forms and is responsible for correctly preparing them for administration on the sterile field (discussed later in the chapter). The following is a representative list of FDA formulations and examples of their use in surgery. The list appears in alphabetical order. Table 12.2 shows a complete list.

Cement: When used in orthopedic surgery, cement is most commonly available as a powder that must be mixed with a chemical liquid **diluent** on the sterile field. This is done with a closed mixing device to prevent exposure to hazardous vapor, which is a byproduct of the mixed components.

Film: A film is a very thin sheet of transparent or semitransparent solid material. It is mainly used where there is a need to seal tissue leaks, such as in the lung, dura mater, and vascular structures. Thin bio-absorbable film may be cut to size as a patch and left in place over tissue, which absorbs the material over time. An additional use for biofilms under research is a film barrier that prevents the formation of adhesions (scarring between the abdominal wall and internal organs).

Graft: A graft is a natural or synthetic substance used to replace tissue, fill in defects, or bridge a defect in tissues. Synthetic graft materials are commonly used for tissue repair (e.g., mesh graft to repair hernia defects) and in the manufacturing of blood vessel replacements. Bioactive tissue grafting materials are actually incorporated into the tissue during the healing process, providing a strong permanent bond.

Implant: Synthetic and biological implants are used in many different specialties. Examples are joint replacement components and in reconstructive surgery to provide replacements where bone or tissue loss have occurred. Electronic implants are important in cardiac medicine and in neurosurgery for the restoration of hearing. Tissue implants are available in many different forms. Tissue may be autologous (from the patient) or a transplant from another individual. For a full discussion on tissue implants, refer to Chapter 18.

Irrigant: Fluids are commonly used to irrigate the surgical wound. Sterile saline for irrigation is used to flush tissues and prevent them from drying during surgery and to remove tissue debris.

Packing: This is gauze or other soft material, usually impregnated with an antibacterial drug. The material is folded and compressed into a hollow cavity to control postoperative bleeding, such as in nasal surgery, or to pack an incision that must remain temporarily open during healing.

Powder: Powdered formulas are used in their dry state or are *reconstituted* (reformulated) into a liquid drug by adding a diluent. Some antibiotics are marketed dry and must be reconstituted with sterile water or saline solution for injection.

Solution: This is a water-based liquid to which one or more substances have been added.

Solution for slush: This is a solution for the preparation of iced saline, which is used to irrigate tissue and induce regional hypothermia. This preparation is used in selected cardiac and kidney procedures.

Sponge: This formation is a porous matrix of soft absorbable or non-absorbable material. Medication may be injected into the sponge by the manufacturer. In surgery, absorbable gelatin sponges are used plain or may be soaked in thrombin and used as a surface coagulant to stop capillary bleeding.

Spray: Drugs are formulated as sprays to facilitate covering a tissue surface quickly and efficiently. Examples are anesthetic spray used on throat tissue before the insertion of endoscopes, and spray-on tissue sealants used to control bleeding capillary surfaces such as on the liver or spleen.

Tincture: A tincture is any solution that is formulated with alcohol. Examples include the skin prep solution used on the operative site before surgery and alcohol antiseptic used in hand asepsis.

HOW DRUGS WORK

When a drug enters the body by any route, *both the body and the drug undergo changes.* That is, the drug is broken down (a change in the drug), and the drug has a physiological effect on the patient (a change in the body).

PHARMACOKINETICS

Pharmacokinetics is the study of the movement of drugs through the body and the changes that occur in the drug. Once inside the body, the drug moves through different chemical and physical pathways. As it moves, it undergoes breakdown and attachment to different cells and molecules in the body along the kinetic path. Finally, it reaches the target tissue, is metabolized, and at the end of the process is excreted out of the body in its transformed state.

In general, there are four main processes or events that occur in the pharmacokinetic pathway. These are as follows:

1. Absorption
2. Distribution
3. Biotransformation (metabolism)
4. Excretion (elimination)

Absorption is the process by which a drug enters the body tissues after administration. The rate of absorption and the amount of drug that actually reaches the target tissue depend on many factors, such as the chemical structure of the drug, the method of administration, and the condition of the patient. Absorption involves chemical and physical breakdown of the drug. For example, oral drugs must dissolve before passing through the wall of the small intestine and

TABLE 12.2 Pharmaceutical Dosage Forms

Form	Description
Aerosol	A product that is packaged under pressure and contains therapeutically active ingredients that are released on activation of an appropriate valve system; it is intended for topical application to the skin as well as local application into the nose (nasal aerosols), mouth (lingual aerosols), or lungs (inhalation aerosols).
Capsule	A solid oral dosage form consisting of a shell and filling.
Cement	A substance that produces a solid union between two surfaces.
Concentrate	A liquid preparation of increased strength and reduced volume that is usually diluted before administration.
Cream	An emulsion, semisolid dosage form used for external application to the skin or mucous membranes.
Emulsion	A dosage form consisting of at least two immiscible liquids, one of which is dispersed as droplets within the other liquid.
Film	A thin layer or coating.
Gel	A semisolid dosage form that contains a gelling agent to provide stiffness to a solution or colloidal solution or dispersion.
Graft	A slip of skin or other tissue for implantation.
Implant	A material containing drug intended to be inserted securely or deeply in tissue for growth, slow release, or the formation of an organic union.
Inhalant	A class of inhalations consisting of a drug or combination of drugs that are carried into the respiratory tract, where they exert their effect.
Injection	A sterile preparation intended for parenteral use. Five classes of injections are defined by the USP.
Irrigant	A sterile solution intended to bathe or flush open wounds or body cavities; used topically, never parenterally.
Packing	A material usually covered by or impregnated with a drug that is inserted into a body cavity.
Patch	A drug delivery system that often contains an adhesive backing that is applied to an external site on the body.
Pellet	A small, sterile, solid mass consisting of a highly purified drug intended for implantation in the body.
Pill	A small, round, solid dosage form containing a medicinal agent intended for oral administration.
Plaster	Substance intended for external application of consistency to adhere to the skin and attach to a dressing, intended to afford protection and support.
Powder for solution	A mixture of dry drugs or chemicals that on addition of a suitable vehicle yields a solution.
Solution	A clear, homogeneous liquid that contains one or more chemical substances dissolved in a solvent.
Solution for slush	A solution for the preparation of an iced saline slush, which is administered by irrigation and used to induce regional hypothermia (in conditions such as certain open heart and kidney procedures) by its direct application.
Sponge	A porous, interlacing, absorbent material that contains a drug.
Spray	A liquid minutely divided as by a jet of air or stream.
Suspension	A liquid dosage form that contains solid particles dispersed in a liquid medium.
Swab	A small piece of flat, absorbent material that contains a drug.
Tablet	A solid dosage form containing medicinal substances.
Tincture	An alcoholic or hydroalcoholic solution.

liver. The substance then enters the bloodstream, where it is carried to the target tissue. Drugs that are injected directly into a blood vessel do not require absorption and thus reach the target tissue almost immediately, whereas one injected into the muscle or connective tissue usually takes 15 to 30 minutes to take effect. Many drugs contain components or additives that enhance (increase the rate or amount) or delay absorption.

Distribution takes place after the drug enters the bloodstream. In this phase, the drug is carried (distributed) to body tissues, where it exerts its pharmacological effect. Not all of the drug administered reaches the target tissue. The amount of drug available and the rate of availability are called the **bioavailability.** For example, some drugs may become tightly bound to blood proteins and are released to the target tissue very slowly. Fat-soluble drugs move rapidly across cell membranes and take effect quickly but tend to accumulate in fatty tissue, which prolongs their effect. Water-soluble substances are much slower to act, because they stay in the bloodstream longer than those that are fat soluble. In all cases, only the free unbound drug is available to tissues for pharmacological effect.

Biotransformation, or drug metabolism, is the chemical breakdown of a drug in the body. Most drugs are broken down into smaller, less complex chemical components by enzymes. This mainly occurs in the liver. Biotransformation prepares the drug for *excretion*, or elimination, from the body. Because most biotransformation occurs in the liver, conditions that decrease liver function can alter drug metabolism, resulting in toxicity. Liver disease and advanced age are two causes of altered liver metabolism, which can affect drug metabolism.

In pharmacology and medicine, it is critical to know how long a drug remains active. This is related to its rate of biotransformation, which is measured by the drug's half-life. The **half-life** is the time it takes for one-half of the drug to be cleared from the body. Some drugs, such as antibiotics, have a short half-life and must be given repeatedly over a short period of time so that the therapeutic amount stays constant for the duration of treatment. Other drugs have a long half-life and can be given less frequently to maintain therapeutic levels.

Excretion is the elimination or clearance of a drug from the body. Most drugs are eliminated through the urinary tract. A small percentage are excreted through the biliary tract, breast milk, saliva, and intestine. Volatile drugs and anesthetics are excreted through the lungs during exhalation. Just as liver disease can alter drug metabolism, kidney disease can severely retard or block drug elimination and result in life-threatening toxicity.

Drugs are mainly eliminated as the byproducts of metabolism. In this process, chemical reactions cause the drug to break down into smaller molecules or components. The metabolic components of the drug are called *metabolites.* In a healthy individual, the entire drug is excreted—in its intact form, or as metabolites—as smaller components resulting from the breakdown of the drug.

PHARMACODYNAMICS

The point in time when the drug first takes effect is called the **onset**. The point when the drug has the greatest effect is called the **peak effect**. From that point, the effects diminish until the drug is cleared from tissues. The total time that the drug is active for is called the duration of action. Changes in the body (both intended and unintended) as a result of a drug are called **pharmacodynamics.** These changes occur with most drugs because of their ability to "lock on" to certain receptor sites on the cells. Normally, the receptor sites receive the body's own (endogenous) chemicals (e.g., hormones and neurotransmitters) that cause specific physiological changes. However, when the drug occupies these sites, the endogenous chemicals are blocked. The drug is then called an **antagonist.** The drug may not have any other function except blocking the site. An increased dose of the drug results in many more receptor sites being taken, and this severely affects the cell's ability to receive the endogenous chemical. A drug or substance that blocks endogenous substances is called an *antagonist.*

Some drugs lock on to the receptor site and increase the efficiency of that site's normal uptake of chemical receptor. These drugs are called **agonists.** Agonists do not create new biological events; they only increase the effect of the receptor by locking on to more receptors or increasing the amount of chemical available to the receptors.

THERAPEUTIC WINDOW

Drug action is related not only to the amount of time it is in the body but also to the amount of drug administered and its **concentration**—the amount of actual drug per unit dose. Although the drug may have a positive effect at a certain level, increasing the amount of drug beyond the therapeutic or effective level can result in toxicity. The practical application of drug therapy is to give only the amount of drug that brings about the desired effect without causing toxicity.

The **therapeutic window** is the highest and lowest amount of a drug needed to produce the desired effect without causing toxicity. Some drugs have a very narrow therapeutic window, meaning that the difference in drug amounts between therapeutic effect and toxicity is very small. This is very important for the surgical technologist who handles dose-dependent drugs on the surgical field. Some drugs handled in surgery are extremely toxic and even lethal at high levels. This is why there is so much importance placed on the identification of the drug strength and on the amount being delivered.

Drug *synergy* occurs when drugs given simultaneously cause an effect that is greater than any one of the drugs would have by itself. Drug synergy allows certain synergistic drugs to be given in lower doses, which is safer for the patient. However, drug synergy can work in the opposite direction, making a combination of drugs more toxic or lethal than any one of the substances by itself.

UNIT SYSTEMS OF MEASUREMENT

The drug process requires precise measurement using the correct measuring devices and delivery systems. This process often involves making calculations involving the strength of the drug, the amount needed, and the amount already administered. For example, the total amount of drug, such as a local anesthetic given intermittently, must be recalculated each time more is administered to prevent overdose. Drugs formulated as a combination of more than one substance (e.g., local anesthetic with epinephrine added) may require separate calculation of each component to prevent overdose of either drug.

Historically, three measurement systems were used in pharmacology: the metric, apothecary, and household systems. The now obsolete "household system" is not used in any branch of medicine because it lacks precision and can cause drug errors. *This system must not be used for any medical measurement.* The apothecary system is also obsolete (see later discussion).

NOTE *Liquid OTC drugs meant to be taken at home may specify a spoon measure for calculating dosage. In these cases, the drug will be packaged with a measuring device to prevent over- or underdosing.*

METRIC SYSTEM

The metric system of weights and measures is an international system. It is commonly used for all measurements in every country except the United States. *It is the universally accepted*

TABLE 12.3 Metric Equivalents

%	Ratio	g/L	g/dL	mg/mL	mg/dL	mcg/mL
10	1:10	100	10	100	10,000	100,000
1	1:100	10	1	10	1000	10,000
0.1	1:1000	1	0.1	1	100	1000
0.01	1:10,000	0.1	0.01	0.1	10	100
0.001	1:100,000	0.01	0.001	0.01	1	10
0.0001	1:1,000,000	0.001	0.0001	0.001	0.1	1

BOX 12.3 Metric System: Mass and Volume

UNITS OF MASS
1 kilogram (kg) = 1000 grams (g)
1 gram (g) = 1000 milligrams (mg)
1 milligram = 1000 micrograms

UNITS OF VOLUME
1 liter (L) = 1000 milliliters (mL)
1 mL = 1000 microliters

standard for scientific measurement, including medicine. The United States also conforms to this standard. It was introduced in 1960 to standardize world trade and science. The system is based on units or powers of 10 (Table 12.3), which are applied to each type of quantity measured (volume, mass, and length). Box 12.3 shows mass and volume equivalents in the metric system.

Prefixes are used to express multiples of the metric system. Therefore, to arrive at an amount, the base unit is multiplied by the amount associated with its prefix. The prefixes are as follows:

Kilo: 1000
Hecto: 100
Deca: 10
Deci: 0.1 (one-tenth)
Centi: 0.01 (one-hundredth)
Milli: 0.001 (one-thousandth)

Examples:
1 *kilo*meter = 1000 meters
1 *kilo*gram = 1000 grams
1 *milli*gram = 1/1000 of a gram
1 *milli*liter = 1/1000 of a liter
5 *milli*liters = 5/1000 of a liter

APOTHECARY SYSTEM

The apothecary system is obsolete and rarely encountered. It has been replaced in all countries by metric measurements and is mentioned here only for historical interest. The system employs Roman numerals to represent measurements and symbols to represent units of measure. The basic units of weight in the apothecary system are grains (not to be confused with *grams*) and ounces. Volume is expressed in drams and minims. The apothecary measure *drop* is applied to liquid medications for instillation in the eye, ear, and nose. In this case, the actual amount depends on the container opening, which has been calibrated to equal the correct amount. The precise equivalent of one apothecary drop is 0.064853 milliliters (mL).

INTERNATIONAL UNIT

The International unit is based on the effect or activity of a specific drug and will only be encountered with those drugs. Penicillin, insulin, and heparin are examples of drugs that carry an International unit value. Drugs that are measured by International unit are prescribed according to the expected result when the measured amount is administered. Because the results are different according to what the drug is, the International unit is only standardized for that drug. For example, if the vial contains 400,000 International units of a drug, the prescriber must multiply the amount in the vial to increase the dose. Remember that when handling dry formulations of drugs that are measured in International units, adding liquid diluent only changes the concentration of the drug, not the amount of drug. To administer the exact number of units stated on the vial, the patient must receive all the dry contents no matter how much liquid is added. The recommended quantity of liquid diluent is always stated on the vial.

ROMAN NUMERALS

Roman numerals were used in the past for writing prescriptions. This system has been phased out in medicine but is still used in some types of general numerical communication. Roman numerals are based on units of 10 and use *letters* to represent numbers. The numeral is a symbol that represents a number in the Arabic system (0 to 9), as shown in Table 12.4.

When numerals are printed in succession, they are added:

III = 3

XXX = 30

When a smaller value is positioned ahead of a larger one, the smaller one is subtracted from the larger one:

IX = 9

IV = 4

Other rules apply for subtracting numerals:

- Subtract only powers of 10 (e.g., XLV = 45).
- Subtract only a single numeral from another single numeral (e.g., 19 = XIX, not IXX).

TABLE 12.4 Roman Numeral to Arabic Number Conversion

Roman Numeral	Arabic Number
I	1
V	5
X	10
L	50
C	100
D	500
M	1000

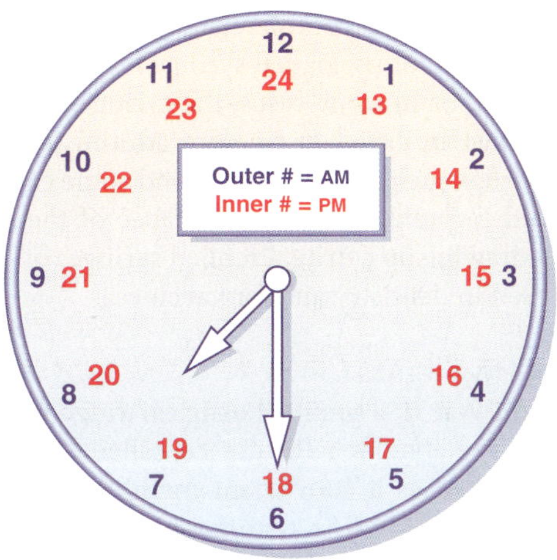

FIG. 12.2 Using international time. (From Kee J, Hayes E, McCuiston L. *Pharmacology*. 5th ed. Philadelphia: WB Saunders; 2006.)

- Do not subtract a numeral from one that is more than 10 times greater.

INTERNATIONAL TIME

International time is used in health care to prevent errors that occur when the same number is used for night and day. International time is based on a 24-hour clock. When international time is written, the colon (:) and abbreviations AM and PM are omitted.

In this system, the 24 hours of the day begin with 0100, "zero one hundred hours," which corresponds to 1 AM, and end at 2400, "twenty-four hundred hours," or 12 midnight. To convert to international time, remove the colon from customary time and use the total number of hours and minutes elapsed from 1200 for daytime and 2400 for nighttime (Fig. 12.2). Note that the term *international time* has replaced its older name "military time."

DEVICES FOR DRUG PREPARATION AND DELIVERY

SYRINGES

In surgery, medications pass through several processes before they are administered to the patient. Specialized equipment is

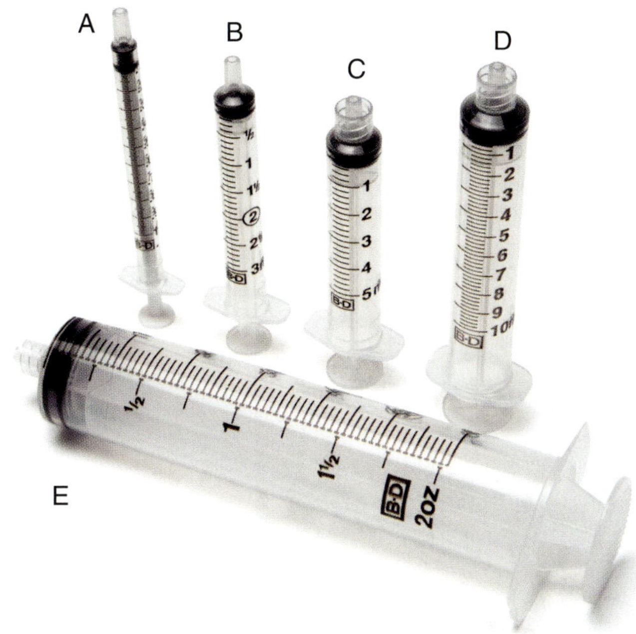

FIG. 12.3 Slip tip and Luer-Lok syringes. (A and B) Slip tip, (C, D, E) Luer-lok. (Courtesy and copyright Becton, Dickinson and Company.)

used to facilitate delivery while also keeping the drug sterile. Liquid drug preparation devices used in surgery include needles and syringes, tubing, stopcocks, and other devices. The physical connection of one device to another is standardized. There are two types of universal fittings. These are the **Luer-Lok** (also called lock tip) and **slip tip** (also called a plain tip). The lock tip is the more secure of the two: it requires a twist to seal it in place or remove it. This prevents accidental separation of the two ends and is used for high-pressure infusion. The male slip tip is attached to a female slip tip by simply pushing the two ends together. A slight twist provides an additional seal. This creates a firm but unlocked connection that can be pulled apart. This type of connection is used for low-pressure connections where leakage is not critical. When connecting two devices, such as tubing and syringe, both fittings must be the same type; that is, both must be Luer-Lok and slip tip. Both types have female and male configurations.

A needleless access port for connecting a patient's intravenous line uses a one-way valve located inside the connection. The connection is made with a counterpart Luer-Lok tip. These are used in emergency situations and in critical care. Fig. 12.3 shows several types of syringes with Luer-Lok and slip tip attachments.

Syringes are used for the injection of fluid medication and for measuring drugs. There are many different types used in medicine, industry, and science laboratories. The most commonly used syringe in the health care environment is the graduated plastic syringe. However, glass syringes are also used when smooth injection is critical, such as the infiltration of tissue with anesthetic or for liquids that are unstable in contact with polypropylene or rubber. Syringes are available with or without a needle attached, in graduated sizes from 1 mL to 60 mL. Smaller syringes are used for administering injections

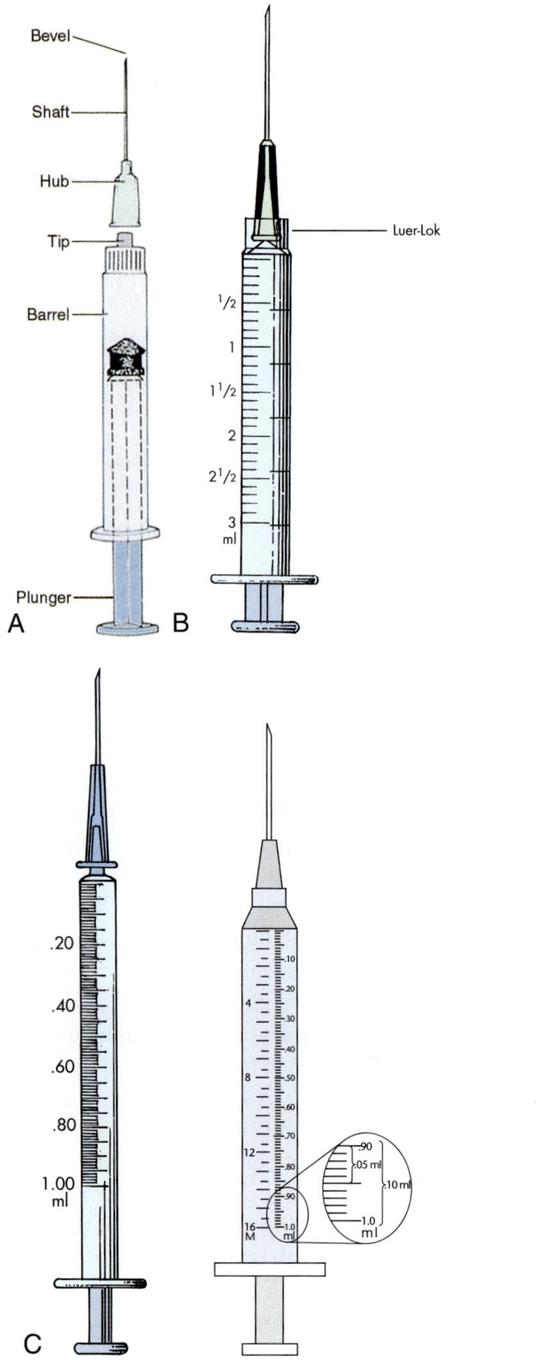

FIG. 12.4 Syringe calibrations. (A) Catheter tip syringe. (B) Luer-Lok syringe. (C) Left, tuberculin syringe; right, normal syringe showing incremental subunits contained with the entire tuberculin syringe. (A, From Elkin M, Perry A, Potter P. *Nursing Interventions and Clinical Skills.* 2nd ed. St Louis: Mosby; 2000; B, From Potter PA, Perry AG. *Fundamentals of Nursing.* 5th ed. St Louis: Mosby; 2001; C, From Clayton B, Stock Y. *Basic Pharmacology for Nurses.* 12th ed. St Louis: Mosby; 2001.)

and measuring. The 60 mL size is used for flushing and irrigation, not for measuring small amounts of drugs, because the increments are too wide for safe calculation. The component parts of a syringe are the *tip* with a slip or Luer-Lok fitting, *barrel, and plunger.* All syringes are calibrated in milliliters (mL), with increment hashes inscribed on the barrel (Fig. 12.4). The tuberculin syringe is the smallest syringe and has a total volume of 0.5 or 1 mL calibrated down to 0.01 mL; it is used for doses equal to 1 mL or less.

The 1 mL *insulin* syringe and needle is a one-piece unit, calibrated in both insulin units and milliliters. This syringe is intended for use with insulin only and carries an orange safety cap to distinguish it from the tuberculin syringe.

NOTE *It is critical that the insulin syringe not be confused with the 1 mL tuberculin syringe, which is used in the measurement of very small amounts of high-alert drugs. The calibrated insulin unit marks on the syringe are not equivalent to metric milliliter calibration. Substituting insulin unit measurement for milliliter measurement can result in patient injury and even death.*

Prefilled syringes are commercially available for selected drugs. The prefilled or preloaded syringe is packaged with the needle attached, or in some cases, the syringe is capped, and the needle must be fitted just before administration. Many emergency drugs such as epinephrine and some cardiac drugs are produced in prefilled syringes because of the extra time involved in drawing up a drug. Prefilled syringes of local anesthetic are used in dentistry and for vaccines.

Historical Highlights

During World War II, a prefilled drug cartridge was designed for use with a metal holder. The device, called a *Tubex syringe*, was manufactured as a convenient method of dispensing a variety of drugs quickly. The system was replaced after WWII with a similar system called the *carpuject*, which is a plastic cartridge holder equipped with a plunger. This device is mainly used by dentists and for patients who self-inject for emergency conditions such as epilepsy and allergy.

NEEDLES

Hypodermic needles are classified by their length and by the diameter of the needle. The needle diameter is measured as the *gauge*. The larger the gauge, the smaller the needle size. For example, an 18-gauge needle has a larger lumen than a 22-gauge needle.

The parts of the needle are the hub, the shaft, and the point. The point has an additional identifier—the bevel. This is the slanted side of the point and is important in **drug administration.** The exact size of the needle required for a procedure depends on the density of the tissue or material it will penetrate, the depth of the target tissue relative to skin (for percutaneous injection), and on the viscosity of the fluid to be injected. Needle length is measured in inches. Table 12.5 shows common needle sizes associated with target tissue.

Because of the risk of blood-borne diseases, the National Institute for Occupational Safety and Health (NIOSH) requires that syringes have some feature that allows the needle to be retracted or protected so that personnel are not punctured during or after use. There are many safety designs, including the needle and syringe combination, in which the needle retracts into the syringe barrel automatically after use, and the needle shield, which can be deployed by a single finger action close to the barrel.

TABLE 12.5 Injection Technique

	Location	Needle Length	Needle Gauge
INTRAMUSCULAR (PERCUTANEOUS)			
Pediatric >18 months	Deltoid; ventrogluteal; vastus lateralis	7/8″–1¼″	22–25
Adult >18 years	Deltoid; ventrogluteal; dorsogluteal	1″–1½″	19–25
SUBCUTANEOUS (PERCUTANEOUS)			
Pediatric to adult	Anterolateral thigh; upper outer triceps; upper buttocks; abdomen	½″–⅝″	26–30
INTRADERMAL			
Pediatric to adult	Anterior forearm; upper chest; upper back; posterior upper arm	⅜″–¾″	26–28

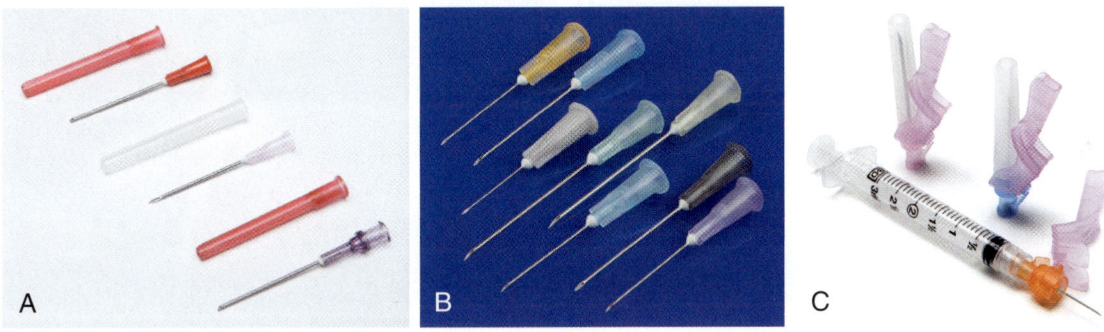

FIG. 12.5 (A) Blunt-tipped needle. (B) Filter needle for use with glass ampoules. (C) Safety needles. (Courtesy and copyright Becton, Dickinson and Company.)

A number of devices are available to allow recapping without handling the needle or hub. A recapping device holds the cap in a rigid container, and the needle and syringe combination is pushed down vertically into the cap. It is also acceptable technique to place the cap on the table and scoop it up with the point of the needle. *Needles should never be recapped using two hands.* The *filter straw* or *filter needle* is used to withdraw medicines from glass ampoules. After the glass ampoule is broken open, the filter straw is lowered into the drug, which can then be withdrawn while excluding any glass shards. Filter straws can be used on the sterile field. A filter needle uses the same principle—one end fitted with a needle and filter for drawing medication safely into a syringe.

The *blunt-tip needle* is used to transfer an injectable drug to the sterile field. This is important when the scrub is taking medication from a vial held by the circulator. The blunt needle prevents needlestick injury to the circulator. Blunt filter needles are also available for use with medications in ampoules. Fig. 12.5 shows the different types of needles discussed here.

DISPENSERS, TUBING, AND PUMPS

A *fluid dispenser* (also called a *medicine decanter*) is a curved, hard plastic tube containing a plastic spike at one end and a rounded spout at the other. This is used to dispense fluid from a sterile container to a receptacle on the sterile field (Fig. 12.6). This system allows the circulator to safely pour liquids into a sterile receptacle on the instrument table without reaching over the sterile field. The *spike* is a short, hard plastic tube with single- or double-ended sharp, beveled tips. One beveled end of the spike is inserted into the rubber stopper of a glass vial container. The other non-beveled end may be fitted with a length of connector tubing or a fluid dispenser/decanter. The double spike is used to connect two rubber-stoppered medication vials when pre-mixing is required.

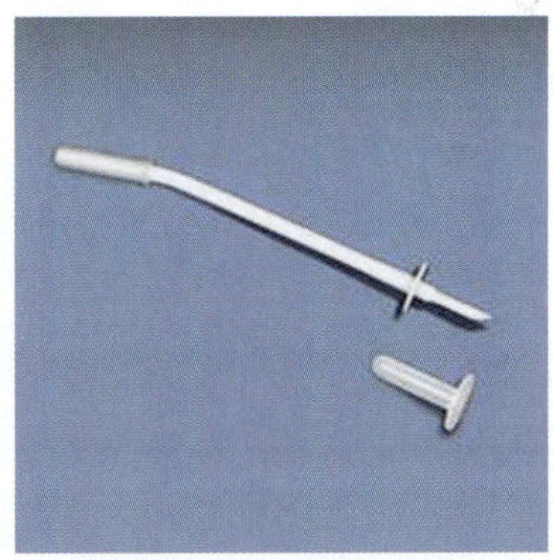

FIG. 12.6 A fluid transfer decanter distributed by DeRoyal Industries, Inc. (Copyright 2016, DeRoyal Industries, Inc. All rights reserved.)

Intravenous tubing has many uses on the sterile field. It can be used to provide a flexible connection between the incision and a syringe when drugs are injected into structures such as blood vessels or ducts within the surgical wound. Short tubing allows flexible handling of the syringe and a more precise directional flow of the contents. A two-way or three-way *stopcock* is used in conjunction with the syringe and tubing to open

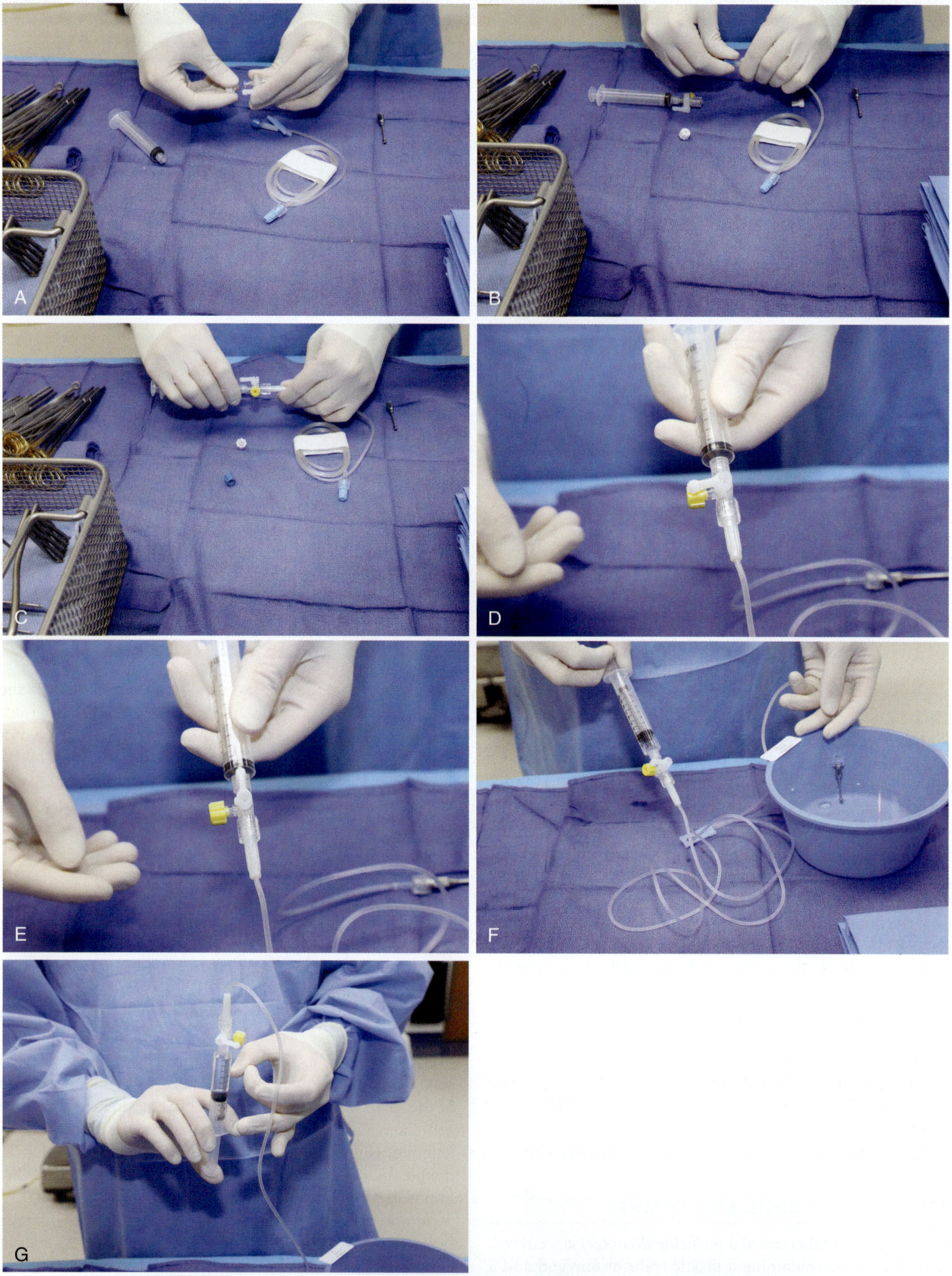

FIG. 12.7 Setting up a syringe, stopcock, and intravenous tubing. (A) Remove the caps from the stopcock. (B) Remove the tubing cap. (C) Fit the stopcock to the syringe and tubing, matching the fittings (Luer-Lok or catheter tip). (D) The closed position of the lever is at a right angle to the tubing. (E) To allow fluid to be drawn into the tubing and syringe, point the lever in the same direction as the tubing. (F) Here, a stainless steel irrigation tip has been placed on the end of the tubing, and the medication can now be drawn into the syringe. (G) Remove any bubbles from the syringe or tubing by flicking the syringe and then pushing the bubbles ahead of the fluid.

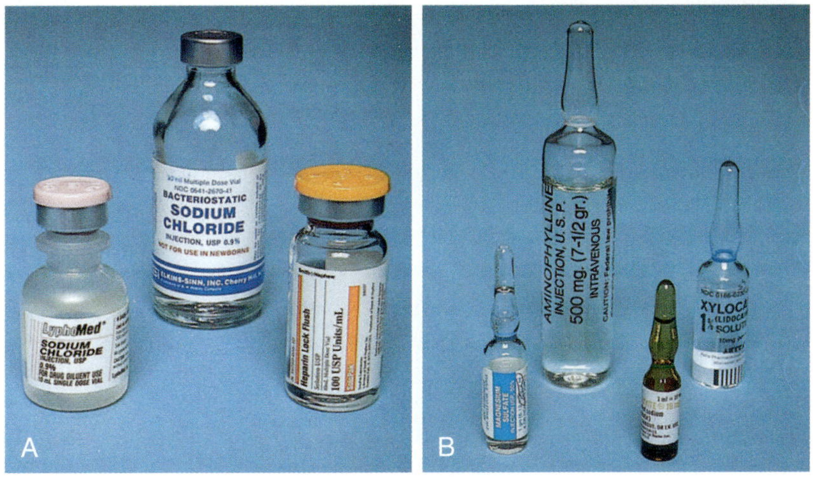

FIG. 12.8 (A) Glass vial. (B) Glass ampoule.

or close the flow of drug. A three-way stopcock also allows two syringes to be attached to one delivery tube for alternate injection of two drugs. Fig. 12.7 demonstrates how to set up a syringe, stopcock, and IV tubing assembly. Note the open and closed positions of the stopcock.

The anesthesia provider administers intravenous drugs to the patient through an *intravenous catheter*—also called an intravenous *cannula*. One or more cannulas are routinely inserted in the peripheral veins before the start of surgery to keep the veins open for routine or emergency drug administration.

The *infusion pump* is an electronic device that delivers a programmed amount of intravenous solution over a designated time period. The infusion pump is managed by the anesthesia provider or nurse circulator. The *intrathecal pump* is used to administer medication, including anesthetic, into the subarachnoid space along the spinal cord. Epidural anesthesia may be delivered through an intrathecal infusion pump.

When there is a need to keep a vein open for medium- or long-term intermittent therapy, a *central line* is placed. This is a narrow-gauge venous catheter that is inserted into one of the major veins of the upper body and sutured in place. A central line is rarely needed for surgery but often used for the treatment of chronically ill patients. See Chapter 30 for more details on central line equipment and procedures.

During surgery, drugs and pharmaceuticals are maintained on the sterile field in various kinds of sterile *medicine containers*. These may be plastic or stainless steel in sizes appropriate for dispensing.

IMPORTANT TO KNOW *Local anesthetics should be placed in plastic or glass containers, as metal ones may react with the drug. The container for any drug must be non-tipping and protected in a specific area of the instrument (back) table. Calibrated medicine cups and containers must never be used to measure a drug because the calibrations are too wide to be accurate.*

DRUG PACKAGING

Drugs are packaged in a variety of ways, with the following objectives:

- Protect the drug from microbial contamination
- Protection from environment-related chemical breakdown
- Prevent tampering
- Ease of dispensing
- Promote environmental *(green)* sustainability
- Economic considerations

Drugs and pharmaceutical substances are packaged in such a way that they can be distributed to the sterile field aseptically. Some packaging requires dispensing and mixing devices to deliver them to the sterile field aseptically.

The *glass vial* (Fig. 12.8) is a common system for packaging liquid drugs. This delivery system is available as single-dose or multiple-dose vials. However, standards agencies recommend using only single-dose vials because of the risk of disease transmission. Glass vials are packaged with a removable rubber stopper and aluminum cap or plastic "flip-off" disc to protect the sterility of the stopper. Glass vials present a problem for dispensing to the sterile field aseptically. The recommended practice is to use a transfer device (described above) whenever a liquid drug must be delivered to the sterile field. It is never acceptable to remove the aluminum cover and rubber stopper and pour the liquid directly into a sterile container, because there is no way to ensure the sterility of the lip of the vial (guidelines published by the Association of periOperative Registered Nurses [AORN], the Association for Professionals in Infection Control and Epidemiology [APIC], and the Institute for Safe Medication Practices [ISMP]). The nurse circulator may transfer a liquid from the vial into a container held by the scrub using a sterile syringe and needle. This method is acceptable as long as there is no spray-back, which could contaminate the liquid as it is injected into the sterile receptacle. An alternate method approved by the Association of Surgical Technologists (AST) is for the circulator to hold the vial while the scrub inserts the needle into the rubber stopper and draws up the liquid. This must be done carefully to avoid injury to the nurse's hand.

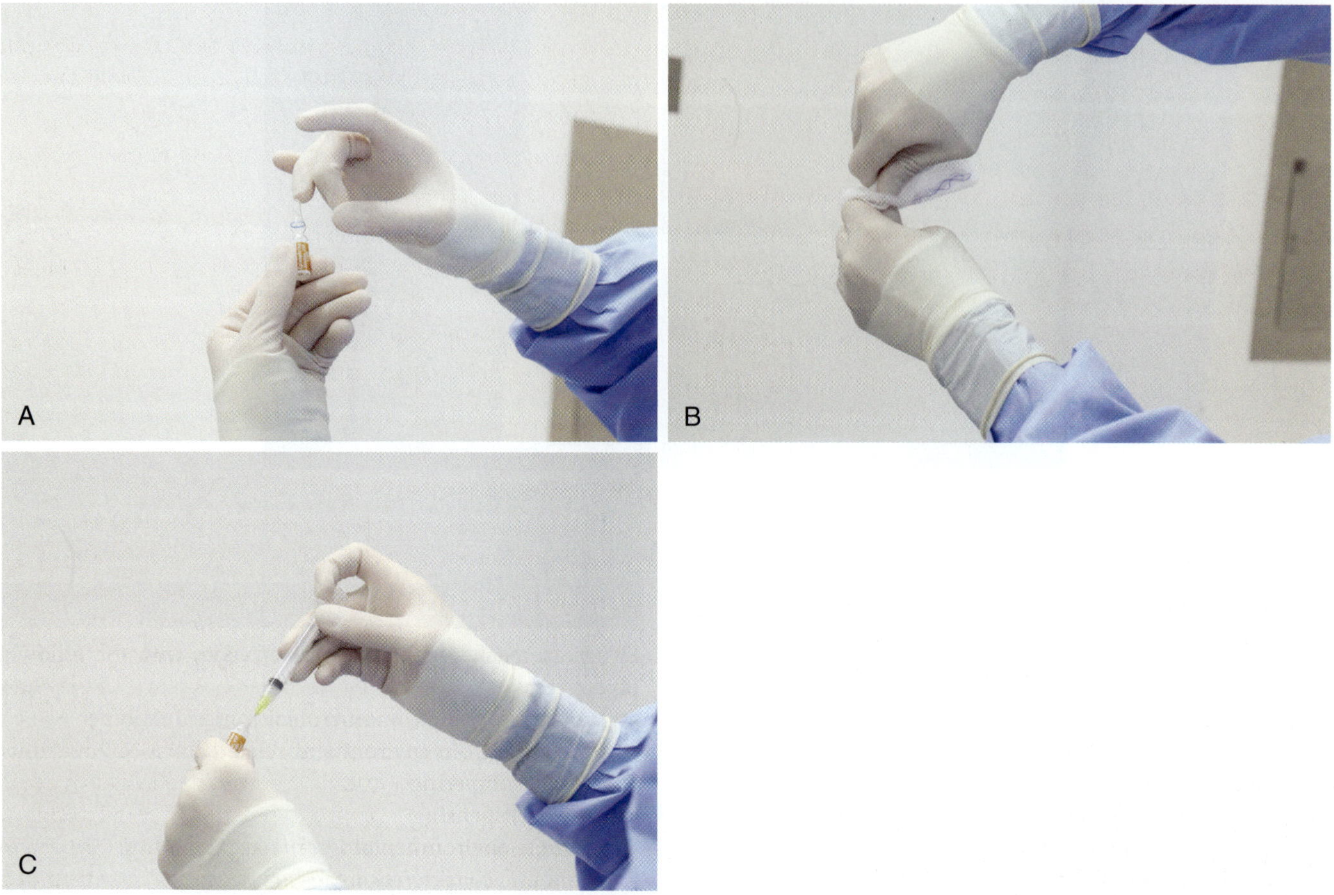

FIG. 12.9 Method for handling a glass ampoule. (A) Remove any air bubbles trapped in the neck of the vial by flicking it a few times. Do not shake the vial. (B) Grasp the top of the vial with a sponge and snap it off away from your face. (C) Use a filter needle to withdraw the contents from the vial.

The *glass ampoule* is a one-piece, hollow glass container with a narrow neck. The ampoule is often used for emergency drugs and others that are dispensed in small amounts or are unstable in other types of containers. A *sterile* ampoule can be distributed unopened to the sterile field. In this case, the scrub opens the vial using the following technique:

1. Note that the neck of the ampoule has a dark band at the narrowest part. This is where the top will separate from the vial during opening.
2. Using the sponge, grasp the top of the ampoule above the banded area and break the top off sharply away from you.
3. Deposit the top into a dry sharp's receptacle on the back table, being careful to contain any shards in the process.
4. Remove the sponge from the sterile field, alerting the circulator that it may contain shards of glass.

It is mandatory to use a *filter needle* to withdraw the fluid into a small syringe. After drawing up the drug, replace the filter device for a needle and inject the liquid into a medicine cup. Label the drug immediately. Never use a filter needle to inject a drug. The filter device is placed in a designated sharps area of the instrument table *separate* from other needles to prevent it from being reused. The empty vial can be placed in the same receptacle as other glass pieces. Do not discard the vial into the kick bucket or trash receptacle, where it could cause injury to others or become lost. Remember that all drug containers must be retained until the patient has been discharged to the recovery unit. Fig. 12.9 illustrates the technique for withdrawing a drug from a glass ampoule on the sterile field.

Prefilled cartridges are used to contain various dry and liquid tissue coagulants, glues, and cements. These cartridges are often capped at one end and contain a plunger at the other. The entire cartridge system is delivered to the sterile field as a single item. Some drugs and an activating ingredient are contained as a double-chambered cartridge leading to a single outlet, which allows simultaneous mixing and dispensing.

Pouches are common packaging for sterile devices and nonliquid pharmaceuticals. Many different products, including suture and some types of dry hemostatic agents, are packaged in this way. To dispense these substances, the circulator opens the pack by peeling back one or both sides of the outer wrap. The scrub then grasps the material and removes it from the pack. This technique is illustrated in Chapter 18.

The duplex container provides a method of mixing a dry drug component with a liquid diluent together without the need for any other device. A flexible pouch contains both components in a dual chamber. Bending the pouch releases the diluent into the dry component, and further manipulation of the pouch mixes the two drugs. The pouch can then be fitted with a dispensing device for immediate use. This type of system is often used for antibiotics, which have a dry powder and liquid diluent.

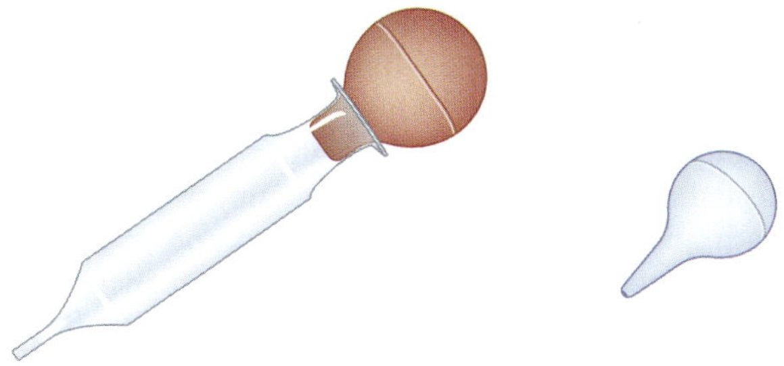

FIG. 12.10 The Asepto syringe and bulb syringe are commonly used for irrigation of the surgical wound.

Irrigation fluid is used during surgery to clear away blood and tissue debris in the surgical wound and to keep tissues moist. The irrigation used in body cavities and large surgical wounds is 0.9% sodium chloride. The most common general irrigation devices for this purpose are the *asepto, Toomey,* and *bulb* syringes (Fig. 12.10).

Irrigation solutions are maintained at body temperature to prevent hypothermia. This is especially important for pediatric, older, and very thin patients. Sterile saline for irrigation is kept at a controlled temperature in a solution warmer. Chilled solutions for cardiac, kidney, and transplant surgery are maintained as sterile ice slush.

Sterile irrigation fluids are delivered to scrub directly into a large stainless-steel basin. When irrigation fluids are poured, the flow is never interrupted. *The entire contents of the container must be delivered at one time.* The rationale for this is that the lip of the container cannot be guaranteed to be sterile once the container has been recapped.

SECTION II: THE MEDICATION PROCESS

In this section, the medication process is discussed, with particular attention to the scrub's role.

The entire process is defined by the following events:

1. A prescription or order is issued by an authorized prescriber such as the surgeon or anesthesia provider. The correct drug is identified and selected by the nurse circulator.
2. The nurse circulator prepares the drug as necessary off the sterile field (e.g., mixing or combining drug components). Mixing may also be performed by the scrub.
3. The scrub receives the drug from the nurse circulator and labels it.
4. The surgical technologist prepares the drug for use on the sterile field, including calculating the dose, measurement, mixing, and placing the drug in a transfer device.
5. The technologist dispenses the drug in its transfer device to the surgeon as required.
6. The surgeon administers the drug to the patient.
7. The anesthesia provider, nurse circulator, or surgeon assesses the effect of the drug on the patient.
8. The surgeon, anesthesia provider, and nurse circulator documents the drug process.

IMPORTANT TO KNOW *The anesthesia provider and circulator are responsible for documenting all drugs used during the surgical procedure in the patient's intraoperative chart.*

PRESCRIPTIONS AND DRUG ORDERS

In the first step of the drug process, a prescription is issued by a licensed health care provider.

The elements of an order are as follows:

- Patient's name
- Prescriber's name
- Date and time that the prescription was issued
- Name of the drug
- Strength of the drug
- Dose (amount)
- Route of administration
- Time or frequency of administration

In the clinical setting, the written prescription that the patient receives from the health care provider is replaced by a *drug order.* A drug order may be verbal, written, emailed, given over the phone, or faxed. Whatever the method used, the drug order must be communicated clearly and precisely. Hospital policy determines which health care professionals (by professional title) may receive and fulfill a drug order. The types of orders are the following:

- *Verbal order:* A verbal order contains the same information as a written order. The order may be given in person or by phone. It is provided by the licensed health care provider and directed to the person who will fill it.
- *Written order:* This can be in longhand, typed, or submitted electronically.
- *Standing order:* An order that remains in effect until the prescriber withdraws it. In the surgical context, standing orders are those included in the surgeon's preference cards, which are maintained electronically or written by hand for a particular surgical procedure. The elements of a drug order are the same as the prescription, except that the name of the patient may be omitted for standing orders, where it is understood that the surgical patient will receive the drug.
- *Stat order:* The drug is to be administered *immediately.*
- *PRN order:* The drug is to be given *as needed.*

SELECTION OF DRUGS

Once a drug order has been issued, the medication is selected from the operating room stock or obtained from the facility's pharmacy. This is a critical step in the medication process, because some drugs have "look alike" labels or "sound alike" names. The name, amount, strength, and expiration date of the drug are verified at this time. The package and contents are checked for any signs of leakage, damage, unusual particles, or discoloration. After this initial check, the drug is delivered to the patient care area, where it will be dispensed and administered. Errors can occur even when the drugs are stored in a computer-controlled system that is stocked and accessed through a code or scanning system. The drug could be stocked in error or the code mismatched to the drug; therefore health care staff must never assume that the correct drug has been delivered by the electronic system.

DRUG PREPARATION AND TRANSFER TO THE SURGICAL FIELD

Before passing a drug to the scrubbed surgical technologist, the nurse circulator must prepare the drug for the transfer. This may involve reconstitution of a powder with a liquid diluent or combining drugs as required by the order. The circulator must then select a delivery device for aseptic transfer to the sterile field.

IMPORTANT TO KNOW *Drugs should never be transferred to the sterile field without the participation of the scrub.*

To receive drugs from the circulating nurse, the scrub must assemble plastic and stainless medicine containers or bowls, drug labels, and a marking pen. He or she must also prepare dispensing devices suitable for the types and amounts of drugs to be received.

Drugs that are needed close to the start of surgery may be prepared during the surgical setup. Those that will be used later are prepared and dispensed to the field after the surgery is underway. This is done to ensure that drugs are prepared close to the time that they will be used.

The scrubbed surgical technologist is responsible for all drugs transferred to the sterile field. He or she must know the generic name of the drug, its effect, the dose limit of each drug, the strength or concentration of the drug, and how much has been used as the surgical case progresses. As an intermediary in the drug-dispensing process, the surgical technologist shares responsibility for drug errors, whether or not there is injury to the patient.

IMPORTANT TO KNOW *Empty drug containers, vials, and cartons are held in the operating room until the patient has recovered. These may be needed for verification in the event of an actual or near-miss drug error.*

Guidelines • Drug Transfer

Specific guidelines for drug transfer have been developed to reduce errors and patient injury.

1. Immediately before receiving a drug, the scrub selects an appropriate size and type of sterile container for the drug. These will have been provided in the sterile setup.
   Rationale: The scrub must not be distracted while receiving drugs on the sterile field. He or she must be ready. Both the nurse and scrub must participate in the transfer process.
2. The nurse shows the drug in its original container to the scrub. Both the nurse and scrub scan the drug for alterations such as discoloration, leakage, unusual sediment, or other impurities. If there is any doubt about the safety of the drug, it must be returned to the facility's pharmacy.
   Rationale: A drug that shows signs of deterioration or contamination must not be transferred to the sterile field, as this may result in patient injury.
3. The circulator holds the drug container so that the scrub can read the label. The nurse reads the name of the drug, the strength, amount, route of administration, and expiry date. The scrub acknowledges the information concurrently with the circulator. Both verbal and visual verification is necessary for both scrub and circulator.
   Rationale: All drugs transferred to the sterile field pose a risk because they are no longer in their original containers. Reading out loud confirms the name of the drug and other critical parameters.
4. The circulator dispenses the drug into a sterile container held by the scrub, using sterile technique and a sterile transfer device (Fig. 12.11). The circulator again shows the drug container to the scrub, and both acknowledge the information a second time.
   Rationale: Drug transfer must be carried out under sterile conditions. Both scrub and circulator re-enforce the drug information to avoid error.
5. The circulator or anesthesia provider confirms the maximum dose limit of the drug.
   Rationale: All members of the team must know the dose limit of the drug to avoid error.
6. The scrub immediately labels the medicine container and any transfer devices used to contain or administer the drug on the sterile field.
   Rationale: Drugs transferred to new containers on the sterile field must be clearly labeled (see description below) to prevent administering the wrong drug.

PREPARING DRUGS ON THE STERILE FIELD

Management of drugs and other pharmaceutical materials on the surgical field requires labeling, organization, and care of the materials and measuring, mixing, and transferring the drug to the surgeon. These roles should be carried out systematically to prevent drug error. Concentration on the task at hand is an important part of the role.

LABELING

Removal of a drug from its commercial container and transfer to an unlabeled container makes the drug unidentifiable. Despite many warnings and methods to encourage surgical personnel to label drugs, unlabeled drugs and incorrect labeling are still the primary causes of patient harm and death. To reduce drug error, every drug container on the sterile field and its delivery device must be labeled as shown in Fig. 12.12. Labels are made as soon as a drug is received, never in advance of receiving the drug. This is to eliminate the possibility of drug error during dispensing. Commercially prepared labels are available for most drugs used on the sterile field, and this is the preferred method of labeling. Other information required can then be added when the drug is received. All drugs and their delivery devices are labeled, *even if there is only one.* The minimum information needed on a label is as follows:

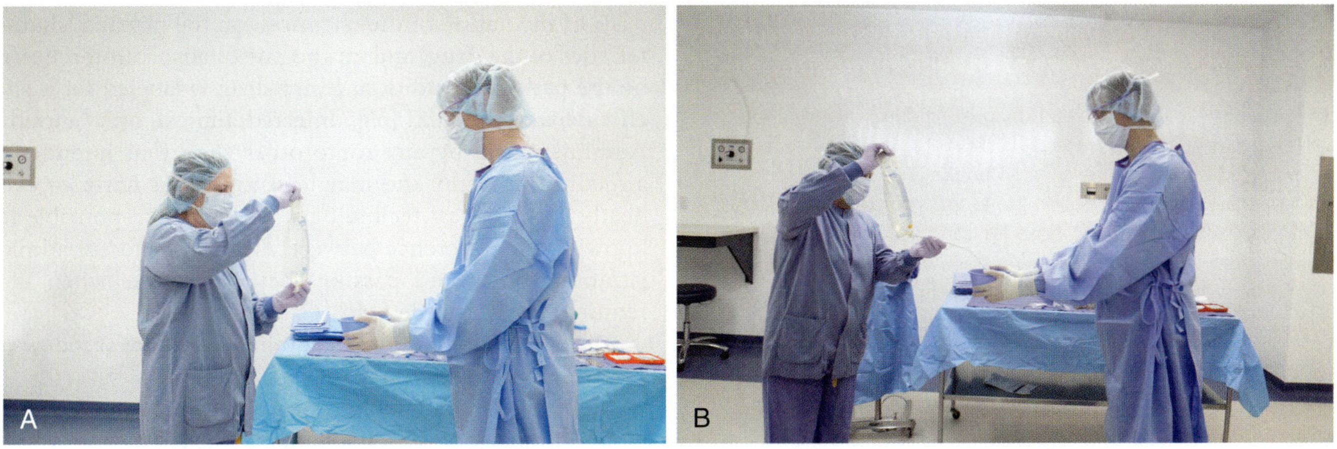

FIG. 12.11 Protocol for receiving drugs on the sterile field; drug delivery to the field. (A) The circulator shows the drug to the scrub for verification. (B) The circulator distributes the drug into a sterile container using a fluid decanter. After distribution, the circulator again shows the label to the scrub.

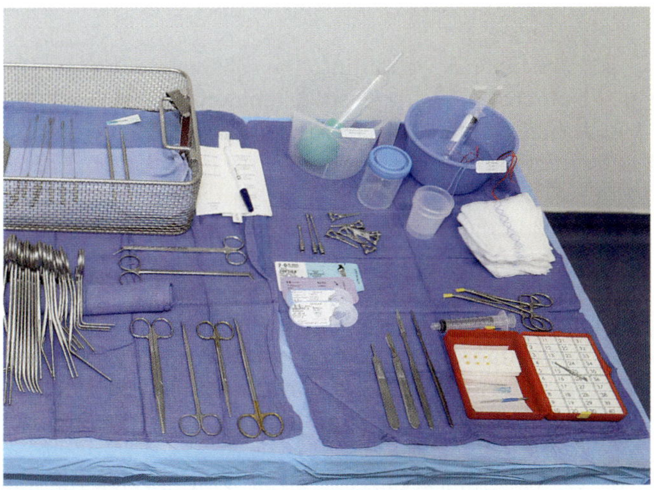

FIG. 12.12 Drugs are labeled immediately after they are received. Note that transfer devices must also be labeled to prevent them from being used with more than one drug.

1. Medication name
2. Strength of the drug
3. Concentration of the drug

Some facilities also require the total amount of drug received in each container and the date and time received.

Labels must be printed using a sharp waterproof marker. Write legibly, and follow The Joint Commission's ruling on "do not use" abbreviations (see Chapter 3). If any doubt exists about the identification of a drug, *the drug must be discarded,* and a fresh drug distributed to the sterile field. Whenever there is a change of scrub personnel during a case, both people must verify the identity of each drug.

Following distribution to the sterile field and labeling, the scrub places the drugs in an area of the back table (see Fig. 12.12). Each drug should have its own labeled delivery device. When there are two formulations of the same drug, do not place them next to each other, where one may be accidentally mistaken for the other. Use two different types of containers for these drugs to further separate them.

MEASURING AND MIXING DRUGS ON THE STERILE FIELD

It is helpful to clear away a space on the back table to provide easy access to devices needed for mixing drugs and preparing drugs for transfer to the surgeon. Non-reactive plastic cups should be used for small amounts of medication received, especially local anesthetic, which may undergo a chemical reaction in contact with metal.

Combination drugs are measured by drawing up the components separately and putting them in a *dry* basin or medicine cup of appropriate size. A new delivery device must be prepared for the combination drug, whose properties are not the same as its individual components. Drug components less than 1 mL must be measured using a *tuberculin syringe* to achieve accuracy. The newly mixed drug must be labeled as soon as it is mixed. Calculations must be performed accurately and checked before releasing the drug to the surgeon. If necessary, the scrub may ask another person on the team to validate the calculation, and this may be a requirement in some facilities.

IMPORTANT TO KNOW *Do not use an insulin syringe to measure drugs other than insulin. When preparing liquid drugs for injection, exclude air from the delivery device. This is very important for precise measurement and to prevent the release of air bubbles in the vascular system and tissue ducts. Box 12.4 provides methods to prevent the introduction of air into a syringe or other delivery device.*

TRANSFERRING A DRUG TO THE SURGEON

Drugs are passed to the surgeon when requested or when their need is anticipated by the scrub. When passing the drug, the concentration and amount must be verbally stated by the scrub and acknowledged by the surgeon. This is particularly important for high-alert drugs but should be carried out each time a drug is passed. This not only

BOX 12.4 Tips for Preventing the Introduction of Air Into a Syringe or Other Delivery Device

- It is much easier to prevent air from entering a device than to remove it once it is there.
- Before drawing up the solution, make sure that the tip (catheter, needle, irrigation tip) of the syringe is attached tightly to the syringe. A loose tip can allow air to be aspirated into the device.
- Ensure that the tip attachment of the delivery device (catheter tip, needle, transfer device) is inserted into the liquid and remains in the liquid while withdrawing the drug. Remember to withdraw the needle slightly as the level decreases to prevent air from entering the syringe.
- When mixing dry and liquid drugs in a vial, do not shake the vial. This creates foam. Instead, hold the vial between your palms and gently roll it back and forth.
- When mixing a dry component with a water-based diluent, do not use force to inject the diluent into the dry component. Instead, inject the fluid slowly.
- To remove air from a delivery device before using: Gravity allows the air to float to the top of the fluid. Gently eject the air. If this does not work, gently tap or flick the tubing or syringe tip. It is very difficult to remove air from small-bore tubing or a syringe. It may be necessary to remove the needle or syringe tip to break the surface tension and release air.
- Be aware that when air is removed, a small amount of drug may be accidentally ejected. This may require recalculation of the total amount required.

provides a safety check but also informs the anesthesiologist and circulating nurse that a drug is being administered for assessment and documentation purposes. Note that the maximum safe dose of a drug is determined by the patient's individual condition, and also by weight. The surgical technologist should validate the maximum dosage with the anesthesia provider and nurse circulator before surgery.

Liquid drugs are passed to the surgeon in a syringe with or without connection tubing. The size of the syringe depends on the amount to be administered. As a general rule, the syringe size will be included in the surgeon's preference card. Many liquid drugs used in eye, ear, and other types of microsurgery are manufactured to accept a small irrigation tip at the top of the bottle. These tips are included in the instrument setup for that specialty.

Solid pharmaceutical products such as hemostatic materials are prepared according to their application on specific tissue.

DRUG ADMINISTRATION

Drug administration is the introduction of a drug into the patient. There are many different methods and routes used for drug administration. The route of administration is indicated on the drug label. It is important to remember that drugs are administered through a specific route on the basis of the nature of the chemical, on the physical characteristics of the drug, and on the rate of absorption required by the patient's condition. Every drug is labeled for a specific delivery method (e.g., injected, topical, or by mouth). Administration by any route other than that intended is a medication error and may lead to serious harm or even death. The surgical technologist is directly responsible for knowing the difference between drugs of different administration routes and passing the correct one when it is required on the sterile field.

The usual clinical routes of administration are as follows:

1. **Parenteral:** By injection
   a. Intravenous (IV): Injection directly into a vein
   b. **Intraosseous** (IO): Injection into the bone marrow; used when an intravenous line cannot be initiated or maintained
   c. Intramuscular (IM): Injection into a muscle
   d. Subcutaneous: Injection into the connective tissue directly beneath the skin
   e. Intradermal (ID): Injection between the dermis and epidermis
   f. Intraspinal: Injection into the subarachnoid space **(intrathecal)** or epidural space (epidural injection)
   g. Intraperitoneal: Injected into the peritoneal cavity
2. Oral (enteral): By mouth (PO, *per os*)
   a. Ingestion: Swallowed
   b. Buccal: Tablet placed between the gum and mucous membrane of the cheek
   c. Sublingual: Tablet placed under the tongue
3. **Topical:** On surface tissue
   a. Instillation: Administration of drops into the eye or ear
   b. **Transdermal:** Drug is absorbed through a skin patch
   c. Rectal: Topical effect or systemic absorption through the rectal mucosa
   d. Vaginal: Topical effect or absorption through the mucous membrane
   e. Nasal: On nasal mucosa
   f. Inhalant: Drug is inhaled as an aerosol and absorbed through the bronchial tree and lungs

ASSESSMENT

After the administration of a drug, the patient is assessed for physiological changes, including adverse reactions. In all clinical situations, assessment is made by the medical or nursing staff, who can quickly respond to the medical needs of the patient in the event of emergency.

Adverse Reaction to a Drug

Whenever a drug is administered, physiological changes take place in the body. Some of these are therapeutic (desirable) effects, whereas others may be undesirable or potentially harmful. Precautions against taking a drug under circumstances known to be harmful are stated as **contraindications.** An **adverse reaction** is an undesirable or intolerable reaction to a drug administered at the *normal dosage*. Adverse reactions are *unexpected*, although they may be predictable in certain individuals. When a drug is

BOX 12.5 Allergic Reactions

- *Type I*: Characterized by tissue inflammation caused by the release of histamine in the body. This causes increased permeability of blood vessels and constriction of bronchioles, leading to difficulty breathing. The most extreme form of sensitivity is anaphylactic shock, which can lead to death.
- *Type II*: Called a *cytotoxic reaction*, the results of interaction between two antibodies and cell surface antigens. Results in the activation of powerful immune defense mechanisms, causing injury or death. Mismatched blood transfusion reactions and hemolytic disease in newborns are type II reactions.
- *Type III*: Caused by antigen–antibody complexes, which cause tissue damage when they trigger immune response. Allergy to antibiotics is an example of a type III response. Symptoms include itching, rash, severe tissue swelling, and fever. This type of reaction usually resolves in several days.
- *Type IV*: Cell-mediated reactions (not related to antibodies) that occur 24–72 hours after exposure to the agent. An example of this type of delayed hypersensitivity is a positive reaction to the tuberculin skin test, in which a small amount of killed *Mycobacterium tuberculosis* is injected.

tested before its release, adverse reactions are documented, and this becomes part of the drug information available to clinicians and patients. Examples of mild adverse effects include nausea and dizziness. This type of effect is usually transient and ceases when the drug is stopped. More serious adverse reactions may include difficulty breathing or increased heart rate.

Medical and nursing personnel are trained to recognize the clinical signs and symptoms of an adverse drug event. Allied health personnel such as surgical technologists have two important roles in this process:

1. Keen observation of a patient's normal behavior and appearance
2. Immediately reporting to medical or nursing personnel any signs and symptoms that seem abnormal

When reporting a suspected drug reaction, follow these guidelines:

- What sign or signs do you observe that you believe are not normal for that patient?
- When did it start?
- What does the patient report (if applicable)?
- What comfort measures did you initiate (e.g., providing warmth or reassurance)?

Drug Allergy

True **allergy** to a drug is mediated by the immune system and requires previous exposure to substances in the drug or a genetic predisposition to allergy. An immune response that causes irritation, respiratory failure, or death is called **hypersensitivity.** Hypersensitivity can be mild, producing only a rash or wheezing, or it can be severe, resulting in respiratory failure and death caused by anaphylactic shock.

Allergic reactions are characterized as immediate or delayed. Delayed sensitivity can occur up to 12 hours after exposure to a drug and is mediated by T lymphocytes. Immediate reactions are mediated by antibodies. All allergic reactions are divided into the categories shown in Box 12.5.

DOCUMENTATION

Documentation is required after administration of any drug or pharmaceutical (including implants). Documentation may be included in the patient's electronic chart, written surgical report, or anesthesia record, depending on the situation. All elements of the drug administration must be included:

- The name of the drug
- Dose (strength)
- Amount
- The route (e.g., intravenous or intraperitoneal) and location in the body
- Time of administration
- Name of the person who administered the drug
- Results of the patient assessment following administration

SECTION III: PREVENTING DRUG ERRORS

A drug error is a mistake made at *any stage* in the medication process. In general, the medication process involves many different steps and involves multiple health care workers. Medication errors are often attributed to fatigue, stress, and distraction in the workplace—all prevalent in the surgical environment. Some of the more common errors made in surgery are negligence in labeling drugs or inability to read the label, incorrect knowledge about the drug, misidentification, and passing the wrong drug to the surgeon. Some of these errors have resulted in death or severe injury to patients.

The problem of medication errors is so serious that recent changes have been made in standards and guidelines to try to reduce the number and severity of drug errors in all areas of care.

IMPORTANT TO KNOW *Increased pressure for surgical technologists to become involved in the medication process now places them in a position of individual responsibility and accountability for patient outcomes, including drug errors that occur during surgery.*

NOTE *Surgical technologists have a responsibility to become familiar with drug alert information provided by the ISMP. This can be obtained through the ISMP website and email alerts.*

The ISMP, in coordination with The Joint Commission's National Patient Safety Goals, has published a list of 10 elements that have the most influence on drug errors:

1. Patient information: including age, weight, height, allergies, and lab results that can affect routes of administration and dosage.
2. Drug information: lack of knowledge about the drug, its action, its intended use, appropriate dosage individualized according to the patient, and drug interactions.
3. Communication of drug information: A common cause of drug errors. Communication "barriers" must be eliminated for communication to flow.

4. Drug packaging, labeling, and nomenclature: Including look-alike and sound-alike drugs, confusing labels (including those made by the scrub during surgery), and indistinct packaging.
5. Drug stock, storage, standardization, and distribution: Standardizing these systems reduces the risk of errors.
6. Environmental factors: Including poor lighting (e.g., when operating room lights are dimmed during endoscopic or minimally invasive surgery), loud conversation, music, and other distracting environmental conditions that prevent concentration.
7. Drug device acquisition, use, and monitoring: Including any devices used for drug delivery. These must be proven safe and monitored in the clinical area to prevent device errors.
8. Staff competency and education: All staff must focus on new medications being used at their health care facility; high-alert medications; and protocols, policies, and procedures related to medication use.
9. Patient education on medications: Remains the responsibility of the licensed primary health care provider.
10. Quality processes and risk management: Focuses the attention on improving practice as a means of attaining a greater reduction in drug errors.

DRUG RIGHTS

One method that has proven successful in reducing drug errors is the drug "rights." This is a verification tool that is used to guide health care workers in the medication process. It is important to note that this method is only partially effective, because it does not account for errors outside of the administration process when the drug is given to the patient. The seven rights have evolved from an original five. Recently added was "the right indication," because a number of serious incidents have involved health care personnel not knowing what a drug's actions were and why it was being given. "The right documentation" was also added recently to remind all health care workers that they must communicate detailed information about drugs they administer so that the next person in the care team has a complete picture of the patient's condition. Deaths in this area have occurred when improper or inadequate documentation was performed during surgery, and the next health care worker in the chain of care gave similar or the same drugs, resulting in overdose.

THE SEVEN RIGHTS

1. *The right drug* is the one that has been ordered by the surgeon or other health care provider. This means that the correct drug must be selected from the operating room or pharmacy stock. Verbal orders are repeated back to the surgeon to verify accuracy. The scrub receives drugs from the circulator at the start of surgery or during the procedure. During this exchange, the drug is verified again. After receiving the drug on the sterile field, the scrub labels the drug and then again selects the correct one when it is requested by the surgeon. Many drug errors made in surgery occur at this point and are related to a lack of labeling or poor labeling.
2. *The right patient* means that the surgical patient is identified on entering the surgical holding area and again when the individual is brought into the surgical suite. Before surgery begins, patient identification is again verified during the TIMEOUT (see Chapter 18).
3. *The right dose* means the correct **dose** (amount and strength of drug) is administered for that particular patient. Throughout the medication process, the dose is checked by each person handling the drug. Verifying the correct dose and strength before the drug is administered to the patient is one of the most important responsibilities of the surgical team. The surgical technologist must also keep track of the amount of drug given throughout the surgical procedure.
4. *The right route* is the one intended for that drug and is labeled accordingly (e.g., "for topical use only" or "not for use in the eyes"). A drug may not be administered by any route other than the one approved and labeled. Some drugs are formulated for different routes but have the same name. The route must be verified by the label.
5. *The right time* refers to a schedule of administration according to the prescription or order.
6. *The right indication* of a drug is the condition for which the drug is intended. This right has been added by patient safety advocate organizations in recent years because of numerous drug errors committed when the person administering the drug lacked the appropriate knowledge about indications, resulting in injury or death of the patient. The Joint Commission and other standards organizations recognize that patients are cared for by teams of individuals who are jointly responsible for patient safety. In the case of drug administration, drugs are contraindicated (must not be administered) under specific conditions.
7. *The right documentation* means that drug administration must be documented in the patient chart. Drugs used by the anesthesia provider are documented in the anesthesia record, whereas those used in or on the operative site are documented in the surgical report (see details of documentation, later). All documentation must identify the name of the drug, the strength, who administered the drug, the time, and the route and include a report of patient assessment after administration.

"DO NOT USE" ABBREVIATIONS

The Joint Commission has developed a list of abbreviations that can lead to drug errors. The "do not use" abbreviations are shown in Table 12.6. Health care facilities are also advised to make additions to their own "do not use" list. This list applies to any documentation, including prescriptions, patient charts, and order transcriptions.

LOOK-ALIKE, SOUND-ALIKE DRUGS

A significant number of adverse drug events have been caused by drugs whose names look or sound alike. The ISMP has

TABLE 12.6 The Joint Commission's "Do Not Use" Symbols in Documentation*

Do Not Use	Potential Problem	Use Instead
U (unit)	Mistaken for "0" (zero), the number "4" (four) or "mL"	Write "unit"
IU (International unit)	Mistaken for IV (intravenous) or the number 10 (ten)	Write "International unit"
Q.D., QD, q.d., qd (daily) Q.E.D., QOD, q.o.d., qod (every other day)	Mistaken for each other	Write "daily" Write "every other day"
Trailing zero (X.0 mg)† Lack of leading zero (.X mg)	Decimal point is missed	Write "X mg" Write "0.X mg"
MS MSO_4 and $MgSO_4$	Can mean morphine sulfate or magnesium sulfate Confused for one another	Write "morphine sulfate" Write "magnesium sulfate"

*Applies to all orders and all medication-related documentation that are handwritten (including free-text computer entry) or on preprinted forms.
†Exception: A "trailing zero" may be used only where required to demonstrate the level of precision of the value being reported, such as for laboratory results, imaging studies that report the size of lesions, or catheter/tube sizes. It may not be used in medication orders or other medication-related documentation.

BOX 12.6 High-Alert Medications

Epinephrine, subcutaneous
Epoprostenol (Flolan), IV
Insulin U-500
Magnesium sulfate injection
Methotrexate, oral, non-oncological use
Opium tincture
Oxytocin, IV
Nitroprusside sodium for injection
Potassium chloride for injection concentrate
Potassium phosphates injection
Promethazine, IV
Vasopressin, IV or intraosseous

From Institute for Safe Medication Practices. *http://www.ismp.org/*. Refer to Publications and Alerts.

published a list of more than 100 of these drugs on their website at http://www.ismp.org. It is best to visit the site frequently to remain up to date on surgical drugs recently released by the FDA. Each health care facility is also required to produce its own look-alike, sound-alike list of drugs used in that particular organization.

HIGH-ALERT DRUGS

High-alert drugs are those that have been implicated in an extraordinarily high number of errors—many of them with *fatal consequences*, as reported to the National Medication Errors Reporting Program. The drugs on this list are those that are frequently cited in drug errors and are those that carry a great risk of adverse consequences when errors are made. High-alert drugs in the perioperative area include the different formulations of heparin, thrombin, epinephrine, and local anesthetics. Box 12.6 lists high-alert drugs.

SECTION IV: SURGICAL DRUGS

In the United States, drugs are classified through the AHFS. This is a tiered system based on the therapeutic action of the drug and is used throughout the health care system.

Drug categories and their subcategories are assigned a code number that can be researched easily. The first-tier categories are shown in Box 12.7; these are the major classifications of drugs. These can also be found on the AHFS website, along with other useful information about drugs and medical devices (http://www.ahfsdruginformation.com/pt-classification-system.aspx).

The surgical technologist is required to handle and deliver a number of different categories of drugs. Naturally, these categories are only a fraction of all drugs. In practical terms, the surgical technologist should give priority to learning these particular drug categories and agents and those that are encountered in the surgical facility where they work or study.

The following section discusses drug categories, their agents used in surgery, and their method of action. Other drugs are discussed in the section to follow.

LOCAL ANESTHETICS

Local anesthetics are used in regional anesthesia to block sensation with or without sedative drugs that relieve anxiety and induce relaxation. These drugs are formulated for a variety of applications, including the following:

- *Infiltration injection:* The drug is injected directly into the operative site in small increments.
- *Regional nerve block:* A major nerve is anesthetized to affect a larger region.
- *Topical:* Anesthetic is applied to the skin or mucous membrane for short-term superficial procedures.
- *Spinal or epidural:* Anesthetic is injected into the spinal canal or epidural space for regional blockade of the lower body.

Some local anesthetics are formulated with epinephrine. As an adrenergic agonist, epinephrine causes vasoconstriction and increased heart rate. It is used in conjunction with local anesthetic to prevent the anesthetic from entering the vascular system, which would shorten the peak effect of the drug.

IMPORTANT TO KNOW *Epinephrine injection directly into blood vessels can be fatal. Therefore extra attention must be*

BOX 12.7 First-Tier Drug Categories

No.	Drug Category
4:00	Antihistamine Drugs
8:00	Antiinfective Agents
10:00	Antineoplastic Agents
12:00	Autonomic Drugs
16:00	Blood Derivatives
20:00	Blood Formation, Coagulation, and Thrombosis Agents
24:00	Cardiovascular Drugs
26:00	Cellular Therapy
28:00	Central Nervous System Agents
32:00	Contraceptives (foams, devices)
34:00	Dental Agents
36:00	Diagnostic Agents
38:00	Disinfectants (for agents used on objects other than skin)
40:00	Electrolytic, Caloric, and Water Balance
44:00	Enzymes
48:00	Respiratory Tract Agents
52:00	Eye, Ear, Nose, and Throat (EENT) Preparations
56:00	Gastrointestinal Drugs
60:00	Gold Compounds
64:00	Heavy Metal Antagonists
68:00	Hormones and Synthetic Substitutes
72:00	Local Anesthetics
76:00	Oxytocics
78:00	Radioactive Agents
80:00	Serums, Toxoids, and Vaccines
84:00	Skin and Mucous Membrane Agents
86:00	Smooth Muscle Relaxants
88:00	Vitamins
92:00	Miscellaneous Therapeutic Agents
94:00	Devices
96:00	Pharmaceutical Aids

given to labeling and keeping track of the amount injected throughout the procedure.

When the scrub dispenses local anesthetic to the surgeon, he or she shares responsibility for ensuring that the maximum dosage is not exceeded. The maximum dosage is therefore confirmed with the anesthesia provider before the case, and incremental amounts injected are documented in real time by the circulator.

Local anesthetic agents are formulated as short or long acting, with or without added epinephrine or other vasoconstrictors. The safe maximum dosage for agents depends on the patient's specific condition and its exact use.

Topical anesthetics are used on surface tissues such as mucous membranes, the surface of the eye, and the urogenital tract. These agents do require an order by a licensed primary care provider. This includes instillation of lidocaine gel to the urethra before catheterization. Topical cocaine is frequently used in nasal surgery to block pain receptors in the mucous membrane before injection with regional anesthetic. Cocaine is never injected—to do so can be fatal. It is a controlled substance, and protocols for handling it are guided by hospital policy and state law. Table 12.7 lists common local anesthetics.

BLOOD AND BLOOD DERIVATIVES

Blood and blood derivatives (also called *blood products*) are used in the treatment of blood loss or for specific blood disorders that result in the loss or destruction of a blood component. Whole blood replacement may be used if a significant amount of blood has been lost because of trauma or disease. It is normally used only when the patient's blood loss exceeds 30% of their total blood volume (approximately 1500 mL in an adult).

Whole blood and blood products are packed in collapsible bags that are labeled to include the type, amount, and number. When blood and blood products are used, an exact protocol must be followed. Cross-checking of products that are ABO-Rh specific is performed by two people (medical or nursing staff) before administration. Blood products must be stored at temperatures between 33.8°F and 42.8°F (1°C and 6°C). External temperature tape may be used to monitor the temperature of individual units. Units must be used within 30 minutes. Unused blood and blood products are returned to the blood bank.

TYPES OF BLOOD PRODUCTS

- *Whole blood* contains serum and blood cells, plus anticoagulant and preservative. Whole blood is not commonly given because it can be broken down into components that can be administered separately. This prevents waste of blood products that are not needed.
- *Red blood cells* (RBCs) are stored in units; one unit of RBCs contains 150 to 210 mL of red cells plus a small amount of plasma and preservative. Packed red blood cells (PRBCs) are administered to increase the oxygen-carrying capacity of the blood. A combination of PRBCs and plasma expanders is effective in increasing the total intravascular volume and oxygen-carrying capacity. All cell transfusions must be ABO-Rh compatible with the recipient. Packed cells are handled and monitored in the same way as whole blood.
- *Washed red blood cells* are normal RBCs that have been washed to remove the plasma and are administered to patients who demonstrate repeated hypersensitivity to blood or blood components.
- *Leukoreduced red blood cells* contain leukocytes in reduced volume within RBCs. Leukoreduced RBCs are used in patients with a history of nonhemolytic febrile transfusion reactions.

TABLE 12.7 Local Anesthetics for Infiltration

		PLAIN SOLUTION		EPINEPHRINE ADDED	
Drug	**Conc %**	**MAX. DOSE (MG)**	**Duration (min)**	**MAX. DOSE (MG)**	**Duration (min)**
SHORT DURATION					
Procaine	1–2	500	20–30	600	30–45
Chloroprocaine	1–2	800	15–30	1000	30
MODERATE DURATION					
Lidocaine	0.5–1	300	30–60	500	120
Mepivacaine	0.5–1	300	45–90	500	120
Prilocaine	0.5–1	350	30–90	550	120
LONG DURATION					
Bupivacaine	0.25–0.5	175	120–240	200	180–240
Ropivacaine	0.2–0.5	200	120–240	250	180–240

From Miller RD, et al. *Miller's Anesthesia*. 8th ed. Philadelphia: Saunders; 2015.

- *Platelets* are essential for blood coagulation and contain coagulation factors, RBCs, and white blood cells. Platelets are administered to patients with bleeding disorders such as thrombocytopenia and platelet dysfunction.
- *Granulocytes (neutrophils)* are obtained from an ABO-Rh-compatible donor and are used in the treatment of severe neutropenia.
- *Fresh-frozen plasma* is extracted from whole blood and contains normal amounts of coagulation factors. This blood product is used in patients who have coagulation disorders and active bleeding and require invasive procedures.
- *Cryoprecipitate* is a concentration of several hemostatic proteins that have been prepared from whole blood. The hemostatic proteins contained in cryoprecipitate are factor VIII, von Willebrand factor, factor XIII, and fibrinogen. Cryoprecipitate is used in patients with significantly decreased fibrinogen who are actively bleeding or require invasive procedures. Cryoprecipitate is also used in the preparation of fibrin glue, orthopedic procedures, and ear, nose, and throat and neurosurgical procedures.
- *Factor concentrates* contain factor VIII, IS, and antithrombin III. This product is used in patients with hemophilia who require invasive procedures.

HEMOSTATIC AGENTS

Management of bleeding is one of the most important goals in surgery. Pharmaceutical agents are used, along with conventional means of hemorrhage control (e.g., suture ligature or electrocoagulation). To understand the mechanism of drugs used to control bleeding, it is important to study coagulation as it occurs in the body.

PHYSIOLOGY OF COAGULATION

The natural (physiological) coagulation process takes place through a series, or *cascade*, of complex events, each triggered by the one preceding it. The *extrinsic* mechanism begins when a blood vessel is injured. The subsequent events are as follows:

1. *Vasospasm:* The blood vessel retracts and constricts. This reduces blood flow through the vessel.
2. *A platelet plug forms:* Platelets aggregate in the area and form a plug. The presence of platelets initiates the release of coagulation factors in the plasma.
3. *Coagulation begins:* A meshwork of fibrin strands forms around the blood platelets, creating a clot. This process is initiated by coagulation *factors* (organic substances present in the blood). Coagulation is activated by two pathways, the *extrinsic pathway* and the *intrinsic pathway.* The intrinsic pathway is activated by factors present in the blood. The extrinsic pathway occurs in the tissues.

Coagulation involves many chemicals that interact in an elaborate feedback mechanism. If any of the factors are missing, through genetic anomaly or disease, hemostasis is altered. Severe hemorrhage may overwhelm the body's natural mechanisms for controlling bleeding, leading to shock and eventual death if the bleeding cannot be controlled.

Many different types of hemostatic agents have been developed in the past decade for use on bleeding surfaces during surgery. These include purified animal and human derivatives and newer synthetic agents. Tissue sealants are a newer category of agents that are used as a coating over raw tissue surfaces to prevent capillary bleeding and in lung tissue to prevent air leakage. There are now several categories of topical agents available with which the surgical technologist should become familiar (refer to Table 12.8 for a complete list of hemostatic agents and tissue sealants). These are the following:

- Active hemostats
- Flowables
- Fibrin sealants

ACTIVE HEMOSTATS

An active hemostat stimulates the body's own coagulation process that converts fibrin to fibrinogen. These agents include topical (human) thrombin, bovine thrombin, and recombinant thrombin. *Topical thrombin USP* is commercially prepared as a dry powder or solution derived from bovine or human sources

TABLE 12.8 Tissue Sealants and Hemostatics

	Dosage Form	Use	Components	Qualities
THROMBIN/FIBRINOGEN USP				
Topical Thrombin USP (Thrombin, Evithrom, Recothrom)	Solution or dry requiring saline diluent	Active hemostasis for topical use on bleeding tissues	Bovine or human origin thrombin	May cause severe coagulation disorder related to development of antibodies
Evicel	Solution	Active hemostasis	Fibrinogen concentrate and thrombin derived from pooled human plasma	Effective as spray or drip application
GELATIN HEMOSTATICS				
Gelfoam Surgifoam	Dry sponge sheets, powder	Mechanical hemostasis on tissue surface or vascular anastomosis	Gelatin sponge used with thrombin solution or saline	Can be soaked in thrombin; partially resorbable but usually removed to prevent granuloma
COLLAGEN HEMOSTATICS				
Avitene EndoAvitene Instat MCH	Dry powder	Mechanical hemostasis	Collagen powder hemostat	Used in dry form
OXIDIZED CELLULOSE HEMOSTATICS				
Surgicel	Gauze fiber tuft or sponge	Mechanical hemostasis	Cellulose	Swells on contact with fluid Absorbs in 1–6 weeks
FIBRIN COMBINATION SEALANTS				
Tisseel	Gel	Capillary hemostasis Prevents air leaks; used to seal lung, liver; also in plastic surgery and skin grafting	Fibrinogen, CaCl, aprotinin, thrombin	Low bonding strength Requires 20 minutes' preparation time
Floseal	Gel	Flowable topical hemostat	Bovine-derived gelatin matrix, human thrombin in CaCl solution	Resorbed in 6–8 weeks postop
Surgiflo	Gel	Flowable topical hemostat for use in surgery	Porcine-derived gelatin, also available with thrombin	Effective with or without thrombin
Crosseal	Gel	Flowable topical hemostasis	Cross-linked gelatin granules and thrombin	Cross-linked gelatin swells on application
Omnex	Liquid/gel	Vascular anastomosis site sealant	100% synthetic cyanoacrylates	Remains in place during healing
CoSeal	Liquid/gel	Used to mechanically seal vascular reconstruction sites	100% synthetic; polyethylene glycol polymers	Remains in place during healing
Dermabond	Liquid	Used to close the skin (incisions and lacerations)	Synthetic cyanoacrylate	Fast setting with high strength; non-absorbable
OTHER				
Platelet gel	Gel	Augments hemostasis, provides additional platelets and growth factors	Autologous preparation from patient's plasma	Must be prepared for each individual patient
Ostene	Putty	Hemostatic agent used on bone surface	Combination of synthetics: ethylene oxide and propylene oxide	Safer than prototype bone wax made from beeswax combinations
BioGlue	Liquid	Tissue sealant used to seal leaks in vascular anastomoses	Bovine serum albumin plus glutaraldehyde	Creates flexible seal independent of suture anastomosis
Silver nitrate	Fluid or applicator	Creates thick eschar; stains tissue	Caustic chemical	Seldom used; used only for superficial bleeding

(recombinant human thrombin). When applied to oozing tissue, it combines with the body's fibrinogen to promote coagulation. This group of drugs actively takes part in the body's coagulation mechanism when the patient's ability to coagulate is hampered by a coagulation disorder.

Topical powder is applied directly to an oozing surface or mixed with injectable isotonic saline for use as a spray, by drop, or for soaking hemostatic sponges.

Topical thrombin is available as a sterile powder in vials containing 5000 or 20,000 International units for reconstitution with sterile saline. Frozen thrombin *solution* is available at 800 and 1200 International units per mL. When labeling these drugs on the sterile field, it is necessary to include the strength in International units per mL.

NOTE *Thrombin is never injected into blood vessels. It is a high-alert medication that must be carefully managed on the sterile field.*

MECHANICAL HEMOSTAT

Mechanical hemostatic agents enhance the normal coagulation (clotting) process by mechanical means, by providing a mesh, granular, or fluff matrix that promotes platelet aggregation on bleeding surfaces. These are formulated from gelatin, collagen, cellulose, and polysaccharides. They are manufactured without natural or synthetic drugs. However, some are prepared in combination with thrombin solution on the sterile field. The mechanical agent promotes hemostasis by forming a barrier on oozing surfaces. In contact with body fluid, they instantly swell and form a physical matrix for coagulation. The mechanical hemostat is *passive* because it does not actually participate in the body's coagulation mechanism.

ABSORBABLE GELATIN

Absorbable gelatin is a dry sponge or film material derived from porcine tissue. When applied to tissue, it absorbs blood quickly and enhances clot formation. The clot is the result of the mechanical rather than chemical action of the material. Absorbable gelatin is most commonly supplied under the proprietary names *Gelfoam, Gelfilm,* and *Surgifoam*. These are available in squares, which are cut to size as needed. The usual size used during surgery is ¼- to 1-inch square or rectangular pieces. Absorbable hemostatic agents are not left in place over neural or bone tissue, because tissue injury can result.

The scrubbed surgical technologist prepares the gelatin sponge on the surgical field. If thrombin is used as a soaking agent for the gelatin, the circulator dispenses injectable saline diluent (liquid) and dry thrombin powder mix to the scrubbed technologist, using aseptic technique. The liquid drug is immediately labeled and used during the case to soak the hemostatic gelatin.

Gelatin sponge is dispensed in 2- or 3-inch squares for cutting into smaller patches as requested by the surgeon. The pieces are placed in liquid topical thrombin or isotonic saline, or they may be used in their dry form. After soaking, gelatin should swell and become soft. If this does not occur, the pieces can be removed from the solution and compressed to remove the air. They are then returned to the solution and kept there until use. The technologist can dispense the sponge pieces to the surgeon in a small basin. All gelatin sponge squares are removed from the surgical wound after use. The technologist should collect these and remove them from the sterile field so they do not fall back into the wound.

OXIDIZED CELLULOSE

Oxidized cellulose USP is available in mesh, fluff, and powder forms. It is always applied to tissue in the dry form. On contact with blood, it rapidly forms a clot that is absorbed by the body during the healing process. Oxidized cellulose is manufactured as *Surgicel.*

It must be kept dry until it is used on tissue. If allowed to become wet, it is difficult to handle and loses its shape. It is available in small strips or squares, which may have to be cut with suture scissors. The pieces can then be dispensed to the surgeon in a small basin or container. Any discarded material should be cleared from the surgical site so that it does not enter (or reenter) the wound accidentally.

COLLAGEN ABSORBABLE HEMOSTAT

Collagen absorbable hemostat is manufactured from bovine collagen and supplied in the dry form as powder, sheets, and sponges. *Avitene* is approved for use in all surgery and is supplied in preloaded applicators for endoscopic use. In its powder form, it is applied directly to capillary surfaces. The strips may be wrapped around the anastomosis connecting two vessels or hollow structures to form a hemostatic seal. This product is not approved for all surgical tissues. The preparation and use of collagen absorbable hemostat are the same as those for oxidized cellulose. It must be kept dry before use.

BONE HEMOSTAT

Hemostasis in bone is achieved by applying a substance, commonly called *bone wax,* onto the surface of a bleeding bone. This material, traditionally made from a combination of beeswax and other additives, has been replaced by more biocompatible agents. The current formulation of bone wax is derived from ethylene oxide and propylene oxide *(Ostene)*. Bone hemostatic materials must be warmed slightly before use. This is done by kneading small pieces between gloved fingers. They are dispensed by mounting them on the edge of a small basin or container that can be placed on the sterile field.

FLOWABLE HEMOSTATS AND SEALANTS

Flowable hemostats are composed of porcine or bovine gelatin. They have a viscous quality (approximately the same as honey) and are used in areas that are difficult to access. Some products such as FloSeal (Baxter, Deerfield, IL) and Surgiflo

(Johnson & Johnson, New Brunswick, NJ) also contain pooled human thrombin.

Fibrin sealants are applied to the surface of tissues to bind them together or to prevent air or blood leakage. A few sealants such as natural fibrin have been marketed for some time. Newer combination products and synthetic polymers are now formulated for use as sealants.

Common uses of sealants and adhesives include the following:

1. To close air leaks on lung surfaces and to close bronchial tubes after anastomosis
2. On liver and spleen surfaces that cannot be sutured easily
3. In vascular surgery, sealants are used to bind together vessels in conjunction with sutures that connect blood vessels together *(anastomosis)*
4. In the esophagus in the treatment of bleeding esophageal varices, and in endoscopic surgery for hemostasis
5. Collagen-based sealants are used to close dura mater leaks

Handling tissue sealants on the field is relatively straightforward. Components that must be mixed are dispensed in their own cartridges, and all are packaged as systems, including single-use applicators with easy-to-use directions.

ANTICOAGULANTS AND THROMBOLYTICS

This category of drugs includes coagulants and anticoagulants used systemically and topically in medical treatment and surgery. These are high-alert drugs that must be very carefully handled on and off the sterile field to avoid drug error. An *anticoagulant* is a drug that inhibits blood clot formation but does not dissolve clots. There are several types of anticoagulant drugs. A *coagulant* induces blood coagulation.

HEPARINS

These are used for the prevention of venous thromboembolism.

- *Unfractionated heparin* has been largely replaced with safer low-molecular-weight heparin.
- *Low-molecular-weight heparin* is administered by injection to prevent venous thromboembolism after major orthopedic and gynecological surgery. It is also used in the prevention of coagulation during renal dialysis and cardiac surgery.

WARFARIN (COUMADIN)

Oral anticoagulant therapy using vitamin K antagonists (warfarin) is used in the treatment of venous thromboembolism, pulmonary embolism, and cardiac abnormalities that increase the risk of embolism in conditions such as valve disease. Patients on warfarin are usually required to stop therapy before surgery and then resume it on the first postoperative day.

THROMBOLYTICS

Thrombolytic drugs are used for the immediate breakdown of systemic blood clots, particularly in myocardial infarction, ischemic stroke, and pulmonary embolism. These drugs are usually administered in combination with heparin therapy. Common fibrinolytic drugs are as follows:

- Recombinant tissue plasminogen activator, alteplase
- Urokinase

CENTRAL NERVOUS SYSTEM AGENTS

Knowledge about nerve transmission is basic to an understanding of how anesthetics and other CNS drugs work. The following basic description of how stimuli are transmitted provides useful background for the study of anesthetic drugs.

The transmission of nerve impulses (signals) is a complex biochemical process. In simple terms, impulses are chemical and electrical. Chemicals that carry impulses from nerve cell to nerve cell are called *neurotransmitters*. The biochemical work of the neurotransmitter is to transport the signal from one nerve cell to the next until the signal reaches the target tissue.

Each nerve cell (neuron) is separated from an adjacent nerve cell by a synapse (also called the *synaptic cleft*). The synapse is the small space in which the neurotransmitter passes from one nerve cell to another. For the neurotransmitter to transport a signal, it must be released from the presynaptic neuron (the neuron before the synapse) and received by the next neuron in line (the postsynaptic neuron). The neurotransmitter is contained in small vesicles (cell sacs). The receptor for a particular neurotransmitter is a specific molecule in the postsynaptic neuron (Fig. 12.13).

The body has many different types of neurotransmitters, each carrying a different type of impulse. About 30 known neurotransmitters occur in specific tissues of the body.

One type of neurotransmitter can be blocked without affecting the others. For example, the neurotransmitter for motor control can be inactivated by a neuromuscular blocking agent, whereas the neurotransmitter for pain remains unaffected. This would result in the ability to feel pain but the inability to move in response. Likewise, sedation or loss of consciousness can be achieved without reducing the sensation of pain.

One method of blocking neurotransmission is to administer a competitive antagonist drug that has an affinity for the postsynaptic receptor. These drugs limit the number of receptors available for the neurotransmitter molecule. When the drug attaches to the receptor site, the neurotransmitter cannot continue on its path because no unbound receptors are available. The neurotransmitter remains in the space between the two neurons (the synapse) and is eventually reabsorbed by the presynaptic cell or broken down by enzymes. In this way, the path of transmission is broken. Antagonist CNS drugs increase the availability of postsynaptic receptors and the movement of neurotransmitters by increasing the release or uptake (or both) of a particular neurotransmitter.

ANESTHETICS

CNS anesthetics provide the physiological conditions necessary for surgery. This category of drugs causes the loss of primary CNS functions such as consciousness, sensation (including pain), some autonomic responses, and recall of

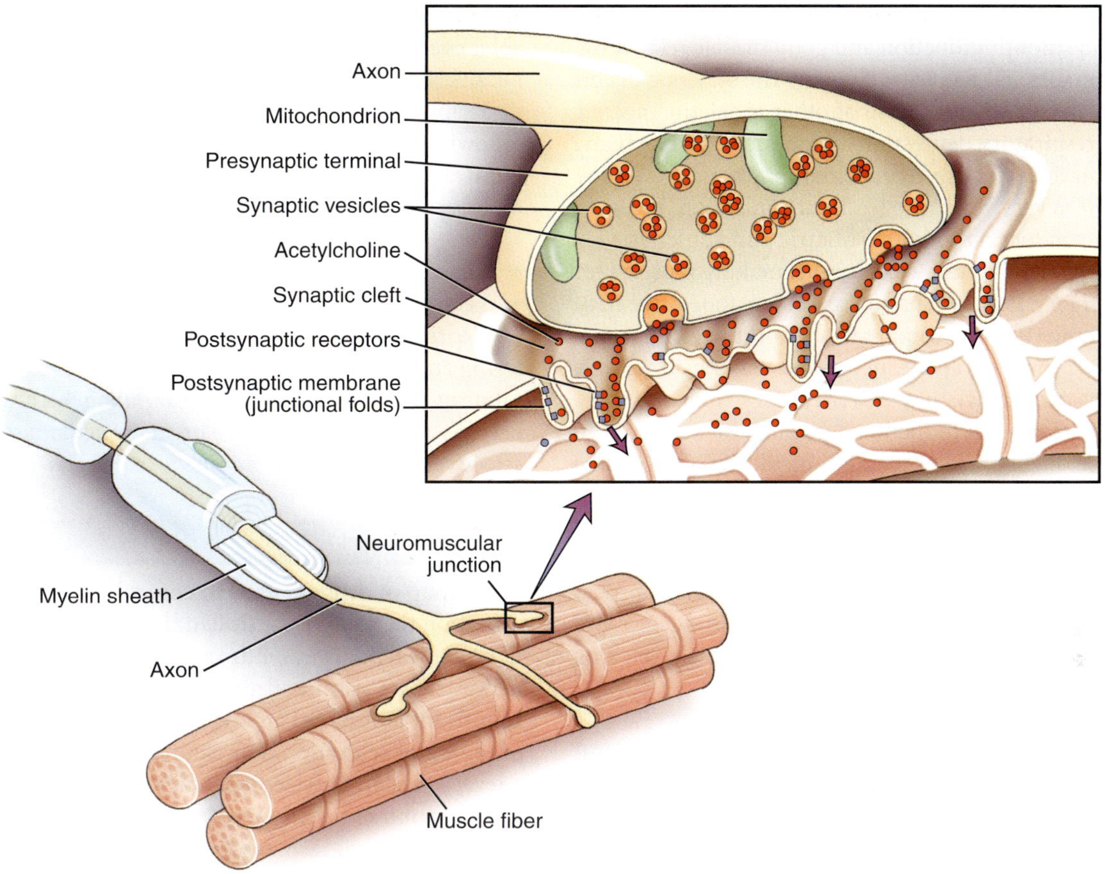

FIG. 12.13 Neuron junction and neurotransmitter molecules. (From VanMeter K, Hubert R. *Microbiology for the Healthcare Professional.* 2nd ed. St Louis: Elsevier; 2016.)

events that occur while the drug is present in the body. The depth of the effect is dose dependent. However, selected adjunct agents are administered during general anesthesia to produce a more profound effect while protecting the patient from the risk of high-dose anesthetic.

Inhalation Anesthetics

Inhalation (volatile) anesthetics are formulated as liquids and administered as a vapor (gas). Only nitrous oxide is both formulated and delivered in gaseous form. All other agents must be vaporized in the anesthesia machine for administration by mask or through an artificial airway inserted into the patient's own upper airway. The agent enters the lungs, where it crosses the alveoli, enters the circulatory system, and is made available to the nervous system, producing deep sedation and unconsciousness.

Inhalation anesthetics are used to *maintain* a surgical level of anesthesia after a fast-acting intravenous anesthetic (discussed later) has been used to induce unconsciousness. Induction (the process of becoming unconscious) by gas anesthetic is slow and can result in delirium and other adverse reactions. However, this method is sometimes used in pediatric patients for whom an intravenous injection might be difficult.

In the past, anesthetic gases such as cyclopropane and vaporized ether were commonly used during surgery. These agents are highly flammable and explosive. Conductive shoes, anti-static flooring, and high environmental humidity were necessary to prevent surgical fires, which were relatively common compared with today. These potent agents caused serious **side effects**. Flammable anesthetic agents are no longer permitted in surgery, and modern agents have created a much safer environment for patients and personnel. However, extended exposure to small amounts of modern vaporized (gas) anesthetics is unsafe, so all anesthetic machines are manufactured with scavenging systems that collect and remove waste anesthetic gas from the operative environment.

Nitrous oxide is a colorless, odorless gas in its natural state. It has low potency, but adjusting its concentration provides a range of anesthetic effects. It has strong analgesic properties and is quickly dissipated from the body, usually within minutes. Nitrous oxide is not flammable, but it supports combustion.

In some patients, nitrous oxide can cause severe cardiovascular depression, leading to shock. It does not affect the respiratory system or the action of neuromuscular blocking agents. It can be used for induction but is commonly mixed with other agents. The main advantages of nitrous oxide are minimal incidence of nausea and rapid absorption and clearance from the body. Disadvantages are low potency and lack of muscle relaxation.

Isoflurane is widely used in many different types of surgery. It causes rapid smooth induction and good muscle relaxation. It is nonflammable and has a strong odor. The systemic effects of isoflurane are superior to those of other inhalation agents. Cardiac and respiratory depression are minimal. Unlike many other agents, it does not cause bronchial spasm.

Sevoflurane is very similar to isoflurane in action. It can be safely used for induction in both pediatric and adult patients. Patients emerge rapidly from sevoflurane, making it useful for outpatient surgery. It does cause increased postoperative nausea and vomiting (PONV) compared with other agents.

Desflurane provides rapid emergence, making it suitable for outpatient surgery when a short recovery time is important. It can be used as an induction agent in adults, but not in pediatric patients, because of the high incidence of bronchial spasm and laryngospasm associated with it. Desflurane must be heated during vaporization.

Enflurane (Ethrane) is used for induction and maintenance. It can also be used in low doses for short surgical procedures that do not require unconsciousness. It produces rapid induction and emergence and has excellent muscle-relaxing properties.

NEUROMUSCULAR BLOCKING AGENTS

Neuromuscular blocking agents are used in conjunction with general anesthesia to paralyze skeletal muscles, an essential component of general anesthesia. Even during profound general anesthesia, autonomic muscle responses can interfere with the manipulation of tissues such as during intubation and mechanical ventilation. Neuromuscular blocking is a complex, controlled process that is chemically reversed at the close of surgery or whenever necessary during an emergency. These drugs cause paralysis of the respiratory muscles, and mechanical ventilation is required during their use. The effect of neuromuscular blocking drugs is adjusted during surgery according to the level of relaxation needed.

Nerve transmission to striated muscles occurs at the neuromuscular junction where the motor neuron (nerve cell to the skeletal muscle) and muscle cell communicate. The nerve cell and muscle (motor endplate) do not touch. They are separated by a small gap called the *synaptic cleft*, as described earlier. Activation of the muscle cell occurs when the neurotransmitter acetylcholine (ACh) is released by the nerve cell where it crosses the cleft and binds to the ACh receptors at the motor endplate. This causes depolarization (electrochemical change necessary for cell activation) of the muscle cells and muscle contraction.

Neuromuscular blocking drugs interfere with normal muscle cell depolarization, which results in muscle relaxation. Two types of drugs are used to prevent muscle contractions. Both types attach to the ACh binding sites and prevent ACh from attaching. An agonist (depolarizing) drug has some of the properties of ACh but does not permit the electrochemical changes (particularly the resting phase of the muscle fiber) necessary for muscle activation. A non-depolarizing agent (antagonist) also binds to the motor endplate but works by simply blocking ACh. Only one depolarizing agent is available, succinylcholine, which is used primarily for intubation because it is short acting.

Examples of non-depolarizing blocking agents are the following:

- Atracurium
- Cisatracurium
- Pancuronium
- Rocuronium
- Vecuronium

Neuromuscular blocking agents are reversed by administering an anticholinesterase. *Neostigmine* is the primary reversal drug and has replaced *edrophonium*, which was previously used as a reversal agent in surgery. *Sugammadex* is used to selectively reverse rocuronium.

ANALGESICS

This group of drugs is used to control pain. Pain is a complex sensation that can be controlled through a number of different neurological pathways. It is important to note that in terms of nerve transmission and the use of analgesic drugs, there are significant differences among analgesia (lack of pain), sedation (sleep), and relaxation. For example, it is possible to produce a level of sedation (sleepiness or somnolence) while retaining the sensation of pain.

OPIATES

Opiates are among the most common drugs used for moderate and severe pain control. All opiates (also known as *narcotics*) produce analgesia by altering the perception of pain. Because they reduce the work of the heart, morphine is often given in specific cardiac emergencies.

Opiates are derived directly from the natural psychoactive substance in the opium plant, whereas opioids are synthetic or semisynthetic drugs that resemble opiates in pharmacological action. The most common opiate used in health care is morphine. Other opiate drugs are often described by their relative strength as an analgesic when compared with natural morphine sulfate.

Examples of natural opiates are the following:

- Morphine
- Codeine

The semisynthetic opiates include the following:

- Hydromorphone
- Hydrocodone
- Oxycodone
- Oxymorphone
- Sufentanil
- Alfentanil
- Remifentanil

Completely synthetic opiates include fentanyl, pethidine (also known as meperidine), and tramadol. All opiates are addictive and, in high doses, cause depression of the CNS, hypotension, respiratory depression, profound sedation, and coma.

Opiate antagonists are used to treat opiate toxicity and overdose. These include naloxone, nalmefene, and naltrexone.

NON-OPIATE ANALGESICS

Non-opiate drugs are used for mild and moderate pain. These may be prescribed for mild postoperative pain after superficial procedures under local anesthesia. Ibuprofen and diclofenac are non-opiate antiinflammatory agents. Acetaminophen is used for mild pain and as an antipyretic.

SEDATIVES AND HYPNOTICS

Sedative or hypnotic drugs are used in a variety of medical and surgical situations to depress consciousness and induce drowsiness. Most do not have analgesic effects. Categories of sedative drugs include the sedative-hypnotics, barbiturates, and benzodiazepines. Sedatives are used to relax patients in the acute care setting and in behavioral emergencies. Oral sedative-hypnotic drugs are prescribed for short-term insomnia and to reduce anxiety in the preoperative period. They are also used during the induction of general anesthesia to allow intubation (placement of an artificial airway) at the start of general anesthesia or in emergency situations requiring intubation.

Intravenous sedatives are used with or without analgesics for procedural sedation or *moderate sedation* for short procedures when profound anesthesia is not required. Under mild and moderate sedation, the patient can respond to verbal commands, and respiratory and cardiovascular functions remain intact. However, a deeply sedated patient cannot be easily roused, and ventilation may be decreased. Modern sedatives are rapidly cleared from the body, making them ideal for procedural sedation and anesthesia. Propofol is the most common intravenous sedative used for the induction and maintenance of general anesthesia and also as a general sedative.

Examples of sedatives are the following:

- Propofol
- Etomidate
- Dexmedetomidine

DISSOCIATIVE ANESTHESIA

Ketamine is a rapidly acting sedative that produces isolation of the sensory parts of the brain, resulting in a trance-like state *(dissociative anesthesia)* and amnesia. Ketamine is valuable for sedation requiring profound short-term analgesia, such as during the debridement of burns. However, it has distinctive adverse effects such as increased intracranial pressure (ICP), delirium, and hypertension. It is generally not used in adults because it may precipitate emergence delirium.

BARBITURATES

This group of drugs was among the first to be used in clinical situations requiring profound depression of the CNS. Oral barbiturates are still used in the treatment of seizure disorders. Intravenous barbiturates are commonly used for the induction of general anesthesia. They are rapidly effective, causing unconsciousness within 10 to 20 seconds. Recovery from thiopental, which is the most commonly used agent, is 20 to 30 minutes. Barbiturates cause dose-related respiratory depression and apnea (absence of breathing), which is transient during initial administration. Laryngospasm and bronchospasm can occur with thiopental.

Examples of intravenous barbiturates are the following:

- Thiopental
- Methohexital

BENZODIAZEPINES

Benzodiazepines have many clinical uses because of their versatility. This category of drugs is anxiolytic (reduces anxiety) and provides muscle relaxation. They cause desirable *anterograde amnesia* (loss of recall of events) for up to 6 hours from the onset of drug action.

Examples of benzodiazepines are the following:

- Midazolam
- Lorazepam
- Alprazolam
- Diazepam

The benzodiazepine antagonist *flumazenil* is used to reverse the effects of this category of drugs.

CONTRAST MEDIA

Contrast media are diagnostic agents injected into tissue or hollow spaces of the body in conjunction with imaging studies. These substances enable clinicians to observe and document the interior margins or path of a hollow organ, vessels, or ducts. In many cases, a radiology technologist is responsible for handling and administering these substances in a diagnostic clinic or unit of the health care facility. The surgical technologist may be asked to assist in these procedures. Contrast media are also used occasionally in surgical procedures to verify the patency of a duct, organ, or vessel.

An *iodinated contrast medium* (ICM) is a clear, injectable liquid that is *radiopaque* (opaque on radiographs). ICMs are commonly used in radiography, computed tomography, and fluoroscopy. Agents differ in *osmolality* (the amount of solute, in this case, iodine, by weight in solution). Contrast media with high levels of iodine are associated with increased adverse effects, whereas those with lower levels of iodine are safer. Allergic reaction can occur, and patients must be monitored during use. The patient may experience allergy or sensitivity to contrast media, but this is not related to shellfish. Modern ICMs are generally very safe compared with prototypes used in the past.

NOTE *There is no scientific basis for the association of shellfish allergy with an adverse reaction to ICMs.*

As with all drugs used in surgery and interventional radiology, the surgical technologist must keep track of the total amount and concentration (dose) of contrast medium used. There are literally hundreds of types of contrast media available for use in medicine. The main categories for safety purposes are whether the substance is *high molecular weight* or *low molecular weight*. The lower-molecular-weight substances are much safer. Examples of ICMs are diatrizoate and metrizoate.

Gadolinium-based contrast media are used for magnetic resonance imaging and magnetic resonance angiography. These agents work by intensifying the magnetic field of protons, which, in turn, creates more contrast.

Perfluorocarbon microsphere contrast media are used in echocardiography and ultrasound. These consist of compressible shells filled with gas that resonate at the frequency of the ultrasound waves.

Barium sulfate is an opaque contrast medium used in radiological studies of the GI tract (barium enema or barium swallow). These studies are performed in the GI clinic or interventional radiology department and are not part of a sterile procedure. However, the surgical technologist may occasionally work in these areas of the health care facility and should be familiar with the use of barium. Barium is supplied as a liquid for oral administration or rectal infusion. After ingestion or infusion, barium radiographs reveal well-defined areas where the substance has filled the GI tract, including small surface irregularities, outpockets of tissue, strictures, and other anomalies. Barium is not absorbed through the tissues but is excreted through the normal GI tract in its intact form.

COLORED DYES AND STAINS

Colored tissue dyes and tissue stains are used in microbiology and in tissue specimens for observation under the microscope. In medicine and surgery they are used to distinguish certain types of tissues (e.g., lymph nodes) and to determine patency (an open passageway) through tissue.

A dye is a colored substance that can be infused into a duct or natural passage such as the fallopian tube or into a tract such as that created by infection (called a *sinus tract*); the path is followed by simply observing the colored liquid as it passes through the tissue or opening. Another common use of tissue dye is in the manufacturing of skin-marking pens used to delineate or identify the location of a skin incision and in plastic and reconstructive surgery to create landmarks that may be obscured once the incisions have been made.

Colored dyes are usually dispensed to the sterile field in glass ampoules. The most common types are the following:

- Gentian violet
- Methylene blue
- Indigo carmine

A *stain* is used as a diagnostic tool to differentiate normal cells from abnormal ones. Clinical laboratories use a variety of staining agents. In the surgical setting, several types of stains are used to enable surgeons to see areas of diseased tissue appropriate for destruction or excision. Stains are typically applied under direct visualization with a sterile sponge or cotton-tipped applicator. The stain is generally absorbed by the abnormal cells, giving these cells a different appearance from that of the surrounding healthy cells.

- Lugol's solution is used to perform Schiller's test to identify cervical dysplasia.
- Monsel's solution is used to identify abnormal tissue cells in gynecological and urogenital procedures.
- Acetic acid is used to enhance the detection of cervical neoplasia during colposcopy.

ANTIINFECTIVE AGENTS

This category includes all drugs used in the treatment of infectious diseases caused by pathogenic organisms. Many drugs are differentiated in their second tier of identification by the type of organism they affect, such as antifungal, antiretroviral, or antibiotic. The categories are listed in Appendix B. The largest category of antiinfective agents is the **antibiotics,** which are used to treat bacterial infections. There are many types of antibiotics, which differ in their action against bacteria. The indication of one antibiotic over another is based on the type of infection, the drug resistance of the bacteria, and the condition of the patient. Many antibiotics developed decades ago are no longer effective because the microbes are resistant to the effects of the drug. As a result, newer drugs are in constant development. Antiinfectives are used in the perioperative setting in several ways:

- As a preoperative medication in selected cases. The patient may be started on intravenous antibiotics a few hours before surgery to prevent postoperative infection.
- As an irrigant in the surgical wound. Topical antibiotics such as bacitracin may be used to irrigate tissues of body cavities and spaces.
- Bacteriostatic agents (those that arrest the proliferation of bacteria) are impregnated into some types of dressings, such as gauze strips and packing material, used in a body cavity after surgery.
- Postoperatively, many patients are prescribed antibiotics to prevent infection.

Antiretroviral medications are in the antiinfective group of drugs. These are used in the treatment of human immunodeficiency virus/acquired immunodeficiency syndrome (HIV/AIDS) and are prescribed as part of postexposure prophylaxis (PEP) immediately after exposure to body fluids, such as a sharps injury in the medical workplace.

The *mechanisms* of antibacterial action can include but are not limited to the following:

- Inhibition of synthesis of the cell wall
- Alteration in the permeability of the cell membrane
- Prevention of the synthesis of cellular proteins
- Inhibition of the cell's genetic material, deoxyribonucleic acid (DNA) and ribonucleic acid (RNA), which is needed for replication
- Interference with cell metabolism

PENICILLIN

Penicillin was developed during the early 1940s. It was the first true antibiotic, and many different categories of penicillin have emerged, all arising from the prototype. Penicillin is divided into two types: broad spectrum (effective on gram-positive and some gram-negative bacteria) and narrow spectrum (effective only on gram-positive bacteria). Other classes of penicillin are distinguished by their ability to target specific bacterial defense mechanisms or groups of bacteria.

Examples are the following:

- Procaine penicillin
- Benzathine penicillin
- Penicillin V potassium
- Ampicillin
- Piperacillin

CEPHALOSPORINS

Cephalosporins were first developed in the 1960s. Each subsequent group has been broader in spectrum than the previous group. These groups are called **generations** of cephalosporins, because they emerged from the previous parent prototype. First-, second-, third-, and fourth-generation cephalosporins have been developed.

MACROLIDES

Macrolides are bacteriostatic at low levels and bactericidal in high doses. These are broad-spectrum drugs, but they are most active against gram-positive bacteria. They are most commonly used to treat respiratory tract infections and sexually transmitted diseases.

Examples are the following:

- Azithromycin
- Clarithromycin
- Erythromycin

LINCOSAMIDES, VANCOMYCIN, AND KETOLIDES

Lincosamides, vancomycin, and ketolides have similar actions. They are bacteriostatic and bactericidal, and they inhibit protein synthesis in bacteria. Vancomycin was used extensively in the 1950s, but its use is now limited because it can cause auditory and cranial nerve damage.

Examples are the following:

- Clindamycin
- Vancomycin
- Telithromycin

TETRACYCLINE

Tetracyclines are broad-spectrum antimicrobials that inhibit bacterial protein synthesis. They are supplied almost exclusively for oral administration against specific microbes such as rickettsiae and mycobacteria.

Examples are the following:

- Doxycycline
- Minocycline
- Tigecycline

AMINOGLYCOSIDES

Aminoglycosides are effective against gram-negative bacteria, in which they inhibit protein synthesis. This group of antibiotics is used selectively and carefully because of adverse reactions.

Examples are the following:

- Gentamicin
- Paromomycin
- Amikacin

QUINOLONES

Quinolones are broad-spectrum antibacterials that inhibit DNA synthesis. They are used in a variety of infections, including respiratory, arthritic, urinary tract, and GI conditions.

Examples are the following:

- Ciprofloxacin
- Levofloxacin

SULFONAMIDES

Sulfonamides were first introduced in the 1930s. They are bacteriostatic only. Because of their limited use and the emergence of increasingly drug-resistant bacterial strains, they have been replaced by drugs that are more effective. Sulfonamides are most commonly used to treat acute urinary tract infections.

An example is as follows:

- Sulfamethoxazole–trimethoprim

ANTIFUNGALS

Antifungal drugs are used for treating superficial and systemic fungal diseases. Skin infections are treated mainly with OTC topical medications, although resistant strains may require oral administration. Systemic fungal infections are difficult to treat and can be fatal. Intravenous administration is required for systemic infection.

Examples are the following:

- Amphotericin
- Miconazole
- Flucytosine

ANTINEOPLASTIC AGENTS

Cancer treatment may include the use of antineoplastic (anticancer) drugs that are occasionally used in the surgical setting. Intravesical treatment for urinary bladder cancer is a common procedure in which the antineoplastic drug is instilled directly into the bladder using a urinary catheter. This may follow tumor resection or as a stand-alone procedure. Intravesical instillation may also be performed in surgery or in the postanesthesia care unit (PACU).

Health care personnel can be injured through exposure to hazardous antineoplastic drugs. Risks include a higher incidence of leukemia and lymphoma, DNA damage, and miscarriage. Pregnant care workers are excluded from procedures in which there is a risk of contamination.

Safety precautions and standards for the handling and storage of antineoplastic drugs include the following:

- Storage of hazardous drugs
- Appropriate personal protective equipment (PPE)
- Disposal of equipment contaminated by hazardous drugs

- Staff teaching on topics related to the safe handling of hazardous drugs

Antineoplastic drugs are normally mixed by the facility's pharmacist and prepared ahead of the procedure.

DRUGS THAT AFFECT THE AUTONOMIC NERVOUS SYSTEM

Autonomic drugs affect neurotransmission in the autonomic nervous system. This category of drugs is used therapeutically in many different specialties to alter nerve transmission, especially in cardiac, respiratory, and ophthalmic medicine. A review of the autonomic nervous system explains the basics of how these drugs work.

The *CNS* is composed of the brain and spinal cord. To exert action in the body systems, nerve impulses are sent from the CNS to the peripheral nervous system (PNS). The PNS is composed of major nerve pathways and their divisions, which extend into all tissues outside the brain and spinal cord. The PNS is divided into two separate systems: the somatic and autonomic nervous systems.

The *somatic nervous system* is under voluntary control. For example, nerve transmission to the striated muscles is somatic. However, the *autonomic nervous system* is involuntary. Stimuli to these nerves produce specific responses in body organs and tissues, such as the heart, smooth muscle, and glands. Examples of autonomic responses are changes in heartbeat, the release of glandular secretions (e.g., insulin in the pancreas), and intestinal contractions (peristalsis).

The *autonomic nervous system* can produce two different types of responses: *sympathetic* and *parasympathetic.* They are often referred to as fight-or-flight responses. However, a more accurate description would be related to stress and nonstress responses. During physiological and emotional stress, the sympathetic system takes priority, so digestion activity is delayed, but the heart rate is increased to supply more oxygen to the tissues. The parasympathetic system is most active when the body is at rest. For example, under the parasympathetic system, the heart rate is slower and cardiac output is decreased, but digestion increases to allow greater storage of energy. The two parts of the autonomic system are constantly at work balancing body systems and physiology.

Separate neurotransmitters and receptors are responsible for the sympathetic and parasympathetic responses. *Noradrenalin* is the primary neurotransmitter for the sympathetic system. Certain receptors can also receive *adrenaline* and *dopamine. ACh* is the primary neurotransmitter of the parasympathetic system.

Receptors at the cellular level bind and interact with specific neurotransmitters. There are two main types of sympathetic (adrenergic) receptors: alpha (α) and beta (β). These are further classified into a number of different subtypes. Receptors for the parasympathetic system are called *cholinergic* receptors.

Autonomic drugs are classified according to the type of receptor and neurotransmitter with which they interact. To understand a specific drug, it is necessary to know where the receptor is located in the body (which tissue), its subtype, and whether it is an agonist (acting to increase the effect of the neurotransmitter) or an antagonist (blocking the effect of the neurotransmitter).

- *Adrenergic* agonists increase the effect of the sympathetic neurotransmitter (includes alpha and beta agonists)
- *Adrenergic* antagonists block the effect of the sympathetic neurotransmitter (includes alpha and beta blockers)
- *Cholinergics* increase the effect of the parasympathetic neurotransmitter ACh
- *Anticholinergics* block the effects of ACh

ANTICHOLINERGICS

Anticholinergic drugs are frequently used during general anesthesia. In the past, potent anticholinergics such as scopolamine and atropine were given routinely to all surgical patients. In modern surgery, these agents are used more selectively and can be administered intravenously during surgery for rapid results. They are used to control airway secretions and to regulate the heart rate in selected patients. In ophthalmic surgery, they are used to produce mydriasis (dilation of the pupil) and cycloplegia (paralysis of the ciliary muscles). Examples of anticholinergic agents include the following:

- Atropine sulfate
- Scopolamine
- Glycopyrrolate

The effects of anticholinergics include the following:

- Increase in heart rate
- Relaxation of smooth muscles in selected ophthalmic procedures
- Reduction of GI, bronchial, and nasopharyngeal secretions
- Emergency treatment of cardiac conduction block and sinus bradycardia
- Prevention of bronchospasm

ADRENERGICS

Adrenergic (also called *sympathomimetic*) drugs are used in many different specialties. In the respiratory system, the smooth muscles of the airways contain adrenoreceptors activated by adrenaline, which causes relaxation of the muscle fibers and dilation of the airways. Adrenergics are therefore used in the treatment of asthma and during respiratory emergencies such as anaphylactic shock. Some drugs are adrenergic to both the lungs and the heart, resulting in increased heart rate and expansion of the airways.

FLUID BALANCE AND ELECTROLYTES

Approximately two-thirds of the body mass is made up of water. Water is normally gained through ingestion (eating and drinking) and lost through normal physiological processes, trauma, or disease (vomiting, diarrhea, burns, and hemorrhage). Surgery and anesthesia also result in shifts in fluid balance. Although surgery does not directly alter fluid balance, the anesthesia process can suppress some autonomic responses that do. Total body water is contained in three spaces: the intracellular spaces (inside the cells), interstitial spaces (between the cells), and intravascular spaces (within the blood vessels). Fluid shifts from one compartment (space) to another as the body maintains homeostasis. This is controlled by oncotic pressure (movement controlled by the presence of large molecules such as plasma proteins) and by the process of osmosis. The total volume of body fluid must remain stable to sustain life.

In surgery, fluid loss is monitored by measuring urine and blood loss. If fluids are needed, the choice is very specific according to the patient's physiological state at the time. Errors in fluid administration can result in fluid overload and heart failure. Administering the wrong dilution (osmolality) of an electrolyte solution can cause serious injury or death related to the chemical reactions caused (or prevented) by the presence of the electrolytes.

Intravenous fluids are administered routinely in surgery and medicine. There are two general categories of intravenous fluids: crystalloids and colloids.

CRYSTALLOIDS

Crystalloids are solutions that contain a small amount of electrolyte solutes (dissolved substances). These solutions are mainly administered to correct physiological imbalance related to electrolytes and blood pH and to restore fluids lost through disease (dehydration).

Crystalloids are classified as follows:

- *Isotonic:* Solute concentration equal to the physiological environment
- *Hypertonic:* Solute concentration higher than that of the physiological environment
- *Hypotonic:* Solute concentration lower than that of the physiological environment

Commonly used crystalloids are 0.9% saline solution (also called *normal saline*) and dextrose solution. Another crystalloid that is frequently used is lactated Ringer solution, the chemical composition of which is close to that of human plasma. Other crystalloids contain specific electrolytes such as potassium and calcium, which are prescribed according to the patient's electrolyte needs.

Alterations in blood pH can occur with trauma, shock, and disease. *Acidosis* is lower than normal blood pH. Respiratory acidosis occurs with hypercapnia (buildup of carbon dioxide), which can be caused by head injury, some anesthetics, and pulmonary diseases. Metabolic acidosis can be the result of kidney disease or low production of bicarbonate. *Alkalosis* is higher than normal blood pH. This can occur as respiratory alkalosis from elevated carbon dioxide concentration or as metabolic alkalosis caused by decreased hydrogen ion concentration. Crystalloids may be used in severe cases of pH imbalance.

COLLOIDS

Colloids are crystalloid-based water and electrolytes. However, they also have additional components that cause the fluid to move into and out of body spaces in a specific way. A colloid is a particle or substance that is dispersed throughout the fluid but not dissolved in it. In medicine, colloids are administered to prevent fluids from escaping the closed vascular system across the cell membrane. Patients who require intravascular fluid replacement may be administered a colloid; however, their use is somewhat controversial. This solution increases the intravascular (oncotic) pressure, but the colloid particles do not allow the fluid to escape into other body compartments.

Common colloids are blood, plasma, and synthetic substances that have large *macromolecules* to prevent the escape of the fluid outside the vascular system. A colloid may be given, for example, as a lifesaving measure when blood is not immediately available. In this case, normal saline cannot be used because it would quickly become dispersed among the other body compartments and would not exert oncotic pressure in the vascular system. During massive blood or plasma loss (as occurs during trauma or in burn patients), the oncotic pressure of the vascular system must be raised to enable the heart to move the blood through the body effectively. Colloids are vascular volume expanders. *Dextran* solutions have properties similar to those of human albumin. *Hetastarch* is a hypertonic synthetic starch. These colloidal fluids increase osmotic pressure, which controls the movement of water into and out of intravascular spaces.

IRRIGATION FLUIDS

Irrigation fluids (described earlier) must be compatible with the physiological environment in which they are used. All irrigation solutions are saline based, and they are labeled as *topical* or *intravenous. A topical solution must not be used in or around open blood vessels.* Only intravenous solutions are used to irrigate blood vessels or near open blood vessels. Differences in osmolality among irrigation solutions can result in abnormal movement of fluid across the cell membrane. Ophthalmic and otology solutions are also specifically labeled to be compatible with these delicate tissues.

CARDIAC DRUGS

Cardiac drugs are divided into categories according to their action (pharmacodynamics). Some are used for acute cardiac conditions, whereas others are part of a long-term treatment plan for patients with heart disease. Cardiac drugs used during surgery are given as needed to regulate heart muscle, maintain arterial pressure, and prevent thromboembolus. Emergency cardiac drugs are also found on the emergency *crash cart*, which is a self-contained unit with drugs and equipment immediately available for physiological emergencies including cardiac or respiratory arrest. Common cardiac drug categories include the following:

- *Inotropes:* Increase (positive inotrope) or decrease (negative inotrope) heart contractility
- *Chronotropic drugs:* Affect heart rate
- *Antiarrhythmic agents:* Used to treat abnormal cardiac rhythm
- *Antianginal drugs:* Used to treat *angina*, which is chest pain associated with decreased oxygen supply to the heart muscle. Blood flow to the heart is supplied by the

coronary arteries. Antianginal agents increase oxygen supply by decreasing the cardiac demand for oxygen or by vasodilation
- *Diuretics:* Increase urine output to balance sodium and intravascular volume
- *Antilipemics:* Cholesterol-lowering drug used in the long-term treatment of hypercholesterolemia
- *Antihypertensives:* Lower blood pressure

DIURETICS

Diuretics stimulate the production of urine by the kidneys. This creates a shift of body fluids. They are most commonly used in the treatment of hypertension and pulmonary edema. However, they are also used for the emergency treatment of intraocular pressure and increased ICP. Diuretics reduce the total vascular volume by depressing reabsorption of sodium in the kidneys and increasing water excretion from nephrons. This results in increased *diuresis* (urinary excretion).

Specific classes of diuretics function differently. Some produce excess excretion of potassium, an electrolyte necessary for cardiac and cell function. Potassium-sparing diuretics are preferred for this reason. Loop diuretics are extremely potent and cause rapid diuresis and loss of electrolytes. The osmotic diuretics are also very potent and are used to reduce intraocular pressure and cerebral edema. This class of diuretics is given during neurosurgical procedures. Carbonic anhydrase inhibitors are used specifically for reducing intraocular pressure in patients with open-angle glaucoma. They inhibit the enzyme carbonic anhydrase, which partly controls the acid–base balance in the blood. Thiazide diuretics are weaker and do not cause immediate diuresis. They are used in the treatment of hypertension because they cause arteriolar dilation and reduce cardiac output.

Examples of diuretics are the following:
- Hydrochlorothiazide
- Bumetanide
- Furosemide
- Mannitol
- Acetazolamide

GASTROINTESTINAL DRUGS

The stomach contains glands that secrete substances to maintain a healthy stomach lining and contribute to the digestion process. Mucoid cells produce protective mucus; the parietal cells secrete hydrochloric acid (HCl); and the chief cells produce pepsinogen, which is converted to pepsin on exposure to HCl for the breakdown of proteins. Activation of the glands is a complex process mediated by the autonomic nervous system.

Neutralization of stomach acid is an important goal during surgery to prevent lung damage in the event of regurgitation and aspiration during general anesthesia. Normally, the pyloric sphincter and cardiac sphincter prevent regurgitation. However, the action is suppressed with unconsciousness (e.g., during general anesthesia). Regurgitation and aspiration are particular concerns in high-risk cases such as emergency trauma, pregnancy, morbidly obese patients, and those with gastroesophageal reflux disease (GERD). To prevent potentially fatal aspiration, gastric drugs are administered selectively in the preoperative and intraoperative periods. These drugs reduce the volume and acidity of the gastric fluid.

HISTAMINE-2 RECEPTOR ANTAGONISTS AND PROTON-PUMP INHIBITORS

Histamine-2 receptor (H_2 receptor) antagonists reduce gastric acidity by blocking the release of gastric acid in the parietal cells. These drugs do not change the acidity of the contents already in the stomach. Examples of H_2 receptor antagonists are the following:
- Cimetidine
- Famotidine
- Ranitidine

Gastric proton-pump inhibitors suppress the action of the parietal cells that release hydrogen ions for the production of HCl. Examples are the following:
- Lansoprazole
- Omeprazole
- Rabeprazole
- Pantoprazole
- Esomeprazole

ANTACIDS

Antacids reduce gastric fluid acidity and volume. These are given on the day of surgery as preoperative medication. Calcium, aluminum, and magnesium salts that are available as OTC antacids are *not* used because they can cause an increase in acid secretion and are contraindicated in renal disease. Instead, prostaglandin drugs such as *misoprostol* are used to suppress acid secretion by the parietal cells. This drug may be used only in nonpregnant patients, because it is an abortive agent. *Sucralfate* is administered to increase the production of mucosal prostaglandin and form a barrier over the stomach lining. It does not influence the production of gastric fluid.

ANTIEMETIC AGENTS

Postoperative nausea and vomiting is a significant problem in the immediate postoperative period. Antiemetic agents are used to prevent or reduce vomiting. These drugs are administered in the PACU. Medications used to control PONV include the following:
- Dolasetron
- Granisetron
- Metoclopramide
- Ondansetron

HORMONES AND SYNTHETIC SUBSTITUTES

Hormones are naturally occurring substances produced by the endocrine system. Their function in the body is to regulate specific cellular and systemic functions. Natural and synthetic hormones are used to treat specific deficiency diseases, to enhance certain processes such as the antiinflammatory

BOX 12.8 Classification of Hormones and Synthetic Substitutes

Adrenal corticosteroids
Contraceptives
Estrogens
Estrogen agonists/antagonists
Gonadotropins
Antidiabetic drugs (insulins, oral hypoglycemics)
Parathyroid substances
Pituitary agents
Progestins
Thyroid agents
Antithyroid agents

response, to counteract neoplasms sensitive to hormonal control, and to maintain reproductive health. There are many hundreds of hormones used in long- and short-term therapy. Recognizing drug groups is important to an overall understanding of pharmacology.

Hormone substances are classified by their origin and action. The major groups are shown in Box 12.8.

CORTICOSTEROIDS

This group of drugs is used to reduce the body's immune response, especially in the treatment of autoimmune disease manifestations, asthma, and adrenal insufficiency. However, they are associated with many serious side effects, such as adrenal cortex suppression, decreased immune response to infection, and muscle atrophy, when used long term.

Examples of corticosteroids are the following:

- Dexamethasone
- Prednisone
- Betamethasone
- Methylprednisolone
- Triamcinolone

ANTIDIABETIC DRUGS

Diabetes mellitus is a metabolic disease in which the beta cells that produce natural insulin are destroyed by an autoimmune disorder (type 1), or natural insulin is not regulated in the body and cells are resistant to insulin (type 2).

Diabetes treatment includes the administration of insulin (for type 1 and often type 2) and drugs that increase the cellular uptake of insulin as needed, usually in type 2. Exogenous insulin for injection is available in different strengths and differing durations of action.

There are eight types of oral hypoglycemic drugs used in the treatment of type 2 diabetes:

- Sulfonylureas: Includes *glipizide* and others
- Alpha-glucosidase inhibitors: *Acarbose* and *miglitol*
- Biguanides: Includes *metformin* and others
- Glitazones: Includes *pioglitazone* and *rosiglitazone*
- Meglitinides: Non-sulfonylureas *repaglinide* and *nateglinide*
- *Dipeptidyl peptidase-4 inhibitors:* Includes *sitagliptin* and others
- *Bile acid resins:* Includes *colesevelam*
- *Dopamine agonists:* Includes *bromocriptine*

PROSTAGLANDINS

Prostaglandins are not endocrine hormones. That is, they do not originate from the endocrine glands. Instead, they are chemicals that are synthesized within the cell, and their effect is within the same cell.

There are many types of prostaglandins that mediate various effects in the body, such as the following:

- Vasodilation
- Platelet and leukocyte aggregation
- Smooth muscle contraction
- Vascular permeability
- Softening and effacement of the cervix during labor

DRUGS USED IN OBSTETRICS

Specific drugs used in obstetrics are administered to induce uterine contraction or maintain the tone of the uterus.

- *Dinoprostone* pessary tablets are used to induce labor.
- *Oxytocin* is used for the augmentation of labor.
- *Ergometrine* is used for the treatment of postpartum hemorrhage.

GONADAL STEROIDS

The gonadal steroids include estrogen in the female and testosterone in the male. In females, estrogen, progesterone, and synthetic substitutes are used for contraception.

EMERGENCY DRUGS

A special group of drugs used in response to physiological emergencies include mainly those that affect the autonomic nervous system and others used in cardiac and respiratory arrest. These drugs, along with intubation and airway equipment, electrocardiograph, defibrillator, and other devices, are maintained on a department crash cart that is checked at each shift for completeness and maintained in all departments of the health care facility.

KEY CONCEPTS

- The manufacturing of drugs is a complicated process that is highly regulated and monitored. Drugs are derived from many different sources using increasingly complex technologies. The source or origin of a drug can be related to adverse reactions such as patient allergy and sensitivity.
- Drug regulations protect the public from harm by establishing quality standards in manufacturing, packaging, storage, transport, dispensing, prescribing, and administration. All health care workers involved in these practices must be familiar with the rules and regulations associated with their specific role in the drug process.
- The identification (naming) of drugs follows rigorous international standards that contribute to public safety and establish a common language among health professionals worldwide.

- The drug process involves many people in multiple health care settings. Surgical technologists have a significant role in preventing errors in surgery. Knowing and practicing the protocols is part of a collaborative process with other members of the surgical team.
- Identification and interpretation of drug labels is one part of the drug process. Surgical technologists must be familiar with the drug label, its package insert, use, and the precautions associated with any drugs they handle.
- Prescription drug errors are responsible for more than 7000 deaths per year in the United States. Methods to prevent drug errors have been established at every stage of the drug process.
- Drug errors most commonly relate to miscommunication and a lack of knowledge on the part of health care workers who handle drugs. Errors are preventable by a conscious effort to learn and act on strategies that have been specifically developed to prevent death and disability from drug errors.
- Inaccuracy in basic drug computation is a significant cause of drug errors. Health care workers must be able to perform conversions among units of measure used in medicine and demonstrate accuracy in drug computation.
- Drug prescriptions or orders are provided by health care providers licensed to do so. To deliver the correct drug, in the correct strength and dosage, and in the correct form to the right patient, the surgical technologist must be familiar with the process and terminology of drug orders.
- A specific protocol (method) is used to receive and deliver drugs to the sterile field. This protocol has been created to reduce the risk of drug errors and is followed strictly for every drug in every situation.
- Drug delivery devices such as syringes are calibrated in small increments to provide a high level of accuracy. Devices not specifically calibrated for exact dosages must not be used in the drug process.
- The role of the surgical technologist in the medication process must be precisely identified by the health care facility and be in accordance with state law, especially state practice acts. Surgical technologists in every state deliver medications to the surgeon after receiving them from the licensed circulating nurse.
- As a participant in the drug process, surgical technologists are mandated to demonstrate competence and knowledge in the specific tasks and roles that they perform.
- The route of administration for any drug is critical knowledge for all health care workers involved in the drug process. An error in the route of administration can have fatal consequences.
- An understanding of pharmacokinetics and pharmacodynamics demonstrates advanced knowledge about how drugs work and their specific effects on the body. Even if this knowledge is not directly applied to a particular phase of the drug process, an understanding of the principles demonstrates the advanced professional capacity required to participate in the entire process.

REVIEW QUESTIONS

1. What particular drug policies are regulated by The Joint Commission?
2. What is a generic drug?
3. If the surgical technologist suspects that a patient is having an adverse reaction to a drug, what information is most important to give the surgeon or nursing personnel in the room?
4. What is an allergy?
5. Outline the headings of the medication process and describe them briefly.
6. How does the surgical technologist ensure that a drug is given by the right route?
7. What units are marked on an insulin syringe?
8. What is the rationale for pouring all of a liquid from its sterile container when it is distributed to the scrub?
9. What is the difference between a contrast medium and a dye?
10. As the scrub, how might you collaborate with the circulator to keep track of the amount of irrigation solution used during a surgical procedure?

CASE STUDIES

CASE 1

Discuss how the concepts of team cooperation, shared communication, and adhering to required protocols for drug handling in the operating room could have changed the outcome of the following *real case scenarios:*

- A pediatric patient undergoing surgery was injected with pure epinephrine during the procedure, because neither the medicine cup nor the syringe were labeled. The child died.
- A pediatric patient underwent surgery under local anesthetic with epinephrine added. The correct dose was calculated and administered in the operating room. At the close of surgery, the child was admitted to the postanesthesia care unit (PACU) for observation. However, during her stay in the PACU, she required additional administration of epinephrine. The patient died in PACU as a result of epinephrine overdose. The surgical team had failed to correctly document the administration of anesthetic with epinephrine during surgery.

CASE 2

One of the most common sources of drug error is failure to correctly label syringes and other drug delivery devices. The Joint Commission's "do not use" list of documentation errors was created to ensure that transcription of drug names and amounts are accurate. Analyze the case of a surgical technologist who labeled his medicine containers "heparin 100 u" and another "heparin 10 u." The actual labels should have been 100 units per mL and 10 units per mL, respectively.

1. What possible consequences might there be?
2. Why does The Joint Commission require "units" to be spelled out rather than just using "u?"

REFERENCES

1. Federal Food. *Drug, and Cosmetic Act.* Sec. 201. [21 U.S.C. 321] Chapter II—Definitions 1. Available at http://www.fda.gov/Drugs/default.htm.
2. Genyk Y, Kato T, Pomposelli JJ, Wright Jr JK, Sher LS, Tetens V, et al. Fibrin sealant patch (TachoSil) vs oxidized regenerated cellulose patch (surgical original) for the secondary treatment of local bleeding in patients undergoing hepatic resection: a randomized controlled trial. *J Am Coll Surg.* 2016;222:261.
3. U.S. Food and Drug Administration (FDA). *Sec. 201. [21 U.S.C. 321] Chapter II - Definitions 1.* https://www.fda.gov/media/80384/download. Accessed June 23, 2019.

BIBLIOGRAPHY

American College of Radiology. *Manual on contrast media*; 2018. version 10.3. https://www.acr.org/Clinical-Resources/Contrast-Manual. Accessed June 23, 2019.

Association of periOperative Registered Nurses (AORN). *Guidelines for Perioperative Practice.* Denver: AORN; 2015.

Hendrickson T. Verbal medication orders in the OR. *AORN J.* 2007;86(4).

Krunic AL, Wang LC, Soltani K, Weitzul S, Taylor RS. Digital anesthesia with epinephrine: an old myth revisited. *J Am Acad Dermatol.* 2004;51(5):755–759.

Hilal-Dandan R, Brunton L. *Goodman and Gilman's Manual of Pharmacology and Therapeutics.* 2nd ed. New York: McGraw-Hill Education; 2014.

Nielsen LJ, Lumholt P, Halmich LR. Local anaesthesia with vasoconstrictor is safe to use in areas with end-arteries in fingers, toes, noses and ears. *Ugeskr Laeger.* 2014;176(44).

Porth C. *Pathophysiology: Concepts of Altered Health States.* 9th ed. Philadelphia: Lippincott Williams & Wilkins; 2013.

Wanzer L. Perioperative initiatives for medication safety. *Aorn J.* 2005;82(4).

13 ANESTHESIA, PHYSIOLOGICAL MONITORING, AND POSTANESTHESIA RECOVERY

KNOWLEDGE AND SKILLS REVIEW

The following skills and knowledge should be reviewed before you start this chapter:
Surgical pharmacology

LEARNING OBJECTIVES

After studying this chapter, the reader will be able to:

1. Explain important anesthesia concepts
2. Identify anesthesia personnel
3. Describe the components of an anesthesia evaluation
4. Discuss the anesthesia selection process
5. Explain the preparation of the patient for anesthesia
6. Describe the components of physiological monitoring
7. Describe basic anesthesia equipment and its use
8. Describe the concepts of airway management
9. Define general anesthesia and describe induction, maintenance, and emergence
10. Discuss the difference between dissociative anesthesia and conscious sedation
11. Explain how regional anesthesia is used
12. Define common types of regional anesthesia
13. Define the role of the surgical technologist during the use of regional anesthesia
14. Describe the layout of the postanesthesia care unit (PACU)
15. Discuss the elements of a handover from the circulating nurse to the PACU nurse
16. Describe the Glasgow Coma Scale
17. Discuss unanticipated PACU outcomes
18. Define the purpose of discharge planning

TERMINOLOGY

Airway: The anatomical passageway or artificial tube through which the patient breathes.

Analgesia: The absence of pain, produced by specific drugs.

Anesthesia: The absence of sensory awareness or medically induced unconsciousness.

Anesthesia machine: A biotechnical device used to deliver anesthetic and medical gases.

Anesthesia provider (AP): A professional who is licensed to administer anesthetic agents and manage the patient throughout the period of anesthesia.

Anesthesia technician: An allied health professional trained to assist the anesthesia care provider.

Anesthesiologist: A physician specialist in anesthesia and pain management.

Term is defined and discussed in previous chapter.

Amnesia: The inability to recall events and sensations. In anesthesia, the patient's inability to recall events that occur after the administration of specific drugs. After the drug is metabolized and cleared from the body, normal recall returns.

Anxiolytic: A drug that reduces anxiety.

Apnea: Absence of breathing.

Aspiration: Inhalation of fluid or solid matter into the lungs.

Bier block: Regional anesthesia in which the anesthetic agent is injected into a vein.

Bispectral index system: A method of monitoring the patient's level of hypnosis during surgery to prevent intraoperative awareness.

Breathing bag: The reservoir breathing apparatus of the anesthesia machine. Gases are titrated and shunted into the breathing bag, which is connected to the patient's airway.

Bronchospasm: Partial or complete closure of the bronchial tubes resulting from spasm.

Central nervous system (CNS) depression: This refers to a decrease in sensory awareness caused by drugs or a pathological condition.

Coma: The deepest state of unconsciousness, in which most brain activity ceases.

Consciousness: Neurological state in which a patient is able to sense environmental stimuli such as sight, sound, touch, pressure, pain, heat, and cold.

Certified registered nurse anesthetist (CRNA): An advance trained and certified nurse licensed to provide anesthesia.

Delirium: A state of confusion and disorientation.

Discharge against medical advice (AMA): Self-discharge by a patient who has not necessarily met discharge criteria.

Emergence: The stage in general anesthesia at which the anesthetic agent is withdrawn and the patient regains consciousness.

Endotracheal tube: An artificial airway (tube) that is inserted into the patient's trachea to maintain patency.

Esmarch bandage: A rolled bandage made of rubber or latex that is used to exsanguinate blood from a limb.

Extubation: Withdrawal of an artificial airway.

Gas scavenging: The capture and safe removal of leaked anesthetic gases from the anesthesia machine.

General anesthesia: Anesthesia associated with a state of unconsciousness. General anesthesia is not a fixed state of

TERMINOLOGY (CONT.)

unconsciousness, but rather ranges along a continuum from semi-responsiveness to profound unresponsiveness.

Glasgow Coma Scale (GCS): A standardized method of measuring a patient's level of consciousness.

Handover (hand-off): A verbal and written report from one nurse to another to provide updated patient information.

Homeostasis: A state of balance in physiological functions.

Hypothermia: Subnormal body temperature.

Induction: Initiation of general anesthesia with a drug that causes unconsciousness.

Intraoperative awareness (IOA): A rare condition in which a patient undergoing general anesthesia is able to feel pain and other noxious stimuli but is unable to react.

Intravascular volume: Fluid volume within the blood vessels.

Intubation: The process of inserting an invasive artificial airway.

Laryngeal mask airway (LMA): An airway consisting of a tube and small mask that is fitted internally over the patient's larynx.

Laryngoscope: A lighted instrument used to assist endotracheal intubation.

Laryngospasm: Muscular spasm of the larynx, which may result in obstruction.

Malignant hyperthermia: A rare state of hypermetabolism that occurs in association with inhalation anesthetics and neuromuscular blocking agents. In extreme cases, the condition causes hyperpyrexia, seizures, and cardiac arrhythmia.

Moderate sedation: Defined by the American Society of Anesthesiologists and The Joint Commission as sedation during a diagnostic or therapeutic procedure that goes no deeper than the moderate stage or lighter. Under moderate sedation, the patient must be able to control his or her own airway.

Monitored anesthesia care (MAC): Defined by the American Society of Anesthesiologists as sedation at a level appropriate for managing a patient's needs and includes close physiological monitoring. The anesthetist/anesthesiologist must be able to convert to general anesthesia as needed. See moderate sedation for differentiation.

Nasopharyngeal airway: Artificial airway between the nostril and the nasopharynx; used in semiconscious patients or when an oral airway cannot be used.

Neuromuscular blocking agent: A drug that blocks nerve conduction in striated muscle tissue.

Oropharyngeal airway (OPA): Artificial airway that is inserted over the tongue into the larynx; used in patients in whom endotracheal intubation is difficult or contraindicated.

Perfusion: Circulation of blood to specific tissue, organ, system, or the whole body. Perfusion is necessary to maintain life in the cells.

Physiological monitoring: Assessment of the patient's vital metabolic functions.

Pneumatic tourniquet: An air-filled tourniquet used to prevent blood flow to an extremity during surgery.

Postanesthesia care unit (PACU): The critical care area in which patients recover from the sedation of general anesthesia.

Preoperative medication: One or more drugs administered before surgery to prevent complications related to the surgical procedure or anesthesia.

Protective reflexes: Nervous system responses to harmful environmental stimuli, such as pain, obstruction of the airway, and extreme temperature. Coughing, blinking, shivering, and withdrawal (from painful stimuli) are protective reflexes.

Pulmonary embolism (PE): An obstruction in a pulmonary vessel caused by a blood clot, air bubble, or foreign body. Causes sudden pain and loss of oxygen to the tissues that are served by the obstructed vessel.

Pulse oximeter: A monitoring device that measures the patient's hemoglobin oxygen saturation by means of spectrometry.

Regional block: Anesthesia in a specific area of the body, achieved by injection of an anesthetic around a major nerve or group of nerves.

Sedation: A state of consciousness in which an individual is only partially aware of sensory stimuli. Depression of the central nervous system. Deep sedation results in loss of sensory awareness.

Sedative: A drug that induces a range of unconscious states. The effects are dose dependent. At low doses, sedatives cause some drowsiness. Increasing the dose causes central nervous system depression, ending in loss of consciousness.

Sensation: The ability to feel stimuli in the environment (e.g., pain, heat, touch, visual stimuli, sound).

Topical anesthesia: Anesthesia of superficial nerves of the skin or mucous membranes.

Unconsciousness: Neurological state characterized by complete inability to respond to external stimuli. Unconsciousness can be induced with drugs or may be caused by trauma or disease.

PART I: ANESTHESIA

Anesthesia means "without sensation." The goal of *surgical anesthesia* is to allow the patient to tolerate surgery and maintain the body in a balanced physiological state, called **homeostasis**. The anesthesia team performs anesthesia and is responsible for physiological management of the patient before, during, and after surgery. They work closely with the other members of the surgical team to maintain safety in techniques such as moving and positioning the patient.

The anesthesia provider (AP) uses highly technical physiological monitoring devices to provide continuous feedback on vital physiological mechanisms that are affected by drugs used in the anesthesia process, the surgery, and the patient's condition coming into surgery. Continuous monitoring provides information on physiological changes that require immediate attention, including emergency situations.

ANESTHESIA CONCEPTS

Anesthesia is achieved by altering the patient's *level of consciousness*, by *interrupting nerve pathways that transmit sensation*, or a combination of the two. The following terms are very important in our understanding of anesthesia, how it works, and what happens during an anesthetic emergency.

Consciousness is a state of awareness in which a person is able to *sense the environment and respond to it*. In a fully conscious person, all autonomic and sensory functions are intact. Consciousness must be considered on a continuum from fully conscious to *completely unresponsive.*

Sensation is the *awareness of stimuli*. The nervous system is capable of many sensations, including hearing, sight, smell, taste, touch, temperature (heat and cold), pressure, and pain.

Analgesia is loss of pain sensation. Specialized nerves transmit signals from the source of pain to the brain. Analgesic drugs interrupt these pain nerve pathways. The neurons that transmit pain are separate from those for pressure or temperature.

Sedation is a state of consciousness described along a continuum. At one end, a person is fully aware of their surroundings and able to respond to stimuli. At the other end is **unconsciousness**, in which the patient is not aware of their environment and cannot respond to external stimuli, including those that are noxious (e.g., pain, cold, heat).

Central nervous system (CNS) depression refers to diminished mental, sensory, and physical capacity. It is another way of expressing sedation.

Deep unconsciousness, such as that achieved during general anesthesia, results in the absence of *protective mechanisms*, such as swallowing, coughing, blinking, and shivering. General (surgical) anesthesia produces reversible unconsciousness.

Coma is the deepest state of unconsciousness, in which most brain activity ceases.

Amnesia is the loss of recall (memory) of events. Drugs that produce amnesia are used during the process of anesthesia.

ANESTHESIA PERSONNEL

Anesthesia professionals, like medical, surgical, and nursing professionals, are licensed according to their academic level, knowledge as demonstrated through examination, and skills as proven through internship and residency.

ANESTHESIA PROVIDER

- The **anesthesia provider (AP)** administers anesthetic agents, performs physiological monitoring, and responds to anesthetic and surgical emergencies. This is the general term indicating the anesthesia professional who delivers the anesthesia and manages the patient's physiological response to the anesthetic and all other drugs related to anesthesia.
- The **anesthesiologist** is a medical doctor with specialist training in anesthesia (MDA).
- The **certified registered nurse anesthetist** (CRNA) is licensed to deliver anesthesia after achieving a master of science degree in nursing and obtaining certification in anesthesia. Specialty areas in the field of anesthesia care include chronic pain management and clinical anesthesia specialties, such as obstetrical, cardiac, pediatric, and ambulatory anesthesia.

The primary role of the AP is to provide an adequate level of anesthesia while assessing and managing the patient's physiological responses to the surgery and anesthesia. The primary role of the AP includes the following:

- Protects and manages the patient's vital functions during surgery
- Manages the patient's level of consciousness and ability to sense pain and other external stimuli
- Provides an adequate level of muscle relaxation during general anesthesia
- Provides sedation as needed during regional anesthesia
- Communicates with the surgeon about the patient's responses to intraoperative stimuli. This includes information on hemodynamic changes, fluid and electrolyte balance, level of muscle relaxation, and level of consciousness
- Reports and responds to any physiological or anesthetic emergency
- Provides psychological support to the patient throughout the perioperative experience

The AP monitors the patient from the time he or she enters the surgical suite until discharge from the hospital. Intraoperative care begins when the patient arrives in surgery and continues through the duration of the procedure and into the next phase, postoperative care. This begins when the patient is transported to the **postanesthesia care unit (PACU)** where he or she is carefully monitored to ensure a safe recovery and continues until discharge from the PACU. The AP is available to respond to medical problems related to the anesthesia, including management of postoperative pain.

CERTIFIED ANESTHESIA ASSISTANT

The certified anesthesia assistant (CAA) assists the AP in tasks that are delegated according to the individual's practice skills and knowledge. The CAA, who has a master's degree, performs a variety of functions on the anesthesia care team. These include obtaining the patient history and performing the presurgical examination of the patient. During surgery, the CAA performs invasive and noninvasive procedures such as drawing blood samples, administering medications, and placing invasive and noninvasive physiological monitoring devices. The CAA may also apply and interpret electroencephalographic spectral analysis, evoked potential, and echocardiography. The CAA also performs and monitors regional anesthesia such as spinal, epidural, intravenous (IV), regional, and other techniques under the direction of the supervising anesthesiologist and according to state law.

CERTIFIED ANESTHESIA TECHNOLOGIST

The certified **anesthesia technologist** is an allied health professional trained to assist the AP. This includes maintaining anesthesia and physiological monitoring equipment, preparing drugs and supplies, and assisting the AP during anesthesia delivery. He or she is knowledgeable about anesthetic agents and adjunct drugs, advanced pharmacology, all airway and related anesthesia equipment, emergency response techniques, clinical monitoring, and anesthesia procedures.

PREOPERATIVE PATIENT ASSESSMENT

Before surgery, the surgeon and AP or other qualified personnel (e.g., nurse practitioner, physician assistant, certified anesthesia assistant) performs a complete assessment of the patient, including history and physical examination. This usually takes place 1 week to 3 days before the date of surgery. The purpose of the preoperative assessment is to determine the patient's specific medical needs and risk factors for anesthesia based on any history of anesthesia and on his or her current physical and physiological status. The decision on the type of anesthesia to be used (general, sedation, regional) may also be discussed with the patient at this time.

During the preoperative evaluation, patients have the opportunity to discuss specific concerns about their physical or psychological well-being as it relates to the anesthesia and postoperative care. Patient education during the assessment often resolves many fears and misconceptions about the effects of anesthesia and pain control. The preoperative assessment is modified according to the type of surgery and known risks such as difficult airway, sensitivity or allergy to particular drugs, and previous anesthetic complications.

IMPORTANT TO KNOW *In an emergency, the assessment is performed just before the procedure and may be done in the patient holding area. Anesthesia risks may increase without an adequate patient assessment and history. At the very least, the patient's baseline vital signs and airway risk are assessed preoperatively.*

ANESTHESIA CLASSIFICATION

A review of systems and screening for specific conditions reduces the risk of complications related to anesthesia and provides the basis of the *anesthesia classification.* This system, created by the **American Society of Anesthesiologists (ASA),** categorizes patients according to their anesthetic risk (Box 13.1). The preoperative evaluation includes a current or past history of the most significant systemic disorders. These are shown in Table 13.1.

BOX 13.1 Classification of Patients by Risk of Anesthesia-Related Complications (American Society of Anesthesiologists [ASA])

ASA 1: The patient is normal and healthy.
ASA 2: The patient has mild systemic disease that does not limit the individual's activities (e.g., controlled hypertension or controlled diabetes without systemic sequelae).
ASA 3: The patient has moderate or severe systemic disease that does limit the individual's activities (e.g., stable angina or diabetes with systemic sequelae).
ASA 4: The patient has severe systemic disease that is a constant potential threat to life (e.g., severe congestive heart failure, end-stage renal failure).
ASA 5: The patient is morbid and is at substantial risk of death within 24 hours, with or without intervention.
E: Emergency status; any patient undergoing an emergency procedure is identified by adding "E" to the underlying ASA status (1–5). Therefore a fundamentally healthy patient undergoing an emergency procedure would be classified as E-1.

MEDICATIONS AND ALLERGIES

The patient's current medications include prescription and over-the-counter medications and herbal remedies. Drugs and agents that the patient takes routinely may interfere with, block, or increase the effect of drugs used during surgery. The patient's normal medications may be altered (decreased or increased) before surgery. Known allergies are very important, and these are clearly documented according to facility protocol. The patient is also asked about substance abuse, including drugs and alcohol, and about tobacco use.

PREVIOUS ANESTHESIA

A history of previous anesthesia is important, especially if the patient experienced any adverse event during the procedure or postoperatively. A history of poor drug clearance, cardiovascular problems, difficult airway, or drug sensitivity is significant to the choice of drugs and anesthesia methods under consideration. Attempts are made to determine the cause of the complications and plan the anesthesia accordingly. All findings are documented in the patient's chart so that other caregivers are aware of possible risks.

AIRWAY EVALUATION

Any abnormality of the **airway** or potential obstruction can create an anesthesia emergency. All patients receiving general anesthesia and selected patients receiving procedural sedation require an airway evaluation. The purpose of the evaluation is to assess conditions that may lead to an airway obstruction or make insertion of an artificial airway difficult. The airway evaluation is performed by the AP. A dental examination may also be required. Example features of the airway exam are shown in Table 13.2.

Mallampati Assessment and Score

The Mallampati assessment is used to predict the patient's relative risk for difficult intubation and airway obstruction. The score is related to the size of the tongue relative to the available space in the airway when the mouth is open (Fig. 13.1). This is directly related to the risk of a difficult endotracheal intubation. The scores are rated as follows with the higher score predicting greater risk.

I: The soft palate, uvula, and pillars are visible.
II: The soft palate and uvula are visible.
III: The soft palate and only the base of the uvula are visible.
IV: Only the hard palate is visible.

MUSCULOSKELETAL ASSESSMENT

Impaired mobility, skeletal injuries, and other structural problems can result in restricted range of motion during surgical

TABLE 13.1 Comorbid Conditions Important to Risk Assessment in Anesthesia

Category	Conditions
Cardiovascular disease	Hypertension Ischemic heart disease Heart failure Murmurs and valve deformities Hypertrophic cardiomyopathy Prosthetic heart valve Rhythm disturbances
Pulmonary disorder	Asthma Chronic obstructive pulmonary disease Restrictive pulmonary disorder Dyspnea Pulmonary hypertension Smokers (and secondhand smokers)
Endocrine disorder	Diabetes mellitus Thyroid or parathyroid disease Hypothalamic pituitary adrenal disorder
Renal disease	Acute renal failure
Hepatic disease	Hepatitis Obstructive jaundice Cirrhosis Remote history hepatitis
Hematological disorder	Anemia Sickle cell disease Coagulopathies von Willebrand disease Thrombocytopenia Thrombocytosis Polycythemia Risk of thromboembolism
Neurological disease	Cerebrovascular disease Asymptomatic bruit Seizure disorder Multiple sclerosis Aneurysms Parkinson disease Muscular dystrophies Neuromuscular junction disorder
Musculoskeletal or connective tissue disorder	Rheumatoid arthritis Ankylosing spondylitis Systemic lupus erythematosus Systemic sclerosis
Cancer or tumor	Carcinoid tumor Mediastinal mass

positioning. The AP therefore documents any joint replacements, previous skeletal injury, disease, and areas of nerve damage. This information is available in the patient's chart, and the AP may provide specific information to other perioperative team members before or during patient positioning.

NEUROLOGICAL STATUS

An evaluation of the patient's mental and neurological status, including cognition, speech, gait, and motor and sensory functions, is important for the diagnosis and also for establishing a baseline before surgery. Baseline evaluation allows comparison of neurological deficit before surgery to assess adverse events during or after the procedure.

TABLE 13.2 Features of the Airway Evaluation

Focus of Evaluation	Risk
Condition of the teeth	Check for loose or cracked teeth—could dislodge or break off. Look for infection. May require dental exam.
Absence of teeth	Difficulty in performing mask ventilation (cheeks are not supported by teeth).
Tongue size	May interfere with ventilation.
Head and neck range of motion	Poor ROM may prevent intubation.
Ability to advance the mandible	The mandible must be advanced to apply mask ventilation, necessary during general anesthesia.
Neck circumference	Patients with large neck circumference are at greater risk for airway problems because of compression of the airway by muscle and other connective tissues.
Dental implants, malocclusion, bridgework	Injury may occur during intubation.
Piercings in the tongue, lips, cheeks, teeth, or nose	Piercings create an airway obstruction risk as they become dislodged and fall into the upper respiratory structures.
Patient weight-to-height ratio (BMI)	Increased difficulty to perform mask ventilation in obese patients.

PSYCHOLOGICAL AND EMOTIONAL STATUS

Many patients fear anesthesia and pain more than the surgery itself. Common concerns are that they will have inadequate medication for pain or that they will become addicted to pain medication. Misinformation from various media sources and lack of knowledge about the pharmacology of analgesics often contribute to these fears. The AP or perioperative registered nurse can answer the patient's questions about the action and duration of postoperative medication, which frequently allays the patient's fears.

SOCIAL ASSESSMENT

The patient's social environment is important to recovery. The AP interviews the patient about care after the surgery and whether a caregiver or helper will be available after surgery. This affects not only the physical care of the patient but also the psychological support available in the postoperative period. Patients who are fearful or anxious about their surgery and the possible consequences for work, family, and social environment may have a higher threshold for sedation and **anxiolytic** (anxiety-reducing) medications.

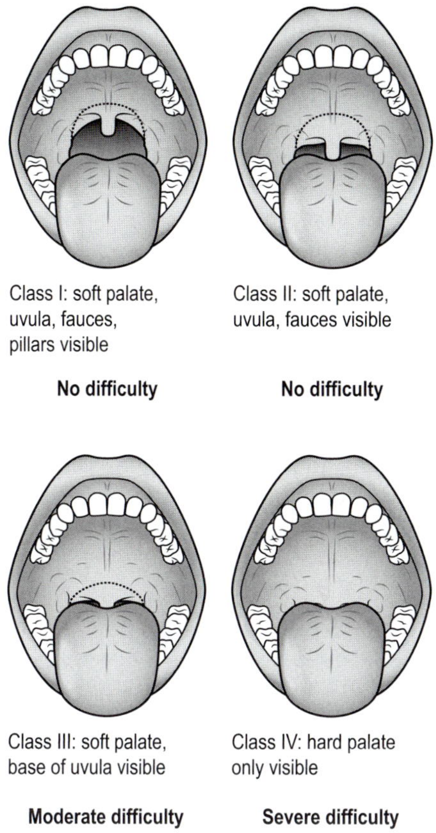

FIG. 13.1 Mallampati assessment for risk of difficult intubation. (From Cameron P, Little M, Biswadev M, et al. *Textbook of Adult Emergency Medicine*. 5th ed. St Louis: Elsevier; 2020.)

PREOPERATIVE INVESTIGATIONS

Diagnostic testing to determine the patient's risk level has been routine for many decades. In current practice, fewer investigations are performed than previously. This has been influenced by managed care and the streamlining of hospital stay and preoperative routines. Institutions vary in their requirements for preoperative assessment, and the rationale for ordering investigations is generally based on the patient's ASA classification. In these cases, the tests are intended to confirm or elaborate on a finding or diagnosis rather than to discover an abnormality. The ASA has determined that "routine" lab tests or other diagnostic screening is unnecessary. Instead, specific tests may be performed to establish a baseline for known risk factors such as cardiac, respiratory, and renal disease. Basic tests may be performed on high-risk patients. These include electrocardiography (ECG), complete blood count, kidney function tests, and specific electrolyte tests.

TYPE AND METHOD OF ANESTHESIA

During the patient evaluation, an appropriate type and method of anesthesia are selected. This is a cooperative and informed decision made by the AP, the surgeon, and the patient. The decision is based on the following:

- The patient's assigned ASA classification
- The patient's physiological status
- The presence or history of metabolic disease
- The patient's psychological status
- The type of surgery, including positioning requirements
- The length of the procedure
- Any history of adverse reactions to anesthetics and drug allergies

The patient's safety and well-being are always the primary considerations in the selection of the method of anesthesia. The medical and surgical goals are to provide the appropriate level of anesthesia without compromising the patient's safety. This means that not only the patient's physical condition and past history are considered but also the requirements of the surgical procedure. The surgeon may participate in the decision based on his or her knowledge of the time required for surgery and the extent of the procedure.

Patients participate in their own anesthesia care by expressing preferences. However, these must be informed choices based on safety and environmental considerations. The AP helps the patient choose among the "best choices." This is especially important for patients who have moderate or high risk factors to consider. Patients differ in their desire to be awake during the procedure, fully sedated, or only partly conscious. An informed consent to anesthesia, including risks and alternatives, is necessary for surgery to take place.

The choice between general anesthesia and regional (local) anesthesia often depends on the anatomical extent of the surgery and the anticipated anesthesia time required. Very long procedures and those involving the abdominal and thoracic cavities are not conducive to regional anesthesia. Superficial procedures and those of the limbs may be performed using regional anesthetics.

PATIENT PREPARATION: ONE DAY BEFORE SURGERY

One week or more before surgery, the patient will have had a consultation with the surgeon, AP, and others on his or her care team. Any investigations such as routine blood tests and other investigations will have been completed. The day before surgery, the patient prepares for the procedure at home, following the directions of the anesthesia team.

MEDICATION

Patients who take medications (including herbal products) on a regular basis must review these with the AP before surgery. This is to include or exclude certain medications from their normal routine in preparation for surgery as some may interfere with the anesthesia planned. The patient is then advised which medicines to take and which to temporarily stop.

PERSONAL HYGIENE

Patients will be advised to bathe the night before and the day of surgery. Scalp and hair are also washed to remove skin flakes and sebum. Depending on the surgery, the patient may be advised *not to shave* around the area of the procedure as this can increase the risk of infection postoperatively (see Chapter

17, Surgical Skin Preparation and Draping, for more details on shaving).

MAKEUP

Makeup of any kind must not be applied before surgery. The AP must be able to observe the skin. Also, makeup can interfere with airway and monitoring devices. Some procedures such as ophthalmic surgeries require patients to refrain from using eye makeup for 5 days or more before the procedure. This is to prevent any small particles of the base substance and pigments from entering the delicate eye tissues during surgery.

Nail polish must also be removed before surgery so that the nail bed can be observed. If the procedure involves the hand or foot, it is especially important to remove artificial nails and coatings as these may contaminate the surgical site and cause infection.

BOWEL PREP

Many surgical procedures require evacuation of the bowel the day before surgery. This can be done at home using a proprietary product or one that is prescribed by the surgeon.

ALCOHOL, TOBACCO, AND RECREATIONAL DRUGS

Patients must not use alcohol, tobacco, or recreational drugs at least 12 hours before surgery. This is to prevent adverse events in connection with the anesthetic agents and other medications required in the perioperative period.

PREOPERATIVE FASTING

Preoperative fasting is required to minimize **aspiration** (inhalation) of gastric contents during procedural sedation or general anesthesia. In the past, all liquids and food were withheld after midnight of the day of surgery. However, protocols have become less stringent for some patient populations. Strict fasting in pediatric and geriatric patients may lead to dehydration and electrolyte imbalance, especially when surgery is delayed. A safer and more realistic fasting period is now determined by the type of surgery and the patient's age and condition. A summary of the current (2011) fasting recommendations by the ASA is shown in Table 13.3.

TABLE 13.3 Summary of Preoperative Fasting Recommendations for Healthy Patients

Ingested Material	Minimum Fasting
Clear liquids	2 h
Breast milk	4 h
Infant formula	6 h
Non-human milk	6 h
Light meal	6 h

From American Society of Anesthesiologists, 2011.

IMMEDIATE PREOPERATIVE PREPARATION OF THE PATIENT

Every precaution is taken to ensure the patient's safety in the perioperative period. When the patient arrives in surgery, the surgical checklist is used to ensure that all preoperative procedures have been completed. This includes any special procedures, such as evacuation of the bowel (bowel prep), before surgery. The admission procedure is also important to the patient's emotional well-being. Reassurance and physical comfort are critical in this first encounter.

In the ambulatory setting, patient education is carried out before the day of surgery, and the patient is made aware of special precautions and procedures. Inpatients are prepared in the ward. Hospitals and other surgical facilities have individual check-in protocols. However, specific details are always verified.

PREOPERATIVE VERIFICATION

- *Patient identity* is meticulously checked. The health care provider asks the patient his or her name and verifies this with the patient's unique identifiers, the surgery schedule, and the medical records at hand.
- *Correct procedure, side, and site* are validated with the patient, the medical record, the surgical schedule, and the consent form. Preoperative procedures include the surgeon's skin markings on the operative side showing the location of the incision. These are matched with all other information available.
- *Surgical and anesthesia consent forms* must be signed according to facility protocol. (Details on legal aspects of the consent are described in Chapter 3.)
- *Resuscitation orders* and any other legal documents are checked.
- *Patient allergies* must be noted on all medical records, and the patient is asked about allergies again in the holding area.
- ***Preoperative medications*** are documented in the patient's medical and preoperative records. Any medication ordered but not yet given may be administered in the holding area as directed by the surgeon or AP.
- *Prostheses,* including dentures and hearing aids, must be removed before surgery whenever possible. In the event that the prosthesis is removed in the holding area, extreme care is taken to protect it from loss or misidentification.
- *Jewelry,* including body-piercing jewelry, is removed before anesthesia or any procedure in which electrosurgery is used. Any jewelry removed in the holding area is placed in a container, labeled, and placed in a secure location until it can be safely returned to the patient. A wedding ring may be taped in place.
- *Medical records* accompanying the patient are noted. Diagnostic results accompanying the patient, such as radiographs or other imaging studies, are clearly labeled.

TABLE 13.4 Physiological Monitoring Devices and Use

Type of Monitoring	Parameters Measured
Pulse oximetry	• Blood oxygen saturation • Heart rate
Automatic blood pressure cuff	• Blood pressure
• Electrocardiography	• Heart rhythm • Heart rate • Myocardial ischemia
• Capnography	• Adequacy of ventilation • Airway pressure
• Oxygen analyzer	• Delivered oxygen concentration
Ventilator pressure monitor	• Ventilator disconnection during general anesthesia and assisted ventilation • Monitor airway pressure
Temperature-monitoring probe (Foley type)	• Core body temperature
Urine output using Foley catheter	• Gross indication of renal perfusion and intravascular volume
Central venous catheter	• Measures central venous pressure • Rapid administration of fluids and blood • Drug administration
Weighing surgical sponges Use of a blood loss analogue	• Total blood loss
• Arterial catheter	• Measurement of arterial blood pressure • Obtain samples of arterial blood for analysis
• Precordial Doppler	• Detects air embolism
• Transesophageal echocardiography	• Evaluates myocardium • Assess valve function • Assess intravascular volume • Detection of air embolism
Esophageal Doppler	• Assessment of descending aortic flow • Assessment of cardiac preload
• Transpulmonary indicator dilution	• Cardiac output • Cardiac preload
• Esophageal and precordial stethoscope	• Auscultation of breathing and heart sounds

Historical Highlights

In the past, preoperative drugs were given routinely while the patient was awaiting surgery in the hospital ward. Patients were heavily sedated, and most arrived in the operating room disoriented and even unresponsive because of the sedative drugs. Heavy preoperative sedation can prolong anesthesia recovery, cause **delirium** and increase cardiovascular and respiratory risks, and produce many unpleasant side effects. For these reasons, *heavy sedation* in the preoperative period is no longer used.

SELECTIVE PREOPERATIVE MEDICATION

The current practice in anesthesiology is *selective* preoperative medication for patients with specific risks or conditions that can be mitigated by drugs, rather than a single drug routine for all patients. Adjunct drugs are given in all phases of the surgery to maintain physiological balance in cardiac, respiratory, and hemodynamic function as well as other metabolic states that require immediate pharmacological intervention. These functions are continually assessed through physiological monitoring.

GENERAL ANESTHESIA

General anesthesia is the *reversible loss of consciousness*, which is accompanied by the *absence* of the following:

- Pain
- Sensory perception
- Cognition (awareness, ability to interpret the environment)
- Memory of experiences during the period of unconsciousness
- Some autonomic reflexes

Inhalation (gas or vapor) anesthetic is the primary agent used in general anesthesia. However, many other drugs and agents are also used to maintain homeostasis and support the transition between the conscious and unconscious state.

ANESTHESIA EQUIPMENT AND DEVICES

Modern anesthesia practice requires highly complex devices and equipment. The advancements in technology have resulted in more refined methods for the delivery of anesthesia and physiological monitoring. Like the surgical technologist's instrument table, the anesthesia technologist and AP are very protective of their work area, devices, drugs, and equipment.

The following discussion includes basic devices and equipment used during general anesthesia.

ANESTHESIA WORKSTATION

General anesthesia requires the use of an anesthesia workstation, also referred to as the **anesthesia machine** (Fig. 13.2). This is a complex biotechnical device used primarily to deliver inhalation anesthetics and oxygen during surgery. All inhalation anesthetics except nitrous oxide are administered in the form of a volatile liquid that is converted into a gas using a vaporizer. The workstation is also equipped with a respirator and patient monitoring devices.

The basic mechanism for medical gases and anesthetics is a return flow system that includes the patient's inspiratory and expiratory functions. Important components are the vaporizer, ventilator, and breathing apparatus.

The anesthesia machine allows the patient to be mechanically ventilated or hand-ventilated with a **breathing bag,** which is part of the ventilator and valve system. Gases enter the bag

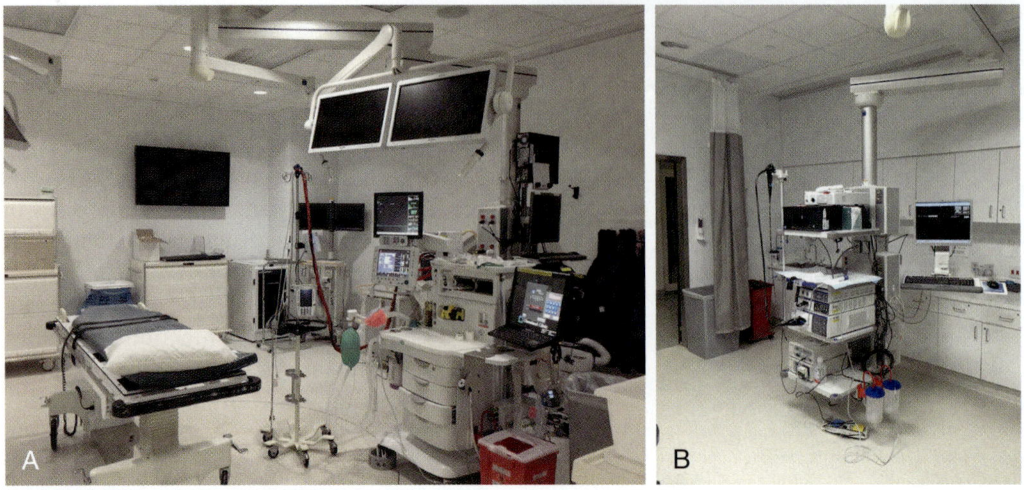

FIG. 13.2 A, Anesthesia workstation (anesthesia machine) Lower right. B, Endoscopy tower with light source, digital imaging controls, energy device controls, and suction. (From Bhavani S. Non–operating room anesthesia in the endoscopy unit. *Gastrointestinal Endoscopy Clinics of North America*. 26:3; 2016:471–483. https://doi.org/10.1016/j.giec.2016.02.007.)

and are then delivered to the patient through a tube, which is connected to an invasive airway or face mask. Exhaled carbon dioxide is captured from the system, measured, and absorbed by a soda lime reservoir.

SCAVENGING SYSTEM

Escape of anesthetic gas into the surgical suite is an environmental hazard for health care workers. **Scavenging** systems capture escaped gases and vent them through a vacuum line. The National Institute for Occupational Safety and Health (NIOSH) and the Occupational Safety and Health Administration (OSHA) regulate the allowable percentage of environmental anesthetic agent in the air. Scavenging equipment can reduce health care worker exposure by up to 95%.

More information on the hazards of environmental exposure to anesthetic gas is available at http://www.cdc.gov/niosh/docs/2007-151.

DRUG AND EQUIPMENT CARTS

The anesthesia team maintains and stocks their devices and drugs in closed carts, which are positioned near the patient for access during surgery. Each cart has a set of drawers with compartments to separate the items and prevent them from contamination. The devices and equipment contained in the carts *are not to be used by anyone except the anesthesia team.* It is common practice to have one cart reserved for airways and others for drugs or injection devices such as syringes, needles, catheters, and spinal sets.

MEDICAL GASES

Medical grade gases include oxygen, nitrogen, air, and nitrous oxide. These are available in the operating room through an inline hose from wall outlets or overhead booms (Fig. 13.3). Portable oxygen cylinders are maintained as backup for use during surgery or during transportation of patients recovering from general anesthesia.

NOTE *A complete discussion on gas and vapor anesthetics can be found in Chapter 12.*

SODA LIME CANISTER

When a closed ventilation system is used during general anesthesia, carbon dioxide remains trapped in the circuit using soda lime or lime. The soda lime absorbs the carbon dioxide and transforms it to water and metal bicarbonate. The soda lime remains contained in a disposable pack or canister. Dyes are added to the soda lime, which cause it to turn color (usually pink) as the carbon dioxide is absorbed. When the maximum amount of carbon dioxide has been absorbed, the self-contained pack is discarded and a fresh pack installed. In some systems, the soda lime is poured directly into the canister and replaced as needed.

AIRWAY DEVICES

Managing the patient's airway is a primary concern during general anesthesia or an emergency in which the patient is unable to maintain ventilation. During an emergency, such as cardiac or respiratory arrest, securing the patient's airway is the first priority. During surgery, the unconscious patient requires an invasive artificial airway to provide a sealed connection between the source of air, oxygen, and anesthetic gases and the patient's lungs. It also supports the patient's natural airway structures.

ANESTHESIA MASK

The anesthesia face mask is used to deliver positive-pressure ventilation with anesthetic gas and oxygen. An anesthesia face

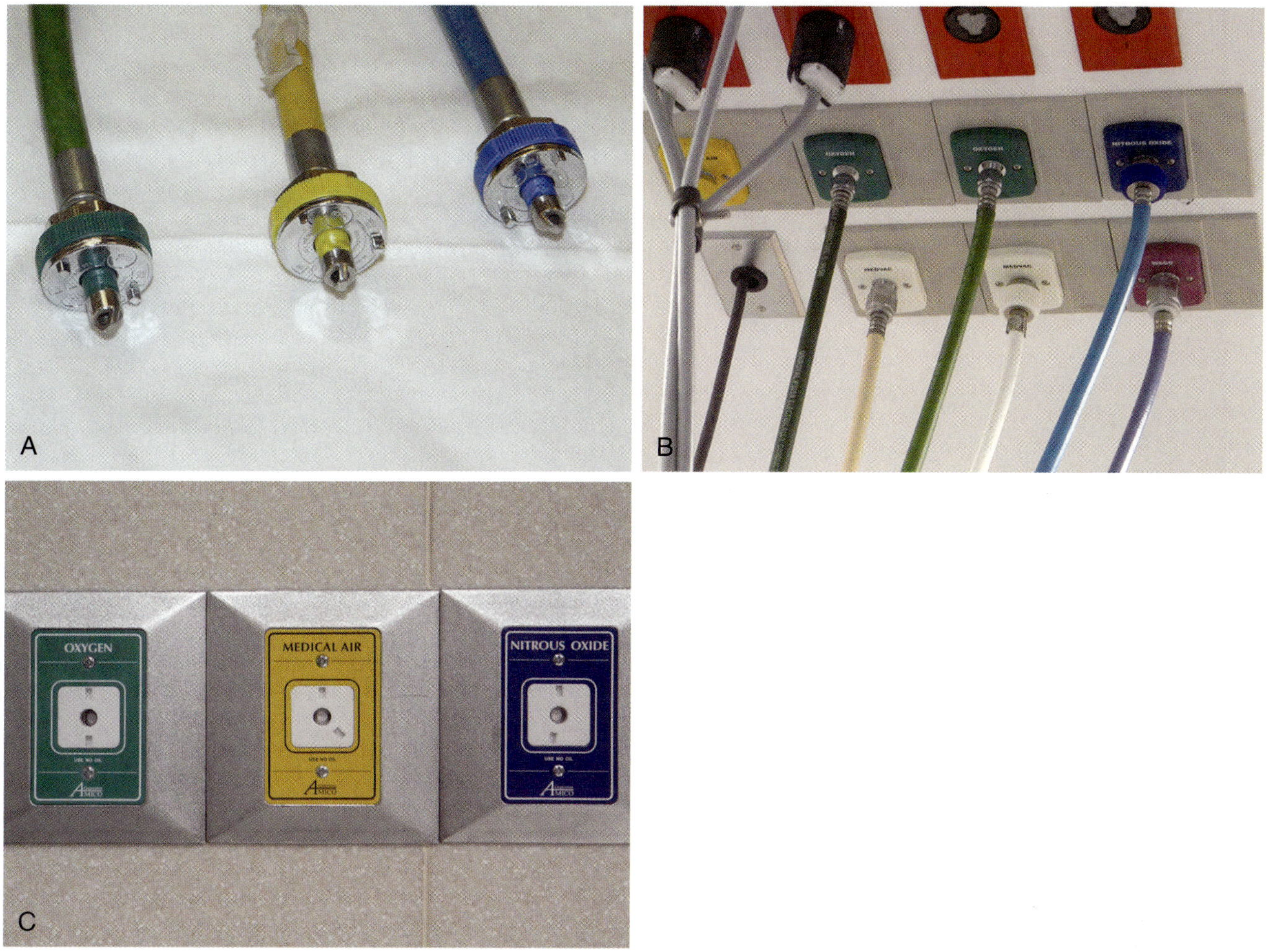

FIG. 13.3 Gas supply lines. (A) Ceiling hose drops. (B) Quick couplers. (C) Wall connections. (From Ehrenwerth J, Eisendraft J, Berry J. *Anesthesia Equipment: Principles and Applications.* 2nd ed. Philadelphia: Saunders; 2013.)

mask is generally not used in place of an invasive airway device except for administration of oxygen during brief sedation or to induce anesthesia in pediatric patients (Fig. 13.4).

ENDOTRACHEAL TUBE

The **endotracheal tube** (ET tube) is an invasive airway that extends from the mouth to the trachea. It is inserted orally or, less commonly, through the nose. The tube has a balloon cuff at the tip that acts as a seal against the tracheal wall (Fig. 13.5). The ET tube is used to convey anesthetic gases and oxygen to the unconscious patient. It is also used to ventilate patients who cannot breathe without mechanical assistance. The procedure for inserting the endotracheal tube is described below.

LARYNGOSCOPE AND ACCESSORIES

The ET tube is inserted with the aid of a rigid or flexible **laryngoscope,** which is a lighted instrument that is inserted into the trachea during intubation (Fig. 13.6). The tube may be guided by placing a flexible rod or *stylet* through the lumen of the tube to add rigidity. Once the tube is in place, the stylet is withdrawn. **Magill forceps** may also be used to grasp the tube during intubation (see illustration under Endotracheal Intubation below).

LARYNGEAL MASK

The **laryngeal mask airway (LMA)** is inserted without the aid of a laryngoscope and fits snugly over the larynx. The LMA may be used in patients with a difficult airway condition. However, it does not protect against aspiration (Fig. 13.7). The LMA is approved for use during cardiac arrest and is useful in prehospital emergency situations.

OROPHARYNGEAL AIRWAY

The **oropharyngeal airway (OPA)** is inserted over the tongue to prevent the tongue or epiglottis from falling back against the pharynx (Fig. 13.8). The OPA is commonly used when the patient is semiconscious, such as during the recovery period or during an airway emergency. The OPA is used in patients who have respiratory function but need upper airway support.

NASOPHARYNGEAL AIRWAY

The **nasopharyngeal airway** provides a passage between the nostril and the nasopharynx. This type of airway is used in semiconscious patients when an OPA causes gagging or when

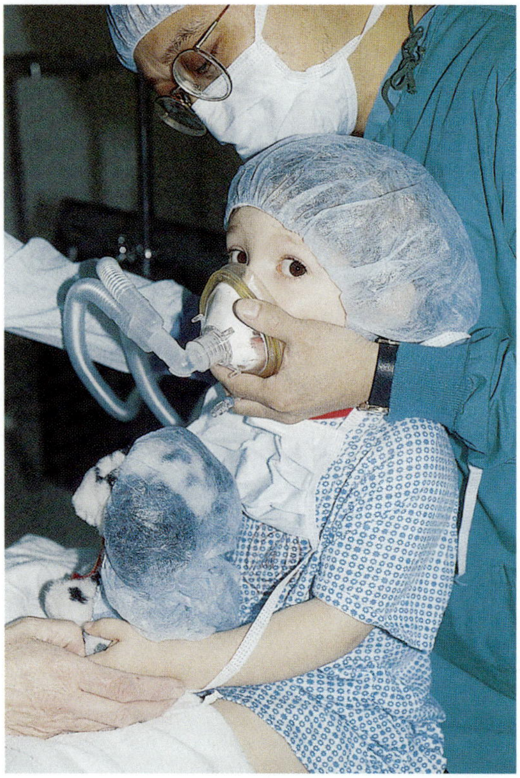

FIG. 13.4 Pediatric patient with an anesthesia mask. (From Leibert PS. *Color Atlas of Pediatric Surgery*. 2nd ed. Philadelphia: WB Saunders; 1996.)

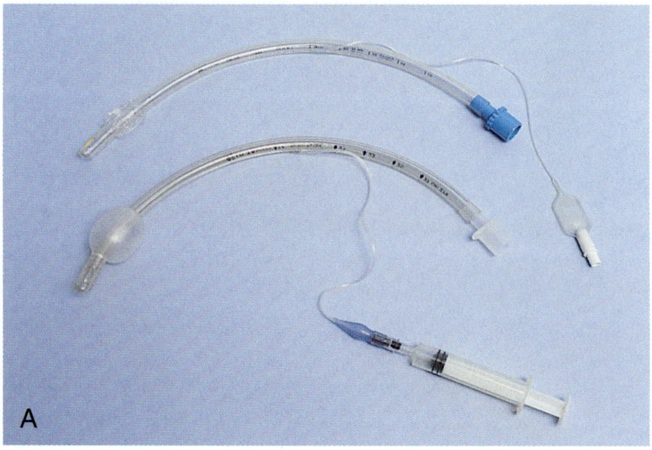

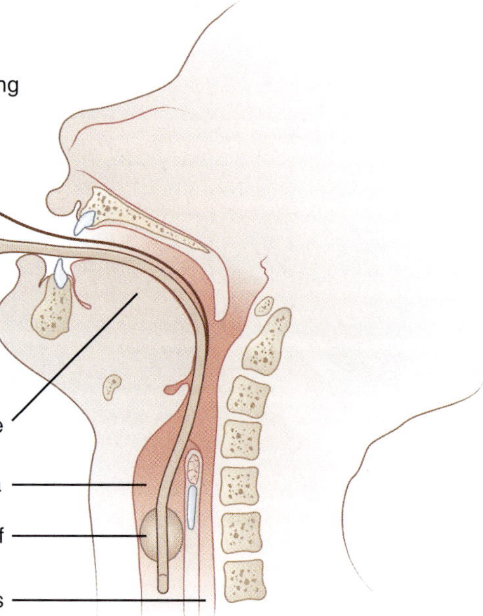

FIG. 13.5 (A) Endotracheal tubes—with and without cuff. (B) Endotracheal tube in position. (A, From Elkin MK, Perry PA. *Nursing Interventions and Clinical Skills*. 3rd ed. St Louis: Mosby; 2004.)

a mouth injury (e.g., fracture) prevents insertion of an oral airway (Fig. 13.9).

AIRWAY TUBING

Corrugated tubing is used to connect the artificial airway with the breathing circuit of the workstation. The tubing structure prevents kinking or bending and blockage of gases. A one-way valve can be attached so that gases cannot flow backward. A bacterial filter is also attached to the circuit to prevent bacterial contamination of the machine and possible cross-infection to other patients.

OXYGEN MASK AND CANNULAS

Patients who do not need assisted ventilation receive oxygen via a non-occlusive mask or nasal cannula (Fig. 13.10). These systems deliver a small amount of oxygen combined with room air. Face masks cover both the nose and mouth and can be adjusted to regulate the ratio of oxygen to air. This is passive delivery of oxygen, because the patient retains respiratory function. The oxygen level is controlled by a flow valve, which can be adjusted to increase or decrease oxygen-air ratio. This type of oxygen delivery system is used in the postoperative recovery unit and in other patient care units.

CARE OF ARTIFICIAL AIRWAYS AND VENTILATION SYSTEMS

Cleaning, disinfection, and basic troubleshooting of the airway circuit is the responsibility of the anesthesia provider and certified anesthesia assistant. Maintenance and testing of the machine are performed by the bioengineering department. All equipment that comes in contact with the patient must be decontaminated to prevent cross-contamination. Standard Precautions are followed whenever equipment is handled and used. The hoses, soda canister, masks, and airways are sources of high bacterial contamination. The intricate valve mechanisms may also harbor large colonies of pathogenic bacteria. The use of disposable patient air hoses, masks, and airways is preferred whenever possible. Nondisposable items are decontaminated and sterilized before use.

STAGES OF GENERAL ANESTHESIA

The most prominent physiological effect of general anesthesia is reversible loss of consciousness, which is maintained while the anesthetic agent is administered. When the anesthetic is withdrawn, the patient regains consciousness. The time- and event-related phases of general anesthesia are as follows:

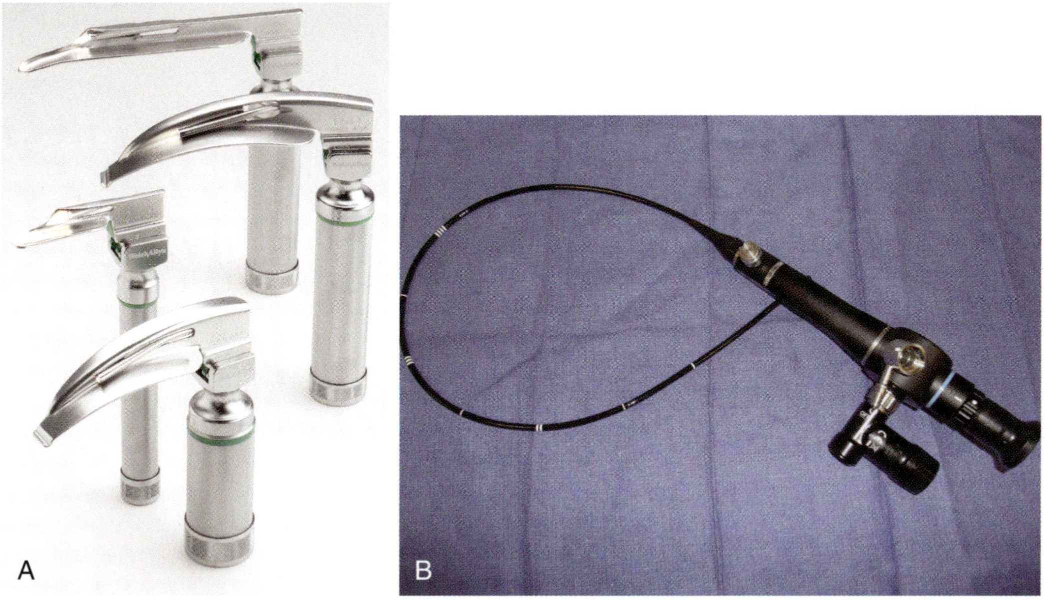

FIG. 13.6 Laryngoscopes. (A) Rigid laryngoscopes. (Courtesy Welch Allyn, Skaneateles Falls, NY.) (B) Fiberoptic laryngoscope. (From Ehrenwerth J, Eisendraft J, Berry J. *Anesthesia Equipment: Principles and Applications*. 2nd ed. Philadelphia: Saunders; 2013.)

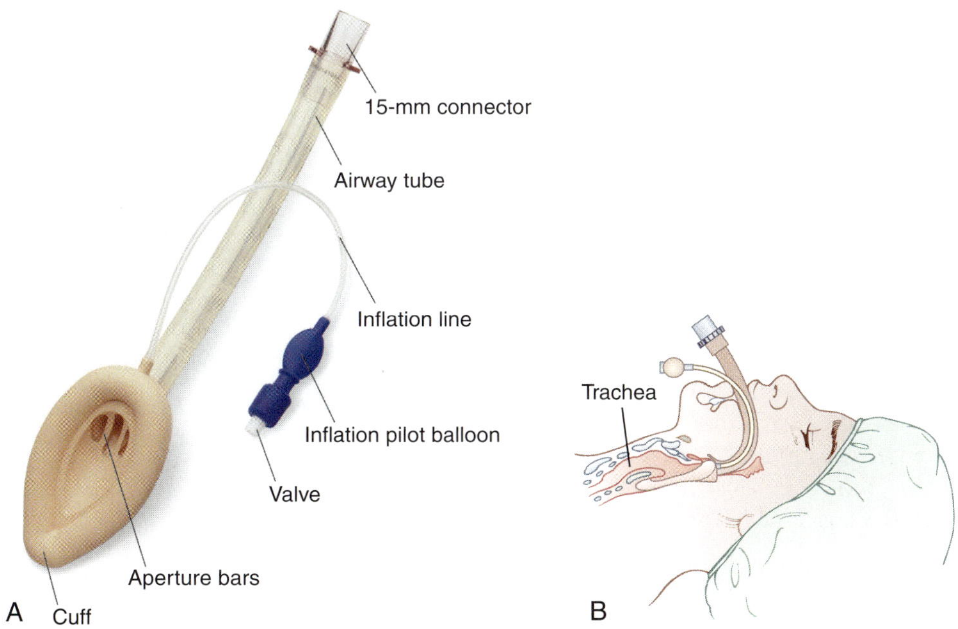

FIG. 13.7 (A) Laryngeal mask. (B) Laryngeal mask in place. Note the position over the larynx. (A, Courtesy LMA North America. B, Redrawn from Phillips N. Berry and Kohn's *Operating Room Technique*. 10th ed. St Louis: Mosby; 2004.)

1. ***Induction:*** General anesthesia begins with loss of consciousness. An induction agent (IV drug, inhalation gas, or combination of the two) is administered.
2. ***Maintenance:*** This phase involves continuation of an anesthetic agent; unconsciousness is maintained with the inhalation agent and adjunct agents.
3. ***Emergence:*** This phase is the cessation of the anesthetic. Reversal drugs may be administered, and the patient regains consciousness.
4. ***Recovery:*** Postanesthesia care is provided in this phase, which ends with the clearance of the anesthetic drugs from the body.

PRE-INDUCTION

The process of general anesthesia starts when all perioperative team members are present and preparations to start surgery have been completed. The patient is brought into the surgical suite, and noninvasive monitoring devices are put in place. If the patient does not have an IV line, the AP inserts one when the patient arrives and ensures that the patient is comfortable and relaxed. The patient is positioned supine (lying face up). If the surgical procedure requires a different position, the patient will be positioned after induction and intubation.

General anesthesia begins only after patient monitoring devices are in place and the operating team is present. The AP

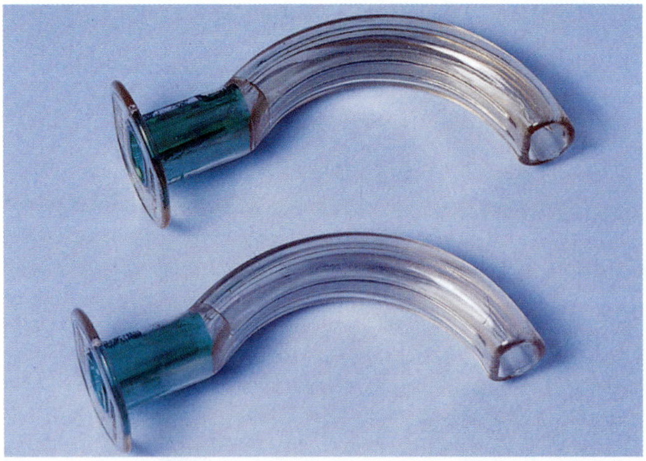

FIG. 13.8 Oropharyngeal airway used in conscious patients who require support of the pharynx. (From Elkin MK, Perry PA, Potter PA. *Nursing Interventions and Clinical Skills*. 4th ed. St Louis: Mosby; 2007.)

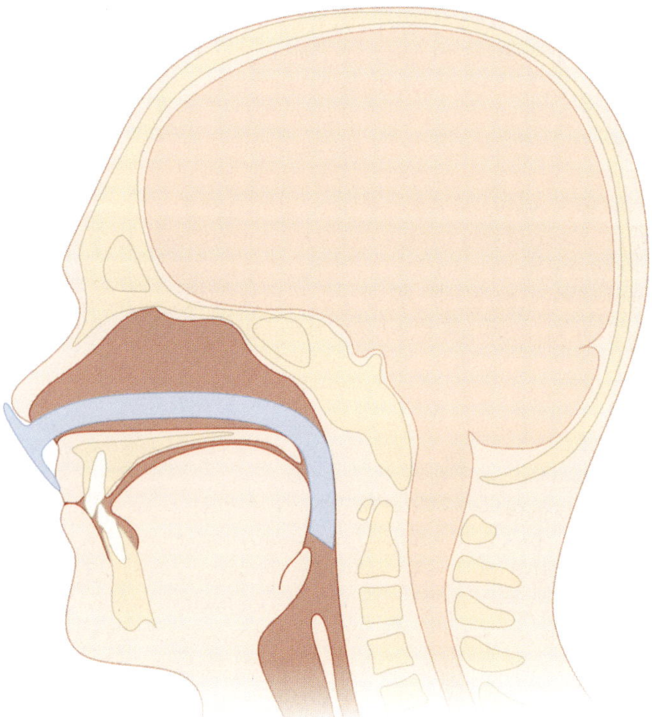

FIG. 13.9 Nasopharyngeal airway. (From Miller R, et al. *Miller's Anesthesia*. 8th ed. Philadelphia: Saunders; 2012.)

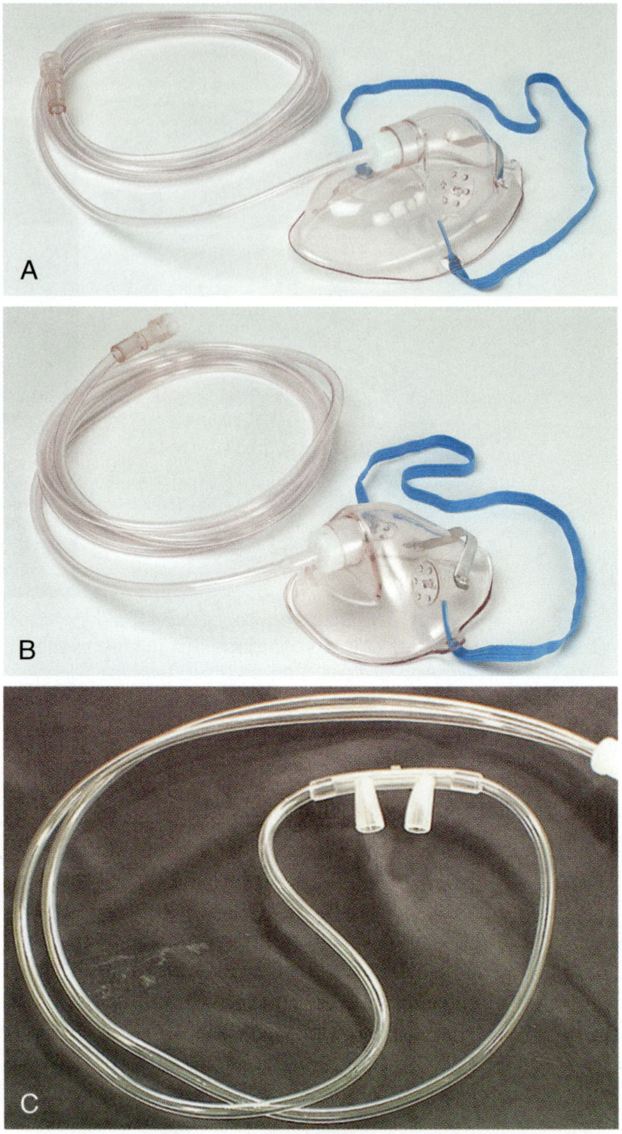

FIG. 13.10 Low-flow oxygen delivery. (A and B) Adult and pediatric masks. (C) Nasal cannula. (From Al-Shaikh B, Stacey S. *Essentials of Equipment in Anaesthesia, Critical Care and Perioperative Medicine*. 5th ed. St Louis: Elsevier; 2019.)

assembles all needed drugs and equipment and reassures the patient while evaluating the individual's physiological status. Preoperative drugs that provide sedation and reduce anxiety may be given during this period.

Suction must be available to the AP at all times. As long as the patient is in the operating suite, suction must remain operative. Inline suction is available from ceiling posts, cables, or wall outlets. When connecting suction cables, match the two ends of the connector, push, and turn the connector to secure it. This locking mechanism prevents the cables from separating.

Just before induction, the AP may administer 100% oxygen to the patient through a face mask. The purpose of this is to ensure that tissues are fully oxygenated during the next steps, induction and intubation. If a temporary airway obstruction occurs, the reserve oxygen will be available in the circulatory system.

IMPORTANT TO KNOW *The procedure for universal protocol in which the team validates the correct patient, correct side, correct surgery should take place before the patient is induced. However, surgeons are not always present in the room before induction. Because the entire team is required to participate in in the protocol, it should be delayed until the surgeon is present.*

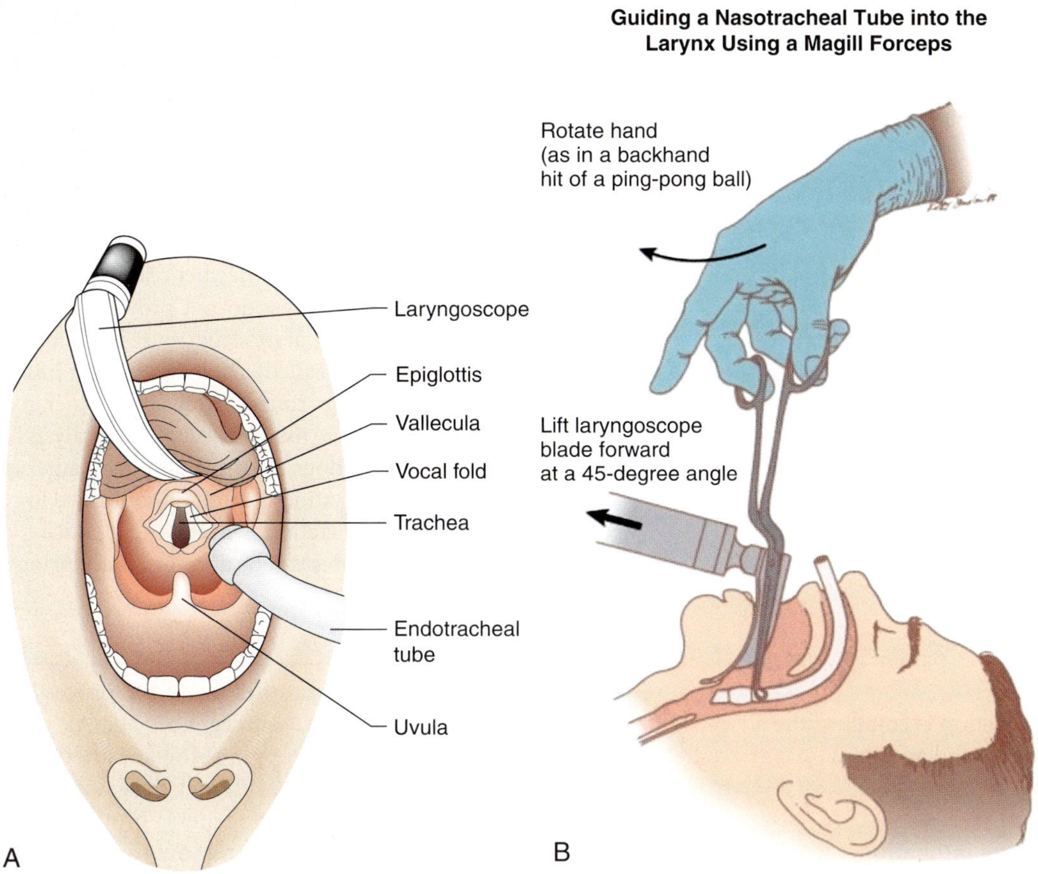

FIG. 13.11 (A) Endotracheal intubation is performed immediately after induction of general anesthesia. The airway is inserted with the aid of a laryngoscope. (B) Nasotracheal intubation with a Magill forceps. (From Miller R, et al. *Miller's Anesthesia*. 8th ed. Philadelphia: Saunders; 2012.)

INDUCTION

Induction is the transition between consciousness and unconsciousness. Three stages or levels of consciousness and a potential fourth have been identified on this continuum. Modern anesthetics and adjunct drugs allow the patient to pass through the stages very quickly, and they are seldom distinct. However, the surgical technologist must be aware of the stages, which may be pronounced under certain circumstances. The stages are the following:

- *Stage 1:* Begins with the administration of the induction drug and ends with loss of consciousness (usually within moments)
- *Stage 2:* The delirium stage, marked by unconsciousness and exaggerated reflexes. The airway remains intact and under the patient's control. The pupils are dilated. In this stage the patient is physiologically unstable.
- *Stage 3:* Surgical plane. The patient is relaxed, and protective reflexes (gagging, blinking, and swallowing) are lost. The patient is unable to maintain an open airway, and the respiratory response fails.
- *Stage 4:* Anesthesia overdose resulting in severe respiratory and circulatory collapse. This stage is never purposefully induced because of its lethality.

IMPORTANT TO KNOW *When the anesthetic agents are withdrawn, the stages occur in reverse order.*

The patient is induced with an inhalation anesthetic by mask or with an IV **sedative** or barbiturate, which causes unconsciousness within seconds. During induction, perioperative staff members must carry out their tasks as quietly as possible. Although induction takes place very quickly, the patient is able to hear well into the induction period. Conversation should stop, and care should be taken to minimize noise. The patient can easily misinterpret sounds and verbal exchanges during induction, because the ability to interpret the environment accurately recedes. Immediately after induction, the patient is intubated.

ENDOTRACHEAL INTUBATION

Intubation is the insertion of an artificial airway to support the natural airway and allow the administration of anesthetic gases and oxygen. Intubation is a routine procedure during general anesthesia and is performed in an emergency to establish and maintain the airway. Endotracheal intubation is illustrated in Fig. 13.11.

During general anesthesia, the patient is intubated immediately after induction. Intubation is a critical process, because the patient's respiratory status may be unstable. During general anesthesia, the circulating nurse or anesthesia

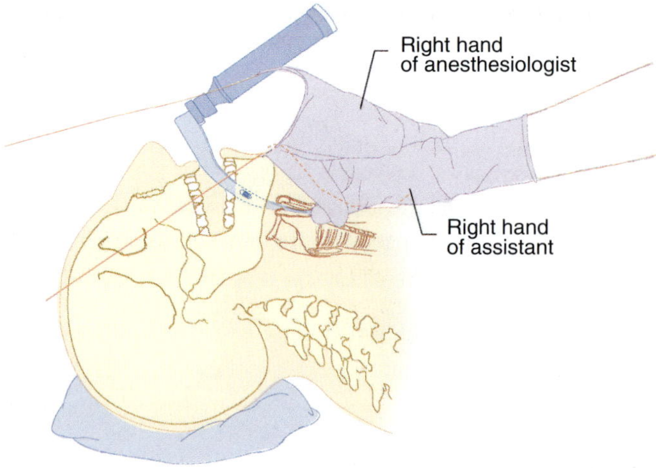

FIG. 13.12 Optimal external laryngeal manipulation (OELM) technique to enhance visualization of the trachea during intubation. (From Miller R, et al. *Miller's Anesthesia*. 8th ed. Philadelphia: Saunders; 2012.)

assistant stands at the patient's head and assists as needed during intubation.

As soon as intubation is complete the airway is attached to the connecting hoses and anesthesia-oxygen outlets.

Manipulation of the Larynx

Occasionally during intubation, the AP may require manipulation of the larynx to facilitate insertion of the airway. Three anterior neck maneuvers for manipulating the larynx are recognized as beneficial for successful visualization of the throat structures and intubation in patients with difficult airways. *All three require training,* which anesthesia and nursing personnel undertake as part of perioperative study. Performed blindly without training, the maneuvers can result in poor patient outcomes. Poor technique that is ineffective can result in the loss of precious time, which quickly leads to hypoxia, hypercapnia, and brain damage. Other adverse outcomes include rupture of the tracheal structures.

Three techniques used to assist the AP during intubation are the backward, upward, rightward (BURP) technique; direct *cricoid pressure* (CP or Sellick maneuver) used in emergency intubation; and the *optimal external laryngeal manipulation* (OELM) technique. In this maneuver, the assistant places his or her hand over the hyoid while the AP applies the correct amount of pressure to advance the laryngoscope as shown in Fig. 13.12.

MAINTENANCE

Anesthesia maintenance begins when the patient's airway is secured and inhalation drugs can be administered. During maintenance, which represents the period of surgery itself, the AP *titrates* (calculates and measures) the appropriate ratio of anesthetic agents and oxygen. These are delivered into the ventilatory system of the anesthesia machine and delivered to the patient via the airway. The levels of consciousness, analgesia, and sedation are continually monitored, along with physiological parameters. All drugs and procedures are documented in the anesthesia record throughout the procedure.

NEUROMUSCULAR BLOCKADE ("MUSCLE RELAXATION")

Adequate muscle relaxation is necessary during general anesthesia to allow manipulation of the body wall and other tissues in the operative site. Anesthetic agents vary in their effect on skeletal muscles. Most do not provide sufficient relaxation for surgery, and a separate drug must be administered. A muscle relaxant drug is called a **neuromuscular blocking agent.** This category of drugs causes paralysis by blocking neurotransmission to the muscle tissue. The level of paralysis is monitored continually throughout the procedure with a nerve stimulator, and the level of relaxation is carefully controlled to prevent overdose. If increased relaxation is needed (e.g., during deep retraction), incremental doses can be administered during surgery.

EMERGENCE

Termination of anesthesia and the process of regaining consciousness is called **emergence.** The AP controls emergence by withdrawing (stopping) the anesthetic agents and reversing the effects of the adjunct drugs as necessary. When the patient regains consciousness, protective airway responses resume, and the AP may remove the artificial airway. Removal of the airway is called **extubation.** A nasal or oral airway may be inserted at this time. Emergence can occur quickly and generally proceeds smoothly. Reversal drugs may be administered to hasten emergence. Occasionally, the patient (especially a child) may enter a state of temporary delirium during emergence. The older person may experience persistent reversible delirium that may require several days to resolve. However, this is a postoperative complication, not a routine occurrence.

RECOVERY

When stable, the patient is transferred to a gurney and transported to the PACU. During transportation, oxygen may be administered from a portable tank. Patients who require continuous cardiac monitoring are transported with a portable monitoring unit. The Joint Commission policy states that any patient requiring continuous cardiac monitoring must be accompanied to the PACU by a licensed perioperative nurse or physician.

PHYSIOLOGICAL MONITORING DURING SURGERY

In a state of well-being, the body responds to specific stimuli in the environment to maintain life. Many complex biochemical, physical, and metabolic processes control the balance between stimuli and responses. Examples are *shivering* (uncontrollable muscle tremor) when the body's temperature drops and *vasoconstriction* (constriction of blood vessels) when blood pressure falls.

During surgery, anesthetic drugs, position changes, and the trauma of surgery can alter normal body functions. Drugs that suppress the central nervous system, including general anesthetics, also suppress the body's **protective reflexes** such as spontaneous breathing, gagging, swallowing, and withdrawal from pain. Rapid physiological changes can occur during positioning (e.g., tilting the patient's body, placing the legs in stirrups). Many types of anesthetic agents cause changes in blood pressure and heart rate. Sedating and analgesic drugs depress respiratory function.

During surgery, the AP monitors the patient's vital physiological processes to quickly respond to potentially dangerous alterations. The complexity and type of monitoring depend on the type of anesthesia, the patient's physical condition, the known risks, and the anticipated complications. Basic and special monitoring devices and their use are shown in Table 13.4.

VENTILATION, OXYGENATION, AND PERFUSION

Methods of monitoring ventilation, oxygenation, and perfusion include the following:

- **Capnography:** Measures the partial pressure of carbon dioxide expired during ventilation.
- **Arterial blood gas (ABG):** Blood gases are measured using a sample of arterial blood.
- **Pulse oximetry:** The **pulse oximeter** detects oxygen saturation in the hemoglobin by spectrometry. The device is placed on a highly vascular area of the body (digit or earlobe) and provides continuous readings.

FLUID AND ELECTROLYTE BALANCE

The AP maintains **intravascular volume** and pressure using adjunct drugs, IV solutions, and blood products as indicated. Fluids are replaced using an IV infusion pump, which delivers the amount of fluids at a programmed rate. The selection of fluids depends on specific physiological parameters measured by rapid blood tests and physiological monitoring of circulatory and respiratory function. Electrolyte balance is measured by a blood test, and fluid volume is indicated by arterial blood pressure and blood loss. Blood loss is calculated during surgery by measuring the amount of total fluids (blood and irrigation fluid) suctioned from the wound and subtracting the total amount of irrigation fluids used. Blood loss is also estimated by weighing surgical sponges or by inspection of the surgical sponges.

CIRCULATORY FUNCTION AND PERFUSION

Circulatory assessment includes monitoring of heart function and peripheral circulation. Two types of methods are used to monitor circulation: direct (invasive) methods and indirect (noninvasive) methods.

- **Electrocardiography:** ECG measures the electrical activity of the heart, which is projected into a waveform. ECG leads are placed on the thorax in a pattern that accurately detects and transmits the electrical impulses of the heart to the monitor (Fig. 13.13).
- **Arterial blood pressure monitoring:** Blood pressure is measured manually with a sphygmomanometer and blood pressure cuff or automatically using a digital blood pressure monitoring system. Noninvasive hemodynamic monitoring is used in selected patients.
- **Transesophageal monitoring:** A transesophageal stethoscope may be used to monitor the heart's rhythm, intensity, pitch, and frequency during general anesthesia. Respiratory sounds and rate may be monitored through the stethoscope, which is attached to a small earpiece worn by the AP.
- **Intravascular monitoring:** Hemodynamic monitoring is used to measure central venous pressure, mean arterial pressure, stroke volume, and cardiac output. Noninvasive electronic systems are now used that replace the older style PACs used in the past (see next item).
- **Pulmonary artery catheter:** The PAC is used for critical care monitoring in selected patients. The catheter provides direct assessment of pulmonary artery pressure and indirect assessment of the left ventricular filling pressure. The PAC is inserted into the pulmonary artery via the subclavian, internal jugular, or femoral vein. Multiple ports (openings) are used for withdrawing blood or injecting drugs. Internally, the catheter measures pressure through a transducer and temperature via a thermistor. The PAC is used to assess the following:
    - Central venous pressure
    - Mean pulmonary artery pressure (PAP)
    - Pulmonary capillary wedge pressure
    - Cardiac output
    - Mixed venous partial pressure of oxygen (Svo_2)

RENAL FUNCTION

Kidney function can be measured by observing renal output during surgery. More specific tests such as blood urea nitrogen (BUN) are used to measure substances in the blood that are not effectively filtered by the kidneys. Selected surgical patients are catheterized before surgery so that fluid balance (input and output) can be measured during lengthy procedures.

BODY TEMPERATURE

Normal body temperature is 97° to 99.5°F (36° to 37.5°C). The body can tolerate environmental temperatures outside this range, but only with protection. The core temperature must be maintained within a range compatible with life.

During *general anesthesia*, the body temperature is measured with various types of internal devices. During cardiac surgery, probes can be inserted into the myocardium to monitor the temperature of the heart. A temperature sensor called a *thermistor* may also be contained within the PAC and used for direct measurement of arterial pressure.

Core temperature is also measured with a thermistor or coupler. Common monitoring sites used during general anesthesia include the esophagus, pulmonary artery, and nasopharynx. Other sites are less reliable. In particular, the rectal probe is generally only used with caution as it does not respond appropriately during **malignant hyperthermia** crisis.

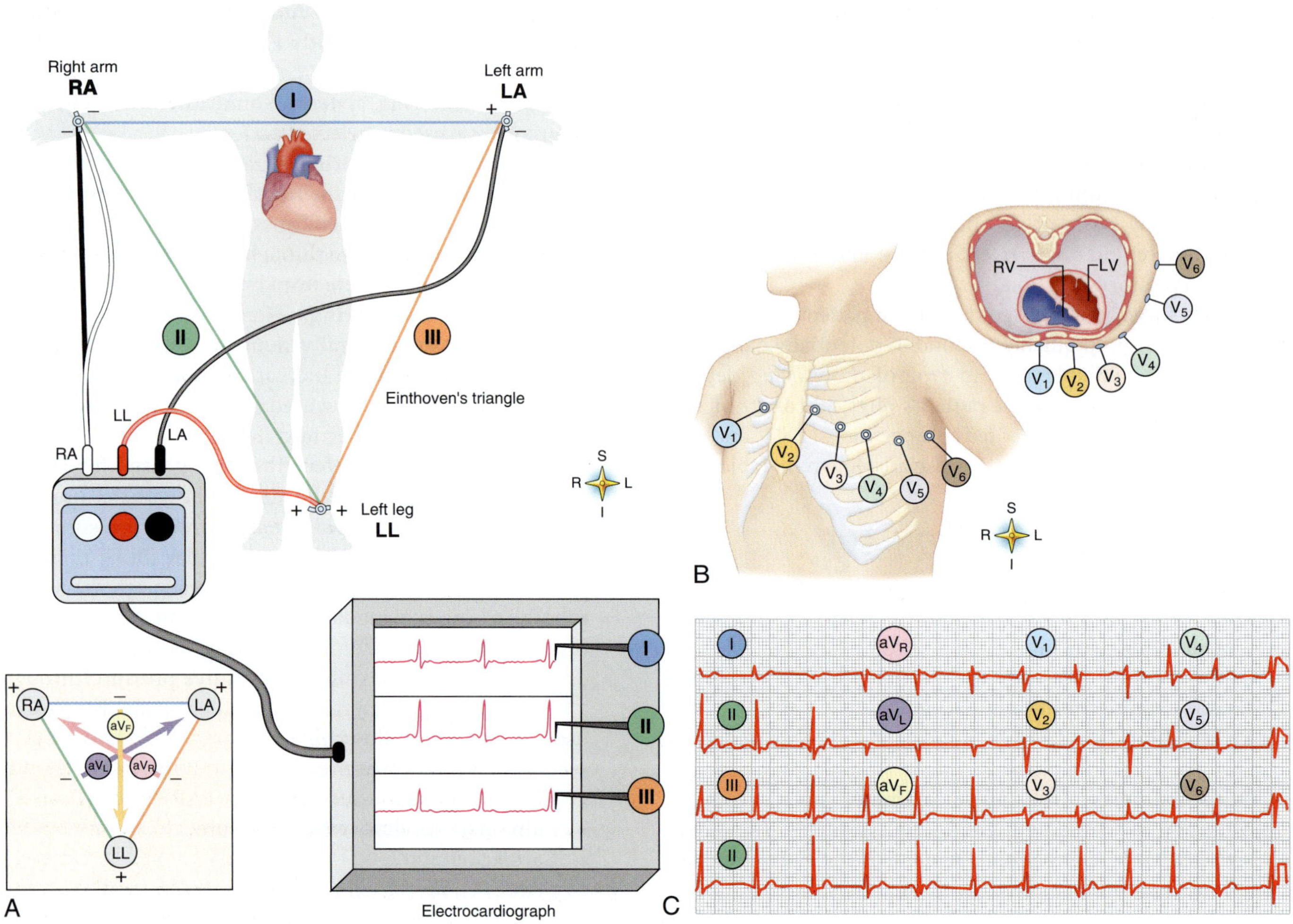

FIG. 13.13 Electrocardiogram (ECG) leads and output. Electrocardiography maps the electrical activity of the heart through electrodes placed on the skin. (A) Electrodes are strategically placed to record, amplify, and display voltage (potentials). Here, the limb leads form a triangle that reflects the basic pattern of electrical potential generated by the heart's pacemaker cells. (B) The chest leads produce a three-dimensional picture of electrical activity represented by the ECG pattern. (C) Each pair of leads is represented as specific patterns on a graph. Heart rate, rhythm, strength of conduction, location of impulses, and other information from the readout is interpreted to assist in diagnosis. (From Thibodeau GA, Patton KT. *Anatomy and Physiology*. 3rd ed. St Louis: Mosby; 2007.)

Maintaining Normothermia

The patient's normal temperature (normothermia) is maintained using medical devices that provide convectional heat. The most common method is with a forced air (Bair Hugger) blanket. This is a baffled air mattress that rests lightly on the patient's body. Warmed air is pumped into sections of the blanket via a flexible hose. The warm air blanket must be monitored to prevent burns. The temperature setting and the air hose-to-blanket connection should be checked before the unit is activated and thereafter at regular intervals throughout the surgical procedure.

The device should be activated only after the correct temperature has been verified with the AP. If the connection is loose and the air hose becomes detached during surgery, the patient's skin may be exposed to a direct stream of heated air. This may go unnoticed under the surgical drapes. Pediatric and geriatric patients and patients who are thin or debilitated are at particular risk for burns. Meticulous attention to any device that creates heat is the collaborative responsibility of everyone on the surgical team.

Other methods are also used to prevent heat loss from the patient's body during surgery. Irrigation solutions are warmed to a safe temperature before use in the body cavities. In the preoperative and postoperative periods, the patient is kept warm using conventional linen blankets.

Deliberate Hypothermia

Deliberate **hypothermia** (lowering of the patient's core body temperature) is used during an episode of **malignant hyperthermia** (MH). This is a physiological reaction to specific anesthetics and neuromuscular blocking agents, in which the body temperature is critically elevated (discussed later in the chapter). Hypothermia may be initiated in selected cardiac and neurosurgical procedures. Controlled hypothermia may be used to lower the body's requirement for oxygen.

Methods of Producing Hypothermia

Hypothermia can be achieved by a number of methods. Blood may be diverted to a cooling system, as during cardiopulmonary bypass. Other methods include IV administration of a cold solution and irrigation of body cavities with a cold fluid. During cardiac surgery, saline ice slush is packed around the heart to produce localized cooling. Target temperatures are no lower than 78.8°F (26°C).

Complications of induced hypothermia include cardiac arrhythmia, which occurs when normal conduction is interrupted. This can lead to heart block and cardiac arrest. Other organs of the body may also suffer damage as a result of inadequate blood supply.

Rewarming is achieved with a heating blanket, heating mattress, warm IV fluids, and warm cotton blankets. Shivering, which increases the body's requirements for oxygen, is controlled with muscle relaxants, selected analgesics, and further rewarming. The patient is rewarmed slowly to reduce the risk of circulatory collapse or sudden dilation or constriction of blood vessels.

IMPORTANT TO KNOW *Intravenous and irrigation solutions are warmed in a solution warmer. This is a thermostatically controlled cabinet that maintains fluids at a constant, safe temperature. Other devices and supplies such as blankets must not be placed in the cabinet unless the manufacturer's guidelines specifically state that it is safe to do so.*

NEUROMUSCULAR RESPONSE

During general anesthesia, neuromuscular blocking agents are administered to relax skeletal muscles. Without adequate muscle relaxation or paralysis, retraction of the body wall and other tissues is difficult, and this prevents adequate exposure of the operative site. Controlled ventilation by mechanical or manual means is required whenever a neuromuscular blocking agent is used, because the respiratory muscles are paralyzed. Neuromuscular blocking agents are discussed in Chapter 12, Perioperative Pharmacology.

A peripheral nerve stimulator is used to monitor the level of neuromuscular blocking. The stimulator delivers a series of painless electrical impulses. Muscle twitching in response to the stimuli produces a means of evaluating the degree of neuromuscular blockade.

LEVEL OF CONSCIOUSNESS

The patient's level of consciousness is monitored to prevent **intraoperative awareness (IOA).** This is a rare phenomenon in which the patient retains some degree of consciousness (including sensory awareness) but lacks motor ability. The **bispectral index system (BIS)** is used to prevent patient recall of pain perceived during surgery. BIS electrodes are attached to the head to measure the level of hypnosis during anesthesia. Although IOA is rare, the psychological consequences are serious and include post-traumatic symptoms.

PROCEDURAL SEDATION

Procedural sedation is a general term that refers to the administration of one or more drugs that suppress the central nervous system, alleviate pain, and reduce anxiety. Many recently approved sedative-hypnotics and opioids such as remifentanil and propofol are now used routinely, especially in the outpatient setting. They do not require an anesthesia machine, and the patient recovers more quickly than from general anesthesia.

LEVELS OF SEDATION

Sedation is measured on a continuum. Because patients are unique in their exact physiological response to the combination of drugs used during procedural sedation, the "correct" level is determined by its effect. Table 13.5 describes the physiological differences between levels of sedation and a comparison with general anesthesia.

WEBSITE BOX *The American Society of Anesthesiologists' website is an excellent source for information on anesthesia. The website is open and does not require registration: https://www.asahq.org/standards-and-guidelines.*

CLARIFICATION: MAC AND MODERATE SEDATION

Monitored anesthesia care (MAC) is a specific service provided by an AP. If a patient is considered high risk, the surgeon may request monitored anesthesia care by an AP who is qualified to "rescue" a patient who has entered an unintended (deeper) level of sedation or requires emergency lifesaving interventions. These professionals include the certified registered nurse anesthetist (CRNA), anesthesiologist, other physicians, dentists, and oral surgeons who have been qualified to administer sedation. **Moderate sedation** can be administered by the same group of professionals but also includes the registered nurse who has been trained and certified.

DISSOCIATIVE ANESTHESIA

Dissociative anesthesia is induced with the drug *ketamine,* which blocks sensory neurotransmission and associative pathways. The patient's eyes remain open, and the person appears to be awake, but he or she is unaware of the environment. The drug also produces amnesia of events that occur while the drug remains active in the body. Ketamine is administered intravenously or intramuscularly and is used for short procedures. It is used mainly in pediatric surgery in combination with other drugs to produce anesthesia and reduce side effects such as excessive salivation and delirium during emergence. Muscle relaxants are often used in conjunction with ketamine because the drug produces muscle *tetany* (rigidity).

The advantages of ketamine are rapid induction and metabolism. The disadvantages are related mainly to cardiac stimulation.

HISTORICAL HIGHLIGHTS

Neurolept analgesia and neurolept anesthesia are two methods of pain control and anesthesia introduced in the late 1940s. This

TABLE 13.5 Levels of Sedation and Comparison With General Anesthesia

	Minimal Sedation Anxiolysis	Moderate Sedation/ Analgesia ("Conscious Sedation")	Deep Sedation/ Analgesia	General Anesthesia
Responsiveness	Normal response to verbal stimulation	Purposeful response to verbal or tactile stimulation*	Purposeful response following repeated or painful stimulation*	Unarousable even with painful stimulus
Airway	Unaffected	No intervention required	Intervention may be required	Intervention often required
Spontaneous ventilation	Unaffected	Adequate	May be inadequate	Frequently inadequate
Cardiovascular function	Unaffected	Usually maintained	Usually maintained	May be impaired

**Reflex* withdrawal from pain stimulus not considered a purposeful response.
From The American Society of Anesthesiologists, Quality Management and Departmental Administration, 2014. https://www.asahq.org/standards-and-guidelines/continuum-of-depth-of-sedation-definition-of-general-anesthesia-and-levels-of-sedationanalgesia.

technique involved a combination of drugs (anxiolytics and powerful analgesics) that suppressed the autonomic nervous system and resulted in immobility. The method was retired from human medicine many years ago as much safer and more predictable drugs were developed for conscious sedation.

REGIONAL ANESTHESIA

Regional anesthesia provides reversible loss of sensation in a specific area of the body without affecting consciousness. Regional anesthesia is also called *conductive* or *local anesthesia*. The term *regional* is preferred, because it describes the process more accurately. This type of anesthesia can be used in a small superficial area of skin and subcutaneous tissue or in an entire region of the body, such as during spinal anesthesia. Patient monitoring is always performed during regional anesthesia. The level and scope of monitoring depend on the patient's condition and whether sedation is required during the procedure.

The most common uses of regional anesthesia are the following:

- Limb surgery, in which complete nerve block is possible
- Procedures in which consciousness is desirable or required (e.g., obstetrical procedures)
- Minor superficial procedures
- Patients for whom general anesthesia poses a significant physiological risk

Regional anesthesia can be provided to a single nerve, to a group of nerves, or to an area of the spinal cord. When sensory nerve transmission is interrupted, tissues that transmit signals along that nerve are unable to receive pain signals.

Patients undergoing regional anesthesia are monitored according to their age, and any pre-existing conditions that put them at risk for the procedure.

DRUG DOSAGE

The effective dosage of anesthetic is calculated according to the individual patient's ability to absorb and metabolize the drug. The "normal" or safe dosage depends on many factors. Therapeutic ranges for all local anesthetics are considered with knowledge of the patient's physical condition, especially the presence of cardiac disease, concurrent use of other drugs, and the patient's age, weight, and vascular status.

The rate of metabolism and response to the drug determine whether toxic levels are being reached. External monitoring is an objective method of detecting signs of toxicity. This is especially important in patients who require large amounts of anesthetic.

TOPICAL ANESTHESIA

Topical anesthesia is used on skin, mucous membranes, and superficial eye tissues. Topical anesthetics are used before insertion of endotracheal and LMA devices and before laryngoscopy and bronchoscopy to prevent reflexive gagging. During regional cystoscopy procedures, transurethral instruments may be coated with a topical anesthetic gel to ease insertion. Topical agents are readily absorbed through the mucous membranes. Although the amount of agent applied is limited, the patient is monitored for toxic reactions.

LOCAL INFILTRATION

Local infiltration is injection of an anesthetic into superficial tissues to produce a small area of anesthesia. The combination of an anesthetic and epinephrine is sometimes used to constrict blood vessels at the infiltration site and prevent dissipation of the anesthetic through the vascular system. Epinephrine also facilitates entry of the anesthetic into the nerve cell. Examples of procedures performed with local infiltration are excision of a skin lesion and insertion of a chest tube.

Role of the Surgical Technologist in Local Filtration

Local infiltration takes place after the patient has been prepped and draped as part of the surgical procedure. The scrubbed technologist assists the surgeon during infiltration at the start of the procedure and at intervals during the surgery as increased anesthetic is requested by the surgeon. The required supplies and procedure for assisting during infiltration anesthesia are shown in Box 13.2.

RISKS The ST's responsibilities during local infiltration are very specific and are carried out using strict standards. Anesthetic

BOX 13.2 Procedure for Assisting During Local Infiltration Anesthesia

1. Prepare supplies:
   At least two 25-, 26-, or 30-gauge needles 1-to 1-½-inch length
   Two 10 or 20 mL Luer-Lok syringes
   Radiopaque sponges ("Raytecs")
   Medicine container for anesthetic agent
   Labels (preprinted are preferred)
   Waterproof marker
2. Receive the anesthetic drug.
   Verify the amount and strength using proper technique (described fully in Chapter 12).
   Immediately label the medicine container.
   Draw the anesthetic up into a syringe. Fill to capacity. A second syringe may be prepared for extensive infiltration.
   Do not load syringes partway. This may cause confusion about the amount of anesthetic used during the procedure.
   A small-gauge needle is used to begin infiltration. A larger one is used to complete it.
   Label the syringes immediately.
3. Separate all syringes and needles used for infiltration from others on the instrument table.
4. When the anesthetic is requested by the surgeon, state the name and strength by its percent.
5. When using managing anesthetic + epinephrine, you must know and label the exact ratio on the medicine container and syringes.
   Note the total amount of anesthetic used and report this to the circulating nurse as required for documentation.

drugs used are relatively safe. However, as the amount of drug injected increases, the risk for adverse events also increases.

The addition of epinephrine to the anesthetic also raises the risk for adverse events.

IMPORTANT TO KNOW *Epinephrine is a high-alert drug. Deaths related to lidocaine with epinephrine in which the surgical technologist was involved have been related to incorrect labeling, no labeling, failure to report the correct amount of drug used during surgery, and the wrong drug passed to the surgeon.*

PERIPHERAL NERVE BLOCK

A peripheral nerve block provides anesthesia to a specific area of the body supplied by a major nerve or nerve plexus (group). This results in blockade to a single nerve and its branches. Anesthetic agent is injected into the adjacent tissue, not into the nerve itself.

The peripheral block is performed after a surgical skin prep of the injection area. The nerve block may be performed as part of the surgical procedure or separately before the surgical skin prep and draping. The procedure for injection is similar to infiltration anesthesia. The scrub assists when the nerve block is carried out as part of the surgery.

INTRAVENOUS (BIER) BLOCK

Intravenous regional anesthesia is often referred to as a **Bier block** (Fig. 13.14). In this procedure, blood is temporarily displaced from a limb and replaced by a local anesthetic drug. To displace the venous blood, an air-filled **pneumatic tourniquet** is placed around the proximal end of the limb. The AP then displaces blood in the limb using a latex-free bandage **(Esmarch bandage).** The bandage is wrapped around the entire length of the extremity, starting at the distal end and extending to the proximal end. This flushes the blood in a proximal direction. The tourniquet is then inflated, and the Esmarch bandage is removed. Anesthetic is injected into the major vein through a previously placed IV catheter. Double tourniquets may also be used, one proximal and one distal. The tourniquet "time" starts at the beginning of inflation and continues until the tourniquet is released. The safe tourniquet time and pressure depend on the patient's age, general condition, size, and the surgical site.

Role of the Surgical Technologist

The surgical technologist assists in a Bier block by having the necessary supplies and equipment prepared. The Bier block is an IV procedure and is performed using aseptic technique, including skin prep and draping as described in Chapter 17. The hand may be excluded from the prep with an occlusive drape. The scrubbed technologist assists in draping the patient's arm and preparing the sterile equipment. The AP usually directs and performs the procedure. The surgeon or surgical technologist assists as needed. The scrub may be required by hospital policy to regown and reglove after the Bier block is performed and before the surgery begins.

SPINAL ANESTHESIA

Spinal anesthesia is the injection of anesthetic into the *intrathecal* (subarachnoid) space. To help facilitate correct placement of the anesthetic in the spinal canal, dextrose is added to the agent. This makes the drug heavier than the cerebrospinal fluid. In relation to the patient's position, the drug settles in the dependent areas (those affected by gravity) and is absorbed at a specific site along the spinal cord.

Conduction along the nerve roots that emerge from that location is blocked, and anesthesia is achieved. The anesthetic can be directed up, down, or laterally by tilting the operating table. Spinal anesthesia can be used for many procedures but is most often used for gynecological, obstetrical, orthopedic, and genitourinary surgery.

Patient Preparation

To facilitate exact placement of the spinal needle for injection, the patient must be positioned in a way that widens the intervertebral space. Two positions are used to achieve this: lateral (side-lying) or sitting. A lateral position is used with the patient's knees drawn up to facilitate exposure of the intervertebral spaces. The circulator stabilizes the patient's shoulders with one hand while providing support behind the patient's knees

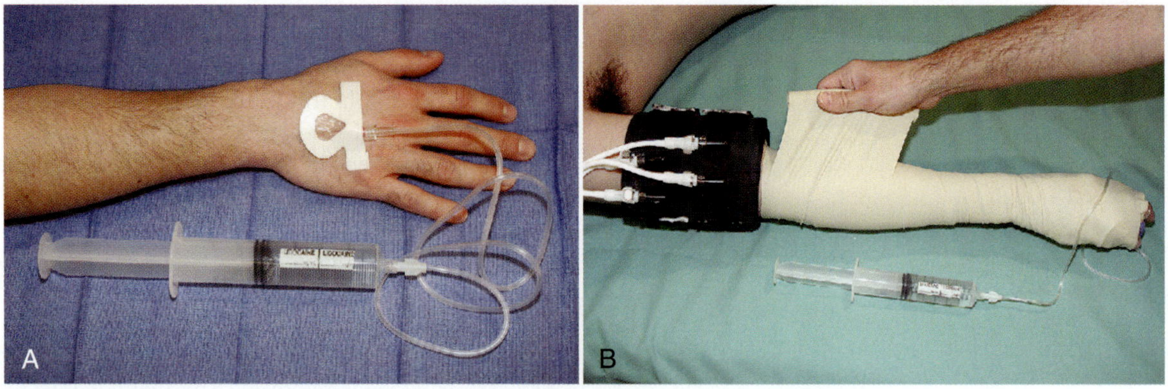

FIG. 13.14 Intravenous vascular anesthesia (Bier block for surgery of the arm using a double cuff tourniquet. (A) The vein is cannulated and the anesthetic syringe attached via connection tubing. The deflated tourniquets are placed around the arm, which has been encircled with soft cotton wrap. B, The arm is exsanguinated using an Esmarch bandage, which is wrapped sequentially from hand to arm. The tourniquet is inflated and the anesthetic injected into the vein. (From Gropper MA. *Miller's Anesthesia*. 9th ed. St Louis: Elsevier; 2020.)

with the other, as shown in Fig. 13.15. The patient may also sit on the edge of the operating table and bend forward to create a rounded back. In this case, the circulator should support the patient as shown in Fig. 13.16. The patient may be covered with a blanket or sheet so that only the injection area is exposed. This provides warmth and protects the patient's modesty.

Procedure

When the patient has been positioned correctly, the AP prepares the injection site with antiseptic and applies a small sterile drape. The spinal injection site is infiltrated with a small amount of local anesthetic. A spinal needle is then inserted into the intervertebral and subarachnoid spaces, and the anesthetic is injected. The patient is placed in the supine position with a slight downward tilt (Trendelenburg position) to maintain a safe level of anesthesia. Patients given spinal anesthesia receive continuous physiological monitoring throughout the procedure and are given adjunct drugs to provide mild sedation and relaxation.

Role of the Surgical Technologist

The circulating surgical technologist assists in the procedure by preparing the spinal tray and the correct size of the spinal needles, prep solution, and drapes as needed. The circulator helps the patient maintain his or her position during the procedure and verifies the type and strength of anesthetic used.

Risks of Spinal Anesthesia

Risks associated with spinal anesthesia include the following:

- *Hypotension:* A severe decrease in blood pressure may occur, resulting in pooling of blood in the lower extremities.
- *Postspinal headache:* This condition is related to decreased cerebrospinal pressure resulting from a leak in the dura mater at the injection site.
- *Total spinal anesthesia:* This occurs when the hyperbaric spinal anesthetic blocks the nerves controlling the diaphragm and accessory breathing muscles.

EPIDURAL AND CAUDAL BLOCK

Epidural anesthesia is produced when the anesthetic agent is injected into the epidural space that surrounds the dural sac. The space contains connective tissue, an extensive vascular system, and the spinal nerve roots. Caudal and epidural anesthesia target the epidural space. However, in epidural anesthesia, the approach is through the lumbar interspace, whereas in caudal anesthesia, the caudal canal is used. A caudal epidural blockade produces analgesia of the perineum and groin.

After injection, the anesthetic agent is very slowly absorbed into the cerebrospinal fluid through the dura mater. It spreads both caudally (toward the feet) and cephalad (toward the head). For a single-injection epidural, the patient's position and the molecular weight of the anesthetic have no effect on its distribution. However, when a continuous epidural is administered, the position of the patient may affect the spread of the local anesthetic. Epidural anesthesia is often used in obstetrical, gynecological, urological, and rectal surgery. It is also used for postoperative pain control.

Procedure

The patient's skin is prepped as for spinal anesthesia. A thoracic, lumbar, or caudal puncture site is used, depending on the target site of the anesthesia. The epidural needle is advanced through the skin until it enters the epidural space, and the anesthetic is injected. Continuous or intermittent epidural anesthesia is provided through a small catheter placed in the epidural space for the duration of the surgery. This technique is also used for postoperative pain relief and for chronic pain management in selected patients.

RISKS ASSOCIATED WITH EPIDURAL ANESTHESIA In contrast to spinal anesthesia, epidural anesthesia requires a much larger amount of anesthetic agent. Accidental puncture of the dura mater can cause total spinal anesthesia. This is paralysis of the respiratory muscles. Also, because the epidural space has an extensive network of veins, overdose by accidental venous injection is a risk. If this occurs, the patient is immediately intubated and ventilated. Although the risk of hypotension exists with epidural anesthesia, the onset is slower than with spinal anesthesia and therefore easier to control and correct. All regional anesthetics are absorbed into the body and metabolized. If absorption is more rapid than metabolism, the risk of toxic reaction increases.

The role of the circulating surgical technologist is the same as for spinal anesthesia.

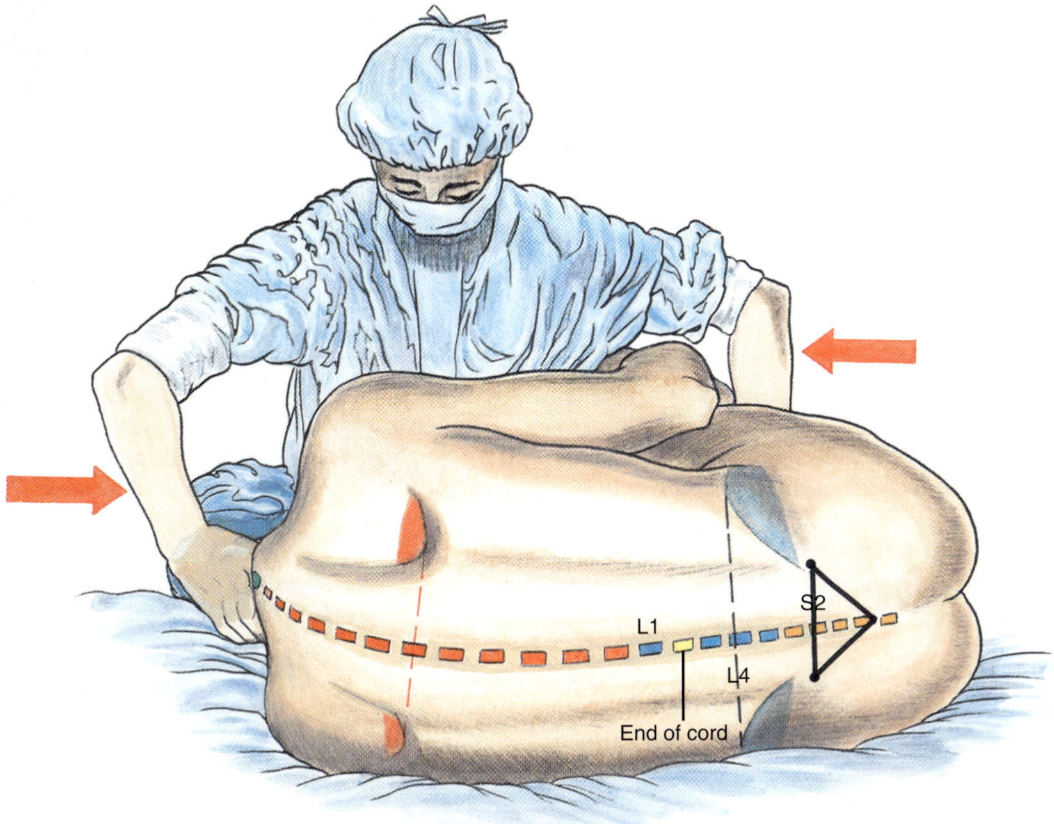

FIG. 13.15 Assisting in spinal block with patient in lateral position. (From Farab E, Mounir-Soliman L. *Brown's Atlas of Regional Anesthesia*. 5th ed. Philadelphia: Elsevier; 2017.)

EMERGENCIES

The role of the surgical technologist at all times during an emergency is to protect the surgical field and assist as directed. The surgical technologist may also be required to assist in cardiopulmonary resuscitation (CPR). However, CPR is meant to be a stopgap measure until biomedical intervention and medical care begin. Because these interventions are already in place in surgery, the patient is in the best location possible for a positive outcome.

REGIONAL DRUG TOXICITY AND ALLERGIC RESPONSE

Toxic reactions to local anesthetics arise most often during **regional block** and epidural anesthesia. This is due to the large amount of drug administered and the proximity to the vascular system. Toxic reactions related to regional anesthetics occur in two forms: CNS toxicity and cardiovascular toxicity.

Central Nervous System Toxicity

CNS toxicity occurs in three phases. The *excitation phase* produces lightheadedness, restlessness, confusion, perioral tingling (tingling around the mouth), a metallic taste, tinnitus (ringing in the ears), and a sense of impending doom. The patient may become talkative. This phase is followed by the *convulsive phase*. Seizures can occur in this phase. The *depressive phase* is characterized by drowsiness, respiratory depression, and **apnea** (loss of respiration).

Cardiovascular System Toxicity

The first phase of cardiovascular toxicity is the *excitation phase*. The patient develops tachycardia, hypertension, and convulsions. This is followed by the *depressive phase,* which is characterized by decreased blood pressure, bradycardia, and possibly cardiac arrest.

Allergic Reaction

A true allergic reaction, which differs from reactions caused by toxicity, ranges from local skin irritation and itching to severe anaphylaxis, which produces life-threatening changes in the cardiovascular and respiratory systems. Maintaining verbal contact with the patient helps in the identification of symptoms. (Chapter 12 presents a complete discussion of drug hypersensitivity.)

Resuscitative equipment must be immediately available whenever a local anesthetic is administered. During any emergency, surgical technologists respond according to their training and scope of practice. CPR is the minimum requirement for emergency response. Beyond this, the resuscitation team is responsible for the administration of resuscitative drugs, airway maintenance, and advanced life support procedures.

CARDIOPULMONARY ARREST

All health care workers must maintain current certification in CPR and be able to respond in case of a cardiac or respiratory arrest. Personnel may not be employed in an accredited health care facility without this certification. The goal of CPR is to support and restore oxygenation, ventilation, and circulation. Restoration of intact neurological function accompanies this process. Return of spontaneous circulation is accomplished with basic life support (BLS) or advanced cardiac life support (ACLS) measures. These follow distinct algorithms that depend on the nature of the emergency. Airway, breathing, and circulation are the most basic priorities, followed by the administration of cardiac drugs and defibrillation as required. In the clinical setting, the defibrillator is immediately available on all crash carts. Automated external defibrillators are located throughout the health care facility for emergency treatment of specific conditions.

Certification in CPR is the required method of ensuring complete knowledge and understanding of the procedure. All health care professionals and students are provided the opportunity for certification before beginning clinical work.

DIFFICULT AIRWAY

A difficult airway is one in which the usual methods of providing ventilation—placement of an artificial airway and mask ventilation—are extremely difficult. In the worst case, the outcome is failure to ventilate, even after many attempts. Adverse events related to a difficult airway are hypoxia leading to brain injury or death.

Patients undergoing elective surgery who are known to have or are at risk for a difficult airway are critically evaluated by the AP before surgery to determine the extent of the

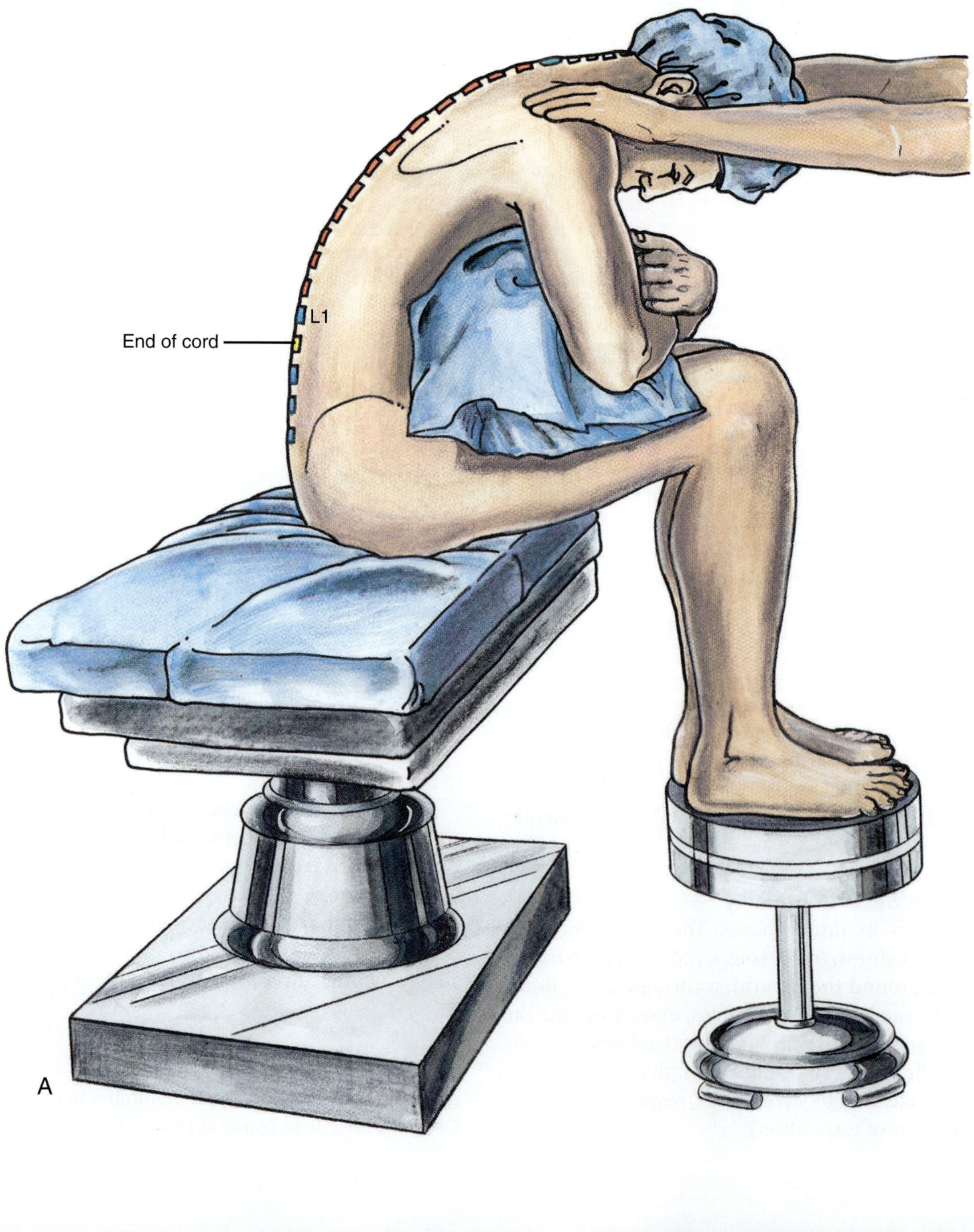

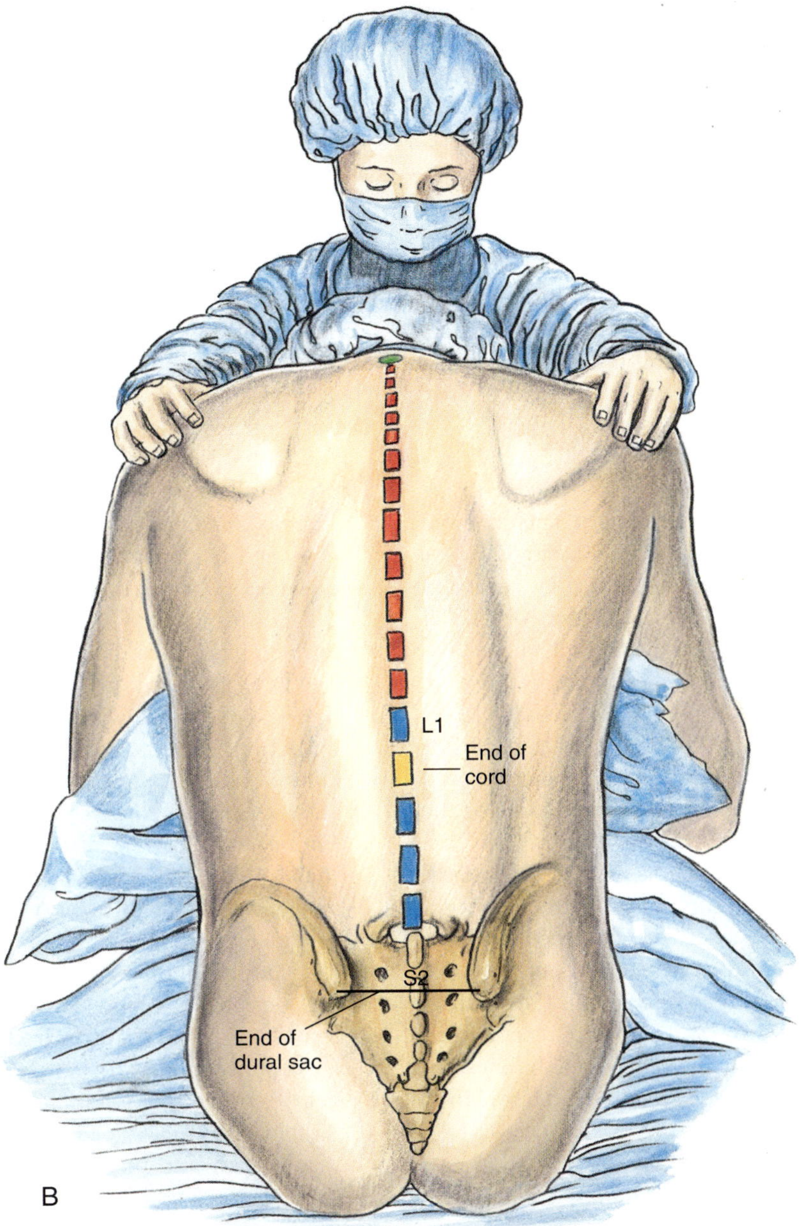

FIG. 13.16 Assisting in spinal block with patient in sitting position. (A) Lateral view. (B) Posterior view. (From Farab E, Mounir-Soliman L. *Brown's Atlas of Regional Anesthesia*. 5th ed. Philadelphia: Elsevier; 2017.)

risk and to prepare for interventions in the event of airway blockage. Preparations include having extra trained personnel available to assist and an emergency airway cart close to or in the operating room suite. Positioning devices that provide hyperextension of the neck are placed near the operating table before induction. The airway cart is managed by the AP, anesthesia technician, and circulator, who must be familiar with the types, names, and sizes of all equipment on the cart and also the emergency drugs that might be needed. The ASA has developed a grading system for airway difficulty and provides algorithms (stepwise decision tree for medical intervention) for establishing an airway in emergency situations. In the case of unexpected difficult airway, there may not be time to secure expert assistance. Having the emergency crash and airway carts available at all times decreases the risk of a poor outcome.

A difficult airway is usually related to the patient's specific neck anatomy. Patients with heavy muscle and fatty tissue in the throat and neck regions are prone to a difficult airway because of the pressure from these tissues collapsing on the airway during anesthesia induction or deep sedation. These conditions are most common in obese patients and in those who are of short,

> To obtain information about ACLS courses and certification, students should contact the American Heart Association or consult the organization's website at http://www.heart.org/HEARTORG/CPRAndECC/CPR_UCM_001118_SubHomePage.jsp.

heavy stature. Other predisposing factors are neck and throat pathology, including facial fractures. Patients who lack most of their teeth may also be difficult to intubate because without the support of teeth, the cheeks tend to collapse inward.

AIRWAY EMERGENCY

An airway emergency is one in which the unconscious patient cannot be intubated. In this case, an artificial airway cannot be established as described earlier because of a difficult airway. The window of treatment to prevent hypoxia and subsequent brain damage is several minutes. The exact time depends on whether the patient was given extra oxygen before induction.

Emergency Response

Emergency response may include repeated attempts by more than one individual to intubate the patient either by ET tube or LMA. An emergency airway cart containing all necessary equipment is maintained by the anesthesia department. If repeated attempts fail, transcutaneous tracheotomy or tracheostomy can be performed to establish the airway. In this case, the surgical technologist should be prepared to assist.

Emergency tracheostomy is an incision over the anterior wall of the trachea through the skin and strap muscles and insertion of a tube to provide immediate access to air or the anesthesia circuit. Refer to Chapter 27 for a description of a tracheostomy. An alternative treatment is the cricothyrotomy, in which an opening is made through the cricothyroid structures and a tracheotomy tube inserted. The procedure may have fewer complications than the tracheotomy and be faster to perform than the standard tracheotomy. In this procedure, a 10-gauge needle is inserted across the cricothyroid membrane. The needle is used to ventilate the patient through the anesthesia circuit by *jet* or *high-velocity ventilation* (often referred to as transtracheal jet ventilation).

LARYNGOSPASM

Spasm of the larynx is usually associated with airway secretions or stimulation of the laryngeal nerve during intubation or extubation. The condition may lead to complete airway obstruction. It is treated with mechanical ventilation or, in severe cases, administration of succinylcholine to paralyze the muscles. Laryngospasm constitutes an emergency when an airway cannot be immediately established by positive-pressure ventilation. Patients with a difficult airway are at the highest risk for laryngospasm.

ANAPHYLAXIS

Anaphylaxis is a true allergic reaction to a substance or drug that can lead to shock (see next section). In surgery, this is most commonly associated with regional anesthesia. Signs and symptoms include rash, abnormal lung sounds detected during auscultation, wheezing, and difficulty breathing. In the event of anaphylaxis, the AP, nurse, or surgeon immediately administers multiple doses of epinephrine. Other respiratory drugs and antihistamines are administered as needed. Airway assistance may be required. The on-call resuscitation team is alerted if no physician is in the room, and an airway and oxygen administration are quickly established. The preoperative examination and pre-anesthesia evaluation can often predict allergic response to substances or drug groups.

SHOCK

Shock is a potentially life-threatening, complex physiological event involving many systems. The primary effect of shock is that blood (and oxygen) is shunted away from the organs (hypoperfusion). This leads to cellular death. Shock can be caused by many other events. Treatment is based on the cause.

Types of Shock

- *Hypovolemic shock* is the depletion of the intravascular volume. This can be due to external fluid loss from vomiting, diarrhea, polyuria, or blood loss. It can also be caused by the redistribution of fluids in the body as a result of trauma or burn injury. Capillary flow diminishes or is shut down. The body tries to conserve fluid by reducing renal blood flow and increasing water retention in the kidneys. Urinary output is diminished or ceases. Eventually, multiple organ failure occurs as a result of oxygen and nutrient starvation at the cellular level.
- *Cardiogenic shock* is caused by decreased cardiac function such as occurs with myocardial infarction. The vascular system is disabled because blood cannot be pumped adequately throughout the body.
- *Distributive shock* is the result of vascular dilation in the peripheral blood vessels, which reduces vascular resistance. This is characterized by very low blood pressure. Distributive shock can be caused by sepsis, anaphylaxis, neurogenic shock, or adrenal insufficiency.
- *Anaphylactic shock* is caused by true allergy, resulting in vasodilation and pooling of blood, which slows or halts normal circulation.
- *Neurogenic shock* is caused by failure of the autonomic nervous system to maintain vascular tone. This type of shock can be caused by specific drugs, brain injury, anesthesia, or spinal cord injury.
- *Septic shock* is caused by severe infection, which results in hypovolemia. Bacterial infection is most often the cause of septic shock, which can be rapidly fatal. Disseminated intravascular coagulation (DIC) is a complication of septic shock in which microcoagulation occurs in the cells. This depletes the body's platelets and other clotting factors, leading to continuous hemorrhage and death.

Emergency Response

Treatment for shock is targeted at restoring circulatory function, electrolyte balance, and oxygenation of the tissues. The immediate emergency response is related to the cause. However, in all cases, anaphylaxis circulatory balance is a priority. This may necessitate administration of fluid or blood components and drug therapy to improve the systemic blood pressure.

MALIGNANT HYPERTHERMIA

Malignant hyperthermia is a rare physiological response to all volatile anesthetic agents and succinylcholine. MH causes severe immediate or delayed hypermetabolism. The patient exhibits an extremely high core temperature, tachycardia, tachypnea, and increased muscle rigidity. Metabolic crises accompany the physical signs and include an increase in intracellular calcium ions, respiratory acidosis, metabolic acidosis, and hemodynamic instability, which may lead to cardiac arrest and death.

MH is related to a familial genetic trait. Patients with family members known to have experienced MH usually report this to the AP during the preoperative evaluation. However, no method has been devised for predicting MH when the patient has no family or personal history of the condition.

Emergency Response

An MH cart is maintained in the surgical department so that all emergency equipment and drugs can be brought in immediately. The cart contains cooling equipment, including Foley catheters, plastic bags, tubing, peritoneal lavage equipment, and nasogastric tubes. Emergency drugs for MH treatment include dantrolene and agents to treat specific metabolic disorders.

If MH symptoms occur during surgery, the AP alerts the team immediately. Treatment requires immediate cessation of anesthesia and drug therapy to treat the adverse metabolic symptoms. The scrub remains sterile to help protect the surgical incision. When immediate body cooling is required, the surgeon and AP may initiate cold irrigation in open body cavities, ice packs, and a cold IV solution. The scrub receives sterile equipment, ice, and fluids to assist in lowering the body temperature. Therapy is continued until the patient is stabilized. The surgical wound is closed quickly when surgery must be halted. The patient is transported to the intensive care unit for further treatment and observation.

SEVERE HEMORRHAGE

Cause of catastrophic hemorrhage during surgery are end-stage renal disease, liver disease, and blood disorders such as disseminated intravascular coagulation (DIC).

Emergency Response

Emergency response is based on the cause. If the hemorrhage is due to unintended surgical injury to a large blood vessel or pre-existing trauma, the immediate response is location of the injury and immediate hemostasis.

Blood volume is restored by giving blood substitutes, blood components, or autologous blood (the patient's own blood previously banked or harvested at the surgical site). Allogeneic (donor) blood transfusions may also be provided.

Packed red cells are mostly commonly used for transfusion, because the patient's immediate need is oxygen-carrying capacity. All blood products must be matched with the patient's blood type. A precise protocol has evolved to prevent the administration of blood of the wrong type. Whether the patient's own blood or banked blood is used, meticulous attention is given to patient identification, blood group, registration number, and date of expiration. Blood is usually brought from the blood bank shortly before surgery; in an emergency, it is brought immediately. Blood must be stored in a location known to all personnel and protected from direct heat. Unused blood must be returned to the blood bank as soon as possible.

Intraoperative cell salvage (autotransfusion) is the immediate harvesting of blood on the surgical field and reinfusion into the patient. This may be planned in advance of a high-risk surgery or implemented in an emergency. Special equipment is required for this procedure. The prototype autotransfusion system is the Cell Saver. However, other systems have now been developed. Surgical technologists must be familiar with the cell salvage device used in their facility, because special training is required.

HEMOLYTIC REACTION

Hemolysis is the rupture of red blood cells. It is associated with ABO factor incompatibility during blood transfusion. Before any transfusion, the ABO and Rh systems are tested and cross-matched against the donor blood. However, mistakes in recording and reading blood registrations do occur, with serious consequences. Patients under anesthesia do not show the signs and symptoms seen in a fully conscious patient. ABO mismatch during transfusion outside of surgery produces the following symptoms:

- Back pain
- Chills
- Hypotension
- Dyspnea

These can lead to complete vascular collapse or renal failure. In surgery, the only symptoms likely to appear are oliguria (cessation of renal output) and generalized bleeding. Treatment requires stopping the transfusion and immediate hydration with IV fluids and forced diuresis.

DEEP VEIN THROMBOSIS

An embolus is any moving particle within the vascular system. Risk factors for emboli include trauma, orthopedic fracture, burns, surgical procedures involving flexion and rotation of the hip, and the use of a pneumatic tourniquet. Venous stasis, or "pooling," occurs when the patient is immobile for long periods, which can lead to clotting. A thrombus may form in proximal deep veins and subsequently break loose, preventing circulation to a vital organ such as the lung **(pulmonary embolism [PE]).** Symptoms may become apparent at any point in the perioperative period. Prevention of deep vein thrombosis (DVT) includes preoperative application of antiembolic stockings, use of a sequential compression device (SCD), and prophylactic medication when appropriate. Other preventive measures include slow, deliberate movement of limbs during positioning and following DVT and PE protocols according to hospital policy. Treatment for DVT includes drug therapy to prevent further embolization and treatment for the specific emergency condition, such as shock and respiratory arrest.

IMPORTANT TO KNOW *The SCD is usually fitted to the patient in the preoperative stage. The patient may be transported to the operating room with the device, or it may be applied by the circulator when the patient arrives. Fig. 13.17 illustrates the SCD. The device requires a doctor's order.*

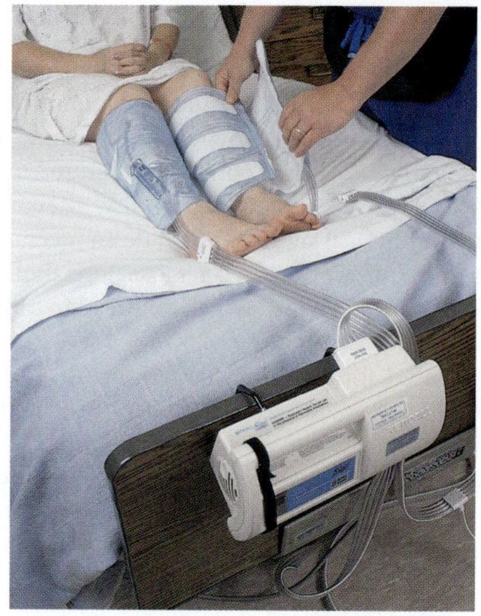

FIG. 13.17 Sequential compression device (SCD). This device is used on patients undergoing long surgeries or those at risk of thrombosis for medical reasons. Compression is sequentially applied to maintain return blood flow to the upper body. (From Sorrentino S. *Mosby's Textbook for Nursing Assistants*. 8th ed. St Louis: Elsevier; 2012.)

PART II: POSTANESTHESIA CARE UNIT (PACU)

After surgery, patients are transported to the postanesthesia care unit (PACU) for recovery. Postoperative patients are at risk for postoperative complications that may require an emergency medical response. The PACU is staffed by critical care nurses who are trained in postoperative recovery and emergency medicine. The unit is equipped with all necessary physiological monitoring equipment, drugs, and emergency supplies. The PACU is close to the surgical suites for rapid transfer of patients after surgery. In some facilities, the PACU also functions as an ambulatory patient recovery area. Even though the surgical technologist does not work in the postoperative recovery unit, it is important for the ST to understand the continuity of care required immediately after surgery.

DESCRIPTION OF THE PACU FACILITY

The floor plan of the PACU is usually one large room with separate patient stations along two or more perimeter walls. Patient beds are positioned in individual care areas (or *cubicles*) on the perimeter wall within view of a central nursing station (Fig. 13.18).

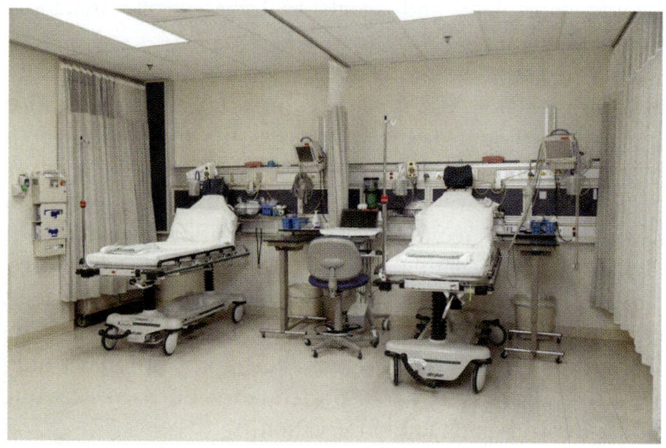

FIG. 13.18 Postanesthesia care unit (PACU) showing two patient bays, telemetry equipment, and patient care supplies.

This arrangement allows the staff to attend to patients quickly and efficiently. Stretchers (gurneys) can be easily moved within the unit and around the cubicles. Because there are no walls between patients, diagnostic equipment such as portable x-ray machines, 12-lead electrocardiograph equipment, and emergency crash carts can be brought to the bedside quickly with minimal maneuvering. The central nursing station is equipped with patient telemetry monitors, phones, and computers. Each patient cubicle or bay has outlets for suction, oxygen, power, and high-level lighting. Individual patient monitoring is transmitted through the department telemetry system so that staff members at the central nursing station can view each patient screen individually. Medication and supplies are dispensed from designated areas attached to the main patient area. Emergency airway equipment, including a tracheostomy tray, is kept in an easily accessible area and on crash carts.

The PACU is fully equipped with patient care supplies that would normally be found on any nursing unit. These include dressings, catheters, airways, and medication administration devices.

In addition to individual patient cubicles, an isolation area provides barrier protection for selected patients, such as those with an active infection. The PACU may also have a designated area for pediatric patients.

If ambulatory patients recover in the same department as inpatients, a designated area is provided with changing rooms, a lounge, and an ambulatory discharge area. Side rooms provide space for dictation, patient and family conferences, and staff lockers.

PACU PROCEDURES

ADMISSION

After surgery patients are transported to the PACU only when the anesthesia care provider has determined that it is safe. The American Society of Anesthesiologists, which determines the clinical standards for the profession, requires the patient to be transported by a member of the anesthesia team (anesthesiologist, registered nurse anesthetist, or licensed anesthesia technologist). The circulating registered nurse must also accompany the patient and anesthesia team member whenever the patient must be transported during cardiac monitoring.

Upon arrival in the PACU an assigned nurse receives the patient. Patients who are recovering from general anesthesia or monitored sedation must be immediately connected to a heart monitor and pulse oximeter. Vital signs are measured, and oxygen and suction are immediately engaged. The patient's level of pain and consciousness, airway, circulatory status, oxygen perfusion, and temperature are then assessed.

HANDOVER (HAND-OFF)

Once all monitoring devices are in place and the patient is stable, the AP performs a **handover** (also called a *hand-off*) to the PACU nurse. The AP communicates all information needed to update the PACU nurse on the patient's physiological status before and during surgery. The AP provides specific orders for the continuation of care and a smooth recovery. The AP remains with the patient until the handover is complete. The following verbal and written information is provided in the handover:

1. A brief patient history. This follows standard nursing and medical protocol and includes the patient's age, allergies, current medications, and existing pathology. This is the patient's preoperative status.
   Rationale: This information is relevant to the proper assessment of current signs and symptoms and for continuity of nursing care.
2. The exact surgery that was performed, including the side and site (e.g., right colectomy with colostomy).
   Rationale: This is reported so that the PACU staff know exactly where the surgical wounds are and the extent of the surgery for continuous postoperative care, monitoring, and assessment.
3. The total length of time anesthesia was delivered, the anesthetic agents, fluids, and drugs given during that time. The amounts and routes are also reported.
   Rationale: Drugs given during the preoperative and intraoperative phase have a direct pharmacological effect on those administered postoperatively. The cumulative effect and drug interactions must be considered when additional medications are administered. The PACU nurse must know what drugs were given to know what physiological changes were caused by the drugs. This information is well documented in the intraoperative anesthesia record; however, the information is passed on verbally by the AP.
4. Estimated blood loss and the amount and type of intravenous (IV) fluids or blood administered. If blood products were administered, the type and amount are reported.
   Rationale: The estimated blood loss is needed to determine the need for further action, such as transfusion. Total fluids given during surgery are balanced against output. Blood loss or fluid imbalance explains specific physiological signs that trigger a nursing or medical response in the postoperative period.

IMPORTANT TO KNOW *Estimation of blood loss requires training and considerable experience. Blood loss is calculated and reported by the anesthesia team.*

5. Condition of the wound, drains, and other devices. If the surgical wound contains drains or a drainage device such as suction or closed water-seal drainage, this is reported in detail. The amount, color, and consistency of the drainage fluid are noted.
   Rationale: Wound assessment and care are of primary importance during the postoperative period. A baseline assessment provides information against which subsequent evaluations are compared. Changes in wound drainage may indicate a problem, which requires an immediate medical response.
6. American Society of Anesthesiologists score. The ASA score reflects the patient's overall health status (see previous discussion in this chapter).
   Rationale: The ASA score is reported on postoperative records and is used in patient care planning.
7. Any surgical or medical complications that occurred during surgery.
   Rationale: This alerts the PACU staff to the patient's current condition and further complications. The information is also needed in case follow-up measures are required, such as x-rays or blood tests.
8. Information about family members (e.g., contact numbers or location) who may be waiting in the family room.
   Rationale: The PACU staff maintains contact with the family during the postoperative period to update them on the patient's progress, condition, and discharge plans.

PATIENT ASSESSMENT AND CARE

After accepting the handover, the PACU nurse performs a patient assessment. This can be either a focused assessment or a head-to-toe assessment. The focused assessment, as the name implies, focuses on specific criteria, such as respiration, circulation, pain, and level of consciousness. The *head-to-toe assessment* covers all or most body systems. Standard procedures are used to assess specific functions. General assessment procedures are carried out to obtain baseline information. This may lead to more complex methods of testing, such as blood tests, a 12-lead ECG, or x-rays. All findings are documented in the PACU record (Fig. 13.19).

RESPIRATORY SYSTEM

- The airway is assessed by *auscultation* (listening with a stethoscope) and by observation for signs of airway obstruction.
- The respiratory rate and rhythm (patterns) are measured by observation of the thorax and accessory muscles during breathing.

CIRCULATION

- **Perfusion** (flow of blood to tissue) is measured by pulse oximeter. Note that *cyanosis* (blue-gray tinging around the

mouth) is a *late sign* of low oxygenation and is not used to evaluate the patient.
- The heart is monitored for rate and rhythm using ECG leads and the cardiac monitor, which produces a digital waveform.
- Heart sounds are assessed with the stethoscope and may be amplified by the cardiac monitor.
- The arterial pressure is measured directly with an arterial line or indirectly by taking the patient's blood pressure with a digital sphygmomanometer.
- Arterial blood gases (ABGs) (the ratio of oxygen to carbon dioxide and the blood pH) may be measured by taking a blood sample from an artery. In the modern PACU, the sample can be analyzed immediately.
- The central venous pressure may be measured with an inline catheter or subjectively by observing the jugular veins.
- The presence or absence of a peripheral pulse is determined by palpation or by Doppler.

TEMPERATURE

- The patient's temperature is assessed continuously or intermittently using a digital thermometer or temperature probe.
- Hypothermia is a serious postoperative complication. The patient is continually monitored for this.

ABDOMEN

- After abdominal surgery, the abdomen is assessed for distention (which may indicate the presence of fluid, including blood, or air). This is done by observation, palpation, and radiographs.
- Bowel sounds are assessed by auscultation. A persistent lack of bowel sounds may indicate surgical paralytic ileus—cessation of peristalsis in the bowel leading to obstruction. Persistent paralytic ileus is a serious postoperative complication.

FLUID AND ELECTROLYTE BALANCE

- Fluid shifts from the vascular space to the intracellular space can occur after surgery, and the patient must be evaluated carefully for this.
- Assessment for dehydration includes physical signs and symptoms. Replacement fluids are administered intravenously as needed.
- Electrolyte imbalance is assessed through blood tests and specific physiological signs of imbalance, such as alteration in consciousness or cardiac dysrhythmia.

NEUROLOGICAL FUNCTION (LEVEL OF CONSCIOUSNESS)

The patient's level of consciousness is assessed using the **Glasgow Coma Scale (GCS).** In this system, points are assigned to the response to specific stimuli (shown in Box 13.3). The GCS score is calculated as the total of all parameters. A score of 15 indicates the best prognosis (medical outcome), whereas a minimum score of 3 indicates a poor prognosis. Table 13.6 shows responses in the non-verbal child.

RENAL FUNCTION

Urinary output is measured in milliliters per hour (includes intraoperative measurements). Urinary retention may be caused by neurological deficit and requires more complex assessment and treatment.
- Appearance of the urine
- Selected blood tests

WOUND ASSESSMENT

- Drainage amount, color, and consistency
- Incision assessment
- Swelling noted and measured for baseline reference

CATHETERS AND TUBING

- Drainage amount, color
- Drains and catheters intact, open
- IV lines intact

PSYCHOSOCIAL

The PACU staff provide continual emotional support to the patient. Patients often need reassurance and orientation to their environment while emerging from general anesthesia or heavy sedation. Patients may be fearful of their diagnosis or the results of the surgery. Although not fully conscious, they may return emotionally to the preoperative state of anxiety. Patients need to know that, although they may not be fully functioning, they are being cared for, and they need to know who is caring for them. In some cases, the surgeon may see the patient briefly and explain the results of the surgery.

Family awaiting the results of the surgery and the patient's emergence from anesthesia also need contact with the PACU staff. The nurse may visit the family (which includes friends) in the waiting area to let them know the patient's progress and estimated time of discharge from the unit.

POSTOPERATIVE COMPLICATIONS

Postanesthesia complications occur because patients are physiologically unstable during the immediate postoperative period and may react to the procedure or drugs administered intraoperatively. They are vulnerable to pain, hemorrhage, reaction to the anesthetic agents, and rapid changes in homeostasis. The PACU staff are specially trained in critical care monitoring and response. Note that the physiological complications discussed in Chapter 13 can occur during the postoperative period.

PAIN

Although pain is expected in the postsurgical phase, not all patients respond to pain in the same way. A patient's response

FORREST GENERAL HOSPITAL
POSTANESTHESIA CARE UNIT RECORD

POSTANESTHESIA RECOVERY SCORE		MINUTES in	30	60	90	out
Activity						
Able to move 4 extremities voluntarily or on command	= 2					
Able to move 2 extremities voluntarily or on command	= 1					
Able to move 0 extremities voluntarily or on command	= 0					
Respiration						
Able to deep breathe and cough freely	= 2					
Dyspnea or limited breathing	= 1					
Apneic	= 0					
Circulation						
BP ± 20 of Preanesthetic level	= 2					
BP ± 20-50 of Preanesthetic level	= 1					
BP ± 50 of Preanesthetic level	= 0					
Consciousness						
Fully Awake	= 2					
Arousable on calling	= 1					
Not Responding	= 0					
O_2 Saturation						
Able to maintain O_2 Sat > 92% on room air	= 2					
Needs O_2 to maintain O_2 Sat > 90%	= 1					
O_2 Sat < 90% even with O_2	= 0					
TOTAL						

Pre-op B.P. ______

Allergy

Airway: On Adm.

Jawthrust ______

Chin Hold ______

Endotracheal ______

Oral Airway ______

Mask Oxygen ______

Nasal Oxygen ______

Trach ______

T-Tube ______

Nasal Airway ______

Ventilator Settings ______

Addressograph

Time In ______ Time Out ______

Accompanied by ______

Type of anesthesia ______

Surgical Procedure:

PULSE - RESPIRATION - BLOOD PRESSURE

	15	30	45	15	30	45	15	30	45	15	30	45
240												
220												
200												
180												
160												
140												
120												
100												
80												
60												
40												
20												
O2 Sat.												
PAP												

CODES: ⊥ A-line, T B.P. — V Manual or Λ NBP — Pulse • Resp. ○ — Siderails: Yes No — Restraints: Yes No

IV Type ______

Total IV in OR ______ cc

Blood in OR ______ units

Urinary Output in OR ______ cc

Est. Blood Loss ______ cc

Foley Cath. ______

Suprapubic ______

Ureteral ______

Levine ______

DRAINS

RN Signature

RN Signature

MEDICATIONS AND TREATMENTS

	AMT.	ROUTE	TIME
Demerol			
Morphine			
Phenergan			
Droperidol			
Zofran			
Toradol			

FORREST GENERAL HOSPITAL

DATE	TIME	DESCRIPTIVE NOTES (SIGN EACH ENTRY)

Report to Family:
Time:

GU IRRIGANT		FOLEY OUTPUT	
TOTAL INFUSED:		TOTAL OUTPUT:	

FIG. 13.19 Sample PACU patient care record.

BOX 13.3 Glasgow Coma Scale

EYE OPENING
No eye opening 1
Eye opening to pain 2
Eye opening to sound 3
Eyes open spontaneously 4

BEST VERBAL RESPONSE
No verbal response 1
Incomprehensible sounds 2
Inappropriate words 3
Confused 4
Oriented 5

BEST MOTOR RESPONSE
No motor response 1
Abnormal extension to pain 2
Abnormal flexion to pain 3
Withdrawal from pain 4
Localizing pain 5
Obeys commands 6

PAIN (DOES NOT CONTRIBUTE TO GCS SCORE)
Alertness: Asleep to hyperalert
Level of calmness: Calm to panicky
Movement: No movement to vigorous movement
Facial expression: Face relaxed to contortion or grimacing
Blood pressure: Baseline or below to 15% or more elevation
Heart rate: At or below baseline to 15% or more elevation
Vocalization: No vocalization to crying out
Note: Refer to Table 13.6 for pain assessment in the preverbal child.

TABLE 13.6 FLACC* Pain Scale for Infants

	SCORING		
Categories	**0**	**1**	**2**
Face	No particular expression or smile	Occasional grimace or frown, withdrawn, disinterested	Frequent to constant quivering chin, clenched jaw
Legs	Normal position or relaxed	Uneasy, restless, tense	Kicking, or legs drawn up
Activity	Lying quietly, normal position, moves easily	Squirming, shifting, back and forth, tense	Arched, rigid, or jerking
Cry	No cry (awake or asleep)	Moans or whimpers	Crying steadily, screams or sobs
Consolability	Content, relaxed	Reassured by occasional touching, hugging, or being talked to	Difficult to console or comfort

The total score ranges 0–10 with 0 representing no pain.
From National Hospice and Palliative Care Organization.
*FLACC – Face, legs, activity, cry, consolability.

to pain is affected by previous experience, level of anxiety, the drugs used during surgery, and environmental factors. Patients also respond to pain according to what is acceptable in their culture. For example, in some cultures, crying out is acceptable, whereas in others, it is not. Pain management requires assessment and planning to ensure a smooth recovery. Analgesics are administered according to the patient's level of consciousness, cardiopulmonary status, and age.

RESPIRATORY SYSTEM

Respiratory problems are the most frequent life-threatening postoperative complication. Inadequate ventilation can be related to the effects of anesthetic drugs, pain, muscle relaxants, or fluid-electrolyte imbalance. Inadequate intake of air and oxygen results in the accumulation of carbon dioxide in the blood. Normally, a high carbon dioxide level triggers the autonomic nervous system to stimulate breathing. However, drugs administered during the intraoperative period suppress this reflex. Pain at the operative site is another cause of *hypoventilation*, resulting in low oxygen saturation. For example, patients with abdominal or thoracic incisions do not breathe deeply because of the pain in the muscles of respiration.

Airway Obstruction

Airway obstruction is most often caused by anatomical structures or aspiration of fluids. The tongue or soft palate can obstruct the airway in a state of deep relaxation related to anesthetic agents and adjunct drugs.

Contraction of the laryngeal muscles **(laryngospasm)** can occur whenever the larynx is irritated or stimulated by secretions, intubation, extubation, or suctioning. **Bronchospasm** is partial or complete closure of the bronchial tubes. It can be triggered by airway suctioning, aspiration of fluid, or allergy. Both laryngospasm and bronchospasm can be caused by particular anesthetic agents.

Aspiration

Inhalation of secretions or stomach contents is associated with a weak gag reflex related to the use of narcotics, sedatives, and anesthetic agents. Aspiration of gastric contents after vomiting can result in an obstructed airway and chemical pneumonia.

Atelectasis

Atelectasis is the collapse of the lung, which can occur suddenly (as in the case of trauma to the chest wall or pulmonary obstruction). Trapped mucus or fluid in the bronchial tree can result in pulmonary obstruction postoperatively. Smokers are particularly vulnerable to atelectasis in the postoperative period. The patient is encouraged to take deep breaths and to cough frequently in the immediate postoperative period to prevent obstruction.

Pulmonary Embolism

Pulmonary embolism is the blockage of a pulmonary vessel by air, a blood clot, or other substance (e.g., fragments of atherosclerotic plaque). This results in *anoxia* (decreased oxygen to the lung tissue), which can cause death of lung tissue and right heart failure. The risk of pulmonary embolism is increased in patients with a history of deep vein thrombosis (DVT). Patients are assessed for signs of DVT and pulmonary embolism in the immediate postoperative period. The patient and family are also provided with information about the signs and symptoms of DVT and pulmonary embolism so that monitoring can continue at home after discharge.

CARDIOVASCULAR COMPLICATIONS

Many anesthetic agents are cardiac irritants that can sensitize the heart muscle to disturbances in rhythm, rate, and cardiac output. Hypotension and hypertension can occur as a result of fluid or electrolyte imbalance.

Hemorrhage

Hemorrhage can occur during surgery or in the postoperative period. The patient is continually monitored for signs of hemorrhage, which include pallor, hypotension, an increased heart rate, diaphoresis (sweating), cool skin, restlessness, and pain. Hemorrhage may be caused by the loss of a ligature placed during surgery, inadequate hemostasis, leakage from a vascular anastomosis, or a clotting disorder. If hemorrhage is suspected, emergency assessment measures are initiated, and the patient may be returned to surgery.

HYPOTHERMIA

Hypothermia is a persistently low core body temperature (less than 98.6°F [37.5°C]). Older, pediatric, and frail patients are the most vulnerable. Hypothermia can result in a longer postoperative recovery period, surgical wound infection, cardiac ischemia, and reduced ability to metabolize drugs. Most patients undergoing general anesthesia experience some level of hypothermia. However, persistent or extreme hypothermia can occur as a result of the following:

- Exposure of the body cavities to the cold, ambient temperature of the operating room
- Administration of cold IV fluids
- Patient exposure before draping
- Vasodilation related to medications administered during surgery
- Decreased metabolism
- Cold irrigation solutions

Risks related to hypothermia are due mainly to physiological stress. These include the following:

- Shivering, which increases oxygen demand and consumption by 400% to 500%
- Excessive demand on body energy
- Decreased immune response, leading to postoperative infection
- Increased risk of adverse cardiac events, especially in patients with coronary artery disease
- Depression of the coagulation pathway
- Decreased tissue healing

Treatment for hypothermia includes the use of a forced-air heating mattress or placement of warm water pads under the patient. Further loss of body heat is prevented by warming IV solutions. Patients who are hypothermic during the intraoperative period may be difficult to warm postoperatively. Preoperative and intraoperative care are essential to prevent complications related to this condition.

MALIGNANT HYPERTHERMIA

MH is a rare condition that causes an extremely high core body temperature, cardiac dysrhythmia, tachypnea (increased respiratory rate), hypoxia, and hypercarbia. The condition is potentially fatal and occurs most commonly at the time of administration of the anesthetic. However, symptoms may appear in the postoperative period. MH can be triggered by inhalation anesthetics and succinylcholine, an anesthetic adjunct used for muscle relaxation.

MH is an extreme emergency during and after surgery, and all perioperative staff members are trained to respond appropriately according to facility protocol. *Dantrolene sodium* is administered as soon as the diagnosis is made by the AP. Additional management includes total body cooling with extracorporeal ice or a hypothermia blanket, iced IV saline, and iced irrigation fluid in an open body cavity (surgical wound site). Surgery is interrupted and the incision closed as quickly as possible. The patient is transferred immediately to the intensive care unit (ICU) for continuous care and monitoring.

NAUSEA AND VOMITING

Postoperative nausea and vomiting (PONV) is both a discomfort and a risk for the patient (see discussion of aspiration). PONV is controlled with medications in the preoperative period (as prevention) and in the postoperative period.

ALTERATIONS OF CONSCIOUSNESS

Anesthetic agents, adjunct medications, and environmental factors may cause patients to become disoriented, confused, or delirious during the immediate postoperative period. Preexisting psychiatric illness or drug abuse may contribute to these effects, which may also be due to organic causes such as electrolyte imbalance. Postoperative delirium is more common in pediatric patients and older patients. Risk factors include the following:

- Cognitive impairment
- Sleep deprivation
- Immobility
- Sensory impairment (e.g., vision, hearing)
- Advanced age
- Electrolyte imbalance
- Dehydration
- Substance abuse
- Depression

ELEMENTS OF DISCHARGE PLANNING

Before an ambulatory (day case) patient is discharged to home or to an extended care facility, the PACU staff, AP, and surgeon must determine that the patient will be safe. The patient must be able to perform the activities of daily living (ADLs) with some degree of independence or have help in dressing, eating, mobilizing, and toileting. Discharge planning is needed to prepare the patient and caregivers for possible problems.

Discharge planning and implementation follow established roles and tasks according to hospital policy:

1. *Discharge criteria:* These are conditions that must be met for the patient to be safely discharged.
2. *Transport or transfer plans:* Safe patient transportation is arranged, and an escort is identified.
3. *Home nursing care:* Home care objectives for the patient's recovery are established, and those who will be involved in the care are identified.
4. *Patient education:* Patients are informed and educated about their own care so that they can fully participate in their recovery. The family is instructed in specific care objectives and how to meet the patient's physical needs.
5. *Referral and follow-up:* The patient is informed of follow-up appointments. Referral numbers for emergencies or further advice are provided on a written document.
6. *Documentation:* Nursing care documentation is completed and signed off. Discharge checklists are prepared and completed.

DISCHARGE CRITERIA

Discharge criteria are physiological, psychological, and social conditions that serve as a measure of the patient's readiness for discharge. Patients are discharged from the PACU only when they meet discharge criteria. These are primarily physiological objectives, which are necessary to ensure patient safety outside the critical care unit. The health care facility establishes the discharge criteria. A number of organizations have written suggested criteria; however, the *Aldrete scale* is often used to determine whether a patient is ready for discharge to the hospital ward or unit. This is a numerical scale used to evaluate activity, respiration, circulation, consciousness, and oxygen saturation. Box 13.4 shows an example of a scored discharge criteria system. Modified versions of the scale have been developed for special circumstances.

Criteria for discharge include physiological criteria and the patient's psychosocial status.

BOX 13.4 Modified Postanesthesia Discharge Scoring System

VITAL SIGNS	
Within 20% of the preoperative value	2
20%–40% of the preoperative value	1
40% of the preoperative value	0
AMBULATION	
Steady gait/no dizziness	2
With assistance	1
No ambulation/dizziness	0
NAUSEA AND VOMITING	
Minimal	2
Moderate	1
Severe	0
SURGICAL BLEEDING	
Minimal	2
Moderate	1
Severe	0

GENERAL PLANNING

Arrangements for discharge are sometimes complex. PACU nurses must not only care for the patient during the recovery period but must also ensure that care is in place and that safe transport has been arranged.

Patients deserve a safe discharge and transfer from the providing facility. Discharge planning must be started at the time of admission to ensure a safe and event-free return home at the end of the recovery period. Home health service providers are notified, and a preoperative conference may be held with the family and discharge nurse.

When the patient is to be transferred to another care facility, a verbal and written hand-off is provided to a designated person at the receiving facility. The hand-off includes all information about the patient's physical and psychosocial status, the details of the surgery, and the care plan, including prescriptions, dressings, and drainage. Fig. 13.20 shows a basic discharge summary.

Physiological Criteria

1. Vital signs are stable and reflect the patient's baseline normal.
2. Nausea and vomiting are controlled.
3. The patient is mobile with assistance or by self (the patient must be able to walk without signs of dizziness or weakness).
4. The patient is able to void (this establishes that no evidence exists of urinary retention).
5. The skin color reflects the patient's baseline normal.
6. The incision site is dry, and drainage is absent or within expected limits.
7. The patient is oriented to time, place, and person.
8. Pain is controlled (patients are discharged when the level of pain is acceptable to the patient).
9. The patient is able to drink fluids.
10. Discharge orders have been written and signed by the AP and surgeon.

PACU DISCHARGE SUMMARY

VITAL SIGNS ON DISCHARGE	PACU OUTCOME	COMFORT LEVEL
B/P: P: R: T:	UNEVENTFUL ☐	PAIN FREE ☐ PAIN CONTROLLED ☐ SLEEPING BUT C/O PAIN WHEN AWAKEN ☐
OXIMETER: PAR SCORE:	COMPLICATIONS ☐	

REPORT TO: TIME:	SKIN CONDITION: WARM COOL DRY MOIST	COLOR: PINK PALE JAUNDICED DUSKY

DRESSINGS / SURGICAL SITE / PUNCTURE SITE

X-RAYS TAKEN IN PACU	LABS DRAWN IN PACU	O_2 ORDERED YES NO ______ L/MIN PER ______ O_2 TRANSPORT YES NO

TOTAL IV IN PACU

TOTAL BLOOD IN PACU

TOTAL PO INTAKE IN PACU

TOTAL OUTPUT IN PACU

URINARY	LEVINE	DRAINS

IV SITE:

______ cc LTC

ORDERS FAXED TO PHARMACY YES NO	EQUIPMENT ORDERED	TRANSPORT BY: AMBASSADOR RN LPN TECHNICIAN

DIAGNOSIS (Circle number of any diagnosis made)	GOAL	Goal Achieved YES	Goal Achieved NO
1 Alteration in neurological status			
2 Alteration in comfort level			
3 Alteration in emotional status			
4 Alteration in circulation			
5 Alteration in fluid volume			
6 Alteration in mobility			
7 Alteration in respiratory function			
8 Alteration in skin integrity			
9 Alteration in temperature			
10 Alteration in elimination			
11 Alteration in gastrointestinal function			
12 Alteration in injury			
13 Alteration in bleeding			
14 Other			

RHYTHM STRIPS

FIG. 13.20 Sample discharge summary.

Psychosocial Status

1. The patient has transportation home (not public transport).
2. A responsible escort is available.
3. Home care is available as needed.
4. The home environment is suitable for the recovering patient.

Transport

Patient transport to home or another care facility is arranged before surgery whenever possible. The patient is not discharged to public transportation, and a responsible escort must accompany the patient.

Home Nursing Care

In the past, patients anticipated a long recovery period, both in the hospital and at home. Because of advanced surgical technology and health care economics, patients are now discharged as soon as possible after surgery. Many procedures that used to require days of hospitalization are now performed as day surgery with discharge within 1 or 2 hours of recovery. Home care during the immediate postoperative period is now more focused and has specific outcome objectives.

Discharge planning includes specific written instructions for home care and goals for the patient. This new health care philosophy has shifted the responsibility of recovery from inpatient nursing to the patient and family. In the event that the patient has no assistance available, community resources, including social services and professional home nursing services, must be brought in.

Patient Education

Patient teaching is the responsibility of trained nursing personnel. Current surgical practice with same-day discharge and fast tracking requires that patients understand all aspects of their recovery. In theory, this allows them to be active participants in their recovery. However, the postoperative patient may not be able to understand or remember new information. Therefore, patient teaching takes place before surgery and may include the family members who will assist in care.

The elements of patient teaching include both verbal and written instructions. In some facilities, video demonstration and education are available. Access to electronic information via the Internet has transformed the field of consumer medicine. However, not all patients have access to these types of resources or the ability to interpret them. Also, many more patients are too sick to achieve a level of self-education. For these reasons, patients' family members (when applicable) are taken through the recovery process, step by step, with thorough explanations of what to expect and what to do. This is especially important for patients who will have drains, dressing changes, and surgical appliances to maintain.

Written information is intentionally simple and easy to understand. It is written in lay language, often with illustrations for clarification. It may include information about the surgery, what it entails, and exactly what anatomical changes were made (if any). All anticipated and unanticipated events are explained. Signs of infection or other complications are written out so that patients can refer to them. Knowing the expected effects of surgery helps give the patient confidence and eases anxiety when they occur.

Patients are fully educated about their prescriptions and how to take them. *Polypharmacy* is a clinical scenario in which patients are prescribed many different medications, sometimes by different primary health care providers who have no knowledge of the other drugs that the patient is taking. It is not unusual for a patient with a chronic disease to be taking 15 or 20 prescribed medications. Therefore it is very important that education about drugs is thorough.

The patient's ADLs are discussed in full. These ADLs often determine the patient's quality of life. Even if the recovery period is rapid, patients must be able to cope with activity restrictions, special toileting needs (or problems), and meal preparation.

Patients who require dressing changes or have appliances, drains, or catheters need particular assistance and teaching to prevent infection. Patients and family may be given supplies to take home with them at the time of discharge.

Patients and family receive referral numbers for emergency care or further information. Upcoming appointments for surgical follow-up are clearly written, along with any preparation for further testing or treatment.

UNANTICIPATED PACU OUTCOME

FAILURE TO MEET DISCHARGE CRITERIA

Some patients may not meet discharge criteria after ambulatory or inpatient recovery. Further observation and care may be required, especially if the patient entered the PACU in a deteriorated condition or an adverse event occurred during recovery. Examples of such individuals are patients who are hypothermic or posthemorrhagic, or those whose vital signs cannot be stabilized. Inpatients are transferred to the ICU for critical care observation and nursing. Ambulatory patients may be admitted to the ICU or surgical unit for overnight care (or longer if necessary).

DISCHARGE AGAINST MEDICAL ADVICE

Occasionally, a patient may opt for self-discharge against the advice of medical and nursing personnel; this is known as **discharge against medical advice (AMA).** Patients have a right to leave the health care facility as long as they do not pose a threat to themselves or others.

Unless evidence exists of potential harm, patients must be allowed to leave. However, if possible, the facility tries to obtain a signed waiver from the patient and explain the possible outcomes of both the surgery and the consequences of early discharge. The waiver states that the consequences of early discharge have been explained, that discharge was not advised, and that the patient takes responsibility for the consequences.

DEATH IN THE PACU

Death of a patient during surgery is unusual. In the event of impending death or a rapidly deteriorating patient, surgery may be terminated and the patient taken to the PACU. Death may be pronounced (formally) in the PACU after resuscitative means have been exhausted. The patient's family is notified, and PACU staff members arrange for an immediate conference with the family and surgeon. A designated staff member stays with the family to provide emotional support. Further care may be implemented through hospital chaplaincy and social services. Chapter 14 presents a complete discussion of death and dying.

KEY CONCEPTS

- Anesthesia is a subspecialty of medicine. Within the practice, there are a number of different professional roles performed by physicians and non-physician specialists.
- The anesthesia evaluation is a critical assessment of the patient's physiological fitness for surgery.
- Anesthesia equipment and devices used in physiological monitoring are becoming increasingly complex. These are needed to ensure patient safety throughout the surgical procedure.
- Airway management is the first of three (airway, breathing, circulation) critical interventions in a physiological emergency and in routine care of the patient.

- Induction of general anesthesia is achieved primarily with the use of intravenous barbiturates. Manipulation of the patient's level of consciousness, sensory awareness, and physiological processes is possible using a combination of drugs and methods of anesthesia.
- The surgical technologist is directly involved in certain types of regional anesthesia. He or she must understand how the drugs are used, when they are used, and how they are delivered.
- The phases of general anesthesia include induction, maintenance, emergence, and recovery.
- Anesthesia emergencies are those that occur as a direct result of the drugs used, or due to a physiological emergency that occurs while the patient is under anesthetic. Some emergencies require action by the entire surgical team. Individual roles depend on the type of emergency.
- The surgical technologist has distinct roles during some types of emergencies. The ST must know what to do, when to do it, and what equipment is needed.
- The postanesthesia care unit (PACU) is designed for immediate access to patients recovering from anesthesia. The open space design allows patient gurneys and large equipment to be positioned quickly and efficiently.
- Equipment and supplies used in the PACU are similar to those used in other intensive care units. Inline oxygen, suction, and monitoring equipment are available in each patient bay for immediate use.
- As patients are admitted to the PACU, care of the patient is transferred from the anesthesia care provider to the PACU nurse. The handover is a formal procedure that requires concise information and clear communication among professional staff.
- The Glasgow Coma Scale (GCS) is a basic assessment tool that can be used to determine the level of consciousness.
- Postoperative complications can occur at any time in the recovery period. Emergencies are handled according to hospital protocol using the normal emergency system. Acute hemorrhage may require the patient to be returned emergently to the operating room for wound exploration.
- Some health care facilities use the PACU for outpatient recovery and discharge. In this case, discharge planning must take place on the unit.
- Patient education is an important phase of discharge planning that requires thorough understanding of the patient's condition, healing process, and attention to the individual needs of the patient.
- Unanticipated, usually uncommon patient outcomes include failure to meet criteria for discharge from the PACU, death of a patient, and discharge against medical advice.
- Early discharge is the patient's right, but they must sign a self-discharge release.

REVIEW QUESTIONS

1. Under what medical circumstances may regional anesthesia be used?
2. What is the purpose of the ASA risk assessment classification?
3. Why is a musculoskeletal assessment necessary for the preoperative patient?
4. What are some considerations in selecting an appropriate method of anesthesia?
5. Define homeostasis.
6. What is physiological monitoring?
7. What is the normal core temperature range for an adult?
8. What are protective reflexes? Describe four or more protective reflexes.
9. Describe commonly used methods of regional anesthesia.
10. Into what specific tissue is a spinal anesthetic administered? An epidural anesthetic?
11. Briefly describe deep vein thrombosis and pulmonary embolism. How are these conditions prevented?
12. Why are the patient's vital signs taken immediately on arrival in the PACU?
13. What is the rationale for providing the PACU nurse with the names and amounts of all drugs administered to the patient in the preoperative and intraoperative periods?
14. What is the Glasgow Coma Scale? What is its application in the postoperative recovery phase for a patient who has had general anesthesia?
15. Hypothermia is one of the most serious complications of surgery. What procedures are necessary during the intraoperative period to prevent hypothermia in the postoperative period?
16. How does the scrubbed surgical technologist contribute to preventing patient hypothermia?

CASE STUDIES

CASE 1

A patient arrives in the operating room for surgery to be performed under general anesthesia. You have been assigned to assist the perioperative registered nurse circulator during the case. The anesthesiologist assists in settling the patient and preoperative medications are administered. The team is ready to start, and the patient is induced. Immediately after intubation, the anesthesiologist hands you the patient's dentures, which she has just removed, and asks you to take care of them. What should you do with these? Should the dentures have been removed before the patient arrived in surgery?

CASE 2

You are assigned to assist in circulator duties on a procedure requiring spinal anesthesia in your teaching hospital. Your immediate task is to help position the patient for the spinal and help the patient maintain the position while the spinal is administered. The patient states to you that she is afraid, but you reassure her that there will be little discomfort. The anesthesia care provider and anesthesia resident state that the patient should be placed in a side-lying position. The anesthesia procedure begins:

1. The anesthesia care provider tells the resident that he or she should go ahead and perform the procedure. The resident steps forward and applies a cold prep solution to the injection site. The patient flinches and moves out of position. What do you do?

2. The local anesthetic has been injected into the spinal injection site, and the resident searches for the correct insertion site for the spinal needle by palpating the intervertebral spaces. The patient asks you quietly if the needle is in yet. What do you reply?
3. Now the resident has made four attempts to enter the subarachnoid space. Fresh spinal needles have been brought into the room for more attempts. The patient is now very uncomfortable and feeling the pain of the repeated insertions of the spinal needle by the resident. Two more attempts are made without success. What should you say to your patient, who is visibly upset and trying to remain still?
4. What, if any, is your dialogue with the resident during these attempts?
5. Finally, after many attempts, the anesthesia care provider takes over and is able to insert the spinal needle at first attempt. Everyone is relieved. Think carefully about what you would say to the patient at this point.

CASE 3

You are assigned to scrub on a case requiring local infiltration anesthetic with monitored sedation for the removal of a skin lesion on the leg. The patient is positioned on the operating table, and the anesthetist applies monitoring devices and administers light sedation. The surgeon arrives and states that he will inject the local anesthetic and then go out to scrub. You have prepared the local anesthetic, and the surgeon puts on gloves and infiltrates the surgical site. He then leaves the room. You have completed your setup and are ready for the case. The circulator has left the room to check on the surgical schedule. The anesthetist states that he needs to step into the hallway to speak to a colleague and asks you to keep an eye on the patient. Within moments, the patient appears restless. You note that the patient's heart rate has increased dramatically, as tracked by the cardiac monitor. The patient mumbles something, and without contaminating your gown and gloves, you come closer to try and understand what he is saying. You are alarmed to see that the patient is quite pale.

1. What should you do?
2. This scenario may be the beginning of an emergency. Was there any violation of patient care responsibilities? Think carefully about this.
3. After the situation is resolved, you mention to the circulator that it may be necessary to fill out an incident report. He replies, "Oh, that's not necessary, nothing bad happened." What is your response to this?

CASE 4

You are asked to transport a fully conscious and alert patient who has just undergone minor surgery under local anesthetic to the PACU. The handover will be provided by the circulating nurse, who will be delayed by a few minutes. When you arrive with your patient, you recognize that there is code (cardiac arrest) in the PACU and most of the staff is engaged in full resuscitation procedures. What should you do? What are the important considerations in this scenario? Think carefully about patient protection, priorities, and the emotional impact on your patient.

CASE 5

At the end of the surgical procedure, the surgeon injected the area around the incision with a long-acting local anesthetic. You realize that you haven't yet reported the amount to the circulating nurse. The AP and circulating nurse have already left the operating suite and are transporting the patient to the PACU. What should you do?

CASE 6

Hospital policy states that patients who are transported with active cardiac monitoring in place must be accompanied to the PACU by a licensed perioperative nurse and anesthesia provider. What do you think is the rationale for this? Among other things, think about patient safety and response in case of medical emergency during transport.

REFERENCES

Ali Algadiem E, Aleisa AA, Alsubaie HI, Buhlaiqah NR, Algadeeb JB, Alsneini HA. Blood loss estimation using gauze visual analogue. *Trauma Mon*. 2016;21(2):e34131.

Mace SE. Challenges and advances in intubation: airway evaluation and controversies with intubation. *Emerg Med Clin North Am*. 2008;26(4):977.

Miller R, Eriksson L, Fleisher L, et al. *Miller's Anesthesia*. 7th ed. Philadelphia: Churchill Livingstone; 2009.

BIBLIOGRAPHY

Agency for Healthcare Research and Quality. *The Inside of a Timeout*; 2008. Available at https://psnet.ahrq.gov/webmm/case/177/The-Inside-of-a-Time-Out. Accessed June 28, 2019.

American Society of Anesthesiologists (ASA), American Society of Anesthesiologists (ASA) Committee on Standards and Practice Parameters:

American Association of Nurse Anesthetists, Postanesthesia Care Standards for the Certified Registered Nurse Anesthetist. https://static1.squarespace.com/static/579770cd197aea84455d6908/t/57d6f8d7bebafb8f2ebe5e1b/1473706200039/PPM+PACU+Standards.pdf. Accessed June 26, 2019.

American Society of Anesthesiologists. *Standards for Postanesthesia Care*; 2014. https://www.asahq.org/standards-and-guidelines/standards-for-postanesthesia-care. Accessed June 25, 2019.

Association of periOperative Registered Nurses (AORN). *Guidelines for Perioperative Practice*. Denver: AORN; 2019.

Farab E. *Brown's Atlas of Regional Anesthesia*. 5th ed. Elsevier; 2017.

Gropper M A. *Miller's Anesthesia*. 9th ed. Elsevier; 2020.

Hemmings H, Hopkins P. *Foundations of Anesthesia*. 2nd ed. St Louis: Saunders; 2006.

Porth C. *Pathophysiology: Concepts of Altered Health States*. 9th ed. Philadelphia: Lippincott Williams & Wilkins; 2013.

The Joint Commission: Preventing and Managing the Impact of Anesthesia Awareness. http://www.jointcommission.org/assets/1/18/SEA_32.PDF. Accessed December 31, 2015.

Thibodeau G, Patton K. *Anatomy and Physiology*. 6th ed. St Louis: Saunders; 2007.

DEATH AND DYING 14

LEARNING OBJECTIVES

After studying this chapter, the reader will be able to:

1. Define the end-of-life period and brain death
2. Describe Kübler-Ross's stages of dying
3. Discuss ways to provide comfort and support to patients in the dying period
4. Understand the conflicts and stress that families face during the dying period
5. Discuss significant ethical issues surrounding death and dying
6. Define cultural competence as it applies to the dying patient
7. Discuss the concept of determination of death and the physical changes in the body immediately after death
8. Give examples of a coroner's case
9. Discuss principles of organ recovery

TERMINOLOGY

Advance health care directive: A written document stating an individual's specific wishes regarding his or her health care to be enacted in the event the person is unable to make decisions.

Coroner's case: A patient death that requires investigation by the coroner as well as an autopsy on the deceased.

Cultural competence: The ability to provide support and care to individuals of cultures and belief systems different from one's own.

Determination of death: A formal medical process to determine brain death.

DNAR: "Do not attempt resuscitation." Emphasizes the patient's desire to refuse intervention to resuscitate.

DNR: "Do not resuscitate." An official request to refrain from certain types of resuscitation, usually cardiopulmonary resuscitation.

End of life: A period within which death is expected, usually days to months.

Heart-beating cadaver: A cadaver maintained on cardiopulmonary support to provide tissue perfusion. This is done to maintain viability in organs for donation.

Kübler-Ross, Elisabeth: A Swiss psychiatrist who proposed a theory of developmental or psychological stages of the dying experience.

Living will: A legal document signed by the patient stating the conditions and limitations of medical assistance in the event of near death or a prognosis of death.

Non–heart-beating cadaver: A cadaver in which perfusion at and after death was not possible. Only certain tissues may be procured for donation.

Postmortem care: Physical care of the body to prepare it for viewing by the family and for mortuary procedures.

Required request law: A law requiring medical personnel to request organ recovery from a deceased's family.

Rigor mortis: The natural stiffening of the body that starts approximately 15 minutes after death and lasts about 24 hours.

Although death in the operating room is a relatively rare event, training in death has returned to the curriculum of health care workers. All allied health personnel benefit from a structured study on death, with the main focus on the psychosocial and procedural aspects.

This chapter is not intended to provide a course in death and dying. It is the basis for further study and exploration. This chapter discusses basic social, personal, ethical, legal, and medical perspectives on death. An understanding of the process of death and the events triggered by it can aid the surgical technologist in providing compassionate care to patients and their families. Knowledge and understanding also contribute to the health professional's beliefs and values.

The procedural aspects of death and the protocols that must be followed may seem "clinical" in nature; however, they are necessary to ensure dignity, order, and professionalism.

DEFINING THE END OF LIFE

Death and the end of life can be defined from many perspectives. The study and experience of different perspectives assists health professionals in their support of the dying patient and family.

From a medical point of view, the **end of life** is the period when death is expected. Most clinicians pronounce the patient's entry into a dying state when death is expected within days, weeks, or months. The dying period is marked by the inability to provide or the cessation of attempts to prolong life. However, this does not mean that comfort care is not provided in the dying period. It simply means that death cannot be avoided.

The diagnosis of *brain death* is used when the entire brain ceases to function without life support mechanisms in place. Some functions such as respiration and heartbeat can be maintained artificially, even during brain death. However, in the United States, brain death means *real death*, and no other distinction is used for legal or medical purposes.

CAUSE OF DEATH

From a medical perspective, the cause of death is determined by the Centers for Disease Control and Prevention *International Classification of Diseases*, which is required for coding all medical cases, including trauma (intentional or unintentional). This coding system provides extensive guidelines for how to register the cause of death on the death certificate and also has implications for the recovery of insurance. The system includes the direct as well as the indirect cause. For example, the individual may have the underlying cause of death as kidney disease, but the direct cause of the death is cardiac arrest.

From a nonmedical or social perspective, the cause of death can influence the family and community's response to death. *Sudden death* is often the most devastating, as it is unexpected regardless of the actual cause. *Accidental* death is a type of sudden death that is referred to by insurance carriers. It is caused by an activity or event caused by the deceased or another person or persons. Examples are motor vehicle accidents, accidents occurring in the workplace, and intentional violence by another person. Death resulting from *terminal illness* is by definition usually expected by the family and community. This includes death related to *chronic illness*, in which the deceased has succumbed to a long-term condition.

MODELS OF DEATH AND DYING

News that oneself or a loved one has begun the dying process triggers a cascade of emotional and psychological events. In the past few decades, a number of models have been presented that explain these events and processes. The best-known model was developed in the 1960s by Swiss psychiatrist **Elisabeth Kübler-Ross**, who described the stages of death. In her model, the stages of death are not discrete, nor are they predictable in all people of all cultures. The Kübler-Ross model proposed the following stages of grief and dying:

- **Denial:** The patient denies that he or she is dying. This is described by mental health professionals as a natural response to shocking events. Denial is a defense mechanism that forestalls the full impact of the fact of death until the mind is ready to accept it.
- **Anger:** Feelings of anger may be projected onto the family, oneself, health workers, or a spiritual entity. Some patients feel great anger and remorse that they did not heed warnings to change lifestyle habits they knew were harmful. Others express anger at those who care for them or become very demanding in their care. Patients may express anger at themselves by refusing treatment or nutrition. These coping strategies may be an attempt to gain control over the environment.
- **Bargaining:** Kübler-Ross describes this stage as a way of postponing death. The patient may make an inner attempt to bargain with a spiritual entity, such as, "I just want to experience one pain-free day with my family" or "If I pray daily, maybe I will live."
- **Depression:** True clinical depression may occur during the dying process. In recent years, there has been a trend away from accepting depression as a natural result of dying and to treat it clinically.
- **Acceptance:** In Kübler-Ross's theory, death is "accepted." The idea and interpretation of death are no longer a source of psychological conflict.

Critics of Kübler-Ross's model believe that the stage theory is too constricting and does not allow for individualism in the experience of death. However, the stages model provided a framework for psychologists and social workers to look at the process of dying in a way that had not been previously studied.

Many modern models have been developed since Kübler-Ross conducted her research. These appreciate individuals according to their situation, personality, culture, and life experiences. For example, William McDougall, a well-known social psychologist, emphasized the need to integrate the dying process into existing life experiences. Rather than focusing on particular tasks or psychological stages, he advocated maintaining a sense of self-awareness in relation to the environment. Social psychologist Charles Corr encouraged the dying to try different individual strategies and coping mechanisms based on their uniqueness as individuals and was a strong critic of the stage theory of death.

SUPPORT AND COMFORT FOR THE DYING AND BEREAVED PATIENT

Perioperative caregivers may have only brief encounters with the dying patient in the surgical environment, whereas contact between patients and palliative care specialists is frequent and the relationships can last weeks or months. Perioperative staff members should always be aware that no matter how brief their contact with the dying patient, all encounters provide an opportunity to support and care for the patient in the dying process.

Communication with the dying patient requires keen listening and observation skills. It is important to recognize and acknowledge the fact of death and what this means to the patient in that moment and time. As a surgical technologist, you should focus on what the patient is experiencing in the operating room or holding area. Observe facial expressions and gestures. Be alert to any changes in mood or signs of anxiety and fear related to death and isolation. Avoid communication that attempts to minimize, rationalize, or deny death. However, this does not imply blunt or insensitive communication. Focus on immediate physical and emotional comfort and acknowledgment, and above all, listen to the patient. Listening is sometimes the most effective source of comfort (but not always the easiest). A response may not be needed and should not be forced. Respect the patient's individuality and uniqueness in the present. Use the patient's verbal and physical cues as a guideline rather than making assumptions about what the patient feels or needs.

Never imply that a surgical procedure may "cure" the patient, but offer the possibility of a good outcome. Perhaps the patient is having surgery to reduce the size of a tumor or for treatment of intractable pain. These procedures offer hope for a longer survival period or one that is physically tolerable.

FAMILY

Families and friends react to dying and death in many different ways. Not only must they cope with the emotional and psychological impact of death, they must also make many significant decisions. They have a central role in the dying patient's emotional environment, and in sudden death, they often need the assistance and guidance of health professionals.

The family's reactions of grief and sadness may be accompanied by bouts of anger and frustration with the health care system, each other, and even the dying family member. Death triggers large and sometimes unmanageable emotions, and these cannot always be contained in ways that are considered socially acceptable. This may be disconcerting to family members as they participate in the death and observe their own reactions as a family unit. The wise health professional recognizes when tensions are mounting and provides validation for these strong emotions. At the same time, the health professional can guide family members toward coping strategies to help defuse the tension and add order to the experience (e.g., support groups).

Families usually face many complex events associated with death and dying. The death may impose a financial burden. The dying patient may have children or other family members who rely on the individual for support, and these responsibilities must be shifted to other family members. Difficult decisions may have to be made about palliative care or "do not resuscitate" (DNR) status. The administrative requirements, such as signing release forms or attending to the details of funeral arrangements, often seem too clinical or cold in the midst of grieving. Professionals who routinely care for the dying provide ongoing support in many areas. This includes not only management of the patient's medical needs but also emotional support and even referral for counseling outside the medical and nursing environment.

SUDDEN, UNEXPECTED DEATH

When death is sudden and unexpected, family and friends have many needs. In the clinical environment, these immediate needs are addressed by nurses, physicians, and spiritual counselors. Early reactions often focus on information about the cause and details of death. The need for cloistered privacy is usually very strong in the initial stages of shock and grief.

The surgical technologist should refrain from providing information to family or friends about the patient's medical condition. This is the responsibility of the physicians and nurses, and any discussions must be deferred to them. The surgical technologist may offer acknowledgment of the loss. He or she may also facilitate communication between the family and other professionals, such as showing the way to the consultation area and making sure that the environment is appropriate.

ETHICAL CONSIDERATIONS IN DEATH AND DYING

The ethics of care and decision making in death and dying are highly personal, and there are many conflicting viewpoints. Beliefs and culture influence the decisions people make about how they want to die or how they would like others to go through the dying process. These beliefs are not universal. This means that whenever possible, an individual's personal wishes for his or her own death should be documented and validated by individuals and their families.

SELF-DETERMINATION

Self-determination is the right of every individual to make decisions about how he or she lives and dies. Advance care planning provides an accepted method for individuals to define their needs and wishes about death and dying. Patients may refuse treatment at any point in the dying process. They may select which palliative measures are performed and which are withheld. Decisions can then be communicated and made official for health care providers. Ethical issues arise when the patient is not competent to communicate. Decisions about end-of-life care fall to the family when the patient is not able to communicate his or her wishes. In these cases, health care workers help provide information about choices, as well as ongoing support throughout the decision-making process. Ethical decisions that cannot be resolved by the family and health care professionals may be brought before the hospital ethics committee for review.

RIGHT TO DIE

An individual may believe that he or she has a "right to die" and may refuse treatment to fulfill this right. However, *not treating a dying patient* is a completely different process from *treating with intent to harm.* Assisted suicide is perceived by many as intent to harm and is rejected on that basis. *Assisted suicide* is intentional harm to a person, at their request, to promote or cause death. The arguments for and against assisted suicide continue in many states and countries. The states that allow assisted suicide include Oregon, California, Washington, Vermont, and Montana. The process involves stringent preconditions and extensive review by an ethics committee.

ADVANCE HEALTH CARE DIRECTIVES

The **advance health care directive** is a document in which an individual states his or her wishes with regard to health care. The document is used in the event that the person is unable to communicate those wishes. This and other documents such as a *living will* that instruct others on how health care is to be delivered, as well as who should act on the patient's behalf and oversee that person's care, are generally referred to as a *power of attorney*. However, the names of the documents that reflect one's wishes regarding health matters differ according to state laws.

"Do not resuscitate" **(DNR)** and "do not attempt resuscitation" **(DNAR)** are two types of health directives that express the patient's decision to decline lifesaving efforts. In some cases, the family makes this decision for the patient who is incompetent to do so at the time. The request not to resuscitate is made official when the patient signs a DNR order, which is charted in the patient's medical record. Explicit forms that define precisely the procedures that can and cannot be performed during resuscitation have been designed to alleviate ambiguity. However, ethical conflicts arise in spite of protocol. These usually occur when no DNR status has been stated and the decision is left for the family. The definition of *resuscitation* may also cause ambiguity. Active measures to prolong life are ethically different from those that do not halt the progression of death.

The individual's DNR status must be verified throughout the period of patient care. In most facilities, the DNR status must be renewed with each hospital admission. Health care providers may not realize that the patient has redefined his or her wishes at some point during his or her illness. Admission to the surgical unit always includes verification of the DNR status.

CONFLICTS IN PALLIATIVE CARE

Palliative care is the medical and supportive care provided to the dying patient. Numerous types of surgical intervention may be included as a component of palliative care, such as debulking of a tumor or debridement of a pressure wound. Procedures for the implantation of biomedical devices, such as a gastric feeding tube or renal dialysis access, require anesthesia in the interventional radiology department or operating room. Medical interventions for the dying patient include extreme measures, such as respiratory support ("artificial respiration"), intravenous feeding, dialysis, drugs to maintain and regulate failed metabolic processes, and many others.

The ethics of palliative care involve reasoned arguments about the definition of particular interventions. Many patients have signed a **living will,** which specifies the exact nature of palliative care that they accept. In the absence of a living will, clinical decisions are sometimes made by consensus among the patient (when able), the family, and care providers. Most people intend to do the "right thing." They try to resolve the conflicts about quality of life. However, families may have trouble deciding when to prolong life by supportive measures and when to discontinue them based on the suffering they may cause. These decisions are extremely difficult and often fraught with emotion and conflict within the family.

An ethical discussion that often arises is whether withdrawal of care constitutes suffering. Intravenous maintenance (hydration) and feeding are often the most sensitive areas for families to resolve. In these cases, the health professional makes every attempt to inform the family about the effects of withdrawing care without interfering with their right to decide.

Health care workers often face personal conflict about the decisions made by their patients or the families of patients. They may not agree with the decisions, but they are obliged to honor them. In extreme cases of ethical conflict, the health professional may ask to be excused from participation in the care of the patient. Although this resolves the conflict temporarily, it does not offer long-term relief from an environment that frequently challenges beliefs and values. At some point in their careers, health care professionals usually need to define their own ethics and accept that others have differing perspectives.

CULTURAL RESPONSES TO DEATH AND DYING

SPIRITUAL AND RELIGIOUS CONCEPTS

Death, as perceived across cultures, is often defined through spiritual values and beliefs. Meaning in life and death are often linked to spiritual hope. The rituals and practices that people of different cultures observe are vital to the fulfillment of their duty to the dying person. In the United States, great efforts have been made to honor and respect the beliefs of others, but there is still a long way to go. Health care workers may question the validity of a belief or an expression of a patient's faith, often comparing it to their own. By definition, spiritual beliefs are valid for the believer and do not require approval or justification by others.

Support and care across cultures is called **cultural competence.** It is learned through experience and active learning. It begins with acceptance and respect. In many cultures, death is considered a natural phenomenon, a possible conclusion of serious illness and not a battle with the cause. Although grief and other deep emotions are present in all families at the time of death, these feelings are often mitigated by ritual and ceremony, which comfort as well as heal the living. In many cultures, they are also believed to comfort the dead.

Handling of the body, especially its preparation for viewing by the family, may require special knowledge about the practices of certain cultures. As long as these practices do not conflict with health and safety standards, they should be carried out with dignity and respect. Notification of death to chosen religious clergy is generally left to the family.

DEATH IN THE CLINICAL SETTING

DETERMINATION OF DEATH

When death occurs in surgery, the surgeon and anesthesia care provider must verify that brain death has occurred; this is called **determination of death.** Death is determined by specific medical criteria, which have legal implications. To determine brain death, specific medical assessment may be carried out on the patient to determine the absence of breathing, response to painful stimuli, and the presence of cranial reflexes. More complex tests can be performed if necessary, such as electroencephalography or computed tomography (Box 14.1).

BOX 14.1 Medical Assessment Criteria for Determining Death

Complete and irreversible cessation of the cardiovascular system
Irreversible respiratory failure that is not a result of drugs or hypothermia
Absence of any response to external stimuli
Cessation of cranial nerve reflexes
Cessation of all brain activity

EXTENDED TESTS FOR BRAIN DEATH

1. Electroencephalography, which registers electrical (functional) brain activity
2. Cerebral radionuclide injection, which demonstrates uptake of radioactive substance in the presence of brainstem function
3. Computed tomography scan to determine massive hemorrhage, edema, or other evidence of critical pathology

When death has been determined, the operating room supervisor communicates with other key individuals to prepare the morgue (or coroner, in some cases) or the supervisor of the postanesthesia care unit (PACU). The deceased may be transported to the PACU for postmortem care. Arrangements are made for the family to meet with the surgeon or a designee in a quiet area near the surgical department or PACU.

The surgical wound is closed appropriately and dressed. Drapes are removed from the patient (if they were not removed during resuscitation), and instruments and supplies are prepared as they would be at the close of any case. The patient may then be transported to the PACU or another location in the surgical department for postmortem care.

Documentation for the surgical procedure is completed as usual, with accurate recording of the chain of events. Operative records for patient care, anesthesia, sponge counts, and all usual forms must be completed as for any case. Documentation related to the death of the patient is completed by the attending physician and anesthesiologist. Registration of the death is a separate legal document that is completed by the attending physician. Because death in the operating room is a sentinel event, the circulator must initial all forms as for any sentinel event. If death was pronounced in the operating room, members of the surgical team are named in the sentinel event documentation.

POSTMORTEM CARE

Postmortem care prepares the body for viewing by the family and assists in further handling procedures carried out by the morgue and mortuary. The exact protocol for postmortem care is carefully defined by every health care facility. All staff members who perform postmortem care must be completely familiar with the protocol, and there should be no ambiguity about the process. The protocol for coroner's cases is different, and this procedure is also clearly documented in each health care facility. General care of the body is based on the process of death.

NATURAL CHANGES IN THE BODY AFTER DEATH

Immediately after death, the body begins to cool. All sphincter muscles, including those controlling feces and urine, immediately lose tone. The eyes remain open, and the jaw drops down. Dependent areas of the body (those under pressure from body weight or gravity) begin to collect fluid, and the areas around the ears and cheeks may turn purple or red (a condition called *livor mortis*). The pooling of blood in these regions cannot be reversed in the embalming process. The sacrum and other pressure areas fill with fluid, possibly resulting in tissue rupture. **Rigor mortis,** the natural stiffening of the body, begins approximately 15 minutes after death and peaks at 8 to 10 hours. The exact time depends on the tissues and environmental temperature. At 18 hours, the process regresses, and the body is usually relaxed after 24 hours. Rigor mortis begins at the head (eyelids) and progresses to the feet. When relaxation begins, it follows the reverse order of progression.

GENERAL POSTMORTEM PROCEDURES

All health care facilities have a postmortem kit that contains the supplies needed to perform aftercare. During the aftercare procedure, the body is handled gently and with respect at all times. Postmortem care that conflicts with the patient's religious affiliation is not performed. In some facilities, when death occurs during surgery, the body must remain on the operating table, intact, until a decision is made about a coroner's investigation.

CORONER'S CASES

The circumstances of the patient's death determine whether the coroner must investigate the death; this process includes mandatory autopsy, and such a case is called a **coroner's case.** Most states have similar criteria for establishing coroner's cases, and the criteria may include the following circumstances of death:

- Death in the operating room or emergency department
- Unwitnessed death
- Death after admission from another facility
- Death in which criminal activity is suspected (the deceased may have been the perpetrator or the victim)
- Suicide
- Death of an incarcerated individual
- Death as a result of an infectious disease that may pose a public health risk

Other criteria may also apply, depending on state law. Coroner's cases require that the conditions of the body remain intact for examination and investigation. In the medical environment, all implanted or invasive devices are left in place. The patient's property may also be transferred to the coroner rather than returned to the family. Meticulous care and identification of specimens are always required, regardless of whether the specimens become part of the investigation. After a death in surgery, any specimens produced during surgery become the property of the coroner. They must be transferred directly from the operating room, as specified by hospital protocol, following universal precautions.

BOX 14.2 Organ Recovery and Tissue Bank Organizations

- American Society of Transplant Surgeons
- The Organ Recovery and Transplantation Network (OPTA)
- United Network for Organ Sharing (UNOS)
- American Association of Tissue Banks

ORGAN RECOVERY

Organ recovery is the removal, preservation, and use of human organs and tissue from a recently deceased person for transplantation into a living individual. Once the decision has been made for organ recovery, exacting clinical protocols are followed to ensure the vitality of the organs.

Permission for Recovery

Before the issue arises, a person can make the decision to donate tissue or whole organs. In many states, this permission may be verified on an individual's driver's license or other identification card. Some states have a **required request law,** which requires medical professionals and other caregivers to ask the family for permission to recover organs from the deceased.

Protocols

The process of recovery is administered through tissue banks and organ recovery agencies, which locate donors, register recipients, and organize recovery. Many organizations are involved in the process, which requires a high level of coordination and data exchange.

Donors are registered in different regions of the country, and the data are exchanged with recovery organizations (Box 14.2). The protocols for medical recovery, care of tissue, and identification of tissue are formulated by the American Association of Tissue Banks, a nonprofit, scientific organization that accredits tissue banks and recovery organizations to ensure professional standards of practice.

Organs are collected and stored by regional organ banks and provided to facilities as needed. Services are available on call 24 hours a day. Data are constantly exchanged between tissue banks and the organ recovery registries to match donor organs with compatible recipients.

Organ recovery takes place as soon as possible after death because the vitality of some tissues is time dependent. Actual recovery takes place at the hospital or in a tissue bank organization. When recovery occurs at the host hospital, a transplant coordinator from the regional tissue bank arrives on site to ensure that medical, administrative, and supportive services are carried out according to set standards. The recovery team travels to the hospital as soon as possible after the death of a donor when time-sensitive tissue is to be procured.

Medical Criteria for Tissue Recovery

Different types of tissue require specific medical maintenance to remain viable after death. Donor cadavers are generally divided into two categories: heart-beating and non–heart-beating.

HEART-BEATING CADAVER A **heart-beating cadaver** is one in which tissue perfusion can be maintained during and immediately after death to preserve the life of the tissue. Cardiopulmonary support provides intact circulation to organs suitable for recovery. The availability of cardiopulmonary support depends on the exact location of death; it is usually restricted to the emergency department, operating room, or critical care unit, where equipment, supplies, and trained personnel are immediately available. The physiological parameters for recovery include renal output, vascular pressure, temperature, and perfusion.

NON–HEART-BEATING CADAVER Tissues from a **non–heart-beating cadaver** are restricted to those that do not need perfusion to sustain viability for later transplantation. These include the cornea, blood vessels, heart valves, bone, and skin.

Controlled Organ Donation After Death

Even though medical associations, ethics organizations, and state legislatures have established criteria and rules for determination of death, it remains a controversial topic. It is beyond the scope of this textbook to discuss the issues at great length. However, one principle is important for health professionals to be familiar with: the controlled organ donation after death. This is the practice of maintaining a patient's vital functions after death to preserve the organs.

Below are two websites that may assist students who wish to research determination of death further. https://www.ncbi.nlm.nih.gov/pmc/articles/PMC4889813/ https://www.asahq.org/standards-and-guidelines/statement-on-controlled-organ-donation-after-circulatory-death

Ethical Dilemmas in Organ Recovery

Organ and tissue donation arise as an ethical issue when the patient has not left a clear directive before death. When no verifiable permission has been granted by the patient, the family may act as a surrogate for the patient.

Many cultures and faiths forbid organ removal after death, and these cases are usually straightforward for the family and patient. However, individuals often leave the question unresolved at the time of death. If no decision has been made by the patient, the attending physician must, *by law*, ask the patient and family to consider organ donation. In cases of sudden death without clear directives, conflicting views may be held by family members about organ donation. The ethical problem is whether the family can and should make such a decision for the deceased. Some families may feel very strongly opposed to organ donation, whereas others feel that it is a way of providing life.

HEALTH PROFESSIONALS CONFRONTING DEATH

The emotional and psychological events triggered by the sudden death of a patient vary in health care workers. The reactions and coping skills available to these professionals are often influenced by the following factors:

- Previous experience with death
- Support available in the environment
- The health care professional's beliefs and values
- Knowledge about the process of death
- The health care professional's emotional well-being

The types of emotions or even severe psychological events that health care workers experience may be similar to those of the dying patient. Shock and denial are common in sudden death, especially when the patient is young or the death was violent.

For many health care workers, care of the dying is extremely rewarding and leads to important understanding about one's own values and beliefs. The ability to provide comfort to both the patient and their family often results in the discovery of a special ability to nurture. This quality is the reason why many health care workers begin a career in patient care.

However, some health professionals may experience a crisis in connection with the death of a patient or in the care of the dying. Unresolved emotions related to previous loss or conflicts about beliefs and values may lead to depression or other severe psychological reactions. This is different from normal feelings of sadness, loss, and even frustration, which health professionals experience at various stages when caring for a dying patient. When these feelings arise, they can affect the quality of the health care worker's life and interfere with the individual's ability to cope with stress in the workplace.

A structured response may be required to help health care workers cope with death. This may involve planned "debriefing" periods or spontaneous expressions of support and acknowledgment by individual team members. Organized support groups for team members can provide a forum for discussion and reflection. Health care workers can often benefit from coping skills that other professionals have found helpful:

- Often it is helpful for staff who were involved in the patient's care or death to discuss the details of the death, going over exactly what happened and why. This is not to "medicalize" the death, but rather to discern the limitations of medical care and the fact that medical professionals cannot control all situations. It helps people understand that human intervention has limits, especially in the face of inevitable death.
- Acknowledgment of one's feelings is helpful for many. Sometimes, it is important to express the sadness, shock, and even anger that professionals feel after the death of a patient. It allows others to understand the feelings of their colleagues and to show acknowledgment and comfort. However, many people are not comfortable displaying their feelings or even discussing them, and this must be respected. No one should be coaxed into expressing that which is private and confidential.
- Distraction provides a healthy break from severe stress. The effects of a tragic death in the operating room can linger for weeks, and this can have a serious effect on team morale and individual coping ability. Sometimes, it is good to "lighten the conversation" or plan activities that do not remind people of the death. This does not diminish the meaning or significance of the death; it simply provides time to step away from it.
- The health care worker must attend to self-care. At some point in their careers, all health care professionals must reflect on whether the stress of work is balanced by healthy coping mechanisms. This can be done through self-reflection or speaking to a confidant (e.g., with a mentor or religious figure).

KEY CONCEPTS

- The terms *end of life* and *brain death* are precisely defined in medicine. Although it may seem that scientific definitions are uncompassionate, they are necessary to provide the basis of legal and ethical decisions surrounding the death of an individual.
- The Kübler-Ross stages of dying were among the first psychosocial descriptions of the experience of death. Since these were published in the 1960s, there has been more advanced work showing an appreciation of the individual nature of each person's response to the death experience. However, the Kübler-Ross model is frequently cited as a basic study.
- Surgical technologists may be required to communicate with the family of a patient who has died in care. Although this is a relatively rare occurrence, the surgical technologist should develop a method of communication that is supportive and comforting to the family.
- The families of dying patients face many challenges and difficulties in the end-of-life period. Effective and compassionate communication with the family and the patient is enhanced by understanding some of the more common problems that families face. These not only include the psychological effects of grief but can also be related to the patient's medical care or to the practical aspects of finances and estate issues.
- At some time in their career, nearly all health care workers are confronted with ethical issues involving death. Although they may not be required to make a decision themselves, they do witness others involved in choices and dilemmas. These are not easy topics and often touch on closely held values and traditions. However, awareness of events that may occur and reflection on the issues is worthwhile early on in one's career.
- Death and dying are often accompanied by traditional practices, many of which are based in culture. Cultural competence in the subject of death is extremely important to understanding how others interpret and respond to the experience. The process of learning about the traditions and rituals that are closely held by others helps to define the way we communicate and show empathy. Certain traditions may also directly affect the disposition of amputated limbs or other tissues removed from the body.
- Specific circumstances under which a person dies determine whether a legal investigation, including an autopsy, is required. If the circumstances meet the legal criteria, the death is referred to as a *coroner's case*. Specific postmortem care and protection of evidence are also required in a coroner's case. The criteria and procedures for such a case vary from state to state. However, the surgical technologist

should be aware of the conditions that constitute a coroner's case in his or her state.

- Organ and tissue recovery may be performed after the death of a patient. The criteria for organ donation are previously established, and no organs are removed until the criteria have been met.

REVIEW QUESTIONS

1. Define the end of life from a medical perspective.
2. What are the five stages of death as defined by Kübler-Ross?
3. Name several administrative responsibilities of the family when death occurs in the clinical setting.
4. How can clinicians help families accomplish these administrative tasks while coping with the grief and shock of death?
5. What is self-determination? How does it apply to death and dying?
6. How can a patient express his or her "right to die"? How can this be carried out if the patient is unable to direct medical intervention?
7. Is there a difference between treating a dying patient for comfort measures and treating with intent to prolong life? Explain.
8. How can health professionals honor cultural practices and beliefs in caring for the dying and the dead?
9. What is a coroner's case?
10. What is rigor mortis?
11. What specimens may be collected from a non–heart-beating cadaver?
12. What kinds of self-care are appropriate for you in times of stress? Why is it important to know this?

CASE STUDIES

CASE 1

A patient who developed severe peritonitis after gastric surgery 1 week ago has been returned to the operating room for an exploratory laparotomy. Within the first 30 minutes of surgery, the patient suddenly begins to hemorrhage from multiple sites within the abdomen, including blood vessels that were previously ligated. Although emergency attempts are made to halt the swift progression of this coagulopathy, the hemorrhaging worsens. When all attempts to reverse the condition have failed, the surgeon closes the abdominal wound and the patient is withdrawn from anesthesia. You now realize that the patient has died and will be quickly transported to the PACU.

1. Can you predict how this sudden death of a patient may affect your ability to carry on with necessary duties?
2. What are your initial responsibilities, assuming that you will not be accompanying the anesthesia care provider to the PACU?
3. After you have been relieved for a break, you are just outside the surgical department when one of the patient's family members whom you met just before surgery approaches you. What will you say to her?
4. What particular documentation does the surgical technologist need to complete as a member of the sterile team in which a patient death occurred? Refer to Chapter 3 for additional information on documentation.
5. Research the laws in your state that establish a coroner's death.

BIBLIOGRAPHY

Centers for Disease Control and Prevention, National Center for Health Statistics. Handbooks and guides for use with U.S. standard certificates and reports. https://www.cdc.gov/nchs/nvss/handbooks-and-guides.htm. Accessed July 1, 2019.

Eelco FMW, Panayiostis NV, et al. Evidence based guideline update: determining brain death in adults: report of the Quality Standards Subcommittee of the American Academy of Neurology. *Neurology*. 2010;74:1911–1918.

Kuebler K, Heidrich D, Esper P. *Palliative and End of Life Care*. 2nd ed. St Louis: WB Saunders/Elsevier; 2007.

Grossman S, Porth C. *Pathophysiology Concepts of Altered Health States*. 9th ed. Philadelphia: Lippincott Williams & Wilkins; 2013.

Thibodeau G, Patton K. *Anatomy and Physiology*. 6th ed. St Louis: Mosby/Saunders; 2007.

ENERGY SOURCES IN SURGERY 15

LEARNING OBJECTIVES

After studying this chapter, the reader will be able to:

1. Review the concepts of conduction, frequency, and impedance
2. Describe the uses and components of electrosurgery
3. Distinguish between monopolar and bipolar circuits used in electrosurgery
4. Discuss the safe use of the patient return (dispersive) electrode
5. List the primary hazards of electrosurgery and explain how to prevent accidents
6. Distinguish between capacitive coupling and indirect coupling
7. Describe the materials in a smoke plume and how to reduce exposure to the smoke plume
8. Describe how lasers are used in surgery
9. Recognize different types of laser media
10. Discuss safety precautions used during laser surgery

TERMINOLOGY

Ablation: The complete destruction of tissue.

Active electrode: In electrosurgery, the point of the electrosurgical instrument that delivers current to tissue.

Argon: An inert gas used in electrosurgery to direct and shroud the electrical current.

Bipolar circuit: An electrosurgical circuit in which current travels from the power unit through an instrument containing two opposite poles in contact with the tissue and then returns directly to the energy source.

Capacitive coupling: A specific burn hazard of monopolar endoscopic surgery. It occurs when current passes unintentionally through instrument insulation and adjacent conductive material into tissue.

Carbon dioxide: An inert gas used as a lasing medium during laser surgery.

Cavitron Ultrasonic Surgical Aspirator (CUSA): This instrument destroys tissue through the use of high-frequency sound waves (ultrasound).

Coagulum: A sticky, semiliquid substance that forms when tissue is altered by electrical or ultrasonic energy.

Cryoablation: A method of tissue destruction in which a probe is inserted into a tumor or tissue mass. High-pressure argon gas is injected into the probe, causing the surrounding tissue to freeze and eventually slough.

Cryosurgery: The use of extremely low temperature to destroy diseased tissue.

Cutting mode: In electrosurgery, the use of high voltage and relatively low frequency to cut through tissue.

Direct coupling: The transfer of electrical current from an active electrode to another conductive instrument by accident or as part of the electrosurgical process.

Dispersive electrode: See *patient return electrode.*

Electrosurgery: The direct use of electricity to cut and coagulate tissue.

Electrosurgical unit (ESU): The power generator and control source in the electrosurgical system.

Electrosurgical vessel sealing: A type of bipolar electrosurgery in which tissue is welded together using low-voltage, low-temperature, high-frequency current.

Eschar: Charred tissue created by a high-voltage current.

Excimer: A type of lasing energy that is created when electrons are removed from the lasing medium.

Fulguration: A process of tissue surface destruction used in electrosurgery.

Holmium:YAG: A solid crystal lasing medium that penetrates a wide variety of substances, including renal and biliary stones and soft tissue.

Impedance: The constriction of electrical current by a nonconductive material.

Implanted electronic device (IED): An electronic device that monitors and corrects physiological conditions. Electrosurgery may interfere with the function of such devices, which include pacemakers, internal defibrillators, deep brain stimulators, ventricular assist devices, and others.

Insulate: To cover or surround a conductive substance with nonconductive material.

Laser: Acronym for light amplification by stimulated emission of radiation.

Laser classifications: Industry and international system for grading laser energy according to its ability to cause injury.

Laser head: The component of the laser system that holds the lasing medium.

TERMINOLOGY (CONT.)

Laser medium: A solid or gas that is sensitive to atomic excitation by an energy source, which creates intense laser light and energy.

Monopolar circuit: In electrosurgery, a continuous path of electricity that flows from the electrosurgical unit to the active electrode, through the patient to the patient return electrode, and then back to the electrosurgical unit.

Nonconductive: The quality of a substance that resists the transfer of electrons and therefore electrical current.

Optical resonant cavity: The component of a laser system in which the lasing medium is contained and light is transformed.

Patient return electrode (PRE): A critical component of the monopolar electrosurgical circuit, the PRE is a conductive pad that captures electricity and shunts it safely out of the body and back to the electrosurgical unit. Also called the dispersive electrode.

Phacoemulsification: The destruction of cataracts using ultrasound technology.

Potassium-titanyl-phosphate (KTP): A low-power lasing medium that produces a very small diameter beam well suited to microsurgery.

Pulsed-wave lasers: Lasers that apply the laser light intermittently to the target tissue.

Q-switched lasers: An alternate name for pulsed-wave lasers.

Radiant exposure: In laser technology, the combination of the concentration of laser energy and the length of time tissue is exposed to it.

Radiofrequency: Electromagnetic energy in which the frequency is in the area of radio transmission. In electrosurgery, radiofrequency electromagnetic waves are used to produce the desired surgical effect.

Return electrode monitoring (REM): A safety system used in electrosurgery in which the PRE transmits continuous feedback on the quality of impedance in the electrode and stops the current when it becomes dangerously high.

Selective absorption: The absorption of a lasing medium into tissue being lased, according to its color and density.

Smoke plume: Toxic smoke emitted by tissue during electrosurgery and laser surgery.

Ultrasonic energy: High-frequency energy created by vibration or excitation of molecules. This type of energy destroys tissue by breaking molecular bonds.

The surgical technologist works with complex devices and instruments that have the potential to create serious injury. The modern ST should, at a minimum, understand the basic principles of energy technologies commonly used in surgery to prevent patient injury and meet the required standards of the profession.

Many forms of energy are used during surgery to cut tissue, coagulate blood vessels, and destroy diseased tissue. The most common forms are electrical, **radiofrequency,** ultrasonic (kinetic), thermal, and laser energy. Although electricity may be used to power these advanced medical devices, the energy used to perform the surgical procedure is not always electrical. For example, an instrument that generates ultrasonic waves is used to coagulate tissue. The instrument is powered by electricity, but the effect on the tissue is caused by vibration and friction.

This chapter discusses common surgical devices that use different types of energy. These devices are safe when used appropriately. However, they all carry the risk of serious injury. Surgical team members must understand the source of these risks to prevent serious accidents.

REVIEW OF ELECTRICITY

FREE ELECTRONS

The **electron** is a negatively charged atomic particle that orbits the nucleus of the atom. The outermost electrons of some substances are so loosely held to their nucleus that they move without a particular direction from one atom to another throughout the substance. These are called **free electrons.** Metals give up their outer electrons to create free electrons easily. Metals and other substances that create free electrons and are called **conductive substances.** Substances such as glass and rubber, which do not give up their electrons, are **nonconductive** materials or **insulators.**

CONDUCTION AND CIRCUITS

Free electrons in a conductive substance such as copper or silver can be forced to move in a line as long as there is a continuous path for them to move along. A copper or silver wire is an example of a conductive path. If the wires are twisted together, they can also become a conductive path. The conductive path can become *continuous* if it loops back to itself in a circle. This is called the **electrical circuit.** It is the basis of electricity.

IMPORTANT TO KNOW *The concept of circuits is one of the most important for the surgical technologist to understand fully.*

CURRENT AND IMPEDANCE

Electricity is similar to the flow of water through a tube. The flow can be regulated, stopped, and started. **Impedance** is resistance to the flow of electricity. When the flow of electrons meets a less conductive substance, it will seek a path around the area of resistance. If there is no alternative path available, the *energy used to move those electrons is converted to heat.* For example, an incandescent light bulb contains a tungsten wire, which is resistant to electrical current. Electrical current flows to the tungsten wire, which resists the energy and is converted to heat. The heat causes the tungsten wire to burn and glow.

VOLTAGE

Voltage is the *pressure* that pushes the flow of charged electrons through its circuit. The greater the voltage, the greater is its ability to push more electrons along the circuit. A larger number of electrons pushed through a small area creates greater heat.

ELECTROSURGERY

Electricity is a source of power used to perform work. In surgery, electricity is used to *provide power* to almost every piece of equipment. However, not every instrument uses electricity to modify tissue or to destroy it.

Surgery that uses electricity to heat tissue to modify it or destroy it is called **electrosurgery.**

Electrosurgery is used in nearly every type of surgery. The main uses of electrosurgery are to cut tissue and to coagulate small blood vessels. To understand how to use electrosurgery, the surgical technologist must understand some very basic principles of electricity. These are important to using electrosurgical instruments safely and preventing patient injury.

EFFECTS OF ELECTROSURGERY ON TISSUES

The energy that pushes electrical current along a conductive path is transformed into heat when it meets a nonconductive or less conductive substance. Heat is produced at the point of contact with the active electrode, which can cut and coagulate tissue.

Tissue reacts to electrosurgical energy according to these parameters:

Tissue type: The amount of water and collagen in the tissue and its density

Exposure time: The duration of contact with the electrical current

Current density: As current density increases, tissue response also increases. Current density increases when voltage is forced through a small area

Frequency and voltage: Specific combinations of frequency and voltage produce different effects in tissue

ELECTROSURGERY COMPONENTS AND THEIR USE

POWER GENERATOR

The generator provides radiofrequency power and the controls for all types of electrosurgery (Fig. 15.1). Settings are programmable and controlled by a keypad or by switches on the screen panel. Digital waveforms showing the frequency, wavelength, amplitude, and other information are displayed on the screen.

IMPORTANT TO KNOW *In many facilities the electrosurgery unit (ESU) is referred to as the "bovie"—the precursor to the modern system. The generator may be referred to as the "bovie machine."*

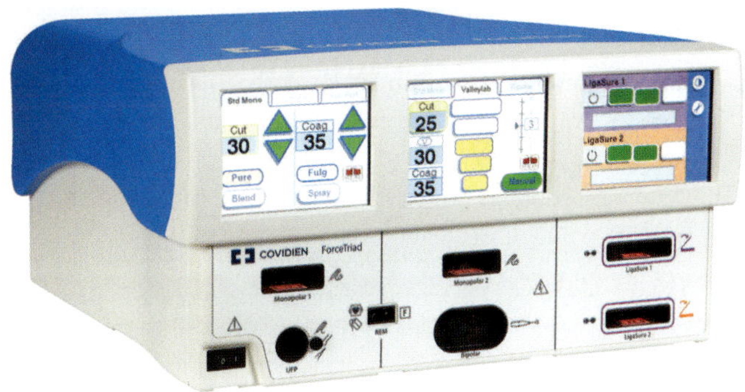

FIG. 15.1 Electrosurgical power unit, also known as the electrosurgical unit (ESU) generator. (Courtesy ConMed, Inc.)

Generator Safety

Generators must be used according to the manufacturer's specifications and within the guidelines of operating room policy. Written instructions and safety guidelines should be kept with the unit or close at hand to prevent misuse.

Alarm systems are designed to alert staff members to safety risks and **should never be turned off or made barely audible.** Loud music in the operating room has been identified as a barrier to the hearing of otherwise audible alarms.

The surgical team must suspect a problem if the surgeon repeatedly requests an increase in ESU power (voltage). This may indicate increased impedance, which can lead to superheating and unintentional patient burns.

Tissue impedance monitoring is available in most modern units. This safety feature provides automatic adjustments in voltage according to the impedance encountered in the tissue. Preprogramming of the automatic settings must ensure that the lowest power setting is used to achieve the desired surgical effect.

Box 15.1 presents safety guidelines for the generator.

ESU HANDPIECE AND ACTIVE ELECTRODE

The ESU handpiece or "pencil" contains a metal extension called the **active electrode** (Fig. 15.2). The active electrode is the point of entry for electrical current from the generator. The handpiece is connected to the generator by a lightweight cable and removable cable plug. The insulated handpiece and cable are contained as one closed unit. Many types of active electrode tips are available according to the type of electrosurgical procedure (Fig. 15.3). The *monopolar* spatula electrode shown attached to the handpiece in Fig. 15.2 is used for most procedures.

Two modes of action—tissue cutting and coagulation—are enabled by depressing the foot pedals. Some ESU handpieces are switched on the handpiece. When these are *not* enabled, the electrical current at the active electrode stops.

Coagulation

To coagulate blood vessels the electrode is held in contact with the tissue or slightly above it. Heating is slower than in cutting mode, and this results in tissue "welding" and coagulation.

BOX 15.1 Safety Guidelines for Use of Electrosurgical Generator

1. Always inspect all power cords and cables before using the electrosurgical unit (ESU) generator.
2. Do not place items on top of the ESU generator. The unit's cooling system may not function properly, and this could result in overheating and malfunction.
3. Always allow the ESU to self-check, if this feature is available, before connecting cables.
4. Always ensure that the ESU generator is approved for the active electrodes and patient return electrodes in use.
5. Keep the generator away from other electronic and power sources because they may cause electrical interference.
6. Keep fluids and fluid sources away from the generator. Never place fluid or solution containers on top of the generator, even if the containers are sealed.
7. Each generator is designed to operate with different waveforms and power settings.
8. Become familiar with your facility's equipment and its capabilities.

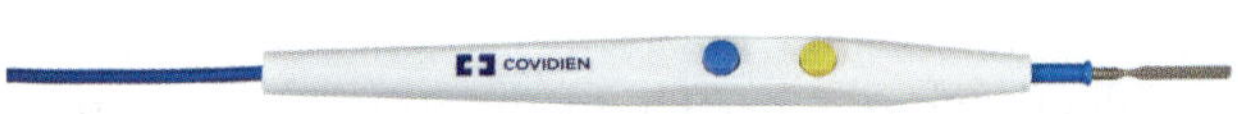

FIG. 15.2 Monopolar active electrode. This handheld unit or "pencil" delivers current to the tissue. Some surgeons may refer to this as a "bovie." (Courtesy ConMed, Inc.)

Cutting Mode

The **cutting mode** is produced by low-voltage energy delivered continuously without interruption. In this mode, the active electrode is held above the tissue and does not make contact. The air between the electrode and the tissue acts as a conductor (called a *spark gap*), allowing the current to flow between the tissue and the electrode.

The cutting mode causes tissue *desiccation* (burning with the loss of water content). When a thin, narrow active electrode is used, the current is very concentrated. The tissue heats rapidly, causing the water in the cells to explode. This releases steam and dissipates the heat. As the superheated tissue releases its water content, it quickly dries.

Cutting electrodes are available in many designs and configurations. These include the standard spatula electrode and others such as wire loops and needle tips.

Active Electrode Safety

Active electrode safety includes precautions to prevent accidental burns at the surgical site and electrical faults that occur between the electrode tip, handpiece, and connecting cord.

Recall that the active electrode is the metal tip of the instrument that conducts energy directly into the target tissue. In monopolar electrosurgery, the tip has the potential to deliver powerful cutting and coagulation properties. The tip is capable of severing dense tissue, including bone. It can cause inadvertent burns to the patient and scrubbed team members when used improperly.

Before surgery, the active electrode and cord must be examined for integrity. The ST is responsible for checking the insulation of the instrument, and the active electrode is seated tightly into the handpiece. Remember that disposable as well as reusable units can have defects. The monopolar active electrode is always used with a patient return electrode which is described in detail below.

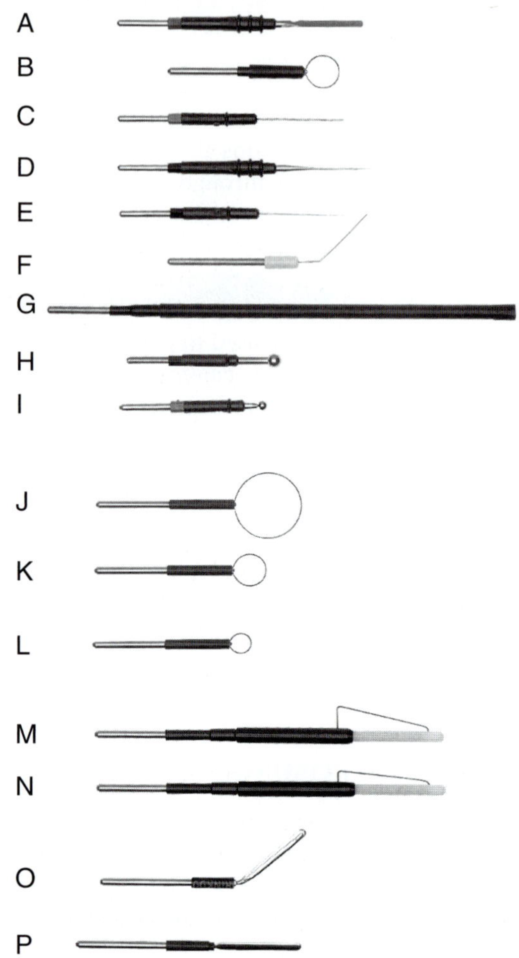

FIG. 15.3 Active electrode tips available for different types of monopolar electrosurgery. (A) Flat tip—general cutting and coagulation. (B) Loop—biopsy and cutting. (C) Fine needle—precise desiccation. (D) Coarse needle. (E) Blunt needle. (F) Angled needle. (G) Flat tip with extension—deep tissue, general use. (H) Ball tip, regular—fulguration. (I) Ball tip, long—deep tissue fulguration. (J to L) Cutting loops, long. (M and N) Conization loop—endocervical cutting and coagulation. (O and P) Straight and angled long flat tips. (Courtesy ConMed, Inc.)

During surgery, the ESU pencil must be kept in a nonconductive safety holster on the surgical field. The holster must be in plain sight of the team, and the ESU pencil must be replaced in it *after each use*. Never leave the pencil on top of the patient or drapes. Place the holster in a position that is convenient to the surgeon's reach so that the pencil can be easily stowed after each use. Do not attach the handpiece to the drapes by wrapping it around metal clamps or twisting the cord. Stray current can escape into the metal clamp. Twisting or tying the cord can break the conductive wires inside and put a strain on the insulation.

IMPORTANT SAFETY INFORMATION: *The buildup of charred tissue on the ESU tip is a hazard. However, the ST should not attempt to remove it using a knife blade or other*

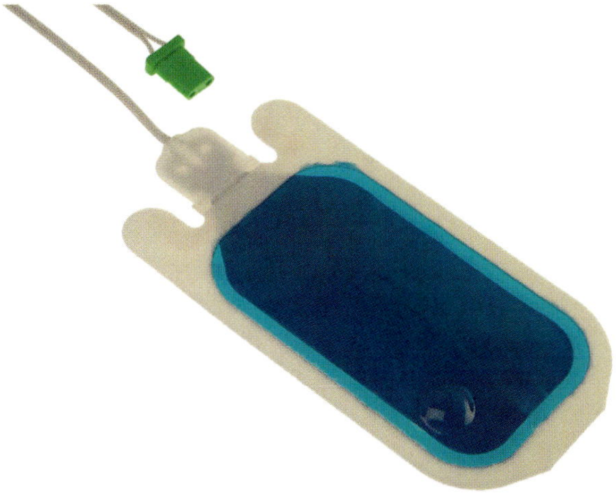

FIG. 15.4 Patient return electrode (PRE) used in monopolar electrosurgery. The PRE is also known as a *patient grounding pad, dispersive electrode*, or *inactive electrode*. The purpose of the PRE is to provide a safe return path for electricity transmitted through the electrosurgical unit pencil and the patient's body. (Courtesy ConMed, Inc.)

metal instrument. Doing this creates scratches and pitting on the surface of the tip. This increases the formation of eschar, causing sparking and excessive heating of surrounding tissues. It is better to use a Teflon pad to remove eschar during surgery.

SMOKE PLUME

During monopolar electrosurgery and laser surgery, tissue is subjected to high temperatures. This process creates toxic smoke called **smoke plume.** Smoke plume contains about 95% water and 5% other products, which include chemicals, blood cells, and intact or fragmented bacteria and viruses. The potential hazards of these substances are infectious disease transmission, toxicity from chemicals, and allergy. The size of aerosol particles ranges from 0.1 to 0.8 μm. These droplets are capable of harboring much smaller viral and bacterial particles.

Smoke plume contains many toxic chemicals in concentrations that can potentially exceed those recommended by the Occupational Safety and Health Administration (OSHA). The chemicals found in smoke plume include toluene, acrolein, formaldehyde, and hydrogen cyanide. Both laser and electrosurgical plumes contain living and dead cells. *Disease transmission through smoke plume is a known risk* to surgical personnel. Other transmissible biological particles, such as cancer cells, at laser and electrosurgical sites are an additional concern.

The dangers of smoke plume have been underreported. In spite of recommendations for the use of local evacuation systems (LEV) for the removal of smoke plume from the surgical environment, fewer than half of all health care facilities recently surveyed have an LEV in place and do not have protocols or guidelines for preventing surgical staff exposure to smoke plume.

Smoke Evacuation System

Normal room ventilation is not sufficient to capture chemical and biological particles from smoke plume. Two methods are used to prevent perioperative personnel from inhaling smoke: inline room suction systems and commercial smoke evacuation devices. Room suction is designed to carry liquids, not smoke. These systems pull at a much lower rate than commercial smoke evacuation systems and must have inline filters attached to be safe. Smoke evacuation systems are specifically designed to extract moist smoke plume from the surgical site.

A smoke evacuation system contains a nozzle tip, suction tubing, filters, absorbers, and a vacuum pump. Smoke plume is evacuated at a rate of about 100 to 150 feet (30 to 46 m) per minute at the site of generation. It then is carried through a high-efficiency particulate air (HEPA) filter and trapped in absorbers. The used filters are biohazardous waste and must be disposed of according to hospital policy. When a smoke evacuator is used, the nozzle tip must be within 2 inches (5 cm) of the surgical site to be effective. Fresh filters and tubing must be used for each patient. Some ESU systems now have intrinsic smoke evacuation systems.

PATIENT RETURN ELECTRODE USED IN *MONOPOLAR* ESU

As explained earlier, the active electrode is the metal tip of the ESU handpiece. This is the point where current is transformed to heat to perform electrosurgery. However, a *second electrode* is needed to attract the current and direct it out of the body. This second electrode is the **patient return electrode** (also known as the PRE or **dispersive electrode**). The PRE is an adhesive patch or metallic plate coated or saturated with conductive electrode gel (Fig. 15.4). The dispersive electrode is connected to the generator by a cable to complete the circuit and prevent unintended heating and burns.

IMPORTANT TO KNOW *The patient return electrode is often incorrectly called the patient "grounding pad." This is not only inaccurate but misleading. The patient is not grounded in the same way we ground appliances with a third wire. The purpose of the PRE is to return the current to the generator to complete the monopolar circuit as shown in Fig. 15.5. A common cause of patient burns during ESU is failure to attach the PRE to* ***both the patient and the generator****.*

Patient Return (Dispersive) Electrode Safety

The return electrode is extremely important for patient safety. Without it, the current that was directed to the surgical site through the handpiece cable will continue to seek an exit path through the patient's body. If any part of the patient is in contact with a conductive surface, the current will exit at that point, seeking a nonresistant path. It is particularly dangerous if the exit point is small because deep third-degree burns can result. For example, patient contact with the steel frame of the operating table can cause severe burns. Burns may also occur at the site of electrocardiogram attachments, which contain metal.

Problems with the dispersive electrode can result when it is improperly attached or attached in a poor location. There may be insufficient electrode gel on the surface of the pad, or the return cable may become accidently detached during surgery. Key safety guidelines are shown in Box 15.2.

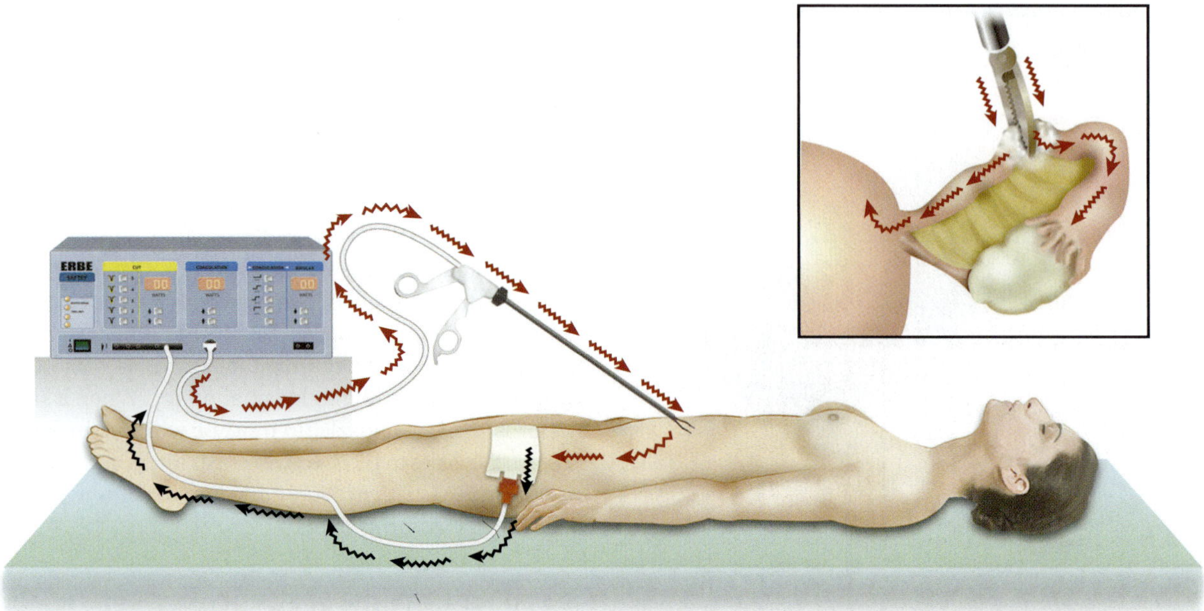

FIG. 15.5 Monopolar electrosurgery circuit. In monopolar electrosurgical units, electrical current flows from the power source to the active electrode, through the patient's body, to the patient return electrode (PRE), which transmits it back to the power unit. This completes the circuit and prevents inadvertent patient burns. (From Baggish M, Karram M. *Atlas of Pelvic Anatomy and Gynecologic Surgery*. 4th ed. Philadelphia: Elsevier; 2015.)

BIPOLAR ESU

Instead of a single active electrode connected to the generator, the surgeon uses *double pointed forceps* or a similar bipolar instrument with *two contact points*. The target tissue is grasped with the forceps. The **bipolar circuit** flows from the generator, through the bipolar cable to one of the tips of the forceps. It then passes through the tissue between the two tines to coagulate or cut. The current then passes through the second tine and returns to the generator through the bipolar cable (Fig. 15.6). The current doesn't pass through the body; therefore no PRE is required. Compare the bipolar circuit shown in Fig. 15.6 with the monopolar circuit shown in Fig. 15.5.

A comparison of monopolar and bipolar electrosurgery is shown in Box 15.3.

FULGURATION

Fulguration, or **spray coagulation,** is performed with pulsed or intermittent application of the active electrode. In this technique the current is pulsed through the active electrode, which is held just above the tissue. The high voltage creates an arc of current that spreads over a relatively large area compared with that seen in direct-contact techniques. The effect is a combination of coagulation and superficial tissue cutting.

ELECTROSURGICAL BIPOLAR VESSEL SEALING

Electrosurgical vessel sealing uses high-frequency *bipolar electrosurgery*, low voltage, and physical pressure to create a weld in tissue. Several vessel-sealing systems are available, such as LigaSure and ENSEAL. The following are elements of a vessel-sealing system:

BOX 15.2 Safety Measures for Use of the Patient Return Electrode

- Always assess the patient's skin before and after applying the patient return electrode (PRE).
- The skin must be dry and free of hair. Moisture under the PRE can cause it to pull away from the skin. Shaving may be necessary for uniform contact with the skin.
- Use only a PRE that has been stored in a sealed package. The moisture content and quality of the conductive gel cannot be guaranteed with prolonged exposure to air.
- Inspect the PRE before applying it and check the expiration date on the package. The electroconductive gel must be moist and should have been stored at the temperature specified by the manufacturer.
- Use the correct size PRE for the patient's surface area. Operating room protocol determines the appropriate pad size.
- Pediatric-size PREs are available. Never cut a PRE to fit the patient's size.
- The PRE must be placed close to the surgical site over a large muscle mass. Muscle has low impedance and is the best conductor. The PRE must not be placed over a prominent bony surface, scar, tattoo, hair, or fatty tissue; these increase impedance and can result in a burn.
- The PRE must be in complete contact with the skin, without tenting or buckling.
- Make sure the PRE cord has adequate slack to prevent pulling and displacement.
- Apply the PRE after final positioning to prevent it from becoming detached.
- Always check the PRE cable to make sure it is intact and undamaged. Check it from end to end, including the attachment clips and the plug or insertion point into the electrosurgical generator.
- Do not assume that single-use items are intact and free of damage. Inspect every device, every time.
- Do not use a PRE *if only bipolar electrosurgery* will be used.

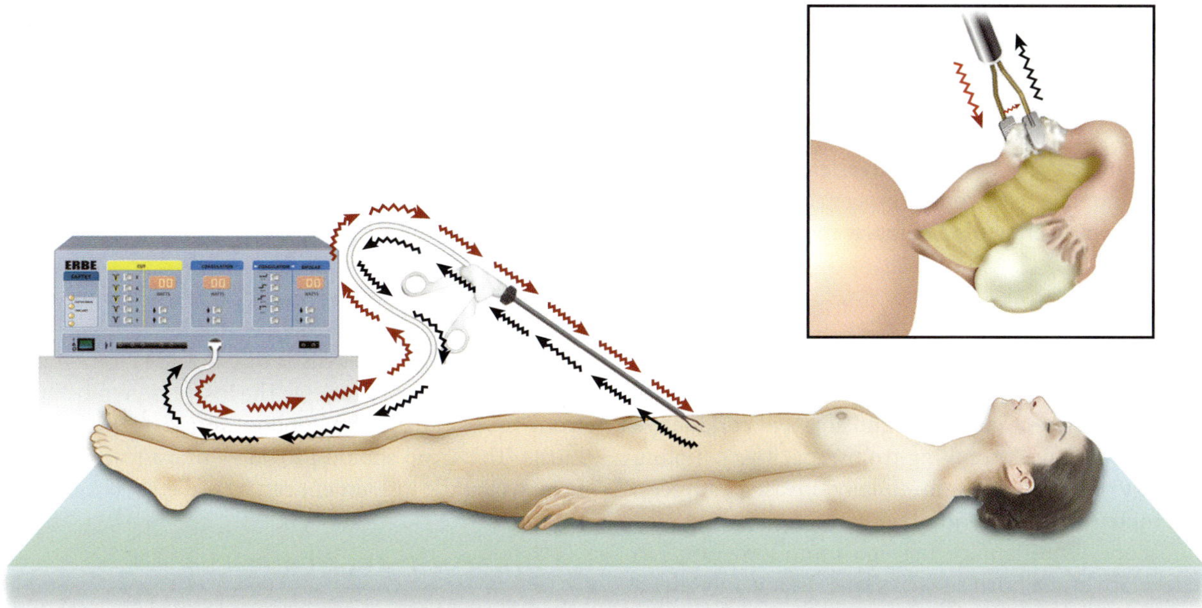

FIG. 15.6 Bipolar electrosurgery circuit. In a bipolar circuit, the electricity flows from the generator directly to the tips of the instrument and then back to the generator. No electricity passes through the patient. No return electrode pad is required. (From Baggish M, Karram M. *Atlas of Pelvic Anatomy and Gynecologic Surgery*. 4th ed. Philadelphia: Elsevier; 2015.)

BOX 15.3 Comparison of Monopolar and Bipolar Electrosurgery

- The voltage in bipolar electrosurgery is lower than that used for monopolar surgery, which makes the bipolar mode a safer technique with fewer risks for patient injury.
- The bipolar unit is used mainly on low-impedance tissue because the low voltage is not strong enough to penetrate effectively through dense tissue such as bone.
- Minimal heat is spread to surrounding tissues, which makes this technique safe for very delicate areas such as the brain and microvascular tissue.
- Bipolar electrosurgery can be used for patients who have an **implanted electronic device (IED)** such as a pacemaker because the current doesn't pass through the body.

- Transmission of radiofrequency waves to tissue through specialized grasping instruments
- Tissue impedance monitoring
- A microprocessor (programmable computer chip) that controls and programs the system
- An alarm system that automatically stops the current when the tissue seal is achieved

The vessel-sealing system is used during resection procedures that traditionally require sequential clamping, suturing, and cutting. Whereas the traditional method of resection requires multiple instruments, the vessel-sealing system accomplishes these tasks with one instrument. The system is for selected gynecology and some general surgery applications. The system operates with low temperatures, which prevent charring and unintentional lateral heating. The instrument tip remains relatively cool, which prevents the tissue from tearing when the tips are released.

ARGON-ENHANCED ELECTROSURGERY

Argon gas is used in some electrosurgical procedures to focus the current during cutting and coagulation. Argon is inert and nonflammable but easily ionized. When a stream of argon gas is directed around the active electrode, it focuses the current and prevents sparking. Argon-enhanced electrosurgery also reduces the smoke plume and displaces oxygen along its path. This increases the safety and efficiency of the procedure. It is particularly useful during long fulguration procedures that require extended electrosurgery.

RADIOFREQUENCY ABLATION

Ablation is the destruction of tissue using radiofrequency energy. This mode has numerous uses, including the destruction of tumors and endometrial tissue in gynecological surgery. During tumor ablation, an electrode is inserted directly into the diseased tissue. The high-frequency energy causes the molecules of the tissue to vibrate, which creates sufficient heat to destroy the tissue.

Bipolar radiofrequency ablation (RFA) is used in conjunction with a conductive fluid medium to destroy diseased tissue in a hollow organ such as the bladder or uterus. The cavity is filled with fluid, and the bipolar probe is used to destroy tissue within the fluid. The specific use of this technology is described more fully in Chapter 23 on gynecological surgery and in Chapter 24 on urological surgery.

ELECTROSURGERY IN MINIMALLY INVASIVE SURGERY

Minimally invasive surgery (MIS) is performed through very small incisions using telescopic instruments. In this technique the surgical field is transmitted to a flat monitor in real time and surgery performed based on the live images projected on the monitor. Electrosurgery is used in all types of procedures, including MIS. However, the electrosurgical instruments used in MIS are telescopic. Bipolar mode is necessary during MIS because of the immediate risk of inadvertent tissue damage inherent in monopolar electronic surgery. There remains a risk of patient burns even with the bipolar mode.

CAPACITIVE COUPLING

Capacitive coupling is a specific burn hazard of monopolar endoscopic surgery. It occurs when current passes inadvertently through instrument insulation and adjacent conductive material into tissue. Burns resulting from capacitive coupling are particularly dangerous in minimally invasive surgery, because the injury most often occurs outside the viewing area of the endoscope. The damage may go unnoticed until an infection develops at the burn site days later. Using only metal cannulas and active electrode monitoring (discussed later in the chapter) can prevent capacitive coupling.

DIRECT COUPLING

Direct coupling is the flow of electricity from one conductive substance to another. This can occur when the insulation protecting the circuit has a defect or when an active electrode comes in contact with another conductive object. During minimally invasive surgery, direct coupling can occur when an active electrode touches the tip of another instrument in an instrument "collision." Direct coupling involving insulation failure can be more dangerous, because the resulting burn may not be detected immediately. In open surgery, direct coupling can occur whenever an active electrode insulator is inserted into a conductive metal sheath, such as a suction catheter. Direct coupling can be prevented by frequent inspection of insulation and proper care and handling of electrosurgical instruments. However, active electrode monitoring is the recommended method of preventing burns from insulation failure.

NOTE *A complete discussion on capacitive and direct coupling in minimally invasive surgery is located in Chapter 20, Minimally Invasive Surgery.*

ULTRASONIC ENERGY

Ultrasonic energy is created when electricity is transformed into mechanical energy generated by high-frequency vibration and the forces of friction. The ultrasonic instrument simultaneously cuts and coagulates tissue by transmitting ultrasonic wave energy through specially designed forceps, scissors, or blades. The instrument vibrates at approximately 55,000 movements per second, and these vibrations cause protein molecules to rupture. One drawback of this type of energy is that it cannot cut tissue without coagulating it. When the instrument is applied, the tissue liquefies and forms **coagulum,** a sticky protein substance that congeals and welds the tissue in the same way that metal is melted to form solder.

Ultrasonic technology uses low temperatures. Electrical current *does not* pass through the patient; therefore no dispersive electrode is required for this type of energy. Examples of ultrasonic energy systems are the SonoSurg (Olympus America, Center Valley, PA) and the Harmonic energy system (Ethicon, Somerville, NJ).

SAFETY PRECAUTIONS

Although the ultrasonic scalpel does not transmit electrical current to the target tissue, the blades *continue to hold heat immediately after use.* This is due to the vibration and friction produced by the instrument. The instrument must be held away from tissue during the cooling period to prevent accidental burns. The scrub should provide a moist towel on the surgical field, where the instrument can be placed between applications.

ULTRASONIC ABLATION

Ultrasonic ablation is used as an alternative to electrosurgery. Tumor ablation is performed by inserting a series of needle probes directly into the tumor under direct fluoroscopic imaging. Other specialties that commonly use this technology are gynecology, endovascular surgery, neurological surgery, and ophthalmology. The **Cavitron Ultrasonic Surgical Aspirator (CUSA)** is commonly used for ultrasonic ablation and aspiration (suction) in tumor surgery. **Phacoemulsification** is a process employing a delicate ophthalmological instrument (phacoemulsifier) that uses ultrasonic energy for the destruction of cataracts.

CRYOSURGERY

Cryosurgery is performed with an extremely cold probe or substance to destroy tissue. Cryosurgery has been used for many years to remove small skin lesions using liquid nitrogen.

In **cryoablation** a probe is inserted into a tumor or tissue mass. High-pressure argon gas is injected into the probe, causing the surrounding tissue to freeze. The tissue is destroyed and eventually absorbed by the body. This surgical technique is often performed in the outpatient setting under guided fluoroscopy.

LASER SURGERY

Laser is an acronym for *light amplification by stimulated emission of radiation.*

LASER STANDARDS AND REGULATIONS

The laser is a powerful instrument that has a variety of applications in manufacturing, engineering, biotechnology, health care, and warfare. However, lasers can also cause irreparable injury and destruction. Because of this, laser standards and regulations have been developed by governmental and nonprofit agencies. In health care, these standards are designed to protect both the patient and those who work with lasers.

In the operating room a *laser team* is established to oversee the training of staff and the implementation of rules and regulations. The *laser safety committee* oversees the planning and implementation of the laser program, including its safety measures. The safety committee is also responsible for teaching and credentialing staff members who undertake advanced courses in laser safety and technology. The laser safety officer is responsible for fielding clinical questions and maintaining the safety standards in the health facility.

HOW LASERS WORK

Light has both particle and wave characteristics. Ordinary light is made up of many wavelengths and colors, which, when combined, emit white light. When ordinary light is generated,

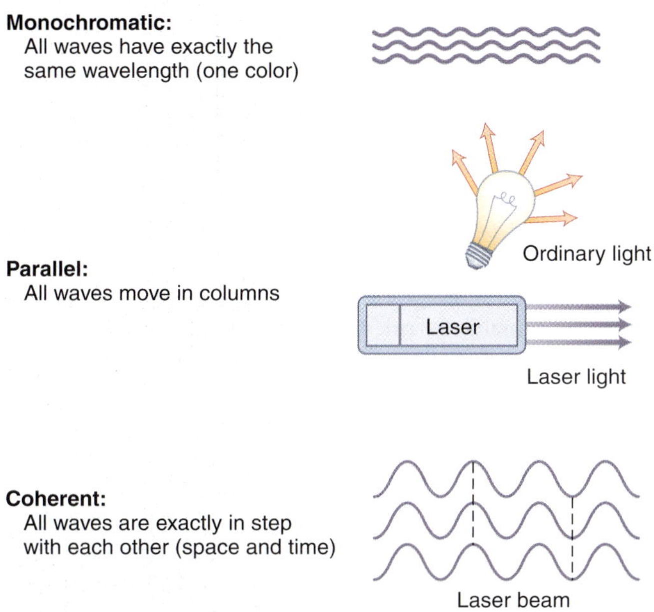

FIG. 15.7 Comparison of normal and laser light. Ordinary light rays are transmitted in all directions. Laser waves are monochromatic, parallel, and coherent. They move in one direction and the waves are lined up, producing an extremely powerful source of energy.

the rays are transmitted from the source in infinite directions. However, laser light is unlike ordinary light. All the waves in the laser light are exactly the same length *and the* waves are lined up so that their peaks and troughs are in exactly the same location, a quality called *coherency* (Fig. 15.7).

The distinctive characteristics of laser energy are created when light is pumped into a sealed chamber and filled with a **laser medium** (i.e., a gas, solid, or liquid). The chamber is called the **optical resonant cavity.** When photons of a specific energy enter the chamber, they stimulate the high-energy atoms in the chamber to vibrate or resonate in duplicate wave patterns. Mirrors in the laser system bounce the photons back and forth through the laser medium in the chamber. This increases the number of resonating parallel photons and is called *amplification* (Fig. 15.8). Laser surgery uses an intensely hot, precisely focused beam of light to cut and coagulate tissue.

Lasers are grouped into two categories according to the duration of the output waves:

Continuous-wave lasers produce a steady stream of light.

Q-switched lasers (also called *pulsed-wave lasers*) emit light in bursts or pulses.

LASER COMPONENTS

The main components of the laser delivery system are the following:

- The *optical resonator* (also called the **laser head**): Contains the lasing medium and mirrors needed to amplify the light waves
- The *excitation source:* Supplies the energy needed to increase the resonance of the lasing medium
- The *delivery system:* The instruments or devices that transmit the lasing energy to the operative site. The system depends on the type of laser and surgery. A laser *fiber* (filament) is commonly used
- The *control panel* and *touch screen:* Contain the control system for the laser functions and operations

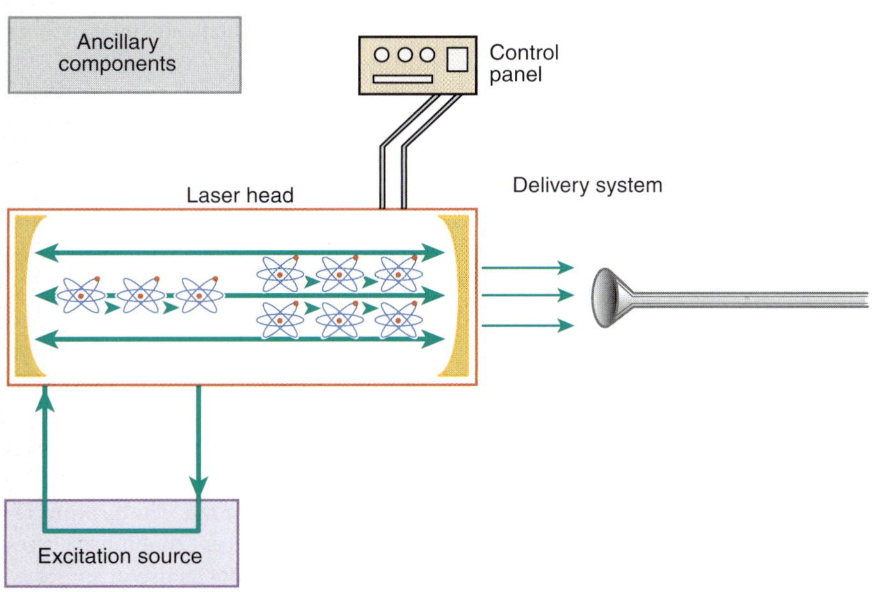

FIG. 15.8 Light amplification in the laser chamber.

- *Accessory equipment:* Includes the cooling system and vacuum pump, if required by the laser type

The modern laser is controlled by microprocessing technology. The optical resonator and control system are contained in a single unit, and accessory equipment is attached according to the requirements of the surgery. The actual laser housing is contained within the laser unit, along with the cooling system and vacuum pump. The controls of the modern laser include a touch panel or screen on which surgical options can be selected and adjustments made. A single foot pedal control is available to the operating surgeon. A registered nurse or surgical technologist is assigned to the console.

EFFECTS OF LASERS

When laser light is directed at a surface, any of the following can occur:

- Absorption
- Reflection
- Scattering
- Transmission

Lasers are distinguished by the functional or biophysical reaction of the target tissue. The tissue reaction depends on the following:

- The laser wavelength
- The power setting
- The absorption quality of the cells (e.g., color, density, and moisture content)

The quality of the laser energy depends on its density, which is determined by the voltage, the diameter of the beam, and the exposure time on the tissue. The sum of these is called the **radiant exposure.**

When certain types of laser light come into contact with the tissue, cells become extremely hot. Just as in electrosurgery, a high temperature causes cell destruction through vaporization. Laser light can also weld tissue.

Selective absorption is an important characteristic of laser energy. This means that some cells absorb the lasing medium, whereas others do not. This characteristic prevents the spread of heat (and damage) outside the target tissue.

The type of gas or other substance used to create specific laser energy determines its absorption by the tissue. The moisture content and density of a particular tissue are important factors in the choice of laser medium.

LASER MEDIA

Lasers are distinguished by the *medium* or the element that is activated to transmit photons. These include the following:

- Gases
- Solids
- Semiconductors (diode lasers)
- Excimers
- Solid-state media
- Liquid dyes

The surgeon selects the correct media and type of laser for specific use in an area of the body and procedure.

Argon (Gas)

Argon gas lasers produce a visible blue-green beam that is absorbed by red-brown pigmented tissue such as hemoglobin. The argon beam is not absorbed by clear or translucent tissue; therefore the beam can pass through the cornea, vitreous, and lens of the eye without burning these tissues. The argon beam is used for coagulation and for sealing or welding tissue.

The argon laser is most often used in dermatological and ophthalmological procedures. In dermatology, it is used to remove pigmented lesions because it is not readily absorbed by light tissue. In ophthalmology, it is used in surgery for retinal tears, glaucoma, macular degeneration, retinopathy, and retinal vein occlusion. The argon beam is delivered through a laser fiber in combination with the surgical microscope, slit lamp, or handpiece attached to an articulated (jointed) arm.

Carbon Dioxide (Gas)

The carbon dioxide laser is invisible to the human eye. The beam has a high affinity for water and functions at a superficial depth. A *helium-neon* laser beam that produces a red light is added to the carbon dioxide laser beam to make it visible. The helium-neon beam is sometimes called the "pilot light" because of its guiding function. The carbon dioxide laser is extremely versatile and is used in many surgical specialties, including microsurgery. *Krypton,* another gas lasing medium, is used for the removal of superficial lesions in dermatology.

Holmium:YAG (Solid)

The holmium:yttrium-aluminum-garnet (holmium:YAG) laser is a crystal containing holmium, thallium, and chromium. Its beam is outside the visible light range and able to penetrate all tissue types. This laser is used to cut, shave, contour, ablate, and coagulate tissue. It is extremely versatile and capable of ablating renal and biliary calculi as well as soft tissues. It has a low depth penetration to a maximum of 0.4 mm. The holmium:YAG laser is used in urological; orthopedic; ear, nose, and throat (ENT); gynecological; gastrointestinal; and general surgery. It also is suitable for use in minimally invasive surgery.

Neodymium:YAG (Solid)

The neodymium:YAG (Nd:YAG) laser is created from a solid-state crystal of neodymium, yttrium, aluminum, and garnet. As with the carbon dioxide laser, a helium-neon beam is used for visibility. The Nd:YAG laser beam has a high affinity for tissue protein but little for water. The beam is near the infrared region of the electromagnetic spectrum and has a penetration of 3 to 7 mm. Of all the laser types, the Nd:YAG has the greatest ability to coagulate blood vessels. Because of its deep penetration, it can coagulate vessels up to 4 mm in diameter. This laser can be used during endoscopic or flexible fiber-optic surgery. It is delivered through a laser fiber or probe in continuous or pulsed mode. The Erbium (Er:YAG) is similar to the Nd:YAG laser, except that it has a stronger affinity for water in tissue, which limits its use in surgery.

Ruby and Alexandrite (Solid)

Synthetic ruby crystals were the first substance to be used as a lasing medium. Initially used in industry and for military purposes, the ruby laser was also used to remove superficial skin defects and tattoos. The Q-switched ruby laser has been replaced with the Alexandrite, a solid lasing material, which is more efficient for use in dermatology.

Potassium-Titanyl-Phosphate (Solid)

The potassium-titanyl-phosphate (KTP) laser is less powerful than the carbon dioxide or Nd:YAG laser, but it is capable of producing a minute beam that is well suited to microscopic surgery. The green laser light is readily absorbed by pigmented tissue and can be delivered by several different methods, including fiber, scanner, or microscope. The beam can also be transmitted through clear solutions. The KTP laser offers two wavelengths; this allows two separate sets of laser characteristics to be selected at any time. These provide hemostatic cutting and ablation as well as deep coagulation. The KTP laser is used in ENT, urological, gynecological, and general surgery and in dermatological procedures. KTP can also be combined with neodymium to double its frequency and increase versatility.

Excimer (Gas)

The excimer laser produces a cool beam by stripping electrons from the atoms of the medium in the chamber. This causes the energy bonds in the atom to break. The resulting shock waves stimulate short bursts of laser light. The light is delivered to the target tissue through fiber-optic bundles.

The beam of the excimer laser creates less heat than other laser types. This reduces damage to nearby tissues and results in less carbonization of lased tissue. Specialized ultraviolet mirrors and optics are required to operate the laser safely. This laser is extremely precise and is commonly used in ophthalmological surgery and dermatology.

Tunable Dye (Solid)

The pulsed dye laser beam (tunable dye laser) is formed when fluorescent liquid or other dyes are exposed to argon laser light. The dye absorbs the light and produces a fluorescent broad-spectrum light. The spectrum of the light is then "tuned" to produce light of a particular wavelength (color). This provides versatility for a variety of tissue types and surgical specialties.

LASER SAFETY

Recall the three specific characteristics of laser energy that distinguish it from ordinary white light:

- It is coherent (peaks and troughs match).
- It is monochromatic (all waves are of the same wavelength).
- Its waves are parallel (waves move in one direction only).

These characteristics make laser light extremely hazardous, because it can concentrate a tremendous amount of energy in one small area.

Surgical lasers pose significant health and safety risks. These risks are manageable but require attention to every detail of safety protocols. All perioperative personnel must know the protocols well and follow them carefully. The specific risks for patients and personnel are eye damage, tissue burns, fire, and smoke plume.

LASER CLASSIFICATION

Laser classifications are based on the safety risks associated with their use:

Class 4: Cause permanent eye damage if viewed directly or if viewed indirectly by reflection. These lasers can also ignite materials and cause skin burns. Most surgical lasers are class 4 lasers.

Class 3b: Cause severe eye injury when viewed directly or by reflection. These lasers do not cause injury when the laser beam is diffused and do not normally present a fire hazard.

Class 3a: Normally do not cause eye injury if viewed momentarily but present a hazard if viewed with collecting optics (e.g., fiber-optic cable, magnification loupe, or microscope).

Class 2: Emit radiation in the visible range of the electromagnetic spectrum. These lasers do not normally cause harm when viewed briefly, although they can be hazardous when viewed for an extended period. Laser pointers and bar code scanners are class 2 lasers.

Class 1: Are not hazardous for continuous viewing, are considered incapable of producing damaging radiation levels, and are exempt from control measures. Laser printers are in this category.

NOTE *Note that class 3b and 4 lasers cause instantaneous retinal injury that may be irreparable. Class 4 lasers can penetrate the sclera and injure the retina. Turning the head away or turning away from the laser does not ensure protection because of the risk of scatter or reflection of the beam.*

PRECAUTIONS AND GUIDELINES

- A laser safety officer is required to manage laser risks and define safety protocols.
- Lasers are key-locked when not in use.
- Lasers are a potent source of ignition in the operating room. All fire safety precautions must be in place before the start of surgery.
- Only personnel trained in and with proven knowledgeable about laser use and precautions are allowed to participate in laser surgery. All reflective surfaces in the laser environment are covered, made nonreflective, or removed from the environment. Nonreflective, black-matte-finished instruments are to be used in laser surgery.
- Laser warning signs must be placed on all entrances to areas where laser surgery is being performed (Fig. 15.9).
- All personnel entering a room in which lasers are in use must wear protective eyewear (see the next section).
- Only flame-retardant drapes are used during laser surgery.

The two most common injuries associated with unintentional laser exposure are eye injury and skin burn. Lasers in the ultraviolet and infrared areas of the spectrum are the most damaging. They can penetrate the sclera and enter the lens, cornea,

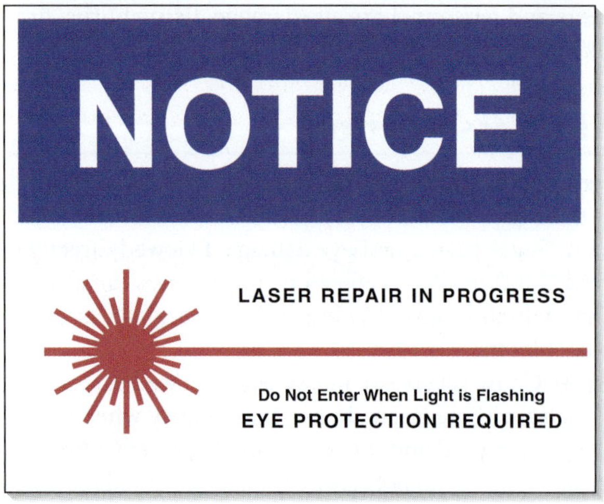

FIG. 15.9 Laser warning sign.

and retina. Eye injury can be permanent, especially if the retina is involved. Injuries range from corneal burns to blindness.

Heat generated by the lasing light beam is the major cause of tissue damage. Intentional use of the laser results in incision or dissection, tissue vaporization, and welding. Unintentional exposure can have the same effects. These range from reddening of the skin to third-degree burns. The following criteria determine the degree of thermal damage:

- Sensitivity of the irradiated tissue
- Amount of tissue affected
- Wavelength of the laser beam
- Energy level of the laser beam
- Length of time the tissue was exposed

EYE SAFETY

The eye is the tissue most vulnerable to accidental laser exposure and injury. To protect the eyes during laser use, personnel must shield them from the *specific wavelength* of light. Protective eyewear of the correct optical density is required for various types of lasers. Eyewear must wrap completely around the eyes, covering the sides, top, and bottom so that no diffuse laser energy can reach the eye. Regular prescription eyeglasses do not offer protection. Only eyewear that is specifically approved for laser use can be used during laser surgery. Protective eyewear is available commercially, and manufacturers offer different styles and lens colors for each type of laser.

The color of the laser lenses is not an indication of the level of protection. The specific *density of the lens, not the color, provides protection.* There is no color code associated with laser type.

The protective eyewear bears an inscription on the lens that details the optical density, and the eyewear must be labeled for the specific laser type. In addition to protective eyewear for staff members, other precautions must be followed to prevent eye injury. These include but are not limited to the following:

- Lens filters are placed over any endoscope viewing port.
- The patient's eyes are covered with wet eye pads or eye cups that are laser-specific. Corneal eye shields are used for patients undergoing laser surgery of the eyelids.
- Appropriate laser backstops, which stop the penetration of laser energy into normal tissue. A titanium quartz rob or guard is used as a backstop. Rhodium or stainless steel mirrors may also be used for backstopping.
- All patients undergoing surgery, while awake, wear protective eyewear.
- The windows to the operating room are covered with barrier material that stops the transmission of the laser beam being used in the room, and warning signs are posted outside to caution against unprotected entry during laser procedures.
- Appropriate protective eyewear is available on the outside of each entryway leading to a room in which lasers are being used.
- The effective danger area where safety precautions must be observed is a closed room, where the laser surgery is being performed, called the *normal hazard zone* (NHZ).

SKIN PROTECTION

Skin injuries result from direct contact with the laser beam. Environmental precautions are necessary to prevent these injuries. In addition, anyone entering a room in which lasers are in use must remove any metallic jewelry, which can reflect the laser beam or absorb heat. The patient's tissues are protected from inadvertent laser injury. Wet towels are placed around the operative site to prevent burns in the area. When endoscopic lasers are in use, the laser fiber must extend more than 1 inch beyond the tip of the endoscope to prevent backscatter of the beam and burning of the endoscope and/or heating of the extension tube, which can damage healthy tissues. Body cavities, such as the nasal cavity or rectal passage, may also be packed with moist sponges to prevent injury during laser use.

AIRWAY PROTECTION

In addition to routine precautions against fire, particular attention is given to anesthesia equipment, especially during laser surgery involving the head and neck. Endotracheal tubes and other anesthesia equipment can easily ignite in the presence of laser energy and oxygen-rich anesthetic agents. To minimize the risk of an endotracheal fire, a special metallic foil is wrapped around the endotracheal tube before laser surgery. Oxygen flow is reduced to a minimum, and combustible gases are avoided.

Although an airway fire is a rare event, the possibility exists during laser surgery. When ignited, the endotracheal tube acts as a blowtorch, and flames may reach 5 to 10 inches (12.5 to 25 cm) within seconds. If a fire occurs, the tube should be removed or flushed with saline. The scrub and circulator should be prepared to offer emergency assistance to both the anesthesiologist and surgeons as needed.

IMPORTANT TO KNOW *Laser safety guidelines are extensive. Surgical technologists must consult the health facilities' standards and guidelines to ensure understanding and compliance not only for themselves but also for the protection of the patient and coworkers.*

KEY CONCEPTS

- The concepts of conduction, frequency, and impedance explain the fundamental properties of electricity.
- Electrosurgery is common in most surgical procedures. It is also one of the most frequent sources of patient injury. The surgical technologist must have a solid knowledge base in this area to protect patients against injury.
- The main components of electrosurgery are the generator, the active electrode, which delivers the electrical energy to tissue, and the return electrode, which captures the current and conducts it safely back to the power unit.
- Incorrect use of the patient return electrode can result in deep third-degree burns.
- Monopolar and bipolar circuitry in electrosurgery gives rise to two very different types of devices, each with its own properties and hazards. Monopolar electrosurgery produces an extremely powerful energy capable of incising all types of tissue including bone. The monopolar current passes through the patient's body before returning to the power unit to complete the circuit.
- Bipolar electrosurgery produces less powerful energy at a lower temperature. The energy passes from the generator, between the tips of the active electrode holding the tissue, and back to the power unit without passing through the patient's body.
- Specific terms are used to describe how electricity works, its behavior, and specific hazards. Examples are capacitive and indirect coupling, smoke plume, active electrode, and many others. Understanding the terms is the first stage of understanding how to handle electrosurgical devices.
- When electricity is applied to the body from an external source, such as during electrosurgery, the voltage and frequency of that source cause alterations in the tissue.
- Smoke plume created by electrosurgical and laser energy contains chemical carcinogens, tissue fragments, and potential bacterial contaminants that can be drawn into the lungs of the operating team. Smoke plume filters and evacuation systems are now required in all devices that create smoke.
- Ultrasonic energy can be used to create mechanical vibrations in a cutting instrument that simultaneously coagulates and severs the tissues.
- Laser energy created when light is passed through particular kinds of media is among the most powerful types of energy used in surgery. Like electricity, it can be contained and directed for beneficial use, but when used incorrectly, it can be a source of injury.
- Anyone working around lasers must have eye protection to prevent retinal damage. Never rely on the color of the eye glasses to determine the correct type; always check the written imprint on the glasses.
- Lasers are the most common cause of patient fires.
- When laser surgery is required for surgery of the neck and upper airway, a light-reflective endotracheal tube is required to prevent ignition of the tube, tissues, and drapes (airway fire) caused by an oxygen-rich environment and extreme heat of the laser.

REVIEW QUESTIONS

1. Discuss the difference between a bipolar circuit and a monopolar circuit.
2. Why do you place the patient return electrode over a large muscle mass?
3. What kinds of electrosurgery require a patient return electrode?
4. What is the effect of impedance of electricity as it flows through a conductive substance?
5. What is cryoablation?
6. Why does eschar on the active electrode create a hazard?
7. What does the acronym *laser* stand for?
8. What precautions are needed during laser surgery of the throat?
9. A colleague asks you why the laser goggles are not color-coded. What would you say?
10. Describe capacitive and direct coupling.

CASE STUDIES

CASE 1

You are in a hurry to pass through a surgical suite where Nd:YAG laser surgery is in progress. You do not use protective eyewear, even though goggles are hanging on the door outside. You enter the room and turn your head away from the patient as you proceed to the other door. Just to be safe, you close your eyes for a few moments until you reach the door. Are you safe?

CASE 2

You are asked to bring a 15-year-old from the holding area for surgery. When you arrive, you see that she has a metal ring through her lip. You explain to her that it is a hazard during electrosurgery. She tells you she cannot take it out because there is no way to remove it. How will you handle this situation?

CASE 3

You are scrubbed during an emergency laparotomy in which monopolar electrosurgery is used extensively. Midway through the case, you notice that the power cord to the electrosurgical unit has been plugged into an extension cord to which the cardiac monitor is also connected. What should you do?

CASE 4

You are at the scrub sink, preparing for an eye procedure in which laser surgery will be used. The surgeon's assistant is next to you at the sink. You notice that he is wearing a metal necklace. Can he tuck it into his scrub shirt?

CASE 5

During surgery in which you are scrubbed, the surgeon asks you to hold a clamp that he has just placed over a vessel bundle. He proceeds to buzz the clamp. You suddenly feel a sharp burning pain on the hand holding the clamp. What caused this? What should you do?

REFERENCES

Lee T, Soo JC, LeBouf RF, Burns D, Schwegler-Berry D, Kashon M, et al. Surgical smoke control with local exhaust ventilation: experimental study. *J Occup Environ Hyg*. 2018;15(4):341–350.

BIBLIOGRAPHY

AORN Guideline Implementation. *Energy-Generating Devices, Part 2 – Lasers*; 2017.

ECRI Institute. *Laser use and safety*; 2018. http://www.ceeducation.org/Documents/3-Lasers/ECRI-SurgAn17.pdf. Accessed July 13, 2019.

Laser Institute of America. *Medical laser safety*. https://www.lia.org/education/medical_laser_safety. Accessed July 13, 2019.

Miller R, Eriksson L, Fleisher L, et al. *Miller's Anesthesia*. 8th ed. Philadelphia: Saunders; 2015.

Occupational Safety and Health Administration. *Use of medical lasers*. https://www.osha.gov/SLTC/etools/hospital/surgical/lasers.html. Accessed July 13, 2019.

U.S. Food and Drug Administration, Medical Lasers, May 14, 2018. https://www.fda.gov/radiation-emitting-products/surgical-and-therapeutic-products/medical-lasers. Accessed July 13, 2019.

MOVING, HANDLING, AND POSITIONING THE SURGICAL PATIENT

16

KNOWLEDGE AND SKILLS REVIEW

The following skills and knowledge should be reviewed before you start this chapter:
Body mechanics
Communication and teamwork
Legal considerations regarding patient abandonment and right to privacy
Risk management

LEARNING OBJECTIVES

After studying this chapter and laboratory practice, the reader will be able to:

1. List and discuss the principles of safe patient transport and transfer
2. Demonstrate professional communication skills with families of patients being transported to surgery
3. Use safe body mechanics during patient transportation, transferring, and positioning
4. Discuss common methods of patient transport and lateral moving devices used in the perioperative environment
5. Describe guidelines for transporting special patient populations
6. Describe the responsibilities of the surgical technologist in patient positioning
7. Demonstrate the use of common operating table accessories and positioning devices
8. Describe how to prevent patient injury during positioning
9. Discuss the principles of safe positioning
10. Demonstrate basic positions used in surgical procedures
11. Discuss the safety precautions for each position

TERMINOLOGY

Abduction: Movement of a joint or body part away from the body.

Compression injury: Tissue injury caused by continuous pressure over an area.

Dependent areas of the body: Areas of the body subject to pressure from gravity and weight. For example, the sacrum is a dependent area when a person is in the supine position.

Embolism: A clot of blood, air, organic material, or a foreign body that moves freely in the vascular system.

Fowler position: In this position the patient is recumbent in a sitting or modified sitting position for exposure to the head, posterior neck and cranium, anterior chest area, face, and shoulders.

Gurney: A patient transport conveyance—a wheeled bed. The word gurney is sometimes used interchangeably with stretcher.

Hyperextension: Extension of a joint beyond its normal anatomical range.

Hyperflexion: Flexion of a joint beyond its normal anatomical range.

Ischemia: Loss of blood supply to a body part either by compression or as a result of a blockage in blood vessels. Prolonged ischemia causes tissue death from lack of oxygen to the tissue.

Kraske position: Also called jackknife position, the patient lies prone with the middle section of the table flexed at a slight angle.

Lateral position: In this position the patient lies on his or her side for exposure to the lateral chest and flank.

Lateral transfer: Transferring the patient from one horizontal surface to another, such as from a bed to a stretcher.

Lithotomy position: Used for exposure to the perineum for gynecological and urological procedures. In this position the patient's legs are elevated and placed in stirrups or leg crutches.

Range of motion (ROM): The normal anatomical movement of an extremity.

Reverse Trendelenburg: A position in which the operating table is tilted downward feet first toward the floor.

Roller board: A lateral transfer device composed of serial rollers covered in heavy plastic fabric.

Shearing injury: Tissue injury or necrosis that results when two tissue planes are forcefully pulled in opposite directions. Shearing usually occurs when the body is pulled or slides by gravity across a high-friction surface, such as a bed sheet.

Transfer board: A thin plastic board that is placed under the patient to perform a lateral transfer.

Trendelenburg position: The position in which a prone or supine patient is tilted with the head down.

Skill in moving and handling patients is required of everyone on the surgical team. This is to prevent injury to the patient and themselves. This chapter covers three important areas of study: patient transport, transfer, and patient positioning on the operating table. Patient *transport* refers to methods and equipment used to move the patient within the health care facility, such as from a hospital ward to the operating room. *Transfer* in the context of patient care refers to moving the patient from a hospital bed to a **gurney** or a gurney to the operating table (discussed below in detail). *Surgical positioning* refers to specific postures or positions the patient is placed in to provide adequate exposure to the operative site while preventing injury and allowing physiological monitoring and administration of anesthesia. The surgical technologist may be required to assist in any of these procedures, which are also collectively referred to as *patient moving and handling*.

Moving patients safely within the health care facility requires proper equipment and training in the operation of the equipment. These principles are coupled with the knowledge of body mechanics and an awareness of specific patient vulnerabilities to injury. The current trends in health care require an increasingly safety-conscious workplace in which patients and care providers can expect detailed attention to all environmental risks. Equipment used to assist in patient movement and handling aims to eliminate patient injury while keeping health care workers healthy. Many health care facilities routinely use a draw (lift) sheet to manually transfer patients. However, the Centers for Disease Control and Prevention (CDC) and the National Institute for Occupational Safety and Health (NIOSH) advise that this method is not as safe because moving and handling equipment should not rely on strength alone.

There are many different brands and types of equipment used to transport and transfer patients in the health care facility. It is the responsibility of every health care worker to become familiar with the equipment and how it works *before* using it.

Transport of the patient within the health care facility is carried out according to facility policy. Safety is the primary consideration. Whether the patient travels by a gurney, critical care bed, or wheelchair and the number and qualifications of people required are decisions based on the patient's history and physical status.

Positioning the surgical patient is one of the primary skills required of the surgical technologist. Study and practice in this area is detailed and exact, requiring knowledge and practice.

SECTION I: TRANSPORT AND TRANSFERS

The surgical technologist may be required to transport patients to surgery either from the patient holding area or hospital ward. **Patient identification is of primary importance in the chain of events leading to the surgical procedure itself.** Because of the critical nature of patient identification, and ensuring the right patient, right site or side, and right procedure, the identification process is discussed at the beginning of the chapter.

IMPORTANT TO KNOW *The following discussions on patient transport and transfers are not intended to replace facility-based in-service demonstrations and classes on safe patient moving and handling. This is a critical area of safety for patients and employees alike, and training must never be treated as "optional." Students and instructors are therefore urged to actively pursue facility-based courses by trained personnel.*

PATIENT IDENTIFICATION

The identity of the patient is verified before transporting and before beginning any procedure. Patient identification is a critical issue in health care. The surgical technologist is responsible for patient identification according to the facility policy and mutual guidelines agreed on by all professional surgical organizations. No patient should be transported and no procedure should be initiated until the protocol for identification has been completed, even if the patient is known to the health care staff.

All patients are identified using at least three methods. The patient's wrist or ankle band is imprinted with the patient's name and other unique identifiers such as birth date and hospital number. If a scan or imprint card system is used, the patient's identification card is used to process all paperwork and matches the patient's identification band. This card must be firmly attached to the chart during transport and must remain with the chart until the patient returns to his or her hospital unit. The patient's chart must accompany the patient whenever the individual is transported from the unit. Errors in patient identification usually occur when the necessary protocol has been bypassed.

Guidelines • Validating a Patient's Identity

To validate a patient's identity, follow these guidelines:

1. Examine the patient's identity band. Compare both the name and the number with those on the patient's chart.
2. Ask the patient to state his or her full name and date of birth. Do not call the patient by name before asking the patient to state his or her name.
3. Ask the patient to state his or her allergies, if any.
4. Ask the patient to tell you what procedure he or she is undergoing and to point to the side on which the surgery will take place.
5. If the patient does not speak English, or seems to have difficulty understanding, you must seek assistance from an interpreter. This information should be determined ahead of time so that an appropriate interpreter is available.
6. Remember that patients may be anxious or worried before surgery and may answer closed-ended questions indiscriminately. It is necessary to question the patient without giving the answer.
7. Always check the chart, the identification band, and hospital ID number for each patient.

EXAMPLES OF VERBAL PATIENT IDENTIFICATION

1. Greet the patient and identify yourself.
   Correct: "Good morning, my name is ____. I'm here to take you for the surgery. Can you state your full name and date of birth for me?"
   Incorrect: "Are you Mr. X? I'm here to take you to the operating room."
2. Verify the procedure and location/side with the patient.
   Correct: "What procedure will you be having today?"
   Incorrect: "I see here that Dr. X is planning to put a plate in your elbow."
3. Verify the operative side of the body.
   Correct: "Can you tell/show me which (arm/leg/side) will be operated on?"
   Incorrect: "So, Dr. X is planning to operate on your right elbow today?"

If the patient's name, hospital identification number, surgery, and surgical site do not match the chart or operative documents, you must report this to the unit charge nurse right away. Do not transport the patient if patient information does not match the chart. Call the operating room to let personnel know about the delay and the reason.

NOTE *If the patient has no identification band, you must report this to the unit charge nurse or nurse manager. Under routine circumstances an identification band must be obtained before the patient leaves the unit.*

SAFETY FIRST

The adult human body is asymmetrical and heavy, and unlike a large inanimate object, the human body cannot always be held close to the health care provider's center of gravity while being moved. Accidents can and do occur. The patient can fall, and catheters and other devices can become entangled or dislodged during transfer. A sudden shift of weight may be required, and this can put unexpected strain on joints and tendons. Hospital rooms are often small and crowded, making movement awkward and sometimes difficult, especially when additional equipment is introduced into a cramped cubicle.

Skeletal injuries also occur in health care workers who must look out for their own well-being while moving and handling patients. Accident and injury to health care staff and patients can be reduced when individuals take responsibility for the possible risks. Here are some of the causes of patient moving and handling injury:

- There are not enough people to perform the required task.
- Specialized moving and handling equipment is not available or is inaccessible at the time it is needed.
- Staff have not been trained adequately for safe moving and handling.
- Staff feel rushed.
- Communication among staff is poor.
- Staff are fatigued.
- Protocols or guidelines are not in place, or they are not followed.
- Staff are distracted.
- Staff are unfamiliar with moving and handling devices.
- Equipment used for moving and handling is in poor condition.

Guidelines • Preventing Injuries During Moving and Handling Patients

The following guidelines can help prevent injuries during moving and handling patients:

1. Prepare yourself and the patient before attempting a move. Assess the situation first. Have all equipment ready before you start.
2. Ensure that you have sufficient help when moving a patient.
3. Know your limits and remain within them while moving and handling patients.
4. Use mechanical, hydraulic, or pneumatic moving and handling devices whenever possible. Maintain the spine in a neutral (natural) position whenever possible.
5. Avoid twisting the spine or other awkward positions.
6. Position yourself as close to the patient as possible; this greatly reduces the spinal load.
7. Keep your feet well apart to provide a wide base of support.
8. When performing **lateral transfers,** such as moving the patient from one surface to another of equal height, *do not bend the knees.*
9. For vertical moves (up or down), *do bend the knees.*
10. Avoid positions that reduce your base of support.
11. Never try to lift or maneuver the patient while reaching forward, away from your center of gravity. Use a transfer device whenever possible.

IMPORTANT TO KNOW *A lift sheet is standard bed linen in many facilities. This is a three-quarter sheet folded in thirds and placed at the torso level of the patient. Previously, mandates for maximum pounds (35 lb) a health worker should lift were set by OSHA; the lift sheet was literally used to lift the patient and perform a transfer. OSHA and CDC have now set standards for the use of lifting and handling devices that aim to greatly reduce the number of skeletal injuries in health care workers. Lifting and handling devices must be used in an integrated program to avoid manual lifting.*

COMMUNICATION AND TEAMWORK COUNT

Teamwork and clear communication are very important when positioning or transferring patients. Members of the health care team work together when transporting a patient, transferring the patient from one type of conveyance or equipment to another, and positioning the patient for surgery. The surgical technologist may be required to assist in all of these procedures.

When the patient is transported from one area of the health care facility to another, teamwork begins even before the transporter arrives to take a patient from the department. To coordinate the move, a call is made ahead of time to the department or ward where the patient is. When the transporter arrives at the patient care unit, he or she notifies the staff. This sets others in action to help prepare the patient and collect required documents. Patients are never removed from a ward or department without notifying the unit manager nurse in charge of that patient's care. She or he is responsible for the whereabouts of the patients and is accountable for their movement to and from the department.

IMPORTANT TO KNOW *Good team relations increase safety in the workplace and reduce job-related stress.*

Teamwork and communication are necessary when transferring the patient from one conveyance to another. An unconscious or immobile patient may require up to six people for a transfer. All actions in the process are coordinated, and communication must be strong so that everyone participating knows their part. Those participating in the transfer are guided by one person. Although there may be a number of people participating in the transfer, all must work as one unit under the direction of the team leader.

Positioning the surgical patient before a procedure requires the joint efforts of several members of the surgical team. During positioning, team members communicate with each other about the details of the position and the safest way to achieve it. Everyone is responsible for making sure that surgical positions are correct and adjusted for each individual patient's anatomical and physical condition.

Communication skills must also be considered when meeting with the patient's family or friends who may be present when the patient is being transported to the operating room. Families are sensitive at this time and naturally concerned for their loved ones. They may accompany the patient on the way to the operating room up to the semi-restricted area. At this point it is best to reassure the family that the patient will be well cared for and that a staff member will communicate with them during or at the close of surgery. Allow family members to express their concern and to speak privately with the patient before he or she enters the surgery doors.

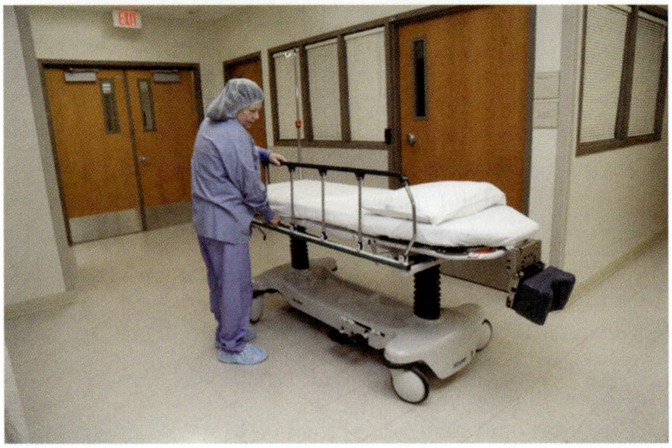

FIG. 16.1 Standard transport gurney. Raising and lowering the side rails.

TRANSPORT BY GURNEY

A *gurney (also known as a stretcher)* is shown in Fig. 16.1. This is a basic method of transporting non-ambulatory patients.

The gurney is equipped with the following:

- *Side rails:* Side rails are the most basic, effective safety mechanism on the gurney. They must be raised at all times when transporting the patient. As soon as the patient has been moved to a gurney, the rails must be raised. The locking mechanism may lock into position automatically (one-handed operation) or require the operator to pull and release the locking mechanism (requires both hands). Always ensure that the patient's hands and arms are well clear of the side rail before raising or lowering it.
- *Intravenous (IV) hanger positioned at the foot:* The IV hanger (pole) is always positioned at the foot of the gurney to prevent patient head injury. The hanger may be raised or lowered in height, and some models can be folded into the frame of the gurney when not in use. Some gurneys have a lock mechanism to remove the hanger completely.
- *Safety strap:* The safety strap is placed 2 to 3 inches above the patient's knees on top of the blanket or sheet. It is secured with three fingers' space between the patient and the strap.
- *Oxygen tank cradle:* A cradle or rack fitted for carrying oxygen is located at the bottom of the gurney between the wheels. The tank should not be placed alongside the patient on the mattress, where it may cause injury or roll off the gurney.
- *Four-wheel brake mechanism:* Modern transport gurneys have four-wheel brakes to ensure safety while the gurney is parked. The brakes are operated by a foot pedal located at the side bottom or front bottom of the gurney. The brakes must be engaged *any time the gurney is at rest* (Fig. 16.2A).
- *Three-phase pedal operation: Neutral, brake,* and *steer* (see Fig. 16.2B): Most gurneys have a three-phase lock and steer mechanism built into the pedal. In *neutral* position, all four wheels turn freely in this position. In *brake* position, the wheels are locked and will not roll. In *steer* position, all four wheels are in the forward position and will not turn.
- *Hand grips for the operator:* Hand grips are used to steer and maneuver the gurney. If possible, avoid using the side rails when pushing or pulling the gurney as they may suddenly disengage.
- *Adjustable upper body and full body Trendelenburg tilt:* The head of the gurney can be raised hydraulically or by using a manual handle according to the needs of the patient and the situation. The gurney bed can also be tilted to **Trendelenburg position** (the whole body is tilted head down) or **reverse Trendelenburg** position for emergency situations.
- *Height adjustment:* All gurneys may be raised and lowered for height adjustment either by hand or using a hydraulic mechanism. When transporting a patient, raise the gurney to the height of your hip.
- *Back board for performing CPR:* All stretchers should have a back board that is usually stowed under the mattress, or

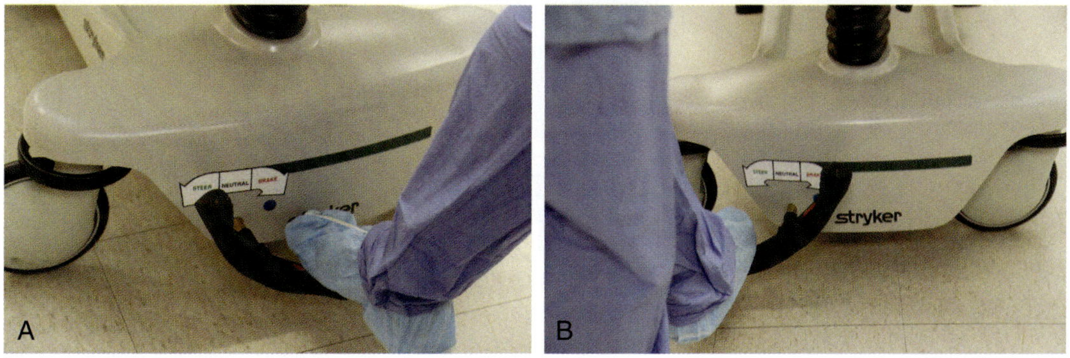

FIG. 16.2 (A) Brake mechanism on transport gurney. (B) Steer mechanism.

it may double as a removable footboard. The back board is used to perform chest compressions during CPR when it is placed directly under the patient's upper body.

- *Removable mattress with cleanable surfaces:* The patient mattress is completely removable for disinfection between patients. The cover is made of heavy synthetic fabric that can withstand cleaning with low-level disinfectants.

IMPORTANT TO KNOW *Under some circumstances, an intensive care unit (ICU) critical care bed may be used for transportation. The ICU bed is used for patients who are unstable (requiring the use of complex medical devices, or particular positioning that are not compatible or safe using a standard transport gurney). In this case, the anesthesiologist or attending physician will provide the order for a critical care bed. Under all circumstances, any patient who is being monitored requires a physician or registered nurse and at least two others to accompany the patient regardless of what type of conveyance is used.*

Using a gurney requires some practice. The weight of the gurney along with an adult patient and any equipment on board can make the load awkward, especially around turns. A gurney equipped with a four-wheel steer mechanism will travel in the direction it is pointed as long as the back wheels are locked facing forward. The wheels steer from the back and not the front. Look toward the direction you want to travel, and this will help in steering.

Always remember to engage the correct steering setting before moving with the patient. When traveling forward, use the *steer* setting. Slight forward pressure to the right or left will assist in turning. When positioning the gurney, such as when maneuvering in tight spaces, use the *neutral* setting. This will allow the gurney to move freely in any direction. Use *brake* whenever the gurney is at rest and always when transferring the patient to or from the gurney from or to another surface such as the bed or x-ray table. The following mnemonic may assist in remembering which setting to use:

Neutral: "No Steering." In neutral setting, the wheels will turn in any direction—used to position the gurney—not used for general steering purposes.

Steer: "Straight ahead." In steer mode, all four wheels are locked in the straight-forward position.

Brake: "Be safe." With the brake pedal engaged, all four wheels are locked.

BED TO GURNEY: BRINGING A PATIENT TO THE OPERATING ROOM

The patient with no movement restrictions can move from the bed to the gurney with limited assistance from staff (Fig. 16.3). Before leaving to transport the patient, prepare the gurney with the required items: safety strap, IV pole, pillow, bed blanket, and sheet. When you arrive on the ward or patient holding area, immediately alert the nursing staff of your arrival. Verify the location of the patient and proceed to the room or cubicle. Collect all the required documents, including charts, test results, and forms, before entering the patient's room or cubicle. After introducing yourself to the patient and others present, verify the patient's identity as previously described.

1. Arrange the furniture to make adequate space for the gurney. Patient rooms and cubicles are often very small. It is easier to make a path for the gurney before entering with it.
2. Lower the bed rail nearest the gurney side and also the gurney rail nearest the bed side.
3. Align the gurney with the bed and lock the wheels on both the bed and the gurney. Align the bed to the height of the gurney.
4. Identify and free up all tubing, drainage bags, or other devices that may restrain the patient or become dislodged during the transfer. Drainage collecting units (e.g., urinary or chest units) must remain lower than the patient's body at all times, and IV lines should be higher than the patient's body. Secure IV bags and other drainage units to the gurney before moving the patient over.
5. Guide the patient slowly across the bed to the gurney. Prevent the bed sheets and other linens from entangling the patient. Maintain the top sheet to protect the patient from exposure.
6. Raise the side rails and secure the safety strap over the sheet or blanket. An additional blanket should be provided.
7. Proceed to the operating room.
8. The fully conscious patient is moved to the operating table with at least two people to assist (Fig. 16.4).
9. After the patient has moved to the table, the safety strap is secured and arm boards are put into place.

Important guidelines for patient transport by a gurney are listed in Box 16.1.

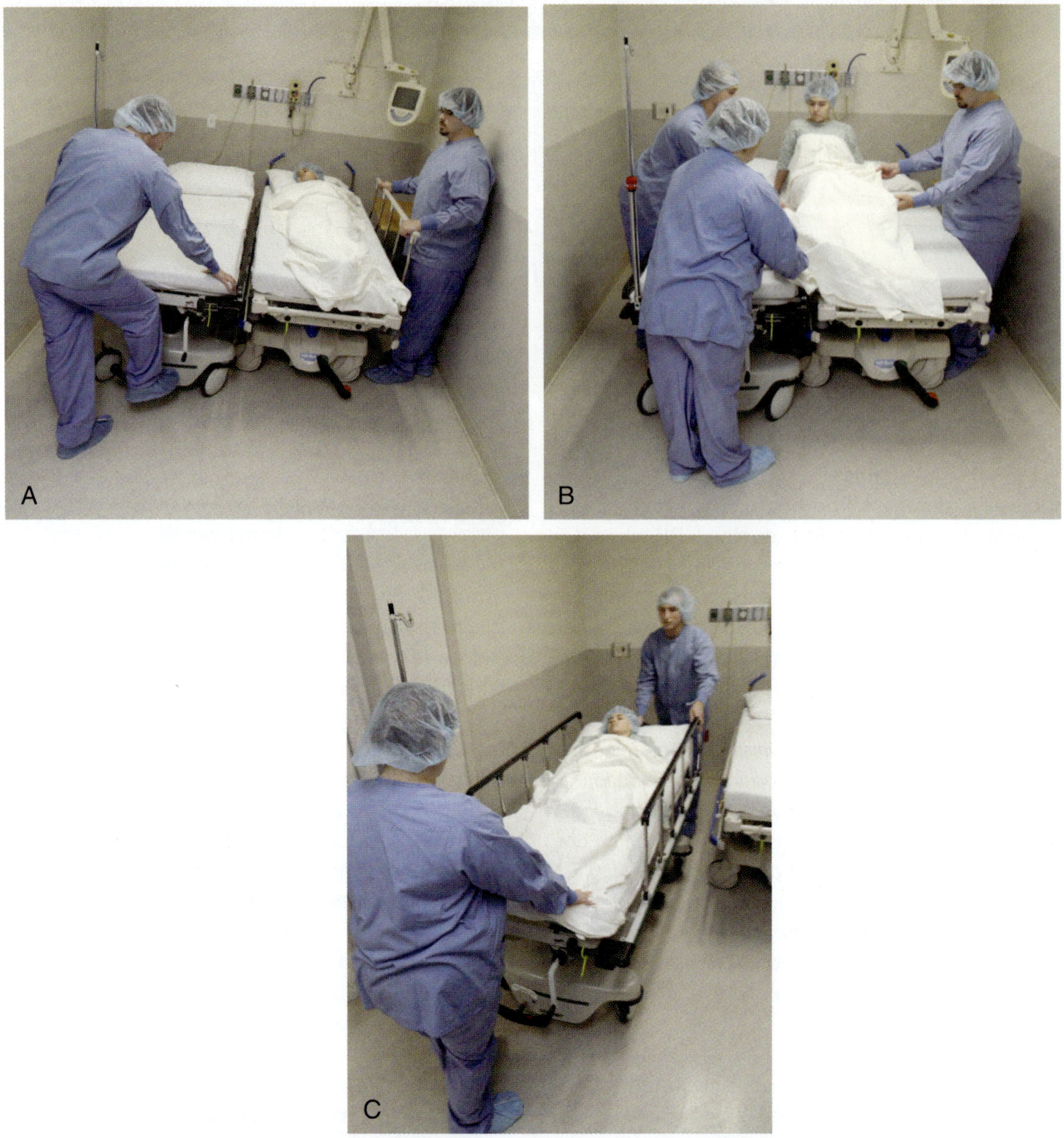

FIG. 16.3 Moving a patient from bed to gurney. (A) Align the gurney with the bed. (B) The patient moves over. Helpers should help move any cover sheets with the patient. (C) Raise the side rails.

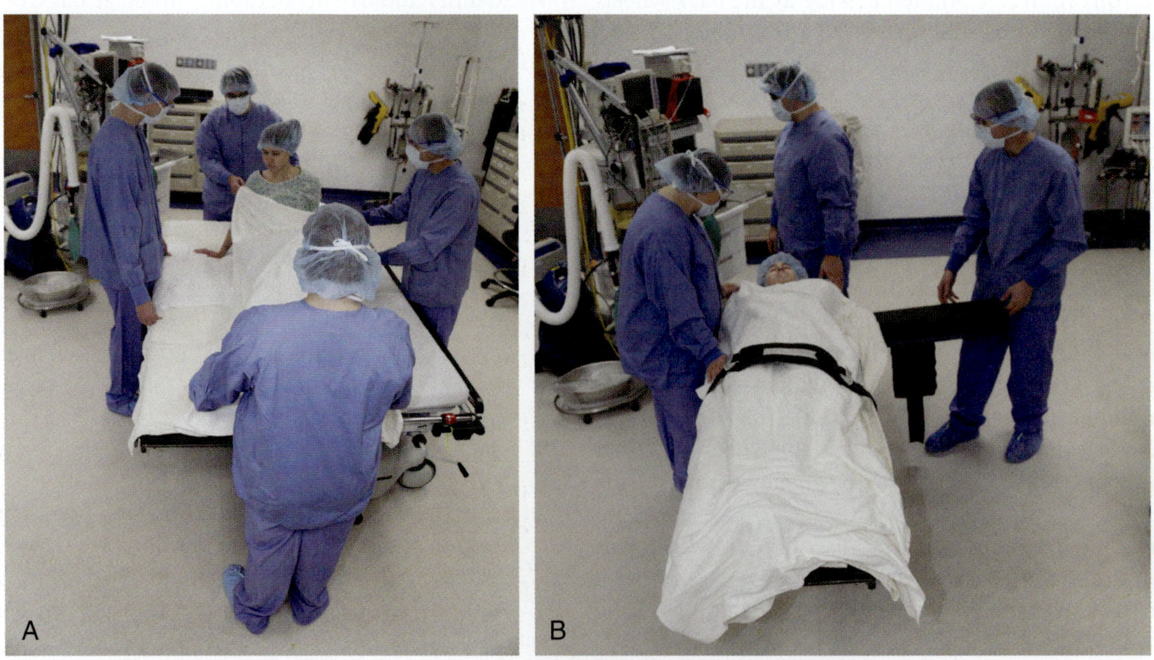

FIG. 16.4 (A) Moving the patient from the gurney to the operating table. (B) As soon as the patient is centered on the table, the safety strap is applied. One or both arm boards should be attached.

BOX 16.1 Important Guidelines for Gurney Transport of the Patient

1. Respect the patient's right to privacy at all times. Ensure that he or she is covered with at least one blanket or sheet.
2. IV bags and bottles must be suspended from an IV hanger (pole) positioned at the patient's feet (not the head) to prevent injury.
3. Keep side rails up and safety strap in place 2 to 3 inches above the knee while the patient is on board.
4. Oxygen cylinders are positioned underneath the gurney on a designated rack. Cylinders should not be laid alongside the patient on the gurney mattress.
5. Try to anticipate obstructions, sudden hallway traffic, and corners. Use ceiling and wall mounted mirrors when approaching corners. Slow down until you know it is safe.
6. When rounding blind corners, be careful of oncoming traffic. Check first before proceeding. It is difficult to stop an occupied gurney, especially when the patient is heavy and medical devices are attached to the frame. If two people are available for transport, one person pushes from the head of the gurney and the other guides the gurney from the foot around difficult obstacles.
7. Use the patient elevator rather than public elevators whenever possible to allow more space for the gurney and needed privacy for the patient. If the patient elevator is unavailable, wait until privacy can be ensured.
8. When entering the elevator, lock the doors in the open position. Then pull the gurney head first into the elevator. Do not unlock the doors until you are certain that the foot of the gurney has cleared the threshold. When exiting, lock the doors open and push the gurney foot first. Remember to unlock the doors after you exit.
9. Be sure to remind the conscious patient to keep the hands and arms within the gurney rails. Anticipation prevents accidents. Gurney rails are not solid and do not protect the patient from injury. The patient can easily bruise or even fracture an elbow, fingers, or wrist on walls and doorways. Observe the patient and maintain verbal contact during transport.
10. Unless the patient is required to remain flat, raise the head of the gurney so that the patient can see where he or she is going.
11. Always warn the patient of bumps or other unfamiliar movements that will be encountered, such as entering or exiting an elevator where there is always a bump.
12. When rolling the gurney down a ramp, do not rely on your strength to hold the gurney against gravity. Seek assistance. One person should stabilize the foot of the gurney while the second is at the head. Traveling up the ramp also requires two people—one to push, the other to pull.
13. When passing through manually operated doors, open the doors first and secure them open. Never use the foot of the gurney to open the doors. This is unacceptable patient care. Push the gurney through the open doors or pull from the head of the gurney.
14. Patients who are on cardiac monitoring devices and are being moved must be accompanied by a registered nurse or physician and two others. This meets normal standards for safety in an accredited health facility. Cardiac monitors are mounted at the foot of the patient gurney. Avoid placing a monitor between the patient's feet.

PERFORMING ASSISTED LATERAL TRANSFERS

Assisted lateral transfer involves moving a patient, in the supine position, from one surface to another of near-equal height, with the aid of a transfer device. In the perioperative environment, patients are transferred from the bed to gurney and from the gurney to the operating table. After surgery, the patient is moved back to the gurney for transport to the postanesthesia care unit (PACU). If the patient is required to go directly to the intensive care unit (ICU) after surgery, he or she will be transferred from the operating table to an ICU bed.

The decision of which lateral device is to be used depends on the patient's weight, physical condition, and level of consciousness. A fully conscious patient with no ambulatory restrictions can move with the guidance and protection of the staff helping him or her with movement as previously described. The *log roll maneuver* is used in the supine lateral transfer, which requires a *friction-reducing transfer device*. In this maneuver, the patient is rolled from supine to a side-lying position while maintaining the patient's spine in neutral position. The transfer device is placed adjacent to the patient, who is then eased back into supine position on top of the device. The device, not the patient, is then pulled from one surface (bed or gurney) to the other.

IMPORTANT TO KNOW *The number of people required to assist in the move depends on the patient's weight, physical condition, and level of consciousness. At least four people are required.*

The **transfer board** is made of durable plastic or similar material, which is semi-rigid and washable. The surface of the board is smooth on both sides, thus reducing the friction between the board surface and transfer surfaces.

The *glide sheet* is made of smooth nylon fabric. It is used in the same manner as the transfer board, eliminating friction between the patient and transfer surfaces.

The **roller board** is a transfer device constructed of serial metal rollers, which are encased in a heavy plastic fabric. The roller board is covered with a clean sheet and placed under the patient. The sheet is then laterally pulled, carrying the patient over the rollers without friction.

The *air-assisted* transfer device uses forced air to lift a baffled mattress off the surface of the transfer surfaces. The bottom surface of the mattress contains multiple perforations, which act as air jets. As air is forced downward on the transfer surface, the entire mattress is lifted slightly, allowing the mattress and patient to be moved easily in supine position in any direction.

An overhead *mechanical hoist* may be used for lateral transfer. This type of hoist is commonly used on patient

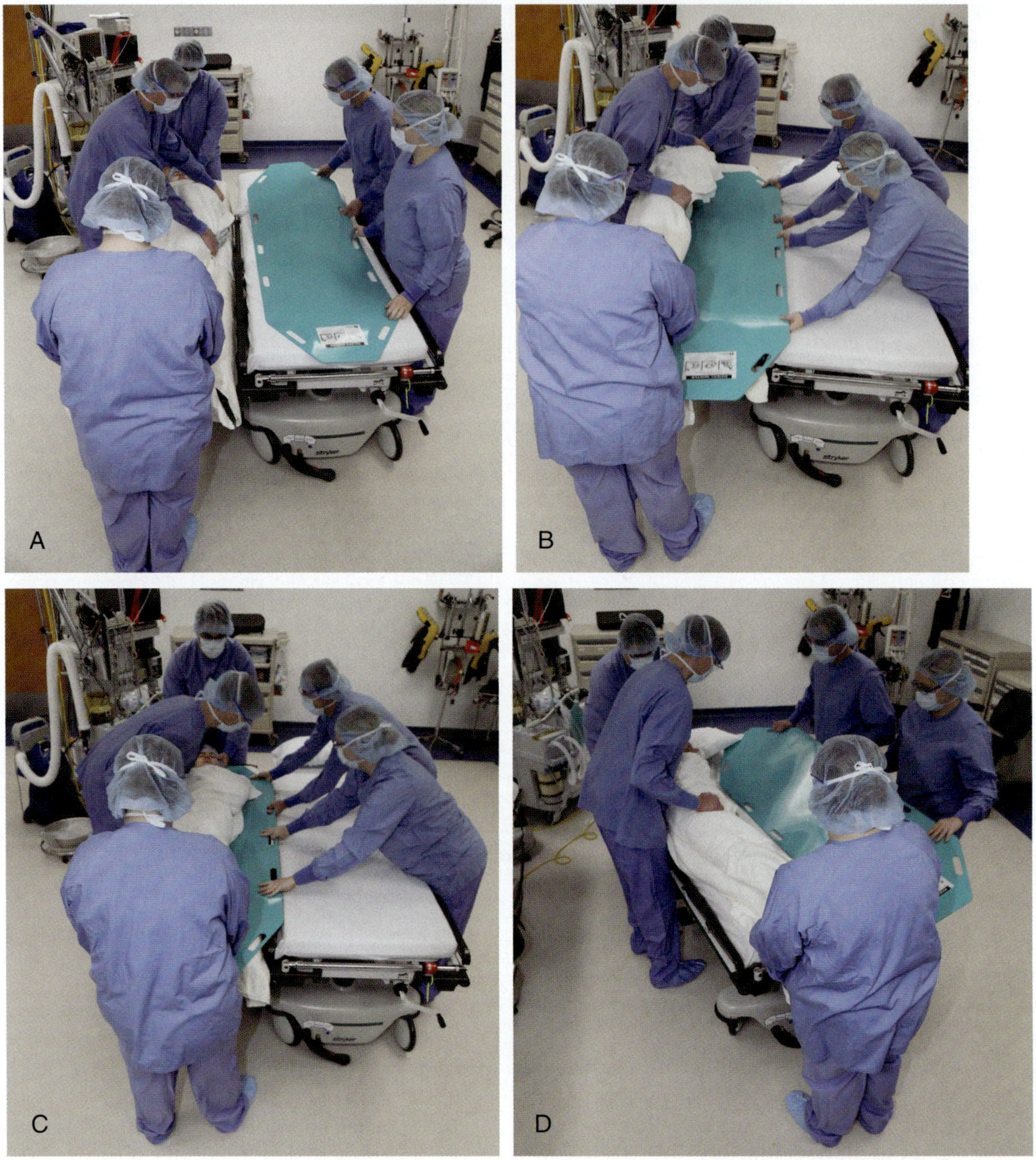

FIG. 16.5 Assisted lateral transfer using a transfer board. (A) Log rolling the patient to position the board under the patient. The log roll is performed with the patient in alignment from head to toe. (B) The patient is lowered onto the board and top sheet, which is then used to pull the board and patient in one or two coordinated moves. (C) The patient is pulled onto the gurney using the transfer board. (D) The patient is log rolled again, and the board is removed.

wards, especially for the care of bariatric patients, and requires detailed skills training.

PERFORMING THE LOG ROLL AND ASSISTED LATERAL TRANSFER

The following steps are used to perform the log roll and assisted lateral transfer. Refer to Fig. 16.5. This move applies to transfer to and from the patient bed or operating table to a gurney.

1. Align both bed and gurney side by side. Lock all wheels on both.
2. Lower the outside rails on both bed and gurney. Raise both bed and gurney to hip height.
3. At least two people are positioned at the open sides of the bed or gurney. One additional person stands at the head to protect the airway and maintain cervical alignment. The anesthesia provider takes this responsibility. Another person should be positioned at the patient's feet.
4. Before moving the patient, free up all tubes, cables, and catheters. These are transferred and secured before the patient is shifted. Remember: Move IV bags, drainage bags, and any other devices first, followed by the patient.
5. The team at the bedside should place their hands at the shoulder, hip, and feet and roll the patient toward themselves into a side-lying position while maintaining the patient's spine in neutral position at all times. The opposite

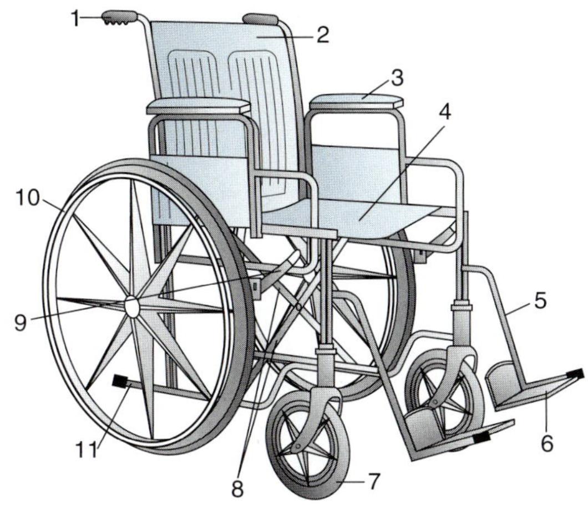

FIG. 16.6 Parts of a wheelchair. The surgical technologist should know how to operate all attachments and moving parts of a standard wheelchair. (From Sorrentino S, ed. *Mosby's Textbook for Nursing Assistants*. 9th ed. St Louis: Mosby; 2017.)

team places the transfer device in position to receive the patient as he or she is rolled back to rest on the device in supine position.

6. The transfer device is pulled gently to the gurney while the patient's head and feet are held in alignment with the body.
7. Immediately fasten the patient safety strap. Check all IV lines, catheters, and other tubing to ensure that there are no kinks or blockage. Also check collection bags, which must be lower than the patient for drainage.

IMPORTANT TO KNOW *Remember that tubing and catheters may be hidden from view by the patient's gown and bed covers. Check carefully before transferring or moving the patient.*

WHEELCHAIR TRANSFER AND TRANSPORT

The basic transport wheelchair (Fig. 16.6) is used to carry patients who need limited assistance during transport within the health care facility. Health care facility policy will determine if all ambulatory surgery patients are required to travel by wheelchair to the procedure room.

Wheelchair designs vary widely. However, all have basic safety mechanisms. There are two foot supports near the front wheels to keep the patient's feet comfortably raised above the floor during transport. These swing away and fold up to allow the patient to access the seat. The transport chair has four wheels, which are rimless. The back wheels are larger than the front. The *brake* mechanism is usually engaged by locking the levers against each of the larger wheels.

The IV hanger is located in the back of the chair. An oxygen tank cradle may be located at the back or under the seat. The side-arm rails can be raised, lowered, or removed. However, during patient transport, they should be locked in the up position. Most transport wheelchairs have a seat belt, which can provide greater security for the patient. A standard wheelchair is steered from the back using the hand grips. The rear wheels provide the drive. To avoid swerving the wheelchair, look ahead toward the direction of travel and allow the chair and your body to follow. To negotiate a turn, add enough diagonal push to turn the front wheels slightly. Too much diagonal push will cause the wheelchair to swerve.

A standard wheelchair can accommodate up to 300 pounds body weight. The bariatric chair is larger in the frame and seat and can carry up to 500 pounds.

SAFETY GUIDELINES FOR WHEELCHAIR TRANSPORT

Transporting a patient by wheelchair requires approximately the same guidelines as those for gurney travel, with some modifications. As with the gurney, never use a wheelchair that is nonfunctional. Both main brakes, foot supports, and arm rests must be operational. If you are unfamiliar with the operation of any part of the wheelchair, seek guidance *before* transporting the patient.

Guidelines • Transporting a Patient by Wheelchair

When transporting a patient by wheelchair, follow these guidelines:

1. Cover the patient with a blanket, taking care to avoid tangling in the wheelchair mechanisms.
2. Avoid piling charts, documents, x-rays, clothes, and other personal items in the patient's lap. Use the racks provided at the back or bottom of the wheelchair or transfer personal items separately. Make sure that the patient's personal items are tagged and identified.
3. Travel facing forward except when entering an elevator or using a ramp.
4. Patients should be transported in elevators designated for patients rather than public elevators.
5. When the elevator car arrives, lock the doors open. *Pull* the wheelchair, back first, fully into the elevator and lock the wheels. Unlock the doors. Keep the wheelchair in locked position while the elevator is in motion.
6. Remind the patient to keep hands and arms within the armrest boundaries at all times.
7. Always lock the wheels when the wheelchair is at rest.
8. When negotiating down a ramp, turn the wheelchair so the back travels first. Guide the chair until the front wheels are well clear of the ramp. Then resume forward-facing travel.

ASSISTING A PATIENT FROM BED TO WHEELCHAIR

Transfer of a patient from a bed to a wheelchair is performed with the patient's participation. During the

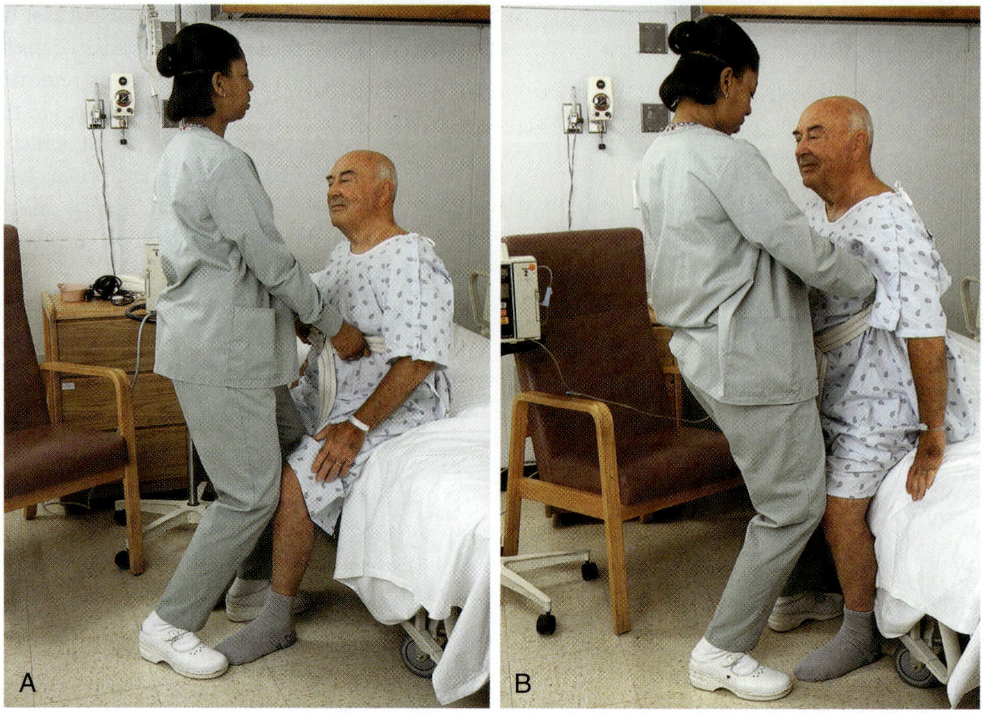

FIG. 16.7 Assisting the patient from sitting to standing position.

transfer, reinforce your instructions and prepare the patient for each step. This increases the patient's confidence and reduces fear. Remember that many elder patients are afraid of falling. Seek help from other staff when transferring a patient who is at high risk of falling (i.e., a patient who is obese, unstable, weak, or encumbered with medical devices).

Before beginning the transfer, familiarize yourself with the equipment. Make certain that the wheelchair's brakes and steering mechanism are functioning properly. The wheelchair must be able to accommodate the patient's size and weight.

Check the patient's identification. Free up any tubes or lines and make certain there is enough slack between the patient and the wheelchair to prevent entanglement or restriction during the transfer.

Always remember to transfer and secure medical devices (tubing, oxygen tank, and fluid collection bags) first, followed by the patient. Assisting the patient to the wheelchair from a lying position requires two separate steps: sitting to standing and standing to moving into the wheelchair.

SITTING TO STANDING POSITION

To help a patient move from a sitting position to a standing position, follow these steps:

1. Standing directly in front of the patient, place your hands around the patient's torso and under the arms.
2. Slightly bend your forward leg while placing your opposite foot in a bracing position (see Fig. 16.7).
3. Slowly rock back and raise the patient to a standing position.

STANDING POSITION TO WHEELCHAIR

To help a patient move from a standing position to a sitting position in a wheelchair and then transport the patient, follow these steps:

1. Taking one small step at a time, rotate your entire body as the patient does the same until the patient's back is lined up with the wheelchair.
2. Slowly lower the patient into the wheelchair. Spread your feet so that they are approximately shoulder-width apart. Use your abdominal muscles to support your back as you lower the patient. Be careful to avoid being pulled downward by the patient's weight.
3. Bend your knees, use the larger thigh muscles, and use your abdominal muscles to support your upper body. Lower the patient when your spine and body are in alignment with the patient and wheelchair (Fig. 16.8).
4. Place the patient's feet on the footrests and cover the patient with a blanket or sheet. Secure the safety strap.
5. Make sure that you have the patient's chart and medical records.
6. Proceed to your destination.

WHEELCHAIR TO BED

To transfer a patient from a wheelchair to a bed or operating table, follow these steps:

1. Place the table or bed at its lowest height.
2. Reverse the steps used to transfer the patient to the wheelchair. Place the wheelchair in line with the bed and lock the wheels.

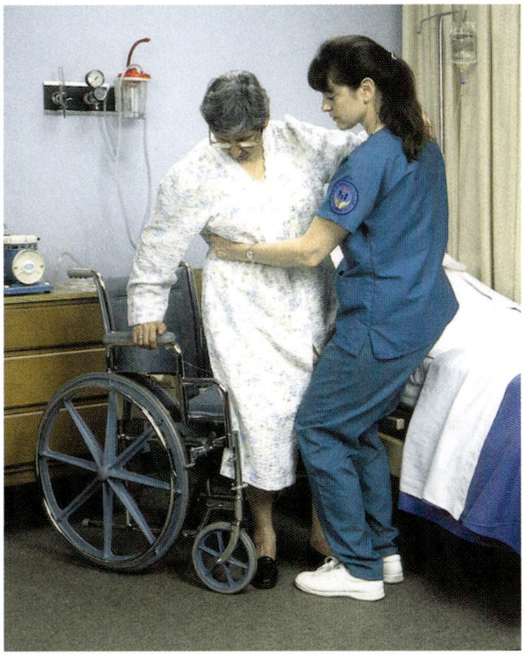

FIG. 16.8 Assisting the patient from standing to sitting in wheelchair or bed.

3. If the patient can put weight on the hands, ask the patient to push down. At the same time, assist the patient by placing your arms under the patient's arms and securing your hands over the patient's shoulder blades.
4. Place your bracing foot back and rotated slightly outward.
5. As the patient stands up, rock back on your bracing foot, and step by step, rotate your body as you move the patient until he or she is positioned squarely at the edge of the bed.
6. Remember to keep your spine and the patient's back in alignment while turning. Ease the patient down to a sitting position on the bed.
7. One person should support the patient's back and head while another assists in bringing the legs to a horizontal position on the operating table or bed. A third assistant should stand at the opposite side of the operating table or bed to prevent the patient from falling.
8. Ease the patient to a lying position. Place a blanket or sheet over the patient and secure the side rails or safety strap.

ASSISTING AN AMBULATORY PATIENT

In ambulatory health care facilities, patients may walk from the holding area to the procedure room according to the health facility policy. The following guidelines are used to assist the patient and prevent falls.

1. Position yourself slightly behind the patient's shoulder while helping the person walk. This places you in a position to support the patient if the individual becomes weak or begins to fall. If the patient seems unsteady, use a wheelchair.
2. Give the patient time to maneuver. Do not rush. Point out or otherwise orient the patient to where he or she is going, rather than simply guiding him or her to the location.

ASSISTING A FALLING PATIENT

In the ambulatory care setting, patients walk or are transported by wheelchair from the holding area to the surgical area, and the surgical technologist may be responsible for assisting them. There is always a risk that the patient may fall while walking. Always anticipate the possibility of a fall, even when the patient is mobile and seems able to walk without assistance.

Patient falls can be dangerous for both the patient and the health care provider. The weight of the falling person can cause you to lose your own balance, which can result in a twisting injury or fracture. Patients who feel unsteady or insecure may take hold of the care provider and pull him or her off balance, causing injury to both.

1. To assist the falling patient, do not try to support the patient's weight. Instead, ease the patient to the floor while protecting the person's head (Fig. 16.9).
2. Spread your feet to create a wide base of support. Bend your knees and use your thigh muscles for support.
3. Follow the patient's movements with your own body to prevent the patient from dropping.
4. Immediately call out for assistance while remaining with the patient. Do not abandon the patient under any circumstances.

SPECIAL PATIENT POPULATIONS

PEDIATRIC PATIENTS

Children are transported to the operating room by a gurney, crib, or bassinet, depending on their developmental age and condition.

It is important to reduce a child's anxiety in the preoperative period because in addition to the emotional effects of distress, a fearful, highly anxious child may experience difficulty during induction and emergence from anesthesia. Health care facilities allow caregivers to accompany the child to the holding area, and in many hospitals, a parent or other caregiver is permitted to stay in the operating suite during the induction of anesthesia.

If the child is unaccompanied by a family member, the separation can be stressful. Most young children, especially toddlers and preschoolers, suffer extreme anxiety when separated from their caregivers.

- Talk with the child during transport and explain the environment in simple, nonthreatening terms. Remember that children understand the meanings of words in their most literal sense. The child's developmental age is critical to communication. Children aged 5 to 9 years are curious about their environment. Preteens want to take part in their care. Teenagers are likely to seem unconcerned but appreciate explanations of the environment.

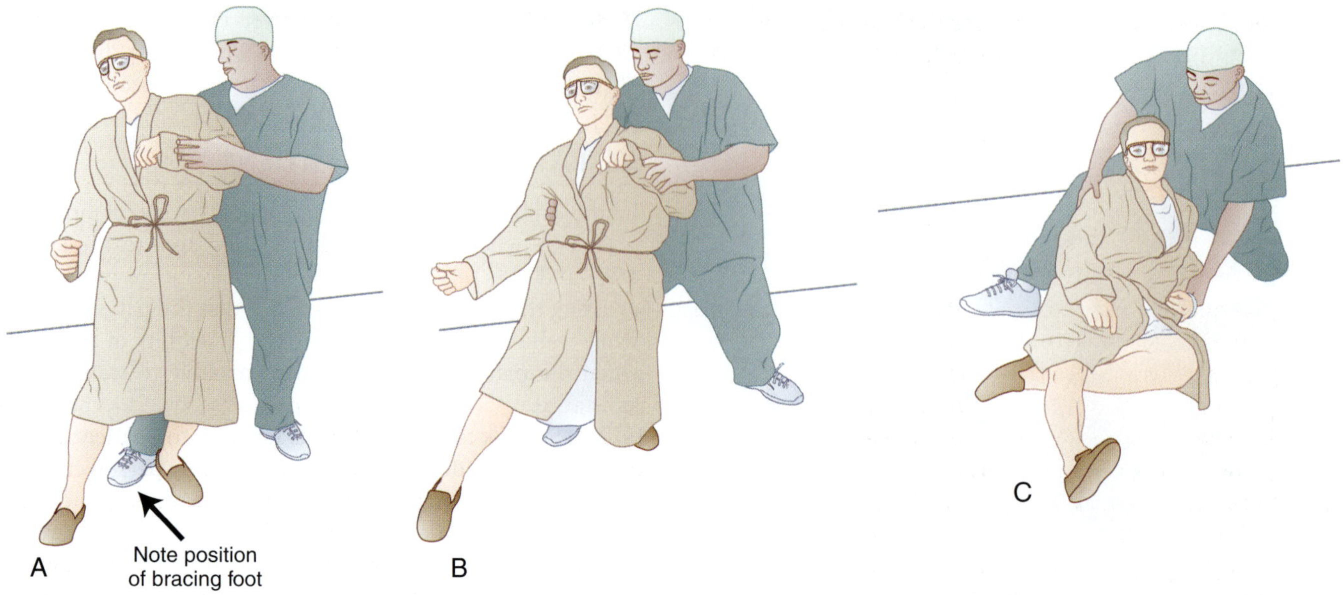

FIG. 16.9 Assisting a falling patient.

- Do not treat the child like a small adult. Provide a calm, supportive presence, showing respect for the child at all times. Children are quick to understand when they are being falsely reassured. Instead of saying, "Oh, don't be afraid; this won't take long," evaluate the child's understanding of what is happening and try to clarify his or her perception in simple, concrete terms. Distraction may also be effective in allaying anxiety.

Cribs should be equipped with a Plexiglas cover during transportation. However, remember that toddlers can climb and move with amazing speed and agility. Even a crib cover may not prevent a small toddler from attempting to climb between the top rail of the side bars and the crib cover. Crib bars can also be a source of danger, especially in health care institutions with older equipment. In recent years, regulations for cribs have become much more stringent. Problems with cribs arise from the width of the bars and from crib bumpers (pads). Deaths from bumpers have occurred in three ways:

- The child becomes wedged against the crib bumper and is strangled by the ties that attach it to the crib frame.
- The child becomes wedged between the crib bumper and the mattress and suffocates.
- The child climbs over the rail and falls to the floor or becomes entrapped by crib bars during the fall and fractures a limb.

The safest way to prevent these kinds of accidents is by checking that the equipment meets safety standards and *never leaving the patient alone*. This cannot be stressed enough.

HEARING- OR SIGHT-IMPAIRED PATIENTS

Transporting the patient with a hearing or sight deficit may require more time and supportive personnel to assist the patient. Patients with profound deafness should have an interpreter present to explain the process of transport to the operating room and the transfer to the operating table. Sight-impaired patients may be able to communicate verbally. However, if hearing is also impaired, an interpreter may be necessary. It is important for the patient to understand each part of any moving and handling procedure. This can be by visual or verbal cues, whichever is appropriate to the patient. When transporting a hearing-impaired patient:

- Allow patients to keep their hearing aids as long as possible.
- Use hand gestures to communicate.
- Speak slowly and articulate your words when speaking to the patient.
- Face the patient during communication.

When transporting a sight-impaired patient:

- Allow the patient to keep glasses as long as possible.
- Provide verbal orientation before attempting any move.
- Explain the environment to the patient and remain in contact.
- Provide increased assistance during moves; the sight-impaired patient may also have problems with depth perception. Be aware of safety implications.

A lateral transfer may be frightening to patients with sensory deficit if performed too quickly or without warning. Make every attempt to communicate comfort to the patient before making any moves. Provide a full handover to the holding area staff on arrival in the operating room so that they understand the extent of the patient's deficit.

BARIATRIC PATIENTS

As the prevalence of morbidly obese or bariatric patients continues to increase in the United States and worldwide, it has become necessary for health care professionals to learn how to mitigate specific risks for this population. The National Center for Health Statistics states that more than 60% of adults in the United States are overweight or obese, and a sizeable number are morbidly obese. Weight categories are defined by the National Institutes of Health using the body mass index, or BMI. This is the relationship between height and weight. The formulas used are as follows:

$$BMI = \frac{\text{Weight in kilograms}}{\text{Height in meters squared}}$$

or

$$BMI = \frac{\text{Weight in pounds} \times 703}{\text{Height in inches squared}}$$

The National Institute of Health defines obesity as a BMI of 30 kg/m^2 or more and morbid obesity as a BMI of 40 kg/m^2 or greater. This figure represents a clinical extreme and presents specific surgical risks that must be considered during their medical care. These complications are also present for the moderately and severely obese patient who may also be classified as high risk on the basis of their BMI and associated (comorbid) disorders.

Certain types of diseases that are associated with obesity can be life threatening. Surgery can compound these risks, and great care is taken to prepare for adverse events related to anesthesia and the surgery.

Airway obstruction is a high risk for obese and morbidly obese patients. Extra tissue in the neck and around the trachea can make intubation difficult. Many obese individuals suffer from a collapsed airway during sleep (sleep apnea) under normal conditions. Administration of general anesthesia complicates this risk even more.

Hemodynamic function (movement of blood through the body and blood pressure) can be greatly altered in the bariatric patient. The heart must work harder to move blood around the body, and severe blood pressure changes can occur rapidly during the positioning and movement required for surgery. The extra work required by the heart results in an enlarged heart and inability to shunt the blood in and out. This often leads to congestive heart failure and hypertension. Kidney disease is a common result of severe hypertension and inability to rid the body of waste products such as urea, nitrogen, and excess salts. Fluid balance is therefore critical in these patients.

Venous stasis is an additional problem of the vascular system that results in edema of the lower extremities and high risk for deep vein thrombosis or thromboembolism. A blood clot that forms in the venous system during surgery may break loose in the postoperative period, causing stroke or pulmonary **embolism.**

Respiratory problems, including difficulty breathing, are common in bariatric patients. The extra effort needed to move air through the lungs is related to increased tissue in the thorax and shortness of breath resulting from overexertion of the heart muscle, which cannot keep up with the oxygen needs of the tissues.

Moving and Handling the Bariatric Patient

The bariatric patient is at high risk for injury during moving, handling, and positioning for surgery. Mechanical devices are available for lateral transfer to the operating table; however, neurological injury, blood pressure shifts, and musculoskeletal complications can occur during positioning. Specialty equipment such as a bariatric operating table, positioning aids, and long safety straps must be prepared before the patient is brought into the operating room.

BOX 16.2 Adult Body Mass Index

Weight Category	BMI (kg/m^2)
Underweight	<18.5
Normal or healthy weight	18.5–24.9
Overweight	25–29.9
Mild obesity	27–30
Obese	>30

Obesity is defined by the BMI. Weight categories, which have been set by the Centers for Disease Control and Prevention, are shown in Box 16.2. The prevalence of obesity in the US population and worldwide has caused a corresponding rise in obese surgical patients. Many specialty health care institutions and surgical centers are trained and equipped to care for the needs of bariatric patients. Moving and handling an obese patient requires training, knowledge of the specific patient, and team planning. The objectives of these are not only to prevent patient and staff injury but also to provide dignity and emotional support during patient care.

Care of an obese patient in surgery is often complicated by comorbid conditions such as diabetes, heart disease, airway obstruction, and airway exchange problems. The lungs do not increase in size as the patient becomes heavier; therefore the patient may have a "resting" hypoxia and hypercapnia. This is because pressure from the abdominal and chest wall restricts full lung expansion, resulting in poor ventilation. Obese patients also have a high incidence of pulmonary hypertension resulting in heart failure. Inability to move blood to all body parts results in poor peripheral circulation. Airway maintenance is a major challenge in surgical settings because an obese patient has little neck flexibility, and the usual landmarks for intubation are obscured by fatty tissue pushing inward on the neck structures. An obese patient is at high risk for deep vein thrombosis (DVT) because of circulatory stasis. All obese patients are fitted with a sequential compression device (SCD) to assist in venous return. Some of the primary challenges faced in the movement and handling of obese patients are practical. That is, patient conveyances, beds, elevators, and lifting equipment must all be capable of handling extreme weight and size.

Equipment needed for an obese patient includes the following:

- Bariatric patient gurney
- Bariatric operating table and accessories for surgical positioning
- Extra-weight-bearing wheelchairs that are capable of tilting the patient to an upright standing position for transfer or ambulation
- Bariatric patient beds
- Slide sheets, which reduce the friction between the patient and bed sheets, for adjusting the patient's position in bed and for moving up the bed

- Extra-large blood pressure cuff
- Extra-large pneumatic tourniquet

Lifting and moving devices require staff training to be used safely and confidently. As with other manufactured devices, the protocol and procedures for the safe use of equipment vary among manufacturers.

PATIENTS IN POLICE CUSTODY

Health care facilities have a duty to cooperate with law enforcement agents and provide appropriate care for patients in custody. Patients who are in police custody while in the health care facility are accompanied by one or two officers at all times. Unless the patient is a minor, the patient may be fitted with hard restraint devices (hand or leg cuffs). Law officers are responsible for protecting the patient from self-harm and harming others.

Communication between law officers and operating room personnel should follow the same protocol as for other staff on duty in the patient care area. Staff in the inpatient ward, emergency room, or other patient holding areas should be notified ahead of time that the patient will be transported for surgery. On arrival in the unit or room, introduce yourself to the custodial officers and patient and explain the procedure for transporting the patient (noting the need to check identity). The custodial police should cooperate with medical procedures, and the health staff has a duty to comply with police procedures. If the patient is in physical restraints, you may expect the restraints to be maintained during transport to the operating room. Most police officers are cooperative. However, they are also required to perform their duties according to strict law enforcement protocol.

Watch Chapter 16: Patient Transfer on the Evolve website: http://evolve.elsevier.com/fuller/surgical.

SECTION II: POSITIONING THE SURGICAL PATIENT

PRINCIPLES OF SAFE POSITIONING

The surgical patient is positioned on the operating table for a specific operative procedure. Positioning begins shortly after the induction of general anesthetic, after the airway is secured but before skin prep and draping. If a regional anesthetic is administered, the patient may be positioned before or after the anesthetic infiltration.

Safe positioning requires the *knowledge of anatomy, physiology, and the individual patient's specific medical condition.* Although each surgical position uses similar techniques with similar results, each patient is unique by age, joint mobility, and disease. *Planning and coordination* promote an organized and efficient effort by everyone involved. *Teamwork and clear communication* are needed to create a safe, purposeful result. *Awareness* of potential injuries is also a component of safe patient moving and positioning.

The following are objectives of positioning:

- Protect the patient's airway at all times.
- Allow access to monitoring sites on the body.
- Provide venous access for the administration of medications.
- Provide adequate exposure to the operative site.
- Maintain and promote homeostasis.

ROLE OF THE SURGICAL TECHNOLOGIST IN POSITIONING

The surgical technologist in a circulating role assists in positioning the patient for surgery. Along with the rest of the team, the surgical technologist is responsible for preventing positioning injury. The following are specific roles of the surgical technologist:

- Become familiar with operating table mechanisms and accessories, as well as their use
- Understand each surgical position and the devices used to support the position
- Know ahead of time the position that will be used for an assigned surgical procedure
- Proactively prevent accident and injury during positioning
- Question any aspect of the patient's position that appears to have risk potential
- Remain alert and focused on patient safety
- Communicate clearly with other members of the team

The scrubbed surgical technologist remains alert during repositioning. When a reposition is called for, equipment and devices must be cleared from the patient. This includes instrument tables, Mayo stand, and surgical instruments (including robotic instruments).

PATIENT SAFETY DURING POSITIONING

Before attempting to assist in patient positioning, know *ahead of time* the patient's particular physiological and anatomical restrictions; this is critical. Even though we have guidelines that tell us how to achieve a particular position, what equipment is needed, and how to move the unconscious patient, ***every patient is an individual.*** The patient may have a skeletal malformation or simple deviation from "normal" structure. These can affect the patient's range of motion and ability to lie in certain positions. Here, the patient's chart, especially the recent medical history and preoperative physical examination, can provide essential information to prevent injury. Positioning may require some creative means of providing support to vulnerable nerves, blood vessels, and bony prominences, while also allowing adequate surgical exposure.

IMPORTANT TO KNOW *Patient positioning is directed by the AP or surgeon. Always follow their directions. They have assessed the patient and know how to proceed safely. Never attempt to position a patient blindly without knowing the details of the patient's physical restrictions.*

Basic Guidelines • Positioning the Patient

1. Equipment needed to position the patient is assembled before the patient is brought into the operating room.

Check all fittings and connections to be sure that they are present and working. Tighten the locking devices of all weight-bearing accessories.
2. Before surgery begins, the surgeon and anesthesia provider discuss the patient's specific physical limitations and vulnerabilities with the circulator. Although this information is available in the chart, members of the team work together to ensure safety.
3. Maintain the patient's cervical spine in neutral position at all times. This prevents injury and maintains the airway.
4. Positioning begins when the anesthesia provider states that it is safe to do so. He or she is in the best position to determine when it is safe to start positioning.
5. An adequate number of trained personnel must be available to position the patient. Each must understand his or her role during positioning.
6. Coordination is best achieved when one person leads the team during positioning.
7. If repositioning is required during surgery, the anesthesia provider usually directs the move. This is because changes in position can cause sudden physiological changes.
8. Ensure that no part of the patient's body rests on the metal frame of the operating table. Padding is used to protect bony protuberances, shallow nerves, and blood vessels. Be aware of catheters, tubing, and other devices attached to the patient. These can be torn away during positioning.
9. Always move the body within its normal range of motion, taking into account the patient's individual limitations.
10. The location of the patient's hands must be confirmed to prevent the fingers from being trapped in the table breaks.
11. Safety straps must not compress the skin or underlying tissues. The safety strap is applied 2 inches above the knee as soon as the patient is moved to the operating table.
12. The heels must not rest on the table surface. This can be achieved by raising the lower legs on a pillow or pad, allowing the heels to extend over the edge.
13. Lower back strain in the supine position can be avoided by placing a pillow under the patient's knees.

NORMAL RANGE OF MOTION

The joints of the human body allow a specific type of movement or **range of motion (ROM).** For example, the elbow joint is hinged; that is, it can move freely in only one direction. Its movement is described by the angle created by the upper and lower arms. The movement of this joint is called *extension* or *flexion*. As the elbow flexes, the angle becomes smaller. Extension results in a larger angle between the forearm and upper arm. Some joints, such as the ball-and-socket joint in the hip, allow rotation of a body part inward toward the long axis of the body and outward away from the long axis. Such inward and outward rotation is called *internal* and *external rotation.*

During patient movement and handling, it is critical not to exceed the limits of a joint. Joint movements are described by direction and in degrees of movement. The surgical technologist may be required to elevate the patient's arm or leg during skin prep or draping. To perform patient movements safely, it is necessary to know the specific limits of that patient's ROM on the basis of a normal baseline. Refer to Fig. 16.10 to study the normal ROM.

POTENTIAL PATIENT INJURIES

Patient safety remains the primary principle on which all positioning activities are based. The normal reflexes that protect the body from injury are blunted or absent in an unconscious or sedated patient. Under general anesthesia and muscle-relaxing drugs, the body can physically be placed in positions that would not be tolerable to a conscious individual. Normal reflexes that are absent in an unconscious patient remain absent. These include the corneal reflex to blink or close the eye and withdrawal from pain. Physiological responses to unsafe positioning may not be witnessed except through monitoring devices.

Some patients are at increased risk for injury because of their medical condition (Box 16.3). The following are potential injuries and unsafe physiological results of positioning.

DECUBITUS ULCER

A *decubitus (pressure) ulcer* is the loss of skin and deep tissue related to continuous pressure over an area of the body. The condition is more common in a debilitated patient but can also occur in a healthy individual. Tissue injury occurs because unrelieved compression blocks the flow of blood in the capillaries of the skin and deeper tissues, causing tissue death. Without skin protection, deep tissues can easily become infected.

SHEARING INJURY

Shearing occurs when a tissue plane such as the skin is pulled in one direction while opposing planes are pulled in the opposite direction. Shearing takes place when the patient is pulled over a high-friction surface such as a bed sheet or blanket. The initial tissue reaction is skin inflammation. However, this can progress to a deeper ulcer because the underlying tissues are also damaged. An elderly patient who is poorly nourished or has poor tissue perfusion often has delicate skin, which can be torn away during an unsafe move.

MUSCULOSKELETAL AND COMPRESSION INJURY

Musculoskeletal injuries include dislocation, tears, and **compression injury** of tendons, ligaments, and muscle. These are avoided with the correct use of padding and soft supports. While moving or positioning the patient, take care to avoid exceeding the patient's ROM as discussed above. *Nerve injury* can occur with continuous pressure on the nerve or its blood supply resulting in bruising or necrosis. **Hyperextension** (greater than normal extension) and **hyperflexion** (greater than normal flexion) can result in a stretching injury. Nerve damage can result in temporary or permanent loss of mobility or sensation.

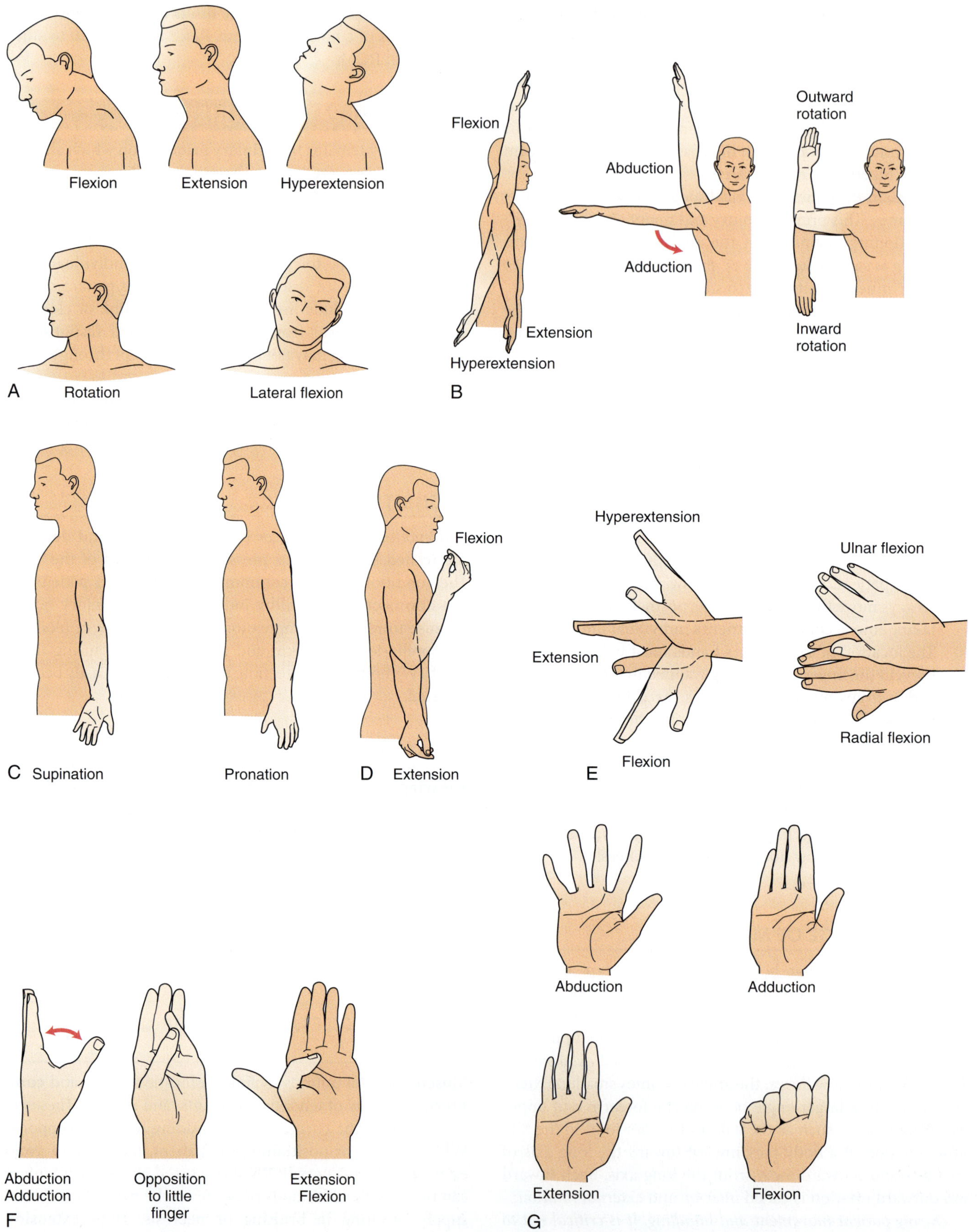

FIG. 16.10 Normal range of movement. When moving and handling patients, it is very important not to exceed the normal range of movement of joints. (From Sorrentino S, ed. *Mosby's Textbook for Nursing Assistants*. 9th ed. St Louis: Mosby; 2017.)

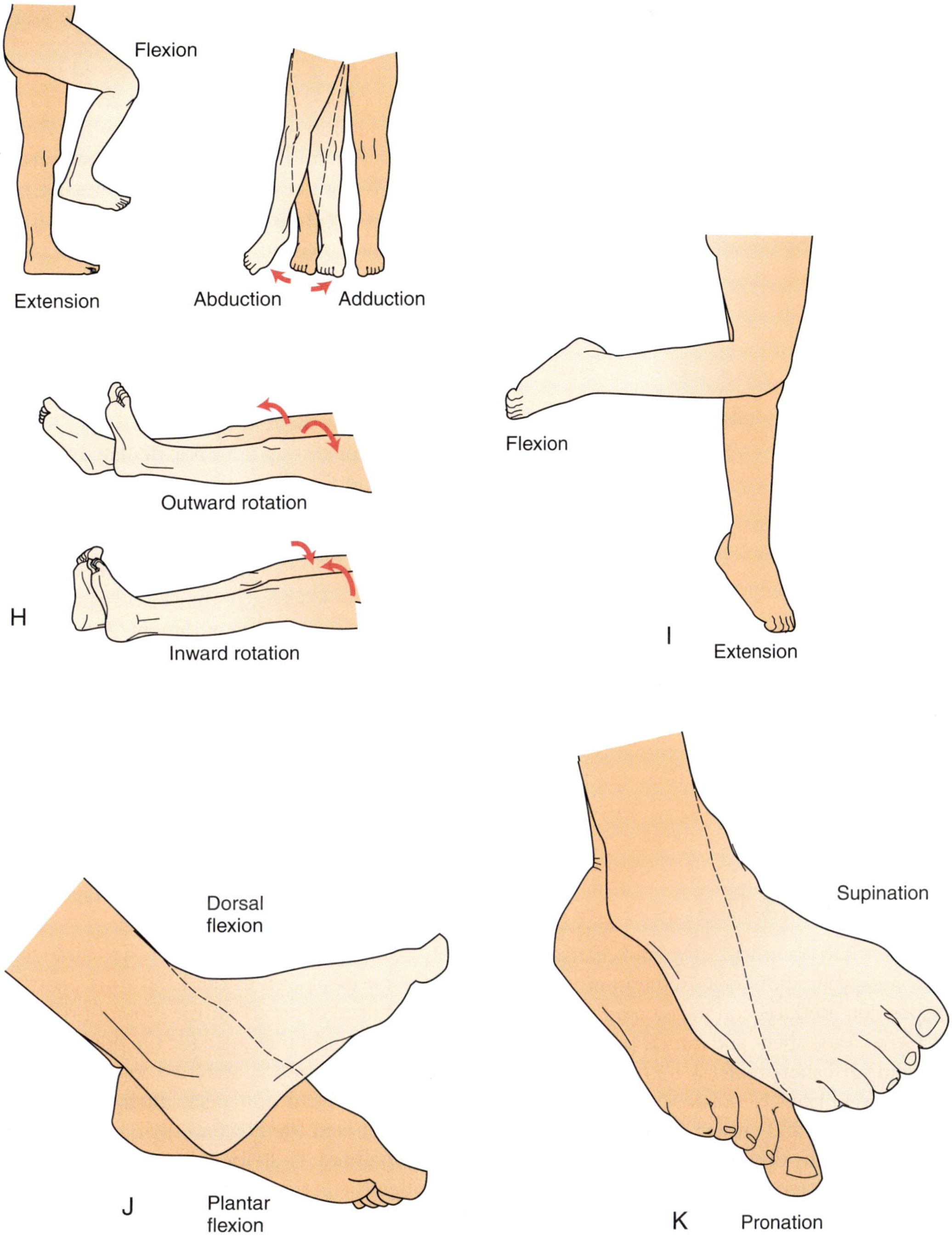

FIG. 16.10—Cont'd

Compression of vessels restricts the blood and therefore the oxygen supply to the tissue, a condition called **ischemia.** Pressure injuries may not be readily apparent because underlying tissues, such as muscle and fascia, are more susceptible to damage than skin. Ischemia is time and weight related. To prevent ischemia and necrosis, all bony prominences and **dependent areas of the body** (areas of the body under gravitational force) must be adequately padded.

EYE AND EAR INJURY

Eye injury resulting in blindness occurs most commonly in the prone position but can also occur whenever the patient is being turned or the eye is unprotected. To prevent eye injury, the patient's eyelids are taped in the closed position during general anesthesia. Further protection includes positioning the head so that no part of the eye is in contact with the head support.

BOX 16.3 Conditions That Increase the Risk of Injury

- Pre-existing nerve compression syndrome
- Diabetes mellitus
- Osteoarthritis (progressive arthritic disease)
- Venous stasis (pooling of blood as a result of inactivity or cardiovascular disease)
- Preexisting decubitus ulcer (pressure sore)
- Previous traumatic injury
- Alcohol abuse
- Smoker
- Vitamin deficiencies
- Malnutrition
- Renal disease
- Hypothyroidism
- Previous joint fractures
- Arthritis
- Corticosteroid use
- Contractures (scar tissue that restricts joint movement)
- Poor skin resilience
- Peripheral edema (intracellular fluid swelling in the legs and arms)
- Reduced range of motion

Ear injury occurs when the patient's downside ear is not protected from folding or compression. These injuries are prevented with a face rest or doughnut, which prevents the ear from bearing the weight of the patient's head.

PHYSIOLOGICAL ALTERATION

Physiological alteration can occur with any rapid change of position and also during specific positions. Respiration is compromised when the position produces compression on the chest and abdominal wall. General anesthetic and muscle paralysis contribute to ventilation and perfusion problems, even when the patient is being mechanically ventilated. Circulatory problems can result in fluid stasis (accumulation) and cardiac distress. All physiological alterations are managed by the anesthesiologist. The risks are minimized by slow, step-by-step positioning and repositioning.

THROMBOSIS AND EMBOLISM

Venous thrombosis and embolism are surgical risks, especially in an obese patient, in a patient with any circulatory disease that interferes with normal circulation, and in a surgery in which large blood vessels are entered or exposed. Antiembolism stockings or an SCD is placed on patients' legs before long procedures or on patients predisposed to clot formation. The SCD wraps around the leg, sequentially fills with air, and then deflates. During the inflation phase, the cuffs push venous blood toward the heart, and during deflation, the vessels refill. This reduces the risk of blood pooling (stasis) and thrombus formation.

NOTE *Refer to Chapter 13 for additional information on antiembolism devices.*

GENERAL OPERATING TABLE

The general operating table is used for most surgical procedures (Fig. 16.11). It can be configured into many positions and accommodates accessories for different types of surgery. The frame is stainless steel and attaches to a hydraulic lift. Weight restrictions for operating tables vary, and it is important to verify the table specifications *before* transfer and positioning. Some bariatric tables have an overall weight capacity of 1200 pounds. The weight capacity of the table articulations must also be strong enough to safely accommodate an obese patient. The table locking device is located near the head and used to secure the table base in position. Operation is by foot pedal and by using the lock feature on the handset.

The operating table is articulated (jointed) at the foot, head, and middle. These are commonly referred to as table breaks. The top of the table can be rotated, flexed, tilted, raised, and lowered. A handset is used to change the height of the table, pitch, and to position individual sections. The base is centered on the frame or may be offset to accommodate x-ray and C-arm fluoroscopy equipment. A wide variety of table attachments are used to create and support the patient in different positions. Attachments vary according to the manufacturer, in operation and configuration. The surgical technologist should become familiar with the safe operation of tables and attachments used in their facility. For uses of the attachments, see Surgical Positions.

The *arm board* is used to extend the arms away from the body at an angle less than 90 degrees. This provides access to the arms for monitoring and intravenous access. The arm is secured by an arm strap or cradle.

Stirrups are used to elevate and abduct the legs for access to the perineal area in the **lithotomy position.** The type of stirrups used depends on the type of procedure and the patient's physiological tolerance for the position (see Lithotomy).

The *headrest* is attached to the operating table and stabilizes the head and neck during a craniotomy or when the patient is in the Fowler (sitting) position. The horseshoe rest is a padded, U-shaped attachment that supports the forehead when the patient is in the prone position. Other attachments, such as the Gardner and Mayfield headrests, penetrate the skull with sterile pins and hold the head in precise position (see Prone).

POSITIONING AIDS

Positioning pads made of gel or foam are used to protect vulnerable areas of the body and to maintain the patient's position. Gel positioning pads are available in all sizes and shapes (Fig. 16.12). Common shapes are as follows:

1. Head *doughnuts* are used to stabilize the patient's head for the administration of anesthesia. The open space in the center prevents pressure on the occipital bone. The prone head pad is a larger device, which cradles the head and frames the face for prone positions. The hollow center provides access to the airway and prevents injury to the eyes, ears, facial nerves, and blood vessels.

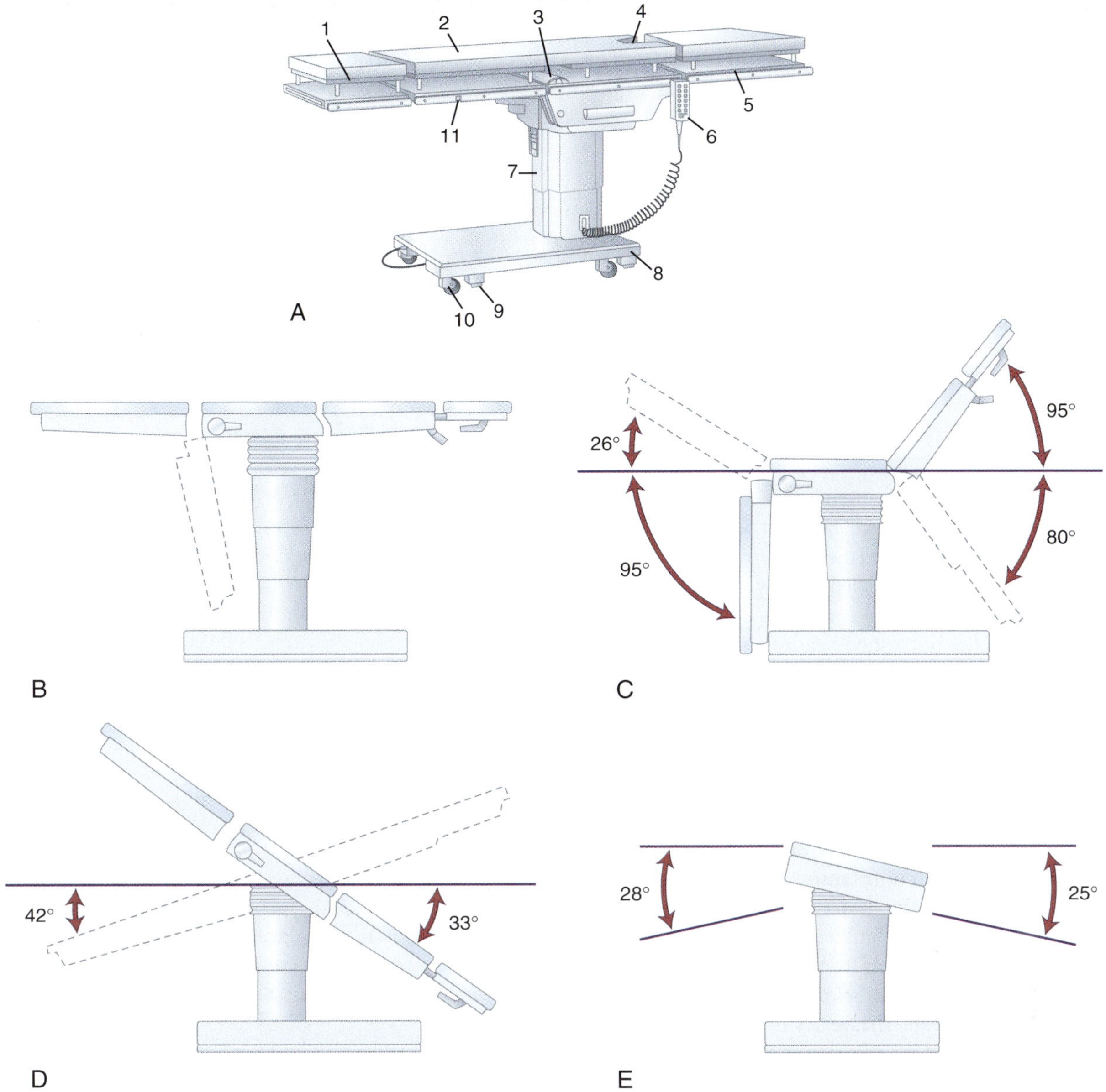

FIG. 16.11 The operating table. (A) Parts of the operating table: *1,* removable head section; *2,* table pad (mattress); *3,* kidney lift; *4,* perineal cutout; *5,* radiolucent top and removable head section; *6,* hand control unit; *7,* hydraulic lift cylinder; *8,* table base; *9,* floor locks; *10,* locking swivel casters; *11,* side rail locking system. (B to E) Positions of the operating table. (Modified from Martin JT, Warner MA, eds. *Positioning in Anesthesia and Surgery.* 3rd ed. Philadelphia: WB Saunders; 1997.)

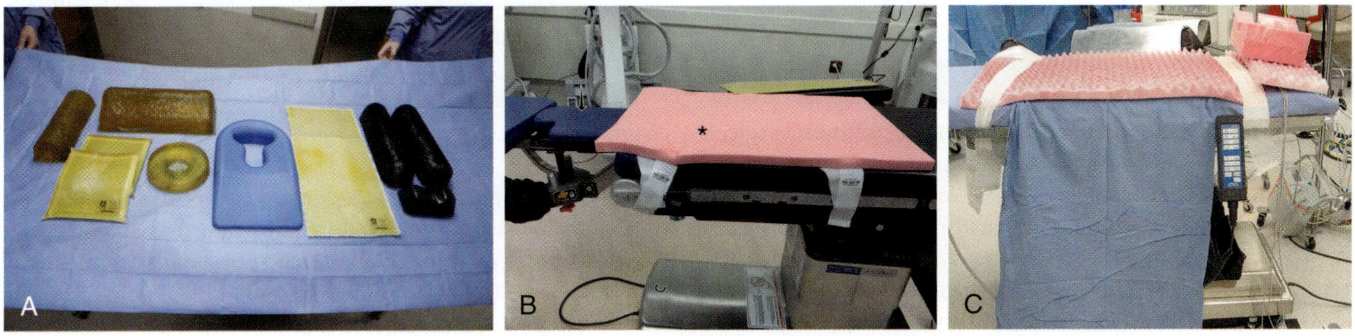

FIG. 16.12 (A) Gel pads and positioning aids. Gel pads are commonly used to protect bony prominences and to support areas on the body that contain shallow nerves and blood vessels. (B) The Pigazzi Pink Pad is a patented anti-skid system that prevents the patient from sliding (skidding) on the table. (C) Egg crate foam to prevent skidding. This system may not have the same safety features as the Pigazzi pad. (B, From Kollmoren C, Ellis T, Lewis BD, Harris JD. Achieving post-free distraction in hip arthroscopy with a pink pad patient positioning device using standard hip distraction tables. *Arthrosc Tech.* 8:4; 2019. https://doi.org/10.1016/j.eats.2018.11.013. C, From Klauschie J, Wechter M, Jacob K, et al. Use of anti-skid material and patient-positioning to prevent patient shifting during robotic-assisted gynecologic procedures. *J Minim Invasive Gynecol.* 17[4]:504–507; 2010. https://doi.org/10.1016/j.jmig.2010.03.013.)

2. Wedges, usually made of foam, are used to tilt the patient from the side or for isolated areas of the body that require elevation.
3. An *abduction pad* is used to separate the legs after hip fracture and postoperatively to maintain **abduction** and prevent dislocation.
4. The *sacral pad* is placed under the sacrum to relieve pressure, especially in the lithotomy position and for emaciated patients.
5. *Arm pads* are used to protect the radial nerve and vessels when the arm is extended on an arm board. A gel *arm cradle* is a more thickly padded arm rest that extends the full length of the arm.
6. The *prone positioner* is used to elevate the thorax and hip region for access to the spine.
7. The *vac pac* ("bean bag") positioner is a sealed pouch filled with small plastic beads. The patient is first positioned, and the pouch is molded loosely around the portion of the body requiring support. Suction is then applied to draw air from the pouch creating a semi-rigid mold, which supports the position.
8. **Head tongs** and the horseshoe headrest support the head for surgery of the cranium. Sterile metal pins are secured to the skull and clamped to the headrest to lock the head in position for neurosurgery and procedures of the cervical spine. The head-up position can also be maintained with a plastic frame and soft straps that support the head in upright position (see section on beach chair position).
9. The *SCD* is used in positions that involve downward flexion of the lower body and in other cases where venous pooling is a potential problem. The device consists of inflatable leg wraps that extend from the ankle to thigh and an insufflator. The leg wraps fill with air from bottom to top, creating sequential pressure and then release, allowing blood to be shunted toward the head. The device is fitted to the patient after he or she has been transported to the operating room, before surgery begins. The anesthesia provider and nurse circulator are responsible for selecting compression settings. Refer to Chapter 13 for a photo of the SCD.

Watch Chapter 16: The Operating Table on the Evolve website: http://evolve.elsevier.com/fuller/surgical.

SURGICAL POSITIONS

The following discussion describes the most common surgical positions the surgical technologist must know and assist with. Each position demonstrates the basic requirements for safety, required supports, and number of staff required.

IMPORTANT TO KNOW *Additional detailed illustrations and photos of patient positions are shown in the context of specific procedures. These demonstrate more advanced techniques according to the procedure and access required. Refer to Part II of the text to study these procedure-based positions, specifically orthopedic surgery, pediatric surgery, and neurosurgery chapters.*

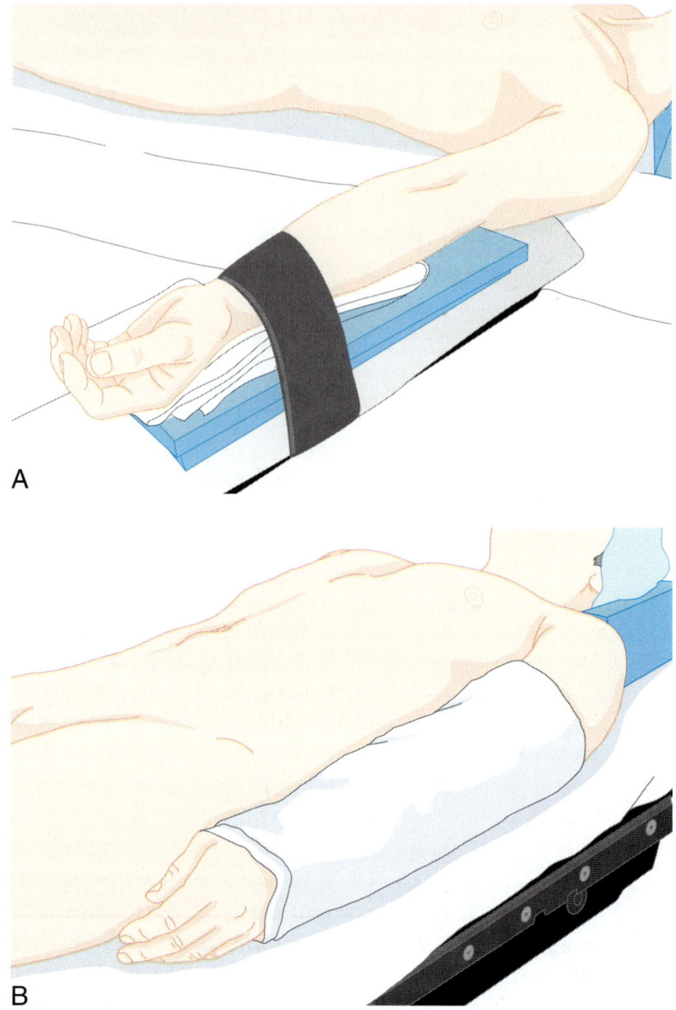

FIG. 16.13 Position of the patient's arm in supine position. (A) Position of the arm in supine position with an abduction of less than 90 degrees. Note that the arm is supinated, and the elbow is adequately padded to prevent ulnar nerve damage. (B) The arm at the patient's side is loosely held within the draw sheet. (From Miller R, Ericksson L, Fleisher L, et al, eds. *Miller's Anesthesia*. 8th ed. Philadelphia: Churchill Livingstone; 2015.)

SUPINE (DORSAL RECUMBENT)

Uses: Procedures of the head and neck, including eye, ear, breast, abdomen, and vascular surgeries and some orthopedic procedures.

Number of people required: Two to four

Safety:

1. Doughnut pad for head; eyes, ears, and superficial facial nerves protected if the face is turned.
2. Arms are extended on padded arm boards at no greater than a 90-degree angle; arms positioned palms up; arm straps in place; elbows slightly bent, with wrist in neutral position (Fig. 16.13A).
3. If arms are tucked at the patient's sides, the hands should face inward (pronated). The arm is wrapped in a draw sheet extended above the elbow (see Fig. 16.13B). Tuck the sheet between the arm and the mattress pad and not between the mattress and the table frame, as

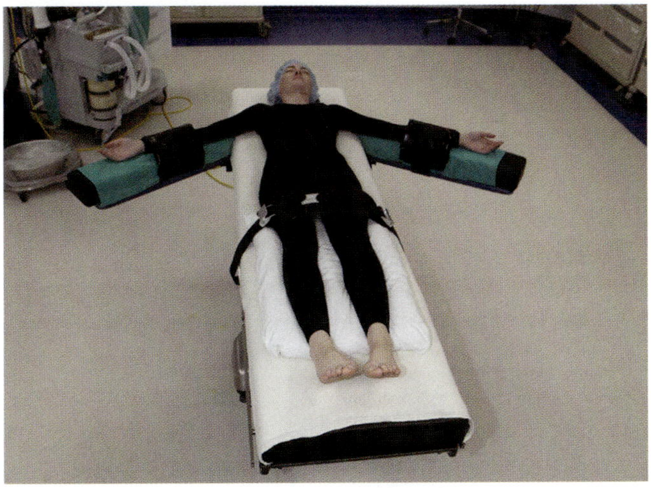

FIG. 16.14 Dorsal recumbent (supine) position. Note that the legs are placed on one or more pillows to lift the heels and feet off the table.

this can cause the arm to drop over the edge of the table and may result in nerve damage.

4. The patient safety strap is secured 2 inches above the knees, allowing two to three fingers' space between the strap and the top sheet.
5. Additional padding for sacrum; pillow under the knees; use padded boots as needed to prevent foot drop.
6. When positioning the pregnant patient, insert a wedge pad under the right flank. This tilts the body to the left and prevents uterine compression on the vena cava, which can cause hypotension and compromise fetal circulation.

See Fig. 16.14 for a demonstration of the dorsal recumbent position.

TRENDELENBURG

Uses: Trendelenburg is a variation of the supine position in which the head of the table is tilted downwards. It is used during lower gastrointestinal and pelvic surgery and during prostatectomy. In this position, abdominal organs shift toward the head (Fig. 16.15).

Number of people required: Two to four for the supine position. Trendelenburg is initiated by the anesthesia provider.

Safety:

1. Use all safety precautions as for the supine position.
2. Prevent the underside of the Mayo tray from contact with the patient's body.
3. Shoulder braces should not be used as they may injure the brachial plexus.
4. Anticipate the possible onset of hypertension during intraoperative positioning from the level supine to Trendelenburg position.

REVERSE TRENDELENBURG

Uses: This is a foot-down variation on the supine position (Fig. 16.16). It is used for procedures of the upper abdomen and neck.

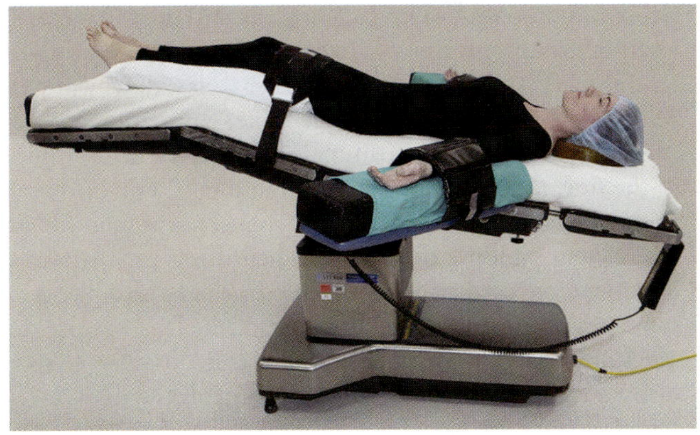

FIG. 16.15 Trendelenburg position. This is a variation of the supine position. The operating table is tilted head down to shift the abdominal viscera away from the incision site. The knees are slightly bent to prevent the patient from sliding.

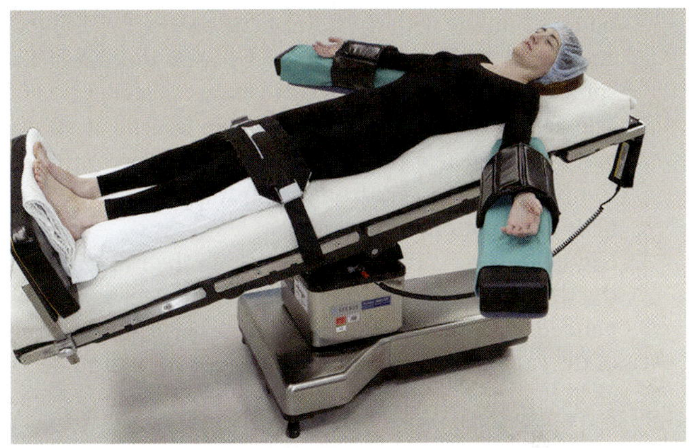

FIG. 16.16 Reverse Trendelenburg position. In this position the table is tipped toward the floor for procedures of the upper gastrointestinal tract. Note the padded footboard. The patient's heels should not rest on the operating table. The lower legs are elevated using a pillow.

Number of people required: Two to four as for the supine position. Reverse Trendelenburg is initiated by the anesthesia provider.

Safety:

1. Use safety precautions as for the supine position.
2. A padded footboard is required to prevent the patient from sliding toward the foot of the table. Padded boots may also be required.
3. The patient's lower legs are supported with a pillow. This prevents the heels from resting on the operating table pad.

The Mayo stand may be moved to accommodate the shift in the patient's position.

LITHOTOMY

Description and use: As a variation of the supine position lithotomy is used during gynecological, some rectal, and urological procedures. Two types of leg holders are available. Knee crutches (commercial name Allen "Yellowfin" stirrups) are the safest method of placing the patient in lithotomy (Fig. 16.17). Cane stirrups (Fig. 16.18) are used to support the legs in elevated position by support to the feet. After positioning the legs, flex downward or remove the lower portion of the table. Numerous injuries are associated with this position. These include crush injury of the fingers, which can be caught in the lower table break as it is raised back into position; peroneal nerve injury from insufficient padding of the foot when using cane stirrups; and increased cardiac output caused by elevation of the legs. Other injuries involve compression of the legs against the vertical portion of the cane stirrup. Lung compliance may also be reduced with increased pressure on the diaphragm when the hips are flexed.

Number of people required: After supine position is achieved, two people are required to raise and flex the legs into stirrups. A morbidly obese patient may require two people for each leg to lift and place the legs in stirrups or crutches.

Safety:

1. The patient is placed in supine position with the patient's buttocks in line with the lower table break. A sacral pad and upper body gel pad should be used to protect the spine. SCDs are used to prevent venous stasis.
2. The arms are placed on padded arm boards at 90 degrees or less. The position of the hands is confirmed to prevent the fingers from being trapped in the lower table articulation.
3. Leg holders require gel padding along the full length of the device. If cane stirrups are used, the feet should be padded to prevent nerve damage. The vertical extensions of the cane stirrup must also be padded for extra safety.

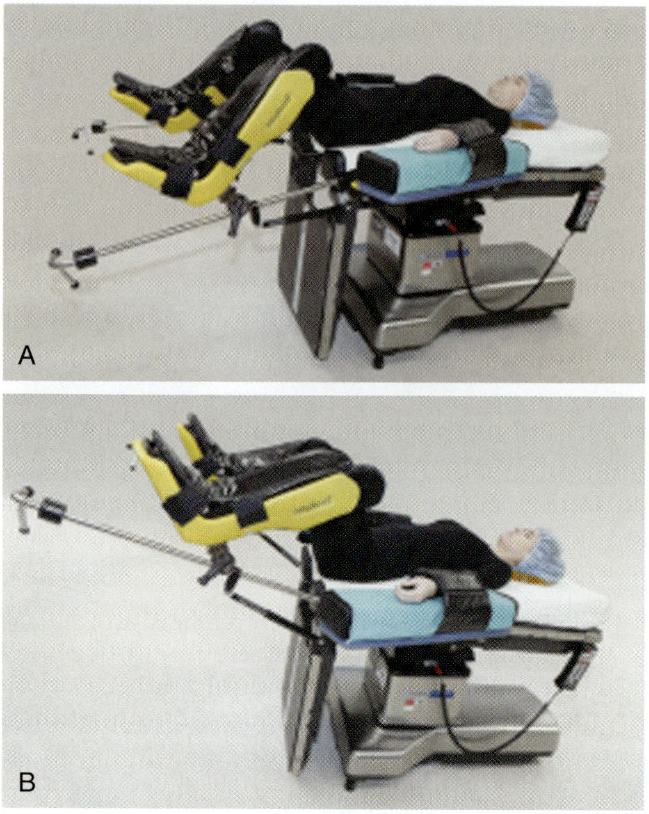

FIG. 16.17 Lithotomy position using crutch stirrups. This type of stirrup is the safest, especially for patients with a high body mass index (BMI). The legs are cushioned with gel pads. Note the position of the arms. See text detail for patient safety measures. (A) Low position lithotomy. (B) High position.

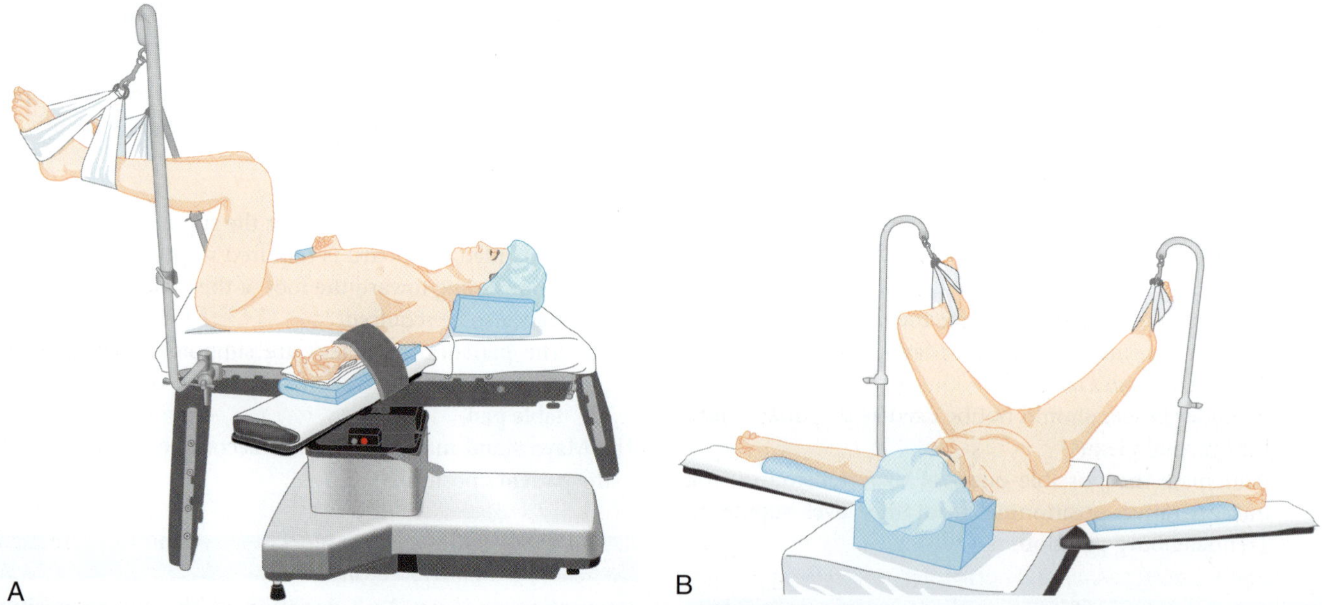

FIG. 16.18 Lithotomy position using cane stirrups. Note the position of the suspension straps. (A) The use of cane stirrups can present several risks including peroneal nerve damage and joint injury to the hips and knees. See text for the details of safety measures. (B) The patient's legs must not rest against the vertical bars of the stirrup as this can result in nerve and vascular damage. (From Miller R, et al, eds. *Miller's Anesthesia*. 8th ed. Philadelphia: Saunders; 2015.)

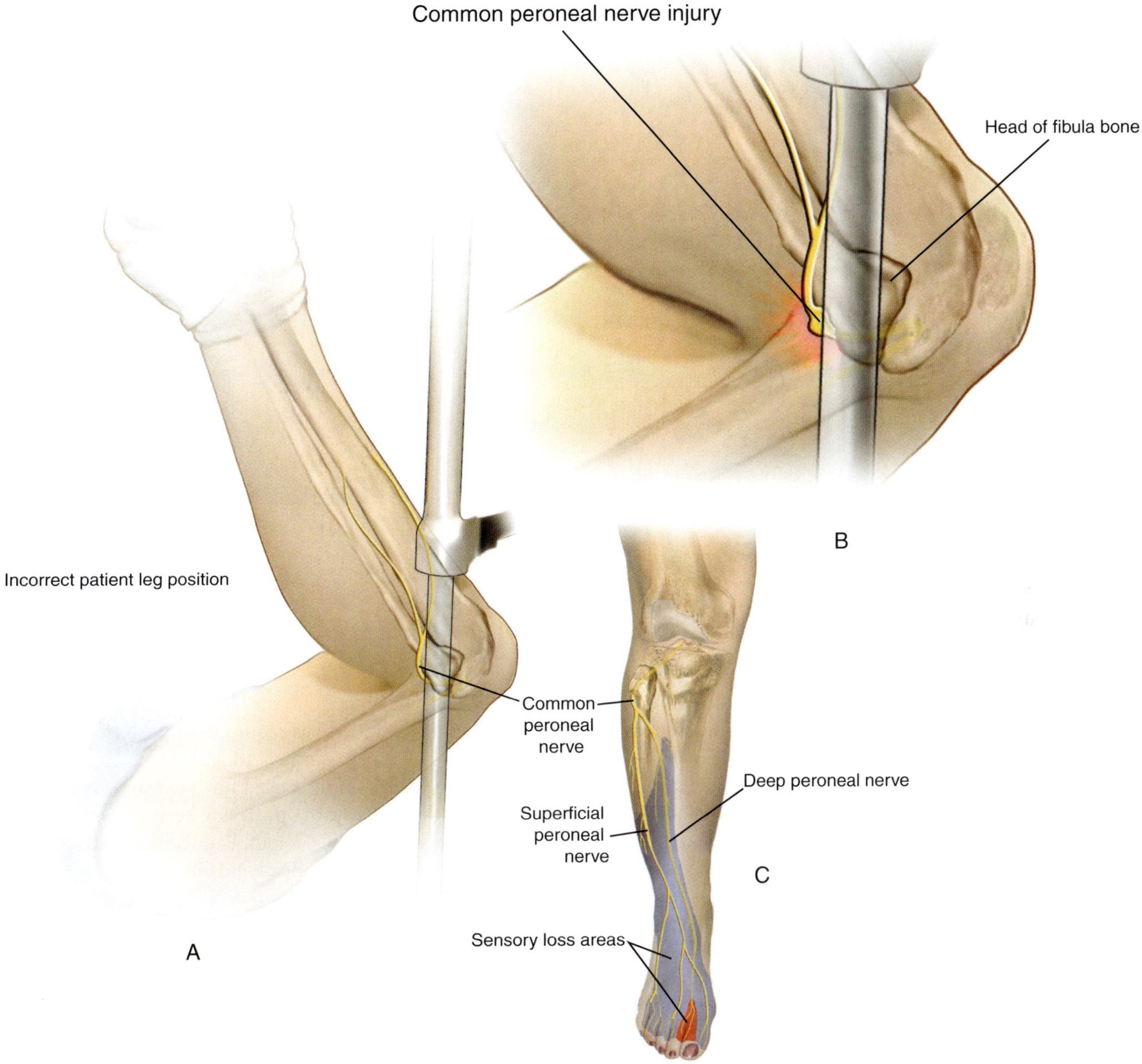

FIG. 16.19 Peroneal nerve damage using cane stirrups. (From Baggish M. *Atlas of Pelvic Anatomy and Gynecologic Surgery.* Philadelphia: Elsevier; 2016.)

4. The patient safety strap is secured 2 inches above the knees until it is safe to raise the legs.
5. The anesthesia provider states when it is safe to raise the legs. At least two people are required to simultaneously lift both legs into stirrups or leg holders. The hips are flexed and the legs are abducted at 30 to 45 degrees. The knees are flexed at 80 to 100 degrees while maintaining them in parallel position. Each leg is then secured in the stirrup or leg holder.
6. The maneuver must be performed very slowly to prevent a sudden shift in blood pressure, hip, or spinal injury.
7. When using cane stirrups, do not place the stirrup slings directly over the Achilles tendon. Distribute the weight of the leg between both slings on the stirrup.
8. The legs must not come in contact with the vertical posts of the cane stirrup attachment. Note the risk of peroneal nerve injury related to pressure from the upright section of the cane stirrup (Fig. 16.19).
9. At the close of surgery, confirm the position of the patient's hands before raising or attaching the lower table section.
10. Release the feet from the stirrups or leg rests, slowly bring the knees together on the midline, and gradually extend the hips and knees.

FOWLER AND MODIFIED FOWLER

Description and use: The **Fowler position** is seated with padding as described previously. The arms are secured

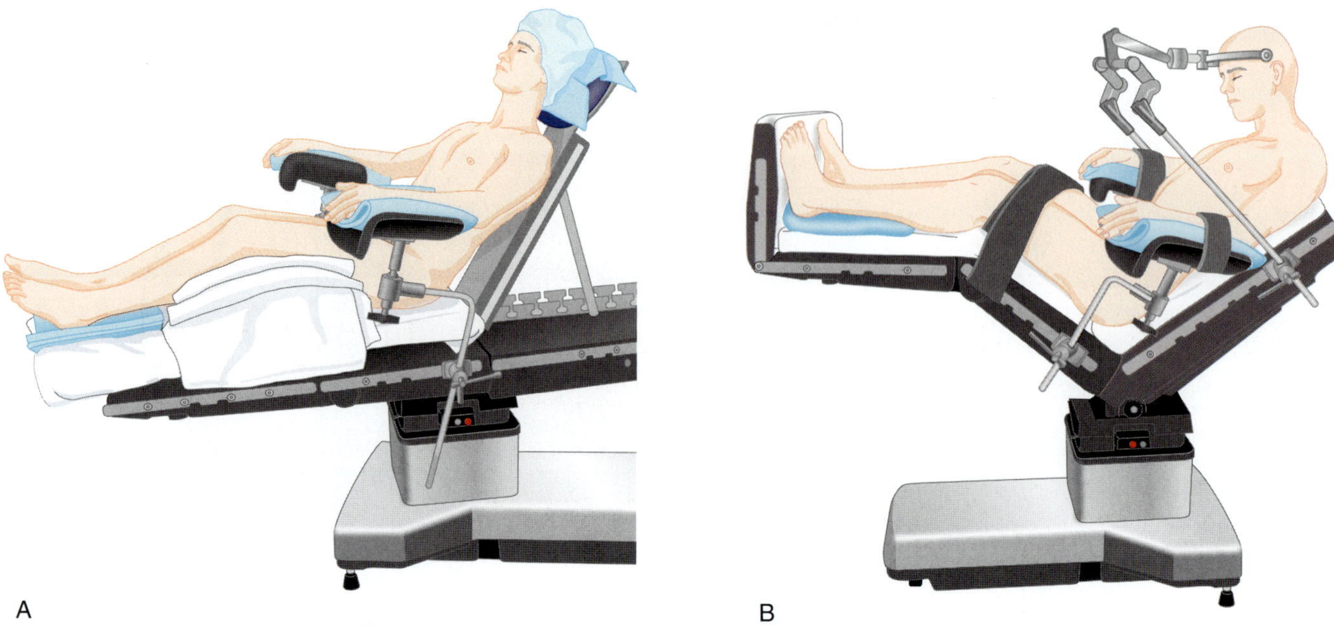

FIG. 16.20 Fowler (beach chair) position. (A) The sitting, reclining, or beach chair position is used for procedures of the breast, shoulder, posterior cranium, and posterior spine. (B) During procedures of the posterior spine or occiput, the head may be secured using Gardner tongs, which penetrate the skull slightly and keep the head safely immobile.

on padded arm boards. The modified Fowler position is a variation of the sitting position into a semi-recumbent or *beach chair* position with the knees flexed, the back nearly vertical, and the table tipped back into Trendelenburg (Fig. 16.20). Further modifications using specialized equipment can be made to change the surgical access to different sites. When used with a cranial (Mayfield) head brace, the back is placed vertically with the head elevated as it provides access to the posterior cranium and cervical spine for posterior craniotomy and craniotomy. With the head supported by soft straps, it can be used for reconstructive breast surgery. Shoulder surgery may be performed in the modified Fowler position using a specialty shoulder chair with a cutaway back support for anterior and posterior access to the shoulder. Double arm rests with padding are used, or the arms may be secured on a pillow on the patient's lap.

Number of people required: After completing supine position, two to three people are needed to achieve Fowler position.

Safety:

1. The patient is first placed in supine position implementing all safety procedures for that position.
2. The patient's arms should be secured on arm rests to maintain IV exposure and access for monitoring devices, or they may be secured in the patient's lap over a pillow.
3. The upper table section is placed vertically, whereas the lower section is flexed downward. The lower legs should be cushioned on pillows, and a padded footboard should be attached. The feet may also be placed in soft foam boots.
4. The patient safety strap is secured as for supine position.
5. For posterior access to the head and neck, the head may then be positioned as required for posterior access and secured by neurosurgical tongs.
6. When the position is used for reconstructive breast or shoulder surgery, the posterior head rest must be padded to support the occiput. Padded safety straps are positioned around the head and chin.

LATERAL DECUBITUS

Description and use: The lateral decubitus or side-lying position exposes the flank and lateral thorax (Fig. 16.21). The patient is maintained in the position with a combination of table accessories and padding, with both arms slightly flexed and extended no greater than 90 degrees on padded arm cradles or holders. When the **lateral position** is described, the side named is the "down" nonoperative side, which rests on the table. For example, in the left lateral position, the patient lies on his or her left side. Flexing the table at the upper break widens the flank area for a greater exposure to the kidney.

Number of people required: Depending on the BMI of the patient, four to six people are needed.

Safety:

1. The patient is anesthetized in the supine position and turned into the lateral position after the airway has been secured.
2. One person is responsible for the lower legs and feet, another for the pelvis, and one for the thorax, including the shoulders. The anesthesia provider maintains the airway and handles the head. The spine is maintained in neutral position at all times, as shown in the schematic diagram in Fig. 16.22.

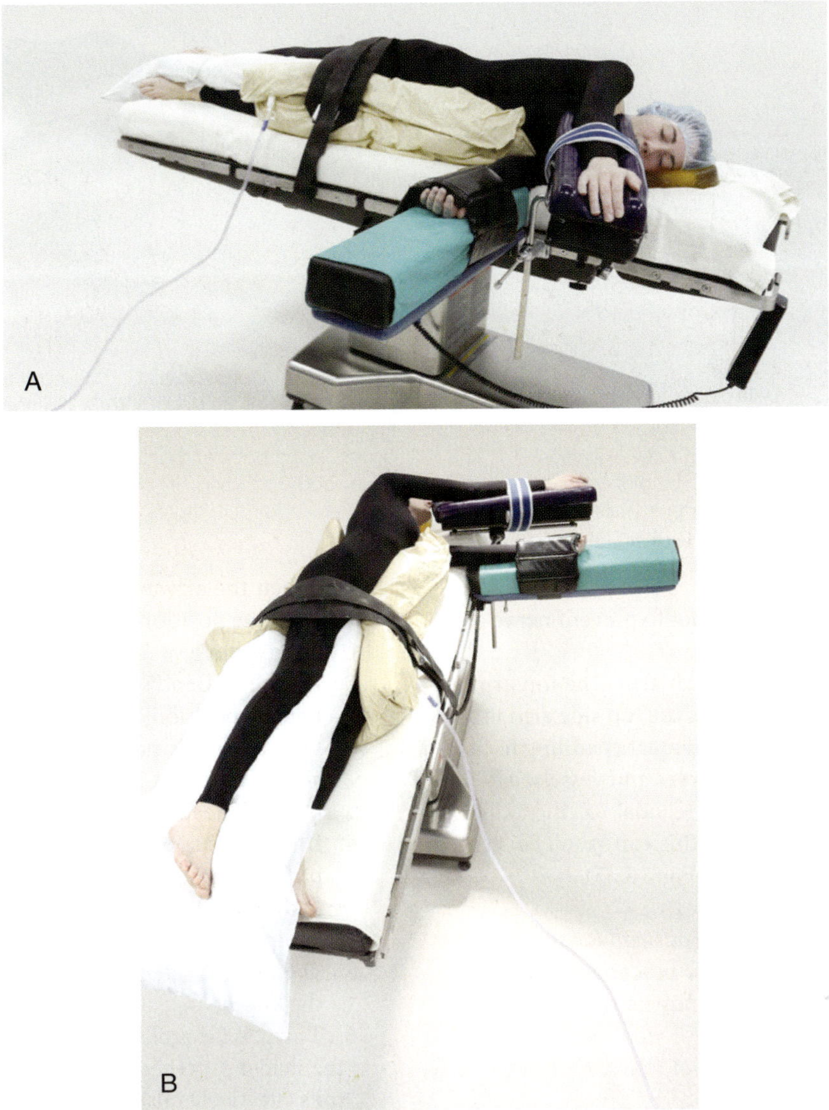

FIG. 16.21 Lateral decubitus position. This position provides access to the flank area, especially for the procedures of the kidney, ureters, and adrenal glands. Note the position of the upper leg, padding between the two legs, and position of the arms. Two arm boards are used and both are well padded. Note also the placement of an axillary pad. This position is supported using an inflatable "bean bag," which is molded loosely to the upper and lower torso. When the positioner is inflated, it provides a semi-rigid cradle, which fits exactly to the contours of the body. The head is supported by a hollow foam pad to prevent contact with the patient's eyes, ears, and face.

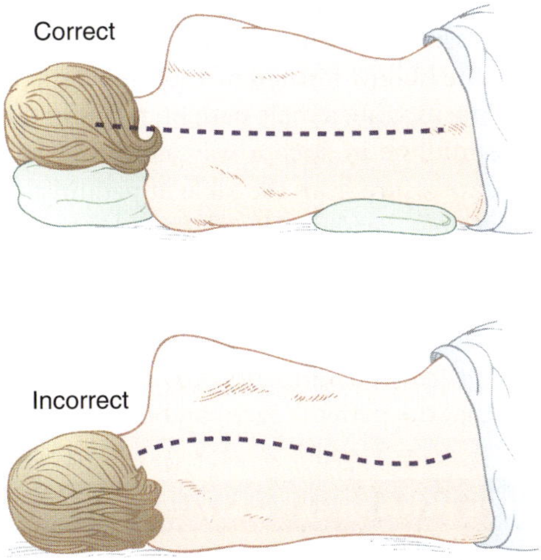

FIG. 16.22 Schematic drawing of the spine in lateral positions. The spine must be kept straight. This is achieved using padding to lift the head and downside flank.

3. The anesthetized patient must be moved as one unit; that is, the head, neck, spine, pelvis, and legs all must be moved together. The spine is maintained in alignment to prevent a torsion injury.
4. The head rests on a horseshoe pad or other cut-away device to protect the ear, eye, facial nerves, and vessels. The eyes must be taped to prevent corneal damage.
5. The patient's body is supported using a vac pac (bean bag) device or table pad attachments positioned anteriorly and posteriorly. A bent downside leg assists in stabilizing the position.
6. The patient safety strap is secured over the hip.
7. The downside leg is flexed slightly at the knee. The upper leg remains extended and rests on a pillow placed between the upper and lower leg.

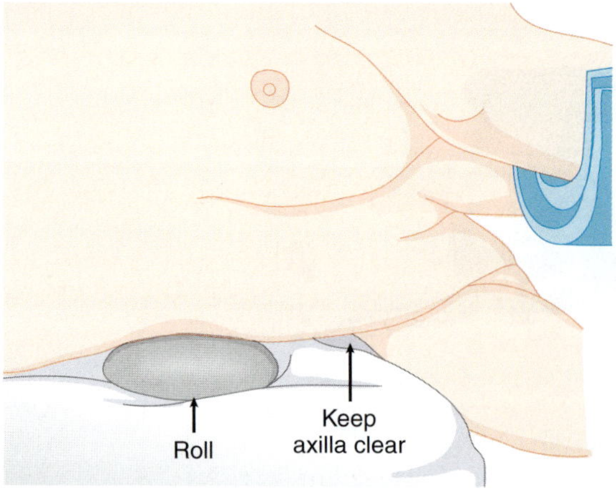

FIG. 16.23 Placement of the axillary roll in lateral position. It is critically important that this elongated roll should be placed below (caudal to) the axillary space to prevent nerve damage. (From Miller R, et al, eds. *Miller's Anesthesia*. 8th ed. Philadelphia: Saunders; 2015.)

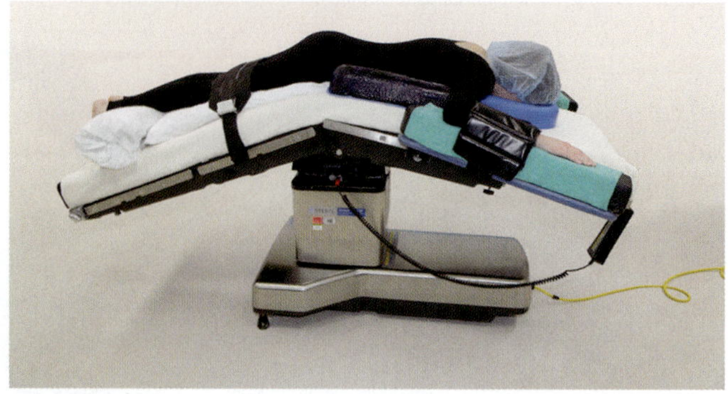

FIG. 16.24 Prone position. This position is used for access to the posterior side of the body. When the hips are flexed at a sharp angle, the position provides access to the anorectal area. It is also used for access to the back and anterior leg. Note the position of the arms and lower body padding. In prone positions, the female breasts must be protected against compression with the use of a foam open chest pad.

8. Padding is placed under each foot to prevent nerve and vessel damage.
9. A safety strap is placed over each arm. The top arm is pronated (palm down), whereas the top side arm is supinated (palm down). Ensure adequate padding to prevent injury to the olecranon nerves and vessels.
10. A gel pad is placed just below (caudal to) the axillary area but *never in the axilla* as this can result in nerve damage to the brachial plexus (Fig. 16.23).

IMPORTANT TO KNOW *The side-lying position is used for medical treatments and some diagnostic procedures such as a colonoscopy. In this case, the position may be referred to as modified lateral recumbent position.*

PRONE

Description and use: In prone position the patient lies recumbent with the front of the body in contact with the operating table. The legs are held in neutral position, and the arms are positioned at no greater than 90 degrees from the midline, with the elbows flexed comfortably. Prone position provides exposure to the perianal region, buttocks, posterior spine, and posterior lower legs. A foam or gel chest lift may be used for access to the spine. The lift has two sloping sides, which are positioned along the contours of the abdomen and hips (Fig. 16.24).

Number of people required: Four to six people are required to turn the patient from the gurney to the operating table. A hydraulic lift may be used to elevate and turn the patient.

Safety:

1. This position is complex and can compromise physiological and structural mechanisms in the body. The pressure exerted on the abdomen and chest may restrict normal ventilation. There is additional risk of injury to the eyes and neck structures.
2. If a general anesthetic is used, the patient is anesthetized and intubated in supine position on the gurney. When the airway is secure, the team turns the patient to prone position while shifting him or her to the operating table.
3. As the patient is turned, the spine is maintained in neutral position, with the airway protected at all times. One person is positioned at the feet and two on each side of the body. The anesthesia provider remains at the patient's head to protect the airway.
4. If a mechanical lift is used to turn and transfer the patient, the entire length of the body is protected by padding; the manufacturer's guidelines for use of the equipment must be followed exactly to prevent injury.
5. The patient safety strap is secured 2 or 3 inches above the knees.
6. Two gel chest rolls are placed at the clavicle and extend to the iliac crest. These must not impinge on the axilla. The rolls effectively raise the thorax to permit chest expansion.
7. The arms are placed on double arm boards with the elbows flexed and resting on gel pads.
8. The legs are bent slightly at the knees, with the lower legs resting on pillows. The feet should extend slightly over the edge of the pillow to prevent the toes from resting on the table.
9. When positioning a female patient, position the breasts within the hollow formed by the two lateral rolls.
10. When positioning a male patient, position the genitalia on the midline in such a way as to prevent impingement or pressure from the table or padding accessories.
11. The patient's head is placed face down on a hollow centered foam rest to protect the eyes, ears, and facial nerves from injury. The hollow core allows the anesthesia provider access to the patient's airway at all times. Some specialty attachments provide an adjustable mirror so that the patient's face can be viewed.

JACKKNIFE (KRASKE) POSITION

Description and use: The jackknife **(Kraske) position** is a modification of the prone position. The middle table break is flexed downward to achieve a simultaneous head-down

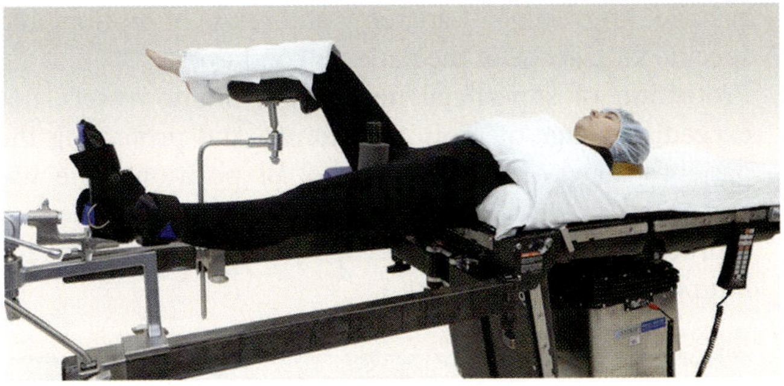

FIG. 16.25 Fracture (hip) table. The fracture table is used to provide complete access to the hip for orthopedic repair. The operative leg can be pulled into traction by placing the foot in a protective boot as shown. Refer to the text for important safety information about this position.

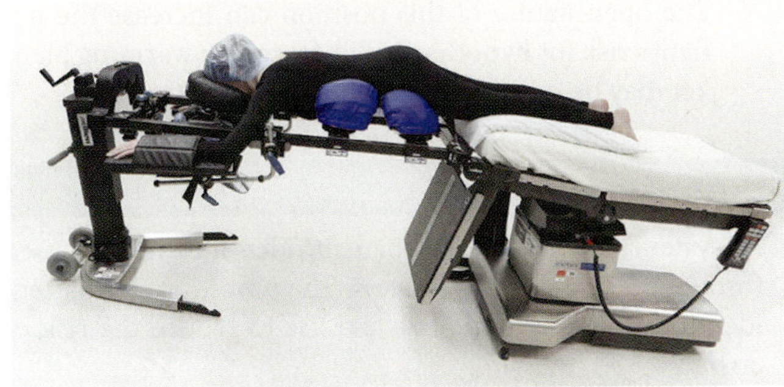

FIG. 16.26 Allen table for procedures of the spine. This table extension is fitted to the regular operating table to provide access to the spine without compromise to the respiratory system. The patient's head is held securely in a hollow frame for protection and free access to the patient's airway. Note the mirror below the head frame, which allows observation of the patient's face during the procedure. Refer to the text description of important safety precautions for this position.

and foot-down posture. This position is used for anorectal surgery. The lower legs are placed on pillows to distribute the weight. The toes extend just over the edge of the pillows. The arms are extended on arm boards as described for the prone position above.

Safety: The safety considerations for Kraske position are identical to those described under Prone.

Watch Chapter 16: Patient Positioning on the Evolve website: http://evolve.elsevier.com/fuller/surgical.

SPINAL TABLE

The spinal or Allen table is a system that attaches to a standard operating table to create positioning used in spinal surgery (Fig. 16.26). The prone position can also be used without this extension. In this case, a simple foam thorax pad elevates the upper body. The Allen table provides many benefits including completely free access to the patient's face and airway. The open design of the table also provides for the expansion of the chest and abdomen to improve respiratory function. The open head rest includes a mirror attachment, which allows the anesthesia provider to observe the patient's face during surgery. The extension is completely adjustable for length and width.

Safety: The Allen table must be carefully assembled to ensure that pressure points are adequately padded. The patient is turned onto the table following induction of anesthesia and intubation to secure the airway. Induction and intubation are performed on the patient gurney or bed. At least six people are needed to turn the patient onto the operating table safely.

1. The patient's arms must be maintained at no greater than 90 degrees, with elbows bent slightly. Arm boards must be padded.
2. The head is positioned on the head rest to avoid any pressure on the patient's eyes, ears, or face.
3. The upper body is suspended on a padded brace with access to the anterior thorax. Note the position of the brace, which must not impinge on axillae or breasts of a female patient.
4. Care must be taken to ensure that the male genitalia are well within the open portion of the brace.
5. The lower body rests on the operating table, which is padded to elevate the toes to prevent them from resting on the table.

ORTHOPEDIC TABLE

Description and use: The orthopedic or fracture table allows the patient to be positioned for hip and other orthopedic procedures of the lower extremities. The table allows circumferential access to the patient's leg (Fig. 16.25). The patient lies in supine position with the upper body supported by the operating table and the operative leg extended and held in a padded boot. The leg may be rotated, pulled into traction, or released as the surgery requires. The unaffected leg rests on an elevated leg holder. The open structure of the table allows intraoperative fluoroscopy. Many different types of attachments are available, depending on the complexity and needs of the surgery.

Number of people required: At least four people are required to position the patient on the orthopedic table.

Safety:

1. When moving the patient from the gurney to the orthopedic table, maintain the spine and head in neutral position at all times.
2. The center post of the orthopedic table must be removed before the patient is moved. The post must be well padded and repositioned to protect the patient's genitalia. The perineal area and genital structures must not rest against the center post.
3. Pressure points on the sacrum, heels, and unaffected lower leg must be padded, and weight must be distributed among all points.
4. Traction on the affected leg is adjusted by the surgeon who directs the positioning team.
5. The arms may be folded over the chest or extended on padded arm boards as described above.

6. The open nature of this position can increase the patient's risk for hypothermia. A forced air warming blanket may be necessary to maintain normothermia.

KEY CONCEPTS

- A systematic method of patient identification is used throughout the surgical process. The procedure for patient identification is intentionally precise to reduce the risk of error.
- Safe transport and transfer begin with knowing how to perform a maneuver, having a plan, and executing the maneuver as per that plan.
- Professional communication with the patient and family is demonstrated by maintaining emotional and social boundaries and by showing respect and attentiveness. One's personal opinions about the health care facility, health care providers, or colleagues should also not be discussed with the patient or family.
- The risk of health worker injury can be mitigated by learning and taking the time to use safe body mechanics and patient lifting devices.
- Surgical patients are transported in the perioperative setting using a standard or specialty gurney or wheelchair. Lateral transfer devices are used to move a patient from one horizontal surface to another, such as the operating table to a gurney.
- Practice in moving and handling patients should include a detailed orientation to moving and lifting devices, how to perform specific maneuvers, and body mechanics. This not only lowers the risk for the patient in real life but also allows feedback from peers.
- When transporting patients, be aware of the special needs of particular patient populations such as children, the sight- or hearing-impaired, obese, and patients with severe physical impairment or injury.
- The following are objectives of surgical positioning:
  - Protect the patient's airway
  - Allow access to monitoring sites on the body
  - Provide venous access for the administration of medications
  - Provide adequate exposure to the operative site
  - Maintain and promote homeostasis
- The surgical technologist may be required to assist in patient positioning. The specific role varies among health care facilities but is always performed under the direction of the anesthesia provider or surgeon.
- Practice sessions in the use of operating table accessories and patient positioning in a controlled environment are valuable learning tools. During practice, the principles of patient safety should be combined with a "dry run" using operating table accessories and equipment.
- Specific techniques and devices are used in positioning to prevent injury. The most common cause of injury during positioning is the inadequate padding of superficial nerves and blood vessels, resulting in paralysis or ischemia. Losing control of a limb during positioning can result in dislocation or fracture. Injury prevention requires attention to the task at hand, knowledge of anatomy and range of motion, and specific knowledge of the patient's condition.
- Protection of superficial nerves and blood vessels, not exceeding range of motion in joints, and protecting the patient's airway are common to all positions; the use of special positioning devices such as limb holders, a thoracic lift (brace), and stirrups compound the risks for injury.

REVIEW QUESTIONS

1. What is a shear injury?
2. How can you best protect yourself from injury if a patient you are escorting begins to fall and leans into you?
3. Describe the proper method for identifying a patient.
4. What are the anatomical risks in the lithotomy position?
5. Why is a sequential compression device used on patients during surgery?
6. Why are patients more prone to skeletal injury when under general anesthesia? What is *thoracic outlet syndrome*?
7. What are the physiological risks of the Trendelenburg position?

CASE STUDIES

CASE 1

You are asked to bring a patient from the medical unit to surgery. When you arrive on the unit, the patient is not in his room or in the hallway. What is the appropriate action?

CASE 2

You are transporting a patient from the medical unit to the operating room. You discover that the patient elevator is out of order. What will you do?

CASE 3

While turning the patient into the lateral position, the patient begins to slide from the table in your direction. What will you do? What precautions can be taken to prevent falls?

CASE 4

You are assigned to circulate in a procedure in which the patient is placed in the lithotomy position. The patient emerges quickly from anesthesia, and she begins to struggle. Her legs are still elevated in stirrups. What are the risks to the patient in this situation? What will you do?

CASE 5

You are scrubbed on a laparotomy case. A number of medical students have been brought in to observe. One of the medical students is scrubbed and is holding a retractor. You notice the student has placed his elbow on the patient's shoulder, and he is resting his weight on the patient. The surgeon has said nothing. What will you do?

BIBLIOGRAPHY

Association of periOperative Registered Nurses (AORN). *Guidelines for perioperative practice, ed 2015*. Denver: AORN; 2015.

AOHP OSHA Alliance Implementation Team. *Beyond getting started: a resource guide for implementing a safe patient handling program in the acute care setting*. 3rd ed.; 2014. https://www.cdc.gov/niosh/topics/safepatient/. Accessed July 16, 2019.

Miller R, Ericksson L, Fleisher L, et al., eds. *Miller's Anesthesia*. 8th ed. Philadelphia: Saunders; 2012.

Porth C, ed. *Pathophysiology: Concepts of Altered Health States*. 6th ed. Philadelphia: Lippincott Williams & Williams; 2009.

U.S. Department of Labor. Safe patient handling. https://www.osha.gov/SLTC/healthcarefacilities/safepatienthandling.html. Accessed July 16, 2019.

Van Wicklin SA. Safely positioning the surgical patient. AORN J. 92(6):703–704.

17 SURGICAL SKIN PREPARATION AND DRAPING

KNOWLEDGE AND SKILLS REVIEW

The following skills and knowledge should be reviewed before you start this chapter:
Aseptic technique

LEARNING OBJECTIVES

After studying this chapter, the reader will be able to:

1. Review the standards of practice for surgical prep and draping
2. Review the guidelines for patient hygiene before surgery
3. Discuss the guidelines for hair removal and skin marking in the surgical prep
4. List the Food and Drug Administration's approved antiseptics for the surgical prep
5. List the supplies needed for skin prep
6. Demonstrate the different procedures for skin prep
7. Discuss the elements of patient safety in regard to skin prep
8. Demonstrate skin prep on the standard prep sites
9. Discuss the rationale and techniques for surgical draping
10. Discuss how to maintain asepsis during draping
11. Demonstrate draping techniques of the surgical site
12. Demonstrate how to remove drapes at the end of a procedure

TERMINOLOGY

Antiseptic: Chemical agent approved for use on the skin that inhibits the growth and reproduction of microorganisms.

Debridement: The removal of devitalized tissue, debris, and foreign objects from a wound. Debridement is performed on trauma injuries, burns, and infected wounds either before surgery or as part of the surgical procedure.

Fenestrated drape: A sterile body sheet with a hole or "window" (fenestration) that exposes the incision site. The fenestrated drape is positioned after other drapes and towels have been placed in keeping with the procedure.

Impervious: Waterproof.

Incise drape: A plastic adhesive drape that is positioned over the incision site after surgical skin prep. The incise drape creates a sterile surface over the skin.

Residual activity: The antimicrobial action of an antiseptic or a disinfectant that continues after the solution has dried.

Retention catheter: A type of urinary catheter that remains in place. Also called an *indwelling* or *Foley catheter.*

Single-stage prep: Also called a *paint prep*. The skin prep is performed using only antiseptic liquid, which is applied to the skin at the operative site.

Solution: Any liquid antiseptic combined with water.

Squaring the incision: Refers to placing four towels in a square around the incision site.

Straight catheter: A urinary catheter used to drain the bladder one time (sometimes called a *Robinson catheter*).

Two-stage prep: Preparation of the skin including washing with antiseptic soap followed by application of antiseptic tincture or solution.

The presurgical skin prep and draping procedures are methods used to prevent surgical site infection (SSI). Bacteria colonize all layers of the skin and its appendages (e.g., sweat and sebaceous glands and hair follicles). Before surgery, the incision site and a wide area around it are cleansed or painted with an **antiseptic** to reduce the number of transient and normal microorganisms to an absolute minimum. After skin prep, the patient is covered with sterile *drapes* that expose only the surgical site and create the center of the *sterile field.* The skin prep and draping procedures described in this chapter take place after the patient is positioned and immediately before surgery starts.

Skin prep and draping are discussed together in this chapter because the events are sequential. The guidelines presented here are presented in a timewise and stepwise way to clarify who does what, and when.

SECTION I: SURGICAL SKIN PREP

PURPOSE OF THE SURGICAL SKIN PREP

Skin is the body's primary defense against infection. A surgical incision provides an entry point for microorganisms. Healthy skin contains colonies of microorganisms, which compete with and usually overcome foreign or transient bacteria. When normal or transient bacteria are introduced into the surgical wound, they can cause an SSI. Skin cannot be sterilized; however, the bacterial load can be reduced significantly with antiseptic cleansing or a coating of antiseptic on the skin.

HAIR REMOVAL

Hair is not removed from the surgical site unless the surgeon determines that it will interfere with the surgical procedure. In this case it is clipped or removed with a chemical depilatory. In the past, the operative site was routinely shaved before surgery. Current research demonstrates that shaving the skin *increases* rather than decreases the risk of SSI. Shaving causes skin abrasions that may not be easily seen. These become a source of bacterial colonization by resident microbes, which are the most common source of SSI. Therefore, unless the patient's hair cannot be kept outside the wound, it is not removed. This recommendation includes craniotomy and facial procedures in which the hair can be braided and secured away from the incision site with elastic bands or water-based gel.

Hair clipping requires a *verbal or written order by the surgeon.* The following guidelines must be followed for this procedure:

- Hair should be removed as close to the time of surgery as possible.
- Hair removal is performed in a nonsterile area.
- Hair is removed with single-use battery clippers or clippers with a head that can be resterilized.
- A chemical depilatory can be used only if the patient has had a skin test to ensure that he or she is not sensitive to the product. This test must be performed at least 12 hours before the start of surgery.
- Hair is removed in an area away from the location where surgery is performed.
- Single-use clippers must be discarded in a biohazard container after use.
- Eyebrows and eyelashes are never removed by other means because they may fail to regrow or may grow abnormally after removal.

PREOPERATIVE SKIN MARKING

The Joint Commission Guidelines for Universal Protocol for preventing wrong site, wrong procedure, and wrong person surgery require skin marking at the surgical site for procedures involving incisions, punctures, and insertions. This is to verify the side, levels (e.g., spinal location), and multiple sites such as fingers. The surgeon is required to mark the site before surgery so that the perioperative team can participate in the verification process from the time the patient arrives in the operating room until the start of surgery.

Surgeons use various types of pens for marking the site. The mark should be made with a surgical skin marker approved for this specific use. Gentian violet ink is the recommended and most effective product because it is antiseptic, does not wash off, and is easily visible. The mark should *not be made with a ballpoint pen* or other inks that are not approved for use on the patient's skin. Nonsurgical inks can wash off during the skin prep, and some (e.g., felt marking pens used in labeling) are not FDA approved for use on skin. If the skin mark has not been made with gentian violet or other long-lasting dye, care must be taken not to wash the mark off during the prep.

BOX 17.1 Appropriate Indications for Indwelling Urethral Catheter Use in the Perioperative Setting

URETHRAL CATHETER USE IN THE PERIOPERATIVE SETTING

1. Patients undergoing urological surgery or other surgery on contiguous structures of the genitourinary tract.
2. Anticipated prolonged duration of surgery (catheters inserted for this reason should be removed in postanesthesia care unit [PACU]).
3. Patients anticipated to receive large-volume infusions or diuretics during surgery.
4. Need for intraoperative monitoring of urinary output.

Centers for Disease Control and Prevention, Infection Control, *Catheter-Associated Urinary Tract Infections CAUTI* 2009 updated 2017. Available at https://www.cdc.gov/infectioncontrol/guidelines/cauti. Accessed July 19, 2019.

URINARY CATHETERIZATION

Urinary catheterization is performed before the skin prep, unless the procedure requires the lithotomy position. In this case catheterization takes place immediately after the skin prep as part of the skin prep.

Catheterization requires an order from the surgeon. The order may be written on the surgeon's preference card and must include the type of catheter to be inserted and the date of the standing order.

Urinary catheterization is performed for specific surgical procedures and circumstances. The Centers for Disease Control and Prevention (CDC) provides the guidelines for appropriate use of indwelling urinary catheters in the perioperative setting. These are listed in Box 17.1.

SUPPLIES

The most common method of continuous drainage is a Foley urinary catheter (Fig. 17.1A). This is a **retention catheter,** which has a small inflatable balloon at the tip. After the catheter is inserted into the bladder, the balloon is inflated with sterile water to prevent the catheter from becoming displaced. The catheter is connected to a drainage tube and collection bag. Two common balloon sizes are the 5 mL and 30 mL. The 5 mL balloon is used for routine continuous drainage. The 30 mL balloon is used mainly for prostatectomy procedures.

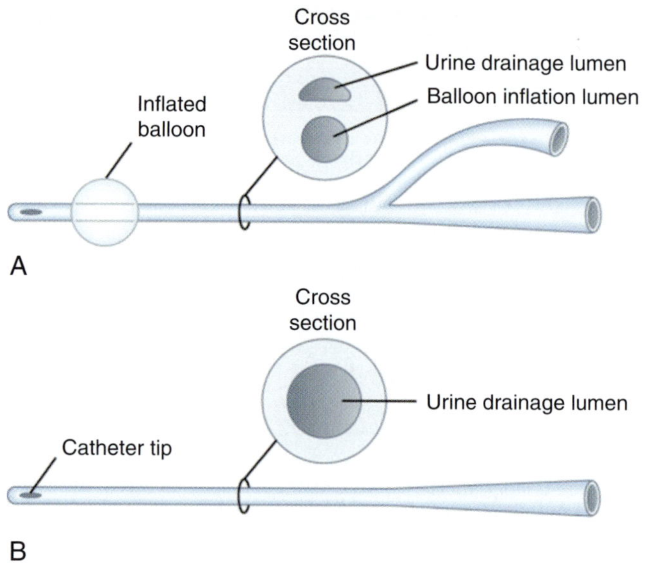

FIG. 17.1 (A) Foley catheter with balloon tip. (B) Straight catheter.

A **straight catheter**, also called a *red, Robinson,* or *intermittent catheter*, is used to empty the bladder before surgery, but continuous urinary drainage is unnecessary (see Fig. 17.1B). Other types of urinary catheters are indicated for specific conditions and circumstances and are discussed in Chapter 24, Genitourinary Surgery.

Prepackaged sterile catheterization kits contain the supplies needed for catheterization. The correct catheter is selected based on the patient's age, size, and gender. A size 14- to 16-French (Fr) Foley catheter generally is appropriate for a female patient; males usually require a 16- or 18-Fr catheter. Pediatric patients require considerably smaller sizes, and this should be assessed by qualified personnel.

The supplies for catheterization must be gathered, checked, and opened before the patient is positioned. A small catheterization table is prepared and moved into place immediately before the procedure.

The following supplies are included in a commercial kit. The catheter may or may not be included:

Foley catheter according to size required
Povidone prep solution (water base)
Sterile lubricant
Sterile gloves
10-mL syringe prefilled with sterile water
Perineal drape
Forceps
Cotton balls to perform the prep
Specimen cup with lid and labels
Drainage tubing and a urine collection unit (may be preconnected)

PROCEDURE FOR CATHETERIZATION

Catheterization is performed only after the ACP has indicated that it is safe. A female patient is positioned with the knees slightly flexed and the hips externally rotated. The male patient is placed in the supine position.

The sterile technique required for catheterization requires the *dominant hand to remain sterile* while the *nondominant hand is nonsterile.* The dominant hand is used to perform the skin prep and insert the catheter. The *nondominant hand* is used to stabilize the genitalia and expose the urethral meatus. The dominant hand remains sterile and contacts only the sterile supplies and catheter.

If the dominant hand becomes contaminated, the procedure must be stopped and the contaminated glove changed. If the catheter becomes contaminated, a fresh sterile catheter must be obtained.

The following guidelines describe the step-by-step procedure for insertion of a Foley catheter. Step-by-step illustrations for catheterization are presented in Fig. 17.2 (female) and Fig. 17.3 (male).

TECHNIQUE

1. Position the patient. If the female patient has not been prepped, an impervious sheet should be placed under the buttocks.
2. Check for body-piercing jewelry on the patient's genitalia. All jewelry must be removed before catheterization. Jewelry is secured in a closed, labeled container and returned to the patient after surgery.
3. Don sterile gloves using the open gloving technique.
4. Moisten the prep sponges with antiseptic.
5. Place a small amount of lubricant gel in the tray or on the tip of the catheter.
6. Note that the drainage end of the catheter must be directed toward a receptacle before connecting it with the drainage system. Urine will begin to flow through the catheter when it is inserted correctly.
7. ***Do not test the balloon before insertion.***
8. If the male patient is in the supine position, place one or more drapes to expose only the genitalia.
9. *Female prep:* With the *nondominant hand*, spread the labia, using the thumb and forefinger to form a C. Then, use the *dominant hand* to cleanse the genitalia. Grasp the prep sponge moistened with antiseptic with the sterile forceps. Cleanse the meatus and internal labia by drawing the cotton prep sponge *downward from the superior apex of the labia majora to the anus.* Drop this sponge into the kick bucket. Do not allow the sponge to touch the area just prepped. Repeat this process several times.
10. *Male prep:* With the *nondominant hand*, retract the foreskin and stabilize the penis just below the glans. Use the *dominant hand* to cleanse the penis. Grasp the prep sponge with the sterile forceps and, starting with the urethral meatus, draw it in a circular direction, widening the circle to include the outer portions of the glans. Do not draw the sponge back over the area just prepped. Discard the sponge and repeat this process several times.
11. Maintaining traction on the genitalia, grasp the insertion end of the catheter and lubricate the tip.
12. Guide the tip of the catheter into the urethra with slow, steady pressure. *Do not force the catheter into the urethra.*

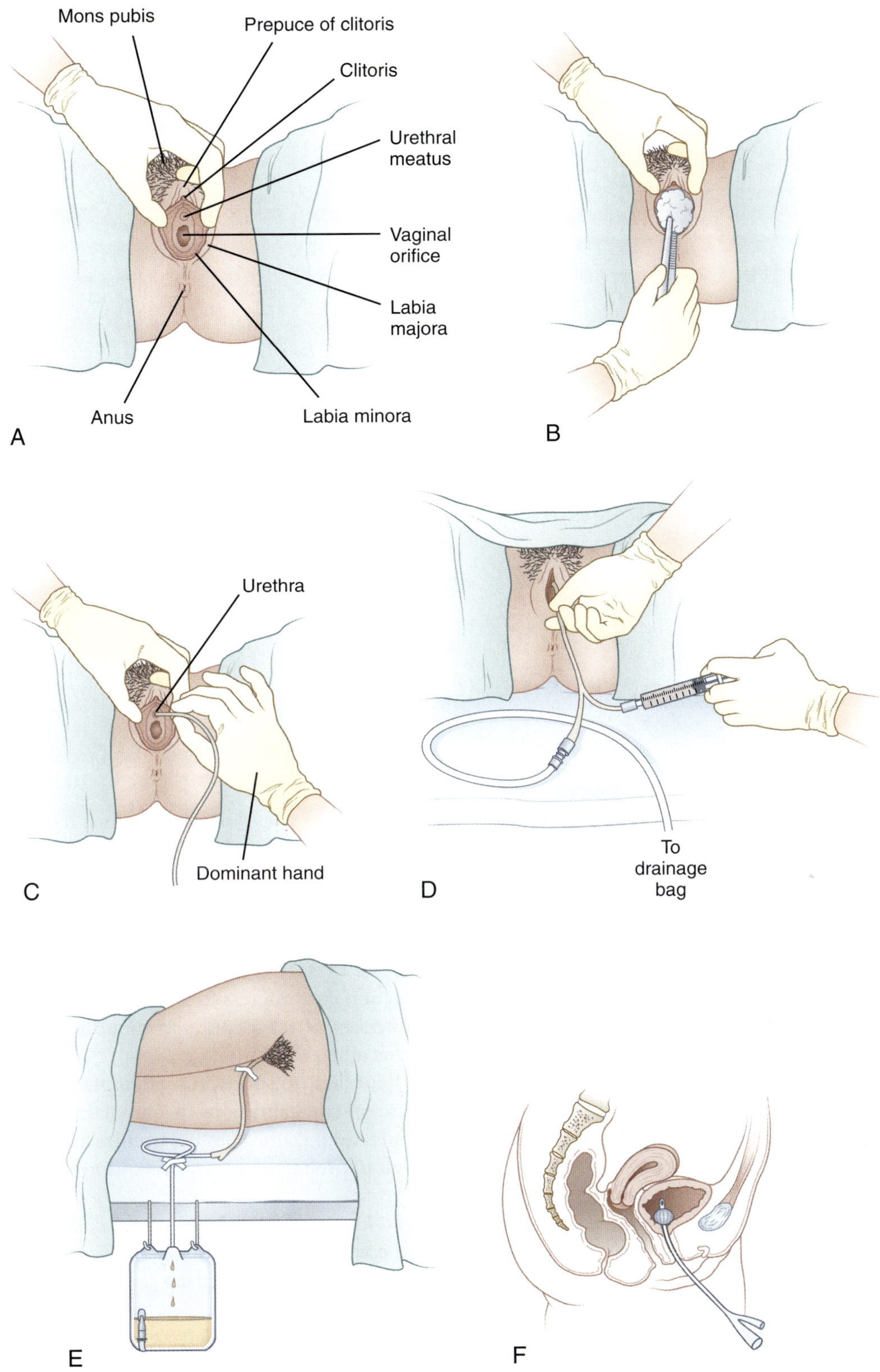

FIG. 17.2 Urinary catheterization of the female. (A) Exposure of the urethra using the assisting hand. (B) Cleansing of the labia using the no-touch technique. (C) Insertion of the catheter. (D) Inflation of the balloon tip. (E) Attachment of the drainage bag. (F) Anatomical position of the catheter.

It should slide easily into place with little resistance. When the tip of the catheter reaches the bladder, urine will begin to flow through the tubing. (In male patients, replace the foreskin into its normal position.) Inflate the catheter balloon by attaching a 10-mL syringe into the Luer-Lok connection of the catheter; inject 10 mL of water and remove the syringe. The balloon will remain inflated. If blood returns through the urethra at any time during insertion, gently retract the catheter and request a medical assessment immediately.

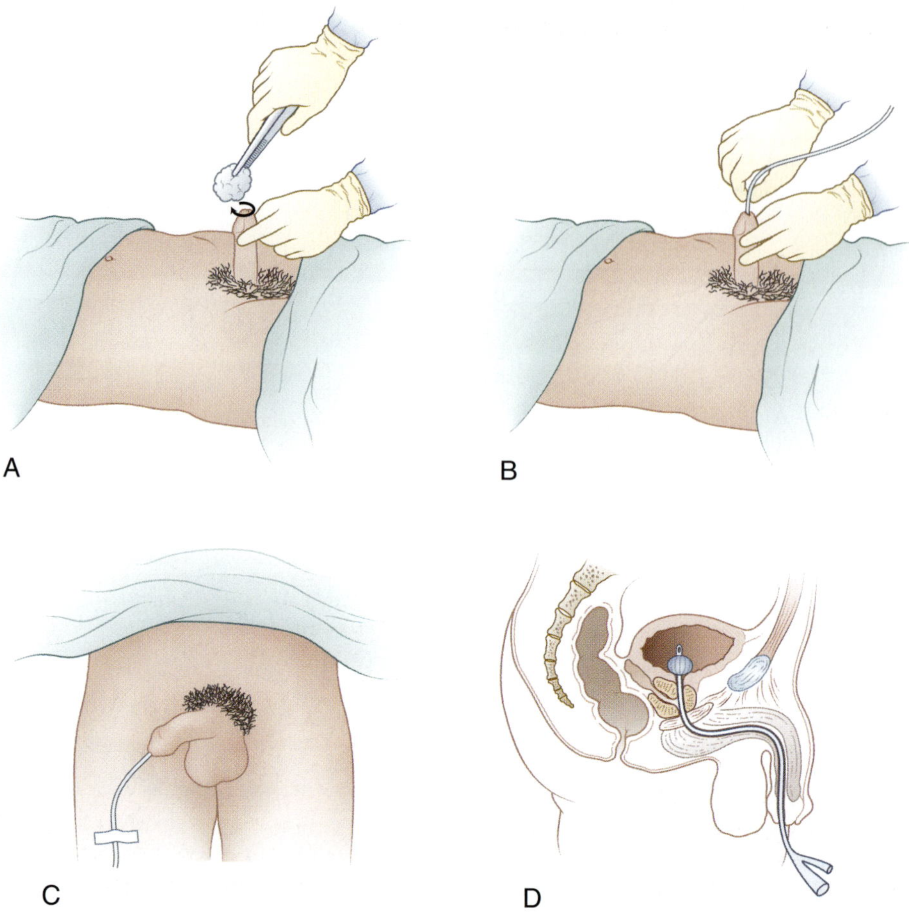

FIG. 17.3 Urinary catheterization of the male. (A) The assisting hand stabilizes the penis and draws back the foreskin. The insertion hand is used to cleanse the urethral meatus and glans. (B) Insertion of the catheter. The assisting hand returns the foreskin to its original position. (C) The catheter is secured to the leg. (D) Anatomical position of the catheter.

13. Connect the distal end of the catheter to the sterile tubing and calibrated urine collection unit. Note that some collection devices may require an adapter.
14. Make sure that the catheter tubing is not under any tension. This can traumatize the bladder neck and proximal urethra. Some institutions require that tape or a special strap be placed on the patient's thigh to secure the tubing.
15. Remove your gloves. Lower the drainage unit to allow gravity drainage. When urine stops flowing, secure the drainage unit to the operating table and measure the baseline amount. Document this amount according to policy.

Patient Safety

Catheterization is performed by trained perioperative personnel; this is usually the circulating nurse. *Urinary catheterization is the most common cause of hospital-acquired infections in the United States.* Two primary risks are associated with catheterization: infection and trauma to the genitourinary tract.

Urinary catheterization is a sterile procedure. The urinary bladder and proximal urethra are sterile, and contaminants introduced by catheterization increase the risk of urinary tract infection. Because of its proximity to the rectum (especially in female patients), the urinary meatus can be easily contaminated with *Escherichia coli,* which may be introduced into the urinary system during catheterization. Urinary tract infection can progress to systemic infection, with serious consequences. Strict aseptic technique is required to safely perform catheterization.

Repeated unsuccessful attempts at catheterization can cause mucosal abrasions that are painful and increase the risk of infection. Damage to the urethra and sphincter muscle can result in prolonged urinary retention (inability to void).

IMPORTANT TO KNOW *Once the catheter has been inserted and connected to the drainage device, the collection unit must remain below the level of the patient because raising it would cause urine to drain back into the bladder. This can result in injury to the bladder or initiate an infection.*

PREOPERATIVE PREPPING AGENTS

The prepping agent is determined by the surgeon based on the surgical site and patient history of sensitivity or allergy to specific antiseptics. Only antiseptic agents approved by the FDA for use on skin may be used for the prep. Some antiseptics cannot be used near the eyes or ears, and others must not be used on abraded skin or burns. Refer to Table 17.1 for a comparison

TABLE 17.1 Surgical Skin Prep Antiseptics

Chemical Name	Product	Action on Gram-Positive Bacteria	Action on Gram-Negative Bacteria	Residual Activity
70% isopropyl alcohol HIGHLY FLAMMABLE	Alcohol	Excellent	Excellent	Little
Chlorhexidine gluconate (CHG)	Hibiclens Exidine	Excellent	Good	Excellent
70% alcohol/chlorhexidine gluconate HIGHLY FLAMMABLE	ChloraPrep	Excellent	Good	Little
Aqueous povidone-iodine	Betadine	Excellent	Good	Good
Iodine povacrylex (7% iodine)/ isopropyl alcohol HIGHLY FLAMMABLE	DuraPrep	Excellent	Good	Good

BOX 17.2 Historical Highlights: Hexachlorophene

Hexachlorophene was popular as an infant bathing soap and anti-acne wash in the 1960s. It quickly became a common surgical prep solution after coming on the market. However, in the 1970s, proven links were found between the active ingredient and central nervous system damage in infants. Hexachlorophene is readily absorbed through broken or damaged skin at all ages. Ingested, it can be fatal, and its use as a surgical skin prep solution *has been officially retired.* However, it is still found in some facilities and ordered by some surgeons. This product is now available by prescription only and is not recommended by any safety agency for use as preoperative skin prep.

of antiseptics. Some agents used in the past are no longer considered safe (Box 17.2).

Antiseptics used for surgical prep are mainly evaluated according to the following criteria:

- Effectiveness on microbes, especially gram-negative and gram-positive bacteria
- Toxicity
- Ability to be used in or around the eyes, ears, mucous membranes, and neural tissue
- Flammability
- Residual antimicrobial action after application and drying

70% ALCOHOL

At 70% concentration, isopropyl alcohol is 95% effective against both gram-negative and gram-positive bacteria, mycobacteria, fungi, and viruses. It is not completely effective against bacterial spores. ***Isopropyl alcohol is extremely flammable and volatile.*** It can be a source of fire in an oxygen-rich environment when lasers and electrosurgery are used. All traces of alcohol must be completely dry on the skin before drapes are applied. See additional information below.

IMPORTANT TO KNOW *Alcohol destroys microorganisms by desiccation (drying) of the cell proteins. For this reason, alcohol is never used on mucous membranes or the eyes or in any open wound. Alcohol preparations must not be used near the eye or ear because they can cause nerve damage or injury to the cornea or tympanic membrane.*

CHLORHEXIDINE GLUCONATE

Chlorhexidine gluconate (CHG) has not been approved as a first-choice skin prep by The Joint Commission or CDC. This antiseptic does provide some **residual activity,** that is, it continues to destroy microorganisms for some time after application. It is not absorbed by the skin. A disadvantage of CHG is that it is not effective in the presence of soap and organic debris, such as skin oils, blood, and body fluids. CHG has been linked to hearing loss when accidentally introduced into the middle ear. Therefore it must never be used during prep of the eye, ear, or face. It is not recommended for use on large, open wounds, such as burns, *or in infants younger than 2 months.*

IODOPHOR

Iodophor is a combination of iodine and povidone (a synthetic dispersing agent). It is commonly used as a surgical antiseptic. When combined with a detergent, iodophor is used for the surgical hand scrub. Iodophor combined with 70% alcohol is commonly used as a commercially prepared prepping agent, which is highly effective. It has some residual activity and retains its microbicidal action in the presence of organic substances.

IMPORTANT TO KNOW *There is no scientific evidence showing a relationship between allergy to fish or shellfish and allergy to iodophor antiseptic.*

PRINCIPLES OF THE SURGICAL SKIN PREP

1. The skin cannot be "sterilized" with antiseptic. However, the *incision site* is prepped to achieve the highest level of microbial reduction possible. A wide margin at the

periphery of the incision site is also prepped as a barrier against contamination of the incision site.

2. During the prep, antiseptic (paint or soap) is applied in a spiral pattern with the incision site at the center of the spiral.
3. The sponge containing antiseptic must not be passed over the areas previously covered as this would draw bacteria from the periphery to the incision site.
4. If the *incision site is more contaminated* than the surrounding area (umbilicus, anus, axilla, open wound, stoma, prepuce), the area of less contamination is prepped first. The incisional site is prepped afterward.
5. A highly contaminated area that lies near the prep site but not within it should be excluded using a plastic or synthetic barrier (adhesive) drape and cloth towels.

SKIN PREP SAFETY

The skin prep exposes the patient to risks related to chemical and thermal burns.

1. Chemical burns can occur when the prepping agent is allowed to pool between the patient and the operating table linens, padding under the pneumatic tourniquet, or beneath the dispersive electrode.

   Towels are placed at the periphery of the prep site to catch any excess antiseptic that may seep between the patient and bed linen, pneumatic tourniquet, dispersive electrode, monitoring leads, or positioning aids. These towels must be removed before draping.

   If the procedure requires the lithotomy position, a waterproof drape must be placed under the patient's buttocks. This prevents the prepping agent from pooling in the gluteal cleft. After the prep solution is dried, the drape is removed.
2. Chemical burns may occur when the prepping agent is not removed from the skin at the end of the procedure. ***This includes iodophor.***

   After the drapes are removed, at the close of surgery use a soft damp towel to remove the prepping agent.
3. Burns may occur when prepping agents are heated.

   Prep solutions must never be prewarmed in a microwave or by other methods. Uncontrolled or unmonitored systems create a risk of thermal burns because the exact temperature is not known. When iodine is heated in a closed container, it combines with free oxygen, causing the iodine to be lost from the solution, which reduces its concentration.
4. Allergy to the prep solution may occur.

   Always check the patient chart for allergies before the surgical prep.
5. Iodophor cannot be used on infants younger than 2 months because the skin of an infant of this age is highly absorbent and may result in high blood levels of the chemical. Some prepping agents can cause severe tissue injury when used on or in the eye, ear, or mucous membranes.

   Always follow the manufacturer's indications and counterindications when prepping the patient.

EXTREME RISK OF FIRE USING ALCOHOL PREPPING AGENTS

As stated above, alcohol prepping agents are highly flammable and create a risk of fire. In the presence of concentrated oxygen in an oxygen-enriched environment such as the operating room, the risk is even greater. Ignition can occur during electrosurgery or laser surgery. Closed cavities, such as the throat, are particularly at risk. Fumes from alcohol-based prep solutions can settle in spaces created by drapes and ignite in these areas.

Prevention of alcohol-related fires requires vigilance and proactive measures on the part of all members of the surgical team. To prevent a fire arising from a prep solution, ensure that the prep area, towels, linens, and operating bed are dry before applying sterile drapes. In some facilities, the team uses a timer to ensure that adequate time is allowed for prep solutions to dry. The prepping agent manufacturer usually indicates the minimum time required for drying. However, safe patient care requires the surgical team to detect any remaining liquid on the skin before applying the drapes.

NOTE *For additional information on patient fires and safety, refer to Chapter 7, Hazards in the Perioperative Environment.*

BASIC SKIN PREP SUPPLIES

Materials used in the skin prep vary according to the type of prep (topical application of antiseptic only for a **single stage** prep, or cleansing plus topical application of antiseptic for a two-stage prep). Prep materials also vary according to the prep site. Basic prep supplies include the following:

Antiseptic prep solution. The prep solution may be contained within a sponge dispenser or in a pre-measured single-use container. Only single-use containers of antiseptic are to be used. Larger stock bottles of antiseptic can harbor microbes and should not be used.
Antiseptic scrub soap (as required)
Small sterile bowls or cups to hold sterile water, normal saline, and liquid antiseptic as required
Prep sponges impregnated with antiseptic soap (two-stage prep)
Gauze sponges as required for the single-stage prep
Forceps for grasping the sponges
Sterile gloves
Sterile towels
Cotton-tipped applicators, as needed

PREPARATION

Commercially prepared sterile prep trays are available that contain all or most of the supplies needed to perform skin prep. Many different types of commercial prep systems are available.

Before the prep is started, the sterile prep kit is placed on a small prep table near the patient, and the outer wrapper is opened using sterile technique. The sterile outside wrapper is folded down over the table, creating a sterile field.

Commercially prepared prep kits contain some or all the sterile materials required. Once the small sterile field has been created, any additional items can be distributed.

NOTE *The skin prep is a sterile procedure; sterile gloves are worn. The circulator must also wear a clean long-sleeved cover jacket during the prep.*

Multiple Prep Sites

When more than one procedure is planned during the same surgery, the circulator must prepare each site separately, using a different prep setup for each site. This can occur in cases of multiple trauma or in grafting procedures when the graft is taken from the patient's own tissues.

IMPORTANT TO KNOW *Two people may prep simultaneously. However, they should not share the same prep supplies.*

More extensive sites such as multiple trauma or prep for cardiac surgery require a different setup. This is described later in the chapter.

Use and Disposal of Non–X-ray–Detectable Sponges

X-ray–detectable surgical sponges are not used to perform the patient prep because they may be confused with the surgical sponges and count. Used prep sponges are discarded according to facility policy to keep them away from the surgical field and out of the incision. In some facilities, the kick bucket is used to collect prep sponges, which are then collected and bagged before surgery begins to keep them separate from surgical sponges.

GENERAL PROCEDURE FOR THE PREP

There are two methods of prepping. In *two-stage prep*, the skin is washed or scrubbed gently with antiseptic soap solution followed by a coating of antiseptic. A **single-stage prep** is performed with antiseptic only. The single-stage prep is used on clean skin. The two-stage prep is used when the surgical site is visibly soiled or likely to be heavily contaminated. The surgeon usually determines the type of prep required.

TWO-STAGE PREP

1. The prep site must be clinically assessed by the circulating nurse before the prep begins. Any lesion, rash, discoloration, or other skin condition must be accurately documented in the patient's chart.
2. If the prep area is grossly contaminated with dirt, debris, industrial chemicals, or other foreign material, the site is cleansed as a separate procedure before the surgical skin prep. This procedure takes place before the patient comes to the operating room.
3. The scrub prep is a sterile procedure. A commercially prepared scrub prep kit contains all needed supplies. These include sterile gloves, towels, antiseptic soap-impregnated sponges, and cotton-tipped applicators. Additional supplies will be required for specialty preps described later.
4. Before starting the prep, it is necessary to verify with the anesthesia provider that it is safe to start.
5. Expose the prep area.
6. Open the scrub kit using sterile technique.
7. Don sterile gloves using the open-gloving technique.
8. Place two or more sterile towels at the periphery of the prep site to absorb any prep solution that may pool between the patient and the operating table. When placing the towels, make a wide cuff in the towel to protect your gloved hands from contamination.
9. Dip a prep sponge in the antiseptic solution and squeeze out any excess. Use one sponge at a time to perform the prep.
10. The prep is performed in a circular or spiral pattern, starting at the incision site and moving outward. As the area of the prep is extended outward, do not bring the sponge back to an area already prepped. A new prep sponge is used to widen the circle as needed or to repeat the pattern. As each sponge reaches the periphery of the prep boundary, it is discarded.
11. After the scrub prep, use a towel to blot the soap from the skin.
12. Antiseptic is applied to the surgical site after the scrub prep. This can be done using a commercially prepared, pre-loaded sponge stick or with individual gauze sponges. Beginning with the incision site, apply paint prep in a circular motion from the center to the periphery. Apply the paint prep solution without allowing the sponge to return to an area previously prepped. When the periphery is reached, discard the sponge.
13. Allow the paint prep solution to air-dry. This enhances its bactericidal effect and is necessary whenever alcohol-based solutions are used to prevent possible ignition. Always follow the manufacturer's instructions for application and drying. The site should be ***visually inspected*** to ensure that the solution is dry. *Timing the drying interval may not be sufficient to ensure patient safety because the dry time is proportional to the amount of solution applied, crevices and folds in the skin, and other geographical features of the skin surface.*
14. Document the skin prep in the patient's chart, including the skin assessment, prep area, solutions, and name of the person who performed the prep.

SINGLE-STAGE PREP

In single-stage prep, the skin scrub is omitted and only antiseptic is applied. Commercially prepared prepping agents are commonly used in most health care facilities (Fig. 17.4). The prepping agent is self-contained (preloaded) in an applicator sponge mounted on a handle. The CDC recommends that pressure be applied during the paint prep. This allows the solution to get into skin crevices, sebaceous glands, hair follicles, and pores more efficiently. The exception to this is the skin

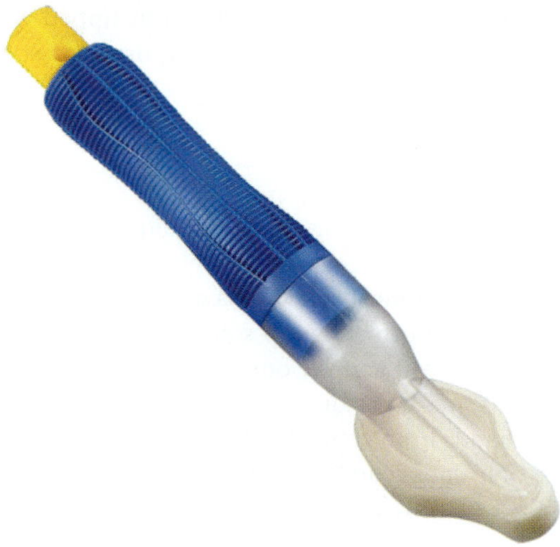

FIG. 17.4 Dura-Prep applicator.

BOX 17.3 Checklist for Starting the Skin Prep

- Prepare the patient. Have you checked the patient's record for allergies? Has the patient been positioned properly? Has the surgical site been verified? Has all jewelry been removed? Has the anesthesia provider given permission to start the prep? Are the surgeons present and available to start surgery?
- Prepare the supplies. Note which items are not included in the prep kit. Are sterile gloves available? Have the prep solutions been poured? Is the prep table positioned close to the patient? Is a receptacle at hand for soiled prep sponges? Do you have adequate light on the prep area? Have you checked the surgeon's preference card for the use of specific antiseptics?
- Prepare yourself. Do you have a plan? Do you know the exact boundaries of the prep area? Is your clothing contained so that it does not touch the prep area? (A loose cover jacket or baggy sleeves may drag across the prep area.)

prep for suspected tumors (see below). The person performing the prep should have ample applicators available for large prep areas. The same rules apply with regard to the application pattern described above.

NOTE *Before starting the skin prep, ensure that you have prepared the patient, the supplies, and the procedure. Refer to Box 17.3 for guidelines.*

EYE

Surgical prep of the eye is performed after the patient has been anesthetized (if a general anesthesia is used). If a regional block is used, the prep may be continuous with the regional anesthetic procedure. Only prep solutions that are safe to use around mucous membranes, including the eye, can be used in the prep. Dilute (5% or less) povidone-iodine is currently approved for eye prep. The eye prep includes the eyelid, inner and outer canthus, brow, and face to the chin line, starting at the eyelid and working outward. When the patient is being prepped for an orbital injury, the prep solution must not come into contact with the open orbital wounds. The surgeon usually performs the prep.

The eye prep usually includes irrigation of the eye with balanced saline solution for ophthalmic use. Other drugs may also be instilled according to the surgeon's orders.

IMPORTANT TO KNOW *Among approved preoperative skin antiseptics, only one is approved for use around the eyes and ears: dilute povidone-iodine.*

SUPPLIES

Adhesive barrier drape
Lint-free cotton balls
Small basins with saline solution and prep solution
Towels
Bulb syringe
Eye sponges

NOTE *Eye prep solutions must be diluted according to the surgeon's orders.*

TECHNIQUE

1. Explain the procedure to the conscious patient. Advise the patient not to touch the face during and after the prep.
2. Turn the patient's head slightly toward the operative side. Prevent solution from entering the patient's ear. Place a cotton ball at the ear canal opening and an adhesive barrier drape at the side of the face to prevent solution from draining into the ear.
3. Start the prep at the eyelid. Prep in a circular pattern around the eye to within 1 inch (2.5 cm) of the hairline, including the nose, cheek, and jaw on the affected side. If the procedure includes both eyes, prep both sides of the face.
4. Discard each sponge after reaching the periphery of the prep area.
5. Repeat the prep at least three times, using fresh sponges each time.
6. Rinse the prepped area using warm saline and cotton balls. Discard each used cotton ball and obtain a fresh one. Rinse the area at least twice.
7. Use balanced salt solution according to the surgeon's order to flush the conjunctiva. Using one finger, pull the conjunctival sac slightly downward while flushing with normal saline solution or a solution ordered by the surgeon.

EAR

SUPPLIES

Occlusive towel drape
Cotton balls
Cotton-tipped applicators
Prep solution according to the surgeon's order
Prep towels

TECHNIQUE

1. Use a sterile plastic drape to exclude the eye on the affected side.
2. Exclude the hair using sterile plastic drapes or cloth towels secured with tape.
3. Place absorbent cotton in the external ear canal.
4. Cleanse the folds of the pinna (external ear) with cotton-tipped applicators.
5. Extend the prep area with sponges to the edge of the hairline, face, and jaw.
6. Remove the absorbent cotton from the external ear canal.

FACE

Patients are advised to remove all makeup before surgery. Any residual products should be removed because they can interfere with the antiseptic properties of the prep and may contaminate the surgical wound. Trauma procedures may require debridement (discussed below) and removal of embedded foreign material as part of the prep or just before it with the patient under sedation. In all cases, an antiseptic solution that is safe around the eyes is ordered by the surgeon. Only nonalcohol solutions are used.

The hair contains a high concentration of bacteria and is a contaminated area. Therefore the hairline must be completely excluded from the prep and draping area. If the patient has long hair, it must be excluded using elastic bands (not metal hair pins) or non-alcohol water-soluble gel to hold it away from the face.

SUPPLIES

Non-alcohol prep solution (e.g., dilute povidone-iodine)
Normal saline
Cotton swabs
Cotton-tipped applicators
Towels
Nonsterile comb and water-soluble hair gel

TECHNIQUE

1. Use elastic bands as necessary to separate and contain hair strands away from the face and ears. Cotton balls may be placed at the external ear canals.
2. One or more occlusive towel drapes are placed at the hairline. The surgeon may require a cap or towel placed over the patient's hair and secured with tape.
3. The prep includes the neck or chin upward to the hairline. The ears may be included in the face prep as ordered.
4. Place absorbent cotton at the external ear canal. Cleanse the folds of the pinna using cotton-tipped applicators. Do not allow prep solution to drain into the ear canal.
5. Prep the face from the incision area outward. Prep the incision site again with fresh sponges.

Any prep sponge that touches the hairline must be discarded. Rinse the skin with cotton swabs dipped in warm normal saline solution.

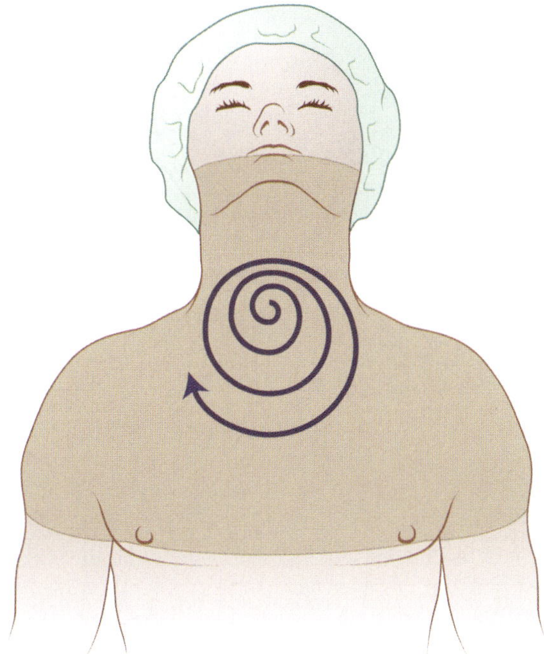

FIG. 17.5 Skin prep for neck and throat procedures.

NECK

The neck, including the external throat area, is prepared for thyroid surgery, tracheotomy, carotid artery surgery, lymph node biopsy, or radical dissection of the mandible, shoulder plexus, and mediastinum. If radical dissection is anticipated or scheduled, the prep area extends from the chin to the nipple line or waist and around the side of the body to the operating table on each side (Fig. 17.5). Standard prep supplies are used.

TECHNIQUE

1. Place sterile towels at the periphery of the prep site.
2. An occlusive towel drape may be placed at the upper boundaries of the prep to exclude the face and airway.
3. Begin the prep at the incision site, applying prep solution in a circular motion to the periphery of the site.

BREAST

The boundary of the prep area for breast surgery depends on the extent of the surgery and the patient's position. The prep area for radical breast surgery extends from the chin to the umbilicus and includes the lateral thorax on each side.

When the surgery involves removal of a mass without the possibility of more extensive surgery, the breast is prepped from the clavicle to the midthorax and from the midline, including the sides of the thorax, to the operating table on the affected side. The prep area is extended into the axilla for lesions in the upper lateral quadrant of the breast.

Surgery that includes both biopsy of a mass and the possibility of mastectomy requires a much wider prep area. A radical mastectomy requires a prep boundary that encompasses the neck, shoulder of the affected side, thorax to the operating table surface, and midpelvic region (Fig. 17.6).

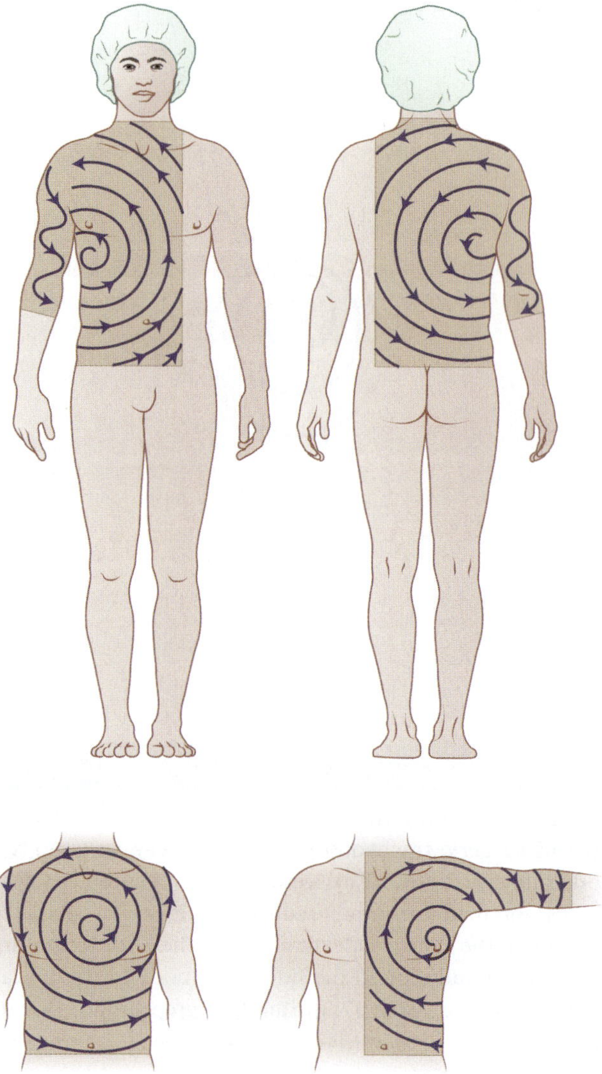

FIG. 17.6 Skin prep for the breast and thorax.

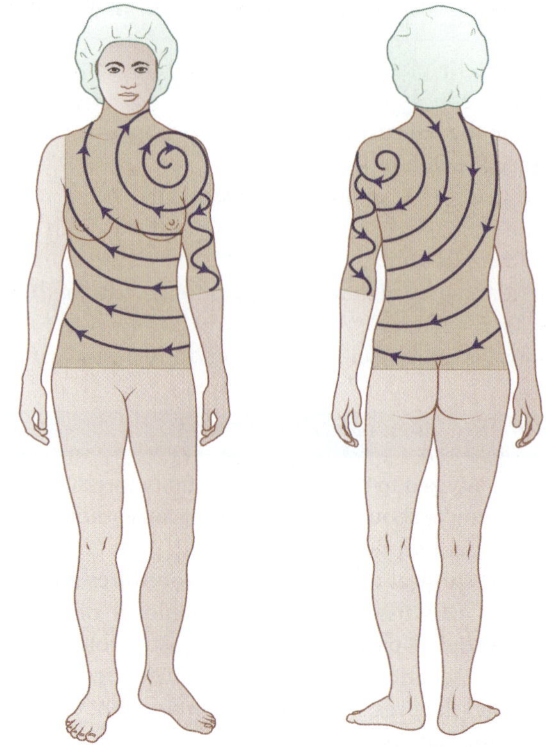

FIG. 17.7 Shoulder prep.

IMPORTANT TO KNOW *In patients who have undergone an image-guided needle location procedure, take great care to prevent dislodging the needle, which is used to guide tissue excision during surgery.*

Tissue that is suspected of being cancerous must be prepared gently. The prep solution should be applied with as little friction and pressure as possible to prevent tumor cells from seeding the surrounding tissue. Skin prep for surgery of the thoracic cavity includes a bilateral extension of the boundaries for radical breast surgery.

TECHNIQUE

1. Square the prep boundary with sterile towels.
2. If the umbilicus is included in the prep, clean it with cotton-tipped applicators.
3. Prep the operative area, starting at the incision site.
4. If the shoulder is included in the prep, an assistant should abduct the arm so that solution can be applied circumferentially.

SHOULDER

The shoulder prep includes the neck, shoulder, upper arm, and scapula on the affected side (Fig. 17.7). One assistant is required to elevate the patient's arm. The subscapular and midback areas also may be elevated on a gel pad.

TECHNIQUE

1. Remove the patient's gown to the umbilicus.
2. Place sterile prep towels at the periphery of the prep area.
3. Place an impervious sheet between the operating table and the subscapular area.
4. Have a gloved assistant elevate the arm.
5. The hand may be excluded from the prep. Some surgeons wrap the hand in an occlusive drape after the prep.
6. Do not pull the patient's shoulder laterally to expose the scapular area. This can cause injury. Seek guidance from the surgeon about the exact nature of the injury or repair to prevent damage.
7. Begin the prep at the incision site and extend it to the periphery.

ARM

Depending on the incision site, the arm is prepped in total or in one section. If a nerve block anesthesia will be performed, the entire arm is usually prepped. The hand, especially in the webs of the fingers and subungual area, is usually heavily contaminated with transient and resident bacteria. It may be prepped but then excluded from the operative site by an occlusive drape. If the operative site is on the forearm, the prep extends several inches above the elbow and may include the shoulder.

In all cases, the arm or hand is prepped circumferentially. An assistant supports the arm and hand while another person performs the prep. If a pneumatic tourniquet is in use, it is important to prevent prep solutions from becoming trapped between the tourniquet and the patient's skin.

TECHNIQUE

1. Elevate the patient's arm carefully, keeping it in anatomical alignment.
2. Place an impervious sheet under the arm, covering the operating table and the patient's torso.
3. Place sterile towels at the periphery of the prep site and under the shoulder.
4. Begin the prep at the incision site and move to the periphery.
5. When the prepped area is dry, remove the impervious sheet.
6. Continue to elevate the arm during draping.

HAND

The routine hand prep begins at the fingernails. A nail cleaner is used to cleanse the subungual area. After the hand is cleaned, prep solution is applied as usual, beginning at the incision site and moving outward and circumferentially. The upper boundary is a few inches above the elbow. If Bier block anesthesia is used, upper arm prep is required to the level of the tourniquet.

SUPPLIES

Nail cleaner
Foam scrub sponges
Impervious sheet
Sterile gloves

TECHNIQUE

1. Elevate the patient's hand carefully, keeping it in anatomical alignment.
2. Place an impervious sheet under the arm and hand.
3. Clean the subungual areas with a nail cleaner.
4. Beginning at the incisional area, prep the hand in the usual manner, moving outward. Include the interdigital spaces, fingertips, and all four sides of each finger.
5. Extend the prep to the arm, covering all sides.
6. Blot excess antiseptic soap and paint with antiseptic.
7. Remove the impervious drape.
8. Support the hand until draping begins and the surgeon takes control of it for draping.

ABDOMEN

The abdominal prep extends from the nipple line to mid-thigh and both sides of the body to the operating table (Fig. 17.8). If a pelvic laparoscopy is planned, a vaginal prep may be included, and two separate preps are necessary.

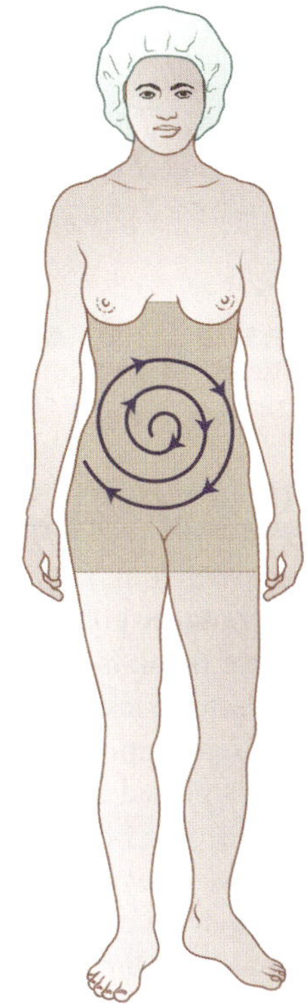

FIG. 17.8 Abdominal prep.

TECHNIQUE

1. Square the abdomen with sterile towels. The upper towel is placed at the nipple line and the lower towel at the pubis.
2. Begin the prep at the umbilicus. Cleanse the umbilicus using cotton-tipped applicators dipped in prep solution to remove loose dead skin.
3. Prep the abdomen, starting at the incision site and moving to the periphery.
4. If soap solution is used, blot dry and then apply antiseptic paint. Allow the prep liquid to dry before applying drapes.

FLANK AND BACK

The flank and back areas are prepped in the same manner as the abdomen, starting at the incision site and moving outward. The sides of the body are prepped to the operating table. The back prep extends from the neck to the sacrum.

TECHNIQUE

1. Square the periphery of the prep site with sterile towels.
2. Begin at the incision area and apply antiseptic in a circular pattern, continuing to the periphery. Complete this pattern at least twice, beginning again at the incision site and working outward to the surface of the operating table.

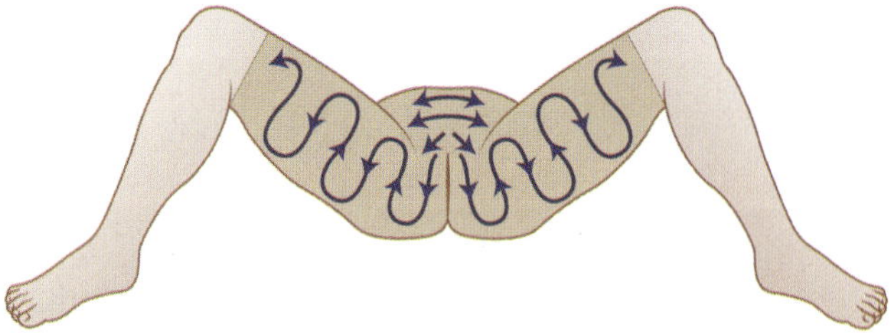

FIG. 17.9 Vaginal prep.

VULVA, PERINEUM, AND VAGINA

Procedures of the vulva, perineum, and vagina are performed with the patient in the lithotomy position. After the patient is positioned, the lower table break is flexed downward. Before beginning the prep, place the kick bucket at the foot of the table to catch run-off antiseptic and used sponges.

An impervious drape is placed under the buttocks to prevent prep solution from seeping between the coccyx and the table. If a single impervious sheet is used, place the tail of the sheet in the kick bucket to drain excess prep solution. A perineal barrier drape with a self-adherent edge is placed across the perineum between the vagina and anus. This is done to prevent prep solution from seeping into the gluteal cleft. Place a prep towel above the pubis.

The vaginal prep is performed in two stages. The pelvis, labia, perineum, and thighs are prepped first as one stage, and the vagina is prepped separately (Fig. 17.9). Sponge forceps are used to prep the vaginal vault. The rationale for the two-step procedure is to ensure that bacteria from the external genitalia and perineum are not introduced into the vagina. If urinary catheterization is required, this is performed after the prep is completed.

IMPORTANT TO KNOW *For combined abdominal-vaginal procedures, such as pelvic laparoscopy, the vaginal prep is completed first, followed by the abdominal prep.*

TECHNIQUE

1. Start the pelvic prep at the pubis, using back-and-forth strokes. This area is prepped to the level of the iliac crest.
2. Apply prep solution at the labia majora, using downward strokes only and including the perineum. Do not return to the area previously prepped.
3. Using clean sponges, prep the inner aspects of the thighs. Start at the labia majora and move laterally, using back-and-forth strokes. Discard the sponge as it reaches the periphery.
4. Prep the vaginal vault last. Use sponges mounted on forceps and ample prep solution to reach the folds of the vaginal rugae. Discard the sponges and repeat.
5. Use a dry-mounted sponge to blot excess fluid from the vaginal vault and remaining prep area.

MALE GENITALIA

Surgery of the male genitalia requires skin preparation of the penis, scrotum, thighs, and inguinal areas. Minor procedures may require prep of only the penis and scrotum, excluding the peripheral areas. The patient is prepped in the supine position.

SUPPLIES

Non-alcohol prep solution, sterile saline, or water
Cotton balls
Sponge forceps
Sponges impregnated with prep solution or plain sponges

TECHNIQUE

1. Place absorbent sterile towels on each side of the hips and under the scrotum. A barrier drape should be placed over the towel to prevent prep solution from seeping underneath the scrotum or legs.
2. If the patient has not been circumcised, the foreskin is retracted. The prep begins at the glans.
3. Using soft sponges or cotton balls and forceps, prep the external urethral meatus first and then extend the prep to the circumference of the penis to the base. This step is repeated with fresh cotton balls. Once the penis has been prepped, return the foreskin to its normal position.
4. Prep the scrotum, ensuring that prep solution enters all folds and skin crevices.
5. The thighs and inguinal area are prepped beginning at each side of the groin, moving outward. The pelvis is prepped separately, beginning at the lower margin of the pubic bone and extending bilaterally to the iliac crest.

PERIANAL AREA

The perianal prep is performed with the patient in the prone position, with a break in the operating table. Because the anus is a contaminated area, the surrounding area is prepped first and the anus last. The anus is exposed by separating the buttocks with wide adhesive tape.

TECHNIQUE

1. Remove the patient's gown and the cover sheet to expose the lower trunk. Keep the patient's legs and upper body covered.
2. Begin the prep outside the anal mucosa and extend the prep area outward about 12 inches (30 cm) in all directions.
3. Prep the outer anus. In some institutions, the anal prep is omitted.

IMPORTANT TO KNOW *For abdominoperineal resection, the patient is placed in the lithotomy position. The technique requires separate abdominal and perineal preps.*

LEG AND FOOT

The leg prep is similar to that of the arm. The prep extends from the ankle to the groin (Fig. 17.10). The limb must be elevated by an assistant or placed in a leg-holder. Use only leg-holders known to be safe. If the leg-holder is not strong

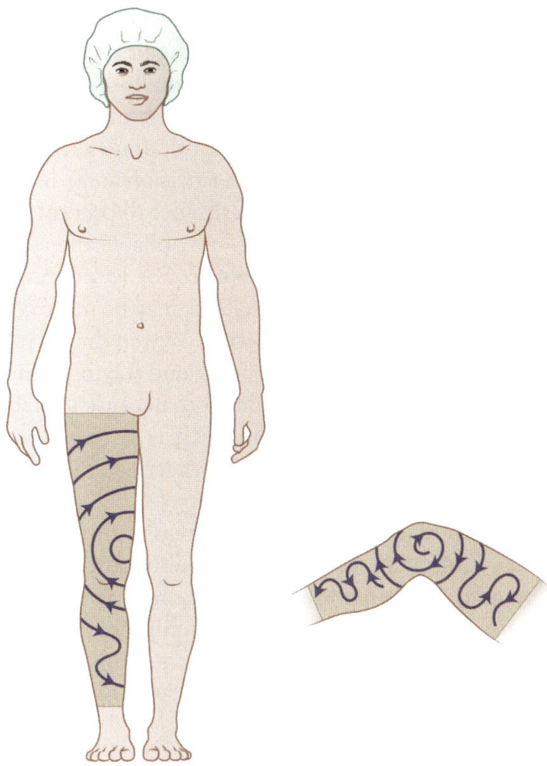

FIG. 17.10 Leg.

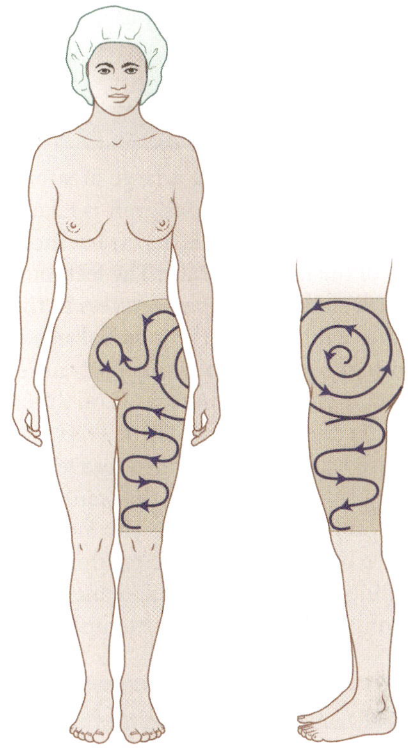

FIG. 17.11 Hip prep.

enough to support the leg, it can rotate or slip, causing injury. For knee surgery, the entire leg is prepped and the foot is wrapped in a separate drape. If a pneumatic tourniquet is in place, prevent prep solutions from seeping under the tourniquet cuff by wrapping a surgical towel proximal to the tourniquet cuff. Remove this towel when the prep is complete and check carefully for any seeping under the cuff.

Hip surgery requires a circumferential prep from the waist to the knee and may include the groin (Fig. 17.11).

TECHNIQUE

1. Place a towel between the groin and the fold of the upper leg.
2. Elevate the leg.
3. Place an impervious sheet over the operating table and the patient's nonoperative leg.
4. If the foot is to be included in the prep, scrub it as you would a hand. Remember that because the leg is elevated, the prep must begin at the highest level and move to the lowest level.
5. If the foot is excluded from the prep, perform wide-skin prep around the operative site.

Watch Chapters 17: Patient Prep on the Evolve website: http://evolve.elsevier.com/Fuller/surgical.

TRAUMA AND DEBRIDEMENT PROCEDURE

Trauma wounds are almost always contaminated because they are caused by external forces and often occur in environments that are mildly or heavily contaminated. These wounds are usually prepped by the surgeon. Penetrating traumatic wounds may contain small pieces of bone and foreign material that must be removed from the wound. A low-pressure water system may be used to clean the wound with the patient under sedation. This requires specialized drapes with drain pockets to collect and drain runoff solution. During the cleansing process, the surgeon removes all foreign material and trims away devitalized tissue (called **debridement**). Preliminary debridement is performed on a stable patient and takes place in the emergency department or in a separate treatment room to prevent gross contamination of the surgical environment. All tissue and foreign material are retained as specimens. After debridement, the wound can be prepped and draped. The prep area for traumatic wounds is larger than normal, and the draping procedure is usually led by the surgeon.

Debridement is used not only for wounds that are contaminated with foreign material but also for infected wounds, including pressure sores and other chronic conditions resulting in dead tissue in and around the wound. If debridement is performed in the operating room, a minor plastic surgery set is needed. This includes several surgical blades of different sizes (15, 20, and possibly 11), plastic surgery scissors, and toothed pickups. An infected wound is usually cultured at the time of surgery (refer to Chapter 8 for details).

AUTOGRAFT

A tissue autograft is a graft that is removed from one site on the patient and grafted to another site. This requires two separate preps. Clear prep solutions are used on the donor site. This is necessary to maintain a clear view of the vascular bed of the graft. It is important to maintain an aseptic barrier between the donor and recipient sites.

CARDIOVASCULAR PREP

Cardiovascular surgery requires a large area of exposure. In cardiac cases in which a saphenous graft is taken from one or both legs, a complete body prep is necessary, including the full circumference of the legs bilaterally. The feet may be excluded from the surgical site after full prep. Access to the deep femoral veins requires a full prep of the inguinal area.

In all cases requiring full body prep, it is necessary to prepare the environment and solutions used on the patient to prevent hypothermia during the procedure. Prep solutions (saline and water), if used, are warmed in an approved device. Do not warm antiseptic solutions because this can alter their effect. The operating room temperature must be monitored to ensure the maintenance of a normothermic environment. This is the joint responsibility of the circulator and anesthesiologist, who continually monitor the patient's core temperature.

SECTION II: DRAPING THE SURGICAL SITE

PRINCIPLES

Draping is performed immediately after the skin prep. The purpose of draping is to provide a wide sterile area around the surgical site. Drapes act as a barrier surface between nonsterile objects and the sterile field. They allow the sterile team to work in relative freedom without risk of contaminating the wound. The center of the sterile field is defined by the position of the drapes. The incision site is the center of the sterile field. Draped tables and equipment are moved into position close to the patient, and scrubbed team members work within the sterile area.

LEARNING TO DRAPE

Draping the surgical patient is one of the more difficult skills for surgical technologists to master. The principles of draping are not difficult to understand. However, the actual handling of drapes while maintaining aseptic techniques is sometimes problematic. Drapes are folded in a specific way before sterilization so that they can be positioned over the operative site and unfolded in a way that prevents their contamination. The orientation of the drape as it is first placed over the incision site is critical because once it is placed, it cannot be moved again without contaminating the site (which has just been prepped). There are many variations on basic draping materials based on slightly different designs. However, all drapes and all draping procedures are based on the same principles. Understanding these principles can help clarify the practice.

DRAPING FABRICS AND MATERIALS

Drapes are made of woven material (cotton or cotton-synthetic blend), nonwoven material (bonded synthetics), or flexible plastic sheeting.

Nonwoven drapes are made from spun synthetic polymers as disposable, single-use items. They are impervious or semi-impervious to moisture. They may be less expensive to use as they do not require laundering or repair. However, they may not be environmentally sound.

Woven cloth drapes are made of sewn cotton and synthetic materials such as polyester. Woven cloth drapes are reinforced around the fenestration (incision area) and chemically treated for moisture resistance to prevent strike-through contamination. They are more pliable and easier to handle than synthetic drapes but require laundering, repair, and reprocessing after use. This may be more costly than purchasing single-use materials. Woven drapes must be carefully inspected for tears, holes, and fraying, which may become sources of contamination. Because the fabric is not waterproof, extra precautions, such as increased layers, are needed to prevent penetration with irrigation solutions, blood, and tissue debris during surgery.

Plastic drapes are used on contoured areas of the body and complex equipment, such as the operating microscope and imaging equipment that must be draped during a sterile procedure. Plastic drapes for equipment are custom designed for specific types of equipment. Those used for patient draping are adhesive on one side or on the edge that adheres to the patient's skin.

TYPES OF DRAPES

Manufacturers of drapes have developed many different types and styles to fit the needs of the draping technique and contours of the patient's body while providing asepsis on the surgical field. Although there are many variations on basic styles, the principles of their application remain the same. Even a complex draping technique uses individual layers, each positioned following the rules of asepsis. The following section discusses commonly used drapes.

SURGICAL TOWELS

Towels are standard for most draping techniques. The cloth surgical towel is soft, pliable, and very absorbent. Their primary use in draping is to "frame" the incision site and create the base layer for the larger drapes, which are placed over them. This is called **squaring the incision** site. Towels are held in place using an adhesive incision drape, towel clips, or surgical skin staples. Sterile towels are also used to exclude the pneumatic tourniquet and hand or foot during arm and leg procedures.

The *plastic towel* drape has a 1-inch strip of adhesive on one edge. It is often used to exclude areas of the sterile field. For example, during ear surgery, a plastic towel drape may be placed along the anterior border of the ear, to exclude the nose, mouth, and eyes. It also prevents prepping solutions from draining into these areas. In gynecological surgery, a plastic towel drape is placed across the perineum on the posterior border of the vaginal vault to exclude the anus from the surgical site. Additional draping layers are added to re-enforce the exclusion.

Impervious (waterproof) towels made of synthetic woven material are also used. Regardless of the material, their purpose is the same. Synthetic towels are adhesive along one border to maintain contact with the patient's skin.

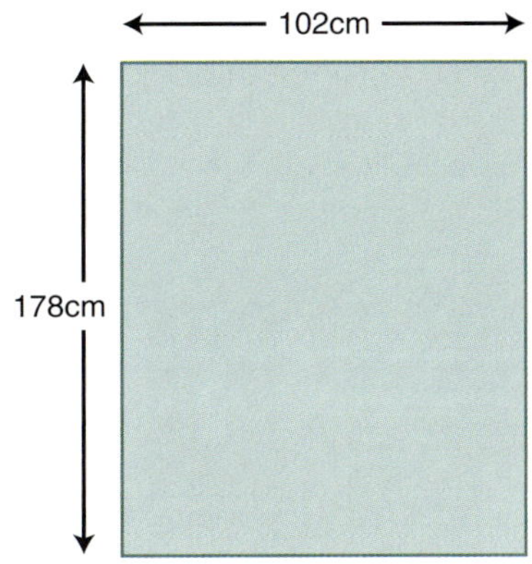

Plain sheet

FIG. 17.12 Plain sheet.

PLAIN SHEET

The *plain sheet* (Fig. 17.12), also called a *utility drape*, is a ½, ¾, or full sheet. It is a simple rectangle or square used as a general-purpose drape. It is commonly used to cover large areas of the body. For example, two plain sheets can be used to cover the upper and lower sections of the body when the incision is at the flank or abdomen. It is also used during orthopedic surgery to drape portions of the operating table on which the limb rests during surgery.

FENESTRATED DRAPE

The **fenestrated drape** is one sheet with a hole or "window" that exposes the operative site. It is used in areas such as the abdomen, back, flank, and perineum. The fenestrated drape exposes the operative site while covering the rest of the body to form a continuous sterile field. Commercially prepared fenestrated drapes are often identified by the manufacturer according to a specific surgical site such as laparotomy, thoracotomy, thyroid, ear, and eye drape.

SPLIT AND U-DRAPE

The *split* and *U-drape* are large rectangles with a split at one end (Fig. 17.13). The U-drape (Fig. 17.14) is commonly used in orthopedic surgery. The split ends are referred to as the "tails."

IMPORTANT TO KNOW *The draping technique may require "tails up" or "tails down," referring to the orientation of the drape to the body and the leg or arm. The tails are draped around the limb, while the opposite end is used to cover the rest of the body.*

Extremity Drape

The *extremity drape* is often used in conjunction with the split drape. It has an elasticized fenestration that fits over the arm or leg (Fig. 17.15).

INCISE DRAPE

The plastic **incise drape** (generic name) is placed over the entire surgical site on top of the towels and any bottom sheets that form the fenestration.

IMPORTANT TO KNOW *The 2019–2020 guidelines for sterile technique and infection control mandate the use of iodophor-*

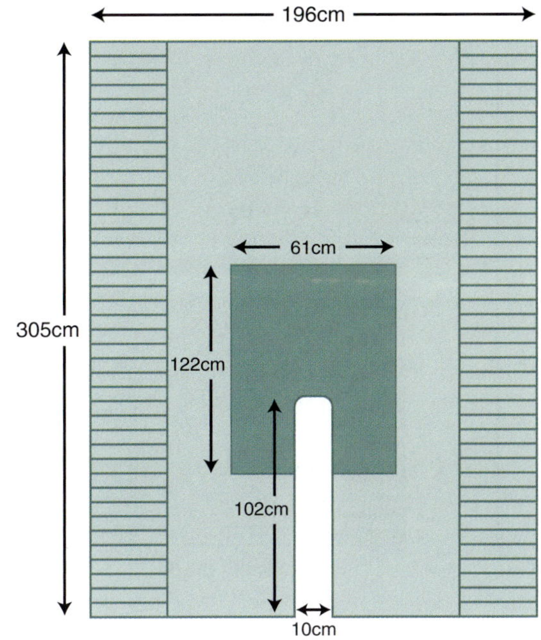

Split drape

FIG. 17.13 Split sheet.

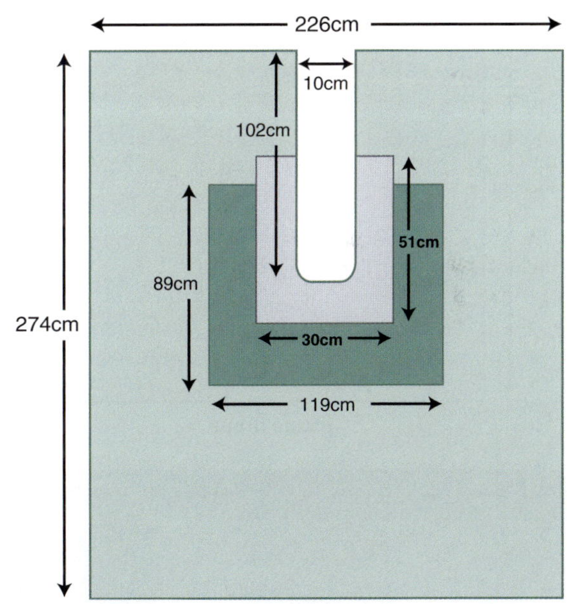

U-drape

FIG. 17.14 U-drape used in shoulder draping and hip draping.

impregnated incise drapes. Incise drapes that do not contain iodophor should not be used as an occluding drape. This guideline applies only to incise drapes and not to towel drapes.

The incise drape is impregnated with iodophor and coated with adhesive on one side with a paper backing. The drape is packaged as one fan-folded piece. To position the drape, the surgeon holds one edge while the assistant or ST slowly pulls the paper backing away while maintaining mild tension on it. This prevents the drape from tangling and sticking to itself. This exposes the adhesive side, which is pressed over the incision site. A folded towel may be used to smooth the drape in place (Fig. 17.16).

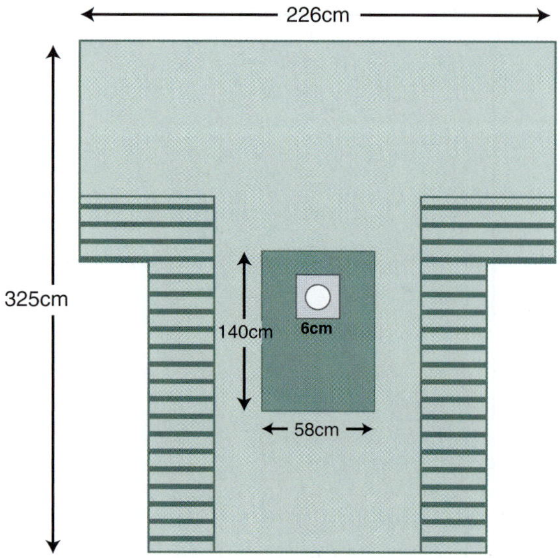

FIG. 17.15 Extremity drape. The limb is placed through the fenestration.

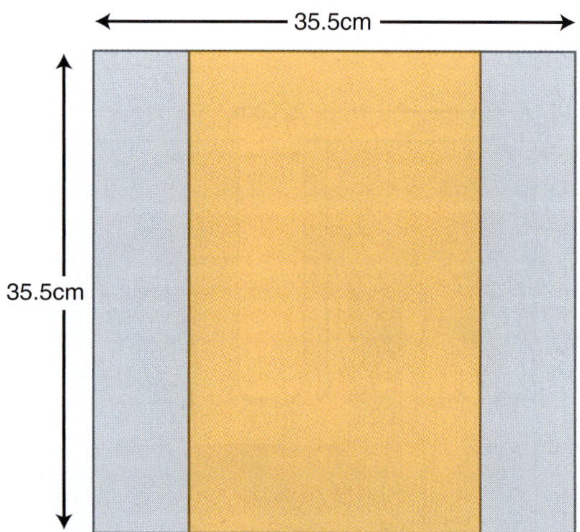

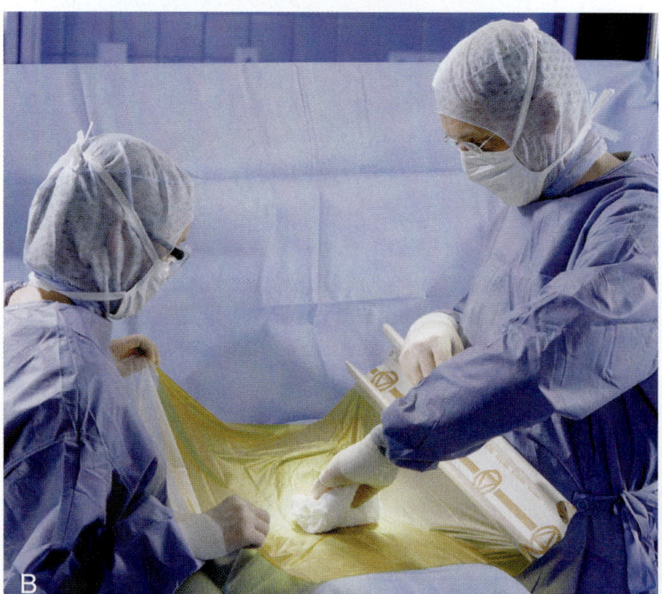

FIG. 17.16 Incise drape. (A) The orange section is impregnated with iodophor and is full adhesive on one side. (B) Once the drape is in place, it may be smoothed down with a towel. (Courtesy 3M.)

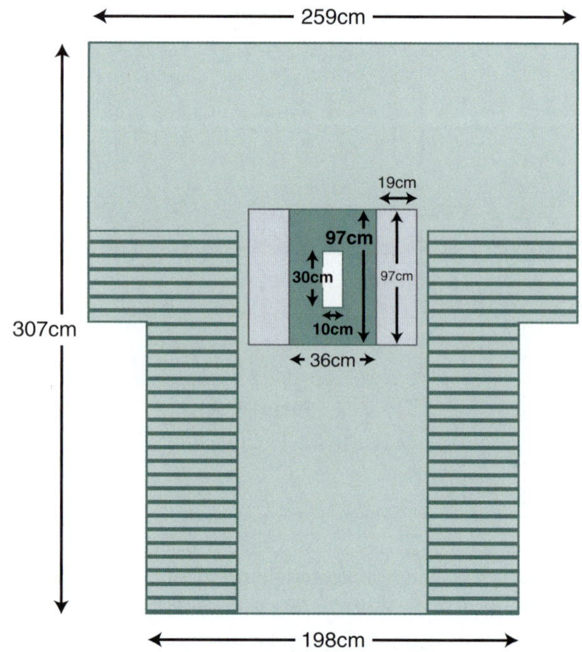

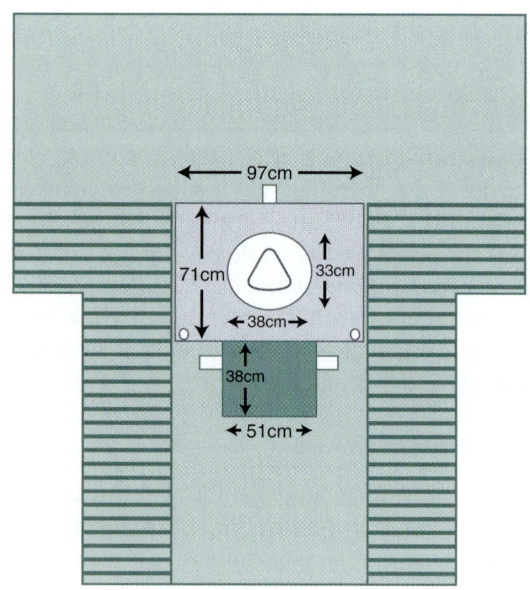

FIG. 17.17 (A) Laparotomy drape. (B) C-section drape.

LAPAROTOMY DRAPE

The *laparotomy* drape (Fig. 17.17A) is a full-size sheet with fenestration (a "window" in the drape which exposes the skin in position for an abdominal incision. The C-section drape (Fig. 17.17B) is similar to the laparotomy drape but also contains a fluid collection system. The C-section drape may be further customized for a Pfannenstiel lateral incision in which the fenestration is positioned over the lower abdomen.

FLUID POUCH

The *fluid pouch* (Fig. 17.18) is used to collect and channel excess fluid. This drape can be used in any procedure in which large amounts of fluid and blood are anticipated.

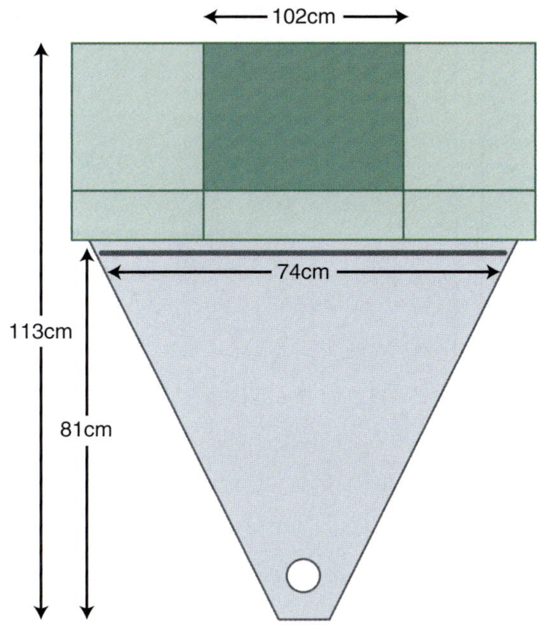

Under buttocks fluid pouch drape

FIG. 17.18 Fluid pouch drape.

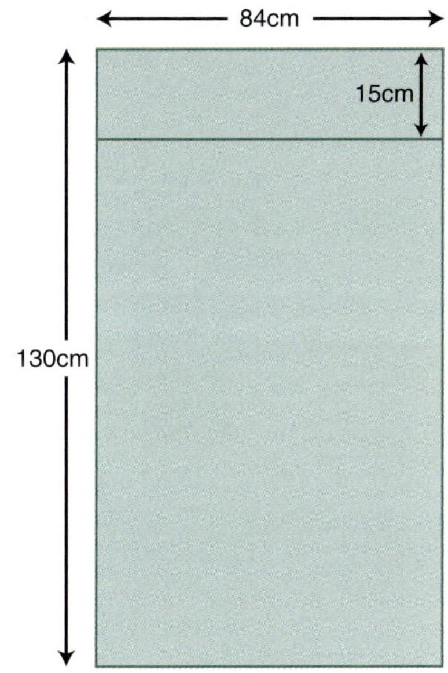

Leggings

FIG. 17.20 Leggings.

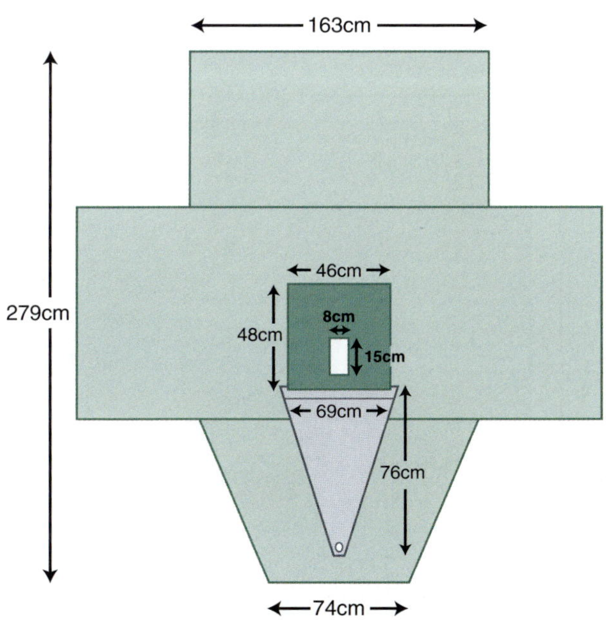

Perineal drape

FIG. 17.19 Perineal drape.

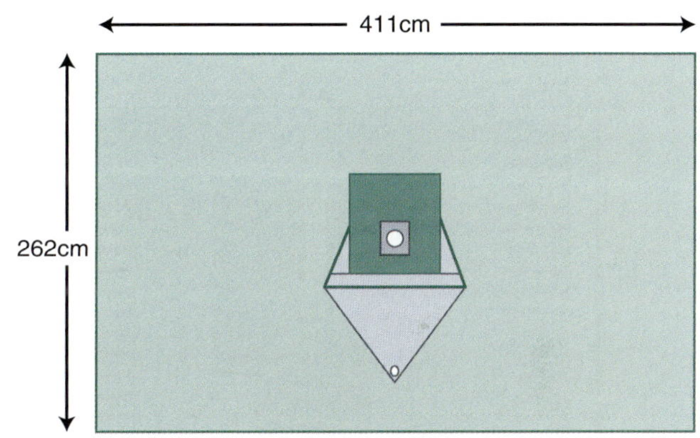

Shoulder drape

FIG. 17.21 Shoulder drape.

Examples are orthopedic procedures, craniotomy, gynecological, and urological surgery. The pouch is fitted with one or more exit ports for removing fluid from the pouch intraoperatively.

PERINEAL DRAPE AND LEGGINGS

The *perineal drape* is a T-shaped full-body drape used to accommodate the patient in the lithotomy position with two arm boards (Fig. 17.19). It is also equipped with leggings that fit over each foot and leg. A fluid collection pouch may be part of the drape or a separate component. *Leggings* (Fig. 17.20) are available separately or as an integral part of the body drape.

ROLLED STOCKINET

The rolled *stockinet* is a tubular drape closed at one end and covered with flexible impervious synthetic material. It is used to exclude a portion of the arm or leg during limb surgery.

SHOULDER DRAPE

The *shoulder* drape (Fig. 17.21) is a full-body drape with round or oval fenestration to accommodate the operative arm and shoulder with the patient in the beach chair (reclining) position. Note that for many shoulder procedures, the U-drape is used in conjunction with the shoulder drape.

THYROID DRAPE

The *thyroid* drape is a full-body drape with a small transverse fenestration near the head end (Fig. 17.22).

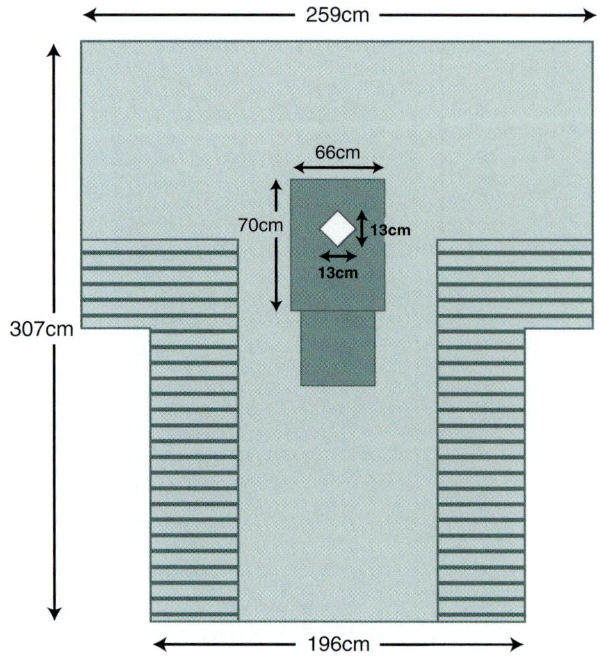

Thyroid drape

FIG. 17.22 Thyroid drape.

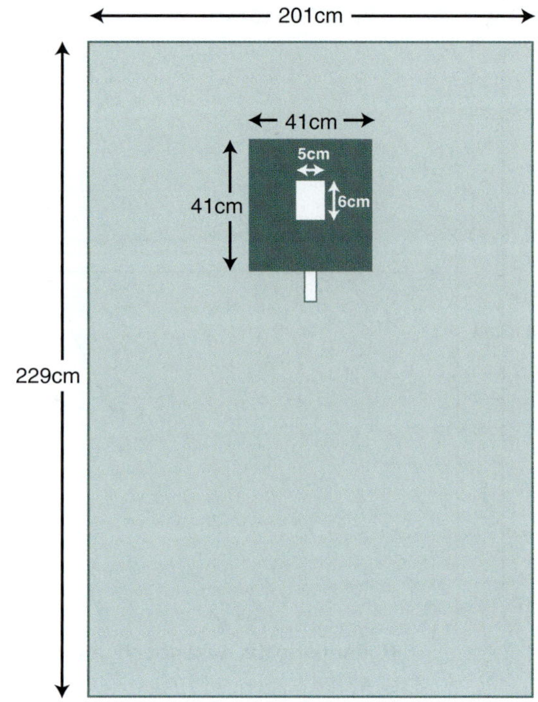

Ear drape

FIG. 17.24 Eye or ear drape.

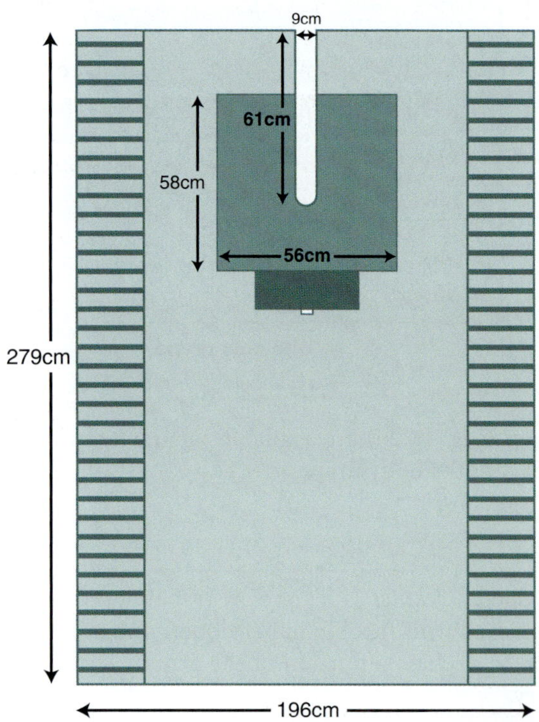

ENT split drape

FIG. 17.23 ENT drape.

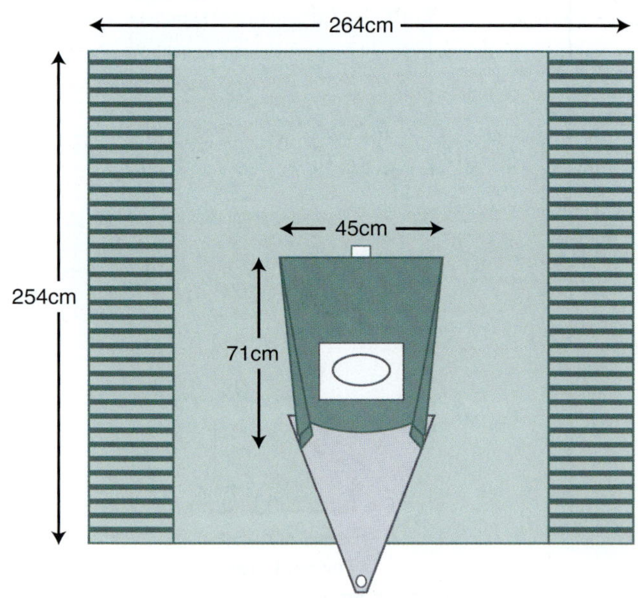

Craniotomy drape

FIG. 17.25 Craniotomy drape.

ENT DRAPE

The *ENT* drape is a full-body sheet with a small split at one end, which can be wrapped at the chin or below the nose for procedures of the nose, throat, or ear (Fig. 17.23).

EYE OR EAR DRAPE

The *eye* or *ear* drape is a ¾-size procedure drape with a small fenestration for exposure of the eye or ear (Fig. 17.24).

CRANIOTOMY DRAPE

The *craniotomy* drape is a full-body top drape with a round fenestration near the head end. It also includes a fluid collection pouch attached at the fenestration (Fig. 17.25).

TECHNIQUES USED IN DRAPING

Techniques used to drape are based on two principles:

1. All drapes are fan folded. The folded drape should be placed strategically so that it can be unfolded, one fold

at a time. This allows the drape to be controlled during application. When positioned correctly while still folded, the rest of the drape will also be in the correct position.

2. Each drape in the process is one of several layers. The order of the layers is standard—the first layer starts at the incision site and subsequent layers extend to the periphery. Fig. 17.26 illustrates, in schematic style, one method for applying drapes for a laparotomy incision.

All disposable procedure drapes (the uppermost drape) have printed instructions on the drape to indicate their correct orientation. Arrows and figures are shown plainly to help the user differentiate top from bottom, head end, and foot end. Utility drapes are used for general purposes and have no directional marks.

The rules of asepsis are followed throughout all draping procedures. When draping, visualize the drape as having two surfaces or sides. One side is in direct contact with the patient and nonsterile surfaces. The other side can come into contact only with other sterile surfaces, such as the gloved hand or sterile instruments. This principle follows the rules of asepsis.

The methods and materials used during draping depend on the anatomical site. Like many other areas of surgical practice, the exact methods and drapes used for an area of the body differ somewhat among surgeons. However, the basic principles are used universally. Methods described in this chapter are commonly used. Students should be aware of regional and facility variation and individual surgeons' preferences.

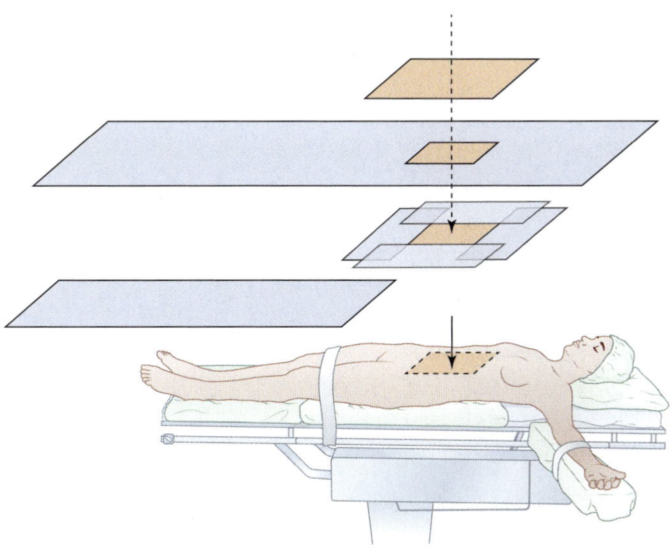

FIG. 17.26 Basic draping layers shown in order of placement, starting at the patient and moving upward on the figure. The first drape to be placed is the half sheet (also called *bottom sheet* or *plain sheet*). Next, four surgical towels frame the incision site. The first towel to be placed is the one closest to the person placing it. The next layer is the procedure drape with the fenestration (opening) placed directly over the exposed area created by the towels. Last to be placed is the transparent incise drape, which is self-adhering on the skin side. This stabilizes the top drape.

GUIDELINES FOR HANDLING DRAPES

The following guidelines support the principles of sterile technique during draping:

- *Handle drapes with as little movement as possible. This reduces the risk of contamination and prevents release of airborne particles that can become vehicles for bacteria.*
- When placing a drape, do not touch the patient's skin or any other nonsterile surface. Remain a safe distance from the patient to avoid contamination of your gown by an undraped area.
- After a drape has been placed, do not shift or move it. To protect the gloved hand during draping with flat sheets, *grasp the edge of the sterile sheet and roll your hand inward.* This forms a cuff. Position the drape and release the edge of the cuff, keeping your hands on the sterile side of the drape or towel.
- Use only nonpenetrating towel clamps for securing drapes. A hole in a drape creates a passageway for bacteria to contaminate the sterile field. When drapes are stapled to the patient's skin, the stapled area should be covered by an impervious (plastic) drape.
- To pass four towel drapes for squaring the incision, fold down the top edge about 4 inches. Present the first three folded towels by grasping the top corners with both hands and the folded sides facing away from the surgeon. The fourth towel is passed with the fold facing the surgeon. Adhesive towels are usually passed with the adhesive side facing away from the surgeon. After the surgeon has grasped the top edge, peel away the backing to expose the adhesive strip.
- After a drape has been placed, any portion that falls below the edge of the operating table is considered contaminated. If an area of the drape is suspected of being contaminated, the area may be covered with another impervious drape or the contaminated drape can be removed and a new sterile drape used. Keep your hands positioned above the level of the operating table during draping.
- After a drape has been placed, the edges are considered nonsterile.
- Do not reach over the prepped surgical site to place a towel or drape. Instead, move around the table to position yourself.
- *Strike-through* contamination occurs when a drape becomes soaked during surgery and solution penetrates to a nonsterile surface. Whenever possible, use only impervious drapes on areas likely to become soaked during surgery.
- Aluminum-coated drapes are used whenever laser surgery is planned. These deflect laser energy and prevent ignition in an oxygen-rich environment, especially in head and neck surgery.
- Plan ahead for draping. Verify the surgeon's procedure at the start of the case and stack drapes on the back table in reverse order of application. Have extra sterile towels and sheets available.

ABDOMEN

The procedure for draping the abdomen is the most basic technique and can be used to drape many other surgical sites, including the back, flank, and thorax (Fig. 17.27).

DRAPES REQUIRED

1. Four towels
2. Bottom sheet (half, ¾, or full plain sheet)
3. Top sheet (half, ¾, or full plain sheet
4. Laparotomy drape with or without arm board extensions
5. Incise drape (optional)

TECHNIQUE

1. A plain sheet is placed over the patient's lower body with the superior edge at the pubis and the lower edge allowed to fall over the foot of the operating table.
2. Four towels (folded cloth, disposable nonwoven material) are placed in a square to frame the operative site. These may be held in place with nonpenetrating towel clamps. Note that some surgeons prefer to place the towels first, and then the bottom sheet. Either technique is acceptable. A plastic incise drape may be applied over the towels as described above. Center a **fenestrated** body drape over the incision site and unfold it to provide a sterile field. The fenestrated drape (with a window) exposes only the surgical site while providing a wide area of sterile field around it.

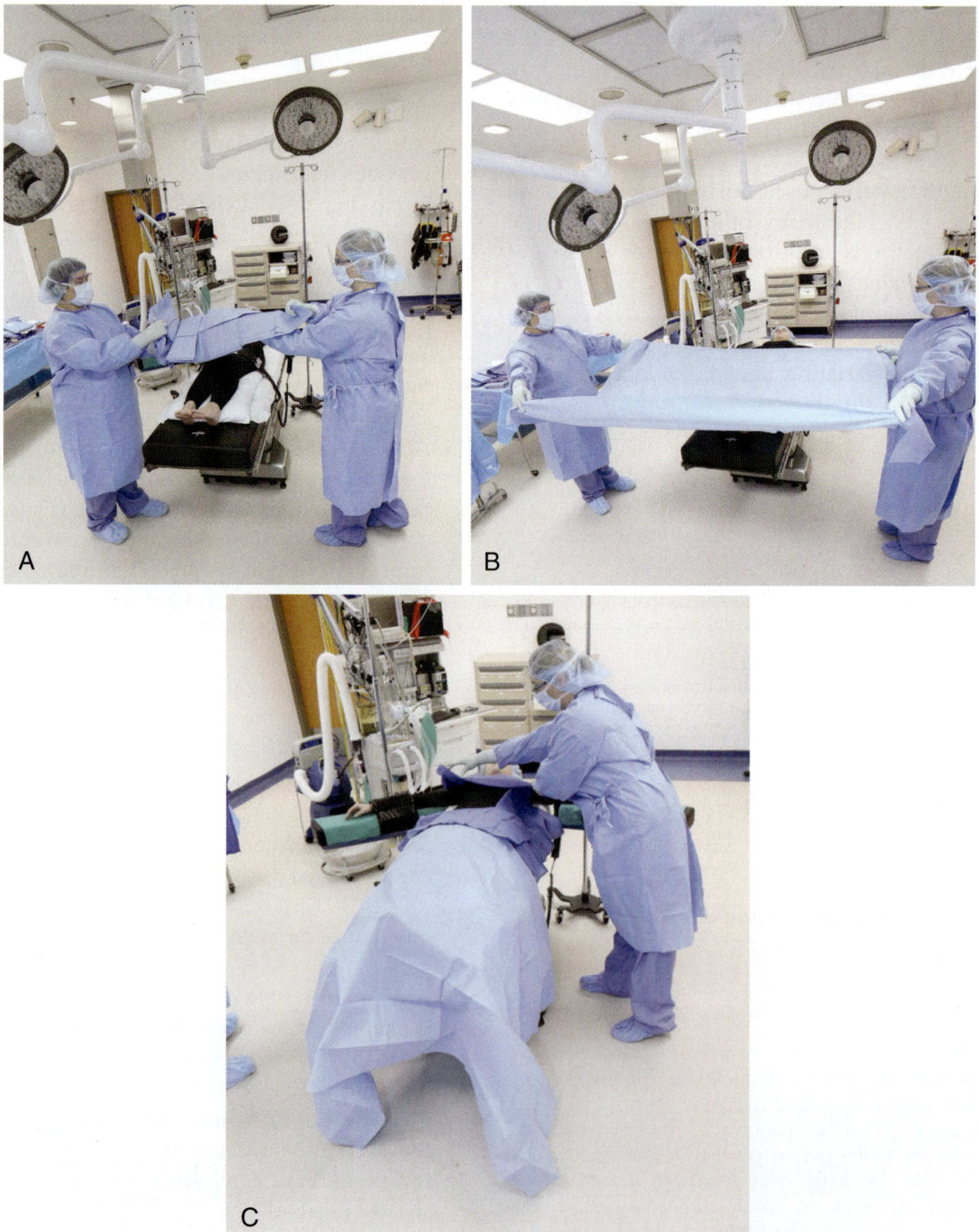

FIG. 17.27 Draping the abdomen. (A) The bottom sheet is applied. The drape is unfolded while keeping it suspended just above the patient. (B) The drape is extended. (C) Four surgical towels are used to square the incision site. Note the technique of cuffing the hand with the drape.

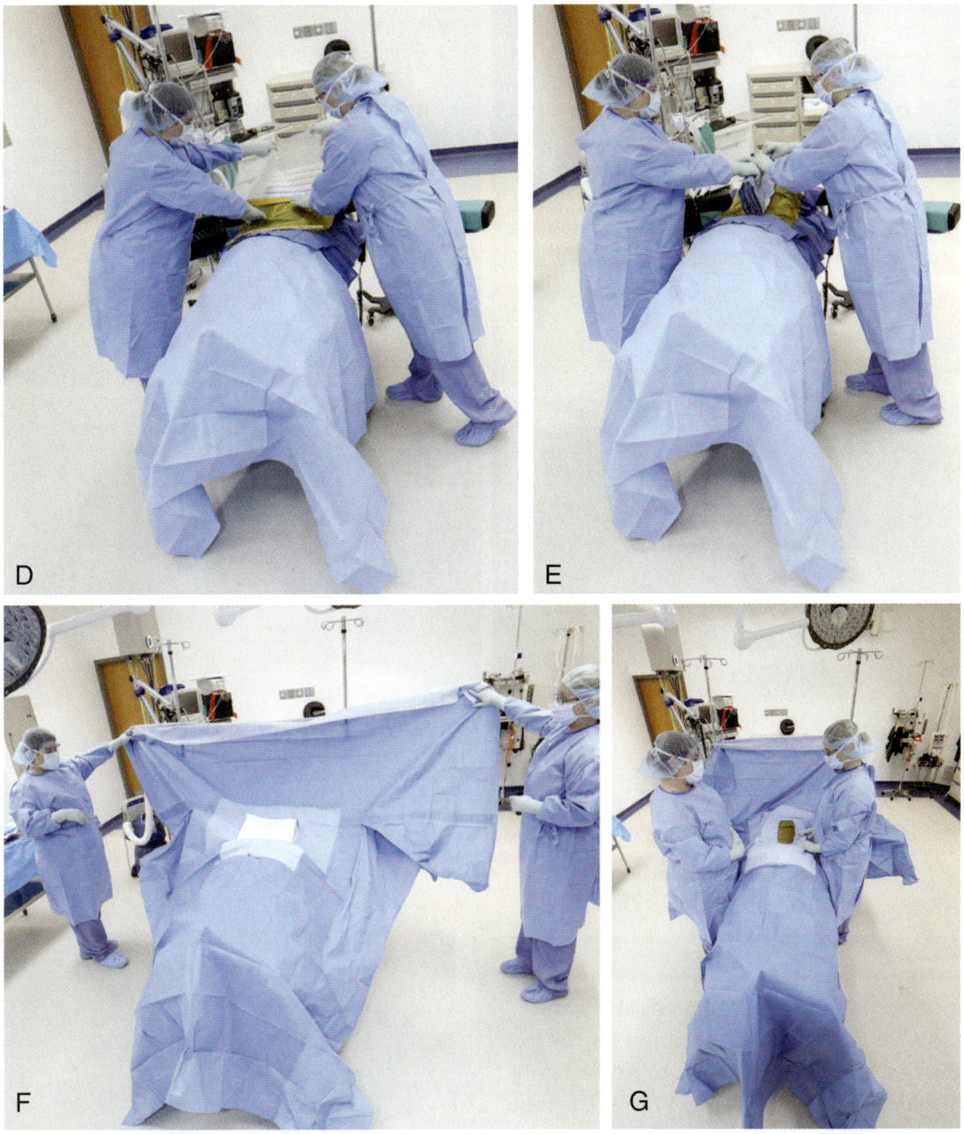

FIG. 17.27, cont'd (D) The adhesive drape is applied. The paper backing is peeled back as the drape is placed. (E) The laparotomy drape is centered over the incision site. (F) The top of the drape is extended to form the anesthesia screen. (G) Completed draping.

3. The anesthesia provider grasps the upper edges of the drape to form the anesthesia screen, which excludes the patient's head from the sterile field and allows access to the patient's airway.

LITHOTOMY (PERINEAL) DRAPING

Lithotomy, or perineal, draping is used for gynecological or transperineal surgery of the prostate and combined abdominal-perineal resection of the colon (Fig. 17.28).

DRAPES REQUIRED

1. Plastic towel drape for perineum
2. Under-buttocks drape or fluid collection drape
3. Four towel drapes for each incision site
4. Top sheet (half, ¾, or full plain sheet)
5. Perineal procedure drape or double-fenestration drape for abdomen and perineum

TECHNIQUE

1. For gynecological surgery, a barrier is necessary between the anus and the vulva. Apply an adhesive towel across the perineum midway between the vulva and anus.
2. Cloth or synthetic towels may be used to square off the perineum.
3. Drape the patient's legs and stirrups using leggings (or the perineal drape may have inserts that extend over the stirrups and the patient's legs).
4. Center a perineal drape over the incision site and extend it upward over the patient's abdomen and upper body.
5. For a combined abdominal-perineal resection or pelvic laparoscopy with uterine manipulation required: Square the abdominal incision site. A plain sheet may be used to cover the upper body. A procedure drape with two fenestrations is used.

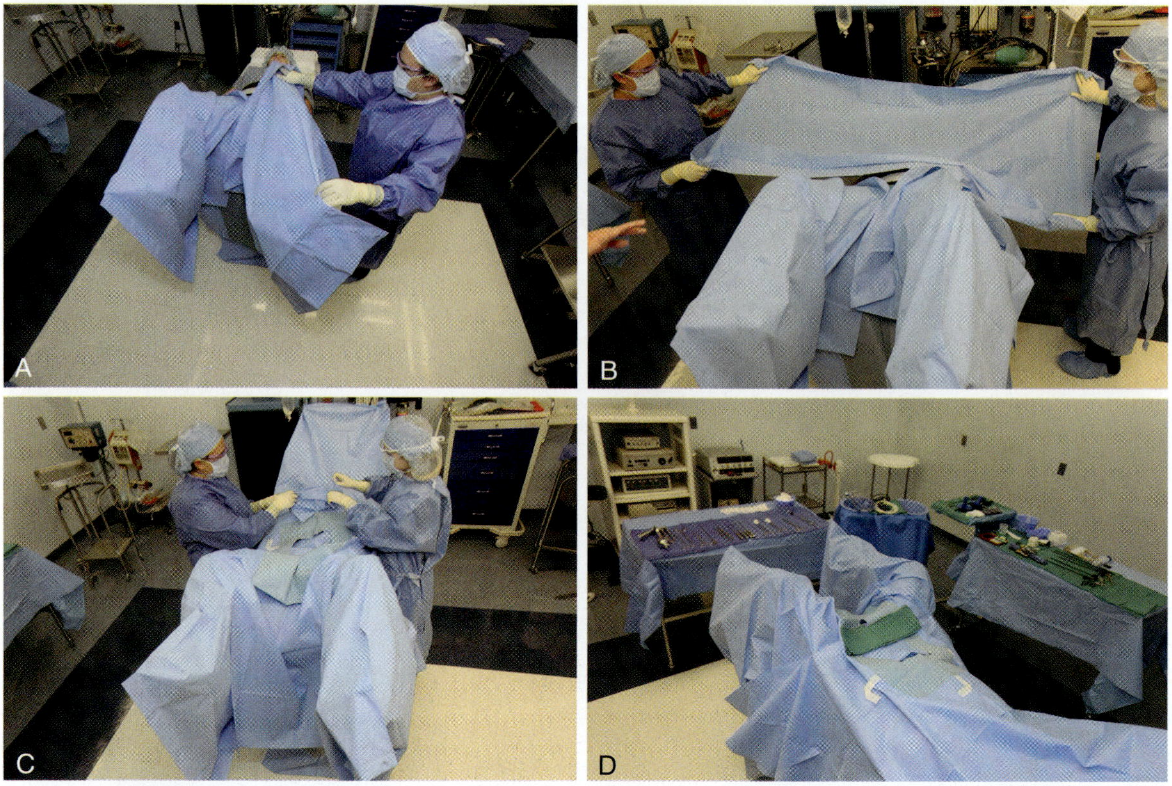

FIG. 17.28 Combination abdominal perineal drape, low lithotomy. (A) The leggings are applied. (B) The upper half sheet is unfolded and placed. (C) The fenestrated drape is centered and unfolded. (D) Draping completed with perineal cover in place and abdomen exposed.

LEG/HIP

The leg may be draped to expose only the upper or lower areas. A split drape can be used or one with a fenestration for the leg to be passed through. The hip may be draped to expose only the acetabulum and a wide area around it (Fig. 17.29). The foot is normally excluded from draping. In this case it is enveloped with towels or impervious drapes and wrapped with a flat or rolled adhesive drape.

DRAPES REQUIRED

1. Bottom drape to place under the elevated leg and foot
2. Impervious tube stockinet to fit over the foot if excluded
3. Surgical towel to cover tourniquet if used
4. Two split or U-drapes
5. Fenestrated top sheet

TECHNIQUE

1. A towel is wrapped around the pneumatic tourniquet and secured with a towel clip.
2. While the circulator suspends the leg to protect the prep site, a ¾ or half plain sheet is placed over the lower section of the operating table, extending from the patient's hips to the foot of the table.
3. The surgeon places the rolled stockinet over the patient's foot while taking it from the circulator. He or she unrolls the stockinet up to the edge of the incision site.
4. A split drape is positioned to expose the incision site with tails down.
5. The limb is inserted through the fenestration of an extremity drape, which is extended over the head of the table and attached to the anesthesia screen.

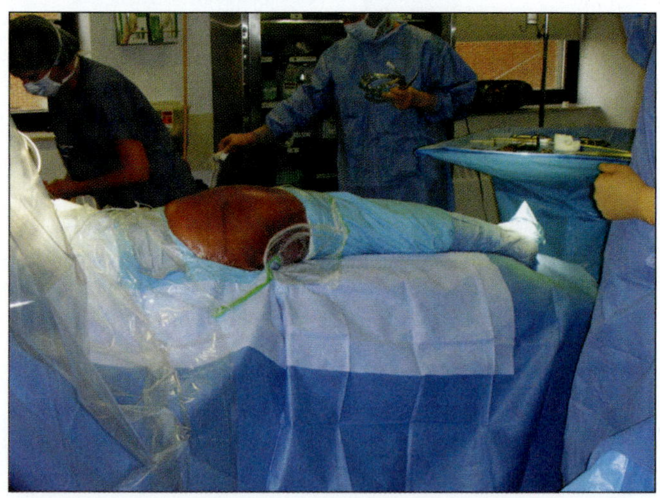

FIG. 17.29 Hip draping. Here the hip has been draped with the patient positioned on a standard operating table. A fenestrated drape with iodophor adhesive drape has been used. (From Schemitsch E, McKee M, eds. *Operative Techniques: Orthopedic Trauma Surgery*. Philadelphia: Saunders; 2010.)

KNEE

Draping for the knee is the same as the leg technique. The lower leg and foot are excluded. See Fig. 17.30.

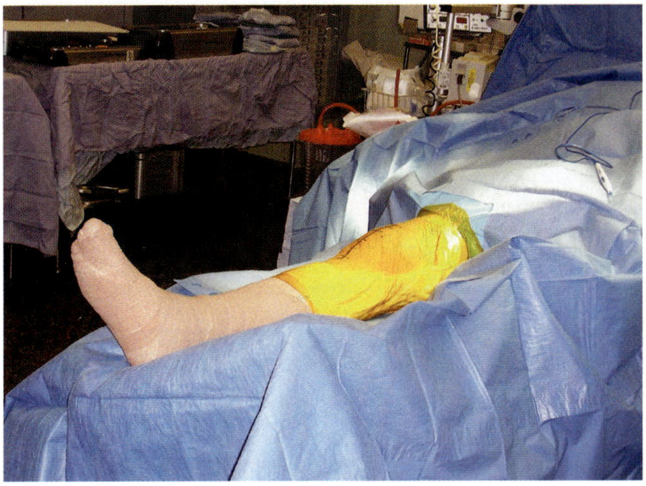

FIG. 17.30 Knee draping. The patient is in the supine position. The foot has been excluded with sterile impervious drapes and rolled bandages. A fenestrated drape has been placed over two split drapes. (From Canale S, Beaty J, eds. *Campbell's Operative Orthopaedics*. 12th ed. Philadelphia: Mosby; 2013.)

HAND

Hand procedures are often performed with the surgeon and assistant seated at a hand table. At the end of the skin prep, the circulator continues to suspend the operative hand above the hand table until the surgeon takes it for draping. A mechanical suspension device may also be used for this purpose.

DRAPES REQUIRED

1. Table drape—full or half sheet
2. Surgical towels to cover tourniquet
3. Tube stockinet (if hand is excluded from the sterile field)
4. Body drape—full or ¾ sheet
5. One or two split sheets
6. Extremity drape

TECHNIQUE

1. With the patient's prepped hand and forearm suspended, a plain half sheet is placed on the surgical arm board to cover it.
2. A surgical towel is wrapped around the proximal arm to cover the pneumatic tourniquet.
3. A tube stockinet may be used to cover the arm (optional).
4. A split sheet may be positioned at the forearm with the tails draped down toward the patient's hand.
5. The hand is placed through an extremity drape up to the forearm. The extremity drape is unfolded to cover the patient's body, with the upper edges forming the anesthesia screen (Fig. 17.31).

NOTE *The procedure for draping the arm is identical to that for the hand, with exceptions. The hand is excluded from the prep and draped with a towel and impervious stockinet. The extremity drape is positioned at the proximal side of the incision site with the remainder used to drape the patient's body.*

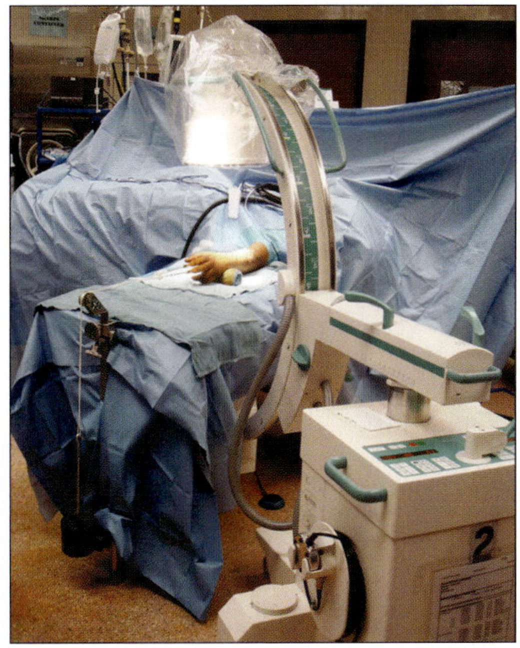

FIG. 17.31 Draping for the arm or hand using a hand table. The arm has been placed through the fenestrated drape and a full-body drape applied. Here traction has been applied to the hand. (From Schemitsch E, McKee M, eds. *Operative Techniques: Orthopedic Trauma Surgery*. Philadelphia: Saunders; 2010.)

SHOULDER

The shoulder is draped with the patient in the beach chair position or with the use of a shoulder chair. The patient's head is secured in a padded head rest. The arm is suspended away from the body, with the hand and lower arm excluded from the surgical site. The arm is draped free so that it can be manipulated during surgery. In this draping procedure, the entire shoulder, including the posterior aspect, is exposed to allow full manipulation of the joint during surgery (Fig. 17.32).

DRAPES REQUIRED

1. Full plain sheet
2. Incise drape
3. Four surgical towels
4. Two U-drapes
5. Extremity (shoulder) drape

TECHNIQUE

1. With the circulator suspending the arm by holding the patient's hand, an impervious sheet is positioned over the patient's torso up to the axillary line.
2. An impervious tube stockinet is threaded over the hand and arm up to the lower edge of the operative site.

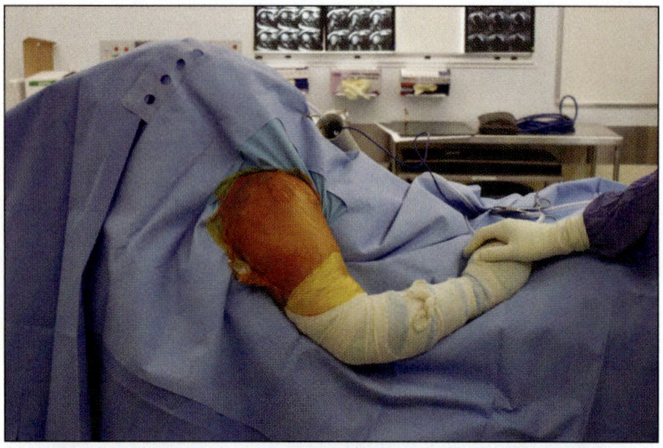

FIG. 17.32 Shoulder draping. The patient is in the beach chair position. The lower arm has been wrapped and excluded. Two U-drapes have been placed around the surgical site, followed by a fenestrated shoulder drape with impervious insert. This was followed by an iodophor impregnated adhesive drape. (From Lee D, Neviaser R, eds. *Operative Techniques: Shoulder and Elbow Surgery*. Philadelphia: Saunders; 2011.)

3. An impervious U-drape with adhesive edge is positioned at the axilla with tails up. The adhesive border of the U is then exposed by removing the paper tabs, and the U is pressed into place. The entire shoulder, front and back, is encircled with the adhesive edge of the drape.
4. A second adhesive U-drape is positioned at the top of the shoulder with tails facing down. This drape is pressed into place, again encircling and exposing the entire shoulder. The long extension of the drape is used to cover the torso and anesthesia screen.
5. A third impervious U-drape with fluid collection pouch is placed over the edges of the previous U-drape, and the long end is positioned over the patient's torso and lower body. If the lower body is not covered, a plain sheet can be placed over the exposed area to extend the sterile field.

Watch Chapter 17: Draping on the Evolve website: http://evolve.elsevier.com/Fuller/surgical.

FACE

The *head drape* is used for exposure of the face, nose, and throat.

DRAPES REQUIRED

1. Full or ¾ plain sheet
2. Half plain sheet
3. Two surgical towels
4. Optional plastic towel drapes
5. Split drape

TECHNIQUE

1. A plain sheet is draped over the patient up to the chin.
2. The patient's head is slightly elevated and a half plain sheet is placed under the head.
3. Two surgical towels are placed over the plain sheet under the head.
4. The corners of the top towel are crossed over the patient's eyes to cover them. These are secured with a nonpenetrating towel clip. Note: a plain sheet may be used in place of the surgical towel.
5. A split drape may be positioned at the patient's chin, with tails up. These are secured with a towel clip. Fig. 17.33 illustrates the head drape.

EYE

The eye is draped to exclude the entire face and head, exposing only the operative eye. The hairline may be excluded with a head drape before the eye itself is draped. Fig. 17.34 illustrates the eye drape with lashes held away from the surgical site.

DRAPES REQUIRED

1. Full or ¾ plain sheet
2. Optional head drape
3. Optional spilt drape
4. Fenestrated plastic eye drape

TECHNIQUE

1. A full-body or ¾ plain sheet is used to cover the patient's upper body.
2. A head drape may be applied as described above, or a plain sheet with adhesive edge may be positioned over the hairline.
3. A fenestrated plastic eye drape is placed over the operative eye. This drape adheres to the patient's eyelids and holds the eyelashes away from the surgical field.
4. A split sheet may be applied at the patient's neck. However, the eye drape extends over the face, excluding the airways and nonoperative eye.

CRANIOTOMY

Draping for a cranial procedure is similar to that for other routines that require a large body sheet with a fenestration. Cranial access is usually obtained with the patient in the prone position using a Mayfield headrest or in the beach chair position. This allows the anesthesia care provider access to the patient's airway while providing access to the cranium. Draping for a craniotomy can be performed with one specialty drape, which is designed for this purpose, and one or two plain sheets to ensure body coverage.

DRAPES REQUIRED

1. Optional ¾ body sheet
2. Fenestrated craniotomy drape

TECHNIQUE

1. Position a body sheet at the neck and extend it to the lower edge of the operating table (optional).

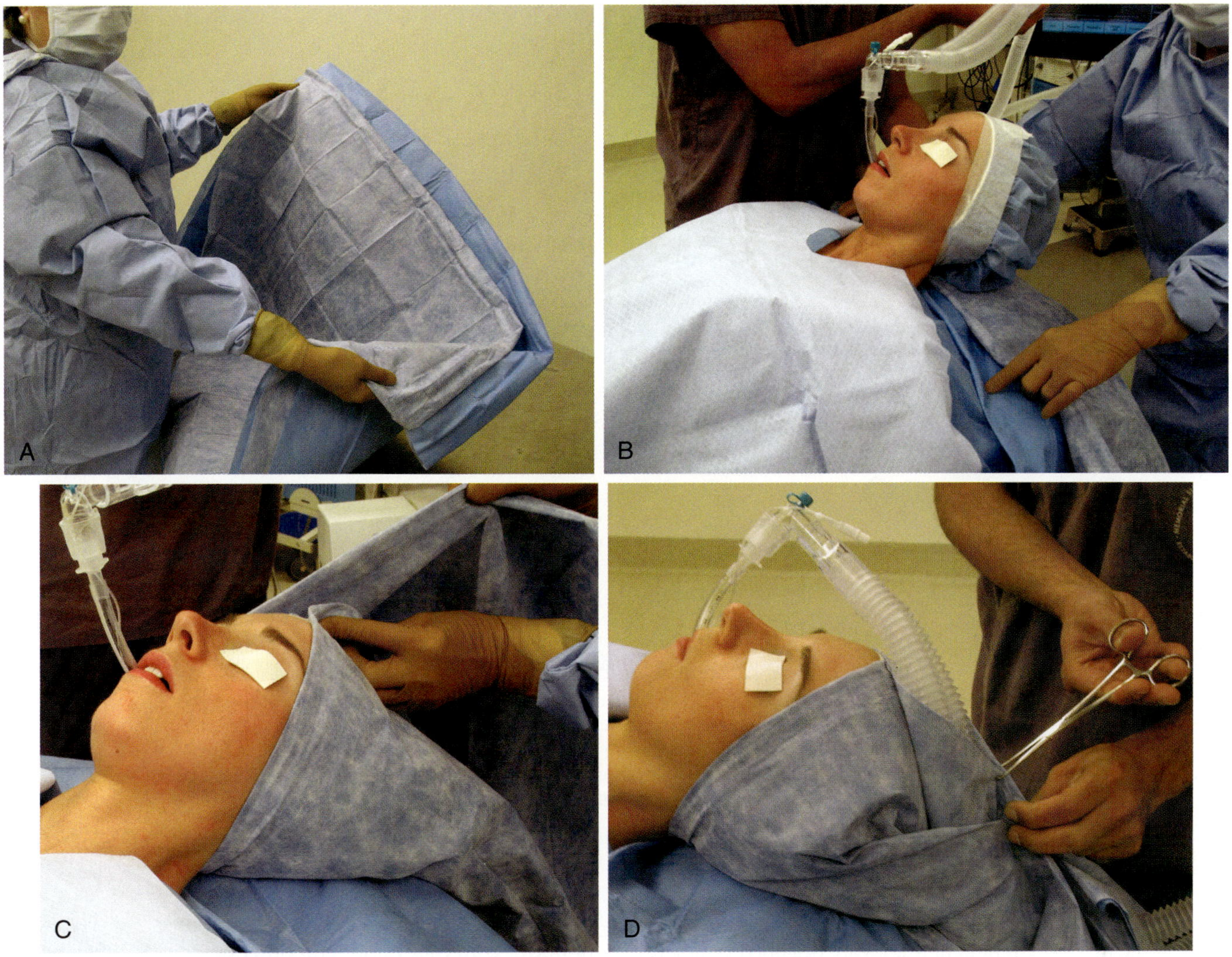

FIG. 17.33 Head drape for exposure to the face. (A) Two folded sheets are placed over each other. (B) Both sheets are placed under the patient's head while the anesthesia provider lifts the head. (C) The top sheet is brought over the patient's forehead and clamped. (D) The anesthesia tubing is secured. (From Shah J, ed. *Jatin Shah's Head and Neck Surgery and Oncology*. 4th ed. Philadelphia: Mosby Elsevier; 2012.)

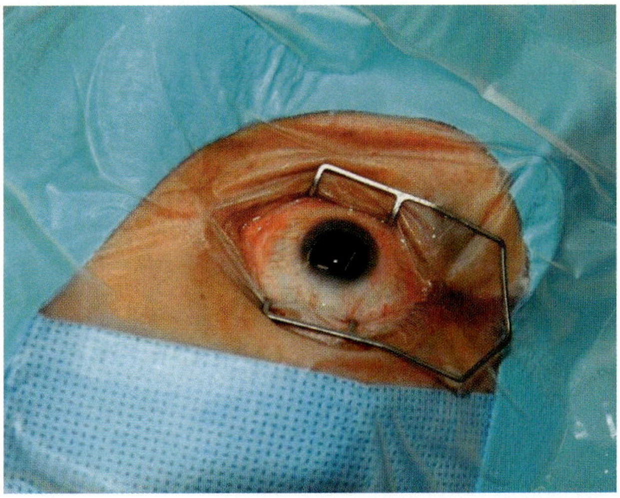

FIG. 17.34 Eye drape. A fenestrated eye drape and full-body cover have been placed. An adhesive eye drape has been placed over the top to secure the patient's eyelashes. (From Spaeth G, Danesh-Mayer H, Goldberg I, Kampik A, eds. *Ophthalmic Surgery Principles and Practice*. 4th ed. Philadelphia: Elsevier; 2012.)

2. Observe the orientation marks on the drape. Remove the adhesive backing from the first portion and place the drape with the plastic portion centered over the incision site. Press the adhesive section gently over the cranium.
3. Slowly unfold the drape to cover the neck area.
4. Some craniotomy drapes contain an adhesive section that is positioned over the patient's upper torso to increase stability. Remove the paper backing over this adhesive square and press the square into place at the chest (patient in beach chair position) or upper back (patient in prone position).
5. Unfold the drape to completely cover the patient.
6. Position the fluid collection pouch.
7. An additional plain sheet may be required to attach to the anesthesia screen.

DRAPING EQUIPMENT

Large equipment, such as the operating microscope, C-arm, and robotic components used within the sterile field, are draped

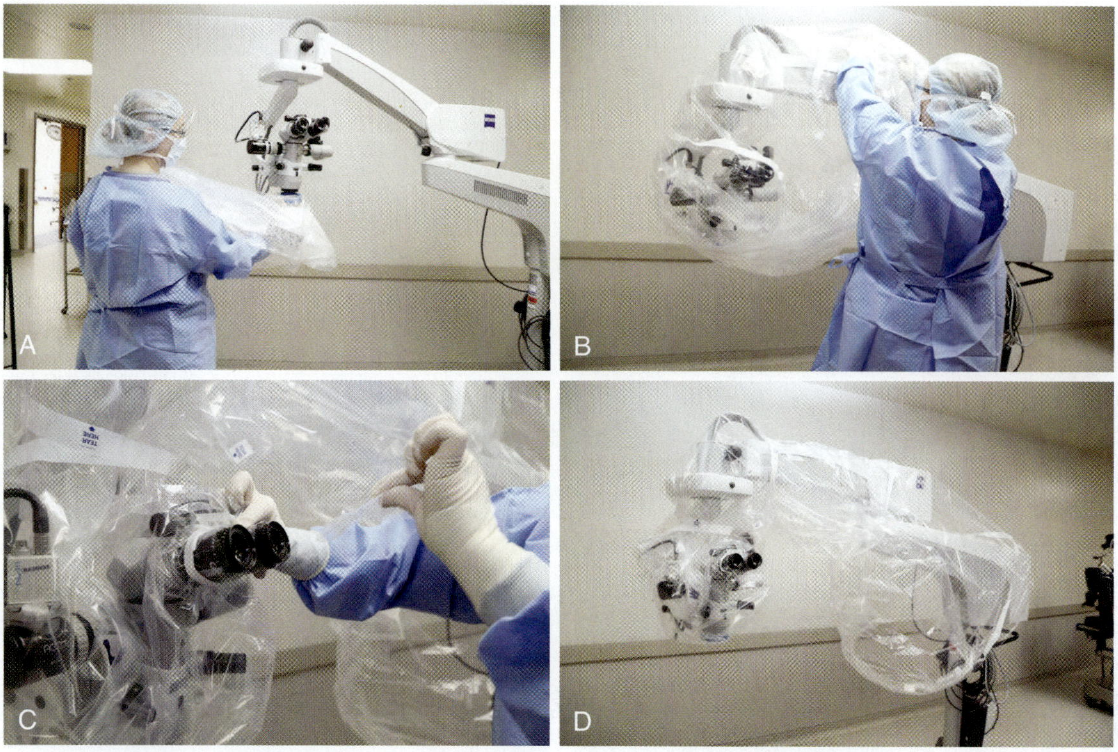

FIG. 17.35 Microscope drape. (A) With hands and arms protected under a wide cuff, the surgical technologist slips the drape over the uppermost area of the microscope. The circulator may assist by grasping the inner side of the drape and advancing it further. (B) The drape is further advanced while the wide cuff is maintained. (C) The ocular fittings are placed over the eyepieces and pulled back to expose the eyepiece. The adhesive strips are wrapped around the eyepiece to hold it in place. (D) The completed draping.

before surgery. Most equipment drapes are designed to fit with cutouts and ample material to allow smooth draping. Adhesive strips and drape openings are imprinted with arrows and directions. The circulator assists during equipment draping by grasping the nonsterile edges of the drape and pulling it into place.

When the operating microscope is to be used immediately during a case, it is draped before the patient prep. If it will not be used for an hour or more after the case begins, it can be draped during the procedure.

The single-use microscope drape is a continuous plastic sleeve that is fan-folded for easy application. The drape has "pockets" that cover the protruding parts of the scope. The scrub starts the draping. The circulator assists by pulling the drape down by holding the bottom portion, which will be outside the sterile field after the drape is in place. The ocular portions and optics of the microscope are not covered. The drape is secured over the lenses with sterile caps. After the drape is in place, it is loosely bound to the body of the microscope with adherent tapes that are an integral part of the drape itself (Fig. 17.35). The C-arm drape, like the microscope drape, is made of clear plastic and has a tubular design.

REMOVING DRAPES

At the close of a procedure, all instruments and equipment are removed from the top drape, including the sterile sections of power cords, air hoses, and other devices that may become tangled in drapes as they are removed. One or more layers of dressings are placed over the incision and any drain sites. One member of the sterile team holds the dressings in place while the drapes are slowly removed. When removing drapes, pull them carefully away from the patient. Drapes should be contained and removed with as little air disturbance as possible to prevent the release of airborne contaminants. As all the drapes are removed, disposable materials are placed in a designated biohazard bag.

KEY CONCEPTS

- *The surgical prep and draping process follows specific standards, which have been set by the Centers for Disease Control and Prevention in coordination with other professional agencies. The primary focus of practice relates to the use of specific antiseptics to perform the skin prep.*
- *It is not possible to sterilize the skin because it is living tissue. Skin and mucous membranes harbor resident bacteria, which are beneficial to the immune system, and nonresident flora, which are potential causes of surgical site infection. Before surgery, the incision site must be made as clean as possible to reduce the risk of postoperative infection.*
- *The materials needed for urinary catheterization must be assembled before the procedure and maintained on a small sterile field during the process. The exact type and size of*

catheter system is determined by the age and gender of the patient and by the surgeon's orders.
- *Some surgical procedures require decompression of the bladder or intraoperative monitoring of urinary output. In these cases, urinary catheterization is performed just before or during the surgical skin prep.*
- *Patient safety and risks associated with catheterization include injury to the urethra, damage to the sphincter muscle, and urinary tract infection. Prevention of these outcomes requires thorough knowledge of the anatomy, familiarity with the equipment used, and use of strict aseptic techniques.*
- *Hair is not removed from the surgical site unless there is no possible way to exclude it from the surgical wound.*
- *It is required practice for the surgeon to mark the skin site of the incision before surgery. This documents the correct side and location of the incision for comparison with the patient records to prevent wrong-site surgery. These marks must be preserved during the skin prep.*
- *Antiseptics are labeled for use on skin. However, not all antiseptics can be used on all surface tissue or mucous membranes. Labeling includes warnings and contraindications that clearly indicate the safe and unsafe uses of the antiseptic.*
- *Supplies for the skin prep include the prescribed antiseptic (contained in a single-patient container), sterile towels, and gloves; they may also include other items such as cotton balls, cotton-tipped applicators, or scrub sponges according to the type of prep.*
- *When the skin is prepped correctly, the area is antiseptically cleaned from the center of the incisional site to the periphery. Application of prep antiseptic in a spiral or circular pattern is used to prevent contamination of the prepped area by microbes in the area not yet prepped.*
- *Elements of the skin prep include obtaining and setting up sterile supplies, draping the prep site, and applying prep solution according to standards of practice. Specific details that may not be standard are prescribed by the surgeon.*
- *Skin burning and blistering occur when prep solution pools between the patient's skin and the operating table surface. This is prevented by the placement of sterile towels at the periphery of the prep area, making a conscious effort to prevent the solution from pooling on the skin.*
- *Surgical drapes are put in place after the prep antiseptic has dried thoroughly. The drape forms a sterile covering over the patient's body, leaving the incision site accessible through an opening in the drape.*
- *Drapes extend far beyond the incisional site so that sterile equipment, instruments, and the sterile team members have freedom of movement within the sterile field.*
- *Elements of the draping technique include preparation of the sterile drapes on the back table, delivering the drapes to the surgeon in the correct order, assisting in correct placement of each drape, and maintaining sterility.*
- *Draping is a sterile process that is performed according to the rules of aseptic techniques. It is important to remember the sterile boundaries that are consistent with any sterile surface.*
- *If a drape becomes contaminated within the sterile boundary during its placement, it must be discarded and a new sterile drape obtained. Likewise, if the sterile gloved hand comes into contact with a nonsterile surface, the glove must be changed.*
- *Drapes are removed at the close of surgery in a particular way to prevent contamination of the incision side and to contain blood and body fluids.*

REVIEW QUESTIONS

1. Describe the risks of urinary catheterization.
2. Why is continuous urinary drainage required during surgery?
3. Explain how to maintain sterility while inserting the catheter.
4. Explain the rationale for surgical skin prep.
5. During the skin prep for a contaminated region, the area of highest contamination is prepped last. Why is this?
6. What is the rationale for surgical draping?
7. What is the purpose of aluminum-coated drapes?
8. What parts of a drape are considered nonsterile after the drape is in place?
9. What techniques are used to prevent contamination of the gloved hands while draping the patient?

CASE STUDIES

CASE 1

You are assisting in the circulator role and have been asked to perform the patient skin prep for a laparoscopy. When you expose the surgical site to begin the prep, you see that a body-piercing stud is embedded in the patient's umbilicus. You do not see any wire or post attached to the stud. You have not encountered this type of body-piercing jewelry before and are unable to ascertain how to remove it safely. The patient has already been anesthetized. Using skills and knowledge learned in this and other chapters, what is your course of action? Consider carefully patient safety with regard to electrosurgery, aseptic techniques, legal issues, and care of the patient's property.

BIBLIOGRAPHY

Association of periOperative Registered Nurses. *Guidelines for Perioperative Practice.* Denver: AORN; 2015.

Association of periOperative Registered Nurses (AORN). Recommended practices for preoperative patient skin antisepsis. In *2015 Perioperative Standards and Recommended Practices.* Denver: AORN; 2015.

Barnes S. Surgical site infection prevention in 2018 and beyond. *AORN J.* 2018;107(5).

Centers for Disease Control and Prevention. *Catheter-Associated Urinary Tract Infections (CAUTI); 2009. Edited 2017. https://www.cdc.gov/infectioncontrol/guidelines/cauti/. Accessed July 19, 2019.*

fur6Cowperthwaite L., Holm R.L.. Guideline implementation: preoperative patient skin antisepsis. *AORN J.* 2015;101(1):71–77.

Healthcare Infection Control Practices Advisory Committee. *Recommendations From the CDC Guideline for Hand Hygiene in Healthcare Settings.*

18 SURGICAL SKILLS I: PLANNING A CASE, OPENING, AND START OF SURGERY

KNOWLEDGE AND SKILLS REVIEW

The following skills and knowledge should be reviewed before you start this chapter:
Sterile technique
Documentation
Surgical instruments

LEARNING OBJECTIVES

After studying this chapter, the reader will be able to:

1. List and define common terms used in surgical technique
2. Discuss the elements of a case plan
3. Explain surgical objectives and how they can be grouped into types
4. Discuss the purpose of preoperative case preparation
5. Describe the correct procedure for performing a count
6. Discuss the guidelines for preventing lost and retained items

TERMINOLOGY

Blunt dissection: The technique of separating tissue layers by teasing them apart with a rough sponge dissector, blunt instrument, or manually.

Case planning: Systematic preparation for a surgical procedure.

Count: A systematic method of accounting for items that may be retained in the patient during surgery.

Dissecting sponge: A small compact sponge used to dissect soft tissue planes; also referred to as a sponge dissector. The dissecting sponge is always mounted on a clamp for use in the surgical wound.

Event related: An activity or process linked with an event.

Graft: An implant used to replace or augment existing tissue. A graft may be obtained from the patient, another person, an animal source, or synthetic or biosynthetic materials.

Implant: Any medical device placed in the body with the intention to be permanent or semi-permanent.

Radiopaque: Any object that is not penetrable by x-rays.

Raytec: A surgical sponge folded to 4 inches by 4 inches. The Raytec derives its name from one of the companies that manufactures surgical sponges.

Sterile setup: The process of organizing and arranging sterile supplies and equipment before surgery to create the sterile field.

Surgeon's preference card: A database or card system listing the methods, materials, and techniques used by each surgeon for specific procedures.

TIMEOUT: Time set aside before the start of surgery to allow implementation of Universal Protocol. During TIMEOUT, all other activities are suspended to allow each member of the surgical team to participate in the Protocol.

Universal Protocol: A procedure for verifying the patient's identity, correct surgical procedure, site, and side and other important information. The procedure is initiated as a TIMEOUT and takes place after the patient has been positioned, prepped, and draped but before the first incision.

This chapter and the next are focused on the skills of the surgical technologist, in a time-related sequence. This chapter begins with case planning, relating the surgery to the instruments, equipment, and supplies needed for that specific surgery. Case planning flows into the nonsterile skills in *opening a case* and then to the *sterile setup,* which occurs just before surgery begins. Table 18.1 shows the responsibilities of the surgeon, the scrubbed surgical technologist, and the circulator *from case planning to the start of surgery*.

Chapter 19 focuses on the principles and basic *surgical assistance skills* and management of the surgical wound. The sequence begins as the surgery starts and finishes at the close of surgery, patient transfer, and decontamination of the OR suite. Chapter 19 also includes an important section on the management of surgical sponges, including types and uses during a surgical procedure.

IMPORTANT TO KNOW *Many of the tasks and procedures carried out in surgery are coordinated between the registered perioperative nurse and the surgical technologist. Guidelines and requirements for the perioperative nurse have been established for specific tasks that she or he has a responsibility to carry out. Likewise, the ST is accountable for specific tasks carried out in the sterile role during surgery. Coordination and communication during surgery are key to ensuring compliance with all professional guidelines for the surgical technologist and the registered perioperative nurse.*

SURGICAL TERMS

Throughout the history of surgery, specific terms have evolved that describe the techniques used during the surgical procedure and the surgical environment. Surgical technologists should learn these basic terms because they are the common language of surgery used in every operating room. Increasing their surgical vocabulary also enables students to understand teaching videos in which a surgical procedure has been filmed with an audio description.

- **Amputate:** Usually refers to the surgical removal of a limb or digit. When other body parts are referred to, the term *remove* or *surgical removal* is used: for example, "The tumor spread to the spleen, which required surgical removal."
- **Anastomose (verb), anastomosis (noun):** The joining of two hollow anatomical structures (vessels, ducts, tubes, or hollow organs) using sutures, surgical staples, or other means. For example, "An anastomosis was created between the distal jejunum and colon." An anastomosis is performed to restore continuity, usually after a section has been surgically removed. When the term is used, it is preceded by the anatomical structures involved: for example, an arteriovenous anastomosis (between an artery and vein).
- **Approximate:** In surgical terms, to "bring together" tissues by suturing or other means. For example, "The skin edges are approximated using fine nylon sutures." We *approximate* bone fragments in a fracture, tissues (especially the edges), and edges of hollow ducts and vessels.
- **Blunt dissection:** Separation of tissue without using sharp instruments. Blunt dissection is used to tease apart delicate tissue layers using a **dissecting sponge,** which has a relatively rough surface. The fingers are also used in blunt dissection to manually separate tissue bands or fibers when sharp dissection is unnecessary or may result in excessive bleeding.
- **Debridement:** The use of sharp surgical instruments such as a scalpel and scissors to cut away dead tissue or remove debris embedded in a wound. Water under pressure called is also used for this purpose. Traumatic wounds generally require debridement to heal. Debridement is also performed on infected wounds to remove nonviable tissue.
- **Dog ear:** In suture technique, an undesirable pucker in the skin as a result of poor suture placement. A dog ear must be corrected because the puckered edges do not come together during healing and can lead to infection.
- **Debulk:** In cancer surgery, to remove a large portion, but not all, of a tumor. This is done to relieve pressure on nearby tissues and before chemotherapy or radiotherapy to enable a reduction in these treatment modalities.
- **Dissect:** Carefully separate anatomical structures with instruments, small firm sponges, or the fingers. For example, surgery on large blood vessels requires meticulous separation of the vessels away from the surrounding connective tissue. Sharp dissection is performed with scissors, whereas blunt dissection is performed with the fingers or dissecting sponges mounted on a clamp.
- **Elevate:** To raise or lift an anatomical structure, sometimes without removing it. Occasionally, during surgery, it is necessary to lift a structure using a retractor or other instrument to pass sutures or instruments underneath, or for better visualization. Instruments called *elevators* are often used to peel away superficial tissue. For example, a periosteal elevator is used to lift away a portion of the periosteum that covers the long bones of the body. This is necessary before cutting the bone. Elevators used in neurosurgery are used for fine separation but not for cutting neural tissue. In facial reconstruction, fine-tipped elevators are used to separate delicate tissue layers such as the nasal submucosa from the underlying cartilage.
- **Excise:** To remove tissue, usually a small lesion, using cutting instruments or electrosurgery. For example, "The tumor was excised using scissors and a #15 scalpel blade." This term generally applies to small or superficial lesions. For example, moles and small skin tumors are excised, but lobes of the lung are *removed.*
- **Expose (verb), exposure (noun):** To enable precise viewing of an anatomical area. For example, a retractor is used to move or hold tissue aside so that other structures underneath can be *exposed.* During surgery, the surgeon may say, "I need better exposure here." This may mean more effective retraction to see the tissues deep in the surgical wound.
- **Exteriorize:** To bring a tissue structure partially outside the body. For example, during bowel surgery, a section of intestine may be temporarily brought out of the surgical wound (exteriorized) for suturing or other surgical maneuvers. During cesarean section, the uterus may be exteriorized briefly to repair the muscle incision.

TABLE 18.1 Responsibilities of the Scrubbed Surgical Technologist, Circulator, and Surgeon

Scrubbed Surgical Technologist	Circulator	Surgeon
BEFORE SURGERY		
Receives case cart for surgery and selects additional items needed from instrument and supply rooms. Assembles all items needed for surgery according to the surgeon's case information. Orients furniture in the room in accordance with surgery. Opens sterile equipment and instruments using sterile technique. Protects the sterile equipment from contamination. Performs surgical hand antisepsis. After hand antisepsis, the surgical technologist is a "sterile" team member.	Positions the operating table and prepares positioning devices and accessories according to the surgery. Assembles needed equipment. Connects suction canisters to ceiling or wall mounts. Tests suction pressure. Keeps the operating room doors closed. Obtains imaging output or other diagnostic reports needed during surgery. Opens sterile supplies. *Selects medications and drugs for use during surgery. *Reviews operative checklist. Witnesses signing of operative or anesthesia permit. Checks all permits. Notes operative side and surgeon's mark or signature on operative side. *Assesses patient's psychosocial condition. *Measures vital signs and performs assessment. *Answers patient's questions about surgery and postoperative care. Transfers patient to operating room. Transfers patient to operating room bed using safe technique. Applies safety strap over patient. Provides warm blankets for patient.	Greets patient in holding area. Orients patient and family. Answers patient's questions. Ensures that permits are signed and witnessed. Identifies operative side and site. If patient is to be placed in complex position, assists after anesthesia induction. Along with surgical assistants, performs surgical hand antisepsis or may scrub after positioning patient following induction.
BEFORE THE SKIN INCISION IS MADE		
Participates in the surgical count. Gowns and gloves self-using sterile technique. Drapes Mayo stand. Places sterile instrument trays in position on back table. Separates sharps (e.g., scalpel blades, needles) from other equipment to avoid injury during setup. Sorts drapes and surgical gowns in order of use. According to the specific surgery, prepares instruments, sutures, devices, solutions, and medications. Protects the surgical setup from contamination. Performs the initial instrument, sponge, and needle count. Receives medications from circulator using correct technique. When setup is complete, waits *within the sterile field*. Hands each surgeon/assistant a sterile towel to dry hands. Gowns and gloves each sterile team member. Hands individual draping materials to surgeon and assistants. Participates in draping, maintaining sterility. Moves Mayo stand into position. Secures suction tubing and power and light cords to top drape. Hands off cords for attachment to power sources. Provides light handle covers to the surgeon.	Participates in the surgical count. Secures scrubbed surgical technologist's gown. Secures surgeons' gowns. Performs the instrument, sponge, and needle count with the scrubbed surgical technologist. *Distributes medications to scrubbed surgical technologist. Prepares nonsterile equipment. *Assists anesthesiologist during anesthesia induction and intubation. Assists in the correct positioning of the patient for surgery. *Carefully applies grounding pads to the patient for use of electrosurgical device. May perform skin preparation. Completes connections to suction, power, electrosurgical unit, and other energy devices sources to be used. Advocates for patient safety during the procedure.	May perform skin preparation. With assistants, enters operating suite from scrub area. Along with assistants, is gowned and gloved by surgical technologist. With assistants and surgical technologist, drapes patient.
Participates in Universal Protocol (TIMEOUT).	Leads Universal Protocol (TIMEOUT).	Leads and participates in Universal Protocol (TIMEOUT).

*Licensed Registered Nurse responsibility.

- **Ligate:** To constrict a vessel or duct using a suture tie. The most common use of this term is ligation of blood vessels. However, the surgeon may also ligate a duct or tissue bundle containing blood vessels.
- **Resection:** A surgical procedure in which a large portion or segment of tissue is removed. The term is often associated with the accompanying reconstruction or repair of the remaining tissue. Bowel resection is the removal of a section of bowel and joining the resulting segments by anastomosis. Resection of a tumor can mean simply removing the tumor and then using surgical means to repair the tissues involved in the dissection.
- **Surgical field:** The physical space occupied by the draped patient, draped instrument tables, and equipment and the scrubbed, gowned, and gloved sterile team members.
- **Surgical wound:** The spaces and tissues that are accessed through the surgical incision.
- **Undermine:** To separate one tissue plane (such as the skin or fascia plane) from another to increase the space between the two. The scissors are laid flat between the tissue planes and gently opened and closed, creating a space between the tissues. For example, the skin can be lifted from the fascia layer below by undermining it.
- **Visualize, direct visualization:** In surgery and medicine, "see in detail." For example, "The surgeon was able to visualize the tumor in the right fossa." Direct visualization means without magnification—that is, with the naked eye.

SURGICAL CASE PLAN

The surgical technologist develops a *case plan* before surgery. **Case planning** is preparation for a surgical procedure. The ST must think strategically about the instruments, supplies, and equipment required for the surgery. A checklist ensures that all needed supplies are ready and available. Keep in mind that no one expects a new graduate ST or student to correctly identify what is needed for every case. This knowledge is developed through experience.

The case plan is based partly on the information contained in the surgeon's preference card (described later). However, the surgeon's preference card is somewhat limited. Specific information based on the details of a procedure, patient profile, and other case-specific details are needed to complete the case plan. For example, a patient with a very high body mass index (BMI) may require mechanical moving and handling equipment, a high-capacity operating table, and extra-long instruments.

ELEMENTS OF A CASE PLAN

Specific information about the patient and the procedure helps to develop the case plan:

- Operative procedure
- Anesthesia planned
- Open or minimally invasive procedure?
- O-arm, C-arm required?
- Preoperative diagnosis as stated in the record
- Patient BMI or weight category
- Patient age category (infant, child, adult)
- Position and incision or entry site
- Special skin prep or draping routine?
- Implants planned, type, specifications if known
- Sutures, surgical staples, or tissue adhesives required
- Special dressings required

However, the patient's condition and special needs are unknown factors. In a busy operating room with little time for preparation between cases, case planning may be difficult, but without planning, some elements of the preparation may be overlooked, resulting in unnecessary delay or a disorganized case.

TYPES OF SURGERY BY OBJECTIVE

There are a number of different ways to categorize surgical procedures for learning purposes. This and other textbooks usually focus on the anatomical specialty such as abdominal, genitourinary, or orthopedic surgery. This is a logical way to learn the regional anatomy, instruments, and techniques.

Another method is to look at the surgical *objectives* or goals. The following categories are simply a tool for learning. There are obvious crossovers from one category to another (e.g., insertion of a pacemaker is a kind of implant; it does not replace an existing anatomical structure but may replace a nonfunctioning implant battery). Understanding categories can aid case planning, because surgical procedures of a specific type require common skills and techniques.

Suggested categories are the following:

1. Diagnostic
2. Reconstruction or implant
3. Repair
4. Removal

UNDERSTANDING THE NAME OF THE SURGICAL PROCEDURE

The first step in case planning is to obtain a copy of the surgical schedule. The name of the surgery provides information needed to start the case plan.

DIAGNOSTIC PROCEDURE

The results of a diagnostic procedure provide information about the nature of a medical or surgical problem and the options available for treatment. Diagnostic procedures may be performed as a part of surgery or as a standalone procedure. In many health care facilities, diagnostic procedures are performed in the *interventional radiology* department, which is equipped with advanced imaging equipment. The surgical technologist may be assigned to assist in surgical diagnostic procedures on a case-by-case basis in this setting.

Invasive diagnostic procedures may include biopsy, in which a portion of tissue is removed and prepared for microscopic examination, or injection of contrast medium, which produces images of tubes, ducts, or vessels. The common factor in diagnostic procedures is that the outcome is tangible and often visible. The process is almost always multidisciplinary—involving clinicians from other departments to assist or consult in the process.

Refer to Chapter 6 for more information on diagnostic procedures.

Questions for Planning

- What is the target structure or tissue? What technique will be used to perform the diagnosis (e.g., biopsy, dye study, magnetic resonance imaging, x-ray)?
- What special equipment or drugs are needed for the planned technique? Will there be tissue samples taken? Do they require any special handling?
- How will the information be documented (e.g., pathologist's report, video record, fluoroscopic image)?
- Is the procedure scheduled to take place in a special procedure room or in the operating room? Have other clinicians involved, such as the pathologist, been notified?
- Are previously performed imaging results available in the room or uploaded to the computer?
- What type of anesthesia will be required?

REPAIR

The goal of repair is to restore function to a structure, organ, or system. Repair can involve any type of tissue. The type of repair and the tissue involved determine which instruments or special equipment is needed. For example, repair of heart structures in the pediatric patient requires, at minimum, extensive cardiac equipment and pediatric chest instruments. Another example of soft tissue repair is hernia surgery, which may require synthetic mesh. Orthopedic repair usually involves implants of some type, even if just a simple plate or screw system. Imaging equipment will be used, and special dressings may be required for external stabilization after the repair.

Questions for Planning

- What will be repaired?
- What special instruments are needed?
- What materials will be used to perform the repair (e.g., sutures, plates, synthetic mesh)?
- How will the repair be held in place (e.g., sutures, screws, fibrin glue)?
- Is the repair related to disease or injury? Does the patient have recent injuries and mobility limitations? If so, what specific techniques should be used in positioning?
- Will imaging be required?

REMOVAL

Removal may involve tissue, an organ, or a foreign body. Extensive cancer surgery practiced in the past often included radical removal of multiple structures. With modern diagnostic, chemotherapeutic, and radiological interventions, these surgeries, which included the radical Whipple, radical mastectomy, and pelvic exenteration, are seldom performed. However, the removal of a single anatomical structure (e.g., gallbladder, appendix, or prostate gland) is common. Removal of a foreign body may include procedures after an industrial or workplace accident when items such as metal shards, wood, or glass are driven into the soft tissues. Forensic surgery involves the removal of ballistic items such as bullets or shrapnel, or sharp weapons such as knife blades.

Questions for Planning

- What will be removed?
- What surgical approach will be used (e.g., abdominal, thoracic)?
- Will a specimen be taken for frozen section analysis (immediate tissue analysis to determine malignancy)?
- Is the wound contaminated? (Procedures involving the removal of foreign bodies are contaminated.)
- What special procedures must be followed to submit forensic items removed from the patient?

RECONSTRUCTION

Reconstruction surgery is performed to remodel or replace tissue for functional or aesthetic reasons. The procedure may be performed in a single operation or may be a multiple-stage procedure. This type of surgery often requires specialty instruments. For example, a maxillofacial reconstruction (reconstruction of a portion of the jaw and other facial structures) could require plastic surgery, oral, and fine orthopedic instruments.

Questions for Planning

- What specialty instruments are needed for the surgery? Are they immediately available?
- Will intraoperative imagining be required?
- Has the surgeon requested special intraoperative precautions, such as to reduce the risk of infection?
- Are implants or grafts needed? Is the implant available? Does the implant require special handling techniques?

IMPLANT SURGERY

A medical **implant** is a manufactured device that is placed in or on the body. An implant may replace all or a portion of the body, provide structural or mechanical support, monitor body function, deliver medication, or provide aesthetic enhancement. Implants are used in nearly every medical-surgical specialty. Implant technology is in a constant state of change as new materials and the means to use them in are developed. The surgical technologist must keep up with new implant technology to provide optimal assistance in surgery. There are many learning resources available to the ST. The manufacturers of implants want their products to be used safely and efficiently. In-service training, intraoperative assistance by a representative of the company, and web-based tutorials are available.

The following discussions are the basis for learning about the types of implants, implant safety, and surgical guidelines associated with implants. The U.S. Food and Drug Administration (FDA) regulates medical implants and sets strict standards for their use in the patient.

TABLE 18.2 Types of Implantable Medical Devices

Cardiovascular	Orthopedic	Other
Pacing devices: cardiac resynchronization devices; cardioverter-defibrillator; cardiac pacemaker	Joint replacement: knee; hip; shoulder; elbow; ankle; hand	Otolaryngology implants: cochlear implant; airway stents
Cardiac stents and grafts: coronary stent; synthetic grafts; vena cava filter	Trauma implants: internal fixation devices; craniomaxillofacial implants	Ophthalmic implants: intraocular lenses; glaucoma and other lenses
Structural cardiac implants: heart valves and accessories; ventricular assist device; implantable heart monitors	Orthobiologics: bone substitutes; bone growth factors; bone cement	Neurostimulators
	Spinal implants: thoracolumbar implants; intervertebral spacers; cervical implants	
		Drug implants: hormonal implant, brachytherapy products; implantable drug pump

PLANNING FOR IMPLANT SURGERY

"Branded" implant systems have been developed in the orthopedic surgery and other specialty markets. These systems are usually not compatible with other manufacturers' devices. Branded sets are frequently leased rather than sold to health care facilities. This is related to the rapid development of new systems and methods.

Information about implant surgery, including the type of system to be used, is often included at the time the surgery is booked. This information is useful to the ST and circulator for case planning. It is important to ensure that all the instruments and devices associated with that implant are available on the day of surgery. If multiple surgeries using the same instruments are scheduled, be sure to allow enough time for re-sterilization between surgeries. Orthopedic equipment and implants can require extra time for cooling after steam sterilization.

IMPORTANT TO KNOW *Recall that all implants require the use of a biological monitor during sterilization. Refer to Chapter 10 to review biological monitoring devices.*

SYNTHETIC IMPLANTS

Many implants are derived from synthetic or biopolymer materials. Examples include artificial heart valves, pacemakers, and artificial joints. Implants must meet certain criteria for a successful surgical outcome. They must be:

- Compatible with body tissue
- Available as a sterile product or able to withstand a sterilization process
- Proven safe and nonpathogenic
- Able to provide adequate tissue coverage and vascularization around the implant
- Able to provide adequate stability for the intended use

IMPLANT MATERIALS

Synthetic polymer implants composed of polylactic acid (PLA) polymer are used in orthopedic and maxillofacial surgery. The newer generation of biopolymers manufactured using recombinant DNA technology has been approved for surgical use, including implants.

Porous *polyethylene* implants are often used in facial reconstruction. The porous nature of the implant allows for both soft tissue and vascular ingrowth. As collagen grows into the implant, the framework of the implant becomes stronger.

Methylmethacrylate is synthetic bone cement used to secure prosthetic implants into bone and, less commonly, for remodeling during cranioplasty. Bone cement is mixed on the sterile field using two components, methylmethacrylate powder and a volatile liquid. Because the fumes created by the chemical mixture are toxic, the cement must be mixed in a special closed container (refer to Chapter 29 for details). The manufacturer's recommendations for mixing and safety precautions should be followed.

Silicone and Silastic are two very common implant materials. They are relatively inert and durable. Implants are available in many forms, including gel, sponge, film, tubing, liquid, and sheets.

IMPORTANT TO KNOW *Silicone and Silastic implants should not be handled with bare hands, and care should be taken to ensure that they do not pick up lint or dust, because any foreign material can cause an inflammatory reaction around the implant.*

Vascular grafts are made from a number of woven synthetic materials. These include Dacron, polytetrafluoroethylene (PTFE), and polyester.

Stainless steel, vitallium, titanium, and other alloys have been used in the manufacture of orthopedic implants for many years. The materials are strong, resilient, and inert. Polyetheretherketone (PEEK) polymer reinforces the implant and prevents leakage and wear. Table 18.2 lists common medical implants across different specialties.

TISSUE GRAFTS

A **graft** is tissue taken from a distant site on the patient, another person, or animal and used to replace tissue lost

TABLE 18.3 Engineered Skin Grafting Materials

Name	Description	Use
Biobrane	Biosynthetic composed of silicone-nylon matrix. Encourages blood clotting between the fibers.	Clean burns not requiring surgical excision.
TransCyte	Temporary skin substitute derived from fibroblasts, which secrete collagen matrix material. Stored frozen to halt cellular activity while structural proteins remain intact.	Temporary skin dressing for full-thickness and deep partial-thickness burns.
Integra Bilayer Matrix	Semipermeable silicone layer with a porous matrix of bovine collagen; controls fluid loss and provides flexible, adherent covering; promotes capillary growth.	Partial- and full-thickness soft tissue injuries and chronic wounds.
Integra Dermal Regeneration Template	Thin silicone film over cross-linked fibers that provide a scaffold for skin regeneration.	Third-degree burns when allografting is not possible.
Epicel	Cultured epithelial autograft generated from skin taken from the patient.	Deep dermal or third-degree burn sites.
Apligraf	Contains two layers – a human-derived epidermis and bovine collagen dermis.	Deep partial- or full-thickness wounds.

from disease or injury. Tissue loss can be caused by trauma or injury, congenital deformity, surgical excision and resection, and degenerative diseases. Many of these tissues can be replaced or substituted with biological dressing, implanted materials, or synthetic prosthetic materials. Tissue grafts usually are obtained from a registered tissue bank (central location in the health care facility or community) unless the tissue is from the patient's body. In this case, it may be removed and stored in the health care facility for a period or used immediately.

IMPORTANT TO KNOW *The Joint Commission (TJC) requires all tissue banks and health care facilities to have an electronic or manual tracking system that details the donors and recipients of all tissues. TJC also sets the precise storage conditions of grafts and requires facilities to have a program in place for receiving, storing, and managing all tissues.*

Below are important terms that relate to grafts:

- **Allograft:** A tissue graft derived from human tissue. Allografts are tested for infectious disease and infection before distribution from the tissue bank.
- **Autologous autograft:** Tissue obtained from the patient's body and implanted into another site, such as a bone graft taken from the hip for implantation into the spine.

SKIN GRAFT

Skin grafts are used to replace skin that has been destroyed by disease or injury. The skin is a critical barrier against infection and fluid loss. A skin substitute is needed to protect deep tissues from injury and contamination. Traditionally, skin grafts were taken only from the patient's own body, because these were the most successful. Now, other biological materials are available that can provide excellent protection against infection while reducing scarring and preventing fluid loss. Some grafting materials also aid the formation of granulation tissue in wounds. (The surgical techniques used in skin grafting are discussed fully in Chapter 28.)

PORCINE DERMIS

Porcine (pig) dermis is used to temporarily cover a full-thickness injury. The graft does not develop vascularization and sloughs after 1 to 2 weeks. Porcine grafts are available in sheets and rolls and may be frozen, fresh, or dried.

AMNIOTIC MEMBRANE AND UMBILICAL CORD

Amniotic membrane from human placentas can be used as a biological dressing for burns, skin ulcers, and infected wounds. This type of graft may also be used to cover spina bifida defects and in corneal surgery. The placenta has two layers or membranes: the *amnion*, which is used primarily in partial-thickness wounds, and the *chorion*, which is used primarily in full-thickness wounds. The amnion may be used fresh, frozen, or dried. Both membranes may be obtained from a tissue bank.

Human umbilical cord is used in vascular surgery to replace an artery when saphenous autografting is not feasible.

ENGINEERED SKIN SUBSTITUTES

Engineered skin substitutes (artificial skin) were created because of the lack of available human skin to cover large defects and wounds. All artificial skin has an outer layer that creates a barrier to infection, and many products include a dermal element that guides the cell during epithelialization. In addition to providing a barrier to infection, artificial skin reduces the severe pain associated with frequent dressing changes. It also decreases the risk of scar **contracture,** which is extreme tightening and shrinking of scar tissue that leads to loss of function and severe cosmetic defect. Table 18.3 lists engineered skin substitutes, their content and use.

BONE GRAFT

Bone grafts are used for structural support and to stimulate new bone growth in a defect caused by trauma or a congenital anomaly. Two types of bone are used for grafting: cancellous bone and cortical bone. Cancellous bone is porous, and tissue fluid can reach deep into it, allowing most of the bone cells to live. Cortical bone is very rigid and strong. It typically is used to repair skeletal defects because of its strength. Cortical bone is fixed into position with metal sutures or plates and screws. Many types of bone grafts are used in modern surgery:

- *Autologous grafts:* Made from the patient's body
- *Allogenic grafts:* Made from nonliving cadaver bone
- *Composite grafts:* Made of a combination of cadaver bone, morcellated allograft bone, and marrow
- *Demineralized bone matrix (DBM):* Processed material made from collagen, protein, and growth factors. It is used as granules, chips, putty, or gel
- *Ceramic materials:* Provide structural support only
- *Graft composites:* Contain combinations of DBM and marrow, ceramic-collagen, and ceramic-autograft-collagen combinations

PREOPERATIVE CASE PREPARATION

SURGICAL SCHEDULE

Scheduled surgical cases are usually assigned to nurses and technologists the day before surgery. Emergency surgeries are added in as needed. In most facilities, assignments are posted on a schedule board (e.g., a whiteboard), which lists cases and assigned personnel. This is usually located near the entrance to the restricted area. Information on the schedule board includes the following:

1. Patient's initials (names are not used)
2. Surgical procedure
3. Operating room designation
4. Surgeon
5. Anesthesia provider
6. Circulator
7. Surgical technologist or scrub nurse
8. Type of anesthesia planned (sometimes posted)

Many operating rooms provide a printout of the schedule for each staff member. It is important to check the master schedule periodically during the day, as changes are often made as cases are canceled, moved up, or postponed.

After receiving the schedule, the surgical technologist plans his or her time and tasks so that all instruments, supplies, and equipment are available and ready close to the time of surgery. Sometimes the surgeon will notify the surgical technologist or circulator of special instruments or equipment required for a case. This information should be passed on to others on a *need-to-know* basis (Box 18.1).

BOX 18.1 Historical Highlights: What Is the Name of That Procedure?

The names of surgical procedures are often inconsistent among surgical texts, academic journal articles, and Internet sites. The evolution of surgical procedure names dates back to the late 1700s when scientists were honored by having their name attached to their discoveries or developments. In the 1800s this practice was extended to surgeons and surgical procedures. Examples are *Marshall-Marchetti-Krantz procedure* (cystopexy) and *Shirodkar procedure* (cerclage). This trend was slowly replaced by the use of Greek roots, prefixes, and suffixes to name or describe a surgical procedure. Examples are *hernio**rrhaphy*** (repair of hernia) and *anterior cystocele and posterior rectocele colpo**rrhaphy*** (A & P repair). This system is still in use today along with the older names associated with the surgeon who developed the procedure. However, a procedure named after its founder can be confusing. One surgeon may have developed a number of different procedures, but all may be referred to by his or her name, perhaps followed by a number. The current trend is less formal; we are more likely to see an abbreviation of the procedure (e.g., dacryocystorhinostomy [DCR] or a simple description such as *cleft lip repair*).

SUPPLIES AND INSTRUMENTS

The method used to gather supplies for a case depends on the system established by the health care facility. The process is called "picking a case" or "pulling a case." The case cart method is most commonly used. In this system, some or all of the wrapped sterile supplies are assembled in the central processing department and sent to surgery on a closed stainless steel *case cart* (introduced in Chapter 4). Prepared case carts are kept in the substerile area to protect them from contamination. Instrument sets may or may not be added by the central processing department because many facilities keep their sterile instruments in the surgical department's sterile supply rooms. Pre-assembly of case carts helps to decrease room turnaround time (the time between the end of one case and the start of another). After the case cart is received in the operating room, the surgical technologist is responsible for checking it for completeness and adding equipment and supplies as required. Selected case carts are kept ready for emergency cases, such as abdominal trauma, craniotomy, aneurysm, and cesarean section (C-section). These are high-priority emergencies in which every minute must be used efficiently to get the case underway. Basic items, such as instrument sets and linen packs, are preassembled on the emergency setup. Special items may be quickly added shortly before surgery.

If case carts are not prepared by the central processing department, cases are picked the night before or on the day of surgery. This may be the responsibility of the night staff (surgical techs and nurses). However, a busy night shift may not allow time for cases to be picked. In this case, the day staff must complete the carts.

SURGEON'S PREFERENCE CARD

The **surgeon's preference card** is an electronic document or paper version of the specific supplies and methods used by each surgeon for cases he or she performs routinely in the facility. Electronic or paper documents are kept on file in the clean work area where instrument trays are assembled and in the central processing department where case carts are prepared. Each preference card contains a list of the specific instruments, equipment, drugs, suture, and other items that a particular surgeon uses on a specific surgery. The preference card also shows the surgeon's glove and gown size, draping routine, and other technical information.

The rationale for keeping preference cards is to have the surgeon's requirements ready *before* they are needed. This allows efficient use of time and prevents delays during the procedure. In general, surgeons are intolerant of delays caused by poor planning. Delays result in increased anesthesia time, which adds to patient risk, can upset the surgery schedule, and are measured in financial cost. Many facilities have adopted elaborate computer programs to create and archive surgeon preference cards that can be modified as needed and are linked to patient billing and scheduling.

Surgeon preference cards in any form may contain information that is misleading or even wrong. Their accuracy depends on updating and making sure that the information applies to all or most cases of that type—not just some. Good case planning is often directly related to the team effort in keeping preference cards updated and accurate.

NONSTERILE ROOM PREPARATION

In the immediate preoperative period, the operating room and all equipment are prepared for surgery. This usually occurs 10 to 15 minutes before surgery. More time may be required, depending on the complexity of the case. In the first stage, nonsterile equipment is prepared. Note that a clear path between the door and operating table must be maintained to allow the patient to be brought in and transferred to the table.

1. Position the operating table according to the type of surgery, ensuring that there is space for anesthesia and monitoring equipment. The operating table is positioned directly under the overhead surgical lights.
2. Arrange the room in a manner that prevents contamination of sterile surfaces by traffic from doorways and nonsterile equipment.
3. The electrosurgical power unit must be placed close enough to the operating table to accommodate the cables and patient connections so that it can be moved into exact position after the start of surgery.
4. Suction canisters are positioned near the operating table. Final positioning takes place after the patient has been draped.
5. Kick bucket liners and trash receptacles should be in place. Usually, this is done by the housekeeping team, but it should be checked by the surgical team ahead of time.
6. Place instrument tables and other surfaces that will be draped (sterile) **no closer than 12 inches (45 cm) to nonsterile surface, equipment, or walls.** It is important to anticipate the need for additional tables and sterile covers for instrument trays or equipment.
7. Place clean linen on the operating table and ensure that arm boards and other attachments are available in the room. Secure one end of the patient safety strap to the table.
8. Have specific positioning devices and aids available according to the scheduled procedures, paying particular attention to patient size.
9. Connect suction tubing to canisters, making sure that the connections are tight. Pre-test the suction lines for adequate and safe pressure.
10. Have imaging output data available in hard copy or uploaded to the computer.
11. If pneumatic power equipment is to be used during surgery, the inline or tank gas sources must be tested and the gauges set according to the manufacturer's recommendations. If a gas cylinder is used, ensure that the tank is ***at least 50% full.***
12. Other equipment such as portable imaging systems must be checked to ensure that all connections and leads are available.
13. Any other special equipment must be available in the room. Specialty carts must be available in the sterile core or corridor.
14. If lasers are to be used, make sure that warning signs are posted outside the room and all protective equipment is available and ready.

Watch Chapter 18 Preparing the Operating Room for the Patient on the Evolve website: http://evolve.elsevier.com/Fuller/surgical.

OPENING A CASE

After sterile supplies have been gathered for a surgical case and the room has been prepared with the needed equipment, the next step is *opening the case*. In this process, sterile instruments and equipment are opened using sterile technique to prevent their contamination.

Sterile supplies are usually opened within 30 minutes before the case. The surgical technologist participates in this activity until it is time to perform the surgical hand antisepsis (10 to 20 minutes before surgery, depending on the complexity of the case, or less in emergency cases). Sterile supplies are opened in logical sequence from large to small while avoiding a pyramid of supplies that can topple over and become contaminated.

Refer to Chapter 9 to review the boundaries of the sterile field and rules of sterile technique.

The basic pack containing linens (towels, drapes, and surgeons' gowns) is centered on the back table and opened using sterile technique. As the wrapper(s) is(are) unfolded, the inner surface is exposed. This provides a sterile surface on which other items can be opened (Fig. 18.1). Small items are opened by removing the outer wrapper using sterile technique. The item is then *gently but purposefully* ejected from the package onto the sterile table without allowing the item to touch the edge of the wrapper (Fig. 18.2).

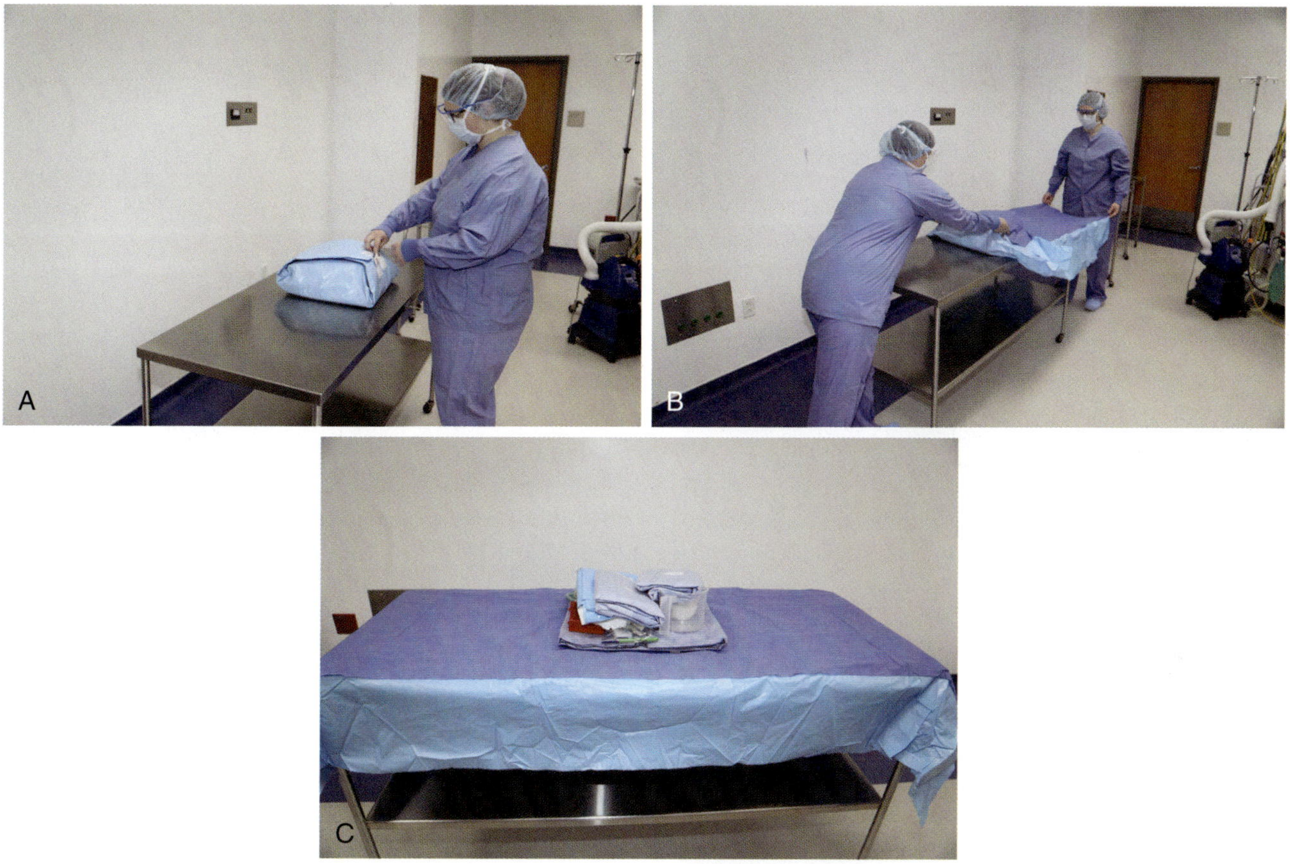

FIG. 18.1 (A) The pack is centered on the back table. (B) Two people grasp the edges of the wrapper and unfold the wrapper. (C) The sterile contents of the pack are now exposed.

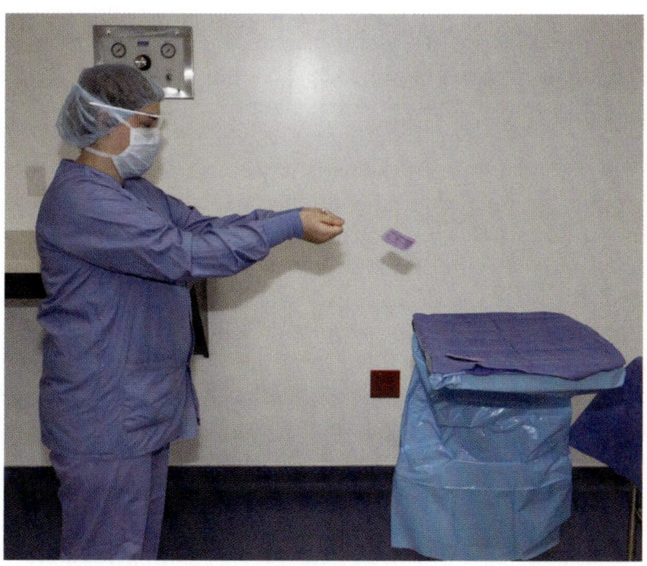

FIG. 18.2 Flipping a suture package onto the Mayo.

Guidelines • Opening a Case

- Always maintain at least 12 inches from sterile surfaces to avoid contamination, but stand close enough to project the item you are opening accurately.
- Before opening sterile packages, check for tears, holes, water marks, or other imperfections that may indicate that the item is contaminated. The process indicator must also be checked to ensure that the item was processed correctly.
- While opening sterile goods, place clean, single-use wrappers in clean paper trash receptacles. ***Do not use kick buckets or biohazard bags for clean waste.*** This creates additional work for the circulator, who must remove the wrappers and place them in the appropriate clean waste bags before surgery begins.
- When opening packages sealed with tape, break the tape rather than tearing it or removing it. This prevents the outer wrapper from ripping.
- Packages wrapped in sealed pouches may contain an inner wrapper. Open the outer pouch and distribute the item with its inner wrapper intact. If the inner wrapper becomes contaminated while removing the outer wrapper, open the inner wrapper and directly offer the contents to the surgical technologist.
- Extra sutures, special equipment, and implants should be held unopened until it is clear that they will be needed. This prevents waste.
- Sharps are opened onto a conspicuous location on the back table during the setup or held until the ST can receive them directly out of the package (preferred method). This prevents the surgical technologist from unexpectedly encountering a sharp item. The circulator opens the outer package and the scrubbed technologist removes them and immediately places them in a magnetic container.

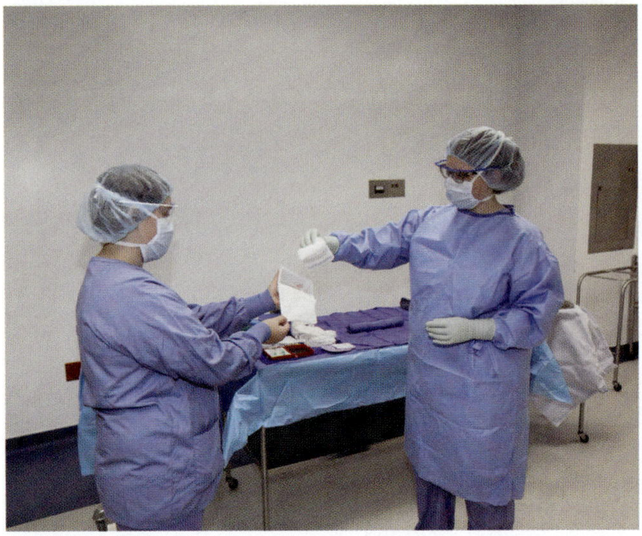

FIG. 18.3 The surgical technologist receives 4 × 4 (Raytec) sponges from the circulator.

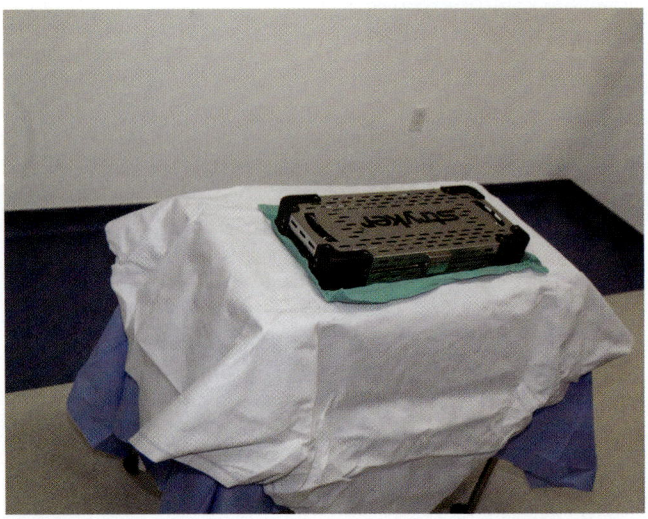

FIG. 18.4 A heavy tray is opened on a separate table. The ST may leave it on the table during the case or transfer it to the back table during the sterile setup.

- Before performing surgical hand antisepsis for the case, the ST opens gowns and gloves onto a small table away from where sterile items have been distributed (never on the back table) to prevent possible contamination of other supplies. Gloves should not be opened on top of the gown. This prevents water from dripping onto the gown (if a surgical hand scrub was performed rather than hand antisepsis).
- When opening supplies, remember that the edge of any sterile wrapper is considered nonsterile (Fig. 18.3).
- Very heavy or large items can be opened on a separate table and transferred to the instrument table by the surgical technologist (Fig. 18.4).

IMPORTANT TO KNOW *The surgical technologist in the scrub role must perform hand antisepsis, allowing sufficient time for the sterile setup. This may mean that not all the sterile supplies are opened before the patient arrives and the circulator's responsibilities shift to patient care. The amount of time needed for the sterile setup depends on the skill of the surgical technologist and the complexity of the case. At least 20 minutes should be allowed for a major case.*

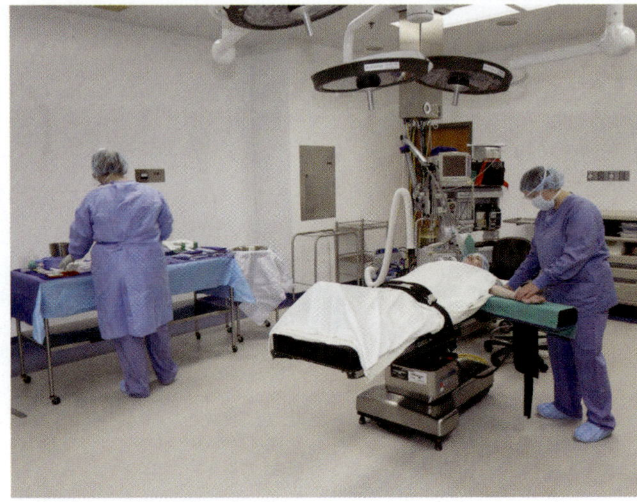

FIG. 18.5 Receiving the patient. The ST should hold requests for other sterile supplies until the circulator has completed checking the patient in and providing direct care.

RECEIVING THE PATIENT

The patient is usually received in the operating room suite during the sterile setup (Fig. 18.5). The circulator and anesthesia care provider (when present) are responsible for the care of the patient. Noise should be kept to a minimum at this time, including conversation between team members, which could be misinterpreted or upsetting to the patient.

The circulator greets the patient, who is assisted during the move to the operating table by the circulator and one other person (anesthesia team or assistant circulator). The patient safety strap is secured as soon as the patient is centered on the table. The patient's medical history and complete documentation, including operative permits, will have been checked in the surgery holding area. However, the circulating nurse will again check the patient's preoperative checklist. This includes the site and side of the surgery, permits, and preoperative orders.

Any mobility restrictions are noted, as well as areas requiring special attention such as stoma sites and skin alterations. Maintaining normothermia (normal core body temperature) is an important activity after the patient arrives, because anesthetic and adjunct drugs can lower the core temperature and lead to physiological complications. This is especially true for pediatric, debilitated, and elderly patients. *The circulator therefore provides one or more additional blankets to the patient.* When the anesthesia care provider (ACP) arrives, the circulator may continue with preoperative tasks, including assisting the ACP as needed, opening supplies, and preparing intraoperative documents.

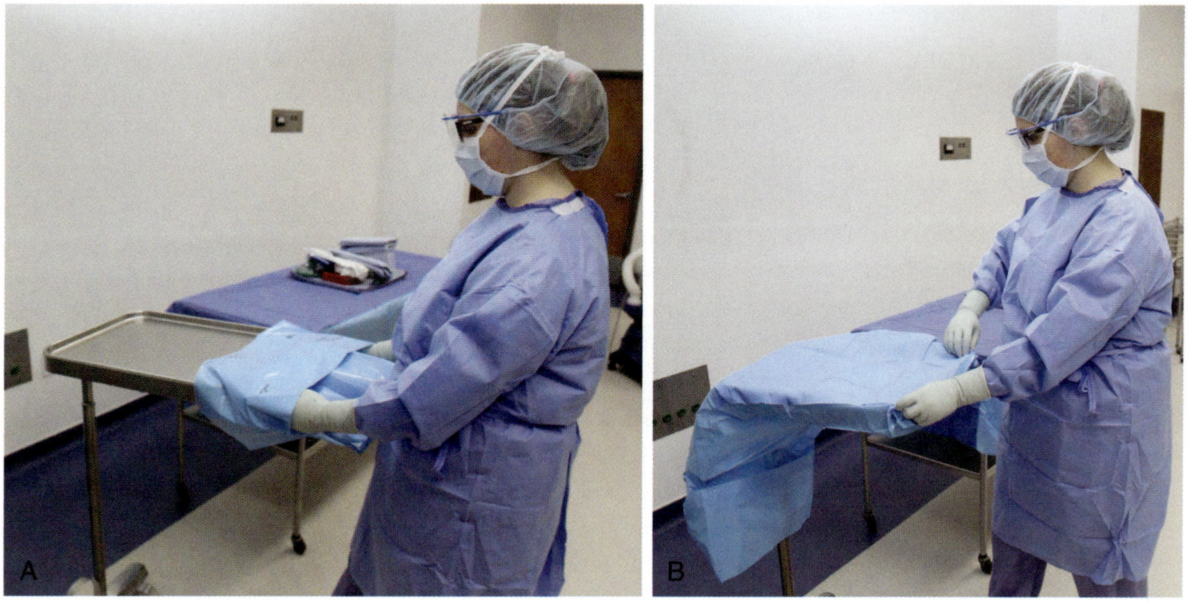

FIG. 18.6 Draping the Mayo. (A) The ST places her hands well inside the cuff and eases it over the open end of the Mayo. (B) The drape is advanced. The circulator may assist by pulling the lower section down by grasping the lower edge. Note that the underside of the draped Mayo and the vertical section at or above the height of the operating table are considered sterile.

The ACP starts an IV in one or two sites. External physiological monitoring devices are put into place, and preoperative drugs are administered to the patient at this time. (In the past, preoperative medications were administered before the patient arrived in the operating room.) These drugs may include a sedative, anticholinergic to control oral secretions, drugs to reduce gastric acidity, and others according to the physiological needs of the patient.

After the surgeon and any assistants arrive and the patient is stable, induction takes place (for general anesthesia). If moderate sedation and local anesthesia are to be used, intravenous (IV) sedative drugs may be administered.

STERILE SETUP

Immediately after performing hand antisepsis, gowning, and gloving, the surgical technologist must organize the sterile items on the back table, Mayo, and other instrument tables. This is called the **sterile setup** or *setting up a case.*

Students and newly graduated surgical technologists can feel overwhelmed by the amount of equipment that must be organized and ready by the time the surgeons arrive to start a major case. Using a methodical method for all setups improves efficiency and greatly decreases stress and errors in the learning stages.

As you first approach the pile of sterile equipment, do not begin moving things around aimlessly. This increases the chance of contamination and does not actually move the process forward. The following are general guidelines that can increase efficiency and decrease stress:

- ***Increase the size of the sterile working area.*** Before organizing and preparing supplies, increase the size of the sterile area. Drape the Mayo stand early on in the setup (Fig. 18.6). After draping the Mayo, place one or two towels over the tray on top of the Mayo cover. This provides some cushioning for the instruments and also helps decrease the possibility of penetrating the tray cover with a sharp instrument or needle.
- ***During setup for microsurgery, ophthalmic, or ear surgery, lint-free nonwoven materials are used to cover the Mayo.*** This prevents the instruments from snagging. Micro instruments are often arranged on a slotted tray; this keeps the instruments stable and protects their tips.
- If you need additional work space for instrument sets or other sterile equipment, this should be arranged before the sterile setup. For example, power equipment or other specialty items can be opened on a separate table and transferred to the instrument table or left in place during the case. If multiple tables are used, they should be placed close to the back table so that a continuous sterile field is created. This saves steps and excess motion.
- ***When opening instruments in closed sterilization trays, the circulator checks the external process indicator first.*** The tamper-proof seals and latches are checked for integrity. The circulator breaks the seals and lifts the top straight up and away from the tray. Remember that the edges of the tray are not sterile. The filter disk of sterilization trays is checked for water marks or perforation at the time they are opened to ensure that the contents have not been contaminated (Fig. 18.7). A damp or improperly positioned filter indicates contamination. After these checks, the surgical technologist lifts the inner instrument tray by its handles straight up and away from the outer nonsterile container.
- ***Check the sterilization indicators inside all instrument trays before removing and handling the contents of the tray.*** If any indicator has not detected the sterilization process, the tray and all contents are considered nonsterile and must be removed from the sterile field. Any equipment

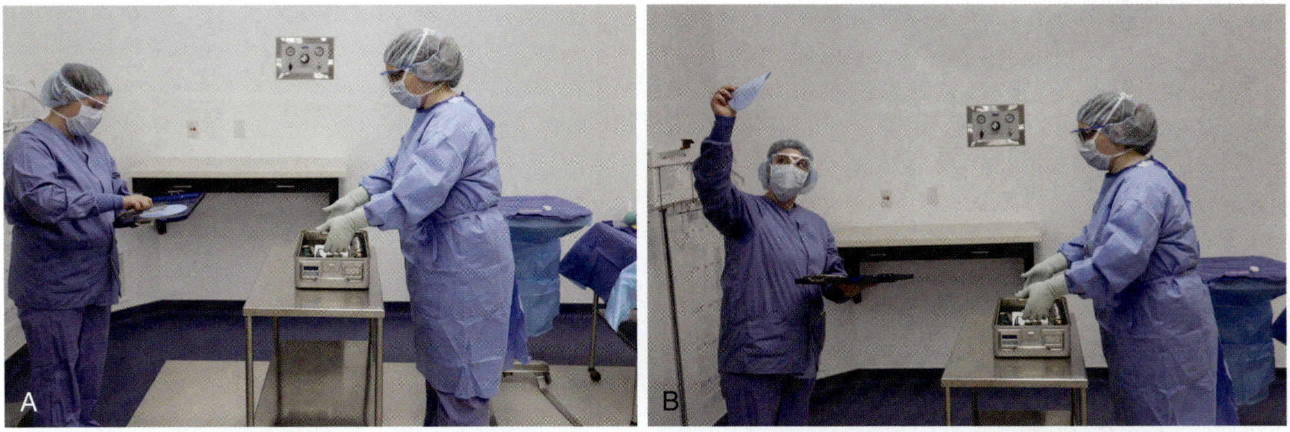

FIG. 18.7 Removing instruments from a sealed sterilization container. The outer container is not sterile. (A) The ST grasps the handles of the sterile instrument tray and lifts it straight up to avoid contamination by the outside container. (B) It is necessary to check the filter on sealed trays to look for any puncture or water marks, which can indicate contamination.

in contact with the tray must also be removed. This may require the ST to change gloves and gown.

- ***Avoid shifting the same items around from one place to another during the setup.*** Try to handle an item only once or twice. Shifting items from one location to another without purpose is not productive. Instead, start to build zones on the back table intended for specific types of equipment such as drapes, sutures, drugs, sharps, and instrument stringers. Retrieve the item you need and place it in its final location once. Even if you have to push other things aside to make space for the item at hand, you will have started to establish zones (Fig. 18.8).
- ***Try to avoid doing several things at once.*** Think and act strategically. Perform one task and then proceed to the next.
- When preparing sutures and other small, wrapped supplies, use the waste bag provided in the setup to dispose of wrappers and suture ends.
- ***Do not discard wrappers in the kick bucket, which is reserved for sponges.***

IMPORTANT TO KNOW *Some facilities require a standardized setup. This method is used to ensure that during a change of shift or breaks when more than one person uses the same setup, everyone is familiar with the arrangement and location of instruments and supplies.*

ORDER OF USE

During the sterile setup, it is useful to focus on items that are needed at the beginning of the surgery and prepare them first. This serves two purposes: it helps in mental preparation for the case and if there is insufficient time to complete the setup before surgery starts, the supplies needed at the start are ready. This is particularly useful in emergency cases when the patient may be brought in very quickly, with little time for the sterile setup.

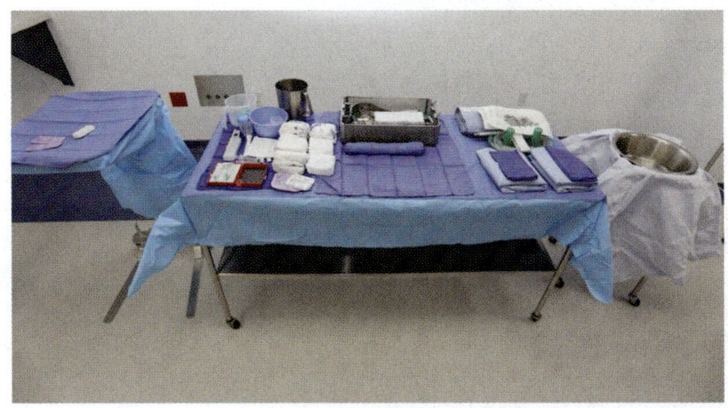

FIG. 18.8 The ST has started setting up the back table by creating zones for specific items such as sharps, sponges, and instruments. Using the same setup for cases greatly increases efficiency and prevents items from being "lost."

The following list is the usual order of items needed on a routine case:

1. *Towels, gowns, gloves, drapes:* Pull the gowns out from the pile and stack them *in order of use* from the top down (e.g., towel, gown, towel, gown). Stack drapes with the first used on top and the last used on the bottom of the stack.
2. *Light handles or covers, suction tubing, ESU pencil, and holster:* You may place these in a dry instrument basin or on the Mayo stand. They will be placed on the field as soon as the patient is draped.
3. *Starting instruments:* These are two lap or 4 × 4 Raytec sponges, knife, scissors, clamps, shallow retractors, sharps receptacle for scalpel, and suture ties. Locate knife handles, dissecting scissors, forceps, and superficial retractors. Mount knife blades. Place these, along with a few necessary instruments, on the Mayo stand. Prepare the ESU pencil and holster along with their holding clamp. These will go up on the surgical field as soon as the patient is draped.
4. *Sponges, sutures, sharps:* Put all sponges except those on the Mayo in one location on the back table, organized by type, so that you are ready to count when the circulator is free to

do so. Do the same with suture packets and sharps. Sharps are placed on a magnetic board or sharps receptacle ready for counting and are safely stored. Suture packets may be placed in a small bowl or square tray on the back table.

5. *You now have all the priority equipment you need to start a case.* All other equipment can be set up as "secondary preparation."

Watch Chapter 18 Preparation of the Sterile Field on the Evolve website: http://evolve.elsevier.com/Fuller/surgical.

Watch Chapter 18 Monitoring the Sterile Field on the Evolve website: http://evolve.elsevier.com/Fuller/surgical.

SUTURE PREPARATION

Suture material needed for a case is listed on the *surgeon's preference card.* If there is no preference card, it is possible to ask the surgeon at the start of the case. Although many different types of suture materials and needles may be opened during a case, not all of them must be immediately available on the Mayo. Sutures are kept on the back table and transferred to the Mayo as needed. After working in a particular facility, you will become familiar with specific sutures required by individual surgeons. It may be helpful to know that students, whether they are surgical technologists or interns starting surgical residency, are not expected to have complete competency in sutures.

Methods of Organizing Sutures on the Mayo

- *Suture ties* (strands) can be removed from their package, separated by size, and placed on the Mayo stand between the folds of a towel, called a "suture book" (Fig. 18.9). Ties may also be maintained in the package, which is placed on the Mayo or in a small basin.
- *Suture reels* can remain on the Mayo, and individual ties removed as needed. Suture-needle combination packages can be placed in a small basin on the back table and brought to the Mayo as needed. Suture packets are designed to be opened quickly and easily. The needles are secured so that they can be grasped from the package using the needle holder. Sutures attached to swaged needles should follow the needle smoothly as it is removed from the package.

A complete discussion of sutures and suture use during surgery is located in Chapter 19.

ORGANIZING THE INSTRUMENTS

Complex surgical cases require many instrument trays. This is why it is important to think about what instruments you need, locate them among all the supplies, and then put them in a specific place. If instrument trays must be stacked, place heavier ones on the bottom. The number of instruments available in the instrument sets usually far exceeds those needed on

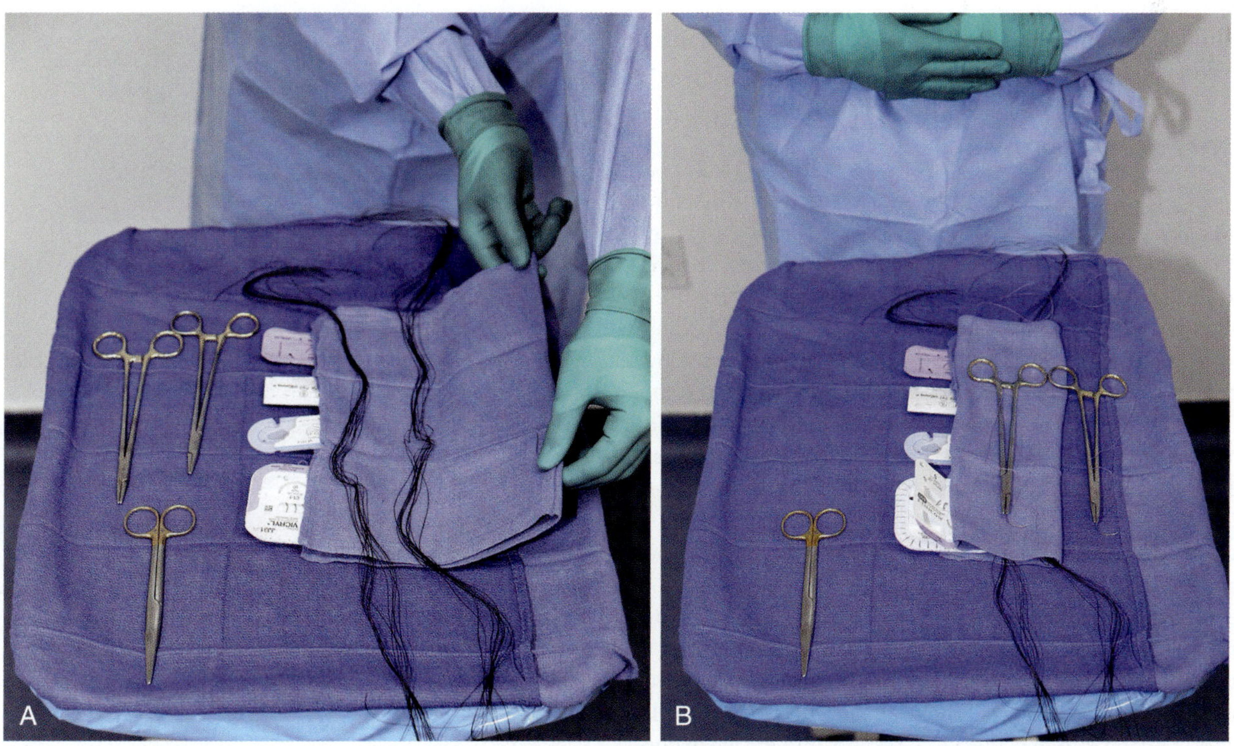

FIG. 18.9 A suture book can be created at the start of surgery and brought up to the Mayo as needed. The folds of the towel keep suture ties separated. Suture-needle combinations can be tucked inside other folds ready for use. Here, the ST has mounted two suture-needle combinations on the appropriate-size needle holders.

the case. The selection of instruments to have available on the back table, or Mayo, is based on experience and guidance from others with experience. During the first months of scrubbing, no one is expected to know exactly which instruments will be needed. Regardless of the method you use to learn, make sure you know each instrument's specific or general location on the back table to avoid delay during surgery. Your scrub mentor will help you locate what you need to prevent unnecessary delay during the case.

MAYO SETUP

The Mayo tray (called the *Mayo*) is the surgical technologist's personal workspace for the rapid exchange of instruments, suture, and other supplies during surgery. It is reserved for items needed immediately and frequently throughout the procedure. Part of the surgical technologist's expertise is in knowing what is immediately needed during the procedure. Ideally, there is a seamless exchange of items from the surgical field to the Mayo. As the case progresses, new instruments are added to the Mayo, and those not needed are placed on the back table or in the water basin; they must be within easy reach in case they are needed again.

The Mayo setup is *personal*, and unless the health care facility requires a standard setup, surgical technologists are free to develop a system and arrangement of items that works best for them. Regardless of the system used, the Mayo stand should be kept neat and orderly, because a disorganized Mayo can lead to surgical errors such as lost needles, needlestick injury, and a sluggish response to needs on the field. Fig. 18.10 shows several classic Mayo setups. However, students should try different setups to see what feels efficient and comfortable.

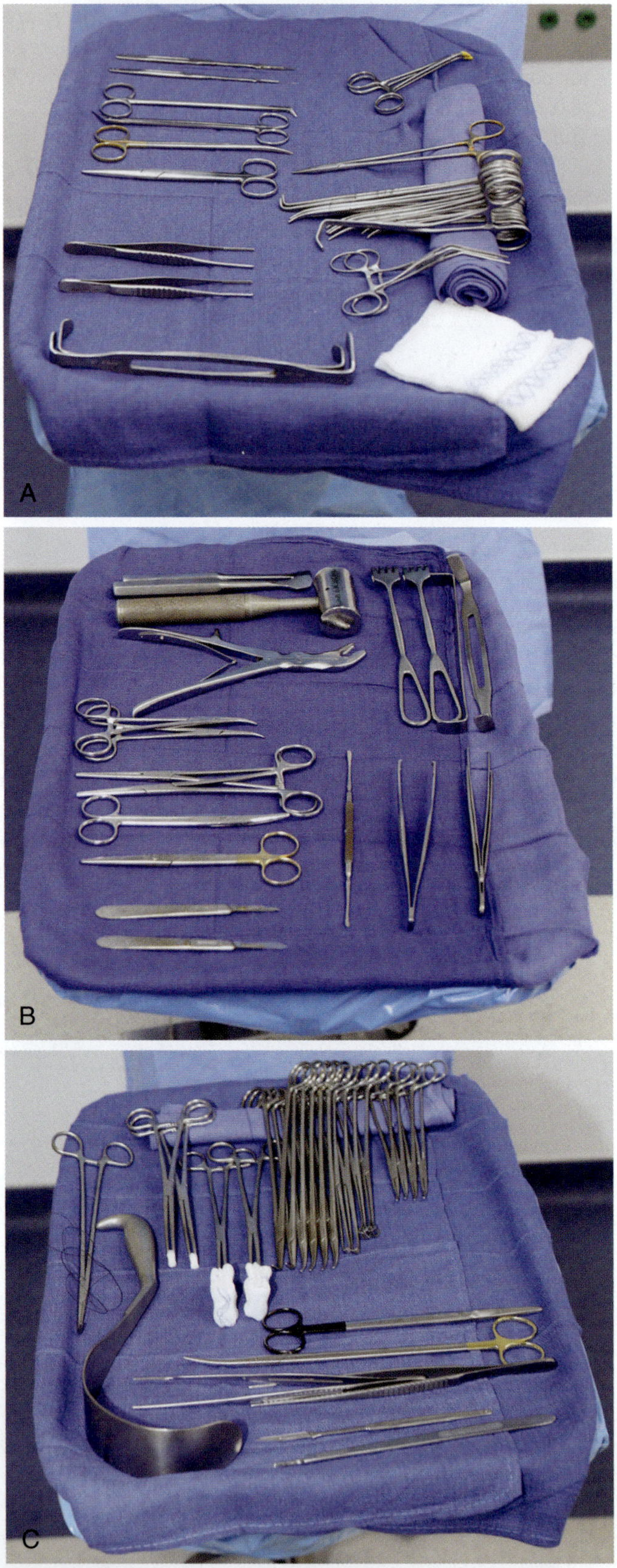

FIG. 18.10 Three examples of Mayo setups. (A) Minor vascular case. (B) Minor orthopedic case. (C) Laparotomy with long instruments.

SOLUTIONS AND DRUGS

Sterile saline for irrigation and sterile water are usually distributed after the case is underway or just before the case begins, *but only when the surgical technologist is present to receive them.* Solutions are distributed into basins or a temperature-controlled basin unit (Fig. 18.11). The wound irrigation solution is kept separate. All irrigation fluid must be measured by the surgical technologist and recorded as it is used so that total blood loss can be calculated accurately. One basin of sterile water is reserved for soaking instruments. Instruments must not be soaked in saline solution as it is corrosive to stainless steel.

Drugs are distributed to the sterile field as close to the time they are needed as possible.

The protocols for receiving medications from the circulator and drug management are discussed in detail in Chapter 12.

A zone for labeled drugs and labeling materials should be created on the back table so that they can be protected and well organized. During surgery, the ST is responsible for all drugs on the back table. He or she must know the name, strength, calculations required for mixing, correct delivery device, and amounts used for each drug.

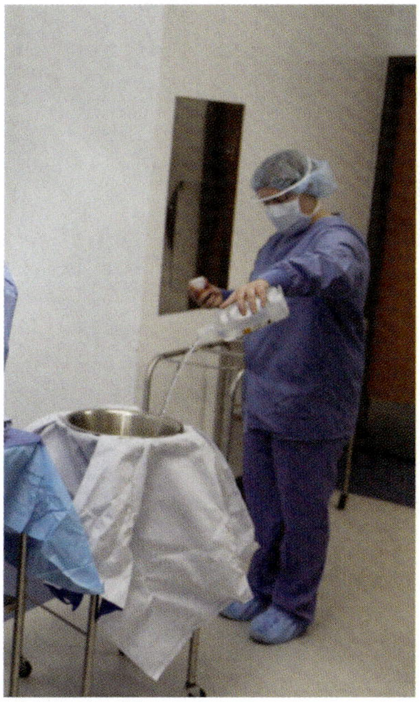

FIG. 18.11 The circulator distributes sterile water to the ST during setup. Note that the entire contents of the bottle must be poured at one time as re-capping can contaminate the lip of the container.

COMPLETING THE SETUP

Once the Mayo and back table have been set up for the start of the case, the remaining supplies can be arranged and prepared. After the setup is complete, instruments and supplies should be handled as little as possible because this increases the risk of contamination.

SURGICAL COUNT

Items that *may be* lost in the surgical wound are counted *in a precise way* before, during, and after the surgery to prevent any object from being left behind in the patient. The problem of *retained surgical items* (RSIs) during surgery was introduced in Chapter 3 as having safety, legal, and financial consequences.

Any item that can be retained in the surgical wound is included in the **count.** This includes sutures, surgical sponges, sharps, instruments, instrument parts, retraction devices (e.g., umbilical tapes, elastic vessel loops), instrument tip covers (shods) , suture reels, and any other small items used on the sterile field.

RSIs continue to be among the most common sentinel events contributing to patient injury. A retained item can cause pain, infection, perforation of an organ, obstruction, and scarring. Repeat surgery for a retained item causes trauma, a longer recovery period, and additional expense. Severe infection or injury may result in death. Loss of an item is a sentinel event that may result in a negligence charge against *any member of the surgical team.*

Research shows that RSIs are often caused by not following established procedure. Excessive noise, lack of organization by the surgical technologist, and pressure to hurry through procedures were found to be the features of an operative environment incompatible with correct counts. The study also identified poor communication among surgical team members as a cause of poor counting and patient risk (Norton et al., 2012).

RESPONSIBILITY FOR THE COUNT

Health care facilities create and enforce policies on the methodology or procedure for counts and documentation. The law does not state how counts are taken or who is to take them. The law *does* state that items not intended to remain in the patient must be removed before the wound is closed. All team members are responsible for ensuring that no items are left in a patient. The scrubbed technologist or nurse and circulator normally perform the count together. In turn, they report the count to the surgeon, whether it is correct or incorrect. Action to resolve an incorrect count is then the entire team's responsibility. During surgery, the scrubbed technologist should know *at all times* how many sponges, instruments, and other items are inside the patient and the location of counted items on the back table and Mayo.

WHEN TO PERFORM THE COUNT

In general, counts are performed on all surgical or invasive procedures. Anyone on the surgical team may request a count at any time.

The health care facility determines policy for counting instruments, sharps, and miscellaneous items. All sponges are counted in the following circumstances:

1. Before surgery begins, to establish a baseline count
2. Any time additional sponges or other counted items are added to the sterile setup
3. Before closure of any body cavity or cavity within a cavity, such as a hollow organ, and again before the body cavity is closed
4. At the start of wound closure
5. At skin closure or when counted items are no longer used on the sterile field
6. Whenever permanent relief staff enter the case (e.g., during a shift or other personnel change in either the scrub or circulator role)

Instruments, sharps, and miscellaneous items are counted according to facility policy.

PROCEDURE FOR THE COUNT

Items are counted in the order usually determined by facility policy:

1. Items on the immediate sterile field (i.e., those on or in the patient)
2. Items on the Mayo stand
3. Items on the back table
4. Items that have been discarded or dropped from the field

The count is performed in a systematic manner. Items should be counted according to their type. For example, count all laparotomy sponges, and then count all 4 × 4 Raytec sponges, sponge dissectors, and so on.

Count suture needles, blades, other small items, and instruments (and their loose parts) as separate groups. The items

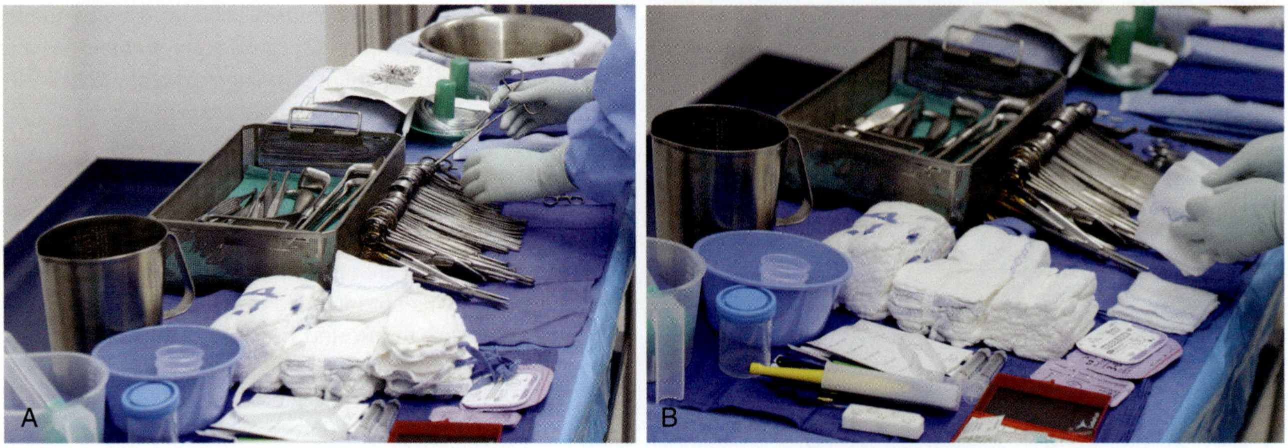

FIG. 18.12 The scrubbed surgical technologist and circulator participate in the surgical count together. (A) An instrument can be used as a pointer during the count. Here, the ST and circulator count the instruments. The circulator records the counts on a count sheet, which remains part of the surgical record. (B) The surgical technologist separates each sponge as it is being counted.

being counted should be grouped together and accessible for the initial count.

The count is performed audibly, with the circulator and the scrubbed ST. Both people participating in the count must *see the items* as they are counted (Fig. 18.12). The circulator and scrub person are required to sign the count on the patient's operative record. This is a legal document that attests to the outcome of the count. Anyone who performs a count, including relief personnel, must sign off their count.

The standard procedure for the count is shown in Box 18.2.

INCORRECT COUNT: PACKAGED ITEMS

Occasionally the pack of sponges or other items normally counted contains an incorrect number of the number of items stated on the package. The current standard of practice for this situation is as follows:

1. Exclude the sponges from the count.
2. Remove the sponges from the field.
3. Isolate the sponge from other countable items in the operating room.
4. Label the sponges.
5. Remove the items from the room *before the patient arrives* (AORN, 2019).

COUNTING SYSTEMS

The most commonly retained item is the surgical sponge. Systems used to collect (confine) and count sponges prevent errors. These include multipocketed bags that can be suspended from an IV stand (Fig. 18.13). Counts may be recorded during surgery using a whiteboard. Electronic technology used for the count includes bar coding and radiofrequency tagging, in which a chip is embedded in each sponge and can be tracked using a tracking device. These devices are rapidly gaining the approval of professional organizations and may become mandatory in the future.

For recommendations on counts published by The Joint Commission, refer to http://www.jointcommission.org/assets/1/6/sea_51_urfos_10_17_13_final.pdf.

WAIVED COUNTS DURING A SURGICAL EMERGENCY

There may be extreme emergency cases in which the life of the patient is immediately endangered and a count is waived. The amount of time between the announcement of an incoming emergency and the arrival of the patient in the operating room may be less than 10 minutes. In these few minutes, the surgical team must prepare the operating room, open the case, perform hand antisepsis, and receive the patient. If an initial count is waived, an *incident report* stating the rationale must be submitted. During the case, counts are performed as usual, as the situation permits. Imaging may be performed at the conclusion of the case to demonstrate that no item was seen. Each facility is responsible for publishing protocols and policies regarding waived counts.

Refer to Chapter 3 for a discussion on incident reporting.

HOW TO DOCUMENT THE SURGICAL COUNT

All counts are documented in the patient record. The documentation includes the names of the individuals who participated in the counts (including relief staff) and their signatures attesting to a correct or incorrect count. Count sheets on which counts are documented in real time may become part of the permanent record, according to facility policy.

LOST AND RETAINED ITEMS

Loss of sponges, needles, instruments, or other surgical equipment extends anesthesia time, increases patient risk, raises costs, and increases stress on the surgical team. If a surgical sponge or other item is left behind in the patient, it may be

BOX 18.2 Standard Procedure for the Surgical Count

WHAT
- Soft goods (textiles) including radiopaque sponges of all types, surgical towels, and packing material (e.g., material used in the nasal cavity to absorb blood)
- Individual suture packages
- Sharps, including intact knife blades, hypodermic needles, suture needles, trocars, and fragments, if broken
- Instruments
- Miscellaneous items such as electrosurgery tips, cranial (Raney type) clips and their cartridges, umbilical and vessel loops, electrosurgery cleaning pads, small bottles and their caps, medical device parts, and any other object that can be lost in the surgical wound

WHEN
- Before the procedure (to establish a baseline)
- Whenever additional items are introduced to the sterile field intraoperatively
- At the start of wound closure
- Before closing any hollow organ
- Before closing a body cavity
- During closure of skin or other final tissue layer
- Whenever permanent relief personnel join the surgical team
- At the request of the surgeon or any other team member

HOW
- According to the health care institution's policy
- In a systematic, deliberate way, without distraction or interruption
- Without deviation from policy and protocol
- In an established sequence by the type of item being counted (e.g., instruments, sponges, sharps)
- By separating or pointing to each and every item and counting them individually
- Audibly and visually; both people performing the count do so aloud, as they see the items being counted

WHO
- As designated by health care facility policy
- The circulator and scrubbed technologist or nurse
- Other members of the sterile team and circulator

DOCUMENTATION
- As soon as a count is taken, it is documented on a count sheet and/or whiteboard.
- Whenever new counted items are added to the sterile field, they are immediately entered on the count sheet and/or whiteboard.
- All scrub and circulating personnel are required to sign off the count, validating the numbers and who participated in the counts during surgery.

spotted on x-ray or by radiofrequency (RF) alert if an RF system is in place.

How Items Are Lost

The most recent studies on RSIs show that specific scenarios in surgery are more likely to lead to lost items and incorrect counts:

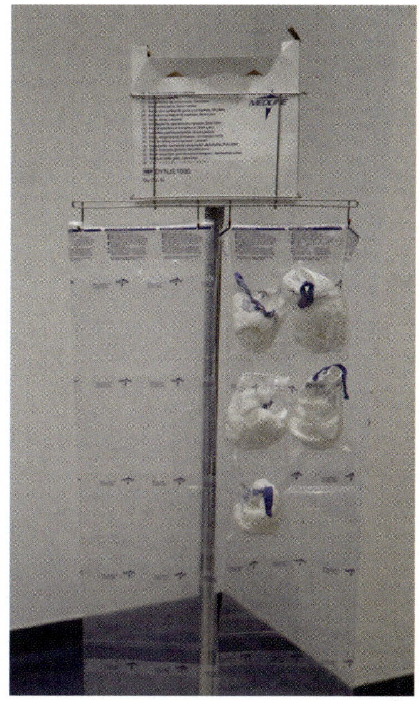

FIG. 18.13 Used sponges are contained using a pocket sponge rack.

- The procedure lasts for more than 8 hours.
- There is multiple staff turnover during a procedure.
- A sponge is used inappropriately (i.e., outside of the usual protocol). For example, a **Raytec** (4 × 4) sponge is not mounted on a clamp for use in a body cavity.
- There is failure to document items added to the field during surgery.
- The team has not kept track of sponges as they are used.
- The surgical field is cluttered or disorganized.
- The sponge count is performed incorrectly, not following standard procedure.
- Excessive noise from music, equipment, talking, and cell phones may make it difficult to hear the count.

The surgical technologist must be accountable for sponges as they are used. This requires focused attention to the operative site and concentration on what items are in use. Sponges (and instruments) can easily become "lost" in the body cavity of a deep-bodied or obese patient. Sponges are often found in the folds of drapes, under basins, among the skin prep sponges, or on the floor under the operating table. Small needles are lost when they snag on drapes or other linen and spring off the field. Small items, such as instrument parts, can easily drop into the surgical wound.

HOW TO SEARCH FOR A LOST ITEM

If the count is incorrect, the surgeon is notified and the count is repeated. If the count is still incorrect, a search is initiated. Nonsterile team members search nonsterile areas, while scrubbed team members search the wound and sterile field. Normally, the surgical technologist is responsible for searching the back table, Mayo, and any other instrument tables. All trash and waste receptacles are emptied onto an impervious drape, and each piece is searched. As each bag is searched, the contents are again bagged systematically. Equipment on the back table must be shifted to allow a search under instrument trays and basins. The floor around the operating table is thoroughly examined, and team members are asked to step slightly away from the field, because sponges are often found between the team member and the table or patient. A magnetized roller is used to search all floor spaces for metal items. Team members must show the soles of their shoes for inspection, another place where lost needles can be found. The smallest microsurgical needles cannot be seen on x-ray and may be very difficult to spot on or around the surgical field.

If a lost item is not located, an x-ray is usually ordered. If the item is lost during closure, the procedure may be halted until the x-ray is read. However, not all retained items are easily seen on an x-ray. If a lost item is neither found in the room nor revealed on an x-ray, it may still be retained in the wound. In such a case, all layers of the surgical wound may be reopened and searched. If the surgeon is confident that the item has not been left in the wound and the risk of extended anesthesia does not outweigh the risk of a retained object, the x-ray may be ordered in the PACU.

PREVENTING RETAINED ITEMS

The problem of retained items and the health consequences are of such significance that safety and professional organizations have instituted conferences, new research studies, and awareness campaigns to try and decrease their incidence. Among the most important messages to operating room teams are the following summary guidelines on preventing retained items, which are derived from both the Association of Surgical Technologists and Association of periOperative Nurses recommended practices:

- During the count, unnecessary activity and distraction should be curtailed to allow the surgical technologist and RN circulator to focus on the task at hand.
- Standardized procedure should be used during all counts. Items are counted by type (e.g., sponges, instruments, needles).
- Sharps must be contained within a magnetic box or board.
- **Radiopaque** soft goods (e.g., sponges, towels, textiles) should be accounted for during all procedures in which soft goods are used.
- If the surgical sponge pack is banded, the band should be broken and discarded before the count.
- Items are counted as they are added to a case.
- Radiopaque sponges must not be used as wound dressings or in the patient prep.
- All *counted* items should stay in the operating room or procedure room until the close of surgery.
- The final count is not complete until all sponges used in the closing wound are accounted for.
- Sponges or other counted items dropped on the floor should be retrieved by the circulator and the item shown to the surgical technologist.
- Sponges and other radiopaque items must not be cut for use in the wound.
- Broken instrument parts are isolated from the setup and accounted for.
- Trash and linen bags must remain in the operating room until the patient has left the room.

START OF SURGERY

The start of surgery begins *officially* with the onset of anesthesia. The events that occur immediately before and after can take place in succession or simultaneously.

Patient positioning begins after intubation of the patient under general anesthesia and only when the patient is stable. The surgeon and ACP may provide guidance during complex positioning. The ACP protects and maintains the patient's airway while coordinating the positioning to ensure patient safety. If the surgeons participate in positioning, they perform hand antisepsis immediately afterward. They will then return to the room for gowning and gloving.

The circulator performs the patient skin prep as soon as the patient position is secure and the ACP has verified that the patient is stable. Draping follows immediately afterward. The surgical technologist assists in draping by providing the correct draping layers in the correct sequence; he or she assists the surgeon as the drapes are positioned. As soon as the drapes are secured, the Mayo and instrument tables are brought into position to complete the sterile field. Suction tubing, the ESU and holster, light cords, and tubing are secured to the top drape using one or more *nonpenetrating clamps*, allowing sufficient slack between the instruments and the edge of the sterile field. The technologist places one or two sponges on the field. At this point, all activity stops so that Universal Protocol can be performed.

Refer to Chapter 17 for detailed information on draping the patient.

UNIVERSAL PROTOCOL (TIMEOUT)

Universal Protocol is a process used to prevent serious errors in patient identification, wrong site, and wrong surgery. Statistics from The Joint Commission indicate that wrong-site surgery accounts for 13.1% of all sentinel events and represents the largest number of sentinel events reported. In human terms, this represents needless trauma and suffering for many patients. In response to these and other errors, The Joint Commission released the first Universal Protocol for preventing wrong-site surgery in 2004. Since that time, additional surgical checklists have been developed, and facilities are able to design their own checklists according to specific needs. The protocol establishes a **TIMEOUT** period for all surgical procedures.

Universal Protocol is performed before the first incision to allow the entire surgical team time to verify patient identity, surgical side and site, and other information critical to the procedure. Basic surgical checklists have been developed by the World Health Organization (WHO) and The Joint Commission. The AORN has compiled a comprehensive list that includes all lists in one tool (Fig. 18.14).

NOTE *that The Joint Commission does not stipulate which team member initiates any section of the checklist. However, the surgeon in charge is usually appointed to lead the process.*

Comprehensive surgical checklist

Blue = World Health Organization (WHO) Green = The Joint Commission - Universal Protocol 2016 National Patient Safety Goals Teal = Joint Commission and WHO

Preprocedure check-in	Sign-in	Time-out	Sign-out
In preoperative ready area	Before induction of anesthesia	Before skin incision	Before the patient leaves the operating room
Patient or patient representative actively confirms with registered nurse (RN):	RN and anesthesia professional confirm:	Initiated by designated team member: All other activities to be suspended (except in case of life-threatening emergency)	RN confirms:
Identity ☐ Yes Procedure and procedure site ☐ Yes Consent(s) ☐ Yes Site marked ☐ Yes ☐ N/A by the person performing the procedure RN confirms presence of: History and physical ☐ Yes Preanesthesia assessment ☐ Yes Nursing assessment ☐ Yes Diagnostic and radiologic test results ☐ Yes ☐ N/A Blood products ☐ Yes ☐ N/A Any special equipment, devices, implants ☐ Yes ☐ N/A Include in preprocedure check-in as per institutional custom: Beta blocker medication given ☐ Yes ☐ N/A Venous thromboembolism prophylaxis ordered ☐ Yes ☐ N/A Normothermia measures ☐ Yes ☐ N/A	Confirmation of the following: identity, procedure, procedure site, and consent(s) ☐ Yes Site marked ☐ Yes ☐ N/A by person performing the procedure Patient allergies ☐ Yes ☐ N/A Pulse oximeter on patient ☐ Yes Difficult airway or aspiration risk ☐ No ☐ Yes (preparation confirmed) Risk of blood loss (> 500 mL) ☐ Yes ☐ N/A # of units available ________ Anesthesia safety check completed ☐ Yes Briefing: All members of the team have discussed care plan and addressed concerns ☐ Yes	Introduction of team members ☐ Yes All: Confirmation of the following: identity, procedure, incision site, consent(s) ☐ Yes Site is marked and visible ☐ Yes ☐ N/A Fire risk assessment and discussion ☐ Yes (prevention methods implemented) ☐ N/A Relevant images properly labeled and displayed ☐ Yes ☐ N/A Any equipment concerns ☐ Yes ☐ N/A Anticipated critical events Surgeon: States the following: ☐ Critical or nonroutine steps ☐ Case duration ☐ Anticipated blood loss Anesthesia professional: Antibiotic prophylaxis within 1 hour before incision ☐ Yes ☐ N/A Additional concerns ☐ Yes ☐ N/A Scrub person and RN circulator: Sterilization indicators confirmed ☐ Yes Additional concerns ☐ Yes ☐ N/A RN: Documented completion of time out ☐ Yes	Name of operative procedure: ________ Completion of sponge, sharp, and instrument counts ☐ Yes ☐ N/A Specimens identified and labeled ☐ Yes ☐ N/A Equipment problems to be addressed ☐ Yes ☐ N/A Discussion of wound classification ☐ Yes To all team members: What are the key concerns for recovery and management of this patient? ________ ________ ________ ________ Debriefing with all team members: Opportunity for discussion of – Team performance – Key events – Any permanent changes in the preference card January 2019

The joint commission does not stipulate which team member initiates any section of the checklist except for site marking. The joint commission also does not stipulate where these activities occur. See the universal protocol for details on the joint commission requirements.

AORN SAFE SURGERY TOGETHER

FIG. 18.14 Universal Protocol to prevent wrong-side, wrong-site, wrong-patient, and other surgical accidents. This checklist is used during a TIMEOUT before every surgical procedure before the first incision is made. All team members participate in TIMEOUT. (From AORN Correct Site Surgery Tool Kit.)

SITE MARKING

Marking the surgical site and side is a *regulatory requirement* to prevent wrong-site surgery. The guidelines for implementation are as follows:

- The patient's identity, procedure, and procedural site including [side] must be verified and the site marked.
- The site marking process must be consistent throughout the health care organization and not open to interpretation.
- The procedure site must be marked before the procedure begins.

Normally the patient should take part in identifying the site and side. Marking should therefore take place in the patient holding area and verified with the surgical team after the patient is brought to the procedure room. An indelible skin marking pen is used. The surgeon marking the site must include her or his initials at or near the site.

KEY CONCEPTS

- A surgical case plan is a method for improving efficiency and accuracy in preparation for a surgical case. It is a way of thinking and doing that can enhance the surgical technologist's organizational skills and increase his or her ability to anticipate the technical requirements of the procedure.
- A surgical case plan contains distinct elements related to the technical and patient care requirements of the procedure. The elements may vary in complexity according to the type of procedure planned and the specific needs of the patient. The case plan elements can be formulated as distinct questions (e.g., Do I need…?) or simply a list of points that must be considered to prepare for the procedure.
- Tasks can be separated into preoperative, intraoperative, and postoperative. Planning ahead of time for each phase is one way to approach case planning.
- The sterile setup can seem difficult at first but can be made manageable by organizing each part of the setup into a sequence that can be used for most cases.
- The nonsterile case setup is the preparation of the operating room for a specific procedure. This includes positioning of furniture and nonsterile devices, correcting room temperature as needed, and the testing and connection of energy and suction sources.
- The surgical count is performed at specific times using prescribed technique to decrease the risk of any surgical device, instrument, or sponge being left behind in the

wound. The count is both time and event related. For example, a count is always performed before surgery begins, before a hollow organ or body cavity is closed, and at the close of surgery before the skin incision is closed.

- Specific practices have been established to prevent retained surgical items. The surgical count is the primary method of prevention. Other important standards identify the proper use, confinement, and detection of items that can be easily lost in the surgical wound.
- The surgical Universal Protocol has been developed in response to the high rate of wrong-site and wrong-patient surgeries. The protocol is specific, precise, and mandatory in all accredited health care facilities.

REVIEW QUESTIONS

1. What do you think is the most difficult part of setting up a surgical case? What steps are you taking to overcoming this challenge?
2. What is the rationale for opening large, heavy items first when preparing for a surgical case?
3. What is the rationale for handling sterile items as little as possible during the setup?
4. Who can perform a count?
5. When are counts performed?
6. Who is legally responsible for the surgical count?

CASE STUDIES

CASE 1

You have been assigned to surgical technologist for an *exploratory laparotomy*. You have received the case cart from the central processing department and have the surgeon's preference card to pick the rest of the supplies noted on the card. You have about 30 minutes before the scheduled case, and it normally takes you about 15 minutes to do the sterile setup for a laparotomy. After opening the case, you proceed to the scrub area to perform the surgical hand antisepsis. When you return to the suite, the anesthesiologist assistant is in the room preparing equipment and drugs. You proceed to gown and glove. *Consider the following events and describe your problem-solving approach:*

1. After approximately 15 minutes, you are finished with the setup; the patient has not arrived, and you are left alone in the room with the setup. The assistant arrives and states that the surgery is delayed. What will you do? Consider the options, the guidelines for a delayed case, and the uncertainty of the situation.
2. You have decided to wait, still scrubbed, with the setup. The circulator arrives in another 15 minutes to tell you that the case has been canceled but another patient is coming in after a motor vehicle accident. The case is scheduled to begin in 30 minutes. How can you use the sterile setup and still prepare for an orthopedic case? You have previously scrubbed only one minor orthopedic case. What is your *strategy* for case planning?

CASE 2

Universal Protocol was developed because of the high rate of medical errors made in surgery, including wrong site, wrong side, and even the wrong patient. The protocols for sponge and needle counts (the *count*) and for the medication process were similarly created because of the number of deaths and injury related to these activities. Based on what you have learned and observed about human nature, job stress, and the causes of surgical errors, *what are the most important advantages to having such protocols?* Try to think about "near misses" you may have witnessed and what strategies you use to prevent errors.

REFERENCES

1. Association of Surgical Technologists. *Standard of practice V. In Standards of Practice for Creating a Sterile Field*; 2011.
2. Association of periOperative Registered Nurses (AORN). *Autologous tissue Management in: Perioperative Standards and Recommended Practices*. Denver, CO: AORN, Inc; 2015.
3. Joint Commission. Facts about the universal protocol https://www.jointcommission.org/standards_information/up.aspx. Accessed July 28, 2019.
4. Norton E, Martin C, Micheli A. Patients count on it: an initiative to reduce incorrect counts and prevent retained surgical items. *AORN*. 2012;95(109).
5. Rowland A, Steeves R. Incorrect surgical counts: a qualitative analysis. *AORN*. 2010;92:410.

BIBLIOGRAPHY

Association of periOperative Registered Nurses (AORN). Policy and procedure retained surgical items. In: *Perioperative Standards and Recommended Practices*. Denver, CO: AORN, Inc; 2016.

AORN. Retained Surgical Items, Guideline Essentials, Policy and Procedure, 2019. https://www.aorn.org/essentials/retained-surgical-items.

Barfield WD. Committee on Fetus and Newborn: standard terminology for fetal, infant, and perinatal deaths. *Pediatrics*. 2011;128:177.

Kallis PJ, Friedman AJ, Lev-Tov H. A Guide to Tissue-Engineered Skin Substitutes. *J Drug Dermatol*. 2018;17(1):57–64.

Occupational Safety and Health Administration (OSHA): Formaldehyde, Regulations (Standards – 29 CFR). https://www.osha.gov/SLTC/etools/hospital/lab/lab.html. Accessed July 28, 2019.

SURGICAL SKILLS II: INTRAOPERATIVE AND IMMEDIATE POSTOPERATIVE PERIOD

19

KNOWLEDGE AND SKILLS REVIEW

The following skills and knowledge should be reviewed before you start this chapter:

Management of surgical specimens
Sterile technique
Surgical pharmacology—solutions used in surgery, wound adhesives, hemostatic agents
Transport of soiled instruments, environmental cleaning
Electrosurgery
Ultrasonic energy

LEARNING OBJECTIVES

After studying this chapter, the reader will be able to:

1. Define the role of the surgical technologist during the intraoperative period
2. Discuss Halstead's principles of surgery
3. Discuss different methods of hemostasis used during surgery
4. Demonstrate how surgical sponges are managed during surgery
5. Discuss the use of absorbable and non-absorbable sutures
6. Demonstrate suture-handling techniques
7. Identify different types of wound drains
8. Identify commonly used wound dressing materials
9. Discuss postoperative wound complications

TERMINOLOGY

Absorbable suture: Suture material that is broken down and metabolized by the body.

Adhesion: An abnormal band of tissue that binds abdominal structures together. Adhesions may form as a result of infection or surgery.

Anastomosis: A connection between two tubular organs such as blood vessels, intestine, tubes, or ducts. An anastomosis can be natural or created by a surgical procedure.

Approximate: To bring tissues together by sutures or other means.

Biopsy: Removal of tissue for examination and interpretation. A biopsy is often performed to rule out malignancy.

Capillary action: The ability of suture material to absorb and wick fluid.

Dehiscence: Separation of the edges of a surgical wound during healing.

Detachable suture: A suture-needle combination in which the suture can be easily removed from the needle by pulling it sharply.

Evisceration: The displacement of tissue(s) outside their normal location in the body. For example, abdominal evisceration in which abdominal contents are displaced out of the body by trauma to the abdominal wall.

Frozen section: A method used to flash freeze, slice, and examine a tissue specimen using the microscope. This procedure is used when an immediate diagnosis is required.

Hematoma: An abnormal blood-filled space in tissue that prevents wound healing and may result in infection.

Hemostasis: Absence of bleeding.

Inert: Causing little or no reaction in tissue. Used to describe a material used in the manufacturing of suture or a surgical implant.

Interrupted sutures: A technique of bringing tissue together by placing individual sutures close together.

Non-absorbable suture: Suture material that resists breakdown in the body.

Primary intention: The wound-healing process after a clean surgical repair.

Reverse cutting needle: A suture needle containing a sharp edge along the inside curve.

Swage: The area of an atraumatic suture where the suture strand is fused to the needle.

Tensile strength: The amount of force or stress a suture can withstand before breaking.

Tie on a passer: A strand of suture material attached to the tip of an instrument.

This chapter introduces essential surgical skills for the surgical technologist from the beginning of surgery to the final closure, and immediate postoperative period. Recall that Chapter 18 covered the following skills in sequence:

1. Development of a surgical case plan
2. Preoperative case preparation
3. Nonsterile room preparation
4. Opening a case
5. Sterile setup
6. Surgical count
7. Start of surgery and Universal Protocol (TIMEOUT)

This chapter continues with the *elementary* skills of surgical assisting as well as management of the sterile field and surgical wound. Each topic includes theory and practice.

HALSTEAD'S PRINCIPLES OF SURGERY

Wound management during surgery involves practices that achieve the surgical objectives while protecting exposed tissues. During surgery, tissues within the surgical wound are vulnerable to drying, lateral heating from electrosurgical instruments, bruising, and blood loss. Local tissue ischemia (poor circulation leading to oxygen deprivation) can also occur as tissues are retracted, clamped, or handled roughly. Effective wound and tissue management prevents postoperative surgical site infection and promotes rapid healing.

Modern techniques in wound and tissue management are based on essential principles that were developed more than 100 years ago by the famous Johns Hopkins University surgeon William Halstead (also spelled Halsted). Halstead shocked his colleagues by criticizing their lack (or complete absence) of sterile technique. At the time Halstead was teaching, surgeons did not use gloves and operated in their street clothes. Halstead also advocated for gentle handling of tissue and the use of very fine sutures placed close together with minimal tension on the tissue edges. The principles of surgical wound and tissue management that he developed are still considered to be the foundation of good surgical practice. As an essential member of the surgical team, the surgical technologist can benefit from studying these principles. Halstead's principles of surgery are as follows:

1. **Handle tissues gently**. Living tissues can be easily bruised, abraded, or crushed during surgery. Following Halstead's principles, gentle handling of tissues is one of the most important goals of wound and tissue management. Rough handling of deep tissues (e.g., bowel, blood vessels) and other delicate structures can cause extensive bruising, tissue swelling, and ischemia. This can result in an increased inflammatory response and delayed healing.
2. **Control bleeding.** Hemorrhage reduces total blood volume. Small bleeding vessels can create blood clots or hematomas that prevent healing and lead to postoperative infection. Careful control of bleeding (**hemostasis**) allows good visualization of the anatomy and a better surgical outcome.
3. **Preserve blood supply.** Meticulous tissue dissection sacrifices as few blood vessels as possible. Without blood supply, tissues cannot heal.
4. **Keep tissues moist.** Body tissues are normally surrounded by fluid that lubricates and protects them. During surgery surface fluid on exposed tissues and organs can become dry. Surface drying increases tissue vulnerability to abrasion and bruising.
5. **Observe strict sterile technique.** This should not need emphasis in today's surgical environment. However, even in modern operating rooms, compromises in sterile technique can be observed when staff are rushed, stressed, or tired.
6. **Minimize tissue tension.** In reference to suturing techniques, tissue tension must be avoided. Tension on suture lines creates trauma, swelling, and compression on capillaries at the tissue edge. All of these prevent healing, cause pain, and may result in a surgical site infection.
7. **Eliminate dead space.** Dead space is a gap between tissue layers that normally lie in close contact. Dead space results in the development of hematomas and serum pockets, leading to infection or the necessity for a second surgery to drain the fluid. Dead space is minimized by careful suturing, hemostasis, and, if necessary, insertion of a surgical drain to prevent the formation of fluid pockets.

INTRAOPERATIVE ROLE OF THE SURGICAL TECHNOLOGIST

This discussion describes the general role of the surgical technologist in the intraoperative period from the time the first incision is made after the TIMEOUT period to implement the *Universal Protocol* until the close of surgery. Expanded topics such as surgical assisting (e.g., retraction techniques, management of sutures, irrigation, and hemostasis) are covered separately because these discussions are lengthy. Table 19.1 is a continuation of Table 18.1 (previous chapter), which describes the roles of the different members of the surgical team in time sequence.

SKIN MARKING AND THE INCISION

Skin marking was discussed in the previous chapter. This procedure may take place in the surgeon's office, or in the preoperative holding area, After the Universal Protocol is completed, the anesthesia care provider must signal to the surgeon that the skin incision can be made. This ensures that the patient under general anesthesia has entered the surgical plane of unconsciousness. The surgeon may request a skin marker to indicate landmarks or further define the incision lines as shown in Fig. 19.1A.

TABLE 19.1 Responsibilities of the Scrubbed Technologist, Circulator, and Surgeon

Scrubbed Surgical Technologist	Circulator	Surgeon
FROM INCISION TO END OF SURGERY		
Places two sponges on incision site. Passes marking pen or scalpel to surgeon. Gives retractors to assistant after skin incision. Participates in all instrument, sponge, and needle counts with circulator. Passes sterile equipment to surgeons and assistants using correct orientation and technique. Listens for direction and anticipates each step of the surgery. Maintains a sterile field, notifying others when sterile technique is broken. Deposits soiled sponges in designated receptacle. Maintains a safe surgical field by exercising all precautions when electrosurgical devices, lasers, and sharps are in use. Requests additional equipment as needed. Secures intraoperative tissue and fluid specimens delivered by the surgeon. Obtains grafts and implants as required by the surgery. Prepares dressings and begins to separate soiled from clean instruments. Participates in final instrument, sponge, and needle count. Notifies surgeon if count is incorrect. If count is incorrect, searches for missing item. Applies sterile dressings as directed by surgeon. Maintains sterility until patient leaves the room. Keeps basic instruments on Mayo stand in case of emergency. Prepares instruments on back table for decontamination.	*Records time of incision on patient record. *Distributes sterile solutions and medications to scrubbed person. Provides additional equipment as needed by the surgical technologist and surgeons. Operates nonsterile equipment. Adjusts lighting. Flash sterilizes instruments as needed. Answers surgeon's pages and relays messages. Anticipates flow of surgery and equipment needs of surgeon and surgical technologist. *Monitors urinary output. Responds to medical emergencies. Directs instrument, sponge, and needle counts at appropriate times. *Labels specimens obtained from the scrubbed person for the pathology department. Wearing gloves, separates sponges and places them in counting area or isolates them in groups of 5 or 10. Maintains safe environment. Keeps doors closed; maintains quiet. Replaces equipment that is unsafe or malfunctions. Assesses the patient's physical status and assists ACP as needed. Near completion of surgery, calls for next patient. Checks on equipment for next procedure. Participates in count. Notifies surgeon if count is incorrect. At completion of surgery, assists in removing drapes and disconnecting hoses and tubing. Suction remains connected until the patient leaves the room. Applies tape to dressings and connects nonsterile ends of drainage devices. *Removes dispersive electrode pad and assesses site. *Completes intraoperative record. Transfers patient to stretcher. Calls for room turnover. *Accompanies patient and ACP to postoperative recovery unit and gives report to PACU nurse.	Marks incision area or begins skin incision. Performs surgery according to plan and intraoperative events. Directs the surgical team during emergency. If count is incorrect and missing item is not found, takes responsibility for further action (e.g., x-ray, reopening of wound). Removes gown and gloves, signs patient care documents, and gives any instructions to RN and ACP. Assists in transferring patient to gurney.
AFTER THE PATIENT LEAVES THE OPERATING ROOM		
Separates single use from reusable items. All soiled disposables are placed in biohazard bags. Linens are also placed in biohazard bags.	Checks on equipment for next case. May begin to open the next case after the operating suite is cleaned. Receives next patient in the holding area.	Notifies the family of the patient's condition. Dictates the operative report.

Continued

TABLE 19.1 Responsibilities of the Scrubbed Technologist, Circulator, and Surgeon—cont'd

Scrubbed Surgical Technologist	Circulator	Surgeon
Aspirates all solutions in closed suction containers. Removes containers from room. Places sharps in secure, closed sharps container. Places all contaminated materials in biohazard bags. Removes soiled gown and gloves and places them in biohazard waste bag. Removes mask by handling only strings. Removes face shield without touching bare skin. Puts on nonsterile gloves to transport covered equipment to decontamination area. Follows hospital policy for equipment decontamination. Is responsible for correct destination of instruments and supplies. Assists with cleaning of operating suite.		

*Licensed registered nurse responsibility.

IMPORTANT TO KNOW *The skin should have been marked to indicate the side of the body and the surgeon's initials in the patient holding area. Fig. 19.1A and B shows two different patients with relevant skin marking. Note the surgeon's initials and the initials YES, which means the surgeon has validated the correct operative side. His or her initials identify who validated the operative side. Skin marking often includes the incision line or lines, anatomical landmarks, and other graphics to provide visual guidance during the procedure.*

At the start of the procedure the ST places two dry sponges on the field along with the receptacle for the scalpel. Raytec sponges can be used for superficial surgery. Lap sponges are used during surgical procedures involving the body cavities (thoracic, abdominal, retroperitoneal, pelvic) and during major orthopedic surgery.

NEUTRAL SHARPS ZONE

Recall from Chapter 9 that a neutral zone for sharp instruments such as the knife and suture needles is established at the start of surgery. The receptacle is set directly on the field in reach of the surgeon who picks up the knife, uses it, and replaces it in the receptacle. This prevents injury, which can occur when the knife or other sharp item is passed hand to hand. This technique is referred to as the *neutral zone* or *hands-free technique* and is the recommended method to prevent injury. The surgical technologist should remove the scalpel tray from the field after the surgeon has finished making the initial incision.

EXTENDING THE INCISION

Once the skin incision has been made, the surgeon increases the depth using the electrosurgery unit (ESU). This allows small bleeders to be managed while the incision is carried through the tissues underlying the skin. The surgical assistant uses a sponge to retract the skin and superficial tissues away from the ESU tip and expose the deeper tissue layers.

The ST should have curved hemostats ready in case of bleeding that cannot be controlled by the ESU or during biopsy procedures in which the ESU would distort the cellular structure of the biopsy tissue.

PACKING THE SURGICAL WOUND

Packing the surgical wound refers to the placement of several surgical sponges inside the incision to displace tissues and organs that would otherwise obstruct the surgeon's working space inside the wound. Large incisions, such as those of the abdomen and thoracic cavity, are packed routinely before placing large retractors. Packing prevents direct contact between large retractor blades and tissues. In this case the sponges act as a cushion or bumper. Packing can also prevent blood from pooling, as the sponges apply wide, gentle pressure on the tissues.

IMPORTANT TO KNOW *The surgeon needs smooth dressing forceps and at least three moist lap sponges to pack a wound cavity. The surgical technologist should select the correct length of the forceps according to the depth of the surgical wound (e.g., adult regular, extra-long, or pediatric patient).*

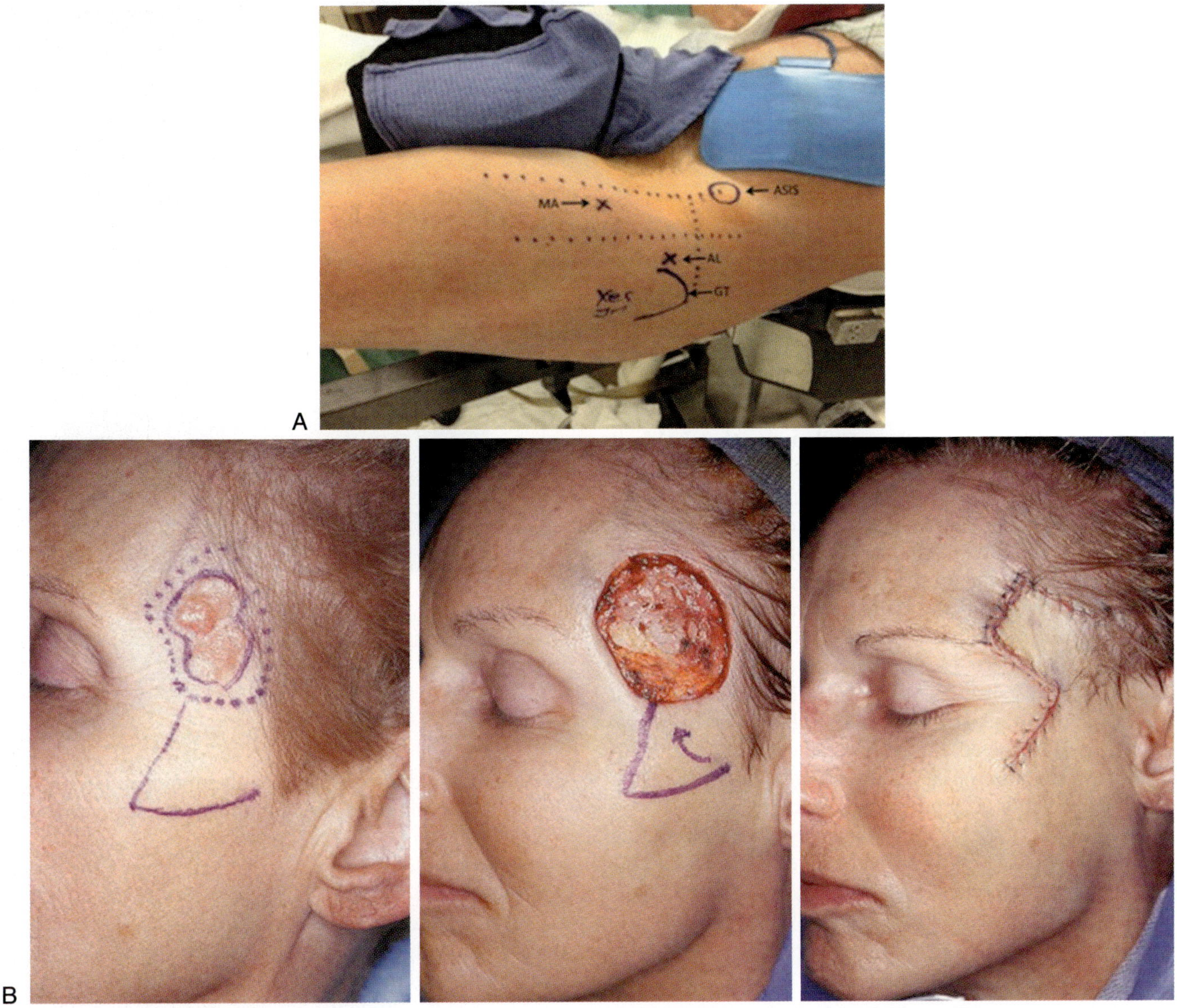

FIG. 19.1 (A) Skin marking to indicate the side of the body and the surgeon's initials is required. The surgeon may make addition marks and measurements to indicate the incision line and anatomical landmarks. (B) Skin marking for excision of a skin lesion. The *solid line* represents the extent of the lesion. The *dotted line* indicates the incision, which has been determined by measuring the distance out from the lesion. The V-shaped marking is the incision required to create a flap necessary for wound closure. (A, From Menge TJ, Chahla J, Soares E, et al. The Quebec City SLIDER: a technique for capsular closure and plication in hip arthroscopy. *Arthrosc Tech.* 2016;5[5]:e971-e974. B, From Baker SR, Little S. *Local Flaps in Facial Reconstruction*. Philadelphia: Elsevier Saunders; 2014.)

IMPORTANT TO KNOW *The ST must count and identify the location of all sponges placed in the wound as they are placed. This includes lap sponges and 4 × 4 Raytec sponges. Raytec sponges are not permitted on the sterile field in procedures involving a body cavity unless they are mounted on a sponge forceps. However, the surgeon may pack one or more Raytec sponges in a superficial wound as a tamponade to control bleeding. This can occur when the ESU cannot be used as such as during biopsy procedures (e.g., breast biopsy). In this instance the ESU is not used because it may distort the margins of a suspected malignancy. All sponges placed as packing should be reported to the circulator during placement and documented on the sponge sheet or white board.*

RETRACTION

Tissue retraction is needed in nearly every type of surgery. Unless the focus of the procedure lies in superficial tissues, access must be obtained by separating tissue planes and, in some cases, dividing them surgically.

There are two basic types of retractors: *handheld* and *self-retaining*.

Handheld: As the name implies, these are held in the hand by the surgical assistant or surgical technologist in the assistant role. Examples are the Richardson retractor and the USA or Army Navy retractors, both common in general surgery. Refer to Chapter 11 for images of these retractors.

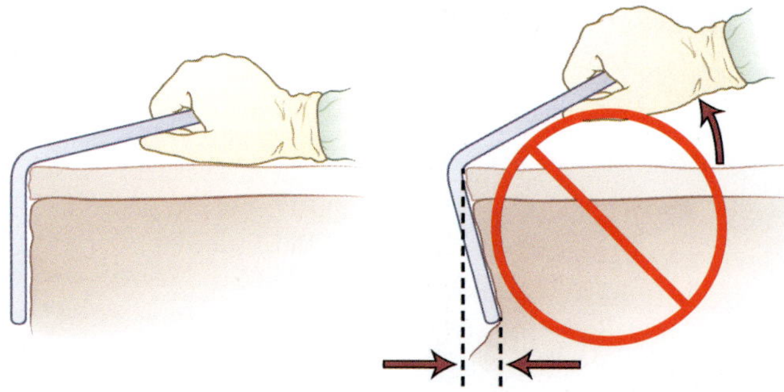

FIG. 19.2 Correct technique for wound retraction using a lateral retractor.

Self-retaining (designed with a mechanism that holds it open): The self-retaining retractor may be spring loaded to remain open (much like a safety pin) or placed in the wound and mechanically held in place. Common self-retaining retractors include the Balfour and Omni used in abdominal surgery, the Finochietto used in some thoracic incisions, and the shallow Weitlaner retractor, which is often used in hernia repair. These are shown in Chapter 11.

Retractors are selected according to the depth of the retracting blade (the distance between the horizontal and vertical parts of the instrument), by their tips (blunt, curved, sharp, claw-like, gently tapered), and by overall size and weight. All of these variables are considered according to the type of tissue being retracted and the depth of the surgical wound.

Retractors are passed with the tip angled down, toward the wound. Self-retaining retractors with a ratchet mechanism are always passed in the fully closed position, ready for positioning and opening in the wound.

RETRACTION TECHNIQUE

The surgical technologist may be required to retract during surgery. The usual method of retraction is for the surgeon to place the retractor and the ST to hold it in place. All but the most delicate retractors are normally held "overhand" rather than "underhand." This provides maximum control and prevents wrist fatigue.

It is very important to maintain the position of the retractor just as the surgeon places it. Do not toe the blade inward unless instructed by the surgeon (Fig. 19.2). If toeing is required, the surgeon will ask for "toe-in."

Retraction for a long period of time can cause stress on the operative hand and arm, which must be kept still the entire time (more so for delicate retraction). This can lead to distraction and slippage of the instrument. If you are required to retract, do not try to manage instruments on the Mayo at the same time. This distraction may cause the retractor to slip or tear tissue. Remember, the retractor is in contact with living, vital tissues. Excessive pressure on these tissues with the blade of the retractor is poor technique that leads to bruising and edema.

Retraction using *skin hooks* or *small rakes* requires focused concentration on the pressure at the tip to prevent accidental tearing of the tissue (Fig. 19.3). Skin hooks or sharp rake retractors should be held between the thumb and two or three fingers in the middle of the instrument for maximum control of the tip.

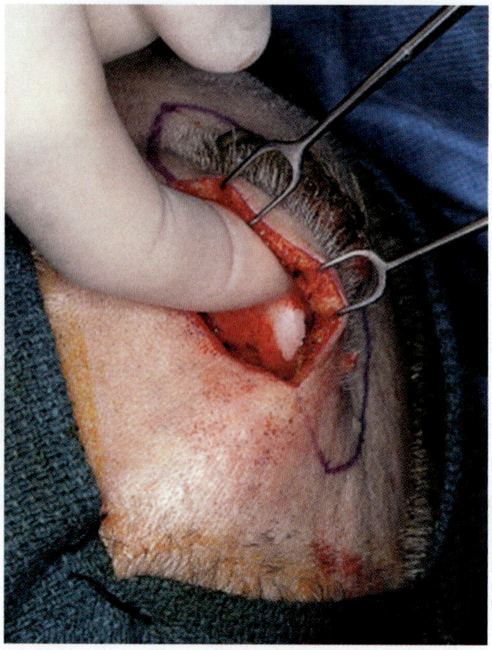

FIG. 19.3 Skin hooks used on superficial tissue. These require close attention to the amount of pressure applied to the tissue to prevent the sharp points from causing injury. (From Shah JP, Patel SG, Singh B. *Jatin Shah's Head and Neck Surgery and Oncology*. 4th ed. Amsterdam: Elsevier; 2019.)

When the surgeon requires a retractor, he or she may not indicate the exact name or size of the retractor. An experienced surgical technologist is able to determine this information by following the progress of the surgery and what tissue layers must be retracted. This skill is acquired with time and not expected of a student.

WOUND IRRIGATION

Tissues must not be allowed to dry out during surgery. Dry tissues cannot withstand handling and may slough during the healing phase. Intermittent wound irrigation is used to protect delicate tissues. Signs of dehydration in internal tissues are surface dullness, loss of surface elasticity, and tissue fraying. At the close of surgery before the incisions are closed, the wound is irrigated to flush out any blood clots, tissue debris, and bits of suture that may have fallen into the wound.

Normal saline (0.9%) irrigation fluid is commonly used in body cavities. The surgical technologist should maintain a basin of ***warm, clean saline*** for this purpose. Antibiotic irrigation solution is sometimes used to prevent infection in selected cases. A large wound is irrigated using an Asepto or bulb syringe, or the solution may be simply poured into the wound using a pitcher. Irrigation solution is removed from the wound using the inline suction with the appropriate suction tip, which is a part of most instrument setups. When large amounts of saline are required, such as during orthopedic procedures or surgery of the major body cavities, a large suction tip such as the Yankauer (tonsil) or Poole suction is used. The Poole suction tip has a removable guard with multiple perforations that distribute the suction pressure and prevent damage to delicate tissue such as the spleen, lung, and intestine. When large amounts of irrigation fluid are used, the surgical technologist must keep track of the volume so that the estimated blood loss can be calculated.

Microsurgery, or any other small wound area such as eye and ear procedures, may not require suction, and only irrigation solutions labeled for these tissues are used. Irrigation during eye procedures is crucial to maintaining the cornea. Balanced salt solution (BSS) is used for irrigation. It is supplied commercially in small plastic bottles to which an ophthalmic irrigation tip is attached. This procedure is discussed more fully in Chapter 25.

Continuous irrigation is used in specific types of surgery such as the joint capsule, genitourinary tract, and uterus. In these cases, the irrigation fluid is used as a medium through which surgery is performed. In bladder, uterine, and prostate surgery, in which tumor tissue is removed piecemeal, continuous irrigation flushes the tissue specimens from the wound. In arthroscopic joint surgery, continuous irrigation increases the joint space, providing better visualization through the arthroscope. (Refer to specific specialty chapters for a complete discussion.)

HEMOSTASIS DURING SURGERY

Hemostasis is the body's physiological mechanism to control bleeding. The body's clotting mechanism is effective for minor injury and bleeding. However, major bleeding from large vessels or highly vascular tissue can overwhelm this system.

Hemostasis is a necessary component of good surgical technique. Pooling of blood and serum in the wound in the postsurgical period can increase the risk of infection. A fluid pocket can also prevent healing, because it forms a physical barrier between tissue edges that must be in close approximation during healing. Uncontrolled oozing or insecure hemostasis can lead to a hematoma.

IMPORTANT TO KNOW *Do not confuse hemostasis with homeostasis, which is physiological equilibrium across all body systems, controlled by the central nervous system.*

The ST must watch the field carefully during surgery, even while preparing supplies and passing instruments. This is required to anticipate the need for specific instruments, equipment, and supplies, including those needed for hemostasis.

METHODS OF HEMOSTASIS

Bleeding in the surgical wound is expected. The ST should be ready to provide the correct instrument, sutures, hemostatic materials, and other supplies required to control bleeding.

BOX 19.1 Historical Highlights: Surgical Sponges

- Before the manufacture of commercial surgical sponges, and even for some years after, a fabric loop was sewn into the corner of the laparotomy sponge. The scrub nurse or technologist attached a heavy metal ring (called a lap ring) to this loop as the sponges were prepared. During surgery, when a sponge was inserted into the wound, the ring and loop were left hanging outside the incision. The purpose of the ring was for x-ray detection in case a sponge was retained. After surgery, the rings were removed, and the sponges washed and resterilized to be used in the next procedure.
- Today, we occasionally refer to laparotomy sponges as "lap tapes." The name comes from laparotomy sponges manufactured in the 1940s and 1950s, when sponges were not square, but long and rectangular—hence the name tape.

Direct Pressure

Direct pressure on bleeding tissue compresses the vascular supply and allows the body's natural clotting mechanism to take effect. This method is occasionally used during surgery. Sponges are placed over the tissue and manual pressure is applied.

Clamps

Hemostatic clamps are designed to grasp individual blood vessels or a small portion of the tissue surrounding the blood vessel. The overall design of the clamp determines how it is used. Short curved and straight hemostats such as the small mosquito clamp and larger Crile or Kelly clamps are used for superficial tissue, while longer curved and right-angled clamps are used in deep tissues. Clamps can have very delicate or heavy tips to grasp a section of tissue and its blood supply to control bleeding. After placing a hemostatic clamp, the surgeon may require a suture tie or suture and needle combination to ligate the vessel. This is discussed and illustrated later in the chapter.

Electrosurgical Coagulation

Electrosurgical coagulation has been discussed in detail in Chapter 15, including a necessary explanation of the technology and patient safety considerations. Electrosurgical coagulation is achieved by passing electrical current through tissue, including small blood vessels. This causes the tissue to desiccate (dry), vaporize, or char, which stops blood flow. The technique can be focused to a pinpoint size with high accuracy.

Ultrasonic Coagulation

This device produces high-frequency vibration concentrated in the instrument tip. No electricity is involved except that which powers the device. The vibrations of the ultrasonic tip cause tissue to liquefy and coagulate, which effectively clots any blood vessels in the area of the vibrations. Very low heat is produced, which is the result of the vibrations. This device, safety features, and further explanation of its use are described in Chapter 15.

Ligature

A ligature is a suture tie that is placed around a blood vessel or other structure and secured with two or more knots. Before the invention of electrosurgery, ligatures were used throughout the surgical procedure to achieve hemostasis in all areas of the body. Now, the ligature is more commonly used on medium and larger blood vessels that cannot be safely occluded using electrosurgery or other means. When a larger blood vessel must be severed, two clamps are placed across the vessel that is divided. Each segment is then ligated.

Hemostatic Agents

A large number of *hemostatic agents* and adjunct drugs are available to control bleeding during surgery. Some agents influence the blood-clotting mechanism, while others work mechanically to provide a scaffolding for clotting to occur. The surgical technologist will encounter these in a variety of different surgical specialties and also in general surgery. A table is also available to provide quick reference (Table 12.8).

MANAGEMENT OF SURGICAL SPONGES DURING SURGERY

Surgical sponges are used in nearly every type of surgical procedure. They are used for the following purposes:

1. They maintain a dry wound by soaking up blood and fluids.
2. They are used to retract tissue in body cavities and as cushioning against instruments used to retract as described previously.
3. Dissecting sponges are used to separate tissue planes by flaying the tissue gently with the tip or edge of the sponge.

Surgical sponges are available in a variety of sizes, shapes, and materials (Fig. 19.4).

Refer to Box 19.1, which provides historical background information on surgical sponges.

IMPORTANT TO KNOW *Because of their compatibility with human tissue and their pliability when wet, sponges can become lodged in the surgical wound and become difficult to differentiate from tissue. As explained in the previous chapter, care of sponges on and off the sterile field is crucial to ensuring that no sponge is left behind in the wound.*

All sponges used during surgery contain radio-opaque band that can be seen on x-ray. Sponges and surgical towels that do not contain radio-opaque material must not be used in the wound. The *surgical count* is the systematic counting of all items on the sterile field as discussed in the previous chapter. The guidelines and recommendations for preventing the loss of an item in the patient are included in that discussion. The surgical technologist is accountable and responsible for making sure that no item is left inside the patient.

RAYTEC 4 X 4 SPONGE

The Raytec sponge (also called a "four by four") is a large square of loosely woven gauze folded into a 4-inch–square pad. When used in a body cavity or in a deep incision, the Raytec sponge is ***always mounted on sponge forceps. This is commonly called a sponge stick.*** To mount a 4 × 4 sponge, fold it in equal thirds in one direction and in half in the other direction. Mounted Raytec sponges and sponge dissectors are shown in Fig. 19.5. Mount the sponge with the folded edge exposed at the tip of the sponge forceps. An alternative method of folding a sponge is shown in Fig. 19.6.

LAPAROTOMY SPONGE

The laparotomy sponge, or *lap sponge,* is used in major surgery, including procedures in which the abdominal or thoracic cavity is opened, during major orthopedic surgery, and in procedures in which large blood vessels are encountered. Laparotomy sponges are used to absorb blood and fluids and for padding the blades of large retractors as described above.

Lap sponges usually are moistened before use. A basin of warm saline is used for this purpose. Before passing a lap sponge, immerse it in saline and wring it dry unless the surgeon specifically asks for a "sloppy wet" sponge or similar description.

SPONGE DISSECTOR

A sponge dissector is a small round or oval sponge covered with gauze and secured with an x-ray–detectable thread. The sponge dissector is used to separate or dissect tissue by *blunt dissection*. Sponge dissectors are packaged in groups of five or ten and contained in a foam holder, making them easy to grasp with an instrument on the sterile field. Because of their small size, sponge dissectors must be mounted on an instrument or secured in their holder. **They should never be loose on the Mayo, instrument table, or any area of the surgical field.** There are many different names attached to sponge dissectors based on their size, which ranges from ½ inch to ¾ inch in diameter. These include *peanut, kitner, cherry,* or *pusher.*

ROUND STRING SPONGE

A round string sponge *(tonsil sponge)* is covered with gauze and has a string attached for retrieval. This sponge is commonly used in throat surgery and often is used to control bleeding in the tonsillar fossae after tonsillectomy. The string is draped outside the patient's mouth. Use of round sponges without strings is extremely dangerous in throat surgery. Such sponges can easily drop into the trachea and cause complete airway blockage. When the round sponge is retrieved after use, always make sure the string is attached.

The *surgical cotton ball* is specially manufactured to resist shredding and is commonly used in neurosurgical procedures, especially on brain and spinal cord tissues. Each cotton ball is attached to an x-ray–detectable string. These are almost always used wet. The ST can maintain them in a small bowl of normal saline or topical thrombin and saline for immediate use in the surgical wound to aid in hemostasis of very fine vessels in the cranial cavity. These must be handled with care

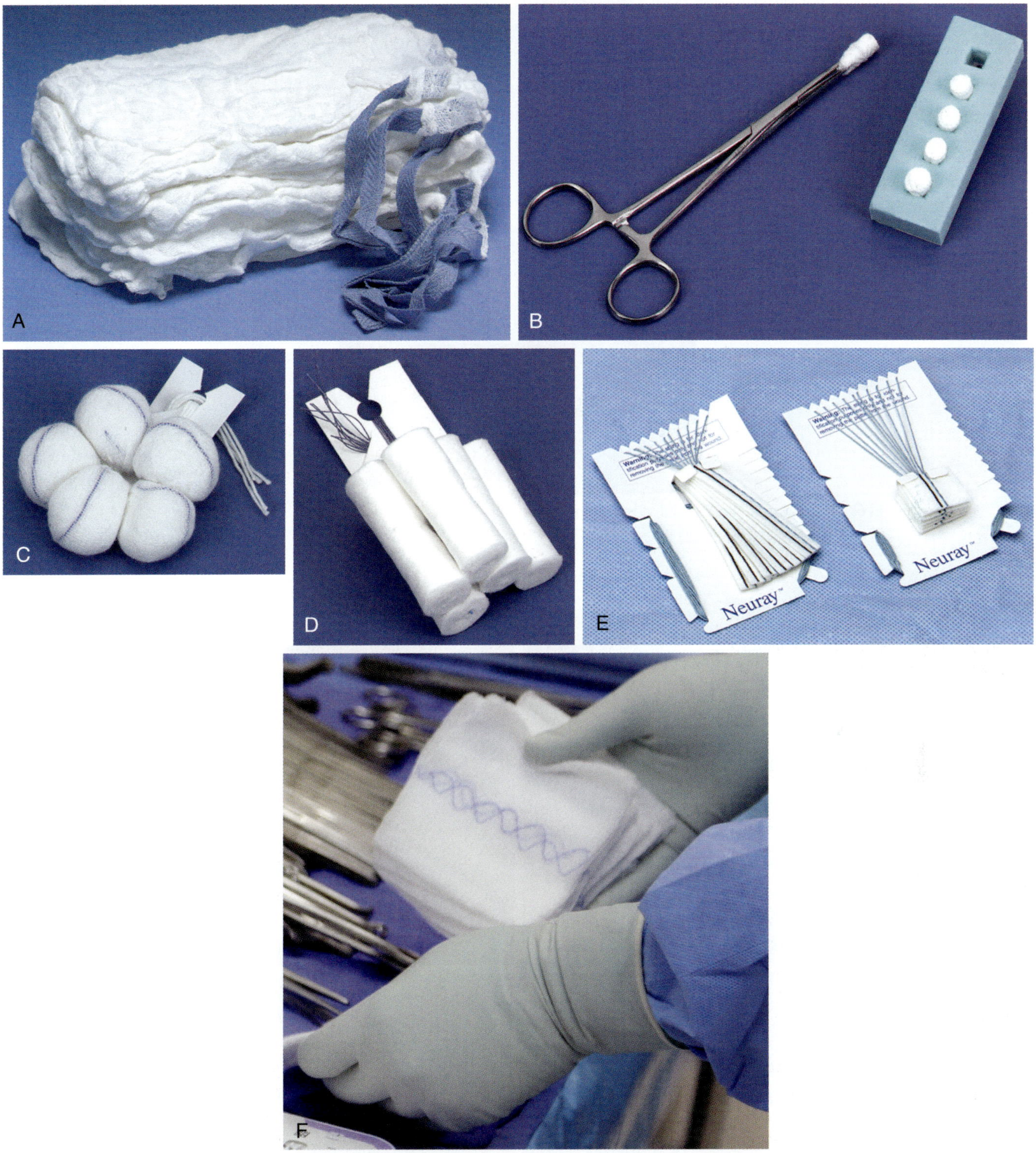

FIG. 19.4 Surgical sponges. (A) Laparotomy sponge. (B) Small dissector (also called a *kitner, peanut,* or *pusher*). (C) Tonsil sponge with string. (D) Cotton roll. (E) Neurosurgical patty. (F) Raytec sponges (also called 4 × 4s). (E, Courtesy DeRoyal Industries, Powell, TN.)

to prevent fraying. They can be floated in solution and maintained on the back table.

FLAT NEUROSURGICAL SPONGES

The flat sponge, also called a *cottonoid* or *patty*, is a compressed square of synthetic or cotton material with an x-ray–detectable string attached. Flat sponges are available in many different sizes for use during neurosurgical, ear, and vascular procedures. They usually are offered to the surgeon moistened with saline or topical thrombin rather than dry. The flat sponge is used to maintain hemostasis or as a filter over delicate tissue requiring fine-bore suction. When flat sponges are exchanged on the field, make sure

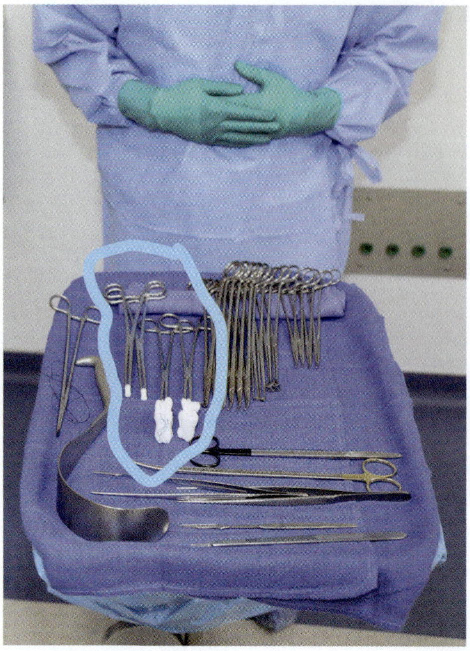

FIG. 19.5 Sponge sticks and dissectors. Raytec sponges should be folded in thirds and then doubled in half. Small sponge dissectors must be mounted on a clamp when introduced on the sterile field.

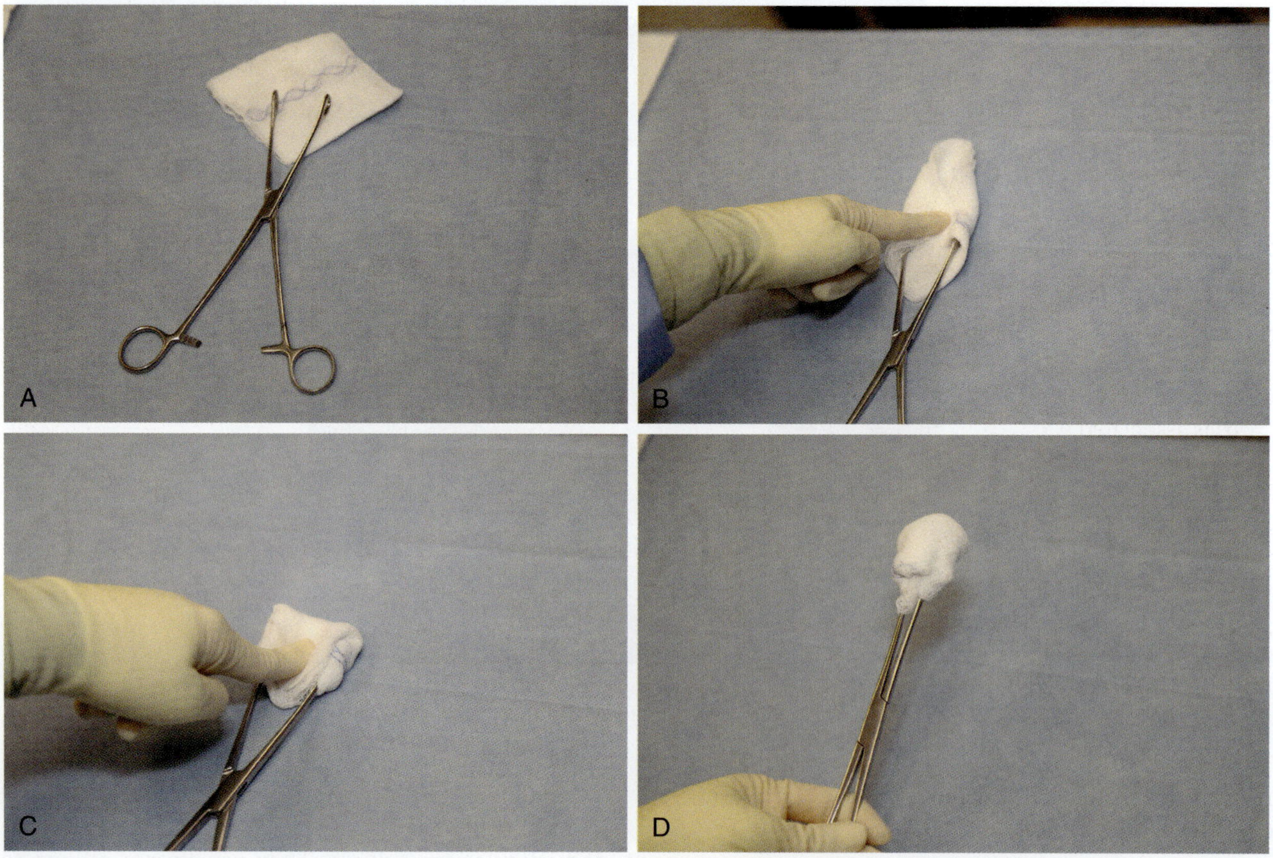

FIG. 19.6 Alternative method for making a sponge stick. (A) Position the open sponge forceps on the Raytec 4 × 4 as shown. (B) Fold two corners over the end of the forceps. (C) Fold the top corner down. (D) Close the forceps.

every sponge is returned intact with the string attached. Never cut the strings as these may become lost in the surgical wound.

MANAGEMENT OF THE STERILE FIELD

The surgical technologist is responsible for managing the sterile field throughout the procedure. It is important for students to know why specific skills are required as well as how to perform them.

Maintain a clean sterile field. The sterile field includes the draped patient, equipment and instrument tables (also draped), and the scrubbed members of the surgical team. The exact boundaries of the sterile field, including the sterile and nonsterile areas of the surgical gown, are indicated in Chapter 9. The sterile area immediately adjacent to the surgical wound is the working space for the surgeon and assistant surgeon. Instruments, surgical sponges, tissue debris, and bits of suture can accumulate in this area of the sterile field. The ST should remove these periodically. However, this should be done with a minimum of movement. A pause in the procedure may provide the opportunity to retrieve instruments and remove debris. However, remove only those items that are not in use. If the surgeon is using an instrument consistently, she or he may set it down momentarily. Do not remove the instrument from the field until you are certain that it is not needed.

Rationale: The field is kept clean to prevent instruments from dropping into the wound or falling to the floor. Tissue and suture debris are removed to prevent them from being introduced into the incision.

Remove blood and tissue from instruments as they are retrieved from the field. Dried blood and tissue that accumulate on instruments can be extremely difficult to remove even with an automated washer-sterilizer system and ultrasonic washer. Use sterile water and sponge to clean blood from the surface of instruments. Rasps and other instruments with rough surfaces should be soaked briefly in water and cleaned as soon as possible after use.

Rationale: Debris remained trapped in box locks, ratchets, and rasps is associated with cross-infection to the next patient exposed to it.

Keep suction tips clear of blood and debris. Suction is used during surgery to draw up blood and fluid from the surgical wound. Suction tips become clogged when blood is allowed to coagulate inside the lumen of the instrument. It is important to prevent this by periodically suctioning sterile water through the tip and tubing. Small-bore suction tips such as those used in plastic surgery can also be cleared with a stylet, which is normally included in the instrument setup.

NOTE *Avoid using instruments such as the ESU tip to clear the suction. This may result in scoring the ESU tip as this causes the tip to overheat.*

Rationale: Suction must be effective and immediately available. Routine clearing prevents delays caused by a solid blockage.

Stay ahead of supply needs. As the surgery progresses, additional sterile supplies such as sponges, sutures, and other devices may be needed. Request these items from the circulator before they are needed but request only what is required. Avoid stockpiling supplies on the sterile tables. This is wasteful and unnecessary. Newly graduated surgical technologists often request abundant quantities of sponges, sutures, and additional instruments out of concern that supplies already on the sterile setup will be depleted before additional ones can be obtained from the circulator. This should be avoided by trusting the circulator and by working in coordination with him or her.

Rationale: Securing items before they are needed maintains the flow of the procedure. Opening too many items is wasteful and almost always unnecessary as long as the ST and circulator have good communication.

Protect the field from contamination. Everyone on the surgical team must be conscious of the sterile field and watch for any breaks in technique. The ST has additional responsibility to watch for *potential* as well as actual contamination. The most common occurrences of contamination are caused when sterile team members move away from the sterile field or come too close to nonsterile areas. Contamination occurs most commonly in the following circumstances:

- When receiving sterile supplies or handing items off to the circulator
- When team members change position (e.g., moving from one side of the OR table to the other or shifting positions to facilitate retraction)
- Inadequate draping (e.g., drapes are too small or not placed correctly)
- During large cases in which there are many draped tables and large equipment—crowding of equipment and team members

The ST must act immediately when contamination has occurred. *The contaminated area must be contained and removed from the field.* Recall from Chapter 9 that there are four categories of breaks in sterile technique, and the correct action to take following contamination is based on the category. This may be a team decision.

The contaminated item (e.g., glove, instrument) must be removed from the field. If the contamination arises from a cut or puncture of both the inner and outer glove, both the gown and gloves must be replaced because there is no effective way to self-glove using closed technique. The cuff of the gown is no longer sterile once the glove is removed.

NOTE *Refer to Chapter 9 for guidelines on what to do when contamination occurs.*

Use the kick bucket for used sponges. The kick bucket is reserved for used surgical sponges. It should be placed close to the surgical technologist so that sponges can be dropped (not thrown).

Rationale: Blood and body fluids must be contained to prevent cross-contamination. The kick bucket allows the circulator to retrieve used sponges easily for transfer to a counting system. The kick bucket is placed close to the ST to prevent sponges from being dropped on the floor.

MANAGEMENT OF SURGICAL SPECIMENS

Among the most important skills of the surgical technologist is the management of specimens removed from the patient during surgery. Nearly all tissues and devices removed during surgery must be submitted for analysis to the pathologist. This includes tissues that are suspected to be malignant. *Critical medical decisions* are made based on specimen analysis. The consequences of negligence involving surgical specimens can be devastating. These include incorrect diagnosis, repeated or needless surgery, delayed treatment for malignancy, or cancer treatment that was unnecessary. In addition to ethical issues and patient safety, there is also a legal responsibility. Specimen loss, misidentification, or a damaged specimen can rapidly result in litigation.

Specific procedures and materials are used to preserve tissue from the time it is removed until it reaches the pathology department for analysis. Not all tissue removed from the patient is submitted for analysis. Exclusions are allowed, unless the surgeon specifies otherwise. These are listed in Box 19.2. Remember that even if tissues or materials removed during surgery do not require analysis by pathology, their removal is still documented. Note that items removed for forensic purposes require documentation before they can be released to law enforcement authorities.

IMPORTANT TO KNOW *The specific role of the ST is the care and transfer of specimens in the intraoperative period (during surgery) from the time they are removed from the patient until they are handed off the sterile field. The ST must coordinate all activities involving specimens with the circulating nurse, who has specific responsibilities and accountability for specimen management. It is the perioperative nurse's decision whether to delegate responsibilities, according to health facility policy and state practice acts.*

BOX 19.2 Tissues Normally Excluded From Pathology Analysis

1. Bone donated to the bone bank
2. Bone fragments removed during corrective or reconstructive orthopedic procedures (e.g., rotator cuff repair), excluding large specimens (e.g., femoral heads) and knee, ankle, or elbow reconstructions
3. Cataracts removed by phacoemulsification
4. Dental appliances
5. Fat removed by liposuction
6. Foreign bodies (e.g., bullets) or other medicolegal evidence given directly to law enforcement personnel
7. Foreskin from circumcision of a newborn
8. Intrauterine contraceptive devices without attached tissue
9. Medical devices (e.g., catheters, gastrostomy tubes, myringotomy tubes, stents, sutures) that have not contributed to patient illness, injury, or death
10. Middle ear ossicles
11. Orthopedic hardware and other radiopaque medical devices
12. Placentas from uncomplicated pregnancies that do not meet the criteria for pathology examination and appear normal at the time of delivery
13. Rib segments or other tissues removed for the purpose of gaining surgical access, provided the patient does not have a history of malignancy
14. Saphenous vein segments harvested for coronary artery bypass
15. Skin or other normal tissue removed during a cosmetic or reconstructive procedure (e.g., blepharoplasty, abdominoplasty, rhytidectomy), provided it is not contiguous with a lesion and the patient does not have a history of malignancy
16. Teeth when there is no attached tissue
17. Therapeutic radioactive materials
18. Normal toenails and fingernails that are incidentally removed

STANDARDS

The College of American Pathologists (CAP) sets standards for specimen management, including handling and preservation. The surgical technologist is responsible for following the current standards and practices that are included in the health facility policies manuals.

Specific topics that are usually covered by policy are the following:

1. General management of specimens
2. Specimens excluded from submission or submitted for *gross examination* (not under the microscope) only
3. Management of amputated digits and limbs
4. Explanted (surgical removal from the patient's body) medical devices
5. Explanted orthopedic hardware
6. Breast cancer specimen
7. Management of radioactive specimens
8. Forensic specimens

The CAP and National Society of Histotechnology publish a guide to handling specimens online. Students are advised to read the guide and bookmark it for future reference. The latest version can be downloaded from https://documents.cap.org/documents/practical-guide-specimen-handling.pdf.

CULTURAL CONSIDERATIONS

The patient's cultural practices involving body tissues are considered and addressed in the preoperative period. Any deviation from normal pathology protocols may require the patient's signature and plans made to fulfill the patient's and family's needs in the matter. Most facilities can accommodate the patients' requests while also complying with public health standards. Arrangements for final disposition of a specimen are usually discussed with the surgeon, and the nurse circulator and pathology department follow up.

PREPARATION FOR RECEIVING SPECIMENS

Preparation for receiving specimens begins before or during surgery. The surgical technologist's case planning should reflect the need for specimen containers. These can be distributed when the case is opened. Under normal circumstances, the circulating nurse prepares the documents required to transport the specimens to the pathology department. This is a specific responsibility of the perioperative nurse.

If the surgical procedure is scheduled to include a **frozen section** (see later in this chapter), the pathology department will have been contacted at the time the procedure was scheduled. The circulator contacts the pathology department at the start of the surgery to notify the pathologist that surgery has begun.

HANDLING SPECIMENS ON THE FIELD

The scrubbed surgical technologist may receive specimens on the field, or the surgeon may pass the specimen directly to the circulating nurse. When specimens are received on the sterile field, they must be immediately identified and protected from damage or loss.

The exact role of the surgical technologist during specimen removal depends on the type of tissue and the surgical procedure used for removal. Before studying these methods, the ST should learn the general guidelines:

1. Do not remove a specimen from the sterile field without the surgeon's specific permission to do so.
2. *Do not use surgical sponges* or towels to wrap a specimen. This is a common cause of specimen loss because the tissue can be disposed of accidentally. Place the specimen in a container in a conspicuous protected area on the instrument table until it can be passed off the field to the circulator.
3. Maintain the specimen in a condition conducive to pathological examination as per the facility's protocol.
4. Never use water to preserve a specimen or keep it moist during surgery. Water can cause cell distortion. Use sterile saline instead.
5. Do not use bone clamps, hemostats, or other crushing instruments on tissue specimens, because this can damage the tissue and interfere with analysis. Use smooth tissue forceps and handle tissues gently.
6. To prevent dropping or losing a specimen during surgery, the ST should place it in a container in a separate protected area of the back table. This is called *sequestering* the specimen.
7. After the surgeon approves it, the specimen should be handed off the field to the circulating nurse ***as soon as possible.***
8. When a specimen is passed off the sterile field, the surgeon must give verbal clarification of the specific anatomical origin, side (right or left), type of tissue, and any other special identifiers. The ST or circulating nurse must repeat the information back to the surgeon for full verification.

PRESERVATIVES, CONTAINERS, AND LABELING

Specimens are prepared for transport according to type. Formalin is the most common permanent tissue preservative. However, there are many different types of specimens that must be handled and preserved according to CAP and facility guidelines.

IMPORTANT TO KNOW *Specimens for frozen section are never placed in formalin and must be kept moist with saline.*

If formalin is required, the container must be large enough that all surfaces of the specimen are covered with preservative. Toxic preservative solutions including formalin *must not be brought into the operating room.* Formalin should be handled only in a well-ventilated environment and with protection to prevent exposure to the skin, eyes, and respiratory tract. It is the responsibility of the health care facility to provide a safe environment for the use of formalin.

The OSHA standard for occupational safety and formalin is located at https://www.osha.gov/pls/oshaweb/owadisp.show_document?p_id=10075&p_table=STANDARDS.

PREPARATION FOR TRANSPORT TO PATHOLOGY

1. All specimen containers must be leak-proof and placed in an impervious bag for transport. *Biohazard labeling is used on all specimens.*
2. When preparing specimens for transport, always place the label on the container, not on the lid, which could become separated from the container after arrival.
3. Information on the label must be legible and written with indelible ink.
4. Before sending a specimen, check that the information on the label matches exactly with that on the requisition form and other documentation to be sent and that these match the information on the patient's chart.
5. Documents sent with the specimen must not be placed inside the bag in which the specimen has been placed.
6. Documentation is usually placed in a clear pouch attached to the leak-proof bag used to hold the specimen container.

DOCUMENTATION

Specimen handling requires documentation at all points in the specimen chain of custody. Before surgery begins, the appropriate laboratory and pathology requisition forms are obtained according to the type of specimen anticipated, and the department will be responsible for analysis. Forms are specific to the type of analysis.

Specimen documents must include the following information or according to facility policy:

- Patient name and two unique identifiers, such as hospital number and Social Security number
- Patient's date of birth and gender
- Tissue of origin
- Preoperative diagnosis as stated by the surgeon
- Analysis required
- Date and time of collection
- Side of the body (right or left)
- Unique tissue identifiers or orientation markers such as sutures, clips, or dye
- The surgeon's name and contact number
- The name of the person preparing and documenting the specimen

NOTE *The CAP cautions against pre-labeling the contents of specimen containers. This helps prevent misidentification and mislabeling at the time that the specimen is obtained.*

TISSUE BIOPSY

Tissue **biopsy** is the removal of tissue or cells for gross identification and microscopic analysis. Microscopic analysis results in a definitive diagnosis, such as malignancy, or is used to determine the nature of an abnormality. Biopsy is performed during endoscopic, image-guided surgery or as part of an open procedure.

- *Excisional biopsy* is "a surgical procedure in which a cut is made through the skin to remove an entire lump or suspicious area so it can be checked under a microscope for signs of disease. A small amount of healthy tissue around the abnormal area may also be removed" (National Institute of Health, National Cancer Institute, available at https://www.cancer.gov/publications/dictionaries/cancer-terms).
- *Incisional biopsy* is "a surgical procedure in which a cut is made through the skin to remove a sample of abnormal tissue or part of a lump or suspicious area. The tissue is then checked under a microscope for signs of disease" (National Institute of Health, National Cancer Institute, available at https://www.cancer.gov/publications/dictionaries/cancer-terms).
- *Fine-needle aspiration (FNA)* uses a long, fine needle to aspirate (suction) small pieces of tissue from a mass.
- *Core needle biopsy* is similar to FNA, but a large-bore, hollow trocar or needle is used to collect the tissue. The needle is inserted into an organ, such as the liver, and tissue is removed for analysis.

Small specimens removed for biopsy should be carefully maintained on the back table because they can easily be lost. Small samples of tissue also dehydrate rapidly. To prevent this, the surgical technologist should dip a Telfa strip in sterile saline and place it in a small specimen container. Tissue specimens are removed during endoscopic procedures using biopsy forceps. To collect the specimen, the surgeon removes the tissue with forceps and withdraws it from the endoscope. The surgical technologist must steady the end of the instrument and collect the tissue using a needle or fine stylet. According to the surgeon's directions, the specimen may be transferred to a container partially filled with saline or Telfa saturated in saline. Core needle and fine-needle biopsy tissue are extruded into the specimen container onto a saline Telfa, or floated in saline, according to the surgeon's request or directions from the pathology department.

FROZEN SECTION

During surgical procedures that require immediate analysis of tissue for malignancy, a **frozen section** is performed. This is done by flash-freezing the suspect tissue and then making sectional slices that can be examined immediately under the microscope. Tissues for frozen section are managed differently than routine specimens. The pathologist must examine the tissue within a short time after it is removed. Therefore it is not preserved in fixative. The tissue is strictly protected from cellular damage to prevent misdiagnosis. Specifically, the tissue must be protected from mechanical damage caused by instruments, rough handling, or drying either by exposure to air or by placing the tissue on a dry surface.

Frozen section analysis is scheduled ahead of the surgery to ensure that the pathologist is available during surgery. Once the pathologist has been scheduled, the circulator notifies him or her when the specimen is close to removal during surgery. To verify the boundaries of a malignant lesion, the specimen may be taken in sections, which are marked according to their orientation to the entire site.

Frozen section specimens are received on the surgical field in a small basin or bowl and kept moistened with a saline-soaked Telfa strip. Do not float the specimen in saline unless directed to do so by the surgeon. Always communicate clearly and precisely about the tissue origin and exact location, because this is critical information.

Frozen section specimens are usually passed off the sterile field immediately after they are surgically removed. Once the specimen has been transported to pathology, it usually takes 20 or 30 minutes for preparation and analysis. The pathologist may come into surgery to speak with the surgeon directly about the findings or communicate through a speaker call to the operating room. The scrubbed technologist should be prepared for further dissection after the initial specimen has been analyzed.

STONES

Stones are removed from the urinary tract, salivary ducts, and gallbladder. The technologist receives these in a small, dry basin. They should be maintained and transported in a dry container.

AMPUTATED LIMB

The surgeon passes an amputated limb to the ST to pass off the field. In all cases, the patient under local anesthesia must be protected from witnessing this. The limb can be wrapped in a paper drape and placed in a protected location on the back table until the circulator is prepared to receive it. It is then wrapped in a plastic bag or according to hospital policy. Final disposition of the limb may be influenced by the patient's wishes and cultural practice. Initially, the limb must be registered and sent for analysis, like other specimens. Special disposition is noted in the patient's record and the documents accompanying the specimen.

CELLS (CYTOLOGY)

Endoscopic procedures often include the collection of epithelial cells for cytological examination. Cells are removed using a soft biopsy brush, which is passed over the epithelium with the aid of the endoscope. The procedure is called a *brush biopsy*. As the surgeon withdraws the biopsy instrument, the ST assists by directing the brush end of the biopsy instrument into a small container of sterile saline. The tip is agitated slightly in the saline to release the tissue and cells, which may not be visible with the naked eye. Some surgeons may clip the brush end and submit it in solution as the specimen. Several containers should be prepared to receive the specimens. These must be clearly identified and labeled.

Cytology slides for microscope examination are prepared by the practitioner (usually in a clinic setting) and sprayed with a *fixative* before being sent to pathology. A fixative is a solution that stabilizes the cells for examination. An example of this type is a cervical smear that is fixed with fixative (98% alcohol). The patient's name is penciled on the slide before it is sent to pathology along with the appropriate documentation.

PRODUCTS OF CONCEPTION

Embryonic and fetal tissue are registered and documented as *products of conception* and are treated with respect and dignity. States have individual reporting requirements for fetal death, and hospital policy is established around these requirements. Surgical technologists must become familiar with appropriate dispensation and specific documentation of fetal tissue for their facility and state.

FORENSIC SPECIMENS

A *foreign body* is a non-tissue item obtained from the patient's body. Forensic specimens are those that may be required by a court of law as evidence. These include weapon fragments such as bullets and knife blades, or any item used as a weapon. These specimens must be handled carefully to prevent scratching, pitting, or scoring. They should not be handled with metal instruments or wiped clean, because these can damage the specimen and obscure analysis. They should be submitted in a dry container with a tight seal unless the surgeon states otherwise. Other items, such as fragments of metal, glass, or wood, may also be retained as forensic specimens. Clothes required for forensic analysis are removed from the patient by cutting only along the seams. Holes and tears should not be divided or cut because they may be significant for evidence. Fabric surrounding the weapon or fragment should also be submitted intact along with the fragment. Items that may be part of forensic evidence are submitted to the pathology department or handed over directly to the police for analysis. These must be registered according to hospital policy related to forensic evidence. No forensic specimen can be released without specific documentation issued by the facility.

MEDICAL DEVICES

Medical devices that were previously implanted are removed from the body because of failure, including breakage or fragmentation. The procedure for removing a previously implanted device is called *explantation*. All pieces of the device are kept dry and sent together in a dry container. The device is examined for identification, and the manufacturer is notified. The device serial number or other identifiers should be included in specimen labeling and documentation along with the packaging, if it is available.

CULTURES

Tissue and fluid are cultured as described in Chapter 8. In this process, a small fluid sample is collected from the wound and transported by culture tube.

The surgical technologist assists in collecting the culture sample. Sampling is performed with a specialized culture tube containing one or two sterile swabs and specific transport medium for that type of test. When the surgeon is ready to take the culture, the circulator removes the top of the culture transport tube, exposing the ends of the swabs. The technologist carefully removes them from the container and passes them to the surgeon, who swipes them across the tissue to be tested. The surgeon returns the swabs to the technologist, who places them carefully back into the culture tube, which is still held by the circulator. Always use Universal Precautions when handling tissue and cultures. Two types of bacterial cultures are commonly taken during surgery: *aerobic* and *anaerobic* (discussed in Chapter 8). *Each requires a designated type of transfer tube.* Anaerobic sampling can be performed with a needle and syringe or using a Dacron swab as described earlier. Using the swab technique, more commonly performed in surgery, the transfer tube contains a small amount of preservative medium that is released into the swab when the tube is compressed.

BODY FLUIDS

Sampling body fluids is usually performed in the clinical setting. However, occasionally, the surgical technologist may be asked to assist in a procedure to obtain fluid samples, such as pericardial or synovial fluid sampling, which require sterile technique. Fluid samples obtained by percutaneous methods (puncturing the skin) are removed using a needle and syringe. The fluid can be transported in the syringe, which is capped after the needle is removed. *Never send a needle attached to a syringe,* because these samples will likely be rejected by the pathology department as a safety hazard. Fluid samples may also be injected into a transport tube with a stopper.

MUSCLE BIOPSY

Muscle biopsy is a specific procedure for the diagnosis of muscle or systemic disease. In this procedure, a small section of muscle is removed from the *vastus lateralis* or other large muscle. However, the site depends on the pathology and whether there has been previous trauma to the area that may obscure analysis. The biopsy is performed routinely, like any small tissue excision. However, no electrosurgical instruments are used for cutting or coagulation.

Muscle tissue is ideally transported quickly to the pathology department on Telfa with saline—not floated in saline and never in formalin. The sample *must be kept cold* and the container (not the specimen) packed in ice. If the specimen cannot be transported within 30 minutes, it may require flash freezing. The method used for this will be directed by the pathology department according to their protocol.

CORD BLOOD, UMBILICAL CORD, AND PLACENTA

Blood remaining in the umbilical cord after birth is collected for simple laboratory analysis or for biobanking. Blood for laboratory analysis is collected in a small basin at the time the cord is severed during delivery. It is then transferred to the appropriate blood tubes according to laboratory requirements.

Cord blood banking is becoming increasingly popular and is performed to preserve hematopoietic stem cells, which may be beneficial in the treatment of blood-related diseases. The umbilical cord may also be preserved for use in the regeneration of organ tissues. Both blood and cord products are preserved in a tissue bank after they have been removed. Cord blood is removed after birth, before the placenta is removed. A blood collection kit containing a collection bag, clamps, and tubing is used on the surgical field. After collection, the blood is sent to the pathology department according to facility protocol. The umbilical cord is removed and also transported according to facility policy. Placenta samples are collected and transported according to facility policy and disposition of the samples—whether for research or other use.

RADIOACTIVE SPECIMENS

Patients who have undergone surgery to implant radioactive seeds or injection of radioactive material (e.g., sentinel lymph node biopsy) will have implants or tissue removed when the exposure time has ended. Special precautions are required for the handling and transport of radioactive tissue and implants. Each health care facility determines which departments may receive radioactive material and how it is to be transported there. Specimens are handled on and off the field using universal precautions. Radioactive implants have very low toxicity beyond the immediate area of the implant. However, precautions must be observed during transport and disposal. These procedures will be approved and published by the facility's radiation safety officer.

AUTOLOGOUS TISSUE FOR IMPLANTATION

Autologous (patient's own) tissue may be removed, preserved, and implanted in the patient later in the same surgery, or during a separate surgery. These tissues must be handled according to specific protocols provided by the pathology department and facility specialists. Examples of autologous specimens are bone grafts, including cranial flaps, skin, amputated digits, and saphenous veins. Protocols for preserving autologous tissue vary among facilities and according to the most recent medical research on this topic. In general, autologous tissue must be protected from damage, including contamination, and preserved during surgery to maintain viability. It is best to consult with the surgeon about immediate preservation of the tissue during surgery. A moist, saline environment is the most common method, but does not apply to all tissue types. In general, autologous grafts should not come in contact with any dry, absorbent surface, as these may stick to the graft.

Autologous tissue to be preserved and implanted in a different patient requires registration with the Food and Drug Administration (FDA). The protocol specifically addresses the recovery process, packaging, labeling, storage, and tracking mechanisms.

Contaminated Autologous Graft

Protocols for handling autologous tissue for implantation that has been contaminated (e.g., dropped on the operating room floor) are available from CAP for adoption by the surgical facility. The most commonly dropped tissue is the bone graft.

IMPORTANT TO KNOW *No guideline recommends steam sterilization for contaminated bone grafts because the process damages the graft and increases the risk of infection and absorption of the bone.*

Precautions can be taken to prevent a graft from being dropped: as the bone is removed, the surgeon places him- or herself on the same anatomical side as the graft so that it falls on the drapes rather than the floor.

- The graft is placed directly on the Mayo or back table rather than handing it off to the ST.
- Avoid handling the graft unless necessary.
- During a change of scrub personnel during the surgery, the ST must point out the location of the graft as part of the handover.

SUTURES

Suture materials are used to **approximate** tissues (i.e., bring tissue edges together by suture or other means) and to ligate blood vessels or tubal structures while healing takes place. In surgery, the term *suture* can refer to a length of suturing thread or a suture thread-and-needle combination. Packages of suture material are simply called "sutures." Suture material is made from synthesized chemicals, animal protein, metal, and natural fibers.

Like medications, suture materials used in the United States must be approved by the U.S. Food and Drug Administration (FDA) and the U.S. Pharmacopeia (USP), discussed in Chapter 12. All substances, including suture products that bear the USP label, must meet minimum standards. The standards for suture materials include size conformity, tensile strength, and sterility. Additional standards cover packaging, dyes used in the suture, and the integrity of the needles. The European Pharmacopoeia (EP) sets standards for sutures used in European Union (EU) countries, including those sutures manufactured and distributed by US companies.

MODERN TISSUE CLOSURE TECHNOLOGY

Tissue closure technology has advanced rapidly since the early 2000s. The role of suture, which used to be restricted to keeping tissues together during healing, has progressed to other functions and advanced features in the wound healing process:

- Suture as a vehicle for the release of antibacterial substances into the wound
- Mechanical features such as one-way barbs, which prevent suture from backing out of the wound
- Suture material as a component of orthopedic anchoring devices to provide extra strength in tissues under extremely high pressure, such as the shoulder joint
- Suture jacketing and coating to ensure smooth passage through tissues during the suturing process
- Synthetic tissue staples that provide rapid tissue closure combined with absorbability
- Staple line reinforcement (SLR) technology to prevent staple line leakage in gastrointestinal anastomosis procedures
- Incision adhesives, which glue tissue edges together

Some innovative technologies become standard practice, while others fall out of use. The surgical technologist will be exposed to trends and obtain training through company representatives assigned to their surgical facility.

STUDYING AND LEARNING SUTURES

Learning the types and uses of sutures is one of the most challenging skills for students in surgery. Familiarity with the types of sutures and needles and techniques for handling them are acquired over time with repetition and study. Suture manufacturers recognize that the surgical technologist and circulator need to identify a suture type quickly. Packages are color coded by suture type, and needles often are pictured on the label for rapid selection and delivery to the sterile field. However, color coding is not always consistent among manufacturers.

When first faced with the number and variety of sutures available, it seems an impossible task to become familiar with each one. However, putting sutures into the context of their use decreases the learning curve. Certain tissues can be associated with suture types. Surgeons normally have a preference to suture sizes and type. These will be noted specifically on the surgeon's preference card.

Many sutures are made synthetically, and the name of each type reflects their chemical composition, in the same way that drugs have chemical names. Some sutures are very easy to become familiar with because their generic types are simple. Examples are silk, nylon, polyester, and polypropylene. Sutures developed from polymers (long chain molecules) from resins and plastics have very long chemical names, which are not helpful for differentiating one from another. In this case it is probably easiest to become familiar with the trade names and their basic composition.

IMPORTANT TO KNOW *Health care facilities usually maintain a contract with one suture company to purchase its products in bulk. It is useful to become familiar with that company's suture products, with focus on those used in your facility. With time and exposure to different sutures, you will become familiar with their names and even develop the ability to recognize the size simply by sight or feel of the suture.*

The properties and characteristics of sutures contribute to the surgeon's choice and application of a suture. The following section describes the important characteristics of sutures. The ST must become familiar with these.

PHYSICAL STRUCTURE OF SUTURES

Structurally, sutures are broadly divided into three categories:

Monofilament: A single continuous fiber made by extruding and stretching a synthetic material

Multifilament: Many filaments together form one strand of suture. A multifilament suture in turn is divided into two types:

Twisted: Multiple fibers are twisted in the same direction.

Braided: Multiple fibers are intertwined.

Composite or coated: A core strand of one suture material is jacketed with another of a different or the same type.

Sutures are coated to add a technical property to the suture. Coatings reduce tissue drag and fraying. Antibacterial substances are infused into the coating of some sutures to reduce the risk of postoperative infection.

SUTURE SIZE

The size of the suture is based on the diameter of a single strand. The USP numbering system indicates the suture's outside diameter and ensures that a stated size is the same across all suture materials. For example, size 2-0 silk suture has the *same diameter* as size 2-0 nylon suture. Although size contributes to strength, there are other factors involved.

Selection of a particular size is based mainly on the type of tissue and the load or tension that will be placed on the sutures. Sutures range in size from 12-0 (thinnest) to 5 (thickest). The greater the diameter, the larger the designated size. For example, ***size 2 is thicker than size 0.*** Sutures smaller than 0 are designated by additional zeros. For example, size 2-0 is an average size for abdominal wall tissue. Size 11-0 is used in microsurgery. This suture is light enough to remain suspended in the air. Sutures of this size naturally are very delicate and expensive and must be handled with care.

Stainless steel suture historically has used the *Brown and Sharp (B & S) sizing system* rather than USP sizes. These numbers begin with size 38/40 gauge (the thinnest) up to 18 gauge (the thickest). Stainless steel is now sized according to USP standards. However, some surgeons may request the B & S number, which is printed on steel wire packages.

The B & S sizes and their corresponding USP sizes are as follows:

B & S gauge	40	35	32	30	28	26	25	24	23	22	20
USP size	6-0	5-0	4-0	3-0	2-0	0	1	2	3	4	5

CHARACTERISTICS OF SUTURES

Tensile Strength

The **tensile strength** is the amount of force needed to break the suture. Tensile strength is one of the most important qualities of a suture. Breakage during the process of suturing is frustrating and time-consuming. Breakage in the wound during healing can lead to complications.

Uniformity (A Quality Control Factor)

Sutures must be uniform in diameter to maintain tensile strength. Poorly manufactured sutures can vary in uniformity along the length of the suture strand.

Capillary Action (Wicking)

Sutures made of multifilament strands absorb moisture and hold body fluids (called *wicking* or **capillary action**). If bacteria are present, suture materials with high capillarity are able to retain and spread infection by means of the suture fibers. Sutures with *low capillarity* are preferred in procedures in which the risk of infection is high. Sutures are generally not used in the presence of infection. However, wounds that may be prone to infection are sutured with low-capillary action sutures such as nylon or polypropylene.

Most multifilament sutures are coated with a synthetic polymer to reduce tissue drag and wicking. In the past, **absorbable sutures** were coated with a material such as beeswax or paraffin. These materials were irritating to tissue, so modern sutures are coated with chemicals that are similar in composition to the suture, making them more biocompatible and lowering the risk of tissue reaction. Synthetic coating materials such as polytetrafluoroethylene (PTFE, also used to coat nonstick cookware) and other complex synthetic polymers decrease suture drag and resist absorption.

Self-Directed Learning: An excellent video that demonstrates how sutures are expertly made can be accessed at https://www.youtube.com/watch?v=Z1-wAK1kZmk.

HANDLING QUALITIES

The handling qualities of a suture determine its ease of use and may affect the technical quality of the wound closure. For these reasons, surgeons are careful to balance the handling qualities of a suture with its other characteristics.

Compliance (Pliability)

Compliance or *pliability* is the ease of handling or softness in the hand. Pliability makes the suture material easier to manipulate. The knots lie flat and remain secure. Silk sutures have traditionally been considered the gold standard of all suture materials for their pliability, tight knots, and ease of use. More inert suture materials have replaced silk sutures through the years, but silk's other qualities rank it high for handling and strength for size.

Memory

Memory describes the suture's tendency to retain its original shape or configuration after it is removed from the package. High-memory suture is springy and tends to tangle during preparation and use. This also correlates with the ability of a suture to stay knotted. Material that is stiff or retains memory tends to loosen easily, and the knots can back out. This is annoying and time-consuming for the surgeon. Extruded monofilament sutures have greater coil memory than that of braided or twisted fiber sutures. Fiber sutures such as silk and polyester have the least memory and greatest pliability.

Plasticity

Plasticity refers to the material's ability to stretch and retain a new shape. Elasticity can be advantageous as long as the suture retains its strength when stretched. Increased plasticity contributes to secure knots. Polypropylene sutures have high plasticity.

BIOACTIVITY

Bioactivity is the body's response to suture. The immune system reacts to suture as it would to any foreign material. The bioactivity depends on the chemical structure of the suture material and the condition of the patient. Sutures that cause little or no bioactivity are said to be highly **inert,** causing little or no inflammation. Stainless steel, titanium, and polypropylene sutures are the most inert of all materials. Natural fiber and protein-based sutures cause the most tissue reaction.

IMPORTANT TO KNOW *A particular suture's medical-surgical advantages and disadvantages are mainly the concern of the surgeon, unless the surgical technologist is a consultant for a suture company.*

ABSORBABILITY

Suture materials are classified as absorbable or non-absorbable. Some suture materials such as those made of collagen (e.g., surgical gut) are absorbed very quickly, whereas others remain in their original state indefinitely. Modern suture technology has contributed to a wide variety of suture materials of differing *rates of absorption*. This technology allows the surgeon to select a suture that is absorbable over an extended period of time, giving tissues a chance to heal before the sutures break down.

Absorbability of a suture is affected by its environment in the body. For example, most sutures break down very quickly in the presence of infection. This is related to a heightened inflammatory response in and around the infection. For this reason, *infected tissues are not sutured.* Instead the infection is treated medically until the infection is resolved and the wound can be closed.

Refer also to Chapter 34.

SELECTION OF SUTURE

The selection of suture and needle for a particular tissue is based on the tissue type, wound category, the age and medical condition of the patient, and the healing prognosis. Surgeons have a large selection of suture materials, needle sizes and types, and specialty products designed for specific surgical needs. The surgeon's choice depends on these specific requirements, on practice and experience with previously used suture materials, and on tradition. People tend to use materials with which they are familiar. Many new materials have been introduced in the past few decades. Some show definite advantages over previously used materials, but with few exceptions, substances that have been used for many years, such as silk and nylon, remain in use with good results.

The following are important considerations that may determine which type of suture to use in a particular tissue:

- *Critical nature of the tissue:* Sutures placed in critical tissue or areas of the body such as the heart, blood vessels, and certain structures of the respiratory tract require nonabsorbable suture.
- *Healing time:* Absorbable suture can be used on *noncritical* tissue that heals very quickly. Examples are the mouth and other mucosal tissue, subcutaneous tissue, and epithelial tissue.
- *Required strength during healing:* Some tissues (usually connective tissues) are under high stress in the body. These areas require nonabsorbable suture or suture in larger sizes (size 0 and up). Examples are abdominal fascia, tendon, and ligament.
- *Scar formation:* A successful surgical outcome sometimes depends on almost complete absence of scarring. In some locations of the body, any scarring or granulation tissue around knots can result in a decrease or loss of function. Repair of structures of the hand, such as tendon and nerve, requires inert suture materials. Internal structures of the eye also require inert suture materials. The suture must pass through the tissue with no resistance or tissue fraying, even at the microscopic level. Stainless steel (reserved for connective tissue), nylon, and polypropylene are the most inert.
- *Urinary tract:* Suture knots or remnants that may come in contact with urine or kidney filtrate can become the source of stones or other mineral deposition. For this reason, absorbable sutures are used in these tissues.
- *Risk of infection:* Some surgical procedures carry a high risk of infection either because of their classification (see earlier discussion) or because of the patient's condition. In these cases, a strong suture line with resistance to absorption is needed. A nonabsorbable suture or absorbable suture with long absorption time may be used. Wounds that are actively infected are not sutured.
- *Cosmetic closure:* A cosmetic closure is one that has the least negative effect on the patient's body image. Naturally, skin closure of the face and other exposed areas of the body is the focus of cosmetic closure. Sutures selected for cosmetic closure are inert and usually monofilament to cause the least tissue injury as the suture is drawn through.

Table 19.2 describes commonly used sutures, their use, and physical characteristics. Images of the packages of prominent companies that manufacture sutures are also shown as a visual cue for memory. The colors used in suture packaging (not the sutures themselves) are for the most part standard in the industry.

SURGICAL NEEDLES

Surgical needles are made from high-quality steel alloy or titanium. The combination of metals used in the manufacturing process renders the needles strong and inert. Needles are available in many types, according to their shape or curvature, and point style. Surgical needles have three distinct parts: the point, the body, and the eye (or swage).

SWAGED (ATRAUMATIC) SUTURE

Most commercial needles are now manufactured with the suture pre-attached. This is called a *swaged* or *atraumatic suture.* During manufacturing, the suture is inserted into the hollow lumen of the needle, and the area is crimped and sealed. This produces a nearly seamless connection between the needle and the suture and allows faster suturing with minimal tissue trauma.

A **detachable suture** (Fig. 19.7) is one in which the suture can be detached from the needle by pulling it straight back from the **swage.** These are referred to by their proprietary names, such as *de-tach* and *control-release.* De-tachable sutures are used when the surgical procedure calls for rapid placement of multiple interrupted (individually tied) sutures, such as during **anastomosis.**

A *double-armed suture* is one with a needle swaged to each end. This type of suture is used for circular incisions, such as in ophthalmic surgery, or for hollow lumens, such as blood vessels or the intestine (Fig. 19.8).

EYED NEEDLES

Few surgeons use eyed needles. However, the surgical technologist must be familiar with their use. The conventional *closed-eye needle* resembles a sewing needle but is round in shape, and the eye hole is round, rectangular, or square (Fig. 19.9).

The *French-eye* (or spring eye) needle was used before swaged sutures became available, and some surgeons still use them. When the spring-eye needle is threaded, the end of the suture is pressed down over the top of the spring, which causes it to snap into the eye (Fig. 19.10). The suture should not be pulled through the eye after it is in place, because this strips the suture and may break it.

TABLE 19.2 Common Sutures by Type

Suture Type	Notes
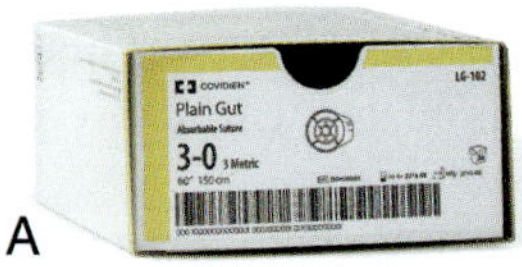 A 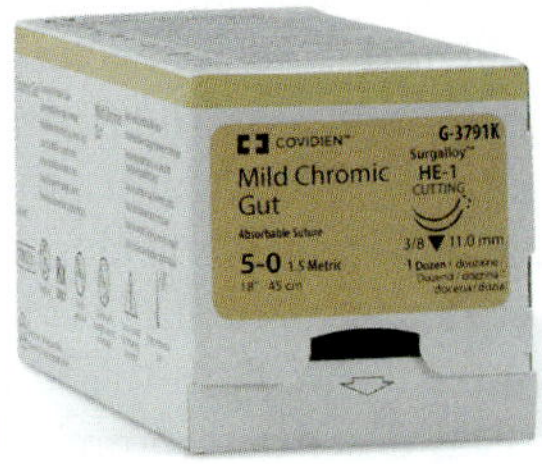 B SURGICAL GUT: Plain, Fast Gut, Chromic Gut, Mild Gut Composition: Natural Absorbability: Absorbable Short-term Structure: Monofilament or braided (chromic only) Color: Plain gut: yellow; Chromic gut: Tan or Brown Handling: Stiff unless moistened; frays easily Primary uses: Mucous membrane, especially the oral cavity Composition: Naturally occurring protein collagen beef or sheep	**Surgical gut** is one of the few sutures made of natural materials used in the United States. Surgical gut has been widely replaced by synthetic absorbable sutures but may be occasionally used by oral surgeons. Plain surgical gut is digested quickly and absorbed by tissues, but this rapid reaction can also cause inflammation. Chromic gut is treated with chromic salts to resist digestion and absorption. Both types of gut are rapidly broken down in the presence of infection. Gut requires special handling to preserve its strength and pliability. The sutures are packaged in an alcohol-and-water solution, which can be a source of fire on the surgical field. Packages must therefore be opened away from the surgical wound. Gut dries out quickly and can be dipped in saline just before use. This prevents the suture from breaking. However, gut should not be soaked, because it absorbs water readily and becomes soggy and weak. Dipping the strands in saline softens them so that the coils can be removed. This is done by grasping the ends of the strand and pulling them gently. It is important to pull on the strands gently, especially when they are wet, because they can overstretch and become weak. Gut should be handled as little as possible, because contact with gloves causes the strands to fray.
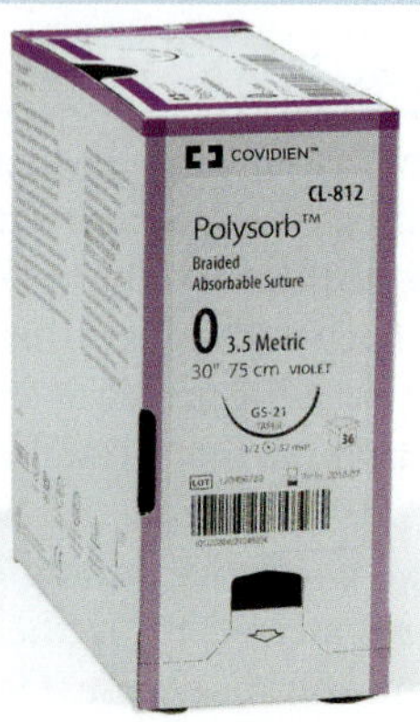 POLYGLACTIN AND DERIVATIVES : Vicryl, Vicryl Plus, Vicryl Rapid, Polysorb, Velosorb, Caprosyn Composition: Synthetic Absorbability: Absorbable—short-term use Structure: Braided, monofilament Color: Violet, natural Handling: Excellent Primary uses: Soft tissue, ligation, ophthalmic, OB-GYN, general surgery	**Polyglactin 910** came on the market in the 1970s and replaced surgical gut because of its superior handling qualities, uniform absorption, and strength. It remains popular, but many other absorbable synthetic sutures are now available with varying absorption rates and reliability. Vicryl Plus is impregnated with triclosan for antibacterial action. Many manufacturers market their own brand of Polyglactin 910 as a generic suture. Newer synthetic polyester sutures made from similar chemicals are comparable in absorbability and handling.

TABLE 19.2 Common Sutures by Type—cont'd

Suture Type	Notes
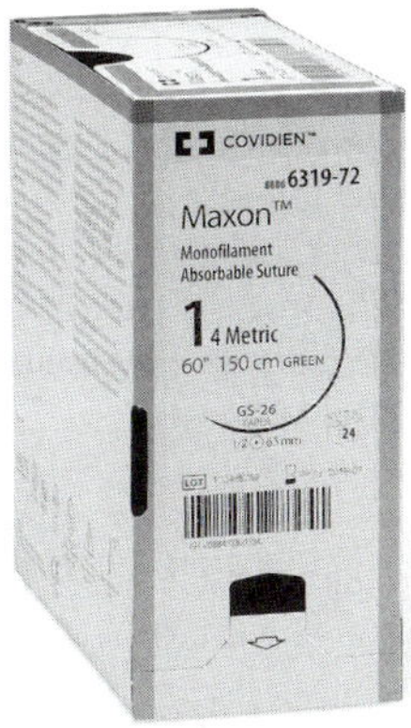 POLYGLYCONATE: Maxon Composition: Synthetic Absorbability: Absorbable—medium term Color: Clear or green Structure: Monofilament Handling: Excellent Primary uses: General, OB-GYN	**Modified polyglactin (glyconate)** suture is used when healing time is expected to be up to 6 weeks. Maxon is available for general use, but Maxon CV (cardiovascular) is indicated for specific use. It is comparable to PDS suture but may provide greater tensile strength initially.
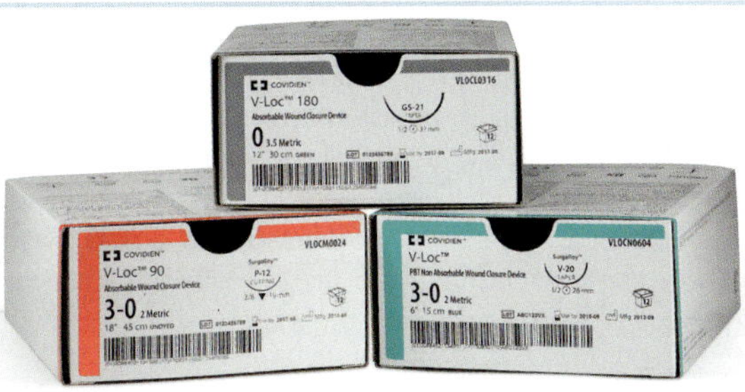 POLYDIOXANONE PDO: PDS, PDS II, Duracryl, V-Lok 90 Composition: Synthetic Absorbability: Absorbable—short- to medium-term Structure: Monofilament, barbed Handling: Excellent Primary uses: General soft tissue, pediatric cardiovascular tissue, microsurgery, orthopedic surgery	**Polydioxanone** suture is superior in strength and produces minimal tissue reaction. It is used in soft tissue and in pediatric cardiovascular, and microsurgery. This suture is known for its high tensile strength and minimal tissue reaction. Note: PDO is available in barbed configuration, which allows it to be implanted in the incision without knots. This format prevents the suture from backing out of tissues during the healing process. The technology mimics the natural defense mechanism seen in porcupines. This is explained in the following short video: Porcupine Barbs for Better Healing, available at https://www.npr.org/sections/health-shots/2019/04/09/711050307/porcupine-barbs-for-better-wound-healing or on YouTube.
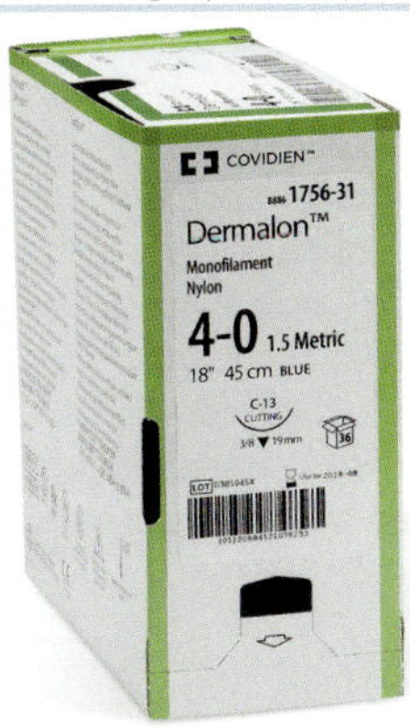 NYLON: Ethilon/Monosof/Dermalon, Dafilon, Surgilon, Monosof Composition: Synthetic Absorbability: Non-absorbable – degrades over time Structure: Monofilament or braided Color Black, white Handling: May be stiff in larger sizes, superior knot formation Primary uses: Intestine, vascular system, ophthalmic, and neurosurgical	**Nylon** was the first synthetic suture material available (1940) and is still widely used. It is available in braided or monofilament strands. The most outstanding feature of nylon is that it causes little or no tissue reaction and passes very easily through delicate tissues of the eye or blood vessels. Nylon has very high tensile strength; however, in larger sizes it is stiff, difficult to handle, and may cut through tissue. Nylon suture loses its tensile strength over time. It is used when long-term strength is not required and is available in black, blue, green, and clear in braided or monofilament strands, coated or uncoated.

Continued

TABLE 19.2 Common Sutures by Type—cont'd

Suture Type	Notes
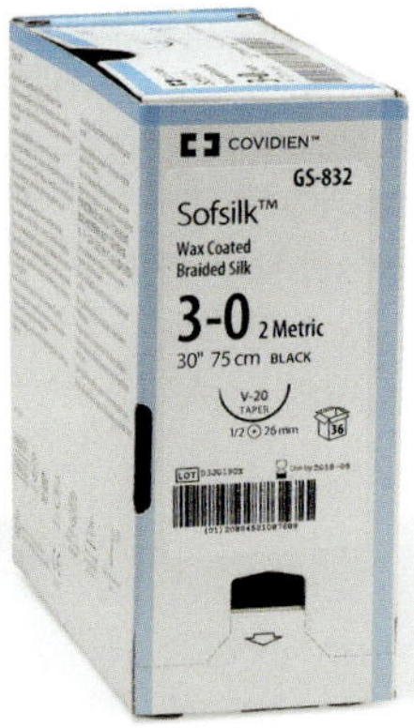 **SILK: Perma-Hand, Sofsilk, Demesilk, Silkam** Composition: Natural fibers spun by silkworm Absorbability: Non-absorbable; degrades over time Structure: Braided, twisted available coated Color: Black, white Handling: Soft, pliable, superior knot formation Primary uses: Intestine, vascular system, ophthalmic, and neurosurgical	**Silk** suture is very soft and pliable, which makes it easy to handle. It also has excellent tensile strength. Silk knots stay tied and remain secure and flat in tissues. It is available in braided or twisted forms. Silk used in most surgical procedures is coated to reduce wicking. However, virgin silk without coating is available. Silk is often classified as a non-absorbable suture. However, it does degrade over time.
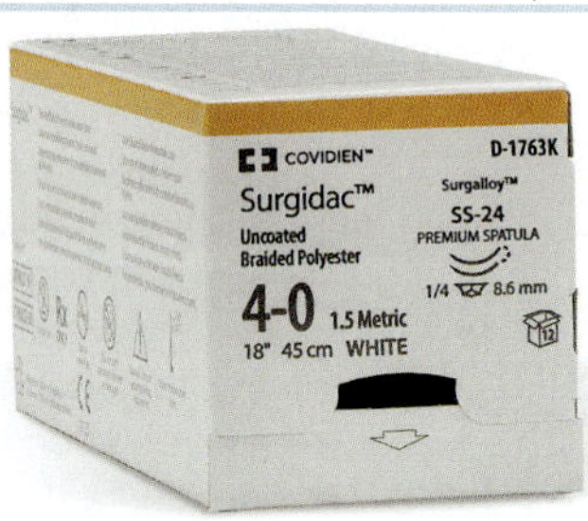 **POLYESTER: Ti-cron, Surgidac, Merselene, Surgidac, Cottony, Polydek, Tevdek, Ethibond (Monofilament brands): Vascufil, Novafil** **Composition: Synthetic** Absorbability: Permanent Structure: Braided and coated Color: Green, blue, white Handling: Excellent Primary uses: Cardiovascular, orthopedic	**Polyester** suture is extremely strong, easy to handle, and relatively inert in tissue. It is braided and is available coated or uncoated. The coated form is widely used for cardiovascular surgery, especially when grafts are used, because of its strength-to-size ratio. There are three types of polyester-based sutures: the PET-based, PBT-based (see Table 21.3 for chemical name), and polybutester-based sutures. Polyester suture is green, blue, or white.
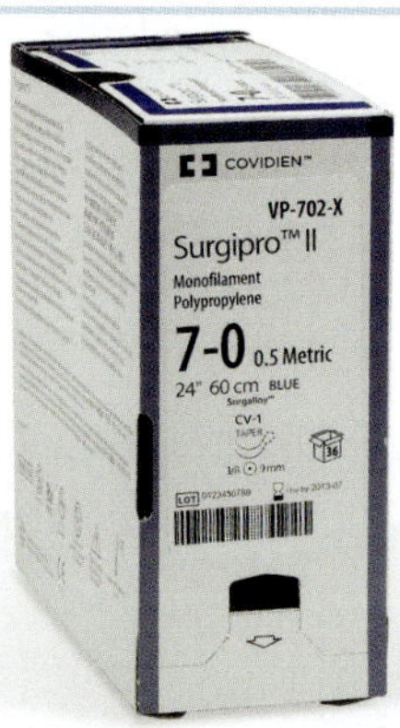 **POLYPROPYLENE: Prolene, Deklene, Surgipro, Surgilene, Premilene, Optilene** Composition: Synthetic Absorbability: Non-absorbable Permanent Structure: Monofilament Color: Blue, clear, pink fluorescent Handling: Fair Primary uses: Plastic surgery, cardiovascular, neurological, ophthalmic surgeries	**Polypropylene** is an extremely inert monofilament suture. Its smooth surface makes it popular for plastic, ophthalmic, and vascular surgery. Because of its high tensile strength, it is used for retention sutures, particularly in abdominal wall closure. Polypropylene knots are flat and do not back out when placed properly. It is somewhat difficult to handle in larger sizes. This is related to its strong coil memory. A number of companies have developed packaging systems that decrease coil memory.

TABLE 19.2 Common Sutures by Type—cont'd

Suture Type	Notes
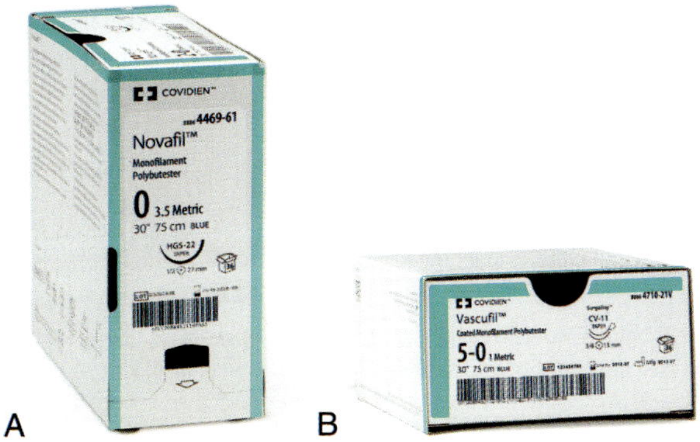 A B POLYBUTESTER: Novafil, Vascufil Composition: Synthetic Absorbability: Non-absorbable Permanent Structure: Monofilament Color: Blue Handling: Good Primary uses: General and cardiovascular	**Polybutester** suture is used where permanent high tensile strength is required during healing. This suture is fibrous and flexible. A unique characteristic of this suture is its ability to stretch during tissue swelling and resume normal configuration as swelling subsides. **Novafil** suture is uncoated, whereas **Vascufil** is coated to reduce tissue drag. It is also approved for use in cardiovascular surgery.
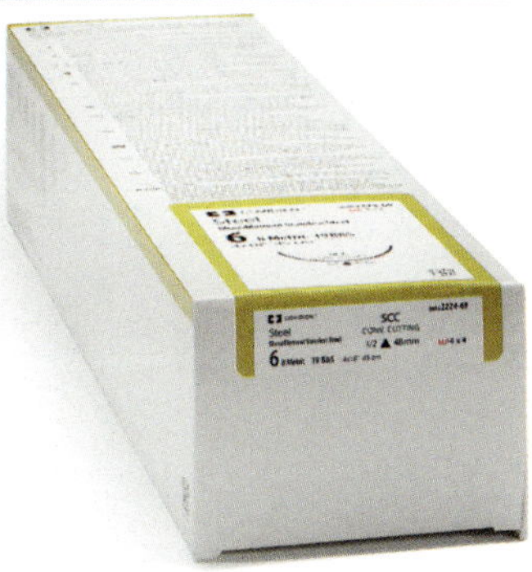 STAINLESS STEEL Composition: Steel alloy Absorbability: Non-absorbable Permanent Structure: Monofilament Color: Silver Handling: Difficult in larger sizes Primary uses: Orthopedic surgery, maxillofacial procedures	**Stainless steel** suture is widely used in maxillofacial surgery during repair and reconstruction of bone and during jaw wiring procedures. Smaller gauges may be used in tendon repair. It is highly inert in the body and keeps its tensile strength. It is, however, difficult to handle (see text for further information).

NEEDLE SHAPE AND SIZE

Needles are available in many different shapes and sizes. The curvature of a needle relates to the body and radius of the needle. The curve is measured as a circumferential fraction in a complete circle. Curvature designations are ¼, ⅜, ½, and ⅝. For example, a ½-curve needle is exactly one-half the circumference of a circle.

In general, deep tissue in a confined space requires a more extreme curve. The shape and characteristics of a needle are shown in Fig. 19.11.

Needle size is measured by the diameter of the shaft and the dimension from tip to eye. Historically, suture needles were identified by their curvature and name. These names are seldom used, and many have been replaced by common manufacturer codes. This is useful for cataloging needles but not for learning and memorizing. Surgical technologists acquire familiarity with needle codes by being exposed to specific preferences of the surgeons in their facility. Most large suture companies provide online tables that cross-reference the stock numbers of their sutures with those of other companies.

NEEDLE POINT

Many different types of needle points are available. However, all are variations of the three basic types:

Blunt: This needle has a round shaft with a blunt tip. It pushes tissue aside as it moves through it. It does not puncture the tissue, but rather slides between tissue fibers. It is the least traumatic and safest needle point. The blunt needle traditionally has been used only for suturing tissues and organs that are highly vascular, such as the liver, spleen, and kidneys. The blunt needle now is advocated for general suture use because it significantly reduces the risk of needlestick injury and transmission of blood-borne diseases.

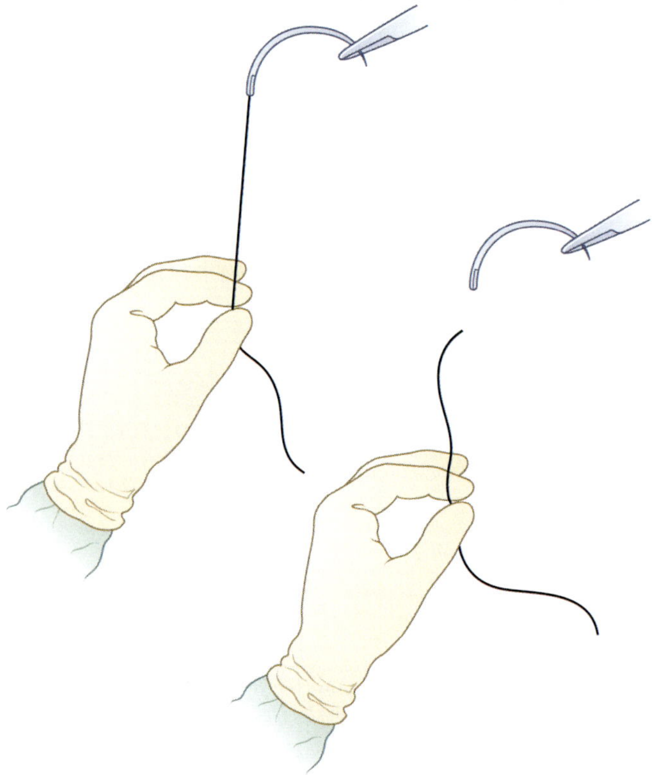

FIG. 19.7 Detachable swaged suture. The suture is released from the needle by pulling it straight back from the swage.

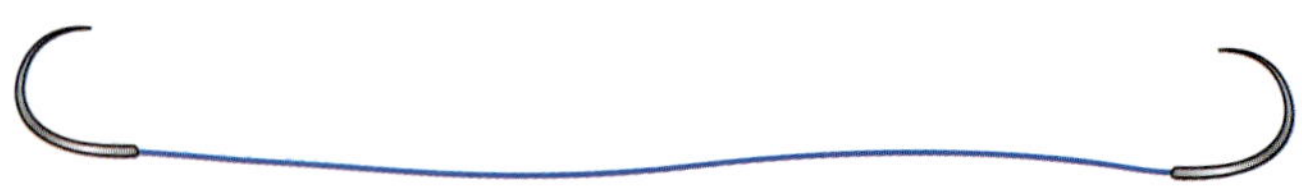

FIG. 19.8 Double-armed suture used for anastomosis or suturing of circular structures (e.g., ophthalmic or in gastrointestinal and vascular surgery).

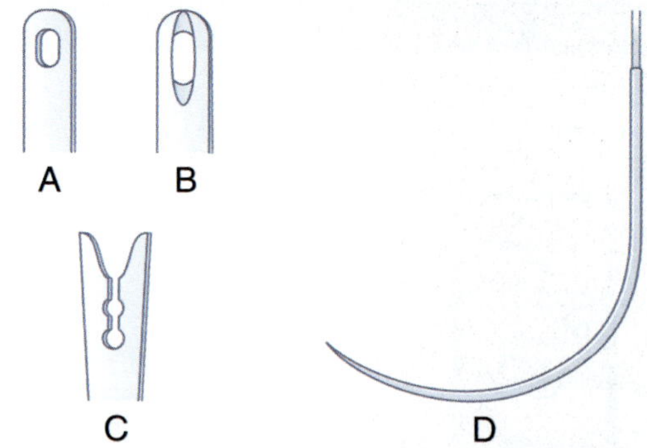

FIG. 19.9 Eyed needles are seldom used in modern surgery. However, the surgical technologist should be familiar with their use. (A and B) Closed eye. (C) French eye. (D) Atraumatic eye. (Redrawn from Phillips N. *Berry and Kohn's Operating Room Technique*. 13th ed. St Louis: Elsevier; 2017.)

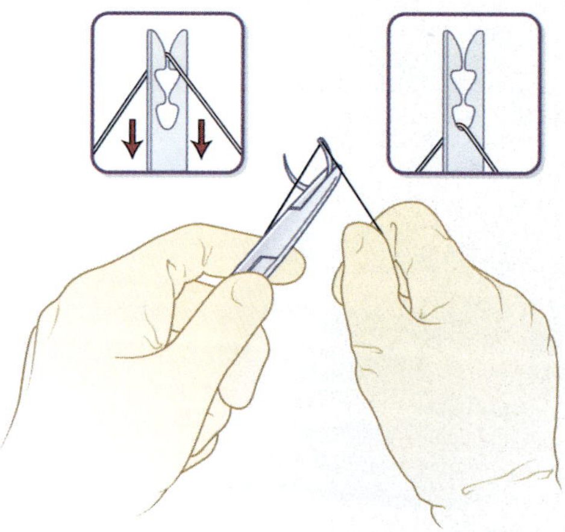

FIG. 19.10 Technique for mounting suture on a French eye needle. (Redrawn from Phillips N. *Berry and Kohn's Operating Room Technique*. 13th ed. St Louis: Elsevier; 2017.)

Tapered: The tapered needle has a round body that tapers to a sharp point. It punctures tissue, making an opening for the body of the needle to follow. Its primary use is for suturing soft tissue, such as muscle, subcutaneous fat, peritoneum, dura, and gastrointestinal, genitourinary, biliary, and vascular tissue.

Cutting: The cutting needle has a sharp edge along its shaft. This type of needle is used on fibrous connective tissue, such as the skin, joint capsule, and tendon. The conventional cutting needle has a triangular shaft. As the needle is drawn through tissue, the curve slices the tissue in an upward direction, allowing the needle to pass through the tissue easily without force. However, tension on the cutting needle may damage the tissue. The **reverse cutting** needle solves this problem by locating the cutting edge on the outside of the curve, away from the direction of tension during suturing. It is stronger than the conventional cutting needle and produces minimal scarring.

Taper-cut: This needle has a reverse cutting edge at the tip and a round body. Taper-cut needles are used for suturing dense fibrous connective tissue, such as the fascia, tendon, and periosteum.

Spatula: This needle is side-cutting with a flat surface on the top and the bottom. These are used in ophthalmic surgery to separate corneal and scleral tissue.

Fig. 19.12 shows the most commonly needle points and the tissues with which they are associated.

Self-Directed Learning: An excellent video on how surgical needles are made can be accessed at https://www.youtube.com/watch?v=tBoeRt9O3js.

SUTURE STORAGE, PACKAGING, AND DISPENSING

Sutures are stored in individual boxes containing multiple suture packs; individual packets contain one suture-needle combination or multiple needles and sutures of the same type. Suture carts and racks may be kept in supply storage areas

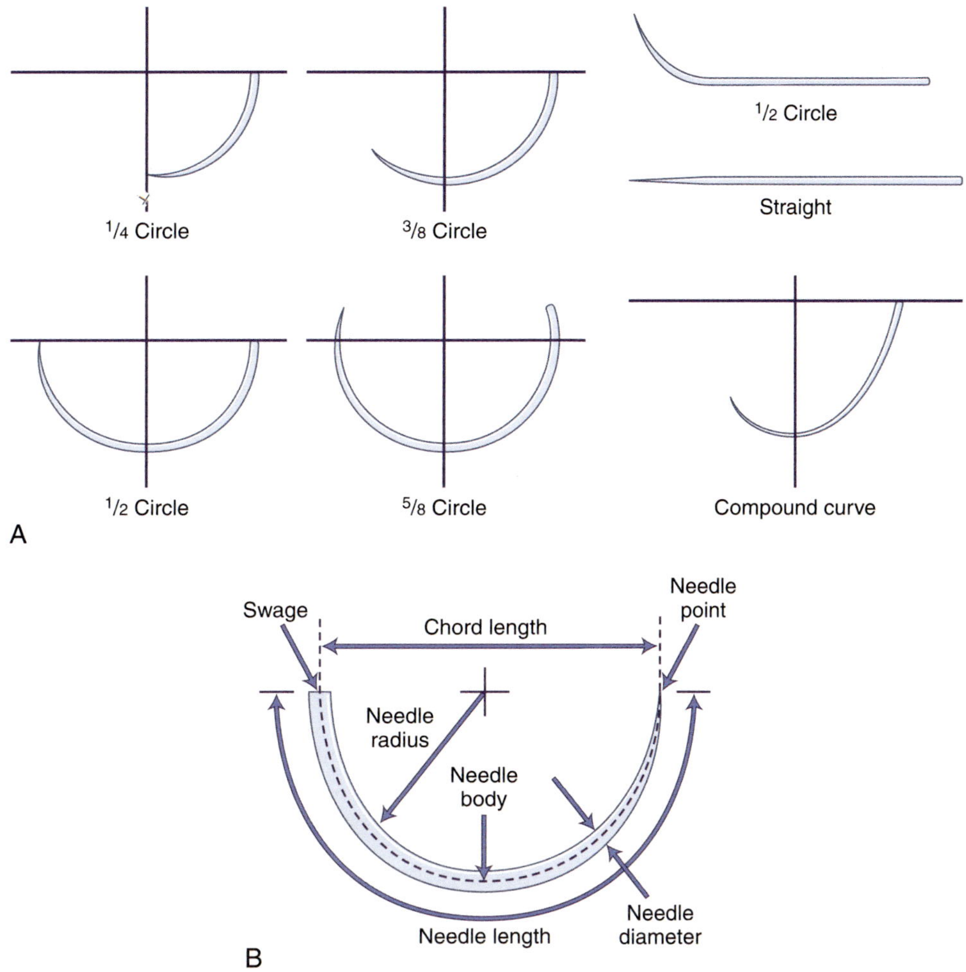

FIG. 19.11 (A) Needle shape and curvature. (B) Characteristics of the needle.

and in closed cabinets in the operating room. Large health care facilities often have a room dedicated to sutures. Suture carts should not be brought into the operating room, where they can become contaminated with blood and body fluids. At the start of surgery, only the minimum number needed are opened.

PACKAGING

Suture manufacturers have developed innovative methods of packaging that are important to surgeons, surgical technologists, and nurses. In recent years, suture manufacturers have adopted a color-coding system according to the composition of the suture. Although this system is not completely reliable, it can be helpful in the learning process.

The following are important features of a packaging system:

- ***Product protection:*** The package must maintain sterility and protect sutures and needles from damage during storage and dispensing.
- ***Efficient dispensing:*** The design of the packaging system must ensure that the suture can be withdrawn rapidly and smoothly without tangling or knotting.
- ***Labeling:*** Package labeling should be easy to associate with a specific suture. Rapid selection is desirable.
- ***Efficient packaging:*** A packaging system that produces minimal waste is desirable. Excessive wrapping and packaging are time-consuming to dispose of and create clutter on the surgical field.
- ***Environmentally responsible:*** Packaging should reflect an effort to promote the use of biodegradable materials.

Suture packages contain information that the surgical technologist needs to know when selecting suture. In Fig. 19.13A and B, note the name, size, and color of the suture; type and size of the needle (when applicable); lot number; and bar code.

PRESENTATION

Suture presentation varies among manufacturers. However, the products themselves are standard.

- ***Suture-needle combination:*** One suture-needle combination is provided per pack.
- ***Multiple suture strands:*** One suture package contains multiple precut strands of suture (Fig. 19.14) without needles. Precut suture lengths are used mainly for ligating blood vessels.
- ***Suture reel:*** A spool of suture material is wound into a round reel. The reel is used when multiple ties are needed in quick succession.

POINT/BODY SHAPE	APPLICATION
Conventional cutting (Point; Body)	Skin, sternum
Reverse cutting (Point; Body)	Fascia, ligament, nasal cavity, oral mucosa, pharynx, skin, tendon sheath
Precision point cutting (Point; Body)	Skin (plastic or cosmetic)
PC PRIME needle (Point; Body)	Skin (plastic or cosmetic)
MICRO-POINT reverse cutting needle (Point; Body)	Eye
Side-cutting spatula (Point; Body)	Eye (primary application), microsurgery, ophthalmic (reconstructive)
CS ULTIMA ophthalmic needle (Point; Body)	Eye (primary application)
Taper (Point; Body)	Aponeurosis, biliary tract, dura, fascia, gastrointestinal tract, laparoscopy, muscle, myocardium, nerve, peritoneum, pleura, subcutaneous fat, urogenital tract, vessels, valve
TAPERCUT surgical needle (Point; Body)	Bronchus, calcified tissue, fascia, laparoscopy, ligament, nasal cavity, oral cavity, ovary, perichondrium, periosteum, pharynx, sternum, tendon, trachea, uterus, valve, vessels (sclerotic)
Blunt (Point; Body)	Blunt dissection (friable tissue), cervix (ligating incompetent cervix), fascia, intestine, kidney, liver, spleen

FIG. 19.12 Needle points. (From *Wound Closure Manual*. Somerville, NJ: Ethicon Inc.; 1999.)

- ***Multiple suture-needle combinations:*** One package contains multiple suture-needle combinations in detachable format (Fig. 19.15).
- ***Double-armed suture:*** One pack contains a single suture strand with a needle attached at each end (demonstrated later).

SUTURING AND LIGATION TECHNIQUES

The primary use of sutures is to bring tissue edges together. The process of suturing two opposing tissue edges together is called *approximation*. Suture is also used to tie, or ligate, bleeding vessels. Sutures are tied using special techniques to ensure that the knots are secure. Each loop of the knot is referred to as a throw. When requesting a suture-needle during a procedure, the surgeon may refer to it as a *stitch*.

The surgical technologist must learn to anticipate the need for sutures and pass them in the accepted manner. The general principles and techniques for each use of sutures can be applied to all surgeries.

A suture technique is the method and pattern of the suture through the tissue. Two general types of suturing technique are used: continuous and interrupted.

CONTINUOUS SUTURE

The continuous or *running suture* has a knot at the beginning and at the end. It is composed of one continuous strand of suture. The needle is alternated from one side of the tissue edge to the other, as one would when sewing (Fig. 19.16). This suture technique is rapid and uses relatively little suture material. Compared with interrupted sutures, a running suture is easier to place but is not as strong.

LOCKING STITCH

The locking stitch provides added strength to a running suture line. As the needle is passed through each side of the wound edges, it is passed underneath one loop. This equalizes the tension between each loop of the suture and provides increased hemostasis on the wound edges (Fig. 19.17). This stitch requires the assistant to maintain traction on the suture a short distance (2 to 4 inches) from the point where it exits the tissue. This traction keeps the suture from backing out or becoming loose while the next stitch is being placed.

BARBED SUTURE

"Self-locking" or *barbed suture* contains intermittent projections that grip tissue in one direction, not allowing the suture to back out. (See Table 19.2.) The technology mimics the natural defense mechanism seen in porcupines. This is explained in the following short video: "Porcupine Barbs for Better Healing" available at https://www.npr.org/sections/health-shots/2019/04/09/711050307/porcupine-barbs-for-better-wound-healing or on YouTube.

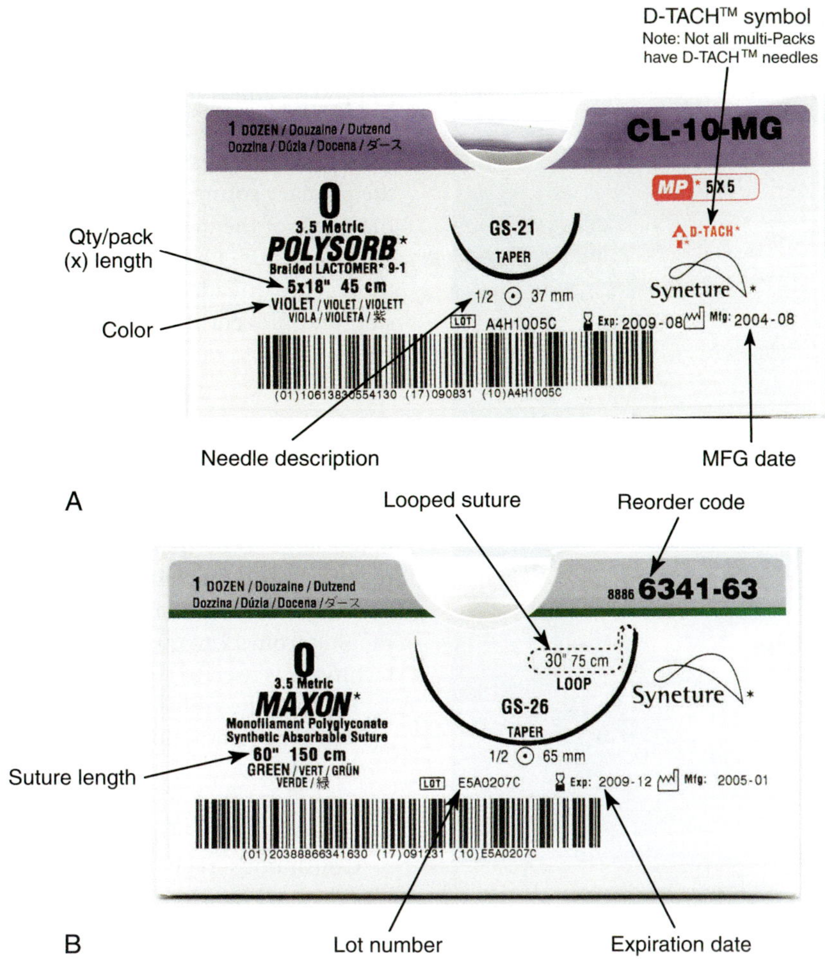

FIG. 19.13 Important information needed to identify the correct suture is printed on the box. (A) Single-suture package details. (B) Multiple-suture pack. (Copyright 2008 Covidien. All rights reserved. Reprinted with permission of Covidien.)

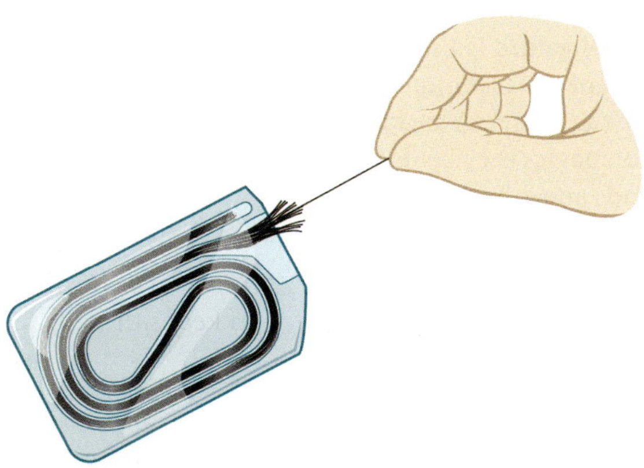

FIG. 19.14 Labyrinth-type packaging for single suture strands.

SUBCUTICULAR SUTURE

The subcuticular or buried suture is a type of running suture, used for cosmetic closure and in pediatric patients. The needle is placed within the dermis from side to side (Fig. 19.18). In this technique the sutures are placed in the dermis, under the epidermis. This brings the skin edges together while burying the sutures themselves. The technique produces a very fine scar or no scar.

PURSE-STRING SUTURE

The *purse-string suture* is a special continuous suture technique for closing the end of a tubular structure (lumen), such as the appendix, its most common application. In this technique, one end of the suture is anchored, and stitches are placed around the periphery of the open lumen. The suture then is drawn tight around the neck of the lumen and tied (Fig. 19.19).

INTERRUPTED SUTURE TECHNIQUE

Interrupted sutures are individually placed, knotted, and cut (Fig. 19.20). The finished suture line is very strong, because the tension of the wound edges is distributed over many anchor points. Many interrupted stitches produce a secure suture line with minimal scarring. Buried interrupted suture (Fig. 19.21) and mattress sutures (Fig. 19.22) provide extra security to the suture line.

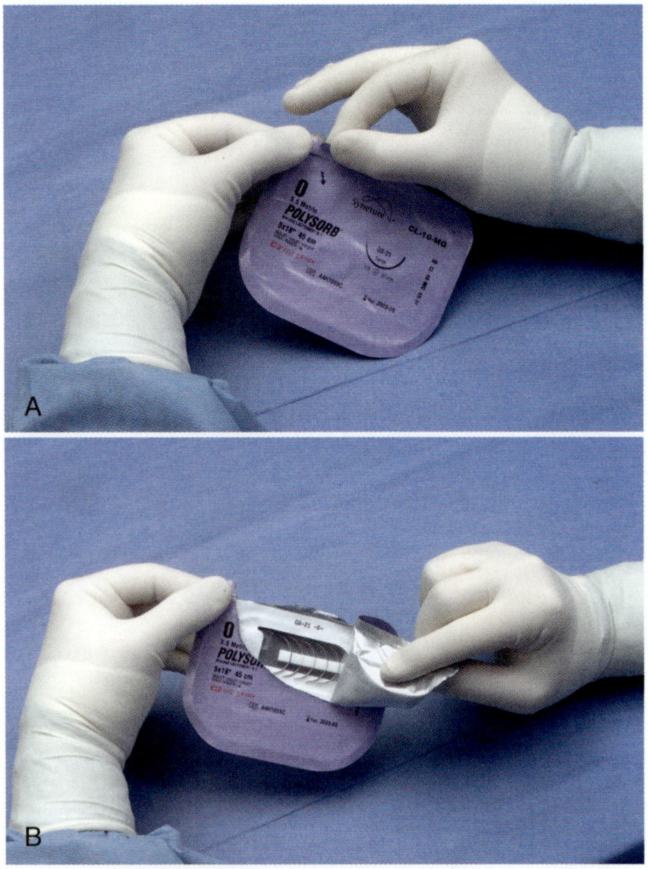

FIG. 19.15 Multiple detachable needles in a single pack. (Copyright 2008 Covidien. All rights reserved. Reprinted with permission of Covidien.)

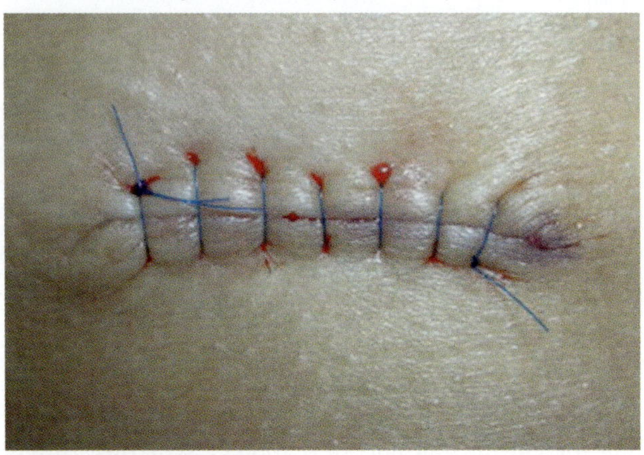

FIG. 19.16 Continuous (running) suture. (Tyers AG, Collin JR. *Colour Atlas of Ophthalmic Plastic Surgery*. London: Elsevier; 2018.)

RETENTION SUTURES

Retention sutures are a type of interrupted technique used to provide additional support to wound edges in abdominal surgery. In this technique, heavy sutures are placed though all the tissue layers of the body wall several centimeters from the primary suture line. As each suture is drawn tight, it pulls the edges of the incision into approximation without cutting into the tissue. Plastic or rubber *bolsters*, or small lengths of tubing, are threaded through the suture to distribute the tension and prevent it from cutting into the patient's skin (Fig. 19.23).

FREE TIES AND REELS

Suture ties are pre-cut lengths of suture used to ligate a bleeding vessel, called a *bleeder*. The tie is used when the bleeder is too large to be managed with the ESU. The surgeon may request "free tie" or simply "tie."

Suture strands are available in pre-cut or full-length strands ranging from 12 to 60 inches (30 cm to 1.5 m). The following technique is used to cut full-length suture into thirds:

1. Remove the coiled suture from its package. Place the coil over one hand and pull the free end slowly to uncoil the strand.
2. Grasp each end of the strand and pull the center into thirds (Fig. 19.24).

Continuous reels or rolls of suture are also used for blood vessel ligation. The reels contain 54 inches (135 cm) of suture material. When suture reels are used, the entire reel is passed (placed in the surgeon's palm). The surgeon usually replaces the reel in the Mayo after use. **Reels must not be left loose on the field because they may fall into the wound.**

SUTURE LIGATURE

A suture ligature is used to ligate a large bleeding vessel. The purpose of the technique is to prevent the ligature from sliding off the vessel. A needle-suture combination is used. The surgeon passes the needle through the midsection of the vessel and adds an additional wrap around the outside. The needle is removed, and the ligature is tied snugly. A suture ligature may be referred to as a *stick tie* (Fig. 19.25).

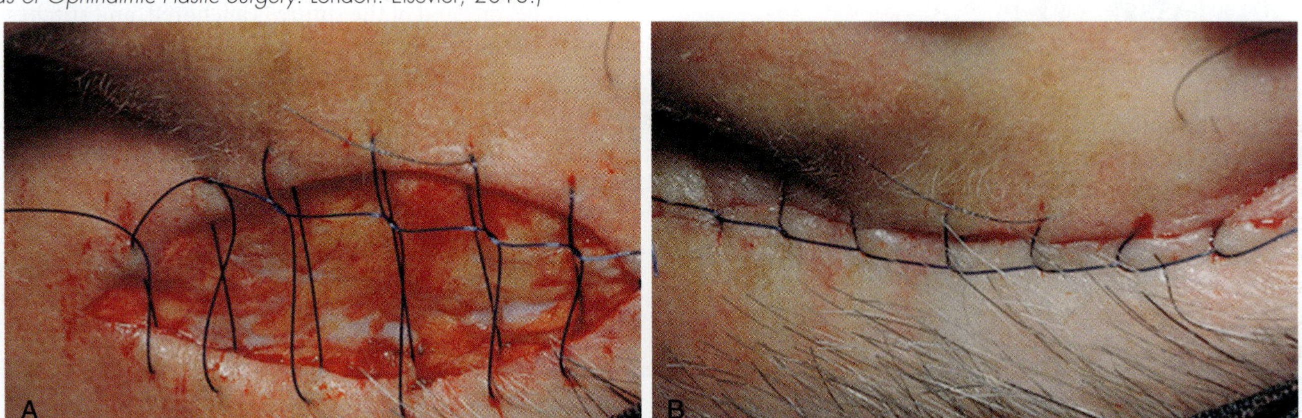

FIG. 19.17 (A) Interlocking (locked) running suture. (B) Suture closed. (From Tyers AG, Collin JR. *Colour Atlas of Ophthalmic Plastic Surgery*. London: Elsevier; 2018.)

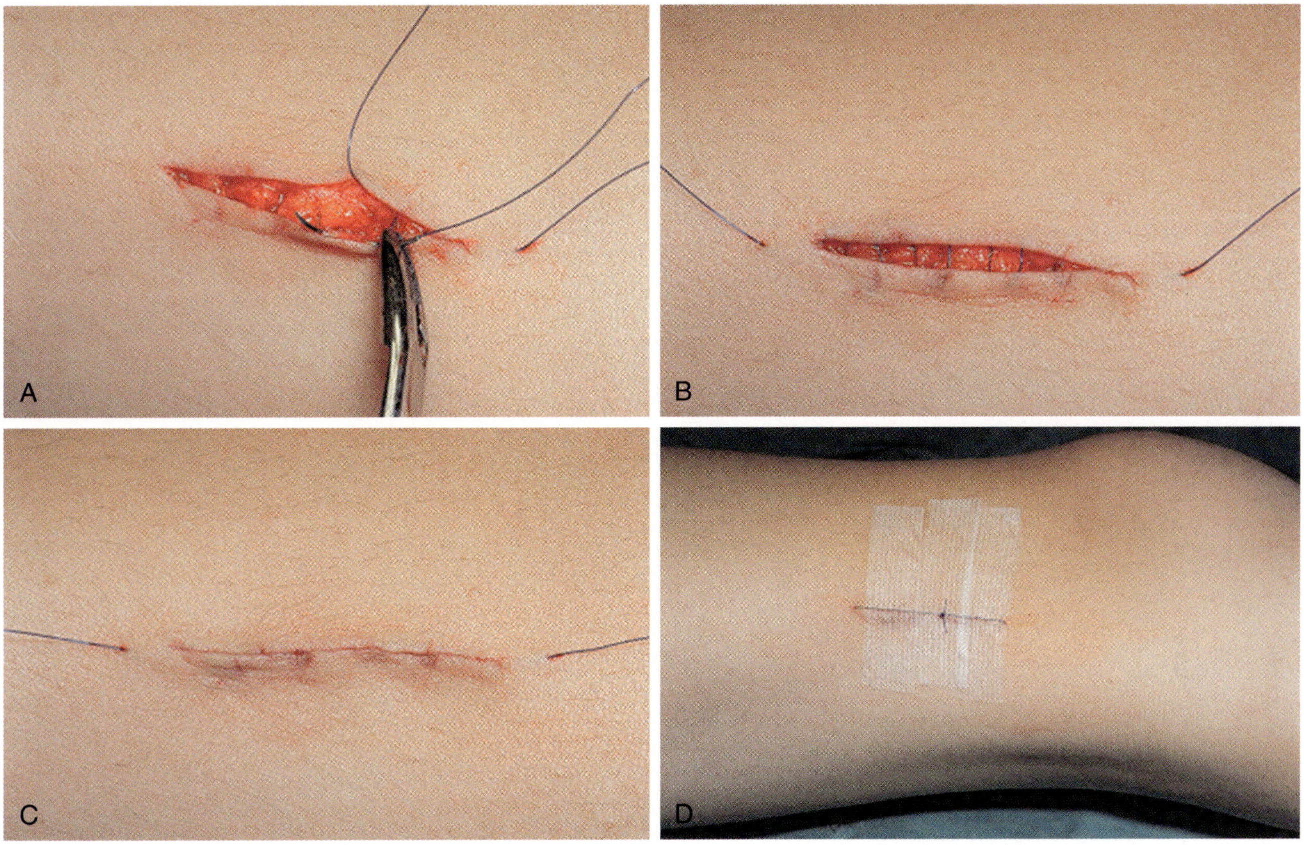

FIG. 19.18 Subcuticular (intradermal) suture. (A) Open. (B) Wound edges closing. (C) Wound edges closed. (D) Closed incision with dressing. (From Tyers AG, Collin JR. *Colour Atlas of Ophthalmic Plastic Surgery*. London: Elsevier; 2018.)

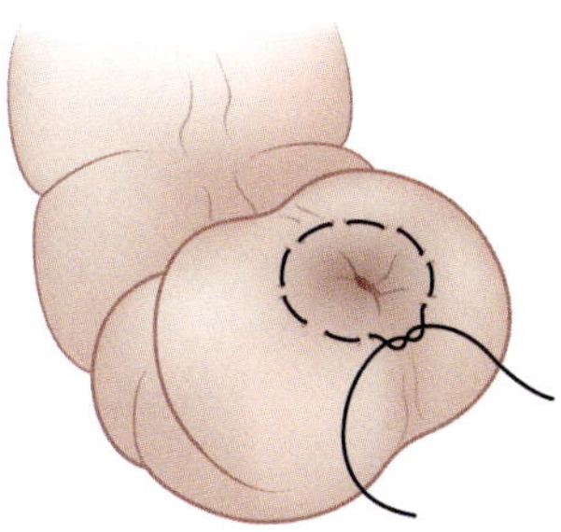

FIG. 19.19 Purse-string suture. (From Robinson J, Hanke C. *Surgery of the Skin, Procedural Dermatology*. 3rd ed. St Louis: Saunders; 2015.)

TIE ON A PASSER

When suture ties (without a needle) are required deep in the wound, they must be passed on a right-angle or curved clamp. The tip of the suture tie is grasped by the tip of the clamps. This allows the surgeon to slip the instrument tip under the vessel or other structure to be ligated. The tie is then released and clamped again as it emerges from the other side of the vessel. The two ends of the suture are then tied. The clamp is passed in the normal manner, but the suture length should be draped over the back of the ST's hand to prevent it from being caught in the surgeon's palm. If this type of tie is needed during a procedure, the surgeon may ask for a **tie on a passer** or simply a tie.

TRACTION SUTURES AND TAGS

A suture tag is a hemostat placed at the ends of a suture tie or ligature. Tagging is used to apply traction on the long ties or to maintain control of the ligature in case further ligation is required. Traction sutures are placed in tissue to provide retraction. This technique is used in many different specialties. When a traction suture is required, the surgeon will usually state the size of suture and needle. This information should also be on the surgeon's preference card. An example of a traction suture is shown in Fig. 19.26.

INTRAOPERATIVE SUTURE MANAGEMENT

One of the primary skills of the surgical technologist is the management of sutures during surgery. Surgeons are accustomed to receiving sutures from the ST in a prescribed manner for safety and efficiency of movement. Good technique in handling sutures prevents the loss of a needle in the surgical wound and helps to prevent needlestick injury.

1. The surgical technologist must know at all times where loaded and free needles/sutures are on the Mayo and back table.
2. Keep suture packs organized. Know where each type of suture is.
3. As soon as a free needle is returned, immediately place it on the magnetic board or sharps holder. *Needles should*

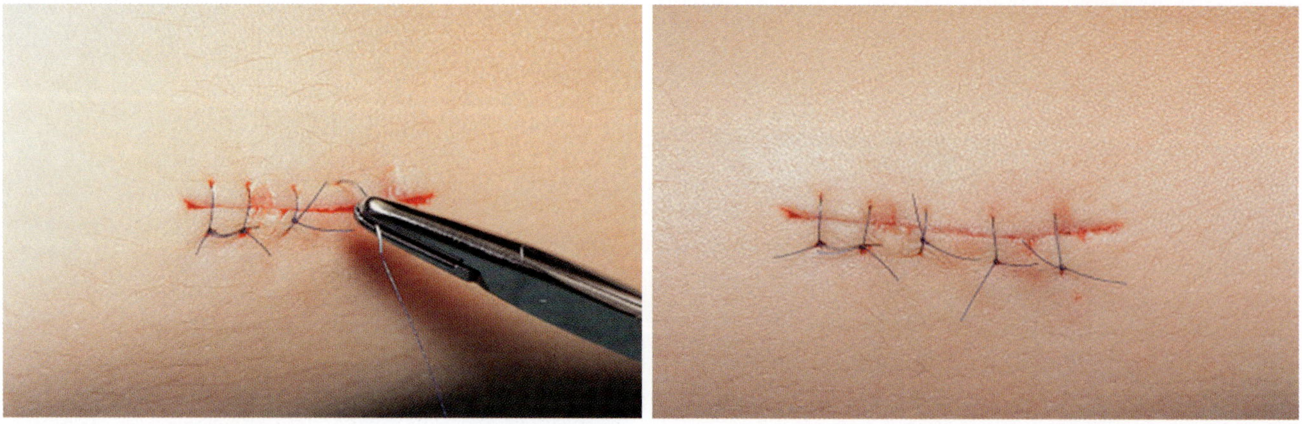

FIG. 19.20 Interrupted sutures. (From Tyers AG, Collin JR. *Colour Atlas of Ophthalmic Plastic Surgery*. London: Elsevier; 2018.)

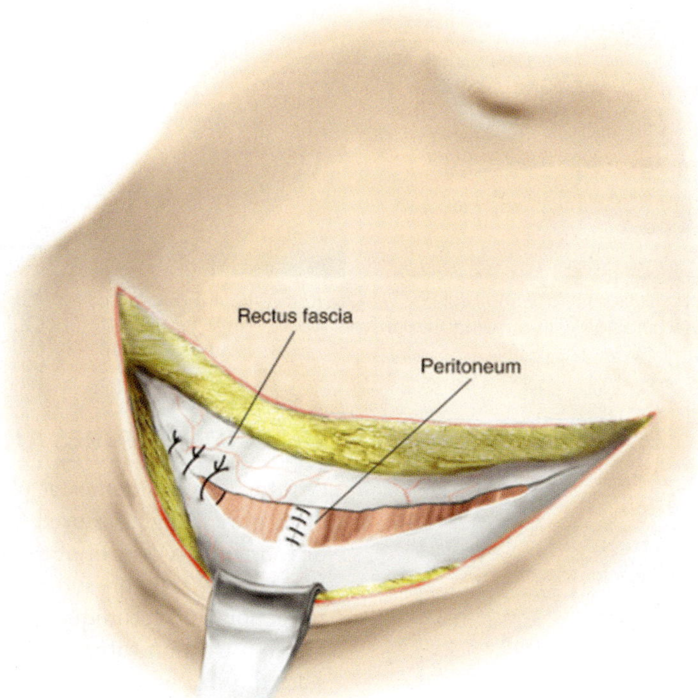

FIG. 19.21 20 Buried interrupted sutures in pelvic fascia. (Baggish MS, Karram MM. *Atlas of Pelvic Anatomy and Gynecologic Surgery*. Philadelphia: Elsevier; 2016.)

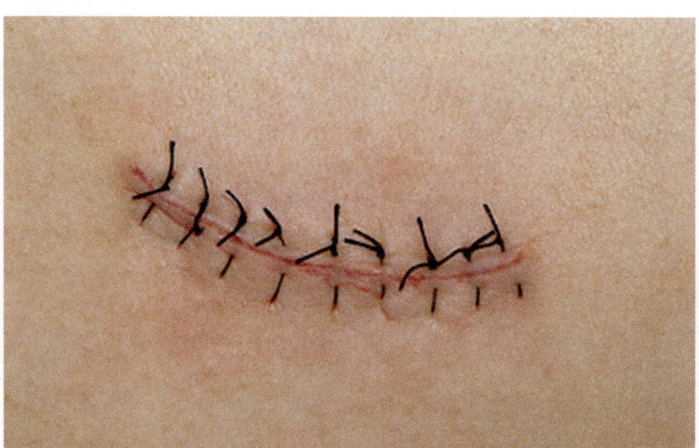

FIG. 19.22 Vertical mattress sutures. (From Tyers AG, Collin JR. *Colour Atlas of Ophthalmic Plastic Surgery*. London: Elsevier; 2018.)

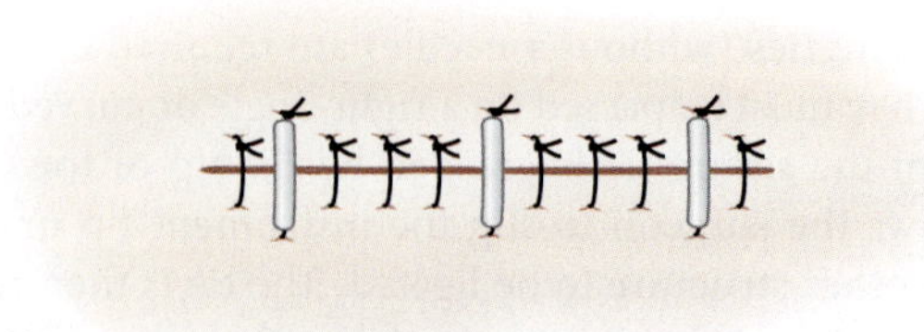

FIG. 19.23 Retention sutures.

never be loose on the field or instrument tables. They should be mounted on a needle holder or secured in a magnetic holder.
4. Sutures are passed on an exchange basis. Have a loaded needle prepared at all times. As the surgeon releases a suture, another one is passed.
5. Load the needle holder before removing the entire needle-suture from its package.
6. Avoid grasping needles with the gloved hand. Use a needle holder.

IMPORTANT TO KNOW *Do not use the kick bucket for suture wrappers. A needle may be lost among the sponges, and it is extra work for the circulator to pick out the wrappers. Instead, use the trash bag provided in the surgical setup.*

SUTURING INSTRUMENTS

Curved suture needles are mounted on a needle holder (also called a *needle driver*) for use. The straight *(Keith)* needle is used like a sewing needle—no needle holder is used. Select a needle holder that is the correct length for the depth of the wound and the correct weight (heavy or delicate). The jaws of the needle holder must be selected according to the delicacy of the needle. Many types of needle holders have diamond or carbon steel inserts over the portion that holds the needle. This prevents the needle from slipping or rotating. The type and size of the needle holder are adjusted to the size of the needle (Fig. 19.27).

Tissue forceps are used to stabilize the tissue while suturing. The ST selects the forceps by length, weight, and type of tip according to the tissue to be sutured. Examples of tissue forceps used for suturing are shown in Fig. 19.28.

- *Smooth forceps* are used on mucous membrane and organ tissue (e.g., the spleen and kidneys) and on any tissue that bleeds easily.
- *Toothed forceps* are used on fibrous connective tissue, such as skin, tendon, and fascia.

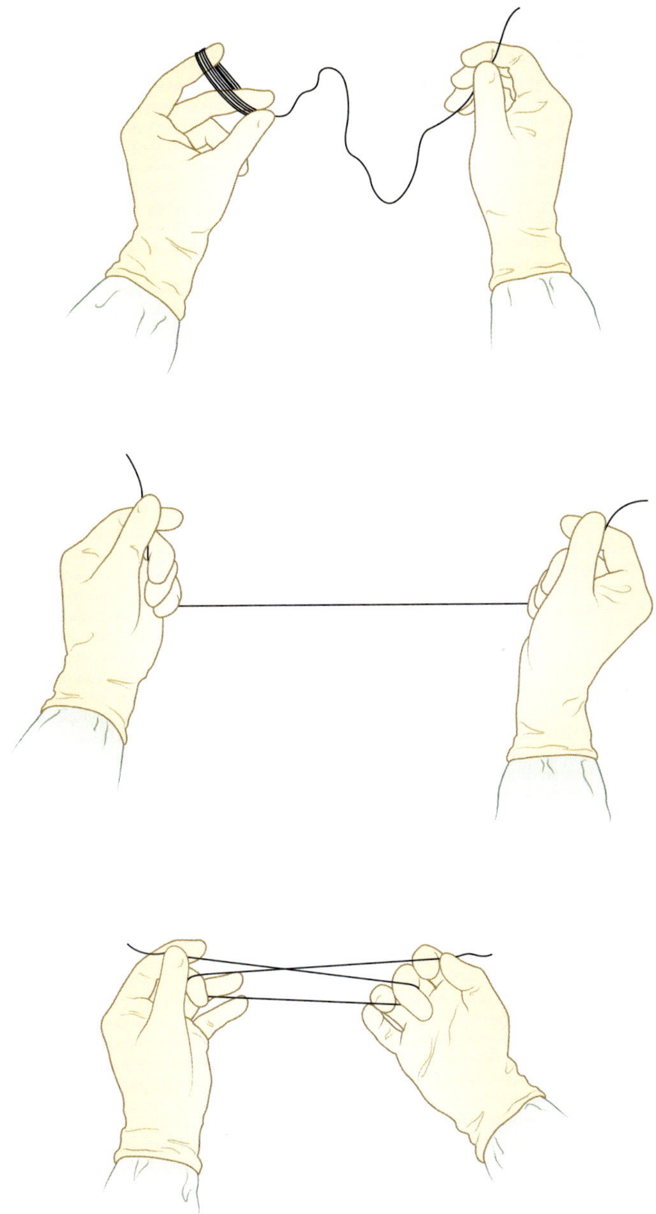

FIG. 19.24 Dividing long suture into thirds. (Redrawn from Phillips N. *Berry and Kohn's Operating Room Technique*. 13th ed. St Louis: Elsevier; 2017.)

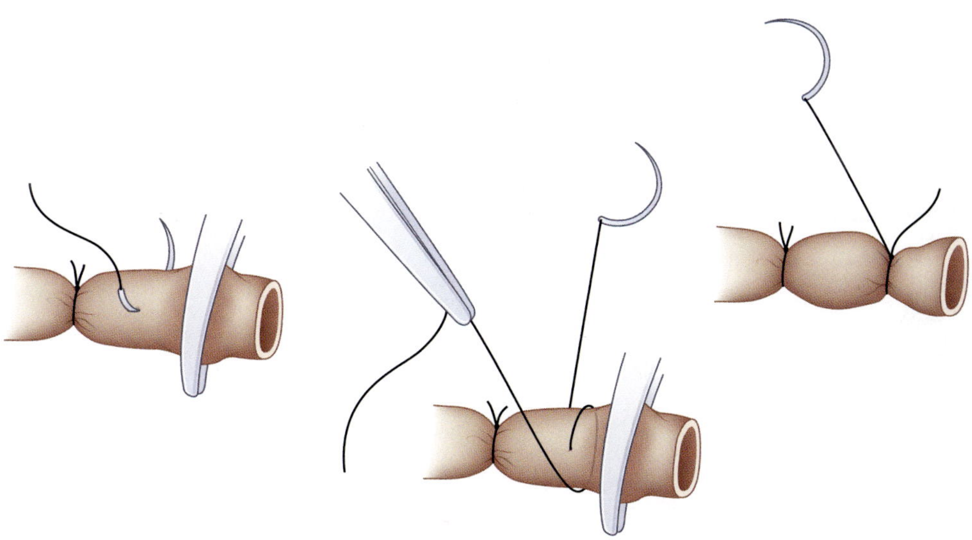

FIG. 19.25 The suture ligature *(stick tie)* is used to secure the ligature. The suture is passed through the body of the blood vessel and looped around the vessel before tying it.

- *Vascular forceps* are specially designed with a scored insert at the working tip; this prevents puncturing of the blood vessel but provides sufficient friction to hold.

PASSING SUTURES

Mount the needle about 0.5 mm from the end of the swaged section. Do not clamp the swage, because this weakens it and places the needle holder too far back for correct balance (Fig. 19.29). Grasp the needle using the needle holder. Draw it carefully from the package. Adjust the needle holder's grasp as needed (Fig. 19.30A). Drape the suture end over the back of your hand or maintain loose contact with the suture as you pass it (Fig. 19.30B). This prevents it from becoming caught in the surgeon's hand as he or she receives the suture. The "armed" needle holder must be passed so that the surgeon does not have to reposition it in the hand or look up from the surgical site. The position of the needle holder in relation to the suture needle depends on:

- Whether the surgeon is right-handed or left-handed
- Whether the surgeon stands opposite the ST or next to the ST
- Whether the suture is requested as "back-handed"

A left-handed surgeon places sutures by driving the needle into the tissue in a counterclockwise direction. A right-handed surgeon drives the needle clockwise. *An exception to this is the back-handed suture, in which the direction is reversed.* With the curved needle positioned at a right angle to the needle holder, the surgeon normally presents his palm to the ST with the thumb pointed upward. The ST should deliver the needle holder in the flat of the surgeon's palm so that the point of the needle is directed toward the surgeon (Fig. 19.30C).

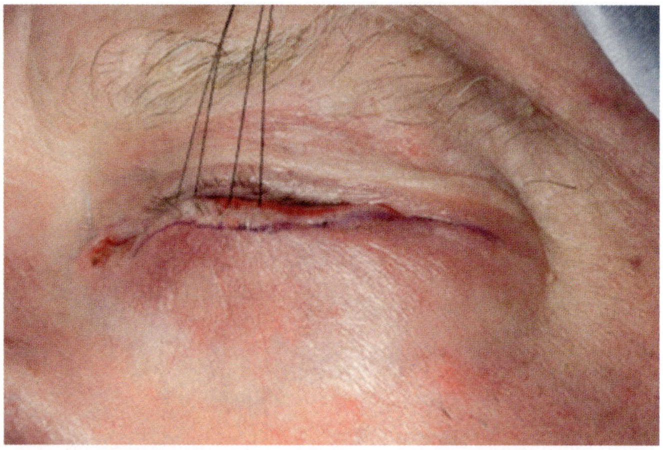

FIG. 19.26 Traction suture—used to retract tissue without using an instrument. In this photo, traction sutures have been placed in the lower eyelid so that it can be pulled upward. (Tyers AG, Collin JR. *Colour Atlas of Ophthalmic Plastic Surgery*. London: Elsevier; 2018.)

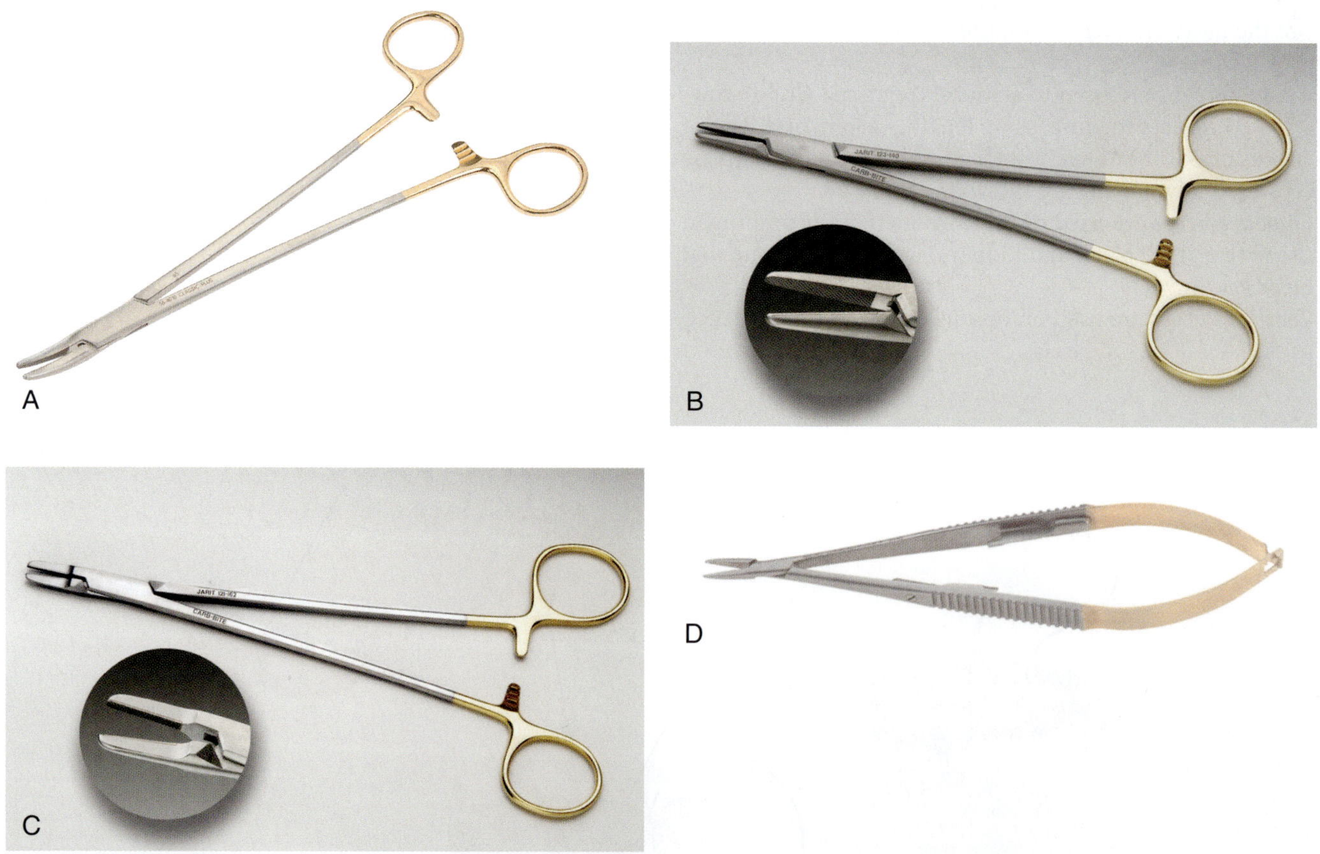

FIG. 19.27 Assorted needle holders. (A) Heaney: OB GYN surgery. (B) Mayo-Hegar: (C) Ryder. Vascular (D) Castroviejo. Microsurgery (C, From Nemitz. *Surgical Instrumentation: An Interactive Approach*. 3rd ed. St. Louis: Elsevier; 2019; D, Photos courtesy Millennium Surgical Instruments.)

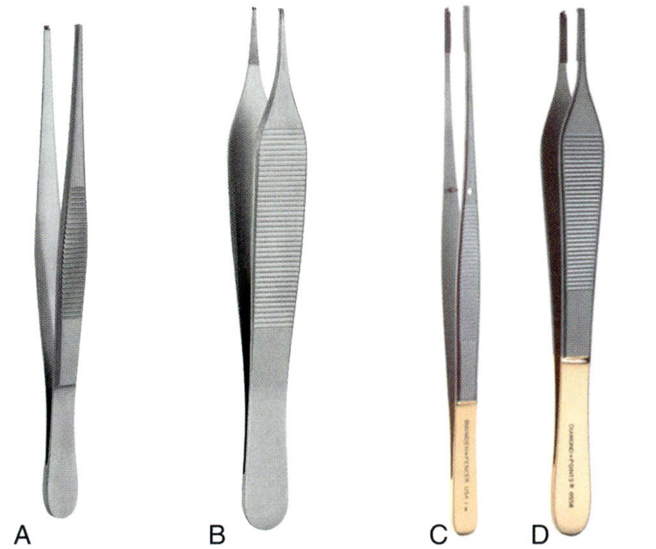

FIG. 19.28 Assorted tissue forceps *(pickups)*. (A) Single tooth. (B) Toothed Adson. (C) Semkin. (D) Adson vascular. (Courtesy V. Mueller Instruments.)

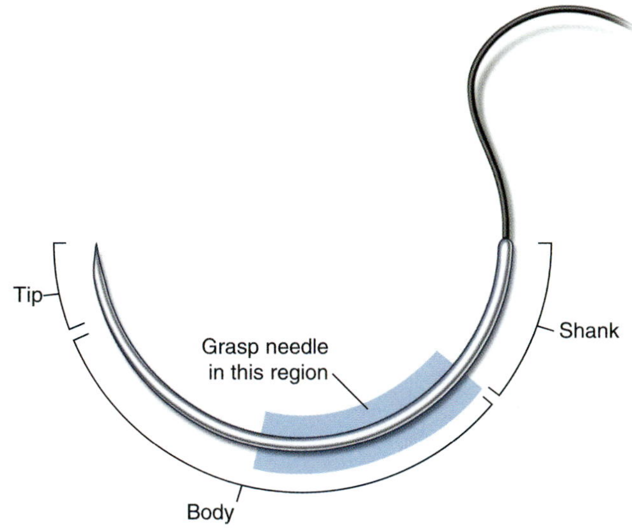

FIG. 19.29 Correct area to place the needle holder. (From Robinson J, Hanke C. *Surgery of the Skin, Procedural Dermatology.* 3rd ed. Philadelphia: Saunders; 2015.)

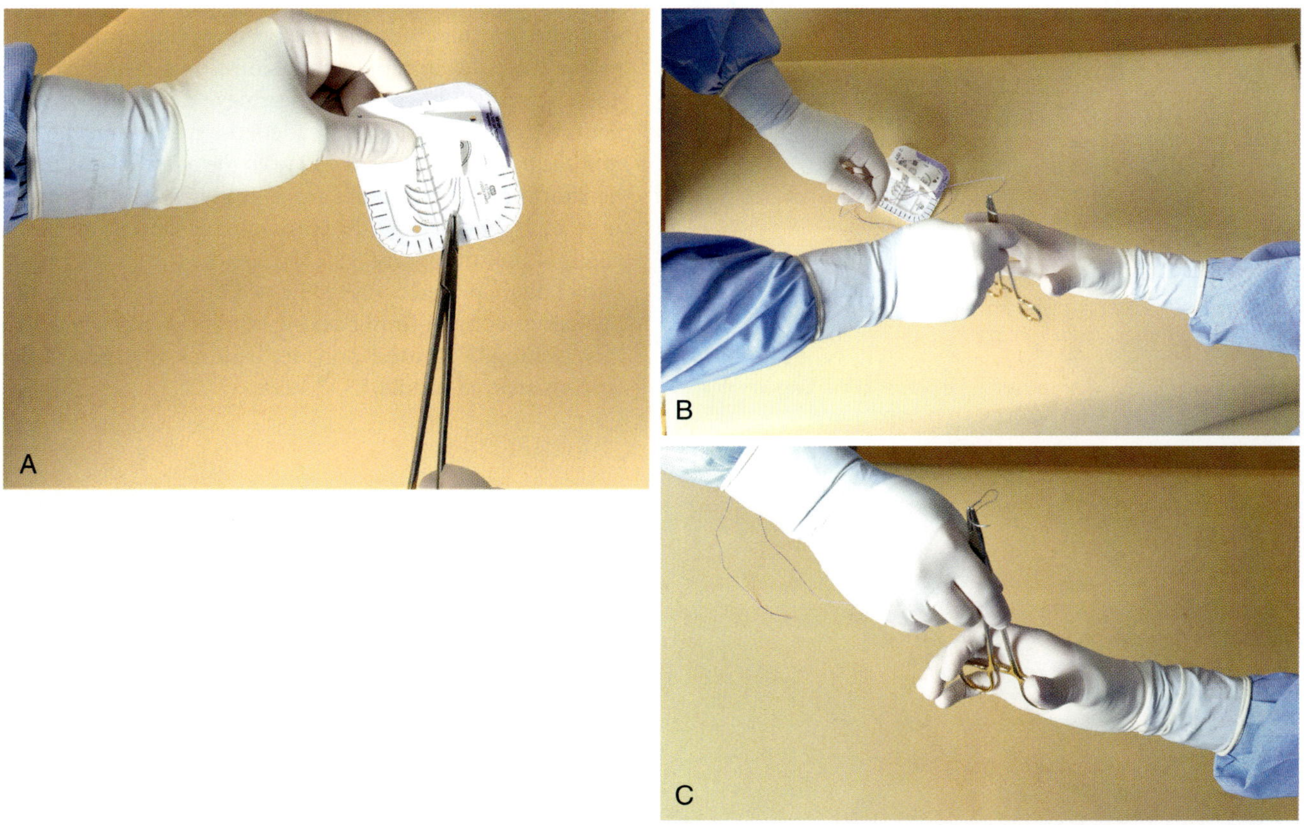

FIG. 19.30 Technique for passing a suture. (A) Grasp the needle at the correct position while it is still in the package. Remove it and re-position it as necessary. (B) Orient the needle so that the tip is facing up, maintaining the suture away from his or her palm. (C) Place the needle holder firmly in the surgeon's hand.

One method of learning the correct orientation of the mounted needle holder is to practice the movements with another person as if one of you were suturing. Work with a colleague and position yourself as the surgeon would be. The logic of presenting the suture in correct spatial orientation will be immediately apparent. Be sure to practice with the surgeon on the same side of the table as the ST as well as on the opposite side. Practice passing with both the right and left hands.

To arm the *Castroviejo* locking needle holder, squeeze gently on the bowed section of the handles to unlock the tips. Grasp the suture as described above, and again compress the handles, to close the locking clip (Fig. 19.31). When passing double-armed sutures, the second needle can be mounted on a small hemostat with shods. Take care when passing the double-armed suture as it can easily become snagged on drapes and sponges, causing them to break away from the suture.

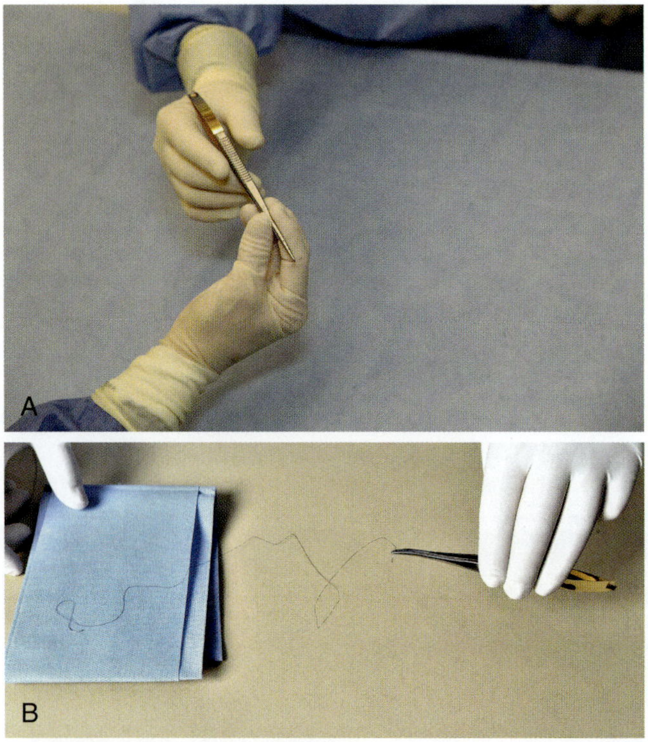

FIG. 19.31 Technique for passing a locking Castroviejo type needle holder. (A) Note position of the hand and placement on the instrument. Not all needle holders of this type have a locking spring. When passing these, be sure to maintain light pressure on the handles to prevent the needle from dropping. (B) The second needle of the double armed suture should be visible when passing the suture to the surgeon this is an example of a needle being placed on a paper towel for visibility.

RAPID-SEQUENCE SUTURING

Since the adoption of swaged needles in surgery, the technique of rapid-sequence threading has been replaced by multiple needle-suture packs. The manner in which the needle is packaged often determines how quickly and safely sutures can be passed to the surgeon. More paper and many more needles are generated than in the past, increasing the risk of a lost or retained needle and increased expense.

THREADING EYED NEEDLES

Most surgical technologists will never work with loose needles that must be threaded. However, it is a skill that should be studied in the event the need arises. Threading and passing eyed needles in rapid succession is not difficult but does require considerable practice to achieve rapid, smooth movement. When the needle is threaded, the suture must be passed *from the inside of the needle curve to the outside.* This prevents the short end of the suture from pulling out of the eye. The short end should extend approximately one-third the total length of the suture (Fig. 19.32A). Before the suture is passed, both ends are placed between the two tips of the needle holder. This prevents them from backing out of the eye (Fig. 19.32B). This technique is used only for sutures that are threaded through an eyed needle.

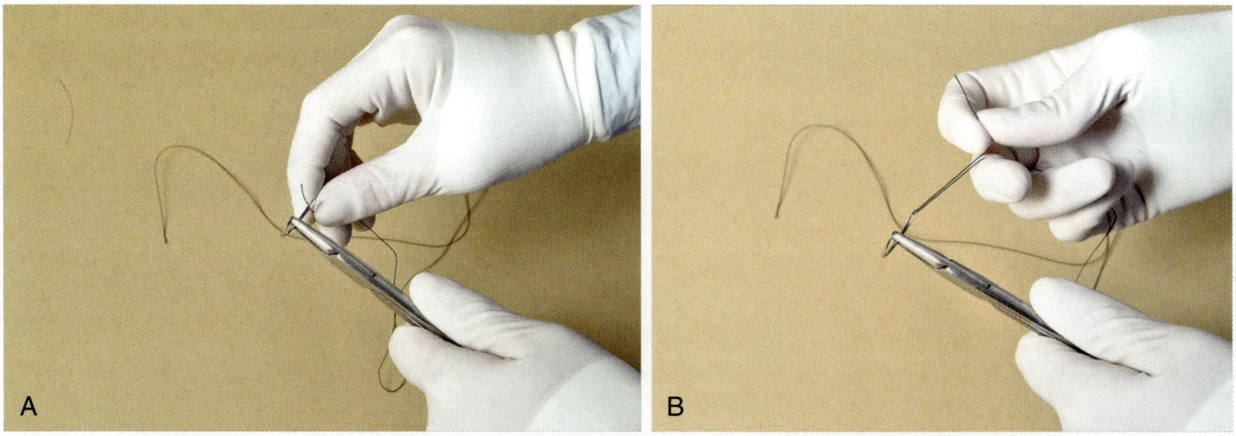

FIG. 19.32 Eyed needle. (A) Pass the suture through the needle eye from the outside to the inside of the curvature. The short end of the suture should be approximately one-third the distance of the long end. (B) After passing the suture through the needle, loop both ends back through the jaws of the needle holder loosely to keep the suture from backing out while being passed.

HOW TO CUT SUTURES

The ST is frequently asked to cut suture ends after a knot is tied, especially on skin sutures. When sutures are cut, the ends must be long enough that the knot does not untie but short enough to reduce the amount of foreign material in or around the wound. When the suture is cut too short, the knot may actually be cut. If this happens, the suture must be removed, and another suture placed. A straight hemostat (Crile or Kelly type) is the best instrument for extracting the remains of a cut suture. Box 19.3 describes the correct technique for cutting sutures. Fig. 19.33 illustrates the technique. If the ST is required to cut sutures while performing other tasks, he or she can "palm the scissors" as shown in Fig. 19.34. To remove a suture, it is important to cut below the knot *on one side only* as shown in Fig. 19.35. If both sides are cut, the suture will be drawn inside the wound, where it may be irretrievable without opening the wound.

BOX 19.3 How to Cut Sutures

1. Use only sharp suture scissors; never use tissue scissors on suture material.
2. To cut the suture, open the scissors slightly. Use the tip of the scissors to cut.
3. Hold the scissors as shown in Fig. 19.33.
4. Place your index finger over the top of the scissors to steady the blades. Turn the scissors at a 45-degree angle. This creates a small "whisker." Cut the suture ends while keeping the scissors at an angle.
5. When cutting sutures and performing other tasks at the same time, it is convenient to "palm" the scissors in one hand (Fig. 19.34).
6. Remove any cut suture ends from the wound area to prevent them from falling into the wound.

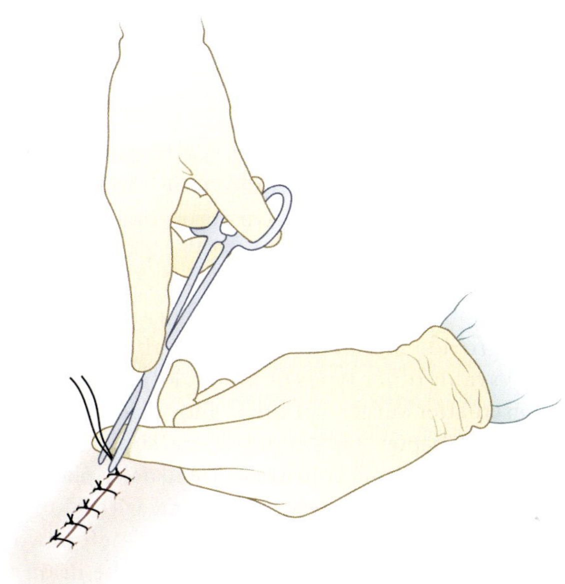

FIG. 19.33 Cutting sutures. Note the use of the ring finger through the ring handle. This provides the best control.

REMOVING EMBEDDED SUTURES

When the surgeon needs to remove deep sutures from a previous surgery, the knots usually are embedded in scar tissue and may be difficult to grasp and cut. A *straight, fine-tipped hemostat works best* for pulling out old sutures. The ST should place a folded surgical towel on the field so that the extracted suture pieces can be isolated so that they do not drop back into the wound. The towel is then removed from the field.

VESSEL CLIPS AND STAPLES

The vessel clip or Hemoclip is a stainless steel, titanium, or synthetic clip that is placed over a blood vessel to occlude it. Clips are an alternative to the suture tie described above. They are available in many different sizes. These are implanted with a clip applier whose jaws match the configuration of the clip (Fig. 19.36).

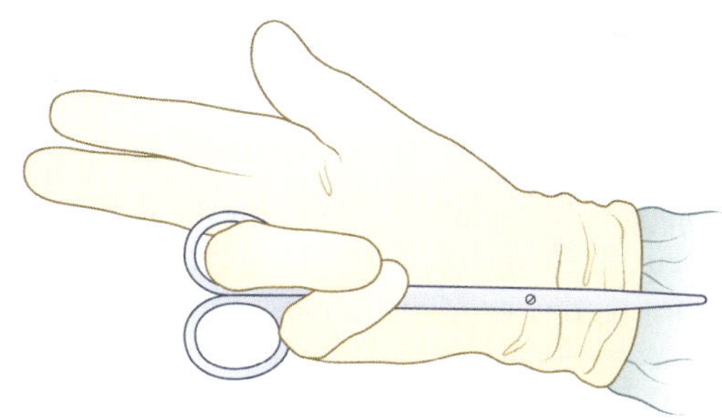

FIG. 19.34 Palming the suture scissors.

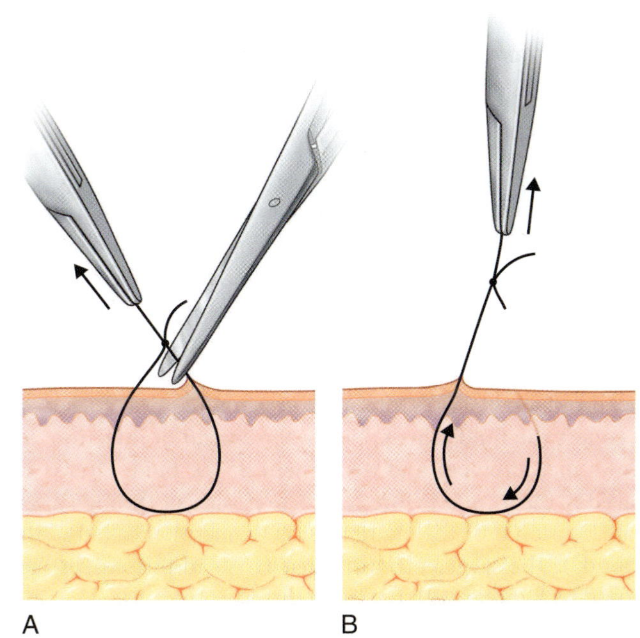

FIG. 19.35 Technique for suture removal. Note that the suture is elevated away from the tissue using a straight clamp. The suture is cut on one side of the knot and then pulled through. (From Robinson J, Hanke C. *Surgery of the Skin, Procedural Dermatology*. 3rd ed. Philadelphia: Saunders; 2015.)

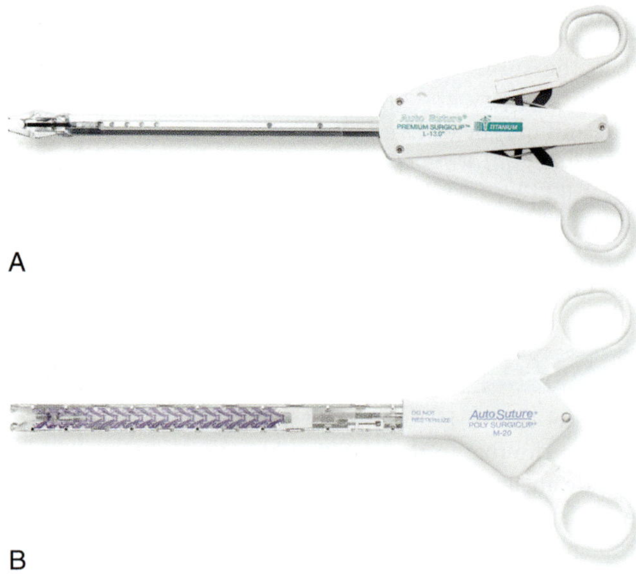

FIG. 19.36 Vessel clip appliers.

Surgical stapling devices have replaced sutures in many different types of surgery, both open and minimally invasive procedures. They are available as single-use items or as stainless-steel instruments. Staples are available in metal and synthetic absorbable material, commercially prepared in cartridges that load into the stapler. Refer to Chapter 11 for a more complete description and illustrations of stapling devices.

IMPORTANT TO KNOW *Surgical stapling devices are manufactured by a number of different companies. The devices require in-service training for surgical technologists. Each company's products feature different mechanisms and safety features, which can be somewhat complex. To ensure patient safety, the surgical technologist should rely on hands-on training from the device manufacturer for stapler assembly, preparation, and use in surgery.*

WOUND DRAINAGE

Fluid sometimes accumulates in the wound after surgery. This is related to the inflammatory process and oozing from small capillaries. The accumulation of *serosanguinous fluid* (blood and serum) can become a medium for microbial growth. To prevent this, a drain may be placed in the wound before closure.

All but very simple drainage systems require a reservoir to collect the fluid. This prevents the spread of infection and allows measurement and assessment of the fluid. Drains are placed in the wound before complete closure or through a separate incision near the main incision (sometimes called a "stab wound"). The surgical technologist assists in this process and should be familiar with common drainage systems.

PASSIVE DRAIN

A passive drain creates a passage from the tissue inside the wound to the outside of the body. These are used when drainage is minimal. The *Penrose* drain is a simple tubular length of nonlatex material similar to surgical glove material. Before closing, the surgeon places the drain loosely in the wound and secures it with non-absorbable sutures. A gauze dressing is placed over the drain to collect fluid from the wound. No reservoir is required. Fig. 19.37 is the Penrose drain. Other types of passive drains include the *T-tube, Pezzer, Malecot,* and *Foley* catheters. The T-tube is used specifically for bile duct drainage and is connected to a bile bag by a length of clear tubing. The *Foley* catheter and *Malecot* drain provide continuous drainage after genitourinary surgery. Various other types of ureteral drainage tubes may also be used after surgery of the kidney or ureter; these are discussed in Chapter 24. Wound drains such as the Pezzer, Malecot, mushroom, and Penrose are usually placed in the wound by positioning the proximal end with blunt-nosed forceps such as a Mayo or Pean clamp. One or two non-absorbable sutures may be used to secure the drain to the tissues as necessary. Some passive drains are connected at the distal end to a collection system for measurement and emptying of the drainage fluid.

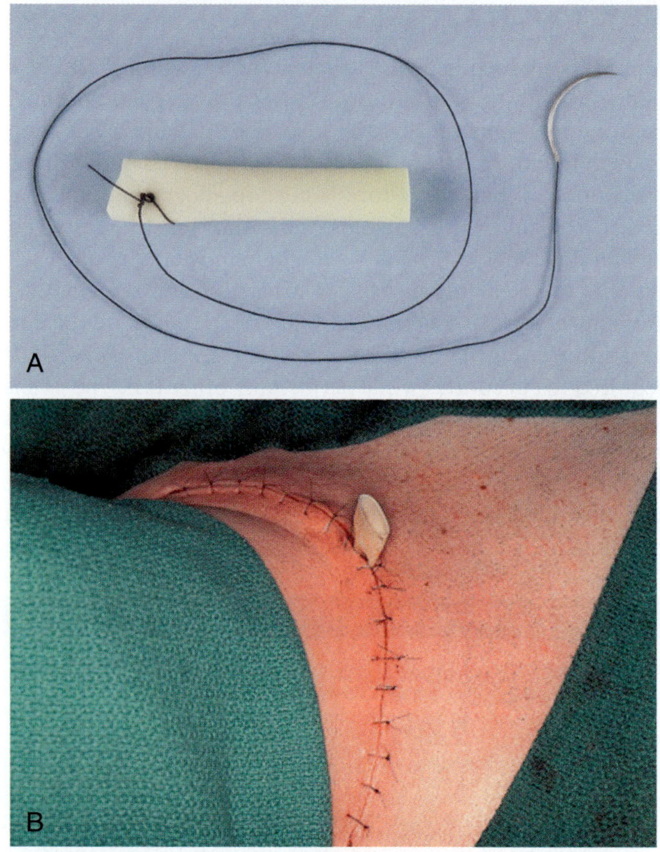

FIG. 19.37 Penrose drain. (A) The Penrose drain is a thin-walled tube, available in different widths and lengths. (B) The drain is placed in the wound before the wound is closed. A small portion remains outside the wound for external drainage. (A, From Hupp JR, Ellis E, Tucker MR. *Contemporary Oral and Maxillofacial Surgery.* 7th ed. Philadelphia: Elsevier; 2019. B, From Shah J, Bhuvanesh S. *Jatin Shah's Head and Neck Surgery and Oncology.* 4th ed. Philadelphia: Mosby; 2019.)

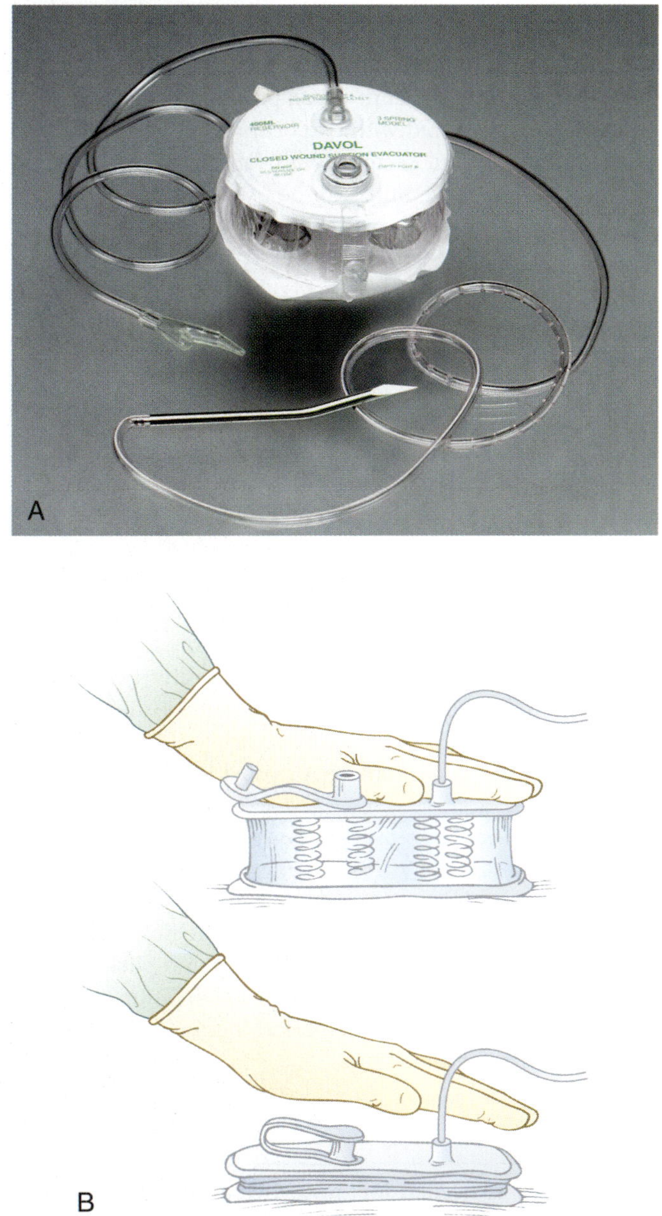

FIG. 19.38 Hemovac suction drain. (A) The proximal end of the drain tubing is placed in the open surgical wound. The distal end is attached to the metal trocar. This is used to make a stab wound for the tubing. (B) The tubing is connected to the reservoir. After wound closure, the reservoir is compressed and the tab is closed, creating suction within the wound and drawing fluid out. (A, From Rothrock JC. *Alexander's Care of the Patient in Surgery.* 13th ed. St Louis: Mosby; 2007. B, Redrawn from Phillips N. *Berry and Kohn's Operating Room Technique.* 13th ed. St Louis: Elsevier; 2017.)

SUCTION DRAINS

A suction drain pulls serum and blood from the wound by a negative-pressure device. A tube is placed in the center of the wound and connected to a one-way valve in the drain reservoir. Air is evacuated from the container by squeezing it to activate the negative pressure, and the wound tubing is attached to the deflated reservoir. As the reservoir returns to its normal shape, it pulls fluid from the wound in the same way a bulb syringe is used to pull fluid. Two common suction drains are the Hemovac (Fig. 19.38) and the Jackson-Pratt (Fig. 19.39).

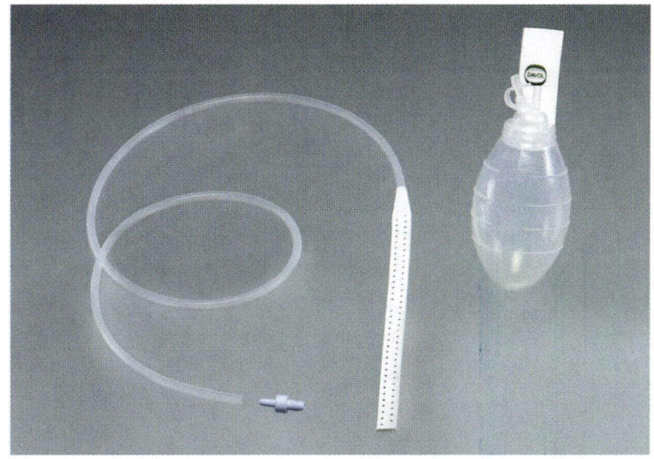

FIG. 19.39 Jackson-Pratt suction-reservoir drain. The perforated tubing is placed inside the surgical wound, and the distal end is connected to the hand suction device. (From Rothrock JC. *Alexander's Care of the Patient in Surgery.* 13th ed. St Louis: Mosby; 2007.)

WATER-SEALED DRAINAGE SYSTEM

A water-sealed drainage system is used to pull fluid or air from the thoracic cavity after thoracic surgery or trauma to the thorax. The thoracic cavity is normally under negative pressure. The difference between atmospheric pressure and thoracic pressure allows the lungs to expand easily. Loss of negative pressure causes the lung to collapse. After surgery or a penetrating injury to the chest wall, negative pressure must be restored. The underwater drainage system removes fluid and air to restore negative pressure.

The drainage system has three separate water chambers sealed in a plastic unit. One or more chest drainage tubes are placed in the thorax and connected to the drainage system. When suction is applied to one of the chambers, air or fluid is pulled into the collection system. Each of the remaining chambers contains a small amount of water, which prevents the loss of negative pressure in the thoracic cavity. Fig. 19.40 illustrates the water-sealed drainage system.

When any drainage system is in use, the collection unit must remain below the level of the insertion tube. This prevents fluids from reentering the drainage space. Chest drainage systems must never be allowed to back up into the thorax, because this can cause immediate collapse of a lung. The drainage system must be kept upright at all times.

STOMA POUCH

A stoma pouch or bag is used to collect body fluids after stoma surgery in which an artificial orifice to the outside of the body is created surgically. The stoma site progresses through a period of remodeling during healing. However, in the first days after surgery, the objective of the pouch is to provide a leak-proof system to collect fluid while maintaining a healthy wound around the stoma opening.

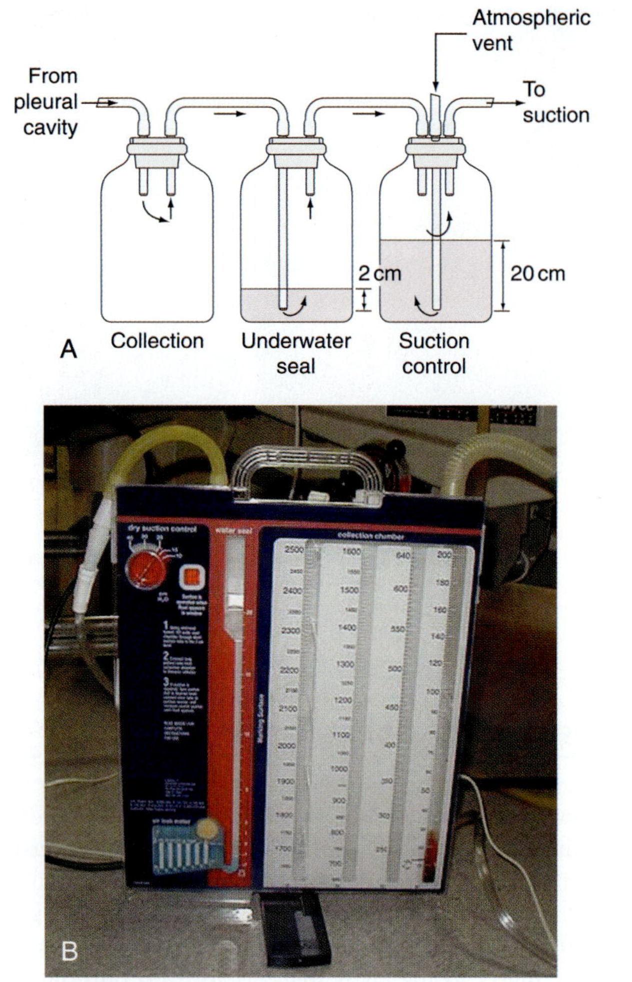

FIG. 19.40 Underwater sealed chest drainage. (A) Schematic of sealed chest drainage system. The first bottle is connected to the drain and tubing and is the collection chamber. The second bottle functions as a one-way valve and forms the underwater seal. The third chamber is connected to suction. (B) Commercial sealed chest drainage system. (A, From Bersten AD, Handy JM. *Oh's Intensive Care Manual*. Oxford, United Kingdom: Elsevier; 2019. B, From Jose M Velasco MD, FACS, FCCM, Rana Ballo MD, Keith Hood MS MD, Jennifer Jolley MD, Daniel Rinewalt MD and Benjamin Veenstra MD *Essential Surgical Procedures*. Elsevier Science Health Science; Oxford, 2016.)

DRESSINGS

Sterile wound dressings are placed over the incision site at the close of surgery. The purpose of the dressing is to:

- Prevent environmental contamination and injury to the wound
- Provide an ideal environment for wound healing
- Absorb exudate from the wound
- Provide mechanical support of the operative site

Most dressings applied at the close of surgery are fairly simple, unless mechanical support is required such as after orthopedic surgery. Fig. 19.41 shows common types of dressings. Ointment is not usually applied on a surgical wound. However, the primary layer of the dressing may be impregnated with sterile ointment alone or combined with a bacteriostatic agent to prevent the other layers from sticking to the wound. A common dressing impregnated with an antibacterial agent is *Xeroform gauze*.

FLAT DRESSING

The flat dressing is composed of a Telfa pad or single-layer mesh impregnated with petroleum-based products or bacteriostatic agent. These are covered with two or three gauze squares (not surgical sponges) and secured with tape. If additional padding is required, gauze fluffs can be used. A *fluff* is packaged as a flat-folded pad. Before applying them to the wound, the layers of the pad are teased out to add bulk and absorbency. Absorbent dressings are layered over the primary dressing and designed to isolate wound exudate. The abdominal *(ABD)* pad is a large absorbent dressing used on draining wounds.

ROLLED DRESSING

Rolled dressing materials are used for wrapping a limb or the head. They may be plain gauze or an elasticized material. *Kling* gauze is very pliable and soft and can be molded over a limb to provide uniform coverage. Elastic roller bandage is used when compression is needed. *Elastoplast* roller bandage is a highly adherent dressing that provides compression and mild support to the wound. *Coban* dressing is protective, elastic, and self-adherent. It is commonly used as an outside dressing layer for a limb. *Tube stockinet* is a woven sleeve that fits over the limb to protect a gauze bandage or provide protection under a plaster cast.

PACKING

Gauze packing is used in a cavity such as the nose or an open wound. It is available in a long, thin strip and packaged in a bottle or similar container. This type of dressing usually is removed early in the recovery period, because it can rapidly become a source of infection.

TAPE

Adhesive tape is needed for most dressings. Tape is used to secure a flat dressing. Paper or "silk" tape is lightweight and has minimal adhesive properties. Plastic tape is pliable and has more adhesive strength. Cloth tape is seldom used for surgical wounds because it is difficult and painful to remove. Commercially available dressings that resemble a large Band-Aid (gauze surrounded by silk or paper adhesive) are also available. This type of dressing may be referred to as an *Owens dressing*. Liquid or spray skin adhesives such as benzoin and Mastisol are used as glue to increase the adherence of tapes and adhesive dressings.

Steri-Strips are used to approximate small incisions and protect the wound. These are used in superficial closures (Fig. 19.42). A small amount of biological adhesive, such as benzoin liquid or spray, may be applied to the skin for extra adhesion before the strips are applied. In some minor wounds, Steri-Strips serve as a dressing.

A simple occlusive film dressing *(OpSite)* prevents most environmental exposure. The film is semipermeable to air but prevents direct contact with the incision site.

Table 19.3 provides a list of dressings used in the immediate postoperative period and during the healing process.

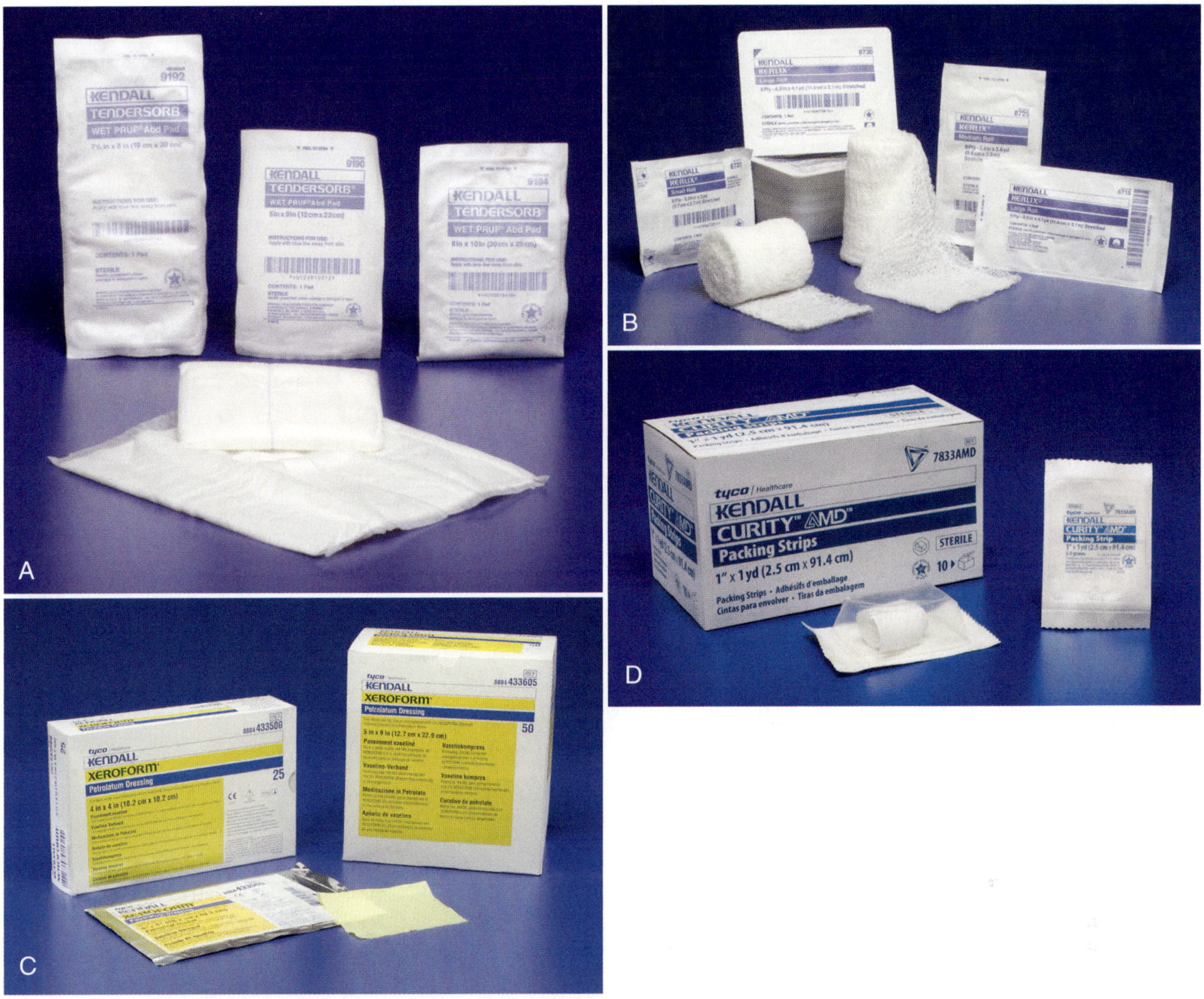

FIG. 19.41 (A) ABD pad used for draining wounds. (B) Rolled dressing material. (C) Dressing with antibacterial agent. (D) Gauze packing strips. (Copyright 2008 Covidien. All rights reserved. Reprinted with permission of Covidien.)

IMPORTANT TO KNOW *Specialty procedures such as those in orthopedics, ophthalmic, and reconstructive surgery requires specific dressing routines. These are discussed in those chapters in Part II of the text.*

WOUND CLOSURE AND THE COMPLETION OF SURGERY

Before closure, all excess instruments are removed from the operative site. Closure materials are placed on the Mayo, along with suture scissors and clean sponges. The ST prepares drains and drain tubing at this time.

FINAL COUNT

The final count begins during the closure of a body cavity such as the peritoneum or thoracic cavity. The ST must prepare for the final count by noting the location of *all the items included in the count.* If the sterile field including the instrument and Mayo tables have been maintained in an orderly way, the final count can be implemented efficiently. The final count is critical because it establishes, with certainty, that nothing has been left behind in the wound. The count must not be rushed; it should be performed with the ST and circulator focused and without distraction. When the count has been completed, the circulator must inform the surgeons that all items have been accounted for. If the count is wrong, the team must immediately implement a search for the missing items.

DRESSINGS

After the final count, the wound dressings are applied. The surgical technologist in the ST role assists the surgeon during the application of dressings at the close of surgery.

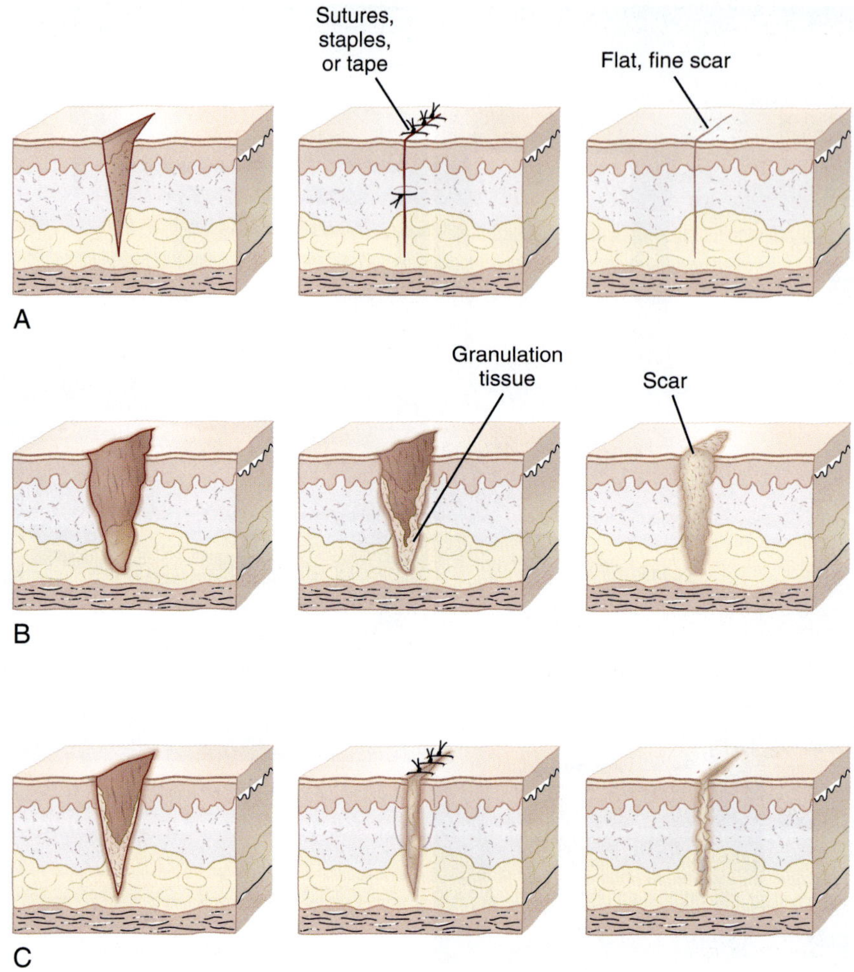

FIG. 19.42 Process of wound healing. (A) Healing by first intention. Wound edges are brought together with sutures, staples, or tape. (B) Healing by second intention. The wound is left open because of infection that would quickly dissolve suture materials and cause further tissue reaction. The wound heals from the bottom up by continuous laying of granulation tissue. (C) Healing by third intention. Infection is no longer present in the previously open wound, which is now closed with sutures.

As the last few sutures or staples have been placed in the skin closure, the ST should remove instruments from the Mayo, except those needed for the last sutures.

IMPORTANT TO KNOW *Dressings are not brought to the Mayo stand until the superficial wound layers have been closed and the final sponge counts have been completed.*

A clean surgical towel should be placed over the Mayo to receive clean dressings. The ST should assemble all needed dressings on the Mayo along with suture scissors and skin forceps. Dressings should be kept as clean as possible.

Before applying the dressings, the surgeon wipes any blood, dried prepping solution, and tissue debris from the incision site. This is done with a clean, wet laparotomy sponge or surgical towel. The incision is then blotted dry. The first layer of the dressing is placed over the incision to protect it while the surgical top drapes are shifted away from the incision site. The remaining dressings are put in place using sterile technique. The dressing is then taped in place.

WITHDRAWAL OF ANESTHESIA

The withdrawal of general anesthesia produces the physiological stages of emergence. The patient regains normal reflexes. The patient is extubated when normal breathing returns and before leaving the operating room.

IMPORTANT TO KNOW *The surgical technologist must maintain sterility until the patient has been transferred out of the operating room.*

POSTOPERATIVE TEAM DEBRIEFING

Many health care facilities now implement a postoperative debriefing as a safety measure and to improve team communication. The debriefing takes place before the patient leaves the operating room. The topics of the debriefing can be tailor-made by each organization. However, certain elements should be included. These are shown in Box 19.4. The postoperative

TABLE 19.3 Dressings and Specialty Wound Care Products

Name	Other Names	Type	Description	Uses
SURGICAL DRESSINGS				
Sterile gauze square	Gauze sponge Flat dressing Gauze dressing "Flat" "Topper"	Flat surgical dressing	Lightweight gauze folded into squares; sterile	For an uncomplicated surgical incision with no drainage. Used in combination with nonadherent layer and surgical tape.
Telfa pad	Telfa	Nonadherent flat fabric pad	Square of compact, felted material with an outer covering of Telfa; used for its nonstick properties	Clean surgical wound. Also used in surgery for care of specimens.
Clear Telfa	Clear Telfa	Nonadherent flat wound covering	Single-layer clear Telfa	Used to cover delicate incisions when a nonadherent surface is required (e.g., burns, skin grafts).
Gauze fluff	Fluffs "Bulky dressing" Kerlix fluff	Diamond weave, flat wound dressing folded many times	Diamond weave, crimped, soft gauze square of synthetic material folded into squares; can be unfolded and "fluffed" to increase loft	Used to provide soft padding and drainage in simple draining wounds or in delicate surgical repair (e.g., hand surgery).
Transparent film dressing	Film; also, various brand names	Film dressing	Single-layer clear adhesive square	Used primarily for intravenous (IV) sites; also used for donor skin graft sites, ulcers.
Cotton sponge	Dermacea Cotton prep sponge	100% cotton flat sponge	Flat gauze sponge with wide "crimped" diamond weave; 100% cotton for lint-free use	For lint-free prepping and wound packing.
ABD pad	Combined dressing "Bulky dressing" ABD	Nonwoven, padded dressing	Oversize square pad; nonwoven material is contained in a lightweight, smooth outer covering that may be water repellent	Used for draining wounds when absorption is required.
Vaseline gauze	Petrolatum gauze	Impregnated nonadherent gauze	Gauze strip impregnated with Vaseline or similar petrolatum substance	Used to cover delicate incisions where tearing of tissue would disrupt repair (e.g., hand, face, minor burns, skin graft, circumcision).
Xeroform gauze	Xeroform dressing	Impregnated nonadherent gauze	Gauze strip or square impregnated with 3% bismuth tribromophenate	Used as for other nonadherent dressings; has bacteriostatic properties*; promotes moisture.
Webril	Webril Rolled cast padding	Rolled bandage; nonsterile	Soft, felted 100% cotton	Used under pneumatic tourniquet and casts for padding and protection.
Roll gauze	Rolled gauze Roller gauze Bandage Rolled bandage	Sterile rolled gauze bandage	Gauze bandage roll, small to medium-size weave made of synthetic or 100% cotton; molds easily to shape	Used to overwrap surgical wound on a limb. Also used in conjunction with flat dressings and other padded dressings.

Continued

TABLE 19.3 Dressings and Specialty Wound Care Products—cont'd

Name	Other Names	Type	Description	Uses
Kerlix rolled gauze; soft roll	Kerlix Kerlix roll Kerlix roller gauze	Sterile rolled gauze bandage	Crimped, rolled gauze bandage with a wide diamond weave	As for *roll gauze*. Diamond weave permits ease of conforming around limb.
Gauze packing	Adaptic Packing strips Gauze packing	Gauze packing material	Narrow, fine-weave gauze in a continuous strip; may be impregnated with a bacteriostatic agent* or petrolatum	Used for packing sinus structures, fistula tracts, or wounds healing by third intention. Single long strip allows for incremental placement in the wound.
Tube gauze	N/A	Tubular gauze	Tube gauze is packaged on a continuous roll or as individual dressings. The weave is somewhat elastic.	Tubes are used to fit over a limb to secure dressing.
Compression bandage	Stretch bandage Ace wrap Elastic bandage Coban self-sticking	Nonsterile rolled compression bandage	Elasticized roller bandage can be supplied as lightweight stretch gauze or heavier stretch cloth; secured with clips or tape or may be self-adhering	Used as a pressure dressing for limbs. Used over a gauze dressing or other type of dressing in direct contact with surgical wound.
Montgomery strap	N/A	Abdominal dressing	Large adhesive straps cover the gauze dressing and can be pulled aside to allow for dressing changes. The straps are simply tied over the gauze pads.	Used for wounds that need frequent or long-term dressing changes.
SPECIALTY WOUND CARE				
Hydrocolloid	Hydrocolloid; also known by brand names	Hydrocolloid occlusive gel dressing	Contains gel-forming agents in a foam or film; self-adhesive and occlusive; adheres to wet or dry wound	Used in clean, granulating wounds with little drainage. Promotes healing by providing moisture and barrier to bacterial invasion. Also, absorbs moisture. May be used in conjunction with sterile maggot therapy.
Intersorb mesh	Intersorb	Wide mesh burn dressing	Layered, wide-mesh gauze made of 100% cotton for lint-free surface	Used as a specialty dressing for burns.
Hydrogel gauze	Hydrogen dressing	Hydrogel-impregnated dressing	Gauze square or strips impregnated with Hydrogel	Hydrogel provides moisture in the wound and supports natural lysis and absorption of necrotic tissue. Can be conformed to fit the wound.
Moist gauze	Sodium chloride dressing Wet-to-dry dressing Wet dressing	Wet-to-dry dressing	Saline-moistened, loosely woven gauze squares	Used to pack the wound and mechanically debride tissue. When gauze packing has dried, it is removed, pulling away necrotic or devitalized tissue.
Foam dressing	Foam	Padded, nonadherent dressing	Soft foam material covered with smooth, nonadherent coating	Used to cushion and protect chronic wounds and absorb exudate. Commonly used for pressure sores.

TABLE 19.3 Dressings and Specialty Wound Care Products—cont'd

Name	Other Names	Type	Description	Uses
Alginates	Alginate dressing	Protective gel dressing	Gel dressing made from seaweed that is highly absorbent and biodegradable; rinses easily with saline solution	Used in deep wounds, fistulas, venous and diabetic ulcers, burns, and pressure ulcers. Provides moisture and enhances epithelialization.
Negative Pressure Wound Therapy (NPWT)	Wound VAC	A closed system applies negative pressure over the wound	System includes specialty foam and vacuum pressure.	Removes exudate. Provides moist environment. Reduces edema.

*Antibiotic ointments (e.g., "triple antibiotic") are no longer recommended for use on surgical wounds. Bacteriostatic agents are preferred, and these are indicated only in selected cases.

BOX 19.4 Sample Postoperative Team Debriefing

Name of operative procedure:
Completion of sponge, sharp, and instrument counts Yes N/A
Specimens identified and labeled Yes N/A
Equipment problems to be addressed Yes N/A
Discussion of Wound Classification Yes
To all team members:
What are the key concerns for recovery and management of this patient?
Debriefing with all team members:
Opportunity for discussion of
- Team performance
- Key events
- Any permanent changes in the preference card

From AORN Comprehensive Surgical Checklist: https://www.aorn.org/guidelines/clinical-resources/tool-kits/correct-site-surgery-tool-kit/aorn-comprehensive-surgical-checklist.

debriefing provides time that is set aside to verify information that is required for documentation and validation.

PATIENT TRANSFER

When the patient is stable, he or she is prepared for transfer to the PACU or another unit such as the ICU. The anesthesia provider is required to accompany the general anesthesia patient to the recovery area. The registered nurse circulator accompanies the patient and anesthesia care provider whenever physiological monitoring devices remain active or if oxygen is being administered during transport.

NOTE *After the patient has left the operating room, the surgical technologist prepares instruments and supplies for transfer to the decontamination area. The procedures for preparation, transfer, and decontamination are found in Chapter 10 along with the procedure for cleaning the OR between patients and terminal cleaning, which occurs at the end of each workday.*

DOCUMENTATION AND SIGNATURES

The operating team, including the surgical technologist, must sign off on all documentation requiring their signatures *before leaving the room.* This ensures that all signatures have been obtained and provides time for verification of supplies, special procedures, identification of the surgical specimen, and reporting of any drugs and solutions used during the procedure (coordinated with the circulating nurse).

DISPOSITION OF THE SPECIMEN

In cases in which the specimen is transported after surgery, the circulating nurse may communicate with the surgeon about the destination of the specimen and any special notes required for the pathology department. Any specific protocols that are out of the ordinary, such as the patient taking custody of a specimen, are verified.

WOUND HEALING AND COMPLICATIONS

CLASSIFICATION OF SURGICAL WOUNDS

Surgical wounds are classified at the time of surgery, according to the risk of infection as shown in Box 19.5. This classification affects how the wound will be managed in the postoperative phase.

Surgical wounds are further classified according to the type of closure. These are illustrated in Fig. 19.42. A clean, uninfected surgical wound that is sutured together heals by **primary intention.** This means that the cut tissue edges are in direct contact.

A wound that is not sutured must heal by *secondary intention.* This type of wound heals from its base. In this process, granulation tissue forms in the base of the wound and slowly fills the gap. It is much slower, and the resulting scar can be large compared with that resulting from primary intention closure. Sometimes a skin graft is necessary because the wound is too large to heal without risk of contamination and infection. Wounds that are infected or grossly contaminated (e.g., those caused by a traumatic injury) also require secondary intention healing.

Third intention healing, or *delayed closure*, is a process in which an infected or a contaminated wound is treated, and the wound space is packed to prevent serum accumulation and to protect it against environmental exposure. When sufficient granulation tissue has filled the wound, it is sutured.

PROCESS OF WOUND HEALING

The permanent cells of the body do not regenerate or divide when they are injured. Permanent cells make up muscles (including heart muscle) and nerves. Tissues that cannot regenerate or repair themselves are replaced by connective tissue after injury. This connective tissue is commonly called *scar tissue*. Scar tissue has few of the characteristics of the original tissue. It has none of the special functions of the permanent cells, such as nerve transmission or secretion. It simply fills the gap left by the injury. The process of tissue repair involves the growth and modeling of scar tissue.

IMPORTANT TO KNOW *Contaminated wounds caused by severe trauma that require delayed closure require specific materials and management.*

The healing process, which involves the growth of new cells and replacement with connective tissue, is divided into three primary phases: the inflammatory phase, the proliferative phase, and the remodeling phase. Under normal healing conditions, these phases progress naturally from the moment of injury until the wound is healed.

INFLAMMATORY PHASE

The *inflammatory phase* of healing begins as soon as tissue is injured. The natural process of hemostasis described previously begins the healing process. Inflammation, platelet aggregation, and the formation of a scab are followed by the cellular phase.

During inflammation, phagocytes migrate to the wound site and digest excess fibrin, bacteria, and cell fragments, a process that usually takes 3 to 4 days. The phagocytes are replaced by macrophages, which remain in the wound for a much longer period. Macrophages attract fibroblasts and release growth factors, which initiate the proliferation of epithelial cells and the growth of new blood vessels. During this period, tissue debris is continually removed by the macrophages.

PROLIFERATIVE PHASE

The *proliferative phase* begins on about day 4 or 5 and continues for approximately 2 weeks. During this phase, fibroblasts synthesize *collagen* and other cell matrices. These form the ground substance of the new tissue, providing support and strength. This new tissue is called *granulation tissue*. Epithelial cells begin to form at the edges of the wound and migrate to the middle, forming a new wound surface. When sufficient epithelial cells have filled in the wound, the scab sloughs away, leaving the new layer. Wound strength increases steadily, and sutures are removed at the end of this phase.

BOX 19.5 Wound Classification

CLEAN WOUND (1% TO 5% RISK OF POSTOPERATIVE INFECTION)

Example
Total hip replacement, vitrectomy, nerve resection

Characteristics
Uninfected
Clean
No inflammation
Closed primarily (all tissue layers sutured closed)
Respiratory, gastrointestinal, genital, and uninfected urinary tracts were not entered
May contain closed drainage system

CLEAN-CONTAMINATED WOUND (3% TO 7% RISK OF POSTOPERATIVE INFECTION)

Example
Cystoscopy, gastric bypass, and removal of oral lesions

Characteristics
Respiratory, gastrointestinal, genital, or urinary tracts were entered without unusual contamination
No evidence of infection or major break in aseptic technique
Includes surgery of the biliary tract, appendix, vagina, and oropharynx

CONTAMINATED WOUND (10% TO 17% RISK OF POSTOPERATIVE INFECTION)

Example
Removal of perforated appendix, removal of metal fragments related to an explosion

Characteristics
Open, fresh, accidental wound
Major break in aseptic technique occurred during the surgical procedure
Gross spillage from the gastrointestinal tract occurred
Presence of acute, nonpurulent inflammation

DIRTY OR INFECTED WOUND (>27% RISK OF POSTOPERATIVE INFECTION)

Example
Incision and drainage of an abscess

Characteristics
Old traumatic wounds with devitalized tissue
Existing clinical infection
Perforated viscera

REMODELING STAGE

The remodeling stage of wound repair begins after about 3 weeks. During this phase, which lasts 22 days to 1 year, the collagen is continually replaced and absorbed in stress areas. As the wound heals, it contracts slightly. However, large wounds (e.g., those caused by a burn injury on the back, buttocks, or posterior neck) are prone to contracture.

Some wounds, even small ones, produce excess amounts of collagen. The resulting scar is called a keloid.

WOUND COMPLICATIONS

The body's ability to heal depends on many different metabolic and environmental factors. A person in good health should recover from surgery without complications as long as the wound is kept clean and protected from injury. However, diseases or conditions that affect metabolism and flow of blood (and therefore oxygen) to the wound site can cause a delay or breakdown in the healing process.

Complications can occur at any time in the wound-healing process but usually are evident in the first week after surgery. Wound complications can occur at the surface incision or in deep tissue, resulting in delayed healing or breakdown of the wound.

SURGICAL SITE INFECTION

Postoperative (surgical site) infection can occur at any time in the healing process. The first signs of infection are excess inflammation and serous discharge from the wound.

A variety of debriding agents and dressings, in addition to meticulous care of the wound, contribute to treating a surgical site infection. However, if the infection threatens to become systemic, the patient is prescribed antibiotics and may require aggressive wound care. This includes continuous wound irrigation, debridement and holistic care to improve the patient's overall health.

SEROMA AND HEMATOMA

A *seroma* is a collection of serous fluid that develops in the wound during healing. This is caused by tissue trauma incurred during the surgery or bleeding inside the wound for another reason. The seroma acts as a physical barrier between the wound's edges and prevents healing. A **hematoma** is a collection of blood that forms in a surgical wound because of incomplete hemostasis during surgery or persistent capillary bleeding. In addition to the dangers arising from an unsecured blood vessel, a hematoma increases the risk of wound infection. With seromas and hematomas, surgery may be required to resolve the problem.

DEHISCENCE

Tissue breakdown at the wound margins that causes the wound to open up is called **dehiscence.** Inflammation is evident, and some serous fluid or pus may be present. Dehiscence can occur at the skin margins or may extend to deeper tissue layers.

Wound breakdown can lead to abdominal wall defects that require surgery. Scars formed after wound breakdown have little strength compared with healthy tissue, and the anatomical planes are disrupted. This can lead to a hernia or rupture in the body wall.

EVISCERATION

Evisceration is dehiscence with protrusion of the abdominal contents outside the wound. Although rare, evisceration requires immediate action to replace and hydrate the extruded tissues and prevent necrosis. Abdominal evisceration can involve a portion of the bowel or omentum. If the dehiscence is small, the viscera may slide through the defect or become trapped by it, resulting in necrosis.

ADHESIONS

An **adhesion** is a band of scar tissue between the abdominal or pelvic organs and the peritoneum. Adhesions usually are associated with infection or multiple abdominal surgeries. Adhesions can cause pain and discomfort. They also increase the risk of injury to organs during surgery.

KEY CONCEPTS

- An uncomplicated surgical outcome is influenced by management of the wound during surgery. This includes maintaining the sterile field, gentle handling of tissues, keeping tissues irrigated, appropriate use of instruments and sutures, and maintaining hemostasis.
- Tissue viability is promoted by good technique, whereas poor surgical technique results in tissue bruising and edema, avoidable hemorrhage, and increased risk of infection.
- The surgical technologist participates and assists in many roles associated with wound management. Some tasks require direct assistance such as retracting tissue, sponging, and irrigation, whereas others need indirect assistance such as preparing sutures, assembling surgical devices, and maintaining the sterile field.
- Tissue retraction is necessary to provide exposure to anatomical structures within the wound. The surgical technologist is often required to retract delicate tissues or organs that can be easily injured though poor technique. Important points of technique are applying the correct amount of tension on tissue without causing injury and maintaining consistent traction on tissue to prevent slippage of the retractor.
- The Halstead principles of surgery were developed more than 100 years ago by the famous surgeon William Halstead. These principles revolutionized the way surgery was conducted, and his teachings on surgical wound management are still considered to be essential in surgical practice.
- The principles and practice of wound management are based on the care and handling of tissues in a way that minimizes tissue damage, promotes healing, and prevents postoperative wound complications.
- Hemostasis is an essential element of wound management. Techniques used to control bleeding in the surgical wound include the use of the electrosurgery unit to coagulate bleeders, biochemical and mechanical hemostats, clamping (occluding) a blood vessel, and

tissue ligation with sutures. Blood replacement or fluid resuscitation is required when the techniques of hemostasis are inadequate to maintain the level of circulating blood.

- Surgical sponges are used for absorbing fluids in the surgical wound, for dissecting tissue, for cushioning tissue during retraction, and for packing—applying pressure to bleeding tissue. Surgical sponges are available in specific sizes and configurations. Specific techniques are used to prevent the loss of a sponge in the surgical wound.
- Learning the many types of suture materials and suture-needle combinations is a gradual process that evolves as new materials are developed. The selection of a specific type and size of suture to be used in a surgical procedure is the surgeon's responsibility. The technologist's role is to deliver the required suture at the required time during the procedure.
- A universal system is used to indicate a suture's size, regardless of the type of material or configuration. The system relates to the diameter of the suture strand.
- Specific suture types and sizes are associated with the strength and type of tissue in which they will be used, the suturing technique, and the classification of the wound. Surgeons generally know what kind of suture they will require before surgery. This information will be listed along with the tissue type and layer associated with it. The surgical technologist is responsible for recognizing the tissue type and layer and then providing the correct suture at the correct time in the procedure.
- Surgical needles are identified by thickness and shape of the shaft, degree of curvature, and type of point. Many combinations of these elements are possible. The surgical technologist is generally required to prepare specific needle and suture combinations as indicated on the surgeon's preference card and make them available at the appropriate time.
- Suture is packaged in a way that facilitates rapid delivery in a tangle-proof system. The system varies by manufacturer and according to the type of suture.
- The use of a specific suturing technique depends on the type of tissue, strength of the closure required, condition of the patient, and wound classification.
- Sharps injuries increase the risk of blood-borne infection in health care workers. Specific techniques are used to prevent injury during surgery. These include confining sharps to a magnetic sharps pad or other sharps device, passing sutures on a "one given–one received basis," and disposing of sharps in a designated container after surgery.
- Surgical specimens are tissue or objects removed from the patient's body as part of the surgical procedure.
- A wound drainage system draws fluid from within the surgical wound in the postoperative phase. This is done mechanically using a suction device or passively by gravity drainage.
- Accumulated fluid in the surgical wound retards healing because it prevents contact between tissue edges during healing.
- A water-sealed drainage system is used following thoracic surgery to reestablish normal negative pressure in the chest cavity, which allows lung expansion.
- The surgical technologist is responsible for preparation of and assistance in applying wound dressings.
- Dressings protect the incision site, acting as a barrier to environmental contamination. A dressing may also provide external support after orthopedic procedures.
- The surgical technologist has specific duties at the close of surgery once the patient has been transported from the operating room. The primary duties include care of specimens, documentation, and preparing soiled instruments and other equipment for reprocessing. Cleanup and room turnover are performed using Standard Precautions for the confinement of body fluids and tissue.
- The physiological process of healing is influenced by many factors that the surgical technologist should understand as part of wound management.
- Surgical wound complications in the healing period are associated with the patient's general medical condition, age, and surgical technique.

REVIEW QUESTIONS

1. Explain how suture is sized.
2. Name four types of surgical needles.
3. How are sutures regulated in the United States?
4. What is the function of a double-armed suture?
5. What is the purpose of a suture ligature?
6. What are the specific responsibilities of the scrubbed surgical technologist in handling tissue specimens?
7. Discuss the consequences of (a) losing a specimen; (b) misidentifying a specimen.
8. Define *allograft, autograft, xenograft, autologous,* and *allogenic.*
9. List the functions of a dressing.
10. What is the purpose of a surgical drain?
11. Explain negative pressure in the thoracic cavity and how water-sealed drainage is used to restore this after surgery.
12. What is dehiscence? How is it different from evisceration?

CASE STUDIES

CASE 1

You placed a package of surgical gut in a basin to rinse it and make it more pliable. You forgot that the suture was in the basin, and now it is very limp and waterlogged. Is it safe to use?

CASE 2

While you are passing a double-armed suture, the free needle snags on the drapes and breaks. What is the next step?

CASE 3

You have been working on a vascular case for 3 hours. You are completely out of ties. When should you have requested more ties? Now you have three packages of ties in three different sizes. The ties are mixed up on top of the Mayo stand in no particular order. What problems can this cause, and how should you have prevented this problem?

BIBLIOGRAPHY

Leong KBMSL, Hanskamp-Sebregts M, van der Wal RA, et al. Effects of perioperative briefing and debriefing on patient safety: a prospective intervention study. *BMJ Open*. 2017;7:e018367. https://doi.org/10.1136/bmjopen-2017-018367.

Porth C. *Pathophysiology Concepts of Altered Health States*. 9th ed. Philadelphia: Lippincott Williams & Wilkins; 2013.

Shirey C, Perrego K. Standardizing the handling of surgical specimens. *AORN J*. 2015;102:516.e1–516.e10. https://doi.org/10.1016/j.aorn.2015.09.012.

Thibodeau G, Patton K. *Anatomy and Physiology*. 6th ed. St Louis: Saunders; 2007.

Zervakis Brent MA. OR specimen labeling. *AORN J*. 2016;103:164–176. https://doi.org/10.1016/j.aorn.2015.12.018.

20 MINIMALLY INVASIVE SURGERY

KNOWLEDGE AND SKILLS REVIEW

The following skills and knowledge should be reviewed before you start this chapter:

Energy sources in surgery

LEARNING OBJECTIVES

After studying this chapter, the reader will be able to:

1. Describe the preparation of the patient for minimally invasive surgery (MIS)
2. Describe the function of each component of the imaging equipment used in MIS
3. Describe the surgical technique used for insufflation in laparoscopy
4. Describe the trocar-cannula system used in MIS
5. Describe the specific electrosurgical risks of direct and capacitative coupling
6. Describe the structure and function of a flexible endoscope

TERMINOLOGY

Active electrode monitoring (AEM): A method of reducing the risk of patient burns during monopolar electrosurgery. AEM systems stop the electrical current whenever resistance is high anywhere in the circuit.

Arthroscopy: Endoscopic surgery of a joint.

Auxiliary water channel: A channel in the flexible endoscope used to deliver irrigation fluid at the tip.

Biopsy channel: A channel that extends the full length of a flexible endoscope and is used to retrieve biopsy tissue.

Camera control unit (CCU): The main control source for the video camera. The unit captures video signals from the camera head and processes them for display on the image system.

Cannula: In minimally invasive surgery, a cannula is a slender tube inserted through the body wall and used to receive and stabilize telescopic instruments.

Capacitative coupling: In minimally invasive surgery, the unintended transmission of electricity from the active electrode to an adjacent conductive pathway, sometimes resulting in a patient burn.

Control head: The proximal section of a flexible endoscope where the controls are located.

Direct coupling: In minimally invasive surgery, the transmission of electricity directly from one conductive path to another, such as from the electrosurgical tip to a conductive instrument.

Elevator channel: A channel that extends the full length of a flexible endoscope for biopsy forceps or other instruments.

Endocoupler: A device that connects the telescope to the camera.

Gain: In electronics, the intensity of the signal.

Haptic feedback: Tactile feedback, conveyed from tissue to the hand when a surgical instrument is used.

High-definition (HD): A type of video format. The clarity of the image is based on the number of signals (pixels) emitted by the camera. HD format has a 16:9 aspect ratio, which is seven times greater than standard definition.

Imaging system: The combined components of the minimally invasive surgery system, which create the image captured in the focal view of the telescope.

Insertion tube: The long, narrow portion of the flexible endoscope that is inserted into the body.

Instrument channel: A channel that extends the full length of a flexible endoscope and receives instruments during flexible endoscopy.

Insufflation: In minimally invasive surgery, inflation of the abdominal or thoracic cavity with carbon dioxide gas.

Intravasation: The unintended absorption of irrigation fluids into the body.

Light cable: The fiber-optic cable that transmits light from the source to the endoscopic instrument; sometimes called a light guide.

Light source: A device that controls and emits light for endoscopic procedures.

Optical angle: The angle at which light is transmitted at the distal end of a fiber-optic telescope.

TERMINOLOGY (CONT.)

Pixel: The smallest unit of color displayed as a computer image. The entire image is made up of many pixels.

Pneumoperitoneum: Distension of the abdomen with carbon dioxide gas during laparoscopy. This is necessary to visualize the surgical anatomy.

Port: In minimally invasive surgery, an opening in the body created by a sharp trocar or blunt obturator and maintained with a cannula that remains in place to receive MIS instruments during surgery.

Resectoscope: A surgical endoscope that has the capability of morcellation or tissue fragmentation.

Standard definition (SD): A type of video format. The clarity of an image is based on the number of signals (pixels) emitted by the camera. A standard definition format displays 640 × 480 pixels in a rectangular image.

White balance: A procedure for adjusting the light color of the video camera to other components of the system.

This chapter covers the principles and technology used in minimally invasive surgery (MIS) and endoscopic procedures. *MIS* is performed with the use of a lensed telescope and long instruments, which are introduced into the body through very small incisions at the operative site. Images that are captured by the telescope are transmitted to a digital monitor. Surgery is performed from outside the body by manipulating and working the long instruments using the monitor view instead of direct visualization. Box 20.1 lists commonly performed minimally invasive surgical procedures by specialty.

Endoscopy is performed with a flexible, semi-rigid, or rigid endoscope, which is inserted into the body through a *natural orifice* such as the esophagus, colon, or urethra. The lens system, channels for introducing small instruments, and light system are contained in one single tube, which is sometimes referred to as the *insertion tube.*

IMPORTANT TO KNOW *The terms endoscope and telescope may be used interchangeably by health facilities and by instrument manufacturers. Terminology used in this text is drawn from modern medical reference terms used by surgical equipment manufacturers. In this text, the term endoscope refers to a lensed tube with channels built into it for biopsy, irrigation, and suction, all housed together in one tube. It is inserted into a natural body orifice or opening. The term telescope refers to the rigid lensed system inserted through an incision and used to visualize the anatomy and other instruments inserted through one or more additional incisions.*

SECTION I: MINIMALLY INVASIVE SURGERY

TECHNOLOGY AND TECHNIQUES

IMAGING SYSTEM

One of the most important differences between open surgery and MIS is how access to the surgical anatomy is achieved. Open surgery requires a larger incision and is performed directly on the tissues through that incision, without an interface. Minimally invasive surgery (MIS) requires a complex **imaging system** to translate what the lensed instrument sees to a computer monitor. The surgeon operates by viewing the images rather than viewing the anatomy directly. The imaging system must produce a clear view of the anatomy in real time to achieve the surgical goals while supporting safe surgery. The surgical technologist may be responsible for setting up the imaging system and assisting in troubleshooting when there are problems.

The components of the imaging system include the following:

- Surgical telescope (or endoscope)
- Camera head
- Camera control unit (CCU)
- Light source
- Light cable
- Video cables
- Monitor screen
- Image management system

Light Source and Fiber-Optic Cable

The **light source** transmits light to a fiber-optic **light cable**, which carries the light to the telescope (Fig. 20.1). The light source control panel is used to adjust the modes and light intensity. The automatic mode of the light source controls the brightness of the image. However, if more light is required, the **gain** (the signal intensity) is increased rather than the light intensity.

High-resolution video endoscopy requires very intense white light. Xenon or LED lamps are used. Most are similar in design and operation.

The light emitted from the telescope is cool as long as the light cable is attached to the telescope. *Light rays emitted from the end of the cable when it is detached from the telescope are extremely hot.* The lighted end of a cable can ignite drapes, sponges, and other materials, especially in the presence of flammable or ignitable liquids such as alcohol.

IMPORTANT TO KNOW *Always turn the light source to standby mode before disconnecting it from the telescope or light cable. The light source must always be turned to standby when not in use. Never place a disconnected fiber-optic cable that is emitting light on the sterile field.*

The fiber-optic *light cable* (Fig. 20.2) transmits light from the light source to the camera head or telescope. The cable is composed of many thousands of glass or plastic fibers, which are aligned in parallel longitudinal bundles. These fiber-optic

BOX 20.1 Common Minimally Invasive Surgery Procedures by Specialty

GENERAL SURGERY AND GASTROENTEROLOGY
Adrenalectomy
Appendectomy
Esophagectomy
Gallbladder procedures
Gastrectomy
Gastric bypass procedures
Gastric reflux procedures
Hernia repair
Intestinal resection
Lymph node biopsy
Pancreatectomy
Parathyroidectomy
Pyloromyotomy
Splenectomy

GYNECOLOGY
Excision of fibroids
Exploratory laparotomy
Hysterectomy
Ovarian cystectomy
Radical hysterectomy for uterine cancer
Removal of fibroids
Repair of vesicle vaginal fistula
Tubal ligation
Uterine artery embolization for fibroids

ORTHOPEDIC SURGERY
Ablation of bone tumor
Arthroscopy
Carpal tunnel release
Fracture of the pelvis
MIS spine surgery
Periarticular and intra-articular fractures of the extremities
Rotator cuff repair
Shoulder instability repair
Spinal decompression
Spinal fixation
Total hip replacement
Unicompartmental knee replacement
Vertebroplasty

THORACIC SURGERY
Fundoplication for gastroesophageal reflux
Lung procedures
Myotomy for achalasia
Repair of hiatal hernia
Thoracic sympathectomy

CARDIAC PROCEDURES
Atrial septal defect
CABG (off pump)
Coronary artery bypass graft (CABG)
Mitral and tricuspid valve procedures
Patent foramen ovale

OTORHINOLARYNGOLOGY
Removal of nasal and sinus tumors
Sentinel lymph node biopsy for head and neck tumors
Sinus surgery
Transcatheter laser treatment of vascular malformations
Transoral laser resection of peripharyngeal/laryngeal tumors

VASCULAR SURGERY
Ablation of varicose veins
Balloon angioplasty and carotid stenting
Renal and peripheral artery stenting
Repair of abdominal and thoracic aortic aneurysms

UROLOGY
Cystic decortication
Diagnosis and removal of kidney stones
Endoscopic exploration of the urinary tract
Endoscopic tumor biopsy
Nephrectomy
Prostatectomy
Pyeloplasty
Treatment for strictures and tumors of the urinary tract

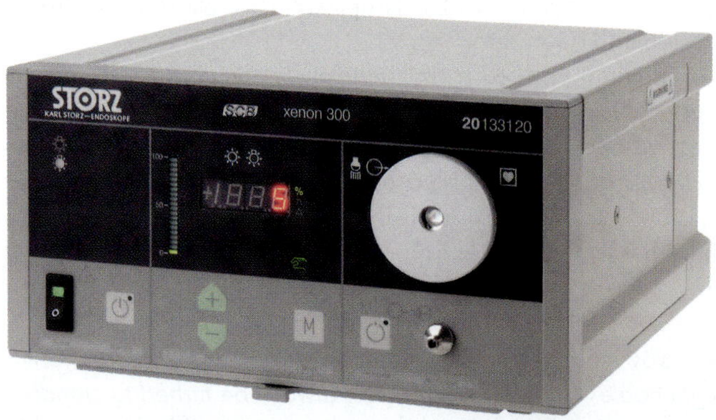

FIG. 20.1 Fiber-optic light source. The light source provides light-emitting diode (LED) or xenon light to the insertion tube or telescope. (Photo courtesy KARL STORZ Endoscopy-America, Inc.)

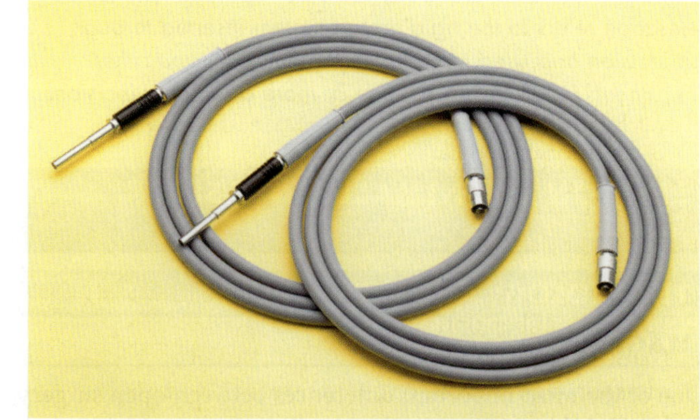

FIG. 20.2 Fiber-optic cable connecting the light source to the endoscope. (Photo courtesy KARL STORZ Endoscopy-America, Inc.)

bundles are delicate and easily broken by sharp impact or over flexing the cable. The fiber-optic cable is securely attached to the light source on the control panel. Because cables of one manufacturer or model are often used with a different model light source, an adaptor may be needed at the connecting point. Adaptors must be available and in place before surgery.

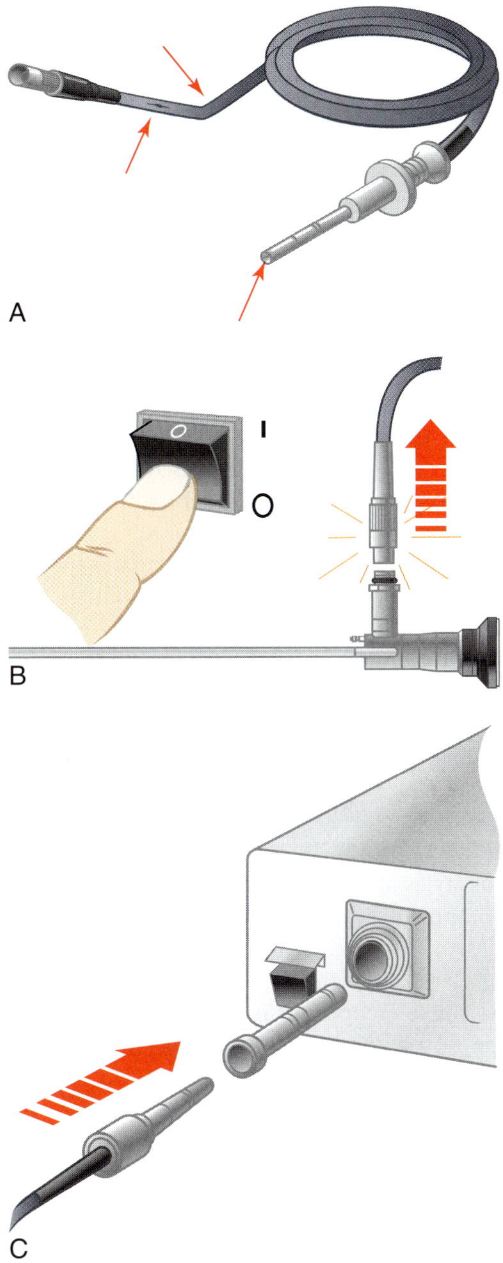

FIG. 20.3 Care of the fiber-optic cable and light source. (A) Fiber-optic light cable: Do not use a cable that is damaged. Look for cuts, nicks, and indentations in the insulation. Make sure the appropriate adaptor tip is used. (B) Power off the light source. Make sure the power switch is off before connecting or disconnecting the light cable. (C) Cable adaptor and plug. Make sure the proper adaptor is used when attaching the cable plug to the power source. (Courtesy Olympus America, Center Valley, PA.)

The care of fiber-optic cables is illustrated in Fig. 20.3.

- Handle fiber-optic cables gently. When storing or transporting the cable, coil it loosely. Do not hang the cable; instead, store it in a flat position.
- Do not allow the cable to strike a hard surface. This can fracture the fiber-optic bundles. Internal fractures are not visible from the outside but produce a distorted image on the monitor.
- Inspect cables for exterior damage before use.

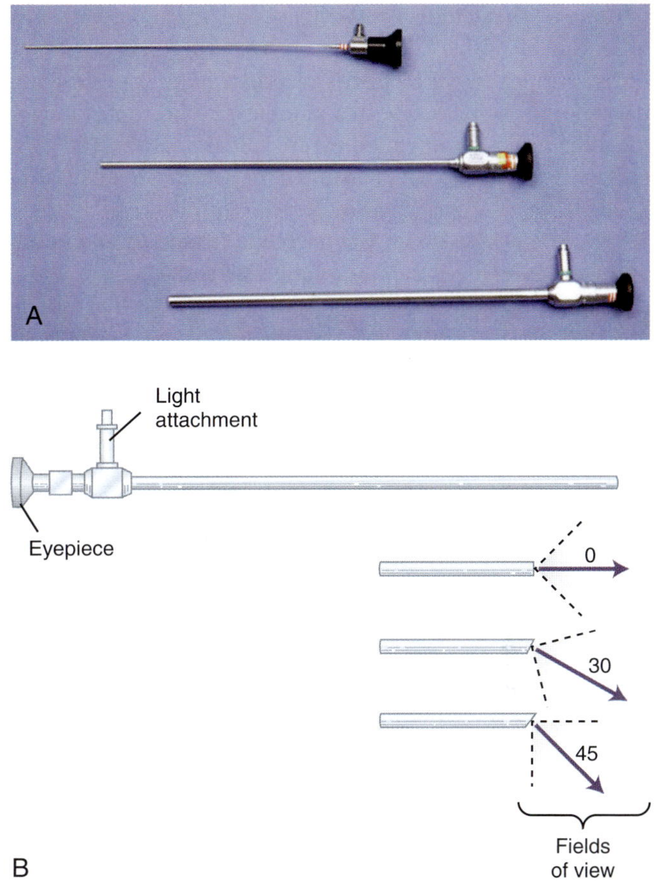

FIG. 20.4 Telescope used in MIS procedures. (A) Telescope diameter: 2 mm, 5 mm, and 10 mm. (B) Lens angles are available at 0 degrees, 30 degrees, and 45 degrees. (*A*, From Goldberg JM, Falcone T, editors. *Atlas of Endoscopic Techniques in Gynecology*. Philadelphia: WB Saunders; 2001. B, Redrawn from Phillips N, editor. *Berry and Kohn's Operating Room Technique. 13th* ed. St Louis: Elsevier; 2017.)

- Power off the light source before connecting or disconnecting the cable. This prevents inadvertent contact between the beam and ignitable materials.
- Do not handle light source bulbs with bare skin. Skin oils can reduce the life span of the bulb.
- Attach the light cable with care. The cable may require an adaptor to fit the light source.
- Keep bulb replacements for the power source immediately at hand during surgery.
- Clean and reprocess the cable according to the manufacturer's instructions for use (IFU).

Rigid Telescope

The telescope contains the serial lens system, which captures the images illuminated at the tip. Light is transmitted to the telescope through the fiber-optic cable, which attaches near the *eyepiece* (Fig. 20.4).

The optical features and dimensions of the telescopes are the following:

- **Optical angle:** This is the direction in which lenses are focused on the image, measured in degrees, usually 0, 30, 45, and 70 degrees
- *Diameter:* The diameter of the telescope shaft, measured in millimeters

- *Length:* The length of the telescope shaft, measured in centimeters

The surgical technologist is responsible for handling and maintaining the telescope in a manner that prevents damage. The following recommendations are guidelines only. The manufacturer's IFU should be consulted for specific detailed care.

1. *Always hold the telescope by its head (heavier) end, never by the tip or shaft.* When the telescope is held by the lighter end, the weight of the headpiece can bend the shaft.
2. *Take care to prevent scratches or dents in the shaft of the telescope.* Contact with heavy instruments or sharps can easily damage the delicate optical system and insulation.
3. *Use only lint-free, soft material to wipe the telescope.* Some woven materials can cause minute scratches on the lens and surface of the instrument. These can lead to blurring and distortion of the transmitted image. Do not allow oils to come into contact with the lens surface.
4. *Never assume that the telescope has been checked by others for damage.* Everyone who handles MIS equipment, from reprocessing to end-user stage, has an equal responsibility to ensure the integrity of the instruments.
5. *Prevent lens fogging during surgery.* When the telescope is introduced into the body, the temperature difference can fog the lens. To prevent fogging, the telescope may be maintained in a warm water bath on the back table before use. Defogging agents may also be used on the lens before use. Be sure to dry the lens before handing it to the surgeon to ensure that there is no distortion resulting from defogging. During surgery, look through the lens to check for a clear view.

Video Camera

The video camera receives visual data from the telescope and allows the surgeon to view structures without looking directly into the telescope. Modern surgical video cameras contain three solid-state silicon chips, which produce electrical signals that are amplified and displayed on the digital monitor. Three-chip cameras produce natural color images, which is important in the identification of pathology. Video chips are located in the camera head, or, in some newer models, they may be located at the tip of the telescope. Each silicon element in the chip represents one **pixel.** The clarity of the image depends on the number of pixels (signals) or silicon units the chip contains. The more units, the clearer the image appears.

The *video format* is the manner in which a video signal transmits information. Individual cameras can use specific formats, and this information is important to the camera's compatibility with other components in the system. Always check the compatibility of the camera with the video system when connecting them.

An important aspect of the video format is the horizontal-to-vertical ratio of the pixels. This contributes to the clarity and resolution of objects transmitted to the monitor. The **standard definition (SD)** format has an aspect ratio of 4:3, which represents 640 × 480 pixels per vertical line. The **high-definition (HD)** format has a 16:9 aspect ratio, which is seven times greater than SD. Modern systems use the HD format.

Camera Head

Numerous styles of camera heads are available, but most have similar components (Fig. 20.5). The telescope mount connects to the telescope through a coupler, lever, or slide control. The *focus ring* clarifies the image. The **endocoupler** connects the camera to the telescope and is specific to the type of camera and scope in use. Options for viewing the surgical anatomy

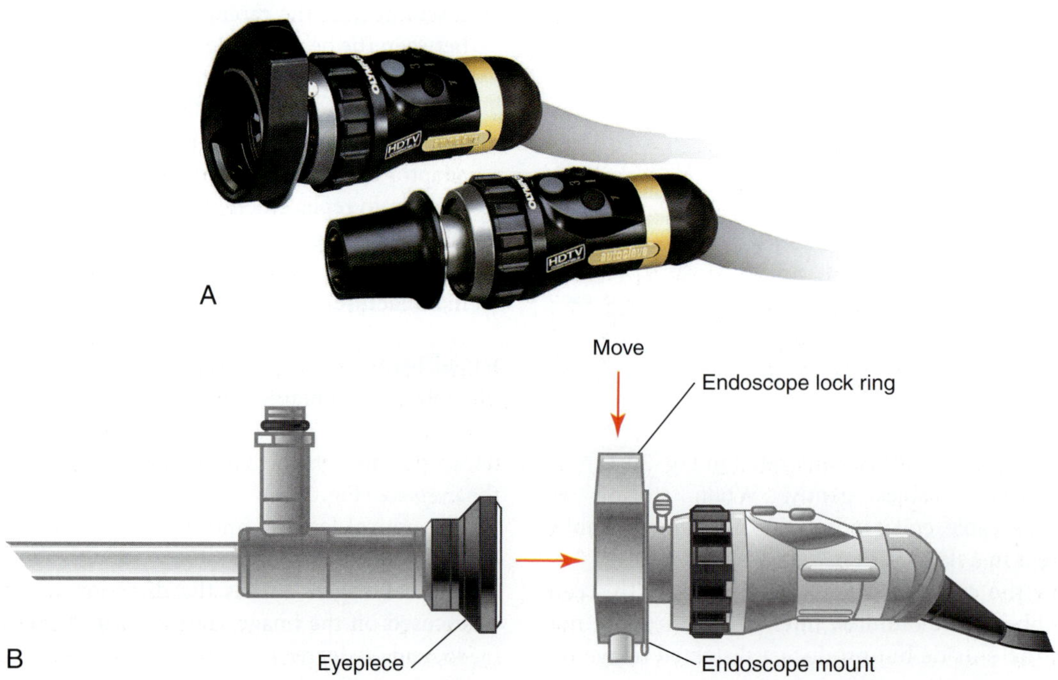

FIG. 20.5 (A) Camera heads that are fitted to the telescope. (B) Camera head with endocoupler. (Courtesy Olympus America, Center Valley, PA.)

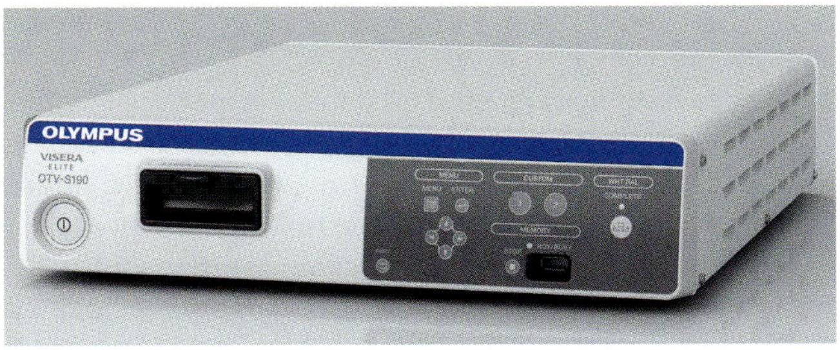

FIG. 20.6 Camera control unit. This unit provides the means of adjusting the quality and appearance of the digital image. (Courtesy Olympus America, Center Valley, PA.)

include the monitor only or a combination of viewing through the telescope with projection to a monitor.

The camera head is delicate and must be handled with care. Always follow the manufacturer's instructions for assembly, reprocessing, and compatibility with other components of the vision system. Following some basic guidelines can help prolong the life of the camera and prevent breakdown during surgery:

1. Hold the camera firmly when transporting it.
2. When connecting and disconnecting the camera head, make sure the lock ring is disengaged. Also make sure the camera is firmly attached to the lock ring after engaging.
3. When connecting the eyepiece, make sure it is firmly engaged. Never try to force or twist these connections. Connect the camera and video plug only when the system is powered off. Do not disengage these plugs with power on.
4. When connecting the camera head to the camera control center, do not bend or twist the camera cable.
5. All connections must be dry before connection.
6. Disconnect the camera cable by grasping the plug, not the cable.
7. After connecting the camera head to the telescope and camera control unit, make sure the light is clearly emitted and is not flickering.
8. Focus adjustment is made before surgery. Make sure the mount is locked during focusing.

Some cameras must be **white-balanced** before each surgery. This is a procedure to adjust the light color to the other components in the system. To white-balance the camera, connect the light cable to the telescope and power up the light on high (or according to the manufacturer's specification). Direct the lens of the telescope 3 to 5 inches away at a solid white object (it is preferable to avoid using porous or woven material, such as a surgical sponge, because this can cause shadows on the image). The white balance usually is recognized and registered automatically by the light source.

Camera Control Unit

The **camera control unit (CCU)** is the receptacle (socket) for the camera. It contains the controls for light intensity, white balance, and resolution (Fig. 20.6). It also receives connections to the power mains and video output remote control. The unit captures video signals from the camera head and processes them for display on the monitor. A computer keyboard may be used for controlling the video display and other functions. The CCU should be able to convert SD to HD signals or vice versa so that images from one format can be viewed by another.

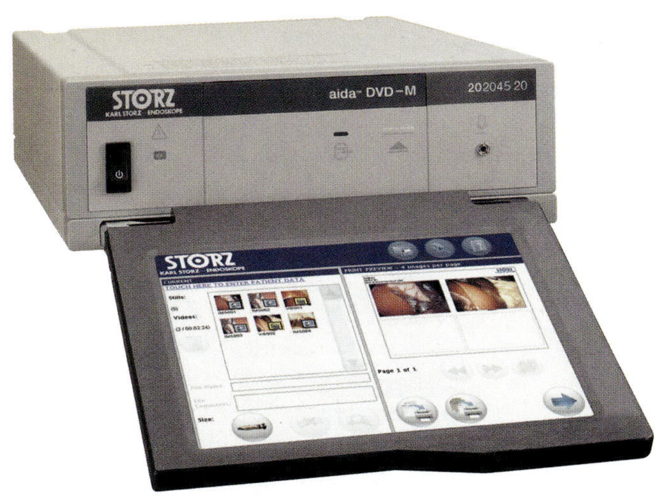

FIG. 20.7 Documentation system for recording and storing images and videos. (Photo courtesy of KARL STORZ Endoscopy-America, Inc.)

Video Cables

The *video cable* transmits digital data from the camera head to the CCU and from the monitor to the documentation system. These high-quality cables use fiber-optic systems, which are necessary for HD signals. Like all fiber-optic cables, the video cable can be easily damaged by rough handling or misuse, and the same care given to light cables should be applied to the video cable.

The video cables are usually patched into the system at the back of the CCU and have dedicated receptacles, which are clearly marked.

Documentation System

During surgery, digital signals captured from the video camera are transmitted to a monitor. The *documentation system* processes these signals (Fig. 20.7). Data can also be transmitted to remote locations, with input from other imaging processes integrated into the camera output.

Monitor

The video monitor shows a projected image of the surgical site in real time. The monitor most commonly used is the flat panel (liquid crystal display [LCD]) monitor. New HD systems are displayed in a widescreen format. Although the image captured by the video is circular, the wide screen covers the entire image by increasing the horizontal field of view and reducing the vertical field. This results in a full-screen image.

The monitor's resolution must be matched to the camera's capabilities to produce the clearest view. The 16:9 ratio monitor is best for displaying HD signals. Because the human eye has a wider horizontal view than vertical, images displayed on the 16:9 monitor are more natural looking and less fatiguing for the eyes.

EQUIPMENT CART

The equipment cart (also called a *tower*) provides shelves for safe storage and transportation of video equipment. Carts contain power strips with dedicated receptacles for video components (Fig. 20.8). Carts allow equipment to be moved safely

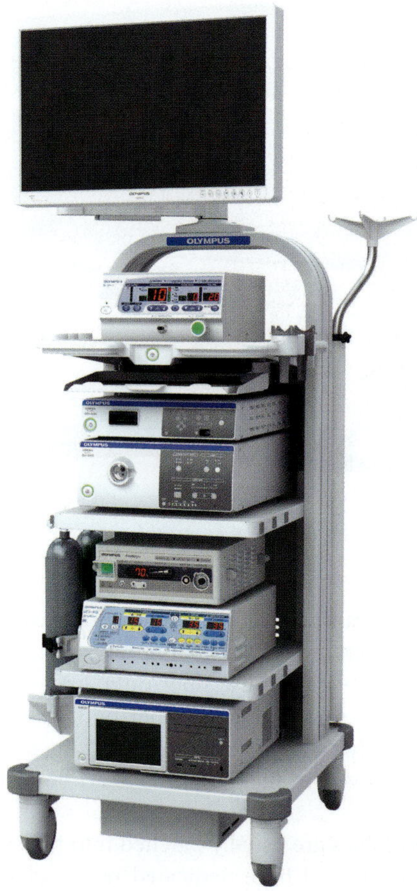

FIG. 20.8 Equipment tower. This system contains space for the digital control units of the MIS system and electric receptacles for the units. In the case of an integrated OR, these units are built into ceiling booms.

and efficiently. An alternative design for equipment is suspension by overhead booms, which are commonly built into integrated operating rooms.

INTEGRATED OPERATING ROOM

The integrated or hybrid operating room provides a method for the delivery and integration of digital technologies to the surgical suite. It provides the most advanced computer and digital technologies, including data management, storage, and transfer required for MIS and robotic procedures. Instead of the equipment cart and individual components, which are portable from room to room, the components are built into overhead booms and controlled by remote control units or voice activation (Fig. 20.9). In addition to these systems, the integrated OR provides an interface for the control of equipment such as the operating table, temperature systems, and lighting. Overhead cameras built into the lighting systems record and transmit surgical procedures for training purposes. Technologies required for diagnostic imaging procedures can be performed through the same systems as those required for MIS. The system allows the video and voice components to be transmitted in real time to locations both in and out of the health care facility. These features bring together specialists for consultation and teaching during the surgical procedures.

TROCAR-CANNULA SYSTEM

A trocar and cannula system is used to create ports or channels through the body wall for the insertion of MIS instruments. This system is commonly used during laparoscopic surgery and thoracic MIS. The trocar is a solid rod with a blunt or sharp end that fits inside a hollow tube **(cannula)** (Fig. 20.10). The trocar and cannula are assembled by the surgical technologist before insertion into the patient. When assembled, the point of the trocar protrudes slightly beyond the end of the cannula. To insert the trocar and cannula, the surgeon makes a small incision in the body wall and advances the trocar and cannula through the tissue. When the trocar is in the correct position, the surgeon withdraws the obturator, leaving the hollow cannula in place. The cannula then receives MIS instruments and is referred to as a **port.**

Trocar-cannula systems can be disposable, reusable, or reposable for a multiple but limited number of uses. Single-use trocars are commonly used, and bladeless obturators are also available (Fig. 20.11). Cannulas and trocars are available in the following sizes:

1. Pediatric: 5 to 8 mm
2. Adult: 5 to 10 mm
3. Large and special-purpose (e.g., specimen retrieval): 10 to 15 mm
4. Microsurgical: 2 mm and 3 mm

It is important that the cannula remain stable in the body wall during surgery. Therefore all cannulas are designed to provide a snug interface and a system for retention in surrounding tissue.

To prevent injury on insertion and provide a seal once they are in place, trocar-cannula systems may have the following features:

- An expanding or dilating tip that provides a seal between the cannula and tissue
- Blunt trocar tips, which do not penetrate tissue but push it aside during entry
- Threaded trocar design to help guide the trocar during insertion
- Perforations or flanges to permit anchor sutures at the proximal end of the cannula
- Fabric or foam interface between the cannula and the body wall
- Optical trocars, which allow the passage of the viewing telescope as the cannula is advanced

Many cannula systems have a reducer ring at the proximal end. This allows a smaller-diameter instrument to be passed through a larger cannula. Variable-diameter seals are also available. A variation on this technique is single-incision laparoscopic surgery (SILS), in which one entry incision is made at the umbilicus to accommodate a single large cannula containing multiple ports.

The number and location of trocar/cannulas needed for a procedure depend on the operative anatomy involved. Abdominal surgery usually requires at least three ports unless SILS surgery is being performed. These are placed according to the type of surgery to be performed. During pelvic surgery the video telescope usually is placed near the midline,

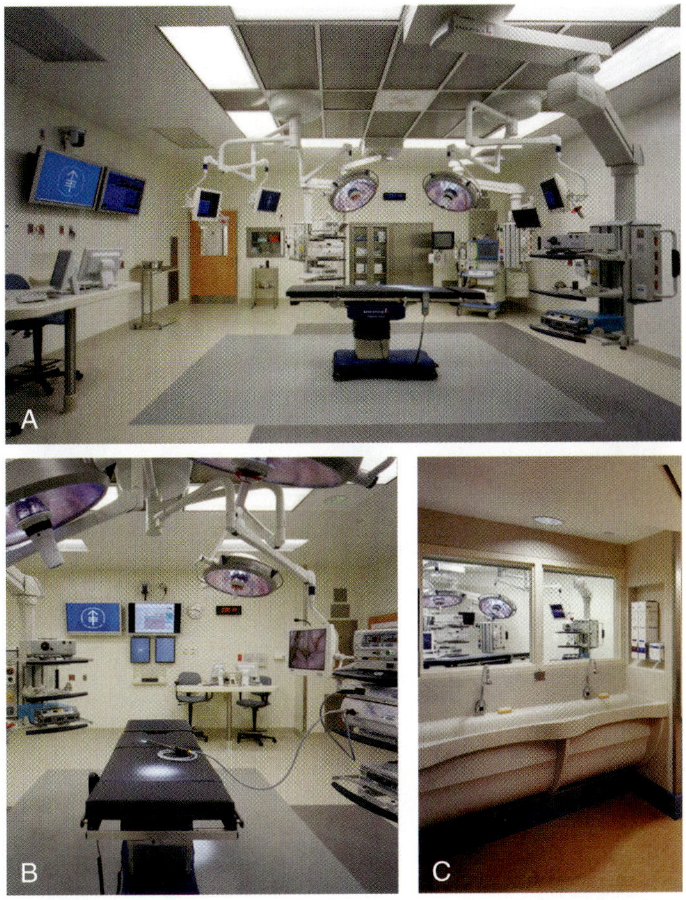

FIG. 20.9 Integrated OR. (From Shah J. *Jatin Shah's Head and Neck Surgery and Oncology*. 4th ed. Philadelphia: Elsevier; 2012.)

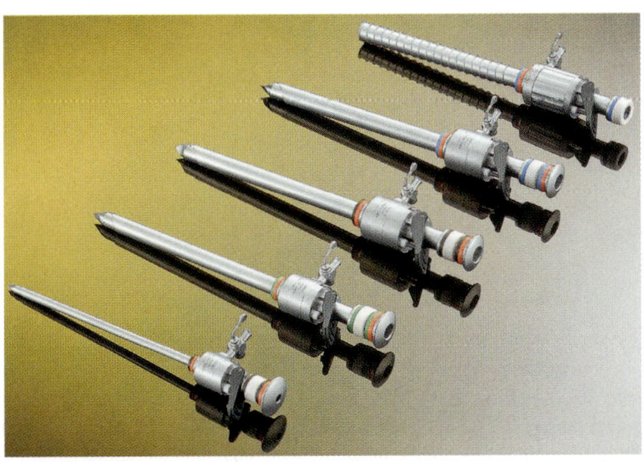

FIG. 20.10 Reusable trocars and cannulas. See text for explanation. (Photo courtesy KARL STORZ Endoscopy-America, Inc.)

approximately 10 inches (25 cm) above the pubic symphysis. This allows for a broad view of the abdominal and pelvic contents. Other trocars are placed at strategic positions at the right or left of the midline. The surgeon may use a ruler to measure the exact locations of the trocar insertion points.

ENHANCING VISUALIZATION DURING MIS

During MIS, the view of the anatomy can be obscured because the tissue planes and spaces are very narrow. A method of expanding the operative space is needed to visualize anatomical structures more distinctly and also provide space for insertion of the trocars. Several techniques are used to accomplish this goal. These are described in the following sections.

Insufflation

Insufflation is a process in which the abdominal and sometimes the thoracic cavities are filled with carbon dioxide (CO_2) gas. This provides a clear view of the anatomy and permits safe entry of the rigid telescope and other instruments during the procedure. CO_2 gas is used because it is nontoxic, readily absorbed by the body, and nonflammable. The CO_2 gas is warmed before insufflation. This maintains the patient's core temperature and prevents lens fogging. To create a **pneumoperitoneum,** the surgeon inflates the abdomen with CO_2 through a large-bore needle called a *Veress needle* or trocar fitted for CO_2 insufflation (Fig. 20.12). The spring is designed to retract the needle when resistance is met at the tip; this alerts the surgeon to possible obstruction during placement. The insufflation control console is adjusted to deliver a steady level of gas through the tubing. Once the abdomen is inflated, the trocars can be inserted. The risks and precautions associated with pneumoperitoneum are listed in Box 20.2.

Continuous Irrigation and Fluid Distention

Continuous irrigation is a technique used in arthroscopic MIS, hysteroscopy, and cystoscopy. Fluid is instilled into a body

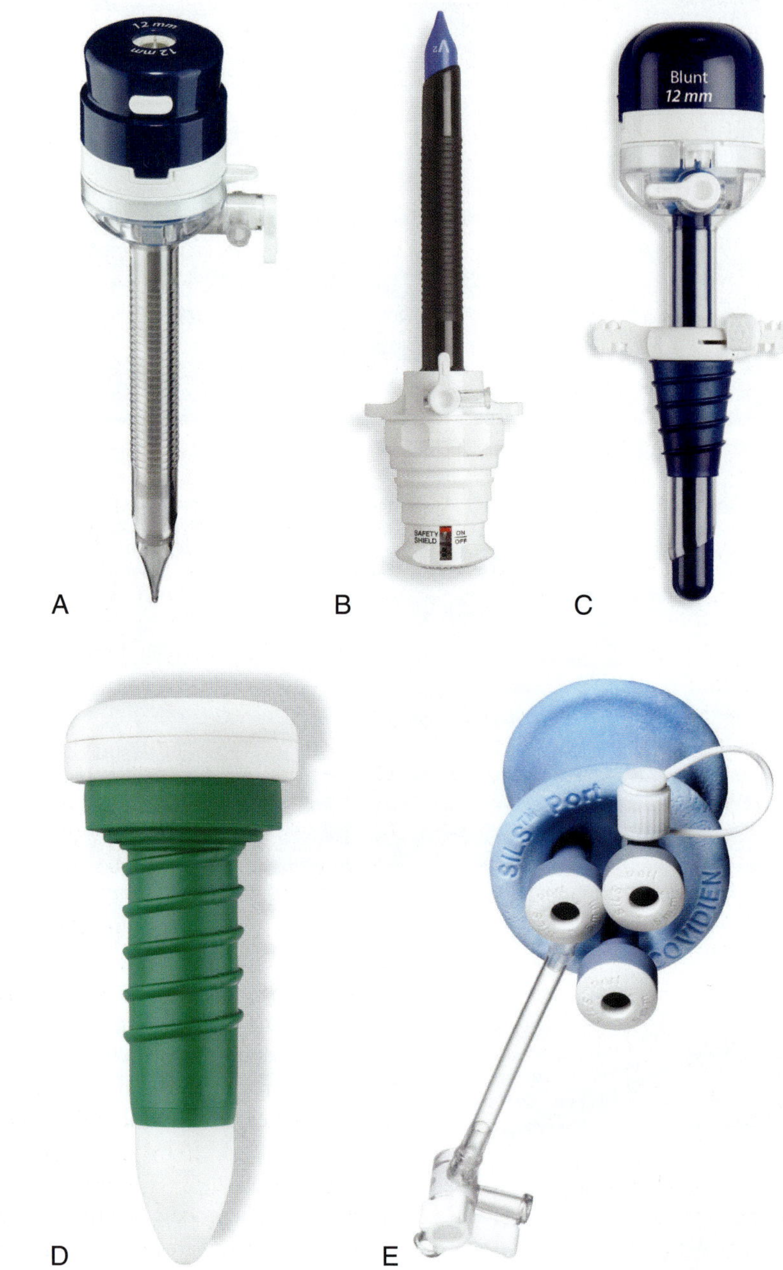

FIG. 20.11 Single-use (disposable) trocars. (A) Bladeless optical trocar allows the surgeon to monitor the entry process as it passes through the tissues using the laparoscope. (B) Bladed trocar with shield. (C) Blunt trocar. (D) Thoracic trocar. (E) Single-incision laparoscopic surgery port. This device can accept up to three trocars through a single incision port. (Courtesy Medtronic. All rights reserved. Used with the permission of Medtronic.)

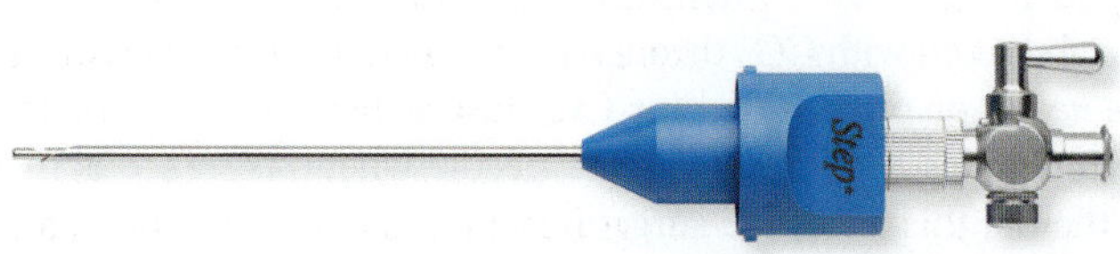

FIG. 20.12 Veress needle. This instrument is used to puncture the abdominal wall. It accepts the insufflation tubing and remains in place until pneumoperitoneum is completed. (Courtesy Medtronic. All rights reserved. Used with the permission of Medtronic.)

cavity or space to expand it and remove small tissue fragments and blood generated during surgery as these can obscure the view through the telescope.

The choice of fluid used for continuous irrigation depends on the electrosurgical instruments used in the procedure. Older electrosurgical systems require nonconductive solutions such as glycine, sorbitol, or mannitol. Some newer systems may be safely used with isotonic saline irrigation. The risk of electrical conduction and fluid balance depend on the solution. The surgical technologist must ensure that the correct solution is used, according to the electrode manufacturer's guideline.

When a body cavity or organ is filled with fluid during surgery, there is a risk that it will be absorbed into the vascular system, causing increasing blood pressure and electrolyte imbalance.

BOX 20.2 Risks and Precautions With Pneumoperitoneum

RISKS

Insufflation presents a number of significant safety risks for the patient:

- Excess pressure can force carbon dioxide (CO_2) into the blood or cause decreased respiration and cardiac output.
- CO_2 can be irritating to nerves and cause severe postoperative pain in the shoulder region.
- Infectious organisms can enter the body from CO_2 tanks.
- Pneumoperitoneum can result in venous system embolism, which can cause death.
- Free gas may obstruct cerebrovascular flow, resulting in cerebrovascular accident.

PREVENTING PATIENT INJURY DURING INSUFFLATION

- Use only medical-grade CO_2 for insufflation (tanks are labeled).
- Replace gas tank cylinders and check levels before the surgical procedure. Extra tanks must be kept on hand during surgery.
- Monitor the insufflator pressure at all times during surgery.
- Position the insufflator above the level of the surgical cavity.
- Always purge tubing of air before insufflation. Air in the tubing can result in a fatal air embolism.
- Replace the gas cylinder before the level is low. This prevents cross-contamination with particles from the tank via the insufflation tubing.
- Before inserting the Veress needle, check the spring action at the proximal end.
- Do not put pressure on the abdominal wall during or after insufflation. Leaning on the patient can create displacement of carbon dioxide and increase intraabdominal pressure.
- Always fit the patient with compression stockings or a sequential compression device before surgery (see the section on preparation of the patient in Chapter 14).

This is called **intravasation.** Fluid is instilled by a pump or by a gravity system (Fig. 20.13). An automated pump is advantageous for controlling and maintaining a specific pressure.

Balloon Dissection

Another method of separating tissue layers is with the balloon dissector. This device is a soft, plastic balloon with a tube and port attached. The tube is inserted into the tissue plane, and the balloon is inflated with air. This pushes the surrounding tissues aside without causing trauma and provides an anatomical space for the telescope and other instruments (Fig. 20.14).

SPECIMEN RETRIEVAL

Tissue specimens are retrieved from the body during MIS using one of several techniques. Large specimens and dense tissue are reduced to small pieces by a process called *morcellation.* The morcellator reduces tissue to pulp, which can be suctioned from the wound.

Large tissue specimens are retrieved through the abdominal wall through a retractable tissue bag inserted into a large

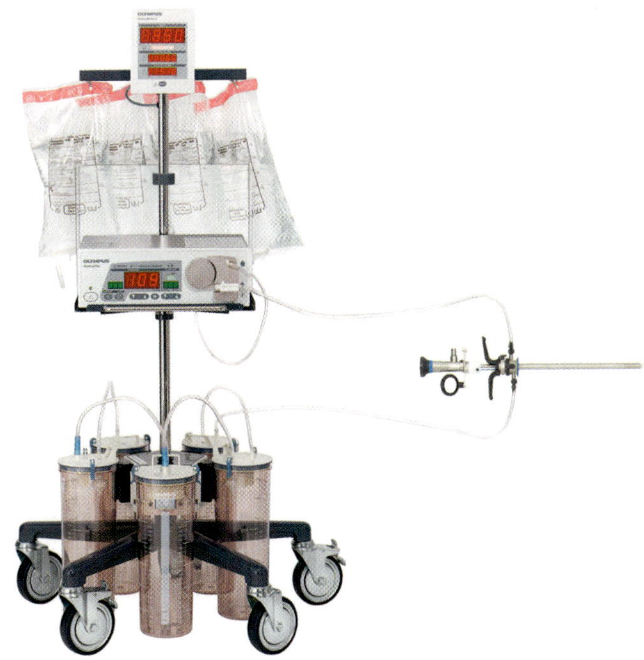

FIG. 20.13 Continuous irrigation system. The system may be controlled by a pump or by gravity. (Courtesy Olympus America, Center Valley, PA.)

cannula port. The surgeon captures the organ into the bag and retracts the open portion to secure the contents. The bag then is withdrawn through the port. For extremely large specimens, an 18-mm port may be required for extraction (Fig. 20.15).

In some procedures, particularly during natural orifice endoscopic procedures, specimens may be delivered through a body orifice, such as the vagina during a hysterectomy.

HEMOSTASIS AND TISSUE APPROXIMATION

The surgical clip appliers and staplers used in open surgery have counterparts in MIS. Disposable delivery systems are the most common. Clips are used in place of suture ligatures to occlude blood vessels or other types of hollow structures, such as the bile ducts. A disposable clip applier can deliver multiple clips in succession without reloading (Fig. 20.16).

Stapling instruments are routinely used in open surgery. They also have counterparts in MIS. Stapling instruments are most commonly used in laparoscopic surgery and video-assisted thoracic surgery (Fig. 20.17).

Suturing in MIS procedures is performed with many different devices and techniques. Electrosurgical and ultrasound modalities have replaced traditional sutures in many procedures. However, needles and sutures remain in use. Various instruments have been designed to tie knots, snug knots, and suture tissue within a confined space (Fig. 20.18). Three types of methods are commonly used: the extracorporeal technique, the intracorporeal technique, and the pre-tied surgical loop. In the extracorporeal suture technique, the knot is tied outside the body cavity and then pushed into place with a knot pusher using the following technique: A swaged suture-needle combination is grasped with a needle holder and passed through the port to the inside of the body. The needle is pushed through

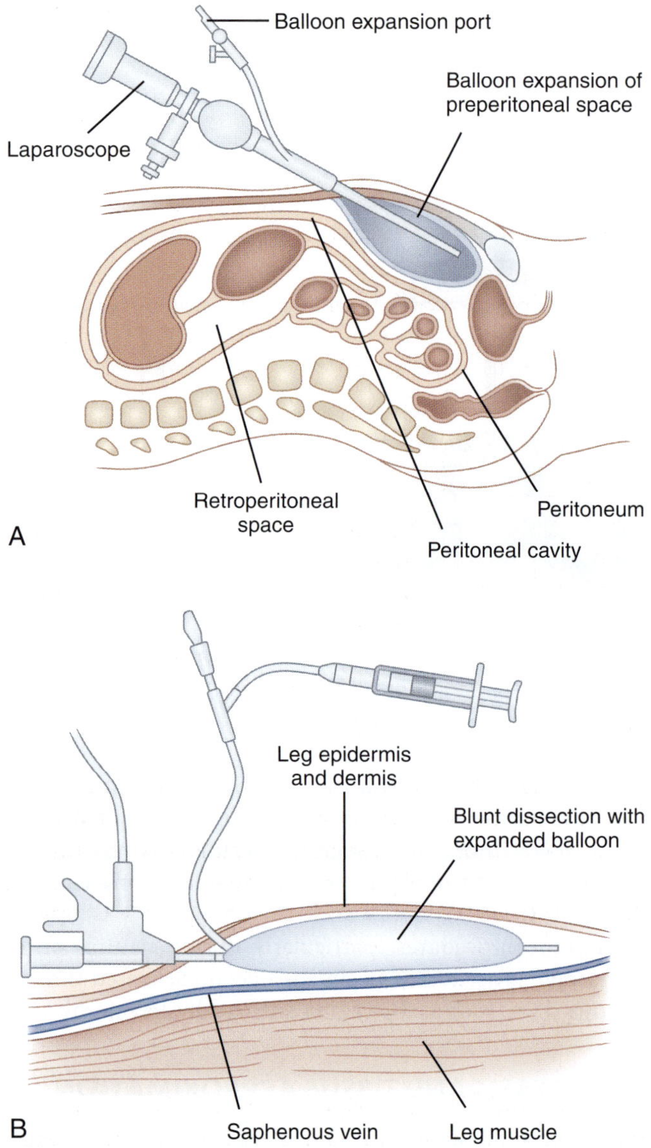

FIG. 20.14 Balloon dissection. (A) Here the balloon dissector has been inserted into the pelvic cavity. The balloon pushes the tissues away from the operative site without causing injury. (B) A dissector is inserted into the tissue space below the superficial tissues to provide increased exposure to the saphenous vein. (Redrawn from Rothrock JC, editor. *Alexander's Care of the Patient in Surgery*. 12th ed. St Louis: Mosby; 2003.)

the tissue with the aid of an additional grasping instrument via a separate cannula. The suture-needle combination is withdrawn, and the needle is removed outside the wound. The knots can then be formed without tightening outside the body and introduced back into the body via the cannula. They are then tightened with the knot pusher.

In the intracorporeal technique, the suture is knotted and tightened inside the body with two grasping instruments inserted into two separate cannula ports.

The suture or pre-tied ligation loop is used when a tissue structure requires ligation rather than suturing. A loop of suture contained in a carrier, similar to a snare, is delivered through the laparoscope and looped around the tissue, such as the appendix. The loop then is tightened, the suture ends cut, and the carrier removed.

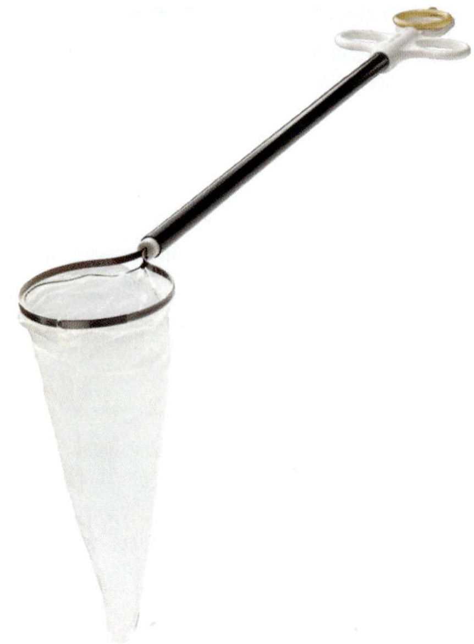

FIG. 20.15 Specimen retrieval. A specimen pouch is used to capture the tissue so that it can be withdrawn from the body through a large-bore cannula. (Courtesy Medtronic. All rights reserved. Used with the permission of Medtronic.)

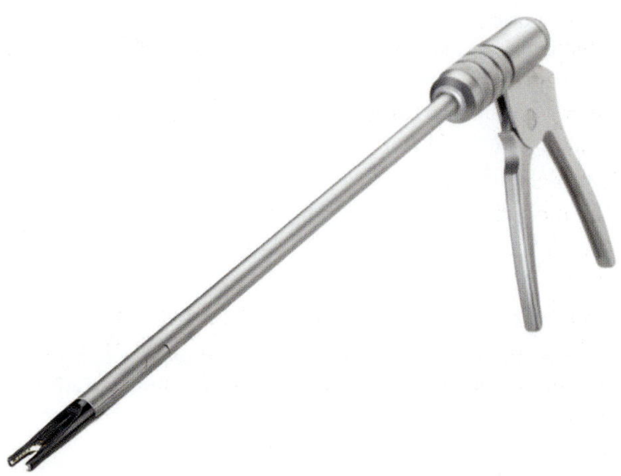

FIG. 20.16 Endoscopic clip applier. Used to ligate blood vessels or small ducts during MIS. (Courtesy Medtronic. All rights reserved. Used with the permission of Medtronic.)

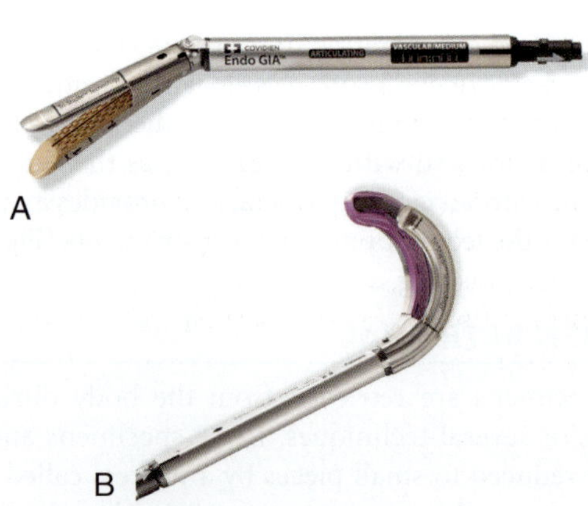

FIG. 20.17 Endoscopic staplers. (A) Linear stapler. (B) Intraluminal circular stapler. (Courtesy Medtronic. All rights reserved. Used with the permission of Medtronic.)

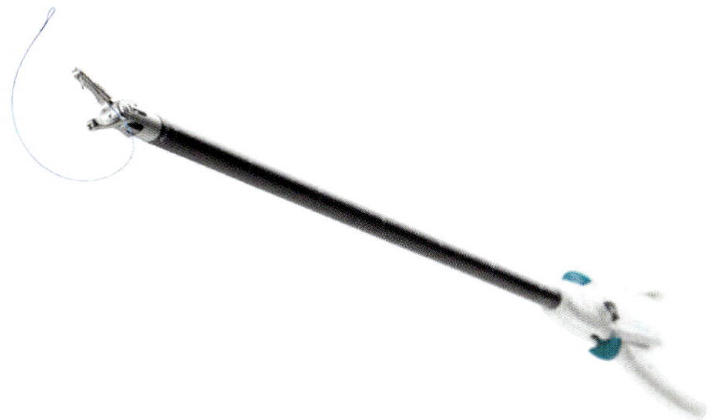

FIG. 20.18 Endo Stitch instrument. (Courtesy of Medtronic. All rights reserved. Used with the permission of Medtronic.)

MIS INSTRUMENTS

MIS instruments are designed to perform a precise surgical task in a confined space. The handles and fulcrums are located at some distance from the working end. Hinges, springs, and valves are very small. A rotational design allows the tip of the instrument to swivel in an arc, increasing the maneuverability of the instruments.

Instruments are supplied in reusable, disposable, and reposable types (only critical components, such as the tips, are disposable). The grip mechanism on MIS instruments is important to the ergonomics and precision of the tool. Lengthy procedures require continuous delicate control. This is enhanced by comfortable handles and good balance between the tips and handles.

The most common handle design is a transaxial type, which has two finger rings at a 90-degree angle to the long axis of the instrument. Because of the short fulcrum and flexibility of the instruments, the amount of applied force is greatly reduced in an MIS instrument. Refer to MIS Instruments (Instrument Table 20.1). Important features of the instruments are the following:

- Retractors use the same principle as open surgery retractors. Because of the limited operating space, retractors extend from the tip of the shaft and flare out or curve at various angles. A probe (rod or hook) is often used to manipulate and retract tissue.
- Scissors are available in straight, curved, and hooked configurations. In open surgery, dissection of tissue planes and cutting frequently are performed with scissors; in MIS procedures, they often are also performed using electrosurgery or ultrasonic shears.
- Grasping (holding) instruments, including clamps and forceps, are commonly used in MIS. Some provide atraumatic grasping, whereas others penetrate the tissue. The working tips of graspers have the same design as those used in open surgery.

CARE OF MIS INSTRUMENTS

The care of telescopes and other MIS instruments requires particular attention to the delicate nature of the instruments and the potential for patient injury. Equipment used in MIS represents a significant cost to the facility. Inferior instruments must never be used, and the chain of care starts before surgery and continues throughout the intra- and postoperative periods.

MIS instruments should be inspected frequently. It is important to examine them during the sterile setup before surgery starts and at the close of surgery. Another inspection should take place before the instruments are assembled for sterilization. Like open surgery instruments, MIS instruments should be examined for mechanical function. Check pins and other mechanical attachments to make sure they are secure. Sight the shanks and shafts of the instrument while rotating it to make sure they are straight. Carefully examine the surfaces of all instruments for defects such as scratches, dents, or nicks. The long shafts of instruments are particularly vulnerable to defects from normal wear. Loss of integrity to the instrument insulation creates a risk for patient burns. Electrosurgical instruments must be checked to make sure there are no breaks in the insulation. Even a small defect may transmit stray current and cause an unintentional burn (Fig. 20.19). A digital insulation tester may be used for this purpose.

Pay particular attention to the lens system, coupling fittings, and shaft. Inspect the distal lens and eyepiece for debris by observing them under indirect light. Look for scratches, chips, and fingerprints.

Look through the eyepiece to check for lens clarity. Rotate the telescope shaft to check all surfaces. If any obstruction appears, the lens may be damaged. Fogging may be caused by moisture trapped between the lens and seal, an indication of leakage. Check for straightness by observing the telescope end to end.

INTRAOPERATIVE INSTRUMENT CARE

During surgery, instruments should be kept as clean as possible. Use a damp sponge to wipe the tips and instrument shafts. Suction tips should be flushed frequently to prevent clogging. Use only sterile water to clean instruments because it is hemolytic and does not erode instruments. As instruments are used, replace them in a specific location on the instrument table or in a specialized instrument rack.

The rigid telescope should be protected by placing it on a lint-free towel or in a warm water bath when not in use. Keep the tip and shaft away from sharp objects and heavy instruments. To prevent the telescope from dropping from the sterile field, make sure cables and tubing are slack. Remember to disconnect cables and tubing when transferring the instruments from the operative field to the instrument table.

After surgery, instruments are processed according to the manufacturer's guidelines and hospital policy. All instruments should ideally pass through a cleaning process within 30 minutes after the procedure followed by and terminal decontamination and sterilization.

SPECIALTY TELESCOPES

Specialty telescopes are designed to fit the anatomical and technical needs of surgical specialties, such as abdominal, orthopedic, thoracic, and gynecological surgery. Design features

TABLE 20.1 MIS Instruments

BIPOLAR FORCEPS	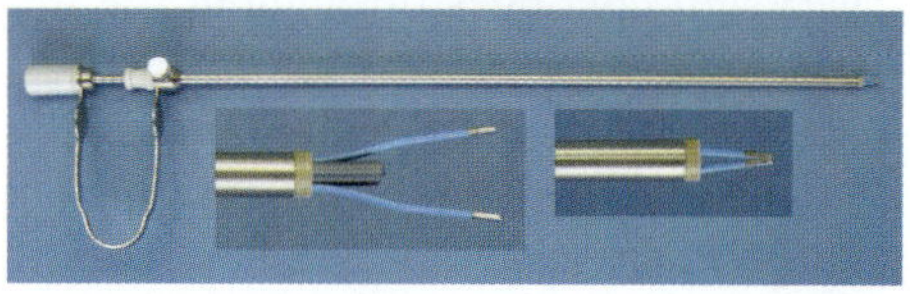 Courtesy Jarit Instruments, Hawthorne, NY.
MARYLAND FORCEPS	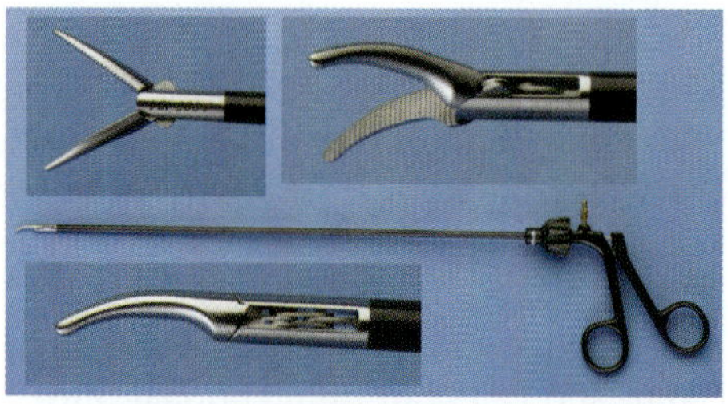 Courtesy Jarit Instruments, Hawthorne, NY.
MIXTER FORCEPS	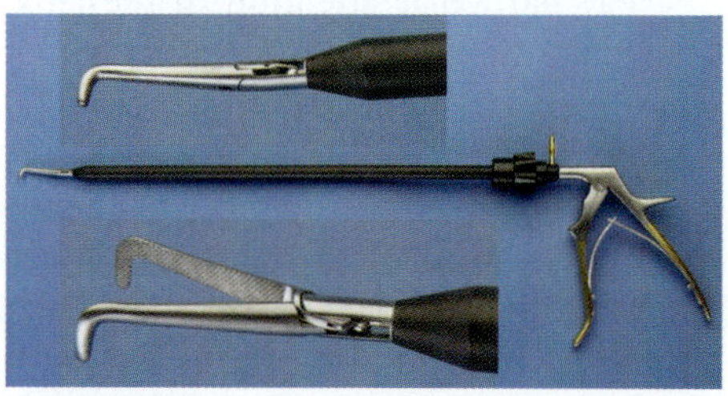 Courtesy Jarit Instruments, Hawthorne, NY.
SUPERCUT SCISSORS	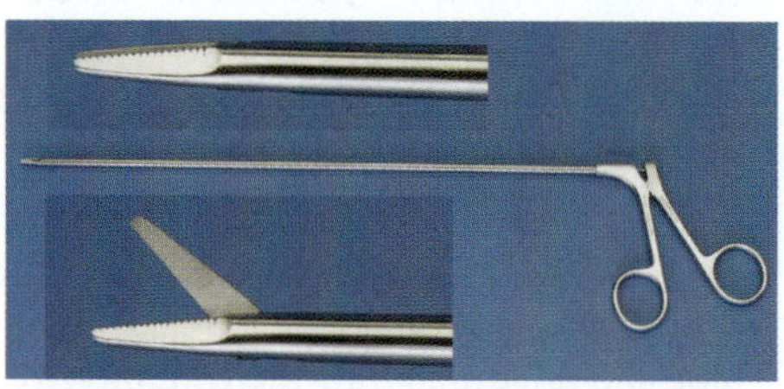 Courtesy Jarit Instruments, Hawthorne, NY.
MICROBIOPSY FORCEPS	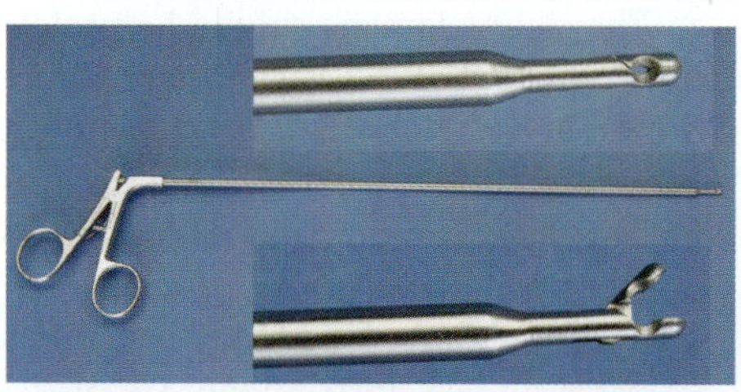 Courtesy Jarit Instruments, Hawthorne, NY.
MARYLAND DISSECTING FORCEPS	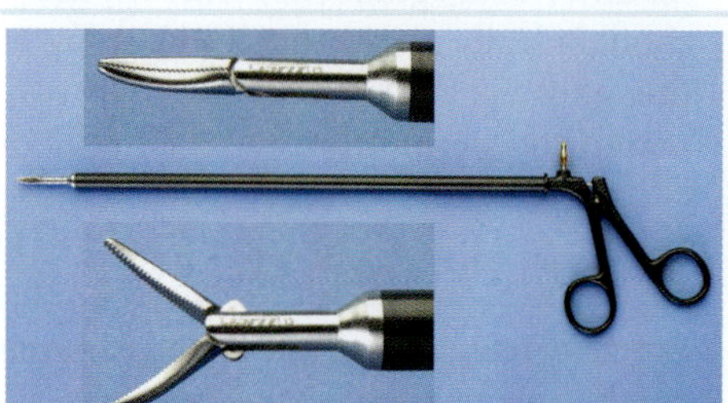 Courtesy Jarit Instruments, Hawthorne, NY.
HOOK SCISSORS	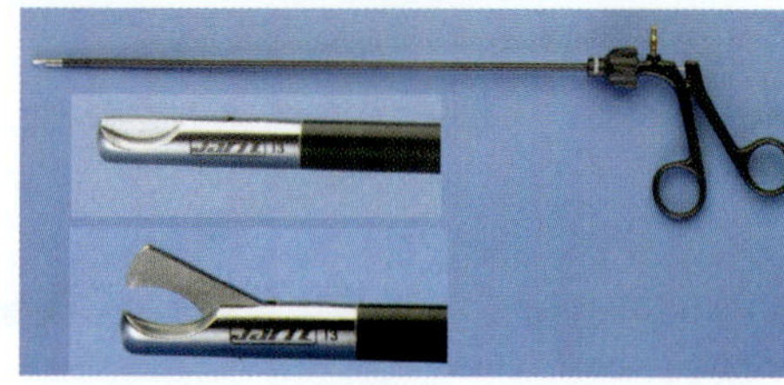 Courtesy Jarit Instruments, Hawthorne, NY.
BIOPSY PUNCH	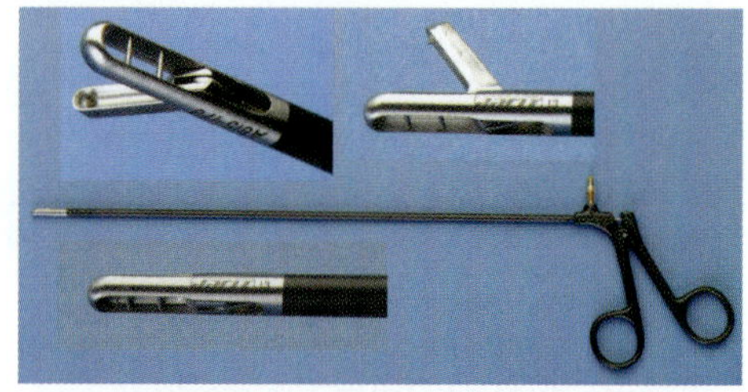 Courtesy Jarit Instruments, Hawthorne, NY.
GRASPER WITH RATCHET	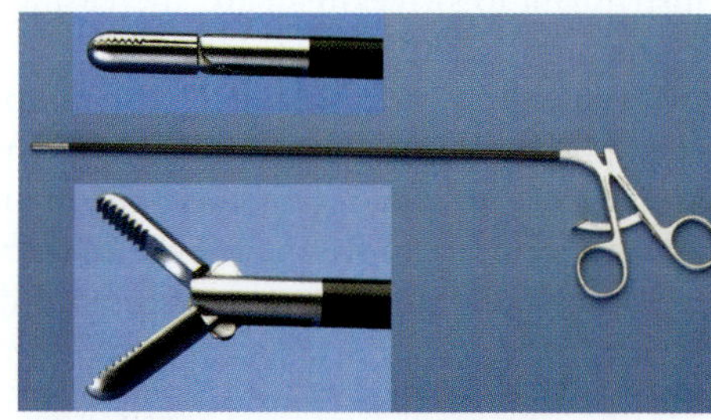 Courtesy Jarit Instruments, Hawthorne, NY.
CLAW GRASPER	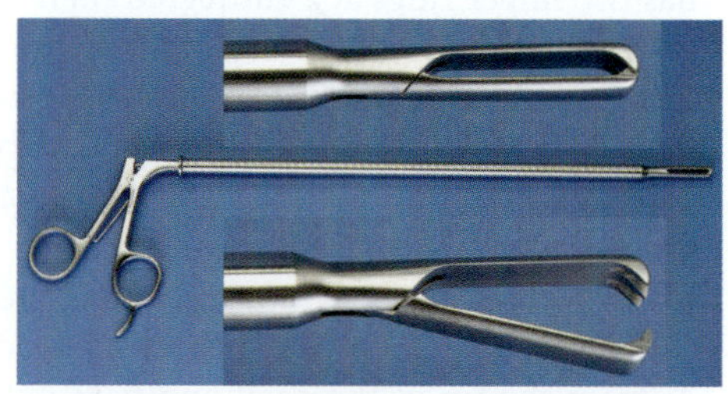 Courtesy Jarit Instruments, Hawthorne, NY.
ALLIS GRASPER	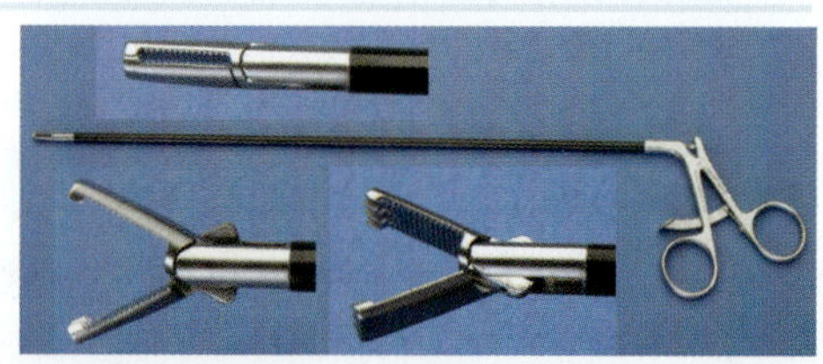 Courtesy Jarit Instruments, Hawthorne, NY.
BIPOLAR MICROGRASPER	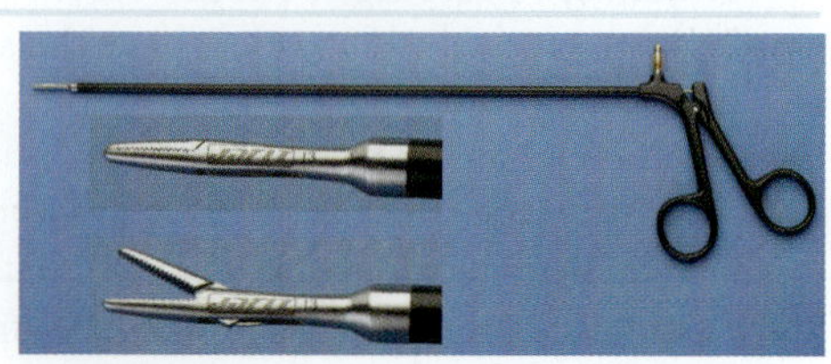 Courtesy Jarit Instruments, Hawthorne, NY.

TABLE 20.1 MIS Instruments—cont'd

ATRAUMATIC FORCEPS	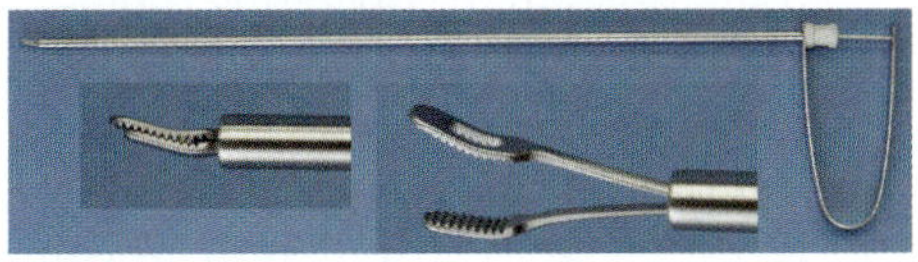 Courtesy Jarit Instruments, Hawthorne, NY.	DUVAL GRASPER	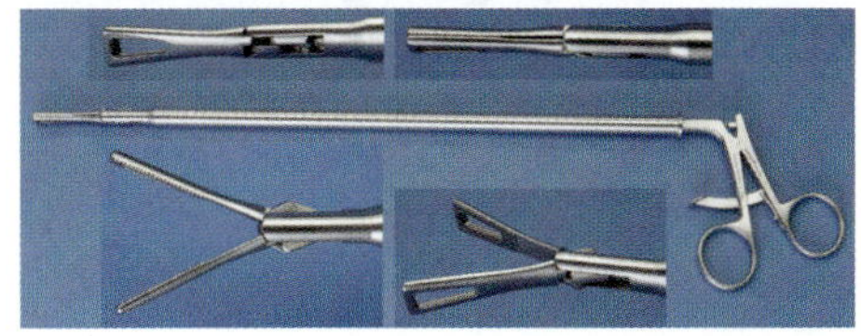 Courtesy Jarit Instruments, Hawthorne, NY.
BIPOLAR TOOTHED GRASPER	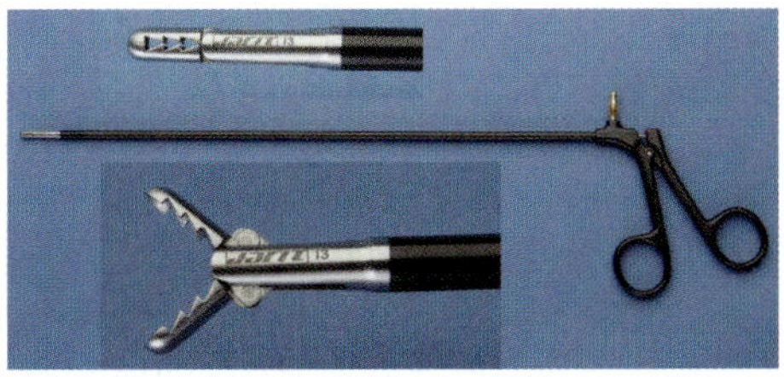 Courtesy Jarit Instruments, Hawthorne, NY.	DEBAKEY FORCEPS	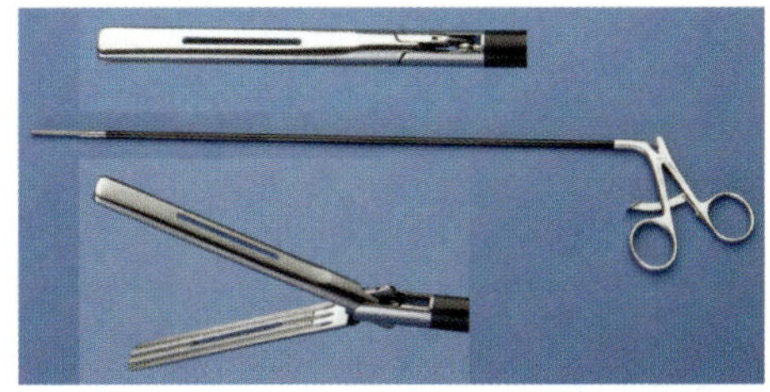 Courtesy Jarit Instruments, Hawthorne, NY.

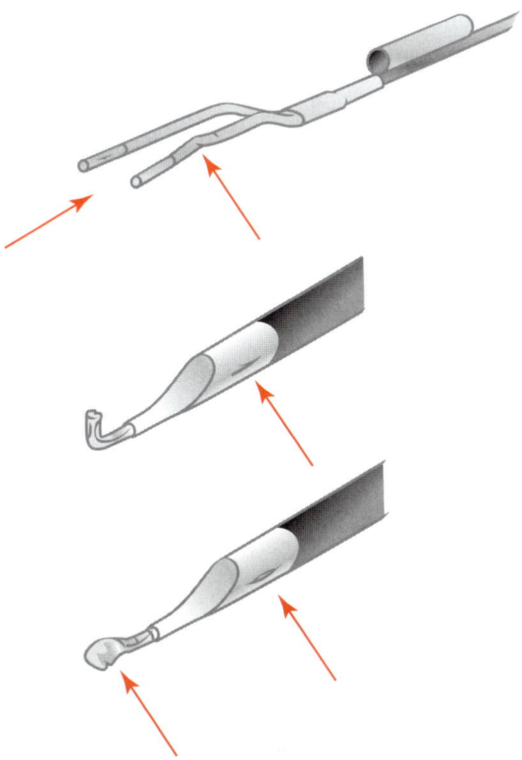

FIG. 20.19 Care of endoscopic instruments. Electrosurgical instruments must be inspected to ensure that there are no breaks in the insulation or distortion of the tips. (Courtesy Olympus America, Center Valley, PA.)

include length, diameter, channels for continuous irrigation, and electrosurgical capability.

A **resectoscope** is a rigid telescope contained within a cutting and coagulating instrument and is used in the sectional removal of tissue (Fig. 20.20). It is commonly used in genitourinary and gynecological surgery to remove tumors of the bladder and uterus and to resect the prostate. The resectoscope is fitted with a cutting tip that uses laser or electrosurgical energy to remove tissue. (Resectoscope techniques are described in Chapters 23 and 24.)

ENERGY SOURCES IN MIS

Energy sources used for tissue coagulation and cutting were introduced in Chapter 15. Electrosurgery, ultrasonic devices, and lasers are used routinely in minimally invasive procedures. The use of these devices in a closed space (within a body cavity or hollow organ) increases the possibility of injury, because although the operative site is accessible through the ports, "blind" spots exist outside the immediate view of the telescope camera. Burns may not be noticed or diagnosed until the signs and symptoms of burned or perforated viscera develop. These can quickly lead to infection. Also, the limited working space for instruments inside body cavities and spaces increases the technical difficulty in using extremely powerful cutting and coagulation instruments. Instrument collisions and inadvertent tissue contact with the device can result in severe injury to the patient.

ELECTROSURGICAL RISKS

Specific risks are associated with electrosurgical techniques used during MIS. The risk may be greater when monopolar instruments are used. The surgical technologist is responsible for checking all instruments and other devices before they are passed to the surgeon for use. The following are known to cause patient injury:

Insulation Failure

All MIS instruments are insulated with materials that do not conduct electricity. However, insulation can be damaged, and poor-quality manufacturing may produce an inferior instrument that is dangerous to use. Insulation failure can lead to patient burns when stray electrosurgical energy seeks a circuit and jumps to an alternative conductive path such as a break in insulation.

Direct and Capacitative Coupling

In **direct coupling,** the active electrode comes in contact with another conductive instrument, causing burns. This effect is

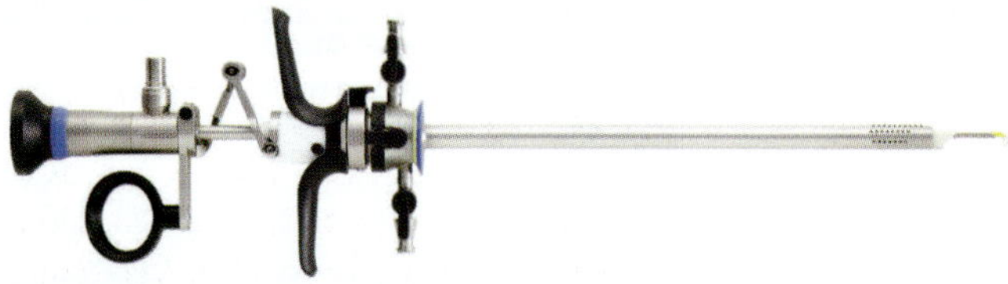

FIG. 20.20 Resectoscope. This is a hollow sheath that fits over the telescope and is used to remove tissue. It is fitted with a trigger device that operates cutting tips. (Courtesy Olympus America, Center Valley, PA.)

used deliberately when the surgeon grasps tissue with a conductive clamp and then touches the clamp with the active electrode.

Unintentional direct coupling is a different matter. Electrosurgical energy can be transmitted from the tip of the active electrode to nearby instruments when they are accidentally touched or are close to each other, causing accidental burns.

Capacitative coupling occurs when stray electrical current is transmitted from an electrosurgical instrument or other conductive material to tissue, even though no break in the insulation may be apparent. Stray current, the cause of capacitive coupling, can be caused by a number of instrument configurations:

- The active electrode is threaded through a metal cannula.
- The active electrode is an integral part of the operating laparoscope.
- The active electrode is threaded through a metal suction-irrigation tube.

In these cases, as mentioned previously, the stray current causes the problem. In MIS, the tubular cannula or the housing of a telescope can act as a capacitor. A *capacitor* is a point in an electrical circuit where energy is built up or stored between insulators. Energy from the active electrode can travel through the cannula or other capacitative areas near the electrode. When a metal cannula is used, the energy is dispersed over a wide area and may not cause a problem. However, plastic cannula anchors can insulate the cannula from the body wall. In this configuration, electricity passes down the cannula and can cause a burn on contact with deep body tissue.

Risk Reduction and Prevention

The risk of patient burns from electrosurgery and MIS can be reduced or eliminated. All perioperative personnel must be alert to potential risks and take an active role in preventing injury.

- The most effective means of preventing burns is **active electrode monitoring (AEM),** a system in which the instruments are self-monitoring during use.
- Continually check instruments and surgical telescopes for damage, especially along the insulated areas and shafts.
- All-metal cannulas are the safest type. Never use hybrid cannulas (those constructed of plastic and metal).
- A constant need to increase the power setting may indicate a problem in the system. Check first before continuing to increase the power.
- Reprocess all instruments, including telescopes, according to the manufacturer's specifications, to prevent damage that can lead to patient injury.
- Do not place electrical cords and fiber-optic cables across traffic areas in the operating room.
- Do not allow kinks and knots to develop; any cord that appears damaged must be immediately removed from service.
- Never allow electrical cords to come in contact with wet surfaces.

ULTRASONIC ENERGY

Ultrasonic technology is used during MIS for coagulation and cutting. Ultrasonic energy coagulates tissue by creating a cool coagulum at the cellular level. No electrical energy and very little heat are involved. Ultrasonic systems include the SonoSurg (Olympus America, Center Valley, PA) and Harmonic scalpel (Ethicon, Johnson & Johnson, New Brunswick, NJ).

HIGH-FREQUENCY BIPOLAR ELECTROSURGERY

High-frequency bipolar electrosurgery is used to coagulate and cut through tissue. Bipolar energy can be an effective method of hemostasis when the combination of low power and high frequency is used. High-frequency energy is transmitted from a power source unit connected to the specialty instruments by a cord, similar to monopolar electrosurgery. Some power sources are capable of producing both bipolar and monopolar energy. However, high-frequency units use a separate, dedicated power source. The PK technology system (ACMI, Southborough, MA) is an example of this type of high-frequency/low-temperature instrumentation. Most commonly, a hook probe is used to simultaneously cut and coagulate tissue. Scissors and grasping instruments are also available. PK technology is also used in the Intuitive robotic system (described later in this chapter).

LASER

Laser technology is used in conjunction with some types of minimally invasive and endoscopic surgery. In these procedures, the lasing fiber is introduced through the cannula or flexible telescope. Advances in digital technology have greatly increased the precision and efficacy of laser endoscopy. However, the hazards related to a small working space and blind areas out of view of the camera also apply to laser surgery. All of the precautions and safety measures presented in Chapter 15 apply to laser use in MIS and endoscopic surgery.

NOTE *Refer to Chapter 15 for a complete discussion of laser surgery, including patient and user safety.*

PREOPERATIVE PREPARATION

Patients undergoing MIS are prepared according to the anatomical location of the surgery. Preoperative preparation for an MIS procedure follows the same or similar protocols as those for open surgery, with additional attention to risks associated with MIS technology.

PATIENT POSITIONING

The positions used for MIS procedures depend on the surgical site and the patient's physiological condition. In general, patient positioning for MIS is identical to that for open surgery. However, some MIS abdominal and pelvic procedures require the patient to be positioned in lithotomy position with Trendelenburg or reverse Trendelenburg.

- *Upper abdomen or lower esophagus:* The patient is placed in reverse Trendelenburg position to displace abdominal viscera. A padded footboard is used to prevent the patient from sliding downward. Intraoperative changes in table position require immediate attention to patient safety. The ST must adjust the Mayo stand and any other overhead tables to ensure that the new position does not create pressure points between the patient and the underside of the Mayo.
- *Pelvic or abdominal laparoscopy:* The patient is placed in the Trendelenburg position. The gynecological patient and those undergoing surgery on the prostate are placed in the lithotomy position. In steep Trendelenburg position, there is a danger of the patient sliding toward the head of the table. A bean bag vacuum positioner or anti-skid device must be used to hold the patient in position and prevent him or her from sliding. Refer to Chapter 16 for a complete discussion of the safety precautions required for lithotomy and Trendelenburg positions.
- *Video-assisted thoracoscopic surgery (VATS):* Procedures of the lungs and bronchi are performed with the patient in the lateral decubitus position.

Arthroscopy of the shoulder is performed with the patient in beach-chair position with the arm free so that it can be rotated and flexed. Knee arthroscopy is performed with the patient in the supine position with the operative leg free so that it can be manipulated in different directions during the procedure.

SKIN PREP AND DRAPING

The skin prep and draping techniques used for minimally invasive procedures allow for the possibility of conversion to an open case. The skin prep is therefore performed as if for an open case. Draping is extended to match the prep area needed for an open incision, as discussed in Chapter 17.

MAINTAINING PATIENT NORMOTHERMIA

The use of carbon dioxide and fluids for distention of body cavities presents a risk of patient hypothermia. Carbon dioxide rapidly cools as it fills the abdominal space, and this can significantly lower the patient's core temperature. Fluid distention used in other body cavities, such as the bladder, uterus, and joint spaces, may have the same effect. Carbon dioxide pumps are equipped with a warming feature, which must be monitored carefully. Fluids for distention are warmed before instillation. Standard means for maintaining core temperature are also employed during MIS. These include the use of warm air blankets and limiting body exposure during the perioperative period.

SURGICAL SETUP FOR MIS

During surgery, the ST should keep MIS instruments in a rack on the instrument table. This maintains them safely and helps in rapid identification. Always separate MIS instruments to protect them from damage by heavier equipment. Telescopes in particular should be maintained on a towel or other soft surface to prevent them from rolling off the table. If a warm water thermos is used for prewarming, it should be kept in an area of the instrument table where it will not be jarred or knocked over.

Nonpenetrating clamps must be used to secure cords and tubing to drapes. Always allow sufficient slack on cord attachments and be alert to changes in table position, which can cause excess tension on them.

When passing an instrument to the surgeon, always orient the instrument so that the working tip points downward. The ST may help position the instrument into a port. In robotic-assisted MIS, the ST helps position and lock the instrument into the robotic arm.

During MIS, the room lights usually are dimmed or powered off. One of the operating lights or an auxiliary light should be positioned over the instrument table to help the ST identify and prepare instruments and supplies. This prevents errors and accidents.

CONVERSION TO AN OPEN CASE

Any minimally invasive procedure has the potential to become an open case. Operative permits are signed with this consideration, and any equipment needed to convert to an open case must be prepared and made immediately available. Some surgeries are scheduled and planned to include both MIS and open stages.

Regardless of whether the conversion is an emergency, it is performed very rapidly. When the MIS procedure is planned, the ST and circulator consult the surgeon's preference card for an open procedure. Sterile supplies are collected and located where they can be opened within minutes of the decision to convert to an open case. During conversion all cords and tubing are released from the drapes and carefully removed from the field to prevent them from becoming tangled in the drapes. Deliberate and purposeful actions help protect equipment during the conversion.

Instruments for the open procedure are quickly distributed and MIS instruments put aside or removed from the surgical field. The ST prepares for immediate incision while receiving other equipment from the circulator. Suction, electrosurgical instruments, and sharps are delivered first so that the open procedure can begin without delay. Sponges, instruments, and sharps are counted as distributed as in all cases.

SECTION II: FLEXIBLE ENDOSCOPY

USE OF THE FLEXIBLE ENDOSCOPE

Flexible and semi-rigid endoscopy are methods of viewing the inside of body passages and hollow organs, such

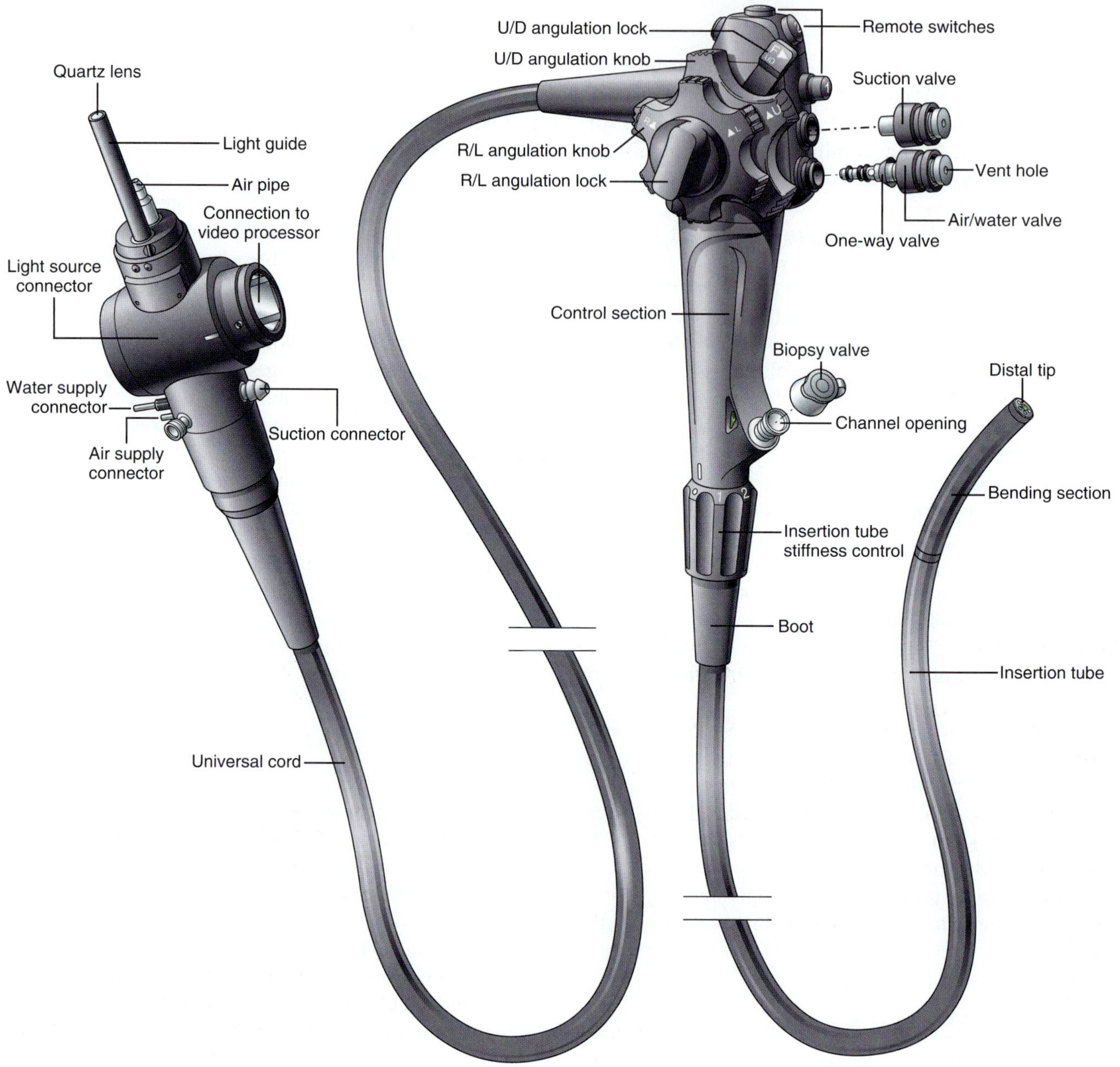

FIG. 20.21 Flexible endoscope external configuration. (From Chandrasekthara V. *Clinical Gastrointestinal Endoscopy: A Comprehensive Atlas*. Philadelphia: Elsevier; 2019.)

as the gastrointestinal system, urinary bladder, uterus, nasal sinuses, bronchial tree, and larynx. During flexible endoscopy, the surgical endoscope is introduced through a natural opening in the body, such as the mouth or nose. The scope is carefully advanced, and the interior tissues are examined with video-assisted technology or directly through the instrument's lens system. The surgeon can remove tissue for biopsy or take cell brushings through the flexible endoscope. Diagnosis is also made by visual examination of the tissues as they appear on the monitor during the procedure.

The flexible endoscope most often is used for examination, visual exploration, and biopsy. Some procedures and specialties use a semi-rigid scope, which is a hybrid form of the rigid endoscope discussed later in the chapter.

FLEXIBLE ENDOSCOPE

The flexible endoscope has two main sections, the head and the insertion tube (Fig. 20.21). The endoscope **control head** connects with the digital camera, optical system control handles, suction, and irrigation. Endoscopes that do not use video technology also have an eyepiece on the control head. The fiber-optic light cable is inserted into the control head to provide illumination. The control head also contains the dials that operate the flexing mechanism at the distal end of the tube. The **insertion tube** is the component of the endoscope that enters the patient's body. The interior of the insertion tube contains the fiber-optic light channel, which terminates at the tip of the instrument.

Inside the endoscope are the optical components and channels for irrigation, air, and biopsy instruments. The **instrument**

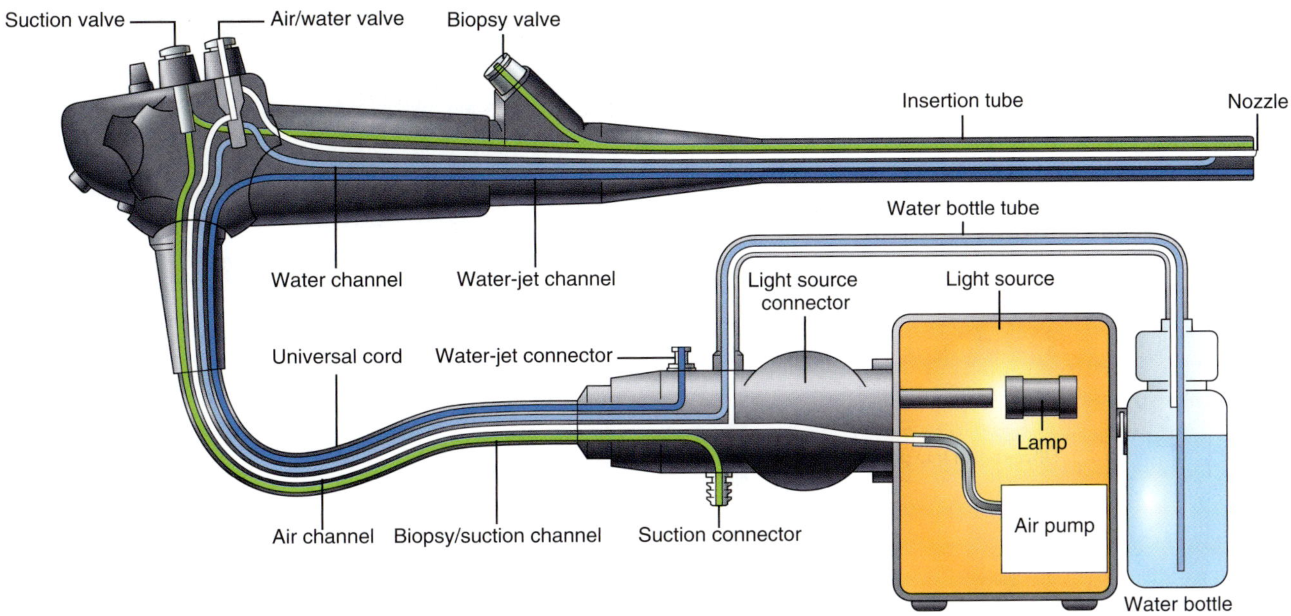

FIG. 20.22 Configuration of the air, water, suction, and lighting system of a flexible endoscope. (From Chandrasekthara V. *Clinical Gastrointestinal Endoscopy: A Comprehensive Atlas*. Philadelphia: Elsevier; 2019.)

channel (also called the **elevator channel**) receives biopsy forceps, brushes, and other instruments used to remove tissue specimens. This channel is the largest one. The **biopsy channel** port is located near the junction of the control head and the insertion tube.

Some endoscopes have an **auxiliary water channel.** The water channel is used to clear blood and tissue debris from the lens. An *air channel* is used to insufflate the lumen of the gastrointestinal tract to create space in the same way as in a pneumoperitoneum. The tip of the insertion tube is operated at the control head to obtain rotational views of the anatomy within the focal area of the lens. Fig. 20.22 shows the design of air, water, light, and suction systems of a flexible endoscope.

ECHOENDOSCOPE

The echoendoscope is similar in structure to the standard endoscope but contains an ultrasound transducer at the tip that is capable of transmitting and receiving ultrasound signals from adjacent anatomy. The signals produce digital images, which can be interpreted and assessed. Fig. 20.23 illustrates the echoendoscope.

CAPSULE ENDOSCOPE

The capsule endoscope is a device for performing endoscopic procedures of the small intestine, esophagus, and large intestine.

The capsule device is the size of a large vitamin and contains a high-resolution camera (in the form of a charged couple device, CCD), lens, light-emitted diode and battery as shown in Fig. 20.24. The device is enclosed in plastic and designed to be swallowed by the patient or placed using routine endoscopic techniques. The images that are captured by the capsule are transmitted to a set of sensors, which are attached to the patient by a belt (Fig. 20.25). The images are then transferred to a computer, where they can be studied and analyzed. The capsule is excreted and therefore does not require retrieval.

IMAGING SYSTEM

The vision system of the flexible endoscope is very similar to that used for MIS. A camera control unit and documentation system perform the same functions discussed previously. Video output is viewed on the LCD or plasma monitor, as in MIS.

MIS may be assisted with a flexible endoscope for increased visibility of the anatomy. In these procedures, the flexible endoscope is managed by a separate team performing MIS through the rigid telescope and instrument ports. Combined procedures of the abdomen and gastrointestinal tract are enhanced with the use of both technologies.

TECHNIQUE

Flexible endoscopy usually is performed in an outpatient setting in a separate unit of the health care facility near the operating room. The procedures are relatively short compared with those for MIS or open surgery. Ambulatory outpatients usually are discharged as soon as they have recovered from the effects of sedation.

After the patient has been sedated and positioned, the surgeon introduces the insertion tube, examining tissue and recording digital images. Biopsies are taken with the aid of forceps, graspers, or biopsy brushes.

The surgeon is assisted by the ST, who helps position the patient and prepares equipment and instruments. During the procedure, the ST maintains suction and irrigation devices and helps place biopsy instruments into the endoscope. The

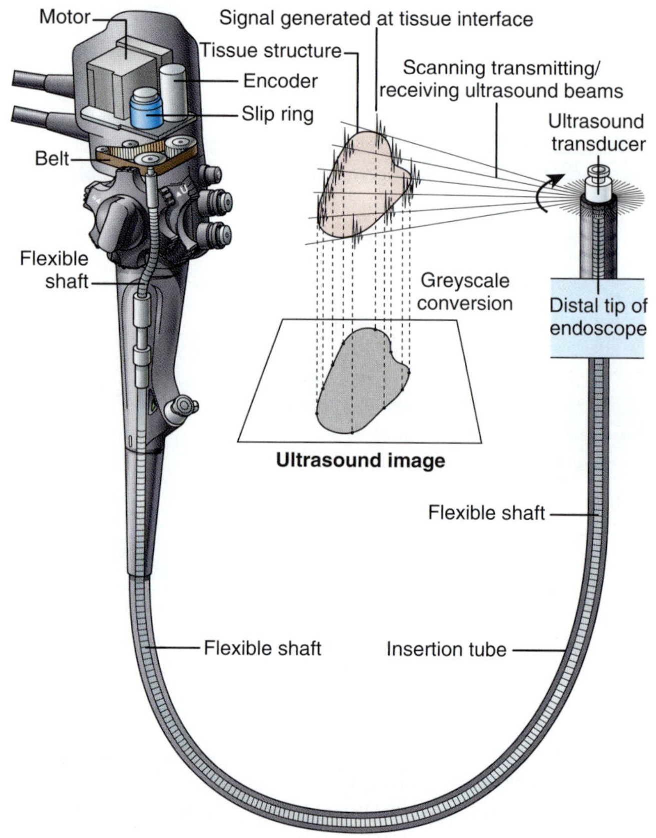

FIG. 20.23 Echoendoscope. The endoscope contains an ultrasound transducer, which receives digital signals from the adjacent tissue. These are then produced as images that can be assessed. (From Chandrasekthara V. *Clinical Gastrointestinal Endoscopy: A Comprehensive Atlas*. Philadelphia: Elsevier; 2019.)

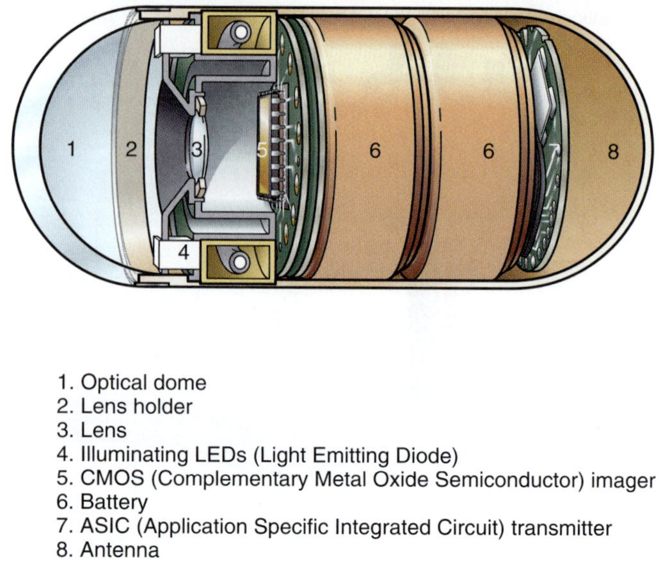

FIG. 20.24 Capsule endoscope internal system showing digital components. (From Chandrasekthara V. *Clinical Gastrointestinal Endoscopy: A Comprehensive Atlas*. Philadelphia: Elsevier; 2019.)

ST also receives specimens as they are withdrawn from the endoscope and properly preserves and documents them. Specimens retrieved during endoscopy are small and easily lost. It is important to have specimen containers ready to receive the tissue. To retrieve tissue from biopsy forceps, the tip of the instrument can be immersed in saline (or according to the surgeon's preference) and moved gently in the liquid. If this does not release the tissue, a needle can be used to remove the tissue from the instrument jaws. Brush biopsy specimens are obtained using a small disposable brush, which is threaded into the endoscope. Suspect tissue is then brushed and the instrument withdrawn. The specimen must be transferred to a glass slide and a fixative applied. The brush may also be clipped from the instrument and sent to pathology as a wet specimen. These techniques differ according to the type of tissue obtained and the specific requirements of the pathology department.

REPROCESSING ENDOSCOPES AND INSTRUMENTS

Disassembly and proper reassembly are critical to safe reprocessing (cleaning, disinfection, sterilization). Reprocessing is discussed in this chapter rather than in Chapter 10, which covers disinfection and sterilization, so that the student can easily refer to discussions and definitions of instrument components in this chapter.

PROTOCOLS AND STANDARDS

The endoscope is a complex instrument with channels, valves, spring fittings, and stopcocks. The endoscope and other instruments often come in contact with areas of the body that have a high level of bioburden. Debris can become trapped in the mechanisms and harbor infectious material. For these reasons, a systematic cleaning process that follows an established protocol is necessary to ensure patient safety.

Hospital policy for reprocessing endoscopes follows guidelines established by the Occupational Safety and Health Administration (OSHA), an agency of the U.S. Department of Labor. All manufacturers of surgical endoscopes provide detailed instructions on the specific care of its equipment. A general overview of reprocessing is presented here.

PRECLEANING OF RIGID ENDOSCOPES

All immersible instruments and rigid endoscopes must be precleaned immediately after use in surgery. Endoscopes and accessories should be disassembled according to the manufacturer's instructions. Manual cleaning removes much of the tissue and body fluid trapped in crevices and fittings. This is done with enzymatic cleaner, a clean cloth, and a soft brush. Endoscopic instruments can be soaked briefly in an enzymatic detergent bath before precleaning.

GUIDELINES FOR PRECLEANING INSTRUMENTS

1. Instruments are best transported in a covered container from the point of use to the cleaning area. They can be transported wet or dry. However, immediate soaking

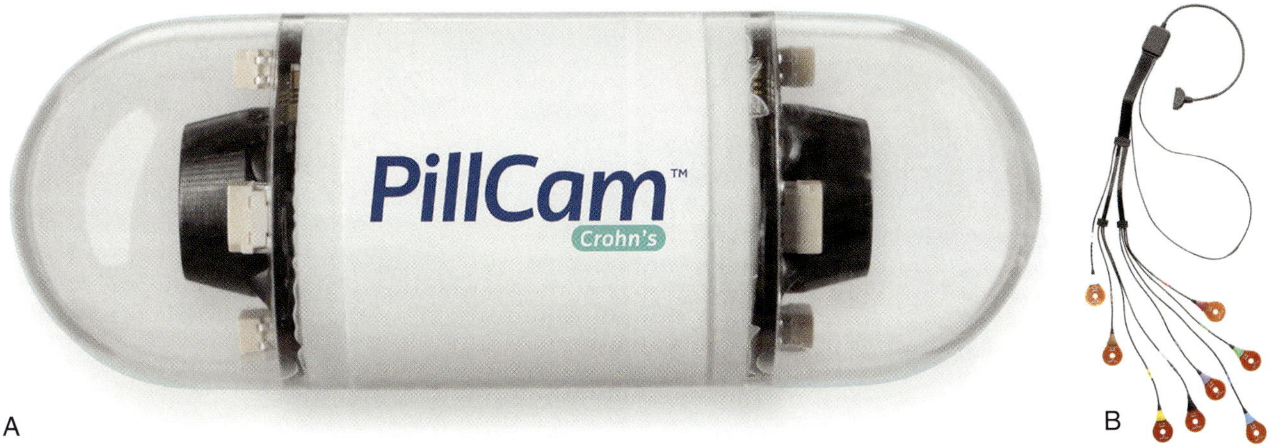

FIG. 20.25 Capsule endoscope and sensor array. (A) PillCam Crohn's capsule. The capsule endoscope is designed to be swallowed by the patient. (B) PillCam sensor array is worn by the patient and picks up signals from the capsule. These are then transformed into images. (All rights reserved. Used with the permission of Medtronic.)

(transport in a wet bath) aids more complete cleaning. Do not soak instruments for longer than 1 hour or as directed by the instrument manufacturer.

2. Before cleaning instruments, make sure to open all stopcocks, ports, and channels.
3. Separate the telescopes from other instruments for individual processing.
4. Follow the manufacturer's instructions for a compatible enzymatic bath. Do not exceed the recommended water temperature.
5. While cleaning, look for defects in the surface of the instrument. Look for any sign that the instrument housing and insulation are damaged. Remember that even small nicks or scratches can create a pathway for stray electricity and cause burns.
6. Use a long brush to clean the inside of tubes and lumens. Irrigate these with large amounts of enzymatic fluid. Reusable brushes must be terminally disinfected and sterilized between uses.
7. Clean air and water channels with forced air or as recommended by the manufacturer.
8. Do not submerge or allow any fluid to enter electrical connections or units! These should be wiped clean with an approved surface disinfectant.
9. Flush all ports with enzymatic solution and make sure all surfaces have been cleaned. Some types of stopcocks may be disassembled for cleaning. Always verify this before attempting disassembly.
10. After cleaning, rinse all surfaces and channels of the instruments with deionized or sterile water. Make sure that every part of the instrument is rinsed to remove detergent and debris loosened during cleaning.
11. Drain the instruments and dry them.

PRECLEANING OPTICAL PARTS AND LENSES

Disassemble the adapter from the light cable. Then proceed as follows:

1. If the endoscope has an eyepiece cap, remove it.
2. Clean the lens surface with a lint-free cloth and ethanol or isopropanol, or as directed by the manufacturer.
3. When cleaning lenses and optical surfaces, take care not to abrade or scrape the lenses. Use a soft cloth to clean the optical surfaces.
4. Check the lenses of the endoscope. Look for any cloudiness or discoloration. Cloudiness may be a sign of leakage. If you suspect that the lens fitting has leaked, remove it from service after decontamination and sterilization according to manufacturer's specifications.

Ultrasonic cleaning is commonly used for stainless steel instruments. However, many instruments are not approved for this type of system, and the process may damage them.

FLEXIBLE ENDOSCOPE REPROCESSING

Flexible endoscopes are particularly difficult to clean. The ports and long tube channels trap debris and biofilm. An automatic reprocessor therefore is used. Several manufacturers have developed enclosed reprocessing machines that terminally disinfect the system as long as precleaning has been correctly performed.

Before disinfection in an automatic reprocessor, several steps must be carried out to ensure patient safety.

1. Pre-clean as soon as possible after the procedure. Thoroughly clean the insertion tube with detergent solution, and clean the channels using dedicated brushes (Fig. 20.26A and B). Then flush detergent solution through the air-water and auxiliary channels and remove it with air suction.
2. The endoscope must be leak-tested after pre-cleaning. This is done to prevent water from entering the system during the remaining steps of reprocessing. Follow the manufacturer's instructions for leak testing. The leak-testing equipment used must be compatible with the individual endoscope.
3. After the leak test, clean the endoscope manually. This is done by submerging the instrument in detergent solution

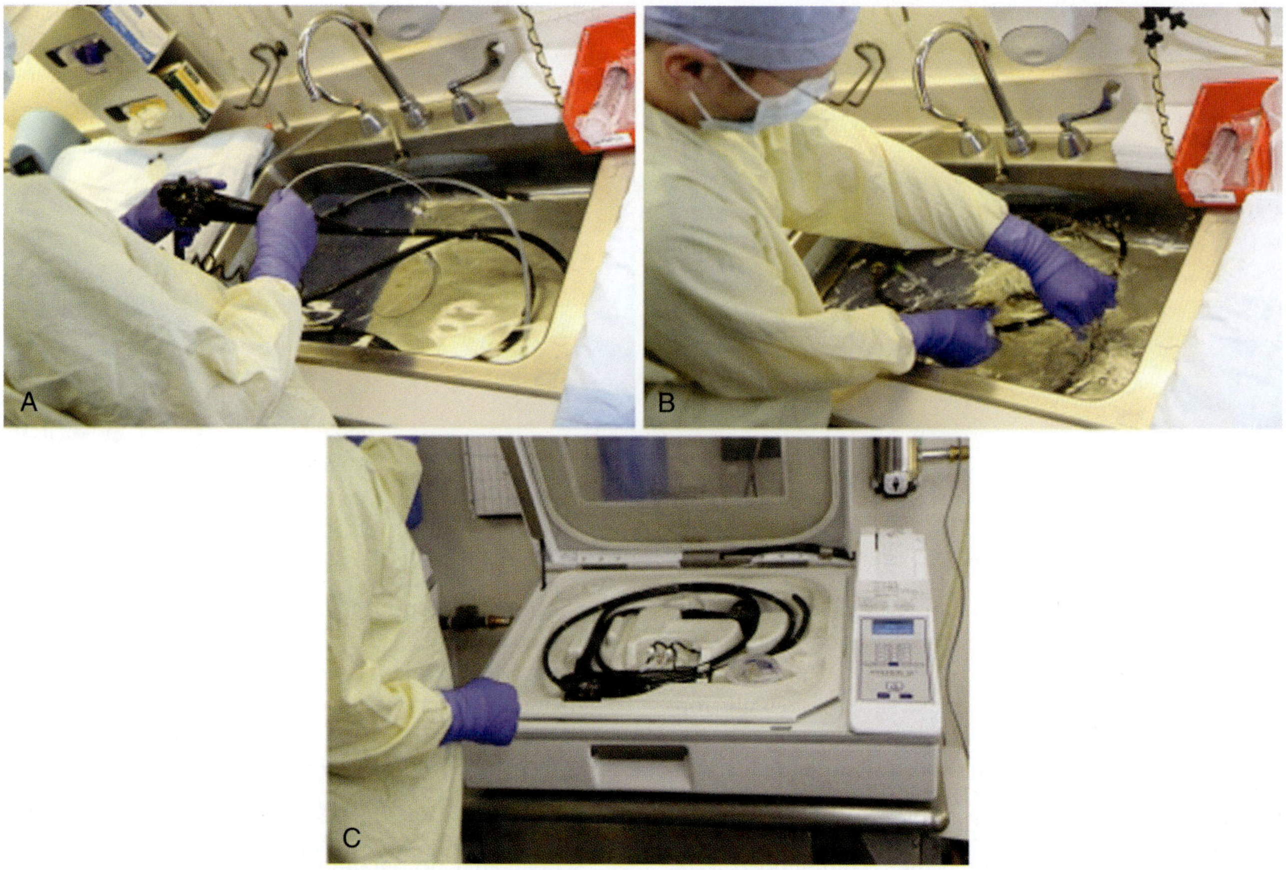

FIG. 20.26 (A and B) Precleaning the flexible endoscope. (C) Sterilization in peracetic acid chamber.

and cleaning all surfaces with a soft cloth. Use a suction pump and syringe to flush detergent through the instrument channels and ports, and insert a soft brush to clean any debris.

4. After cleaning with detergent, completely rinse the endoscope to remove all traces of detergent and debris.
5. Remove all water from the instrument's channels and exterior. The endoscope may then be processed in an automated endoscope reprocessor according to the manufacturer's specifications.

DISINFECTION AND STERILIZATION

After instruments have been thoroughly cleaned, they must be disinfected. High-level disinfection kills 100% of *Mycobacterium tuberculosis*. The process of disinfection is specified by the manufacturer of the equipment. A common method uses peracetic acid in a specially designed container (Fig. 20.26C).

Sterilization methods for endoscopic instruments vary with the type of equipment and the manufacturer's specifications. Instruments used in sterile areas of the body, including the vascular system, require sterilization before reuse. Some equipment, including cameras, may be steam-sterilized, whereas others require ethylene oxide gas or other methods.

KEY CONCEPTS

- Operative MIS involves less tissue trauma and postoperative pain and a shorter recovery time compared with open surgery.
- MIS patients must be carefully screened, because not all patients are good candidates.
- MIS involves complex electronic and imaging systems. All team members must study the technologies involved and remain current with new developments in the specialty.
- The operative principle of MIS is that surgery is performed on internal organs from outside the body using telescopic instruments and an operative telescope, which projects the surgical site onto a monitor.
- The components of the MIS imaging system must be compatible.
- Risks associated with MIS include complications resulting from insufflation, intravasation, and unsafe electrosurgical techniques.
- Preoperative preparation of the patient for MIS is the same as for open surgery, because there is always the possibility that the case will convert to an open procedure.
- MIS is performed in a dimmed operating room to enhance viewing on the video monitor. A dedicated light must be positioned over the instrument table to prevent accidents and errors.

- MIS instruments are extremely delicate and expensive. Care and handling require attention to detail and knowledge of instrument design.
- MIS is practiced in nearly every surgical specialty. The most common applications are in abdominal, gynecological, orthopedic, thoracic, and genitourinary surgery.
- Reprocessing of MIS instruments is performed according to the manufacturer's instructions. Most instruments can be steam-sterilized but require careful cleaning and decontamination before sterilization.
- Because MIS is performed in limited anatomical spaces, various techniques are used to open these tissue planes. Insufflation and fluid expansion are the two most common methods.
- Electrosurgery during MIS can increase the risk of patient burns because the instruments are not always under direct vision of the lensed telescope. Extra caution and vigilance are necessary to prevent patient injury.
- During flexible endoscopy, a flexible tube is inserted into a body cavity for diagnostic assessment, biopsy, and minor surgery.
- The rigid endoscope is used for resection of tumors and more complex surgery of the genitourinary tract and in gynecological procedures.
- Reprocessing of the flexible endoscope is a primary issue in infection control. This is because the endoscopes are used in semi-critical areas of the body and may have a heavy bioburden.
- The protocol for reprocessing of endoscopes is established by health care organizations, guided by safety and accrediting agencies.

REVIEW QUESTIONS

1. Explain how abdominal adhesions can cause injury during MIS.
2. Explain how the view of the surgical site is transmitted to the monitor during MIS surgery.
3. What would be the effect on a fiber-optic light if some of the fibers were broken?
4. In what ways are the physical aspects of minimally invasive instruments different from those of standard instruments used in open surgery?
5. What do you think may be the reasons for converting from an MIS surgery to open surgery?
6. Compare the risks of stainless steel trocars and plastic or nonconductive trocars.
7. Explain the difference between capacitative coupling and direct coupling.
8. What is the role of the surgical technologist in preventing patient burns during the use of electrosurgery in MIS?

CASE STUDIES

CASE 1

The risk of inadvertent thermal injury (burns) to abdominal viscera during minimally invasive surgery of the abdomen (laparoscopy) can be prevented by using risk-reduction measures. Some of these measures are under the direct control of the scrubbed surgical technologist. Using your knowledge of electrosurgery, outline a risk-reduction plan. Use a time-related structure for the plan (preoperative, intraoperative, and postoperative). Use material learned in this chapter and Chapter 15 to formulate the plan.

CASE 2

Flexible endoscopy is often performed as a diagnostic procedure in outpatient clinics. A surgical technologist may assist during the procedure and in care of the endoscopic equipment and instruments. He or she may also be required to provide direct care to the patient in positioning, transporting, and taking vital signs. Based on your current knowledge of communication skills, patient movement and handling, and care of the high-technology equipment used in endoscopy, describe which aspects of this role may be difficult for you personally. In your self-evaluation, explain what you may do to increase your knowledge base and skills.

BIBLIOGRAPHY

Association of periOperative Registered Nurses (AORN). Guideline for minimally invasive surgery. In *Guidelines for Perioperative Practice, 2015 Edition*. Denver: AORN; 2015.

Catalone C, Fickenscher K. Emerging technologies in the OR and their effect on perioperative professionals. *AORN J*. 2007;86:958.

Khraim F. The wider scope of video-assisted thoracoscopic surgery. *AORN J*. 2007;85:1199.

Olympus America. *Reprocessing Instructions*. http://medical.olympusamerica.com/customer-resources/cleaning-disinfection-sterilization/cds-instructions. Accessed February 17, 2016.

21 ROBOTIC-ASSISTED SURGERY

LEARNING OBJECTIVES

After studying this chapter, the reader will be able to:

1. Describe the components of a robotic-assisted surgical system
2. Compare the features of robotic-assisted surgery with standard minimally invasive surgery
3. Describe the movements of wristed instruments
4. Differentiate between open and closed surgeon consoles
5. Describe the patient cart and its functions
6. Describe the features of robotic-assisted optics and vision system
7. Differentiate between the Veress needle technique and Hasson techniques for pneumoperitoneum
8. Discuss the importance of robotic system room layout
9. Discuss the role of the surgical technologist during robotic-assisted surgery
10. Discuss the importance of teamwork and communication during robotic-assisted surgery

TERMINOLOGY

Bedside unit: Component of a robotic-assisted surgical system that holds a surgical instrument and receives signals from the surgeon at the console. In the da Vinci system this is comparable to the *patient cart*.

Docking: Refers to the process of moving the patient cart into position and locking the instrument arms in place (da Vinci systems only).

Hand controllers: Devices located in the surgeon console for manipulating surgical instruments. The surgeon uses his hands to control the devices.

Haptic feedback (force pressure): The sense of touch and pressure. Some robotic systems do not feature haptic feedback in their surgical instruments. In this case the surgeon must use visual cues to sense the instrument pressure.

Modular robotic system: One that features a single instrument and its arm, which is attached to a dedicated movable base.

Near-infrared imaging: The use of an optical instrument such as a specially adapted surgical endoscope to detect near-infrared fluorescence in tissues. See text for full description of this technique.

Port: Refers to an opening in the body created with a trocar and tubular cannula. The port is used for insertion of minimally invasive instruments and endoscope.

Registration (of a digital image): Using computer technology to layer separate digital images of the same subject to create a 3-D composite.

Remote data display: Data such as CT scan images and x-rays located in a remote location is streamed to the screen monitor of the surgeon console.

Reposable: Refers to surgical instruments that can be reprocessed a limited number of times. After that they must be safely discarded.

Robotic-assisted surgical (RAS) system: A device that uses computer technology and software to control and manipulate surgical instruments.

Scaled movement: Translation of the surgeon's normal hand movements on the controller to a much smaller scale, usually in a 5:1 ratio. Some systems can scale to different ratios to suit the surgeon's preference.

Surgeon console: A robotic system component in which the surgeon sits or stands to manipulate the surgical instruments remotely and control other devices used in the system.

Surgical access: A technique used to enter the body to perform surgery.

Wristed instruments: A feature of robotic instruments, which have 7 degrees of freedom, plus allow for opening and closing the jaws of the instrument.

This chapter focuses on robotic-assisted surgical systems that enable the surgeon to perform surgery through the computer-based robotic interface.

The first robotic-assisted surgical systems appeared in hospitals in the mid-1980s. The prototypes were developed by a collaborative group including the U.S. National Aeronautics and Space Administration (NASA), the Department of Defense (DOD), the Stanford Research Institute (SRI), and a number of private companies. The government agencies were interested in the application of remote performance surgery to the battlefield, where it could be applied to wounded military personnel. NASA's interest was also in remote surgery as it may apply to personnel working in outer space. The first U.S. Food and Drug Administration (FDA)-cleared device appeared in 1994, and by 1998 it was used in the first human patient. Robotic-assisted surgery is now a mainstream technology with an ever-increasing number of innovations and applications.

Surgical technologists have a significant role in robotic-assisted surgery (RAS). Learning starts with knowledge and skills in minimally invasive surgery (MIS). Once these have been acquired, the foundation principles and entry-level practice of robotic technology can be applied. Students may be exposed to RAS as observers or assistants to staff STs. Extended training and hands-on learning is provided by individual manufacturers and their experienced trainers. This ensures that all members of the surgical team have the specific knowledge and skills required for safe surgery. However, it is important to know that manufacturers are not responsible for the skills and knowledge of those who use their systems. This is the duty of professional organizations and certifying agencies. They must set the standards for competency and follow through with the means to measure the competency of their members.

This chapter discusses a number of different robotic systems to illustrate the technologies and the role of the surgical technologist. The surgical robotics market is extremely competitive, and manufacturers are naturally eager to promote their products. This chapter does not evaluate or compare the benefits of one system over another.

SECTION I: OVERVIEW

WHAT IS ROBOTIC-ASSISTED SURGERY?

The FDA defines an RAS device as a subtype of computer-assisted surgical (CAS) systems. RAS uses computer technology and software to control and manipulate surgical instruments.

Since 2016, a large number of new RAS systems have been developed, and some have been released for use in the United States. The sudden appearance of new systems occurred when the patents on the only existing system available in the US market expired. This allowed other companies to present their robotic systems for FDA approval. Newer systems combine robotic capabilities with other computer interfaces to plan and perform surgical procedures.

This chapter uses the FDA term **robotic-assisted surgical (RAS) system** to define surgical systems that are enabled by robotic technology. This term is used to avoid confusion and is not intended to redefine new or existing systems.

FEATURES OF ROBOTIC SYSTEMS

RAS has special features and capabilities that are specific to the technology. It is important to note that these features do not *necessarily* affect the surgical outcome. A skilled surgeon remains skilled whether using a robotics platform, MIS platform, or open surgery.

The decision to purchase a system is made by individual facilities based on the requirements of their patients and their health care teams. A system that uses only single-use instruments may not be suitable in all settings. Likewise, the choice between a system that enables haptic feedback may be desirable to some surgeons but not to others. Robotic technology and systems are in rapid development with many new innovative systems on the market.

SCALED MOVEMENT

The robotic system can scale the surgeon's hand movements to varying ratios from 1:2 to 1:5. This **scaled movement** means that the computer interface can translate movement to a much smaller scale, enabling greater precision without demanding greater motor skills. This feature also dampens or removes normal hand tremor.

IMAGE REGISTRATION

Digital image **registration** is the layering of multiple images of the same subject to produce a blended image in three dimensions. In surgery, registration is used to plan a surgical procedure based on preoperative images produced by computed tomography (CT), magnetic resonance imaging (MRI), and ultrasound. Some robotic systems feature image registration. Image-guided surgery (stereotactic surgery) uses a 3-D coordinate system to guide the surgeon to a specific location in the tissue, such as a tumor or lymph node.

AUTONOMY

Robots used in industry are programmed to perform repetitive tasks. Once the system has been programmed, it can perform those tasks autonomously within the digital parameters established. A fully robotic system of any kind is automated. It is not controlled by a human. *Robotic-assisted surgical systems are not autonomous.* Their actions are under the direct control of the surgeon. However, newer systems may have some automated features.

SIMILARITIES TO MINIMALLY INVASIVE SURGERY

RAS evolved from the technology of MIS.

Both systems use minimally invasive techniques for access to the target tissues. These include the following:

- Individual **port** sites or a single port for multiple instruments. An endoscopic camera whose field of vision is captured on a flat-screen monitor.

- An enlarged gas-filled space to accommodate the instruments and perform the surgery (e.g., pneumoperitoneum). (This applies primarily to body cavities.)
- Telescopic instruments, including minimally invasive stapling and suture systems.
- Common energy modalities including monopolar, bipolar, ultrasonic, and combination modalities to coagulate, cut, and dissect tissue.

SECTION II: ROBOTIC TECHNOLOGY

COMPONENTS

RAS uses separate components that are connected digitally. Each component controls specific functions. These are the nonsterile console, one or more bedside carts with attached instrument arm(s), equipment for imaging, and an auxiliary screen for the sterile bedside team. The electrosurgery unit (ESU) and other power modality units are incorporated into one cart or "tower."

NOTE *The components are shown later in this chapter in Types of Robotic and Computer-Assisted Systems.*

SURGEON CONSOLE

The **surgeon console** is a nonsterile control station where the surgeon sits or stands while operating. This unit is connected to the other components, which are activated by the controls in the console. Here the surgeon can manipulate the surgical instruments, adjust the parameters of the optics system, and perform many other tasks.

CONSOLE DESIGN

There are two console designs: *open* and *closed*. The *closed* system is sometimes referred to as *immersive*. This type of system features a cockpit-style viewer. The surgeon activates the unit by positioning his or her head within the console, which displays the endoscopic camera video feed on a stereo viewer. An *open* system has no cockpit or hood. The surgeon views the monitor just as one would a computer screen. See Figure 21.6.

REMOTE DATA DISPLAY

Remote data such as the patient's CT or MRI scans can be displayed on the screen monitor at any time as **remote data display**. Image-guided navigation is used in some systems, especially those developed for orthopedic surgery and neurosurgery. Systems that use image guidance are able to overlay the CT images onto the real-time display for precision tissue modeling. These are discussed in more detail in subsequent sections.

HAND CONTROLLERS

The **hand controllers** are used to move the surgical instruments during the procedure. The controllers are located in an ergonomic position below the monitor. The hand controllers operate in open space so that they can be moved easily through all dimensions. Fully adjustable arm rests decrease muscle strain on the surgeon's shoulders and neck.

FOOT CONTROLS

Foot controls are used on some systems to activate the energy instruments. They may also control the camera and clutch on the bedside cart; on new systems these controls are built into the hand controllers. A clutch controls the instrument arms and may be used for activation and deactivation.

BEDSIDE UNIT AND INSTRUMENT ARMS

The **bedside unit** is the receptacle for the surgical instruments and endoscope, which are inserted into designated arms. The da Vinci system (Intuitive, Inc.), which features multiple arms and instruments on the same base, refers to the bedside unit as a *patient cart*. In this unit the arms are attached to an overhead *boom*. The boom projects from a central column. A single arm multi-port system is also available from Intuitive. This component features one arm mounted on a moveable base. The da Vinci patient cart is heavy and is moved using a motor drive. The cart is managed from the helm located at the back of the unit, which also contains a touch screen to program the cart's movements. The circulating nurse is responsible for its management and positioning during surgery. Operation of the cart is *prescriptive* (ordered by the surgeon). This means that only licensed staff (i.e., the licensed perioperative nurse) may operate the cart during patient care.

Modular robotic systems feature a single instrument and its arm, which is attached to a dedicated base as shown in Figure 21.5. These units are freely moveable and can be transported easily between operating rooms.

OPTICS (VISION)

Just as in standard MIS, the RAS system requires an endoscope (telescope). Using robotic-assisted optics, the endoscopic field of vision can be panned in or out without loss of image quality or light. The image captured with robotic components is 3-D, the same as human binocular vision in which each eye sees the image from a different angle and the brain merges the two into a single 3-D image. Note that the high-definition (HD) image captured with a nonrobotic endoscope is also extremely sharp without shadows. However, it projects in two dimensions only. The robotic endoscope image shows much greater depth than with a conventional endoscope. This allows the surgeon to see structures and other instruments beyond the immediate focal point without moving the scope.

IMPORTANT TO KNOW *Some systems rely on 3-D glasses for the surgeon to perceive a 3-D image.*

EQUIPMENT OR VISION TOWER

An RAS system requires accessory equipment such as energy modalities, system electronics, video controller, and touch screen. These are placed on an equipment tower, and their signals are relayed by fiber-optic cables to the surgeon console so that they can be controlled. The exact configuration of the accessories varies with the robotic system. The layout of the cables in a multi-component system is extremely important to efficiency and safety during a procedure (see Room Layout).

The touch screen is very important to the ST and circulating nurse. It shows which instruments are active in a specific robotic arm. It also allows control of the audio and visual functions of the system.

The da Vinci unit provides a method for contacting on-call technical personnel in the event of a system malfunction. The circulating nurse or robotic coordinator uses a manufacturer's hotline to provide the location and identification number of the specific system in use to a technician at the company end. Using the identification information provided by the surgical team, technical personnel can immediately retrieve intranet-enabled data. These data show the status of the system, including faults, to troubleshoot the system in real time and advise actions to take. Other manufacturers also provide telephone hotlines for person-to-person troubleshooting.

ROBOTIC INSTRUMENTS

Instruments used in RAS have been derived from minimally invasive technology. They feature a long shaft, working tip (called the *end effector*), and head, which attaches to the robotic arm. However, it is important to note that not all RAS systems use **wristed instruments.** Some, like the Senhance system, use standard MIS instruments.

INSTRUMENT DESIGN

Like minimally invasive instruments, robotic instruments are long and slender and may be as small as 3 mm in diameter or up to 10 mm. A standard MIS instrument has 4 degrees of freedom plus opening and closing the jaws. The robotic instrument has 7 degrees of freedom plus opening and closing the jaws. This enables very fine movement in all directions. The term "wristed" has been coined to describe instruments whose tips are multi-directional.

Robotic terminology uses specific names for each type of movement that is expressed in degrees. The degree of rotation is the ability to pivot (rotational turns like a spinning coin). The tips of robotic instruments allow 90-degree rotation. If we picture the movements of an airplane, the other robotic movements become very clear. An airplane that dips its wings in either direction exhibits *roll*. The nose-up and nose-down positions are called *pitch*. Right and left turns in space are called *yaw*. These features all contribute to the robotic instruments' maneuverability, especially important in small spaces. For example, suturing techniques used in robotic surgery would be nearly impossible using conventional MIS instruments because of their limited maneuverability compared with robotic instruments. Fig. 21.1 shows a comparison between wristed instruments and standard minimally invasive instruments.

NOTE *A number of companies and research groups are active in the development of wristed instruments for MIS that do not require a motor or robotic controls.*

The robotic instruments are maneuvered from the surgeon console. However, the surgical technologist and assistant surgeon are responsible for attaching and detaching an instrument from its arm using clutch controls on the arm. Systems also provide a method of manually removing an instrument without using the clutch in case of malfunction.

TYPES OF INSTRUMENTS

Like MIS, RAS requires fewer instruments than open surgery. Many laparoscopic procedures are performed with 6 to 10 instruments, plus stapling and energy instruments. Specialties such as cardiac, ear-nose-throat, vascular, and neurosurgery do require a larger *variety* of instruments for MIS and robotic procedures. This is due to the variety of tissue types and structures.

The most common instruments used in general, urological, and gynecological surgery are shown in Fig. 21.2. These include common categories: graspers, scissors, needle drivers, forceps, and dissectors.

REPROCESSING ROBOTIC INSTRUMENTS

Reposable robotic instruments can only be reprocessed a designated number of times. After that they must be disposed of in the same category as sharps (e.g., blades, hypodermic needles, suture needles). The number of times an instrument can be reprocessed. varies according to the instrument and the manufacturer. A robotic instrument that has reached the maximum number of uses cannot be activated. The number of uses is digitally tracked. Instrument inventory, including the number of uses remaining on each instrument, is managed by a designated member of the robotics team. Electronic monitoring and re-ordering ensures a ready supply of replacement instruments.

The reprocessing procedure must be followed strictly according to the manufacturer's guidance to ensure sterility and prevent damage to the instrument, which may result in patient injury.

HAPTIC FEEDBACK

Haptic refers to the sense of touch. In open and conventional MIS procedures the surgeon relies on a sense of touch to provide cues and obtain information about the tissues within the surgical wound. These cues are transmitted to the surgeon's hand either directly by palpation or through the surgical instruments. The skills needed to interpret the texture, resistance, and size of structures in the surgical wound are developed along with the technical skills needed to perform the surgery.

Some robotic systems such as the da Vinci do not feature **haptic feedback.** Without it, the surgeon must rely on visual cues alone. Some robotic surgeons who have trained on systems without haptic feedback have adjusted to this. Others would prefer to perform robotic procedure *with* haptic feedback. A number of companies and research institutions are actively in development of haptic feedback that does not significantly increase the cost of surgery. At least one robotic system in use does have this feature. Others are researching the need and feasibility.

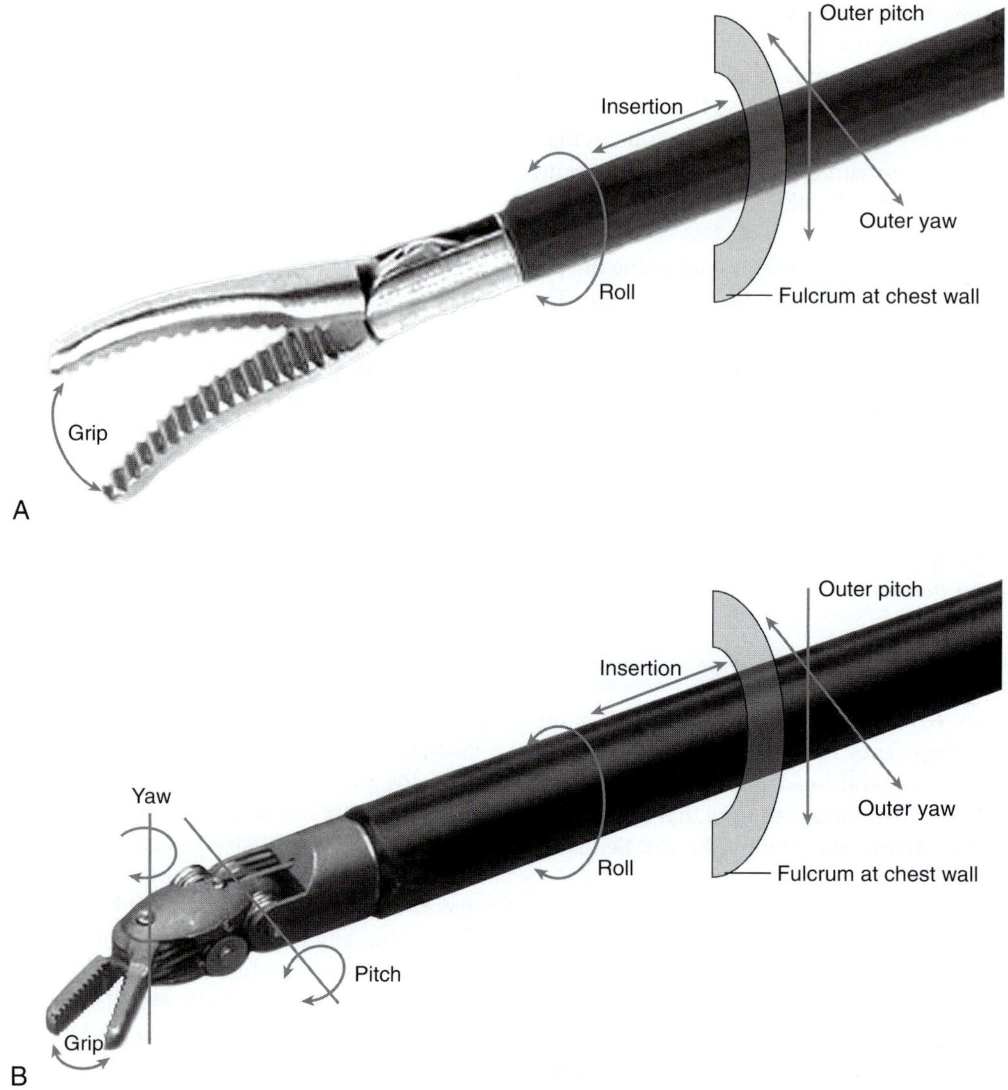

FIG. 21.1 Comparison of robotic and standard MIS instruments. (A) MIS instrument with degrees of freedom. (B) Wristed instruments showing additional degrees of freedom. (Copyright 1999 Intuitive Surgical, Sunnyvale, CA. From Gropper MA. *Miller's Anesthesia*. 9th ed. Philadelphia: Elsevier; 2020.)

RIGID ENDOSCOPE

The rigid endoscope similar to the type used in nonrobotic MIS is available in various lengths, diameters, and viewing angle. The 0-degree and 30-degree endoscopes are used most often. The endoscopic field of vision is displayed in two or three dimensions. This is enabled by both the endoscope and the video equipment, including the display screen. The robotic interface enables a much larger field of vision over standard MIS endoscopes plus the ability to pan in and out.

Endoscope fogging can be a problem during RAS. The ST is responsible for preventing fogging and for troubleshooting fogging problems during surgery. Warmed CO_2 gas used during pneumoperitoneum decreases lens fogging. However, it may be necessary to use a defogging agent, which is applied to the lens. A warm saline bath device may also be used.

NEAR-INFRARED IMAGING

Near-infrared imaging is used during surgery to illuminate anatomical structures. A fluorescing substance (indocyanine dye) is injected intravenously by the anesthesia provider. A near-infrared endoscope is necessary to capture the fluorescent images that are displayed on the monitor. This technique is used to assess local perfusion (blood supply), such as an anastomosis site that the surgeon has just created.

ACCESS

Surgical access refers to the method used to enter the body to perform a surgical procedure. An incision is one form of access. Another form of access is the trocar-cannula (port) system used in MIS. RAS also uses trocars and cannulas compatible with the robotic platform. A robotic platform that uses

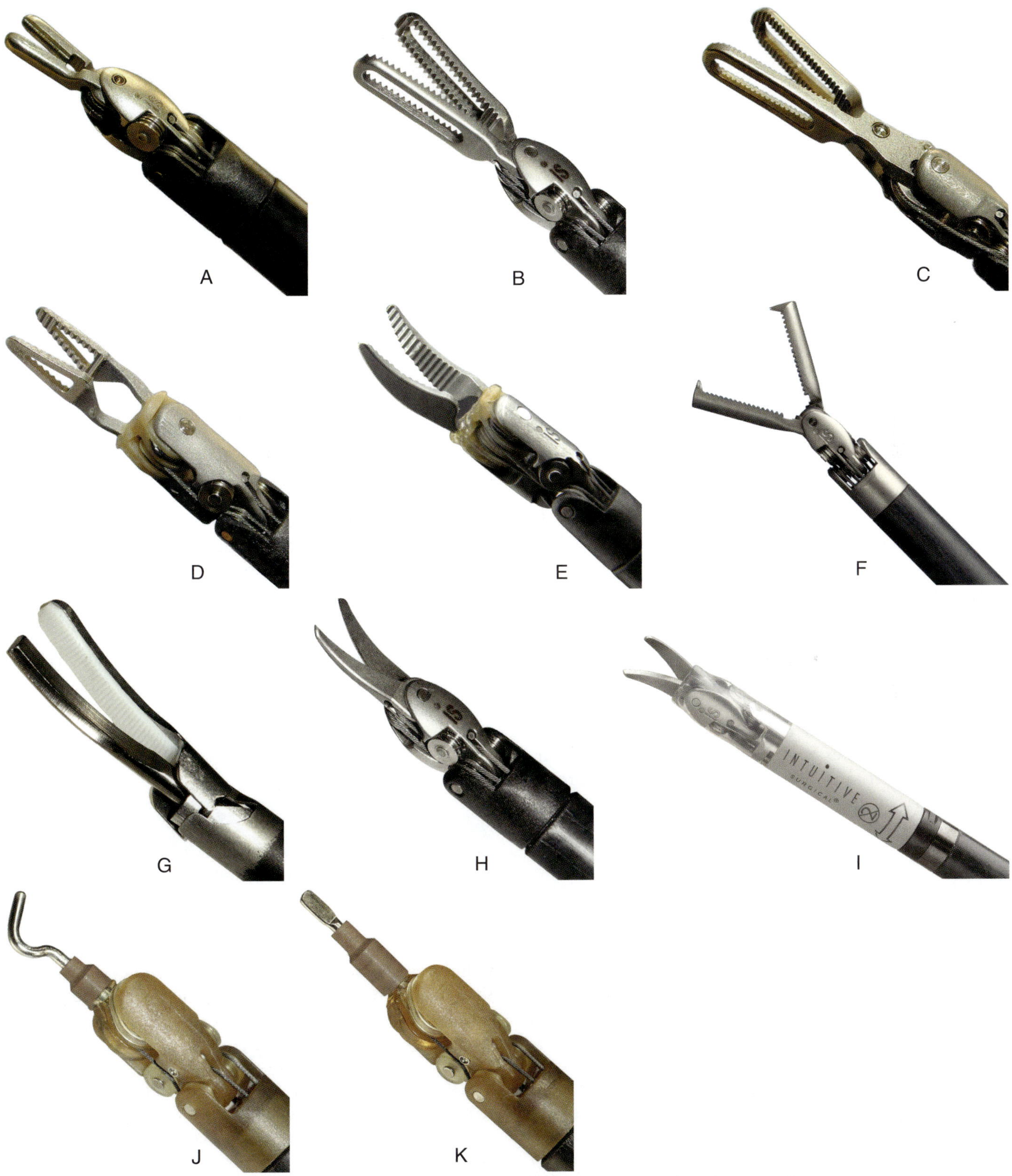

FIG. 21.2 Robotic instruments (da Vinci). (A) DeBakey forceps. (B) Cadiere forceps. (C) Prograsp forceps. (D) Precise bipolar forceps. (E) Maryland bipolar forceps. (F) Toothed forceps. (G) Harmonic shears. (H) Curved scissors. (I) Fine dissecting scissors. (J) Monopolar hook. (K) Monopolar spatula. (Courtesy Intuitive Surgical, Inc., 2007.)

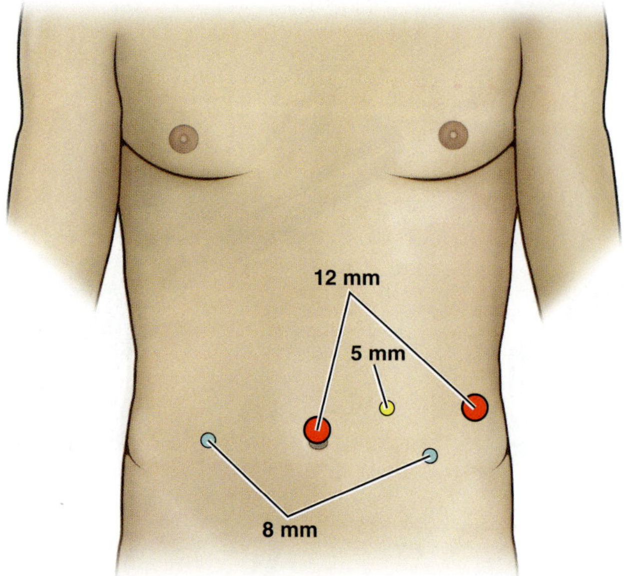

FIG. 21.3 Examples of port placement diagram. This diagram shows the location of two 12-mm ports for the endoscope and robotic trocar (shown in red). Two 8-mm ports and one 5-mm port are placed for additional robotic instruments. (In Partin AW, et al., eds. *Campbell Walsh Urology.* 12th ed. St Louis: Elsevier; 2021.)

nonrobotic, minimally invasive instruments (such as the *Senhance* system) can use any trocar-cannula system.

INITIAL ACCESS

Port placement is performed ahead of robot docking as the first step in a robotic procedure in which a body space is entered. The types, number, sizes, and configuration of the access ports are noted on the surgeon's preference card. Robotics companies also provide illustrated diagrams for port placements. An example is shown in Fig. 21.3. The surgical technologist assists the surgeon and assistant surgeon with port placement.

REVIEW OF PNEUMOPERITONEUM AND PORT PLACEMENT

Pneumoperitoneum is required to enlarge the potential space in the abdomen or thorax to enable MIS and robotic procedures. It prevents injury to the viscera during surgical access and provides working space for the instruments. The steps for pneumoperitoneum and port placement are reviewed here.

Recall from Chapter 20 that the Veress needle is a closed method of establishing pneumoperitoneum. The needle consists of a very small spring-loaded trocar, which is used to puncture the abdominal wall through a small stab incision. Once the needle is inside the body cavity, a small amount of saline is lightly injected or dropped into the needle hub. The abdominal cavity is normally under *negative pressure.* If the Veress needle has not entered the visceral tissues, the saline will be sucked into the abdominal cavity. If the needle has been driven into tissues, the saline will not flow. After the correct position of the needle is validated, the CO_2 tubing

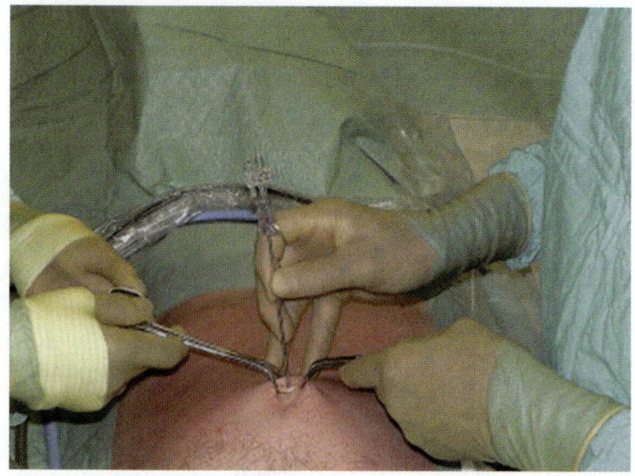

FIG. 21.4 The Veress needle is inserted to initiate pneumothorax. (From Smith R, Singh S. Abdominal access techniques [including laparoscopic access]. *Surgery [Oxford].* 2009;27[6]:237–242. doi:10.1016/j.mpsur.2009.05.002.)

may be attached to the needle and the gas streamed into the abdomen through a calibrated pressure valve. When the desired pressure has been reached, the needle is replaced with a trocar, which is sealed at the body wall to prevent the escape of gas.

The Hasson technique is an *open* procedure. The blunt Hasson trocar is inserted carefully into the abdominal wall through an incision. It is sutured in place and the CO_2 delivered directly into the abdomen through the trocar.

The steps for Veress needle technique are as follows:

1. The abdominal wall is elevated using towel clamps.
2. A stab incision is made and the Veress needle or Hasson trocar is placed in the abdominal wall (Fig. 21.4).
3. The CO_2 tubing is connected.
4. Once the endoscope has been placed, it is used to view the insertion of additional trocars to prevent injury to the viscera.

TYPES OF ROBOTIC AND COMPUTER-ASSISTED SYSTEMS

Robotic and computer-assisted surgical systems are available for many different surgical specialties. Some are used in *hybrid* procedures, in which robotic technology is used for a portion of the surgery or to perform a single task, while standard MIS or open techniques are used for other steps. The surgical technologist should be aware of the types of systems that are available.

VERSIUS (CMR SURGICAL)

The Versius (CMR Surgical) is a robotic-assisted surgical system. Surgery is performed using wristed instruments that are controlled by the surgeon from the console and enabled by a computer interface.

The system features modular (freely moveable) bedside carts for wristed instruments and the robotic endoscope (Fig. 21.5). The vision system features 3-D viewing through special glasses. The surgical non-haptic instruments are reposable, and the system uses compatible energy devices. The system encompasses an open-console design that allows the surgeon to adopt an

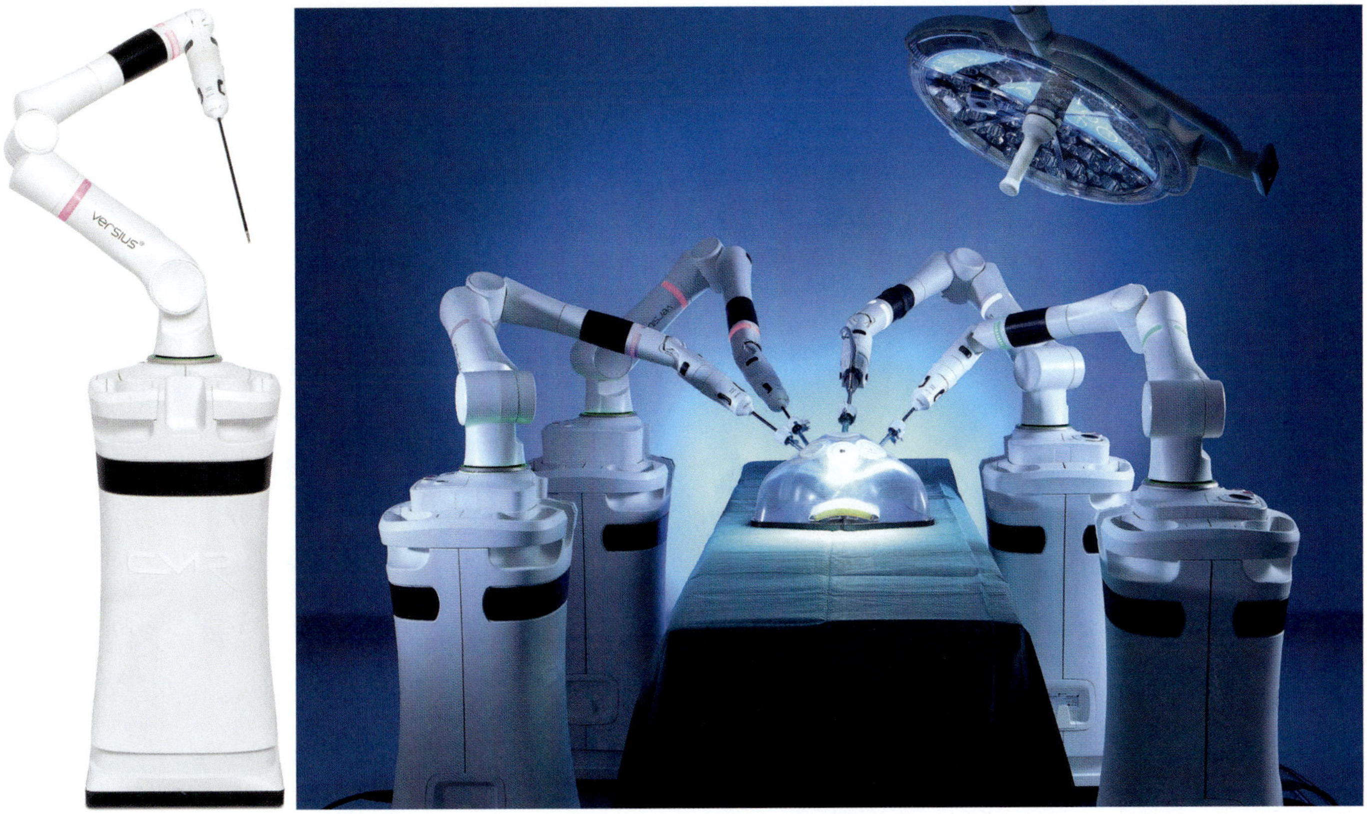

FIG. 21.5 Versius robotic system. This system features modular bedside carts for each instruments. The carts are freely moveable. Setup and turnover time is reduced. (CMR Surgical.)

ergonomically beneficial position throughout the procedure, whether standing or sitting at the surgeon console (Fig. 21.6). The freely moveable bedside carts can be positioned as needed for a particular procedure. Fig. 21.7A and B shows the system in use during surgery. Note that the robotic arms feature color-coded rings. These colors correspond to icons visible on the screen monitor, indicating which instrument is active in a specific arm.

DA VINCI SYSTEMS (INTUITIVE, INC.)

The *da Vinci* system uses similar technology. However, the system uses a single bedside (patient) cart with multiple instrument arms mounted on a boom from a central column (Fig. 21.8A, B, and C). It has a closed surgeon console with 3-D viewing (Fig. 21.8D). The instruments are reposable, and the system uses energy devices compatible with each model. The da Vinci system does not have haptic feedback.

The da Vinci system has been in use for over two decades, and several models have evolved over the years. It received FDA approval for many different surgical specialties. However, since the da Vinci patents have expired, other companies and systems are available, with more to come with different technologies and cost-containment features.

SENHANCE (TRANSENTERIX, INC.)

The Senhance system is labeled as a *robotic-assisted digital system*. The Senhance features an open surgeon console and uses standard minimally invasive instruments and trocar-cannula systems (Fig. 21.9A). It is a modular system with freely moveable bedside carts for each instrument and the endoscope. The instruments are *reusable*. The robotic component provides precise, scaled, tremor-free instrument control and haptic feedback. The endoscopic camera is controlled by *robotically enabled eye-tracking*. The surgeon can shift the camera's field of vision by moving his or her line of sight to the desired direction and point. The camera then follows to the new location. Fig. 21.9B illustrates the system in an operating room.

JOINT ARTHROPLASTY SYSTEMS

Robotic assistive systems used in joint arthroplasty perform specific technical tasks required during surgery. These types of systems can be divided into three categories: *passive, semi-active,* and *active*. A passive system is one in which the robot holds the jig in a pre-planned location on the bone while the surgeon makes the cuts using manual tools. A semi-active system uses haptic feedback to restrict the volume of the cuts. In this type the surgeon is controlling the cuts. Using an active system, the robotic instrument performs the cuts without intervention by the surgeon, although he or she can stop the process at any time.

Orthopedic systems with a robotic interface are used to enable accurate bone preparation and tissue balancing for total or partial joint replacement. The systems produce images of the patient's skeletal anatomy, plan bone cuts required, and execute the plan during the surgical procedure (Fig. 21.10).

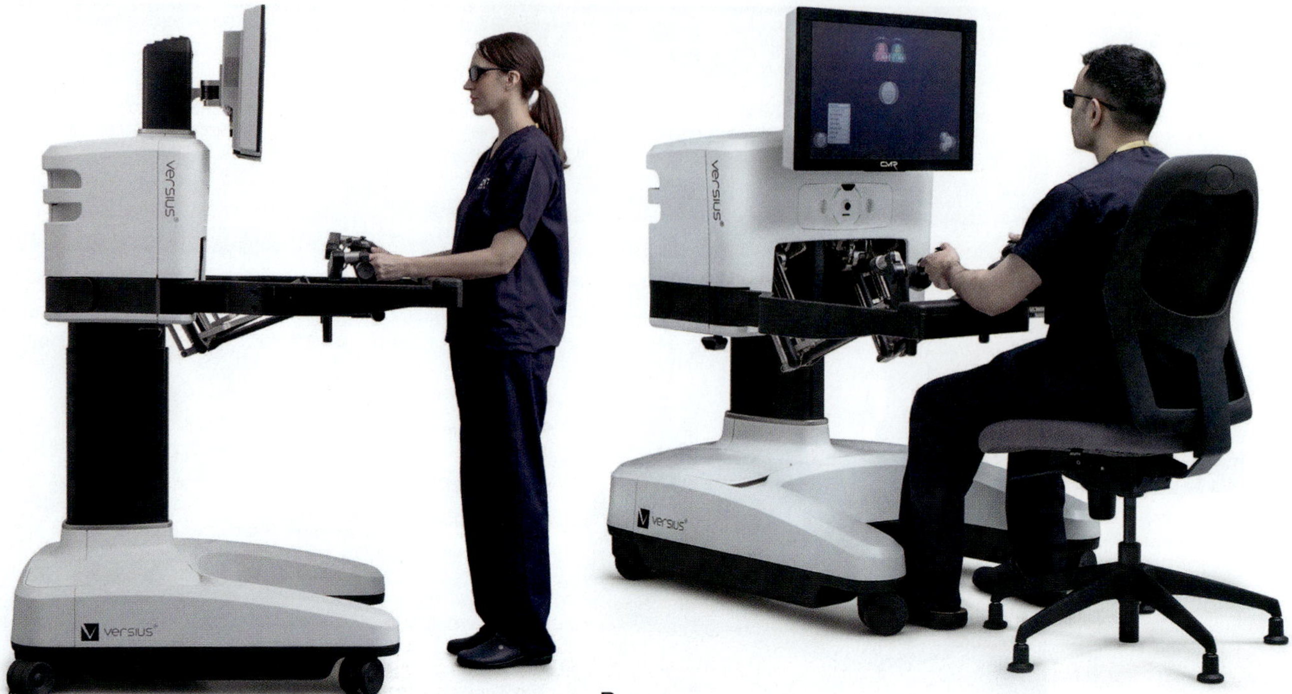

A B

FIG. 21.6 Versius surgeon open console. (A and B) The surgeon can operate standing or sitting. (CMR Surgical.)

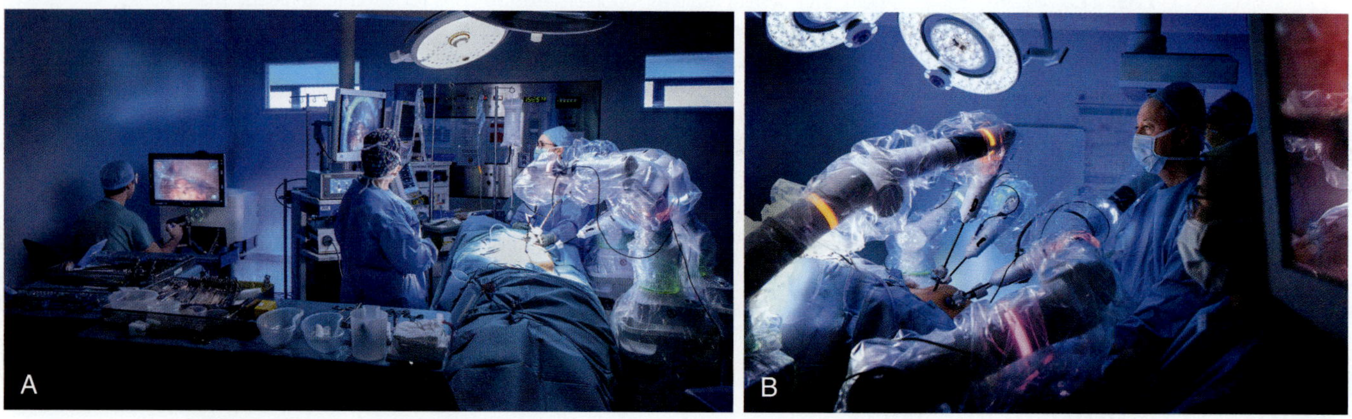

FIG. 21.7 Versius setup. (A) Note the arrangement of the patient carts. (B) The Versius arms feature color-coding to indicate which instrument is attached to a particular arm. This information appears on the monitor in the same color. (CMR Surgical.)

The orthopedic computer controlled system is designed to carry out three distinct tasks:

1. Support preoperative CT and other forms of imaging of the diseased joint.
2. Enable the creation of a surgical plan for bone cutting.
3. Perform robotically controlled bone cuts (called *bone milling*). This step may be autonomous or used as a computer-guided system for the surgeon to perform the cuts.

The most commonly used systems are the following:

- NAVIO PFS (Blue Belt Technologies [Figs. 21.11 and 21.12])
- MAKO Robotic Arm Interactive Orthopedic System (Stryker)
- iBlock robotic cutting guide (OMNIlife Science)

FLEX ROBOTIC DRIVE AND MONARCH PLATFORM (MEDROBOTICS, INC.)

The Flex robotic system is a semi-robotic platform that features a flexible endoscope and robotically controlled instruments. The Flex systems are used in transoral and transanal surgical procedures. The system features an outer tube mechanism and flexible instruments. The outer mechanism is supported and stabilized by the system while the surgeon advances it robotically. The endoscope is extremely flexible and therefore able to navigate around complex anatomy. The surgical instruments are passed through the lumen of the scope and managed robotically with a controller. The optics provide high-definition 3-D vision with video streaming.

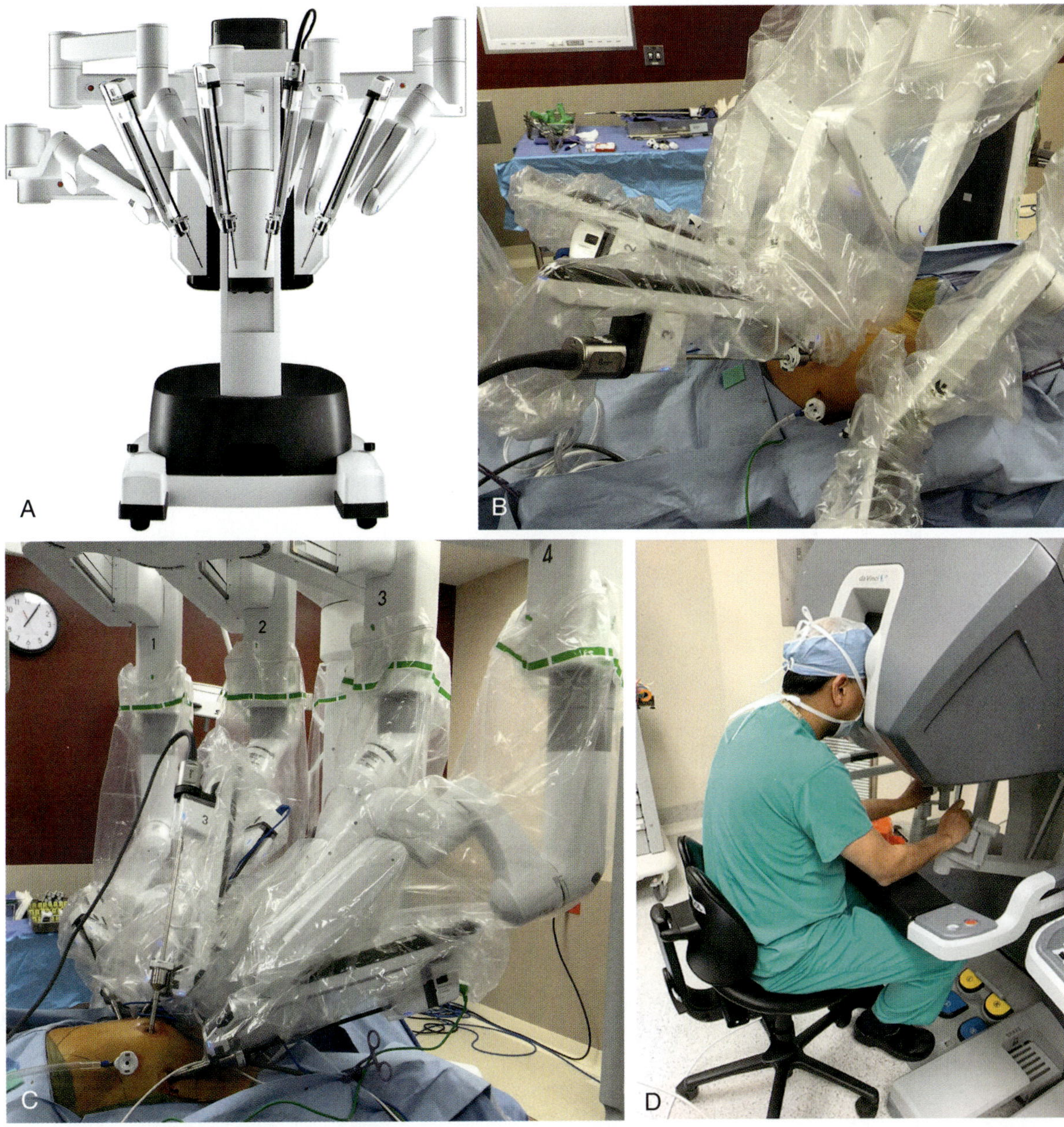

FIG. 21.8 da Vinci system. (A) The bedside cart contains multiple arms (depending on the model) mounted on an overhead boom attached to a central column. The cart is motorized and steered from the back. (B and C) The patient cart is docked in position that provides optimal space for the instruments to be maneuvered during surgery. (D) The da Vinci surgeon console is closed using a cockpit-style viewer. (C, Courtesy Intuitive Surgical. D, From Shah JP, et al. *Jatin Shah's Head and Neck Surgery and Oncology*. Philadelphia: Elsevier; 2020.)

Fig. 21.13 shows the system. The Flex drive is capable of complex procedures including radical resection.

The Monarch Platform (Auris Health) is similar to the Flex systems. The Monarch is a robotically controlled bronchoscope with a high degree of flexibility and HD 3-D vision. The platform is used in peripheral bronchoscopy for taking biopsies and in some therapeutic procedures.

PREPARATION FOR SURGERY

Immediate preoperative preparation for a robotic procedure requires enough time to set up the components and allow the camera to warm. A room design is pre-planned for standardization of each type of robotic procedure. Each component and its connecting cables are considered in the plan.

ROOM LAYOUT

The room layout is a carefully planned map that designates the operative location of each component of the robotic system, connecting cables, and other accessories required for the procedure. The following are considered in planning:

1. Anesthesia care provider access to the equipment, patient's airway, and monitoring sites

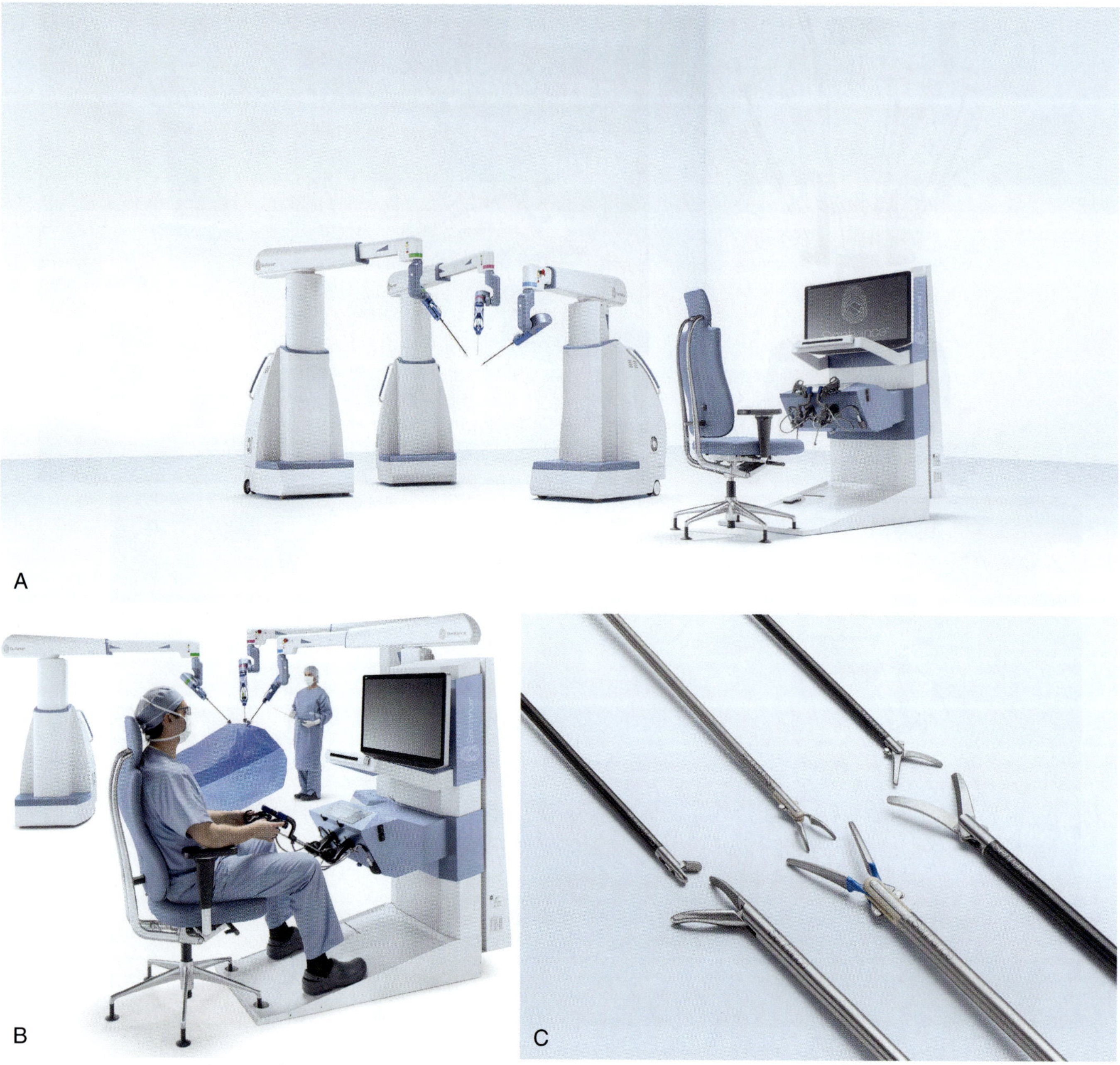

FIG. 21.9 Senhance Robotic System (TransEnterix). (A) The Senhance features modular bedside carts. (B) Open console. (C) The system uses standard minimally invasive instruments, which are reusable. (D and E) Senhance setup. (C, Courtesy TransEnterix. D and E, From Darwish I, et al. A roadmap for robotic-assisted colon resection in diverticular disease using a Senhance surgical robotic system: results and technical aspects. *J Robotic Surg*. 2019;14:297–304. doi:org/10.1007-019-00980-9.)

2. Components and devices that will be part of the sterile field and those that will not
3. Distance between sterile and nonsterile areas and surfaces required to maintain the sterile field
4. Separation between sterile and nonsterile areas of the room
5. Position of sterile equipment in relation to the doors
6. Equipment access to electrical outlets, each component requiring a separate dedicated circuit
7. Cords and cables positioned to prevent trip hazard or damage caused by running heavy equipment over them

HAZARDS ASSOCIATED WITH CROWDING

Crowding of equipment and personnel in the robotic operating room can be a real hazard to the patient and surgical team. During an emergency in which a robotic procedure is converted to an open case, the surgical team must be able to obtain the required equipment quickly and enough space allowed to open supplies while maintaining sterile technique. Robotic components must be moved back from the patient and stowed. This requires a logical plan for room layout from the start of every case. Each facility

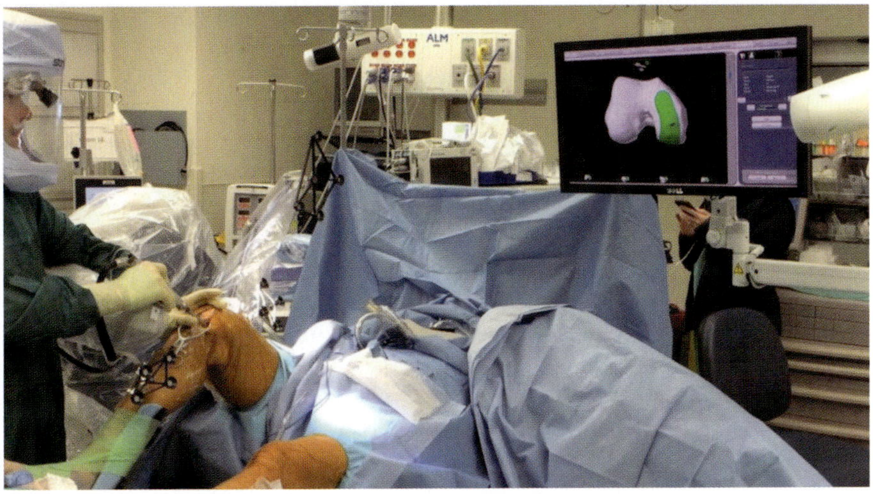

FIG. 21.10 Robotic-assisted knee arthroplasty. (From Roche M. Robotic and sensor-assisted technologies in knee arthroplasty. *Oper Tech Orthop*. 2015;25:[2]:127–149.)

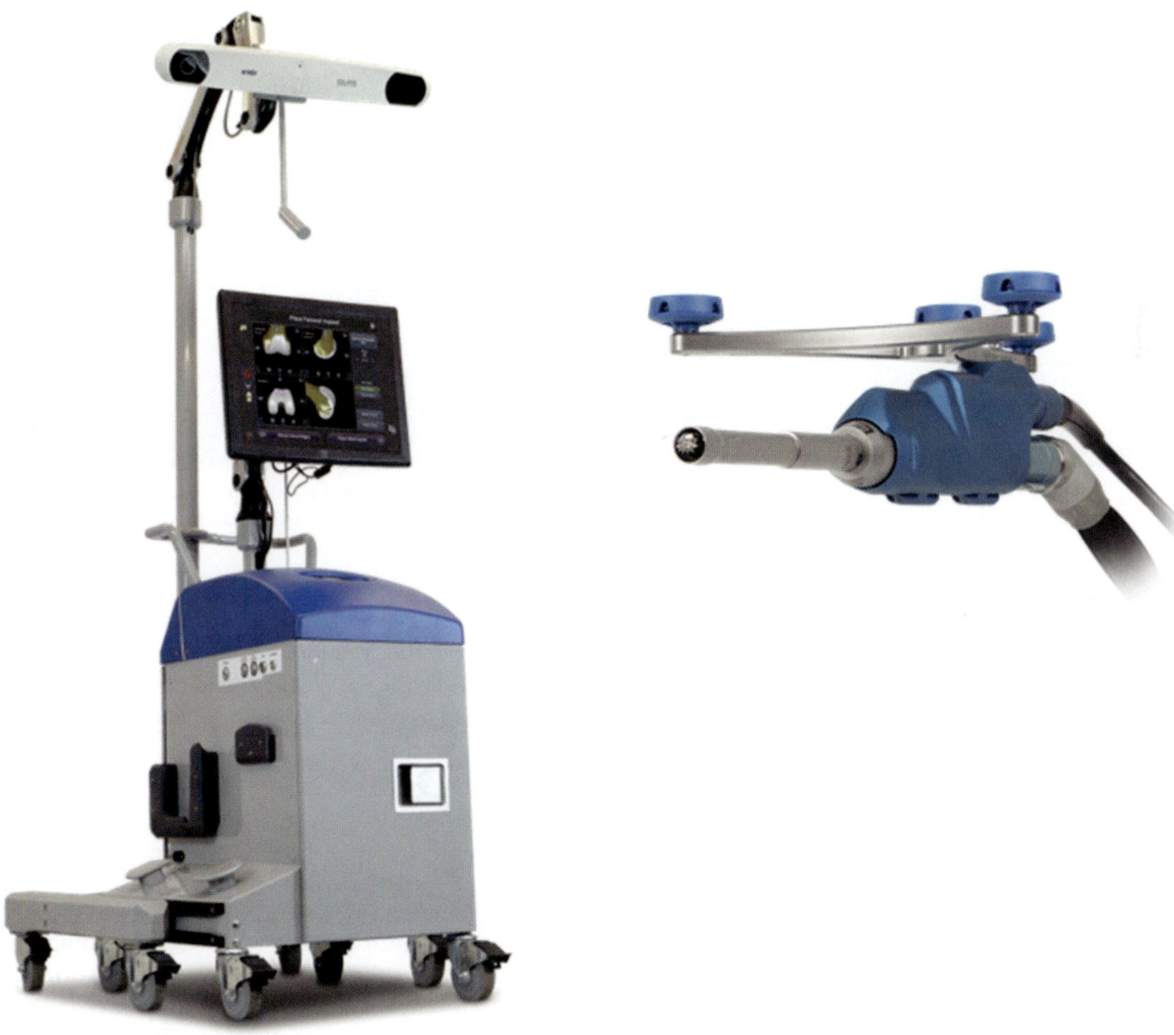

FIG. 21.11 NAVIO system and robotic-assisted tool. (From Mitra R, Jaramaz B. NAVIO Surgical System—handheld robotics. *Handbook of Robotic and Image-Guided Surgery*. Amsterdam, Netherlands: Elsevier; 2020.)

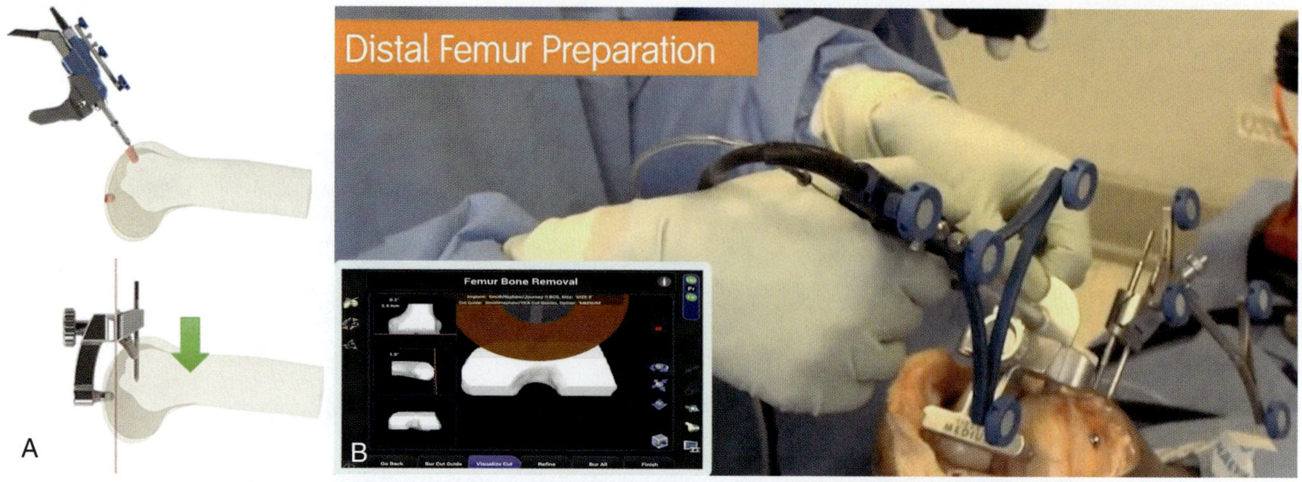

FIG. 21.12 NAVIO system. (A) The system prepares locking procedures on the patient anatomy according to the surgical plan. The locking cut guides are used in preparation for the saw cuts. (B) The surgeon confirms the saw cut using the locators according to the prothesis plan before proceeding. (From Mitra R, Jaramaz B. NAVIO Surgical System—handheld robotics. *Handbook of Robotic and Image-Guided Surgery*. Amsterdam, Netherlands: Elsevier; 2020.)

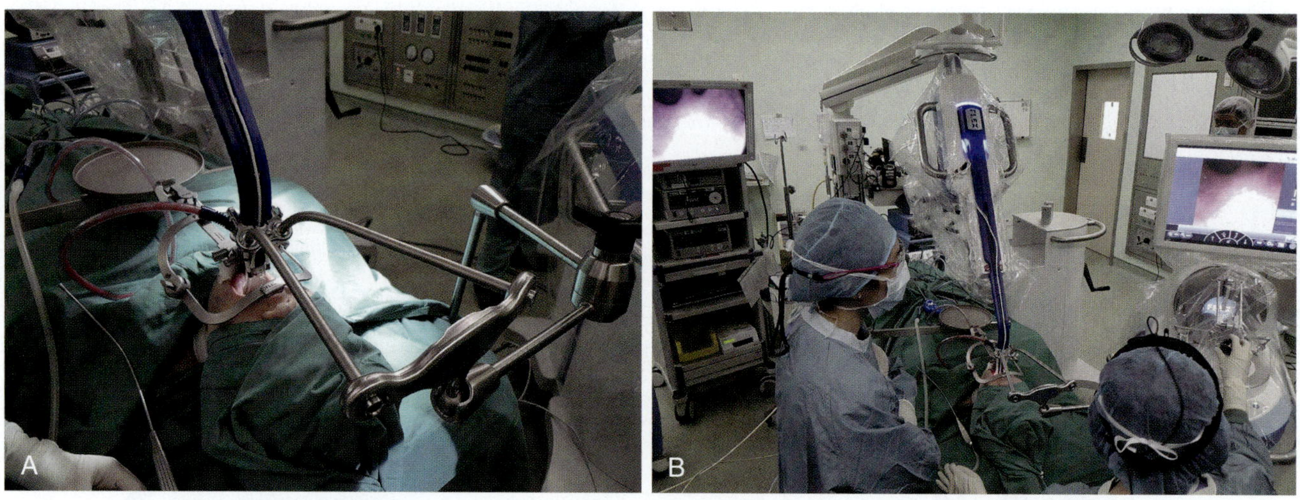

FIG. 21.13 Flex robotic system. (A) Operating room and equipment setup. (B) Flex system retractor. (From Sheng BTW, Wong P, and Hoon CTE. Transoral robotic excision of laryngeal papillomas with flex robotic system – a novel surgical approach. *Am J Otolaryngol;* 2018 39[3]:355-358.)

develops its own layout according to existing design and traffic patterns.

SURGEON CONSOLE

The surgeon console must be positioned where the surgeon can see the sterile field. This is required so that he or she can observe any unintended movements or events such as collisions of the instrument arms. There should be a clear path between the console and the main door so that the surgeon can move quickly to perform surgical hand antisepsis in the event of an emergency requiring the surgeon at the sterile field.

BEDSIDE CART

The *bedside* or *patient cart* is positioned strategically according to the surgical procedure with room to back a cart away from the surgical field in an emergency. Modular carts such as those used in the Versius and Senhance systems are plotted differently from the da Vinci patient cart, which has multiple arms attached to a single column. The anesthesia team must be consulted during planning for the layout to ensure that the equipment does not block access to the patient's airway or monitoring lines.

EQUIPMENT TOWER

The equipment tower connects to other components by cords and cables. *Cord management* is essential for efficient movement of staff and equipment. Cords and cables should never be tangled or knotted. This is both an electrical hazard and a physical impediment to staff. Excess length should be coiled neatly and secured where it cannot trip anyone.

SECTION III: THE PATIENT

PATIENT POSITIONING

Patient positioning for any surgery requires strict attention to detail to prevent injury. Positioning for robotic procedures can multiply the usual concerns because of the exaggerated positions required. In addition, unless an integrated operating table is used (see below) or the system does not require docking, the position cannot be changed once a robot has been docked.

Anti-skid devices must be used for all robotic cases in which there is a risk of the patient slipping in any direction. These are discussed in Chapter 16.

Many robotic transperitoneal and pelvic procedures require lithotomy position as shown in Fig. 21.14. In these cases, Allen Yellofin stirrups are used. A split-leg position may also be used if one of the robotic components is positioned between the patient's legs or if it is necessary for one of the team members to assist from this position. The split-leg position is shown in Fig. 21.15.

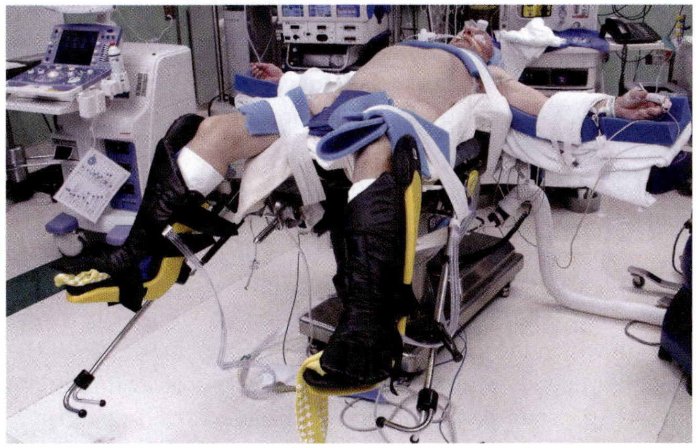

FIG. 21.14 Patient positioning for robotic pelvic surgery. In most procedures, the patient is placed in severe Trendelenburg before starting surgery. (From Corvera C. *Blumgart's Video Atlas: Liver, Biliary & Pancreatic Surgery*. Elsevier Health Science, 2020.)

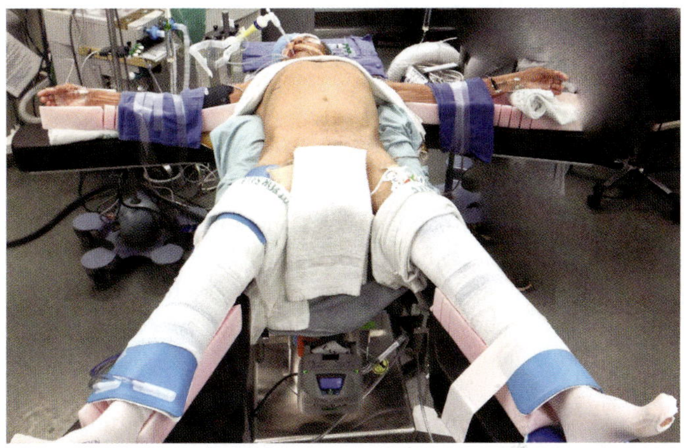

FIG. 21.15 Split-leg position when one of the robotic components is positioned between the patient's legs or if it is necessary for one of the team members to assist from this position. (From Corvera C. *Blumgart's Video Atlas: Liver, Biliary & Pancreatic Surgery*. Elsevier Health Science, 2020.)

REPOSITIONING THE PATIENT DURING SURGERY

During conventional minimally invasive surgery in which robotic instruments are not used, surgery, the operating table can be repositioned as needed within the parameters of safety and according to the patient's condition. During RAS, which requires the instrument arms to be docked and locked in place, the operating table must not be moved, because this would result in patient injury. A robotic-compatible table has been developed to operate with the da Vinci Xi robotic system. The Trumpf Medical TruSystem 7000dV OR Table is integrated with the Xi system to allow the table to move with the instrument arms without undocking the robot. This feature is particularly advantageous in procedures that require lateral tilt, such as low anterior resection of the colon.

The surgical technologist positions the Mayo stand at the side or foot of the operating table. As with all surgical procedures, the ST must prevent devices that are kept on the field during a procedure from falling. Drape pockets should be used at all times.

SKIN PREP AND DRAPING

The skin prep for robotic procedures is similar to *nonrobotic* procedures. Transperitoneal and thoracic robotic surgery may extend beyond the customary prep boundaries to accommodate the trocar-cannula systems. In *nonrobotic* procedures, body hair is seldom removed. However, robotic procedures often require hair removal with clippers. This is performed in the patient preparation area before surgery.

Drapes for robotic procedures are disposable. Equipment drapes are provided by the system's manufacturer and are designed to fit over the contours of the sterile components. All drapes are clearly marked to facilitate the draping process. Robotic patient drapes are patterned in the same configuration as nonrobotic drapes. However, the top drape is fitted with side pockets for stowing energy devices (e.g., ESU, vessel-sealing system, ultrasonic dissector).

EMERGENCIES DURING ROBOTIC SURGERY

RAS presents unique problems with regard to intraoperative emergencies. All minimally invasive procedures, including robotic procedures, are planned with the expectation of converting to an open case in an emergency. Sterile equipment and supplies needed for a conversion are kept just outside the room. As discussed above, the operating room is arranged with a clear path to the doors, and staff are specifically oriented and trained on their responsibilities during an emergency.

TECHNICAL PROBLEMS

Technical problems, which arise from malfunction or failure of an instrument or device, can occur in any surgery. RAS requires complex technical systems, which can fail in spite of the many safety features that are built into the system.

Loss of vision can create extreme risks, especially during highly vascular dissection or suturing. Instrument failure or a system error may not result in patient emergency, but it requires attention and may result in conversion to an open procedure.

SURGICAL PROBLEMS

The greatest cause of concern and most common cause of conversion to an open case is hemorrhage. Unlike open surgery, in which the surgeon can usually locate the source of the bleeding quickly and take measures to control it, minimally invasive procedures are much more problematic. In open surgery, retraction of the body wall and the ability to pack the viscera away from the target anatomy enable quick location of the bleeding vessel. Laparotomy sponges can be placed immediately over the area and pressure applied to temporarily staunch the flow of blood. The closed working space and small instruments used in MIS may not allow effective tamponade (pressure) over the bleeding area, and finding the source of bleeding is more difficult because immediate exposure of the tissues is limited.

PROBLEMS RELATED TO ANESTHESIA

Pneumoperitoneum can cause serious complications during the procedure. These include decreased lung capacity related to the displacement of the abdominal viscera toward the thorax. Extreme Trendelenburg used in many cases can also create edema of the upper body and face.

Large robotic systems can reduce access to the patient's upper body and airway. Monitoring lines may be difficult to maintain because of crowding. A patient cart positioned at the patient's head or shoulder can completely obstruct access to the patient's chest, which may be required for cardiac compression. The large footprint of some systems may also obstruct emergency equipment such as the crash cart and defibrillator.

CONVERSION TO AN OPEN CASE

The decision to convert to an open case is announced by the surgeon. This sets the team in motion for specific tasks and responsibilities. These are established by each facility according to the systems they use and their specific operating room layout.

SCRUBBED SURGICAL TECHNOLOGIST DURING CONVERSION

Surgical technologists, along with the entire team, must know what their responsibilities are during an emergency conversion to an open case. Preparation for emergencies is organized by the robotics coordinator or committee as part of the program planning. Guidelines must be available for all staff members who participate in robotic cases. The procedures are normally discussed in detail during staff orientation and training.

Accuracy is very important during an emergency. This means deliberate movements with purpose and focus to avoid errors, which cost time. In general, the scrubbed surgical technologist must quickly and smoothly receive sterile instruments and supplies, separate those needed immediately, and prepare them for the surgical field as usual. He or she may or may not assist in detaching the robotic instruments from the patient. The assistant surgeon may be required to do this, depending on the emergency plan.

NOTE *Refer to Chapter 18 for a description of waived counts during a surgical emergency.*

SECTION IV: THE ROBOTICS TEAM

The addition of a robotics program in a health facility can involve considerable investment and staff efforts. Facilities that undertake such a program establish a robotics team to coordinate and manage the different activities required. A large program requires a multidisciplinary robotics committee, which provides oversight on training, credentialing, marketing, safety, and administrative tasks. Small programs may only need a group of trained individuals and a coordinator.

ROLES OF THE SURGICAL TEAM

Roles and responsibilities of the robotics surgical team are similar to nonrobotic teams. Team members are identified as *sterile* and *nonsterile* (scrubbed or nonscrubbed). The specific responsibilities of each team member are somewhat modified in RAS.

SURGEON

The surgeon is responsible for the overall plan and supervision of every procedure. She or he leads the team through the different procedural steps and coordinates the team as a whole. However, the surgeon's responsibilities are divided between sterile and nonsterile activities. While operating at the bedside (the patient and operating table), she or he is a scrubbed member of the team. While operating from the nonsterile surgeon console, the surgeon is a nonscrubbed team member. From this position, he or she directs the scrubbed team requesting repositioning of instruments, the addition of new instruments, and assignment of specific instruments to a particular robotic arm. The surgeon directs the assistant surgeon in specific tasks such as retraction and suctioning.

ASSISTANT SURGEON

The assistant surgeon (AS), who works routinely with one or more surgeons who perform RAS, is often the point person for communication about the specific needs and requirements for a case (case planning). In the immediate preoperative stage of a surgical procedure, the AS is active in the preparation of the robotic equipment and selection of instruments. He or she also assists with patient positioning. After performing surgical hand antisepsis, the AS assists in patient draping and alignment of the robotic system with the patient. He or she remains at the patient bedside during the surgery and is also responsible for patient safety at all times.

Most robotic procedures include placement of an assistant's port for additional instruments to be managed by the AS. The surgical technologist and AS work together to swap out robotic instruments during the case. If a problem arises with the equipment, the AS and surgical technologist troubleshoot the problem and resolve it immediately or initiate the next step according to the protocol.

At the close of surgery, the AS remains at the beside during withdrawal of anesthesia and assists as needed.

ADVANCE PRACTICE PROVIDERS

Advance practice providers (APPs) are licensed by states to practice under the supervision of a licensed physician, including surgeons. They are used in rural areas or other regions where there is a shortage of medical doctors and surgeons. The state-licensed physician's assistant (PA) and licensed perioperative nurse practitioner may be trained specifically for this role by the surgeon who has hired him or her and by the robotic company. This role may require the APP to perform the same tasks as the assistant surgeon. At the time of this writing, individual states are responsible for setting the educational standards and legal requirements for the licensed APP surgical assistant.

CIRCULATING NURSE

The usual role of the circulating nurse is not altered during RAS. He or she remains in the nonsterile role as for any other procedure. Above all, the circulator is responsible for direct patient care, protecting the sterile field, and assisting the anesthesia provider as needed. He or she also assists in setting up the robotic equipment and in preoperative testing as needed. Other duties depend on the procedure and robotic system in use. Some systems require **docking** the robotic cart containing the instrument arms (driving the instrument cart or bedside cart into position at the operating bedside). The circulating nurse is responsible for driving the base unit or patient cart into place under the guidance of the surgical technologist.

During surgery the circulator performs all the routine tasks required of the role as described in Chapter 18. This includes extensive documentation of the case, management of nonsterile equipment, obtaining drugs and medications, opening sterile equipment and devices when they are needed, and managing communication between the surgeons and others outside the surgical suite. In an emergency the circulator initiates the appropriate actions as required, including patient care and protection.

Immediately after the end of surgery, the circulator assists in moving the robotic equipment away from the bedside and providing direct patient care. The circulating nurse may accompany the patient to the postanesthesia care unit and complete tasks as outlined in Chapters 18 and 19.

ROBOTICS COORDINATOR

The robotics coordinator is a registered perioperative nurse who is highly trained and experienced in robotic surgery. In a small program she or he is responsible for directing and coordinating the robotics program for the health care facility. The coordinator establishes protocols according to professional guidelines and facility policies. He or she develops the training program for staff and is actively involved in the training. The coordinator also ensures that new staff develop the knowledge and skills required for their responsibilities and that trained staff participate in continued professional development. She or he responds during emergencies that arise during RAS and assists immediate problem solving with backup from the robotic company's emergency hotline.

ROLE OF THE SURGICAL TECHNOLOGIST IN ROBOTIC-ASSISTED SURGERY

The surgical technologist usually assists in RAS in the scrubbed role. However, the exact duties may differ among facilities. An experienced ST who has acquired advanced knowledge and skills in robotic technology may participate in sterile or nonsterile roles within the practice laws of state (refer to Chapter 4), facility policy, demonstrated professionalism, and appropriate supervision where necessary. In general, the ST performs the same tasks as in any type of surgery with variations according to the specific nature of RAS. Box 21.1 provides a list of tasks that may be assigned during RAS.

PREOPERATIVE PREPARATION

During the preoperative preparation for a robotics case, the ST plans for the case with the assigned circulating nurse. Using the surgeon's preference card, all equipment, medical devices, and instruments are pulled in readiness. Supplies to be opened in the immediate preoperative period are separated from those that must be held back for use later in the case or those that must be available in case of an emergency (see later). During preparation the ST checks the robotic equipment with the circulating nurse. Both should also check the room layout, including the cords and cables.

After surgical hand antisepsis, gowning, and gloving, the ST performs the usual sterile preoperative tasks. These include setting up the sterile equipment and supplies and draping the robotic equipment. The first steps of a surgical procedure include placing the endoscope and the other instrument ports. Some systems require programming the alignment of the instrument arms with the central column (da Vinci system) and moving the patient or side carts into position so that the instruments can be attached to the ports. The ST is responsible for guiding the patient or side cart into position, while the circulating nurse manages the cart. From that point forward, the ST works with the assistant surgeon in standard tasks highlighted in Chapter 20.

Tasks that are specific to RAS include swapping out robotic instruments and troubleshooting any faults that occur with the equipment. These may include crowding or collision of instrument arms. The ST must also maintain the sterile field at all times and ensure patient safety.

BOX 21.1 Possible Roles for Members of the Robotics Team

PREOPERATIVE NONSTERILE DUTIES	ST	RN	SA
Picking the case	x	x	
Laying out the case (going over the equipment)	x	x	x
Nonsterile preparation of the robotic components	x	x	x
Nonsterile positioning and calibration of robotic components	x	x	x
PREOPERATIVE STERILE DUTIES	**ST**	**RN**	**SA**
Case setup	x		
Draping the robotic equipment	x	x	
Patient skin prep		x	x
Checking the camera	x	x	
INTRAOPERATIVE STERILE DUTIES	**ST**	**RN**	**SA**
Patient positioning		x	x
Targeting the robot (da Vinci)	x		
Patient draping	x		x
Assisting with access (entry)	x		x
Placing trocars			x
Docking patient cart (da Vinci)	x	x	x
Manage cords and tubing	x		
Establish and maintain sterile field	x		
Troubleshooting robotic faults	x	x	x
Trouble shooting case problems (arm collisions, space problems, etc.)			
POSTOPERATIVE NONSTERILE DUTIES	**ST**	**RN**	**SA**
Ensuring patient safety	x	x	x
Removing tissue debris and prep solution from patient's skin	x		x
Patient transfer to stretcher	x	x	x
Prepare instruments for decontamination	x		
Manage robotic equipment	x	x	

Note: These are *in addition* to standard roles and tasks.
RN, Registered perioperative nurse; *SA*, surgeon's assistant; *ST*, surgical technologist.

COMMUNICATION DURING ROBOTIC SURGERY

Communication between members of the surgical team during robotic surgery is a well-studied subject. Poor communication is a deterrent to team cohesion and, ultimately, patient safety. The problem arises from separation of the scrubbed team and the surgeon who operates from a nonsterile console away from the sterile field. In this position the surgeon is sometimes unable to see the patient or anesthesia provider. The problem is made worse with a periscope-type *closed* console, in which the surgeon places his or her head within the console and is fixed on the stereo viewer. Instead of speaking face-to-face to the team members, the surgeon's voice is projected through speakers. Nonverbal communication ceases and problems are further worsened by ambient noise in the operating room, which is at times loud enough to drown out speech.

Many new robotic system designs, such as the Versius, include an open console, which allows the surgeon eye contact with the assistant surgeon and surgical team. These have been developed following research on team communication using closed console systems. Robotic teams are now more aware of the problems that arise from the surgeon's isolation. Refer to Chapter 2 for a complete discussion on team communication.

ROBOTICS TRAINING

Training in robotics can take place through a number of paths. Private and public institutions now offer training courses, which include hands-on experience with the equipment. Continuing professional development is available from many sources. Manufacturers of robotics systems offer online and on-site courses tailored for all members of the surgical team. This is an important source for training in a specific system. The surgical technologist may receive some training as a student and extended training on the job. It is very important that the ST researches the structure and learning objectives of all courses taught outside of their structured training programs. These include courses outside your school, surgical facility, or programs offered by the robotic system manufacturer. Course sponsors should state not only the *measurable outcomes* of the course but also the methods used to teach the courses.

KEY CONCEPTS

- Robotic surgery is a general term that refers to many different types of systems that use computer technology to perform or guide the surgical procedure. However, the FDA makes a clear distinction of those systems that actually control or manipulate the surgical instruments. A robotic-assisted surgical (RAS) device uses computer technology and software to control and manipulate surgical instruments.
- As surgical technology continues to become more complex, the surgical technologist will be required to acquire more in-depth understanding of complex digital systems.
- Only about 30% of surgical procedures are performed as open surgery. The rest use minimally invasive techniques, including robotic-assisted procedures.
- Robotic-assisted surgery (RAS) uses optical systems, which provide a larger field of vision over conventional minimally invasive procedures. The image captured by the endoscopic camera can be scaled according to the surgeon's requirements.
- Most computer-assisted systems are not autonomous. The surgeon remains in control of the instruments.

- RAS has many similarities with minimally invasive surgery (MIS). A solid grounding in minimally invasive procedures is the first step in assisting in RAS.
- The surgical technologist is an active member of the robotics team. More advanced skills and knowledge are required as compared to MIS.
- One of the main differences between the da Vinci systems and newer technologies is the structure of the "patient cart," which, in the da Vinci model, has multiple arms mounted on a single motor-driven base. A modular system has a separate base for each instrument arm and can be moved easily without a motor.
- The surgeon's console contains all of the controls needed to perform surgery. The closed console is one in which the surgeon must place his or her head inside a hood or cockpit while operating. The open system resembles a computer monitor and is not hooded. The same controls are available on each.
- Wristed instruments are a feature of many robotic systems. The wristed instrument has 7 degrees of movement and resembles a human hand in flexibility.
- Robotic instruments can represent a significant recurring cost. This is because each instrument is designed to fail after a finite number of times it is reprocessed. This is a safety feature required to prevent malfunction resulting from normal wear and tear of the electronics required to operate the instrument. Most instruments can be used up to 10 times, depending on the system.
- Robotic instruments are reprocessed in accordance with the manufacturer's instructions. Steam sterilization is the most common method.
- Haptic feedback is the sense of touch. The technology required to enable the surgeon to feel tissues, suture, and supplies though the computer interface is extremely complex. Some systems feature haptic touch, whereas others do not.
- Surgical access in robotic-assisted systems is identical to those of MIS. However, the trocar/cannula systems must be compatible with the system in use.
- The number and type of surgical procedures that can be performed using RAS and MIS nearly equal those of open surgery. However, complex and high-risk procedures are usually performed as open cases to prevent the risk of emergency conversion.
- Joint arthroplasty using computer guidance and robotic techniques are becoming commonplace in many facilities. These systems provide superior accuracy during bone sculpting (milling) required to fit the prosthesis.
- Room layout is extremely important when planning surgery. Cords and cables must be managed and equipment placed strategically.
- Patient positioning during abdominal RAS requires critical thinking and the use of specific devices to prevent the patient from sliding on the operating table.
- The most common and dangerous emergency during a robotic procedure is hemorrhage.
- It is necessary to have all equipment needed for a conversion to an open case available at the start of an RAS.
- The role of the surgical technologist during RAS involves many skills that are not used in other specialties.
- Specific training in RAS for the surgical technologist is available from a number of different sources. After learning the basics, the ST must continue to upgrade his or her skills with continuing professional development. This requires hands-on training. Reading is important to learning but is not a replacement for skills training.

REVIEW QUESTIONS

1. What are the advantages of an open surgeon console?
2. Why are there fewer instruments required during robotic-assisted surgery as compared to open surgery?
3. In what ways are the wristed instruments different from standard minimally invasive instruments?
4. What are the *advantages* and *disadvantages* to reposable instruments compared with non-disposable instruments?
5. Compare the Veress needle technique with the Hasson technique. Provide at least four points of comparison to demonstrate your knowledge of these systems.
6. What is the saline (drop) test used in the Veress technique? Why is it necessary?
7. The robotic system provides an endoscopic view which is *scaled*. Explain what this means in practical terms.
8. Explain why the room layout is so important in robotic-assisted surgery.
9. What is a modular robotics system?
10. Explain the benefits of *digital registration* used in some robotic procedures.
11. What is your opinion on the use of robotic systems in modern surgery? Demonstrate your knowledge of the advantages and disadvantages of robotic systems, and use these to form your opinion.

BIBLIOGRAPHY

1. Darwish, Ibrahim, et al. A roadmap for robotic-assisted colon resection in diverticular disease using a Senhance surgical robotic system: results and technical aspects. *J Robotic Surg.* 2019;14:297–304. doi:org/10.1007-019-00980-9.
2. Kamath S, Rachana G. LapCap: A novel device to reduce entry complications. *J Minimally Invasive Gynecol.* 2017;25(4):566–568.
3. Liow Ming Han, Lincoln, et al. THINK Surgical TSolution-One® (Robodoc) Total Knee Arthroplasty. *Sicot-J.* 2017;3:63. https://doi.org/10.1051/sicotj/2017052.
4. Jonathan H. Koenig, Matthew S. Hepinstall, available robotic platforms in partial and total knee arthroplasty. *Oper Tech Orthop*, 2015;25(2):85–94, ISSN 1048-6666, https://doi.org/10.1053/j.oto.2015.03.002. (http://www.sciencedirect.com/science/article/pii/S1048666615000166).
5. Mitra R. *NAVIO Surgical System -- Handheld Robotics. Handbook Robotic Image-Guided Surg.* Elsevier; 2020.
6. Nezhat F. Minimally invasive surgery in gynecologic oncology: laparoscopy versus robotics. *Gynecol Oncol.* 2008;111(2).
7. Partin AW, et al. *Campbell-Walsh-Wein Urology.* Elsevier; 2021.
8. Protyniak, Bogdan et al. The use of robotics in colorectal surgery. In: Abedin-Nasab Mohammad H, ed. *Handbook of Robotic and Image-Guided Surgery.* Elsevier; 2020.
9. Roche Martin. Robotic and sensor-assisted technologies in knee arthroplasty. *Operat Tech Orthopedics.* 2015;25(2):127–149.

10. Shah JP, et al. *Jatin Shah's Head and Neck Surgery and Oncology*. Elsevier; 2020.
11. Shah P. *Bladder Surgery for Benign Disease. Campbell Walsh Urology*. Lee Richstone, Elsevier; 2021.
12. Shah S. Robotic surgery and patient positioning: ergonomics, clinical pearls and review of literature. *Trends Anesthesia Crit Care*. 2017;14.
13. Sheng BT, Constance TH. Transoral robotic excision of laryngeal papillomas with flex robotic system - a novel surgical approach. *Am J Otolaryngol Head Neck Med Surg*. 2018;39(3):355–388.
14. Smith JA, et al. *Hinman's Atlas of Urologic Surgery*. Elsevier; 2018.
15. Wong B, et al. Transoral robotic excision of laryngeal papillomas with flex robotic system - a novel surgical approach. *Am J Otolaryngol*. 2018.

GENERAL SURGERY 22

KNOWLEDGE AND SKILLS REVIEW

The following skills and knowledge should be reviewed before you start this chapter:

- ***Techniques and instruments used in minimally invasive surgery (see Chapter 20)***
- ***Techniques and instruments used in robotic surgery (see Chapter 21)***

LEARNING OBJECTIVES

After studying this chapter, the reader will be able to:

1. Identify the anatomical regions and structures of the abdominal wall
2. Discuss specific elements of case planning for abdominal wall hernias, including instruments and repair materials
3. Discuss specific elements of case planning for gastrointestinal surgery
4. Discuss the purpose and procedure of isolation technique
5. Discuss specific elements of case planning for general surgery procedures

TERMINOLOGY

THE ABDOMEN:

Abdominal peritoneum: The serous membrane lining the walls of the abdominal cavity. The retroperitoneum is the posterior aspect.

Adhesions: Strands of scar (connective) tissue that form between the peritoneum and membranes of abdominal viscera. These occur as a result of inflammation or infection. During abdominal surgery adhesions must be released from their attachments to restore the normal position of the tissue planes and organs involved. This technique may be referred to as lysis of adhesions.

Direct inguinal hernia: A hernia that results from weakness in the inguinal floor.

Fistula: An abnormal tract or passage leading from one hollow organ to another or from an organ to the skin; usually caused by infection.

Hernia: A protrusion of tissue or an organ through an abnormal opening.

Incarcerated hernia: Herniated tissue that is trapped in an abdominal wall defect requiring emergency measures to prevent ischemia and tissue necrosis.

Incisional hernia: The postoperative herniation of tissue through a surgical incision during or after the healing process.

Indirect inguinal hernia: A hernia that protrudes into the membranous sac of the spermatic cord—usually because of a congenital defect in the abdominal wall.

Linea alba: A strip of avascular connective tissue that lies on the abdominal midline.

McBurney incision: An incision in which the oblique right muscle is manually split to allow for removal of the appendix.

Ventral hernia: A weakness in the abdominal wall, usually resulting in protrusion of abdominal viscera against the peritoneum and abdominal fascia.

Viscera: The organs or tissue of the abdominal cavity.

GASTROINTESTINAL SURGERY:

Anastomosis: A surgical procedure in which two hollow structures are joined.

Billroth I procedure: A gastroduodenostomy, or surgical anastomosis, of the stomach and the duodenum.

Billroth II procedure: A gastrojejunostomy, or surgical anastomosis, of the stomach and the jejunum.

Exploratory laparotomy: A laparotomy performed to examine the abdominal cavity when less-invasive measures fail to confirm a diagnosis.

Gastrostomy: A surgical opening through the stomach wall connecting to the outside of the body or another hollow anatomical structure.

Isolation technique: A method of preventing contamination of the sterile field during bowel or metastatic tumor resection.

Laparotomy: A procedure in which the abdominal cavity is surgically opened. The techniques used for laparotomy are used for all open surgical procedures of the abdomen.

Morbid obesity: A condition in which the patient's body mass index (BMI) is 40 or higher, and the individual is at least 100 pounds (45 kg) over the ideal weight despite aggressive attempts to lose weight.

-ostomy: A suffix that refers to an opening between two hollow organs. For example, gastroduodenostomy, a surgical procedure that joins the stomach and duodenum.

Stoma: An opening created in a hollow organ and sutured to the skin to drain the organ's contents (e.g., an intestinal or ureteral

TERMINOLOGY (CONT.)

stoma). A stoma may be a temporary or permanent method of bypass.

Stoma appliance: A two- or three-piece medical device used to collect drainage from a stoma. The appliance is attached to the patient's skin and completely covers the stoma. This allows for free drainage into a collection device or bag.

BILIARY SYSTEM, LIVER, PANCREAS, AND SPLEEN:

Cirrhosis: A disease of the liver in which the tissue hardens and the venous drainage becomes blocked. It usually is caused by chronic alcoholism but may result from other disease conditions.

Lobectomy: Surgical removal of one or more anatomical sections of the liver or lung.

Segmental resection: Anatomical resection of the liver in which segments divided by specific blood vessels and biliary ducts are removed.

BREAST SURGERY:

Body image: In psychology, the way a person sees himself or herself through the eyes of others. A negative body image can severely affect a patient's sense of identity as well as social and personal interactions.

Needle wire localization: A technique used to identify a nonpalpable tissue mass, used in preoperative breast biopsy.

Mastectomy: A procedure in which breast tissue, including the skin, areola, and nipple, is removed, but the lymph nodes are not removed (also called a simple mastectomy).

Modified radical mastectomy: A procedure in which the entire breast, nipple, and areolar region are removed. The lymph nodes also are usually removed.

Radical mastectomy: The entire breast, all axillary nodes, and the chest wall muscles are removed.

Resection: Removal of a portion or all of an organ or other structure.

Sentinel lymph node biopsy (SLNB): A procedure in which one or more lymph nodes are removed to determine whether a tumor has metastasized.

Skin flap: A full-thickness mass or flap of tissue containing epidermis, dermis, and superficial fascia, which is attached to an area of the body where tissues have been removed. As the area heals, the blood supply and tissues of the flap integrate into the recipient site.

Subcutaneous mastectomy: A procedure in which the breast is removed, but the skin, nipple, and areola are left intact (also called a lumpectomy).

Technetium-99: A radioactive substance used to identify sentinel lymph nodes.

General surgical procedures include those of the abdomen and its viscera, the thyroid, and some procedures of the breast. The organs and organ systems involved include the following:

- Abdominal wall
- Gastrointestinal (GI) system
- Biliary system (the gallbladder and associated structures)
- Spleen
- Pancreas
- Hepatic system
- Breast
- Thyroid

Although these regional systems remain in the category of general surgery, the trend increasingly is toward specialization. This is particularly true for bariatric (the medical and surgical treatment of **morbid obesity**), breast, and GI surgery.

The general surgeon may also perform surgery of the superficial tissues of the body, (e.g., lipomas, sebaceous cysts).

SECTION I: THE ABDOMINAL WALL

ANATOMY

The body is divided into semi-closed compartments or cavities that contain specific anatomical structures and organs (Fig. 22.1 and Table 22.1). The cavities are separated by membrane, muscle, and other connective tissue. The *abdominal cavity* contains the abdominal **viscera** (organs). The *pelvic cavity* contains structures of the reproductive, genitourinary, and lower GI systems. The *retroperitoneal cavity* contains the kidneys, adrenal glands, and ureters. The anterior abdominal cavity is separated from the retroperitoneal cavity by the *posterior abdominal peritoneum*.

The abdomen is divided into four major sections, or landmarks, called *quadrants* (Fig. 22.2). This terminology is used by health care workers to describe a specific area of the abdominal cavity. The quadrants are named by location:

- Right upper quadrant (RUQ)
- Left upper quadrant (LUQ)
- Right lower quadrant (RLQ)
- Left lower quadrant (LLQ)

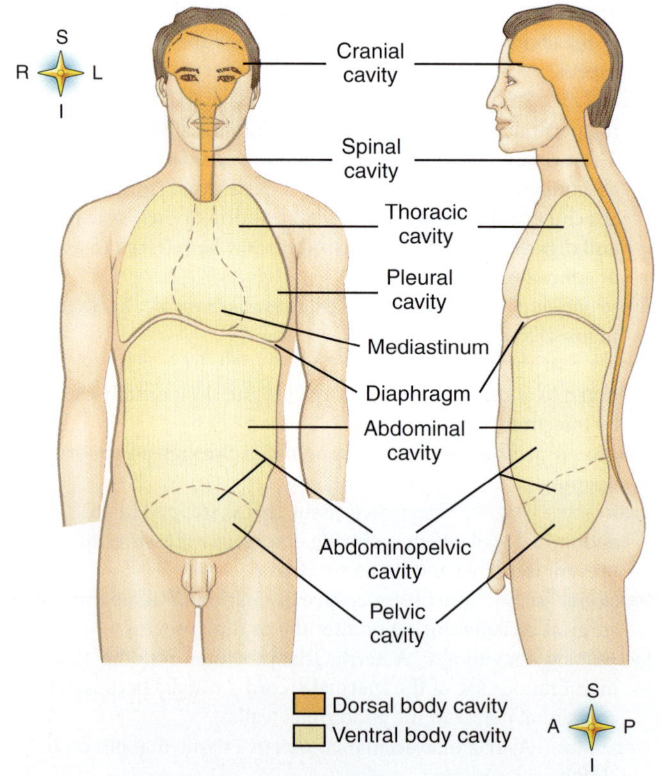

FIG. 22.1 The major body cavities. (See Table 22.1 for the organs contained in individual cavities.) (From Patton K, Thibodeau GA. *The Human Body in Health & Disease*. 6th ed. St Louis: Elsevier; 2014.)

The abdomen is further divided into *nine regions* by an imaginary grid made by two vertical and two horizontal lines (Fig. 22.3):

- Left and right hypochondrium
- Epigastric
- Left and right flank
- Umbilical
- Left and right groin (inguinal)
- Pubic

ABDOMINAL WALL TISSUE LAYERS

The abdominal wall encloses the ventral (front) part of the abdominal cavity and extends from the diaphragm to the pubis. It is composed of distinct tissue layers, which support the abdominal organs (Fig. 22.4). These layers are as follows:

- Skin
- Subcutaneous adipose tissue
- Fascia
- Muscle
- Peritoneum

The *subcutaneous* layer lies directly under the skin. It is composed of lobulated adipose (fat), which varies in thickness from ¼ inch (0.63 cm) to more than 8 inches (20 cm).

The muscles and fascia of the abdominal wall protect the abdominal viscera and move the upper body in flexion and rotation. The muscles also assist in respiration and in "bearing down" during defecation and childbirth. Two longitudinal rectus muscles attach from the pubis to the fifth, sixth, and seventh *costal* (rib) cartilages. Lateral to the

TABLE 22.1 Organs of the Ventral Body Cavities

Body Cavity	Organs
THORACIC CAVITY	
Right pleural cavity	Right lung
Mediastinum	Heart
	Trachea
	Right and left bronchi
	Esophagus
	Thymus gland
	Aortic arch and thoracic aorta
	Venae cavae
	Lymph nodes and thoracic duct
Left pleural cavity	Left lung
ABDOMINAL CAVITY	
Right upper quadrant	Liver
	Gallbladder
	Colon
	Portions of the small intestine
Left upper quadrant	Stomach
	Pancreas
	Spleen
	Colon
	Portions of the small intestine
	Kidneys
	Adrenal glands
	Descending aorta
	Ureters
Pelvic cavity	Ureters
	Uterus and adnexa (female)
	Prostate gland (male)
	Urethra
	Urinary bladder
	Sigmoid colon
	Rectum

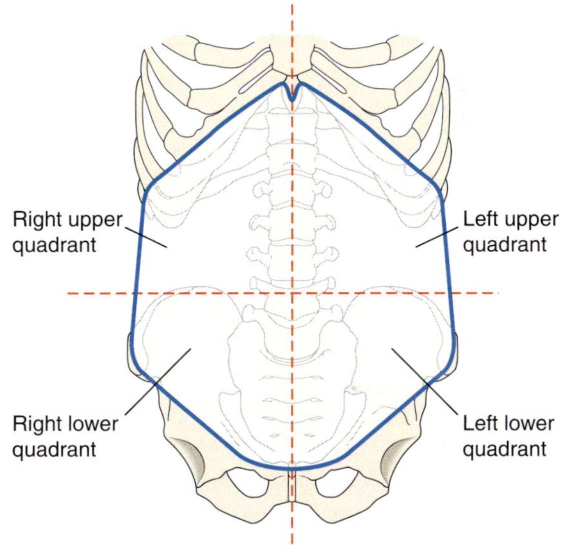

FIG. 22.2 The quadrants of the abdomen. (From Drake RL, et al. *Gray's Anatomy for Students*. 4th ed. Philadelphia: Elsevier; 2020.)

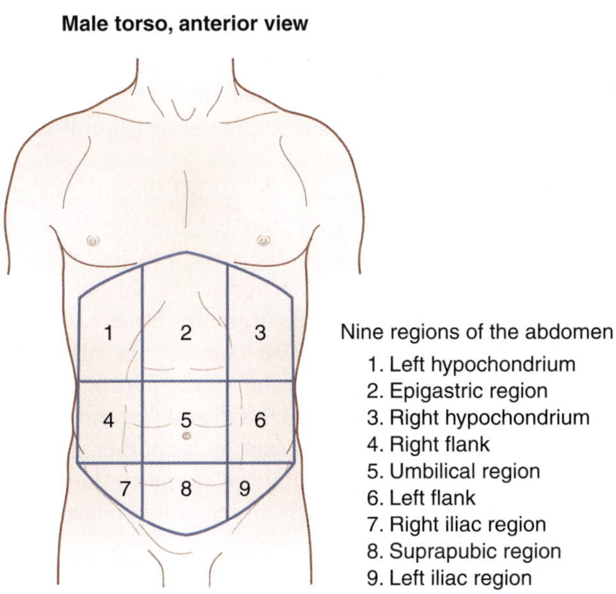

FIG. 22.3 The nine regions of the abdomen.

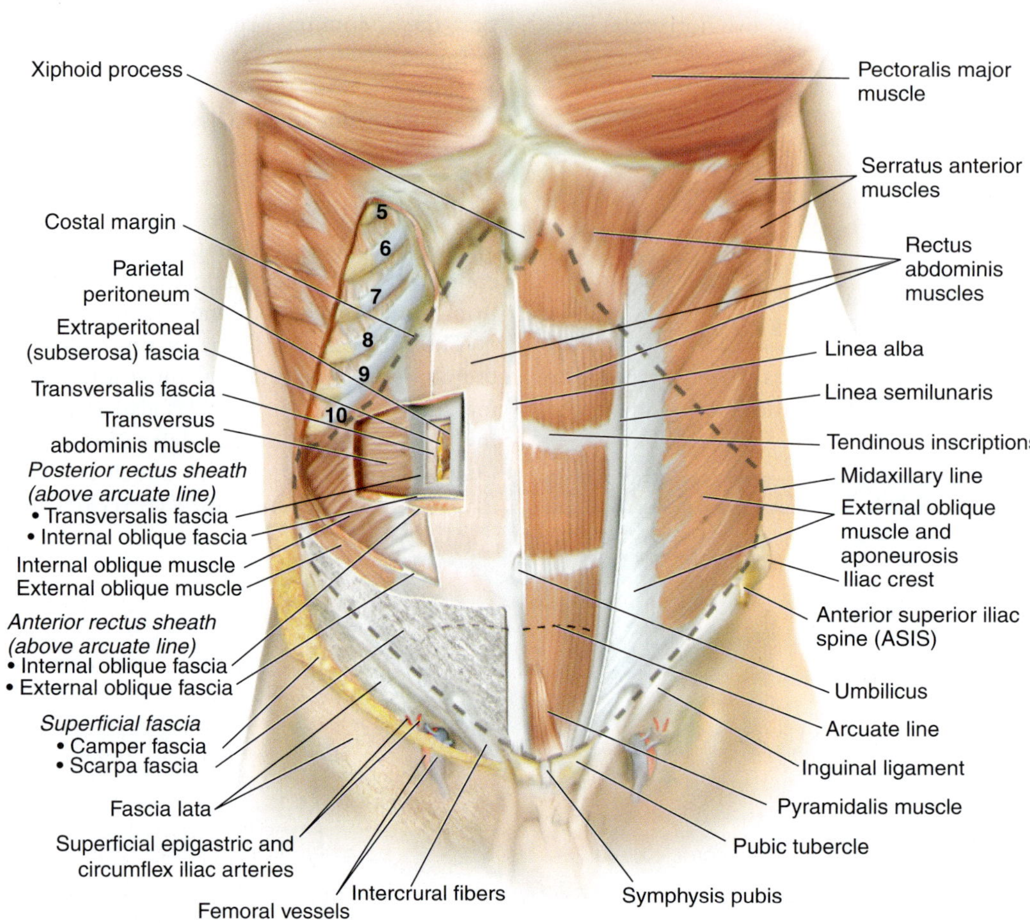

FIG. 22.4 The layers of the abdominal wall. (From Rosen M. *Atlas of Abdominal Wall Reconstruction*. Philadelphia: Saunders; 2012.)

rectus muscles are the three flanking muscles: the transverse external oblique, internal oblique, and transverse abdominis muscles. The muscle groups are interrupted by tendons and surrounded by deep fascia, subserous fascia, and the abdominal peritoneum. The rectus sheath is a broad fascial layer that extends across the abdomen without interruption. The rectus muscles are attached to the rectus sheath close to the midline, or linea alba. This is an avascular band of connective tissue that extends the full length of the midline.

The **abdominal peritoneum** (also called the *parietal peritoneum*) is a strong serous membrane that lines the abdominal cavity. The peritoneum protects the viscera in the abdomen and secretes serous fluid, which lubricates the abdominal structures, allowing them to slide over each other easily. Sections of peritoneum fold back to connect the abdominal organs. The *mesentery* is an extension of the peritoneum that attaches to the posterior abdominal wall and fans out to cover the small intestine. The *greater omentum* is another extension of the serous membrane, covering the stomach, duodenum, and part of the colon. These extensions are often referred to as *peritoneal reflections*.

INGUINAL REGION

The muscles, ligaments, and fasciae of the inguinal and femoral (groin) regions are more complex than those of the central and upper abdomen. A basic understanding of the tissue layers can best be acquired by studying the illustrations included here.

As the fascial layers continue into the pelvis, they pass in front of the two rectus muscles. Here the inguinal canal splits between the muscle layers near the inguinal ligament. The inguinal canal originates at an opening in the transversalis fascia at the deep inguinal ring and continues to the superficial inguinal ring. The *Hesselbach triangle* is the area bounded by the rectus abdominis muscle, the inguinal ligament, and the inferior epigastric vessels. This is the area associated with an inguinal hernia (Fig. 22.5). The space is larger in the male than in the female, which corresponds to the higher incidence of inguinal hernias in males.

The spermatic cord in the male follows the inguinal canal and contains the following structures:

- Ductus deferens
- Artery to the ductus deferens
- Testicular artery

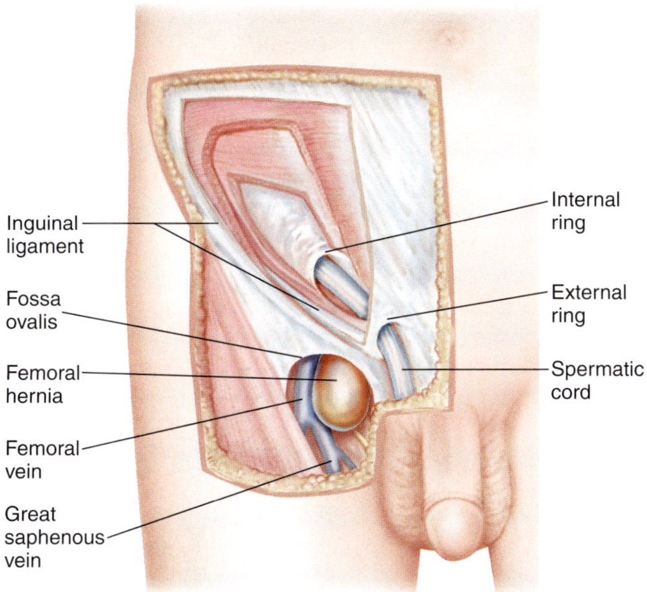

FIG. 22.5 The anatomy of the inguinal region. (From Seidel HM, Ball JW, Dains JE, Benedict GW. *Mosby's Guide to Physical Examination.* 5th ed. St Louis: Mosby; 2002.)

- Pampiniform plexus (testicular veins)
- Cremasteric artery and vein
- Sympathetic and visceral nerve fibers
- Lymphatics
- Remnants of the *processus vaginalis*

ABDOMINAL INCISIONS

Abdominal incisions are named according to their anatomical location (Fig. 22.6 and Table 22.2). Surgical technologists should become familiar with the names of the following incisions:

- Chevron (inverted V and part of the Mercedes-Benz incision)
- Midline (upper and lower)
- Paramedian (right and left)
- Subcostal right and left (also called *Kocher*)
- Inguinal right and left
- Right oblique (also called ***McBurney*** or *appendectomy*)
- Right lower transverse (Rocky Davis)
- Lower transverse (also called *suprapubic* or *Pfannenstiel*)

A variety of sutures can be used on the abdominal wall depending on the patient's BMI and condition as well as surgeon's preference.

Peritoneum: Size 0 absorbable synthetic on a curved needle—running suture.

Fascia: Size 0 or 2-0 synthetic braided suture such as polyester. A cutting or taper needle may be used. Note, however, that if the peritoneum and fascia are closed as one layer, size 0 is preferred.

Muscle: If the incision cuts through muscle tissue, it is closed with synthetic absorbable sutures size 2-0 or 3-0—interrupted sutures.

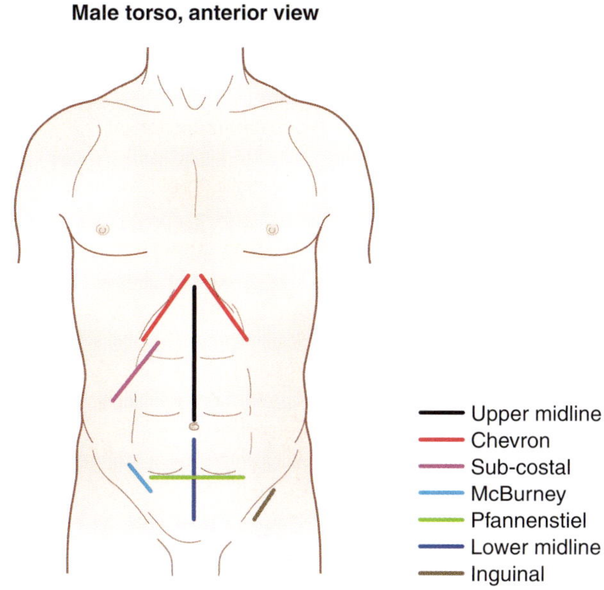

FIG. 22.6 Incisions of the abdominal wall.

Subcutaneous adipose: Synthetic absorbable sutures size 3-0 on a taper needle.

Skin: Staples are used for a noncosmetic closure. Absorbable or nonabsorbable synthetic subcuticular suture is used for a cosmetic closure.

Trocular incisions: The small incisions made to accommodate the trocar/cannulas are closed in two layers. The deep layer is closed with figure-of-8 synthetic absorbable sutures on a cutting needle. Skin is closed with staples or wound strips. Wound adhesive may also be used in combination with Steri-Strips.

GENERAL SURGERY INSTRUMENTS

Many different types of surgical procedures are performed through the abdominal wall. Some of these require instruments that are designed for a surgical specialty, whereas others are used according to tissue type across many different kinds of procedures and anatomical structures. Self-retaining retractors used on the abdominal wall include those that attach to the operating table. A number of systems are available, but all feature right-angle paddles that attach to a frame. These are detachable so that the specific requirements of the surgery and patient profile can be addressed. Commonly used retractor systems are shown in the General Surgery Instruments table.

Open procedures have been replaced by minimally invasive surgery (MIS); at least 70% of procedures are now performed using minimally invasive techniques and instruments. Newly developed technologies, especially in the use of ultrasonic cutting, vessel-sealing systems, and stapling instruments mean that far fewer instruments are required for complex **resection** and anastomosis procedures. Refer to Chapter 20 for minimally invasive instruments used in general surgery.

TABLE 22.2 Types of Abdominal Incisions

Incision	Tissue Layers	Exposure	Details
Midline (upper and lower)	Skin Subcutaneous fat Fascia (linea alba) Abdominal peritoneum	Lower esophagus Stomach Small intestine Liver Biliary system Spleen Pancreas Proximal colon	A midline incision is made through the skin, subcutaneous fat, and the linea alba. This is the center of the fascial layer to which the rectus muscles attach; it is also an avascular area of the rectus sheath.
Paramedian (upper and lower)	Skin Subcutaneous fat Anterior rectus muscles Rectus fascia Abdominal peritoneum	*Right:* Biliary system Pancreas *Left:* Spleen Sigmoid colon	This is a muscle-splitting incision. It is less painful than a subcostal muscle-cutting incision for access to the upper quadrants.
Subcostal	Skin Subcutaneous fat Rectus muscles Fascia Abdominal peritoneum	*Right:* Biliary system Spleen *Bilateral* (chevron): Liver transplantation	This incision follows the lower rib margin in a semicurved shape; it is painful postoperatively.
McBurney	Skin Subcutaneous fat Fascia Oblique and transversalis muscles Abdominal peritoneum	Appendix	This incision is made on the right side, at an oblique angle, in the flank below the umbilicus; it is a muscle-splitting incision and offers only limited exposure.
Inguinal (oblique)	Skin Subcutaneous fat Fascia Muscle Ligaments Peritoneum	Muscles and fascia of the inguinal abdominal wall Spermatic cord Inguinal ring Abdominal ring Inferior epigastric artery and vein	This incision is used to gain access to the inguinal region for hernia repair; it also may be used for internal access to the spermatic cord.
Lower transverse abdominal (Pfannenstiel)	Skin Subcutaneous fat Rectus fascia Rectus muscles	Uterus Adnexa Bladder Access for cesarean section	This incision follows the natural skin folds to achieve cosmetic closure; it is very strong and offers good exposure to the pelvic contents.

GENERAL SURGERY INSTRUMENTS (OPEN)

#3 Bard Parker BP Knife Handle 5″	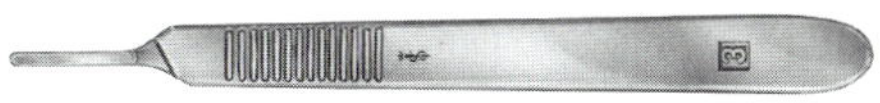 Photo courtesy Aesculap, Inc., Center Valley, PA.	#3-L BP Knife Handle 8″	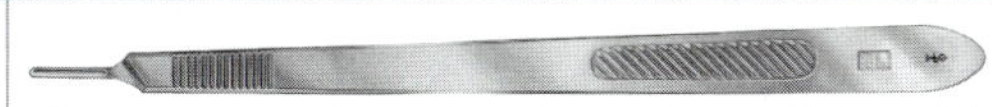 Photo courtesy Aesculap, Inc., Center Valley, PA.
#3- L Angled Knife Handle 8¼″	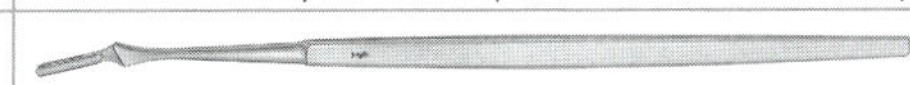 Photo courtesy Aesculap, Inc., Center Valley, PA.	#4 BP Knife Handle 5½″	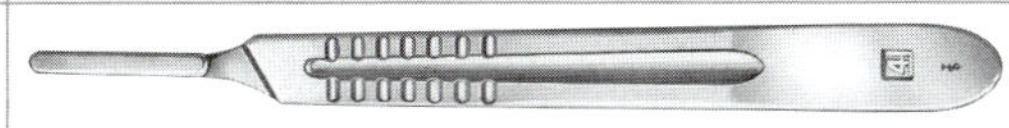 Photo courtesy Aesculap, Inc., Center Valley, PA.
#7 BP Knife Handle 6¼″	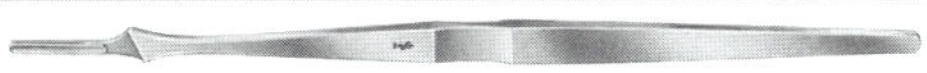 Photo courtesy Aesculap, Inc., Center Valley, PA.	#10 BP Blade	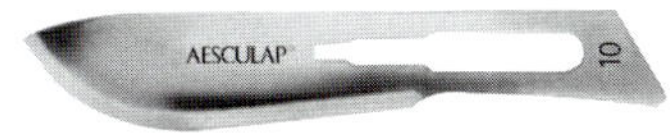 Photo courtesy Aesculap, Inc., Center Valley, PA.
#11 BP Blade	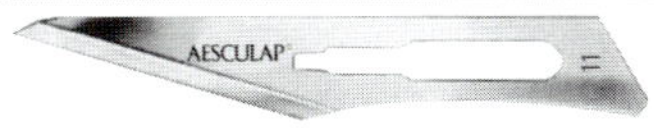 Photo courtesy Aesculap, Inc., Center Valley, PA.	#12 BP Blade	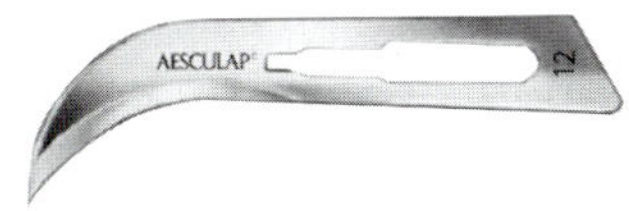 Photo courtesy Aesculap, Inc., Center Valley, PA.
#15 BP Blade	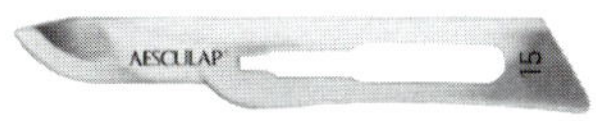 Photo courtesy Aesculap, Inc., Center Valley, PA.	#20 BP Blade	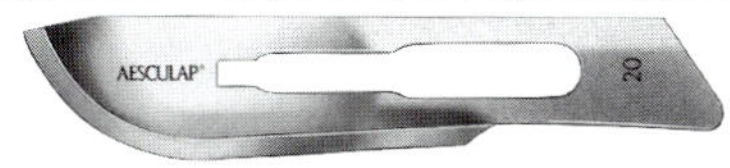 Photo courtesy Aesculap, Inc., Center Valley, PA.
Mayo Curved Scis 5½″	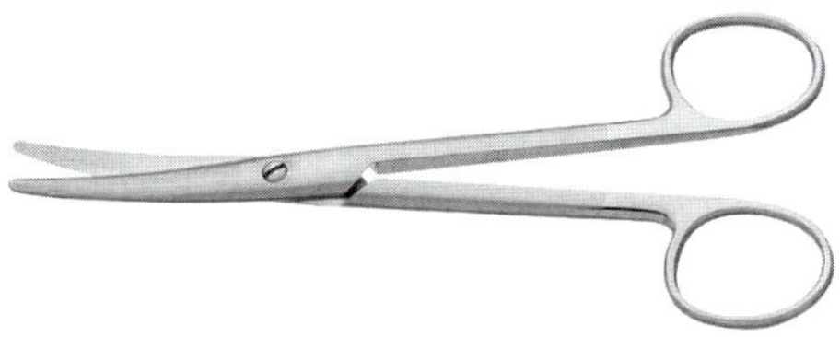 Courtesy and copyright Becton, Dickinson and Company.	Mayo Straight Scis 5½″	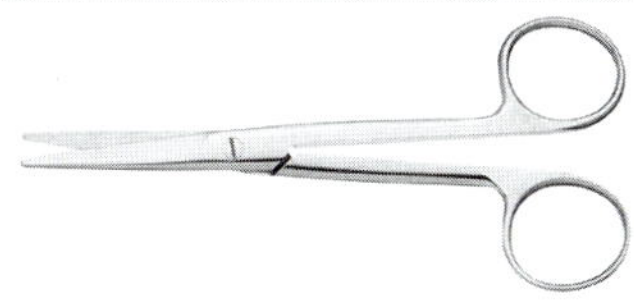 Courtesy and copyright Becton, Dickinson and Company.
Metzenbaum Scis 5¾″, 7″	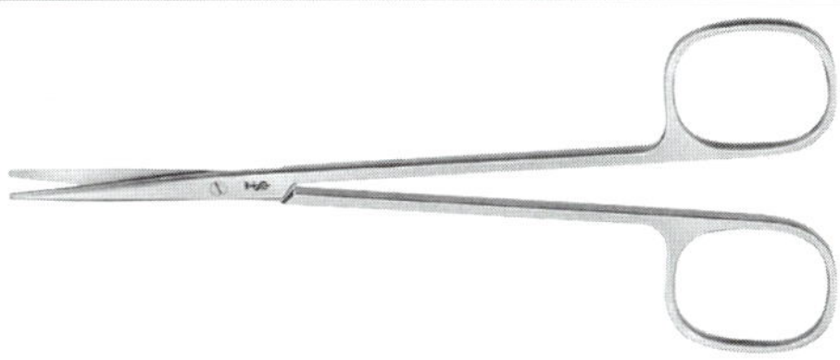 Courtesy and copyright Becton, Dickinson and Company.	Tissue Forcep with Teeth	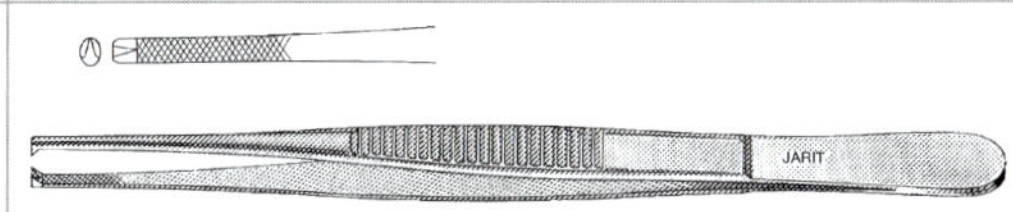 Courtesy Jarit Instruments, Hawthorne, NY.
Short Dressing Fcps Smooth 5½″	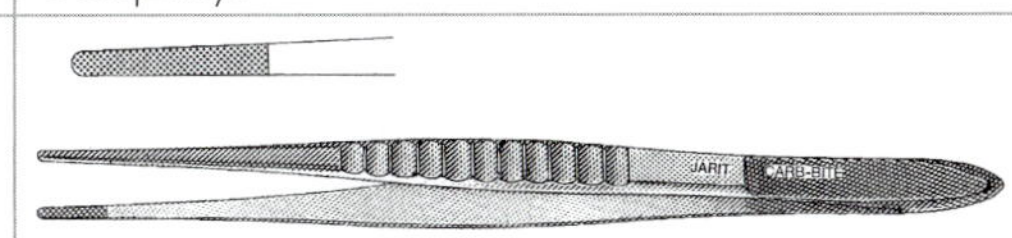 Courtesy Jarit Instruments, Hawthorne, NY.	Dressing Fcps Smooth 10″	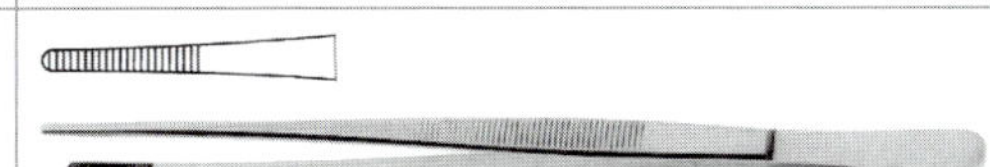 Copyright 2016 Symmetry Surgical Inc.; Photo courtesy Symmetry Surgical Inc.
Adson Fcps 4¾″	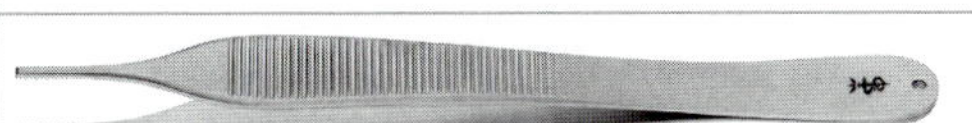 Photo courtesy Aesculap, Inc., Center Valley, PA.	Russian Fcps 6″, 8″	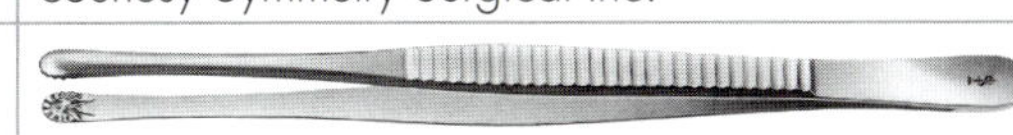 Photo courtesy Aesculap, Inc., Center Valley, PA.
Mosquito Fcps Curved and Straight 5″	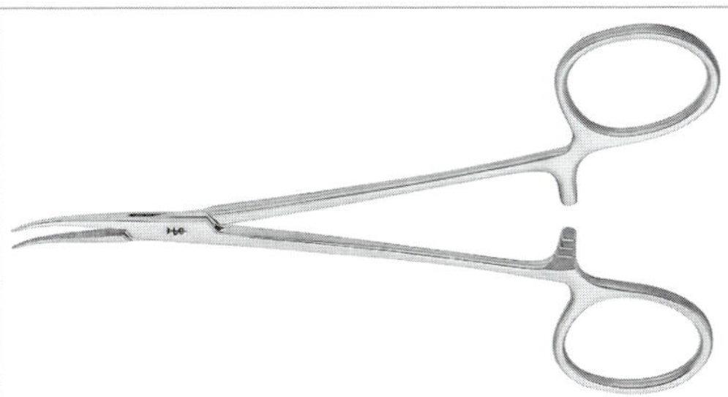 Photo courtesy Aesculap, Inc., Center Valley, PA.	Kelly Fcps Curved 5½″	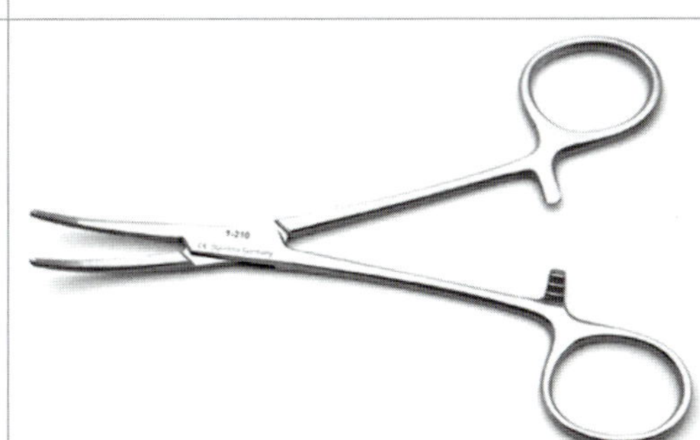 Millennium Surgical Corp.

GENERAL SURGERY INSTRUMENTS (OPEN)—cont'd

<table>
<tr><td>Kelly Fcps Straight 5½″</td><td>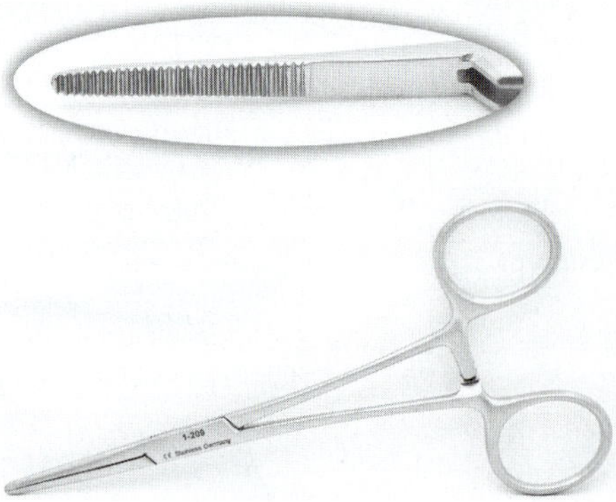
Millennium Surgical Corp.</td><td>Crile Fcps Straight 5½″</td><td>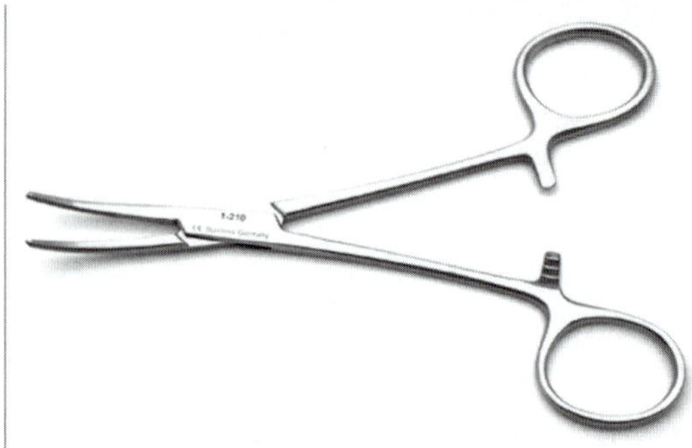
Courtesy and copyright Becton, Dickinson and Company.</td></tr>
<tr><td>Rochester Pean Fcps 8 ⅞″</td><td>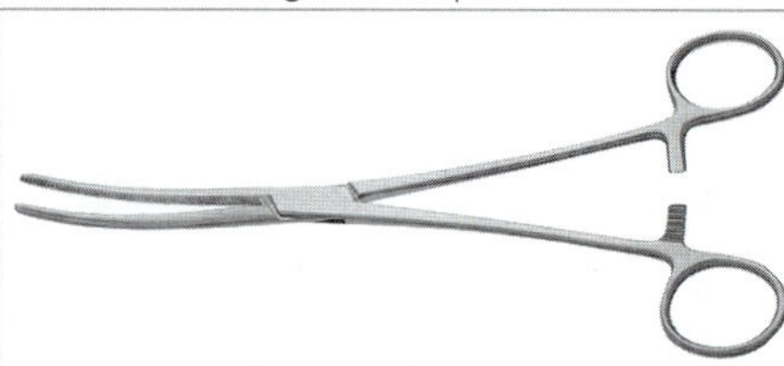
Courtesy and copyright Becton, Dickinson and Company.</td><td>Right angle Mixter clamp</td><td>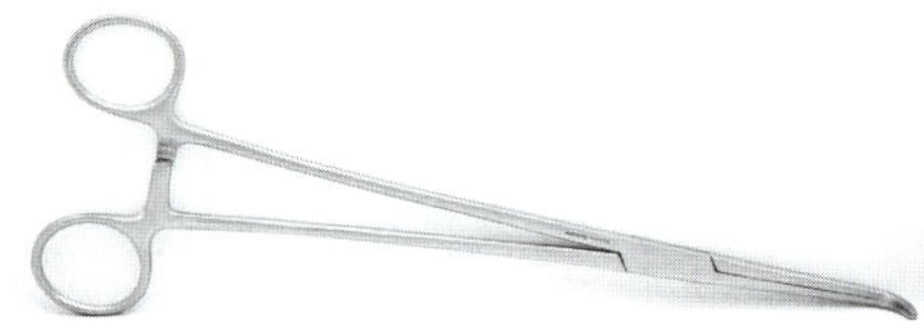
Millennium Surgical Corp.</td></tr>
<tr><td>Kocher Clmp 5 1/2″</td><td>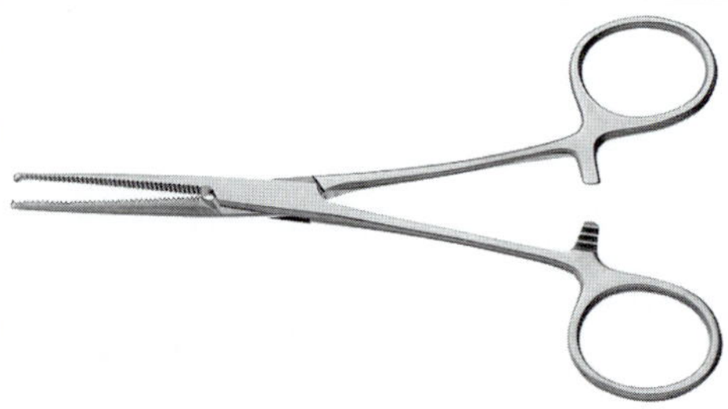
Millennium Surgical Corp..</td><td>Schnidt Clmp 9″</td><td>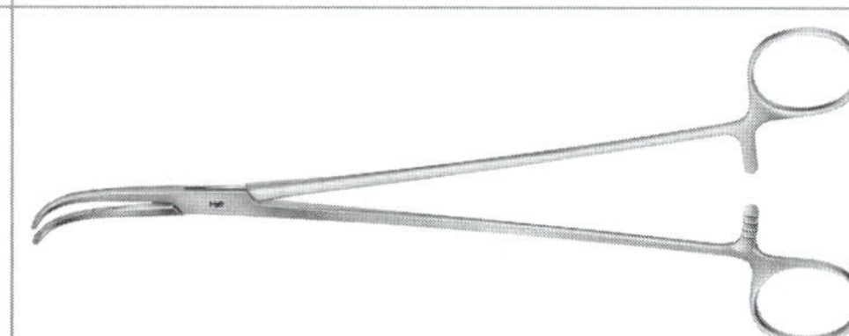
Courtesy and copyright Becton, Dickinson and Company.</td></tr>
<tr><td></td><td></td><td>Allis clamp 7″</td><td>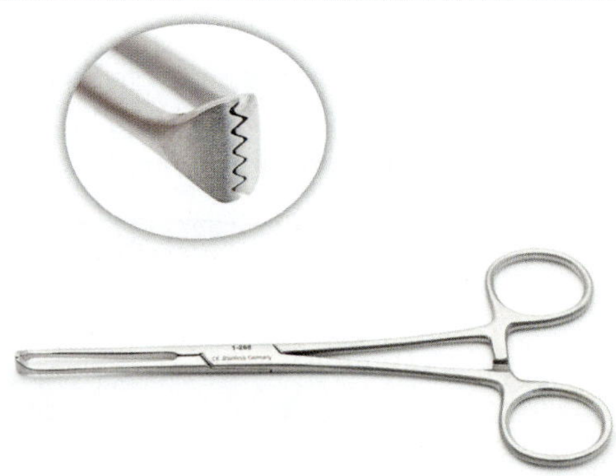
Millennium Surgical Corp.</td></tr>
</table>

GENERAL SURGERY INSTRUMENTS (OPEN)—cont'd

Babcock Clamp 7″	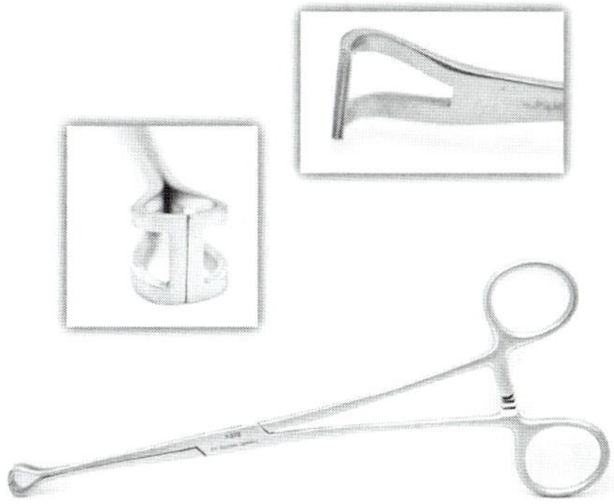 Courtesy and copyright Becton, Dickinson and Company.	Sponge Fcps 7″	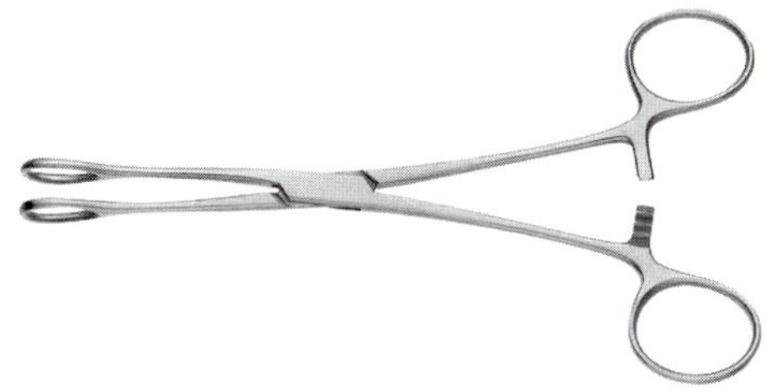 Millennium Surgical Corp.
Backhaus Towel Clmp 4″	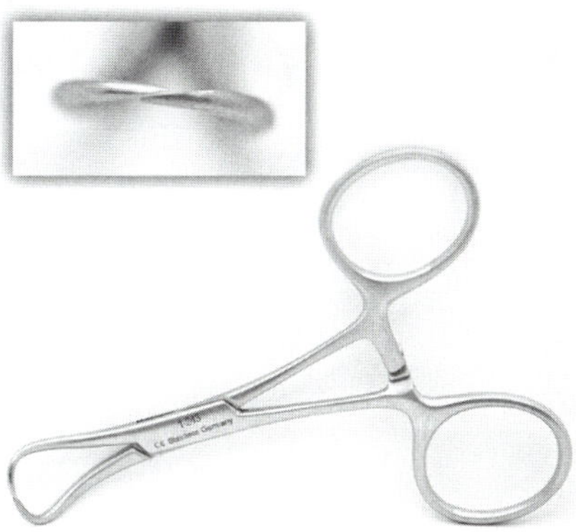 Courtesy and copyright Becton, Dickinson and Company	May-Hegar Needle Holder 9″	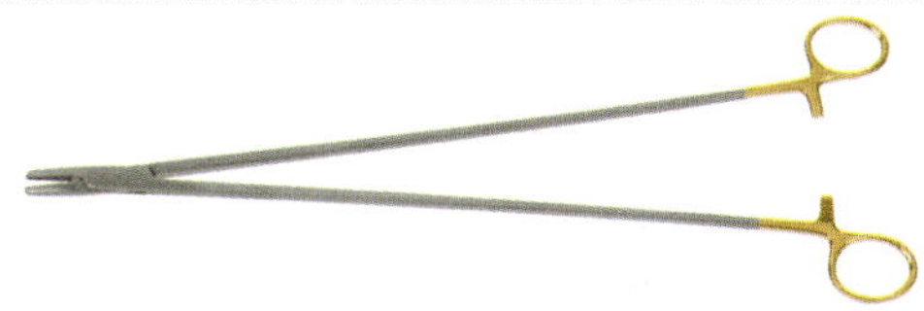 Copyright 2016 Symmetry Surgical Inc.; Photo courtesy of Symmetry Surgical Inc.
Ryder needle holder 5″	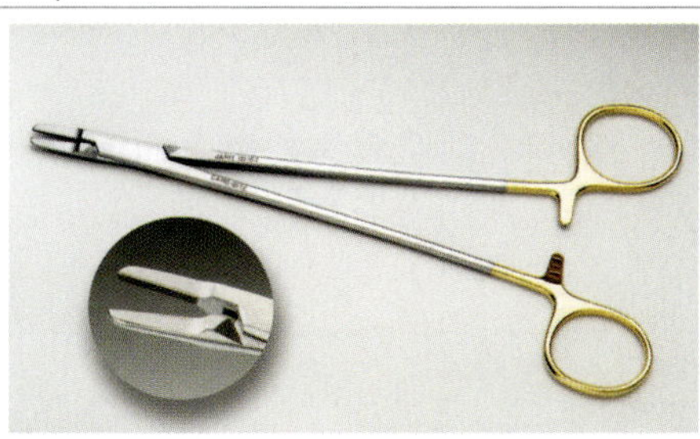 From Nemitz. *Surgical Instrumentation: An Interactive Approach*. 3rd ed. St. Louis: Elsevier; 2019.	Baumgartner Needle Holder 5 ⅜″	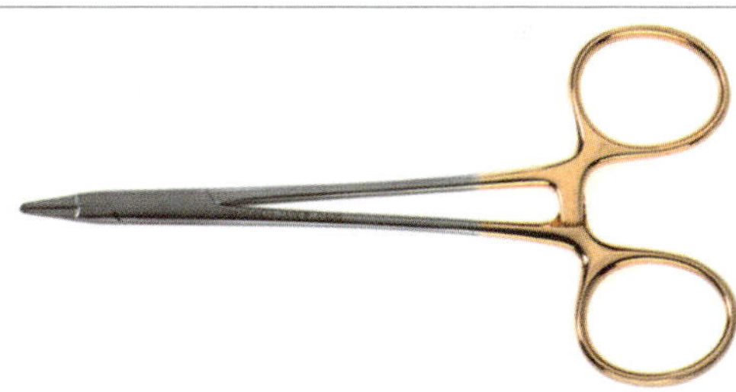 Courtesy and copyright Becton, Dickinson and Company.
		U.S. Army Retractor	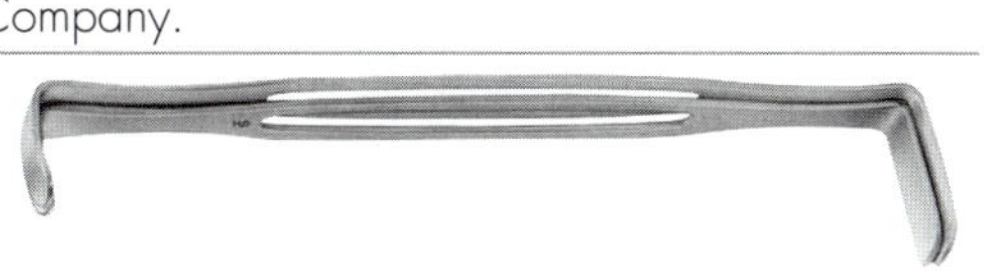 Millennium Surgical Corp.

GENERAL SURGERY INSTRUMENTS (OPEN)—cont'd

Richardson type retractor	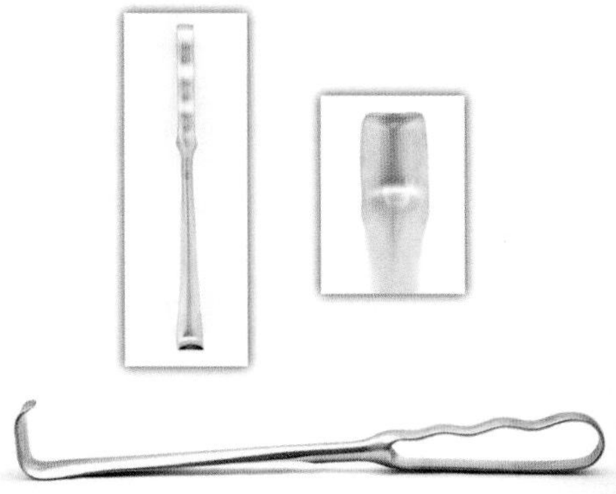 Millennium Surgical Corp.	Deaver retractors	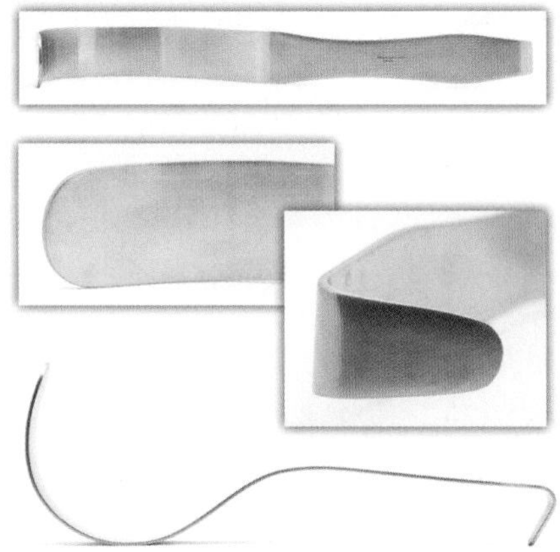 Courtesy Jarit Instruments, Hawthorne, NY.
Goulet retractor	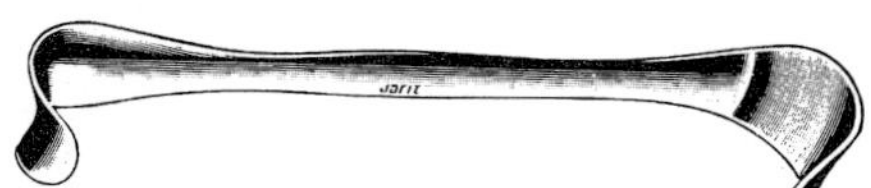 Courtesy Jarit Instruments, Hawthorne, NY.	Harrington retractor	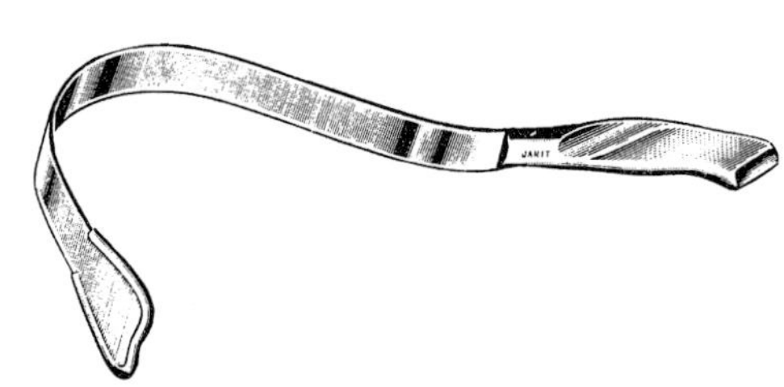 Photo courtesy Aesculap, Inc., Center Valley, PA.
Ribbon Retractor	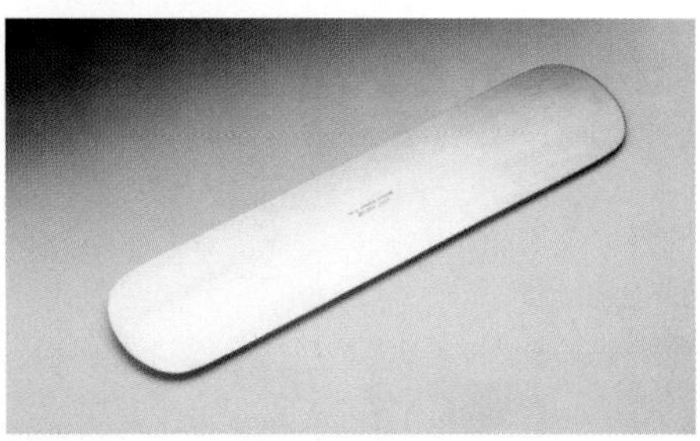 From Nemitz. *Surgical Instrumentation: An Interactive Approach*. 3rd ed. St. Louis: Elsevier; 2019.	Weitlaner retractor	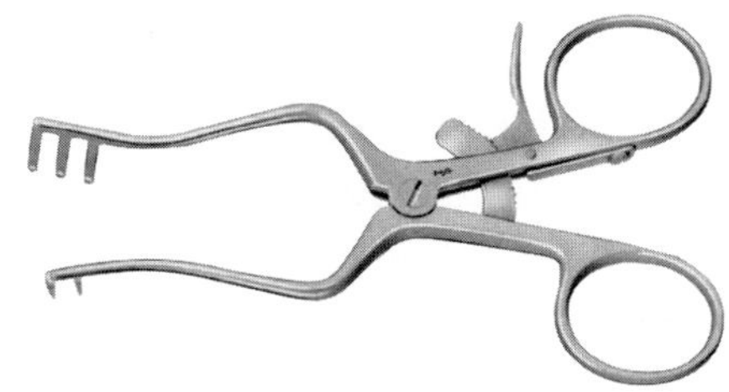 Courtesy Jarit Instruments, Hawthorne, NY.
Balfour retractor	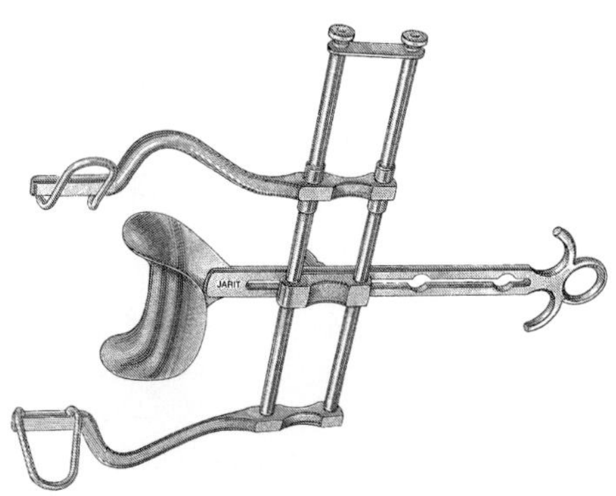 (From Barr J, Brayman K. Development and evolution of self-retraining retractors. *Surgery*. 2015;221[2]:628–634.)	Bookwalter retractor	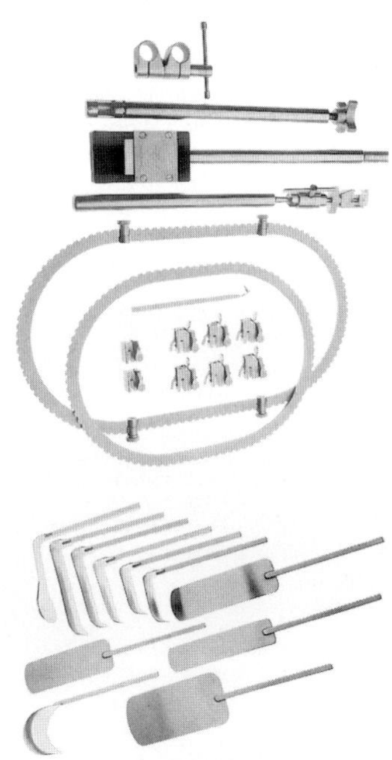 Courtesy and copyright Becton, Dickinson and Company.

Poole abdominal suction	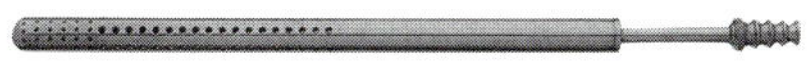 (From Sidawy A, Neville R. *Rutherford's Vascular Surgery and Endovascular Therapy.* 9th ed. Philadelphia: Elsevier; 2019:727–746.e4.)
Yankauer Suct 14″	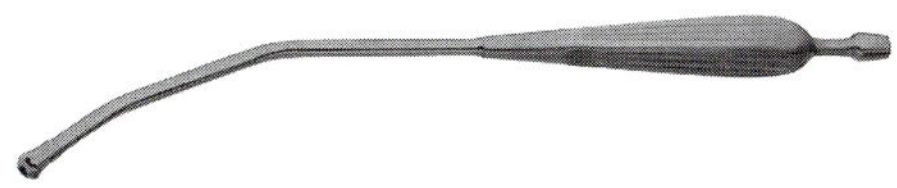 Courtesy and copyright Becton, Dickinson and Company.

GASTROINTESTINAL INSTRUMENTS

Pennington Clamp 6″	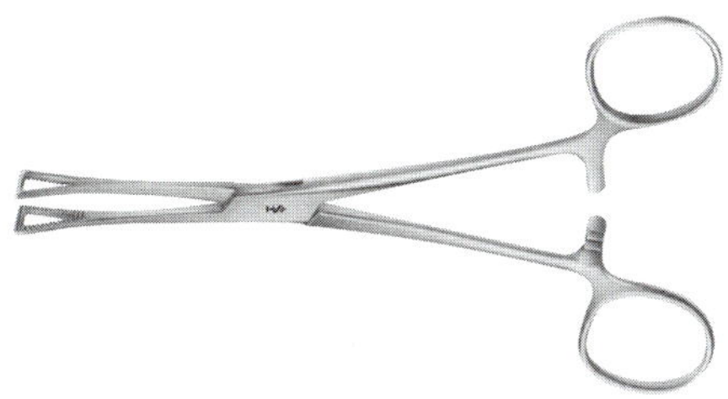 Photo courtesy Aesculap, Inc., Center Valley, PA.	Payr Pyloric Gastric clamp	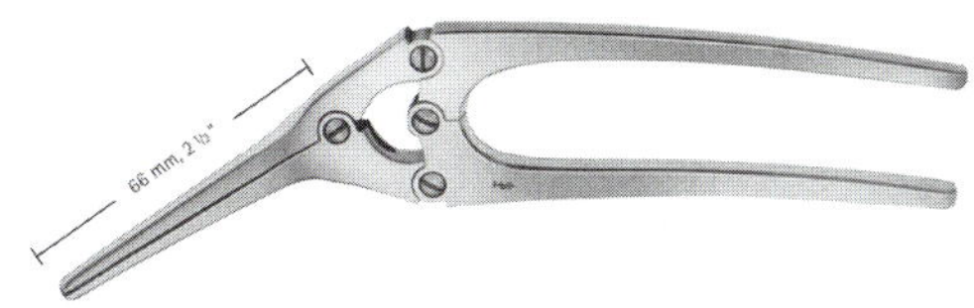 Photo courtesy Aesculap, Inc., Center Valley, PA.
Doyan Intestinal clamp 8″	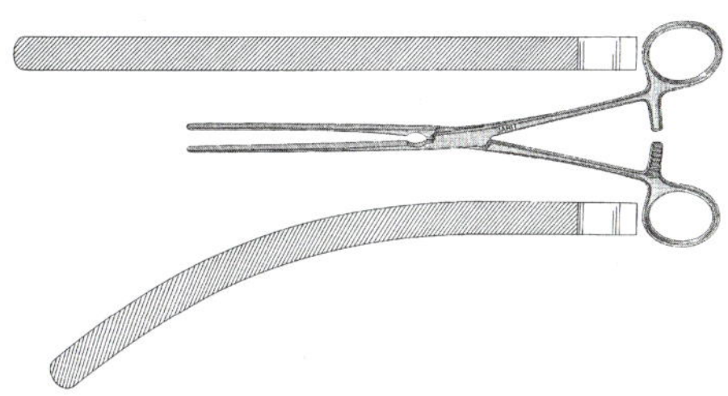 Courtesy Jarit Instruments, Hawthorne, NY.		
Lloyd-David Sigmoid Anastomosis Clmp 12 ½″	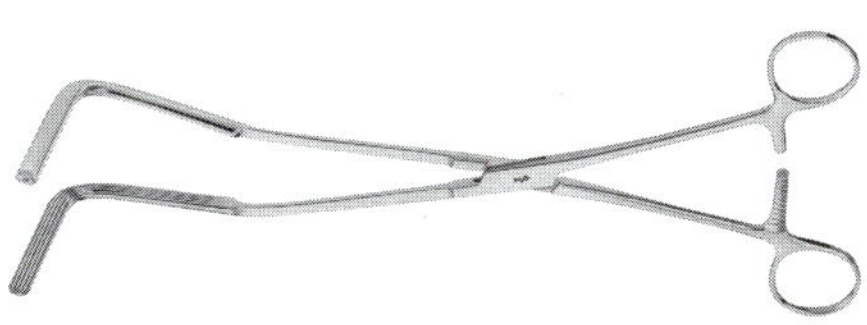 Photo courtesy Aesculap, Inc., Center Valley, PA.	Kelly Sphincteroscope 6 ¼″	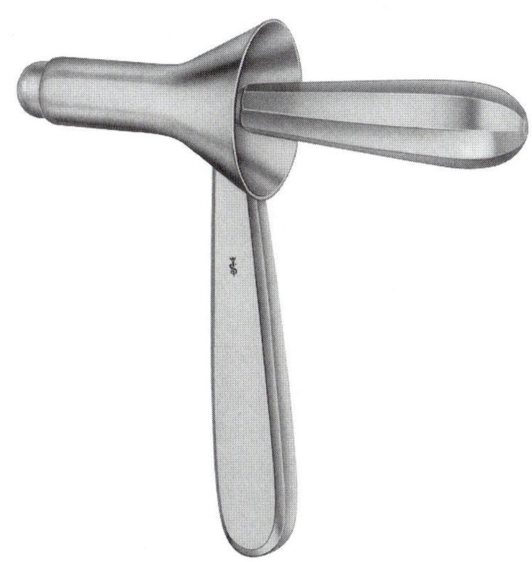 Photo courtesy Aesculap, Inc., Center Valley, PA.
Groove director probe with tongue tie	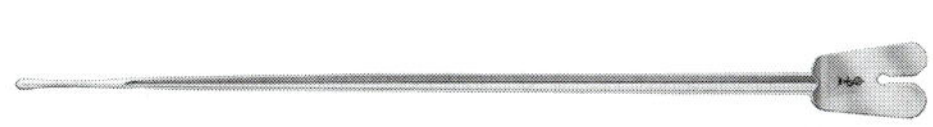 Photo courtesy Aesculap, Inc., Center Valley, PA.		

GALL DUCT INSTRUMENTS

Bakes Gall Duct Dilators 12 ½″	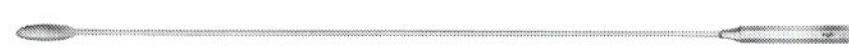 Photo courtesy Aesculap, Inc., Center Valley, PA.	Gall Duct Forceps 8 ¾″	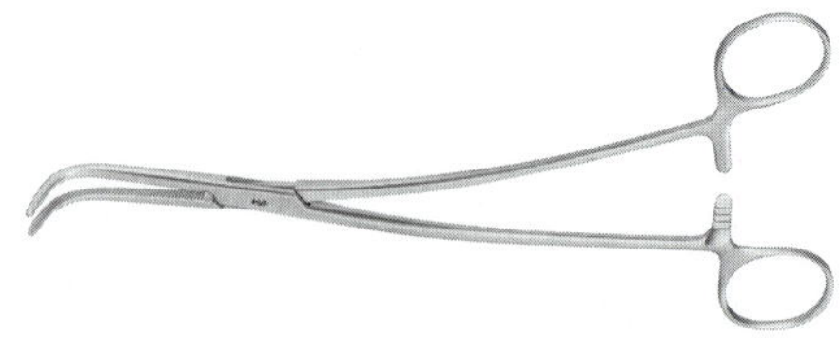 Photo courtesy Aesculap, Inc., Center Valley, PA.
Blake Gall Duct Stone forceps	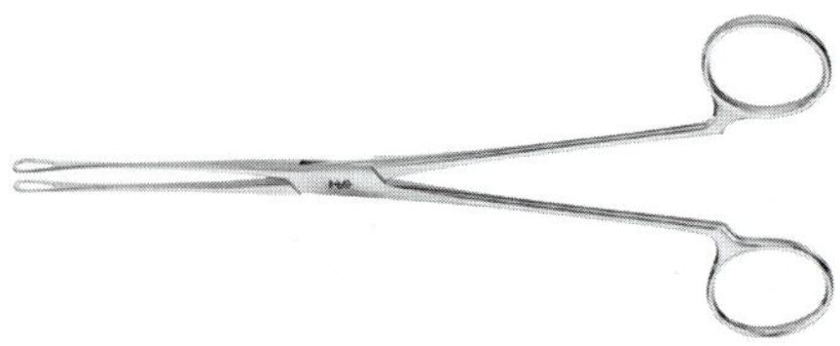 Photo courtesy Aesculap, Inc., Center Valley, PA.		

PROCEDURES OF THE ABDOMINAL WALL

HERNIA REPAIR

Hernia is among the most common pathologies of the abdominal wall. This is a protrusion of tissue through abnormal defect or weakness in the abdominal wall. The weakness may be caused by a congenital anomaly, previous surgery, or injury. Hernias most often occur in the inguinal and femoral regions. A hernia may also occur along the linea alba, umbilicus, or previous abdominal incision.

A hernia may require urgent surgical treatment if the herniated tissue becomes trapped or strangulated by the surrounding tissue; this is called an **incarcerated** or strangulated hernia. This deprives the herniated tissue of its blood supply and may lead to necrosis. Table 22.3 lists common types of abdominal wall hernias.

CASE PLANNING

Surgery for the repair of a simple hernia may be performed in the outpatient setting. Most patients arrive the day of surgery and can be discharged on the same day. Both open and minimally invasive surgical techniques are used. General anesthetic is commonly used; however, in patients for whom general anesthesia is not suitable, local infiltration or spinal anesthesia may also be used.

The patient is placed in the supine position for procedures of the abdominal wall. A Foley catheter may be inserted before surgery to decompress the bladder during repair of an inguinal or a femoral hernia.

Synthetic mesh, which is constructed using the same materials used in the manufacturing of sutures, is used in the repair of many types of hernias. The principle of mesh repair is to provide a strong scaffold over the weakened area of the abdominal wall. This prevents tension on the tissue edges during repair and healing. During the remodeling phase of healing, scar tissue fills the spaces of the mesh in the same way that mesh fabric is used to hold new plant growth in bare soil.

Mesh is available in sheets or patches that are fitted to overlap the edge of the defect. A patch usually is measured and cut during surgery, although pre-cut patches are available.

Sutures used on hernia repair are usually soft, pliable materials, such as polyester and synthetic absorbable sutures, to increase the strength of the weakened abdominal wall and to ensure that the tissues stay in approximation during the entire healing period. Mesh is secured in the wound with a combination of surgical tacks, staples, and sutures. Occasionally, heavy polypropylene sutures may be used to secure a mesh graft. The strength of the closure is increased using interrupted rather than running sutures for the fascia layer. Absorbable synthetic sutures size 3-0 can be used on the hernia sac, which is composed of more delicate peritoneal tissue.

OPEN REPAIR OF AN INDIRECT INGUINAL HERNIA

Open repair of an indirect inguinal hernia is performed to restore strength to the inguinal floor and prevent the abdominal viscera from entering the inguinal canal.

Pathology

An abdominal wall defect is an actual tear, an enlarged opening, or a weakened area in the abdominal wall. Defects can be congenital or acquired later in life. An **indirect inguinal hernia** results in protrusion of the abdominal viscera into the inguinal canal from the deep inguinal ring. In males, the herniated tissue can extend through the superficial ring, within the spermatic cord, and into the scrotum. In females, the tissue can protrude into the labia. Fig. 22.7 shows the steps involved in the repair of an indirect inguinal hernia in a male.

POSITION:	Supine
INCISION:	Inguinal
PREP AND DRAPING:	Laparotomy/laparotomy
INSTRUMENTS:	Laparotomy
POSSIBLE EXTRAS:	Mesh graft, Penrose drain

TABLE 22.3 Hernias of the Abdominal Wall

Condition	Description	Considerations
Incisional hernia	Protrusion of abdominal tissue through one or more abdominal layers. This arises from a previous abdominal incision that failed to heal completely or later broke down because of obesity, infection, or disease.	May require mesh reinforcement to bridge and strengthen the tissue edges
Strangulated hernia Incarcerated hernia	Tissue protruding from the hernia may become swollen and squeezed. This may result in local ischemia or other complications.	Strangulated hernia is an emergency condition requiring surgery to release the tissue and prevent ischemia and necrosis
Indirect inguinal hernia	A hernia in which abdominal viscera slides into the inguinal canal from the deep inguinal ring. Herniated tissue may extend through the superficial ring in the spermatic cord into the scrotum or labia.	Usually caused by a congenital weakness in the inguinal ring. Surgery may be necessary.
Direct inguinal hernia	Protrusion of abdominal or inguinal tissue directly through the transversalis fascia	The condition is usually acquired in older men
Femoral hernia	A hernia arising from a weakness in the transversalis fascia below the inguinal ligament	Occurs mainly in women and may require surgery to prevent tissue incarceration
Umbilical hernia	Abdominal wall defect occurring in the linea alba at the umbilical ring; seen in infants and adults	Rarely requires surgery. Incarceration is more common in obese adults.
Spigelian hernia	Rare hernia occurring between the transverse abdominis and rectus muscles	Rarely diagnosed but seen occasionally during surgery for other reasons

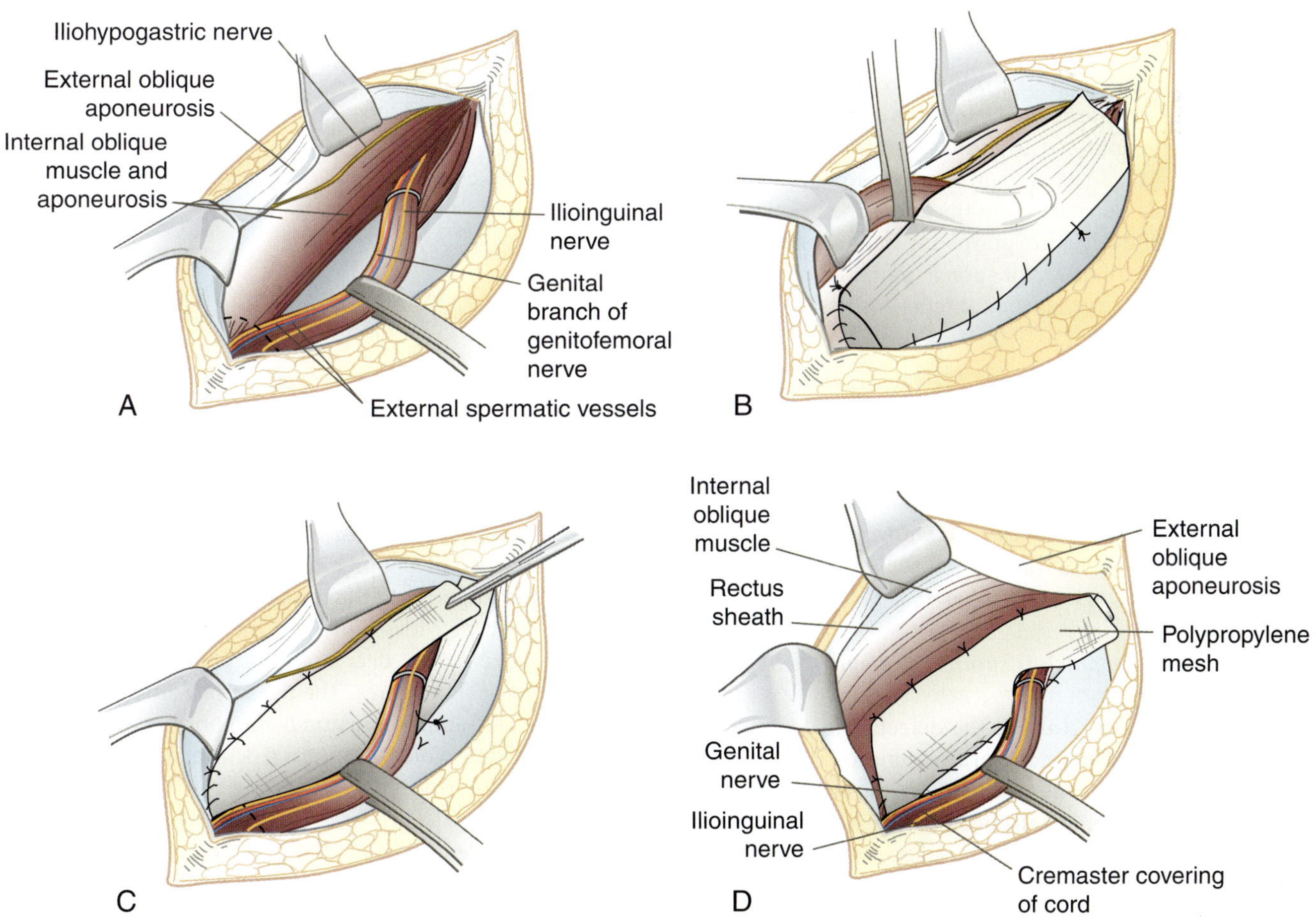

FIG. 22.7 Technical steps in repair of an indirect inguinal hernia.

Technical Points and Discussion

1. ***A right or left inguinal incision is made.***
   The surgeon incises the skin over the groin using the skin knife. Both sharp and blunt dissection are used to separate the tissue layers and expose the hernia.

2. ***The deep layers of the abdominal wall are incised, and the edges are retracted.***
   Several hemostats can be placed on the edges of the fascia to retract it and expose the spermatic cord. An Army-Navy or small Richardson retractor is used on the abdominal wall.

3. ***The spermatic cord is dissected from preperitoneal fat and other surrounding tissue.***
   After identifying the cord, the surgeon carefully separates it from the hernia sac. A dry sponge can be used to bluntly separate the tissues. The electrosurgical unit (ESU) is used to control small bleeders.

4. ***The spermatic cord is retracted with a Penrose drain.***
   A small Penrose drain is looped around the spermatic vessels and vas deferens (spermatic cord). This is seen in the 5 o'clock position in the earlier illustrations. The ST should dip the drain in saline before passing it to the surgeon. A Kelly or Crile clamp is used to hold the two ends of the drain together. This permits soft retraction of the cord during dissection.

5. ***The hernia sac is dissected from the cord and opened. The contents are pushed back into the abdomen.***
   Dissection is continued to the level of the defect in the abdominal wall. Metzenbaum scissors are used to dissect the hernia sac away from the cord. The hernia sac is opened, and the edges are grasped with hemostats. Using a finger or a small dissector sponge mounted on a clamp, the surgeon then pushes the contents of the sac back into the abdomen.

6. ***The hernia sac is ligated with ties or a purse-string suture.***
   If the defect is very small, it can be ligated. For large sacs, a purse-string suture of 2-0 synthetic absorbable material is placed around the neck of the sac. The excess neck tissue above the suture is cut away and removed as a specimen. An alternative method is to invert the sac and imbricate (fold under) the edges with sutures.

7. ***A synthetic mesh patch is sutured or stapled into place over the defect.***
   If mesh is used to reinforce the defect, it is trimmed to match the size of the floor of the inguinal canal, and a small hole is made to allow the spermatic cord to emerge in its normal anatomical position. The ST should provide mesh material and suture scissors to the surgeon. Pre-cut mesh patches are also available. The edges of the mesh are secured with interrupted synthetic sutures or staples.

8. ***The incision is closed in multiple layers and dressed.***
   The abdominal wall is closed in layers and a flat dressing applied to the wound.

LAPAROSCOPIC REPAIR OF A DIRECT INGUINAL HERNIA (TAPP APPROACH)

Laparoscopic direct hernia repair is performed to *reduce* herniated tissue (return the tissue to its normal anatomical configuration) and strengthen the inguinal floor. Most inguinal hernia procedures are performed laparoscopically. The procedure described is the transabdominal preperitoneal (TAPP) approach.

Pathology

A **direct inguinal hernia** arises from a defect behind the superficial inguinal ring in the inguinal floor, through the transversalis fascia. The defect is located in the inguinal triangle, which is sometimes called the *Hesselbach triangle*. This area is located on the inferior (lower) aspect of the anterior abdominal wall. The direct hernia is acquired in the male, usually later in life. Unlike the indirect hernia, the protruding tissue rarely descends into the scrotum. The defect gradually becomes larger with age or obesity. Increased intraabdominal pressure ("bearing down") with heavy lifting or pulling can precipitate a large, painful direct hernia.

POSITION:	Supine
INCISION:	Laparoscopic
PREP AND DRAPING:	Laparotomy
INSTRUMENTS:	Laparoscope, two to four 5-mm trocar/cannulas, one 8- to 12-mm trocar/cannula
POSSIBLE EXTRAS:	Mesh graft, surgical staples, or tacks

Technical Points and Discussion

1. ***Pneumoperitoneum is established, and trocars are inserted into the abdomen.***
   For TAPP laparoscopy, pneumoperitoneum is established using a Veress needle or the Hasson cut-down approach (as described in Chapter 20). The first trocar placed within or just superior to the umbilicus may be an optical trocar, which provides a view of the anatomy as the trocar is advanced. This decreases the possibility of injury to the internal structures. The telescope is inserted into this port. Additional 5-mm and 8-mm ports are placed in the iliac regions. Note: A 12-mm trocar may be used in place of the 8-mm trocar.

2. ***The herniated tissue is identified and grasped.***
   The surgeon explores the tissues in the area of the hernia to identify important landmarks and the extent of the hernia. Exploration may be carried out by means of a probe

and retractor. He or she then grasps the hernia sac with forceps or an atraumatic grasper.

3. ***A transverse incision is made above the direct hernia space.***
   An incision is made in the peritoneum above the direct space with scissors, ultrasonic scalpel, or an ultrasonic dissector. Dissection is continued with the ultrasonic scalpel to release adhesions and manage bleeders. The peritoneum is retracted with right-angle retractors to expose the pelvic floor.

4. ***The weakened area in the pelvic floor is reinforced with mesh.***
   Surgical mesh is introduced through the largest port. Surgical staples are used to attach the mesh to the Cooper ligament and to close the peritoneum.

5. ***The wounds are closed and dressed.***
   The pneumoperitoneum is released, and the fascial and skin layers are closed with 2-0 sutures or skin staples. Single-layer dressings are secured over the incisions.

ROBOTIC REPAIR OF AN INDIRECT INGUINAL HERNIA

The robotic transabdominal preperitoneal (rTAPP) approach is preferred over a robotic totally extraperitoneal approach (rTEP) by most surgeons. A bilateral hernia may be performed without undocking or redocking the patient cart. The following procedure describes robotic inguinal hernia repair using polypropylene mesh. The most common size mesh for an adult is 15 mm by12 mm.

Pathology

The pathology is the same as that described previously (see Open Repair of an Indirect Inguinal Hernia).

POSITION:	Supine using anti-skid system.
INCISION:	3 incisions across the abdomen, first being above the umbilicus, then the other two incisions lateral to the first.
PREP AND DRAPING:	Prep extends from nipple line to pubic symphysis. Laparoscopy draping to provide exposure for placement of trocars.
INSTRUMENTS:	Xi laparoscopy instruments, 8.5-mm 30-degree or 0-degree endoscope; monopolar curved scissors; ultrasonic scalpel, Cadiere forceps, or fenestrated bipolar forceps; needle driver; laparoscopic grasper.

Technical Points and Discussion

1. ***The patient is placed in supine position on an anti-skid device, prepped from nipple line to symphysis pubis; draping follows immediately.***
   The procedure will be performed with the patient in Trendelenburg position. Therefore an anti-skid system must be put in place on the operating table before the patient is positioned. When positioning the patient, ensure that all bony prominences are well padded and that the patient's arms are securely tucked at the sides using a draw sheet. The abdomen is draped for a laparotomy.

2. ***Pneumoperitoneum is established.***
   A small incision is made within or above the umbilicus. The fascia is grasped with two towel clamps and elevated. A Veress needle is inserted through the fascia to perform the saline drop test. After it is verified that the needle is in correct position in the abdomen, the insufflation tubing is attached to the needle and pneumoperitoneum is established. The *Hasson* and *optical trocar* techniques described in Chapter 20 may also be used.

3. ***The first trocar and port are inserted through the periumbilical incision and the endoscopic camera inserted.***
   The Veress needle is removed. An 8.5-mm optical trocar is inserted through the small stab incision performed with a #11 knife. This port is dedicated to the camera. The surgeon may assess the patient's anatomy and hernia defect before inserting the other ports.

4. ***Two or more additional ports are created for the robotic instruments.***
   Addition ports size 8 mm are placed under direct vision through the camera. These will be used for the robotic instruments. An additional 5-mm port may also be created for the assistant's access.

5. ***The patient cart is positioned and docked.***
   Before the patient cart is positioned and docked, the patient is placed in steep Trendelenburg. The ST must ensure that the overhead surgical lights are moved away from the field and that there is ample clearance between the robotic arms and the patient. The patient cart is docked on the side of the hernia *(side docking)*. If the procedure is performed in lithotomy position *(pelvic docking)*, the patient cart is placed between the patient's legs. The cart arms are positioned over the ports and then locked into the position using the clutch system.

6. ***Adhesions are released.***
   Before starting the hernia repair, the surgeon releases tissue adhesions. This is performed using a monopolar scissor and fenestrated bipolar grasper.

7. ***A peritoneal flap is created.***
   The dissection continue s with the creation of a peritoneal flap. In this maneuver the same dissecting instruments are used to dissect the tissues in line with the peritoneum so that the hernia contents can be reduced and the repair initiated.

8. ***The hernia sac is reduced.***
The visceral contents of the hernia are freed up from the sac and allowed to return to normal anatomical position. The peritoneum can then be dissected from the adjacent tissue to allow room for the mesh. The ST should prepare the mesh as directed by the surgeon (split or not split). An additional fenestrated grasper may be required for this.

9. ***Mesh is inserted to cover the defect and sutured in place.***
The ST should verify the type, size, and configuration of the mesh. The mesh is introduced through one of the instrument ports. Two fenestrated graspers are used to manipulate the mesh into position over the defect. Once the mesh is in place, it can be sutured down using size 2-0 absorbable or nonabsorbable material on a curved needle. Interrupted or continuous suture technique can be used. Two needle drivers are used during suturing. One of the needle drivers contains a scissor behind the grasping point so that sutures can be cut without exchanging the needle drivers.

10. ***The peritoneum and port sites are closed.***
The peritoneum is now closed using nonabsorbable barbed suture size 2-0 on a small curved needle. Continuous or interrupted sutures are used. After assessing the repair, the surgeon withdraws the instruments and ports and releases the pneumoperitoneum. The port sites are closed with absorbable synthetic sutures and sterile skin strips.

OPEN REPAIR OF INCISIONAL HERNIA

The goal of incisional hernia repair is to correct a weakened area in the abdominal wall, which allows abdominal tissues to bulge between the tissue planes of the abdominal wall, where they can become entrapped. The noninfected defect is most often repaired using synthetic mesh between the edges of the defect.

Pathology

An **incisional hernia** (a type of ventral hernia) may develop at the site of a previous surgery. The local anatomy can be very complex, with scar tissue integrated throughout the body wall layers. One or more fistulas may also be present. A **fistula** is a tract or tunnel through the tissue and develops an epithelial (skin) lining, which prevents it from healing. The walls of the fistula must be surgically removed for a successful outcome. In extreme cases of incisional hernia, internal structures such as fatty tissue or a portion of the bowel may become entrapped in the hernia.

POSITION:	Supine
INCISION:	Midline or paramedian
PREP AND DRAPING:	Laparotomy/laparotomy
INSTRUMENTS:	Laparotomy
POSSIBLE EXTRAS:	Mesh graft

Technical Points and Discussion

1. ***The abdominal scar (if present) is removed, and the edges of the previous incision are trimmed.***
To begin the surgery, the surgeon places several Allis clamps on the abdominal scar. These are used to apply upward traction on the scar while it is incised, first with a skin knife and then with the ESU. The ST should retain the scar as a specimen.

2. ***Old sutures are removed.***
Sutures from previous surgery are removed with a straight hemostat and scissors. A folded towel placed near the incision is convenient for the surgeon to wipe the suture remnants from the hemostat. The ST should remove the towel and suture remnants from the field to prevent them from re-entering the incision.

3. ***Abdominal adhesions are separated from the viscera and the peritoneum.***
After the sutures have been removed, the surgeon may attempt to re-establish normal tissue planes by trimming and reducing superficial fascia and subcutaneous fat. The edges of the incision, which usually are ragged and poorly defined are then remodeled with Metzenbaum scissors and toothed forceps. Allis clamps may be needed to provide traction on the tissue edges during this step. In most cases it is not necessary to enter the abdominal cavity to repair an incisional hernia unless adhesions must be released or if the hernia originates from within the abdomen. If there are any fistula tracts present in the tissue, these may require identification with a fistula probe. The probe is inserted into the opening of the fistula and advanced. The tissue forming the fistula is then obliterated with ESU.

4. ***Synthetic mesh is secured over the abdominal defect.***
Once the wound edges have been trimmed and the tissue layers clearly defined, the defect can be repaired. A mesh graft is sutured or tacked across the edges of the deep fascia. The ST should provide a mesh sheet and suture scissors to the surgeon, who cuts the graft to the correct size. The mesh is then sutured in place with size 2-0 suture or staples.

5. ***All layers of the abdominal wall are closed.***
The tissue layers are then closed with interrupted sutures and skin staples. Tension on the wound can be relieved by the use of a heavy continuous suture (e.g., polydioxanone suture) through all layers or by the use of retention sutures with bolsters as discussed in Chapter 19. A simple single-layer dressing is applied.

INCISIONAL HERNIA REPAIR (LAPAROSCOPIC)

Pathology

A large **ventral hernia** in the adult is often caused by multiple abdominal surgeries in the same location. The herniated tissue protrudes from within the abdominal cavity in one or more locations and often contains preperitoneal fat or fat arising from the omentum. The repair is performed using synthetic mesh.

POSITION:	Supine
INCISION:	Laparoscopic
DRAPING:	Laparoscopy
INSTRUMENTS:	Laparoscopy, two to four 5-mm trocar/cannulas, one 8-to 12-mm trocar/cannula; laparoscopic forceps, scissors, monopolar hook, Babcock forceps, needle driver, ultrasonic scalpel
POSSIBLE EXTRAS:	Mesh graft; spinal needles; laparoscopic tacking instrument

Technical Points and Discussion

1. ***The abdomen is prepped and draped for a wide operative site.***
   Although a laparoscopic approach is used, a wide area is prepped and draped to accommodate a total of at least four trocars. These are positioned at the far lateral edges of the abdomen to avoid injury to the bowel.

2. ***Pneumoperitoneum is established and trocars placed.***
   A Veress needle or another insufflation device is used to establish pneumoperitoneum (refer to Chapter 20). A 5-mm trocar is placed to accommodate the laparoscope. Before placing the other trocars, the surgeon explores the abdomen. At least two more 5-mm trocars are then placed. Up to five trocars may be placed according to the size of the hernia.

3. ***Adhesions are released, and the contents of the hernia sac are pulled into the abdomen.***
   In a large abdominal hernia, there are typically many adhesions that may involve the bowel and abdominal wall. These are released using blunt and sharp dissection using smooth forceps and curved scissors. Once the adhesions are released, the surgeon enters the hernia sac and pulls its contents into the abdominal cavity using the smooth forceps. If the bowel is near the dissection site, it is examined for any injury.

4. ***The defect is measured.***
   The surgeon now measures the defect. There are several methods for this. One is to release the pneumoperitoneum and directly measure the defect from outside the body. A second method is to insert two 20-gauge spinal needles on either side of the defect while viewing it through the laparoscope. Needle placement allows direct measurement from inside the body. An additional 2 to 4 cm is added to the size to allow overlap of mesh over the edges of the defect. A flexible ruler is inserted through one of the 5-mm ports, and the distance between the two needles is measured.

5. ***The graft is prepared.***
   It is necessary to mark the graft according to its orientation in the body. This can be done using a tissue-marking pen, with sutures, or both. Two different types of sutures may be placed in the graft to show "north-south" and "right-left." The suture ends are left long to attach the graft to the abdominal wall once the graft is positioned. Size 0 nonabsorbable polyester or Gortex sutures are commonly used. After placing the sutures, the surgeon rolls the graft for insertion into one of the 5-mm ports.

6. ***The graft is placed over the defect and tacked in place.***
   The surgeon inserts the graft into the abdomen and carefully unrolls it in the correct orientation. Smooth graspers are used to handle the graft. Now the graft can be positioned and secured in place. The sutures will be tied externally. To do this, small incisions are made at the point of the suture ends with a #11 knife blade. A suture passer is inserted through the incision and used to bring the sutures to the outside of the abdomen. These are tied securely at the fascia layer. Absorbable or nonabsorbable tacks are dispensed from a tacking instrument, which automatically inserts a tack by operating the trigger. Surgical tacks are placed around the circumference of the graft. Additional sutures size 0 or 1 will also be placed every few centimeters to add support to the closure.

7. ***The incisions are closed and the wounds dressed.***
   The cannulas are withdrawn and abdominal wall incisions closed with size 0 synthetic absorbable suture. Skin is closed with adhesive strips. Postoperative pain can be managed by local infiltration of long-acting local anesthetic into the tissues of the abdominal wall before closure. Fig. 22.8 illustrates lysis of adhesions and mesh repair.

UMBILICAL HERNIA REPAIR (OPEN)

Umbilical hernia repair is performed to repair a defect and reestablish continuity of the periumbilical tissues.

Pathology

An umbilical hernia is the result of a defect in the linea alba at the umbilical ring. This hernia is most common in children and usually disappears spontaneously by age 2. In adults, the hernia appears more frequently in individuals with a high BMI. The sac of an umbilical hernia frequently has a small base, which increases the risk of tissue strangulation. An umbilical hernia most often contains fatty tissue that has protruded from within the abdomen.

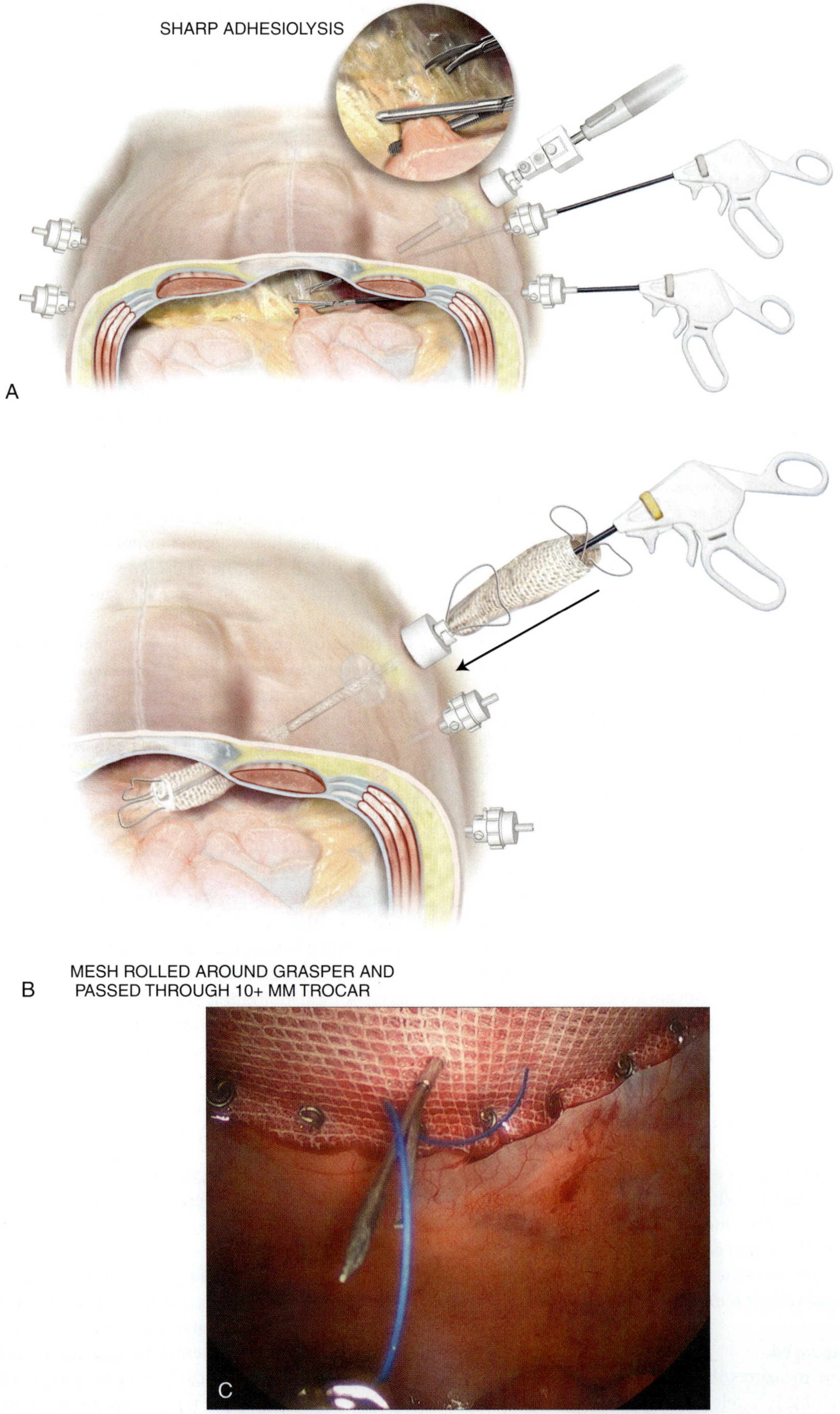

FIG. 22.8 Laparoscopic ventral hernia repair. (A) Sharp dissection of adhesions using ultrasonic scalpel and scissors. (B) Insertion of the rolled mesh graft through the largest port. (C) Mesh graft in place showing tacks. Sutures are placed between the tacks for added support. (From Rosen M. *Atlas of Abdominal Wall Reconstruction*. Philadelphia: Saunders; 2012.)

POSITION:	Supine
INCISION:	Infra-umbilical
PREP AND DRAPING:	Abdominal/laparotomy
INSTRUMENTS AND SUPPLIES:	Laparoscopic
POSSIBLE EXTRAS:	Synthetic mesh

Technical Points and Discussion

1. ***A small incision is made in the umbilicus.***
   A skin incision is made in the umbilicus with a #11 knife. This exposes the fatty tissue and linea alba. A self-retaining retractor such as a Gelpi can be used to hold the skin edges back. Senn retractors may also be used. Bleeders are managed with the ESU.

2. ***The surgeon grasps the edges of the linea alba using Allis clamps.***
   The extent of the defect can now be determined. The ESU is used to coagulate bleeders and sever the fatty tissue from the fascia. The Allis clamps are repositioned as needed to maintain traction on the fascia layer.

3. ***The defect is repaired with sutures or mesh.***
   A synthetic mesh plug is inserted over the hole in the fascia plane and sutured in place with absorbable synthetic sutures, size 2-0 or 3-0, on a taper needle. The mesh bridges the defect without tension and prevents the hernia from recurring. The skin is closed with a subcuticular absorbable suture and dressed with a small, flat dressing.

REPAIR OF UMBILICAL HERNIA (LAPAROSCOPIC)

An umbilical hernia arises from a defect in the abdominal ring, usually in patients with a high BMI. Laparoscopic repair with mesh is commonly performed.

Pathology

A small umbilical hernia can be corrected by open surgery. A more extensive defect may be reduced and closed by laparoscopy.

POSITION:	Supine
PREP AND DRAPING:	Laparotomy/laparotomy
INSTRUMENTS:	Laparoscopic
POSSIBLE EXTRAS:	Mesh graft; spinal needles; tacking instrument

Technical Points and Discussion

1. ***Pneumoperitoneum is established and ports placed.***
   Pneumoperitoneum is established using a Veress needle or Hasson cut-down approach. A 10-mm trocar is used to enter the abdomen. The laparoscope is inserted through this port. Depending on the size of the defect, additional 5-mm trocars are used at the lateral sides of the abdomen.

2. ***The abdomen is explored to determine the extent of the defect and adhesions.***
   An umbilical hernia commonly contains fatty tissue enclosed within a hernia sac. Multiple adhesions may be present in the area of the defect or in areas of previous surgeries. The surgeon examines the abdomen to identify these and to locate any areas where the bowel is involved.

3. ***The hernia contents are reduced and adhesions released.***
   Using a smooth grasper and curved scissors, the surgeon severs the adhesions from the abdominal wall and pulls the contents of the hernia back into the abdomen. The ultrasonic scalpel can also be used to perform this step. The defect can be closed once the contents are fully reduced.

4. ***The defect is closed and supported with mesh.***
   A small incision is made in the umbilicus with a #11 knife blade. This incision is used to pass a size 0 nonabsorbable suture on a curved needle. The needle is passed to the internal abdominal wall and back out again to the level of the fascia several times, catching the defect edges and closing it. After the defect is closed, a mesh graft is sutured to the abdominal wall with size 0 nonabsorbable sutures and tacks using the technique described above.

5. ***The pneumoperitoneum is released and incisions closed.***
   The cannulas are removed and the pneumoperitoneum released. Size 0 synthetic absorbable sutures are commonly used on fascia. The skin is closed using Steri-Strips. Skin adhesive may also be used to seal the skin incisions.

SECTION II: GASTROINTESTINAL SURGERY

SURGICAL ANATOMY

ESOPHAGUS AND STOMACH

The esophagus is a tubular structure that extends from the pharynx to the stomach. Food travels along its length by a combination of voluntary and involuntary muscle actions called *peristalsis*. Reverse peristalsis results in regurgitation of the stomach contents. The esophagus enters the abdominal cavity at the level of the diaphragm. In the adult, it measures approximately 10 inches (25 cm).

The stomach is located just under the diaphragm in the left upper abdomen. The three contiguous anatomical sections of the stomach are the *fundus* (upper portion), the *body* (midsection), and the *antrum* (distal or lower portion). These are shown in Fig. 22.9A.

The wall of the stomach contains an outer serosa, two inner layers of smooth (involuntary) muscles, and a submucosal lining, which lies in folds called *rugae*. The submucosa secretes hydrochloric acid and pepsin for the breakdown of proteins and carbohydrates, which is aided by the mechanical action of the muscle layers. A mucous barrier is also secreted to prevent damage to the stomach tissue by these chemicals. Two orifices (openings) and associated sphincters provide continuity between the esophagus and stomach and the stomach and duodenum. These

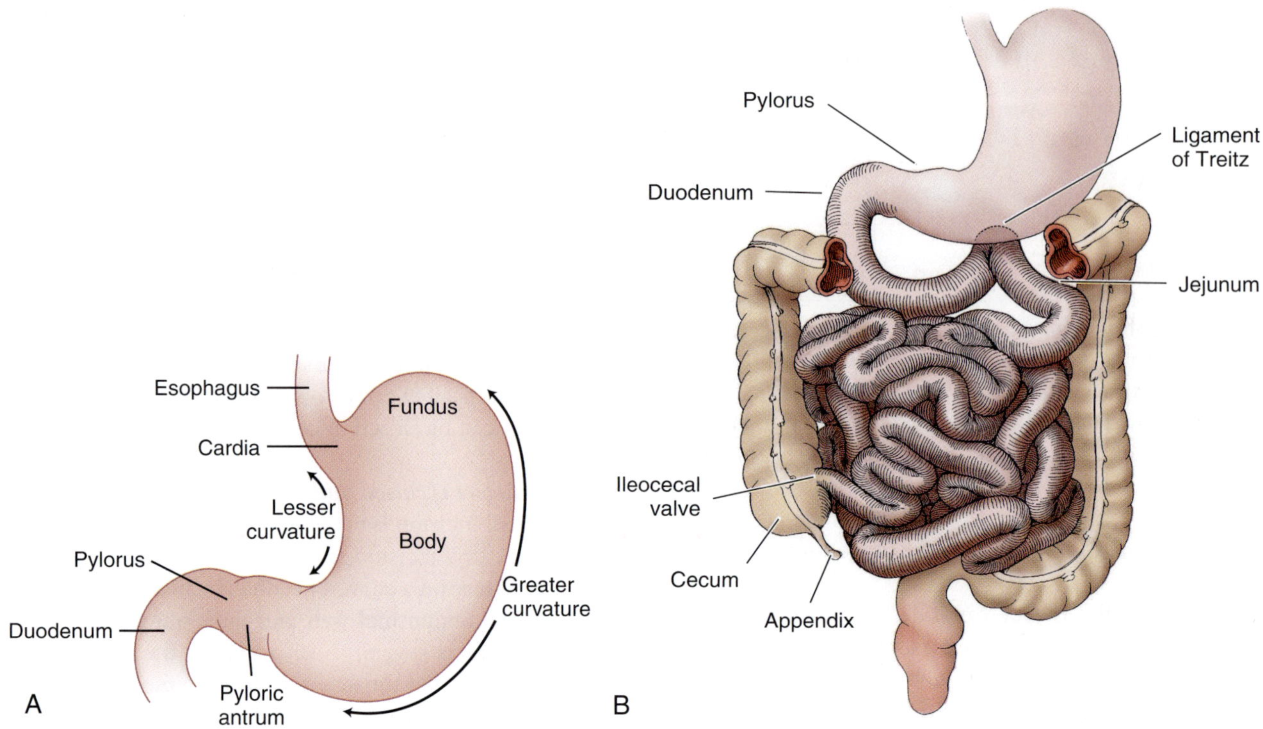

FIG. 22.9 Anatomy of the gastrointestinal tract. (A) The regions of the stomach. (B) The small intestine. (From Townsend C, Beauchamp B, Evers B, Mattox K. *Sabiston Textbook of Surgery: The Biological Basis of Modern Surgical Practice.* 19th ed. Philadelphia: Elsevier; 2012.)

are the *cardia*, which communicate with the esophagus, and the *pylorus*, which opens into the duodenum. Only a few molecules (including alcohol and some simple carbohydrates) are actually absorbed by the stomach. Instead, the stomach's main function is to break down its contents into a liquid slurry called *chyme*.

A sheet of connective and vascular tissue, called *omentum*, attaches to the greater and lesser curvatures of the stomach and covers the intestinal folds, providing warmth and protection to the viscera. This peritoneal sheet also contains fat lobules and may form out pockets, which can become infected. Whenever a portion of the stomach is removed or remodeled, the omentum must be separated from its attachments.

SMALL INTESTINE

The small intestine is the proximal portion of the intestinal tract. It extends from the pylorus of the stomach to the proximal end of the large intestine and contains three anatomical sections known as the duodenum, ileum, and jejunum. The individual tissue layers of the digestive tube are similar to those of the stomach. These are the inner mucosa, submucosa muscle, and serosa. The duodenum is approximately 8 to 10 inches (20 to 25 cm) long. It receives *chyme* from the stomach. The pancreatic duct *(duct of Wirsung)* and the common bile duct from the liver drain digestive enzymes into this section of the intestine.

The jejunum is approximately 9 feet (2.7 m) long. It connects with the ileum, which is approximately 13½ feet (4 m) long. These sections are suspended from the abdominal wall by a sheet of vascular tissue called the *mesentery*, which supplies blood and lymph to the lower sections of the small intestine. During resection of the jejunum or the ileum, the mesentery must be clamped and divided from the intestine.

The tissue layers of the small intestine are similar to those of the stomach and large intestine. The inner surface of the small intestine has small finger-like projections called *villi*, which increase the surface area of the intestinal lumen and contain blood and lymphatic vessels. The small intestine terminates at the cecum, the first portion of the large intestine. Fig. 22.9B illustrates the small intestine.

LARGE INTESTINE (COLON)

The large intestine extends from the distal ileum to the rectum and is divided into five distinct sections: the ascending colon, the transverse colon, the descending colon, the sigmoid colon, and the rectum. The colon measures about 5 feet (1.5 m) in the adult. The long axis of the colon forms a series of puckers called *haustra*, which are formed by contraction of a longitudinal band of muscle called the *teniae coli*.

The first section of the large intestine is a blind pouch called the *cecum*. The terminal end of the cecum has a slender tube, called the *vermiform appendix*, which has no function. The ascending colon extends upward behind the right lobe of the liver. The transverse colon then crosses the abdomen to the left, below the stomach. The descending colon extends downward on the left side of the abdomen and terminates at the sigmoid colon, which lies in the pelvic cavity. The sigmoid colon terminates at the rectum. Fig. 22.10 illustrates the large intestine.

RECTUM AND ANUS

The distal 4 to 5 inches (10 to 12.5 cm) of the intestine form the *rectum*, which terminates at the *anal canal*. This section is lined with folded tissue. Two muscular sphincters in the anal

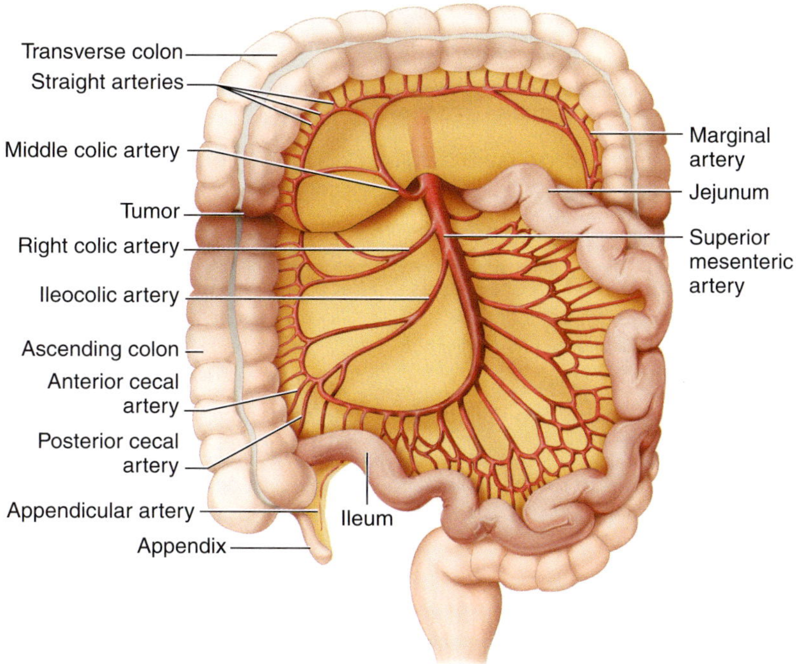

FIG. 22.10 The colon. (From Fleshman J, et al. *Atlas of Surgical Techniques for the Colon, Rectum, and Anus.* Philadelphia: Saunders; 2013.)

canal control the release of feces to the outside of the body *(defecation).* The internal sphincter is composed of involuntary (smooth) muscle. The external sphincter is under voluntary control (striated muscle).

DIAGNOSTIC PROCEDURES

The presence of GI disease is confirmed primarily by imaging studies, blood and metabolic studies, and physical examination. Endoscopy (described later) often is performed before open or laparoscopic surgery. Biopsy and visual examination of the inner surfaces of the intestine and stomach are performed to rule out or confirm carcinoma and provide tissue for further tests. Contrast studies performed under fluoroscopy frequently are done to outline the GI structures. Other important imaging tools are magnetic resonance imaging (MRI), ultrasound, and computed tomography (CT).

CASE PLANNING

During laparotomy and laparoscopy, patients are at high risk for hypothermia. Therefore thermoregulation is a high priority for patient safety during all abdominal procedures. A forced-air warming system is used. Irrigation solutions are maintained in a solution warmer. Exposure of the patient is kept to a minimum in the perioperative period, and the patient is covered with warm blankets before and after surgery. A sequential compression system (see Chapter 16) may be used during laparotomy procedures to prevent deep vein thrombosis.

The patient is placed in the supine position for most laparoscopic and open procedures of the GI system. Exceptions are procedures that require perineal access, such as abdominoperineal resection. In these cases, the lithotomy position is used. The patient's arms are placed on arm boards. The operating table is tilted into normal or reverse Trendelenburg position, depending on the anatomical exposure required during the procedure.

Patients undergoing surgery for morbid obesity require particular attention to safety during positioning. An anti-skid device or vacuum positioning device must be used to prevent the patient from sliding on the table (refer to Chapter 16 for details). The operating table must be able to accommodate up to 800 pounds (360 kg). Extensions must be well padded, and great care must be taken in transferring the patient between the gurney and the operating table.

INSTRUMENTS

A basic laparotomy set is used for GI surgery. GI specials include atraumatic clamps and grasping instruments. Vascular clamps may also be required. Long instruments may be added, depending on the size of the patient. Surgical stapling instruments for both open and laparoscopic procedures are also needed.

Sharp dissection is performed with Metzenbaum scissors, the ESU, and ultrasonic scalpel.

Babcock clamps are used to grasp intestinal tissue. Smooth or vascular forceps are used for suturing the mucosal layers. Resection of the bowel or stomach is performed with atraumatic clamps or with surgical stapling instruments. Atraumatic clamps do not close tightly over the tissue; rather, they leave a small gap between the jaws to prevent crushing. Long intestinal clamps may be covered with soft rubber tubing to provide a snug seal on the tissue; these are generally referred to

TABLE 22.4 Surgical Techniques Used for the Gastrointestinal System

Term or Technique	Definition	Example
Resection (*verb:* resect)	A procedure in which a section of an organ is divided or removed	A portion of the intestine is removed. If one of the free ends is surgically closed as a blind end, it is called a *stump.*
Anastomosis (*verb:* anastomose)	A procedure in which two hollow structures are joined surgically	Placing sutures around the circumference of the two cut edges can join two hollow structures. This applies to portions of the gastrointestinal (GI) system and other hollow systems, such as blood vessels and organ ducts.
Division (*verb:* divide)	In surgery, a procedure in which one section of tissue is cut away from another. This differs from *resection,* in which a portion of the organ is removed.	Recall that the small intestine is attached to the mesentery, a loose connective tissue containing many major blood vessels. When a section of small intestine is removed, the mesentery must be divided from the intestine to free up the section.
Cross-clamp	To place one or more clamps at a right angle to a tube or vessel	The "cross" simply refers to the angle of the clamp in relation to the organ or tissue.
Double-clamp	To place two clamps over a section of tissue to prevent bleeding when the tissue is severed	Double-clamping is performed before a tissue that may bleed profusely is divided or cut. In the case of GI structures, a section of intestine or stomach must be double-clamped before it is cut. This prevents hemorrhage and the release of fluids from the intestine or stomach.
Mobilization (verb: mobilize)	The freeing up of tissue from its attachments before anastomosis or resection	No tissues in the body are free-floating. Blood and lymph vessels, connective tissue, and membranes nourish and protect tissue. To remove tissue or to reconstruct the anatomy, the tissue must be removed from its normal attachments. Mobilization requires dissection or division.
Clamp and divide	To both double-clamp and divide tissue. Because the purpose of the clamps is to prevent bleeding, the tissue inside the jaws of the clamp must be sealed with the electrosurgical unit (ESU) or with suture ties. If surgical stapling instruments are used, the instrument clamps, staples, and cuts the tissue in one process.	During mobilization of the intestine, the surgeon repeatedly applies two hemostatic clamps, divides the tissue, and seals the tissue with the ESU or ties the cut ends. For the ST, the tools needed are: • Two hemostats (e.g., Kelly, Mayo, Crile) • ESU or tissue scissors • Two ties (if the ESU is not used) • Suture scissors (if ties are used)

as *rubber-shod clamps*. Although they are not commonly used, some facilities may include them in a GI set.

When the bowel, omentum, and mesentery have been exposed, a Poole suction tip should be available. This tip is perforated throughout the length, preventing excess suction pressure on delicate tissue.

EQUIPMENT AND SUPPLIES

Special equipment that may be required during GI surgery includes the following:

- Ultrasonic coagulation and cutting systems
- Vessel loops for large vessel dissection
- Ultrasound probe
- Bowel bag (a plastic bag used to enclose the bowel during open surgery to prevent tissue dehydration)
- Temporary ostomy bag
- Wound protector—used for isolation technique to isolate the bowel when it is surgically opened and during resection of metastatic tumor resection (see subsequent illustrations)

TISSUE APPROXIMATION AND HEMOSTASIS

Modern GI procedures, whether open or minimally invasive, rely almost entirely on surgical stapling technology for resection and anastomosis. The newest generation of surgical stapling systems are designed for minimally invasive laparoscopic and robotic procedures. Staple cartridges ("reloads") are color coded by size, easy to install in the staplers, and, for the most part, reliable for their intended use.

Suture closure usually is performed in two or three layers. Fine absorbable sutures (3-0 or 4-0) on a taper needle are used to close the mucosa and submucosa. The outer serosa layer can be closed with fine interrupted sutures of polydioxanone or other synthetic material on a taper needle. Large vessels and vascular bundles are ligated with sutures, surgical clips, or a vessel-sealing system. Large vessels of the omentum and mesentery often are secured with 0 or 2-0 suture ties or stick ties.

SURGICAL TECHNIQUES IN GASTROINTESTINAL PROCEDURES

Special techniques are common to most GI procedures. A surgical vocabulary has been developed that describes these (Table 22.4).

The GI system is a continuous "tube" attached to the abdominal and pelvic wall by a complex system of vascular membranes. These attachments limit the mobility of sections in the abdominal cavity and help prevent intestinal obstruction. To remodel a section of intestine or stomach, the surgeon must free up portions of these attachments (mesentery and omentum). This involves a technique of clamping the tissue, cutting it, and maintaining hemostasis. This is called *mobilization*.

Surgical stapling and use of ultrasonic scalpel and bipolar vessel-sealing systems have, to a large degree, replaced traditional methods of mobilization in which each section of mesenteric mesentery is clamped, ligated, and divided.

Anastomosis is the joining of two hollow structures by sutures, staples, or a combination of both. In GI surgery, anastomosis can be performed between any structures of the system. The suffix **-ostomy** means anastomosis. For example, a gastroduodenostomy is an anastomosis between the stomach and duodenum. A duodenoduodenostomy is the removal of a section of duodenum and rejoining of the two limbs, or open ends of the duodenum. Ileostomy refers to an opening made between the ileum and the outside abdominal wall for drainage. Anastomosis has been historically performed using a technique in which two or three layers of sutures were placed in a circumference around the two hollow structures to join them. Stomach or intestinal clamps were used to bring the two structures together while suturing took place. This technique is still used today, although surgical staples are used more frequently. These techniques are illustrated and described subsequently in the surgical procedure sections.

It is important for the ST to be familiar with surgical stapling instruments in conjunction with the types of anastomosis used in gastrointestinal surgery as many procedures are carried out using staples or a combination of staples and sutures.

If we picture the GI system as a tubular structure, there are several options for joining structures. A *side-to-side* anastomosis is performed by aligning two linear parts of the bowel. For this closure, a linear stapler is required. Two entry wounds must be made into the bowel to position the forks of the stapler, one in each segment of the two bowel sections. This procedure requires an *end-to-end* anastomosis (EEA). EEA is the joining of two ends of the bowel where they terminate. *End-to side* anastomosis is performed by joining the open end of a section of bowel to the side (linear) section of another structure through an opening made surgically. For tissue segments that require cutting and stapling, such as the terminal end of a section of bowel or mesentery at the point of its attachment to the bowel, a combination cutter-stapler is required.

ISOLATION TECHNIQUE

Surgery involving the intestinal tract carries a risk of bacterial contamination of the abdominal or pelvic cavities when the bowel is surgically opened during a procedure. Even though patients are required to undergo a preoperative bowel prep, which clears the bowel contents, and a preoperative course of antibiotics, the risk of surgical site infection remains. The same principles apply to surgical resection of metastatic tumors. During resection cancer cells may be released (seeded) into healthy tissue and thereby the disease is spread. To prevent these situations during surgery, a specific procedure must be used. This is called isolation technique. It may also be referred to in some texts as, **bowel** technique.

The purpose of isolation technique is to *ensure that the sterile field is not exposed to intestinal bacteria or metastatic cells.* In practice, it means implementation of specific techniques during bowel procedures and metastatic tumor resection. To accomplish this, all instruments, drapes, and supplies that *have been* or *could have been* exposed to open bowel or metastatic tumor cells are considered contaminated and must be isolated from the sterile setup. The student should be able to recognize the point where isolation technique must be initiated during surgical procedures described in this chapter.

There are two types of techniques: double setup and single setup. Refer to Table 22.5 for a comparison of single and double setups.

SINGLE SETUP

The single setup requires just one set of instruments and supplies. However, before the bowel or tumor resection is started, instruments and supplies required for this part of the procedure are brought to the Mayo. The back table remains sterile during resection but may not be touched while the resection is in progress. When resection is completed, all contaminated instruments and supplies are removed from the field and isolated in a basin, which is passed off the field to the circulator. The team changes gowns and gloves. The surgical incision is re-draped and the Mayo is covered with sterile towels. Instruments and supplies needed for closure can be brought from the back table to the field as needed. If the Mayo tray has become damp or wet, it must be covered with an impervious drape to prevent strike-through contamination of the sterile instruments.

DOUBLE SETUP

This technique requires one sterile setup used from the beginning of the surgery until the bowel has been closed or the resection is completed including removal of tissue specimens. A second sterile setup is prepared before surgery begins and is used for closure of the surgical wound.

IMPORTANT TO KNOW *In both types of setups a wound protector is placed in the wound before resection begins. This provides a barrier between the bowel segment or tumor and the other organs and tissues in the wound.*

In both techniques the wound is irrigated before the change to a sterile closure.

DIAGNOSTIC AND PROCEDURAL ENDOSCOPY

Endoscopy is the insertion of a flexible tube into a natural opening in the body. When used as a stand-alone procedure, it is most often performed in an outpatient setting, in a dedicated endoscopy clinic, or in a location near the operating room. High-risk patients require intensive physiological monitoring. In all cases, physiological monitoring includes cardiac monitoring and monitoring of oxygen saturation, respiratory function, blood pressure, and level of consciousness. Although not usually painful, endoscopy can be uncomfortable. With light or moderate sedation, patients are able to respond to

TABLE 22.5 Comparison of Single and Double Setups Required for Isolation Technique

Single Setup	Double Setup
Prepare 1 sterile setup for the procedure and closure.	Prepare 1 sterile setup for the procedure. Prepare and cover a second sterile setup for the closure.
Before transection of the bowel or metastatic tumor excision place a wound protector or clean sterile towels around the surgical site.	
Segregate all contaminated instruments and other items that have contacted the bowel lumen or metastatic tumor to a designated area such as the Mayo, or a basin.	N/A
Refrain from touching the sterile back table while the bowel is open or metastatic tumor excision is in progress.	N/A
When the anastomosis/resection is complete, remove the contaminated instruments, wound protector, towel drapes, and any other potentially contaminated items such as ESU pencil, suction, and light handles, from the surgical site and place them in a separate area of the sterile field that will not be touched during closing.	When the anastomosis/resection is complete, remove the contaminated instruments, wound protector, towel drapes, and any other potentially contaminated items such as ESU pencil, suction, and light handles, from the surgical site and place them on the sterile field used during the procedure that will not be touched during closing.
Irrigate the wound and initiate counting procedures.	
Announce the change to clean closure.	
One sterile team member remains at the sterile field, while all other team members change gloves. Gowns may also be changed. The team member who remained at the sterile field should remove the moist counted sponges or towels, then change gloves when the other team members are back at the sterile field.	
Apply sterile light handles.	
Apple sterile drapes to cover the existing drapes, which may be soiled with bowel contents or may have been in contact with the metastatic tumor tissue.	
Secure a sterile ESU pencil and suction to the field.	
Proceed with wound closure using only sterile instrumentation and supplies.	Proceed with wound closure using only sterile instrumentation and items from the sterile field for closure.

From the Association of periOperative Nurses. Guidelines for perioperative practice. Sterile Technique. *Preparing the Sterile Field*. Standard No. 3; 2020.

commands, and the airway is maintained without artificial support.

Preparation for endoscopy includes a period of fasting or dietary restriction, depending on the extent and type of endoscopic procedure. Upper GI studies require limitations on oral intake. Lower GI endoscopy requires dietary restrictions and an enema, which the patient can self-administer the day before the procedure.

NOTE *A complete discussion of the technology, handling, and reprocessing of fiber-optic endoscopes is presented in Chapter 20.*

Gastrointestinal endoscopy is indicated for the following:

- To establish or confirm a diagnosis by direct visualization and biopsy
- To perform selected surgical procedures (restricted to surgery in which bleeding is minimal and the risk for technical complications is low)
- To allow postoperative inspection of the surgical site from within the lumen of the GI tract and for screening

ESOPHAGODUODENOSCOPY

Esophagoduodenoscopy (EGD) is diagnostic endoscopy of the esophagus, stomach, and proximal duodenum. Specific goals are the following:

- Direct diagnostic observation of the inside of the esophagus and duodenum, with biopsy
- Treatment of varices (varices are prone to frequent bleeding and sometimes require emergency treatment)
- Polyp removal (polyps are small, benign mucosal outgrowths in the lumen of the esophagus)
- Endoscopic **gastrostomy** for insertion of a feeding tube
- Placement of a stent for an esophageal stricture
- Dilatation of the esophagus to treat a stricture using gastric bougies such as the Maloney, Savary, and balloon-type dilators

Before the procedure, the ST should ensure that the endoscope, imaging system, and data storage devices are in working order and ready for use.

The patient may be required to remove his or her clothing. In this case a patient gown is provided. An intravenous cannula is inserted. During the procedure, the patient's vital signs will be assessed and documented. Anesthetic spray is applied to the pharynx.

The patient is placed in the left lateral position and intravenous sedative is administered. A small amount of lubricating gel is put on the tip of the scope, and a bite block is inserted into the patient's mouth.

The insertion tube (the distal end of the endoscope) is advanced slowly, and the tissues are examined. Real-time digital imaging is performed to view the anatomy. If biopsy samples are taken, the ST passes biopsy instruments to the surgeon and helps thread the tip into the instrument port. Several procedures may be initiated at this point:

- *Removal of small tumors or benign growths:* The ST is required to remove specimens from the biopsy instruments, place them in an appropriate container, and label the container.
- *Injection of esophageal varices:* The ST prepares the sclerosing agent, which is injected through the endoscope after needle placement in the varicosity.
- *Varicocele banding:* A special banding system is passed through the endoscope, and the varicosity is ligated.
- *Esophageal dilation:* Graduated dilators are introduced over a guidewire under fluoroscopy after endoscopic examination.
- *Insertion of an esophageal stent:* Self-expanding esophageal stent may be inserted to dilate and hold open a stricture caused by tumor. The stent is preloaded into an insertion device, which is threaded to the level of the stricture and released. It remains in place as a palliative measure.
- *Endoscopic laser therapy:* A neodymium-yttrium-aluminum garnet (Nd:YAG) laser may be used to debulk an esophageal tumor.

The ST assists the surgeon by guiding long instruments into the endoscope and receiving them as they are withdrawn. Care must be taken to ensure that all specimens are immediately placed in the liquid specimen container, as directed by the surgeon. The specimen is cleaned from the biopsy forceps with a sterile hypodermic needle or by swishing the tip in the specimen cup liquid.

If laser surgery is planned, all safety precautions are observed to prevent patient fires or burns (see Chapter 15).

Postoperative considerations include monitoring for effective gag reflex, pain, and complete recovery from sedative drugs. The patient is taken to the postoperative recovery unit or a designated area of the outpatient area for observation and monitoring before discharge.

COLONOSCOPY

Colonoscopy is endoscopy of the large intestine. The procedure is used for diagnostic purposes and for minor surgery, such as the following:

- Removal of polyps
- Biopsy or removal of lesions
- Coagulation of small bleeding diverticula
- Laser treatment of small tumors
- Routine screening for colon cancer

Combined colonoscopy and laparoscopic surgery may be used during resection of the lower GI system.

Colonoscopy requires sedation of the patient. The procedure can be uncomfortable and embarrassing for the patient. The ST should offer support throughout the procedure. The technique used to obtain biopsy samples and for other minor procedures is similar to EGD.

The patient is placed in the left lateral position. The individual should be covered with warm blankets, and only the lower back and buttocks should be exposed. A small protective drape can be placed over the pelvis.

The scope is lubricated with water-soluble gel and gently inserted into the anus. It is then advanced slowly. When the proximal colon is in view, the surgeon begins to withdraw the scope slowly while examining the mucosa. Air may be instilled into the colon with a pump attachment. This may cause the patient some discomfort, and the ST should offer reassurance. As the scope is withdrawn, the length of the colon is examined for lesions and abnormalities. Digital photographs of any suspect tissue are taken. Suction and irrigation are controlled at the scope head. The ST should make sure the irrigation reservoir remains full by refilling it as needed.

Cupped or brush biopsy forceps are guided through the scope. As tissue is withdrawn from the endoscope, the ST receives the forceps and maintains control on the tip to ensure that the specimen is not lost. The specimen can be removed from the tip with a hypodermic needle or by swishing the tip in the specimen cup.

Postoperative considerations include observation for pain or bleeding and sensitivity to any medications given during the procedure.

SIGMOIDOSCOPY

Sigmoidoscopy is performed to examine tissue and/or obtain a biopsy specimen of the sigmoid colon and rectum. The patient is placed in the prone or lithotomy position, and the scope is introduced. Biopsy tissue can be obtained, or rectal polyps can be removed with cup biopsy forceps.

SURGICAL PROCEDURES

LAPAROTOMY

A **laparotomy** is open surgery of the abdominal cavity for access to the abdominal organs. A laparotomy to confirm a specific pathological condition is called an **exploratory laparotomy.** The procedure for entering the abdominal cavity is the same for many different pathologies, although the location of the incision may differ. The following detailed description is omitted from individual surgical procedures discussed in this chapter. Note that routines such as sponge and instrument counts, documentation, and care of specimens are not included in each procedure described in this chapter. These are covered in Chapters 18 and 19.

POSITION:	Supine
INCISION:	Abdominal, depending on the region to be explored
PREP AND DRAPING:	Laparotomy
INSTRUMENTS:	Laparotomy or major general set
POSSIBLE EXTRAS:	According to the specific procedure planned

Technical Points and Discussion

OPENING THE ABDOMEN

1. ***An incision is made through all layers of the abdominal wall.***
The skin is incised using a #20 knife blade. A shallow pan should be placed on the field to receive the skin knife, which is removed from the field as soon as the skin incision has been made (no-touch technique). Once the skin is incised, the assistant applies counter-traction on the incision using a folded lap sponge. The monopolar ESU is used to manage bleeders and incise the fatty subcutaneous layer. Large bleeding vessels can be clamped with Kelly or Crile hemostats and ligated with the ESU.

2. ***The incision is carried through to the next layer, the fascia.***
At this level, the ST should have small Richardson or US retractors available for the assistant. The surgeon incises the layer with a #10 knife (called the "deep knife") or ESU and extends the incision as needed with the ESU or curved Mayo scissors. If the incision is off the midline, the muscle layers are separated manually. The abdominal peritoneum is then visible. The ST prepares several moist lap sponges and a self-retaining retractor. Any 4 × 4 Raytec sponges that are *not* mounted on an instrument must be removed before the peritoneum is opened. Refer to Chapter 18 for a complete discussion on the management of surgical sponges.

3. ***The peritoneum is lifted with hemostats, and a small incision is made with the deep knife or Metzenbaum scissors.***
The incision is carried deeper with scissors or the ESU.

4. ***The contents of the abdominal cavity are explored.***
The surgeon now explores the abdomen. A medium or large Richardson retractor should be offered to the assistant during exploration. The patient may be placed in Trendelenburg position at this time. The ST should ensure that there is clearance between the patient and the Mayo tray as the operating table is tilted.

5. ***The edges of the wound are covered with moist laparotomy sponges, and a self-retaining retractor is inserted into the wound.***
From this point on, saline-moistened sponges are used. The ST passes the moistened sponges to the surgeon, who covers the tissue edges to protect them from the self-retaining retractor. The retractor is now secured in position by the surgeon and the assistant. When the area of disease has been located, the surgeon packs the abdominal contents away from the diseased area with several moistened lap sponges. A specific surgical procedure then can be performed.

CLOSING THE ABDOMEN

6. ***The wound is irrigated, and drains are inserted, as needed.***
When the specific procedure is completed, it is common for the surgeon to irrigate the wound with warm saline. This removes tissue debris and bits of suture from the wound. The ST should offer only fresh warm saline, which helps prevent hypothermia. An Asepto syringe or pitcher can be used to deliver the saline into the wound. Abdominal suction such as a Poole tip is used to remove the excess saline from the abdominal cavity. The abdomen is checked for any signs of bleeding before the wound is closed.

7. ***The abdominal layers are closed, and dressings are applied.***
After irrigation, the surgeon and assistant remove all sponges and instruments from the abdomen, and the count is initiated. The incision then is closed in layers. The choice of suture materials (absorbable, nonabsorbable, synthetic, or natural fiber) depends on the amount of tension on the incision, the wound classification, the size of the patient, and the surgeon's preference. The count is completed before the peritoneum is closed.

When all sponges and instruments have been removed from the abdomen, the surgeon's assistant grasps the edges of the peritoneum with several hemostats. The peritoneum usually is closed with a continuous 0 or 2-0 absorbable suture with a taper needle. The fascia may be sutured with the peritoneum as a single layer, and a variety of materials, both synthetic and nonsynthetic, may be used. Nonsynthetic materials currently are favored for their strength and lack of reactivity in tissue. If the fascial layer is closed separately, 2-0 suture is most often used in patients who are not obese.

During closure of the fascia, the assistant retracts the skin and subcutaneous layer with US or Richardson retractors. Toothed tissue forceps are used during closure of the abdominal wall.

Retention sutures may be placed before peritoneal closure in patients who are at risk of wound dehiscence. Size 0 or 1 retention sutures are placed approximately 1.2 inches (3 cm) behind the incision line, catching all layers of the abdominal wall. The suture is threaded through a short length of flexible tubing (bolster) before the knots are tied. This distributes the tension evenly along the retention suture and prevents it from tearing through the tissue (see Chapter 20).

The subcutaneous layer is closed with interrupted sutures of 3-0 absorbable synthetic suture. Fine tapered needles are used. Skin closure often is performed with staples. Alternative methods, such as subcuticular or fine interrupted sutures, may be used in selected patients for a cosmetic closure. If staples are used, the assistant pulls the tissue edges together with two Adson skin forceps while the surgeon places the staples across the incision. At the completion of skin closure, the ST or surgeon places the dressings over the wound. The drapes are then removed, and tape is applied to the dressings by the circulator or surgeon.

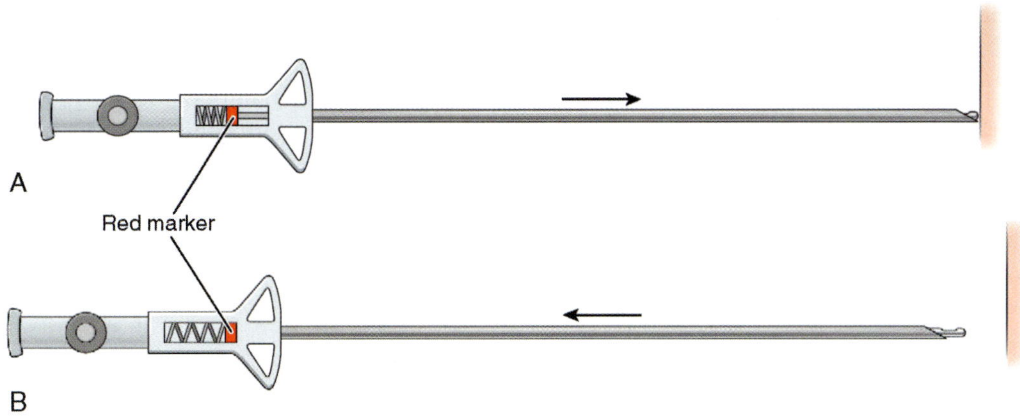

FIG. 22.11 Veress needle used to inflate the abdomen (pneumoperitoneum) during laparoscopy.

LAPAROSCOPY

Laparoscopy is performed as a stand-alone procedure for diagnosis *(diagnostic laparoscopy)* or as a means of performing many different types of procedures across general and gynecological surgery. Chapter 20 describes the supplies, instruments, and safety aspects of laparoscopy. The procedure is described here as a foundation for laparoscopic procedures discussed in this chapter and in Chapter 24.

During laparoscopy, the surgical instruments are placed in the abdominal cavity through small incision (usually 1 to 2 cm long) and surgery performed without opening the abdominal cavity. Access to the abdominal cavity is maintained by first inflating the abdominal cavity with carbon dioxide gas (pneumoperitoneum) as described in Chapter 20, and by inserting a series of cannulas, which receive the long laparoscopic instruments and maintain the pneumoperitoneum.

POSITION:	Supine or lithotomy
INCISION:	Laparoscopic
PREP AND DRAPING:	Abdominal or combined abdominal/perineal
INSTRUMENTS:	Laparoscopic including trocars
POSSIBLE EXTRAS:	Hand port; ultrasonic scalpel; vessel-sealing system; laparoscopic staplers; sutures; others according to the requirements of the procedure

Technical Points and Discussion

1. ***The patient is prepped and draped.***
The surgical prep and draping for laparoscopy will follow the techniques for supine position or lithotomy. Lithotomy is commonly used during gynecological procedures and those involving the sigmoid colon and rectum. In both cases, the abdomen is prepped as for a laparotomy, whereas most gynecological procedures require a complete vaginal prep as discussed in Chapter 19. Draping is carried out in routine fashion for abdominal or combined abdominal-perineal access.

2. ***Peritoneal access and pneumoperitoneum.***
The procedure begins with establishing pneumoperitoneum. The ST should have available sterile CO_2 tubing for insufflation and the surgeon's choice of trocars. There are many different types and designs of peritoneal access devices. The most common methods used for initial entry into the abdomen are the following:

   - Veress needle technique
   - Hasson technique
   - Optical trocar

VERESS TECHNIQUE

The Veress needle device contains a hollow needle with a spring-loaded obturator (Fig. 22.11). The obturator is a blunt tip stylus that retracts to expose the needle when slight pressure is applied. As the needle enters the abdominal cavity, the obturator returns to its normal position ahead of the needle point. This prevents injury to the abdominal viscera during insertion. Before passing the device to the surgeon, the ST should test the tip to ensure that the spring mechanism is working properly. This is done by simply applying light pressure to the tip of the needle. Pressure causes the needle point to retract. The surgeon elevates the exterior abdominal wall either by hand or by placing two penetrating towel clamps into the superficial abdominal layers to elevate the abdominal wall. A short nick is made in the skin using a #11 knife blade. A disposable or reusable Veress needle is then inserted through the incision and advanced through the peritoneum. A saline drop test is performed to ensure that the needle is in position and has not penetrated the viscera on entry. A 10-cc syringe is filled with sterile saline, and several drops are placed into the needle port. Negative pressure in the abdominal cavity pulls the saline into the body, and this is an indication that the needle has been correctly placed. The insufflation tubing is attached to the Veress needle and pneumoperitoneum established. When the abdomen is sufficiently inflated to prevent injury to the viscera, the needle is replaced by a trocar-cannula, which maintains the pneumoperitoneum.

HASSON TECHNIQUE

In this technique, the Hasson blunt trocar is used to establish pneumoperitoneum. A short incision is made in the skin at the site of trocar placement. This incision is carried to the fascia layer with Metzenbaum scissors and ESU. A US Army retractor or S retractor is used to expose the fascia, which is then incised. Two size 0 synthetic stay sutures are placed at either end of the incision. These are used to elevate the abdominal wall. A small incision is made in the peritoneum using Metzenbaum scissors. The Hasson sleeve and obturator are inserted into the abdomen through all layers and secured in place using the preplaced sutures (see Chapter 20). The insufflation tubing is attached to the Hasson trocar, and pneumoperitoneum is established.

OPTICAL TROCAR

The bladeless optical trocar (see Chapter 20) is inserted through the abdominal wall as described for the open Hasson technique without prior insufflation. However, in this technique the laparoscope is attached to the head of the trocar so that the abdominal layers can be visualized as they are penetrated. The insufflation tubing is attached to the trocar and the pneumoperitoneum established.

ACCESSORY TROCARS ARE PLACED

After the pneumoperitoneum is established, the surgeon places the other operative trocars according to the specific needs of the procedure. A 10-mm port is commonly used for the laparoscope, and 5- to 10-mm ports are used for the surgical instruments. Larger ports are required for hand-assisted procedures and for large specimens.

3. ***A specific procedure is carried out.***
When all ports have been placed, a specific procedure can begin. For diagnostic laparoscopy, two instruments are commonly used to manipulate the tissues and organs. These are the dolphin-nose forceps and the probe (refer to Chapter 20 for photos). Retractors such as the fan retractor are also used by the assistant to assist in viewing the surgical anatomy.

4. ***Instruments are withdrawn, the pneumoperitoneum is released, and the wounds closed.***
At the close of the procedure, the instruments are withdrawn and the pneumoperitoneum released. The incisions may be closed using a variety of techniques. Figure-of-8 sutures of absorbable synthetic size 0 or 2-0 are commonly placed to close the superficial layers of the port incisions. The fascia layer and peritoneum may not be sutured if the ports are small. Skin is closed using Steri-Strips with skin adhesive or surgical staples, followed by adhesive strips.

GASTRECTOMY, BILLROTH I AND II (OPEN)

Gastrectomy is removal of a portion of the stomach and anastomosis to the duodenum (**Billroth I**) or jejunum (**Billroth II**) to restore continuity. A gastrectomy may also include vagotomy (severing the vagus nerve) or lymph node dissection. Gastrectomy is nearly always performed using minimally invasive techniques—laparoscopic or robotic. However, in some cases, an open technique is necessary.

Pathology

Partial gastrectomy is most commonly performed for the treatment of gastric carcinoma or obstructive ulcer disease. Obstructive ulcer disease is commonly caused by *H. pylori* bacteria and chronic use of nonsteroidal antiinflammatory drugs. Partial (subtotal) gastrectomy requires reconstruction of the stomach to maintain continuity of the GI tract. The method and location of anastomosis depend on the extent and type of pathology, the patient's overall condition and age, and the surgeon's preferred technique. The gastric pouch (the remainder of the stomach after resection) can be attached to the small intestine, or the divided end of the intestine can be attached directly to the stomach. A full endoscopic exam is performed on the patient before surgery to establish the size and scope of the pathology. This is accompanied by endoscopic ultrasonography.

POSITION:	Supine/low lithotomy
INCISION:	Upper right or midline
PREP AND DRAPING:	Abdominal; laparotomy
INSTRUMENTS:	Laparotomy set: gastrointestinal instruments; long instruments
POSSIBLE EXTRAS:	Longitudinal and circumferential surgical staplers; hemostatic clips; Silastic vascular loops; wound drainage system

Technical Points and Discussion

1. ***A laparotomy is performed through an upper right or midline incision.***
A laparotomy is performed through an upper midline incision. The surgeon examines the abdominal contents to determine the extent of disease and to select a site for anastomosis. The exact lines of resection are determined, and the stomach is mobilized from the ligaments, vessels, and omentum. The ST should be prepared with many Mayo, Crile, or Kelly clamps, vessel clips, and suture ties. Suture ligatures are used on the major vessels of the stomach and omentum.

2. ***The stomach is mobilized from the omentum; the duodenum or jejunum is mobilized from the omentum.***

Allis or Babcock clamps are used to hold traction on the stomach while the omentum is divided from the greater curvature. Large gastric blood vessels are isolated, occluded with vessel clips, and divided separately. After double-clamping the segments of omentum, the surgeon divides the tissue with dissecting scissors, the ESU, or an HF vessel-sealing system. The lesser curvature of the stomach is mobilized using the same technique. Lymph node dissection may be performed at this time. Once identified, the nodes are mobilized and removed using scissors. The ST should immediately label these and pass them off to the circulator.

3. ***The intestine is cross-clamped with two intestinal clamps, and the tissue is divided into two sections.***
When mobilization is completed, the surgeon places two intestinal cross-clamps (Kocher or Allen type) side by side across the duodenum (Billroth I procedure) or the jejunum (Billroth II procedure). An incision is then made between the two clamps. The duodenal or jejunal stump is closed with a stapling instrument or fine sutures. The stomach is cross-clamped and divided.
Hand-suturing and surgical stapling are the two techniques commonly used to join the stomach with the intestine. Although stapling instruments are commonly used, the ST should also be familiar with the traditional two-layer suture closure. Stapling procedures involving the stomach and small intestine are discussed in the next section.
The intestine and stomach are made up of separate tissue layers, the outer serosa, smooth muscle, submucosa, and mucosa. Two suture lines are used to create the anastomosis. The inner suture catches the mucosa, submucosa, and muscle layers. The outer serosa layers of both structures are joined separately. Absorbable suture can be used for the inner closure and absorbable or nonabsorbable sutures for the serosa.

4. ***The stomach is double-clamped and divided. The open stomach edges are sutured or stapled together.***
To begin the anastomosis, the surgeon brings the cross-clamped sections close together. A traction suture is placed at each end. An outside row of sutures is placed, joining the two structures. Next, the surgeon makes two incisions, one on each side of the suture line. This exposes the inner lumen of the intestine (or stomach). The surgeon brings the inner layers together with continuous running or interrupted sutures. Finally, the outer layer is completed circumferentially with interrupted sutures. The double layer of sutures prevents leakage.
Stapling instruments have largely replaced traditional suturing techniques in GI anastomosis. If stapling instruments are preferred, the gastrointestinal anastomosis (GIA) and thoracoabdominal (TA) linear staplers are used to resect the stomach and intestine (see Chapter 11).
Isolation technique is observed, and any instruments or sponges in contact with the open tract are removed from the field. These are not used on the closed GI tract. It is useful to have a second setup ready for the closure.

5. ***If postoperative stomach depression is required, a percutaneous (through the skin) gastric tube is inserted.***
To insert a gastric tube, the surgeon selects a location in the stomach remnant and places a purse-string suture around the point. He or she elevates the stomach wall with Allis or Babcock clamps and incises a small hole at the center of the purse-string suture, which is drawn together around the tube. The gastric tube is then brought through the abdominal wall through a small stab incision. Sutures are placed through the skin and abdominal wall to secure the tube.

6. ***The abdomen is irrigated and closed in layers.***
Before the surgical wound is closed, the abdomen is irrigated with sterile saline. One or more Penrose drains may be placed in the abdomen and brought out through a separate stab incision or the abdominal wound. The abdomen is closed as for laparotomy. A flat dressing including abdominal pad is applied over the incision and drainage sites.
Fig. 22.12 shows important technical highlights of an open Billroth II procedure.

LAPAROSCOPIC BAND GASTROPLASTY

Band gastroplasty is performed in the treatment of obesity. Nutritional intake is restricted by creating a small pouch in the proximal stomach. Food passes slowly into the stomach while creating a feeling of fullness.

The pouch is created by encircling the upper stomach with an inflatable band. The inner part of the band connects with a tube and saline reservoir implanted into the body wall. This allows the band to be filled from an external port embedded in the subcutaneous tissue. Tension on the band is adjusted by the addition or removal of saline, thereby regulating the flow of food out of the pouch and into the stomach. Several different types of bands are available. The Lap-Band is described here, although the more traditional Roux-en-Y procedure is also performed by some surgeons. Fig. 22.13 illustrates the gastric band procedure as described in the following text.

During the procedure, the surgeon is positioned between the patient's legs, which are held in low lithotomy. Care must be taken to ensure that the patient is securely positioned. A bean bag positioner may be used to support the patient as reverse Trendelenburg is used for access to the upper stomach.

Pathology

Obesity is an endemic health problem in the United States. It contributes to cardiovascular disease, cancers of the breast and large intestine, diabetes, stroke, urinary stress incontinence,

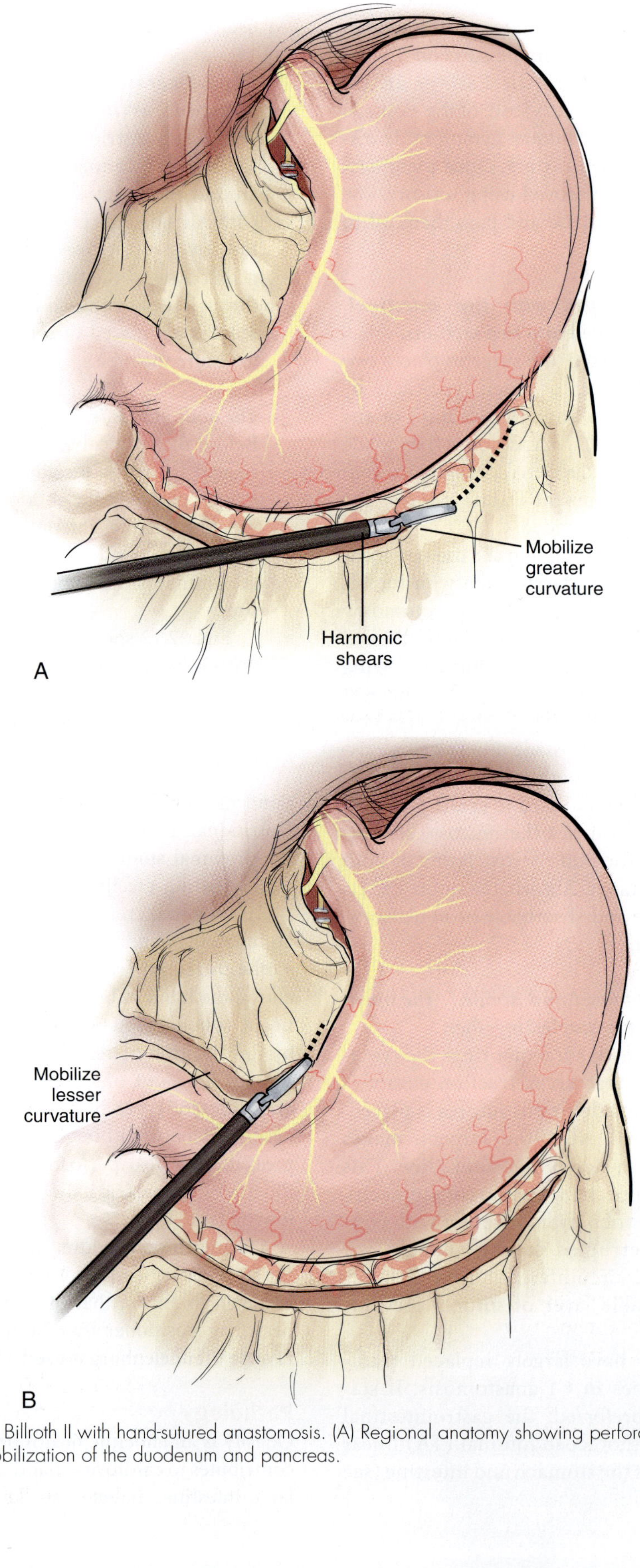

FIG. 22.12 Billroth II with hand-sutured anastomosis. (A) Regional anatomy showing perforated gastric ulcer. (B) Mobilization of the duodenum and pancreas.

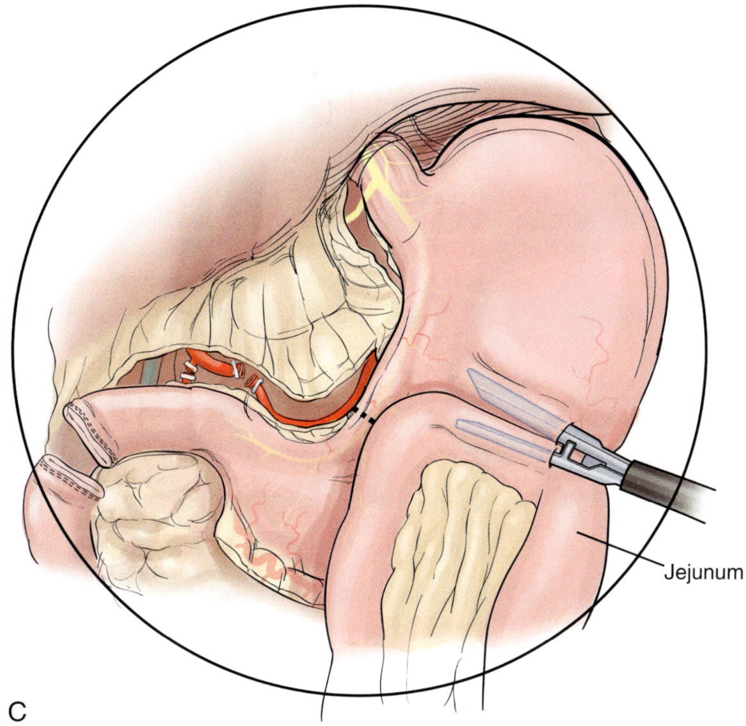

FIG. 22.12, cont'd (C) Gastroduodenectomy has been performed. The end-to-end anastomosis begins with the posterior wall. Sutures are left long until all are placed. The final layer of interrupted sutures is placed in the anterior wall. (From Khatri V. *Atlas of Advanced Operative Surgery*. Philadelphia: Saunders; 2013.)

and depression. Approximately 400,000 people die annually as a result of obesity in the United States.

Prospective patients are screened and usually are required to attempt conservative weight loss measures before surgical intervention. Criteria include the following:

- Motivation and commitment to weight loss
- Abstinence from alcohol and tobacco
- Absence of psychological factors that could hinder a successful outcome

Bariatric surgery has a long history of attempts to restrict food intake or interference with nutrient absorption. Early radical gastric bypass procedures resulted in severe malabsorption and multiple medical problems related to nutrient deficiency. Other techniques, such as vertical band gastroplasty, have been abandoned because the procedures failed to achieve the medical goal (patients alter their eating habits to include high-calorie liquids) or stenosis (narrowing) of the stomach outlet.

Adjustable gastric banding does not result in malabsorption, it is reversible, and it can be performed as minimally invasive surgery. Postoperatively, the patient experiences rapid satiety after eating a small amount of food, which passes slowly from the pouch to the stomach. Patients must be screened preoperatively for suitability for the procedure.

POSITION:	Supine/low lithotomy
INCISION:	Laparoscopic
PREP AND DRAPING:	Abdominal/laparotomy
INSTRUMENTS AND SUPPLIES:	Laparoscopy: two 5-mm trocars; one 5- to 10-mm trocar; one 10-mm trocar; 30-degree laparoscope; laparoscopic instruments extra long; ultrasonic scalpel; bipolar ligation system; standard monopolar ESU; banding system

Technical Points and Discussion

1. ***Pneumoperitoneum is established, and trocars are placed through the abdominal wall.***
   Pneumoperitoneum is established using a Veress needle or Hasson cut-down approach. A 10-mm trocar is used for a 30-degree laparoscope in the left upper quadrant. A 10- to 15-mm trocar is placed at the left axillary line, 5-mm trocars are placed in the right and left midclavicular lines, and a 5- to 10-mm trocar is placed below and left of the xiphoid.

2. ***The stomach is grasped with two smooth grasping forceps, and the gastric ligament is incised.***
   To begin the surgery, the ST should provide two grasping forceps to elevate the fundus of the stomach. This provides traction on the gastric ligament, which is perforated using a monopolar dissecting hook. A liver retractor such as a wide Deaver is also needed at the start of the case.

3. ***The gastric ligament opening is increased to accommodate the band.***

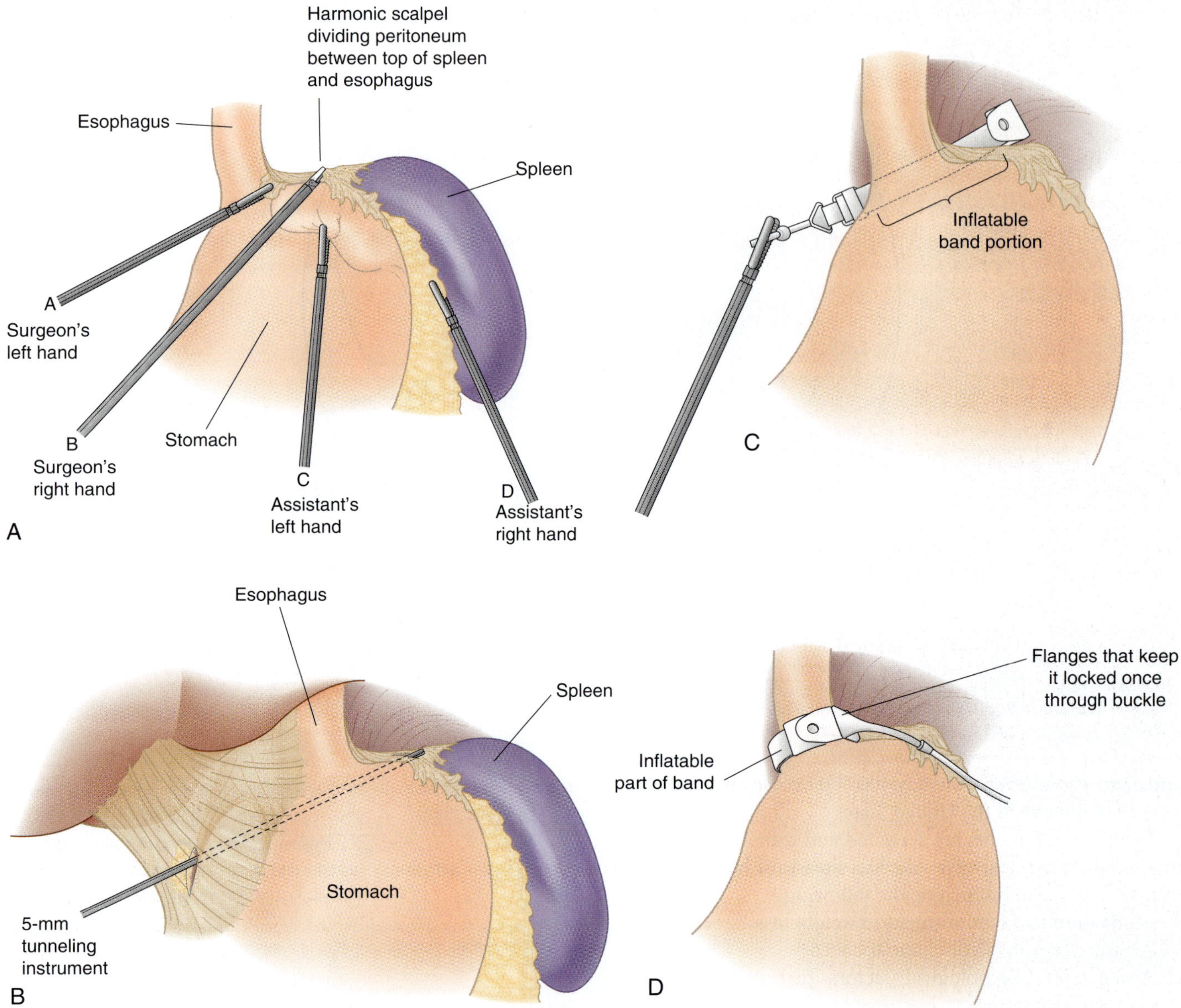

FIG. 22.13 Gastric banding procedure. (A) The visceral peritoneum is divided at the antrum of the stomach (angle of His). (B) A tunneling instrument is placed behind the stomach. (C) An inflatable band is inserted through the tunnel. (D) The band is passed around the stomach. (E) The band is locked in place. (F) A section of the stomach is pulled up over the band. (From Townsend CM. *Sabiston Textbook of Surgery*. 17th ed. Philadelphia: WB Saunders; 2001.)

The attachment to the proximal stomach is released to create a tunnel for the band. An additional opening is made in the tissue attachment at the lesser curvature. Bleeders are managed with the ultrasonic ligation system. The ST prepares the band by testing it for leaks and flushing it with normal saline. After flushing, 5 mL of saline is left in the band and tubing. The ST should place a clamp at the distal end of the tubing prevent saline from leaking from the tube.

4. ***The band is placed around the proximal stomach and secured.***
The ST should dip the band in saline before passing it and a smooth grasper to the surgeon. The band and tube are then passed through the openings. The tip of the band is secured into the lock end of the band. At this point the anesthesia provider will insert a gastric tube with an inflatable 25-mL balloon into the proximal stomach. The balloon is inflated and retracted slightly to position it at the esophageal junction. The band is then locked in place.

5. ***The gastric wall is folded over the band and sutured in place.***
The ST should provide three to four sutures of nonabsorbable suture to secure the stomach to the band. This is done by folding the gastric wall over the band and tacking it in place.

6. ***The saline port and tubing are implanted and tested.***
The larger port is removed, the pneumoperitoneum released, and the Lap Band tubing is brought out through

the incision originally made for the port. It is cut to size and then attached to the injection port. The port is implanted on the fascia layer under the skin using multiple sutures of the surgeon's choice. It may be necessary to decrease the size of the trocar incision around the injection port. This is done with size 0 or 1 Dexon.

7. ***The wounds are closed.***
   The deep tissue at the laparoscopic ports is now closed using figure-of-8 nonabsorbable sutures of size 0. Steri-Strips or staples are used to close the skin.
   Patients usually are discharged the same day they have laparoscopic surgery. The band is adjusted by injecting additional saline into the port percutaneously under fluoroscopy. In the first postoperative year, the band is adjusted three to four times; thereafter, it is adjusted yearly to ensure continued weight control.

ROUX-EN-Y GASTRIC BYPASS (LAPAROSCOPIC)

The Roux-en-Y procedure is performed to bypass most of the stomach, leaving only a small stomach pouch. A section of the jejunum is transected and re-established at the stomach to allow food to exit the pouch. The remaining jejunal limb is attached to the upper jejunum to allow gastric secretions to enter the intestine.

Pathology

The Roux-en-Y procedure traditionally has been used to treat gastric ulcers and gastric carcinoma. It is now also the preferred surgery for long-term weight loss control.

POSITION:	Supine or low lithotomy
PREP AND DRAPING:	Laparotomy with leggings for lithotomy
INSTRUMENTS:	Laparoscopy; extra-long instruments for obese patients; flexible or fan liver retractor; 30-degree telescope; 12-mm port-trocar system, 3, 8-mm port-trocar system; optical trocar or other entry trocar; Veress needle
POSSIBLE EXTRAS:	TA 90 endo stapler; GIA endo stapler; endo clip applier with clips; ultrasonic dissector; small Penrose drain

Technical Points and Discussion

PNEUMOPERITONEUM IS ESTABLISHED

A pneumoperitoneum is established by means of the Veress needle or Hasson cut-down approach. Trocars are then placed. Three 12-mm trocars and two 5-mm trocars are placed in the abdominal wall. A 0-degree laparoscope is used to start the procedure; this will be replaced by a 30- or 45-degree laparoscope later in the case.

1. ***The gastric pouch is created.***
   To form the gastric pouch, the assistant must first retract the liver using a flexible liver retractor or wide Deaver, while the surgeon creates an opening in the lesser omentum at the level of the proposed partition.
   The ST should provide an ultrasonic dissector and a bowel grasper to create the opening. This enables the use of a linear endostapler to form the first part of the pouch.
   Dissection is continued to mobilize the stomach from its attachments. The surgeon may ask the anesthesia provider to insert a 32 Fr bougie or 25-mL balloon catheter into the stomach. This helps identify and size the pouch. The pouch is made using the endo GIA stapler. The surgeon will determine the correct size of staples for this maneuver.

2. ***The jejunum is transected.***
   To create the gastrojejunostomy, the jejunum must be transected (divided and closed). This is done using the linear endostapler. Two small openings are made in the mesentery to accommodate the endostapler. The forks of the stapler are placed across the jejunum and fired. The staple line is oversewn with size 2-0 absorbable sutures. The mesentery perforations are repaired with synthetic or polydioxanone suture.

3. ***A gastrojejunostomy is created.***
   To create a new opening between the jejunum and the stomach, the surgeon makes two stab wounds to accommodate the forks of the GIA stapler—one in the jejunum and one in the stomach. This is done with ultrasonic scalpel. The stapler is inserted into the stab wounds, and the staples are fired. This attaches the jejunum to the stomach. Note that this anastomosis can be double- or triple-sealed with lines of staples. The staple site is oversewn with size 2-0 absorbable synthetic sutures. Any other defects in the mesentery are repaired with size 2-0 polydioxanone or similar suture.

4. ***The wounds are closed.***
   The wound is irrigated with normal saline, and the pneumoperitoneum is released. Trocar incisions are closed with buried size 0 figure-of-8 nonabsorbable suture. Skin is closed using staples and Steri-Strips. Fig. 22.14 illustrates several important steps of the Roux-en-Y gastric bypass.
   Weight loss is more rapid after Roux-en-Y surgery than with band gastroplasty. Patients who did not have the procedure for morbid obesity are followed carefully for adequate nutritional intake.

NISSEN FUNDOPLICATION (LAPAROSCOPIC)

Nissen fundoplication commonly is performed to treat noncomplicated *gastroesophageal reflux disease* (GERD). The term *fundo* refers to the fundus of the stomach; *plication* means to

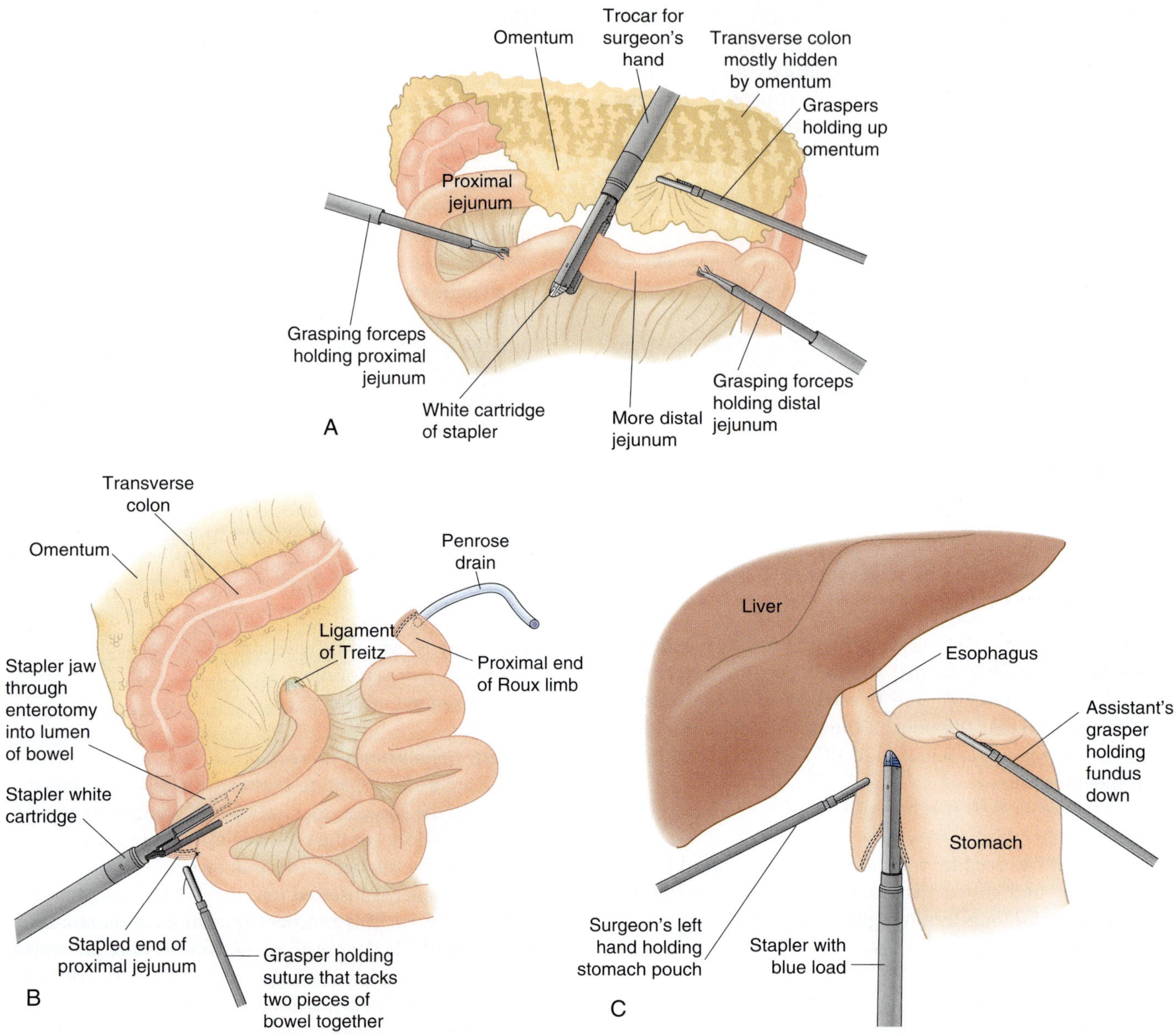

FIG. 22.14 Roux-en-Y gastric bypass. (A) The jejunum is divided with a surgical stapler. (B) The jejunum is measured and positioned for the distal anastomosis. (C and D) Placing the stapler to create the duodenostomy. (E) Firing the stapler to create the proximal gastric pouch. (F and G) Creating the proximal anastomosis. (H) Closure of the defect in the mesentery. (From Townsend CM. *Sabiston Textbook of Surgery*. 17th ed. Philadelphia: WB Saunders; 2001.)

fold. In this procedure, the upper stomach is folded around the esophagus below the hiatus to act as a sphincter. This prevents backflow of the stomach contents into the esophagus.

Pathology

Gastric contents are normally prevented from entering the esophagus by the lower esophageal sphincter, which has sufficient pressure to prevent the backflow of stomach contents into the esophagus. Loss of pressure or tone in the lower esophageal sphincter allows the highly acidic stomach contents to wash into the esophagus, causing erosion of the esophageal mucosa. GERD causes pain, esophageal erosion, and respiratory irritation and can lead to esophageal cancer.

POSITION:	Supine/reverse Trendelenburg
PREP AND DRAPING:	Abdominal/abdominal
INSTRUMENTS:	Basic laparoscopy; two 10-mm trocars; two 5-mm trocars; flexible liver retractor
POSSIBLE EXTRAS:	Ultrasonic scalpel; extra-long instruments; Penrose drain; additional 10-mm trocar for obese patients

Technical Points and Discussion

1. ***Pneumoperitoneum is established, and trocars are placed in the abdomen.***
   Pneumoperitoneum is established using a Veress needle or the Hasson cut-down approach. A 10-mm trocar is placed at the umbilicus, and the abdominal cavity is assessed using a 10-mm, 30-degree laparoscope. Three 5-mm trocars are placed.

2. ***The stomach is mobilized and divided from the omentum.***
   The liver is retracted upward to expose the lower esophagus as it passes through the diaphragm. The assistant uses smooth graspers to lift the fundus upward. Some surgeons wrap a Penrose drain around the stomach for retraction. The assistant may retract the stomach, which can then be divided from the omentum. An ultrasonic scalpel is frequently used for dissection and coagulation.

3. ***The phrenoesophageal membrane and crura are dissected free.***
   The phrenoesophageal membrane and ligament, which adhere to the esophagus under the liver, then are divided with the ultrasonic scalpel or fine scissors. This exposes the crura. If the patient has a hiatal hernia, it is repaired at this stage of the procedure. A gastric bougie is inserted orally by the anesthesia provider, and the hiatus (opening in the diaphragm through which the esophagus passes) is sutured together with three or four nonabsorbable synthetic sutures. The bougie is then withdrawn.

4. ***The upper portion of the fundus is wrapped around the distal esophagus and sutured in place.***
   To perform the fundoplication, the surgeon must mobilize the upper stomach from its attachments to the omentum. The short gastric vessels are ligated using endoscopic clips. The mobilized portion then is grasped with atraumatic forceps and wrapped around the esophagus. The anesthesia provider passes a gastric bougie through the esophagus and into the stomach to gauge the diameter of the gastric sleeve. With the tube in place, the stomach wrap is secured with interrupted sutures through the seromuscular layers of the esophagus and stomach.
   The sleeve is approximated with several interrupted sutures. Synthetic braided suture material is commonly used for fundoplication. The gastric tube is then removed, and the gastric fold is inspected to ensure adequate constriction. The tissues are then irrigated and checked for bleeders.

5. ***The wounds are closed.***
   All cannulas are removed, the pneumoperitoneum is released, and the wounds are closed with figure-of-8 absorbable synthetic sutures and skin staples or sutures. Fig. 22.15 illustrates the Nissen fundoplication.
   Patients usually are discharged the same day as surgery.

SEGMENTAL RESECTION OF THE SMALL INTESTINE (OPEN)

Resection of the small intestine is removal of a section followed by surgical anastomosis to maintain continuity of the intestinal tract.

Pathology

Resection of the small intestine is performed to treat mechanical obstruction, inflammatory disease, or carcinoma.

Intestinal obstruction is a general term that encompasses a number of mechanical or pathological conditions that can block the intestine and require emergency surgery. Obstruction can lead to perforation, necrosis resulting from ischemia, and peritonitis. The most common obstructing pathological conditions include the following:

- *Strangulation* of a loop of bowel by a defect in the abdominal wall (hernia)
- *Volvulus:* Twisting of the bowel on itself
- *Intussusception:* Telescoping of the intestine (this occurs mainly in children and results in ischemia and necrosis of the bowel)
- *Paralytic ileus:* Paralysis of the ileum; this occurs most often as a postoperative complication after abdominal surgery
- A *peptic ulcer* may lead to perforation of the duodenum and requires surgery to prevent peritonitis. A small ulcer may be repaired, or a short segmental resection may be required.

POSITION:	Supine
INCISION:	Midline or paramedian
PREP AND DRAPING:	Abdominal/laparotomy
INSTRUMENTS AND SUPPLIES:	Major laparotomy set; intestinal instruments; vascular forceps; vessel loops; surgical clips and applier
POSSIBLE EXTRAS:	Penrose drain

Technical Points and Discussion

1. ***A laparotomy is performed through a midline incision.***
   The abdomen is entered through a midline incision as described for laparotomy. The abdomen is explored for disease and the intestine inspected.

2. ***The intestinal segment is mobilized.***
   The intestine is mobilized from the omentum along the site of resection with Metzenbaum scissors, an ESU, or a vessel-sealing system. Larger mesenteric arteries are secured with surgical clips or suture ligatures.
   Two methods of resection and anastomosis are used in current practice—surgical stapling and the more traditional method of resection and anastomosis by suturing.

3. ***The intestine is cross-clamped and divided into two sections.***

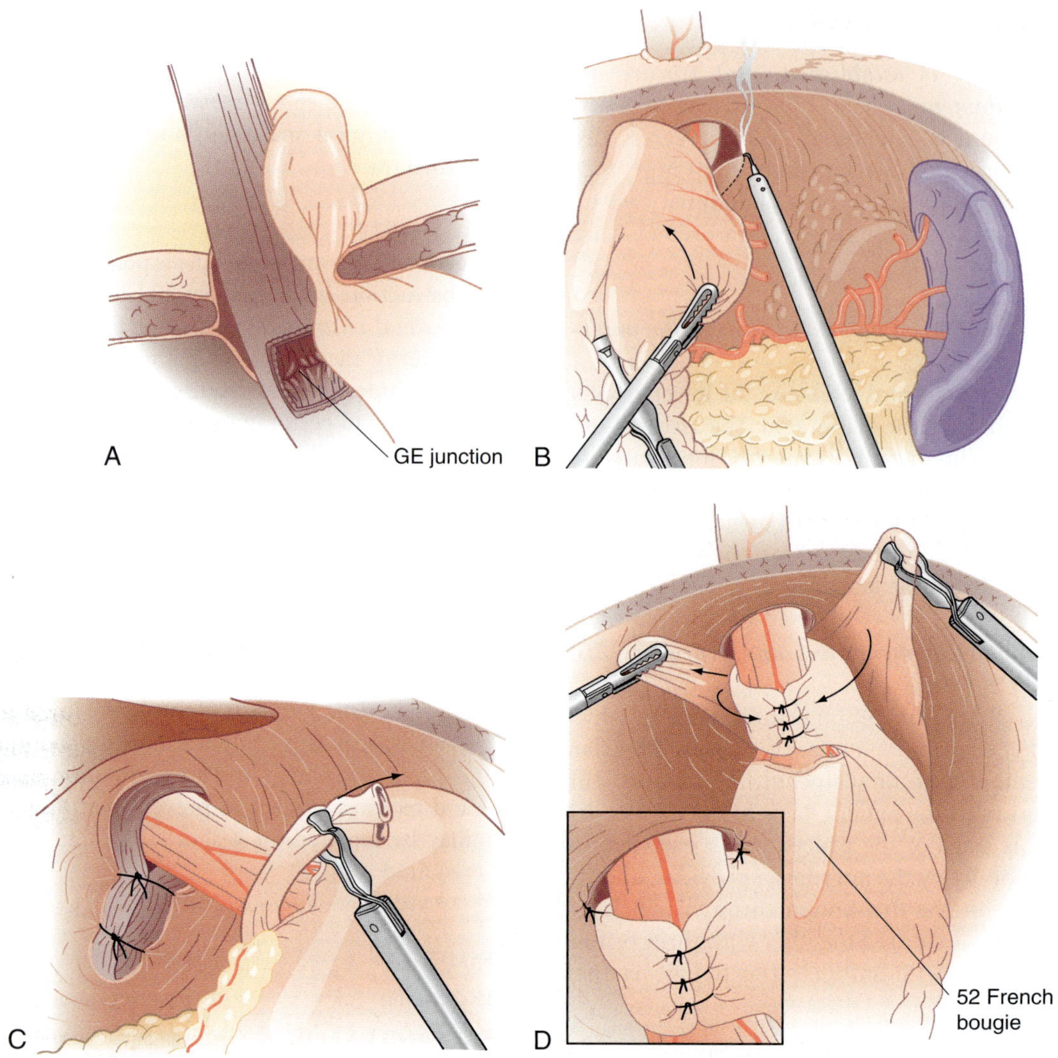

FIG. 22.15 Nissen fundoplication. (A) View of the gastroesophageal junction, with a portion of the stomach protruding through the hiatus. (B) The crura are dissected to expose the hiatus. (C) Sutures are placed through the crura to close the defect. (D) Fundoplication (wrapping) of the stomach around the distal esophagus. An esophageal catheter (bougie) is inserted. (From Townsend CM. *Sabiston Textbook of Surgery*. 17th ed. Philadelphia: WB Saunders; 2001.)

The bowel is cross-clamped with two intestinal clamps placed close together at each incision site in the bowel. The intestine is then incised between the clamps, and the diseased portion of intestine is removed as a specimen. The more common method is to use a linear staple-cutting instrument (see next step).

4. ***The diseased portion of the intestine is removed and continuity restored by anastomosis.***
Resection and anastomosis can be performed using several techniques:
- *End-to-end:* The two intestinal "limbs" are sutured together circumferentially.
- *Side-to-end:* One limb is sutured closed, and the other is implanted into a longitudinal incision in the other limb.
- *Side-to-side:* Longitudinal incisions are made in each limb, and these are joined together.

When surgical stapling techniques are used, the site of bowel resection is identified and the peritoneal covering of the mesentery is incised on each side using the ESU or Metzenbaum scissors. The mesenteric vessels are dissected free, clamped, divided, and ligated with size 3-0 sutures. Alternatively, large vascular staples can be used for ligation. Additional ligatures are often placed adjacent to the staples to ensure hemostasis.

The bowel is transected with a GIA-60 stapler, and noncrushing intestinal clamps are placed at each end of the stapled sections. The ends of the bowel can then be stapled or sutured by hand.

A layered suture anastomosis is performed by aligning the two ends of the intestine and rotating them outward. The inner layer is closed with continuous or interrupted stitches of absorbable sutures (e.g., chromic or Vicryl), and the outer serosa is closed with interrupted 3-0 or 4-0 sutures (e.g., polydioxanone).

The mucosa is closed with continuous or interrupted absorbable sutures. The serosa layer can be sutured with interrupted absorbable or nonabsorbable sutures. The mesentery is repaired with interrupted absorbable sutures.

5. ***The wound is closed in layers.***
The wound is irrigated, all bleeders are controlled, and the incision is closed in layers. The incision is dressed with a single-layer flat dressing.

END ILEOSTOMY

An **ostomy** is a procedure in which a portion of the intestine is divided and the open end is secured to the skin, draining the bowel or urine contents outside the body. The opening is then called a **stoma.** Stoma terminology indicates which area of the intestine is used to form the opening. An ileostomy is created with the ileum, whereas a colostomy is performed on the colon.

A disposable ostomy pouch is used to collect intestinal fluid; this is a **stoma appliance.** The appliance system consists of an adherent skin disc with an opening for the stoma and a collection reservoir that fits tightly into the skin wafer. The patient drains the collection reservoir as needed and changes it every few days. The appliance fits tightly over the stoma and adheres to the contours of the body to prevent leakage and odor. After the disruption of the intestinal tract, the remaining part of the intestinal system becomes nonfunctional but is left intact. A stoma may be permanent or temporary, depending upon the pathology.

Before surgery, the surgeon and the ostomy nurse discuss the exact location of the ostomy, considering the patient's lifestyle and age and protection of the ostomy from the belt line. The site is drawn on the skin before surgery as a reference. The location of an ostomy depends on the section of the intestine to be removed. The patient's psychological and physical adjustments to an ostomy procedure depend on many factors. Body image at the time of surgery, developmental age, level of debilitation before the procedure, and family and professional support affect the patient's ability to accept the change.

Stoma care requires qualified patient teaching by a certified ostomy specialist. Patients require a period of adaptation while learning to care for the ostomy. The stoma nursing team provides psychological and social support as well as technical assistance with stoma fit, cleansing, and emptying procedures.

POSITION:	Supine
PREP AND DRAPING:	Abdominal/laparotomy
INSTRUMENTS:	Laparotomy; intestinal instruments
POSSIBLE EXTRAS:	Temporary stoma pouch; stoma rod

Technical Points and Discussion

END ILEOSTOMY

1. ***A circular incision is made in the abdomen and carried through the peritoneum.***
The surgeon grasps the skin at the location of the proposed stoma with an Allis clamp and makes a small circular incision around the clamp. The skin disc is then removed from the field. The assistant retracts the abdominal wall with a small Richardson or other right-angle retractor. The incision is carried through the deep layers until peritoneum is identified. The peritoneum is grasped with two hemostats and a small incision made. Bleeders are managed with the monopolar ESU.

2. ***The terminal end of the previously mobilized bowel is brought up through the stoma incision.***
The proximal end of the mobilized bowel is pulled into the body wall incision using Babcock clamps. Note that this terminal end will have been sealed with the linear staple-cutting instrument to prevent leakage.

3. ***The bowel limb is opened out and sutured to the skin.***
Before the stoma is created, the mesentery may be attached to the abdominal wall. The previously placed staple line is excised using ESU. The ST should have suction available as soon as the limb is opened. The tissue is removed from the field and retained as specimen. The edges of the now-opened bowel limb are everted, and long sutures are attached near the open edge. These are tacked to the abdominal wall with absorbable sutures. Size 2-0 absorbable sutures on a curved cutting needle are passed through the full thickness of the bowel and the abdominal wall skin. Four sutures are placed to hold the bowel in place. Additional interrupted sutures are placed between the tacking stitches around the circumference of the stoma. An ileostomy drains fluid that is caustic to the skin; therefore the stoma is created as a raised "spigot" so that the contents are emptied into the stoma pouch without touching the skin. The end ileostomy is illustrated in Fig. 22.16.

LOOP ILEOSTOMY

1. ***An incision is made in the abdominal wall to accommodate the stoma.***
Just as for end ileostomy, an incision is made in the abdominal wall using the skin knife. The edges of the wound are retracted with right-angle retractors. The incision is carried through fatty and muscle tissues using blunt dissection. The surgeon grasps the abdominal fascia with clamps and incises it with the ESU. The peritoneum is grasped with two hemostats and perforated with dissecting scissors.

2. ***The selected loop of ileum is grasped and brought out of the abdominal perforation.***
The previously selected portion of ileum is brought through the stoma site using Babcock clamps. The

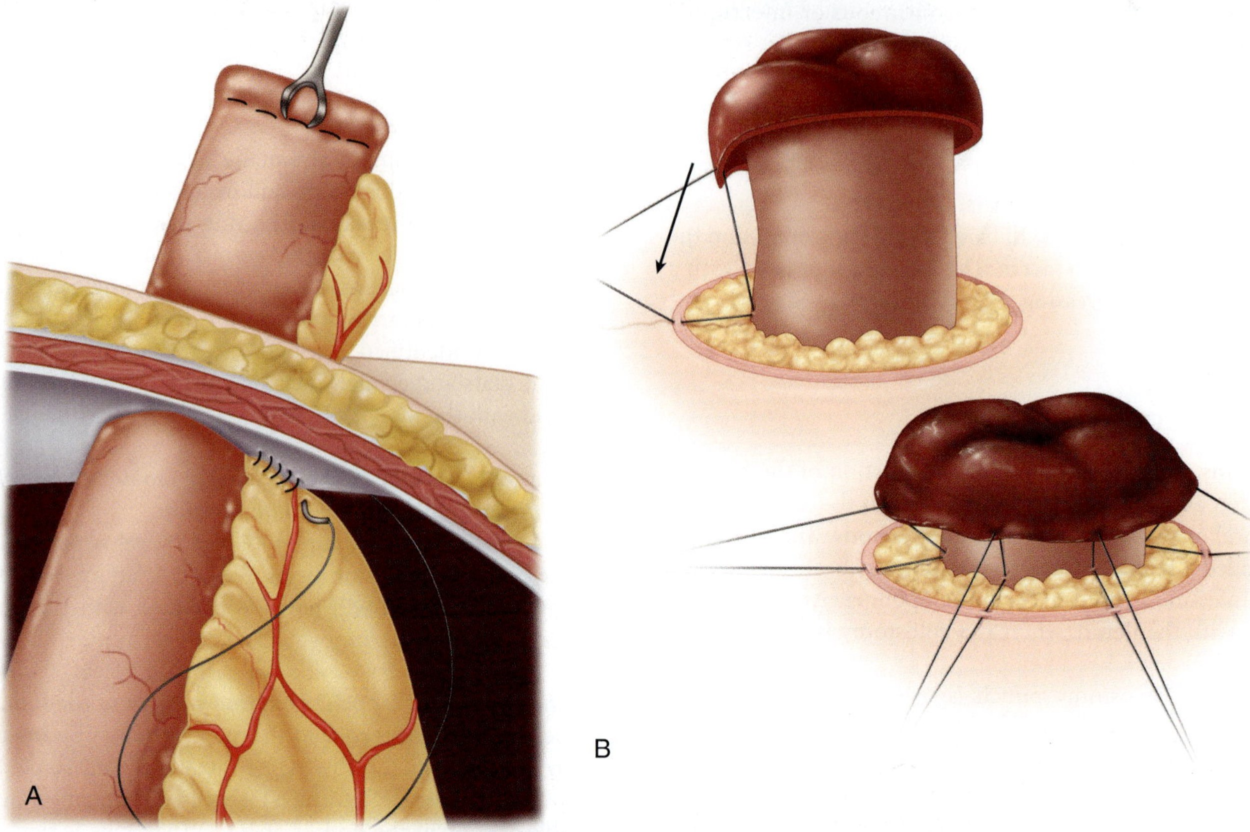

FIG. 22.16 Intestinal stoma. (A) The sutured end of the ileum is brought out of the abdomen and secured to the facia. The sutured end will be severed and the structure everted to form the stoma. (B) The stoma is formed using many interrupted sutures which allow the edge of the stoma to protrude away from the skin. (From Fleshman J, et al. *Atlas of Surgical Techniques for the Colon, Rectum, and Anus.* Philadelphia: Saunders; 2013.)

surgeon may need to enlarge the site. This is done with dissecting scissors.

3. ***A loop appliance is placed between the two limbs of the loop.***
   A stoma rod is used to keep the loop of bowel from slipping back into the abdomen. The rod has two "wings," which can be sutured to the skin to secure it.

4. ***The bowel loop is opened and the edges sutured to skin.***
   A longitudinal incision is made in the bowel loop that exposes both lumens. The edges of the incision are everted and sutured to the skin using interrupted sutures of 2-0 absorbable synthetic material. The rod will be removed at the fifth or sixth postoperative day. A temporary stoma pouch is placed over the wound.

TERMINAL COLOSTOMY

The terminal colostomy is performed using the same technique as for the terminal ileum, with one difference. Drainage from the colostomy is solid and nonirritating to tissue. For this reason, the edges of the colostomy are sutured directly to the skin without formation of the raised spigot.

Closing the Stoma

After the patient has been prepped and draped, a gauze sponge is placed at the opening of the colostomy. This prevents gross contamination of the wound by fecal material. The surgeon then incises the skin around the edges of the colostomy. The incision is carried through the subcutaneous and fascial layers. The peritoneum is dissected free of the colostomy with Metzenbaum scissors. To prevent contamination of the peritoneal cavity, the colostomy is surrounded with one or two lap sponges. The surgeon then trims the skin from the edges of the colostomy.

The surgeon closes the colostomy by inserting two layers of suture through the colostomy edges. The first layer is closed with running or interrupted 3-0 absorbable sutures swaged to a fine needle. A second layer of interrupted 3-0 or 4-0 polydioxanone sutures is placed over the first suture line. The bowel is then allowed to slide back into position in the peritoneal cavity, and the wound is closed in routine fashion.

RIGHT HEMICOLECTOMY (OPEN)

A hemi (partial) colectomy is performed to remove a section of diseased colon and restore continuity to the intestine. This may be performed with or without a stoma. This procedure is frequently performed using a minimally invasive approach with isolation technique. An open approach is illustrated here to demonstrate the anatomy and use of a wound protector.

Pathology

A colectomy is removal of part or all of the large intestine. The colon is removed to treat carcinoma, ulcerative colitis, diverticulitis, and intestinal obstruction. In this description a segment of bowel between the distal ileum and colon is removed.

POSITION:	Supine
INCISION:	Midline or right paramedian
PREP AND DRAPING:	Abdominal/laparotomy
INSTRUMENTS AND SUPPLIES:	Major laparotomy set; intestinal instruments; long instruments; stapling instruments; clips and appliers; vessel loops; wound protector
POSSIBLE EXTRAS:	Penrose drain for retraction; bowel bag

Technical Points and Discussion

1. ***A laparotomy is performed.***
The surgeon performs a laparotomy through a midline incision. If an ileostomy is planned, the paramedian incision on the opposite side of the ostomy often is preferred to separate the stoma from the surgical incision and prevent contamination of the incision site.

2. ***The colon is divided from retroperitoneal structures.***
The dissection begins with separation of the terminal ileum and cecum from the retroperitoneal tissues. Important structures lie in the area, including large blood vessels and the ureter. Careful blunt and sharp dissection is carried out using Metzenbaum scissors and smooth forceps. The ultrasonic scalpel may also be used. Where ligation of large vessels is required, a surgical clip or suture ligature of size 0 or 2-0 polydioxanone can be used. Very large vessels may be divided and sealed using a linear staple cutter. Atraumatic Babcock and Allis clamps are used to grasp the bowel. Systematic dissection of the mesentery, major arteries, and peritoneal reflections is performed until all attachments are eliminated.

3. ***The mesentery of the distal ileum and the right colon is dissected.***
The dissection is carried superiorly (upward) toward the gastrocolic ligament. A medium Penrose drain may be looped around the bowel for retraction. Dissection is carried out to separate all mesenteric attachments between the bowel specimen and its attachments.

4. ***The distal ileum is transected.***
At this stage the distal ileum, which defines the extent of the specimen, is divided and closed. It is most common to use a linear stapler for this procedure. However, for the sake of learning, a hand-sewn closure is described here.
The proximal end of the segment to be transected is held by the assistant using Babcock clamps. The surgeon then places two intestinal clamps a short distance apart, across the ileum at the point where the tissue will be severed. The ileum is then transected using the deep knife. A lap sponge is placed at the base of the divided tissues.

5. ***The transverse colon is transected.***
To release the specimen, the transverse colon is transected. The selected site of division is cross-clamped as with intestinal clamps. Before dividing the colon, the ST should ensure that a closure setup is ready as bowel technique will be used after the colon has been joined to the ileum. The surgeon places a lap sponge at the base on the transection site and severs the bowel between the two intestinal clamps. This releases the specimen, which is brought out of the wound. The ST should have a large specimen basin ready to receive the specimen, including any attached clamps. The specimen may be passed off the field to the circulator.

6. ***The terminal ileum and transverse colon anastomosis are performed.***
The limbs of the bowel will be closed in two separate layers. To do this, the proximal clamp (ileum) and limb are brought into alignment with a cecal clamp at the distal limb. Traction sutures are placed at each side of the anastomosis site. These may be size 2-0 polydioxanone or other nonabsorbable suture on a round needle. The first line of sutures is placed across the deep tissues, including the mucosa and muscle tissue of the bowel. This is performed using size 3-0 absorbable synthetic suture. The suture line is continued until the inner lumen is joined.
The assistant then rotates the intestinal clamps to bring the serosa layers of the two limbs together. These are joined using interrupted polydioxanone sutures size 2-0. The second, distal anastomosis is performed using the same technique. Note that a count must be performed before the anastomosis has been completed. The mesenteric defects are closed using interrupted polydioxanone suture, size 3-0.

7. ***The wound is irrigated and bowel technique implemented.***
Once the anastomosis has been completed, the wound is thoroughly irrigated with warm saline.
Bowel technique is now implemented. All instruments are removed from the sterile field. A new instrument setup is brought in, and the previously used Mayo stand and back table are moved aside. From this point, only fresh instruments and supplies are used on the field. This includes irrigation fluid. The team changes gowns and gloves to complete the procedure. The existing drapes

may be covered with new layers of drapes, including towels, adhesive drape, and laparotomy drape.

8. ***The wound is closed.***
The wound may be again irrigated using fresh saline. The incisional site is then checked for bleeders. The ST should have a medium Penrose drain available, along with closing sutures. The abdomen is then closed in routine fashion and dressed with flat gauze and an abdominal pad secured with tape. The procedure for a right open colectomy is illustrated in Fig. 22.17. In this demonstration, a *wound protector* is used to bring the specimen out of the abdomen.

ROBOTIC ASSISTED LOW ANTERIOR RESECTION (LAR)

In this robotic procedure a large segment of large intestine is removed for treatment of rectal cancer. This is a *sphincter-sparing* procedure, in which the anal sphincter is not removed with the tissue specimen. In the following description, indocyanine green dye (ICG) and the near-infrared imaging endoscope. After the distal stapling of the bowel, ICG is injected intravenously and the near-infrared endoscope is used to assess perfusion (blood supply) at the site of the proposed anastomosis.

POSITION:	Modified lithotomy using a vacuum positioner ("bean bag"). Trendelenburg with lateral tilt using a Trumpf surgical table.
INCISION:	12-mm camera port; three 8-mm instrument ports; stapler port; 5-mm assistant's port; additional instrument port as needed
PREP AND DRAPING:	Nipple line to symphysis pubis Standard robotic laparotomy draping
INSTRUMENTS:	30-degree-down endoscope, 0-degree endoscope; robotic stapler; ultrasonic vessel sealer; monopolar hook, 12-mm stapler cannula set, laparoscopic scope and camera; grasping retractor; Cadiere forceps; monopolar curved scissors; fenestrated bipolar forceps; suction irrigator

Technical Points and Discussion

1. ***The patient is positioned, prepped, and draped.***
The patient is positioned in modified lithotomy position using a vacuum mattress to enable safe lateral table tilt with Trendelenburg during the procedure. Both arms are tucked at the sides. The prep extends from the nipple line to the symphysis pubis. Standard laparotomy drapes with pockets are applied.

2. ***Pneumoperitoneum is established and the endoscope port and endoscope are inserted.***
Pneumoperitoneum is established using the Veress needle. A small incision is made at the endoscope port site using a #11 knife or monopolar ESU. An optical port is placed in the incision. The patient is placed in Trendelenburg position with lateral tilt to the right.

3. ***The remaining port sites are incised and trocars inserted.***

4. ***The robot is docked.***
The robot is ready for docking following the targeting procedure (refer to Chapter 21). The surgeon indicates which ports are docked with a specific robot arm. At this point the surgeon leaves the operating table to work at the console.

5. ***Adhesions are released.***
Adhesions can be released using a variety of ESU monopolar and bipolar cutting instruments such as a hook, scissors, or grasping forceps. **Adhesions** (bands of scar tissue) must be released ("taken down") to differentiate tissue planes and obtain good exposure to the target structures.

6. ***The left colon is mobilized.***
The left and descending colon are mobilized by surgically separating them from the mesentery. This is performed with bipolar and monopolar cutting devices and ultrasonic cutting instruments.

7. ***The inferior mesenteric vein and artery are identified and divided.***
These major vessels are dissected free during mobilization of the bowel. They are individually sealed and divided using robotic linear staples. The mobilization of the bowel is carried along the full length of the planned resection.

8. ***The ileum and colon are resected.***
The ileum and colon are resected using the robotic stapler. The ST should be prepared for several staple loads to complete the resection.

9. ***Indocyanine green (ICG) dye is injected intravenously.***
The anesthesia provider administers an intravenous injection of ICG. The dye is fluorescent, and perfused vessels can be seen with near-infrared endoscope. This allows the surgeon to assess the blood supply (perfusion) at both anastomosis sites. The rectal stump is also checked.

10. ***The anastomosis is performed.***
There are numerous methods used to perform an LAR anastomosis, including end to end, side to side, and end to side. A side-to-side anastomosis is performed by aligning the two limbs and performing an enterotomy using a monopolar hook. The robotic stapler is introduced through the enterotomy and fired. The enterotomy is closed using size 2-0 synthetic absorbable suture.

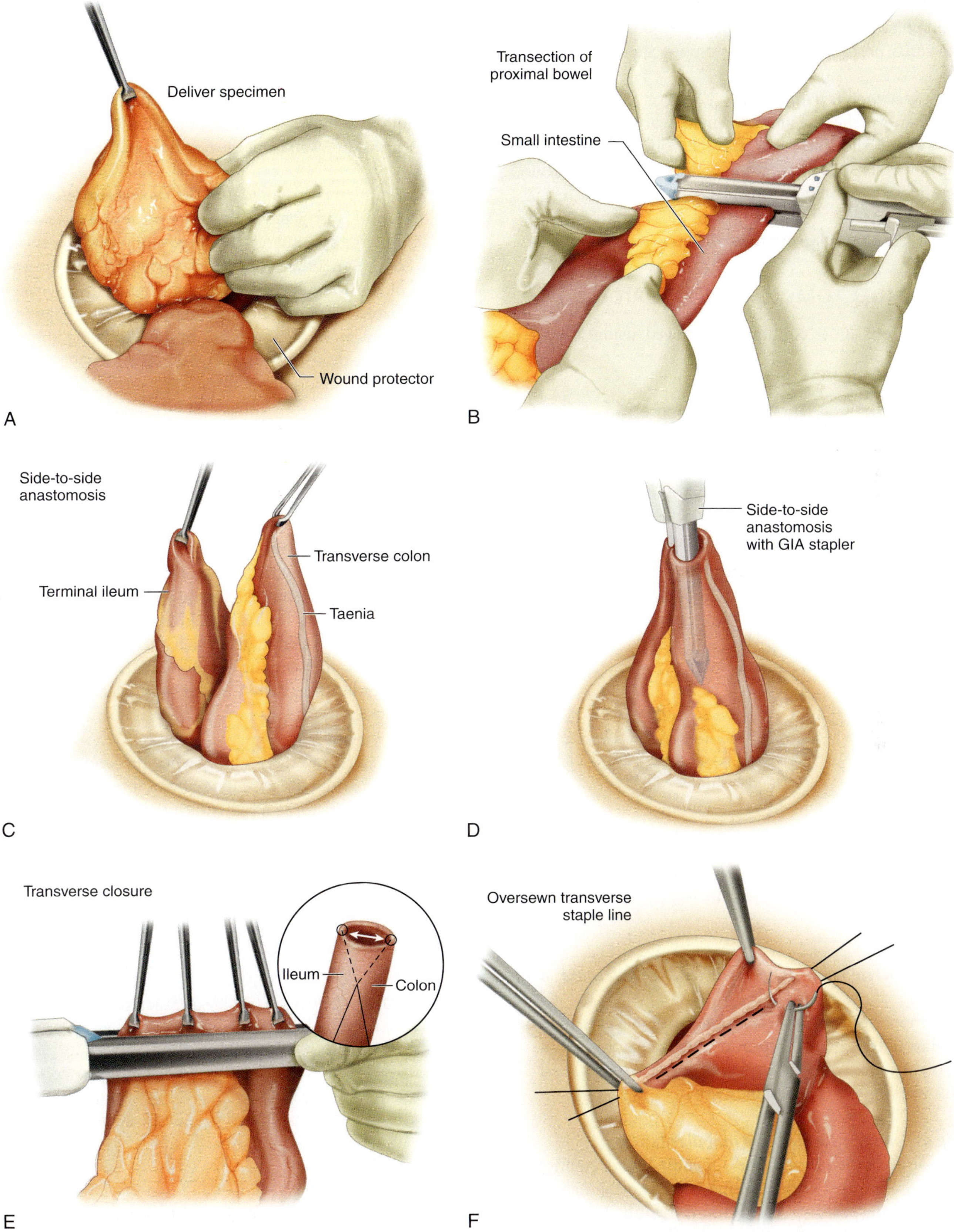

FIG. 22.17 Open hemicolectomy. (A) The bowel is brought out of the abdomen through the wound protector. (B) The proximal large intestine is transected and stapled at the ileum using a GIA stapler cutter. (C) Preparation for the side-to-side anastomosis. Allis or Babcock clamps are shown on the edge of the bowel. (D) A side-to-side anastomosis is created using the GIA stapler. (E) The transverse opening is closed. (F) The closure is oversewn using size 3-0 silk sutures. (From Fleshman J, et al. *Atlas of Surgical Techniques for the Colon, Rectum, and Anus*. Philadelphia: Saunders; 2013.)

Knotless suture material is commonly used (refer to Chapter 19). An additional bolus of ICG may be injected to verify perfusion at the anastomosis site.

11. ***The specimen is withdrawn.***
To remove the specimen a small wound protector is placed in the port used for the robotic stapler. The specimen is grasped with a Babcock clamp and carefully withdrawn through the port.

12. ***All ports are withdrawn and the incisions closed.***

APPENDECTOMY (LAPAROSCOPIC)

The appendix is most commonly removed using a laparoscopic technique.

Pathology

Pathology is the same as for open appendectomy. Contraindications for laparoscopic surgery are pregnancy, ruptured (perforated) appendix, and peritonitis.

POSITION:	Supine; Trendelenburg
INCISION:	Laparoscopic
PREP AND DRAPING:	Abdominal/laparotomy
INSTRUMENTS AND SUPPLIES:	Basic laparoscopy instruments; one 10-mm trocar; two 5-mm trocars; 30-degree laparoscope; ultrasonic cutting and coagulating system, monopolar ESU; hook ESU; laparoscopic clip applier; linear stapler endo GIA, 45 mm; specimen retrieval bag
POSSIBLE EXTRAS:	Laparoscopic hook ESU, endoscopic specimen bag; small Penrose drain

Technical Points and Discussion

1. ***Pneumoperitoneum is established, and trocars are placed.***
Pneumoperitoneum is established using a Veress needle or Hassan technique. A 10-mm trocar is placed within or near the umbilicus for the endoscope. Two additional 5-mm working ports are established.

2. ***The appendix is located and mobilized.***
The surgeon then locates the appendix by systematically moving aside the large intestine with an atraumatic endoscopic grasper, until the cecum is identified. A grasper is used to elevate the tip of the appendix. An entry hole is made in the mesoappendix at the base of the appendix. A vascular endostapler is used to divide mesoappendix. This step can also be performed with a monopolar hook.

3. ***The appendix is amputated from the cecum.***
After the appendix has been mobilized, it can be amputated from the cecum. The endo stapler with a vascular load is used to transect and seal the base of the appendix. A specimen retrieval bag is inserted and the specimen placed inside. The bag is clamped and removed later with the trocar cannula. If signs of contamination are noted, the surgeon takes a culture swab from the free fluid in the abdomen.

4. ***The abdomen is irrigated and the wounds are closed.***
The wound is irrigated with warm saline and checked for bleeders. The specimen is delivered along with the 10-mm trocar. The pneumoperitoneum is released. The deep tissues of the wounds are closed with figure-of-8 synthetic absorbable or nonabsorbable sutures. A small Penrose drain may be placed if the risk of postoperative infection or excessive drainage exists. The skin is closed with staples or nonabsorbable sutures.

EXCISIONAL HEMORRHOIDECTOMY

Hemorrhoids are vascular cushions supported by anchoring connective tissue. They are the terminal branches of the superior rectal artery. They extend along the length of the anal canal and are *normal structures.* External hemorrhoids are covered with skin and can become engorged because of thrombosis. Internal hemorrhoids lie beneath submucosal tissue. Hemorrhoids can become engorged when their connective tissue anchors weaken, allowing the hemorrhoid to descend into the canal. This results in irritation, severe pain, and bleeding. Prolapsed hemorrhoids can also interfere with normal defecation and lead to infection.

Surgical intervention is required when diet and office-based therapies such as banding are inadequate. Two procedures are commonly used in these cases: surgical (sharp) excision and treatment using a bipolar vessel-sealing and cutting device.

The following procedure describes *excisional hemorrhoidectomy.*

POSITION:	Jackknife (Kraske) or lithotomy
INCISION:	At site of hemorrhoid
PREP AND DRAPING:	Anal/fenestrated sheet; lithotomy
INSTRUMENTS AND SUPPLIES:	Minor rectal set; monopolar ESU; depending on procedure, ultrasonic and bipolar vessel-sealing system

Technical Points and Discussion

1. ***The patient is positioned, prepped, and draped.***
The patient is positioned and the buttocks taped apart. A routine skin prep and draping are performed.

2. ***The surgical site is assessed.***
The surgeon first performs an internal and external assessment of the anus.

3. ***The hemorrhoid is grasped and an elliptical incision made.***
The surgeon grasps the hemorrhoid with a Babcock or Allis clamp. A #10 or #15 knife is used to make an elliptical incision up to the apex of the hemorrhoid. Small bleeders may be managed using the monopolar or bipolar ESU.

4. ***The apex is clamped, ligated, and amputated.***
The apex of the hemorrhoid is clamped, amputated, and ligated using absorbable suture ligation size 3-0 or 2-0 on a small taper needle. The ends of the suture may be left temporarily long to locate an area of postoperative bleeding.

5. ***Metzenbaum scissors are used to undermine the epithelium lining the anal canal.***
To ensure a tension-free closure, the epithelium is undermined with Metzenbaum scissors.

6. ***The procedure is repeated for additional hemorrhoids as needed.***

7. ***The wounds are closed.***

SURGICAL TREATMENT FOR ANAL FISTULA

A *pilonidal* sinus is a malformation of the sacrococcygeal region that may become blocked (pilonidal cyst) or infected (pilonidal abscess). An unresolved pilonidal abscess may progress to a fistula *(fistula-in-ano),* a tract (tunnel) that connects an internal opening in the anal canal with an external opening in the perianal skin. The progression of clinical features usually starts with one or more hair follicles in the gluteal cleft. Hair follicles contain glands that secrete sebum, and when blocked, they are prone to abscess. Abscess and fistula can also be caused by blocked anal glands that become infected.

Surgical excision of a fistula involves removing the lining of the tunnel so that the defect can heal by granulation. If the fistula crosses the sphincter, more complex surgery is required to preserve the sphincter and prevent incontinence. The following simple excision procedure can be performed under regional anesthesia with monitored sedation.

POSITION:	Jackknife (Kraske) or lateral
INCISION:	At site of fistula
PREP AND DRAPING:	Anal/fenestrated sheet
INSTRUMENTS AND SUPPLIES:	Minor rectal set including fistula probes; monopolar ESU; depending on procedure, ultrasonic scalpel; curettes

Technical Points and Discussion

1. ***The patient is positioned, prepped, and draped.***
The most common positions used are lateral and jackknife. The buttocks are taped apart as for hemorrhoidectomy.

2. ***The fistula is probed.***
The surgeon uses a lighted retractor and rectal probe to identify each end of the fistula.

3. ***The fistula is cored out.***
The fistula is cored out using the ESU. Tissue surrounding the fistula is excised and the wound left to heal by secondary intention. To maintain drainage during healing, a Silastic vessel loop can be pulled through the tunnel and the ends tied together.

SECTION III: SURGERY OF THE BILIARY SYSTEM, LIVER, PANCREAS, AND SPLEEN

SURGICAL ANATOMY

LIVER

The liver, gallbladder, spleen, and pancreas are located in the midabdominal cavity. The spleen lies in the upper left quadrant, beneath the diaphragm, and posterior to the stomach. The liver occupies most of the upper right abdominal space and a portion of the left upper quadrant.

The liver is a large vascular organ that aids digestion and the filtration of toxic substances from the body. It has many vital functions in the body, including carbohydrate, fat, and protein metabolism, the storage of glycogen and synthesis of glucose, and the storage of vitamins and minerals. The liver is also responsible for the synthesis of clotting factors, immune factors, and plasma proteins. It also filters toxins and bacteria from the blood and metabolizes drugs. It is divided into two major sections, or lobes, the right lobe and the left lobe, which are separated by the falciform ligament. These sections are identified by the *bifurcation* (Y-shaped division of a hollow anatomical structure) of the portal vein with right and left bile ducts. The vascular supply of the liver is derived from the hepatic artery and the hepatic portal vein. The liver is drained by the hepatic veins, which connect to the inferior vena cava.

The two lobes of the liver are further divided into eight subsections, according to their blood supply. The blood supply to each section is carried in a pedicle containing a bile duct, a hepatic artery, and a branch of the portal vein. Because each section is connected to its own pedicle, resection of an entire lobe requires dissection of the pedicle from the lobe and secure ligation of the pedicle, including the specific portion of the hepatic vein.

The liver is encapsulated by a thick fibrous sheath called the *Glisson capsule.* Fibrous sheaths also cover and protect the blood vessels and biliary ducts. These sheaths are continuous with the abdominal peritoneum and must be carefully dissected and mobilized before liver resection or anastomosis of the biliary system to another abdominal structure.

The anterior surface of the liver, which is in contact with the diaphragm, is referred to as the *right* and *left subphrenic spaces.* The *subhepatic space* lies between the peritoneal covering on the liver and the right kidney. These spaces are clinically significant. The subphrenic spaces are common sites of abscesses, and the subhepatic space can trap intestinal contents after a rupture of the appendix and become infected.

BILIARY SYSTEM

The biliary system includes the gallbladder, hepatic ducts, common bile duct, and cystic duct. The gallbladder is a small sac located under the right lobe (ventral side) of the liver. It is composed of smooth muscle and has an inner surface of absorptive cells.

The function of the biliary system is to produce, store, and release *bile*, which is composed of bile salts, pigments, cholesterol, lecithin, mucin (a glycoprotein), and other organic substances. Bile is necessary for the breakdown of cholesterol and helps stimulate peristalsis in the small intestine during digestion. It is formed in the liver and stored in the gallbladder.

Bile formed in the liver is released from the right and left hepatic ducts. These ducts converge to form the common hepatic duct. From the common hepatic duct, bile flows into the gallbladder through the cystic duct. When food enters the stomach, the gallbladder contracts, releasing stored bile into the common bile duct. Bile then enters the duodenum through an opening called the *ampulla of Vater*. This opening into the duodenum is shared by the pancreatic duct, which allows the release of pancreatic enzymes. The release of both bile and pancreatic enzymes is controlled by a sphincter at the ampulla called the *sphincter of Oddi*.

The hepatic and biliary anatomy is shown in Fig. 22.18.

PANCREAS

The pancreas is an elongated, lobulated gland that lies inferior to the liver, behind the stomach. This organ has two landmarks, the head and the tail. The head, which is the broader portion of the gland, lies in the curve of the duodenum and is connected to the duodenal portion of the small intestine. The pancreatic duct (duct of Wirsung), which is the central duct of the pancreas, communicates with the duodenum at the ampulla of Vater, a location shared with the common bile duct. The tail of the pancreas lies near the hilus of the spleen. The pancreas produces insulin and glucagon, which are necessary for digestion of carbohydrates. Insulin and glucagon are synthesized in specific regions of the pancreas called the *Islets of Langerhans*. Insulin is synthesized and secreted directly into the bloodstream by alpha cells, whereas glucagon is synthesized and released by beta cells. Delta cells in the pancreas produce *somatostatin*, which controls the rate of nutrient absorption from the intestine. Gamma cells in the pancreas secrete *pancreatic polypeptide*, which reduces appetite. The pancreas also produces enzymes such as trypsin, chymotrypsin, carboxypeptidase, and elastase, which are necessary for protein digestion.

SPLEEN

The spleen is a kidney-shaped organ that is extremely vascular and relatively soft. It lies under the diaphragm in the left upper abdomen. This organ destroys aged red blood cells, stores blood, filters microorganisms from the blood, and plays a major role in the immune system of the body. Because of its vascularity and location, the spleen may be injured in vehicular and sports accidents. The spleen can be removed safely, without harming the body's ability to function, and this procedure is indicated whenever splenic hemorrhage becomes life threatening. This is because hemorrhage is difficult to control without clamping the splenic arteries, and removal has little or no long-term medical consequences for most patients.

DIAGNOSTIC PROCEDURES

Diseases of the liver, biliary system, pancreas, and spleen have direct consequences on metabolism, digestion, production of blood cells, and blood clotting. The symptoms of disease often are dramatic, and the diagnostic process is initiated when a patient experiences symptoms of pain, jaundice, diabetic pathology, or generalized weakness.

Blood tests can detect substances normally filtered by the liver and pancreas. Liver function tests measure liver enzymes and other chemicals. The liver is responsible for hundreds of physiological processes in the body. Specific blood tests are performed according to the presenting symptoms.

Imaging studies using CT, MRI, fluoroscopy, and ultrasound, including those that use contrast media, are performed to outline organs and observe the movement of bile through the biliary system. Pancreatic imaging is used to detect stones and tumors, and the ducts may also be revealed if a contrast medium is used. Endoscopic retrograde pancreaticoduodenoscopy is performed to explore the ducts directly and for simple endoscopic procedures.

CASE PLANNING

INSTRUMENTS

Open and laparoscopic procedures of the liver, biliary system, pancreas, and spleen require basic general surgery instruments. Vascular instruments are needed for open resection procedures and for major hepatic surgery.

Because these accessory organs contain many ducts and blood vessels, right-angle clamps should be available with all procedures. These clamps allow the surgeon to reach underneath and around the blood vessels, ducts, and connective tissue attachments of the organs.

Procedures of the biliary system and pancreas, including choledochoscopy and endoscopic retrograde cholangiopancreatography (ERCP), sometimes require intraoperative use of flexible fiber-optic endoscopes. These scopes are inserted into the small ducts of the accessory organs to locate stones, tumors, or benign lesions.

SPECIAL EQUIPMENT AND SUPPLIES

The organs of the hepatic system and spleen are highly vascular, and any tear or rupture can result in profuse bleeding that sometimes is difficult to control. Therefore hemostasis is a major technical concern during surgery of the liver or spleen.

Hemostatic techniques must include individual blood vessels and capillary bleeding. The ultrasonic scalpel and ESU may be used to cut and coagulate the tissue. *Skeletonization* (the removal of parenchyma and other connective tissues around a structure) of the hepatic and biliary system requires meticulous care to prevent hemorrhage and to preserve the essential blood supply to the organs. This is performed with dissecting scissors or an ultrasonic system. Vessel loops and surgical clips are frequently used to retract and ligate vessels. An HF vessel-sealing system may also be used.

Hemostatic agents used in surgery include the following:

- Microfibrillar collagen
- Oxidized cellulose
- Topical thrombin
- Absorbable gelatin matrix
- Fibrin hemostatic tissue adhesive

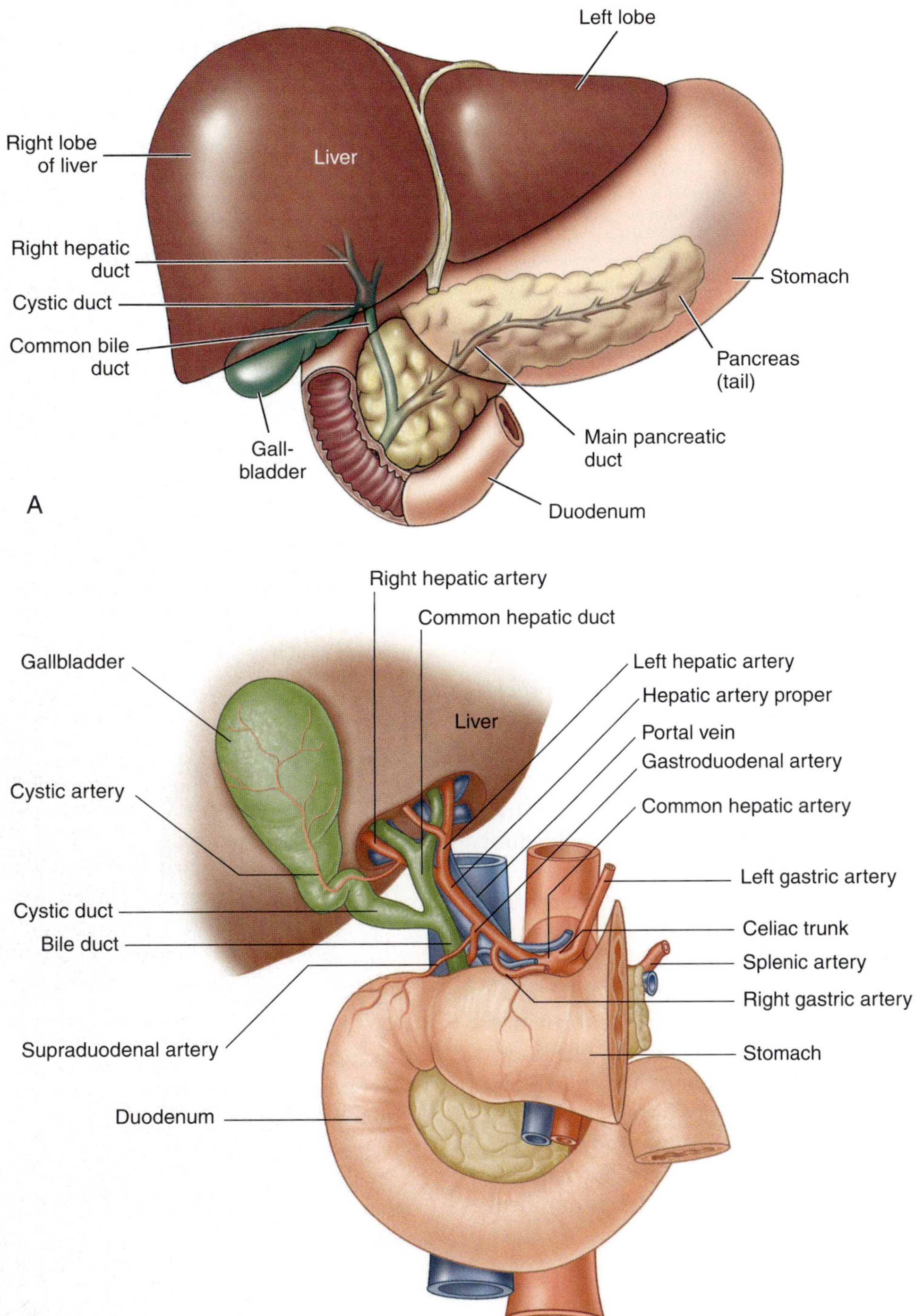

FIG. 22.18 Biliary and hepatic anatomy. (A) Note the position of the spleen and the main pancreatic duct (duct of Wirsung). (B) Details of the biliary system.

Continued

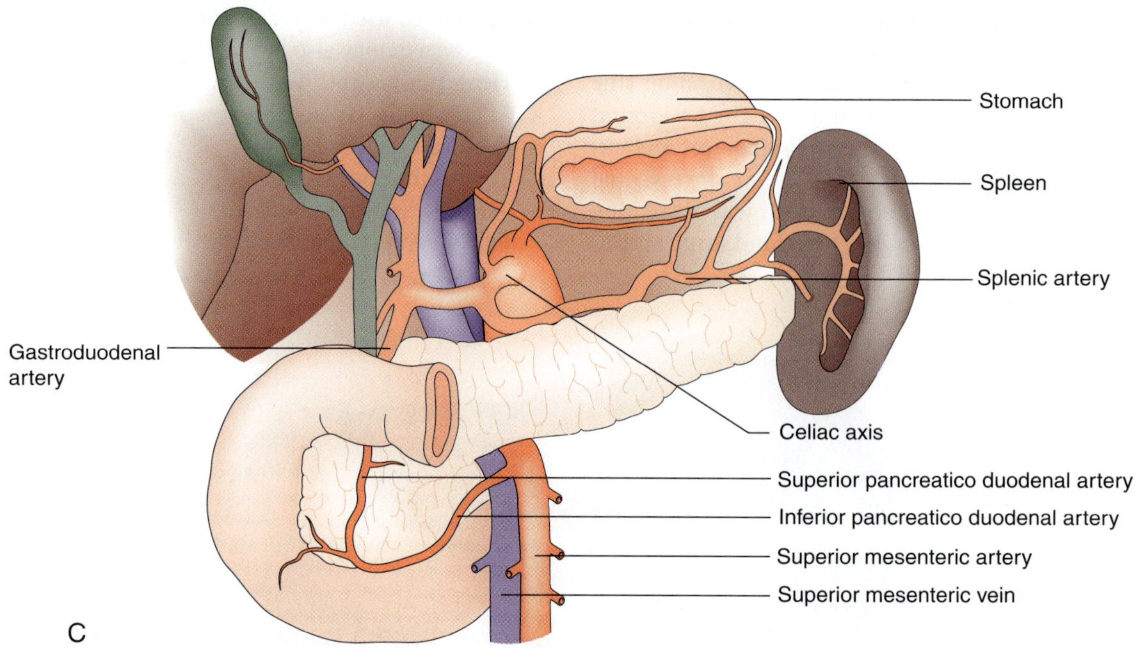

FIG. 22.18, cont'd (C) Anatomical relationship of the spleen and arterial system. (A, Modified from Herlihy B, Maebius NK. *The Human Body in Health and Illness.* 2nd ed. Philadelphia: WB Saunders; 2003. B, From Drake R, Vogl W, Mitchell A. *Gray's Anatomy for Students.* Edinburgh: Churchill Livingstone; 2004. C, From Garden O, Bradbury A, Forsythe J, Parks R. *Principles and Practice of Surgery.* 5th ed. Edinburgh: Churchill Livingstone/Elsevier; 2007.)

SURGICAL PROCEDURES

CHOLECYSTECTOMY (LAPAROSCOPIC)

Cholecystectomy is removal of a diseased gallbladder. A laparoscopic approach is used for noncomplicated procedures and may include cholangiography—intraoperative dye studies of the gallbladder ducts to check for stones. Intraoperative common bile duct exploration (CBDE) and stone removal have been largely replaced by preoperative endoscopic procedures in which stones are removed before surgery.

Two common diseases of the biliary system are *cholelithiasis* (the presence of gallstones) and *cholecystitis* (chronic or acute inflammation of the gallbladder). The main components of gallstones are cholesterol and bilirubin. High blood cholesterol and obesity contribute to the formation of gallstones, which can lead to blockage of the bile ducts. Obstruction increases the concentration of bile and results in swelling, pain, and infection. Jaundice occurs in obstructive biliary disease. Bilirubin, a normal by-product of the breakdown of hemoglobin, is absorbed into normal bile. Biliary obstruction causes increased serum levels of bilirubin, resulting in toxicity.

POSITION:	Supine; reverse Trendelenburg; operating table tilt left
PREP AND DRAPING:	Abdominal/laparotomy
INSTRUMENTS AND SUPPLIES:	Laparoscopy set with gallbladder instruments; flexible tipped or rigid laparoscope; one or two 10-mm ports; two or three 5-mm trocars; ultrasonic scalpel; L hook ESU; endo clips and appliers; specimen retrieval system
POSSIBLE EXTRAS:	Laparotomy instruments; vessel loops; equipment for cholangiography: 10-mL and 30-mL syringes; IV tubing, stopcock; cholangiogram catheter or ureteral catheter; syringe tip; cholangiography dye (surgeon's preference); C-arm and drapes; T-tube and drainage bag

Technical Points and Discussion

1. ***Pneumoperitoneum is established, and trocars are positioned in the abdomen.***

   A pneumoperitoneum is established using the Veress needle or an open cut-down approach. In this procedure, four trocars are placed: an umbilical 10-mm trocar, an additional 10-mm trocar at the midline, and two 5-mm trocars at the axillary line. This procedure usually requires a 30-degree telescope to view the gallbladder, which lies high in the abdominal cavity.

   The patient is placed in the reverse Trendelenburg position. The laparoscope is inserted through a 10-mm port.

2. ***The gallbladder is retracted upward with a grasper.***
A straight locking grasper is inserted through one axillary trocar and used to apply upward traction on the gallbladder. The assistant maintains retraction on the gallbladder. The patient then may be repositioned into the reverse Trendelenburg position as the dissection continues. An additional grasper may be placed on the gallbladder. This exposes the cystic duct and cystic artery.

3. ***The cystic duct and cystic artery are mobilized.***
Sharp dissection with scissors, an additional grasper, and an ESU hook may be used to separate the cystic duct and artery. After the cystic duct and artery have been isolated, surgical clips are used to ligate the cystic duct. Operative cholangiography may be performed at this stage of the procedure.

4. ***Operative cholangiography may be performed.***
The ST should have a cholangiocatheter, contrast medium, stopcock, and 30-mL syringe available. The circulator distributes the contrast medium and injectable saline to the ST. The ST then dilutes the contrast medium according to the surgeon's order. At least 30 mL of contrast medium solution should be prepared. The solution is aspirated into the syringe, which is attached to a stopcock and cholangiocatheter. Refer to Chapter 12 for illustrations on preparing a syringe and stopcock. All air bubbles are removed from both the syringe and the catheter (these appear as solid white spots on radiographs and can be interpreted as stones). The ST then places a clamp across the catheter near its tip to prevent air from backing up into the syringe. The syringe, cholangiocatheter, and its attaching clamp are then passed to the surgeon.
To begin operative cholangiography, a catheter introducer is placed through the abdominal wall in the right upper quadrant. This is done by simply puncturing the abdomen with the introducer sheath with a needle. The needle is removed, leaving the introducer in place to receive the catheter. A small opening is made in the cystic duct with dissecting scissors. The surgeon threads the tips of the cholangiocatheter through the introducer and advances it into the common bile duct using straight forceps. The catheter is secured with a suture tie or vessel clip. All instruments and radiopaque sponges must be removed from the field, and a sterile drape is placed over the sterile field and the incision.
The C-arm then is brought into position, and the surgeon injects the contrast medium. Stones are removed under fluoroscopy. A balloon biliary catheter often is used to remove stones. The catheter probe is advanced beyond the level of the stone, the balloon is inflated, and the catheter is withdrawn, bringing the stones with it. As the stones are removed, the ST receives them as specimens. These should be maintained *dry* on the back table. The technique for this procedure is illustrated in Fig. 22.19.

5. ***The gallbladder is completely mobilized.***
Additional clips may be placed across the cystic duct. The cystic artery is completely mobilized and clipped. These are divided using dissection scissors. The gallbladder is dissected free of the underside of the liver (liver bed). Upward traction is maintained to create tension on the gallbladder and the tissue plane directly underneath and facilitates dissection. The surgeon uses the ESU hook, scissors, or ultrasonic scalpel to separate the connecting tissues and free the gallbladder from the liver completely.

6. ***The gallbladder is placed in a specimen retrieval bag and withdrawn from the abdomen.***
A specimen retrieval bag such as the Endo Catch is inserted into the 10-mm port, and a 5-mm laparoscope is inserted into the upper 5-mm port. The surgeon then uses a large grasper to place the gallbladder into the specimen bag, which is then withdrawn. The 10-mm laparoscope is re-inserted. The ST should receive the gallbladder in a small basin, taking care not to allow its contents to spill onto the surgical field.

7. ***A T-tube is inserted into the common bile duct.***
A T-tube may be inserted at this time to provide for continuous postoperative drainage of the common bile duct. The limbs of the T-tube are trimmed, and the tube is inserted. The limbs of the tube are threaded into the common bile duct, and the long end is pulled through the trocar. The common bile duct is closed with endoscopic sutures. The abdominal cavity then is irrigated, and each trocar incision is closed with absorbable sutures and skin staples. The T-tube is secured to a drainage bag.

CHOLECYSTECTOMY (OPEN)

Pathology

See the cholecystectomy laparoscopic approach.

POSITION:	Supine; reverse Trendelenburg
PREP AND DRAPING:	Abdominal/laparotomy
INSTRUMENTS AND SUPPLIES:	Laparotomy set; gallbladder set; ultrasonic scalpel; bipolar and monopolar ESU; surgical clips and applier; Potts scissors; #11 knife
POSSIBLE EXTRAS:	Long instruments; supplies for cholangiography: 10-mL and 30-mL syringes; IV tubing, stopcock; cholangiogram catheter or ureteral catheter; syringe tip; cholangiography dye (surgeon's preference); C-arm and drapes; T-tube and drainage bag; lead aprons for team

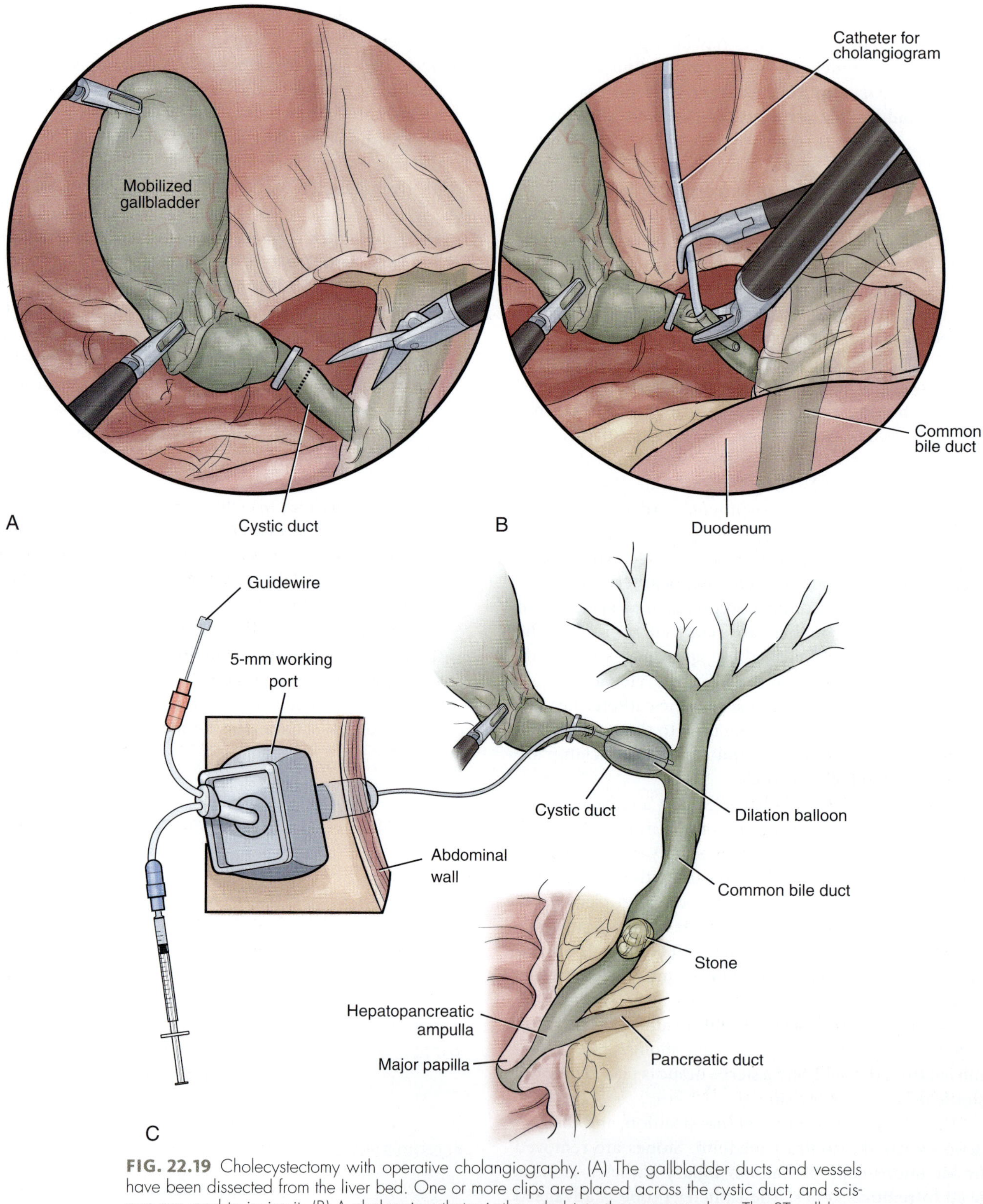

FIG. 22.19 Cholecystectomy with operative cholangiography. (A) The gallbladder ducts and vessels have been dissected from the liver bed. One or more clips are placed across the cystic duct, and scissors are used to incise it. (B) A cholangiocatheter is threaded into the common duct. The ST will have prepared radiopaque dye for injection into the catheter. (C) After fluoroscopic examination of the ducts, a balloon catheter is introduced to remove the stone. The catheter is advanced beyond the stone and retracted, bringing the stone with it.

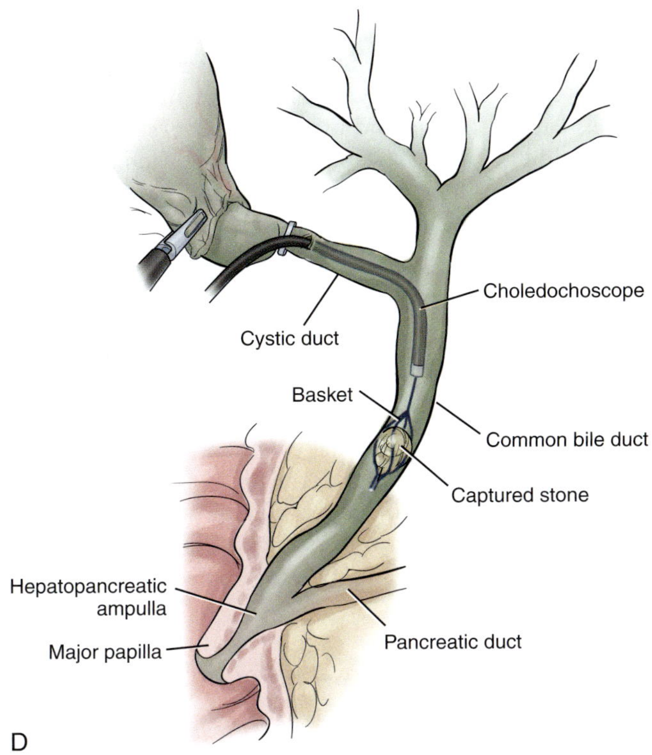

FIG. 22.19, cont'd (D) A stone basket may also be used to remove stones. (From Khatri V. *Atlas of Advanced Operative Surgery*. Philadelphia: Saunders; 2013.)

Technical Points and Discussion

1. ***The abdomen is entered through an upper midline or right subcostal incision.***
An upper midline or right subcostal incision can be used to gain access to the biliary structures. The subcostal incision provides better exposure to the biliary system but is more painful during postoperative recovery. If a subcostal incision is used, the surgeon may inject the incision with long-acting local anesthetic to decrease patient discomfort. The abdominal layers are incised as for a laparotomy. However, the muscle layer is also incised (rather than manually spread) along the costal margin. A self-retaining retractor is inserted in the wound along with lap sponges to protect the wound edges.

2. ***The gallbladder is grasped for retraction and manipulation.***
A Deaver or Harrington retractor is used to retract the liver and expose the gallbladder. Hemostasis is maintained with the ESU. If the gallbladder is distended with bile, the surgeon may drain it with a trocar fitted to the suction tubing or with a large-bore needle and syringe. After the trocar has been withdrawn, a Mayo clamp is used to seal the perforation. The cystic duct and artery are identified and ligated.

3. ***The gallbladder is mobilized.***
To start the dissection of the gallbladder, ducts, and vessels, a Mayo or Péan clamp is placed across the body of the gallbladder, which then is retracted upward. The peritoneal membrane, which covers the cystic duct, artery, and common bile duct, is incised with Metzenbaum scissors. The dissection is continued with scissors, fine-toothed forceps, and small sponge dissectors. Dissection and ligation of bleeding vessels are completed with scissors and right-angle clamps until the cystic duct is exposed and dissected free. Operative cholangiography is performed at this stage of the procedure.

4. ***Operative cholangiography may be performed.***
Operative cholangiography using contrast media and fluoroscopy may be performed at this point in the procedure. The procedure is the same as described previously under laparoscopic technique. However, in the open procedure, the cholangiocatheter is introduced into the common duct under direct vision. Stones located in the duct may be "milked down" into the gallbladder or retrieved using a stone basket or balloon catheter as described previously.

5. ***The dissection is completed and the gallbladder removed.***
When all stones have been removed, an additional clip may be placed across the cystic duct. The cystic artery is clipped and transected. Dissection of the gallbladder is now completed using the ultrasonic scalpel, Metzenbaum scissors, and fine-toothed forceps. With dissection complete, the gallbladder is removed. The ST should receive it in a basin along with any clamps to prevent bile from seeping into the wound or sterile field.

6. ***Drains are placed and the wound closed.***
The liver bed may be closed with fine absorbable sutures. If postoperative drainage is required, a T-tube is inserted into the common duct at this time. The ductal incision then is closed with 3-0 or 4-0 absorbable sutures on a fine tapered needle. The long end of the T-tube is brought out of the wound and later attached to a collection bag. Penrose drains are inserted into the abdominal cavity, and the ends are brought through a stab wound near the main incision. The wound is irrigated with warm saline solution and closed in layers. The peritoneum may be closed separately using size 0 absorbable suture, or sutured with the fascia layer. A separate fascia closure is performed using nonabsorbable 2-0 sutures. The muscle layer is closed using interrupted sutures of nonabsorbable material. The subcutaneous tissue is closed using interrupted sutures of size 3-0 absorbable material. Skin is closed with staples or interrupted nonabsorbable suture such as polypropylene or nylon. The wound is dressed with a bulky abdominal pad and gauze. The individual drains are each secured to the skin with size 3-0 or 4-0 nylon or polypropylene. Each is covered with a flat abdominal pad. If a T-tube was inserted, it is attached to a collection bag.

SPLENECTOMY

The spleen is removed surgically to stop hemorrhage caused by trauma or to treat disease. Severe splenic trauma may be a life-threatening condition that requires immediate operative intervention. However, more conservative treatment is adequate for low-grade trauma cases. CT scanning and ultrasound are now used to grade splenic injury. Conservative nonsurgical therapy is adequate for injuries that do not affect hemodynamic stability. An open procedure for traumatic spleen is discussed here, whereas laparoscopic splenectomy is discussed in Splenectomy (Laparoscopic).

The ST can contribute significantly to a successful outcome in the following ways:

- The surgeon must have access to the hemorrhage site. This starts with a rapid laparotomy.
- Retraction, either manual or self-retaining, must be established quickly. Suction must be available immediately to clear blood and clots. The ST may be required to assist in suctioning and evacuating blood clots while passing other needed instruments.
- Excellent lighting is required to locate and stop the hemorrhage. This is the collaborative duty of the ST and the circulator.
- Clamps are required to occlude the bleeding vessels. The ST must have vascular, pedicle, and other hemostatic clamps immediately available on the field.
- During a surgical emergency, it is important to remain focused on the job at hand. The ST should carefully watch what is happening at the wound site while listening to instructions and act quickly and carefully to decrease errors.

Pathology

In addition to splenectomy to treat traumatic injury, the procedure is performed to treat various types of blood disorders. Immune thrombocytopenic purpura (ITP) is the most common pathology requiring removal of the spleen. In this condition, alterations in the immune system result in loss of platelets, which are critical for blood clotting.

POSITION:	Supine
PREP AND DRAPING:	Abdominal/laparotomy
INSTRUMENTS AND SUPPLIES:	Laparotomy set; assortment of vascular clamps; vascular forceps; kidney pedicle clamp; vascular clips
POSSIBLE EXTRAS:	Extra suction tubing and tip; large specimen basin(s); auto transfusion system; extra lap sponges

Technical Points and Discussion

1. ***A laparotomy is performed.***
An upper midline incision is made. Small bleeders may be clamped but not ligated during abdominal entry. The ESU may be used extensively to quickly gain entry to the abdominal cavity.
Two suctions must be available as soon as the abdomen is opened. These are used to evacuate the blood and clots from the abdomen so that the splenic vessels can be located and manually compressed. The ST should have a large basin available to evacuate and remove large blood clots from the abdominal cavity as soon as the abdomen is opened. Laparotomy sponges are used in rapid succession as the bleeding is controlled.

2. ***Blood and clots are immediately removed from the abdomen.***
The surgeon's assistant evacuates the blood clots. All quadrants of the abdominal wound are packed with lap sponges. A self-retaining retractor is inserted. The lap sponges are removed as each quadrant is systematically examined for sources of bleeding. A blood recovery system (e.g., Cell Saver) may be used immediately to replace blood.

3. ***The splenic ligaments are dissected free and the splenic vessels occluded.***
To gain access to the splenic blood vessels, the ligaments must be dissected. This is done using sharp and blunt dissection. When the splenic vessels are located, a kidney pedicle clamp or a vascular clamp is placed across the splenic artery and vein. The vessels are doubly ligated using size 0 polydioxanone. The gastric arteries are then identified and ligated. After the vascular supply to the spleen has been controlled, the wound can be more carefully cleared of blood and the extent of damage ascertained.

4. ***The wound is explored for other sites of injury.***
The wound is explored for other areas of trauma. The abdominal retractors may be repositioned at this time. The surgeon examines the abdominal cavity again to ensure that all hemorrhage has been controlled and to locate any other areas of abdominal trauma. The ST should be prepared to provide clamps and ligatures. The wound is then irrigated with warm saline. A section drain is placed in the vicinity of the splenic pedicle, and the wound is closed in layers.

SPLENECTOMY (LAPAROSCOPIC)

Laparoscopic splenectomy is removal of the spleen using a laparoscopic approach. After dissection of the splenic attachments, the spleen may be extracted from the abdomen using a mini-laparotomy and wound protector or by using a specimen retrieval bag. In this case, the spleen is morcellated (fragmented) either by hand or using a morcellator instrument.

Pathology

The most common indication for laparoscopic splenectomy is disorders of the blood.

POSITION:	Right lateral decubitus—45-degree tilt
PREP AND DRAPING:	Flank/laparotomy
INSTRUMENTS AND SUPPLIES:	Laparoscopy set; two 10- to 12-mm laparoscopes; three to five 5-mm trocars; specimen retrieval system; ultrasonic system; monopolar ESU; bipolar ESU; linear endo staplers; endo stapler cutter; clips and applier
POSSIBLE EXTRAS:	Morcellation system; minor laparotomy set

Technical Points and Discussion

1. ***Pneumoperitoneum is established and the spleen is mobilized.***
The first operative step of the procedure is to mobilize the spleen from its attachments, including those of the colon and stomach. Dissection is performed using smooth forceps, bipolar ESU, or ultrasonic scalpel, and probe. Surgical clips are used as the larger vessels of the stomach are encountered. The splenic artery is also isolated and ligated.

2. ***The splenic hilum structures are occluded.***
A linear endo stapler is used to occlude the splenic hilum. This seals the vessels within the hilum. Further dissection releases the spleen from its attachments and blood supply.

3. ***The specimen is placed in a retrieval bag.***
The specimen retrieval bag is inserted through one of the larger ports. The spleen is then placed inside the bag. The opening of the bag is completely withdrawn so that no tissue is left behind during morcellation. Morcellation can be done digitally or by using a morcellator instrument. The splenic tissue is now able to fit through the port for extraction. The ST should receive the tissue in a basin large enough to contain the entire organ and specimen bag. An alternative method of extraction is with the use of a wound protector. To use the wound protector, the surgeon opens the abdomen at the 12-mm port and inserts the protector. A seal between the edge of the protector and the abdominal wall prevents loss of CO_2 gas. This technique is called "hand-assisted" splenectomy.

4. ***The splenic tissue is extracted and the surgical site assessed for bleeding.***
At this time the wound may be irrigated with warm saline and explored for bleeders. The ports are removed.

5. ***The wounds are closed and dressed.***
The trocar/cannula wounds are closed with figure-of-8 sutures through the deep layers. If a mini-laparotomy was performed, it is closed in separate layers using absorbable synthetic sutures. Skin is closed with staples and dressed with Steri-Strips and flat gauze dressing (mini-laparotomy).

Patients are usually ready for discharge after the first or second day of hospitalization.

PANCREATICODUODENECTOMY (WHIPPLE PROCEDURE)

Pancreaticoduodenectomy is performed as a curative procedure in the treatment of pancreatic cancer. In the Whipple procedure, the head of the pancreas and duodenum and a portion of the jejunum, distal stomach, distal section of the common bile duct, and gallbladder are removed. The biliary system, pancreatic system, and GI tract are reconstructed. Lymph node staging is also carried out to determine the extent of metastasis. Pancreaticoduodenectomy is a radical operation that requires 5 to 8 hours to complete. Because the procedure includes elements of pancreatic, biliary, intestinal, and gastric procedures, the ST should prepare all instruments normally used in these specialties. Most are included in a major laparotomy set. Vascular instruments should be added to the sterile setup. Extra suction and two ESU sets are sometimes needed. Long instruments and wide retractors (e.g., wide Deaver and Harrington retractors) should also be available. Right-angle clamps are used throughout the procedure.

Much of the procedure includes meticulous dissection, management of bleeding, and anastomosis. The surgeon's preferred sutures staples, and locking clips are made available but should be distributed to the sterile field economically. Additional sutures and other equipment, such as sponges, vessel loops, and scalpel blades, should be held in reserve. Extra surgical towels and half-sheet drapes should be available to keep the operative site orderly and clean.

There are many variations on the Whipple procedure; the exact resection depends on the pathological condition. Reconstruction procedures include the following:

- Gastric resection and gastrojejunostomy (in some procedures the stomach is not resected)
- Intestinal resection and anastomosis
- Choledochojejunostomy or choledochoduodenostomy
- Pancreatojejunostomy

Table 22.6 describes the most common anatomical changes that occur during the procedure.

Pathology

Pancreatic cancer is a rapidly spreading adenocarcinoma that can affect multiple organs early in the course of the disease. The pancreas lies in close approximation to the liver, spleen, duodenum, stomach, and gallbladder. The disease is often not detected until a late stage, by which time it has already metastasized. Diagnostic tests include complete lab workup, MRI, PET, and CT scan. ERCP is also performed, and tissue biopsies are taken.

POSITION:	Supine
INCISION:	Upper midline; bilateral subcostal

TABLE 22.6 Reconstruction Using the Whipple Procedure

Normal Anatomical Structure	Postreconstruction Configuration
The duodenum is continuous from the distal stomach to the jejunum.	The duodenum and a portion of the jejunum are removed. A portion of the proximal jejunum is removed.
The distal stomach is continuous with the duodenum.	The gastric omentum attachments are divided, and the distal (lower) third of the stomach is removed. The remaining gastric section is attached to the jejunum with a side-to-side technique.
The common bile duct is an extension of the common hepatic duct and communicates directly into the duodenum at the ampulla of Vater.	The common bile duct is divided just below the Y-junction of the cystic and hepatic ducts. The common bile duct is anastomosed to the jejunum with an end-to-side technique.
The pancreatic duct communicates with the duodenum at the ampulla of Vater.	The head of the pancreas is removed and the remaining portion is anastomosed to the jejunum with an end-to-end or side-to-side technique.

PREP AND DRAPING: Abdominal—axillary to pubis/laparotomy/continuous urinary drainage (Foley catheter)

INSTRUMENTS AND SUPPLIES: Major laparotomy set: gallbladder instruments; gastrointestinal instruments; vascular clamps and forceps; Silastic vessel loops; surgical clips and applier; linear stapler cutter

POSSIBLE EXTRAS: Topical hemostatic agents; assorted stapling instruments; umbilical tapes; hemostat shods; universal or Bookwalter retractor

Technical Points and Discussion

1. ***A laparotomy is performed through an upper midline incision.***
The abdomen is first entered through a short midline incision. This allows the surgeon to manually explore the abdomen for metastasis in the organs around the pancreas. If metastasis is found, the team may opt to close the incision and recover the patient without further surgery. If there is no evidence of palpable metastasis, the incision is lengthened and the procedure continued.

2. ***The duodenum is mobilized with blunt and sharp dissection.***
The wound is packed with moistened lap sponges, and a self-retaining retractor is placed in the usual manner. Accessory retractors or a self-retaining retractor fitted with attachments (Thompson or Bookwalter) may be used.
The procedure begins with exposure of the head of the pancreas. This involves mobilization of the duodenum, which is attached to the peritoneal reflection (an extension of the abdominal peritoneum). The surgeon separates loose connective tissue from the duodenum with the ultrasonic scalpel, bipolar radiofrequency vessel sealer, monopolar ESU, and Metzenbaum scissors. Babcock clamps may be needed to elevate the duodenum during dissection.

3. ***The porta hepatis is exposed and gallbladder structures mobilized.***
The inferior surface of the liver contains a fissure, which contains important vessels and ducts. This area is called the *porta hepatis*. The structures in the area are now identified and mobilized. These may be retracted using Silastic vessel loops. Surgical clips should also be mounted on a holder and ready to pass. A lymph node normally encountered in this area is removed as a specimen. The ST must receive the node in a small container and immediately label it. The gallbladder is now mobilized completely but left attached.

4. ***The duodenum and stomach are mobilized and the duodenum transected.***
The gastrocolic ligament and omentum are mobilized using sharp and blunt dissection.
The lower third of the stomach is separated from the omentum. Surgical clips, staples, and a vessel-sealing system are also used throughout the dissection and mobilization of the small intestine and stomach. The monopolar ESU, ultrasonic scalpel, and Metzenbaum scissors are used extensively during the mobilization procedures. The duodenum is transected and sealed using a GIA stapler cutter. This line of staples is oversewn with interrupted sutures of 2-0 polydioxanone. The head of the pancreas, gallbladder, and duodenum are now free of attachments and are passed off to the pathologist for frozen section.

5. ***The pancreas is anastomosed to the jejunum.***
A 5-Fr stent is inserted into the pancreatic duct to facilitate anastomosis of the duct into the wall of the jejunum to form the pancreaticojejunostomy. The duodenum is placed in the right upper quadrant during this phase of the procedure. To start the anastomosis of the pancreatic duct, two traction sutures of 3-polydioxanone are placed at the corners of the duct. The anastomosis is performed with size 5-0 synthetic absorbable suture on the inner layer of the duct followed by interrupted sutures of 3-0 polydioxanone on the outer layer and serosa of the jejunum. This completes the attachment of the pancreatic duct to the jejunum.

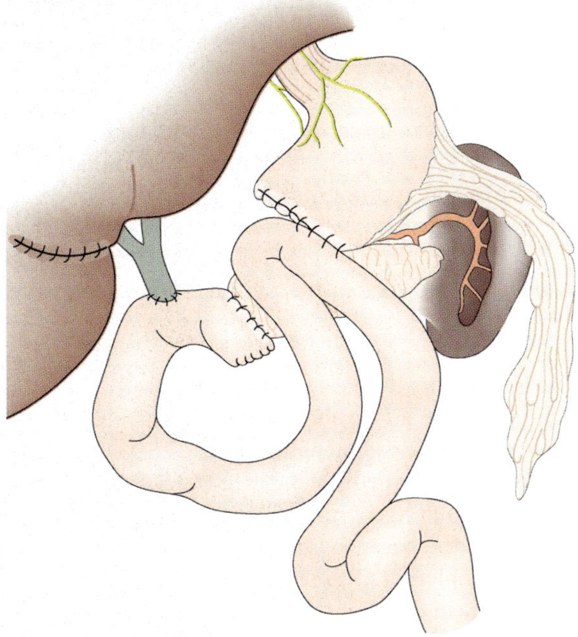

FIG. 22.20 Whipple procedure anastomoses. (From Garden O, Bradbury A, Forsythe J, Parks R. *Principles and Practice of Surgery*. 5th ed. Edinburgh: Churchill Livingstone/Elsevier; 2007.)

6. ***The common bile duct is anastomosed to the jejunum (hepaticojejunostomy).***
A hepaticojejunostomy is now performed just distal to the pancreaticojejunostomy. This will join the common bile duct to the jejunum. As with the previous anastomosis, two traction sutures are placed at the corners of the hepatic duct. Multiple 5-0 synthetic absorbable sutures are placed at the periphery but not tied to complete the anastomosis.

7. ***The stomach is anastomosed to the duodenum (duodenojejunostomy).***
To complete the last anastomosis of the procedure, the surgeon brings the stomach and duodenum into approximation with the jejunum. The previously placed suture line is cut away using the monopolar ESU. A two-layer anastomosis is then performed. The inner layers are joined using 3-0 synthetic absorbable sutures on a curved taper needle. The outer serosa layers are attached with interrupted polydioxanone, size 3-0. Fig. 22.20 shows the completed anastomoses.

8. ***The abdomen is irrigated, drains placed, and closed in layers.***
After checking the wound for any bleeding tissues, the surgeon places two suction drains in the abdomen. These are sutured to the abdominal wall. The wound is closed in layers as for routine laparotomy.

After radical surgery, the patient recovers in the PACU and may be taken to the intensive care unit (ICU) for observation. Complex physiological monitoring is performed throughout the initial phases of postoperative recovery. As normal homeostasis returns, the patient is still monitored for metabolic and renal function, infection, and fluid and electrolyte balance.

Patients remain in the hospital for up to 10 days, depending on the course of healing. Chemotherapy and radiotherapy are usually indicated for 3 to 6 months postoperatively.

SEGMENTAL RESECTION OF THE LIVER (OPEN)

Hepatic resection is performed to remove a portion of the liver to treat a benign or malignant tumor. **Segmental resection** or **lobectomy** is the usual approach for tumor removal. This is the removal of one or more of the nine liver segments. Lobectomy is the removal of one or more of the major lobes of the liver: the right lobe, the left lobe, or the entire right lobe and a portion of the left (called *right hepatic tri-segmentectomy*). Liver resection follows diagnostic studies, including percutaneous needle biopsy performed under MRI or ultrasound guidance in an outpatient setting.

Pathology

The most common indication for liver resection is a malignant liver tumor. The tumor may be primary (the original source of the cancer) or metastatic (cancer that has spread from another location in the body). The most common types of liver tumors are metastatic, especially those arising from primary tumors in which the blood supply is drained by the portal vein. Primary liver tumors are rare. Cancer of the liver usually is well advanced by the time it is diagnosed. Less common indications for liver resection include parasitic disease, infection, and laceration of or trauma to the liver.

POSITION:	Supine
INCISION:	Upper midline; bilateral subcostal
PREP AND DRAPING:	Abdominal – axillary to pubis/ laparotomy/continuous urinary drainage (Foley catheter)
INSTRUMENTS AND SUPPLIES:	Major laparotomy set; vascular clamps and forceps; Silastic vessel loops; surgical clips and applier
POSSIBLE EXTRAS:	Bookwalter retractor

Technical Points and Discussion

1. ***A laparotomy is performed through a right subcostal, midline, or paramedian incision.***
After entering the abdomen, the surgeon examines the liver and adjacent viscera. This may be done before or after a self-retaining retractor is placed in the wound. Because of the size of the liver and the wide exposure required, a self-retaining retractor with accessory attachments such as a Bookwalter retractor is often used. Before placing the

retractor, the surgeon places moist laparotomy sponges over accessory organs surrounding the liver and between the liver and the diaphragm.

IMPORTANT TO KNOW *One of the areas in which sponges often are retained is the subphrenic area (under the diaphragm). The ST counts all sponges placed in the wound, taking special care to note the number of sponges placed in this area of the abdomen.*

2. ***The abdominal cavity is examined for evidence of disease.***
   After all retractors have been placed, the surgeon examines the diseased segment. A sterile ultrasound Doppler probe may be needed to determine the segmental location of the tumor. Removal of liver segments requires identification and dissection of veins, arteries, and ducts that branch into each segment.
3. ***The pedicle segment is identified and individual vessels and ducts (bile duct, hepatic artery, and portal vein branch) are dissected free.***
   To begin the resection, the surgeon dissects the attachments between the liver and abdominal wall, such as the falciform ligament. To perform a segmental resection, the surgeon must locate the correct segment pedicle. These two steps of the procedure are performed with the standard dissecting instruments. The surgeon may need to place an additional retractor at the top of the incision to displace the liver upward. A Harrington retractor or wide Deaver retractor may be used here. The surgeon protects the liver with a moist laparotomy sponge and uses the hand to expose the ligaments that attach the liver to the posterior wall of the abdomen. The ultrasonic scalpel may be used to expose the pedicle, where it branches into the parenchyma.
4. ***Ultrasound may be used, or methylene blue dye may be injected into the pedicle to stain the segment and identify the exact anatomical boundaries.***
   At this stage, the surgeon must identify the exact borders of the segment. If multiple segments are to be removed, all ligament attachments are transected during the procedure. A common method is to begin dissection at the pedicle (at the hilum of the liver) and follow the structures into the parenchyma, using the ultrasonic scalpel or ESU to resect the liver tissue. If this approach is used, the surgeon temporarily stops the vascular supply to the segment by applying vascular clamps across the vessels that supply that segment. This prevents excess bleeding during the dissection.
   An alternative method is to first identify the pedicle structures and then inject methylene blue dye into the pedicle. The methylene blue dye enters the pedicle structures and stains the segment that includes the tumor. If this technique is used, the ST should have methylene blue dye, a 10-mL syringe, and the surgeon's preferred needle for injection. A small Silastic catheter may be attached to the hub of the needle and syringe.
5. ***The pedicle structures are clamped and ligated.***
   When the portal (branches of the portal vein) and pedicle structures and appropriate segment have been identified, the pedicle structures are individually clamped, ligated, and transected. The pedicle and portal structures are ligated with polydioxanone, synthetic nonabsorbable suture, or surgical staples.
6. ***The liver segment is resected.***
   The liver segment can be resected at this point. The surgeon scores the segment using the ESU. Complete resection is performed with the ESU, CUSA or ultrasonic scalpel, or by finger fracture (the surgeon uses the hand to "break" the parenchyma along the lines of resection). At the completion of the resection, the liver bed and raw surfaces must be free of hemorrhage. The argon beam coagulator and ESU are typically used to secure hemostasis.
7. ***The wound is irrigated, drains placed, and closed.***
   The wound is irrigated using warm saline and all tissue debris removed. A suction drain (e.g., Jackson-Pratt or Penrose drain) is placed in the wound, which is closed in layers as for a laparotomy. The incision is dressed with abdominal pads and flat gauze. The drains are secured to the skin and the wound closed in layers as for a laparotomy.

SECTION IV: BREAST SURGERY

SURGICAL ANATOMY

The breasts lie within the fascia of the anterior chest wall from the second to the sixth ribs. The breast is composed of glandular, connective, and fat tissue contained within extensions of fibrous ligaments that radiate from the nipple to the periphery of the breast. Membranes or septal ligaments separate each of these radial sections. Each breast has about 15 to 25 separate sections. The glandular tissue forms clusters or small lobes, which are interspersed with alveoli that contain the secretory cells that form milk (Fig. 22.21).

The lactiferous ducts branch to connect the lobes to the nipple. The nipple contains glandular, vascular, nerve, and epithelial tissue. It is surrounded by the *areola*, a circular area of darkened skin. Small nodes in the areola contain sebaceous glands. Estrogen and progesterone are secreted cyclically and during pregnancy, causing the areola to darken.

Breast tissue changes with development of the individual, hormonal changes, pregnancy status, and nutritional state. The release of breast milk and other secretions from the nipple is controlled by complex hormonal changes.

The upper thoracic lymph drains to the axillary lymph nodes. This is an important anatomical feature, because cancer staging and diagnostic surgery often require biopsy of one

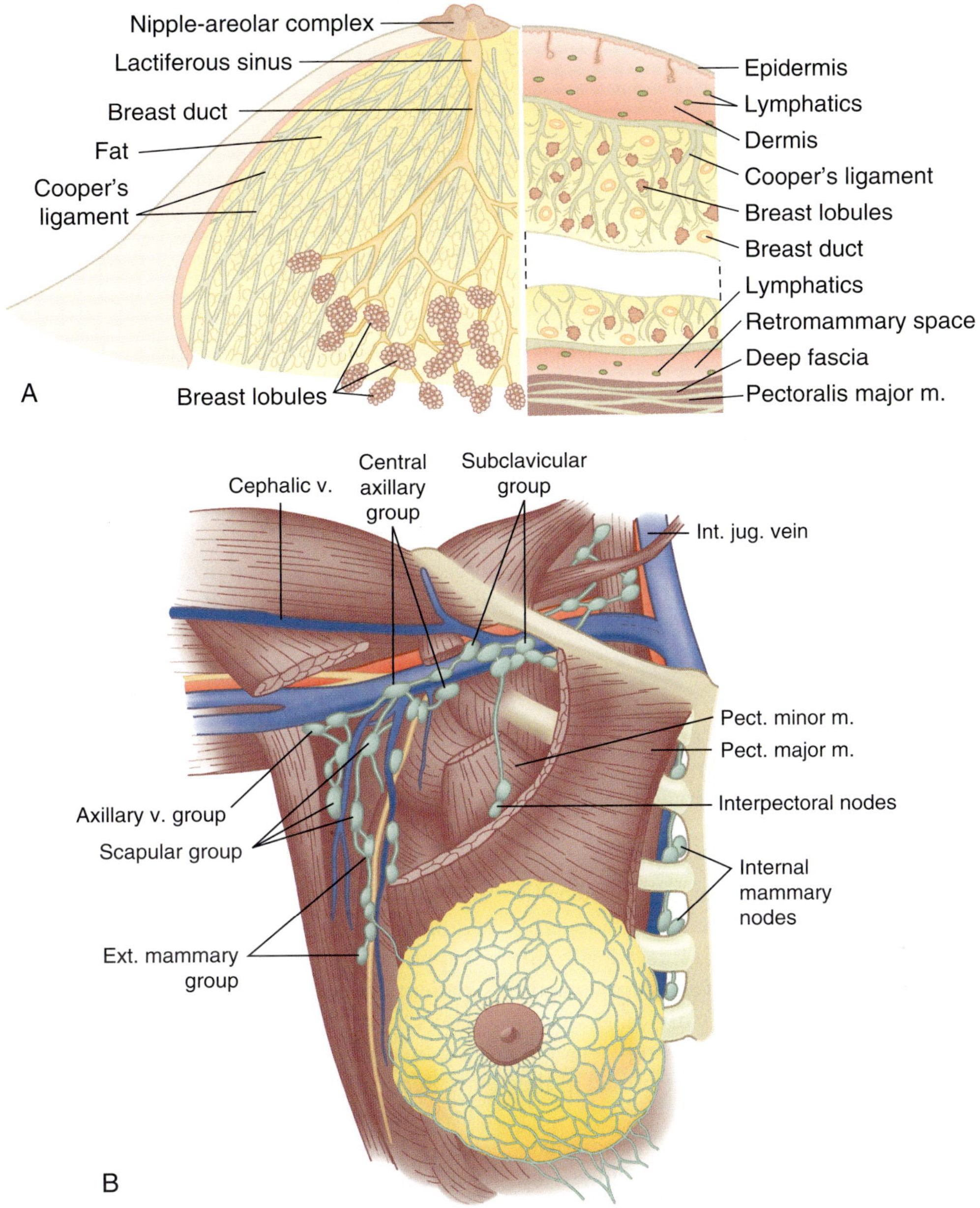

FIG. 22.21 Structures of the breast. (A) Breast anatomy. The cutaway on the right illustrates the tissue layers. The breast is supported by deep fascia and muscle. (B) The axillary anatomy, showing lymph node drainage and the vascular supply. (From Donegan WL, Spratt JS. *Cancer of the Breast*. Philadelphia: WB Saunders; 1988.)

or more axillary lymph nodes. The type and extent of change in the lymph nodes are primary determinants of the disease outcome and survival rate.

BREAST CANCER

Most noncosmetic surgical procedures of the breast are performed for the treatment of cancer. Breast cancer diagnosis and treatment is a surgical specialty that has advanced greatly in the past two decades. Procedures that were common 10 years ago may never be performed in most clinical facilities. However, the psychological and social consequences of a cancer diagnosis have not changed. This aspect of patient care remains a critical concern of those caring for a patient undergoing breast surgery.

Breast cancer is the leading cause of death in women aged 20 to 59 in the United States. Improvements in diagnostic technology and aggressive public health campaigns in the United States have increased the reported number of cases of cancer in the last 10 years because of early detection. Both malignant and some benign breast neoplasms generally present as a mass that is visible on breast ultrasound and MRI. A mass smaller than 0.4 inch (1 cm) usually is not palpable but can be detected with routine mammography. Invasive ductal carcinoma is the most common type of breast cancer. Risk factors include a family history of breast cancer, benign breast disease, and hormonal conditions that result in early menarche and late menopause. Breast cancer in men accounts for 0.8% of all breast cancers. The annual mortality rate for male breast cancer averages 400, compared with 400,000 in women.

TABLE 22.7 Diagnostic Procedures of the Breast

Type	Description	Considerations
Breast self-examination (BSE)	Women and men are taught how to perform BSE by a primary care professional. The procedure for BSE involves systematic palpation of the breast and axillary region and visual examination, starting at age 20.	The patient should be instructed by a qualified health professional who can answer questions and make sure the patient understands the procedure and its importance.
Clinical examination	The clinical examination involves palpation and visual examination of the breasts by a qualified health professional.	Women in their 20s and 30s should have a clinical examination every 3 years.
Mammography	A mammography is a radiological examination of the breasts for detection of masses or other lesions.	Mammography is the only screening method effective for the detection of nonpalpable lesions. A yearly mammogram is recommended for women age 40 or older.
Fine-needle aspiration	A fine-gauge needle is inserted into a suspect breast mass, and tissue (cells and fluid) is withdrawn for examination and diagnosis.	This procedure may be performed in the physician's office.
Stereotactic biopsy	The patient lies prone on the mammography table with the breast isolated. A computer-assisted needle is guided into the suspect mass, and a core sample is withdrawn.	This procedure is less invasive than surgical biopsy. Stereotactic technology provides accurate placement of the needle and has 96% accuracy for detecting cancer.

Cancer *staging* is used to determine the possible outcome and options for treatment. However, the final decision rests with the patient, in consultation with the primary health care specialist, surgeon, and oncologist. Breast cancer treatment has changed radically over the past 20 years, with a tendency toward less radical surgery. Early detection combined with improved chemotherapy and radiological treatment now provide an outcome equal to or better than that achieved with the radical mastectomy performed routinely several decades ago.

A range of procedures are available for surgical management of a breast tumor. These include the following:

- *Needle aspiration biopsy,* which usually is performed in the physician's office to confirm a cystic mass
- *Fine-needle insertion* into the suspect mass, with immediate surgical excision and frozen section. This is followed by breast-conserving surgery (*lumpectomy* or segmental resection), with or without lymph node excision.
- *Sentinel node detection and biopsy* followed by breast-conserving surgery and axillary node dissection
- *Breast-conserving procedures,* such as lumpectomy and segmental resection
- ***Mastectomy*** *(preplanned)* for advanced metastatic cancer or as a prophylactic procedure in high-risk patients

Breast-conserving surgery with sentinel node biopsy is now the choice of most oncologists unless the cancer is advanced at the time of presentation. The prognosis is influenced more by the extent of lymph node involvement than by the size of the breast tumor.

Table 22.7 describes diagnostic procedures of the breast.

CASE PLANNING

PSYCHOLOGICAL CONSIDERATIONS

For most women, the breast reflects reproductive ability and **body image** and secures feminine identity. Surgery of the breast threatens these images and can produce anxiety and depression. Increased public awareness of breast cancer and advanced technology for early detection has increased women's ability to take an active part in breast health.

Although early detection is an important advance in breast medicine, the prospect of surgery remains an emotional and difficult event for the patient. The patient's need for emotional support requires health care professionals to listen to the patient and support and acknowledge her feelings. The clinician's most important roles in providing support are to provide a calm presence and to convey respect for the patient's feelings.

Reconstructive breast surgery may be performed immediately after a mastectomy or as a separate procedure at a later date. The patient may enter a deep grieving period after such radical surgery. Psychological support at this time is critical in restoring the patient's positive self-image.

POSITION AND DRAPING

Noncosmetic breast surgery is performed with the patient in the supine or modified beach chair position. A pad may be placed under the affected side to elevate the surgical site area. The affected arm is prepped and draped free for extensive procedures that require axillary node dissection.

If the arm is draped free, an arm board is used, as in limb surgery. This allows the surgeon to manipulate the arm for exposure to the axilla at various angles.

INSTRUMENTS AND SUPPLIES

Surgery of the breast requires general surgery instruments and a plastic surgery set. Senn, vein, small rakes, and other small retractors are needed for breast biopsy. Surgical clips, absorbable and nonabsorbable sutures, and an ESU are used for hemostasis. Vessel loops are needed for retraction of deep veins, arteries, and nerves. Wound drains include the

Jackson-Pratt, Hemovac, and simpler gravity drains, such as the Penrose drain. The ESU is used extensively in radical breast surgery. The surgeon may require a nerve stimulator to differentiate blood vessels from small nerves during dissection of the chest wall and axilla.

SURGICAL PROCEDURES

WIRE LOCALIZATION AND BREAST BIOPSY

Wire localization (also known as **needle wire localization**) is the insertion of a fine wire into a breast mass using guided imagery such as mammography, ultrasound, or MRI. The needle wire assembly is triggering device that includes a needle or blade trocar. After needle insertion and deployment of the wire into the tissue, the wire remains in position by its hooked, barbed, or J-shaped tip. The wire is taped in place during the imaging process. The patient is transferred to the operating room and a biopsy is performed at the site of the wire.

POSITION:	Supine or modified beach chair
INCISION:	Elliptical at site of the wire
PREP AND DRAPING:	Thoracic including the arm on the affected side
INSTRUMENTS AND SUPPLIES:	Minor set including small skin and superficial retractors, Allis clamps, fine hemostats
POSSIBLE EXTRAS:	Small Penrose drain

Technical Points and Discussion

1. ***A needle wire is placed used guided imagery.***
Wire insertion takes place in the interventional radiology department. The surgical procedure is scheduled to follow immediately.

2. ***The patient is draped for an excisional biopsy of the breast.***
After administration of an anesthetic, the breast is very gently prepped to avoid dislodging the needle or potentially seeding the tissue with cancer cells. A fenestrated body drape is then applied. Care must be taken not to displace the needle during the draping.

3. ***The needle is located and an elliptical incision is made that includes the needle and a 2-cm margin of skin.***
The surgeon begins the procedure by making an elliptical skin incision around the tip of the wire. Metzenbaum scissors are used to increase the depth of the incision. Senn retractors or small rakes are placed at the wound edges. Scissors rather than an ESU are used to complete the dissection to avoid distorting the margins of the mass. Allis clamps may be used to grasp the tissue during dissection.

4. ***The tissue specimen with wire is delivered to the pathologist.***
The specimen, with identification needle intact, is delivered to the pathologist for examination. If the margins of the specimen are *not* clear of tumor, additional tissue is removed and examined. When the margins include a clear area of 0.4 to 0.8 inch (1 to 2 cm), the wound is closed.

5. ***The wound is irrigated and closed.***
The excision site is irrigated with warm saline and closed with several subcutaneous interrupted sutures of absorbable synthetic material. The skin usually is closed with Steri-Strips or subcuticular sutures.

SENTINEL LYMPH NODE BIOPSY

The procedure for **sentinel lymph node biopsy (SLNB)** involves injection of isosulfan blue dye, radioactive material (**technetium-99**), or both directly into the breast mass or nearby. Both materials may be used to track the lymph nodes visually (dye) and by gamma ray emission (technetium-99). The technetium then is tracked with a device similar to a Geiger counter.

If radioactive material is used, it may be injected up to 6 hours before surgery in the nuclear medicine department. Isosulfan is injected at the time of surgery to provide greater visibility of the nodes. Sentinel node biopsy is performed before mastectomy. Fig. 22.22 shows several steps of the procedure.

NOTE *Isosulfan blue may cause anaphylactic shock in some patients. When it is used in conjunction with SLNB, the patient is monitored carefully throughout the procedure. A crash cart must be immediately available in these cases.*

Pathology

Sentinel lymph nodes are usually located at the proximal axillary lymph chain. A metastatic tumor in the breast drains (theoretically) first to these nodes. Excision of the sentinel nodes is an alternative to axillary lymph node dissection, in which 10 or more nodes are removed for preventive treatment. Sentinel node excision may be appropriate only in selected patients with a low risk of metastasis.

POSITION:	Supine with operative side arm secured on arm board
INCISION:	Over the area of a "hot" node
PREP AND DRAPING:	Anterior thorax including axilla on the operative side
INSTRUMENTS AND SUPPLIES:	Minor set with shallow retractors; gamma probe; monopolar ESU; surgical skin marker
POSSIBLE EXTRAS:	Isosulfan blue tissue stain; 5- and 10-mL syringes; fine-gauge needles

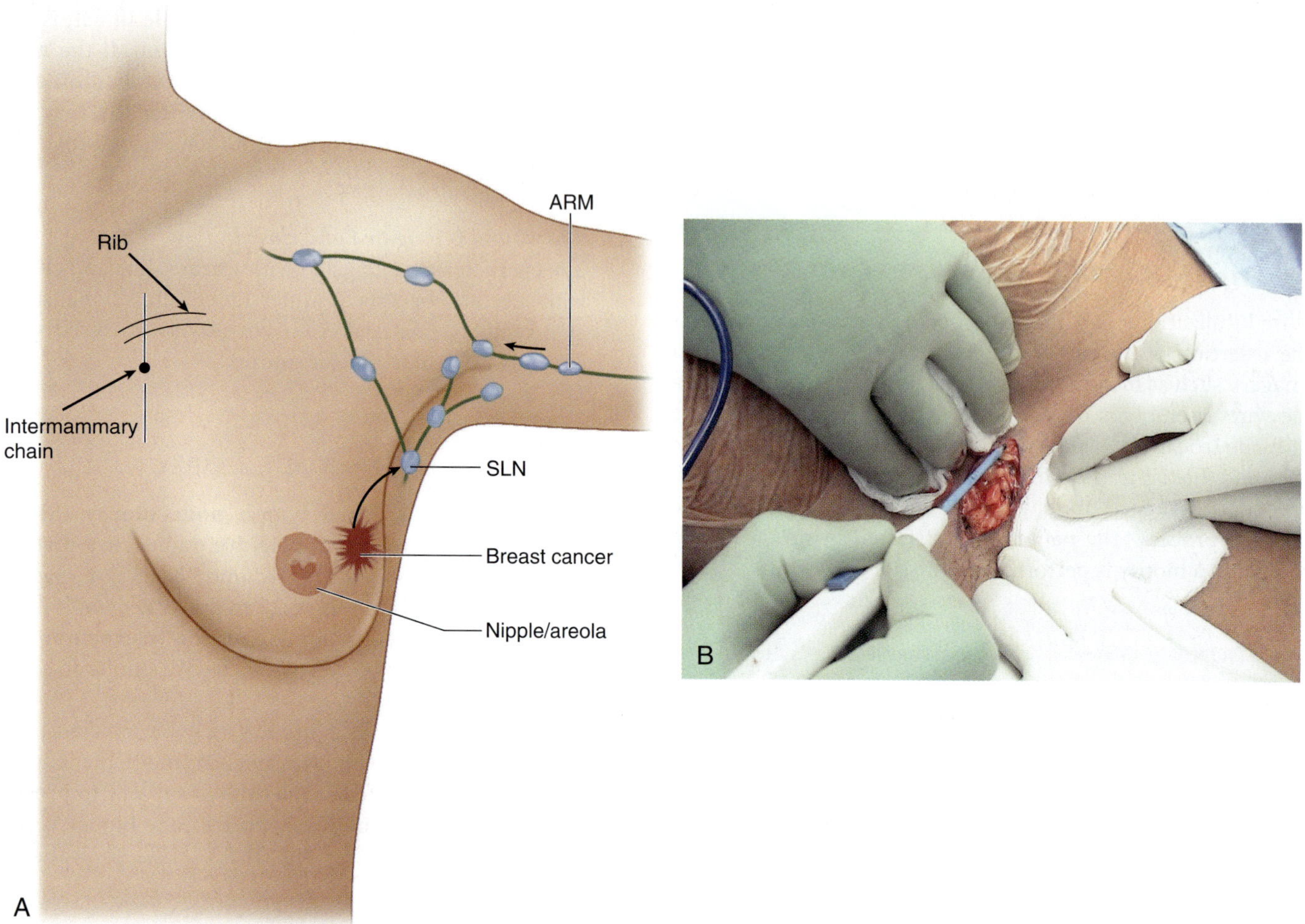

FIG. 22.22 Sentinel biopsy. (A) Surgical anatomy. (B) Incision directly over "hot" area. Lymph node stained blue for identification and removal. (From Klimberg V, Townsend C, Evers M. *Atlas of Breast Surgical Techniques*. Philadelphia: Saunders; 2012.)

Technical Points and Discussion

1. ***The breast mass is injected with technetium-99 4 to 6 hours before surgery, or 3 to 5 mL of isosulfan blue dye is injected near the mass site.***
   The surgeon may choose to use isosulfan blue dye, technetium-99, or both. Technetium-99 is injected 4 to 6 hours before surgery. Isosulfan blue stain is injected at the time of surgery. The ST should have at least 10 mL of stain, a 10-mL syringe, and 1½-inch 22- and 24-gauge needles or smaller.

2. ***The sentinel nodes are detected using a gamma probe.***
   The surgeon drapes the gamma probe. He or she then slowly scans the area around the mass and axilla with the probe. When a "hot" node is detected, the area is marked using a skin marker.

3. ***The node is removed.***
   A small incision is made into the area using a #10 or #11 knife. Dissection is continued using Metzenbaum scissors. Small bleeders are tied with fine polydioxanone sutures or managed with the ESU. The wound edges are retracted in two or three directions using Senn retractors or other small right-angle retractors. A small self-retaining retractor may be used. The tract of the node appears blue and leads to the hot node. The node is removed. The ST must provide a separate container for each node and ensure that they are identified appropriately.

4. ***The incision is explored using the probe.***
   The incision is explored using the gamma probe. The axilla is probed and palpated to search for other hot nodes. These are removed as described.

5. ***The instrument setup is removed from the field.***
   All instruments used for sentinel node biopsy are removed from the surgical field, and a new instrument setup used for breast surgery follows.

6. ***The lymph node incisions are closed when outside the area of breast resection.***
   The deep nodal incision tissues may be closed using fine absorbable synthetic sutures. Skin is closed at the same time as mastectomy incision closure.

BREAST-CONSERVING SURGERY FOR A MASS (LUMPECTOMY, SEGMENTAL MASTECTOMY) WITH AXILLARY DISSECTION

A breast mass is removed to confirm a diagnosis or to treat malignancy. The mass is excised, ensuring that the margins are completely free of cancer cells. Axillary dissection to remove a group of lymph nodes or removal of selective sentinel lymph nodes may be performed during the same procedure. Analysis of the mass by frozen section is done during surgery; this determines the extent of the excision discussed and planned with the patient before surgery. In a skin-sparing **(subcutaneous) mastectomy,** the overlying skin tissue, the areola, and the nipple are not removed. An implant may be placed immediately after the procedure.

Axillary lymph nodes, which drain the breast, can include cancer cells from a malignant tumor. There is a trend away from performing axillary dissection in favor of sentinel lymph node removal as described previously. Axillary dissection is included here for study and discussion.

POSITION:	Supine with arm board on affected side
INCISION:	Elliptical around mass
PREP AND DRAPING:	Thorax and arm on the affected side
INSTRUMENTS AND SUPPLIES:	Basic set; rake retractors; small Deaver retractors; vessel loops; surgical clips and appliers; monopolar ESU; skin marker
POSSIBLE EXTRAS:	Penrose drains

Technical Points and Discussion

1. ***An incision is made at the border of the areola or directly over the tumor mass.***
The skin incision is made along skin lines drawn preoperatively. This incision is carried through the subcutaneous and breast tissue with Metzenbaum or Mayo scissors. Small bleeders are coagulated with a needlepoint ESU tip. A spatula ESU tip generally is not used for en bloc removal of a suspect mass, because this may obliterate the tissue margins and obscure a diagnosis.

2. ***The mass is grasped with one or more Allis clamps and excised using sharp dissection.***
The surgeon grasps the subcutaneous and breast tissue with two or more Allis clamps. The ST should have retractors available as the incision is extended to deep tissue. Small rake or Senn retractors can be used for shallow retraction, and right-angle retractors (small Richardson or Deaver retractors) are needed for deeper excision. Hemostasis is maintained with fine absorbable sutures and an electrosurgical needle. As the excision is extended, 4 × 4 Raytec sponges should be removed from the field and replaced with laparotomy sponges. These can be easily lost inside the breast wound, especially if the excision is deep.

3. ***The specimen may be marked with sutures for orientation and then removed for pathological examination.***
The specimen is removed in one piece. The surgeon may place one or more sutures on the periphery for identification of the margins. These must be carefully preserved. The breast wound may be closed at this time, or closure may be delayed until lymph node dissection is completed. If a frozen section is required, the specimen should be immediately passed off the surgical field to the circulator.

4. ***After a positive pathology report, the wound is extended to include a greater portion of the breast.***
To gain access to the axillary nodes, the surgeon makes an incision just below the upper axillary fold. This tissue plane includes the subcutaneous and fascia layers. The lower flap is tapered toward the chest wall.
After the flaps have been created, right-angle retractors are placed along the edges. The pectoralis muscles are then retracted to expose the axillary vein and its small branches, which are clamped and divided. The axillary vein is ligated with polydioxanone sutures. Small branches may require fine-suture ligation or surgical clips.

5. ***The thoracic and intercostobrachial nerves are identified.***
The surgeon continues to dissect the axillary tissue to expose the two major nerves in this area (thoracic and intercostobrachial nerves). These nerves must be preserved during node dissection. Vessel loops are placed under the nerves with a right-angle clamp. Axillary tissue containing the nodes is then dissected away from the underlying muscle.

6. ***The wound is irrigated, drains placed, and closed.***
Before closing the axilla, the surgeon irrigates the wound with warm saline. The surgeon places a Jackson-Pratt or Penrose drain in the wound. If a closed suction drain is used, the end is brought out through a small stab incision near the main incision. The drain is secured with one or two nonabsorbable sutures. The wounds are closed in two layers. The axilla and subcutaneous breast tissue are closed with interrupted absorbable sutures. The skin is closed with running subcuticular sutures of the surgeon's choice. The incision is dressed with fluffed gauze and abdominal pads.

MODIFIED RADICAL MASTECTOMY

Mastectomy is removal of the entire breast. The extent of the surgery depends on the diagnosis and the patient's medical history.

- In a total (or simple) mastectomy, the entire breast is removed. The axillary lymph nodes are not removed, and the muscles of the chest wall are preserved. Sentinel node biopsy may be performed.

- In a **modified radical mastectomy**, the entire breast is removed, and sentinel node biopsy or axillary dissection performed.
- In a **radical mastectomy** the entire breast, all axillary nodes, and the chest wall muscles are removed. Historically, a radical mastectomy was the only treatment available for a malignant breast mass. This procedure is now rarely performed. Radical mastectomy has been modified, and it is indicated only for late presentation of chest wall metastasis arising from a primary breast tumor.

POSITION:	Supine with arm board on affected side
INCISION:	Elliptical around mass extending into axilla (for axillary dissection)
PREP AND DRAPING:	Thorax, axilla, and arm on the affected side
INSTRUMENTS AND SUPPLIES:	Basic set; rake retractors; small Deaver retractors; vessel loops; surgical clips and appliers; monopolar ESU; skin marker
POSSIBLE EXTRAS:	Penrose drains

Technical Points and Discussion

1. ***The skin and subcutaneous tissue are incised in an elliptical pattern following skin marking.***
To begin the procedure, the surgeon marks both the incision and the extent of the skin flaps. Incising the skin and creating a space between the skin and the underlying tissue creates a **skin flap.** This is called *raising a skin flap.* In this procedure, the skin flaps include subcutaneous tissue. The superior and anterior flaps are extended to the previously marked lines on the skin. Skin hooks are used to elevate the flaps and extend the dissection.

2. ***Lateral edges of the flaps are carried to the edge of the latissimus dorsi muscle.***
The surgeon uses sharp dissection to carry the flaps deeper to the edge of the latissimus dorsi muscle. The ST should have two ESU units available so that one can be cleaned while the other is in use. As large blood vessels are encountered, they are ligated with surgical clips and divided or clamped and secured with polydioxanone ties. The surgeon separates the breast and fascial tissue from the pectoralis major muscle. The skin flaps are retracted gently to preserve their blood supply and to prevent bruising and ischemia at the edges.

3. ***The specimen is dissected free from the lateral chest wall and axilla.***
Axillary dissection, if performed, is a continuous part of this procedure. Rake or Richardson retractors are placed over the axillary edge of the incision. Blunt rakes are preferred to prevent puncturing the skin in this area. An additional right-angle retractor or narrow Deaver or Richardson retractor may be needed for the medial side of the incision.
Tributaries of the axillary vein are exposed and cross-clamped with right-angle clamps; they are then divided, and clipped or ligated. For level III node dissection, the surgeon must sever the pectoralis minor muscle with the ESU. Retraction of the pectoralis muscles with right-angle retractors exposes the axillary tissues. The specimen is dissected from the chest wall and muscles. The apex may be marked with a suture for pathological identification.

4. ***The specimen is removed.***
The surgeon may then pass the specimen to the ST, who receives it in a small basin.

5. ***The wound is irrigated, drains are placed, and the wound is closed.***
Before closing the wound, the surgeon irrigates the area with warm saline. He or she then checks for small bleeders and manages them with the ESU. One or two suction drains such as Jackson-Pratt or Hemovac are placed in the wound and the ends brought out of the skin flaps. The wound is then closed in layers. The ends of the pectoralis minor muscle are sutured together with absorbable sutures. Subcutaneous sutures size 3-0 are placed. The skin is closed with a running subcuticular suture or skin staples. The surgeon may inject local anesthetic into the wound site. The wound is dressed with a nonadherent pad, flat gauze, and gauze fluffs. Fig. 22.23 illustrates a modified radical mastectomy.

NOTE *Cosmetic surgery of the breast is covered in Chapter 29, Plastic and Reconstructive Surgery.*

SECTION V: THE THYROID AND PARATHYROID GLANDS

THYROID GLAND

The thyroid gland is located in the mid-neck and overlies the trachea below the larynx (Fig. 22.24). It has two lobes, which are connected by a central band of tissue called the *isthmus.* A thin strip of thyroid tissue also projects from the superior edge of the isthmus. The thyroid secretes the hormones thyroxine (T4) and triiodothyronine (T3). These hormones are necessary for regulating cell metabolism and growth. Calcitonin, which is also secreted by the thyroid, is necessary for calcium regulation. The parathyroid glands are situated within the lobes of the thyroid. These small glands produce parathyroid hormone (PTH), which influences calcium and phosphate levels in the blood. There are normally four parathyroid glands: two in the upper and two in the lower poles of the thyroid gland.

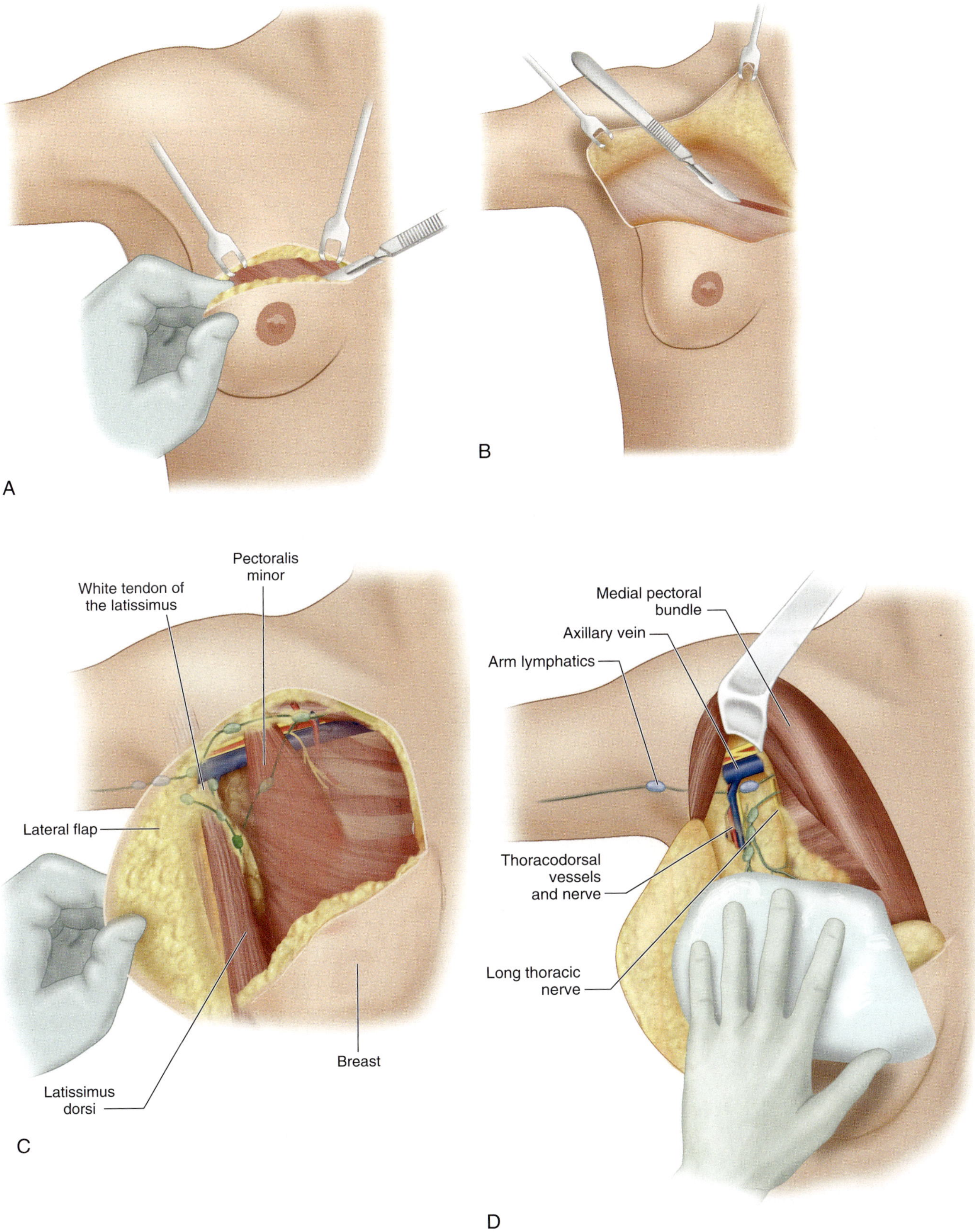

FIG. 22.23 Modified radical mastectomy. (A) Skin sparing incision. (B) Creating the upper flap. (C) Lateral flap is created. (D) En bloc removal.

Continued

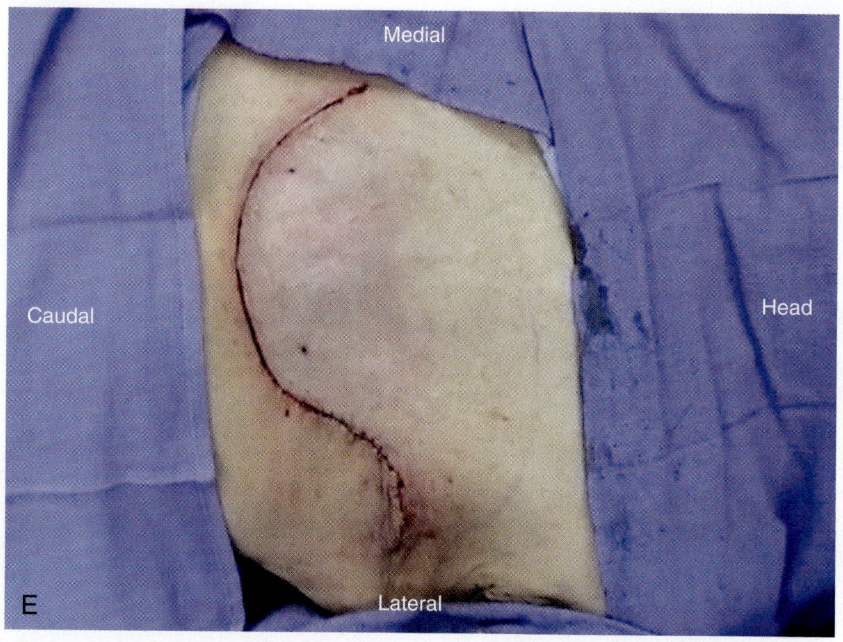

FIG. 22.23, cont'd (E) Wound closure. (From Klimberg V, Townsend C, Evers M. *Atlas of Breast Surgical Techniques*. Philadelphia: Saunders, 2012.)

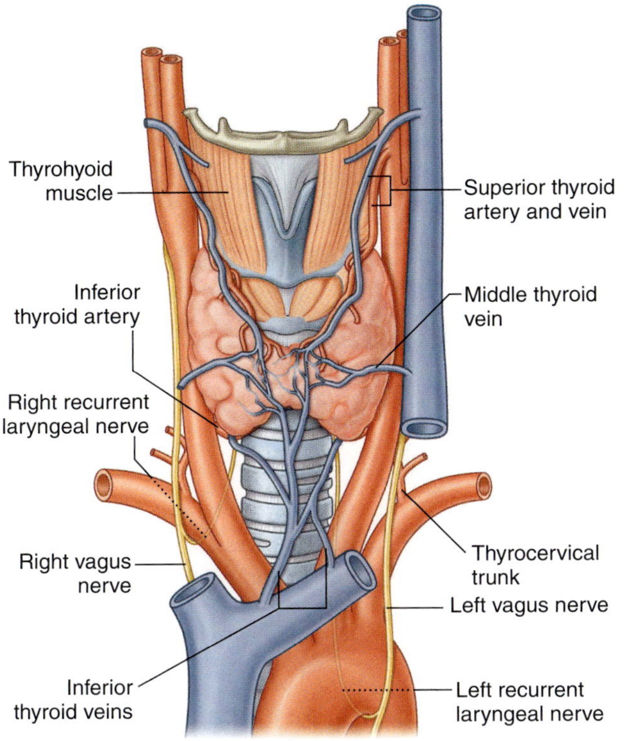

FIG. 22.24 Thyroid gland. Relationship of the thyroid to the trachea and larynx. (From Drake R, Vogl W. *Mitchell Gray's Anatomy for Students.* Edinburgh: Churchill Livingstone; 2004.)

MINIMALLY INVASIVE VIDEO-ASSISTED THYROIDECTOMY (MIVAT)

Thyroidectomy is the surgical removal of one or more lobes of the thyroid gland. The procedure may also include removal of the parathyroid glands.

The standard approach used for open thyroidectomy is through a lateral incision in the neck, which results in a wide scar. Minimally invasive procedures are performed with or without an endoscope. A *totally endoscopic* procedure is carried out using the endoscope with carbon dioxide insufflation of the tissues and special instrumentation. This is a technically demanding procedure not commonly performed. However, minimally invasive video-assisted thyroidectomy (MIVAT) is now a standard procedure. The surgical access is through the neck. However, advanced technology allows alternative access such as transoral and transaxillary. These are in demand by patients who want a cosmetic result. The procedure described below is an MIVAT with access through the neck. Note that two assistants are usually required for retraction. The surgical technologist is positioned opposite the surgeon.

Pathology

Thyroidectomy is performed to treat known or suspected malignancy or for the treatment of hyperthyroidism in selected cases. Benign enlargement of the thyroid *(goiter)* may compress the airway or esophagus. Removal of all or one lobe of the thyroid relieves the obstruction. In hyperthyroid disorders, such as Graves disease, the patient may select partial removal of the hyperfunctioning gland or treatment with radioactive iodine. Selected MIVAT instruments are shown in Fig. 22.25.

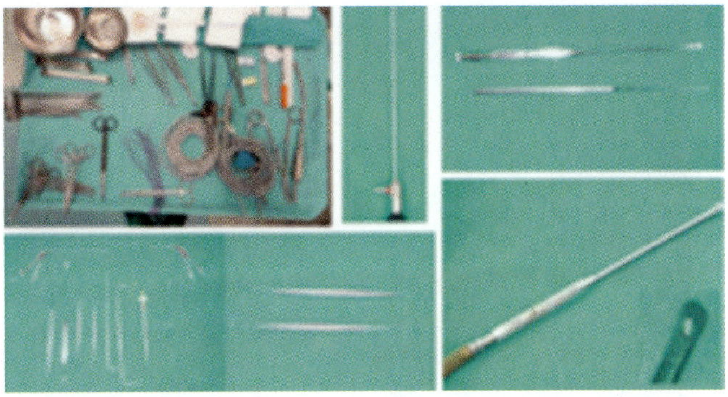

FIG. 22.25 MIVAT instruments. (A) Mayo set-up for open portions of MIVAT. *Lower right,* Note monopolar and bipolar ESU, clip applier, and tonsil suction. *Upper left,* Specimen containers and Farabeuf retractors. (B) 30-degree telescope. (C) Suction-dissector with stylet in place *(top)*. Probe *(bottom)*. (D) Microsurgical scissors and forceps *(top)*. Probe, suction dissector Langenbeck retractors. *Left to right bottom,* Farabeuf right-angled retractors, dissecting scissors, atraumatic tissue forceps. (E) Close-up Langenbeck retractors. (F) Fenestrated suction dissected (see also device tip magnified). (From Randolph G. *Surgery of the Thyroid and Parathyroid Glands.* 3rd ed. Philadelphia: Elsevier; 2021.)

POSITION:	Supine with slight hyperextension of the neck
INCISION:	Mid-neck
PREP AND DRAPING:	Thyroid prep: chin to axilla
INSTRUMENTS:	MIVAT tray: insulated monopolar ESU; ultrasonic scalpel; dissecting spatula; aspirating spatula; suction-dissector, endoscopic scissors and forceps; forward-oblique endoscope, 30-degree viewing angle 5 mm; small right-angle retractors; blunt rake retractors; US retractors; Metzenbaum scissors; vascular forceps; insulated-tip ESU; small vessel applier with clips. A nerve monitoring system may also be needed.

Technical Points and Discussion

1. ***The patient is prepped and draped.***
   After administration of general anesthetic or cervical block, the patient is placed in the supine position with the neck slightly hyperextended. A thyroid skin prep is performed and thyroid draping procedure completed.

2. ***A mid-neck incision is made.***
   A 1.5 cm horizontal skin incision is made above the sternal notch using a #15 blade. The subcutaneous tissue is dissected carefully to avoid bleeding and uses the insulated-tip ESU to manage bleeders. The assistant retracts the tissue layers with small, blunt rake retractors to expose the cervical fascia. The surgeon incises the fascia.

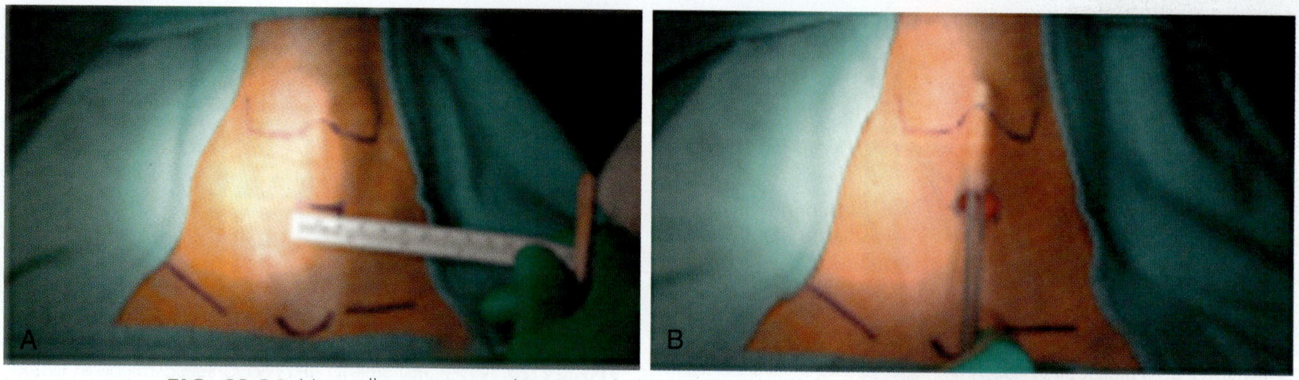

FIG. 22.26 Minimally invasive video-assisted thyroidectomy (MIVAT). (A) Skin incision marking. (B) Preparation of the upper and lower flaps. (From Randolph G. *Surgery of the Thyroid and Parathyroid Glands*. 3rd ed. Philadelphia: Elsevier; 2021.)

3. ***The thyroid gland is separated from the strap muscles.*** The thyroid lobe is dissected bluntly from the strap muscles using small thyroid spatulas. The assistant can be passed larger double-ended retractors such as Farabeuf or US retractors. These will be needed for the endoscopic portion of the procedure.

4. ***A 30-degree endoscope is inserted in the incision and the endoscopic portion initiated.*** The ST should prepare the endoscope for insertion in the wound. The surgeon may require a nerve stimulator to identify the laryngeal nerves during the next portion of the procedure. The ultrasonic scalpel will be used for dissection. A vessel-sealing system should also be immediately available. With the Farabeuf retractors holding back the strap muscles, the endoscope is inserted into the wound. An endoscopic suction dissector and spatula are also inserted to perform dissection of the thyroid lobe from the strap muscles.

5. ***Dissection is extended and hemostasis maintained.*** After the lobe has been dissected from the strap muscles, the deep vessels are dissected with the spatula and aspirator. They are then ligated with clips and divided. The laryngeal nerves and parathyroid glands are identified.

6. ***The thyroid lobe is carefully brought outside the incision to complete the dissection.*** The lobe is separated from the trachea using the ultrasonic scalpel until the dissection is close to the nerve and parathyroid glands, standard non-thermal dissection is used to prevent lateral heating of the tissues. Vessel clips or fine nonabsorbable sutures can be used.

7. ***The opposite lobe is resected using the same technique if a total thyroidectomy is planned.***

8. ***The wound is assessed for hemostasis and closed.*** The wound is irrigated and bleeders controlled using the ESU. The tissue layers of the neck are closed individually. Muscle is closed using size 4-0 absorbable suture, and skin may be closed using a subcuticular absorbable suture or tissue sealant. The incision is dressed with flat gauze. A minimally invasive thyroidectomy is illustrated in Fig. 22.26.

RELATED PROCEDURE: PARATHYROIDECTOMY

Surgical excision of the parathyroid gland is routinely performed as a minimally invasive procedure. The techniques used in removal are identical to a thyroidectomy. The gland is grasped using DeBakey vascular forceps and carefully dissected free using bipolar and ultrasonic systems. The pedicle of the gland is then clipped or ligated with fine nonabsorbable sutures and sharply divided. Closure is the same as a thyroidectomy: the platysma muscle is closed with 4-0 absorbable sutures and the skin with subcuticular absorbable suture or tissue adhesive.

THYROIDECTOMY (OPEN)

Exclusively open thyroidectomy is seldom performed since the development of robotic and hybrid procedures. Selected cases including massive enlargement of the thyroid may require an open approach.

Pathology

Refer to Minimally Invasive Video-Assisted Thyroidectomy (MIVAT).

POSITION:	Supine with neck hyperextended
INCISION:	Mid-neck
PREP AND DRAPING:	Thyroid
INSTRUMENTS:	Thyroid instruments: thyroid tenaculum, spring retractor, short right-angle clamps, fine-tipped hemostats right-angle retractors; minor general surgery set; vascular forceps

Technical Points and Discussion

1. ***The patient is prepped and draped.***
After administration of general anesthetic, the patient is placed in supine position with the neck hyperextended. A thyroid skin prep is performed and thyroid draping procedure completed.

2. ***A mid-neck incision is made.***
The neck is incised with a #10 or #15 blade. The subcutaneous tissue is incised with the ESU, exposing the platysma muscle. The assistant retracts the tissue layers with rake retractors. The surgeon then divides the muscle layer with the deep knife or ESU. The incision is carried deeper with the ESU and Metzenbaum scissors. Numerous bleeders are encountered in the deep tissue, and these are controlled with the ESU and silk ties size 3-0 and 4-0.

3. ***The thyroid gland is exposed.***
As the dissection continues, deeper retractors are used, such as a Green retractor designed for thyroid surgery. When the thyroid gland is exposed, two Lahey spring retractors, or a Mahorner thyroid retractor, are placed in the wound. The surgeon then grasps the gland with one or two Lahey tenacula. As the surgeon dissects the gland from the surrounding tissues, the parathyroid glands, the superior laryngeal nerves, and the recurrent laryngeal nerve are identified and preserved.

4. ***Hemostasis is maintained and the thyroid removed.***
The thyroid gland is an extremely vascular structure. Therefore, to mobilize it, the surgeon successively double-clamps small sections of tissue, divides the tissue between the clamps, and ligates each section. Most surgeons use Kelly or mosquito clamps for mobilization. The ST should have at least 12 to 15 clamps available for dissection of the thyroid. Large arteries of the thyroid are ligated with suture ligatures of 2-0 or 3-0 silk mounted on a fine needle. When mobilization and excision are complete, the gland is passed to the ST. A frozen section may be required for determination of malignancy.

5. ***The wound is irrigated and closed.***
The wound is irrigated, and a Penrose drain is placed in the wound if necessary. The tissue layers of the neck are closed individually. The skin is closed with staples or fine nonabsorbable suture. The incision is dressed with flat gauze. Fluff gauze may be used if a drain has been inserted.

KEY CONCEPTS

- Pathology related to structural weakness of the abdominal wall contributes to the surgeon's overall strategy for repair, which in turn contributes to the surgical technologist's case planning and implementation.
- The surgical technologist's familiarity with common procedures of the abdominal wall contributes to successful preparation before and anticipation during the surgery.
- Knowledge of key anatomical structures and pathology of the gastrointestinal system contributes to the surgical technologist's ability to anticipate the need for instruments, sutures, and other equipment during the surgical procedure.
- Understanding of surgical techniques such as mobilization, anastomosis, sharp and blunt dissection, and resection used in general surgery provide the basis of general surgery proficiency.
- Bowel technique used during intestinal surgery is used to prevent postoperative infection and is a skill in which the surgical technologist is proficient. Other special techniques used in GI surgery include anastomosis of major structures.
- Knowledge of key anatomical structures and procedures of the liver, biliary system, pancreas, and spleen are necessary for case planning and anticipation of the surgeon's needs during a surgical procedure.
- An awareness of breast anatomy and tissue structure is important in selecting the correct instrument during surgery.
- Basic pathology of the breast contributes to the surgical technologist's care of the patient and to case planning.

REVIEW QUESTIONS

SECTION I: THE ABDOMINAL WALL

1. Discuss the importance of knowing the names of the abdominal regions.
2. What are the primary tissues of the abdominal wall?
3. Name five abdominal incisions and the organs associated with them.
4. What is the principle involved in hernia repair with biosynthetic mesh?
5. What is the difference between a direct inguinal hernia and an indirect inguinal hernia?
6. Describe an incarcerated hernia.

SECTION II: GASTROINTESTINAL SURGERY

1. Describe isolation technique and why it is used.
2. When a patient is positioned for bariatric surgery, what special safety precautions are practiced?
3. What is the principle of Nissen fundoplication surgery?
4. Define *anastomosis*, *resection*, and *mobilization*. List several instruments used in these techniques.
5. What is a bowel obstruction?
6. What is a stoma?

SECTION III: SURGERY OF THE BILIARY SYSTEM, LIVER, PANCREAS, AND SPLEEN

1. Why is the spleen removed rather than repaired after severe trauma?
2. What structure drains bile after a cholecystectomy?
3. What are the surgical priorities in emergency surgery for a ruptured spleen?
4. Review and explain the preparation of microfibrillar collagen, oxidized cellulose, and thrombin sealants and fibrin sealants for use in a surgical wound.

5. Which handheld retractors may be used to retract the liver during gallbladder surgery?
6. Why is it harmful for bile to spill into the abdominal cavity during gallbladder surgery?

SECTION IV: BREAST SURGERY

1. Why do women have more options for breast cancer surgery now than they did 20 years ago?
2. What is the difference between needle aspiration and stereotactic biopsy?
3. Why is tissue dye used during sentinel node biopsy?
4. Why is the arm of the affected side draped free during many breast procedures?
5. Describe how you would handle and maintain a breast biopsy sample for frozen section.
6. What is the principle of sentinel node biopsy?
7. What retractors should be available for tissue-sparing mastectomy?
8. Why is the ESU not used for dissection of a breast tumor?

SECTION V: THE THYROID AND PARATHYROID GLANDS

1. What are the advantages of using a minimally invasive approach to thyroidectomy?
2. Why are two surgical assistants required during MIVAT?
3. How is bleeding controlled during open thyroidectomy?

BIBLIOGRAPHY

Allen PJ, et al. *Blumgart's Surgery of the Liver, Biliary Tract, and Pancreas*. 6th ed. Elsevier; 2017.
Bailey HR. *Colorectal Surgery*. Saunders Elsevier; 2013.
Brennan P, et al. *Gray's Surgical Anatomy*. 4th ed. Elsevier; 2020.
Cameron A. *Current Surgical Therapy*. 13th ed. Elsevier; 2020.
Drake RL, et al. *Gray's Anatomy for Students*. 4th ed. Elsevier; 2020.
Hagen-Ansert, S. *Textbook of Diagnostic Sonography*. 8th ed. Elsevier; 2018.
Kademani D, Tiwana PS. *Atlas of Oral and Maxillofacial Surgery*. Elsevier; 2016.
Ozdemir A. Umbilical *Stalk Elevation Technique for Safer* Veress *Needle Insertion in Obese Patients: a Case-Control Study. Eur J Obstet Gynecol Reprod Biol*. 2014;180:168–171.
Porth C, Matfin G. *Pathophysiology: Concepts of Altered Health States*. 10th ed. Wolters Kluwer Health/Lippincott Williams & Wilkins; 2018.
Shackelford RT, Yeo, CJ. *Shackelford's Surgery of the Alimentary Tract*. 8th ed. Elsevier; 2019.

GYNECOLOGICAL AND OBSTETRICAL SURGERY 23

KNOWLEDGE AND SKILLS REVIEW

The following topics should be reviewed before you start this chapter:
Techniques in minimally invasive surgery
Techniques in robotic surgery

LEARNING OBJECTIVES

After studying this chapter, the reader will be able to:

1. Identify key anatomical structures of the female reproductive system
2. Discuss common diagnostic procedures of the female reproductive system
3. Discuss specific elements of case planning for gynecological and obstetrical surgery
4. Discuss surgical techniques used in gynecological and reproductive surgery
5. List and describe common gynecological and obstetrical procedures

TERMINOLOGY

Gynecological and Reproductive Terminology:

Ablate: To remove or destroy tissue.

Adnexa: A collective term for the ovaries, fallopian tubes, and their connective and vascular attachments.

Coitus: Sexual intercourse.

Colposcopy: Microscopic examination of the cervix.

Cystocele: A herniation of the bladder into the vaginal wall.

Dermoid cyst: A mass arising from the germ layers of the embryo that contains tissue remnants, including hair and teeth.

Electrolytic fluid: Fluids that contain electrolytes and therefore can transmit an electrical current.

Episiotomy: A perineal incision made during the second stage of labor to prevent the tearing of tissue.

Fibroid: See leiomyoma.

Hyperplasia: An excessive proliferation of tissue.

Incomplete abortion: Expulsion of the fetus with retained placenta before 20 weeks' gestation.

LEEP: Loop electrode excision procedure. In this technique, an electrosurgical loop is used to remove a core of tissue from the cervical canal.

Leiomyoma: A fibrous, benign tumor of the uterus that usually arises from the myometrium.

Menarche: The onset of menstruation, menses.

Menorrhagia: Excessive bleeding during menses.

Missed abortion: An abortion in which the products of conception are no longer viable but are retained in the uterus.

Obturator: A blunt-nose instrument that is inserted through the sheath of a rigid endoscope or hysteroscope to protect the tissue as the instrument is advanced.

Papanicolaou (Pap) test: A diagnostic test in which epithelial cells are taken from the endocervical canal and examined for abnormalities that can lead to cervical cancer.

Parturition: Birth.

Perineum: The anatomical area between the posterior vestibule and the anus.

PID: Pelvic inflammatory disease, caused by a sexually transmitted disease or some other source of infection. It causes scarring of the fallopian tubes and adhesions in the abdominal and pelvic cavities.

Transcervical: Literally, "through the cervix." In surgery, a transcervical approach means that surgery is performed by passing instruments through the cervix.

Obstetrical Terminology:

Amniotic fluid: Fluid surrounding the fetus during pregnancy.

Amniotic membranes: Two membranes that encase the fetus, amniotic fluid, and placenta during pregnancy.

APGAR score: Method of assessing neonates according to respiratory rate, color, reflex response, heart rate, and body tone.

Birth canal: The maternal pelvis and soft structures through which the baby passes during birth.

Breech presentation: Presentation of the baby in which the buttocks or feet deliver first.

Cerclage: A procedure in which a suture ligature is placed around the cervix to prevent spontaneous abortion.

Cord prolapse: Complication of pregnancy in which the umbilical cord emerges from the uterus during labor and may be compressed against the maternal pelvis or the vagina. This can obstruct the fetal blood supply.

Eclampsia: A seizure during pregnancy, usually as a result of pregnancy-induced hypertension.

Ectopic pregnancy: Implantation of the fertilized ovum outside the uterus.

Epidural: A type of anesthesia in which the anesthetic is delivered through a small tube into the epidural space of the spinal cord.

Fetal demise: Death of the fetus.

Gestational age: The age of the fetus as measured by the number of weeks from conception.

Incompetent cervix: A condition in which previous cervical injury results in repeated spontaneous abortions.

TERMINOLOGY (CONT.)

Labor: The regular uterine contractions that results in birth.

Meconium: A nearly sterile fecal waste that accumulates while the fetus is in the uterus. It is passed within the first few days after birth.

Normal spontaneous vaginal delivery (NSVD): A normal delivery of the fetus, without the need for medical intervention.

Nuchal cord: A complication of pregnancy in which the umbilical cord is wrapped around the neck of the fetus. This may lead to obstructed blood flow to the fetus.

Placenta: The organ that transfers selected nutrients to the fetus during pregnancy.

Placental abruption: Premature separation of the placenta from the uterine wall after 20 weeks' gestation and before the fetus is delivered.

Placenta previa: A complication of pregnancy in which the placenta implants completely or partly over the cervical os. In this position, the placenta begins to bleed as it separates from the cervix during labor.

Prenatal: The period of pregnancy before birth.

Presentation: Refers to the part of the baby that descends into the birth canal first.

STD: Sexually transmitted disease. This acronym is used among *medical practitioners*. The term STI (sexually transmitted infection) is a more socially acceptable term, used more commonly in social contexts.

Suprapubic pressure: Pressure that is applied downward on the patient's abdomen just above the pubic bone.

Uterus: The muscular organ that holds the fetus and the placenta during pregnancy.

Obstetrical and gynecological surgery is a combined medical-surgical specialty. Gynecology focuses on the treatment and prevention of diseases affecting the female reproductive system. Fertility medicine combines gynecology and endocrinology to achieve and maintain pregnancy. Obstetrics relates to the process of pregnancy and birth (**parturition**).

In addition to providing routine surgical assistance in gynecological procedures, surgical technologists are employed in the obstetrical department or free-standing childbirth center. This specialty requires a high level of knowledge about not only anatomy and physiology but also important psychosocial factors that influence the process of childbirth. Normal childbirth is included in this chapter as an introduction to this specialty.

SURGICAL ANATOMY OF THE FEMALE REPRODUCTIVE SYSTEM

UTERUS

The uterus and associated organs of the female reproductive system are located in the anterior female pelvic cavity. The **uterus** is roughly pear shaped, approximately 3 inches (7.5 cm) long and 2 inches (5 cm) deep. It houses and protects the fetus during pregnancy. It is composed of thick muscular tissue and is suspended in the pelvic cavity by ligaments that completely enclose the organ (Fig. 23.1). Two fallopian tubes communicate directly with the interior of the uterus at each lateral "horn" of the uterus. The superior (upper) portion of the uterus, which lies above the insertion of the fallopian tubes, is called the *fundus*. The middle portion is called the *body*, and the lower portion is the *cervix* (Fig. 23.2). The uterus normally tilts forward in the pelvic cavity, with the fundus closest to the anterior abdominal wall. However, variations occur and usually are not significant. The cervix is approximately 0.8 to 1.2 inches (2 to 3 cm) long and communicates directly with the vagina through a small orifice called the *external os*. During labor and childbirth, the os dilates as the cervix thins (*effaces*) to provide an opening for the fetus to emerge.

Structure

The endometrium, which lines the uterus, changes under hormonal influence and with pregnancy. It is continuous with the lining of the fallopian tubes and the vagina. The myometrium is a thick muscular layer that is continuous with the muscles of the vagina and the fallopian tubes. The myometrium contracts during childbirth and menses. The perimetrium, or outer serous layer of the uterus, is a reflection (folding back) of the abdominal peritoneum over the bladder. This forms a pouch called the *cul-de-sac;* the fold is called the *bladder flap*.

The *cervix* is the lower neck of the uterus. It extends into the vaginal vault. The opening of the cervix is called the *cervical os*. The os is dilated for **transcervical** procedures; it also dilates naturally under hormonal influence during childbirth. The os has two anatomical sections, the external os and the internal os. These two openings communicate by means of a short canal.

Uterine Ligaments

The uterine ligaments sometimes are difficult to picture and understand. The broad ligaments suspend the uterus from the pelvic wall. Above the broad ligaments, near the fallopian tubes, lie the round ligaments, which help suspend the uterus anteriorly. The cardinal ligaments lie below the broad ligaments and provide the primary support for the uterus. The uterosacral ligaments curve along the bottom of the uterus and attach it to the sacrum.

FALLOPIAN TUBES

The two fallopian tubes attach directly to the uterus, one on each side. Each fallopian tube has four sections: the *interstitial section*, which connects to the uterus; the narrow *isthmus* in the midportion; the *ampulla*, which is the widened portion of the tube; and the *infundibulum*, the terminal end of the tube. The *fimbriae* are small projections that extend from the end of the tube. These direct the ovum toward the infundibulum during ovulation. The fallopian tube is very narrow (3 to 5 mm wide). It is not connected to the ovary but is suspended from the upper margin of the pelvis by the infundibulopelvic ligament. The lower margin

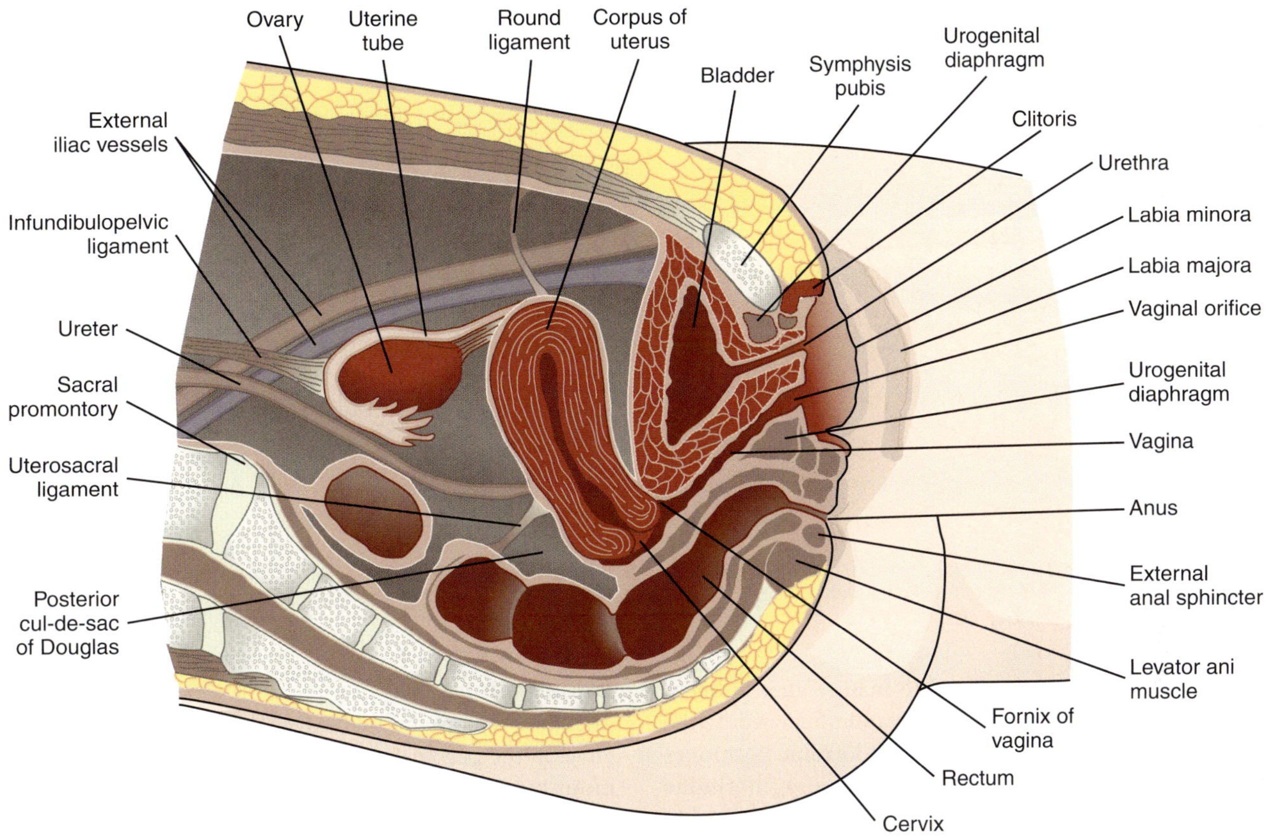

FIG. 23.1 The pelvic cavity. Note the position of the urinary structures in relation to the uterus. (From Lowdermilk DL, Perry SE, Cashion K. *Maternity Nursing.* 8th ed. St Louis: Elsevier; 2010.)

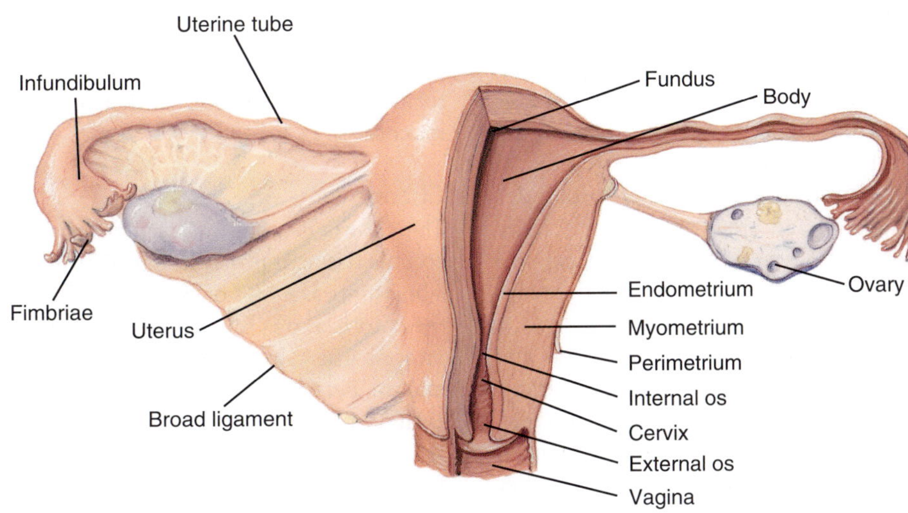

FIG. 23.2 The uterus and adnexa. (From Applegate E. *The Anatomy and Physiology Learning System.* 4th ed. St Louis: Elsevier; 2011.)

is suspended by the mesosalpinx. Surgery of the fallopian tube usually requires dissection of the mesosalpinx, which frees the tube from its attachments. The fallopian tube, the ovaries, and their ligaments are collectively called the **adnexa.**

OVARIES

The ovaries secrete the female hormones—estrogen and progesterone. They lie on each side of the uterus in the upper portion of the pelvic cavity. The ovaries are suspended by the mesovarium, peritoneal tissue attached to the uterus by ovarian ligaments. The ovary is oval and approximately 1½ inches (3.75 cm) long. Each ovary contains approximately 1 million eggs, which are present at birth.

The fibrous outer layer of the ovary, called the *cortex,* contains follicles that hold ova in different stages of maturity. The inner core of the ovary, the *medulla,* is composed of connective and vascular tissue. Vesicles in the medulla hold the

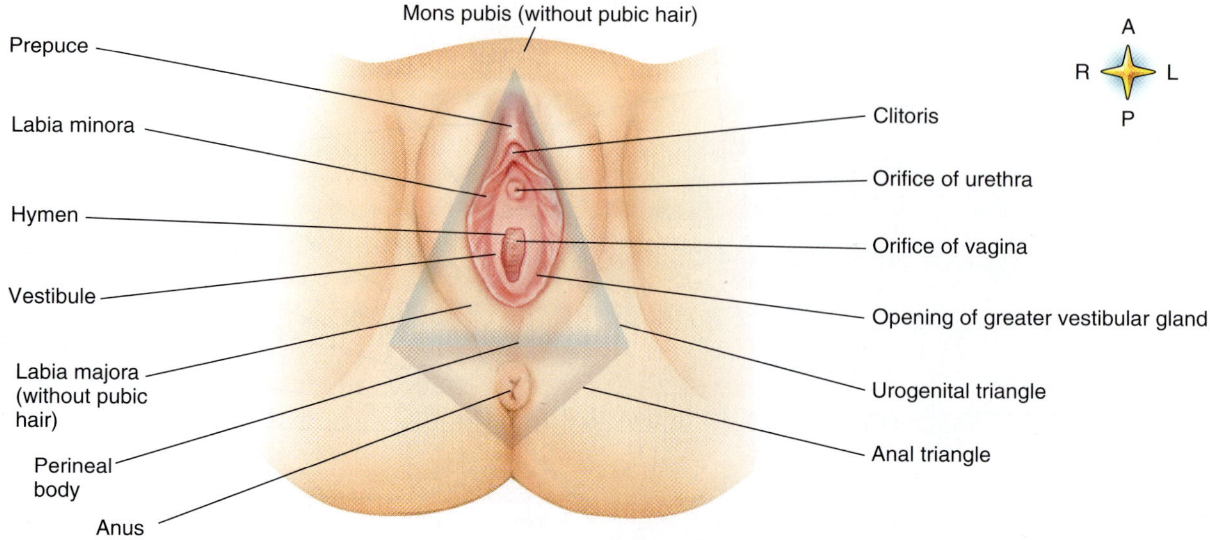

FIG. 23.3 Anatomy of the vulva. (From Thibodeau G, Patton K. *Anatomy and Physiology*. 6th ed. St Louis: Mosby; 2007.)

immature ova, which are stimulated to mature after puberty. The development and release of the ova are influenced by the pituitary gland, which stimulates the gonadotropic hormones luteinizing hormone (LH) and follicle-stimulating hormone (FSH). Ova remain in hormone-secreting follicles and develop in stages until they are released from the ovary. A complete cycle is called the *ovarian cycle.*

VAGINA

The vagina, or vaginal vault, is a muscular passageway that shares a thick fibrous wall with the rectum on the posterior side and the bladder on the anterior side. The vagina extends from the vestibule, or introitus (opening to the outside of the body), to the uterine cervix, which protrudes at the upper vagina. The recessed areas around the cervix are referred to as *fornices.* The function of the vagina is to enable sexual intercourse (**coitus**) and delivery of the fetus during childbirth.

The vaginal lining is composed of thick connective tissue covered with epithelium. The lining has numerous folds, called *rugae,* which can distend during childbirth. The tone, lubrication, and elasticity of the vaginal mucosa are influenced by the level of female sex hormones, especially estrogen. After menopause, a decrease in hormonal levels causes changes in the vaginal pH and dryness of vaginal tissues.

VULVA

The vulva is composed of distinct structures that together make up the external genitalia (Fig. 23.3).

Mons Pubis

The mons pubis is a raised mound of tissue that protects the symphysis pubis. It is covered with skin and contains connective and fatty tissue that is continuous with the lower pelvic wall.

Labia Majora

The labia majora are two external folds of adipose tissue that envelop the perineal area. They are extensions of the anterior mons pubis. They encircle the vestibule and protect the external genitalia.

Labia Minora

The labia minora are bisectional (composed of two sections) and lie directly beneath the labia majora. The two sections come together anteriorly, where they are attached by the frenulum. Anteriorly, they meet just in front of the clitoris to form the prepuce (hood) and are continuous with the vaginal mucosa.

Clitoris

The clitoris is a highly vascular organ that contains sensitive erectile tissue. It projects slightly from the anterior folds of the labia minora. A fold of skin called the *prepuce,* or hood, covers the clitoris and is formed by the superior juncture of the labia minora. The clitoris, which is protected by the folds of the labia majora, becomes engorged and highly sensitive during sexual excitation.

Vestibule

The term *vestibule* refers collectively to all the structures located within the labia minora. The vestibular glands collectively include the *Skene* glands (paraurethral glands) and the Bartholin glands. The Skene glands are two small, paired glands that lie beneath the floor of the urethra, which terminates at the urethral meatus within the vestibule. The Bartholin glands lie on both sides of the vestibule and secrete mucus during sexual intercourse. These glands are homologous to the bulbourethral glands in the male.

Hymen

The hymen is a thin vascular fold of tissue that attaches around the entrance of the vagina. The hymen separates the vagina from the vestibule. In the young female, the membrane is usually but not always intact. The membrane generally is torn during coitus and then remains as a notched membrane, which may be further reduced during childbearing.

Perineum

The **perineum** is located between the posterior vaginal wall and the anus. Incision into the perineum exposes the strong connective tissue and muscles of the pelvic floor. The perineum may be incised during the second stage of labor to prevent tearing when the baby's head emerges through the birth canal. This is referred to as an **episiotomy.**

OVARIAN (MENSTRUAL) CYCLE

The ovarian cycle is characterized by hormonal and physical changes that occur regularly from **menarche** (the onset of menstrual periods) until menopause (cessation of natural childbearing). The cycle is controlled by a complex feedback system involving hormones of the pituitary, hypothalamus, and ovaries. The ovarian cycle is approximately 28 days long, with normal variation. The cycle occurs in distinct phases:

1. *Follicular phase:* This phase lasts from day 1 to day 14. In this phase, the levels of FSH and LH rise, and a small number of Graafian follicles containing the immature ova begin to develop. The fastest-growing follicle secretes estrogen, which blocks FSH and stops continued development of the other follicles. When more than one follicle reaches maturity simultaneously, a multiple pregnancy can occur.
2. *Ovulatory phase:* This phase begins approximately 14 days from the start of the cycle and lasts from 16 to 32 hours. The estrogen level falls, and progesterone is secreted by the follicle (the corpus luteum [CL]). This causes the release of the ovum, which leaves a small, blister-like structure on the surface of the ovary. The ovum is picked up by the fimbriae of the fallopian tubes to enable fertilization.
3. *Luteal phase:* The luteal phase begins approximately on day 16 and lasts approximately 12 days. After ovulation, the corpus luteum secretes estrogen and progesterone. This triggers changes in the endometrium in preparation for implantation of a fertilized ovum. If fertilization does not occur, the FSH and LH levels fall, the CL regresses, and the endometrial lining is shed (menstruation occurs).

DIAGNOSTIC PROCEDURES

PATIENT HISTORY AND PHYSICAL EXAMINATION

Diagnosis of a gynecological condition begins with a history and physical examination. These are completed well before any surgical decisions are made. The physical examination includes a complete review of systems with a manual internal (vaginal) examination. Information for the evidence-based medical assessment is derived from the following:

- *Menstrual history:* The year of menarche, the start of menopause, and the history of any diseases or abnormal menstruation. It also includes the duration and amount of monthly flow, characteristics of blood (clots and size), pain, or other symptoms.
- *Obstetrical history:* The number of pregnancies (called *gravity*) and the course of each pregnancy; the number of successful pregnancies, fetal deaths, and full-term and premature births at 24 weeks' or more gestation (called *parity*); and the number of hours in labor and the weights of infants at birth.
- *Use of contraceptives:* The type used and whether barrier protection was used against sexually transmitted diseases (STDs).
- *History of previous infection:* The type of infection, treatment, and possible or known exposure to the human immunodeficiency virus (HIV).
- *Signs and symptoms:* Abnormal bleeding, such as postcoital bleeding, spotting between periods, **menorrhagia** (excessive bleeding during menstruation), and dyspareunia (painful intercourse); abdominal or genital pain and vaginal discharge (color, odor, and amount); and signs of prolapse or uterine hernia (e.g., pressure on the vaginal wall and irritation).
- *Current medications and allergies:* Current over-the-counter (OTC) medicines, prescription drugs, current or past allergies, and history of substance abuse.
- *Family history:* Family members with cancer, gynecological disease, obstetrical problems, fetal demise, or fetal abnormalities.
- *Social history:* Living situation, stability in the family unit, physical or emotional abuse in the social or family environment, and access to social support.

PREOPERATIVE MALIGNANCY SCREENING

Preoperative testing for malignancy involves a combination of tests, which may include routine blood tests and a serum CA-125 test (tumor marker blood test). These combined assessment tools provide substantial data for estimating the risk of malignancy before surgical intervention. Laparoscopy provides a further means of assessment.

IMAGING TECHNIQUES

Ultrasound and Sonohysterography

Pelvic or transvaginal ultrasound is commonly used to assess the reproductive system and the stages of pregnancy. Ultrasound is also used during pregnancy to detect fetal abnormalities, gender, and gestational age.

A newer technique, called *sonohysterography*, provides greater clarity of ultrasonic images. In this process, normal saline, lactated Ringer solution, or 1.5% glycine is injected into the uterine cavity through a small *transcervical* (through the cervix and into the uterus) catheter before ultrasound testing. This procedure is replacing hysterosalpingography because it is safer, painless, and does not require exposure to radiation.

Hysterosalpingography

In hysterosalpingography, a radiological contrast medium is injected into the uterus and fallopian tubes. Fluoroscopy is then used to visualize the uterus and tubes.

Magnetic Resonance Imaging

Magnetic resonance imaging (MRI) is a more precise tool for diagnosis than either ultrasonography or sonohysterography. MRI reveals the exact location and size of tumors. It can determine the extent of tumor invasion into the myometrium. Congenital anomalies in the reproductive tract are extremely clear with MRI, and the images assist in the preoperative planning for reconstructive surgery.

CERVICAL AND ENDOMETRIAL BIOPSY

The **Papanicolaou (Pap) test** is used to screen for cervical cancer. Superficial endocervical (epithelial) cells are collected from the internal cervical os with a delicate plastic "brush." The brush then is swirled in a prep solution, which is used to prepare a series of microscope slides. Abnormal epithelial cells can indicate early stage cancer or precancerous tissue changes.

Culture of the endocervical and vaginal environment is performed to isolate specific nonresident organisms such as chlamydia, herpes, and *Trichomonas vaginalis.* A test for beta-hemolytic streptococci also is done during pregnancy. Screening for the human papilloma virus (HPV) can be performed during routine cervical cancer screening. Evidence of abnormal epithelial cells or a positive test result for high-risk HPV strains is followed by **colposcopy,** which is the microscopic examination and biopsy of the cervix. During colposcopy, the cervix is painted with acetic acid, which causes preinvasive cells to appear white. These areas are biopsied with forceps.

CONE BIOPSY OF THE CERVIX

Epithelial carcinoma of the cervix or severe dysplasia (abnormal cells) may be treated with cone biopsy. This involves the removal of a circumferential core of tissue around the cervical canal. The cone biopsy encompasses the abnormal cells for a conclusive diagnosis of invasive carcinoma. Conization is most often performed using a local anesthetic and an electrosurgical loop filament. The technique is referred to as a loop electrosurgical excision procedure (**LEEP**). A LEEP may be performed in the outpatient clinic or in the operating room. Laser energy may also be used to perform conization.

PSYCHOSOCIAL CONSIDERATIONS

Psychosocial considerations for the obstetrical or gynecological patient concern reproductive ability as well as social, cultural, family, and community expectations. In many women, body image and identity are closely linked with the patient's ability to reproduce and to care for her children.

The patient's developmental age is an important aspect of clinical care. Younger patients often associate genital surgery with extreme violations of privacy and social taboos. In the perioperative experience, the child is encouraged to yield to examination and touch that she has been culturally and socially trained to resist. Exposure of and focus on the genitals can create feelings of embarrassment, confusion, fear, and uncertainty, all of which require great tact, patience, and empathy on the part of the caregiver. Respect for the patient's modesty is an obvious prerequisite in all cases. Each step of the surgical preparation should be explained to the patient in terms she can understand. Reassurance from the primary caregiver before surgery can ease the fear of surgery.

Patients of childbearing age can be very fearful of reproductive surgery, seeing it as a threat to their reproductive ability. Other patients may feel relieved that long-term medical problems will be resolved. Surgery may also hold the promise of reproductive ability, and patients undergoing procedures to restore reproductive function can experience emotional fluctuations of hope and worry.

Cancer surgery creates feelings of fear and grief. Women of childbearing age may be particularly vulnerable to grieving and depression related to the loss of reproductive ability.

CASE PLANNING

POSITIONING

Gynecological procedures are performed with the patient in the supine or lithotomy position. Cane or Allen (Yellofins) stirrups are used to maintain the lithotomy position. Patient safety considerations for the lithotomy position are fully discussed in Chapter 16. Many surgical facilities favor the use of Allen stirrups because of the risks associated with cane stirrups. However, students must be familiar with *both types* to be competent to assist in positioning the patient when necessary. Important patient care considerations for the lithotomy position are as follows:

1. Protect the patient's modesty and dignity at all times, even when the patient is anesthetized.
2. All patients must wear antiembolism stockings or a sequential pressure device.
3. When the patient is placed in the lithotomy position, raise both legs simultaneously and slowly into the stirrups—this requires two people. No exceptions can be made.
4. When raising the legs into the stirrups, make sure the hips are slightly externally rotated. At no time should the knees or hips be allowed to drop laterally because this can dislocate the knees or avulse the hip joint.
5. Raise or lower the patient's legs only after the anesthesia care provider has advised that it is safe. Placing the patient in the lithotomy position may cause changes in blood pressure.
6. When operating the lower table break, make sure the patient's hands are not near the break.
7. When lowering the legs from the stirrups, follow the same procedure as for raising them: two people are required, and the move must be performed slowly to prevent injury.
8. Patients that will be placed in extreme Trendelenburg or reverse Trendelburg position must be placed on an antiskid device such as a Piggazi Pink Pad system to prevent the patient from sliding during surgery.

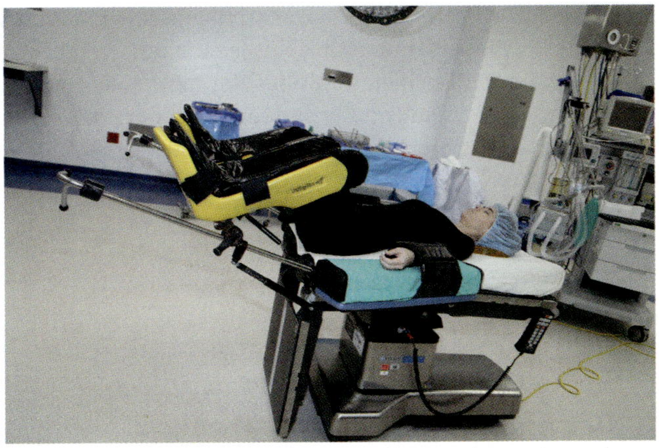

FIG. 23.4 Lithotomy position for perineal procedures. The undraped patient in lithotomy position demonstrates the lack of space for the ST and surgeons. The surgeon and assistant (if there is one) are positioned at the foot of the table facing the operative field. The ST must then stand slightly behind and between the two surgeons. If only one surgeon operates, the ST stands beside him or her.

TEAM POSITIONING

The surgeon may operate from either side of the patient during open procedures. During abdominal procedures, a right-handed surgeon stands at the patient's left side. This allows the best access to the pelvis. The surgical technologist should stand to the patient's right unless otherwise directed. During laparoscopic procedures, the patient is placed in the low lithotomy position, and one assistant is positioned at the foot of the table. A pregnant patient is positioned in a modified left lateral position to prevent hypotension from pressure on the vena cava by the fetus. This position is facilitated by placement of a wedge support between the bed/table and the patient's hip.

During vaginal procedures, the ST is in an awkward position, with the back table placed at the foot of the patient, behind the surgeon, or at the side (Fig. 23.4). This requires the ST either to reach across the front of the surgeon and assistants or pass equipment between them. Neither option is entirely satisfactory; the ST must take care to prevent contamination of the field in either position.

SKIN PREP AND DRAPING

Gynecological procedures are performed with the patient in the supine or lithotomy position. Skin prepping usually includes both abdominal and perineal (including vaginal) prep with insertion of a Foley catheter. A uterine manipulator (internal cervical retractor) is inserted after the vaginal prep for selected laparoscopic and robotic procedures.

The order of prepping for a combined abdominal-vaginal prep is as follows:

1. The perineal prep is performed first. The rationale for this is to prevent possible contamination of the abdomen from splashed droplets during the perineal prep.
2. Always prepare the two sites sequentially, *not simultaneously.*
3. A separate prep kit and gloves are required for each site.

INSTRUMENTS

Tissue of the reproductive system varies from extremely delicate to very strong and fibrous. Procedures of the fallopian tubes require atraumatic graspers and delicate dissecting instruments. A bipolar electrosurgical unit (ESU) is used rather than monopolar, which produces more heat and is less precise. Microinstruments are used to anastomose the fallopian tubes.

The fibrous ligaments that surround the uterus are capable of suspending the pregnant uterus and several quarts of amniotic fluid for many months. These tissues are richly supplied with large blood vessels, which require tight, strong clamps that do not slip during surgery. The uterus itself is composed of strong, thick muscle fibers that require heavy dissecting scissors and toothed or grooved clamps (e.g., Heaney or Kocher clamps) for resection. Laparoscopic instruments are specialized for reproductive structures; they include Babcock or other atraumatic forceps, Harmonic shears, a monopolar hook dissector, graspers, and a vessel-sealing system.

Open gynecological procedures of the pelvic cavity require a general surgery setup with uterine clamps, plus additional atraumatic clamps (e.g., Babcock forceps and vascular forceps) for handling the fallopian tubes, ovaries, and bowel. Long instruments are needed for patients who are deep-bodied and for deep pelvic procedures. Harmonic shears and a high-frequency (HF) vessel-sealing system often are used during uterine surgery. Hysterectomy and resection of uterine neoplasms often are performed with a combination of cutting and coagulating techniques.

Transvaginal pelvic procedures require vaginal speculums and long instruments, including uterine clamps and heavy dissecting scissors. Instruments can easily slip off the surgical field onto the floor during transvaginal surgery. Unlike abdominal surgery, in which the surgical field is flat and contiguous with the instrument tables, during vaginal procedures there is an open gap between the patient (the operative site) and the sterile instrument table. Because of this, various clips, pockets, instrument holders, and magnetic pads are attached to the lithotomy drape to prevent instruments from dropping to the floor. Although these are helpful, it is best to have extra sterile instruments (especially forceps and dissecting scissors) and ESU handpieces available.

Transcervical procedures require graduated cervical dilators, uterine sounds, forceps, sharp and smooth curettes, and an ample supply of sponges. Suction and a monopolar ESU or HF bipolar ESU are needed for all procedures. A variety of active electrode tips is required for selected procedures, such as endometrial ablation or removal of intrauterine lesions.

Procedures of the external genitalia require small (7- to 9-inch [17.5- to 22.5-cm]) plastic surgery instruments, as well as regular dissecting scissors, fine-tipped hemostats, forceps, ESU, and 4 × 4 sponges. Fine scalpel blades (e.g., #15 and #11) are also used. Refer to Gynecological and Obstetrical Instruments to see common instruments used in this specialty.

EQUIPMENT AND SUPPLIES

Equipment for obstetrical and gynecological surgery is divided into categories by type and approach to the procedure. Most abdominal procedures are performed using minimally invasive techniques. Laparoscopic equipment includes appropriate-sized telescopes, trocars, imaging system, and a carbon dioxide insufflation unit. (This technology is described fully in Chapter 20, which describes the minimally invasive instruments, equipment, and techniques used during laparoscopy.) A list of the most common instruments is provided in Table 23.1.

GYNECOLOGICAL AND OBSTETRICAL INSTRUMENTS

Mayo Scis Curved. 5 ½″

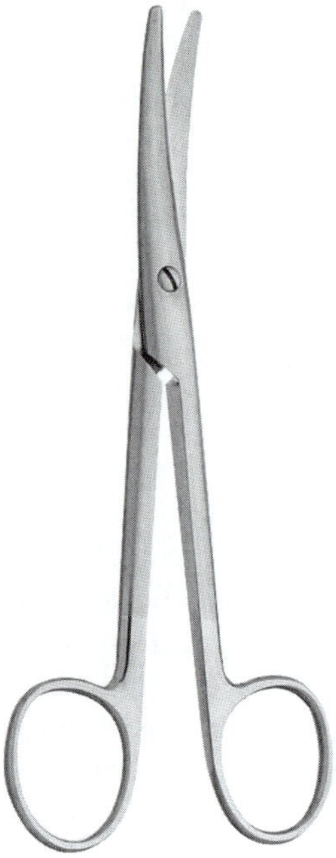

Courtesy and copyright Becton, Dickinson and Company.

Mayo Scis Straight

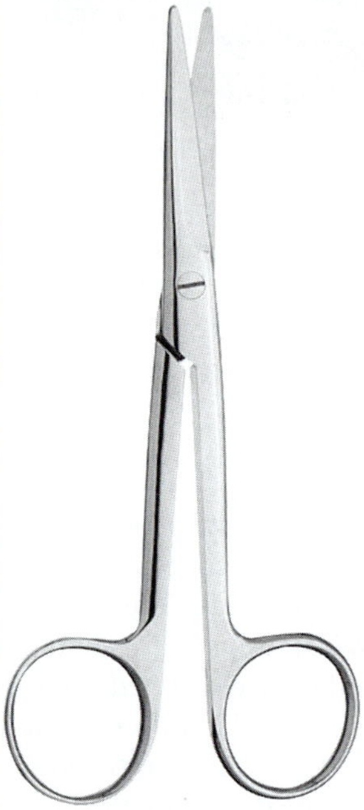

From Baggish M, Karram M. *Atlas of Pelvic Anatomy and Gynecologic Surgery*. Philadelphia: Elsevier; 2016.

Russian Forceps

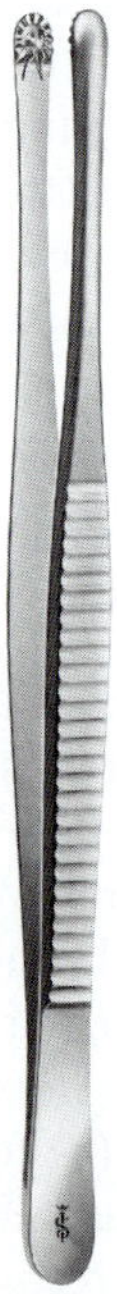

From Nemitz R. *Surgical Instrumentation*. 3rd ed. St Louis: Elsevier; 2019.

Heany hysterectomy fcps 8¾″

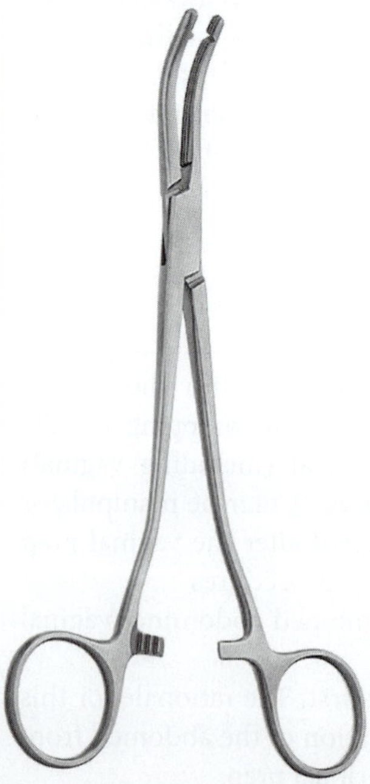

Courtesy and copyright Becton, Dickinson and Company.

GYNECOLOGICAL AND OBSTETRICAL INSTRUMENTS —cont'd

Heaney-Ballentine Hysterectomy Fcps 10½″

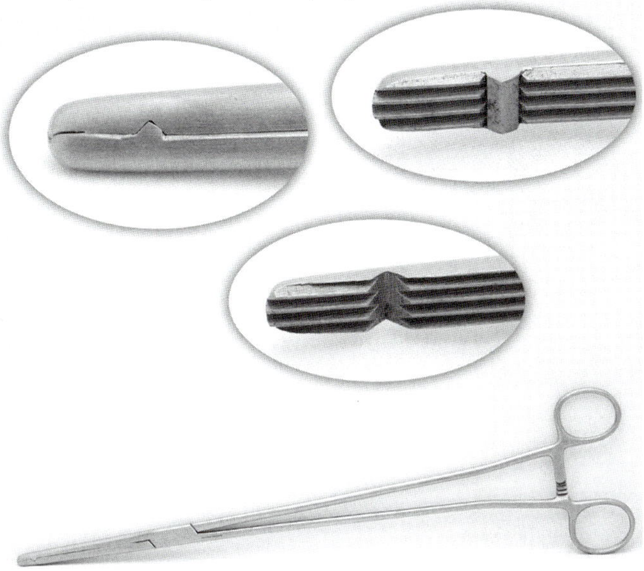

Millennium Surgical Corporation.

Eastman Retractor

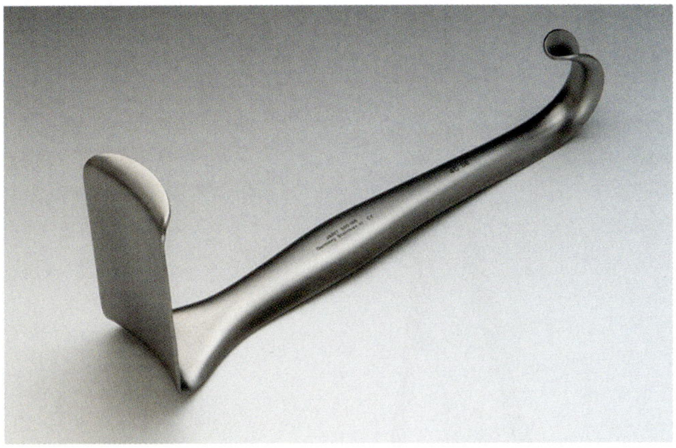

From Nemitz. *Surgical Instrumentation: An Interactive Approach.* 3rd ed. St. Louis: Elsevier; 2019.

Rochester Péan Clamp 8⅞″

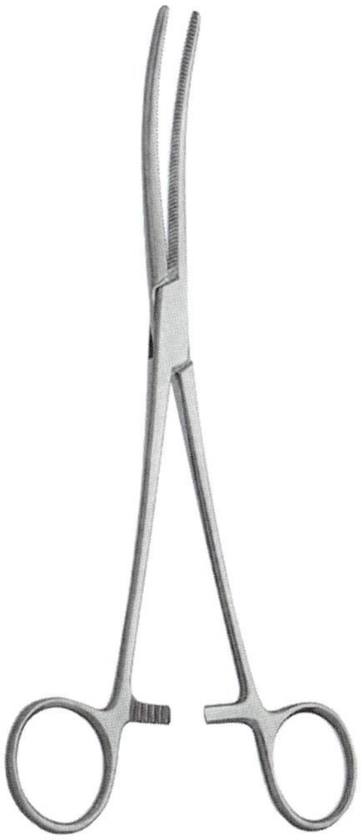

Courtesy and copyright Becton, Dickinson and Company.

Babcock Fcps 5½″, 7″

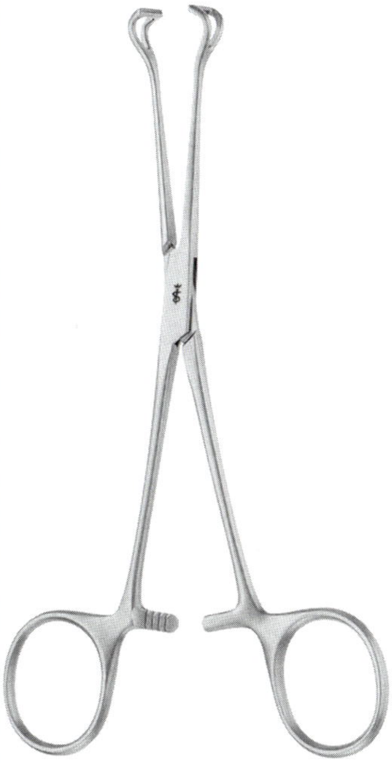

Photo courtesy Aesculap, Inc., Center Valley, PA.

GYNECOLOGICAL AND OBSTETRICAL INSTRUMENTS —cont'd

Mayo-Hagar Needle Holder 8″

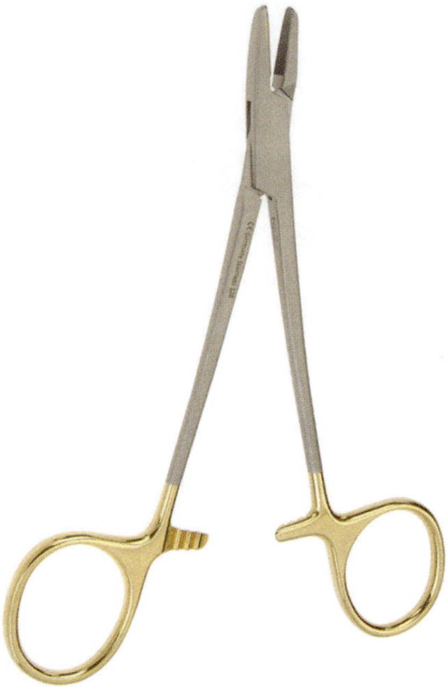

Copyright 2016 Symmetry Surgical Inc.; Photo courtesy Symmetry Surgical Inc.

Heaney Needle Holder 7½″

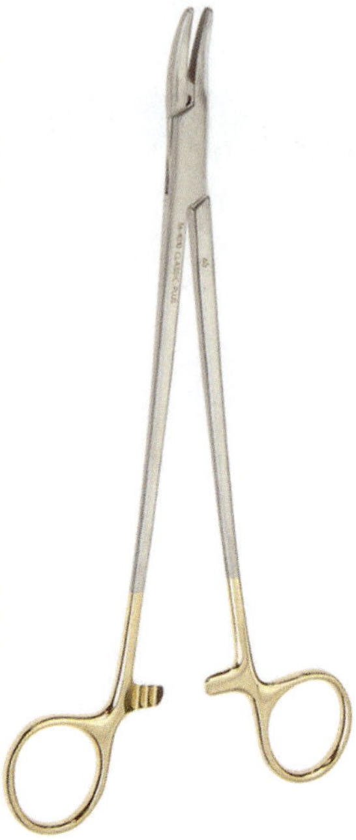

Copyright 2016 Symmetry Surgical Inc.; Photo courtesy Symmetry Surgical Inc.

O'Sullivan-O'Connor Retr

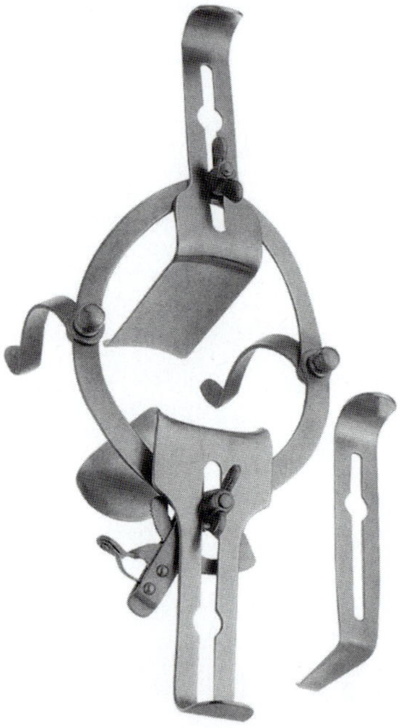

Courtesy and copyright Becton, Dickinson and Company.

Heaney Simon Lateral Retr 7″

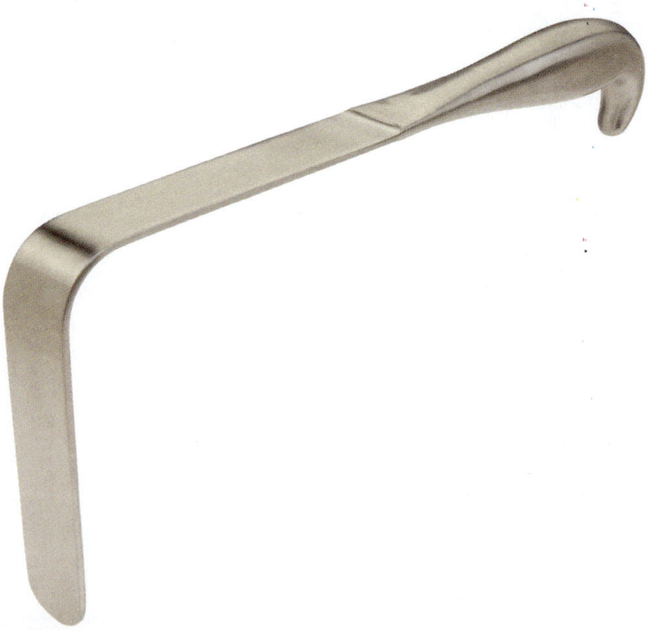

Copyright 2016 Symmetry Surgical Inc.; Photo courtesy of Symmetry Surgical Inc.

GYNECOLOGICAL AND OBSTETRICAL INSTRUMENTS —cont'd

Steiner-Auvard Vaginal Speculum 5½″

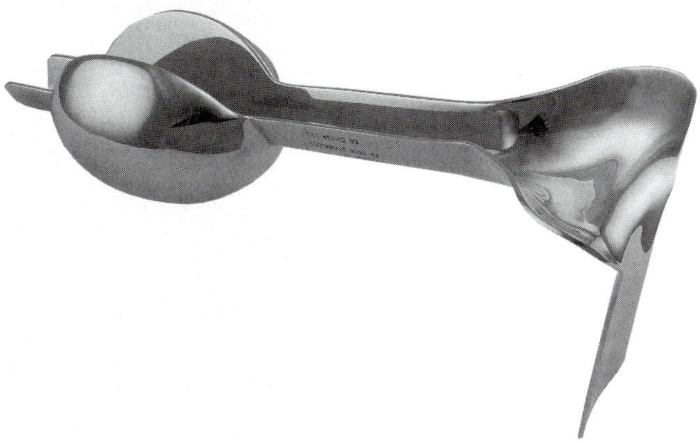

Copyright 2016 Symmetry Surgical Inc.; Photo courtesy Symmetry Surgical Inc.

Somers Uterine Elevator 8¾″

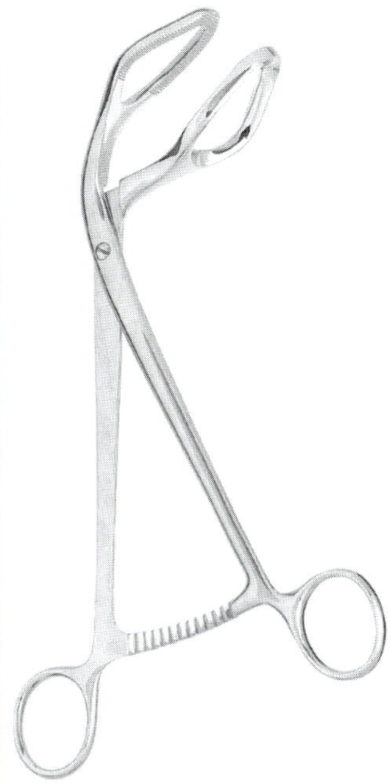

Courtesy and copyright Becton, Dickinson and Company.

Hanks Cervical Dilators 10½″

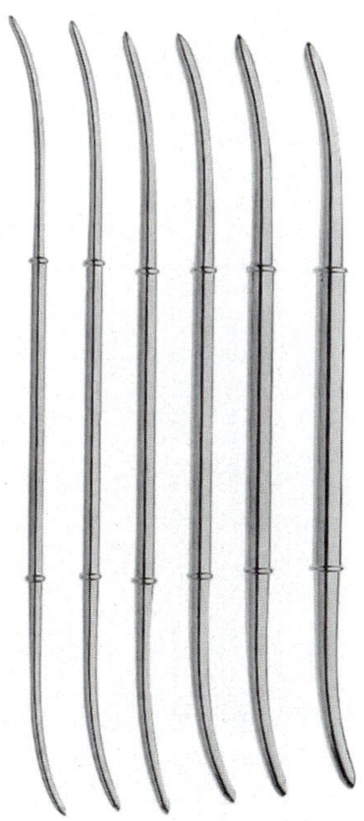

Courtesy and copyright Becton, Dickinson and Company.

Uterine Sound 13″

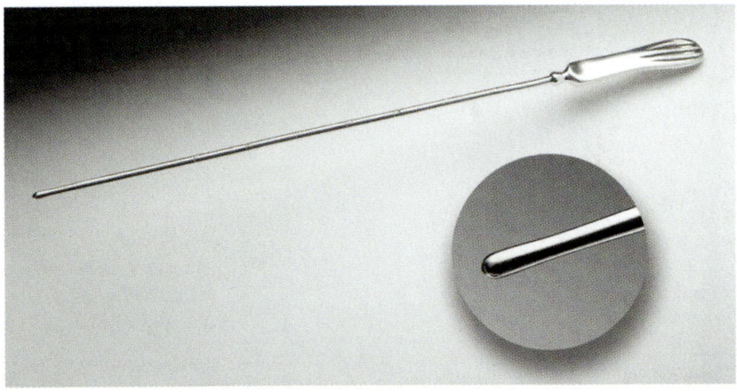

From Nemitz. *Surgical Instrumentation: An Interactive Approach*. 3rd ed. St. Louis: Elsevier; 2019.

GYNECOLOGICAL AND OBSTETRICAL INSTRUMENTS —cont'd

Single Tooth Tenaculum 7⅛″

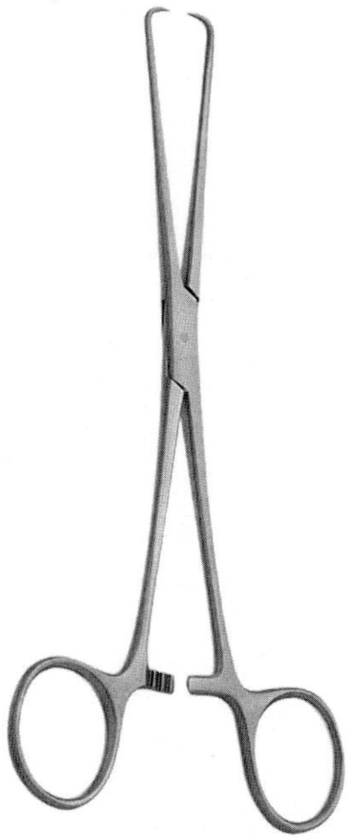

Courtesy and copyright Becton, Dickinson and Company.

Schroeder Vulsellum

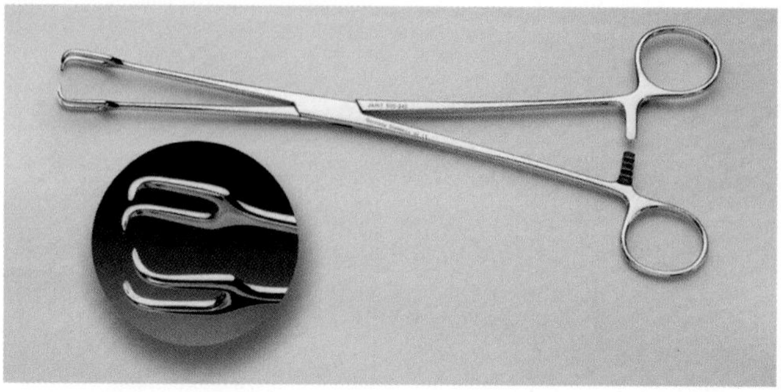

From Nemitz. *Surgical Instrumentation: An Interactive Approach*. 3rd ed. St. Louis: Elsevier; 2019.

Cohen Uterine Manipulator 14½″

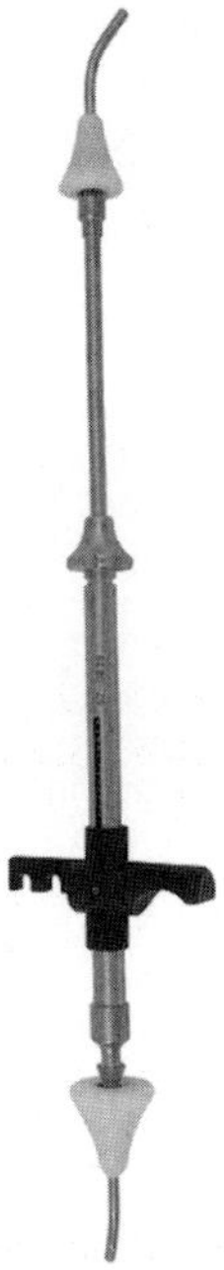

Copyright 2016 Symmetry Surgical Inc.; Photo courtesy Symmetry Surgical Inc.

Laufe Uterine Polyp Forceps 8″

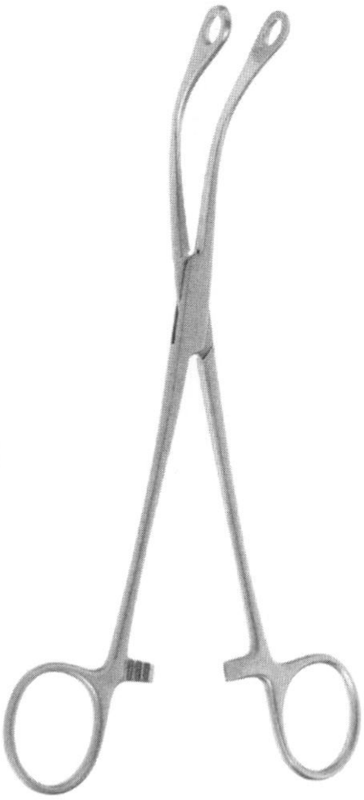

Courtesy and copyright Becton, Dickinson and Company.

GYNECOLOGICAL AND OBSTETRICAL INSTRUMENTS —cont'd

Uterine Curette (Sharp Curette)

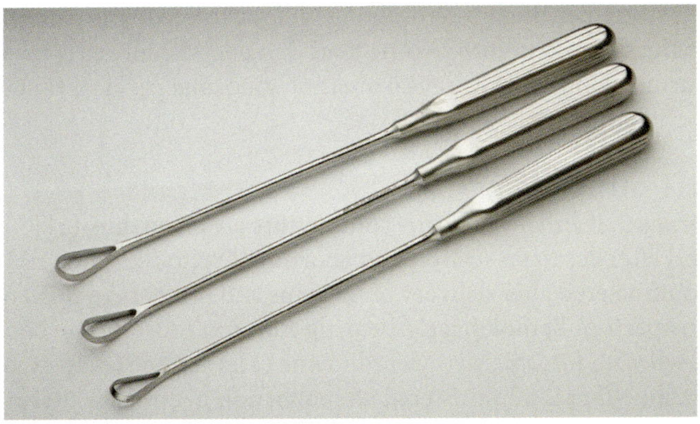

From Nemitz. *Surgical Instrumentation: An Interactive Approach.* 3rd ed. St. Louis: Elsevier; 2019.

Tischler Uterine Biopsy Punch 10″

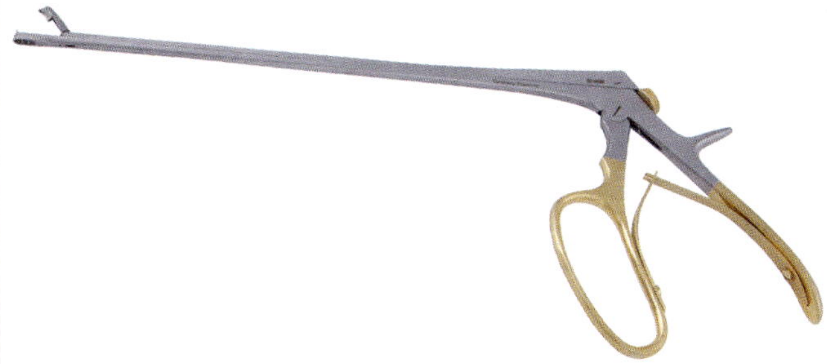

Copyright 2016 Symmetry Surgical Inc.; Photo courtesy Symmetry Surgical Inc.

Delee Obstetrical Forceps 10″

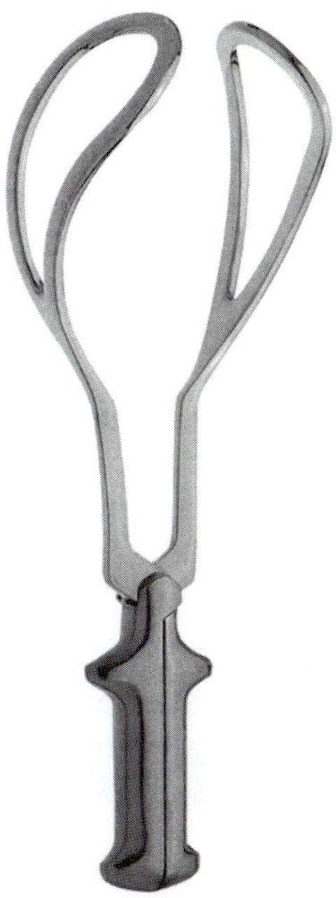

Courtesy and copyright Becton, Dickinson and Company.

TABLE 23.1 Laparoscopic Gynecological Instruments

Instrument	Use
Allis clamp	Grasping the myometrium, large myomas, and large ovarian cysts after drainage Removing specimens from the abdominal cavity
Hook scissors	Cutting through very dense tissue
Metzenbaum scissors with monopolar capability	Dissection Cutting Simultaneous coagulation and cutting
Babcock grasper	Manipulation of the bowel Retraction
Monopolar hook	Incising and coagulating
Biopsy forceps	Removing peritoneal or ovarian specimens
Maryland dissector	Blunt dissection
Standard grasper	Tissue handling Manipulation
Suction-irrigation probe with Poole sleeve. The probe connects to a handle with trumpet valves for separate suction and irrigation. Irrigation is introduced through a plastic tube connected to irrigation fluid.	Hydrodissection Aspiration of fluids and clots Irrigation
Aspiration needle (14 gauge)	Withdrawal of fluid from cysts
Alligator grasper	Grasping myoma tissue Retrieving specimens

Transcervical access to the uterine cavity requires a hysteroscope and components, including tubing, imaging equipment, and distention fluid pump. Other specialty equipment that may be needed during hysteroscopy includes cutting loops, a suction curette, or a vaporization electrode. During hysterectomy, a Koh colpotomy ring or similar device can be inserted over the cervix. This is a blue synthetic "doughnut," which is easily seen on dissection as a landmark and informs the surgeon of the exact level of the cervix.

DRUGS

Numerous drugs are used during reproductive diagnosis, surgery, and labor. Many reproductive drugs are available to control fertility, hormonal dysfunction, and diseases of the reproductive system. Relatively few are used in the intraoperative period or during labor. (Anesthetics and pain medications are discussed in Chapter 12.) Other drugs not classified specifically for use in obstetrical or gynecological surgery may be administered for conditions that arise during labor and delivery (e.g., hypotensive drugs or electrolyte replacement fluids).

Dyes and Stains

Colored dyes are used to identify and trace anatomical structures during assessment. Methylene blue dye or carmine red dye is used during hysterosalpingography to verify the patency of the fallopian tubes. Acetic acid or Lugol's solution is used during colposcopy to reveal areas of abnormal cervical tissue. (Schiller test).

Uterotropic Drugs

Drugs that enhance uterine contractility are given during labor and after cesarean section and abortion. Oxytocin (Pitocin) is administered after delivery of the fetus and placenta to prevent postpartum hemorrhage. The drug *Pitressin* must not be confused with *Pitocin*. Methylergonovine (Methergine) is an ergot alkaline that is administered after abortion to enhance uterine contractions and control uterine bleeding.

SUTURES

Gynecological surgery involves many types of tissue. The following sutures are commonly used:

- *Uterine ligaments and vessels:* Absorbable synthetic 0 to 2-0 taper needle
- *Bladder reflection:* Absorbable synthetic 2-0 to 3-0 small taper needle
- *Ovary:* Absorbable synthetic 3-0 to 4-0 small taper needle
- *Fallopian tube repair or anastomosis:* Inert monofilament or braided 5-0 to 7-0
- *Vaginal vault:* Absorbable synthetic size 0 medium taper needle
- *Plastic procedures of the vulva:* Nylon, Prolene, or other monofilament, 3-0, 4-0; ⅜ circle cutting needle

SECTION I: GYNECOLOGICAL SURGERY

TRANSCERVICAL PROCEDURES

HYSTEROSCOPY

Transcervical procedures are defined as those in which the internal uterus is approached through the cervix. During *hysteroscopy*, a fiber-optic hysteroscope is inserted through the cervix and into the uterus. This technique is used to assess the uterine cavity, the endocervix, and the lower uterine segment and for selected operative procedures. Operative hysteroscopy is performed to assess for intrauterine pathology, such as polyps, leiomyoma, adhesions, and septal defects of the uterus. To obtain a clear view of the uterine wall, the surgeon distends the uterine cavity with fluid or carbon dioxide. This allows small blood clots and other tissue debris to be removed and maintains a clear view. There are several different types of distention fluids. The choice depends on the type of procedure. It is important to note that saline is not used when electrosurgery is anticipated because saline is **electrolytic** (conducts electricity). Distention fluid enters through the hysteroscope via a monitored pump system. Waste fluid is released as fresh fluid enters, which provides continuous irrigation.

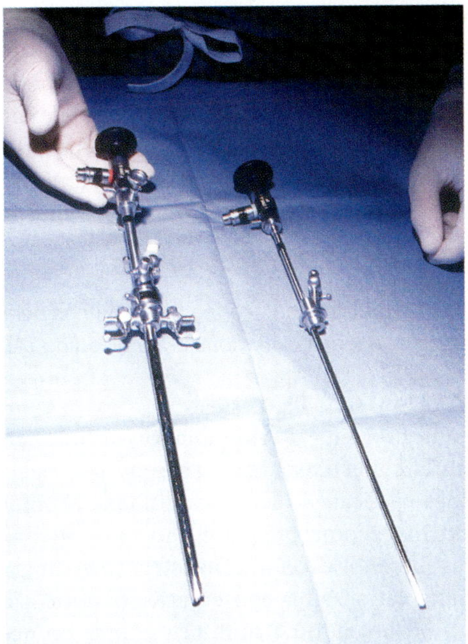

FIG. 23.5 Hysteroscope and bridge. (From Baggish M, Karram M. *Atlas of Pelvic Anatomy and Gynecologic Surgery*. Philadelphia: Elsevier; 2016.)

Examination, biopsy, and surgical procedures are performed through the hysteroscope and operating channels in the same way that cystoscopic surgery is performed through the bladder. Biopsy and resection using a variety of energy technologies (e.g., laser, HF bipolar electricity, and automated ablation) can be performed through the hysteroscope.

HYSTEROSCOPE

The hysteroscope may be rigid or semi-rigid. A rigid scope incorporates a 0-degree and 12- to 30-degree-angled lens at the distal tip (Fig. 23.5). The operative scope has a large sheath to permit the insertion of instruments and a channel for instilling and draining the distention medium. The hysteroscope is inserted into the uterus with the sheath in place. The main operating channel receives the telescope, and side channels, controlled by stopcocks, receive accessory instruments. The main channel is fitted with rubber gaskets that prevent the backflow of distention fluid. Both double- and single-channel sheaths are available. Some models have separate channels for the telescope and the liquid medium, used to flush fluid and debris from the uterus while operating simultaneously.

IMAGING SYSTEM

Fiber-optic light is used to illuminate the surgical site during hysteroscopy. Equipment includes a standard fiber-optic light cable and light source. The digital imaging system, which is similar to the laparoscope, has video components, including a monitor, video cable, and image management system. (Chapter 20 presents a discussion of digital imaging.)

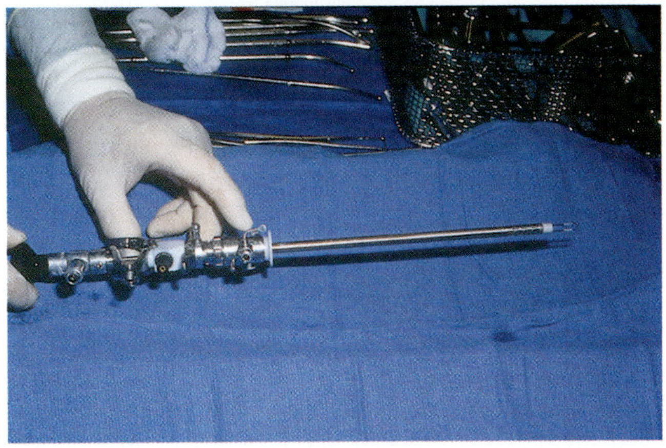

FIG. 23.6 Resectoscope with cutting element. (From Baggish M, Karram M. *Atlas of Pelvic Anatomy and Gynecologic Surgery*. Philadelphia: Elsevier; 2016.)

RESECTOSCOPE

The conventional intrauterine resectoscope is used to remove abnormal tissue and also for endometrial ablation (see later).

The outer diameter of the scope is either 7.3 or 8.7 mm. A 0- or 12-degree telescope is inserted into a separate sheath. A spring-loaded handle retracts and exposes the loop-shaped electrode tip, which shaves and coagulates tissue when activated. As tissue is removed from the uterine wall, it remains free-floating in the liquid medium until it is flushed from the uterine cavity. The advantage of the loop resectoscope is that it can both shave and coagulate tissue bit by bit so that bleeding can be easily controlled.

The resectoscope is equipped with an outer sheath that allows for fluid outflow and an inner sheath for continuous irrigation. A deflector attachment on the sheath is used to bend and direct the tips of flexible instruments. Specimens are morcellated and retrieved through the distention fluid. Other instruments used with the resectoscope are vaporizing and cutting electrodes and microknives. Modern high-frequency resectoscopes can be used in either monopolar (unipolar) or bipolar mode, depending on the unit. Fig. 23.6 shows the resectoscope.

OPERATING INSTRUMENTS

Most hysteroscopic procedures require 3-mm instruments, although 2-mm accessories are available for very fine tissue dissection. Standard instruments include scissors, graspers, biopsy forceps, and ESU. Laser fibers are also used. A variety of tips is available for HF bipolar and standard monopolar ESU. These include the ball tip, spring tip, needle, and loop electrodes used for removing polyps and dense tumors.

Flexible instruments can be fitted into the sheath with or without a deflector. A suction cannula and flexible catheter are used to remove blood clots, debris, blood, and mucus. Rigid and semirigid instruments are inserted directly into the sheath. Figs. 23.5 and 23.6 illustrate the hysteroscope and resectoscope.

TRANSVAGINAL PROCEDURES

HYSTEROSCOPIC ENDOMETRIAL ABLATION

Endometrial ablation is the destruction of the endometrium to render it nonfunctional. Ablation specifically refers to the vaporization of tissue, usually with heat. The procedure is performed only in women who do not want to become pregnant. The endometrial tissue is destroyed by the procedure, thereby making normal implantation impossible.

Current gynecological practice offers numerous safe, effective methods of endometrial ablation. Common procedures are roller ball ablation (electrocoagulation) and global (reaching all areas of the endometrium) endometrial ablation with an intrauterine device. Cryoablation and radiofrequency ablation are also available. Laser ablation is also used but not as commonly as other methods.

Roller ball ablation is performed with a ball tip electrode and resectoscope. This is an electrosurgical procedure and therefore requires all safety precautions associated with electrosurgery. After assessing the uterus with the hysteroscope, the surgeon systematically applies a 3-mm roller ball tip to coagulate and desiccate the endometrial tissue. The surgeon begins with the lower uterine segments and proceeds to the cornual region.

In global endometrial ablation, most of the endometrial surface is ablated. Global ablation procedures are "blind" (i.e., they are not done under direct visualization of the hysteroscope or resectoscope). A variety of methods can be used for global ablation:

- *The NovaSure system* consists of a radiofrequency controller, disposable ablater, CO_2 canister, desiccant, and operating system. This system delivers radiofrequency energy through the device, which is inserted into the uterine cavity. It measures impedance while delivering the energy to **ablate** the tissue. The device automatically stops when impedance reaches a dangerous level.
- *The Hydro ThermAblator* uses a 0.9% sodium chloride solution and a rigid hysteroscope. A D & C is performed, and a rigid scope then is used to fill the uterine cavity with saline. The temperature is automatically raised and measured. The active ablation phase reaches 176°F (80°C) and remains at that temperature for 10 minutes. A cool-down period is then initiated, and the flushing phase is completed.
- *Her Option* uterine cryoablation uses a cryotherapy probe and compressed gas to achieve temperatures below 32°F (0°C) to freeze the endometrium. The procedure is carried out under direct ultrasonographic guidance. The probe is activated sequentially and followed by a short heating cycle.

Most methods of endometrial ablation are performed in an outpatient setting, and the patient is allowed to return home the same day. Severe cramping and watery discharge are expected for several days postoperatively. Patients are provided home care instructions on the danger signs of uterine perforation and infection. Few women experience complete amenorrhea after the procedure, and repeat treatment may be required.

Pathology

The endometrium, which lines the uterine cavity, is made up of two layers. The functional layer lies over the basal layer and proliferates during the endometrial cycle under hormonal influence. It is sloughed off during menstruation and is replaced throughout the endometrial cycle. Abnormally heavy menses (menorrhagia) can result in anemia and abdominal pain.

NOTE *The term dysfunctional uterine bleeding has been replaced by the more precise term abnormal uterine bleeding (AUB).*

Other indications for uterine ablation include certain types of endometrial **hyperplasia** (excessive endometrial tissue) and specific types of localized adenocarcinoma. Women who no longer want to become pregnant and have attempted other types of treatment for excessive menstrual bleeding are offered endometrial ablation after conservative treatment has failed. Destruction of the endometrium prevents or reduces menses and is not reversible. Note that many minor hysteroscopic procedures that were formerly performed in the OR are now performed in the physician's office. This is related to improved technology in instrumentation.

POSITION:	Lithotomy
INCISION:	None
PREP AND DRAPING:	Perineal/vaginal
INSTRUMENTS:	Dilation and curettage (D & C) instruments; vaginal retractors; sterile tubing. According to the method used: hysteroscope and all accessories; electrodes (roller ball, cylinder, or cutting loops) or other ablation device (surgeon's choice)
POSSIBLE EXTRAS:	On standby: laparotomy instruments

Technique and Discussion Points

1. ***The patient is prepped and draped.*** The patient is placed in the lithotomy position, and a vaginal prep is performed. An under-buttocks pouch drape is used to collect and measure fluid as it is flushed from the operative site. The ST should prepare the surgeon's choice of instruments, including the hysteroscope and accessories. The imaging system should be checked before surgery begins.
2. ***Hysteroscopy is performed after cervical dilation.*** The surgeon inserts a self-retaining or weighted vaginal speculum and grasps the cervix with a tenaculum. The cervical os is then dilated progressively using cervical dilators. When dilation is complete, the resectoscope is brought to the field. Distention fluid is then infused into the uterine cavity, and the surgeon performs an assessment of the endometrium.
3. ***A specific ablation technique is applied.***

4. ***The uterine cavity is assessed and distension fluid drained.*** After the ablation procedure, the surgeon again assesses the uterine cavity for any bleeding. The fluid is drained from the cavity and the instruments withdrawn. The ST should carefully collect specimens from the procedure, observing the universal technique. A peri-pad may be applied to the perineum.

MYOMECTOMY

Myomectomy is the removal of a benign leiomyoma (**fibroid**) of the myometrium to control bleeding and prevent pressure on other structures in the pelvis. Submucosal myoma can be removed with the resectoscope power morcellator or during laparoscopy. The power morcellator fragments fibroid tumors and polyps and simultaneously removes the specimen with suction. The procedure described here follows a technique using the resectoscope.

Pathology

A **leiomyoma** is a benign, smooth-muscle tumor of the uterus. These tumors may cause abnormal uterine bleeding and lead to anemia, or they may impinge on adjacent structures, causing pain or dysfunction.

POSITION:	Lithotomy
INCISION:	None
PREP AND DRAPING:	Perineal/vaginal
INSTRUMENTS:	Dilation and curettage (D & C) instruments; vaginal retractors; sterile tubing. According to the method used: hysteroscope and all accessories; electrodes and cutting loops
POSSIBLE EXTRAS:	On standby: laparotomy instruments

Technical Points and Discussion

1. ***The patient is prepared for hysteroscopy.***

2. ***After cervical dilation, a double-sheath resectoscope is inserted.***
The procedure begins as the surgeon dilates the cervix and inserts the resectoscope sheath with or without an **obturator,** which is a blunt-tipped rod that is advanced ahead of the sheath to protect the tissue from injury. If used, the obturator is removed after insertion of the sheath.

3. ***The uterine cavity is irrigated and infused with distention fluid.***

4. ***A resectoscope loop is used to shave and coagulate tumor tissue.***
A resectoscope with a 0-degree or fore-oblique telescope is inserted into the cervix. The resectoscope is surrounded by an 8- or 9-mm sheath, which has an insulated tip to prevent contact between the active electrode and the outer sheath. The outer sheath provides for inflow of the distention fluid. A bridge attachment allows for entry of the electrodes.

5. ***The outer sheath is removed to flush out the sectioned tumor pieces.***
The resectoscope's spring-loaded handle operates the active electrode loop. The surgeon removes sections or slices of tissue by repeatedly looping a small portion of tissue and drawing it into the resectoscope. This cuts and coagulates the tissue and releases it into the uterine cavity, where it is flushed out through the resectoscope sheath.

Bleeding can be controlled by the ball electrode attachment of the resectoscope. The surgeon flushes irrigation fluid and tissue by removing the outer sheath and allowing the fluid to drop into the perineal drape.

The myoma is reduced until it is level with the endometrium. All specimen pieces must be retrieved and collected for pathological examination.

DILATION AND CURETTAGE

Dilation and curettage (D & C) is transcervical removal of superficial endometrial tissue. A D & C is commonly performed for diagnostic purposes.

Pathology

A D & C is most commonly performed to diagnose or confirm endometrial or cervical cancer.

POSITION:	Lithotomy
INCISION:	None
PREP AND DRAPING:	Vaginal/perineal
INSTRUMENTS:	D & C set
POSSIBLE EXTRAS:	Hysteroscope with accessories

Technical Points and Discussion

1. ***The patient is positioned, prepped, and draped.***
The patient is placed in the lithotomy position. The bladder is emptied with a straight nonretention (Robinson) catheter. The patient is then prepped and draped for a vaginal procedure. The surgeon stands or sits at the foot of the operating table. The ST should stand next to the surgeon. To begin the procedure, the surgeon places an Auvard speculum in the vagina. The surgeon then grasps the anterior lip of the cervix with a tenaculum and retracts it slightly forward and downward.

2. ***The uterine depth is measured with a uterine sound.***
A uterine sound is inserted into the cervix to measure its depth and position. This prevents accidental perforation during the procedure.

3. ***The cervix is dilated with graduated cervical dilators.***
The surgeon dilates the cervix with Hagar, Pratt, or Hank uterine dilators. After cervical dilation, the surgeon places a Telfa dressing on the floor of the vagina.

4. ***Curettes are used to remove endocervical and endometrial tissue.***
The endocervix is then curetted, and the specimen is collected on the Telfa. This specimen must be kept separate from the endometrial specimen to follow. The technologist should have several types and sizes of curettes available, including smooth, sharp, and serrated. The specimens are passed to the ST on the Telfa. Each specimen and its Telfa are placed in separate containers.

NOTE *Evacuation of the uterine cavity using suction may be performed in the operating room with the patient under general or local anesthesia. In this case, the procedure is similar to that for a D & C but requires a suction evacuator to perform the evacuation, and the specimen is collected from a gauze trap inside the evacuator.*

VAGINAL HYSTERECTOMY

Vaginal hysterectomy is surgical removal of the uterus using a transvaginal approach. The procedure is often performed using combined laparoscopic-vaginal techniques described later in the chapter. Transvaginal hysterectomy is selected as an approach in selected patients in whom surgical access is adequate to perform surgery safely and in those who are suitable for outpatient surgery or early discharge.

Pathology

Hysterectomy is performed in the treatment of early stage adenocarcinoma, endometriosis, and abnormal uterine bleeding when other techniques have failed.

POSITION:	Lithotomy
INCISION:	Vaginal
PREP AND DRAPING:	Lithotomy
INSTRUMENTS:	Vaginal hysterectomy set

Technical Points and Discussion

1. ***The patient is prepped and draped for a vaginal procedure.***
The patient is placed in the lithotomy position. A wide vaginal-perineal prep is performed and a Foley retention catheter inserted. Routine lithotomy draping with a fluid pouch is used.

2. ***An incision is made in the vaginal mucosa at the base of the cervix.***
The surgeon places a weighted speculum in the vagina and grasps the cervix with a double-toothed tenaculum. A circumferential incision is made in the cervix using a #10 or #15 knife blade. The incision is extended using the monopolar ESU and Mayo scissors. This separates the vaginal mucosa and fascia from the body of the cervix. The incision exposes the first set of ligaments, which are double-clamped with Heaney forceps, divided, and ligated. Size 0 synthetic absorbable suture is used with a taper needle. Mobilization is performed by sequential clamping, ligating, and severing of the vascular pedicles and ligaments at their attachment to the uterus.

3. ***The peritoneal reflection of the bladder (bladder flap) is dissected from the uterus.***
The posterior peritoneum is elevated with toothed tissue forceps and incised with the scalpel or scissors. With the peritoneal cavity open, the surgeon removes the peritoneal reflection of the bladder from the uterus using Metzenbaum scissors. The assistant retracts the bladder upward with a Sims or Heaney retractor. The ST must have long tissue forceps and long dissecting scissors available because the mobilization is carried deep into the pelvis. Multiple sponge sticks are also needed. Sharp dissection continues until the uterus is completely mobilized and removed.

4. ***The bladder flap is reconstructed and the peritoneum closed.***
Before closing the bladder flap and peritoneum, the ST should initiate a sponge count.

The surgeon closes the bladder flap with running suture of 2-0 absorbable synthetic material on a taper needle. The deep vaginal incision is closed with size 0 absorbable synthetic suture. A perineal pad is placed over the perineum to absorb any drainage from the wound.

REPAIR OF A CYSTOCELE AND RECTOCELE (ANTERIOR-POSTERIOR REPAIR)

Herniated tissue of the anterior and posterior vagina is reduced, and the vaginal walls are reconstructed. When both the anterior and posterior walls of the vagina are repaired, the surgery is commonly called an *A P repair*. The more formal name of the procedure is *colporrhaphy*.

Pathology

A **cystocele** (herniation of the bladder) and a *rectocele* (herniation of the rectum) occur when the musculature and connective tissues become weakened and prolapse against the anterior and posterior vaginal walls. The most common cause is multiple pregnancies. The pelvic floor provides support to the intestinal and genitourinary structures, especially during pregnancy, when gravity pulls the fetus downward and stretches the ligaments and muscles. Repair and reconstruction of the supportive structure restore normal function and relieve discomfort and pain.

POSITION:	Lithotomy
INCISION:	Anterior and posterior vaginal walls
PREP AND DRAPING:	Lithotomy
INSTRUMENTS:	Vaginal set with extra Allis clamps

Technical Points and Discussion

ANTERIOR REPAIR

1. ***The patient is prepped and draped.***
The patient is placed in the lithotomy position, prepped, and draped for a vaginal procedure. A retention catheter is inserted at the end of the prep.

2. ***The anterior vaginal mucosa is incised.***
The surgeon inserts a weighted speculum into the vaginal outlet. The cervix is grasped with a tenaculum and retracted. Using the scalpel or curved Mayo scissors, the surgeon makes an incision in the anterior vaginal wall. The edges of the incision are grasped with several Allis clamps. These are fanned out to distend the tissue edges and delineate the plane between the mucosa and the connective tissue underneath. A Sims lateral retractor is inserted.

3. ***Blunt and sharp dissection is used to create a tissue plane between the vaginal mucosa and the submucosal fascia.***
With the tissue planes exposed, the surgeon uses a Raytek 4 × 4 sponge to push the connective tissue off the mucosa. This technique of blunt dissection effectively separates the two tissue layers and creates a flap (the vaginal mucosa) with a minimum of bleeding. The ST should have ample sponges available. As the sponge becomes moist, its surface becomes smooth, and the sponge is less effective for dissection. The curved Mayo scissors are used alternately with sponges to continue the dissection to the level of the bladder. Bleeders are managed with the monopolar ESU.

   During this portion of the procedure, the assistant or ST may be required to retract the superior vaginal vault upward with a lateral (Heaney) right-angle retractor. This elevates the roof of the vagina and exposes the dissection plane. The dissection is continued to the level of the bladder neck.

NOTE *During retraction, the ST should exert gentle, even pressure on the retractor to prevent bruising and hematoma in the vaginal mucosa.*

4. ***The vaginal wall is reconstructed with sutures.***
When the dissection has reached the bladder neck, several sutures of size 0 chromic gut or synthetic absorbable sutures are placed through the fascia and pulled laterally. This tightens the tissue and prevents the bladder from bulging into the vaginal vault. The edge of the vaginal mucosa is measured over the repair, and the edges are trimmed. The mucosa is then approximated with running or interrupted sutures of absorbable material, usually of the same size as that used on the bladder repair. Note that in some cases, a natural graft of fascia lata may be used to reinforce the repair.

POSTERIOR REPAIR

5. ***The posterior vaginal wall is incised, and steps 2 and 3 are repeated.***
To begin the posterior repair, the surgeon places two Allis clamps in the posterior vaginal wall and makes a small transverse incision between them. The assistant provides traction on the clamp as described for the anterior repair.

6. ***The tissue plane is continued to the rectum.***
The techniques used in anterior repair are repeated to the level of the rectum. The levator muscles and fascia then are brought together and tightened with absorbable interrupted sutures, and the vaginal mucosa is repaired. Fig. 23.7 shows the technique used to repair a cystocele.

REPAIR OF A VESICOVAGINAL FISTULA

A vesicovaginal fistula is a small, hollow tract that connects the bladder to the vagina. Fistulous tracts can be caused by infection or trauma. Chronic fistulous tracts are lined with epithelial tissue, which prevents the tract from closing. The surgical goal is to incise the length of the tract and remove this tissue. Healing then can occur normally, and urine is prevented from draining into the vagina. Diagnostic procedures, including instillation of a contrast medium, may have preceded the surgery. Films obtained from the procedure show the route of the fistula. These should be available in the operating room for reference during surgery.

Pathology

A vesicovaginal fistula may be caused by a traumatic penetrating injury, infection, radiation therapy that thins and weakens the pelvic structures, vaginal birth, or chronic inflammation. Urine drains into the vagina, causing irritation and incontinence. The fistula may extend into the urethra. The repair may be approached through pelvic laparotomy or vaginally. A pelvic approach is required when the tract occurs in the proximal vaginal vault. A vaginal exposure is described here.

Technical Points and Discussion

1. ***The patient is prepped and draped for a vaginal procedure.***
A metal probe may be placed in the fistula to identify its course. The surgeon places an Auvard or Sims retractor in the vagina to expose the fistula. A malleable probe is inserted into the fistula. The surgeon then uses dissecting scissors to make a circular incision around the probe and fistula.

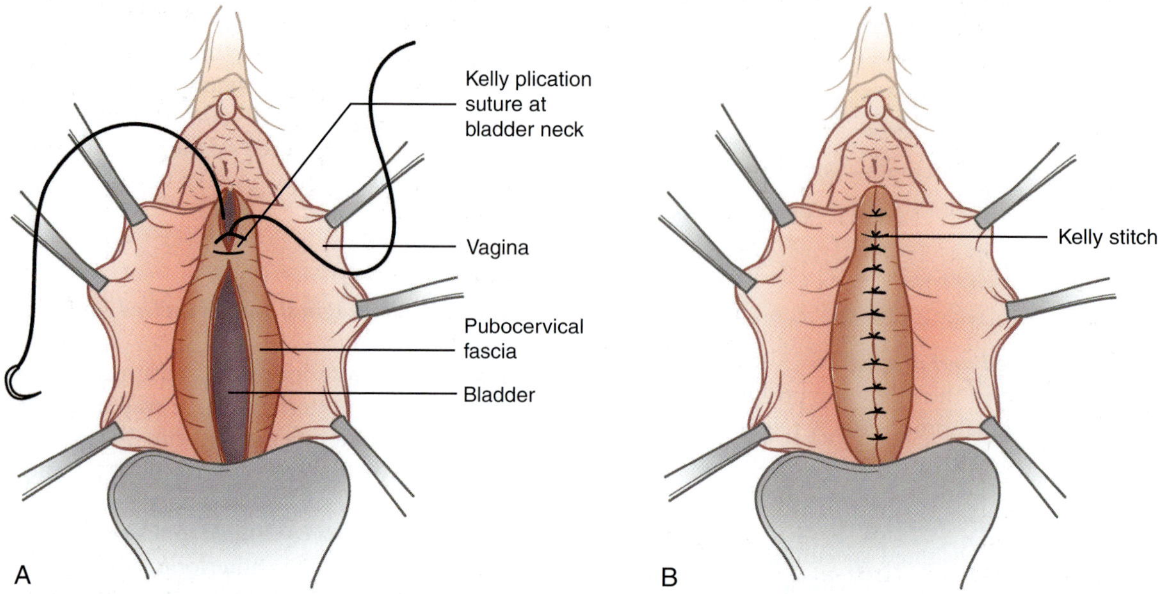

FIG. 23.7 Repair of cystocele. (A) After an incision on the anterior vaginal midline, excess tissue is bluntly separated from the fascia. (B) The fascia is approximated, redundant vaginal tissue removed, and the vaginal incision closed. (From Seidel HM, et al. *Mosby's Guide to Physical Examination*. 5th ed. St Louis: Mosby.)

2. ***The tissue around the fistula is sharply dissected.***
   The surgeon carries this incision the full length of the fistula with dissecting scissors until the anterior bladder wall is exposed. Two lateral retractors may be placed in the vagina for better exposure. The surgeon creates a tissue plane between the bladder and the fistula with sponge dissectors or by sharp dissection.

3. ***The mucosa is inserted, and sutures are placed through the smooth muscular layer and mucosa.***
   When the bladder mucosa and smooth muscle layer have been exposed, the surgeon inverts the bladder tissue layers and approximates the edges with interrupted 3-0 absorbable sutures.

4. ***The vaginal wall is repaired.***
   The vaginal wall is repaired with size 0 or 2-0 synthetic absorbable sutures on a taper needle. A Foley catheter may be inserted into the bladder at the close of the procedure.

Cervical Cerclage

Cervical **cerclage** is the fixation of sutures or Mersilene tape at the cervical os to prevent spontaneous abortion related to spontaneous cervical dilation—*insufficient cervix*—leading to abortion. Surgical intervention to prevent spontaneous abortion may be performed before or during pregnancy. Traditional treatment for early spontaneous abortion historically led to the development of various types of cerclage. The Shirodkar and McDonald procedures are just two of many types of cerclage in which a suture is placed around or through the cervix. These procedures have been modified many times over the decades, and cerclage is now identified by more exact terms. These are high-transvaginal or low-transvaginal cerclage. *Cerclage remains controversial because data are insufficient to prove that the procedure is effective.* The American Congress of Obstetricians and Gynecologists (ACOG) recommends cerclage only for patients with a history of three or four previous unexplained spontaneous abortions. ACOG further states that the procedure should be limited to pregnancies in which fetal viability has been achieved.

PATHOLOGY

Recurrent spontaneous abortion occurs when the cervix dilates spontaneously during the second or third trimester of pregnancy. The cause of **incompetent cervix** has not been identified. It may be associated with cervical trauma, including conization of the cervix, laceration, and previous cerclage. Table 23.2 defines types of spontaneous abortion. In transvaginal cerclage (TVC), a synthetic band is placed around the proximal cervix through a vaginal approach. TVC is performed with the patient in the lithotomy position. The cervix is retracted with sponge forceps, and a circumferential incision is made at the highest (proximal) point of the cervix. A narrow strip of Mersilene tape is then placed around the cervix, and the paracervical tissue is closed with interrupted 2-0 or 3-0 synthetic absorbable sutures.

PROCEDURES OF THE VULVA

REMOVAL OF A BARTHOLIN GLAND CYST

Treatment for a Bartholin gland cyst involves removal of the cyst and gland to prevent future episodes of infection (Fig. 23.8).

TABLE 23.2	Types of Spontaneous (Noninduced) Abortion
Complete abortion	Expulsion of all products of conception. Surgical intervention is not necessary.
Incomplete abortion	The products of conception have been expelled but the placenta retained. Medical intervention may be necessary to control hemorrhage.
Inevitable abortion	The cervix is dilated and there is rupture of the membranes or vaginal bleeding. The products of conception have not been expelled.
Missed abortion	Undiagnosed and undetected embryonic or fetal demise (death); the products of conception are not expelled.
Septic abortion	Severe uterine infection associated with abortion.
Threatened abortion	Uterine bleeding without cervical dilation occurring before 20 weeks' gestation.

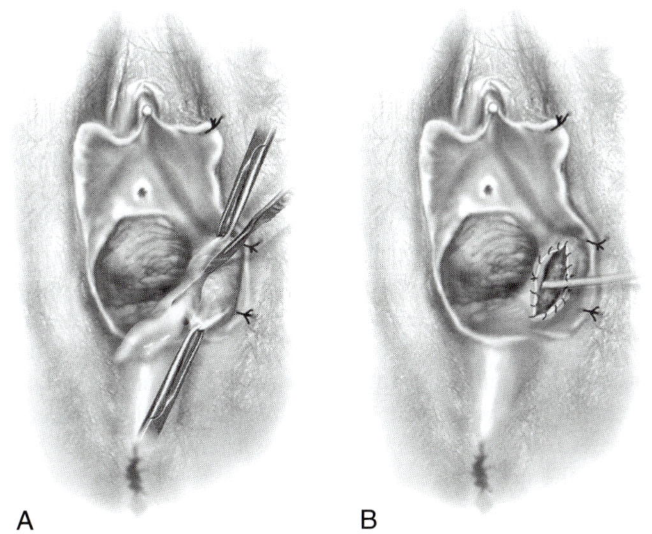

FIG. 23.8 Bartholin gland cyst. (A) The cyst is excised and drained. (B) The edges of the cyst are sutured open (marsupialized). (From Baggish M, Karram M. *Atlas of Pelvic Anatomy and Gynecologic Surgery*. 4th ed. Philadelphia: Elsevier; 2016.)

Pathology

The Bartholin glands are a common site of cyst formation. The cyst may become infected, and in such cases, surgical removal is indicated. Infection of a Bartholin gland is extremely painful, and many patients arrive for surgery in distress.

Technical Points and Discussion

1. ***The patient is placed in the lithotomy position, prepped, and draped for a perineal incision.***

2. ***The labia minora are retracted.***
   The surgeon may begin the procedure by securing the labia minora laterally with sutures or small skin staples.

3. ***The mucosa overlying the cyst is incised.***
   A curved incision is made in the mucosa over the cystic gland with a #15 knife. The incision is lengthened with Metzenbaum scissors. Small bleeders are coagulated with the ESU.

4. ***The cyst and sometimes the gland are removed.***
   The gland and the cyst may be removed together, or the cyst may be dissected away from the gland with dissecting scissors. The wound edges are secured open with sutures to allow secondary closure.

SIMPLE VULVECTOMY

Simple vulvectomy is surgical removal of the labia and other structures of the vulva according to the extent of the pathology. *Skinning vulvectomy*, in which only the skin of the vulva is removed, usually by laser surgery, is the preferred procedure for noninvasive lesions. A *labioplasty* procedure differs from the vulvectomy in that the labia minora are excised for cosmetic reasons. Labioplasty is performed in a clinic or physician's office.

Pathology

Cancer of the vulva represents about 5% of all genitourinary carcinomas. It is more common among women over age 60. Most invasive carcinoma that involves the lymph nodes is seen in this age group. Local vulvar cancer (vulvar intraepithelial neoplasm) appears to be associated with some strains of HPV.

Technical Points and Discussion

1. ***The patient is prepped and draped for a vulvar excision. A skin graft site is also prepped.***
   The patient is placed in the lithotomy position and prepped for a wide vulvar incision. A skin graft site may also be prepped at this time. The outer aspect of the thigh is normally prepared for a split-thickness graft. A Robinson (straight) urinary catheter is used to decompress the bladder before the start of surgery.

2. ***The incisional lines are drawn on the skin using a marking pen.***
   The surgeon begins the procedure by marking out the incision lines of the procedure with a marking pen. The extent of the incision depends on previous biopsy and may or may not include the labia minora, clitoris, and vaginal vestibule. The skin incision is made using a #10 or #15 knife blade following the surgical plan. The incisional lines may be injected with a 1:100 solution of vasopressin to help control bleeding.

3. ***The incision is carried into the fatty tissue.***
   The incision is carried into the fatty tissue using a #10 knife blade. The ST should keep a supply of 4 × 4 sponges on the surgical field. Small rake retractors can be used to expose bleeders. These are clamped with fine right-angle

or curved clamps and ligated with ligatures of 3-0 synthetic suture. Note: ESU coagulation is not used as it creates excess dead tissue, which can lead to necrotizing fasciitis. As dissection continues, the edges of the specimen are grasped with Allis clamps for retraction. The completed dissection results in en bloc removal of the specimen.

4. ***Primary closure of the wound may be attempted.*** Depending on the size of the defect, a primary closure may be possible. This is performed using cutaneous interrupted sutures of size 4-0 nylon or Prolene. A small Penrose drain may be inserted during closure.

5. ***A split-thickness skin graft is taken to cover the defect.*** If primary closure is not possible, a split-thickness graft is taken, usually from the lateral thigh, using the Brown dermatome. The graft is sutured to the defect using the surgeon's preferred suture.

6. ***A Foley catheter is placed, and the wound is dressed.*** At the completion of the procedure, a Foley retention catheter is placed. The wound is dressed first with Xeroform gauze followed by fluffed gauze squares. An abdominal pad may be placed over the gauze and taped into place.

REMOVAL OF CONDYLOMA ACUMINATA

Removal of condyloma acuminata (venereal warts) can be performed in the outpatient clinic or physician's office. Occasionally, when the number and size of the lesions are excessive, the patient may be admitted for their removal under general anesthesia in the operating room.

Pathology

Condyloma acuminata is caused by the human papillomavirus (HPV), types 6 and 11. The virus does not usually progress to a malignancy. However, it can be spread through direct contact including via laser and ESU vapor, blood, and body fluids. Refer to Chapter 9 for further discussion on the use of high-particulate N95 filter masks during laser procedures, including those for obliteration of condylomata.

POSITION:	Low lithotomy
INCISION:	None
PREP AND DRAPING:	Lithotomy
INSTRUMENTS	CO_2 laser; laser speculum

Technical Points

The procedure is performed under the microscope using the CO_2 laser. The patient is positioned and prepped. A very shallow incision is made around the area of excision in the perivulvar area. The laser fiber is then used to vaporize all lesions to the level of the skin. Vaginal and anal lesions are then vaporized using a laser speculum and smoke evacuator. At the conclusion of the case, the lased area is treated with silver sulfadiazine cream.

ABDOMINAL PROCEDURES

DIAGNOSTIC LAPAROSCOPY

Many abdominal procedures of the reproductive system are performed as laparoscopic surgery. Chapter 20 presents a complete description of minimally invasive surgery techniques, including equipment, approach, special safety considerations, and perioperative patient care. The ST should be familiar with these before approaching the gynecological specialty. Chapter 20 contains a description of a diagnostic laparoscopy. A general review of techniques includes the following:

1. The laparoscope (its use and handling)
2. Imaging systems used in laparoscopy (components and how to use them)
3. Instruments (their use and care)
4. Carbon dioxide (CO_2) insufflation (techniques and patient safety)
5. Safe use of a monopolar and an HF bipolar ESU in laparoscopy
6. Use of vessel-sealing systems (e.g., LigaSure)
7. Ultrasonic cutting and coagulating systems (e.g., SonoSurg, Harmonic shears)

The principles of laparoscopic surgery apply to the pelvic and combined vaginal-laparoscopic procedures discussed in this chapter. During laparoscopic pelvic surgery, the uterus is retracted with a uterine manipulator. This instrument is placed through the cervical os after the complete abdominal and vaginal prep and immediately before surgery. The handpiece of the manipulator is accessible outside the perineum, where it is handled (usually by the assistant) under the guidance of the surgeon.

LAPAROSCOPIC TUBAL LIGATION

Tubal ligation is performed to block the passage of ova (egg) through the oviduct and prevent its implantation in the uterus. Tube-sparing techniques may be performed to facilitate reversal. Several methods are currently used in laparoscopic tubal ligation. Three common methods are described here.

Pathology

The fallopian tube receives the female ovum after its release from the ovary. The ovum is moved along the tube, is fertilized there, and eventually implants in the uterine lining. Surgical blockage prevents implantation (pregnancy) and development of a fetus.

Many techniques for tubal ligation have been developed. The most popular are application of Silastic bands and clips to the fallopian tubes, which results in scarring and blockage of the tubes.

POSITION	Low lithotomy
INCISION:	Laparoscopy
PREP AND DRAPING:	Laparotomy or combined abdominal–perineal
INSTRUMENTS:	Two 10-mm trocars; laparoscopic GYN set; uterine manipulator; ESU
POSSIBLE EXTRAS:	Falope ring system; Filshie clips; additional 10-mm trocar for obese patients

Technical Points and Discussion

1. ***The patient is placed in the low lithotomy position. Both the abdomen and vagina are prepped if a uterine manipulator is required.***
The manipulator attaches to the cervix so that the uterus can be tilted and fallopian tubes brought into view of the laparoscope. The manipulator is inserted after the perineal prep.

2. ***Pneumoperitoneum is established and trocars are placed in the abdomen.***
Pneumoperitoneum is established using a Hasson trocar with minilaparotomy or Veress needle. A 10-mm trocar is placed at the umbilicus, and a second trocar is positioned below and lateral to the first one. This is the preferred approach.

3. ***The fallopian tube is brought into laparoscopic view and grasped.***
The assistant uses the uterine manipulator to bring the fallopian tube into view, and the surgeon grasps it using a Babcock clamp.

One of the four methods described below is used to occlude the fallopian tubes.

TRANSECTION AND COAGULATION

The fallopian tube is grasped with a Babcock endoscopic grasper. The HF bipolar unit is used to sever the tube and coagulate the free ends.

FALOPE RING METHOD

Using the Falope ring method, the ST loads a small Silastic O ring into a ring applicator. The surgeon inserts the applicator into the trocar site and withdraws a loop of the fallopian tube into the applicator. The Silastic ring is ejected over the loop, which is then released back into the pelvis (Fig. 23.9A). The loop causes local ischemia and eventual necrosis of the loop of tissue.

HULKA CLIP METHOD

The Hulka applicator is inserted through the operative port. The clip is applied over the fallopian tube and clamped in place (Fig. 23.9B). After the procedure, instruments are withdrawn and the pneumoperitoneum is released. One or two deep sutures are inserted and the skin is closed.

IRVING METHOD

This technique is used following cesarean delivery as an elective serialization procedure. Although it is an older procedure, the Irving technique carries the lowest rate of failure and is favored for postpartum serialization after a cesarean delivery. In this procedure, the fallopian tube is severed and ligated. The proximal stump is buried in the uterine serosa with several absorbable sutures (Fig. 23.10). After ligation, the severed portions of the oviduct are passed to the ST as specimen. The wound is closed in routine fashion.

LAPAROSCOPIC MANAGEMENT OF AN OVARIAN CYST

Exploratory laparoscopy is performed to confirm the pathology of an ovarian mass. Preoperative evaluation of a mass is routine in all procedures. Ovarian cysts are removed to determine their pathology and for cancer staging as explained in Chapter 6. *Oophorectomy* (removal of the ovary) or ovarian cystectomy (removal of an ovarian cyst) may be performed during laparoscopy. The ST should also be prepared for transition to an open case.

Pathology

Normally during the ovarian cycle, several ovarian follicles begin to mature. The dominant follicle continues to form, whereas the others rupture spontaneously; these are referred to as *functional ovarian cysts*. Occasionally these form benign fluid- or blood-filled cysts, which regress normally. Polycystic ovary syndrome (PCOS) is diagnosed in women with persistent multiple cystic follicles. The condition is associated with obesity, diabetes, or other forms of insulin resistance. Persistent cysts may be removed surgically.

A teratoma (also called a **dermoid cyst**) is a common ovarian tumor that arises from one of the germ layers of the developing embryo. The tumor persists throughout development and may contain hair, teeth, sebaceous material, and skin, which are normal components of the germ layer. A teratoma may be malignant but seldom causes symptoms. Most are found incidentally during ultrasound or surgery for other reasons.

The three types of primary ovarian malignancy are epithelial cancer (90% of cases), germ cell cancer, and gonadal stromal tumor. Ovarian cancer is among the most lethal cancers. Metastasis generally occurs before a diagnosis is made. Exploratory laparotomy or laparoscopy is required for definitive diagnosis with staging. Cytological washing with tumor debulking may provide palliative treatment. Laparoscopic management of an ovarian cyst depends on the size and type of cyst and the risk of malignancy. Spillage of a potentially malignant cyst is always avoided to prevent the spread of cancerous cells (seeding).

POSITION:	Lithotomy
INCISION:	Laparoscopic
PREP AND DRAPING:	Abdominal/perineal

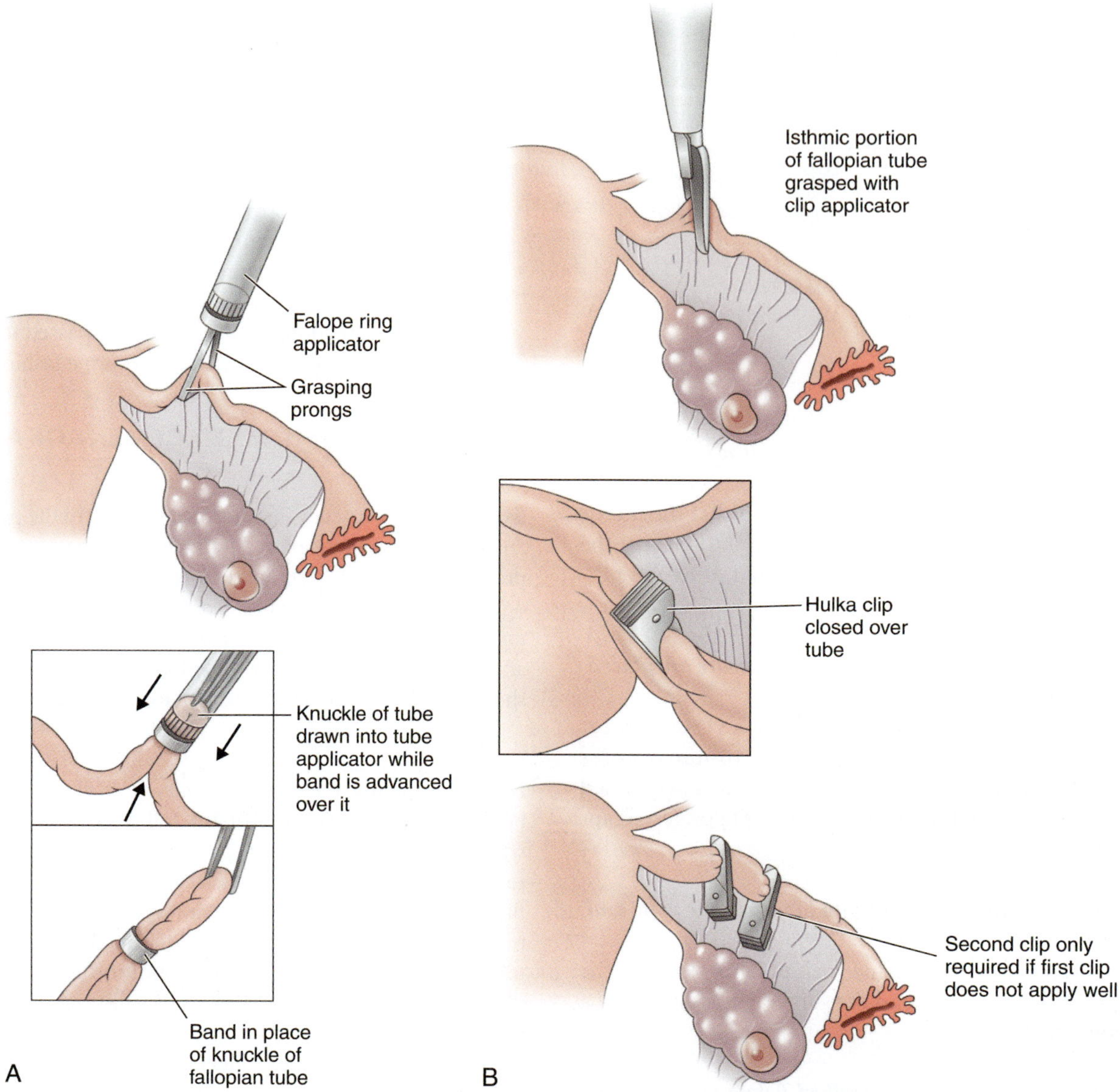

FIG. 23.9 (A) Falope ring and clip technique for tubal ligation. The Silastic ring applicator is used to grasp the tube, retract it, and apply the O ring. (B) The use of Hulka clips to occlude the fallopian tube. (From Falcone T, Hurd W. *Clinical Reproductive Medicine and Surgery*. Philadelphia: Mosby; 2007.)

INSTRUMENTS:	Sizes 10- and 15-mm trocars; laparoscopy set; specimen retrieval system; bipolar ESU; suction irrigator
POSSIBLE EXTRAS:	Linear endostapler; vessel sealing system; Harmonic shears; vascular clips; Endo Stitch and suture; tissue morcellator

Technical Points and Discussion

1. ***Pneumoperitoneum is established and trocars placed.***

2. ***Pneumoperitoneum is established using a Veress needle or the Hasson method.***
   Two 10-mm trocars and one 15-mm trocar are positioned in the abdomen. The abdomen is explored.

   After pneumoperitoneum has been established, the surgeon examines the abdominal contents. The cyst is then identified. If fluid is present in the abdominal cavity, it may be aspirated and removed as part of the specimen.

3. ***The cortex is coagulated and then divided from the body of the cyst.***
   With use of the bipolar ESU, a small area of the cortex is coagulated and the dissection initiated in the area with fine dissecting scissors. The surgeon continues the plane of dissection, coring out the cyst using blunt-nose dissector and suction irrigation. Dissection continues until the cyst is completely mobilized.

4. ***The cyst is prepared for removal.***
   If the specimen is too large for retraction, it can be reduced with a morcellator, and the pieces can be brought out through the bag opening.

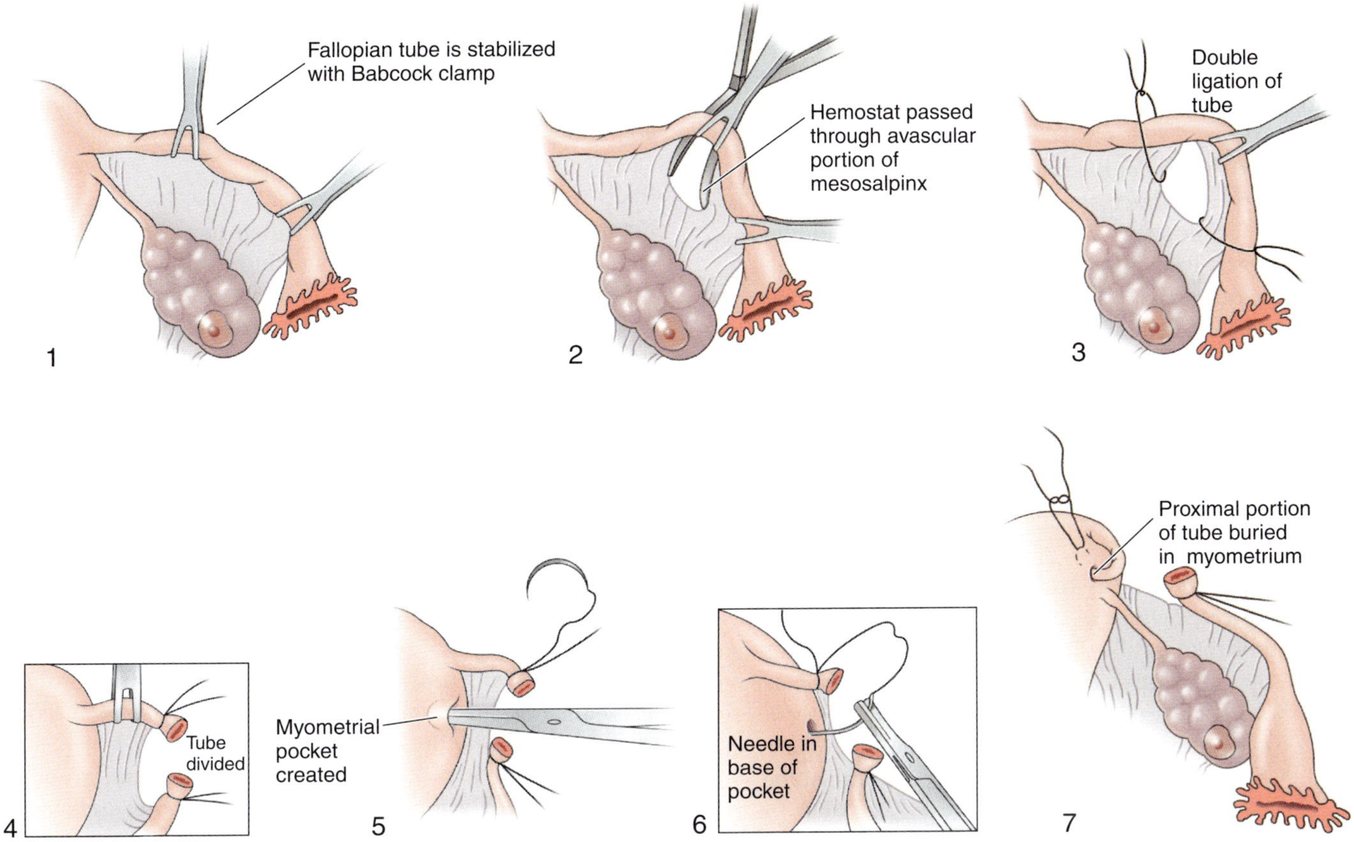

FIG. 23.10 Classic Irving technique of open tubal ligation. (From Falcone T, Hurd W. *Clinical Reproductive Medicine and Surgery*. Philadelphia: Mosby; 2007.)

5. ***The cyst is withdrawn into the specimen bag.***
   The cystic bed is examined and bleeding controlled with the bipolar ESU. If the cyst ruptures within the abdomen, copious amounts of lactated Ringer solution are used to irrigate the abdomen.

6. ***The abdomen is examined for bleeders, and the trocars are withdrawn.***
   The surgeon examines the wound for bleeders, which are managed with the bipolar ESU. The trocars are withdrawn and entry sites closed with deep figure-of-8 synthetic absorbable sutures. The skin is closed with surgical staples or Steri-Strips.

TUBOPLASTY

Tuboplasty is performed to restore continuity to the fallopian tube. There are many causes of tubal stricture, including infection, previous tubal ligation, previous tubal pregnancy, and endometriosis. The exact technique required for tubal anastomosis depends on the situation and patient condition. If the tube is diseased or if the two segments to be joined differ greatly in size, the procedure becomes more complex because the larger segment must be reduced to fit the smaller end.

Before surgery, the patient will have undergone diagnostic laparoscopy, hysterosalpingography, or chromotubation, in which dye is injected into the oviducts to determine patency. Tuboplasty can be performed as a laparoscopic procedure with or without robotic assistance, or as an open procedure.

Pathology

Obstruction of the fallopian tube frequently occurs as a result of an infection that spreads from the lower genital tract to the uterus, fallopian tubes, and ovaries. According to the Centers for Disease Control and Prevention (CDC), approximately 1 million women per year acquire pelvic inflammatory disease (**PID**) as a result of genital tract infections. Of these, 100,000 women become infertile and 150 die. The causal organism usually is *Chlamydia trachomatis* or *Neisseria gonorrhoeae,* both of which cause scarring and loss of fertility. Previous tubal pregnancy can result in excessive scarring of the oviduct. The following technique is used to reconstruct the fallopian tube with occlusion at the uterine junction.

Technical Points and Discussion

1. ***A pelvic laparotomy is performed.***
   The patient is placed in the low lithotomy position for access to the cervix and intrauterine cavity during surgery. The abdomen is entered through a transverse pelvic incision. A self-retaining O'Sullivan-O'Connor retractor is

placed in the wound, and the bowel is packed away from the uterus with moist laparotomy sponges. The patient may be placed in a slight Trendelenburg position to allow for displacement of the abdominal organs.

2. *The proximal fallopian tube is excised.*
The surgeon retracts the uterus with a tenaculum and locates the fallopian tube, mesosalpinx, ureter, and uterine ligaments. To control bleeding, the tube may be injected with vasopressin 1:100. Continuous irrigation may be used to locate microscopic bleeders. A solution of glycine or lactated Ringer solution is used.

The occluded area is grasped with vascular forceps and the serosa incised with an ESU needle. The incision is carried through the tube with the microdissecting rod. Small bleeders are controlled with the microbipolar forceps.

3. *The proximal tube is transected until patency can be demonstrated with dye.*
The tube then is fully transected with iris scissors or other fine-tipped, sharp scissors. This incision is carried deeper with scissors. If patency is not evident, the dissection is repeated. Indigo carmine or methylene blue dye is instilled transcervically to establish patency of the tube.

4. *The distal tube is transected and tested.*
The distal segment of the tube is then dissected from the mesosalpinx, and the outer (peritoneal) tissue of the tube is incised with the bipolar ESU. The segment is divided with iris scissors or other fine-tipped, sharp scissors, using the same technique as for the proximal segment. The surgeon then irrigates the distal segment with indigo carmine dye. The appearance of the dye at the severed end indicates patency.

5. *The limbs of the oviduct are sutured in layers.*
A fine silastic stent may be inserted into the tube and the two segments anastomosed over the stent. Stay sutures are placed and tagged with fine, small hemostats. Nylon or polypropylene 8-0 or 9-0 sutures with a tapered needle are used for the anastomosis. A two-layered anastomosis is performed. The serosa and mesosalpinx of the tube are closed with interrupted 8-0 sutures. The silastic stent is removed before testing the closure.

6. *The oviduct is again tested for patency and the pelvic wound closed.*
Indigo carmine dye is instilled into the tube to confirm that it is patent. The abdominal wound is irrigated and closed in layers.

SURGICAL MANAGEMENT OF AN ECTOPIC PREGNANCY

An **ectopic pregnancy** develops when the fertilized egg implants outside the uterus. The fallopian tube is a common site of ectopic implantation. Abdominal cavity pregnancy outside the uterus is also possible. Tubal rupture requires emergency surgery to control hemorrhage. The surgical goal is to control bleeding and remove the embryo. A laparoscopic or an open approach may be used, depending on the patient's condition.

Pathology

Ectopic pregnancy occurs most often in the fallopian tube (tubal pregnancy). Risk factors include a previous history of pelvic inflammatory disease, smoking (reduces tubal motility), previous tubal surgery, and a history of STD (sexuallyl transmitted disease) infection. Tubal rupture, hemorrhage, and hypovolemic shock can be rapidly fatal. Early tubal pregnancy may be treated with methotrexate, which causes embryonic death. As mentioned, the surgery may be performed laparoscopically or through open surgery. An open approach is discussed in the next section, although techniques are similar for both types of surgery.

Discussion

Two approaches may be used in the surgical treatment of an ectopic pregnancy: salpingectomy (complete removal of the affected fallopian tube) and salpingostomy (removal of the tubal contents with preservation of the tube).

The patient is placed in the supine position, prepped, and draped for a laparotomy. A Pfannenstiel incision is used to open the pelvic cavity. If the ectopic pregnancy has already ruptured, the ST must be prepared for surgical hemorrhaging. The ST should have suction and irrigation immediately available. Clots are removed manually, and the source of the bleeding is identified as quickly as possible. A basin should be placed on the field to receive the blood clots. A self-retaining retractor may or may not be inserted during this stage of the procedure. When the bleeding has been controlled, the embryo (or tube and embryo) can be removed. In all approaches, the ST should have an ample supply of Mayo and Crile clamps available. Suture ligatures of fine absorbable synthetic material or surgical staples may also be required soon after the start of the procedure.

SALPINGECTOMY To control the bleeding, the surgeon may cross-clamp the fallopian tube and mesosalpinx with Mayo or Crile clamps. The tube then is resected with the HF bipolar ESU. Suture ligatures may also be used. (In laparoscopic surgery, Harmonic shears, staples, or pretied ligatures are used.)

SALPINGOSTOMY Tube-preserving surgery requires incision of the tube and removal of the embryo, with irrigation and suction. Reconstruction of the tube is performed at the time of surgery or deferred until a later date. The tube is grasped with Babcock forceps, and a small incision is made with a scalpel, needle electrode, or ultrasonic scalpel. The embryo is removed using irrigation and fine forceps. The ESU is used sparingly to prevent scarring. The tube is irrigated and may be left to heal by secondary intention.

The surgery is complete after the wound has been irrigated and carefully examined for any bleeding. The wound is then

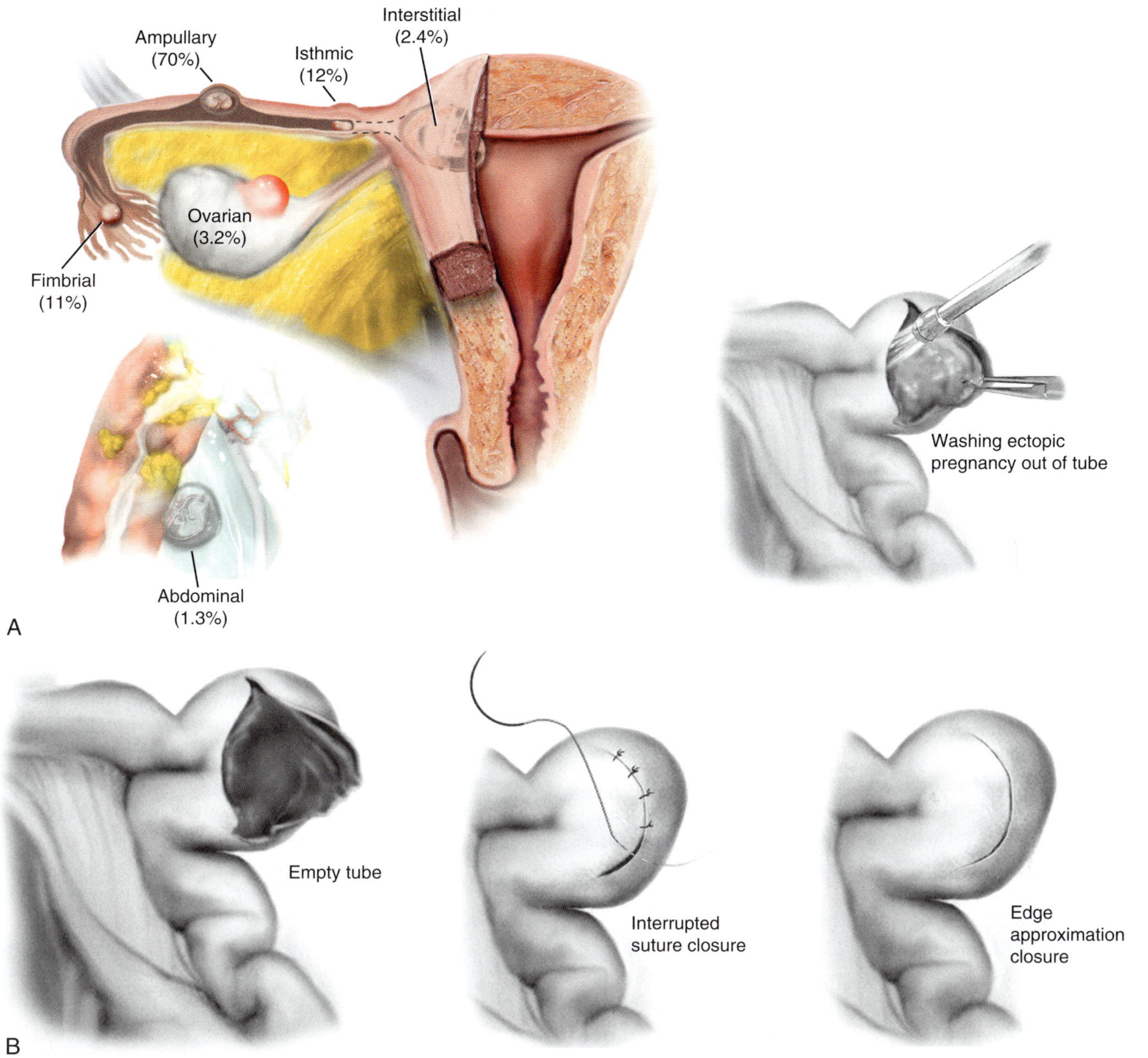

FIG. 23.11 Surgical management of ectopic pregnancy. (A) *Left,* Sites of ectopic pregnancy. Ampullary pregnancy is the most common. *Right,* After incising the tube, the pregnancy may be flushed out using low pressure irrigation. (B) *Left,* The pregnancy has been evacuated from the tube. *Center,* The tube is closed using interrupted sutures. *Right,* A suture-free closure may also be used, allowing the tube to heal by secondary intention. (A and B, From Baggish M, Karram M. *Atlas of Pelvic Anatomy and Gynecologic Surgery.* 4th ed. Philadelphia: Elsevier; 2016.)

closed in layers. The skin is closed with staples or subcuticular suture and Steri-Strips.

Surgical treatment of an ectopic pregnancy is illustrated in Fig. 23.11.

LAPAROSCOPIC-ASSISTED VAGINAL HYSTERECTOMY

Laparoscopic-assisted vaginal hysterectomy (LAVH) is the removal of the uterus by a combined laparoscopic and vaginal approach. The uterine ligaments, adhesions, and any other attachments are released through the abdominal portion of the procedure. The vaginal cul-de-sac is opened, and the specimen is removed vaginally.

Pathology

The LAVH approach for hysterectomy can be performed for early stage uterine malignancy, benign tumors, or endometriosis. *Endometriosis* is a disease in which endometrial tissue develops anywhere outside the uterus, most often on the abdominal viscera. The tissue remains responsive to hormonal changes and causes pain, bleeding, and scarring. Conservative treatment focuses on pain management and hormone therapy. Surgery may be necessary to remove endometrial tissue. The cause of endometriosis is unknown.

POSITION:	Low lithotomy
INCISION:	Laparoscopy
PREP AND DRAPING:	Combined abdominal–perineal
INSTRUMENTS:	Two 5-mm trocars; two 10-mm trocars; laparoscopic GYN set; uterine manipulator; colpotomy ring; bipolar ESU; uterine manipulator; linear endostapler; size 0 absorbable synthetic suture on a taper needle; specimen retrieval system; LigaSure system; Harmonic scalpel
POSSIBLE EXTRAS:	Tissue morcellator

Technical Points and Discussion

1. ***The patient is placed in a low lithotomy position, prepped, and draped for a combined abdominal-vaginal approach.***

2. ***A routine prep of both the abdomen perineum and vagina is performed. A Koh colpotomy ring and uterine manipulator are inserted after the prep.***
   Pneumoperitoneum can be established using the Veress needle or Hasson trocar. At least four trocars are necessary for the procedure. Sizes 10 mm and 5 mm are used. If the specimen is to be removed laparoscopically, a morcellator is required before its withdrawal from the abdomen. In this case, a 10- or 12-mm trocar is required to accommodate the morcellator.

3. ***The uterine ligaments are divided.***
   The surgery begins with a thorough assessment of the abdominal cavity to determine the site of the pathology and exact operative plan.

   Assessment is carried out with a probe and dolphin-nose forceps. The uterine ligaments are located and divided using the Harmonic scalpel or LigaSure vessel sealing instrument. Division is carried to the lower uterine segment to create the bladder flap. The bladder flap is then created.

4. ***The ovarian vessels are located and coagulated. The bladder is dissected from the uterus.***
   The peritoneal reflection of the bladder and uterus is located and the peritoneum separated. Dissection is carried to the vagina. This exposes the colpotomy ring. The uterine arteries may be dissected at this stage using the bipolar cutting device. The procedure is repeated on the opposite side.

5. ***The posterior cul-de-sac is incised.***
   The posterior cul-de-sac is incised using the Harmonic scalpel. This is the start of the colpotomy. In this part of the procedure, the uterus is released at the cervix by creating a circular incision around the colpotomy ring, which maintains the pneumoperitoneum.

6. ***The specimen is moved into the vagina.***
   The colpotomy incision is completed and the uterus is shifted into the vagina for retrieval. The colpotomy ring is replaced to maintain pneumoperitoneum.

7. ***The vaginal cuff is oversewn, and laparoscopic incisions are closed.***
   The vaginal cuff is closed in one or two layers using size 0 monofilament synthetic absorbable suture such as polydioxanone or quill suture.

TOTAL ABDOMINAL HYSTERECTOMY WITH BILATERAL SALPINGO-OOPHORECTOMY

Total abdominal hysterectomy (TAH) is removal of the uterus and cervix. Bilateral salpingo-oophorectomy is surgical removal of the fallopian tubes and ovaries.

Pathology

This procedure is performed in the treatment of endometrial cancer. Unrelated to cervical cancer, endometrial cancer is associated with obesity and high levels of circulating estrogen. All stages of endometrial cancer may also require lymph node excision with radiation therapy. *Brachytherapy* is performed in the clinical setting. In this procedure, a radiation source contained in a cylinder is placed in the vagina for a specified period of exposure. Several treatments may be required.

POSITION:	Supine
INCISION:	Lower midline or transverse
PREP AND DRAPING:	Abdominal-vaginal-perineum
INSTRUMENTS:	Laparotomy with hysterectomy set
POSSIBLE EXTRAS:	Long abdominal instruments; LigaSure; Harmonic scalpel

Technical Points and Discussion

1. ***The abdomen is entered through a transverse pelvic incision.***
   The patient is placed in the supine position. After a routine abdominal and vaginal prep, a Foley catheter is inserted for continuous urinary drainage. A lower midline or Pfannenstiel incision can be used for a hysterectomy. The incision traverses the lower abdomen approximately 3 to 4 inches (7.5 to 10 cm) above the symphysis pubis.

   To begin the surgery, the surgeon makes a transverse skin incision and extends it through the subcutaneous tissue with the ESU. The next layer, the fascia, is entered with the scalpel, and the incision is lengthened with curved Mayo scissors. The surgeon then grasps one edge of the fascial margin with two or more Kocher clamps. Using blunt dissection, the surgeon separates the fascia from the underlying muscle.

This procedure is repeated on the lower fascial margin. The muscle layer is then divided manually. The peritoneum is incised with the scalpel, and the incision is lengthened with Metzenbaum scissors. A self-retaining retractor (e.g., O'Sullivan-O'Connor or Balfour retractor) is placed in the wound. The surgeon packs the bowel away from the uterus with moist lap sponges.

2. ***The round ligaments are clamped, divided, and ligated.***
Mobilization of the uterus begins with the round ligaments. The ST should have at least six heavy uterine clamps available. The round ligaments are double-clamped using Heaney or Ochsner clamps and then divided using the ESU or deep knife. Suture ligatures are placed through each tissue pedicle using size 0 Vicryl or other synthetic absorbable suture on a heavy taper needle. Both round ligaments are divided.

3. ***The incision is carried anteriorly to the peritoneal bladder reflection.***
The surgeon mobilizes the uterus to the level of the bladder. At this point, the bladder is continuous with the uterus; both organs are attached by a peritoneal covering. Using Metzenbaum scissors and long tissue forceps, the surgeon separates the two structures by dissecting the peritoneal covering away from the bladder.

4. ***The infundibulopelvic ligaments and arteries are divided.***
The dissection is carried through the infundibulopelvic ligaments (ovarian arteries and veins), which are triple clamped, separated from the ureter, and ligated.

5. ***The cervix is incised circumferentially and amputated from the vaginal cuff.***
At the level of the cervix, long Allis or Kocher clamps are placed around the edge of the cervix, and it is divided from the vagina.

The surgeon uses long scissors or the long scalpel to divide the tissue. This maneuver completely frees the uterus, which is passed to the ST. All instruments that have come in contact with the cervix or vagina must be kept separate from the rest of the setup. The specimen and isolated instruments should be received in a basin.

6. ***The uterine vessels are mobilized and divided.***
Dissection continues with the uterine vessels on both sides, which are triple clamped, divided with Mayo scissors or the knife. These are also ligated with suture ligatures using 0 Vicryl.

7. ***The cardinal and uterosacral ligaments are clamped, severed, and ligated on both sides.***
This mobilizes the uterus so that it can be retracted upward to expose the vagina. The vagina is clamped and the specimen removed. The ST should have a basin ready to receive the specimen on the field.

8. ***The vaginal cuff is grasped with clamps and sutured and the bladder flap reattached.***
To close the wound, the surgeon first closes the vaginal vault where it was separated from the cervix. Absorbable sutures of the same type used on the uterine ligaments are used. The muscular layer of the vagina is closed with figure-of-8 sutures. After closing the vagina, the surgeon uses 2-0 or 3-0 suture on a small tapered needle to reattach the bladder flap.

9. ***The abdominal wound is irrigated and closed in layers.***
The abdominal wound is irrigated with warm saline and checked for bleeders. To close the abdomen, the surgeon grasps the edges of the peritoneum with several Mayo clamps. The peritoneum is closed with running suture of size 0 absorbable suture swaged to a tapered needle. The muscle tissue may be loosely approximated with three or four interrupted absorbable sutures. The fascial layer is closed with a wide variety of sutures, absorbable or nonabsorbable, usually size 0 or 2-0. The subcutaneous tissue may be approximated with 3-0 interrupted absorbable sutures. The skin is closed with staples or subcuticular running suture.

Abdominal hysterectomy with bilateral salpingo-oophorectomy is shown in Fig. 23.12.

ROBOTIC-ASSISTED HYSTERECTOMY

Robotic hysterectomy can be used for laparoscopic removal of the uterus using the da Vinci system. Robotic technology is discussed in Chapter 21. In this procedure, the technical aspects are described from the point of entry.

Pathology

As described previously.

Technical Points and Discussion

1. ***The patient is prepped for a combined abdominal-perineal approach.***
A routine prep is performed, and a uterine manipulator and Koh colpotomizer are placed in the cervix. This system includes a blue ring, which during dissection of the lower uterine segment can be visualized to delineate the area of excision. A balloon attachment allows the uterus to be inflated toward the end of the dissection, which effectively maintains the pneumoperitoneum, which would otherwise be lost through the vaginal vault after removal of the uterus.

2. ***Pneumoperitoneum is established, and trocars are placed.***
Pneumoperitoneum is established using the Veress, Hasson, or optical trocar system. Two 12-mm and one additional 8-mm instrument ports are inserted.

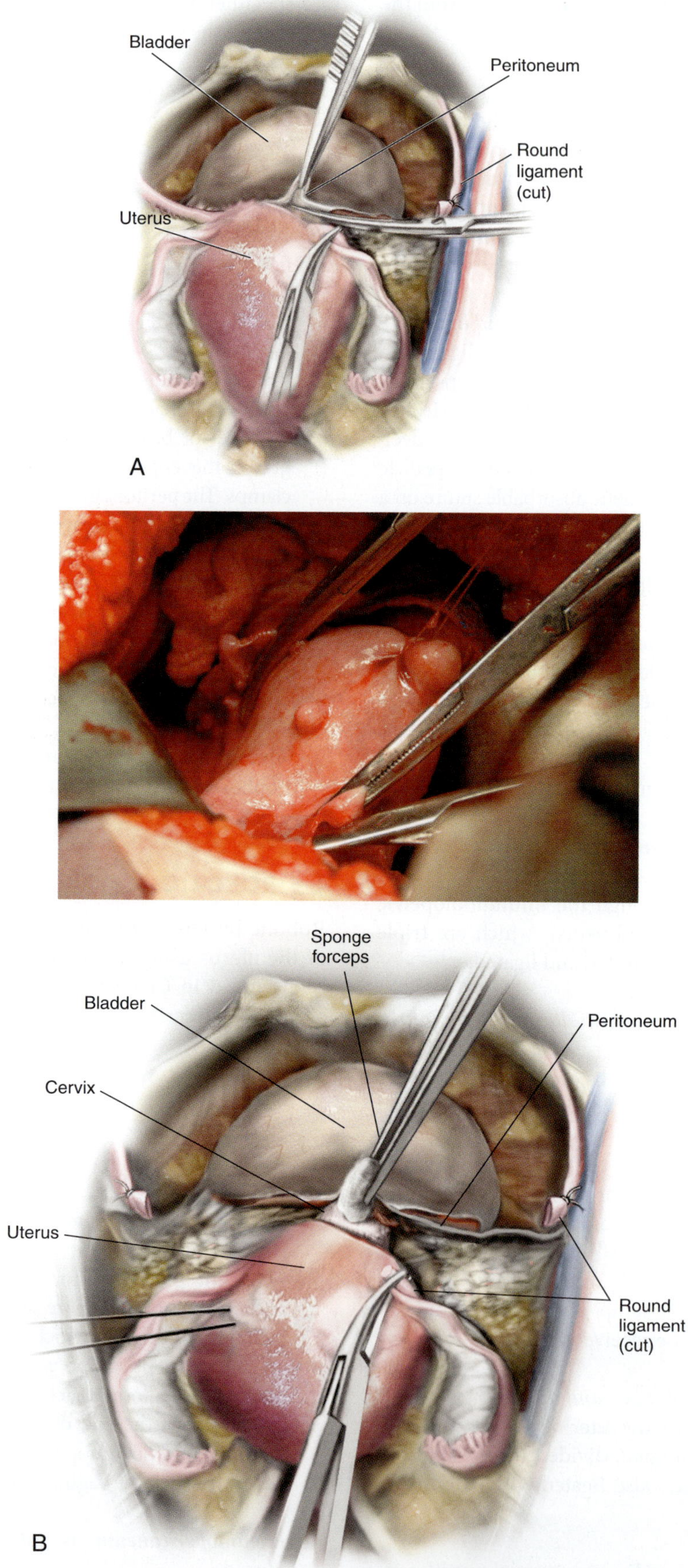

FIG. 23.12 Abdominal hysterectomy with bilateral salpingo-oophorectomy. (A) The peritoneal attachment of the bladder to the uterus is dissected free, creating the *bladder flap*. (B) The bladder is further separated from the uterus with a sponge forceps for blunt dissection.

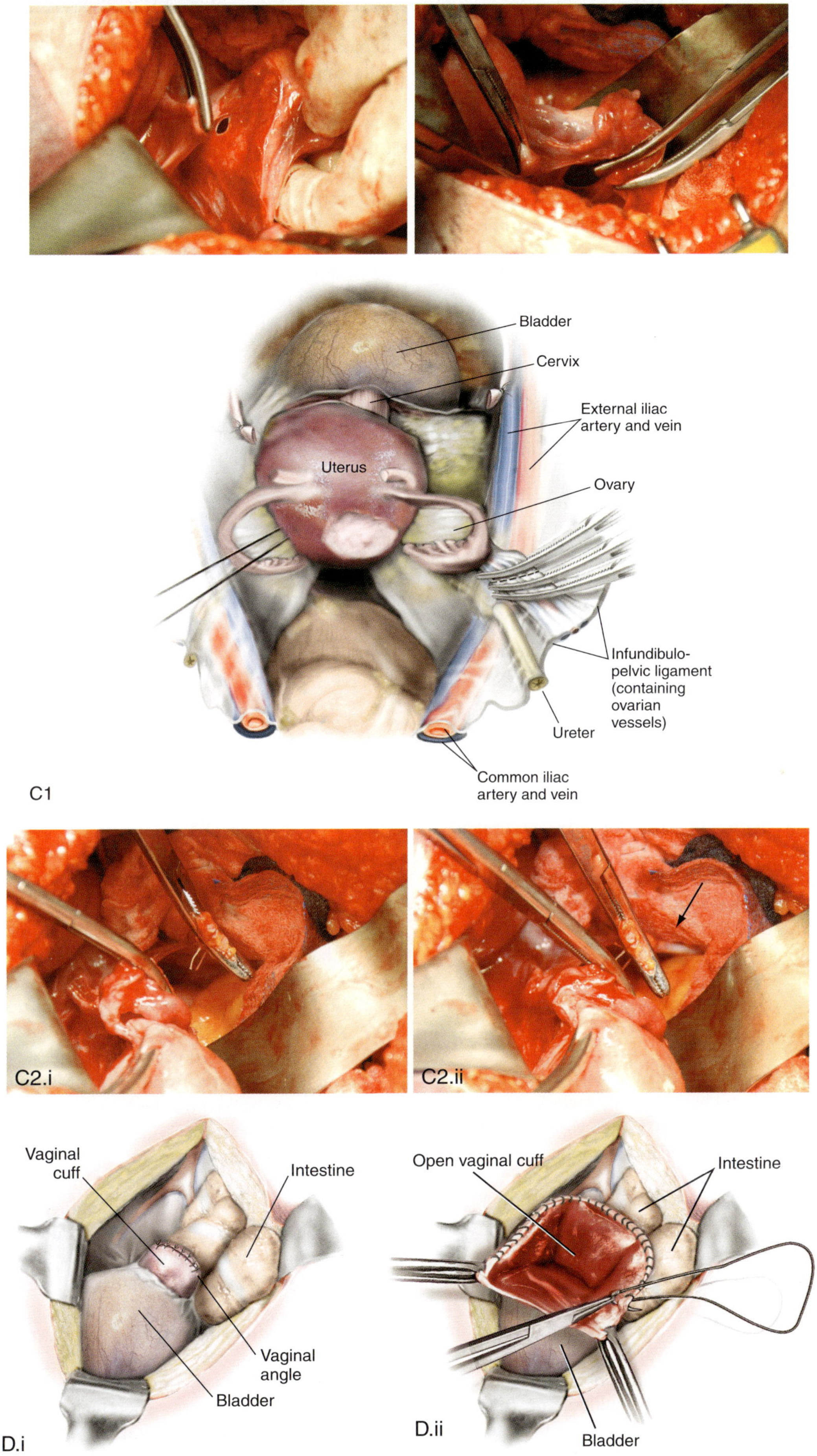

FIG. 23.12, cont'd (C) The ovarian ligament and vessels are triply grasped, cut, and ligated. (D) After the uterus, ovaries, and fallopian tubes have been completely mobilized and removed, the vaginal vault is closed. (From Baggish M, Karram M. *Atlas of Pelvic Anatomy and Gynecologic Surgery*. Philadelphia: Elsevier; 2016.)

3. ***The robot is docked.***
The draped robotic system is brought into place and the surgical arms locked into each port. The primary surgeon goes to the console, and the assistant remains at the sterile field.

4. ***The abdomen is explored.***
The surgeon locates the ureters, ovaries, and fallopian tubes. The assistant places a double-toothed tenaculum into the body of the uterus for retraction.

5. ***The uterine ligaments are dissected free and blood vessels coagulated.***
Dissection is performed using the Metzenbaum scissors, ultrasonic knife, and blunt forceps. As dissection progresses, the surgeon develops the bladder flap (peritoneal attachment to the urinary bladder). Dissection is further developed at the level of the Koh ring, which is visible as the lower uterine segment is separated from the upper vaginal vault.

6. ***The uterus is released from the cervix.***
When dissection is completed, the assistant pulls the uterus *into* the vaginal vault. Placement of the uterus within the vaginal vault essentially maintains the pneumoperitoneum.

7. ***The vaginal cuff is sutured.***
After securing hemostasis, the vaginal vault is closed with figure-of-8 synthetic absorbable sutures, size 2-0.

8. ***The abdominal cavity is flushed with saline, and robotic arms are detached.***
All abdominal ports are withdrawn, and the wounds are closed with figure-of-8 sutures. The skin can be closed with Steri-Strips or skin staples.

RADICAL HYSTERECTOMY WITH LYMPHADENECTOMY

A radical hysterectomy differs from a total hysterectomy in several ways. Whereas total hysterectomy includes removal of the entire uterus and cervix, radical hysterectomy (Wertheim-type procedure) includes the ovaries, fallopian tubes, supporting ligaments, upper vagina, and pelvic lymph nodes. The Wertheim hysterectomy, which has been modified many times in the past century, also includes wide excision of pelvic lymph nodes and differs from the radical hysterectomy only in the sequence of steps in parametrial excision. The exact sequence of steps and extent of the tissue removed depend on each individual case. For example, in radical hysterectomy with lymph node dissection, the ovaries may be left intact. It is important to note that extensive operations such as the radical hysterectomy, Wertheim, and pelvic exenteration (discussed later) proceed anatomically. The ST can prepare for such lengthy cases by watching the sterile field for indications of what technique is being used (e.g., sharp or blunt dissection, hemostasis, suturing, specimen removal, and closure). In the following description, the techniques are explained for each step. However, the order of steps will differ somewhat according to the surgeon's own technique and the requirements of the procedure.

Deep pelvic procedures require extra attention to sponge and instrument counts because items can easily be lost in the wound. In addition to routine counts, the ST should keep track of lap sponges placed inside the wound for retraction or packing. The ST should maintain a clean workspace and ensure that instrument tips are free of tissue debris. A basin of water used for maintaining instruments intraoperatively must be kept fresh.

Pathology

A radical hysterectomy is performed for the treatment of cervical cancer.

POSITION:	Supine
INCISION:	Midline
PREP AND DRAPING:	Abdominal; Foley catheterization; sequential compression device and warming air mattress are usually required
INSTRUMENTS:	Laparotomy; long general surgery set; hysterectomy instruments
POSSIBLE EXTRAS:	Harmonic scalpel; vessel sealing system; vascular loops; linear surgical stapler; bowel bag

Technical Points and Discussion

1. ***The abdomen is opened through a midline incision.***
Refer to the description of an abdominal laparotomy in Chapter 22.

2. ***The retroperitoneal space is entered, and retractors are placed.***
To enter the retroperitoneal space, a self-retaining retractor such as the Bookwalter or Balfour is needed. Lap tapes are packed on the lateral areas of the abdominal cavity. The retroperitoneal membrane lies deep under the abdominal viscera, including the intestine. A bowel (isolation) bag may be used to maintain the intestines in a moist condition while simultaneously isolating them in the surgical wound. The ST should prepare the bag by placing approximately 20 mL of warm saline inside and moistening the outside before passing it to the surgeon.

3. ***The round and infundibulopelvic ligaments are clamped and ligated.***
For these steps in the procedure, the ST should have hysterectomy instruments including Heaney clamps, Russian-type or heavy-toothed forceps, Mayo clamps, and Péan clamps. Numerous stick sponges are required throughout the dissection. Suture ligatures are

needed after clamping and dividing the ligaments. The ST should always keep two suture ligatures of two sizes ready during dissection. The uterine ligaments require size 0 absorbable synthetic sutures on a heavy taper needle. Size 2-0 should also be available.

4. ***The ureter is identified and retracted.***
Here the ureter must be dissected from its attachments along its full length up to the level of the bladder. To accomplish the dissection, light traction on the ureter may be needed. A small Penrose drain or vessel loop can be used to encircle the ureter, and its ends clamped together with a blunt-nose hemostat such as a Kelly or Mayo clamp. The Penrose must be dipped in saline before use in the wound. Dissection of the ureter is performed with long Metzenbaum scissors and atraumatic forceps such as a DeBakey or dressing forceps.

5. ***The iliac artery, obturator fossa, and ureter are dissected of lymph and connective tissue.***
The regions of external iliac vessels and obturator fossa contain fatty tissue and lymph nodes. These are dissected systematically on both sides. Allis clamps can be used to grasp the lymph nodes during dissection. The ST should have several specimen containers ready to receive lymph nodes. The containers should be passed off the field and labeled soon after they are received.

6. ***The uterine artery and vein are clamped, cut, and double ligated.***
Dissection of the uterine artery and vein requires long Metzenbaum scissors and vascular forceps. The vascular bundles can be clamped with Péan or hysterectomy forceps. Suture ligatures of size 0 or 2-0 on a taper needle may be used for ligation.

7. ***The peritoneal reflection of the bladder is dissected from the cervix and vagina.***
Sharp dissection is carried out with Metzenbaum or similar scissors.

8. ***The cul-de-sac is opened, and the uterosacral and cardinal ligaments are resected and ligated.***
The cul-de-sac is grasped with two long hemostatic clamps and incised with Metzenbaum scissors. The exposed uterosacral and cardinal ligaments are grasped with Heaney hysterectomy clamps and transected with the deep knife, Mayo scissors, or ESU. The pedicles are ligated with size 0 synthetic absorbable suture on a heavy taper needle.

9. ***The upper vagina is cross-clamped and divided, and the specimen is removed.***
To remove the specimen en bloc, the upper vagina must be dissected free. It is cross-clamped with Péan or similar forceps and transected with the knife or Mayo scissors. The ST should have a basin available to receive the specimen. This should be kept separate from other specimens received during the case up to this point.

10. ***The vagina is closed with running locked suture.***
The vagina is closed using a synthetic absorbable running locked suture. Long tissue forceps should be available during closure. Note that a sponge count is necessary before the retroperitoneal and vaginal closures are finished. The pelvic incision may also be closed with the same suture, size 0 or 2-0.

11. ***Suction or gravity drains may be placed in the wound, which is then closed.***
One or two suction drains are placed in the wound before closure. The tubes may be brought to the exterior through stab incisions. The abdominal wound is then closed in layers using the surgeon's preference of sutures.

12. ***The incision and drain ports are dressed with flat gauze layers and abdominal pads.***
After radical abdominal or pelvic surgery, the patient is closely monitored for urinary output, hemorrhage, and infection. The patient may recover in the postanesthesia care unit, or she may be taken directly to the intensive care unit, depending on her physiological status at the close of surgery.

PELVIC EXENTERATION

Pelvic exenteration is performed to treat metastatic cancer of the pelvic structures. The surgery involves techniques across three different specializations: gynecology, urology, and intestinal surgery. It includes the complete removal of the rectum, the distal sigmoid colon, the urinary bladder and distal ureters, and the internal iliac vessels and their lateral branches. All pelvic reproductive organs and lymph nodes, as well as the entire pelvic floor, pelvic peritoneum, levator muscles, and perineum, are also removed. These procedures are discussed separately in relevant chapters; radical hysterectomy is included in this chapter; resection of the bowel and bladder are described in Chapters 22 and 24. The student should refer to these procedures for guidance on techniques required for each individual step listed below.

Two approaches are used for the surgery: abdominal and perineal. Two separate teams may work simultaneously, or one team may operate sequentially on each part.

The relative length of the surgery (6 to 9 hours) adds some technical difficulty for the ST and circulating team. Care of the patient requires constant monitoring, and the technical needs for supplying ample sutures, sponges, and other items are demanding. The ST must keep an orderly setup, paying attention to setting priorities. During very long, complex surgical procedures such as this one, the instruments should be frequently wiped down to prevent the buildup of organic material and tissue debris. A basin of sterile water should be kept clean and replenished from time to time to avoid the transfer of tissue debris back into the wound. Bowel isolation techniques will be required during and after the colectomy. The variety and amount of supplies and equipment required may be best handled by using two back tables, each with a designated purpose.

In addition to suture materials, surgical stapling devices (LDS, TA, and GIA) and clips are needed. Instrumentation is drawn from the three surgical specialties mentioned earlier. Basic vascular instruments and sutures should also be available. Throughout the dissection, the ST should have vascular loops, vessel clips, suture ligatures of several sizes, free ties, and dissection sponges ready at all times. Right-angle and long curved hemostatic clamps are also needed during mobilization of the organs and ligation of blood vessels. The dissection is carried out using regular and long Metzenbaum scissors, ESU, and sponge dissectors. The specimen is mobilized in anatomical phases and the entire specimen released en bloc. Lymph node packs are excised and kept separate. After this phase, reconstruction is necessary. A sigmoid colostomy may be performed along with a urinary diversion procedure such as ileostomy or ureterostomy (anastomosis of the ureters to the small bowel).

Because of the length of this procedure, the ST may be relieved for a break at several points in the surgery. It is important that the relieving ST be completely briefed during handover. This includes not only a repeat surgical count but also the location of specific sutures and instruments that may be needed emergently, the identification of all drugs and solutions, and a brief explanation on the status of the procedure. If two teams operate simultaneously, the setups should be separated; instruments and supplies used on the perineal portion should not be used for the abdominal procedure.

Pathology

Pelvic exenteration is performed for recurring carcinoma of the cervix, vulva, or vagina. Cases in which the patient has undergone radiation therapy before surgery present a challenge because of the alterations in the tissues, which may include excessive scarring.

POSITION:	Lithotomy
INCISION:	Midline
PREP AND DRAPING:	Abdominal, extending from the nipple line to mid-thigh. Sequential compression device is required. A Foley catheter is inserted immediately after the prep. A thermal air blanket or underpad should also be available
INSTRUMENTS AND SUPPLIES:	Laparotomy; gynecological (hysterectomy) intestinal; long instruments; vascular instruments; vascular loops; umbilical tapes; bowel bag; suture boots; topical hemostatic agents; ureteral stent; surgical stapling instruments; surgical clips; long ESU monopolar electrode
POSSIBLE EXTRAS:	Vessel sealing system, Harmonic scalpel (ultrasonic), heating apparatus for irrigation solutions

Technical Points and Discussion

ABDOMINAL PHASE

1. ***A long midline incision is made from the symphysis pubis to the umbilicus, and the abdomen is opened.***
   The abdominal incision is made and the peritoneal cavity explored for metastasis to the liver, the nodes of the celiac axis, the superior mesenteric artery, and the para-aortic tissues. The space of Retzius is entered and the pelvis explored for lymph node involvement. If negative findings are noted, retractors are placed and the small bowel is packed with moist lap sponges. Loose connective tissue is separated at the pubic symphysis using sharp and blunt dissection. The ureters and iliac vessels are identified and vessel loops placed around them. The ureters are mobilized and divided, leaving as much length as possible. A ureteral stent is placed in one of the ureters to measure urine output during the procedure.

2. ***Lymphadenectomy and hysterectomy are performed.***
   A lymphadenectomy is performed in the region of the iliac veins. These are ligated in sequence to the level of the vascular pedicles of the bladder. The obturator nerve and its associated vessels are mobilized and a silastic vessel loop placed for traction. A total hysterectomy is performed. The bladder is dissected free from the pubic symphysis, and the urethra, rectum, and vagina are divided.

PERINEAL PHASE

3. ***The structures of the lower pelvic floor are mobilized through a perineal incision.***
   The perineal incision is made circumferentially around the anus, rectum, and vagina. The incision is carried to the muscle complex and along the pubic arch. The vagina and urethra are mobilized. The rectum is divided using the GIA. Any remaining attachments to the pelvic wall are divided. The specimen is then removed and the wound irrigated. The urethra and perineal incision are closed in layers using synthetic absorbable sutures.

RECONSTRUCTION

There are several options to restore continuity to the urinary and intestinal systems. An ileal conduit with ureterostomy is the most common choice (refer to Chapter 24). A terminal colostomy is performed for continuity of the bowel as described in Chapter 22.

Before the reconstruction phase of the procedure is begun, the pelvic cavity and abdomen are irrigated using warm saline. A new setup should be used for the remainder of the procedure. When the stomas have been completed, the wound is closed. Two suction drains (Jackson-Pratt or Hemovac) are installed, and the wound is dressed using gauze and abdominal pads.

Numerous complications may arise after exenteration. These include fluid and electrolyte imbalance, sepsis, hemorrhage, venous thrombosis, and pulmonary embolus. The 5-year survival rate is 23% to 61%.

SECTION II: OPERATIVE OBSTETRICAL PROCEDURES

Birth is a physiological process that seldom requires interventions for a healthy mother. Mother and fetus are linked during pregnancy as the mother's body accommodates the growing fetus. Healthy mothers usually provide a nourishing environment that produces a healthy baby. The placenta plays a major role in the fetus' health by allowing essential nutrients to pass from the mother's blood to the baby. Failure of the placenta to function, for any reason, can be life-threatening to the fetus. Many medical and obstetrical problems are identified before birth. Unexpected problems that arise during **labor,** at birth, or after birth can present as emergencies that threaten the life of the mother or the baby. Surgical technologists may be asked to assist in a variety of roles during emergency situations.

STAGES OF PREGNANCY

Development of the embryo and fetus occurs when the ovum is fertilized by sperm, which normally occurs in the fallopian tube. The combination of chromosomal material from each completes the fertilization process. The egg passes through early embryonic development as it moves into the uterus and implants in the endometrium, about 10 days after fertilization. As the embryo grows, distinct developmental changes occur. The embryonic stage ends at week 8, and the fetal period begins.

During development, fetal circulation begins shortly after conception. Changes in the endometrial cells provide nourishment and protection for the fetus. The **placenta** is a thick organ that adheres to the uterus on the maternal side. The fetal side contains large vessels within the structure's smooth membranes. The umbilical cord, which attaches to the placenta, contains the umbilical artery and vein and communicates directly with fetal circulation.

Fetal membranes surround the growing fetus and are filled with **amniotic fluid.** The two membranes, the *chorion* and the *amnion*, are very close together. The amnion is continuous with the umbilical cord. The fluid-filled sac in which the fetus develops protects it against physical injury and maintains thermoregulation. The watery environment allows the fetus to move and develop without restriction (Fig. 23.13).

Average normal gestation occurs over 40 weeks and is marked by predictable growth patterns that can be measured by ultrasound. **Prenatal** assessment is performed throughout gestation to ensure that fetal development progresses normally and to detect complications early. Abdominal ultrasound is routinely used to assess pregnancy (Fig. 23.14).

COMPLICATIONS OF PREGNANCY

PLACENTAL ABRUPTION

The placenta is the organ that acts as a filter from mother to baby; it allows nutrients to pass from the mother's blood to the fetus and carries away waste products. It is essential to the life of the fetus during the entire pregnancy. The placenta attaches to the uterine wall and grows during pregnancy to accommodate the fetus' needs. **Placental abruption** is a premature separation of the placenta from the uterine wall after 20 weeks' gestation and before the fetus is delivered (Fig. 23.15). A variety of conditions can cause abruption, such as abdominal trauma, abnormalities of the uterus, a short umbilical cord, and hypertension. Abruption of the placenta from the uterine wall can be partial or complete. Abruption of the placenta presents as vaginal bleeding and sometimes concealed bleeding. The fetus has a good chance of surviving if half of the placenta remains attached to the uterus. **Fetal demise** (death of the fetus) results if the entire placenta separates from the uterus. If this happens during labor, fetal distress is evident during monitoring of the fetal heart. The woman may experience increased abdominal tenderness and back pain. If delivery is not imminent, a cesarean section is necessary.

PLACENTA PREVIA

During normal labor, the baby's head is pushed toward the cervix, and the cervix begins to thin. Eventually the cervix dilates to about 10 cm, thins out, and becomes part of the lower uterus. Normally the placenta implants on the uterine wall, far from the uterine opening (cervix). The location of the placenta usually is identified on routine ultrasound scans in the prenatal period. **Placenta previa** occurs when the placenta implants completely or partly over the cervical os (Fig. 23.16). In this position, the placenta begins to bleed as it separates from the cervix during labor. The amount of bleeding is greater when the placenta covers the cervix completely. Sudden hemorrhage is life threatening to both mother and fetus. An immediate cesarean section is necessary to prevent fetal death and maternal hemorrhage. Often, hemorrhage can be prevented if a cesarean section is performed before labor begins.

PREGNANCY-INDUCED HYPERTENSION

Pregnancy-induced hypertension (PIH) is diagnosed as high blood pressure that occurs only during pregnancy after 20 weeks' gestation. PIH may be mild and monitored but not treated, or it may be severe and affect other systems, such as the kidneys (proteinuria), liver (elevated liver enzymes), and blood (low platelets). It also can lead to maternal seizures (**eclampsia**). This disease process is also referred to as *toxemia* and *preeclampsia.* It usually occurs in the first pregnancy, but its cause is unknown. Hypertension can constrict blood flow to the placenta and fetus, resulting in a small fetus and placenta. If this occurs or if symptoms worsen, labor is induced artificially with drugs. During the induction, the mother may receive medicines intravenously to reduce the risk of seizures, although this is rare if the mother is receiving preventive medication. If a seizure occurs, it usually lasts 60 seconds or less, but it may be life threatening to the fetus and mother. Airway maintenance is of primary importance during a seizure; therefore airways usually are within easy reach in each labor room. Once the mother's condition has stabilized after a seizure, a cesarean section can be performed.

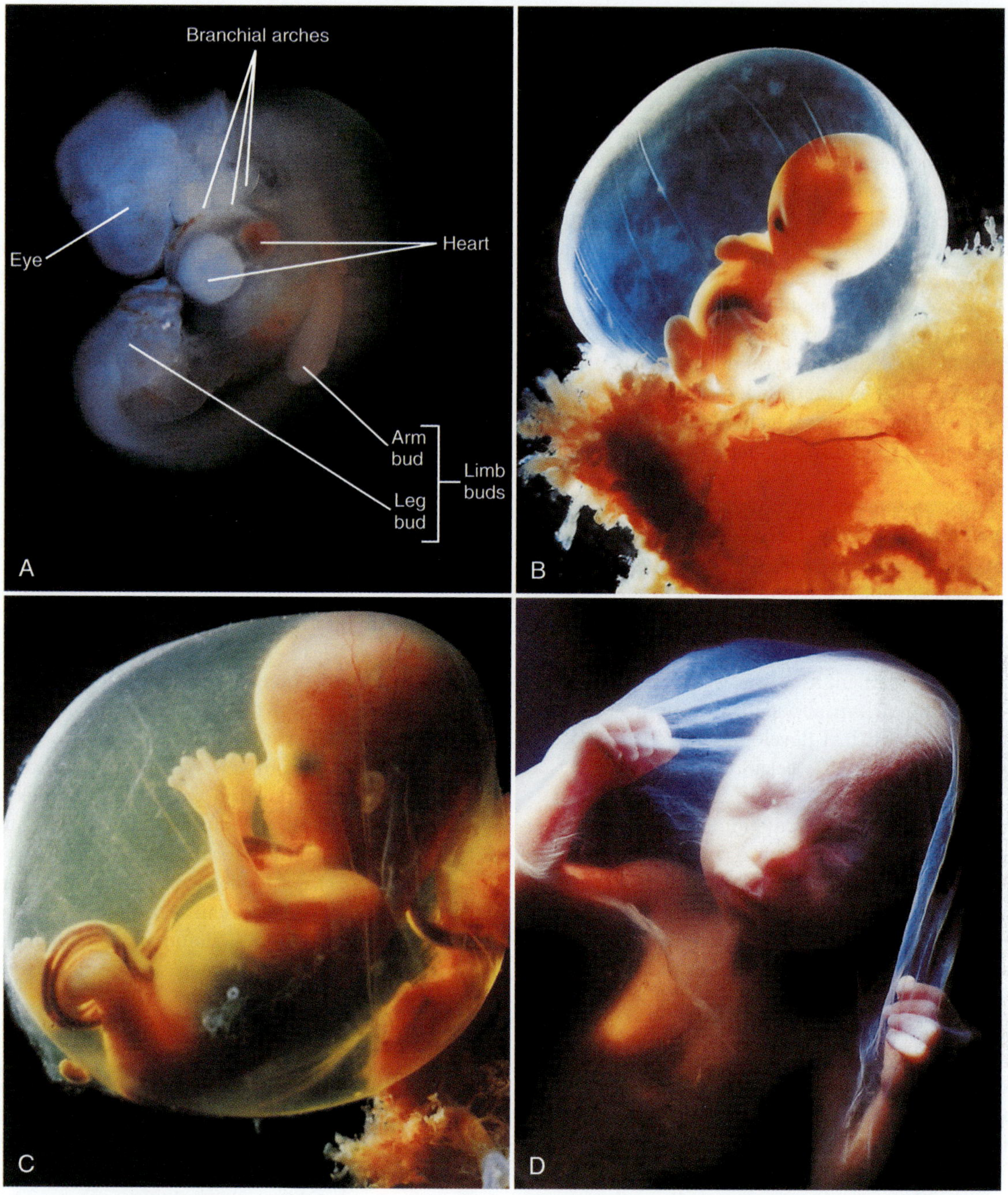

FIG. 23.13 Embryonic life. (A) 35 days. (B) 49 days. (C) 12 weeks. (D) 16 weeks. (From Thibodeau G, Patton K. *Anatomy and Physiology*. 6th ed. St Louis: Mosby; 2007.)

NUCHAL CORD

An umbilical cord wrapped one or more times around the baby's neck is called a **nuchal cord.** This usually occurs with an active fetus in the early months of pregnancy, when there is plenty of room for the fetus to move. A nuchal cord is seldom diagnosed before labor, but it may be suspected if the baby's heart rate decreases markedly during contractions. If the nuchal cord is tight, blood flow through it will be constricted during contractions as the baby moves downward, causing the heart rate to slow markedly. After this, the heart rate may return to a normal range. Usually babies recover from this labor stress and are born with the cord around the neck. However, if the fetal heart rate continues to decrease markedly with every contraction and takes longer to recover to a normal rate, the baby may become too stressed to deliver vaginally. A cesarean section may be an option if delivery is still hours away. If the baby is delivered with a nuchal cord, it usually is not a problem to slip the cord over the head or, alternatively, clamp and cut it before the body is born.

LACK OF LABOR PROGRESS

During labor, the baby is expected to make steady progress through the **birth canal,** maneuvering into appropriate positions that provide the best fit for the baby's head and the maternal pelvis. Various problems can occur to impede this

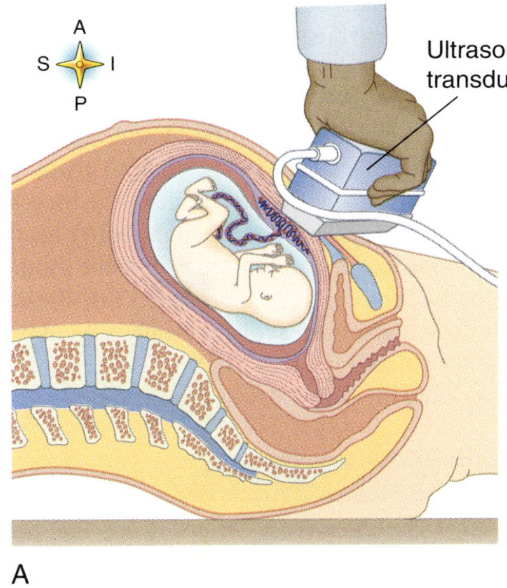

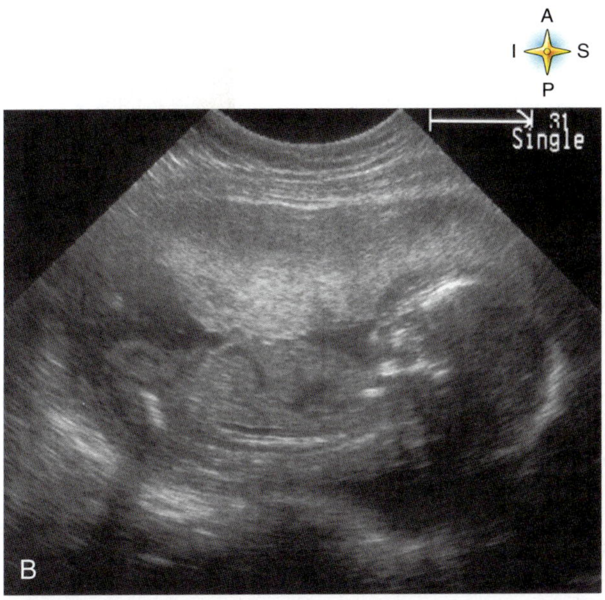

FIG. 23.14 Prenatal testing. (A) Ultrasound assessment of the fetus. (B) Sonogram of the fetus. (From Patton KT, Thibodeau GA. *The Human Body in Health & Disease*. 6th ed. St Louis: Elsevier; 2014.)

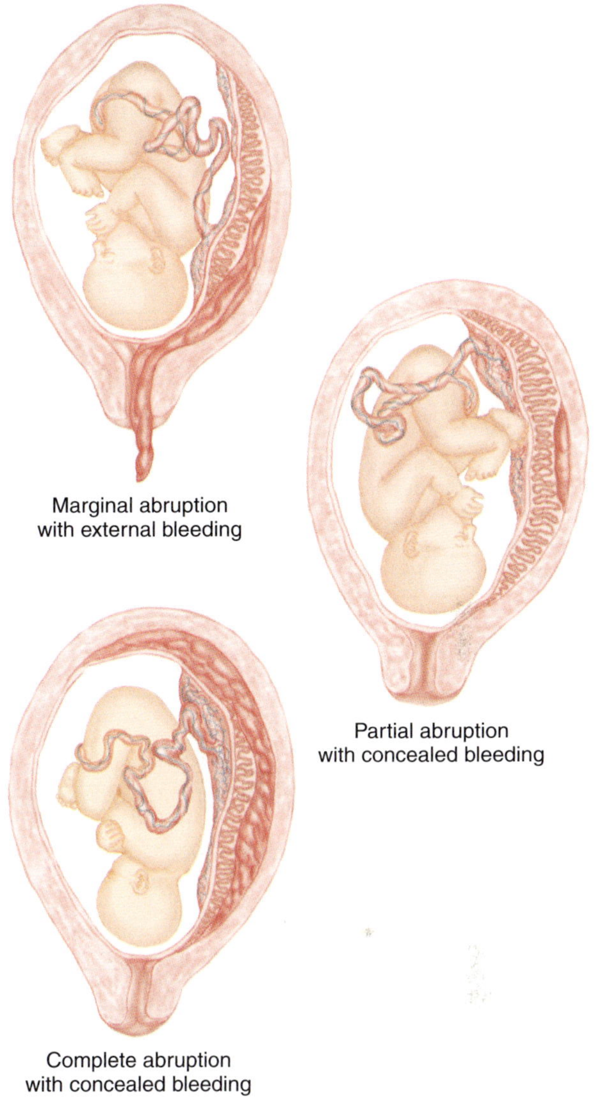

FIG. 23.15 Placental abruption. (From Murray SS, McKinney ES. *Foundations of Maternal-Newborn Nursing*. 4th ed. Philadelphia: WB Saunders; 2006.)

process. These include weak contractions, a fetal head that is not flexed sufficiently or is tilted to the side, or a fetal head that is too large to fit through a narrow maternal pelvis. Some positions of the baby's head require more room in the pelvis (e.g., babies who are "face up"). If diagnosed early in labor, maternal position changes or manual manipulations on the fetal head may help rotate the baby into a better position for descending through the birth canal. If this fails or if the baby is too large (or the mother's pelvis is too small), then progress is impeded and a cesarean section is needed.

CORD PROLAPSE

During pregnancy, membranes extending from the edge of the placenta encase the fetus as it moves in a water-filled environment as described previously. Normally, the amniotic sac remains intact until labor. When the **amniotic membranes** break spontaneously or artificially, the amniotic fluid flows out of the vagina. If the fetal head is not low in the birth canal and the membranes rupture, there is a chance the umbilical cord may be swept in front of the baby's head with the flow of water and may lodge in the vagina or even outside the vagina. When the cord precedes the head, **cord prolapse** has occurred. This rarely happens before labor begins but can persist during labor. This condition is more likely with a breech **presentation** or an excess of amniotic fluid. When the cord precedes the baby in the birth canal, it can be compressed by the baby's head as it presses against the cervix and maternal pelvis. This reduces or stops the flow of oxygen to the baby. This condition requires an emergency cesarean section. In rare cases, the birth may occur vaginally if the cord prolapses suddenly along with the amniotic sac. The baby's head then follows with the next contraction. The nurse, midwife, or physician who discovers this problem puts counterpressure on the baby's head at the vaginal outlet to reduce cord pressure while the woman

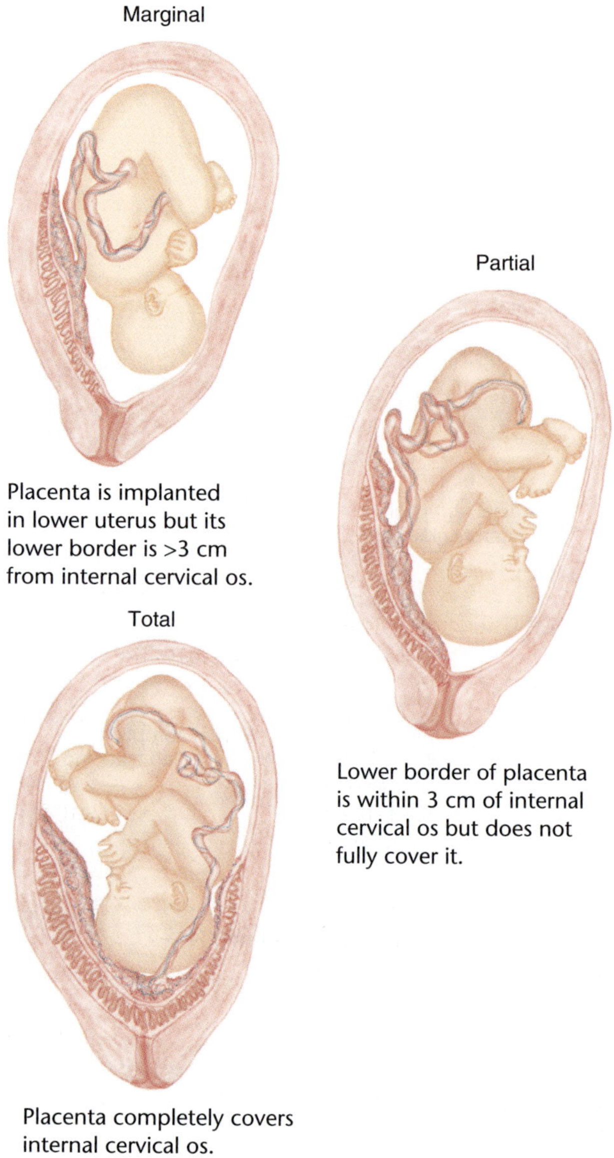

FIG. 23.16 Placenta previa. (From Murray SS, McKinney ES. *Foundations of Maternal-Newborn Nursing.* 4th ed. Philadelphia: WB Saunders; 2006.)

is quickly moved to the operating room. In case of a pending emergency, the operating room staff is notified and a setup prepared. However, there may be little time between the diagnosis of cord prolapse and the start of surgery.

BREECH PRESENTATION

A **breech presentation** occurs when the baby's feet, knees, or buttocks enter the birth canal before the head. This can be a difficult, long labor that stresses the baby and the mother. It usually is diagnosed before labor, but it may be missed. If this position is known in the prenatal period, attempts can be made to change the baby's position so that the head presents first. Before 38 weeks' gestation, the woman can try positions at home to rotate the baby. If these fail, she is likely to be scheduled for a procedure to rotate the fetus. This is called a *version.* If attempts to change the baby's position fail, a cesarean section is scheduled. Few physicians or nurse-midwives conduct planned breech deliveries. Most breech deliveries are unplanned, are imminent, or occur with a twin birth. If the fetus is not too large and contractions are consistent and strong, breech birth is possible. Dangers include a compressed umbilical cord, cord prolapse, and impinged fetal arms or head. Both physicians and nurse-midwives learn maneuvers to facilitate the breech birth, and extra hands may be called for to keep the baby's head flexed (**suprapubic pressure**), to position the bed or the mother, and to resuscitate the baby. Breech babies often are stressed and present with thick **meconium** at birth. Ideally, a good pediatric team is present to attend the birth, but if a delay occurs, assistance for suctioning the baby's airway may be requested.

DIAGNOSTIC TESTS

Pregnancy test: The pregnancy test detects the hormone human chorionic gonadotropin (HCG) either in the blood or the urine. HCG can be quantified in a blood test to assess whether the level is increasing at the expected rate in the first trimester. A pregnancy is confirmed most often by ultrasound or detection of a fetal heartbeat.

Ultrasound scans: Ultrasound is routinely used for a variety of tasks in pregnancy. It is useful for assessing fetal age if the last menses is unknown. Transvaginal ultrasound in the first trimester can determine the **gestational age** within 3 to 5 days. A diagnostic ultrasound performed at 18 weeks may be useful for identifying some types of fetal defects and confirming the gestational age. Ultrasound is commonly used in pregnancy for checking fetal growth, amniotic fluid volume, fetal position, and the location of the placenta.

Routine blood and urine tests: Routine blood and urine tests include tests that may affect the health of the present baby or of subsequent babies. These tests include the following:

- *Maternal blood type, Rh, and antibody screen:* These tests are important in the event transfusion is needed after hemorrhage. A negative Rh factor in the mother may induce her to make antibodies against her baby if she is exposed to the baby's Rh-positive blood (at birth or if bleeding occurs during pregnancy). If the mother is Rh negative, she receives anti-D immunoglobulin at 28 weeks' gestation and again postpartum if her baby is Rh positive. This prevents the formation of antibodies against future Rh-positive babies during gestation. The antibody screen also confirms the presence of antibodies to other blood types.
- *RPR (rapid plasma reagin) syphilis antibody test:* Syphilis is a sexually transmitted infection that can be passed to the baby during pregnancy. It causes a variety of defects or miscarriage, depending on the maternal stage of the disease.
- *Rubella antibody testing:* Rubella can cause severe defects or miscarriage if contracted by the mother in the first 16 weeks of pregnancy.
- *HIV and acquired immunodeficiency syndrome (AIDS) screening:* HIV infection and AIDS can be transmitted to the baby during pregnancy or birth, or through breast milk.
- *Hepatitis B:* This disease can be transmitted to the baby during pregnancy or through breast milk and may cause liver cancer if left untreated in the newborn.

- *Screening for gonorrhea and chlamydia:* These diseases can be passed to the baby during its passage through the birth canal, resulting in respiratory or eye infections and blindness if left untreated after birth. The diagnosis is made by cytological examination of a cervical smear or by a urine test.
- *Complete blood count (CBC):* This test is performed to diagnose anemia, insufficient platelets, or an increased white blood cell count indicating infection.
- *Cervical cancer screening (Pap smear):* The Pap smear is routinely done during prenatal care. It detects abnormal cells and HPV, which can cause cervical cancer.
- *Maternal serum screen:* This blood test is done at 16 to 18 weeks' gestation to screen for three or four biochemical markers in the maternal blood that indicate the baby's risk for Down syndrome, spina bifida, and trisomy 18. If the test is positive, the woman may decide to undergo amniocentesis to confirm the diagnosis.
- *Urine culture:* This culture is routinely done on the first prenatal visit to detect a urinary tract infection. Asymptomatic urinary tract infection may occur during pregnancy, and an untreated infection can lead to pyelonephritis (kidney infection) and preterm labor.

NORMAL VAGINAL DELIVERY

As mentioned, the birth of a term baby is a normal event that seldom requires intervention. The event is called a **normal spontaneous vaginal delivery (NSVD)**. The birth usually occurs in a delivery room or birthing center. In many locations, the mother can choose her position for birth, especially if she is not medicated and able to position herself. More often, she may have an **epidural** to relieve pain that may prolong the pushing phase of labor.

As the baby's head emerges, the tissues around the vagina and perineum stretch. The period for this stretching is longer if this is the mother's first vaginal birth, and lacerations of the vagina, perineum, or labia may result. If the fetal heart rate remains below 100 beats per minute and the baby's head is near delivery but not immediately delivering, the physician or nurse-midwife may incise the perineum to provide a wider opening and hasten delivery. This is called an *episiotomy*, and it requires sutures after delivery. Once the baby is born and has been dried, and the umbilical cord has been cut, the physician or nurse-midwife inspects the perineum for lacerations or extension of the episiotomy.

The placenta usually is delivered within 20 minutes after birth and may be assisted by gentle cord traction, the administration of an oxytocic drug, a maternal squatting position, or breastfeeding. After delivery of the placenta, the perineum is repaired. Lacerations or extensions of the episiotomy rarely go through the entire vaginal tissue to the rectal mucosa (fourth-degree laceration) or into the rectal sphincter (third-degree laceration). It is very common to repair a laceration that involves the muscles between the vagina and rectum (second-degree laceration) or a laceration of the vaginal mucosa (first-degree laceration). Lacerations along the side of the vagina occur less often. Repairs are done with 3-0 absorbable suture (Dexon or chromic on a tapered needle) except for rectal mucosal and labial repairs, which are done with 4-0 absorbable suture.

The ST should have a basic vaginal set and general surgery instruments. Right-angle retractors (e.g., Heaney or Sims lateral retractors) should be included. A simple closure kit includes Allis and Kelly or Crile clamps. Curved Heaney and Metzenbaum scissors, needle holders, Adson forceps, or single-toothed tissue forceps may be used for skin and subcutaneous repairs.

IMMEDIATE POSTPARTUM CARE

Postpartum care includes monitoring the status of the mother and baby during this immediate transition. During the first 2 hours, the mother's blood pressure, pulse, and respirations are assessed every 15 minutes and her temperature is taken hourly. During this time, the nurse also checks her bleeding by giving a firm uterine massage. A firm uterus means that the muscles of the uterus are tight, squeezing the small blood vessels that fed the placenta during pregnancy and thus minimizing bleeding. The mother may receive intravenous medication to increase uterine tone, which prevents postpartum bleeding.

If the mother received an epidural anesthetic, she is monitored for return of sensation and ability to mobilize. Full mobility and ability to urinate are expected within 1 hour after the anesthetic has been discontinued. As soon as she is able, she may eat and drink normally.

NEWBORN CARE

The baby usually is dried and stimulated immediately after birth. If all is normal, and the mother agrees, the baby can remain on her abdomen. The baby is assessed according to the American Pediatric Gross Assessment Record, commonly known as the **APGAR score.** This includes the following assessment parameters:

- Respiratory rate
- Color
- Reflex response
- Heart rate
- Body tone at 1 and 5 minutes after birth

A score of 2, 1, or 0 is given for each parameter. A score of 7 to 10 is considered normal; a score of 4 to 6 indicates mild to moderate depression; and a score of 0 to 3 indicates severe depression. It is important that the baby maintain a temperature of about 98.6°F (37°C). This can be done by drying the baby and providing a warm environment (e.g., a baby warmer or skin-to-skin contact with the mother or father while keeping the baby covered). Respirations, heart rate, and temperature are monitored every 15 minutes in the first hour or two. The baby is most alert in the first hour after birth and eager to suck. Breastfeeding during this time has many benefits, such as augmenting uterine contractions and facilitating bonding between mother and baby. The baby's weight and length can be obtained once the baby is warm and stable.

The immediate postpartum period is an important time for both mother and baby as they transition into a new phase

BOX 23.1 Grades of Perineal Lacerations

First-degree	Superficial laceration of the vaginal mucosa or perineal body
Second-degree	Laceration of the vaginal mucosa and/or perineal skin and deeper subcutaneous tissues
Third-degree incomplete	Second-degree laceration plus laceration of the capsule and part of the anal sphincter muscle
Third-degree complete	As above with complete laceration of the anal sphincter
Fourth-degree	Complete third-degree with laceration of the rectal mucosa

of life. Each health care facility has a set of guidelines for care. The mother's and father's preferences also should be taken into consideration. Hospital personnel can provide a supportive, calm, and private environment to assist the family while gathering critical assessments of the status of mother and baby.

OBSTETRICAL PROCEDURES

EPISIOTOMY

Episiotomy is an incision made in the perineum during second-stage labor to prevent the tissues from tearing as the baby's head and shoulders emerge from the birth canal. Perineal laceration is a recognized complication of childbirth under specific circumstances. There is inconclusive evidence to show that *routine* episiotomy (deliberate cutting of the perineum) prevents later problems of the pelvic floor. However, *selective* episiotomy after a prescribed method is beneficial in preventing sphincter injury. The recommended incision is mediolateral. This discussion explains the repair for third- and fourth-degree lacerations.

Pathology

The incidence of third- and fourth-degree perineal lacerations is associated with medial episiotomy, delivery using stirrups, and the premature use of oxytocin. Secondary associations are prolonged labor, null parity (first-time delivery), and younger age of the delivering woman. Lacerations are classified according to the severity as shown in Box 23.1.

POSITION:	Supine, knees and hips flexed
INCISION:	Mediolateral perineal
PREP AND DRAPING:	Perineal
INSTRUMENTS:	Minor set including Allis clamps, curved and straight Mayo scissors, bandage scissors, Halsted or Crile clamps, Mayo needle holders, vaginal set

Technical Points and Discussion

MEDIOLATERAL EPISIOTOMY

1. ***A mediolateral cut is made through the vestibule and lower margin of the labia major.***
The cut is made with the Mayo scissors with the operator's fingers placed between the vagina and the baby's head to prevent injury to the baby.
2. ***After delivery of the baby, bleeders are controlled.***
While awaiting delivery of the placenta, the operator clamps bleeders with Crile or Kelly hemostats. These are then ligated using 3-0 Vicryl or similar suture. The cut edges of the muscle are grasped with several Allis clamps. The ST should have several abdominal pads or lap tapes available to place pressure on the wound as needed.
3. ***After delivery of the placenta, the episiotomy is repaired.***
The muscle and fascia are closed with size 2-0 or 3-0 Vicryl suture on a taper needle. Subcutaneous tissue and skin are closed with size 3-0 Vicryl on a cutting needle.

THIRD-DEGREE REPAIR

1. ***The tear is assessed and bleeders controlled.***
Before beginning the repair, the surgeon examines the extent of the injury. The assistant or ST may apply direct pressure to the bleeding vessels. These are clamped with mosquito or sharp Crile hemostats. Suture ligatures of size 3-0 Vicryl are used to control the bleeding.
2. ***The edges of the external sphincter are clamped.***
The surgeon places multiple Allis clamps on the edges of the external sphincter. The ST or assistant uses these to apply countertraction while the surgeon assesses the sphincter digitally.
3. ***The sphincter is repaired.***
The sphincter muscle is repaired with size 3-0 Vicryl. Multiple mattress sutures are placed. Following this maneuver, the surgeon will require regloving.
4. ***Superficial tissues are closed.***
The fatty tissues are closed with size 3-0 or 4-0 Vicryl in a running stitch. Skin can be closed with a subcuticular or interrupted suture of size 3-0 Vicryl.

FOURTH-DEGREE REPAIR

1. ***The anorectal mucosa is grasped with Babcock clamps.***
A marker suture of 3-0 chromic or Vicryl is placed through the rectal wall.
2. ***The rectum is repaired using interrupted sutures of size 2-0 chromic or Vicryl.***
The external sphincter is grasped with Allis clamps as described for third-degree tear.
3. ***The fascia, fat, and skin are sutured.***
Final closure of the tissues is completed with size 3-0 Vicryl. Repair of third- and fourth-degree perineal lacerations is illustrated in Figs. 23.17 and 23.18.

CESAREAN DELIVERY

Surgical Goal

A cesarean delivery (commonly called a *C-section*) is the surgical removal of the fetus through an abdominal incision. A

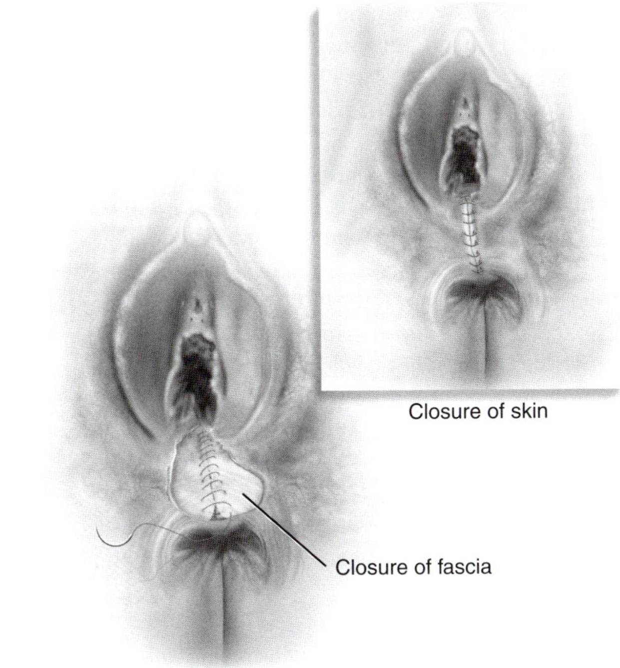

FIG. 23.17 Repair of third-degree perineal laceration. The torn sphincter muscle has been repaired with interrupted sutures of 2-0 or 3-0 Vicryl. Here, the fascia and skin are closed with size 3-0 and 4-0 Vicryl. (From Baggish M, Karram M. *Atlas of Pelvic Anatomy and Gynecologic Surgery*. Philadelphia: Elsevier; 2016.)

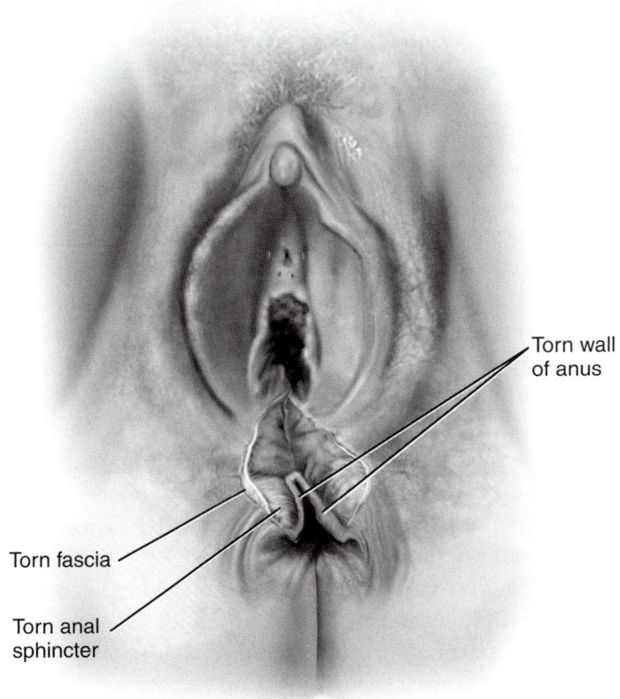

FIG. 23.18 Repair of fourth-degree perineal laceration. The rectal wall may be closed with 2-0 chromic catgut. The external sphincter, fascia, and skin are closed with size 3-0 and 4-0 Vicryl. (From Baggish M, Karram M. *Atlas of Pelvic Anatomy and Gynecologic Surgery*. Philadelphia: Elsevier; 2016.)

cesarean delivery can be scheduled, or it may be done as an emergency procedure. If the procedure is scheduled (e.g., a repeat C-section), a spinal or an epidural anesthetic is administered and a routine setup can be done. An emergency delivery occurs very quickly. If a general anesthetic is given, time is extremely critical to prevent fetal anesthesia and to correct the condition that caused the emergency. In emergency surgery, several instruments are used to start the procedure and safely deliver the baby. In many cases, lack of time may prevent a normal setup.

In emergency cases, fetal monitoring may be in place when the patient arrives, along with trained staff from the obstetrics unit. A newborn resuscitation unit is brought in along with respiratory resuscitation equipment and emergency drugs. A suction line from the operating room must be dedicated to the resuscitation unit.

Pathology

A cesarean section is medically necessary when the mother's life is in jeopardy and for obstetrical conditions that would result in fetal death. Some of these conditions are as follows:

- Transverse, breech, or other malpresentation of the fetus
- Prolapsed umbilical cord
- Ruptured placenta (placental abruption)
- Delivery of the placenta ahead of the fetus (placenta previa)
- Active genital herpes infection
- Previous cesarean section
- Cephalopelvic disproportion (the fetus cannot be delivered through the pelvis because of its shape)
- Failure to progress in labor
- Prolapsed cord
- Toxemia
- Diabetes

Technical Points and Discussion

1. ***The patient is positioned and prepped.***
   The patient is placed in the modified left lateral position. A wedge positioning pad is placed under the right hip to maintain the position and prevent aortocaval compression by the fetus. Such compression can cause hypotension of the mother because of decreased return blood flow to the heart, which may cause fetal hypoxia.

   A Foley catheter is normally already in place. The patient is fully prepped and draped before anesthesia is started. However, physiological monitoring is initiated as soon as the patient enters the operating room suite.

2. ***If the procedure is an emergency, the ST prepares essential instruments.***
   As soon as the technologist has performed hand antisepsis and donned gown and gloves, the following items, which are needed to deliver the baby, should be prepared:

   - Laparotomy drape
   - Scalpel

- Lap sponges
- Mayo clamps (four to six)
- Metzenbaum, curved Mayo, and bandage scissors
- Bladder retractor (DeLee or the bladder blade from a Balfour retractor)
- Hemostats (e.g., Kelly or Crile clamps)
- Bandage scissors
- Abdominal suction (two)
- Bulb syringe

3. ***A low transverse or midline incision is made to the level of the rectus muscles.***
The surgeon enters the abdomen through a midline or Pfannenstiel incision. The incision is carried to the muscles, which are divided by hand. Bleeders are clamped but may not be immediately ligated or coagulated, to save time.

4. ***The peritoneal cavity is entered.***
The surgeon and assistant elevate the peritoneum with two Mayo clamps. The surgeon then makes a small incision between the clamps. This incision is lengthened with Metzenbaum or Mayo scissors.

5. ***The peritoneal reflection of the bladder (bladder flap) is divided from the uterus.***
This is done with Metzenbaum scissors. A bladder retractor is placed on the lower edge of the incision, and the bladder is displaced downward.

6. ***The uterus is entered.***
A small transverse incision is made in the uterus. The ST brings the suction tubing (without its abdominal tip), bulb syringe, and bandage scissors near the wound. The uterine incision is extended with the bandage scissors. Amniotic fluid is quickly suctioned from the open uterus. The assistant applies pressure to the upper abdomen while the surgeon rotates the baby's head into view. The baby's airway is cleared.

7. ***The baby's nose and mouth are immediately suctioned with the bulb syringe or a separate suction catheter (e.g., DeLee suction catheter). The baby is removed from the uterus.***
The surgeon clamps the umbilical cord with two Mayo clamps and severs it with bandage scissors. The ST must have two blood specimen containers in hand to receive cord blood. The surgeon releases one of the Mayo clamps slightly to fill the containers. The ST caps these and passes them to the circulator. The baby is handed to the resuscitation team and placed in the warming unit. The baby is again suctioned and dried, oxygen is administered as needed, and the baby is assessed. The baby is taken to the nursery or intensive care unit.

8. ***The placenta is delivered.***
The surgeon removes the placenta manually. The ST should have a large basin available to receive the placenta. The surgeon will examine the placenta to ensure that it is intact. The remaining fluid and blood are suctioned from the wound. A sponge count is taken.

9. ***The uterus is closed in layers and bladder flap reattached.***
The surgeon controls bleeders with the ESU or suture ties. When the wound is clean and dry, the remaining layers are closed. The surgeon grasps the edges of the uterus with sponge forceps, Duval lung clamps, or Collin tongue clamps. These atraumatic clamps prevent maceration of the uterine tissue during closure. The uterine incision is closed in two layers with size 0 running absorbable suture. The bladder flap is closed with a running suture of 2-0 or 3-0 absorbable suture on a taper needle.

10. ***A tubal ligation procedure may be performed.***
Tubal ligation is described earlier in this chapter.

NOTE *Some surgeons use an intramyometrial injection of oxytocin (directly into the uterine muscle) to control postpartum hemorrhage.*

11. ***The abdominal layers are closed.***
The abdomen is closed in routine fashion. A flat gauze dressing is applied to the incision.

A cesarean delivery is shown in Fig. 23.19.

KEY CONCEPTS

- Pelvic or transvaginal ultrasound is commonly used to assess the reproductive system and the stages of pregnancy. Ultrasound is also used during pregnancy to detect fetal abnormalities, gender, and gestational age.
- Key diagnostic procedures in gynecology are important to patient care and may also involve a surgical procedure.
- Many gynecological procedures are performed laparoscopically, although some require open surgery depending on the condition of the patient.
- Transcervical procedures are performed to access the uterine cavity.
- Transvaginal procedures are performed to access the peritoneal cavity and for surgery of the vagina itself.
- A subtotal hysterectomy is the surgical removal of the uterus but not the cervix.
- Total hysterectomy is removal of the uterus and cervix.
- Radical hysterectomy is removal of the uterus, cervix, fallopian tubes, and ovaries. Lymph nodes may also be removed.
- Most major gynecological procedures require the use of a sequential compression device (SCD) for the patient. All procedures in lithotomy require SCD or antiembolism stockings.
- Many pelvic procedures in gynecology require the use of a uterine manipulator. This is inserted after the vaginal prep.

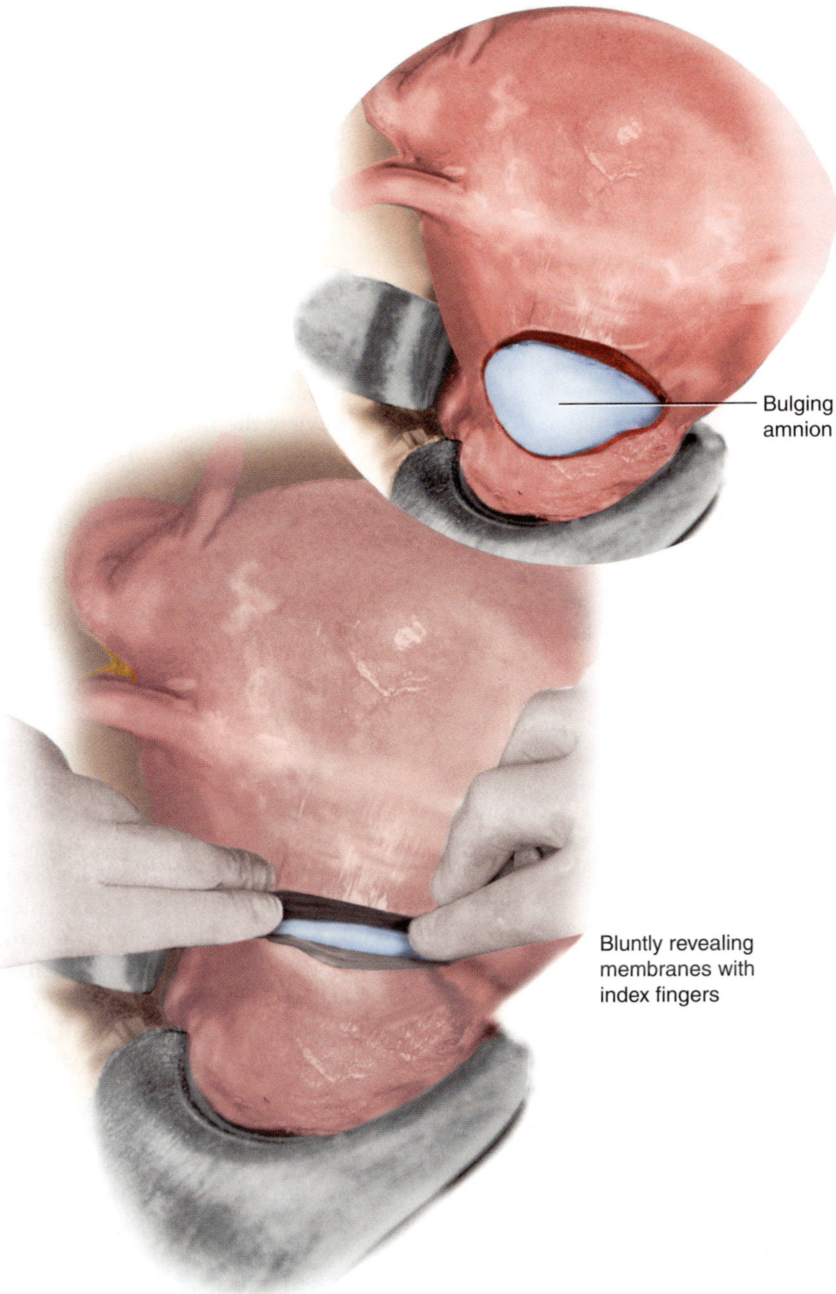

FIG. 23.19 Cesarean delivery. (A) A small incision is made in the lower uterine segment. (B) The incision is extended. (C) The membranes are ruptured and the infant's head is visible. Delivery can be performed. (From Baggish MS, Karram M. *Atlas of Pelvic Anatomy and Gynecologic Surgery*. Philadelphia: Elsevier; 2016.)

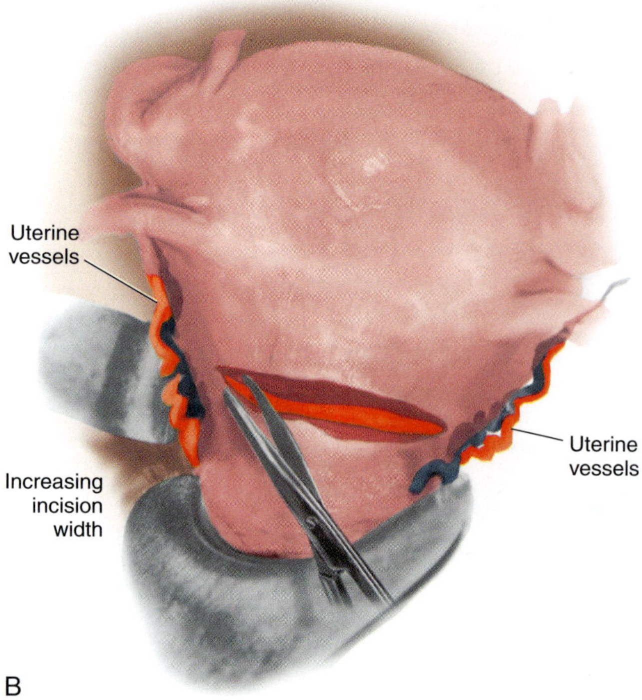

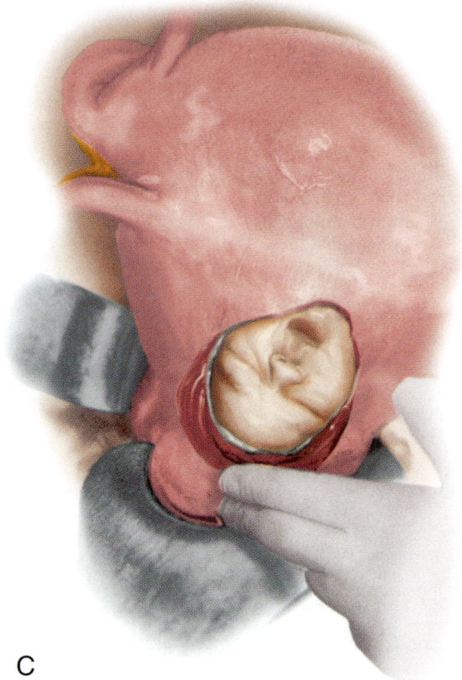

FIG. 23.19, cont'd

- Distention medium is used during hysteroscopic procedures to provide a clear view of the endometrial anatomy and distention of the uterus. The selection of distention fluid is critical to patient safety.
- During emergency gynecological procedures, it is very important to maintain a neat setup so that instruments and supplies can be located and passed quickly and smoothly.

REVIEW QUESTIONS

1. What is the rationale for performing the perineal prep ahead of the abdominal prep in combined access procedures?
2. Discuss uterine distention solutions used for high-frequency bipolar surgery and monopolar surgery. What is the rationale for using nonelectrolytic versus electrolytic solutions in each case?
3. Why does the uterine distention fluid have to be closely monitored during hysteroscopy?
4. List the risks of the lithotomy position and the precautions needed to prevent patient injury.
5. Review the imaging system components for laparoscopy found in Chapter 20. List the components and their basic uses.
6. What is the risk of allowing an ovarian cyst to rupture into the pelvic cavity during surgery?
7. Babcock clamps usually are required for any surgery of the fallopian tubes. Why wouldn't a Kocher clamp be used instead?
8. During laparoscopy and removal of tissue, such as a morcellated tumor or an ovarian cyst, a specimen retrieval bag is used to remove the specimen from the abdomen. What size trocar is needed when a specimen retrieval bag is used?
9. Radical abdominal and pelvic procedures, such as pelvic exenteration and the Whipple procedure, are performed much less often now than they were several years ago. What do you think are the reasons for this?
10. Consider a situation in which you are called to ST for an emergency cesarean section. What is the minimum instrumentation and equipment you should have ready when the mother is brought into the operating room? Assume that your instrument tray is open and the Mayo stand is draped, but you have no instruments on the Mayo stand. The surgeon is ready to start; you have approximately 4 minutes to prepare for abdominal entry and removal of the baby.

REFERENCES

1. Agency for Healthcare Research and Quality. *Cerclage for the Management of Cervical Insufficiency*; 2014, https://www.guideline.gov/summaries/summary/47771. Accessed April 13, 2020.
2. Centers for Disease Control and Prevention. *Sexually Transmitted Diseases Surveillance*. Chlamydia; 2007. http://www.cdc.gov/std/stats07/chlamydia.htm. Accessed April 13, 2020.

BIBLIOGRAPHY

Baggish M, Karram M, eds. *Atlas of Pelvic Anatomy and Gynecologic Surgery*. Philadelphia: Elsevier; 2016.

Murray SS, McKinney ES, Gorrie TM. *Foundations of Maternal–Newborn Nursing*. 3rd ed. Philadelphia: WB Saunders; 2002.

Porth CM. *Pathophysiology: Concepts of Altered Health States*. 9th ed. Philadelphia: Lippincott Williams & Wilkins; 2004.

GENITOURINARY SURGERY 24

LEARNING OBJECTIVES

After studying this chapter, the reader will be able to:

1. Identify key anatomical structures of the genitourinary system
2. Discuss common diagnostic tests and procedures of the genitourinary system
3. Discuss specific elements of case planning for genitourinary surgery
4. Describe common pathology of the genitourinary system
5. List and describe common genitourinary procedures

TERMINOLOGY

Arteriovenous fistula (or AV shunt): Surgically created vascular access for patients undergoing hemodialysis.

Calculi: Stones caused by the precipitation of minerals, such as calcium, and other substances from the kidney filtrate.

Extracorporeal shock wave lithotripsy (ESWL): A procedure in which ultrasonic sound waves are used to morcellate kidney or gallbladder stones.

Foley catheter: A retention catheter with an expandable balloon at the distal end.

Glomerular filtration rate (GFR): An indication of kidney function in which serum creatinine (normally filtered by the kidney) is measured.

Indwelling catheter: A urethral or ureteral catheter that is left in place for continuous drainage.

Meatotomy: A procedure in which a small incision is made in the urethral meatus to relieve a stricture.

Percutaneous: A term for a procedure that is performed "through the skin." For example, in percutaneous nephroscopy, the nephroscope is inserted into the kidney through a skin incision.

Reflux: Flow of a body fluid in the direction opposite its normal path.

Resectoscope: An instrument used to cut and coagulate tissue piece by piece. It is used in conjunction with endoscopic procedures to remove tumors or other tissue, such as the prostate.

Retrograde pyelography: Imaging studies of the renal pelvis in which a contrast medium is instilled through a transurethral catheter. Retrograde refers to flow, which is opposite the normal direction.

Specific gravity: The ratio of the density of a fluid compared to water. The specific gravity of urine is an important diagnostic tool.

Staghorn stone: A large, jagged kidney stone that forms in the renal pelvis.

Stent: A supportive catheter that is placed in a duct or tube to allow fluids to pass through while the duct heals.

Tamponade: A device that puts pressure on tissue to control bleeding.

Torsion: Twisting of an organ or a structure on itself. Torsion may cause local ischemia and necrosis.

Transurethral: Surgical access through the urethral orifice.

Genitourinary (GU) surgery includes procedures of the urethra, bladder, ureters, kidneys, and male reproductive system (i.e., the testicles, penis, and accessory structures). Three common approaches are used in GU surgery:

- ***Transurethral** surgery:* Surgery that is performed through a flexible or rigid fiber-optic endoscope inserted through the urethra. This provides direct access to the lower urinary tract, including the urethra, bladder, prostate gland, and ureters.
- *Open surgery:* Surgery that is performed through an open incision in the abdomen (including the retroperitoneum) or flank. Many procedures that were formerly performed using the open technique can now be performed using minimally invasive techniques.
- *Minimally invasive surgery:* Closed procedures that are performed using **percutaneous** (through the skin) endoscopic techniques, such as laparoscopy and nephroscopy.

NOTE *GU procedures performed exclusively in children are discussed in Chapter 33.*

SURGICAL ANATOMY

RETROPERITONEAL CAVITY

The *retroperitoneal cavity* (also referred to as the retroperitoneal *space*) lies posterior to (behind) the peritoneal cavity. Unlike the viscera of the abdominal cavity, the organs in this space are embedded in dense muscle, fascia, and fatty tissue. These connective tissues support the structures and protect them from injury. The retroperitoneal space is covered on the anterior side by the *retroperitoneum*, a serous (fluid-producing) membrane. Surgical access to the organs in the retroperitoneum is through the abdominal peritoneum or flank.

KIDNEY

The kidneys are the primary organs for filtration of the blood. Normally, two kidneys are located in the retroperitoneal cavity at the level of the 12th thoracic vertebra (Fig. 24.1). The right kidney usually sits lower than the left. The kidneys are supported by dense fascia and fatty tissue.

Two main tissue layers make up the kidney: the outer layer, the *cortex*; and the inner layer, the *medulla*. The cortex is covered with strong fibrous tissue called *Gerota's capsule* and contains portions of the microscopic tubules that filter the blood. The medulla is composed of 8 to 12 large collecting areas called the *renal pyramids*.

A notched area on the medial side of each kidney is called the *hilum*. The ureter, renal artery, and vein emerge from this area. At this point the ureter opens into the *renal pelvis* of the kidney, which branches into sections called *renal calyces* (Fig. 24.2).

Nephron

Although the kidney appears as a dense, continuous tissue, the microscopic structure is extremely complex. Each kidney has about 1 million filtering units, called *nephrons*. Each nephron communicates directly with the vascular system through a capillary structure called the *glomerulus*. The glomerulus is composed of a vast system of microscopic tubules that communicate directly with the capillaries to filter the blood. The capillary network of each nephron is contained within a space called the *Bowman capsule* (Fig. 24.3). This structure is closely related to the nephron tubules where filtering takes place. The juxtaglomerular cells in the Bowman capsule release *renin*, which is necessary for the regulation of blood pressure.

Blood flows into the capillary network through the efferent arteriole of the glomerulus. As the blood circulates through the microscopic capillaries, fluid (glomerular filtrate) moves selectively into the Bowman capsule. Proteins and cells remain in the blood, but other substances cross the arterial membrane and enter the capsule. The filtrate then

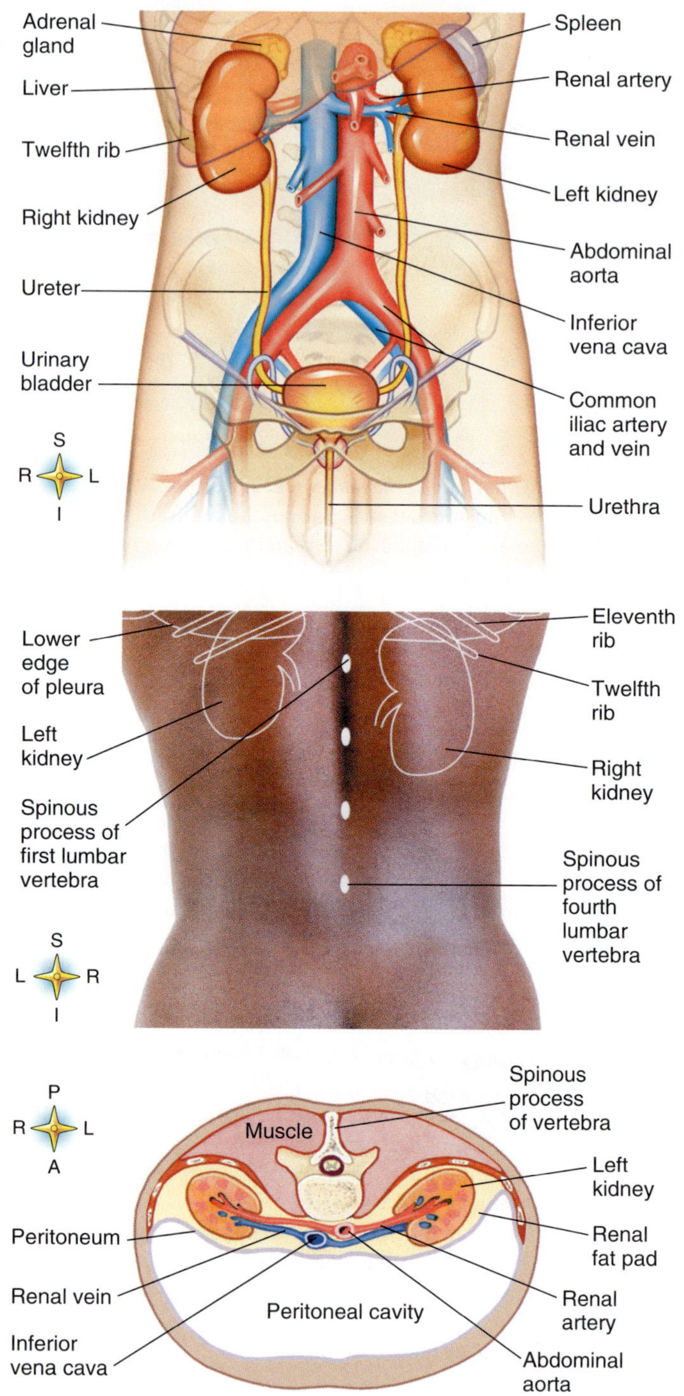

FIG. 24.1 The kidneys, ureters, and associated blood vessels lie in the retroperitoneal cavity. (From Abrahams P, Hutchings RT, Marks SC. *McKinn's Color Atlas of Human Anatomy*, 4th ed. St Louis: Mosby; 1999.)

moves into the nephron tubules. The glomerulus can filter about 125 mL per minute. This is referred to as the **glomerular filtration rate (GFR).**

Formation of Urine

Filtrate is continually refined as it moves through the tubules. Each renal tubule has a parallel capillary. Substances are selectively moved from the blood into the tubules (a process called *secretion*) and from the tubules into the blood (called

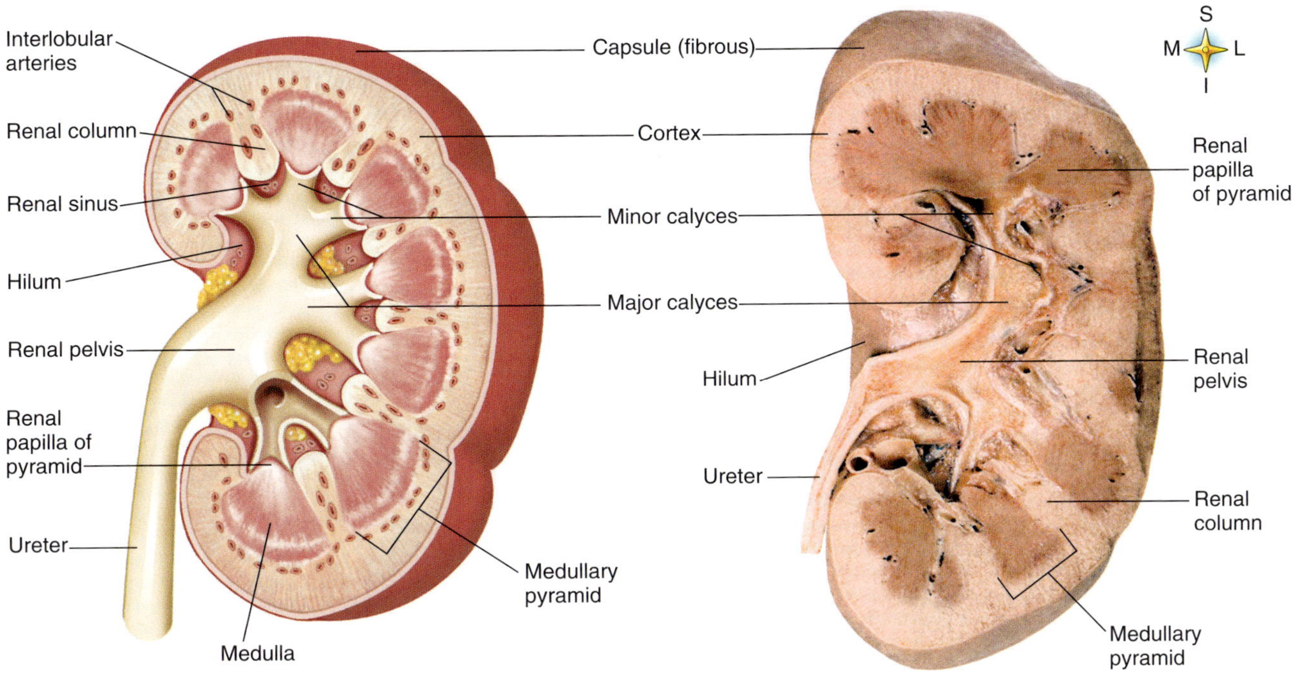

FIG. 24.2 The kidney, showing the layers, pyramids and collecting tubules, and ureter. (From Brundage DJ. *Renal Disorders*. St Louis: Mosby; 1992.)

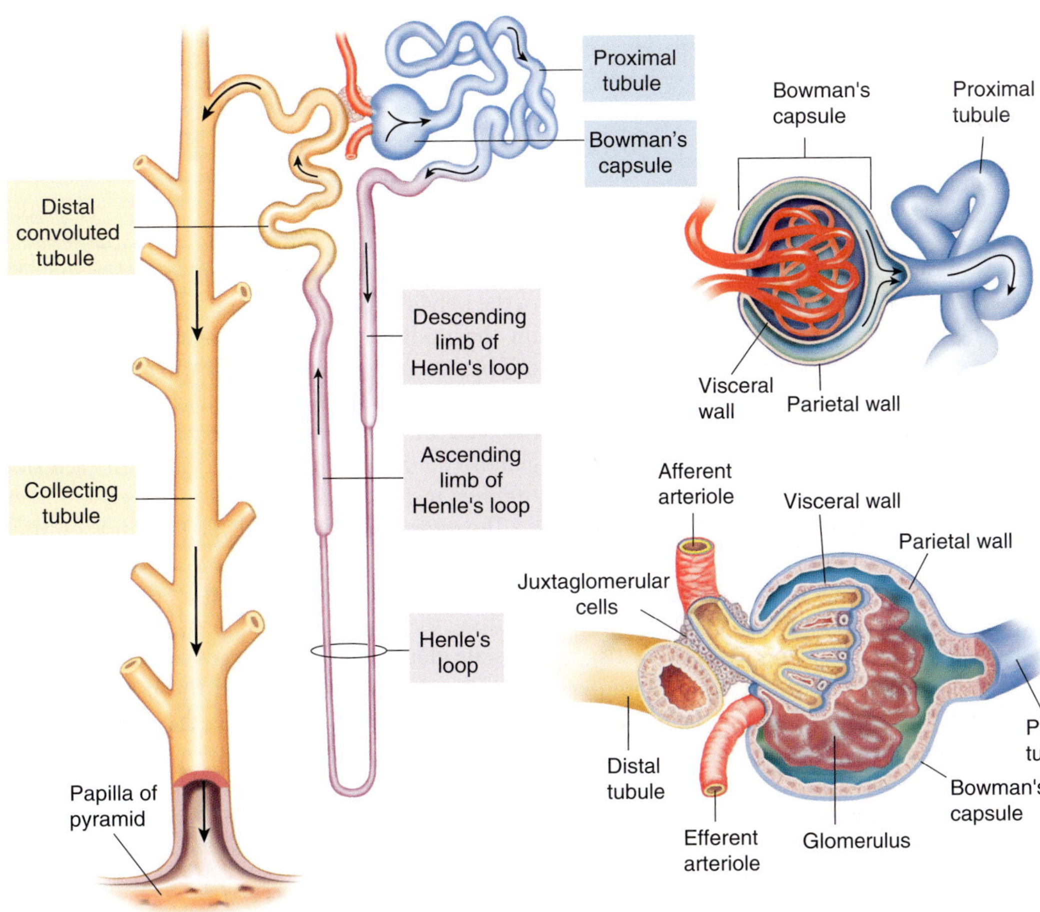

FIG. 24.3 The nephron and Bowman capsule. (From Brundage DJ. *Renal Disorders*. St Louis: Mosby; 1992.)

absorption) according to osmolality (solutes contained in the fluid) and membrane permeability. This is why diseases of the circulatory system, such as hypertension or arteriosclerosis, can affect the kidneys and damage this delicate transport system.

As filtrate moves through the tubules, electrolytes, nonorganic salts, and water, which the body needs to maintain homeostasis, are absorbed from the filtrate back into the circulatory system. The tubule system is divided into specific regions, which filter certain substances. These regions are called the *proximal tubule*, the *loop of Henle*, and the *distal convoluted tubule*.

From the renal tubules, the filtrate enters the *renal calyces* (sing., *calyx*) and renal pelvis, which communicates directly with the *ureters*. The ureters are the collection and transport areas for filtrate. Each ureter carries filtrate into the bladder. Once it enters the bladder, the filtrate is referred to as *urine*. Urine is excreted from the body through the *urethra*. Filtrate and urine are sterile throughout the length of the system; they become *potentially* contaminated by the environment in the periurethral areas, such as the distal urethral orifice (Fig. 24.4).

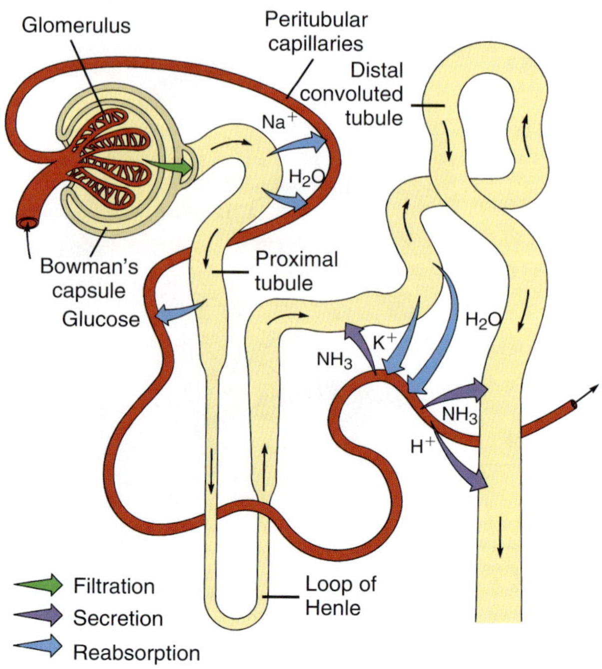

FIG. 24.4 Urine formation. As filtrate moves through the tubules, electrolytes, salts, and water are absorbed from the filtrate back into the circulatory system. The tubule system is divided into specific regions, which filter certain substances. These regions are called the *proximal tubule, the loop of Henle*, and the *distal convoluted tubule*. (From Patton KT, Thibodeau GA. *The Human Body in Health & Disease*, 6th ed. St Louis: Elsevier; 2014.)

ADRENAL GLANDS

The *adrenal glands* are paired organs that lie on the medial side of the upper kidney. The gland has two layers, the outer cortex and the inner medulla. The adrenal glands secrete glucocorticoids, mineralocorticoids, and adrenal sex hormones. Blood is supplied to each gland by the aorta and branches of the renal and inferior phrenic arteries. The adrenal glands are important in the production of norepinephrine and epinephrine, which are necessary for functioning of the autonomic nervous system.

URETERS

In adults, each ureter is about 12 inches (30 cm) long and about 5 mm in diameter. The ureter is a three-layered tubular structure; it has an outer fibrous layer, a middle muscular layer, and an inner mucosal layer. Urine moves along the ureter by *peristalsis*, which is the segmental contraction and relaxation of the ureter's muscular layer.

Each ureter enters the bladder at the *ureterovesical junction (UVJ)*, which is located in the lower bladder.

URINARY BLADDER

The urinary bladder lies behind the symphysis pubis in the pelvic cavity. The wall of the bladder is composed of four tissue layers: the outer serosa, the muscular layer, the submucosa, and the inner mucosa. The distal portion of the bladder is called the *trigone*. This triangular region has both superficial and deep muscle layers. The superficial layer extends into the bladder neck of the female and into the proximal portion of the urethra in the male. The trigone has three corners that correspond with the two ureteral openings and one urethral opening (Fig. 24.5).

Urine is excreted from the bladder by the process of *micturition* (urination), which is activated by sphincter muscles in the bladder neck. These muscles are controlled by the autonomic nervous system, which maintains retention or release of urine.

URETHRA

The *urethra* communicates with the lower bladder to enable excretion of urine from the body. *In the female*, it exits the bladder at the trigone and is embedded in the levator muscles of the pelvic floor. The urethral opening, the *meatus*, is located on the midline of the labia near the clitoris. The proximal urethra is composed primarily of smooth muscle tissue. The periurethral muscles on the pelvic floor support the distal urethra and aid in sphincter control. Two small, mucus-secreting glands (the *Skene glands*) are located on each side of the urethra just inside the meatus.

The *male urethra* exits the bladder and continues to the end of the penis, terminating at the urethral meatus. The male urethra is divided into several distinct parts. The *prostatic urethra* begins at the bladder neck and passes through the center of the prostate gland, which surrounds the urethra distal to the bladder. The midportion is called the *membranous urethra*. The distal, or *cavernous*, urethra is the distal end, which extends the length of the penis.

REPRODUCTIVE STRUCTURES OF THE MALE

SCROTUM AND TESTICLES

The *scrotum* is a layered tissue sac that encases the testicles. The skin of the scrotum contains numerous folds, or *rugae*,

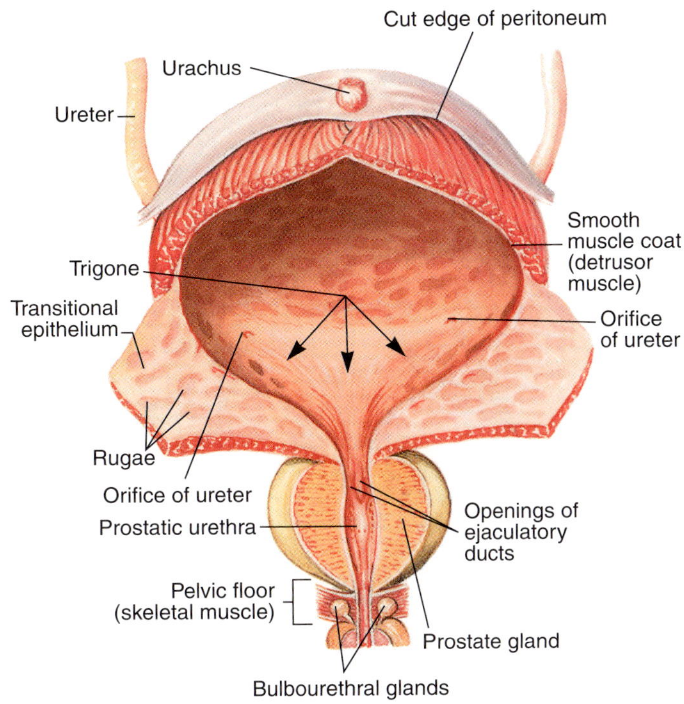

FIG. 24.5 Structures and tissue layers of the bladder in the male. Note the position of the prostate gland, which surrounds the prostatic segment of the urethra. (From Monahan FD et al. *Phipps' Medical-Surgical Nursing: Health and Illness Perspectives*. 8th ed. St Louis: Elsevier; 2007.)

and is continuous with the perineum. The inner layer of the scrotum is composed of fascia and dartos muscle. In cold environments, the dartos retracts the testicles closer to the body; it relaxes when the ambient temperature is warm. This temperature regulation system protects the *spermatozoa* (male reproductive cells) produced by the testicles.

The testicles are enclosed within a fibrous membrane called the *tunica vaginalis*. A septum in the scrotum separates the two testicles. The internal structure of the testicle is composed of tightly coiled tubules and ducts that produce sperm. The smallest units of this ductal system are the *seminiferous tubules*. Testosterone, the primary male sex hormone, is produced in these tubules, which communicate with the larger efferent ductules, epididymis, and vas deferens. The vas deferens exits the testicle at the superior end and joins the ejaculatory structures of the pelvis.

EPIDIDYMIS

The *epididymis* is a convoluted duct that secretes seminal fluid, the liquid substance that gives sperm mobility through the male reproductive tract.

VAS DEFERENS

The *vas deferens* joins the epididymis with the ejaculatory duct. It passes through the inguinal canal in the abdominal wall at the level of the internal ring. At this level, it lies inside the spermatic cord, a strong tubular structure that includes nerves, blood vessels, and lymphatic tissue. The vas deferens continues across the bladder and ureter, where it meets the opening of the seminal vesicle and forms the ejaculatory duct. The paired ejaculatory ducts traverse the prostate gland and terminate at the urethra.

SEMINAL VESICLES

The seminal vesicles are paired structures situated close to the ejaculatory duct at the proximal end. These vesicles (sac-like structures) secrete approximately 60% of the semen (the ejaculatory fluid containing sperm).

PROSTATE GLAND

The *prostate gland* surrounds the urethra and secretes an alkaline fluid that contributes to seminal fluid. The gland is divided into six lobes covered by a fibrous *prostatic capsule*. The function of the prostate is production of some components of seminal fluid. The prostate gland surrounds the prostatic urethra. Consequently, diseases of the prostate are likely to affect the urethra and the process of urination.

BULBOURETHRAL GLANDS

The bulbourethral glands (also called *Cowper glands*) are paired structures that lie just below the prostate on each side of the urethra. These glands secrete mucus, which contributes to the total volume of the semen.

PENIS

The penis is suspended at the pubic arch by fascia. The body of the penis is composed of several columns of tissue. Two dorsal columns, called the *corpora cavernosa* (sing., corpus

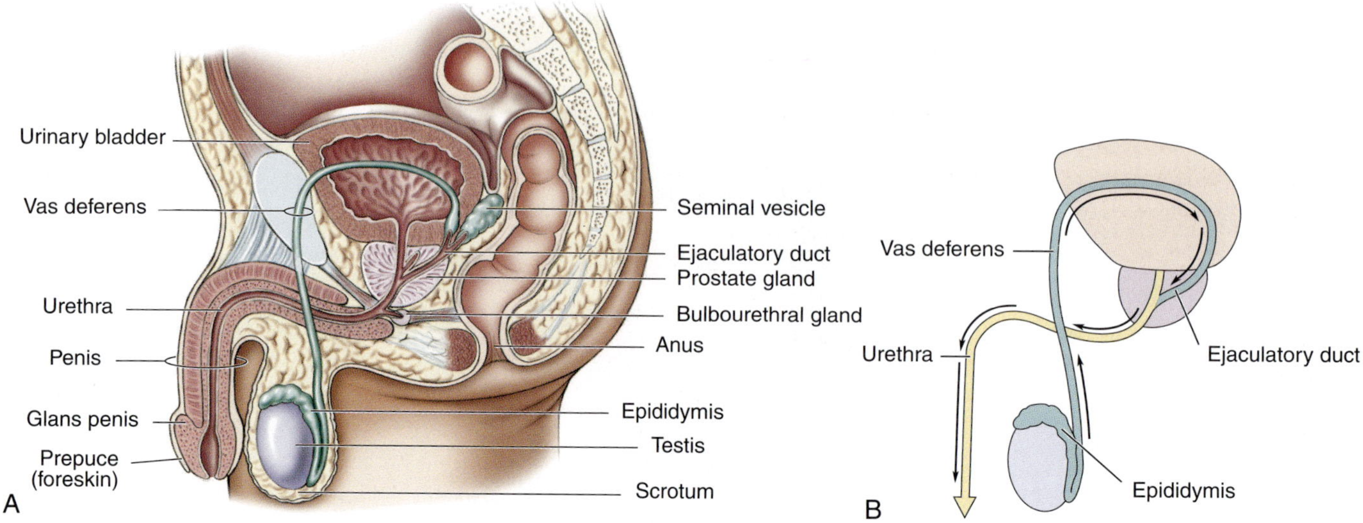

FIG. 24.6 The male reproductive system. (A) Cross-section of the pelvic cavity and male reproductive organs. (B) Schematic showing the path of the ejaculatory duct, vas deferens, and urethra. (From Herlihy B, Maebius NK. *The Human Body in Health and Disease*. 2nd ed. Philadelphia: WB Saunders; 2003.)

cavernosum), are composed of spongy vascular tissue necessary for functional erection of the penis. The columns are separated by a septum and bound together by a fibrous sheath. A third tissue column, called the *corpus spongiosum*, encloses the urethra. The distal portion of the corpus spongiosum forms the *glans penis*, which is covered by skin called the *prepuce* or *foreskin*. Fig. 24.6 illustrates the male reproductive system.

DIAGNOSTIC PROCEDURES

Many laboratory tests in GU disease focus on the presence or absence of substances found in the blood and urine. Imaging tests are performed to outline the structures of the GU system, to observe its function, and to detect tumors. Structural pathology of the genitourinary system is diagnosed by cystoscopy, computed tomography (CT) scanning, and enhanced imagery.

URINALYSIS

In a healthy adult, the kidneys produce about 3.2 pints (1.5 L) of urine per day. The main components of urine are water (95%) and solutes (5%). Urinalysis is performed to detect specific substances, both normal and abnormal, in the urine. Filtrate can be sampled from any location in the upper urinary tract. This is often necessary to detect abnormalities caused by disease in a specific location within the kidney or ureter. Urine is obtained directly through a catheter inserted into the bladder or by collection as it passes from the body; the latter may be a single sample or the amount collected over 24 hours.

Simple urinalysis provides basic information about substances such as the blood, glucose, and white blood cells. The physical characteristics of urine are also important. Odor, color, density, and clarity have specific clinical significance, which can help confirm disease. Microscopic examination reveals the presence of blood cells, cell fragments, and other metabolic substances. Infection of the bladder or other locations in the urinary tract may be detected by the presence of protein or blood cells in the urine. A simple dipstick test can be used for screening purposes, and urine culture and sensitivity (discussed in Chapter 6) may be performed to confirm a diagnosis and determine the appropriate antimicrobial therapy.

The presence of protein in the urine is an important diagnostic sign. Albumin is a primary protein component of the blood. Normally, the glomerulus allows very little protein to cross the capillary system and into the filtrate. Therefore albumin in the urine may be a sign of glomerulus disease. Specific tests for urine albumin are routinely performed when kidney disease is suspected.

The **specific gravity** (the ratio of the density of urine compared to water) is an important indicator of the concentration of solutes in the urine. Dissolved solutes are present after filtration in the kidney. Therefore the specific gravity provides important information about the hydration of the body and also the kidney's ability to maintain fluid balance. The specific gravity is measured with a calibrated hydrometer or urinometer.

BLOOD TESTS

The presence or absence of specific substances in the blood reveals kidney function. Expected values of chemicals and metabolic products in the blood shift in kidney disease. An increase in certain substances can mean that harmful waste products are not filtered out of the blood.

Creatinine is a normal waste product of metabolism in the muscles that is filtered by the kidneys. Serum creatinine levels are therefore measured as an indicator of kidney function.

Glomerular filtration rate (GFR) measures the rate of creatinine clearance from the blood. The GFR is measured as the amount of creatinine filtered per minute. This is an important test of kidney function. Blood creatinine begins to rise when the GFR is about 50% of normal.

Measurement of the *blood urea nitrogen* (BUN) is a test that assesses the elimination of urea from the liver. Urea is a waste product formed in the liver as a product of protein metabolism. Normally it is cleared by the kidneys. The blood urea value may indicate renal failure, but it is also influenced by protein intake, age, and hydration.

IMAGING STUDIES

Imaging studies provide the basis of diagnosis for functional and physiological disease. Imaging provides a permanent record of the shape, location, and density of structures. Selected studies can also detect stones or malformation of the tubes and ducts of the urinary system. The following imaging studies are commonly used:

- *Computed tomography (CT):* CT is the preferred method for imaging tumors of the kidney. Noncontrast helical CT is used to diagnose calculi.
- *Fluoroscopy:* C-arm fluoroscopy (real-time radiography) is used in many imaging studies.
- *Intravenous urography:* This process involves radiographic studies using a contrast medium, which is injected intravenously to obtain serial radiographs of the renal pelvis and calyces. The rate of emptying and the sizes of the ureters are also measured.
- *Kidney, ureter, bladder x-ray (KUB):* This is a radiograph of the kidney, ureters, and bladder. A KUB may be used to outline structures of the urinary system, including any stones larger than 2 mm. However, CT is now preferred for stone imaging, because stones of all types are visible, and even small stones can be seen.
- *Micturating cystourethrogram (MCU):* This study provides images of the bladder (cystography) while it is emptying. A contrast medium is instilled into the bladder via a catheter, and images are obtained during urination.
- *Magnetic resonance imaging (MRI):* MRI provides an extremely detailed assessment and is commonly used in the diagnosis of tumors.
- *Nuclear imaging:* Radioisotope scanning is used in GU studies to detect metastasis arising from a primary tumor of the prostate.
- *Retrograde ureteropyelography:* Retrograde injections are made using a catheter inserted into the ureter. A contrast medium is instilled into the catheter and viewed with fluoroscopy.
- *Ultrasonography:* Ultrasound is one of the first-line imaging techniques used in GU medicine.

KIDNEY DIALYSIS

The kidneys normally remove waste products from the blood. Without this function, the body becomes quickly weakened by toxins produced during normal metabolism. Kidney dialysis is a procedure that performs this function in patients who have lost kidney function. The two types of kidney dialysis are *hemodialysis* and *peritoneal dialysis*. Dialysis is performed regularly, or it can be done as an emergency procedure to remove ingested toxins from the blood that otherwise would lead to immediate kidney failure. Patients receiving dialysis treatment have a restricted lifestyle and frequently are facing a poor disease outcome. The extreme shortage of donor kidneys and the rigorous dialysis schedule, which determines the patient's quality of life, may lead to feelings of hopelessness and depression.

During hemodialysis, the blood is shunted into a heparinized hemodialysis machine, where it passes through a series of membranes and a dialyzing solution that filters waste and then returns the blood to the body. Blood leaves the body through an artery and is returned through a vein. Electrolytes and other substances can be added to the blood during dialysis as required according to the patient's specific physiological requirements. The process normally takes about 3 hours and is performed three or four times a week in a dialysis clinic or at home.

VASCULAR ACCESS FOR HEMODIALYSIS

For access to the vascular system, an **arteriovenous fistula** (or **AV shunt**) is created surgically. In this procedure, a major vein and artery (usually the radial) are anastomosed, or an artificial graft is implanted to connect the artery and vein. The fistula or AV shunt is used to access the vascular system during dialysis. Hemodialysis patients are extremely protective of their AV access sites and need to take precautions to prevent injury at the site. (The procedure for an AV shunt or a fistula is performed by a vascular surgeon and is described in detail in Chapter 30.)

PERITONEAL DIALYSIS

Peritoneal dialysis is performed through a silastic tube implanted into the suprapubic peritoneal space. Dialysis solution is instilled into the catheter. The solution remains in the peritoneal cavity and slowly extracts metabolic wastes using the peritoneum as an osmotic filter. The fluid then is removed. The total dwell time may be 4 to 6 hours, and the entire process can be performed by the patient.

RENAL CALCULI

Kidney stones (**calculi**) are formed by the precipitation of specific salts from kidney filtrate that has become supersaturated. Stones can become lodged in the kidney itself or can migrate into the ureters. Stones rarely form in the bladder. The crystalline structure of stones is jagged and sharp, and they cause severe pain and nausea in the patient. Most small stones pass through the urinary tract without treatment. However, stones in the upper urinary tract can cause obstruction and *anuria* (decreased or no urinary output), kidney abscess, and sepsis. Renal calculi can therefore be considered a medical emergency.

There are four main types of stones, which are identified by their chemical composition:

- Calcium oxalate or calcium phosphate stones derived from many different foods

- Uric acid stones that form when urine is overacidic
- Struvite stones made of phosphate, magnesium, and ammonium—usually related to certain types of urinary infection
- Cysteine stones derived from the natural cysteine, usually related to a genetic disorder

Stones can be removed using extracorporeal (outside the body) or intracorporeal (inside the body) techniques.

Lithotripsy is a procedure in which stones in the urinary tract are crushed so that they can be removed from the body. **Extracorporeal shock wave lithotripsy (ESWL)** is performed without surgery. Shock waves are delivered to the stone during fluoroscopy from outside the body. This fragments the stone without harming the surrounding tissue. This method is used on stones smaller than 2 cm and is less effective on cysteine and calcium oxalate stones.

Ureterostomy is used to remove the stones by an invasive procedure using one of the following methods:

- Ultrasound energy is delivered by a probe through the ureteroscope. Stones are crushed and the particles removed with graspers and irrigation.
- Electrohydraulic lithotripsy (EHL) is performed using an EHL probe. The probe delivers a spark which causes vaporization of the water around the probe and results in cavitation. Stone particles are removed using graspers and irrigation.
- The holmium:YAG laser is used to fragment the stones.
- The ballistic lithotripter uses air to apply a "jackhammer" effect on the stone, which breaks it into small pieces.

TRANSURETHRAL CYSTOSCOPY PROCEDURES

Transurethral cystoscopic procedures take place in a specialized cystoscopy ("cysto") room. This dedicated surgical suite contains the equipment needed to perform diagnostic or therapeutic procedures. Sterile supplies and other equipment are usually stored very near the operating area, and there is often a dedicated area for sterilization of scopes and accessories. The suite may also have full capabilities for general and regional anesthesia.

PERSONNEL

Most facilities employ a *cystoscopy (cysto) assistant.* This is a trained surgical technologist or nurse whose main duty is to work in this specialty. Other perioperative staff in the department may have little clinical time in the cystoscopy room and thus would not have the opportunity to learn about the specialty. The system is efficient as long as the cysto assistant is available at all times. However, if this person is absent, other staff members must take the individual's place. A written protocol is usually available for all staff members.

The *cysto assistant* may perform duties as both a sterile team member and nonsterile circulator. After donning sterile gloves, the assistant sets up the instrument table and all other sterile equipment. The urologist does not always require a scrubbed assistant; therefore, after setting up the supplies, the cysto assistant functions as a circulator during the case.

During cystoscopy, the cysto assistant in the circulating role has the following responsibilities:

1. Remain in the room at all times unless otherwise directed by the urologist.
2. Connect the nonsterile ends of the power cables or tubing.
3. Open sterile supplies for the urologist as needed.
4. Replace irrigation containers as they empty and note the number used.
5. Receive any specimens from the urologist and label them correctly.
6. Monitor the patient's vital signs every 15 minutes if a local anesthetic is used during the procedure.

After a cystoscopy procedure, the circulator has the following responsibilities:

1. Assist in transferring the patient from the cystoscopy table to the gurney and accompany the urologist or anesthesiologist to the postanesthesia care unit.
2. Transfer any tissue or fluid specimens to the designated area and record them in the specimen log.
3. Put away nonsterile supplies used during the procedure.
4. Transfer soiled equipment to the workroom and carry out proper terminal sterilization or decontamination of the equipment.

The surgical technologist may be responsible for maintaining a current inventory of surgical supplies and for communicating with manufacturers' representatives.

NOTE *Cases in which the patient needs general anesthesia or monitored anesthesia care require the presence of a registered nurse circulator. A registered nurse circulator may also be required regardless of the type of anesthesia used, according to facility policy.*

DISTENTION AND IRRIGATION FLUIDS

During cystoscopy, the bladder is distended with fluid to enhance visualization of the internal structures. Continuous or intermittent irrigation is also used to flush blood and tissue debris from the focal site during a procedure. Whenever electrosurgical instruments are used, the irrigation fluid must not contain electrolytes. Electrolytic solutions cause electrical current to disperse throughout the fluid. This reduces the electrode's ability to cut and coagulate. The distention solutions most commonly used *during diagnostic endoscopy* are *sterile water* (nonelectrolytic) and *saline* (electrolytic). Sterile water is used routinely for cystoscopy without electrosurgery. However other nonelectrolytic solutions such as sorbitol and glycine are used when a large amount of fluid absorption is expected. There are other considerations according to the specific patient profile and the procedure.

Sterile distilled water may be used during assessment of the bladder and **retrograde pyelography,** which do not require electrosurgery. Continuous irrigation is provided in 1L and 3L airtight plastic bags and closed-unit tubing. A pumping unit regulates the amount of flow. Pressure is regulated by a combination pump and pressure regulator or by gravity flow. The assistant is responsible for ensuring a continuous flow of fluid during the procedure. The solutions used in surgery are

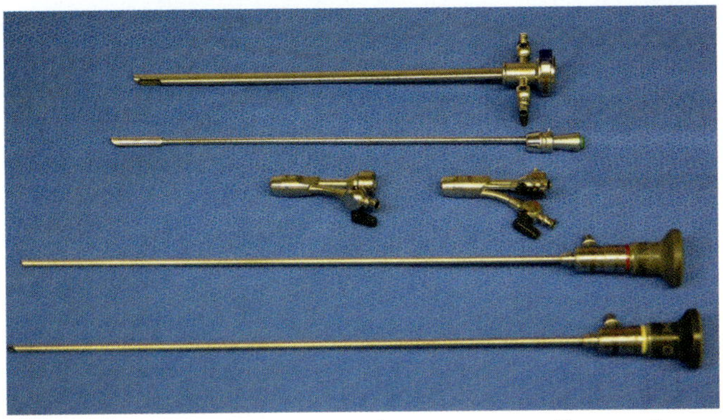

FIG. 24.7 Cystourethroscope and components. *Top to bottom:* Sheath, obturator, bridges, lenses. (From Wein A, Kavoussi L, Partin A, Peters C. *Campbell-Walsh Urology*. 11th ed. Philadelphia: Elsevier; 2016.)

stored in a fluid warmer. The warmer must be carefully maintained and checked frequently to ensure that the temperature is safe. Fluid warmers may contribute to increased hemorrhage, because the warm water suppresses or delays the body's natural clotting mechanism. Bladder spasm or hypothermia may occur when cold irrigation solutions are used. The assistant must verify the surgeon's orders for the solution type and temperature before a procedure.

FLUID WASTE MANAGEMENT

Fluid waste management is considered in the design of the cystoscopy suite because most procedures require fluid distention and irrigation. Automatic fluid waste system disposal units are a relatively recent technology in which waste fluids are channeled directly into a filtering and suction unit. There are no suction canisters, and there is no direct contact between staff and waste fluids. An alternative is a disposable fluid pouch assembly that attaches to the end of the operating table. The pouch collects fluid as it is drained from the patient and feeds it by gravity into tubing that connects directly with the facility waste system.

ACCESS AND DRAINAGE: LOWER URINARY TRACT

Rigid Cystourethroscope

Cystourethroscopy includes endoscopic procedures of the urethra and bladder. The rigid cystourethroscope is made of stainless steel and consists of a telescope (also called the *optical lens*), sheath, obturator, and bridge (Fig. 24.7). The *telescope* is the optical portion of the instrument. It consists of an attachment for fiber-optic light cable and high-quality lens system. Different telescopes vary according to their viewing angle at the tip—from 0 (in line with direct sight) to 120 degrees (backward view). The *sheath* is a hollow tube used when operating instruments or irrigation is needed. The *obturator* is a smooth rod with rounded tip. It is inserted into the sheath before passing. Its function is to dull the tip of the sheath to prevent injury to the ureter during insertion. After the sheath and obturator are in place, the obturator is removed and replaced with the telescope. The *bridge* connects the sheath to the telescope. It also has one or two working channels for carrying wires, stents, and other instruments discussed below. A commonly used bridge is the *Albarrán,* which has a lever for deflecting (bending or curving) the tip of a wire or catheter for accurate placement. The images captured by the lens are transmitted to a flat screen or a separate camera attachment. The surgeon may also directly visualize the surgical field through the lens system; however, modern digital imaging is more common.

The cystoscopy *sheath* is available in a variety of sizes measured in the French system. The diagnostic sheath is size 15 Fr and 17 Fr. Larger sheaths up to 28 Fr are used for therapeutic procedures requiring larger instruments. The rigid cystourethroscope has an irrigation channel that allows for continuous flow and removal of fluid in the bladder. Its working channels that accommodate the instruments are much larger than those of the flexible cystourethroscope discussed below.

Instrumentation for the rigid cystoscope is similar to other types of instrumentation used in surgery. Commonly used instruments are the graspers, scissors, biopsy punches, and electrodes for resection procedures and coagulation.

Flexible Cystourethroscope

The flexible cystourethroscope is similar in design to other endoscopes discussed in Chapter 20. The scope is available in digital and fiber-optic models. The *digital* model has fiber-optic capabilities built into the system, so there is no need for a separate light cable or camera. The camera is located in a digital chip at the distal end of the instrument, which feeds the images onto a flat-screen monitor. The camera is automatically white-balanced and does not require focusing. The *fiber-optic* cystourethroscope requires an external camera, fiber-optic light source, and cable, plus other routine endoscopic imaging as discussed in Chapter 20.

The flexible scope is more comfortable for the patient but is limited in its capacity to perform therapeutic procedures. The working channels are smaller than those of the rigid cystourethroscope, and the water channel is also much smaller, with restricted flow. However, the newer, smaller flexible scopes do not require dilatation of the urethra for passage. The flexible scope is available in sizes 15 to 18 Fr. Instruments used in flexible urethroscopy are generally more limited in type of number as compared with the rigid scope.

Urethral Catheters

A urinary catheter is a flexible tube inserted into the bladder through the urethra. There are many different types of catheters, which are differentiated according to their function and design. They are available in latex rubber, polyvinylchloride, or silicone. The French size of the catheter is printed on its distal end, which also bears a colored ring corresponding to its size. Catheters vary according to the type of *tip* and *design of the holes* (single, multiple). The *Coudé tip* is bent and used to traverse the urethra through an enlarged prostate. The *whistle-tip* catheter has an elongated opening at the tip. It is used for drainage or to instill retrograde contrast medium.

A *retention* or **indwelling catheter** is designed to stay in the bladder for a time period. The most common is the **Foley**

TABLE 24.1 Reference Table of Catheters, Stents, and Their Tips

Name	Characteristics	Function
Council tip catheter	Reinforced tip	Resists buckling during insertion
Coudé tip catheter	Bent tip	Negotiating through the prostate or other stricture
Olive tip catheter	Rounded distal tip larger	Ease of use—male catheterization
Ureteral access sheath	Large single sheath	Accommodates the ureteroscope, stone retrieval system. May be inflating
Ureteral stent	Flexible tube for holding open the ureter	Provides support to the ureter; provides drainage from the kidney; bypass a stone or stricture; used to carry contrast media into the kidney
Urethral catheter	Flexible tube; various tips and shapes	Used for intermittent or continuous bladder drainage; provides support to the urethra during surgery; used to irrigate the bladder; used to instill medication into the bladder
Guidewire	Stainless steel core with nitinol jacket	During ureteral access acts as the inner component of a coaxial system to insert stents, working instruments, and catheters. Types are plain guidewire or house wire, hydrophilic (glide) wire (very slippery, must be exchanged once access is gained, super stiff)
Ureteropelvic junction occlusion catheter	Balloon tip	Occludes the UPJ during lithotripsy to prevent stone fragments from entering the urethra
Percutaneous Malecot	Mushroom tip	Drainage of the renal pelvis
Illuminating catheter	Fiber-optic catheter	Used for transillumination of ureters during open or laparoscopic procedures
Biopsy needle		To obtain core biopsy
Whistle-tip catheter	Elongated opening at tip	For drainage and retrograde pyelogram

catheter. It has one or more holes in the proximal end and a balloon located near the tip. After insertion, the balloon is inflated with sterile water the catheter from backing out of the urethra. The size of the balloon varies with the type and manufacturer. The amount of water to be used in inflation is normally indicated at the proximal end. Within this category of catheters, there are other types with additional features. The 2-way Foley is the simplest retention catheter. It has a double lumen—one for inflation of the balloon, and the other for urinary drainage. The 3-way Foley has a larger balloon, either 30 mL or 75 mL. The larger balloon functions as a **tamponade**—a means of applying pressure at the bladder neck to stop hemorrhage after prostate surgery. The third lumen is used to irrigate the bladder after prostate surgery or to instill medication.

Table 24.1 is a reference that describes the specific features and names of urinary catheters, stents, and their tips.

The *intermittent* (Robinson) catheter (sometimes called a "red rubber" catheter) is used to drain the bladder one time. It has no balloon mechanism for retention. This catheter can be used to obtain a urinary specimen or to drain the bladder for other reasons such as before surgery. Fig. 24.8 shows commonly used urethral catheters.

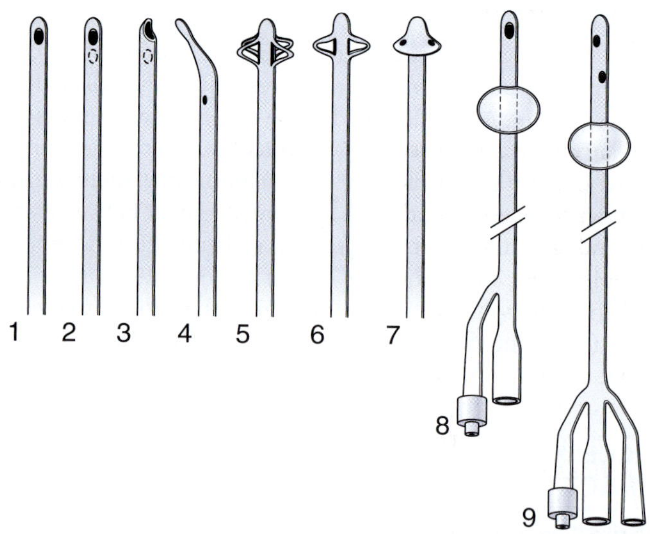

FIG. 24.8 Urethral catheters. *1*, Conical-tip catheter. *2*, Robinson catheter. *3*, Whistle-tip urethral catheter. *4*, Coudé olive-tip catheter. *5* and *6*, Malecot catheter. *7*, Pezzer catheter. *8*, Foley retention catheter. *9*, Three-way irrigation catheter. (Modified from Walsh PC, Retik AB, Vaughan ED, et al. *Campbell's Urology*. 8th ed. Philadelphia: WB Saunders; 2002.)

ACCESS AND DRAINAGE: UPPER URINARY TRACT

Ureteroscopy

The ureteroscope is used to perform endoscopic procedures of the ureter. A flexible ureteroscope ranges in size from 6.9 to 9 Fr. The flexible tip allows the scope to be positioned in the renal pelvis and advanced into the calyces. The ureteroscope has working channels for the insertion of instruments, suction, and irrigation. Irrigation fluid can be delivered through a pump or manually through the channel used for the working instruments. Sterile saline is used for most procedures that do not require electrosurgery. Water or glycine is used when electrosurgery is required. A contrast medium may be added to the irrigation fluid for a fluoroscopic examination.

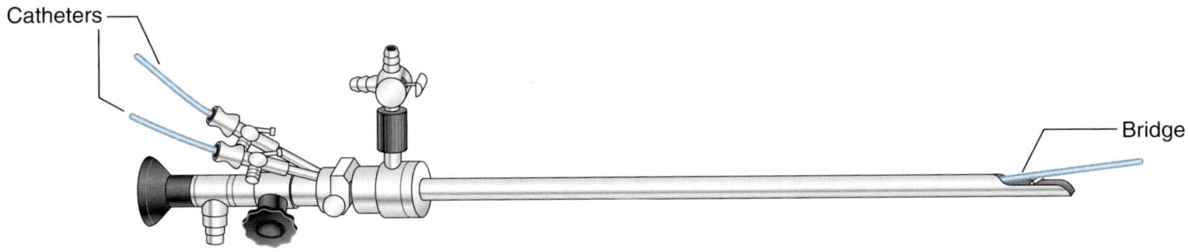

FIG. 24.9 Cystoureteroscope with stents and deflector in place. (From Garden O, Bradbury A, Forsythe J, Parks R. *Principles and Practice of Surgery*. 6th ed. Edinburgh: Churchill Livingstone; 2016.)

BOX 24.1 Ureteroscopy Instruments

- Ureteroscope
- Guidewires
- Cystoscope
- Saline for irrigation
- Connectors and tubing
- 3-way stopcock
- Syringes (20- and 50-mL)
- Contrast media
- Lithotripter (as needed)
- Grasper
- Stone basket
- Double-lumen catheter
- Ureteral dilators
- Active fulgurating electrode
- Luer-Lok connectors
- Specimen containers

The digital ureteroscope is preferred by most urologists for evaluation of the upper urinary tract. It has the same features as other therapeutic endoscopes, including an integrated camera and light source. It is slightly larger in diameter than the flexible urological endoscope.

The *semi-rigid ureteroscope* is designed to accept accessory instruments, and the scope also has designated channels for suction, irrigation, and a telescope. A small-diameter, semi-rigid ureteroscope is narrower than 7.5 Fr. Rigid and flexible scopes often are used in the same surgery, each providing functions necessary to the procedure. For example, the semi-rigid scope is used to dilate the lower ureter to allow passage of the flexible scope. It is also used to implant catheters and stents (Fig. 24.9). Instruments required for ureterostomy are listed in Box 24.1.

The ureteroscope may be inserted with the aid of a guidewire. The guidewire is passed through the scope and advanced into the ureter and renal pelvis under fluoroscopy. The ureteroscope is then advanced over the wire. The ureter may be dilated with a balloon dilator. After the scope is positioned in the renal pelvis, the flexible tip can be deflected to enter the renal calyces. Accessory instruments are threaded into the working channels to perform various types of procedures as described earlier.

Tissue biopsy is performed with cup forceps or with a flat wire basket. Cell biopsy can be taken with the cytology brush. After the specimen is retrieved on the brush, the technologist agitates the brush gently in a prepared specimen container containing normal saline to release the cells from the brush. Tumors can be removed by fulguration using the electrosurgical unit (ESU) or the holmium:YAG laser.

Stone fragments are removed from the ureter or kidney using a stone grasper or wire stone basket. In the past, stones were commonly removed from the proximal ureter and kidney pelvis using this technique. However, the procedure is seldom performed because more modern technologies used to crush stones have made it somewhat obsolete. Although stone baskets are available in many different configurations, they all function similarly. The basket is passed in closed position through the endoscopic sheath, which is passed to the level of the stone. The basket is then advanced ahead of the sheath tip and opened up. It is then used to capture the stone between the fibers of the basket. It can then be withdrawn, carrying the stone out.

Percutaneous Nephroscopy

Access to the kidney can be performed using the cystoureteroscope. However, it is sometimes necessary to perform renal endoscopy through a percutaneous approach using nephroscopy. The rigid nephroscope has a 45-degree or 90-degree offset eyepiece and is operated using standard imaging equipment. The rigid scope can accommodate several different accessory instruments for lithotripsy (stone crushing) and stone retrieval, insertion of stents and catheters, biopsy, and irrigation. Nephroscopy is performed with the patient in the prone position. The flexible nephroscope has a design similar to the ureteroscope. It is used mainly for examination of the renal calyces. Like the flexible ureteroscope, it has limitations of diameter and fluid distention but excels in its ability to reach the narrow angles of the calyces, especially in the upper poles.

Access to and drainage of the upper urinary tract is performed using stents, sheaths, guidewires, and ureteral catheters. The surgical technologist should become familiar with the most common types. This section describes the use of the devices and common names.

Stents

A ureteral **stent** is a slender, hollow tube inserted into the ureter for access to the ureter itself or the kidney. Stents are composed of polyurethane, copolymers, polyethylene, or metal. They are coated to facilitate insertion, reduce encrustation, and prevent irritation. Triclosan and chlorhexidine coatings reduce colonization of bacteria. Hydrogel coating absorbs

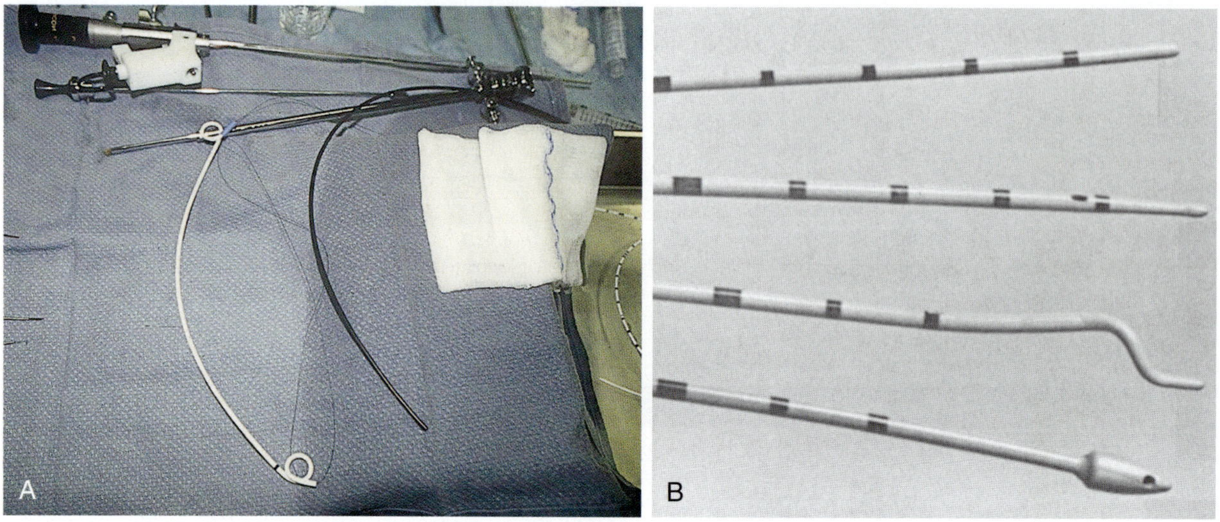

FIG. 24.10 Ureteral catheters. *Top to bottom*: Round tip, olive tip, spiral tip, and conical or bulb tip. (*A*, From Nagle GM. *Genitourinary Surgery: Perioperative Nursing Series*. St Louis: Mosby; 1997; *B*, From Walsh PC, Retik AB, Vaughn ED, et al. *Campbell's Urology*. 8th ed. Philadelphia: WB Saunders; 2002.)

water and increases flexibility of the stent. Various copolymers are also used as coatings. These are similar to the coatings used on suture material.

Stents have many functions. They can be used to relieve obstruction or bypass a stone or tumor to restore continuity in the ureter. Insertion of a stent can be an emergency procedure when both ureters are blocked, or in cases of *hydronephrosis* (swelling of the kidney because of obstruction of the ureter) or infection. A stent can also be used to enable retrograde injection of radiopaque contrast media. During the operative and postoperative phases of ureteral reconstruction, the stent is used as a splint to support the ureter.

A stent may be indwelling or temporary. Indwelling types have a curled tip at one or both ends. These are referred to as *pigtail, J,* or *double J stent*. During insertion, the stent is straightened out over the guidewire. After the stent is in position, the guidewire is removed, allowing the end to curl in the renal pelvis or bladder. This prevents the stent from migrating out of the ureter.

Specialty stents include the illuminated stent, which is composed of fiber-optic fibers. When connected to a light source, they provide transillumination through the tissues so that the ureter can be identified during open surgery. The woven metallic stent is used to support the walls of the ureter and can be left in place for many months.

A stent is inserted using the rigid or flexible cystourethroscope. A guidewire first is inserted under fluoroscopy, and the stent is inserted over it. When it is in place, the guidewire is withdrawn, leaving only the stent in place. Alternatively, the stent may be placed using only fluoroscopy. The guidewire is positioned using the cystoureteroscope. When the guidewire is seated in the correct position, the ureteroscope is withdrawn and the stent inserted over the guidewire. A *stent pusher* can be used to advance the stent along the guidewire. Commonly used stents are shown in Fig. 24.10.

Guidewire

Guidewires are an essential accessory for ureteral surgery. The guidewire is made of steel or nitinol. Some have a nitinol core with steel jacket. Guidewires are differentiated by their stiffness and coatings. Teflon and hydrophilic guidewires are also commonly used. The hydrophilic guidewire is extremely slippery and is commonly called a *glide wire*. As its name implies, the guidewire is inserted under fluoroscopy and other stents or catheters are inserted over the guidewire for precise placement.

Ureteral Dilator

The dilating *ureteral catheter* is used to increase the diameter of the ureter. There are two basic types—the balloon catheter and the solid synthetic dilator. The balloon dilator has an elongated balloon just below its tip, which is inflated once the catheter is in place. The flexible dilator is available in a set of different sizes so that the ureter can be incrementally enlarged. The *filiform* catheter is used with a *follower*. The filiform has a slender proximal end. It is inserted into the bladder. Graduated followers of different sizes are attached to the filiform sequentially. The tip of the filiform softens in the body, and the end curls inside the bladder during dilatation. The *olive tip* has a slightly enlarged bulb at the distal tip. This facilitates insertion and is often used by patients who are required to self-catheterize. These are shown in Fig. 24.11.

Lithotripsy

Lithotripsy is a procedure in which stones in the urinary tract are crushed so that they can be removed from the body. Kidney stones (**calculi**) are formed by the precipitation of specific salts from kidney filtrate that has become supersaturated. Stones can become lodged in the kidney or can migrate into the ureters. Stones rarely form in the bladder. The crystalline structure of stones is jagged and sharp, and they cause

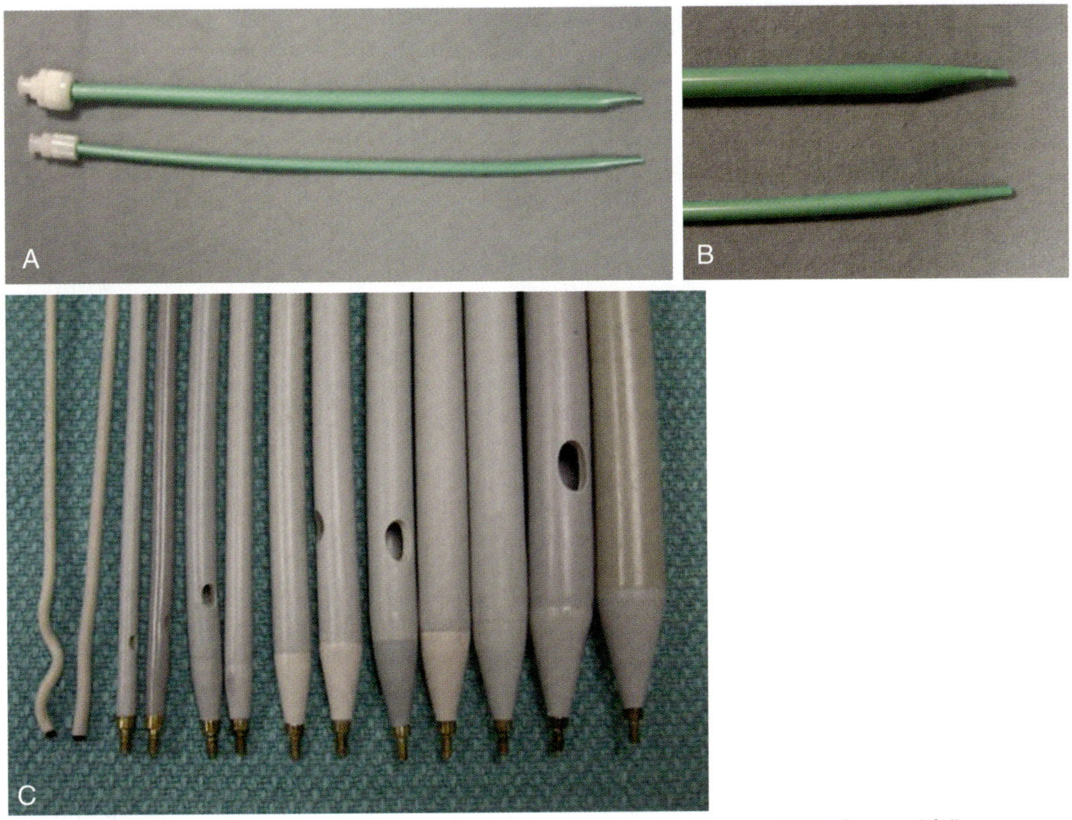

FIG. 24.11 Urethral dilators. (A) Taper tip size 12 and 18 Fr. (B) Close-up. (C) Filiform and followers. (From Wein A, Kavoussi L, Partin A, Peters C. *Campbell-Walsh Urology*. 11th ed. Philadelphia: Elsevier; 2016.)

severe pain and nausea in the patient. Most small stones pass through the urinary tract without treatment. However, stones in the upper urinary tract can cause obstruction and *anuria* (decreased or no urinary output), kidney abscess, and sepsis. Renal calculi can therefore be considered a medical emergency.

There are four main types of stones, which are identified by their chemical composition:

1. Calcium oxalate or calcium phosphate stones derived from many different foods
2. Uric acid stones that form when urine is overacidic
3. Struvite stones made of phosphate, magnesium, and ammonium—usually related to certain types of urinary infection
4. Cysteine stones derived from the natural cysteine, usually related to a genetic disorder

Stones can be removed using extracorporeal (outside the body) or intracorporeal (inside the body) techniques.

Extracorporeal shock wave lithotripsy (ESWL) is performed without surgery. Shock waves are delivered to the stone during fluoroscopy from outside the body. This fragments the stone without harming the surrounding tissue. This method is used on stones smaller than 2 cm and is less effective on cysteine and calcium oxalate stones.

Ureterostomy is used to remove the stones by an invasive procedure using one of the following methods:

- Ultrasound energy is delivered by a probe through the ureteroscope. Stones are crushed and the particles removed with graspers and irrigation.
- Electrohydraulic lithotripsy (EHL) is performed using an EHL probe. The probe delivers a spark, which causes vaporization of the water around the probe and results in cavitation. Stone particles are removed using graspers and irrigation.
- The holmium:YAG laser is used to fragment the stones.
- The ballistic lithotripter uses air to apply a "jackhammer" effect on the stone, which breaks it into small pieces.

ROUTINE DIAGNOSTIC CYSTOSCOPY

Cystoscopy of the lower urinary tract is performed with the flexible or rigid cystourethroscope (also called a *cystoscope*). Basic cystoscopy for assessment is performed as a stand-alone procedure or at the start of any transurethral procedure. As a standalone procedure it can be performed under local anesthetic or without anesthesia. Basic instruments and supplies needed for cystoscopy are shown in Box 24.2.

Indications for cystourethroscopy are shown in Box 24.3.

Technical Points and Discussion

1. ***The patient is positioned on the operating table, prepped, and draped.***
   The patient is placed in lithotomy position. A perineal prep is performed using Betadine solution or chlorhexidine. Alcohol prep solutions cause injury to the genitalia and are not used. Perineal or lithotomy drapes are used.

BOX 24.2 Basic Setup for Cystoscopy

Cystoscopy pack (gowns, towels, drapes)
Sterile gloves
Cystourethroscope
Cystoscopy irrigation tubing
Albarrán bridge
Catheter adapters
Lateral and fore-oblique telescope
Electrosurgical unit
Bugbee electrodes
Penile clamp
Luer-Lok stopcock
Water-soluble lubrication gel
Irrigation solution
Fiber-optic light source
Specimen containers
Lead aprons
Laser units (if required)
Syringes
Assorted catheters

BOX 24.3 Indications for Cystourethroscopy

HEMATURIA

1. Gross
2. Microscopic

MALIGNANCY

1. Urethral cancer
2. Bladder cancer
3. Atypical cytology
4. Upper tract transitional cell carcinoma surveillance

LOWER URINARY TRACT SYMPTOMS

1. Recurrent urinary tract infections
2. Voiding problems
3. Urinary incontinence
4. Chronic pelvic pain
5. Urethral stricture

MISCELLANEOUS

1. Trauma
2. Bladder abnormalities seen on imaging
3. Removal of foreign bodies and small bladder stones

2. ***The urethra is dilated as needed.***
   Before the scope is inserted, a water-based gel containing local anesthetic may be injected into the urethra, which is dilated to at least 2 Fr. Dilation is performed using metal dilators or sounds such as the Van Buren, Otis, or LeFort sounds. Flexible filiform dilators may also be used.

3. ***The scope is inserted and the lower urinary tract assessed.***
   The scrubbed assistant should assemble the rigid scope ahead of its use. After application of anesthetic gel, the scope is lubricated and inserted. A 30-degree and a 70-degree lens may be used. The bladder is distended using water or saline. A systematic evaluation of the urethra and bladder can then be performed. Biopsy tissue may be sampled using cup forceps or biopsy punch or brushes. The ST should remove brush cytology samples by swishing the tip in saline. Each sample is placed in a separate container or according to the surgeon's directions. The bladder can also be flushed with saline and the fluid collected for cytology. During cystoscopy, the ST will assist the urologist by directing instruments into the cystoscope and managing the distal ends to prevent them from becoming contaminated. As working instruments or catheters are removed, the assistant receives them in a way that prevents them from bending or kinking. When the procedure is completed, the instruments are withdrawn.

TRANSURETHRAL RESECTION OF A BLADDER TUMOR (TURBT)

Removal of a bladder tumor using a transurethral approach is limited to those tumors that are visible during cystoscopy. The procedure is the first stage in the diagnosis and staging of a bladder tumor. The technique used is very similar to that described for transurethral resection of the prostate. A cutting loop is used to incise and remove serial sections of the tumor, which are then retrieved from the distention media.

Pathology

Bladder cancer is a common condition, which has the highest rate of recurrence of any cancer. The most common type is that arising from the interstitial cells. However, there are many types of bladder cancer that vary in their ability to progress. Most patients present with hematuria. The disease is diagnosed using bladder washing for cytology, CT scanning, biopsy, and urinalysis.

POSITION:	Lithotomy
INCISION:	None; multiple cuts of the tumor
PREP AND DRAPING:	Perineal
INSTRUMENTS:	Flexible cystourethroscope; rigid cystourethroscope including resectoscope; mono- or bipolar cutting loops; continuous irrigation system

Technical Points and Discussion

1. ***The patient is prepared for cystoscopy.***
   The patient is prepped for a routine cystoscopy in the lithotomy position. A perineal skin prep is performed.

2. ***Flexible cystoscopy is performed.***
   Before starting the tumor removal, the surgeon performs a complete cystoscopy using the flexible cystourethroscope.

3. ***The tumor is resected.***
   Tumor resection is carried out using a 12- or 30-degree lens and **resectoscope** sheath. Continuous irrigation suitable for use during electrosurgery is used at low pressure.

The tumor is sliced piecemeal using the cutting loop at high or low temperature, depending on the size and type of tumor. If the specimen is very small, a cup biopsy forceps can be used to remove it. A specimen evacuator (Ellik or Toomey syringe) is used to remove the pieces of tumor. The ST collects these in the specimen container. After all specimens have been removed from the distention fluid, the surgeon may make a final "cold-cut" without using the ESU to send to pathology separately. This will determine whether the muscle wall is diseased. After resection, the bladder is examined for any bleeding, which is managed with a Bugbee electrode. At completion, the instruments are removed and the bladder is drained.

OPEN GENITOURINARY PROCEDURES

INSTRUMENTS

Open GU procedures require specialty and general surgery instruments. The ureters are extremely delicate and require atraumatic clamps, such as Babcock clamps. Right-angle and Schnidt (tonsil) clamps are frequently used to occlude vessels and for blunt dissection. Silastic vessel loops are commonly used to retract large blood vessels and the ureters.

Kidney procedures may require kidney pedicle clamps, which have right-angle jaws for reaching around the back of the pedicle. Vascular clamps are required for procedures involving the renal vessels or whenever temporary interruption of the kidney's blood supply is necessary. Fine-tipped needle holders and vascular forceps are used for both kidney and ureteral procedures.

Most prostate procedures are now performed using minimally invasive surgery (MIS). However, if open surgery is required, prostate retractors and grasping clamps are needed, as are right-angle clamps and general surgery instruments. Instruments for open GU surgery are shown in Genitourinary Instruments. Surgery of the vas deferens and repair of penile anomalies require plastic surgery or microsurgical instruments.

GENITOURINARY INSTRUMENTS

LOWSLEY PROSTATIC TRACTOR

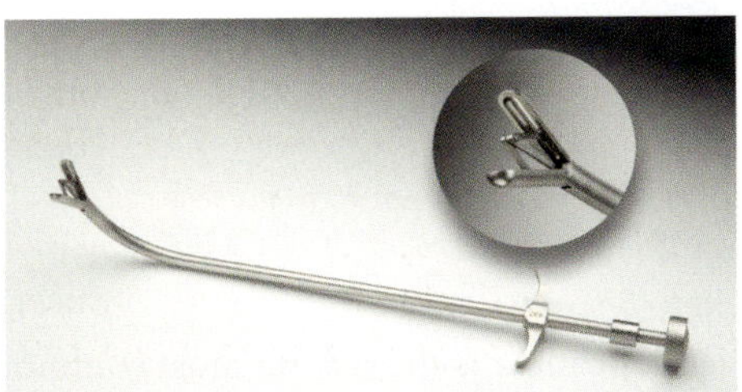

From Nemitz. *Surgical Instrumentation: An Interactive Approach*. 3rd ed. St. Louis: Elsevier; 2019.

ELLIK EVACUATOR

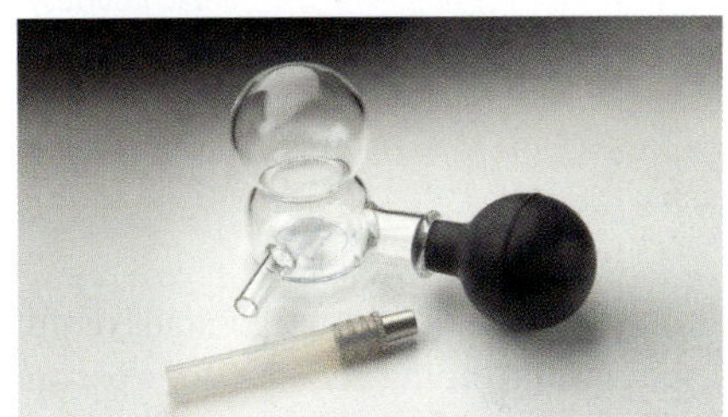

From Nemitz. *Surgical Instrumentation: An Interactive Approach*. 3rd ed. St. Louis: Elsevier; 2019.

STOCKMAN PENIS CLAMP 2¾″

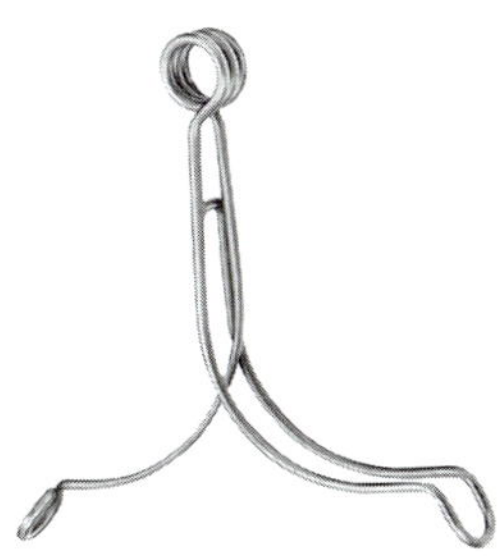

Photo courtesy Aesculap, Inc.

URETERAL ATRAUMATIC FORCEPS 9″

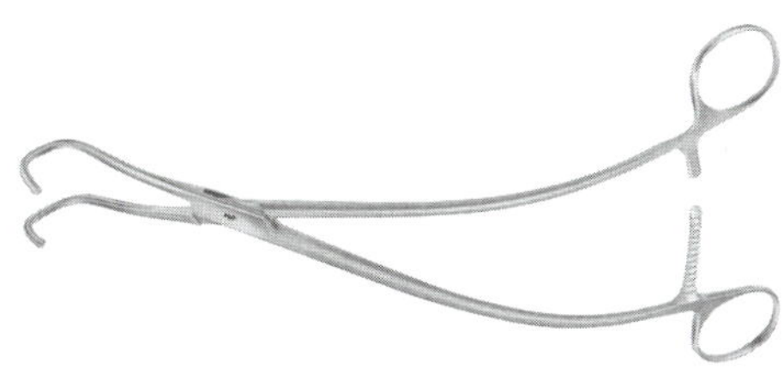

Photo courtesy Aesculap, Inc.

RANDALL KIDNEY STONE FORCEPS 9½″

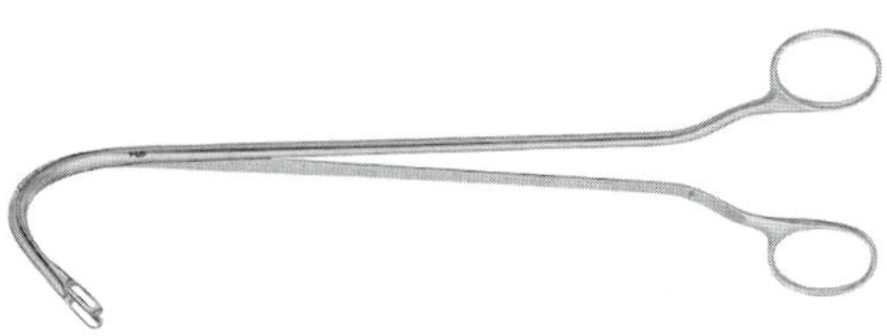

Photo courtesy Aesculap, Inc.

HERRICK KIDNEY PEDICLE CLAMP 9″

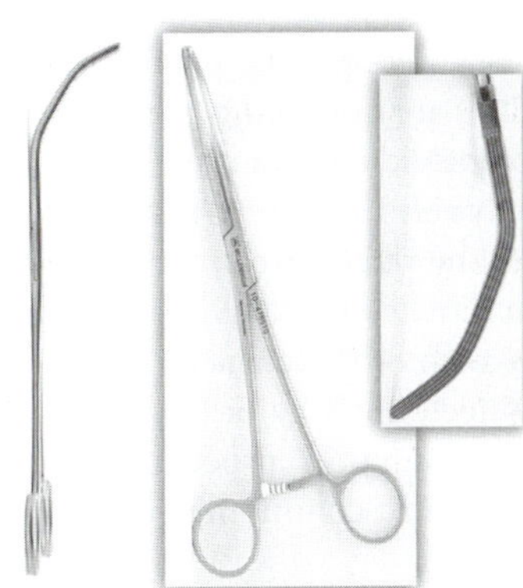

Millenium Surgical Corp.

GENITOURINARY INSTRUMENTS —cont'd

BLADDER SPATULA 10¼″

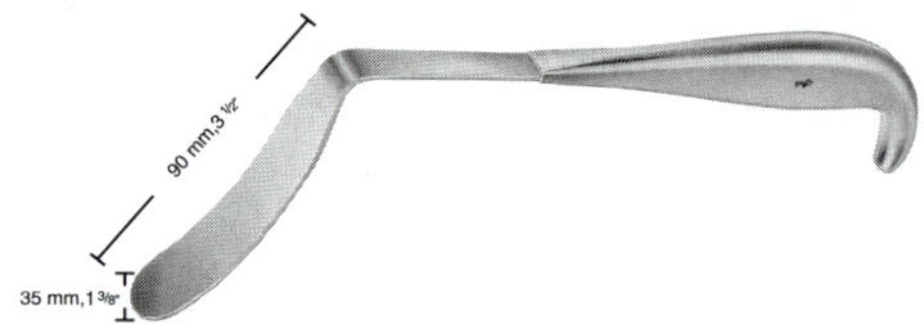

Photo courtesy Aesculap, Inc.

MCDOUGAL PROSTECTOMY CLAMP 9½″

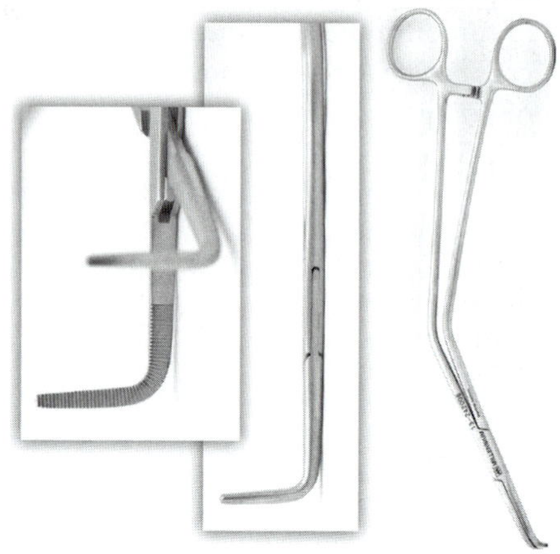

Millenium Surgical Corp.

PROSTATE LOBE GRASPING FORCEPS 9¾″

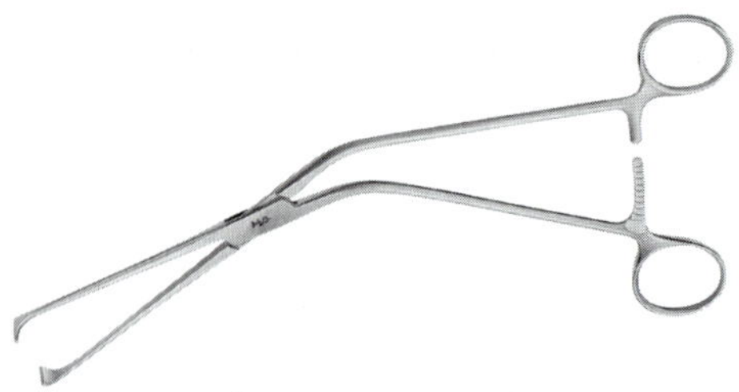

Photo courtesy Aesculap, Inc.

Procedures of the external genitalia require fine plastic surgery instruments, including scissors, forceps, and hemostatic clamps with refined tips. Minor plastic surgery sets are usually adequate for most procedures of the male genitalia. Allis and Babcock clamps are ideal for grasping the tissue layers of the genitalia.

CYSTECTOMY WITH THE ILEAL CONDUIT

Cystectomy is the total or partial removal of the bladder. This procedure is performed for the treatment of bladder cancer. Historically and in current-day practice, radical bladder surgery including lymph node removal has been the standard treatment for bladder tumors that invade the bladder musculature. The procedure carries a high rate of complications, and an increasingly aged population has added to the percent of patients with comorbidities, further complicating treatment. Bladder-sparing procedures with multiple treatment modalities are now being performed. Radical cystectomy with anterior pelvic exenteration is reserved for patients who are medically able to undergo radical procedures. Selected patients who decline radical treatment and whose condition can benefit from more conservative surgery are now offered less radical surgery with other forms of treatment, including chemotherapy. Cystectomy may be performed laparoscopically, robotically, and as an open procedure. The cystectomy with the ileal conduit is most commonly performed as a robotic procedure.

Pathology

Bladder cancer is the second most common cancer of the GU system (prostate cancer has the highest incidence). It arises most frequently from the transitional cells. The diagnosis is made by cystoscopy, which includes tissue biopsy, cytological brushing, or bladder washing to collect cells for pathological assessment. Transurethral resection of a tumor is performed to establish a diagnosis of invasive bladder cancer that has spread to the muscle. Other diagnostic interventions include MRI and combined PET and CT scanning. After a cystectomy, a false bladder may be constructed using a portion of the ileum.

POSITION:	Low lithotomy (women); supine (men)
INCISION:	Lower midline
PREP AND DRAPING:	Abdominal; Foley catheter
INSTRUMENTS:	Laparotomy; kidney set; long instruments for dissection and transfixion; sponge sticks and small sponge dissectors; shods for hemostatic clamps; vessel loops, vessel clips; ureteral stents; Bookwalter or other large abdominal retractor; Deaver retractors

Technical Points and Discussion

1. ***A lower midline incision is made and carried to the bladder.***
To begin the surgery, the surgeon makes a lower midline incision. The abdominal fascia in the midline is identified and the fascia is incised with the ESU. This opens the retropubic space (also called the *space of Retzius*). Blunt dissection is used to separate the bladder from the pelvic sidewall attachments. Large blunt rake retractors or Richardson retractors are used to pull back the edges of the abdominal wall.

2. ***The dissection is carried inferiorly and the peritoneum entered.***
Blunt and sharp dissection is carried out using Metzenbaum scissors, ESU, and forceps to the level of the round ligament (women) or vas deferens (men). The peritoneum is elevated using two curved hemostats, and an incision is made between them.

3. ***The urachus, round ligaments (women), and attachments to the vas deferens are divided.***
The urachus (the fibromuscular attachment at the umbilicus) is clamped with a heavy right-angle clamp and divided with the ESU.

4. ***The bowel is mobilized and the posterior peritoneum incised.***
The bowel is mobilized to gain access to the ureters and large pelvic vessels. Right-angle clamps and long fine curved clamps are used to dissect the bowel attachments to the level of the cecum. Here the posterior peritoneum can be seen. It is elevated using long forceps and entered using the Metzenbaum scissors. This exposes the mesentery of the small intestine, which is incised. A large self-retaining abdominal retractor such as a Bookwalter is inserted, and the bowel is packed with moist lap sponges behind the retractor blades.

5. ***The ureters are dissected free and the superior vesical artery and ureters are ligated.***
Dissection continues with the ureters bilaterally. These are mobilized from their attachments using right-angle clamps and long Metzenbaum scissors. A window is formed in the attachments so that the ureters can be retracted using a vessel loop or narrow Penrose drain. The ends of each vessel loop are tagged with a hemostat. Dissection is continued. The next step is ligation of the superior vesical artery. The vessel is cross-clamped with right-angle clamps, ligated on each side using size 2-0 or 3-0 suture, and divided with scissors. Likewise, the ureter on each side is clamped, ligated using stick ties or suture ties, and divided. Temporary ureteral stents are placed in each ureter, and urine is diverted away from the surgical field. The ureters may also be temporarily ligated to prevent urine from entering the surgical wound.

6. ***A lymphadenectomy is performed.***
Removal of pelvic lymph nodes is performed at this stage or after the bladder specimen has been removed. The lymph nodes are located in "packets" of connective tissue. The extent of node removal depends on previous staging. Nodes are identified, dissected bluntly, and freed using sharp dissection. The ST should maintain these specimens carefully, separating them as directed by the surgeon. The remaining vascular pedicles are now visible and can be controlled with a vascular stapler, surgical clips, or vessel-sealing system.

MALE CYSTECTOMY

7. ***The rectum is dissected free and vesicle pedicles controlled.***
In the male patient, the rectal cul-de-sac is identified and the overlying peritoneum incised. The surgeon creates a dissection plane between the rectum and bladder. Sharp or blunt dissection is continued to the prostate. The posterior vesical pedicles are reached. These are controlled as before using vascular clips, linear stapler, or vessel-sealing device.

8. ***Anterior dissection is carried through the fascia and levator muscles.***
The anterior dissection of the bladder is performed using sharp dissection. This exposes the venous complex and urethra, which are ligated and divided. A frozen section of the urethral margin may be carried out at this time.

FEMALE CYSTECTOMY

9. ***During immobilization of the bowel, the ovarian vessels are managed.***
Immobilization of the bowel is performed as described for the male patient. In the female patient, the ovarian vessels are identified and ligated using 2-0 silk suture. Suture ligatures and ties are used.

10. ***Anterior pelvic exenteration is performed.***
The anterior pelvic exenteration starts with the vaginal cuff. This is incised using long Mayo or Heaney scissors, knife, or ESU. The vaginal canal is entered and the posterior vascular pedicles are controlled with linear staples, clips, or a vessel-sealing system. The urethral meatus is incised and the specimen removed en bloc. The vaginal closure is completed using size 2-0 synthetic absorbable suture. The posterior vaginal wall is dissected from the rectum and the vaginal flap closed with size 2-0 synthetic absorbable interrupted sutures.

11. ***Ileal conduit (male and female). A section of ileum is selected, mobilized, resected, and anastomosed.***
The surgeon selects a 12- to 15-cm section of ileum to be used as the pouch (neo-bladder). This section is then separated from the mesentery using the ESU. The smaller mesenteric vessels are ligated with size 3-0 silk. The mesenteric artery is preserved. The proximal and

distal sections of the selected bowel segment are cross-clamped using four atraumatic bowel clamps—two at each end of the selected segment. The segment limbs are then severed using the knife. The two limbs of the original section of ileum are joined in a side-to-side anastomosis in three layers. Vicryl size 2-0 or 3-0 is used for the seromuscular layer. A linear stapler-cutter is inserted into the open of the limb and fired. Finally, the outer layer of the short staple line is oversewn with silk sutures size 3-0. The selected ileal segment is irrigated.

12. ***The ureters are spatulated and anastomosed to the ileal pouch segment.***
A ureteral stent is inserted at the sites of the ureter anastomosis. The severed edges of the ureter are splayed out (spatulated). The ureters are then anastomosed in layers to the ileal pouch using size 4-0 absorbable suture. The distal end of the selected ileal loop is closed using the linear stapler. During the fine suturing of the ureter, the ST may irrigate the area lightly using a syringe and fine irrigation tip such as that used in microsurgery. The ureteral stents remain in place.

13. ***The ileostomy is created in the abdominal wall.***
To perform the ileostomy, the surgeon first incises a button of skin over the pre-marked stoma site, excising a small disc of tissue from the abdominal wall. Dissection is taken down to the rectus sheath but not through it. The fascia is then incised in a cross, and mosquito clamps are placed at each corner. One ureteral stent is brought through the opening. The open end of the ileal segment is everted and sutured to the abdominal wall using size 3-0 absorbable synthetic sutures.

14. ***Suction drains are placed and the wound is closed.***
The wound is irrigated and checked for any bleeders. One or more suction drains are placed. The wound is then closed in layers. The wound is dressed with flat gauze and an abdominal pad. A temporary ileostomy pouch may be placed over the ostomy site.
The wound is then irrigated, and a suction drain is placed in the abdomen. Closure is routine, as described for a laparotomy. Important points in cystectomy are shown in Figs. 24.12 and 24.13.

NOTE *Refer to Chapter 23 for a complete discussion and illustrations of an ileostomy.*

BRACHYTHERAPY OF THE PROSTATE

Brachytherapy is the implantation of radioactive material into tissue for the treatment of cancer. Brachytherapy of the prostate is performed as an outpatient procedure under regional or general anesthetic. The procedure requires a team including a urologist, radiation oncologist, dosimetrist, radiation safety personnel, and anesthetist. The implantation takes place under transrectal ultrasound and fluoroscopic guidance using iodine-125 or palladium. To place the seeds accurately in the most advantageous positions, a coordinating grid attached to the probe receives needles with the preloaded seeds. The seeds are injected directly into the prostate through the perineum.

The prostate volume is scanned in real time with transrectal ultrasound, and a dosimetrist calculates the exact dose based on special software. After the procedure, the patient may undergo cystoscopy to further verify position of the seeds. The procedure may be repeated over several days or a week.

PROCEDURES OF THE URETERS AND KIDNEY

PERCUTANEOUS NEPHROLITHOTOMY (PCNL)

Percutaneous nephrolithotomy (PCNL) is the removal of one or more kidney stones using a nephroscope. The instruments are inserted through a small skin incision and tunnel created in the fascia into the renal pelvis. The method of lithotripsy depends on the size of the stone and its chemical composition. The procedure is carried out using fluoroscopy. The patient may be anesthetized on the patient gurney, intubated, and then turned onto the cysto table in modified prone position.

Pathology

A percutaneous endoscopic procedure for lithotomy is indicated in the following circumstances:

- The stone (or stones) are extremely large (larger than 2.5 cm), such as a **staghorn stone.**
- Conservative treatment, such as oral medication to dissolve the stones, has failed.
- The patient exceeds the weight limit (300 pounds [135 kg]) for extracorporeal shock wave therapy.
- The stone cannot be reached through the endoscopic ureteroscope.
- The stone is infected (the percutaneous method allows evacuation of infectious material at the time of the procedure).

POSITION:	Modified prone
INCISION:	Flank
PREP AND DRAPING:	Flank
INSTRUMENTS:	Rigid and 24-Fr nephroscope with PCNL instruments, ureteral catheter 5 Fr; 18-gauge access needle; guidewires 0.035, stiff Amplatz wire; fascial dilator; 8/10 coaxial dilator; ultrasonic lithotrite; stone-grasping forceps; nitinol stone basket; ureteral stents as required
POSSIBLE EXTRAS:	Holmium laser fiber, flexible nephroscope; Malecot or Pezzer drainage catheters

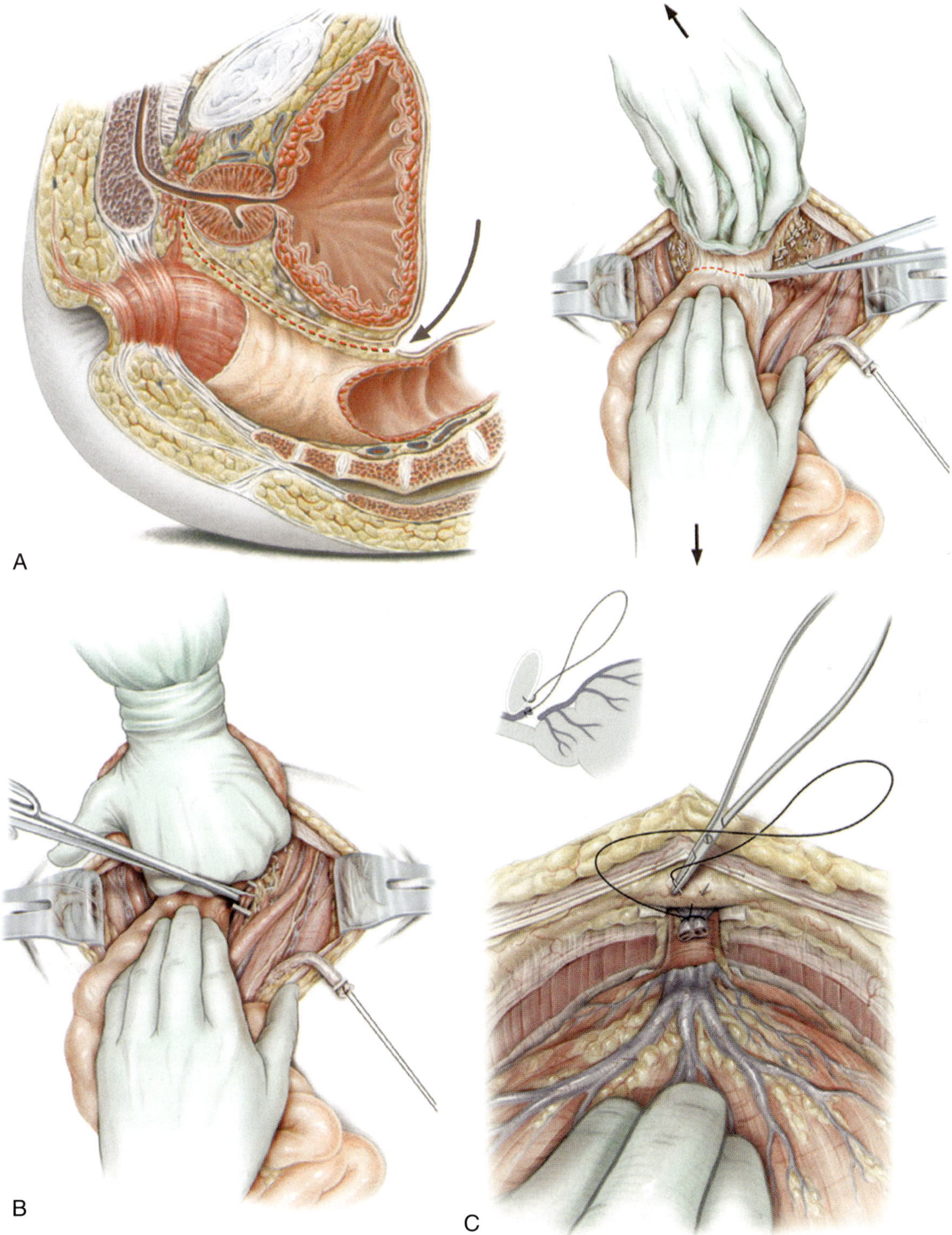

FIG. 24.12 Radical cystectomy. (A) Plane of dissection between the bladder and prostate from the rectum. (B) Separation of the rectum from the bladder using blunt dissection. (C) Dividing and ligating the central venous complex.

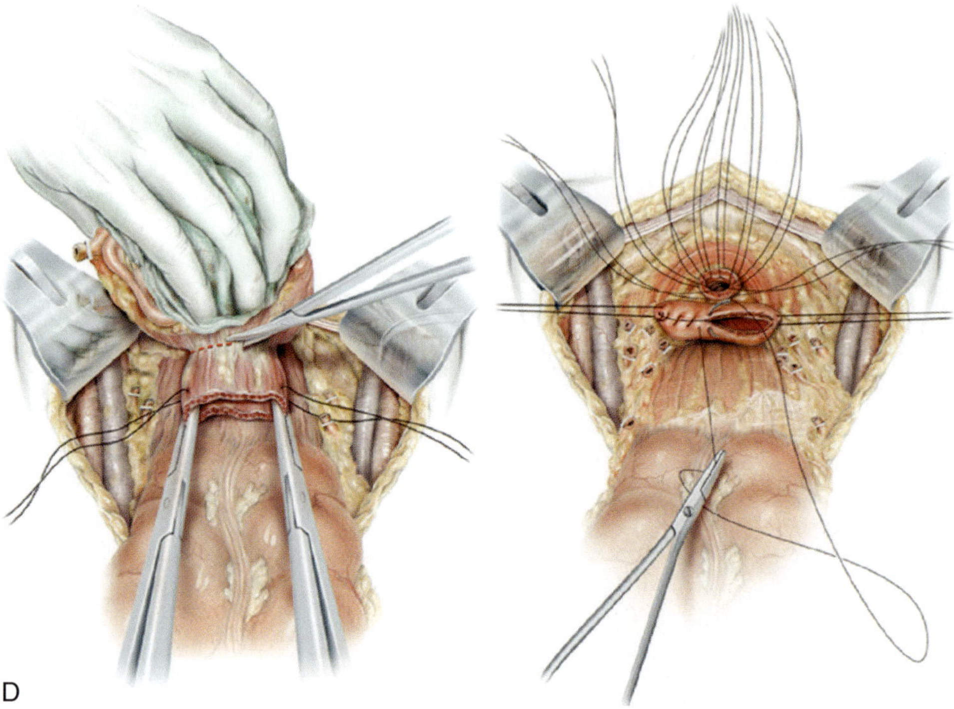

FIG. 24.12 cont'd (D) Division and closure of the vaginal cuff. (From Wein A, Kavoussi L, Partin A, Peters C. *Campbell-Walsh Urology*. 11th ed. Philadelphia: Elsevier; 2016.)

Technical Points and Discussion

1. ***The patient is positioned, prepped, and draped.***
After administration of general anesthesia and intubation, the patient is placed in the prone position with the operative side elevated on a foam wedge. Wide tape may be used to secure the patient in position. The patient is then prepped and draped for a flank incision. Intravenous tubing is attached to the distal end of a previously placed ureteral catheter for access during the procedure.

2. ***A nephrostomy tract is created and dilated.***
To start the procedure, an 18-gauge needle with sheath is passed into the renal calyx under fluoroscopy. When the correct location has been entered, a contrast medium is injected to verify the location. The needle is withdrawn, leaving the sheath in place. An occlusion balloon catheter may be inserted at this point to block the proximal ureter against any stone fragments that may be pushed into the ureter during lithotripsy. A glide wire with Coudé tip is passed into the renal pelvis and an angiographic catheter inserted. The glide wire is then removed, and a working guidewire such as the Amplatz stiff is inserted. An 8/10 coaxial sheath is placed over the guidewire. The coaxial sheath (a tube within a tube) contains an 8-Fr sheath within a 10-Fr sheath. The 8-Fr sheath is advanced into the wound, and the 10-Fr sheath is advanced to provide further dilation. An independent safety wire is now inserted. The function of this wire is to maintain access if there is injury to the ureter or kidney, which would necessitate a change of procedure. The 10-Fr sheath is removed, and a 30-Fr balloon catheter preloaded with a 30-Fr PTFE sheath is inserted and inflated. The sheath is then advanced in the nephrostomy tract and will provide continuous access. The Amplatz stiff wire is removed. The rigid scope can then be used to visualize the kidney.

3. ***The stone is identified, and lithotripsy is performed.***
Lithotripsy can be approached using the rigid or flexible nephroscope. An ultrasonic lithotripsy probe may be inserted through the nephroscope and the stone crushed. A holmium laser or pneumatic lithotripter may also be used to crush the stones. The flexible scope is used to explore the upper calyces, which cannot be viewed using the rigid scope. Stones often lodge in the renal pelvis. These can be accessed through the nephroscope. Stone fragments are removed using graspers, a stone basket, or by flushing them with irrigation fluid. Contrast medium is instilled in the kidney to check for any remaining stones or fragments.

4. ***Nephrostomy drainage catheter is placed and the wound is closed.***
The ureteral Malecot, Pezzer, or a loop drainage catheter is inserted using the Amplatz guidewire. The guidewire and sheath are removed and the drainage catheter sutured in place. If needed, one or two skin sutures can be placed with use of size 3-0 synthetic suture. Important points of the procedure are illustrated in Fig. 24.14.

SIMPLE NEPHRECTOMY (FLANK INCISION)

Flank incisions were performed in the past. The current procedure is to perform an abdominal incision in the modified lateral positioning. Simple nephrectomy is the surgical removal of one kidney. In most cases, this procedure is performed as a laparoscopy or laparascopy with robot.

Pathology

A nephrectomy is performed most often for severe hydronephrosis, obstruction, localized tumor, stones with infection, and trauma to the kidney. A kidney also may be removed from a live donor for transplantation.

POSITION:	Flank
INCISION:	Flank
PREP AND DRAPING:	Flank
INSTRUMENTS:	Kidney set including long GU instruments, bulldog clamps, Satinsky vascular pedicle clamps, vascular forceps, surgical clips; Omni-Tract retractor or Bookwalter retractor; vascular loops; topical hemostatic materials; heparinized saline; irrigation tips
POSSIBLE EXTRAS:	Sterile ice (for donor kidney)

Technical Points and Discussion

1. ***The patient is positioned, prepped, and draped.***
The patient is prepared for a flank incision. A Foley catheter should be inserted before positioning the patient. After administration of anesthesia, the patient is placed in the lateral decubitus position with the operative side up. The middle table break will be used to widen the exposure to the flank, so the patient is positioned with flank area over this break. A vacuum positioner ("bean bag") may be used to hold the patient in position (refer to Chapter 16 for a complete description of the position). The patient is prepped from the axilla to thigh anteriorly and posteriorly. A transverse flank draping procedure is then performed. The incision is made with the knife just above the 12th rib and developed to the level of the fascia and latissimus dorsi muscles. Right-angle or rake retractors may be required at this stage. The ESU is used to incise the muscles. This exposes the fascia. The transverse abdominal muscle is then split digitally. A Bookwalter retractor is inserted with moist laparotomy tapes.

2. ***The renal fascia is dissected to expose the kidney.***
The posterior renal fascia is dissected from the muscles, mesentery, and peritoneum. It is then incised sharply, providing access to the fatty tissue that is dissected from the kidney. This step is performed using both blunt and sharp dissection, including ESU. A kidney that is hydronephrotic may require drainage for further mobilization.

3. ***The kidney is mobilized from surrounding structures.***
Mobilization of the kidney from the surrounding structures begins at the adrenal gland. Scissors, vascular forceps, and ESU are used for sharp dissection. The attachments to the spleen, pancreas, and liver are also released using sharp and blunt dissection. The lower pole of the kidney is now immobilized and the ureter identified and mobilized. A narrow Penrose drain may be slung around the ureter for gentle traction as it is separated from the connective tissues that surround it. The gonadal vein and renal artery are also identified and mobilized.

4. ***The ureter is cross-clamped, divided, and ligated.***
The ureter is cross-clamped using Mayo or right-angle clamps or simply clipped with vessel clips and divided with scissors.

5. ***The kidney pedicle is divided.***
A right-angle clamp is placed across the renal artery, which is then divided. The stump is suture-ligated using nonabsorbable synthetic sutures. The renal vein is cross-clamped with a Satinsky or right-angle vascular clamp and divided. It is then oversewn with size 5-0 Prolene suture. The kidney is removed and placed in a small basin.

6. ***The wound is closed.***
The wound is irrigated with warm saline and checked for bleeders. Before the wound is closed, the table break is closed to release tension on the flank. A Penrose drain is placed in the kidney fossa and brought out through a separate stab wound. The fascia and muscle layers are closed with interrupted absorbable sutures, size 2-0. The skin is closed with staples. The wound is dressed with flat gauze and an abdominal pad. Simple nephrectomy is illustrated in Fig. 24.15.

KIDNEY TRANSPLANT

Kidney transplantation is removal of a kidney from a living or deceased donor and implanting it into the recipient. Currently in the United States there are 100,791 people awaiting a donor kidney. Recipients can expect a waiting period of more than 3½ years. In 2014, 17,107 kidney transplants were performed in the United States. The sources of living donor kidneys include living related donors, living unrelated donors, and altruistic donors (nondirected donors) who volunteer a kidney to anyone needing one. Kidney transplantation is performed by a transplant team, and the routines are well established. In this procedure, surgeons operate on the living donor and recipient simultaneously. However, the kidney can be perfused to preserve the tissues. The operating rooms should connect to minimize contamination if the kidney is removed from a living donor. In this procedure, the donor kidney is placed outside the peritoneal cavity in the recipient. The recipient's own kidney is usually not removed.

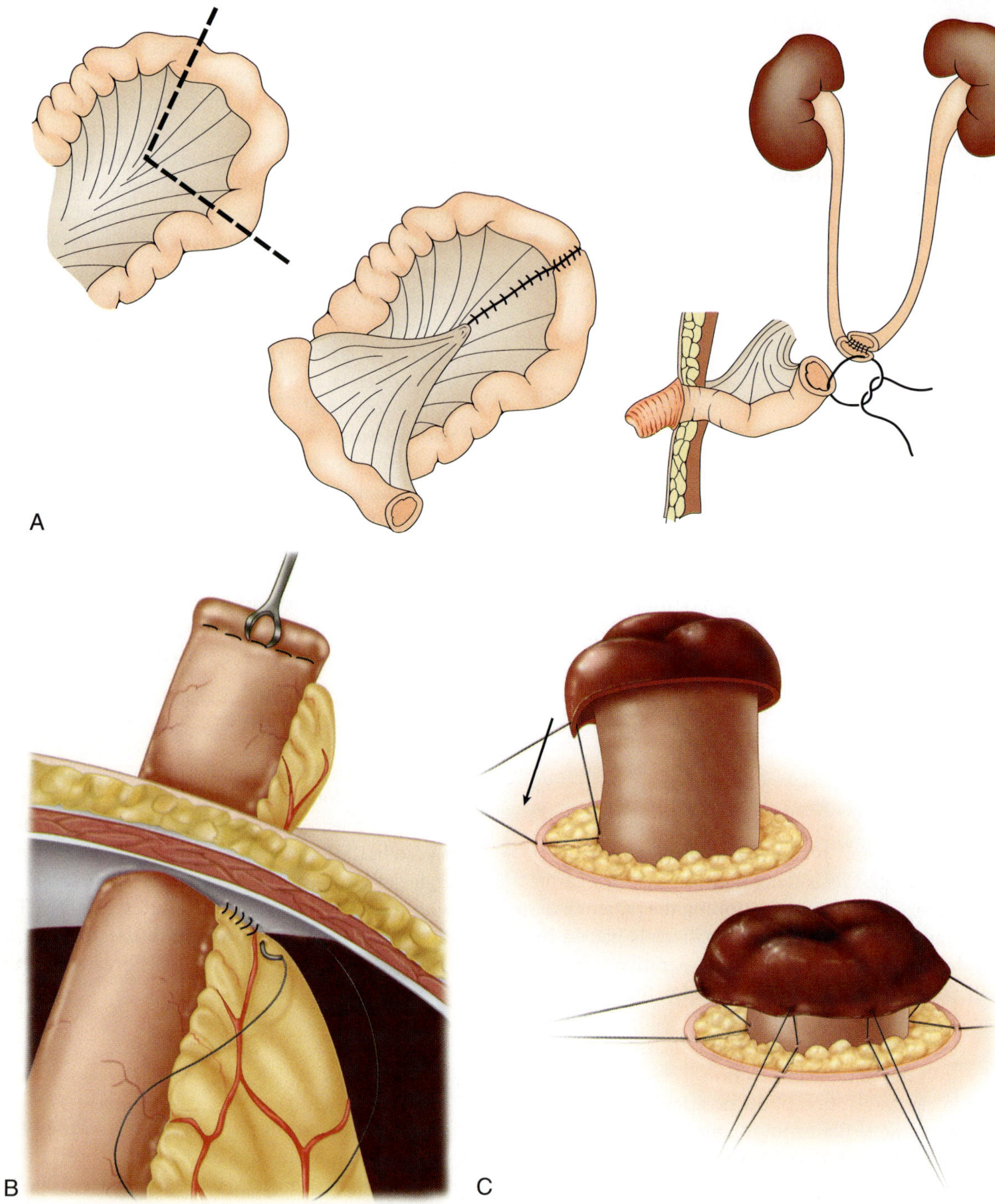

FIG. 24.13 End ileostomy. (A) A section of ileum is removed, and an end-to-end anastomosis is performed to restore continuity. The isolated section of ileum is brought through the abdominal wall in preparation for ileostomy procedure. (B and C) The ileum is everted and sutured to the abdominal wall. (A, From Garden O, Bradbury A, Forsythe J, Parks R. *Principles and Practice of Surgery*. 5th ed. Edinburgh: Churchill Livingstone; 2007. B and C, From Fleshman J, et al. *Atlas of Surgical Techniques for the Colon, Rectum, and Anus*. Philadelphia: Saunders; 2013.)

Pathology

Kidney transplantation is performed for acute or chronic end-stage renal disease. Common causes of ESRD are as follows:

- Diabetes mellitus
- Hypertension
- Glomerulonephritis
- Polycystic kidney disease
- Severe anatomical problems of the urinary tract

Patients awaiting kidney transplant are carefully screened to ensure compatibility and survivability following transplant. Potential medical reasons for excluding a patient for transplant include the following:

- Cardiovascular disease that cannot be treated
- History of metastatic cancer or current chemotherapy
- Active systemic infection
- Substance abuse
- Neurological impairment with no surrogate decision maker

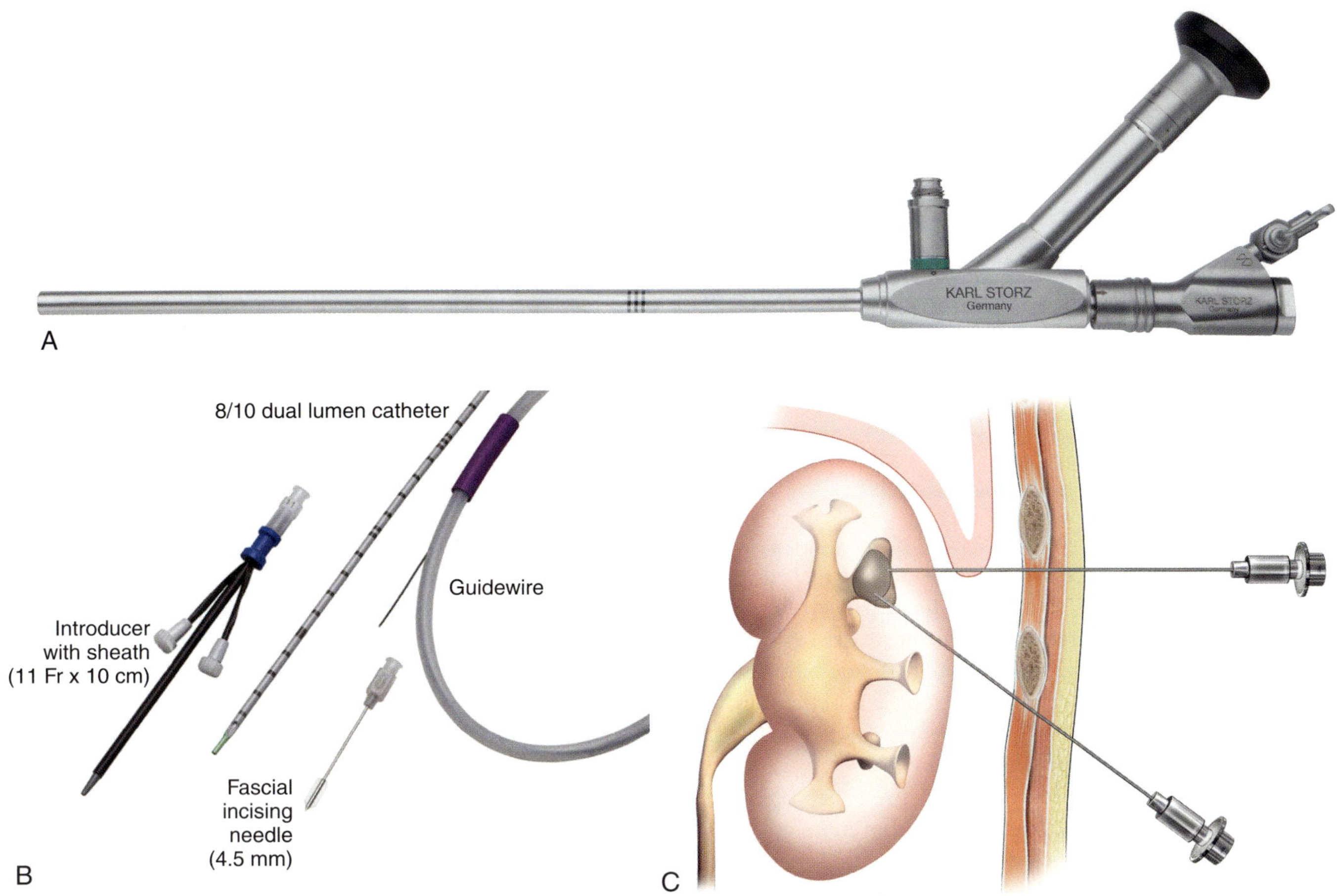

FIG. 24.14 Percutaneous nephrolithotomy. (A) Nephroscope with offset lenses. (B) Percutaneous set with vascular access sheath to accommodate the nephroscope, guidewire, introducer sheath, and fascia incising sheath. (C) Percutaneous access to the kidney during nephroscopy. (*A*, Photo courtesy of KARL STORZ Endoscopy-America, Inc. *B and C*, From Wein A, Kavoussi L, Partin A, Peters C. *Campbell-Walsh Urology*. 11th ed. Philadelphia: Elsevier; 2016.)

POSITION:	Supine
INCISION:	Midline
PREP AND DRAPING:	Abdominal
INSTRUMENTS AND SUPPLIES:	Major laparotomy; abdominal vascular set; fine vascular suction tips; long instruments including right-angle clamps, curved hemostatic clamps; dissecting scissors; bumpers for clamps; vascular loops; long electrode tips for ESU; sterile ice
POSSIBLE EXTRAS:	Bowel bag; topical hemostatic materials

Technical Points and Discussion

1. ***The donor kidney is removed.***
Refer to Simple Nephrectomy (Flank Incision). This procedure can be used, with several differences. The renal pedicle, which contains the vascular supply, is isolated and ligated before the kidney is removed. The Gerota's fascia may be left intact on the donor kidney. After removal, the donor kidney is preserved in a cold solution and perfused with the surgeon's choice of electrolyte solution. When the recipient team is ready to receive the kidney, the surgeon transports it in a covered container, maintaining the correct temperature. The donor wound is closed as previously described.

2. ***The recipient patient is prepped and draped for a right iliac incision.***
The patient is placed in the supine position and prepped for a laparotomy. A 3-way Foley catheter is inserted. Bladder irrigation with a broad-spectrum antibacterial may be instituted during the procedure. The patient is draped for a laparotomy.

3. ***The retroperitoneal space is entered.***
A midline incision is made. A self-retaining Balfour retractor is placed in the wound. The right colon is mobilized using sharp and blunt dissection and moved aside to expose the peritoneal layer, which covers the iliac vessels.

4. ***The iliac vessels are prepared for anastomosis.***
The iliac vein and artery will be anastomosed to the donor kidney renal vein and artery. The recipient vessels are prepared by first isolating them using sharp and blunt

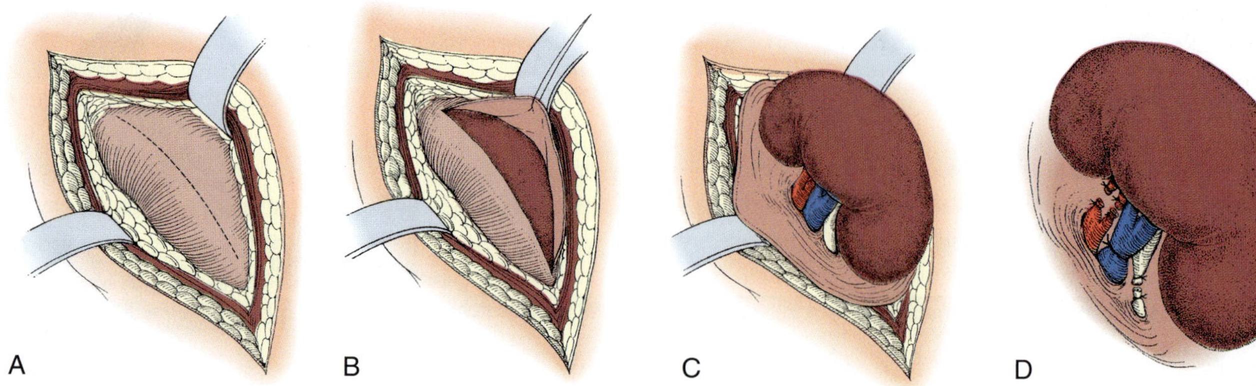

FIG. 24.15 Nephrectomy. (A) Incision line in Gerota's fascia. (B) The fascia is incised with the ESU or #10 knife blade. (C) The kidney is delivered from the capsule. (D) The renal artery and vein, and ureter are ligated. (From Wein A, Kavoussi L, Partin A, Peters C. *Campbell-Walsh Urology*. 11th ed. Philadelphia: Elsevier; 2016.)

dissection. In this process, the lymphatics are ligated and incised. A right-angle clamp and fine-tip Metzenbaum scissors are used to carefully isolate the vessels. A vessel loop is placed around the right iliac vein. A side-biting Satinsky clamp is then placed along the long axis of the vein.

5. ***The donor kidney (allograft) is prepared.***
The donor kidney is received from the other operating team and prepared. The ST should prepare a separate sterile setup for this procedure. The kidney is presented wrapped in moist lap tapes in an ice-filled basin. First, the vascular staple lines are divided on the artery and vein. Vascular clips are replaced with nonabsorbable synthetic suture ties to prevent their becoming dislodged during the transplant phase. The kidney is flushed with heparinized irrigation fluid. The Gerota's fascia is carefully removed using sharp dissection. The donor kidney is again wrapped in the basin with cold moist lap tapes.

6. ***The vascular anastomosis is performed.***
To start the vascular anastomosis between donor and recipient kidneys an incision (venotomy) is made in the iliac vein using right-angle vascular scissors. The incision is extended using Potts scissors.

The donor kidney is brought onto the surgical field. It is oriented in the iliac fossa of the donor with the cold lap sponge in place. The renal vein is then anastomosed end-to-side to the donor iliac vein using a running vascular suture of 6-0 Prolene on a vascular needle. When completed, the anastomosis is tested. To begin the arterial anastomosis two Fogarty clamps are placed distally and superiorly across the recipient iliac artery. An incision (arteriotomy) is made in the artery using a #11 or #15 knife blade. A round aortic punch may be used to make the arteriotomy to accommodate the donor renal artery. The donor renal artery is then anastomosed to the recipient iliac artery using a running suture of 6-0 Prolene on a vascular needle. The anastomosis may be tested at this point.

7. ***The donor ureter is implanted into the recipient bladder wall.***
To begin the ureterocystostomy the recipient bladder wall is divided using the ESU. The mucosa layer can then be incised using fine dissection scissors. The donor ureter is spatulated (the distal end is opened out in petal formation). A ureteral stent is placed into the donor ureter. It is advanced into the rental pelvis and brought out through the urethra. The stent will be removed using a cystoscope 4 to 6 weeks after the procedure. The distal ureter mucosa is then joined to the bladder wall mucosa using absorbable monofilament suture size 4-0 or 5-0. The muscular layer in the bladder is then approximated using size 2-0 absorbable synthetic running sutures. The bladder is irrigated to test the anastomosis.

8. ***The wound is closed.***
The wound is irrigated with warm saline and explored for any bleeders. The abdominal wall fascia is closed with size 0 running absorbable suture. The subcutaneous tissue is closed with size 2-0 or 3-0 interrupted sutures. One or two suction drains may be placed in the wound during closure. The wound is dressed with gauze fluffs and tape.

Patients are monitored closely for acute organ rejection, hemorrhage, and infection in the immediate postoperative period.

PROCEDURES OF THE PROSTATE

TRANSURETHRAL RESECTION OF THE PROSTATE

Transurethral resection of the prostate (TURP) is removal of the prostate gland using a cystourethral approach. In this procedure, continuous irrigation flow is necessary to maintain a clear view of the anatomy. A nonconductive distention fluid is used for monopolar segmental resection. The procedure can be performed using monopolar electrical energy (MTURP) or with bipolar electrodes (BTURP). Bipolar vessel-sealing technology allows for lower-temperature resection in a saline environment.

Pathology

Enlargement of the prostate in men age 40 and above is most often caused by a benign prostatic adenoma. This is a non-malignant tumor of the prostate gland, which can occur in men older than 40 years. The tumor presses on the urethra and bladder, resulting in obstruction and other voiding problems. Obstructive disease may cause **reflux** (backward flow) of urine, infection, and difficulty voiding. Benign prostatic hyperplasia is commonly treated by TURP, retropelvic prostatectomy, or suprapubic prostatectomy.

POSITION:	Lithotomy
INCISION:	Transurethral
PREP AND DRAPING:	Lower abdomen, genitalia, and perineum. Lithotomy draping including fluid collection pouch.
INSTRUMENTS:	Urethral dilators; cystoscope; resectoscope with 24-Fr or 27-Fr sheath; imaging system accessories; cutting electrodes; roller ball electrodes (monopolar or bipolar); Ellik evacuator; 3-way Foley balloon catheter

Technical Points and Discussion

1. ***The patient is positioned and prepped for a transurethral procedure.***
The patient is prepared for surgery. A sequential compression device should be in place and the patient positioned at the edge of the lower break in the operating table. It is important that the patient's buttocks be positioned far down the table so that the table edge does not interfere with access for the scope. Lithotomy prep and draping, including a fluid collection pouch, are then completed. All needed instruments should be assembled and checked before the procedure starts. This includes the imaging system and the surgeon's preference of cutting loops. The ST will be required to assist the surgeon during the procedure, so it is good practice to have the instruments in clear view and organized neatly on the back table.

2. ***The bladder and bladder neck are assessed.***
Before beginning the resection, the surgeon may need to dilate the urethra to allow passage of the cystourethroscope. Dilatation can be performed with balloon dilators or graduated metal sounds. After inserting the scope, the surgeon performs a routine cystoscopy with a 30-degree lens to evaluate the bladder and other structures.

3. ***The prostate is resected systematically.***
After attaching the resectoscope with appropriate cutting device, the resection begins, usually at the middle lobe, and proceeds to the lateral lobes. Fragments are flushed from the bladder and collected as specimens. Arterial and venous bleeding can be controlled using the cutting loop set on fulguration mode. However, if bleeding cannot be controlled in this way, a urinary balloon catheter can be temporarily inserted and used as a tamponade against the bleeding surface.

4. ***Prostatic specimens are collected.***
During the dissection and at the close of the procedure, the specimens are collected using an Ellik evacuator or Toomey syringe. The ST must collect all pieces of the specimen for pathology. At the end of the procedure, a large-bore balloon catheter is inserted into the bladder. The surgeon will determine the volume of fluid required in the balloon, according to the amount of tissue that has been resected. When bleeding has subsided, a 3-way Foley irrigation catheter may be inserted. After a TURP procedure, the patient may remain catheterized for several days to facilitate irrigation of the bladder. The patient can usually be discharged on postoperative day 1.

SIMPLE PROSTATECTOMY (SUPRAPUBIC)

Simple suprapubic prostatectomy is removal of an enlarged prostate (prostatic adenoma) through an incision in the lower abdominal wall through the bladder. In this procedure, the prostate is enucleated (taken out as a whole specimen) rather than through piecemeal dissection. The procedure is indicated when the bladder and urethral openings require excellent visualization during surgery, such as a highly enlarged mid-prostate, if there are bladder calculi or diverticula, or if the patient is obese.

Pathology

Benign prostatic hypertrophy is discussed under Transurethral Resection of the Prostate.

POSITION:	Supine with hyperextension at the umbilicus
INCISION:	Lower midline
PREP AND DRAPING:	Abdominal
INSTRUMENTS AND SUPPLIES:	General surgery; prostate extras

Technical Points and Discussion

1. ***The patient is positioned, prepped, and draped.***
The patient is placed in the supine position on the operating table with the middle table break at the level of the patient's umbilicus to allow for hyperextension. The skin prep is performed to include the abdomen and genitalia. A Foley retention catheter with a 30-mL balloon is placed and inflated with saline before the skin prep.

2. ***A lower midline incision is made and the space of Retzius entered.***
A lower midline incision is made with the knife and extended through the linea alba using the ESU and dissecting scissors. Right-angle retractors such as Army-Navy or Richardson are used on the margins. The rectus abdominus muscles are then manually separated. The transversalis fascia is exposed using the retractors, and this layer is incised, exposing the space of Retzius (retropubic space). At the upper end of the wound, the posterior rectus fascia is incised with the ESU to the level of the umbilicus. The peritoneum is mobilized. The surgeon then assesses the pelvic cavity for abnormalities. A Balfour retractor is placed in the wound and the blades padded with moist abdominal tapes.

3. ***The bladder is incised.***
The bladder wall is identified, traction sutures of 3-0 Vicryl are placed in the bladder wall on the midline, and an incision is made between them using the ESU. The bladder edges are then grasped with Allis clamps and retracted upward. The surgeon extends the incision using Metzenbaum scissors. The ST should have suction available to drain the bladder. Additional stay sutures are placed at the incision angles to prevent tearing of the incision during blunt dissection.

4. ***The prostate is enucleated.***
A Judd or Deaver retractor is placed in the bladder over moist lap tapes. An additional narrow Deaver retractor may be used to retract the bladder neck. Indigo carmine dye may be administered at this point to expose the ureteral openings. An incision is made into the bladder mucosa using the ESU. Metzenbaum scissors are then used to develop the tissue plan between the prostate and capsule. Blunt dissection is used to extend the plane circumferentially and inferiorly. The prostatic urethra is exposed and transected digitally. This allows the prostatic adenoma to be removed en bloc or in separate lobes from their fossae. A Babcock clamp may be used to aid in removal.

5. ***Bleeding is controlled.***
The bladder retractors are replaced. Bleeding in the fossa is controlled using several means. The ESU or size 4-0 Vicryl suture ligatures can be used. The main artery can be suture-ligated with size 0 Vicryl. Capillary bleeding may be controlled using a topical hemostatic agent such as Gelfoam or Avitene.

6. ***The wound is closed.***
The surgeon inspects the wound for any traces of remaining adenoma and removes these. When hemostasis is satisfactory, a 3-way Foley catheter with 3-mL balloon is inserted into the urethra and prostatic fossa into the bladder. An additional Malecot suprapubic catheter may be placed in the bladder, exiting through a stab incision in the side of the upper bladder. The suprapubic tube is then secured with size 3-0 non-absorbable suture. The prostatic capsule is closed using size 2-0 absorbable suture.

The bladder is closed in two layers with absorbable sutures. The wound is irrigated, and a wound drain is placed in the cavity. The Foley catheter must be inflated to capacity to prevent it from migrating into the prostatic fossa. The bladder is irrigated to check for leakage. A Jackson-Pratt suction drain may also be placed through a separate stab incision to prevent hematoma.

The pelvic cavity is irrigated with warm saline. The incision is then closed in layers and the wound dressed using flat gauze and abdominal pads. The technique used in TURP is shown in Fig. 24.16.

PERINEAL PROSTATECTOMY (OPEN)

This procedure is very rarely performed. It has been transitioned to robotic procedures. Perineal prostatectomy is the removal of the prostate through a perineal approach. In the past, prostatectomy often resulted in impotence and incontinence. Nerve-sparing procedures now are practiced to prevent these complications. In this procedure, lymph nodes are removed for cancer staging. Although prostatectomy is commonly performed using minimally invasive techniques including robotic surgery, the surgical technologist should also be familiar with open techniques, which are available for the patient with unusually large adenoma.

Pathology

Perineal prostatectomy may be performed for the treatment of adenocarcinoma of the prostate. Prostatic cancer is usually a slow-growing tumor arising from the prostatic gland occurring in men from age 40 to 60 years. Adenocarcinoma is often symptom free until the late stage of the disease. Prostatic cancer is diagnosed at the early stages using the prostate-specific antigen (PSA) blood test and digital rectal exam (DRE). Routine screening for prostatic disease has greatly improved the survival rate of men with prostate cancer. Biopsy is the standard for establishing diagnosis. Staging is then performed using lymph node biopsy. Localized prostate cancer is treated using radical prostatectomy and brachytherapy (radiation). Cancer that has spread to other organs is rarely curable.

INCISION:	Perineal
POSITION:	Lithotomy
PREP AND DRAPING:	Abdomen, perineum, scrotum, penis, and anus are prepped. Anus is isolated from draping. An under-buttocks fluid collection pouch is placed followed by full perineal draping including anal pouch. Compression stockings and sequential compression devices are required.
INSTRUMENTS AND SUPPLIES:	Major general surgery; urological extras; perineal retractors; Lowsley prostatic retractor; prostate extras; right-angle and fine curved hemostatic clamps; vessel loops
POSSIBLE EXTRAS:	Penrose drains; suction drainage device

Technical Points and Discussion

1. ***The patient is placed in the high lithotomy position.***
The patient is placed in the exaggerated lithotomy position with the legs well above the pelvis and the buttocks brought to the edge of the operating table break. A gel pad is placed under the sacrum. This is an extreme position that puts strain on the lower back, hips, and sacrum. Positioning must be performed with attention to all risk factors (refer to Chapter 16).
The patient is prepped for a perineal incision extending to the abdomen, mid-thigh, penis, scrotum, anus, and lower sacrum. A Foley catheter is placed in the bladder after the prep. This provides a landmark to the urethra and urine output during the procedure. Draping exposes the perineum. An adherent barrier drape with anal pouch is used for the procedure. The pouch provides an inlet through which the surgeon can digitally support the roof of the rectum during dissection.

2. ***An inverted U-incision is made in the perineum and carried through the muscle and fascia.***
To start the procedure, the surgeon passes a Lowsley retractor through the urethra and into the bladder. This pushes the bladder down toward the perineum. A U-shaped incision is made in the perineum with the skin knife. Bleeders are controlled with the ESU. The surgeon then places several Allis clamps on the incision edges for retraction. The incision is extended to muscle and fascia using blunt dissection. The ST should have ample moist and dry sponges plus small sponge dissectors mounted on clamps. The assistant manages the Lowsley retractor, which is maneuvered according to the requirements of the progressive dissection.

3. ***The central tendon is isolated and divided.***
The central tendon and rectourethral muscle are isolated and divided with scissors. Right-angle retractors such as a Richardson or Deaver are used at this stage. The levator muscle is retracted to expose the prostatic capsule and prostate gland. The surgeon may use digital support through the anus to assist dissection. Small sponge dissectors, Metzenbaum scissors, and the ESU are used to extend the dissection and isolate the prostate. The recto-urethral muscles are divided and retracted.

4. ***The prostate is further dissected from the urethra, bladder neck, anterior bladder, seminal vesicles, and rectum.***
This stage of dissection is carried out precisely. Right-angle clamps are needed to isolate the neurovascular pedicles and to divide and ligate them with suture, vessel-sealing system, or ligation clips. Dissection of the vascular system is carefully extended on both sides of the prostate. Vessel loops may be used to provide traction on major blood vessels and the neurovascular bundles. In nerve-sparing procedures, *no electrosurgical coagulation* is used to separate the prostate from the surrounding tissue, which contains the nerves and blood vessels that innervate the penis for erectile function.

5. ***The urethra is isolated.***
The urethra is isolated from the base of the prostate and bladder neck. A vessel loop can be placed around the urethra for traction during dissection. It is then double-clamped and divided, preserving the bladder neck. This leaves a small urethral stump at the bladder neck. The wound is irrigated, and bleeders are controlled with the ESU and fine suture ligatures.

6. ***The prostatic capsule is incised, and the prostate is removed.***
With dissection completed, the prostate can be enucleated from the capsule. The urethral stumps are then anastomosed to bypass the prostate. The anastomosis is completed with fine nylon or another synthetic monofilament suture. The closure is tested by instilling saline into the bladder.

7. ***The wound is closed.***
When bleeding has been controlled, the wound is irrigated with warm saline. Drains are placed in the wound and brought out through the incision or a separate stab incision. Closure is completed in layers with 2-0 and 3-0 absorbable synthetic sutures. The skin is closed with 3-0 or 4-0 subcuticular or interrupted sutures. The wound is dressed with gauze fluff squares and an absorbent pad to absorb drainage.

NOTE *Lymph node dissection is performed before or after the perineal portion of the surgery.*

A perineal prostatectomy is shown in Fig. 24.17.

An indwelling Foley catheter is left in place for 1 to 2 weeks after the procedure. This allows the urethral anastomosis to heal. Recovery from an open procedure takes considerably longer than from laparoscopic or robotic-assisted surgery.

ROBOTIC-ASSISTED LAPAROSCOPIC PROSTATECTOMY (RALP)

Prostatectomy has become an established robotic procedure because of an enhanced nerve-sparing outcome. As with all robotic procedures, the ST must be fully trained in the use of the equipment, including troubleshooting during the procedure. The following description outlines the main techniques of the procedure. Advanced training is required to assist in the procedure. The following procedure includes removal of lymph nodes.

Pathology

See Perineal Prostatectomy (Open).

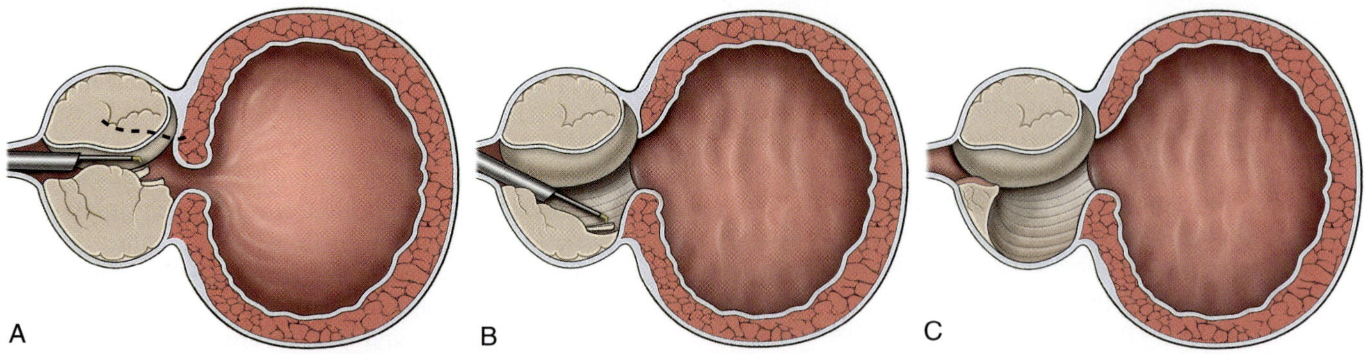

FIG. 24.16 Transurethral prostatectomy. (A) An electrosurgical cutting loop is inserted through the urethra. (B) The cutting loop is drawn back along the resectoscope sheath, cutting and coagulating the hypertrophied prostate. (C) Prostatic capsule with prostate removed. (From Wein A, Kavoussi L, Partin A, Peters C. *Campbell-Walsh Urology*. 11th ed. Philadelphia: Elsevier; 2016.)

POSITION:	Low lithotomy; slight hip hyperextension; arms secured at the sides; sequential compression devices
INCISION:	Laparoscopic
PREP AND DRAPING:	Laparotomy including the groin and perineum.; Foley catheter; laparotomy draping; In addition to the groin, the perineal area needs to be prepped as well.
INSTRUMENTS AND SUPPLIES:	Three- or four-arm robotic setup. 0-degree endoscope; Maryland forceps; curved monopolar scissors; ProGrasp forceps; blunt grasper; ultrasonic scalpel; bipolar forceps; vessel sealing instrument; suction-irrigation device; 12-mm trocars; 8-mm trocars; 0-degree and 30-degree telescope; Veress needle; 5-mm and 12-mm trocars; ligating clips, absorbable and metal; Foley catheters size 22 Fr; specimen retrieval bag

Technical Points and Discussion

1. ***The patient is positioned, prepped, and draped.***
The patient is placed in low lithotomy using a nonskid padding system or vacuum positioning device and prepped from nipple line to pubic symphysis. The abdomen is draped with towels and leggings placed. A laparotomy drape is then applied.

2. ***Pneumoperitoneum is established and ports are placed.***
To start the surgery, a Veress insufflation needle is placed in the midline through the abdominal wall (described in Chapter 20). Insertion of the needle requires minor cutdown instruments, including #11 knife, hemostats, and towel clips to elevate the abdominal wall. After the needle is inserted, a saline drop test is made to ensure correct placement. The insufflation tubing is attached to the needle and pneumoperitoneum established. A 12-mm trocar is placed in the midline incision and the camera inserted. The operating table is lowered and the patient placed in Trendelenburg position. The remaining trocars are inserted under direct vision of the camera as shown in Fig. 24.18. With all ports in place, the robot is targeted and docked.

3. ***The space of Retzius is developed.***
The dissection is started by first releasing adhesions using monopolar curved scissors, fenestrated bipolar forceps, and Prograsp forceps. This is followed by meticulous dissection of the tissue planes to develop exposure to the prostate capsule. This is performed using monopolar curved scissors and Maryland bipolar forceps for sharp and blunt dissection. These are inserted into the appropriate robotic arms and energy cables connected. As the surgeon performs the dissection, the assistant handles the suction to assist in exposure.

4. ***The dorsal vein is suture ligated.***
A suture of 0 polydioxanone is used to ligate the dorsal vein. A slip knot is used to secure the suture. The suture is carried into the pubis to support the bladder and prevent the urethra from retracting after it is transected within the prostate. Some surgeons secure the suture with a locking clip. The urinary catheter is retracted slightly and then moved back in place to ensure that the suture did not enter the urethra.

5. ***The bladder neck is identified and divided.***
Identification of the bladder neck may require manipulation of the Foley catheter to aid in identification. The midline of the anterior and posterior bladder neck is dissected sharply and the anterior bladder neck divided. This exposes the Foley catheter, which is decompressed and brought out of the bladder. The assistant applies countertraction to the catheter, which effectively suspends the prostate. The posterior bladder neck can now be divided. The dissection is carried deeper using the monopolar scissors to the level of the seminal vesicles and vas deferens.

6. ***The seminal vesicles and vas deferens are mobilized and divided.***
At this stage, the surgeon may swap out the 0-degree telescope to a 30-degree down scope. The seminal vesicles and vas deferens are exposed. These are dissected free using the spatula ESU and Maryland forceps. Clips may be used to occlude the vessels. The vessels are grasped

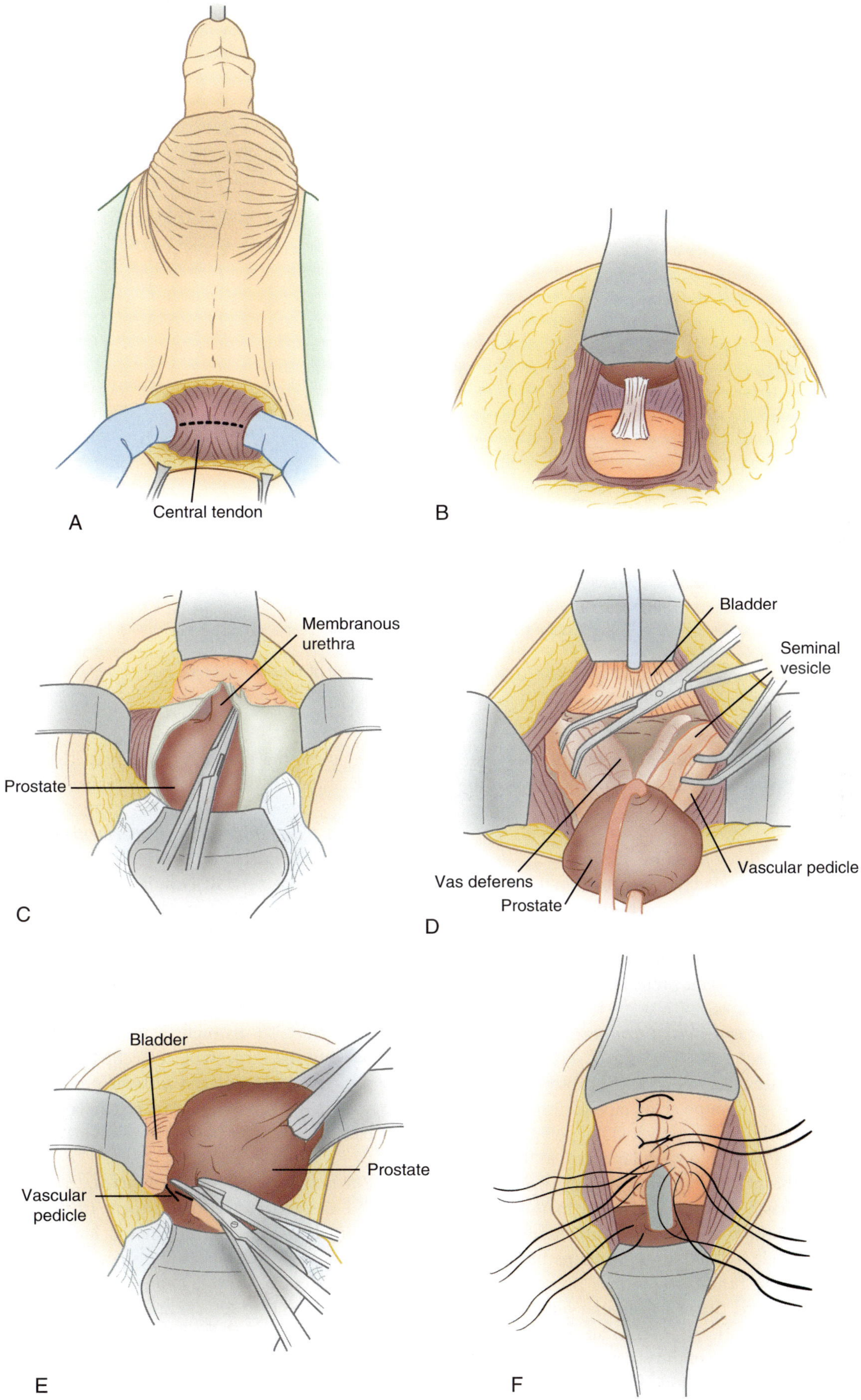

FIG. 24.17 Perineal prostatectomy. (A) Incision through the perineum. (B) Exposure of the central tendon. (C) The periprostatic fascia (gray) has been incised to expose the prostatic capsule. (D) Mobilization of the vascular pedicle. (E) The vascular bundle is severed. (F) Closure of the bladder neck. (From Rothrock J. *Alexander's Care of the Patient in Surgery*. 17th ed. St Louis: Mosby; 2007.)

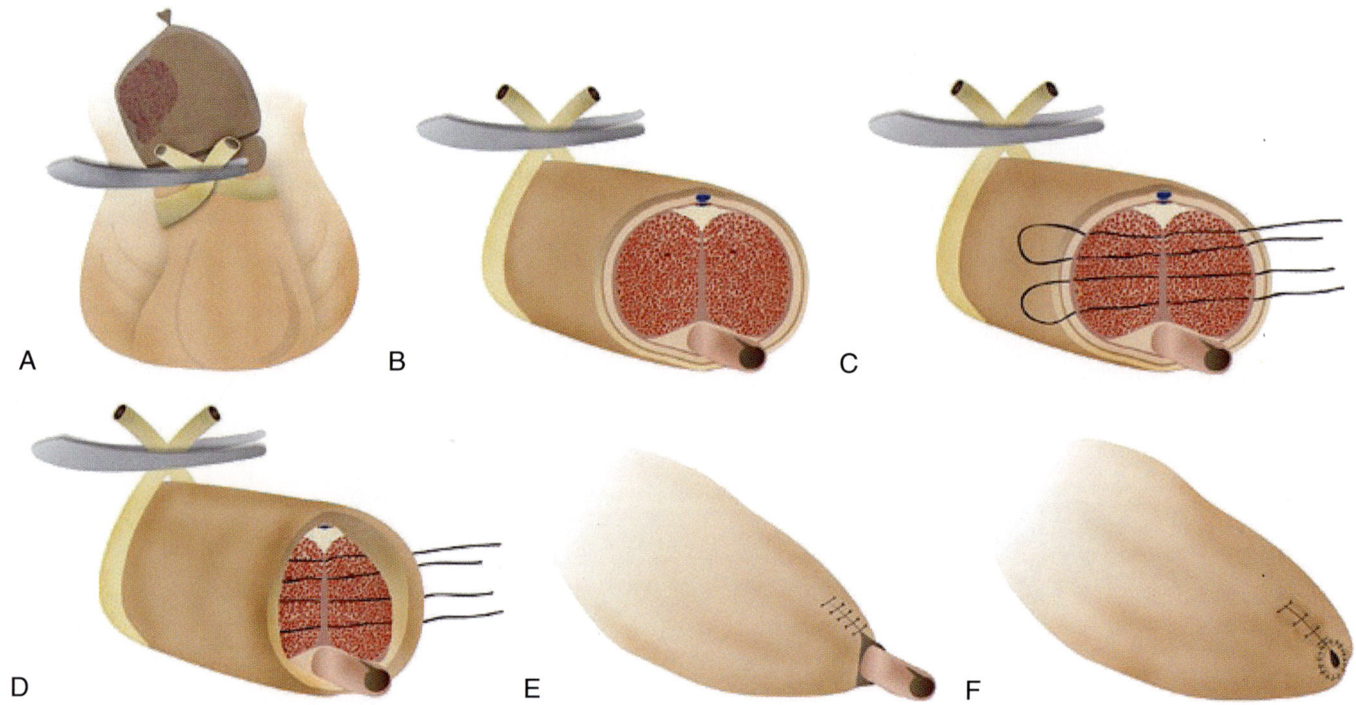

FIG. 24.18 Penectomy. (A) Tourniquet is placed. An impermeable dressing covers the glans and prevents seeding of cancer cells. (B) A circumferential incision is made to the level of the dartos fascia with urethral catheter in place. (C) Mattress sutures are placed. (D) The skin is retracted laterally to provide a tension-free closure. (E) A Y-V plasty is performed around the urethra. (F) Attachment of the urethra to skin using 4-0 sutures. (From Greenberg R. Surgical management of carcinoma of the penis. *Urol Clin North Am.* 2010;37:3.)

and brought out of the opening of the bladder neck and amputated. A grasper is used to remove them from the surgical wound.

7. ***The prostate is mobilized from the rectum.***
The next step is separation of the prostate from the rectum. This involves sharp dissection using ESU scissors and blunt dissection of the fascia between the prostate and rectum. The plane of dissection is continued until the rectal wall is mobilized on both sides to the prostatic apex and pedicles.

8. ***The prostatic pedicle is dissected from the neurovascular bundles.***
Several methods are used to divide the prostate pedicle. Some surgeons use monopolar or bipolar instruments. An alternative method is to apply locking polymer clips. A third method is to apply a vascular clamp to the pedicle, dividing it sharply, and applying a suture ligature after the prostate has been removed. In any method used, the surgeon is careful to protect the neurovascular bundle near the pedicle as the bundle contains the nerves that enable erectile function. In this "nerve-sparing" stage of the procedure, the neurovascular bundle is dissected from the prostatic pedicle. In all cases, thermal energy is avoided. Release of the prostatic pedicle results in nearly complete mobilization of the prostate gland. In the last step of mobilization, the urethra is divided. This frees the specimen. The surgeon inspects the specimen to assess the margins of disease. The prostate is then placed in the pelvic cavity for retrieval later.

9. ***Pelvic lymphadenectomy is performed.***
If lymphadenectomy is planned, it is performed at this time. The extent of lymph node excision depends on the patient's specific profile and risk factors. The lymph nodes are removed by removing the full node packet. This is done using sharp and blunt dissection. Each packet is mobilized, ligated with absorbable hemostatic clips, and divided. Lymph node packets are taken from each side. To distinguish the right- from the left-side packets, the surgeon places a clip in one or the other. The packets are then placed with the prostatic specimen. The specimens can now be placed in a specimen retrieval bag, which is introduced through a 12-mm port.

10. ***The bladder neck is reconstructed.***
The dissection and detachment of the prostate to this point leave an opening in the bladder and a divided urethra. In this stage, these structures are anastomosed. The extent of this stage of the surgery depends on the size of the bladder opening in comparison to the urethral segment. Before the vesicourethral anastomosis is performed, sutures are placed in the posterior fascia supporting the bladder. Size 2-0 barbed or Monocryl suture is often used. The anastomosis is performed using poliglecaprone sutures size 3-0, either running or interrupted. If a running suture is used, a double-armed

suture is used. In this case, the assistant may use the ProGrasp forceps to maintain tension on one arm of the suture. A urethral catheter is passed before completion of the anastomosis. After completion, the bladder is irrigated to check for leaks.

11. ***The specimens are retrieved and the robot undocked.*** After the bladder has been irrigated and any additional sutures placed, the pelvis is assessed for any bleeding. The specimens are then retrieved by transferring the retrieval bag to the telescope port. The pneumothorax is released and the retrieval bag extracted. The robotic arms are undocked.

12. ***The wounds are closed.*** The laparoscopic incisions are closed at the fascia level using size 2-0 absorbable synthetic sutures, and skin is approximated using subcuticular sutures or skin staples and Steri-Strips. A drain may be placed in one of the 8-m ports. The urethral catheter may be left in place for 1 week postoperatively.

SURGERY OF THE MALE EXTERNAL GENITALIA

CIRCUMCISION (ADULT)

Circumcision is the removal of the prepuce (foreskin), which is done to improve genital hygiene and for cultural and religious reasons.

Pathology

An uncircumcised male may develop several conditions that affect the glans and foreskin. Skin detritus can become trapped between the foreskin and glans, leading to infection and scarring. In these conditions, the foreskin cannot be retracted from the glans (phimosis), or it adheres to the base of the glans and cannot be returned to its normal anatomical position (paraphimosis).

Some evidence indicates that uncircumcised males may be at risk for penile cancer related to repeated infection or exposure to human papilloma virus. In general, circumcision is widely practiced. Normally, the procedure is performed on newborns. However, adults who have experienced infection and scarring of the foreskin may seek circumcision.

POSITION:	Supine
INCISION:	Foreskin
PREP AND DRAPING:	Genital
INSTRUMENTS:	Minor plastic surgery set; needlepoint ESU

Technical Points and Discussion

1. ***The foreskin is measured and marked.*** The patient is placed in the supine position, prepped, and draped with a small fenestrated sheet. The coronal ridge is outlined with a skin marker to identify the incision.

A dorsal incision is made in the skin and carried circumferentially.

The surgeon places several Kelly, Crile, or mosquito hemostats on the edge of the prepuce. A longitudinal incision is made on the dorsal side of the foreskin with fine dissecting scissors. The incision is carried circumferentially around the prepuce, and small bleeders are controlled with the needlepoint ESU.

2. ***The foreskin is sutured to the corona and dressings applied.*** The surgeon then sutures the wound edges to the corona with 4-0 or 5-0 interrupted absorbable sutures. The wound is dressed with petrolatum gauze.

PARTIAL PENECTOMY

Penectomy is partial or complete amputation of the penis for the treatment of cancer of the penis and urethra.

Pathology

Penile cancer is rare in Western countries. About 30% of cancers are related to the human papilloma virus (HPV). Squamous cell carcinoma, basal cell carcinoma, and melanoma have also been identified in association with penile cancer. The dissection may be performed using the Mohs technique, described in Chapter 28. In this procedure, the tumor margins are identified and the tissue specimen examined as a frozen section. The excisional margin is then increased until the edges are no longer positive for cancerous cells.

Because of the psychological effects of penectomy, all attempts are made toward conservative surgical treatment. In many patients, circumcision is adequate. The following description describes partial penectomy, which is the most common procedure for invasive squamous cell carcinoma.

POSITION:	Supine or lithotomy
INCISION:	According to the pathology
PREP AND DRAPING:	Genitalia
INSTRUMENTS:	Minor set; ESU with needlepoint
POSSIBLE EXTRAS:	Narrow Penrose drain

Technical Points and Discussion

1. ***The patient is prepped and draped and the skin incision marked.*** The patient is placed in the supine or lithotomy position, and the external genitalia including a wide margin are prepped and draped. A Foley catheter may be placed after the skin prep. The skin incision may be marked to extend over 2 cm of the lesion.

2. ***The skin is incised and the incision carried to the fascia.*** Before the procedure starts, some surgeons place a narrow Penrose drain around the base of the penis to act as a tourniquet. The circumferential skin incision is made using a #15 surgical blade. Small Allis or mosquito clamps are used to grasp the incised skin edges for traction. The penile skin is retracted proximally to enable further dissection of the tissue planes. The incision is carried to the level of Buck's fascia. The fascia is then incised laterally to create a new dissection plane. This may be performed with fine plastic scissors such as tenotomy scissors or other fine-tissue scissors. Small sponge dissectors should be available to dissect the tissue between the tunica albuginea and the neurovascular tissue. Hemostasis is controlled using fine mosquito forceps and size 4-0 suture ties to ligate the penile vessels.

3. ***A skin flap is created.*** The sharp tissue dissection is carried through the two corpora structures to the urethra circumferentially, leaving an additional 1 cm of skin that will be used to cover the defect. The urethra is isolated to extend approximately 1 cm from the two corpora and then divided. The specimen is thus freed and passed to the ST.

4. ***The corpora are sutured and a urethrostomy performed.*** The defects in the corpora are closed using interrupted horizontal mattress sutures, usually of 2-0 or 3-0 Vicryl on a small curved needle. To perform urethrostomy, the urethra is splayed on one side. The skin is then sutured to form a YV-plasty with the urethra everted over the opening. The urethra is secured to the skin using size 4-0 interrupted absorbable sutures. If only the glans is to be removed, the skin flap can be brought over the defect using a buttonhole technique to form the urethrostomy. In this case, a small hole is made in the skin flap to accommodate the urethra, which is secured to the skin as in the YV-plasty. The operative steps are shown in Fig. 24.18.

   The wound can be dressed using Xeroform gauze strips over the incision site covered with plain gauze. The Foley catheter remains in place for 3 to 5 days.

INSERTION OF PENILE IMPLANT

A penile implant is surgically placed to treat impotence caused by organic disease. Many types of inflatable penile implants are available. Each manufacturer provides detailed instructions on the tools and techniques used to place the implant. The technique described here uses an inflatable pump manufactured by Coloplast. As with any implant, the system should be handled as little as possible and steps taken to prevent any lint from adhering to the surface of the components.

This system has three components. Inflatable cylinders are placed in the corpora cavernosa of the penis. A saline reservoir is connected to the cylinders and implanted under the rectus muscle. The pump that inflates and deflates the cylinders is placed in the scrotum.

Pathology

A malfunction in the erectile system of the penis is most often caused by neurological disease, diabetes, vascular disease, or a psychological problem. Patients for whom no organic cause can be found are carefully screened for this procedure.

Technical Points and Discussion

1. ***The patient is prepped and draped for a scrotal procedure.*** The patient is placed in the supine or lithotomy position, prepped, and draped for a scrotal approach. A 16-Fr Foley catheter is placed and capped. A self-retaining Scott ring retractor is placed over the genitalia.

2. ***The scrotum is incised at the penoscrotal junction and carried into the superficial fascia.*** A #15 knife blade is used to make a midline scrotal incision. Small bleeders may be controlled using the needlepoint ESU. The fascia layer is incised and the Scott retractor with hooks is used to hold the tissue edges back.

3. ***The corpus cavernosum on each side is exposed and entered.*** A set of 2-0 Vicryl stay sutures is inserted into the tunica albuginea on each cavernosum. A 1-cm incision is then made into each cavernosum using the knife and deepened with fine-tissue scissors. A Hegar cervical dilator may be used to dilate the spongiosum tract, which will accommodate the cavernosa cylinder. A measurement device is inserted into each side to determine the correct length for implantation. The implant tracts are irrigated with saline using a syringe and soft adapter tip.

4. ***The penile cylinders are inserted into the cavernosa.*** The correct size prosthesis is opened on the field and maintained in a small basin. The cylinders are then primed with saline. A Furlow inserter is used to insert the cylinders into each side. This device passes a traction suture attached to a straight Keith needle at one end and to the cylinder at the other. The device is pushed into the cavernosa space and the needle passed through the glans penis. This allows the cylinder to be pulled into the cavernosa. This step is repeated on each side. The suture ends are tagged with hemostats to prevent them from retracting back into the penis. The incisions in the tunica albuginea are closed on each side with synthetic absorbable running suture. Each cylinder is flushed with saline using a 60-mL syringe.

5. ***The reservoir is implanted.***
An appropriate size reservoir is selected based on the length of the cylinder prosthesis. The bladder is fully drained. A small Deaver retractor is inserted at the superior end of the scrotal incision. The groin area is entered with closed Metzenbaum scissors followed by digital separation of tissue to form a pouch behind the abdominal wall in front of the bladder. The fluid reservoir is placed in the pouch. The retractor is removed and the reservoir filled with saline using a 60-mL syringe and short IV tubing with connectors. The reservoir tubing is trimmed and connected using the plastic connection collars that come with the system.

6. ***The pump is installed.***
Two Babcock or Allis clamps are placed on the edges of the scrotal incision. A small space is created digitally or by using a nasal speculum as shown below between the testicles. The pump is then placed in the space created.

7. ***The incision is closed.***
The scrotal incision is closed in two or three layers using synthetic absorbable suture. A dressing composed of flat and fluff gauze is placed over the wound. The procedure is illustrated in Fig. 24.19.

IMPORTANT TO KNOW *The procedure details, including specifications and instructions for handling and assembly of the system, are available from the manufacturers of implant systems. These are very useful for learning the details of each type of system, including intraoperative steps for the surgical technologist.*

HYDROCELECTOMY

A hydrocele is a benign, fluid-filled sac that develops in the anterior testis. It is drained and removed to prevent rupture and hemorrhage. The procedure can be performed as an open surgery or endoscopically.

Pathology

A hydrocele in the adult may arise from trauma, infection, or tumor, or as a result of peritoneal dialysis.

POSITION:	Supine
INCISION:	Scrotal
PREP AND DRAPING:	Lower abdomen and genitalia
INSTRUMENTS:	Minor plastic surgery set; Allis clamps; Babcock clamps; plastic surgery scissors
POSSIBLE EXTRAS:	Needlepoint ESU

Technical Points and Discussion

1. ***An incision is made in the scrotum over the hydrocele.***
The patient is placed in the supine position and prepped for a scrotal incision. The surgeon makes a small incision in the scrotum using a #15 knife blade and ESU.

2. ***The hydrocele and sac are brought out of the scrotum.***
The hydrocele is brought out from the scrotum and a small opening made with scissors. The ST should have suction immediately available to remove the fluid from the surgical field. The sac is further opened.

3. ***The sac edges are oversewn.***
The edges of the sac are grasped with fine hemostats and retracted outward. The sac tissue is then trimmed and oversewn with size 3-0 synthetic absorbable suture. Alternatively, the sac edges may be brought around the testis and approximated. The surgeon may insert a small Penrose drain in the wound, which then is closed in two layers with fine absorbable sutures. A bulky gauze dressing is applied. Hydrocelectomy is shown in Fig. 24.20.

ORCHIECTOMY

Orchiectomy is the surgical removal of one or both testicles.

Pathology

Removal of one testicle most often is performed in cases of testicular carcinoma or **torsion** (twisting of the testis, resulting in ischemia and necrosis). Bilateral orchiectomy may be performed to control metastatic carcinoma of the prostate.

Rotation of the testicle is related to a congenital anomaly or occurs as a result of vigorous activity in young males. Torsion is a medical emergency, because the testicular blood vessels may be occluded, resulting in ischemia and necrosis of the testicle. Testicular cancer usually arises from the germ (reproductive) cells of the male. It represents 1% of all cancers, but it is the most common cancer among young men. Early screening and vigorous public health campaigns have lowered the incidence in the past several decades.

Orchiectomy can be performed using local anesthesia with sedation or with general anesthesia.

POSITION:	Supine
INCISION:	Scrotal
PREP AND DRAPING:	Lower abdomen, genitalia, perineum
INSTRUMENTS:	Minor set

Technical Points and Discussion

1. ***An incision is made in the scrotum and the testicle mobilized.***
The patient is placed in the supine position, prepped, and draped for a scrotal incision.

The surgeon makes a 1- to 1.2-inch (2.5- to 3-cm) midline incision into the anterior scrotal wall with a #15 blade. Using the ESU, the surgeon separates the testicle from the fascia and dartos muscle. This technique exposes the tunica vaginalis. A sponge is used to separate the tunica vaginalis from remaining attachments until the testicle can be delivered from the wound. The tunica is then incised to expose the testicle.

2. ***The spermatic vessels and vas deferens are clamped and divided.***

The spermatic cord is bluntly separated into several segments with the vas deferens isolated. The vas deferens is separated, double-clamped, cut, and ligated with 2-0 Vicryl ties. A suture ligature may also be placed through each segment. The testicular artery and veins are cross-clamped with Kelly or Mayo clamps. The tissue vessels are divided with the ESU

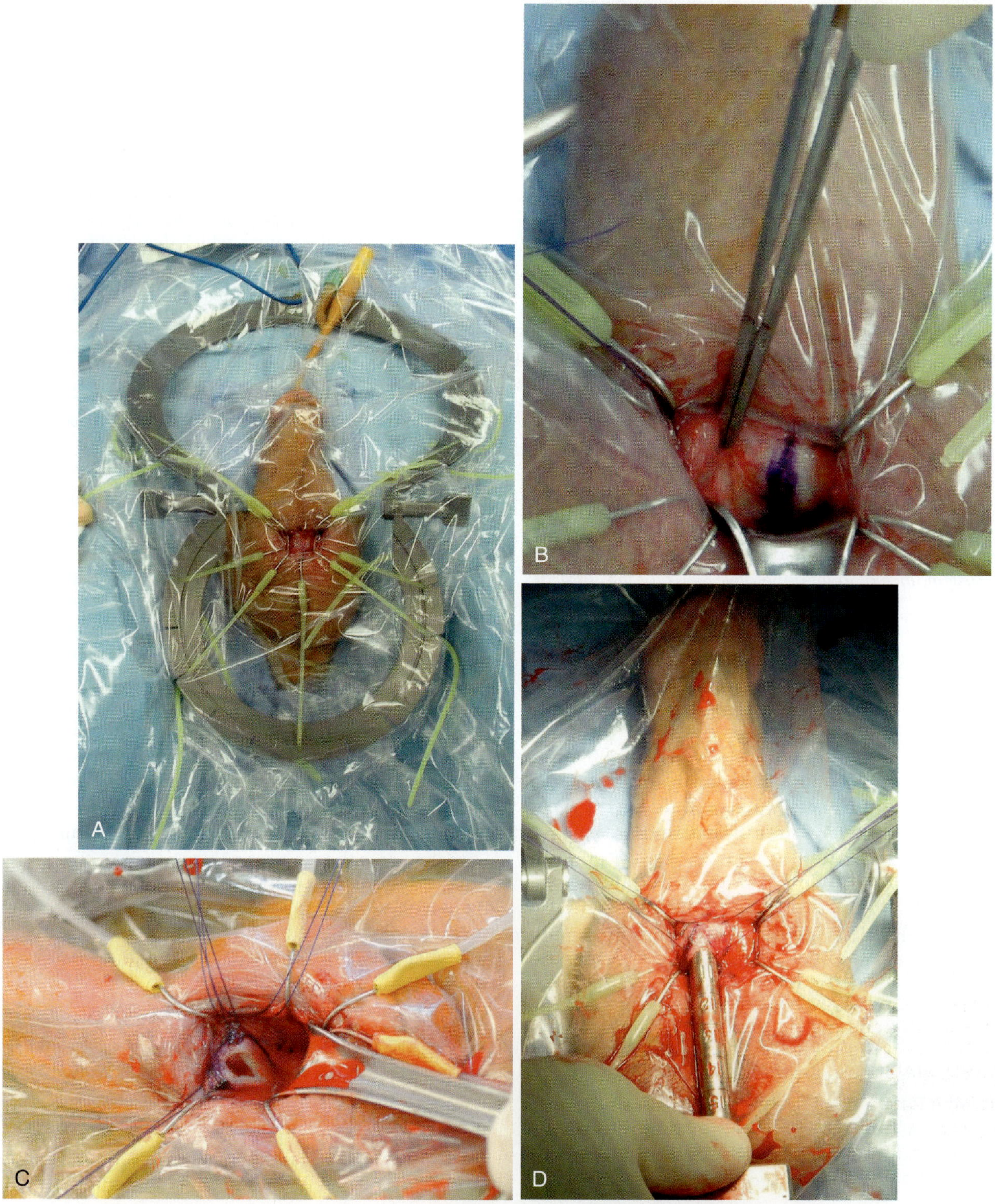

FIG. 24.19 Penile implant. (A) A self-retaining rubber band and hook retractor are placed in the scrotal incision. Here a transparent drape is used. (B) The corpus cavernosum is identified and marked on each side of the urethra. (C) The incision is made into the corpus. Note traction sutures. (D) Hegar dilators are used to create a tunnel in each cavernosum.

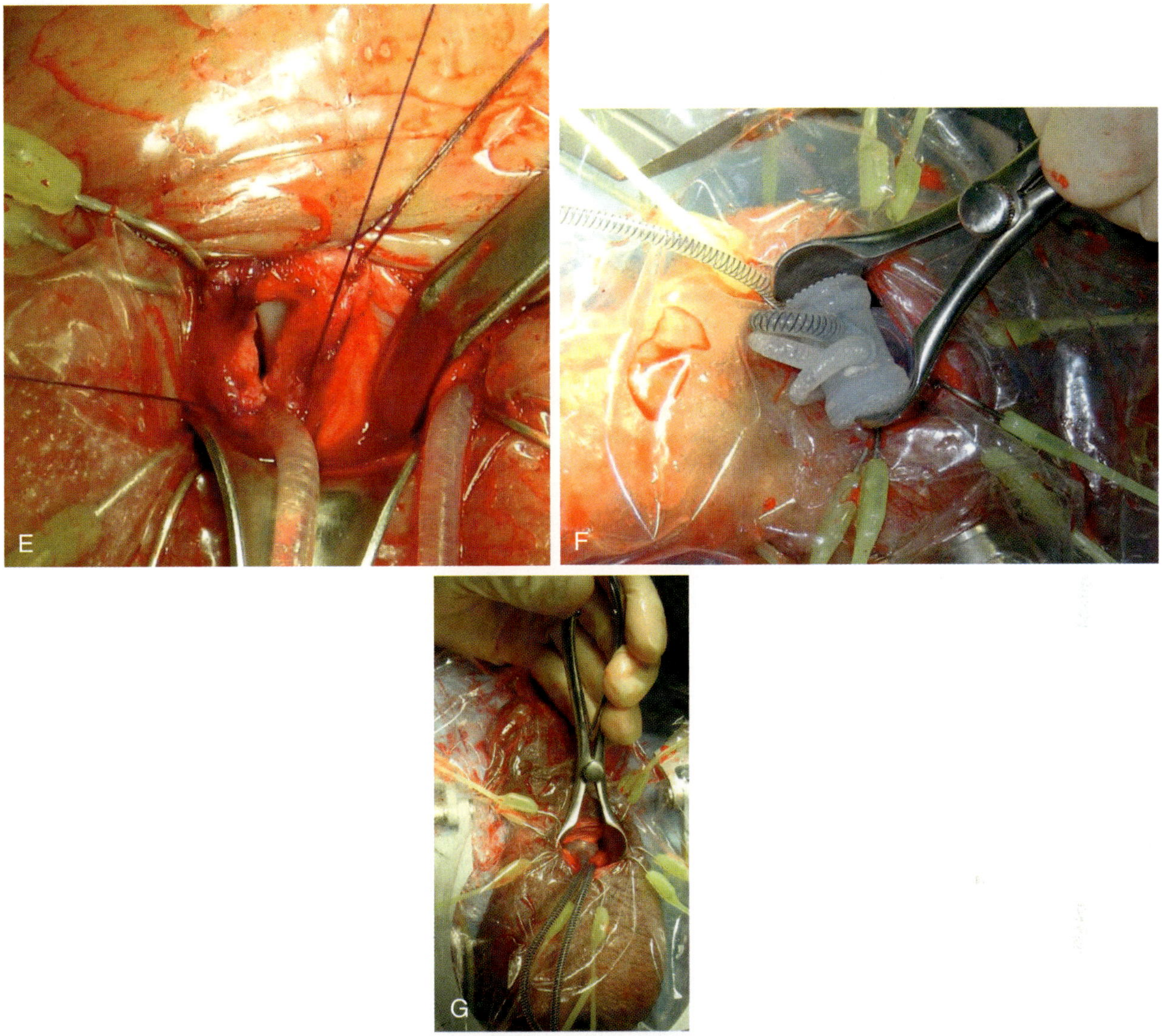

FIG. 24.19 cont'd (E) A suture introducer has been passed through the length of the cavernosa and the cylinders pulled through the tunnel. (F) The pump is placed in the scrotal sac. Here a nasal speculum is used to create the space and place the pump. (G) The reservoir is placed into the space of Retzius. (From Wein A, Kavoussi L, Partin A, Peters C. *Campbell-Walsh Urology*. 11th ed. Philadelphia: Elsevier; 2016.)

and ligated with size 0 absorbable synthetic suture ligatures. A suture ligature is also placed in the vessels.

The suture ends are left long and tagged until there is no risk of hemorrhage.

3. ***The wound is irrigated and closed.***
The wound is irrigated and inspected for any remaining bleeders. The dartos layer is closed with size 2-0 or 3-0 absorbable suture. Skin is closed with a subcuticular suture. Dressing consists of gauze fluffs and a scrotal support. Testicular prosthetics may be inserted at the time of surgery or in a subsequent procedure.

Complications after orchiectomy may include those expected after cessation of testosterone production. These include loss of libido, fatigue, and tenderness of the breasts. Patients are prescribed testosterone postoperatively to prevent these symptoms.

KEY CONCEPTS

- Genitourinary procedures involve the upper and lower urinary tracts and male genitalia.
- Many health care facilities have a designated endoscopic technologist for their urology suite. This position requires a high level of knowledge about the techniques and

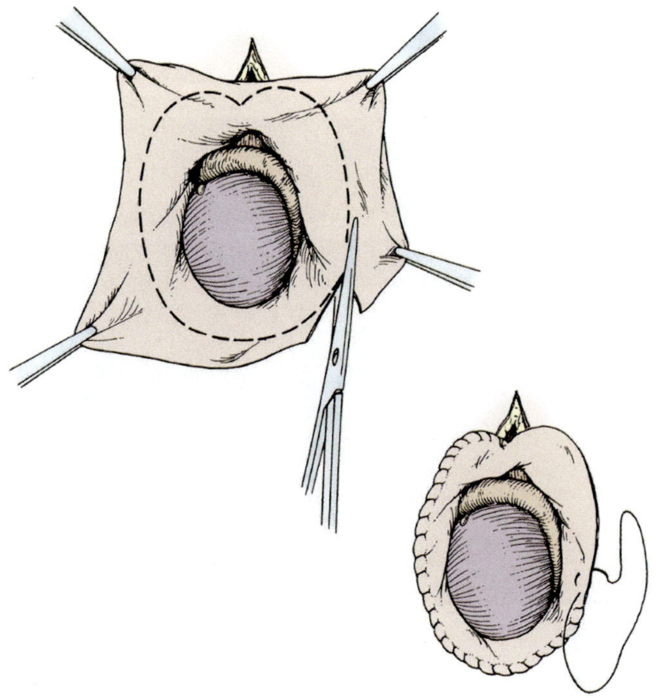

FIG. 24.20 Hydrocelectomy. The hydrocele sac is excised and the edges oversewn. (From Wein A, Kavoussi L, Partin A, Peters C. *Campbell-Walsh Urology*. 11th ed. Philadelphia: Elsevier; 2016.)

equipment used in cystourethroscopy and cystoureteral procedures.

- Transurethral and percutaneous equipment includes a wide variety of catheters and stents. Catheter exchange is a technique used to replace one with another while maintaining the precise position of the tube in the ureter or kidney.
- The cysto suite is designed specifically for endoscopic procedures, including a fluid waste system and specialized operating table.
- Bladder distention solutions used during cystoscopy are selected according to whether electrosurgery is used. Electrolytic solutions are not used when electrosurgery is anticipated.
- Lithotripsy, the crushing of stones, is a common procedure using many different methods. Modern methods have replaced open procedures for removal of stones.
- The French measurement system is used in urology and other specialties to designate the diameter of instruments and devices. In this system, size 1 Fr equals 3 mm.
- Transurethral procedures are commonly performed in bladder and prostate surgery.
- Removal of a kidney in a live donor can be performed as a hand-assisted endoscopic or open surgery.
- The donor kidney is placed outside the recipient's abdominal cavity in the retroperitoneal space.
- Nerve-sparing prostatectomy is routinely performed using robotic and laparoscopic techniques.

REVIEW QUESTIONS

1. Explain the purpose of continuous irrigation during transurethral surgery.
2. Explain how a urethral catheter is used as a tamponade.
3. Explain why testicular torsion is an emergency.
4. The lateral position is used for many procedures of the genitourinary tract. List at least five critical safety considerations for this position. Include specific anatomical locations and risk factors.
5. Many patients undergoing transurethral surgery are older. List four methods you would use to communicate with these patients.

BIBLIOGRAPHY

Arthur D. *Smith's Textbook of Endourology*. 2nd ed. London: BC Decker; 2007.

Graham SD. *Glenn's Urologic Surgery*. 6th ed. Philadelphia: Lippincott Williams & Wilkins; 2004.

Greenberg R. Surgical management of carcinoma of the penis. *Urol Clin North Am*. 2010;37:3.

Hanno P, Guzzo T, Malkowicz S, Wein A. *Penn Clinical Manual of Urology*. 2nd ed. Philadelphia: Saunders; 2014.

Pietrow P, Karellas M. Medical management of common urinary calculi. *Am Fam Physician*. 2006;74:86.

Smith J, Howards S, McGuire E, Preminger G. *Hinman's Atlas of Urologic Surgery*. 3rd ed. Philadelphia: Saunders; 2012.

Tanagho EA. *Smith's General Urology*. 17th ed. New York: McGraw Hill; 2008.

Walters M, Karram M. *Urogynecology and Reconstructive Pelvic Surgery*. 4th ed. Philadelphia: Saunders; 2015.

Wein A, Kavoussi L, Partin A, Peters C. *Campbell-Walsh Urology*. 11th ed. Philadelphia: Elsevier; 2016.

OPHTHALMIC SURGERY 25

LEARNING OBJECTIVES

After studying this chapter, the reader will be able to:

1. Identify key anatomical structures of the eye
2. Discuss common diagnostic procedures of the eye
3. Discuss specific elements of case planning for eye surgery
4. Discuss surgical techniques used in eye surgery, including use of the operating microscope
5. Describe common surgical procedures of the eye

TERMINOLOGY

Accommodation: A process in which the lens continually changes shape to maintain the focus of an image on the retina.

Cataract: Clouding of vision caused by a disease in which the crystalline lens of the eye, its capsule, or both become opaque. This prevents light from focusing on the retina, resulting in visual distortion.

Cryotherapy: A technique in which a cold probe is used to freeze tissue, such as the sclera, ciliary body (for glaucoma), or retinal layers, after detachment.

Diathermy: Low-power cautery used to burn the sclera over an area of retinal detachment.

Enucleation: Surgical removal of the globe and accessory attachments.

Evisceration: Surgical removal of the contents of the eyeball, with the sclera left intact.

Exenteration: Removal of the entire contents of the orbit.

Focal point: The point where light rays converge after passing through a lens.

Glaucoma: A group of diseases characterized by elevation of the intraocular pressure. Sustained pressure on the optic nerve and other structures may result in ischemia and blindness.

Keratoplasty: Surgery of the cornea. The term penetrating keratoplasty refers to corneal transplantation.

Muscle recession: Surgery in which the eye muscle is moved back to release the globe.

Muscle resection: Surgical shortening of an eye muscle to pull the globe into correct position.

Phacoemulsification: A process whereby high-frequency sound waves are used to emulsify tissue, such as a cataract.

Pterygium: A triangular membrane that arises from the medial canthus; the tissue may extend over the cornea, causing blindness.

Refraction: A phenomenon of physics in which light rays are bent as they pass through a transparent medium that is denser than air. In the eye, refraction occurs as light enters the front of the eye and passes through the cornea, lens, aqueous humor, and vitreous.

Spatula needle: A flat-tipped suture needle commonly used in ophthalmic surgery.

Strabismus: Inability to coordinate the extraocular muscles, which prevents binocular vision.

The goal of ophthalmic surgery is to restore vision lost as a result of disease, injury, or congenital defect. Procedures include those performed on the external and internal structures of the eye.

Eye procedures are particularly delicate and precise. Teamwork and attention to detail are critical in ophthalmic surgery. Ophthalmic procedures are performed in a variety of health care settings, including the hospital and outpatient center. Regardless of the setting, preparations and procedures for the patient's safety are fully implemented in the perioperative period. Of particular concern are verifying that the operative site and the implants are correct, positioning precautions, and drug and environmental safety.

SURGICAL ANATOMY

ORBITAL CAVITY

The basic structure of the eyeball, the globe, is contained within the orbital cavity (also called the *bony orbit*). Seven separate bones come together to form the orbit: the frontal, lacrimal, sphenoid, ethmoid, maxillary, zygomatic, and palatine bones. The paired palatine bones form a part of the orbital floor. The cavity is lined with connective tissue, which cushions the eye. Although most of the orbit is composed of thin bone, the rim is particularly thick and therefore more protective. The optic nerve enters the posterior orbital cavity through the optic foramen (Fig. 25.1).

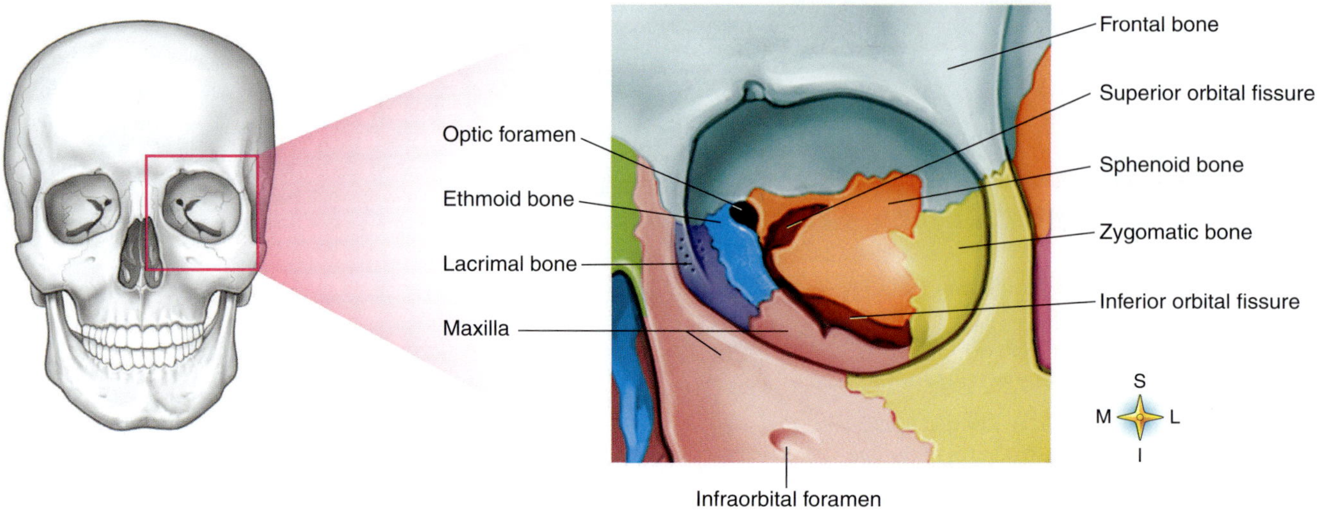

FIG. 25.1 The orbital cavity (bony orbit) showing the composite bones. (From Thibodeau G, Patton K. *Anatomy and Physiology*. 6th ed. St Louis: Mosby; 2007.)

EYELIDS

The eyelids are composed of fibrous connective tissue (referred to as the *tarsal plate*) covered with skin. The lids protect the eye from injury and light. The term *palpebral* refers to the eyelids. The space or interval between the upper and lower lids is called the *palpebral fissure*. Each juncture of the eyelids is called a *canthus*. Sebaceous glands located along the lid margin and in the lacrimal caruncle secrete waxy oil that seals the eyelids when they are closed. The eyelashes, which extend along the tarsus, protect the eye from airborne particles (Fig. 25.2).

GLOBE

The globe has separate cavities, each of which contains functional structures. The posterior cavity lies at the back of the eyeball and contains a gel called *vitreous*. The anterior cavity is divided into two spaces, the anterior and the posterior chamber.

The globe is enclosed by separate tissue layers, each very distinctive in structure and function (Fig. 25.3).

EYE MUSCLES

Six muscles attach the sclera to the bony orbit and move the eyeball around various axes. This allows both eyes to focus on a single point. Each eye has four rectus muscles: the superior, inferior, lateral, and medial. Each eye also has two oblique muscles, the superior and inferior. The visual field is the area we see when the eyes are focused on a single point. Vision normally is binocular; that is, each eye has a nearly separate visual field, and the two are brought together as one image in the brain. The visible area consists of central and peripheral vision (Fig. 25.4).

CONJUNCTIVA

The palpebral conjunctiva is a thin, transparent mucous membrane that lines each eyelid and reflects onto the globe,

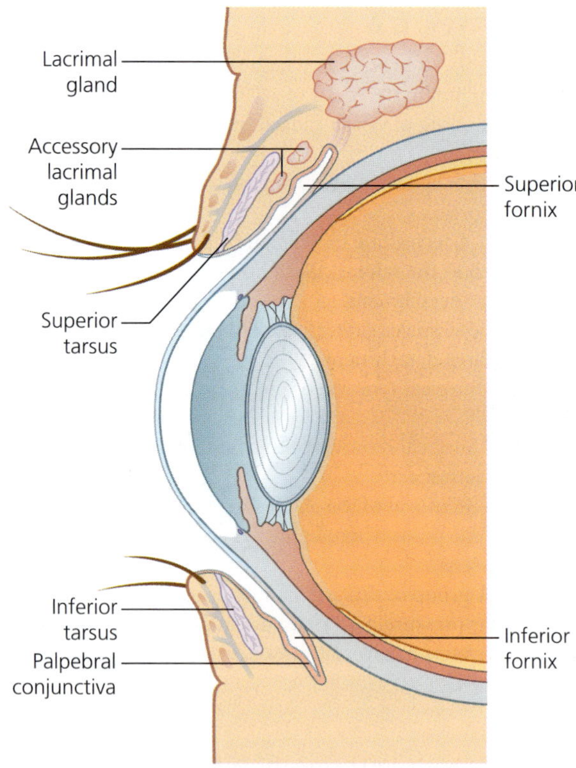

FIG. 25.2 Vertical section of the eyelids and conjunctiva. (From Stein H, Stein R, Freeman M. *The Ophthalmic Assistant*. 9th ed. Philadelphia: Saunders; 2013.)

where it is called the *bulbar conjunctiva*. It moves anteriorly, encompassing the globe up to the anatomic junction of the cornea and sclera at the *limbus* (sclera junction). The bulbar conjunctiva appears white, because the sclera lies directly beneath it.

CORNEA

The cornea is a clear tissue layer overlying the front of the eyeball. Light enters the eye through the cornea and is refracted

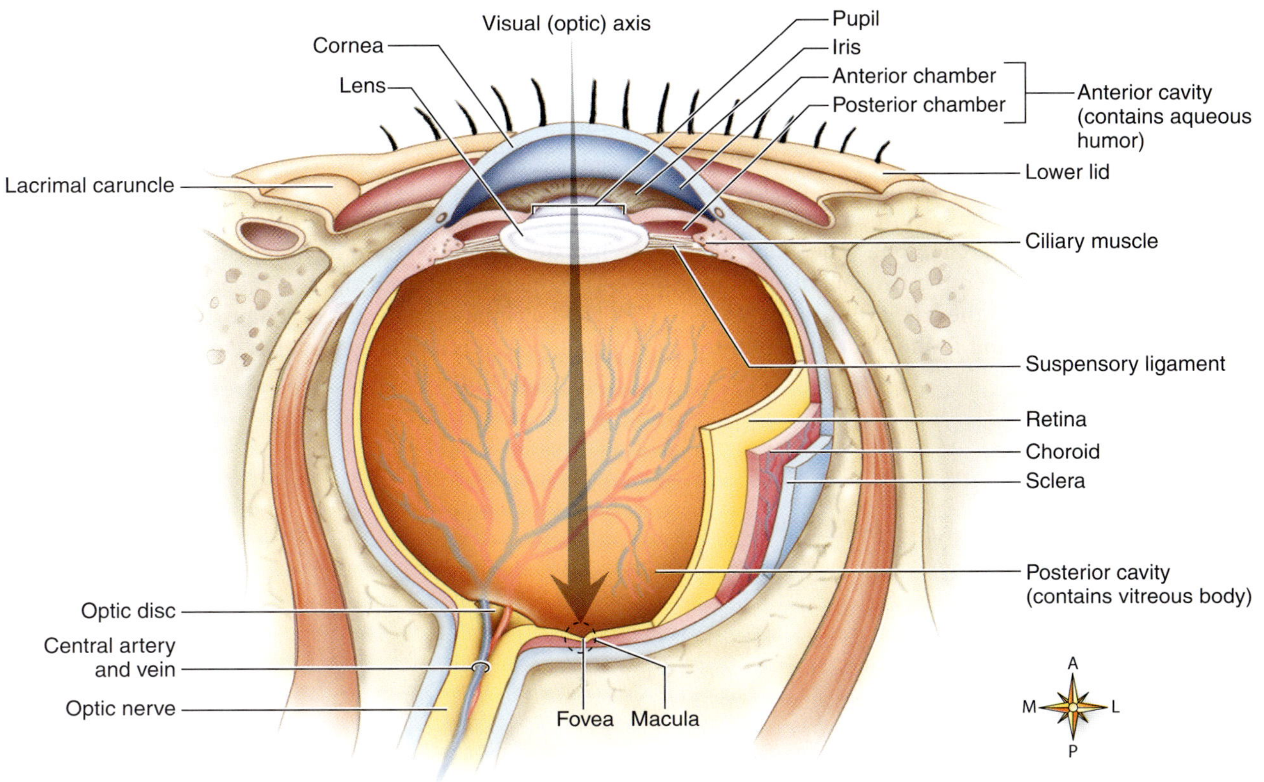

FIG. 25.3 The interior of the globe showing the layers of the inner eye, chambers, lens, retina, and optic nerve. (From Patton KT, Thibodeau GA. *The Human Body in Health & Disease*. 6th ed. St Louis: Elsevier; 2014.)

(bent); this allows images to be focused on the retina. The cornea has no blood vessels. It is composed of three tissue layers: the epithelium (superficial layer), the stroma, and the endothelium. The circular boundary of the cornea extends to the sclera. During cataract surgery, the initial incision is made in the limbus where the two tissues meet.

SCLERA

The sclera is a thick, white, fibrous tissue that encloses about three-fourths of the eyeball. It is the external supporting layer of the eyeball. The sclera is contiguous with the cornea at the front of the eye. The sclera communicates with the optic nerve sheath.

CHOROID LAYER AND CILIARY BODY

The highly vascular pigmented choroid layer lies directly beneath the sclera. The primary function of the choroid is to prevent the reflection of light within the eyeball. An extension of the choroid layer, the ciliary body, is located at the periphery of the anterior choroid. It is composed of smooth muscle tissue to which suspensory ligaments are attached.

IRIS

The iris is a pigmented membrane composed mainly of muscle tissue that surrounds the pupil. The actions of the muscle fibers cause the pupil to close or open, to exclude light, or to admit light into the inner eye. The pupil may appear dilated or constricted, depending on the action of the iris.

RETINA

The innermost layer of the posterior globe is called the *retina*. The retina is the photoreceptive layer of the eye; it receives and transmits images to the brain via the optic nerve. Light projected onto the retina from the front of the eye is converted into nerve impulses that are transmitted to the brain, creating sight. The two types of photoreceptive cells are those that transmit black and white and those that enable color perception. The macula is a distinct area of acute vision that lies near the optic nerve. The center of this structure is called the *fovea centralis*. The optic nerve exits the globe in an area of dense neurons called the *optic disc*. The optic disc has no photoreceptors.

LENS

The lens lies directly behind the iris in the anterior chamber. It is a clear biconvex disc contained in a transparent capsule. The lens is held in place by suspensory ligaments called *zonules*, which are attached to the capsule and ciliary body. The suspensory ligaments change the shape of the lens to bend light that passes through the lens. This focuses the images that are projected onto the retina.

ANTERIOR AND POSTERIOR CHAMBERS

The anterior cavity of the eye is divided into two chambers: the anterior and posterior chambers. The pupil is the only passageway between the two chambers. The anterior chamber lies in front of the iris, whereas the posterior chamber lies behind the iris but in front of (anterior to) the lens. A clear fluid produced by the ciliary epithelium, called *aqueous humor*, fills the anterior chamber. The pupil allows aqueous humor to pass between the two chambers through a space between the lens and the iris. From there, it passes into the canal of Schlemm and is shunted directly into the venous system.

LACRIMAL APPARATUS

The lacrimal apparatus produces tears and provides channels for their drainage. This group of structures includes the lacrimal gland, caruncle, tear ducts, lacrimal sac, and nasolacrimal duct (Fig. 25.5). Tears are produced by the lacrimal gland located laterally in the orbit. Each gland has numerous ducts that drain into the conjunctiva. The lacrimal ducts extend from the inner canthus to the lacrimal sac. The opening of each duct is called the *lacrimal punctum*. The lacrimal sac is an enlarged portion of the nasolacrimal duct, which is a passageway that connects the punctum and the nasal sinus.

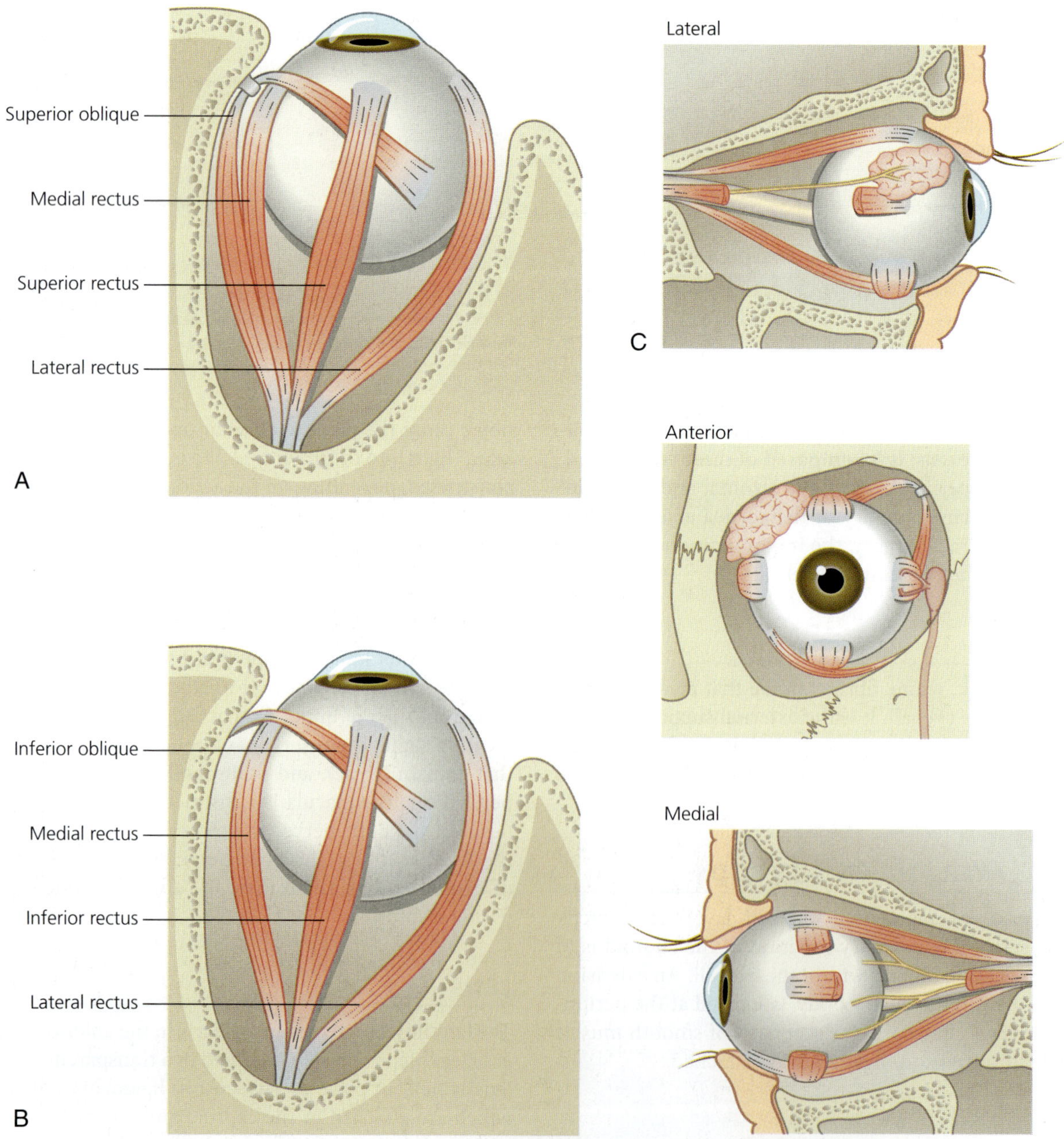

FIG. 25.4 Muscles of the eye. (A) The right eye viewed from above. (B) Muscles viewed from below. (C) Muscles viewed laterally, anteriorly, and medially. (From Stein H, Stein R, Freeman M. *The Ophthalmic Assistant*. 9th ed. Philadelphia: Saunders; 2013.)

Tears are composed of many chemicals, including proteins, mucus, sodium chloride, glucose, and enzymes capable of breaking down the cell membrane of bacteria. Tears continually bathe the eye and protect it from dehydration and infection. Tearing is stimulated by chemical and physical irritants and strong emotion. Tears produced by emotions have a different composition than those arising from irritation and pain.

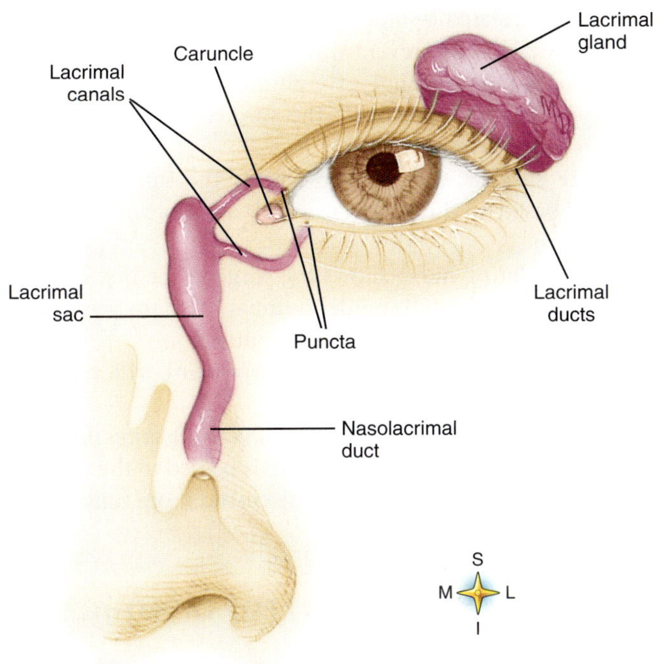

FIG. 25.5 The lacrimal apparatus, including the lacrimal gland and ducts, lacrimal canals and sac, and nasolacrimal duct. (From Abrahams P, Marks S, Hutchings R. *McMinn's Colour Atlas of Human Anatomy*. 5th ed. Oxford: Mosby; 2003.)

REFRACTION

Refraction is the bending of light rays through a transparent medium. Refraction occurs as light enters the front of the eye and passes through the lens. The light rays are refracted as they pass through the cornea, aqueous humor, lens, and vitreous. The rays converge at the **focal point.** The image produced by the light rays is brought into focus by **accommodation.** This is a complex process in which the lens continually changes shape to keep the image focused on the fovea. This enables us to view objects at various distances and keep them in focus (Fig. 25.6).

DIAGNOSTIC TESTING

Refraction is a test for visual acuity, performed using a *phoropter*. This device has a range of corrective lenses that allow the patient to compare different combinations while viewing an eye chart. The term *refraction*, described earlier as the bending of light rays through a transparent medium, is also used to describe this test. A *slit lamp* is used to examine the anterior chamber of the eye. Details of the lid margins, conjunctiva, tear film, cornea, and iris can be studied. The pupil can be dilated and the lens and anterior vitreous examined. Fluorescein is used to stain the cornea and highlight irregularities of the epithelial surface. A *tonometer* is used to measure the intraocular pressure (IOP).

Direct examination of the eyes is performed using an *ophthalmoscope*. This is a handheld instrument that magnifies the focal point, allowing the examiner to evaluate the fundus and

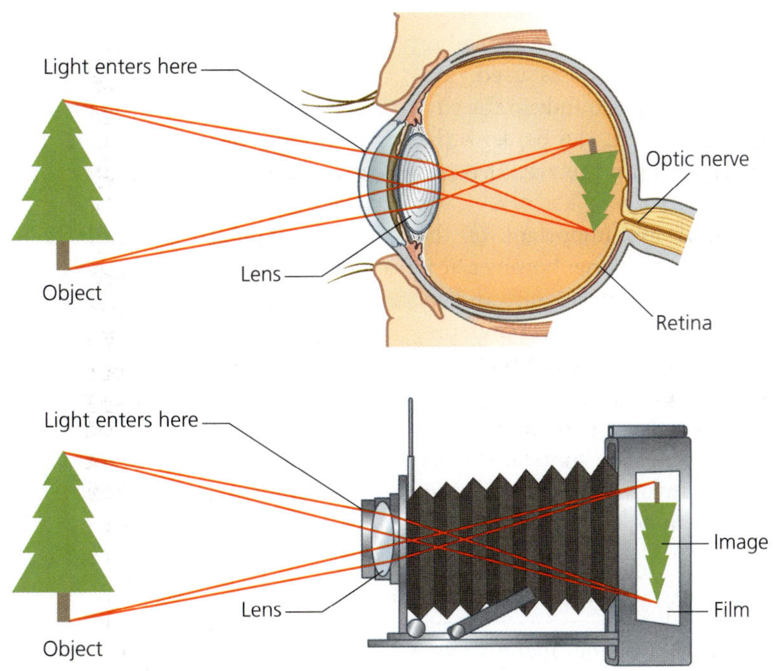

FIG. 25.6 Image created by light passing through the lens, which is similar to a camera. (Courtesy Medline, Inc.)

other internal eye structures. An indirect binocular ophthalmoscope is used to examine the retina and other structures within a wider focal point.

Fluorescein angiography is used extensively in the diagnosis and evaluation of retinal and choroid diseases. It delineates areas of abnormality and is essential for planning laser treatment of retinal vascular disease. In this test, fluorescein dye is injected intravenously. When the dye reaches the retina and choroid, the vessels and epithelium are clearly delineated and images are recorded.

Ophthalmic ultrasonography is used to measure the density of eye tissues and detect abnormalities. Two types of ultrasound can be used, A-scan or B-scan. B-scan ultrasound produces an image of the target tissue that shows a series of spots, the brightness of which corresponds to tissue density. As tissue density increases, the image appears darker. For example, vitreous appears very dark or black on ultrasound. The A-scan ultrasound depicts tissue density as amplitude on two axes. The output is represented in waveform, resembling an electrocardiogram. High-density tissue produces an amplified wave.

Magnetic resonance imaging and computed tomography are used in the evaluation of the orbital and intracranial structures. Computed tomography may have some disadvantages in ophthalmology, because it is unable to differentiate between structures of similar density and those that are very small.

CASE PLANNING

PSYCHOLOGICAL CONSIDERATIONS IN EYE SURGERY

Ophthalmic surgery can be frightening to patients. Although many look forward to correcting medical problems to improve or restore their eyesight, they often have unspoken fears that a poor outcome will result in blindness. In most ophthalmic surgeries, the patient receives a topical or regional anesthetic, and monitored sedation is used. The patient therefore is awake and able to hear sounds in the surgical environment. In addition, the patient can perceive the objects and instruments that are placed in the eye. This can increase preoperative anxiety.

A reassuring environment is always important to the patient's psychological and physical well-being; however, it is particularly important in ophthalmic surgery, because anxiety can result in increased hemorrhage and intraocular pressure. The surgical technologist can help the patient by maintaining a calm, supportive atmosphere. Patients find it reassuring to be given simple explanations of what they will feel or sense as the procedure starts. During the procedure, the surgeon usually warns the patient of any steps that involve pressure or pain, such as the initial sting of an anesthetic or loss of sensation.

VERIFICATION OF THE OPERATIVE SITE

The Universal Protocol for verification of the operative site and side and other critical information was introduced in Chapter 20. In ophthalmic surgery, particular concerns arise because marks around the eye may be covered by drapes before the verification process is started. This means that the team must be especially vigilant during the TIMEOUT. Verification of implants has historically been a problem in ophthalmic surgery. The consequences of implanting the wrong lens implant during cataract surgery are extremely serious. Intraocular implants *must be verified before insertion.* Lens implants are treated in much the same way as a drug distributed to the field. To prevent insertion of the wrong implant, the American Association of Ophthalmologists (AAO) has developed a sample protocol. The surgical technologist participates in this protocol:

1. Before surgery, the surgeon selects the intraocular lens (IOL) based on the patient's records available *in the operating room.*
2. The circulating nurse shows the surgeon the box and verbally verifies the IOL model number and lens power. The surgeon acknowledges this communication.
3. The circulating nurse *repeats this procedure with the surgical technologist.*
4. The scrubbed surgical technologist *verbally states the model number and lens power* as the IOL is passed to the surgeon.

Documentation of implants is discussed more fully later in this chapter.

POSITIONING THE PATIENT FOR OPHTHALMIC SURGERY

Ophthalmic surgery is performed with the patient in the supine position with the head stabilized on a circular gel headrest (sometimes called a *doughnut*). The top of the head may be level with the end of the table, or the patient may be positioned with the head resting on a specialized holder that extends beyond the edge of the table. A wrist rest is attached to the head of the table or the head attachment to support the surgeon's hands during the procedure.

Many health care facilities use a combination stretcher–operating table for transporting the patient and performing surgery. This is because shifting the patient immediately after surgery may result in an increased IOP and eye injury.

If a standard gurney is used, the patient must be transferred cautiously and slowly. The older patient may have difficulty moving across the gurney onto the operating table. The patient should be warned of the narrow table, and the safety strap should be secured as soon as possible. The circulator then can stabilize the patient into a comfortable position with gel or foam supports as needed. The patient should be covered with warm blankets to prevent hypothermia and for comfort.

As mentioned, most eye procedures involve a regional block and monitored sedation. The position of the patient for eye surgery must be safe and comfortable. An uncomfortable patient may become restless during surgery, and this can result in injury to the eye. It is critical that patients remain still. Some patients may benefit from lumbar support and a cushion for the popliteal region. The patient's arms may be tucked at the sides with correct technique to prevent contact with any part of the table frame or attachments.

PREPPING AND DRAPING

The skin prep is commonly performed after the patient has been anesthetized. Because regional anesthesia often is used, the circulator should have all prepping supplies ready before anesthesia is started, to prevent delay. The standard approved eye prep antiseptic is dilute povidone-iodine (5% or as directed by the surgeon). Supplies needed for the sterile prep setup include the following:

- Small basins for the solutions
- Surgical towels
- Plastic towel drapes
- Lint-free gauze sponges
- Cotton balls
- Cellulose eye sponges
- Balanced salt solution (BSS)

The prep area includes the eyelid and margins, inner and outer canthus, brows, and face, ending usually at the chin. Before starting the prep, the circulator secures an adhesive towel drape at the hairline. Surgical towels are placed to absorb any solution runoff. However, runoff can be prevented by squeezing excess solution from each sponge. A small piece of cotton may be placed in the ear on the operative side and the head turned toward the operative side. Irrigation of the eye may be required before the skin prep. BSS or a mild antiseptic of the surgeon's choice is used. The prep is performed starting at the eyelid and extending outward. The eyelid margins are cleansed using cotton-tipped applicators. The canthus is considered a contaminated area, and any sponge that touches this area is discarded. Skin prep of the eye may include instillation of drugs to prepare the eye for surgery.

Several techniques are used to drape the eye. It is important to isolate the hairline and nonoperative side of the face. Some surgeons use a head drape. This usually is followed by a fenestrated drape to expose the operative eye. A body sheet is used to maintain a wide sterile field, or the procedure drape may be large enough to extend over the sides of the operating table.

ANESTHESIA

Most ophthalmic surgery is performed using a regional anesthetic with monitored sedation. A topical anesthetic, local infiltration, peribulbar nerve block, or a combination of these is most often used. A retrobulbar block may be used in selected patients. However, this approach is associated with several serious risks and has more limited uses. Pediatric patients receive a general anesthetic.

For local anesthesia, a dedicated setup is prepared according to the surgeon's preferences. Anesthetic, syringes, infiltration needles (25- to 27-gauge), transfer needles, and sponges are needed.

Commonly used injectable local anesthetics include procaine hydrochloride 1% to 4% and lidocaine hydrochloride (Xylocaine) 1% to 2%. Any of these may be combined with epinephrine to maintain vasoconstriction at the operative site. Topical anesthetic in drop form is instilled onto the cornea. Commonly used topical anesthetics include proparacaine hydrochloride (Proxymetacaine, Alcaine, Parcaine), and benoxinate hydrochloride. A topical anesthetic is applied over the cornea before injection. Patients generally tolerate the local anesthetic procedure well. The circulator is present at the patient's side to assist and to provide reassurance.

OPHTHALMIC DRUGS

Ophthalmic surgery requires the use of many types of drugs, which are administered preoperatively, during surgery, and in the postoperative period. Many of these drugs have potent effects, and a medication error could irreparably damage the eye. Chapter 12 discusses the appropriate protocol for receiving drugs on the sterile field. Important highlights are the following:

- All drugs on the sterile field must be labeled as soon as they are received; this is critical.
- Every drug passed to the surgeon must be identified and acknowledged by the surgeon—no exceptions.
- Preoperative topical drugs may be administered by the surgeon or the circulating registered nurse.
- The amounts of all drugs used must be recorded on the intraoperative report.

A table of ophthalmic drugs and their use is presented in Table 25.1. Adverse reactions to medications used during eye surgery are a serious consideration. Many different drugs are used in combination, and the circulator must be vigilant in watching for signs and symptoms that may indicate allergy or sensitivity. The ST should notify the circulator and surgeon of any symptoms reported by the patient. The technologist does not assess the patient medically but should immediately report any observed changes in the patient's appearance or behavior.

INSTRUMENTS

Ophthalmic instruments are delicate and expensive. All surgical personnel must take special care to ensure that the edges and tips of microsurgical eye instruments are not dulled or damaged. Before the procedure begins, the ST should check all instruments. Sharp items must be smooth, and scissor blades must align properly. Needle holders are particularly susceptible to injury. The ST should make sure that catches and spring mechanisms are working properly. Suction tips should be checked for patency. A neat instrument table is essential. Refer to Ophthalmic Instruments to see photographs of common instruments used in eye surgery.

OPHTHALMIC INSTRUMENTS

DIAMOND KNIFE

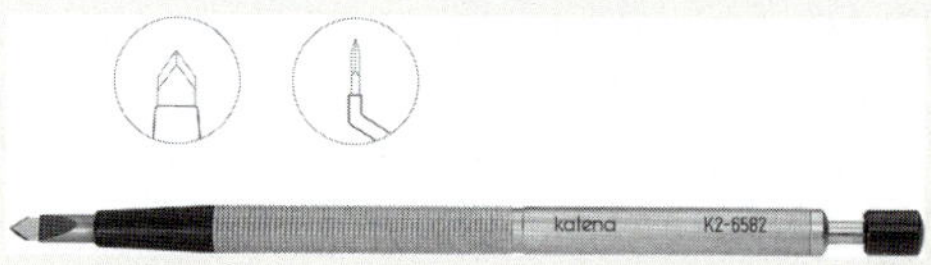

Courtesy Katena Eye Instruments, Denville, NJ.

DIAMOND STEP KNIFE

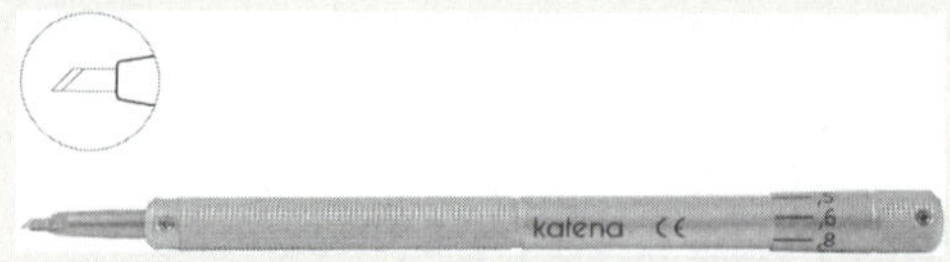

Courtesy Katena Eye Instruments, Denville, NJ.

BARRAQUER IRIS SCISSORS

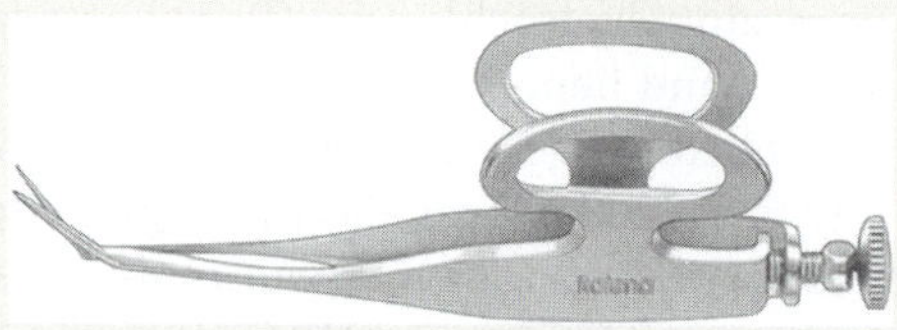

Courtesy Katena Eye Instruments, Denville, NJ.

STEVENS SCISSORS

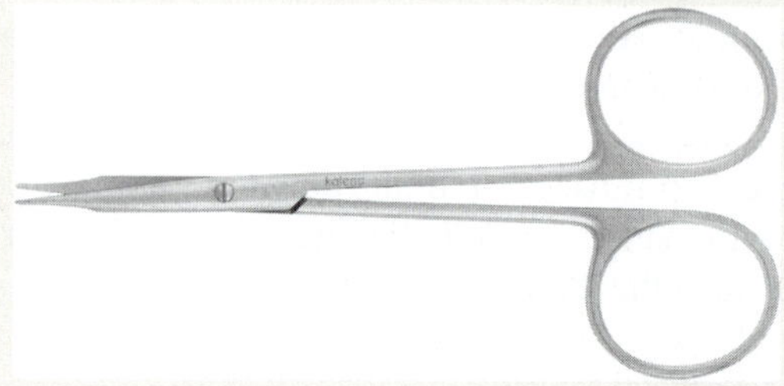

Courtesy Katena Eye Instruments, Denville, NJ.

VANNAS SCISSORS

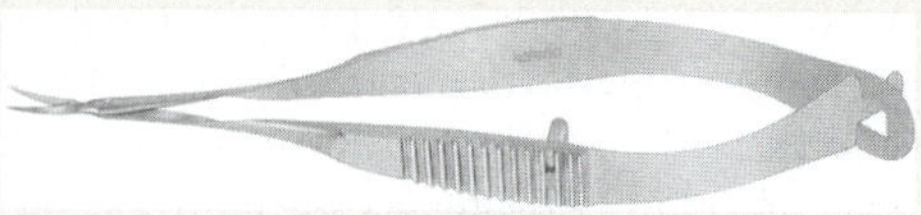

Courtesy Katena Eye Instruments, Denville, NJ.

WESTCOTT STITCH SCISSORS

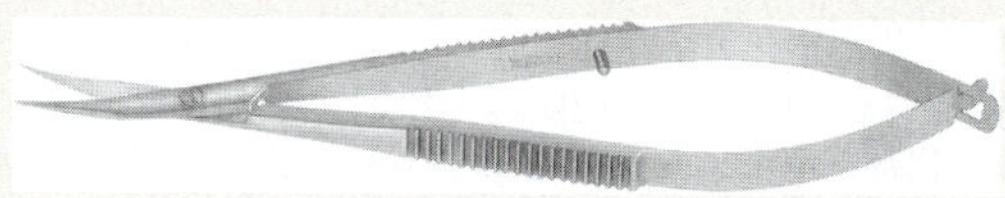

Courtesy Katena Eye Instruments, Denville, NJ.

WESTCOTT TENOTOMY SCISSORS

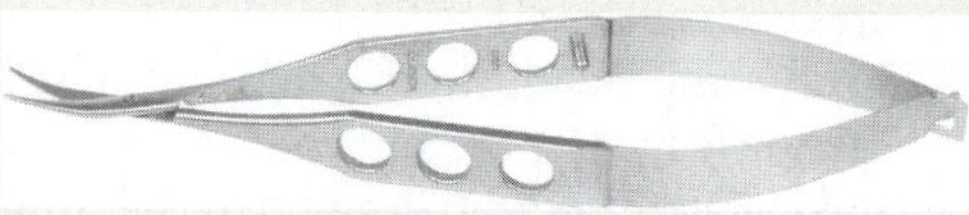

Courtesy Katena Eye Instruments, Denville, NJ.

KATENA-VANNAS SCISSORS

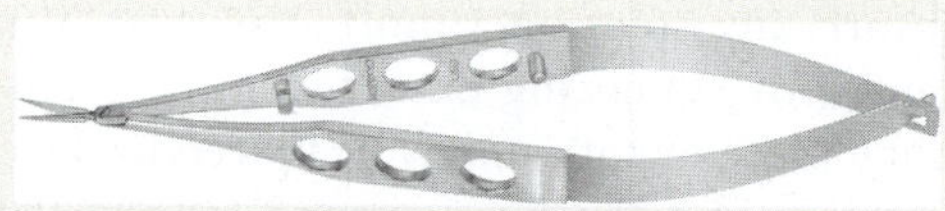

Courtesy Katena Eye Instruments, Denville, NJ.

BARRON VACUUM TREPHINE

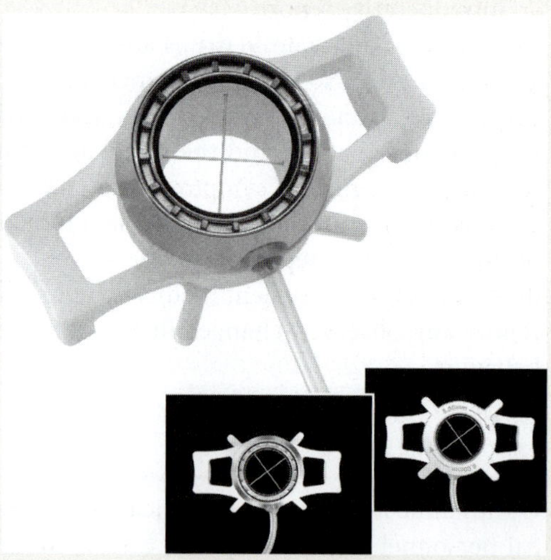

Courtesy Katena Eye Instruments, Denville, NJ.

ENUCLEATION SPOON

Courtesy Katena Eye Instruments, Denville, NJ.

FREER LACRIMAL CHISEL

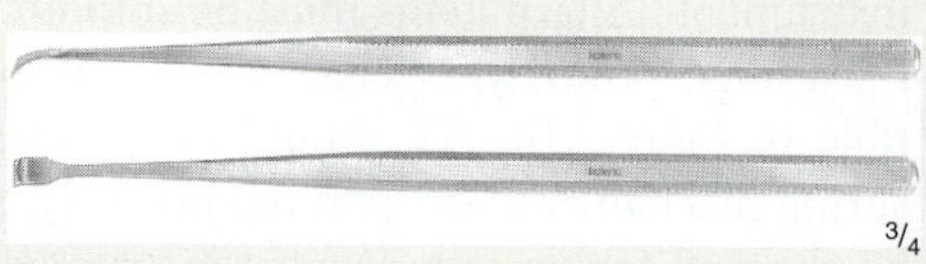

Courtesy Katena Eye Instruments, Denville, NJ.

BIPOLAR FORCEPS

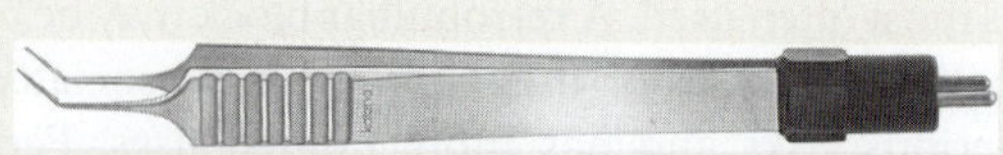

Courtesy Katena Eye Instruments, Denville, NJ.

OPHTHALMIC INSTRUMENTS— cont'd

BISHOP-HARMON FORCEPS

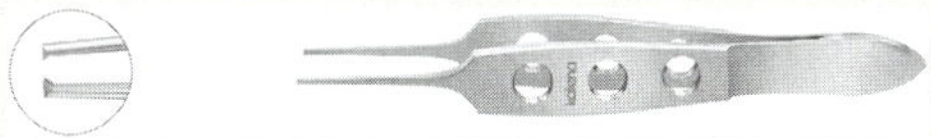

Courtesy Katena Eye Instruments, Denville, NJ.

BONN FORCEPS

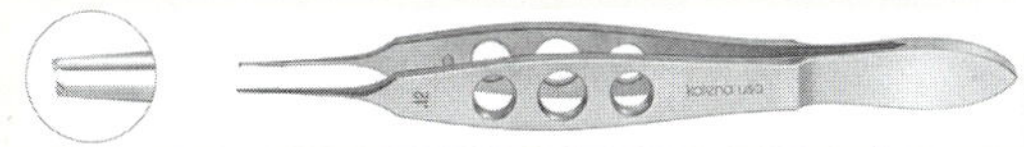

Courtesy Katena Eye Instruments, Denville, NJ.

CASTROVIEJO NEEDLE HOLDER

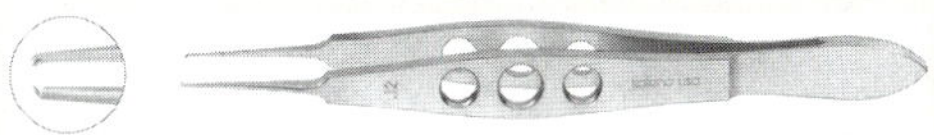

Courtesy Katena Eye Instruments, Denville, NJ.

CLAYMAN LENS HOLDING FORCEPS

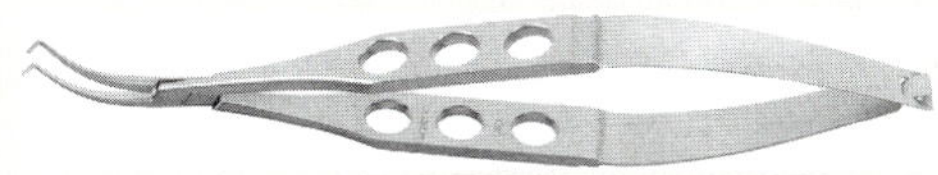

Courtesy Katena Eye Instruments, Denville, NJ.

COLIBRI FORCEPS

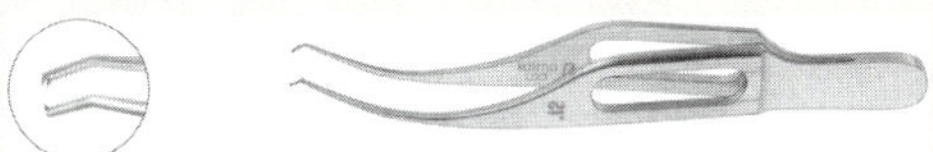

Courtesy Katena Eye Instruments, Denville, NJ.

HARMS-COLIBRI FORCEPS

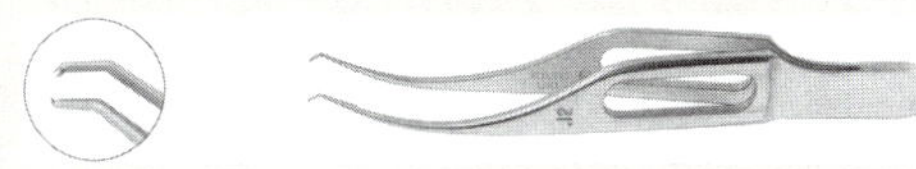

Courtesy Katena Eye Instruments, Denville, NJ.

HUNT CHALAZION FORCEPS

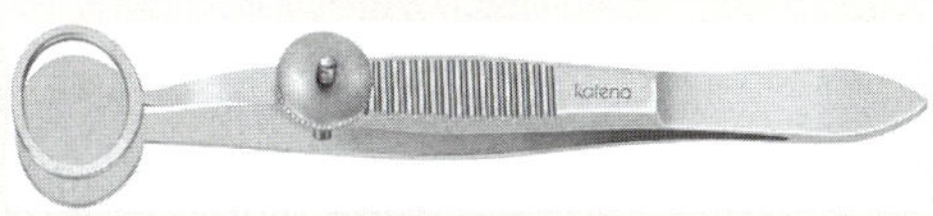

Courtesy Katena Eye Instruments, Denville, NJ.

JAFFE TYING FORCEPS

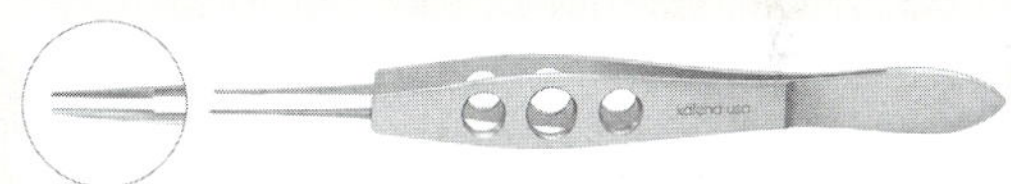

Courtesy Katena Eye Instruments, Denville, NJ.

JAMESON MUSCLE FORCEPS

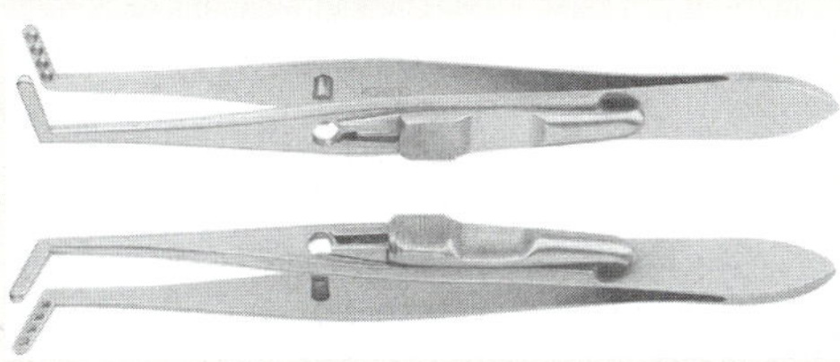

Courtesy Katena Eye Instruments, Denville, NJ.

JEWELER FORCEPS

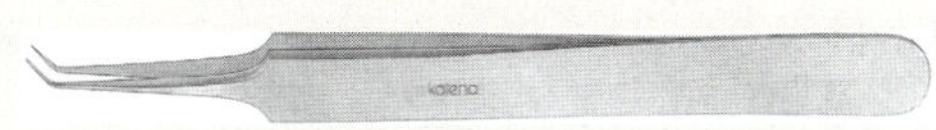

Courtesy Katena Eye Instruments, Denville, NJ.

LESTER FIXATION FORCEPS

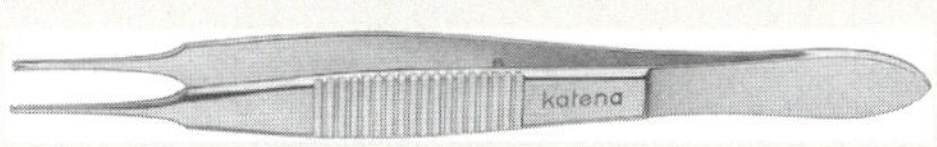

Courtesy Katena Eye Instruments, Denville, NJ.

PIERCE CORNEAL FORCEPS

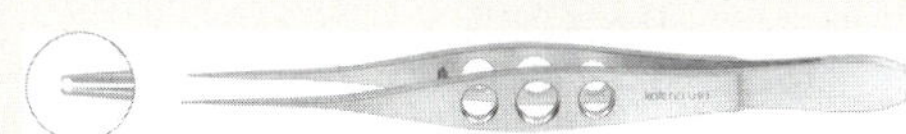

Courtesy Katena Eye Instruments, Denville, NJ.

TROUTMANN RECTUS FORCEPS

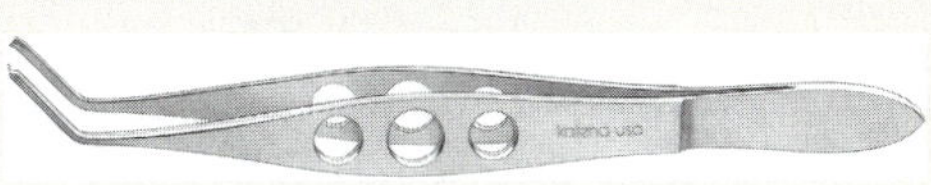

Courtesy Katena Eye Instruments, Denville, NJ.

ULTRATA CAPSULORRHEXIS FORCEPS

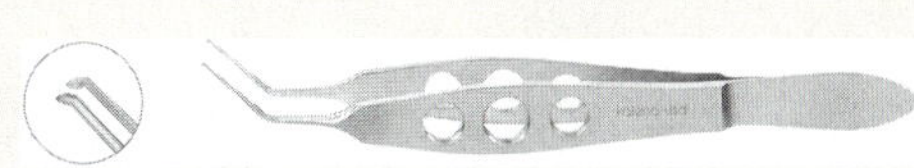

Courtesy Katena Eye Instruments, Denville, NJ.

ENUCLEATION SCISSORS

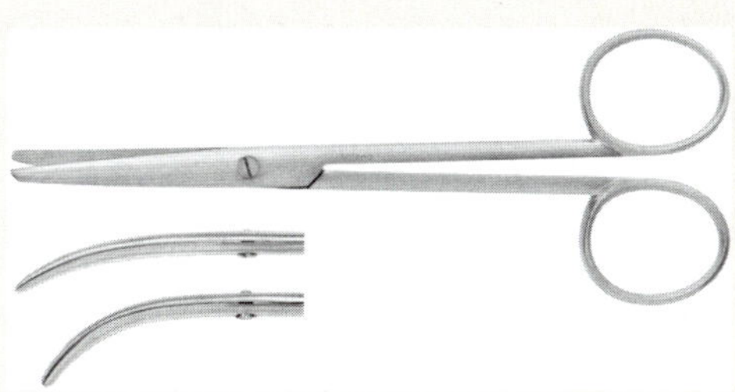

Courtesy Katena Eye Instruments, Denville, NJ.

ANTERIOR CHAMBER CANNULA

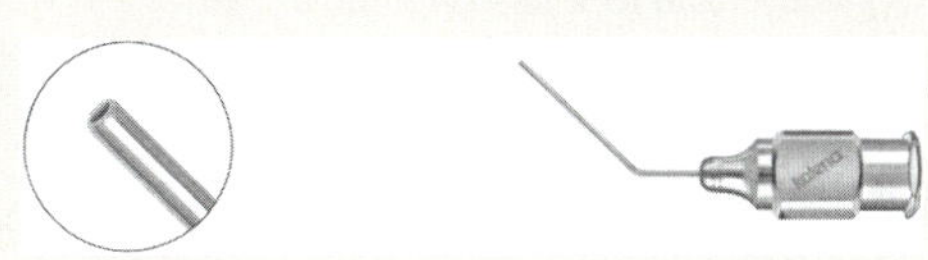

Courtesy Katena Eye Instruments, Denville, NJ.

OPHTHALMIC INSTRUMENTS—cont'd

CRAWFORD LACRIMAL TUBE

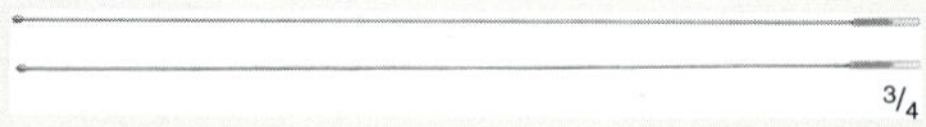

Courtesy Katena Eye Instruments, Denville, NJ.

HYDRODISSECTION CANNULA

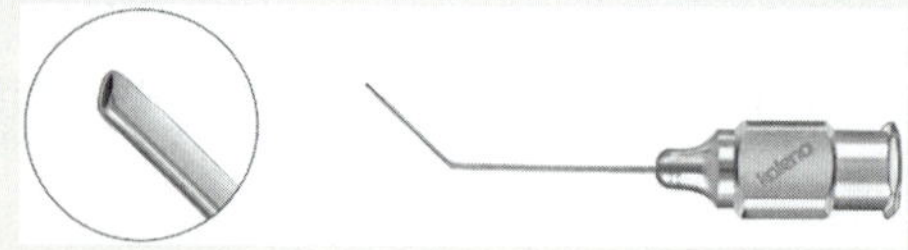

Courtesy Katena Eye Instruments, Denville, NJ.

LACRIMAL CANNULA

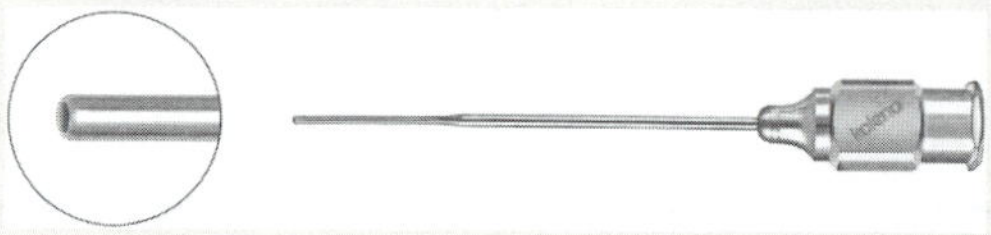

Courtesy Katena Eye Instruments, Denville, NJ.

LESTER INTRAOCULAR LENS MANIPULATOR

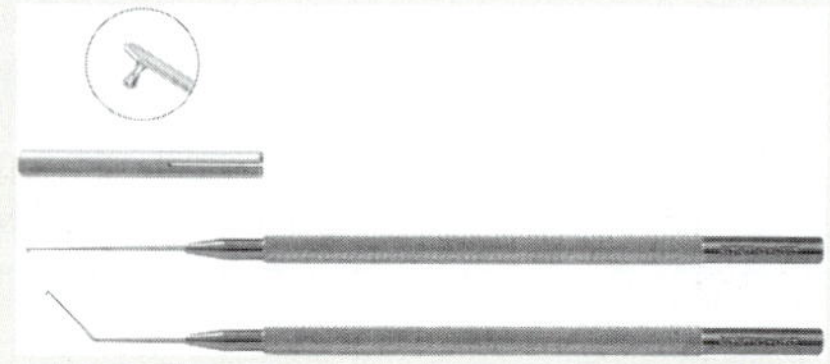

Courtesy Katena Eye Instruments, Denville, NJ.

RANDOLPH CYCLODIALYSIS CANNULA

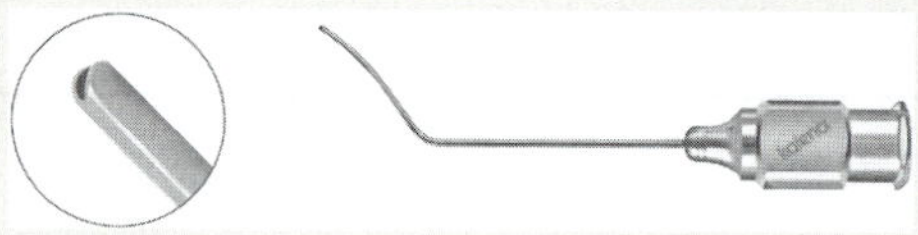

Courtesy Katena Eye Instruments, Denville, NJ.

WELSH OLIVE-TIP CANNULA

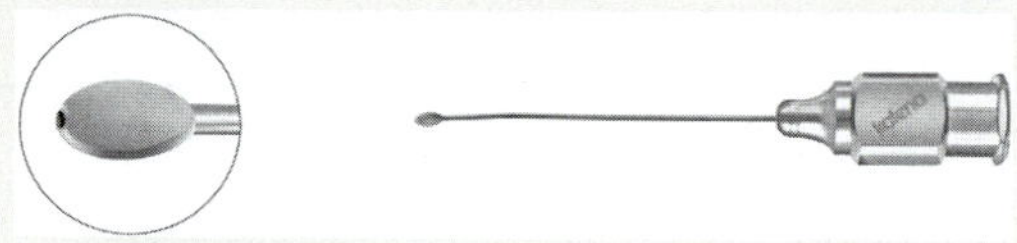

Courtesy Katena Eye Instruments, Denville, NJ.

JENSEN POLISHER

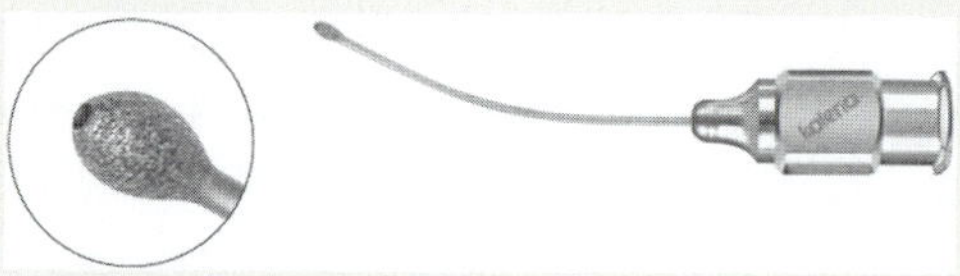

Courtesy Katena Eye Instruments, Denville, NJ.

BARRAQUER IRIS SPATULA

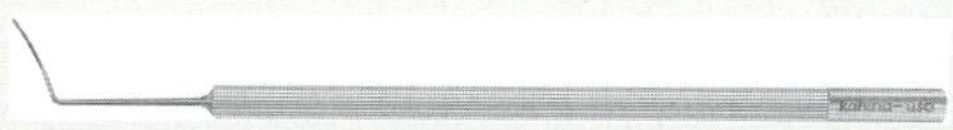

Courtesy Katena Eye Instruments, Denville, NJ.

BISHOP HARMON A/C IRRIGATOR

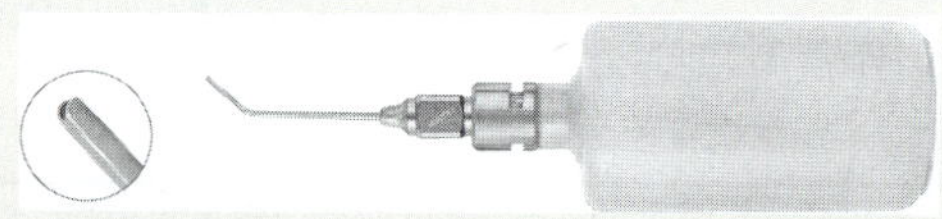

Courtesy Katena Eye Instruments, Denville, NJ.

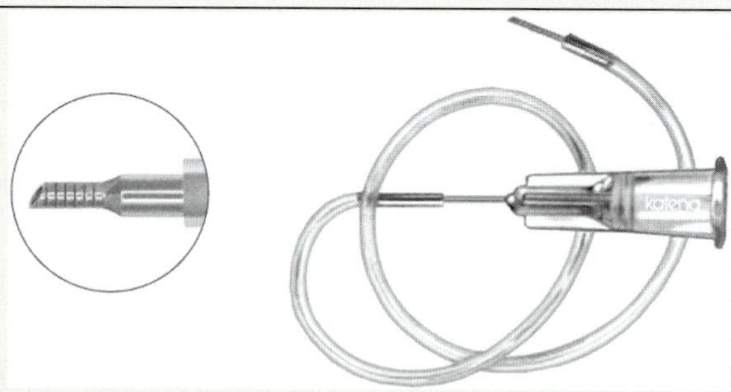

CHAMBER MAINTAINER
Courtesy Katena Eye Instruments, Denville, NJ.

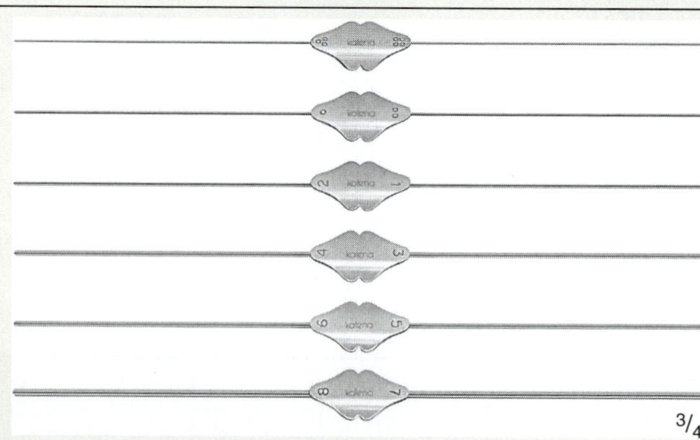

BOWMAN LACRIMAL PROBE SET
Courtesy Katena Eye Instruments, Denville, NJ.

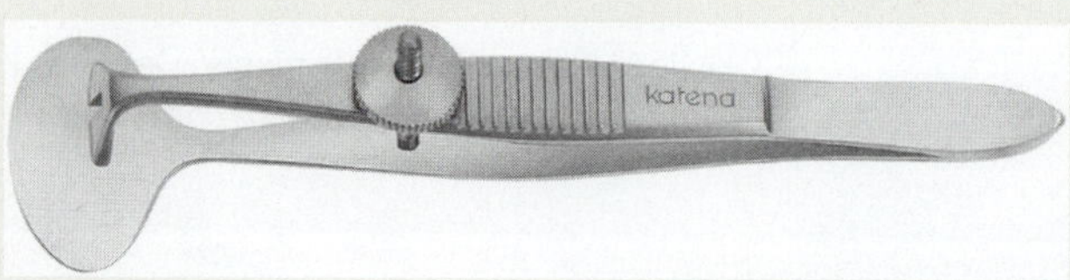

ERHARDT LID FORCEPS
Courtesy Katena Eye Instruments, Denville, NJ.

OPHTHALMIC INSTRUMENTS— cont'd

JAMESON MUSCLE HOOK
Courtesy Katena Eye Instruments, Denville, NJ.

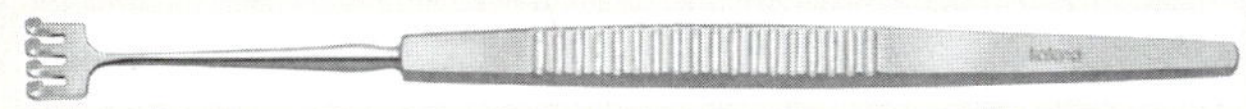

KNAPP RETRACTOR
Courtesy Katena Eye Instruments, Denville, NJ.

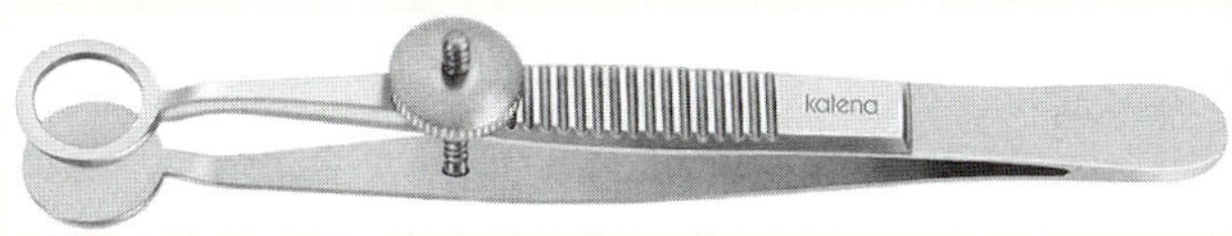

LAMBERT CHALAZION FORCEPS
Courtesy Katena Eye Instruments, Denville, NJ.

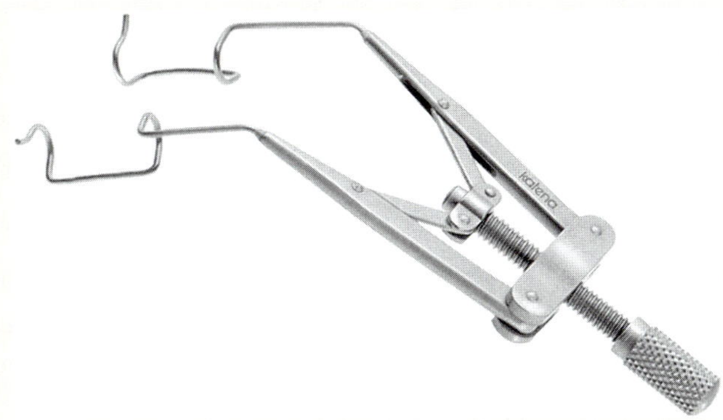

LIEBERMAN SPECULUM
Courtesy Katena Eye Instruments, Denville, NJ.

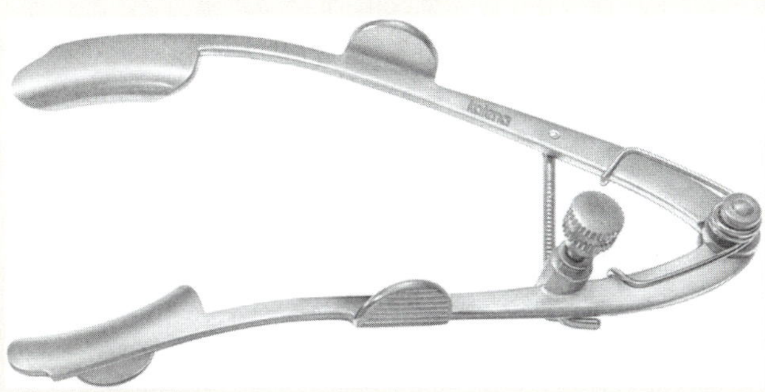

LESTER-BURCH EYE SPECULUM
Courtesy Katena Eye Instruments, Denville, NJ.

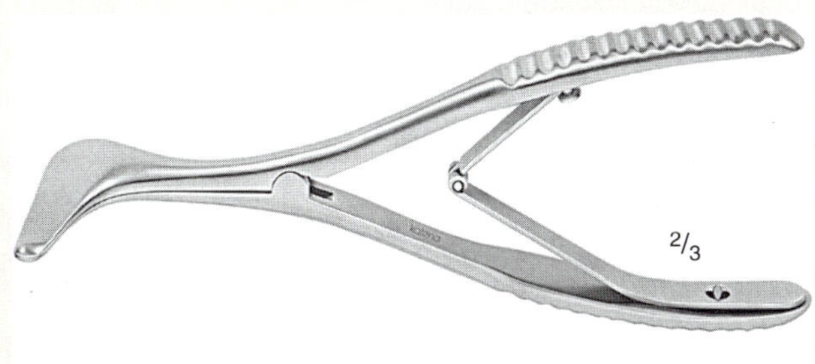

NASAL SPECULUM ADULT
Courtesy Katena Eye Instruments, Denville, NJ.

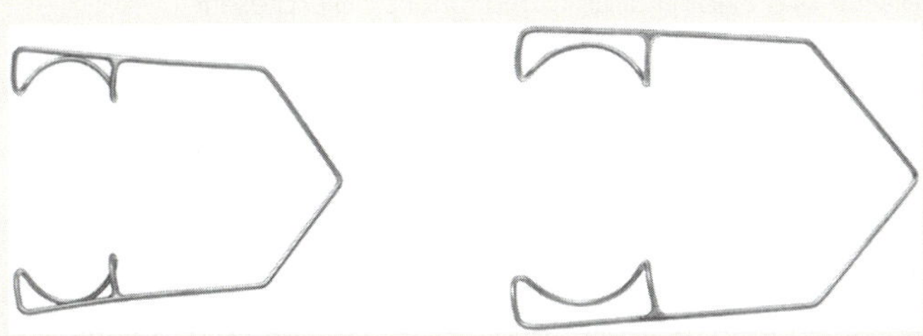

BARRAQUER WIRE SPECULUM
Courtesy Katena Eye Instruments, Denville, NJ.

TABLE 25.1 Mydriatics (Drugs That Dilate the Pupil But Permit Focusing)

Drug (Brand Name)	Description/Uses
Phenylephrine (Neo-Synephrine, Mydfrin), 2.5%, 10%	Objective examination of the retina, testing of refraction, and easier removal of lenses; mydriatics may be used alone or with a cycloplegic drug
CYCLOPLEGICS (DRUGS THAT PARALYZE ACCOMMODATION AND INHIBIT FOCUSING)	
Tropicamide (Mydriacyl), 1%	Anticholinergic, dilation of the pupil, examination of the fundus, and refraction
Atropine, 1%	Dilates the pupil, inhibits focusing; anticholinergic, potent, and has a long duration of action (7–14 days)
Cyclopentolate (Cyclogyl), 1%, 2%	Anticholinergic; dilates the pupil, inhibits focusing
Scopolamine hydrobromide (Isopto Hyoscine), 0.25%	Anticholinergic; dilates the pupil, inhibits focusing
Homatropine hydrobromide (Isopto Homatropine), 2%, 5%	Anticholinergic; dilates the pupil, inhibits focusing
Epinephrine (1:1,000) preservative free (PF)	Dilates the pupil; added to bottles of balanced salt solution (BSS) for irrigation to maintain pupil dilation during cataract surgery or vitrectomy
MIOTICS	
Carbachol (Miostat), 0.01%	Potent cholinergic; constricts the pupil, used intraocularly during anterior segment surgery
Carbachol (Isopto Carbachol), 0.75%, 1.5%, 2.25%, 3%	Potent cholinergic; constricts the pupil, used topically to reduce intraocular pressure (IOP) in glaucoma
Acetylcholine chloride (Miochol-E), 1%	Cholinergic; rapidly constricts the pupil, used intraocularly during anterior segment surgery; reconstitute immediately before using
Pilocarpine hydrochloride, 1%, 4%	Cholinergic; constricts the pupil, used topically to lower IOP in glaucoma
TOPICAL ANESTHETICS	
Tetracaine hydrochloride 0.05%	Applied directly to the eye provides loss of corneal sensation
Proparacaine hydrochloride 0.05%	As above
INJECTABLE ANESTHETICS	
Lidocaine (Xylocaine), 1%, 2%, 4%	Provides anesthesia of the deep tissues. Often given as a nerve block
Methylparaben free (MPF)	Preservative free; adjunct to topical anesthetic
Bupivacaine (Marcaine, Sensorcaine), 0.25%, 0.50%, 0.75%	Long-acting; may be used in combination with lidocaine for block
Mepivacaine (Carbocaine), 1%, 2%	May be used for local infiltration and nerve block
ADDITIVES TO LOCAL ANESTHETICS	
Epinephrine, 1:50,000–1:200,000	Combined with injectable local anesthetics to prolong anesthesia and reduce bleeding
Hyaluronidase	Enzyme mixed with anesthetics (75 units per 10 mL) to increase diffusion of anesthetic through tissue, improving the effectiveness of the block; contraindicated if skin inflammation or malignancy are present
VISCOELASTICS	
Sodium hyaluronate (Healon, Amvisc, Provisc, Vitrax) in a sterile syringe assembly with blunt-tip cannula	Lubricant and support; maintains separation between tissues to protect the endothelium and maintain the anterior chamber intraocularly; removed from anterior chamber to prevent postoperative increase in pressure; should be refrigerated (except Vitrax); allow 30 min to warm to room temperature
Sodium chondroitin–sodium hyaluronate (Viscoat) in a sterile syringe assembly with blunt-tip cannula	Maintains a deep chamber for anterior segment procedures, protects epithelium of cornea, and improves visualization; may be used to coat intraocular lens before implantation; should be refrigerated
DuoVisc	Packages of separate syringes of Provisc and Viscoat in the same box
VISCOADHERENTS	
Hydroxypropyl methylcellulose 2% (OcuCoat) in a sterile syringe assembly with blunt-tipped cannula	Maintains a deep chamber for anterior segment procedures, protects epithelium of cornea, and may be used to coat intraocular lens before implantation; removed from anterior chamber at end of procedure; stored at room temperature

TABLE 25.1 Mydriatics (Drugs That Dilate the Pupil But Permit Focusing)—cont'd

Drug (Brand Name)	Description/Uses
Hydroxyethyl cellulose (Gonioscopic Prism Solution)	Bonds gonioscopic prisms to the eye; stored at room temperature
Hydroxypropyl methylcellulose 2.5% (Goniosol)	Bonds gonioscopic prisms to the eye; stored at room temperature
IRRIGANTS	
Balanced salt solution (BSS, Endosol)	Used to keep the cornea moist during surgery; also used as an internal irrigant in the anterior or posterior segment
BSS enriched with bicarbonate, dextrose, and glutathione (BSS Plus, Endosol Extra)	Used as an internal irrigant in the anterior or posterior segment; must be reconstituted immediately before use by adding part I to part II with the transfer device
HYPEROSMOTIC AGENTS	
Mannitol (Osmitrol)	Intravenous (IV) osmotic diuretic; increases the osmolarity of the plasma, causing the osmotic pressure gradient to pull free fluid from the eye into the plasma, thereby reducing the IOP
Glycerin (Osmoglyn, Glyrol)	Oral osmotic diuretic given in chilled juice or cola; increases the osmolarity of the plasma, causing the osmotic pressure gradient to pull free fluid from the eye into the plasma, thereby reducing the IOP
ANTIINFLAMMATORY AGENTS	
Betamethasone sodium phosphate and betamethasone acetate suspension (Celestone)	Glucocorticoid; injected subconjunctivally after surgery for prophylaxis; also used to treat severe allergic and inflammatory conditions
Dexamethasone (Decadron)	Adrenocorticosteroid; injected subconjunctivally after surgery for prophylaxis; also used to treat severe allergic and inflammatory conditions and intraocularly for endophthalmitis
Methylprednisolone acetate suspension (Depo-Medrol)	Glucocorticoid; injected subconjunctivally after surgery for prophylaxis; also used to treat severe allergic and inflammatory conditions
ANTIINFECTIVE DRUGS	
Polymyxin B/bacitracin (Polysporin ointment)	Topical treatment of superficial ocular infections of the conjunctiva or cornea; also used prophylactically after surgery
Polymyxin B/neomycin/bacitracin (Neosporin ointment)	Topical treatment of superficial infections of the external eye; used prophylactically after surgery
Neomycin and polymyxin B sulfates and dexamethasone (Maxitrol ointment or suspension)	Topical treatment of steroid-responsive, inflammatory ocular conditions or bacterial infections of the external eye
Tobramycin/dexamethasone (TobraDex)	Topical treatment or prevention of superficial infections of the external part of the eye; also has antiinflammatory properties
Cefazolin (Ancef, Kefzol)	Injected subconjunctivally for prophylaxis after eye procedures; also used topically, intraocularly, and systemically for endophthalmitis
Gentamicin sulfate (Garamycin)	Injected subconjunctivally for prophylaxis after eye procedures; also used topically, subconjunctivally, and intraocularly for endophthalmitis
Ceftazidime (Fortaz, Tazicef, Tazidime)	Injected subconjunctivally and intraocularly for the treatment of endophthalmitis
OTHER DRUGS	
Cocaine, 1%–4%	Used topically only, never injected; used on cornea to loosen epithelium before debridement and on nasal packing to reduce congestion of mucosa
5-Fluorouracil (5-FU)	Antimetabolite used topically to inhibit scar formation in glaucoma-filtering procedures; handle and discard in compliance with the regulations of the Occupational Safety and Health Administration (OSHA) and health care facility's policies for safe use of antineoplastics
Mitomycin (Mutamycin)	Antimetabolite used topically to inhibit scar formation in glaucoma-filtering procedures and **pterygium** excision; handle and discard in compliance with OSHA's and health care facility's policies for safe use of antineoplastics
Tissue plasminogen activator (tPA) (Activase)	Thrombolytic agent; used for the treatment of fibrin formation in patients who have had vitrectomy and for the lysis of clots on the retina

Continued

TABLE 25.1 Mydriatics (Drugs That Dilate the Pupil But Permit Focusing)—cont'd

Drug (Brand Name)	Description/Uses
Fluorescein	*IV diagnostic aid:* Used in fluorescein angiography to diagnose retinal disorders *Topical stain:* Fluorescein strip temporarily stains the cornea yellow–green in areas of denuded corneal epithelium
Timolol maleate (Timoptic)	Beta-adrenergic receptor-blocking agent; used in the treatment of elevated IOP in ocular hypertension or open-angle glaucoma
Acetazolamide sodium (Diamox)	Carbonic anhydrase inhibitor; given IV to reduce the secretion of aqueous humor, resulting in a drop in IOP; also has a diuretic effect
Dextrose, 50%	Added to BSS, Endosol, BSS Plus, or Endosol Extra for patients with diabetes during intraocular procedures

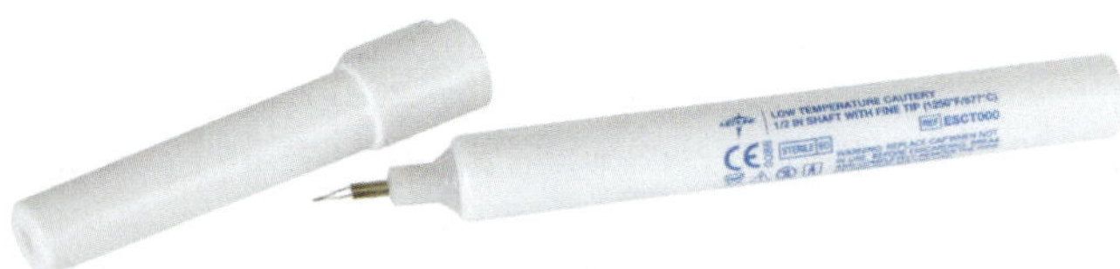

FIG. 25.7 Eye cautery pen. The cautery unit is used to control small bleeders. (Courtesy and copyright Becton, Dickinson and Company.)

EQUIPMENT AND SUPPLIES

ELECTROSURGICAL UNIT

Two types of electrosurgical systems are commonly used in eye surgery, the single-use, battery-powered cautery and the bipolar unit. The handheld battery unit has a very small filament tip that becomes hot when the unit is activated (Fig. 25.7). Unlike monopolar or bipolar electrosurgical units (ESUs), this unit is a true cautery instrument. The filament is used to coagulate very small vessels of the eye; however, it does not have cutting capability. The bipolar or radiofrequency ESU is used for procedures in which fine cutting and coagulation are required. The bipolar unit is used in conjunction with bipolar instruments, which are connected to the unit by a thin cable. (A complete discussion of these technologies and safety precautions can be found in Chapter 17.)

EYE SPONGES

Eye sponges are made of lint-free cellulose or similar material. These are supplied commercially attached to a short plastic rod (Fig. 25.8). Sponges should be separated from supplies that may discharge lint particles. During surgery, the ST may be required to blot blood or fluid from the surgical site. The sponge is never used on the cornea. The sponge absorbs fluid by wicking. This is done by holding the tip of the sponge in contact with the fluid and allowing the sponge to absorb it.

SUTURES

Eye sutures are supplied in a wide range of materials in sizes 4-0 to 12-0. These must be handled gently and carefully. Sutures should be handled as little as possible, and the points of the needles should be protected from damage. Double-arm sutures frequently are used in eye surgery to close circumferential incisions. Ophthalmic needles may be as small as 4 mm at the widest part.

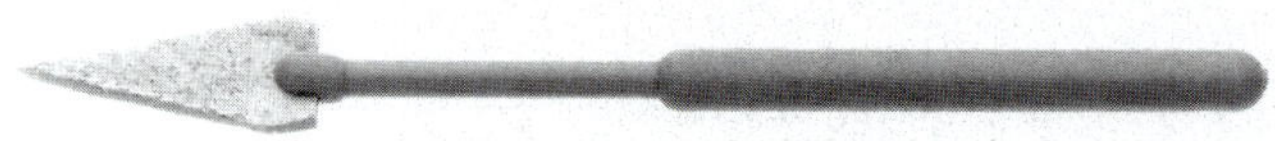

FIG. 25.8 Eye sponge (2½″). Eye sponges (spears) are composed of cellulose, which is lint free. (Courtesy and copyright Becton Dickinson and Company.)

Sutures should not be allowed to come into contact with cloth towels, which can transfer lint to the needle and suture material.

OPHTHALMIC DRESSINGS

A soft dressing or hard shield may be used to protect the eye after surgery. Soft, lint-free gauze eye patches are supplied for a simple dressing that absorbs fluid and prevents debris from entering the eye. A rigid eye shield is taped over the eye to provide protection from bumping or abrasion, which may cause dehiscence of an incision.

SURGICAL TECHNIQUES IN EYE SURGERY

MICROSURGERY

Microsurgery presents challenges to the ST for several reasons:

- The surgeon's field of vision is magnified, but the scope (i.e., the area of vision) is very limited. Special technique is required for passing instruments because the surgeon must not look away from the field to receive them.
- When required to look away from the field, the surgeon loses concentration and the rhythm of the surgery. To prevent such interruptions, the ST should prepare for each step of the procedure. Using the proper method to pass instruments reduces the risk of patient injury.
- The patient and surgical field must be completely still. The ST must prevent even slight movement of the microscope. When passing instruments or preparing items near the field, the ST must have a steady hand and create as little movement as possible. Remember that if the patient raises his or her head or if any instruments are jarred while touching the eye, the patient can be injured.

Operating Microscope

Although the operating microscope is a heavy piece of equipment, it has delicate components. The technologist should become familiar with all components to prevent injury to the

BOX 25.1 Microscope Terminology

Assistant binoculars: A separate optical body with a nonmotorized, hand-controlled zoom.
Beam splitter: A device that transmits an image from the primary ocular to an observer tube, producing an identical picture.
Broad-field viewing lens: A low-power magnifying glass attached to the front of the oculars that produces an overview of the field.
Coaxial illuminator: A light source (usually fiber-optic) transmitted through the lens or body of the microscope. It illuminates the area in the field of view of the objective lens.
Compound microscope: A microscope that uses two or more lenses in a single unit.
Illumination system: The lighting system of the microscope.
Magnifying power: The magnification specification of a lens.
Objective lens: The lens that establishes the working distance and produces the greatest magnification.
Ocular or eyepiece: The component of the microscope that magnifies the field of view.
Paraxial illuminators: One or more light tubes that contain incandescent bulbs and focusing lenses. Light is focused to coincide with the working distance of the scope.
X-Y attachment: A mechanism that allows the scope to move precisely along a horizontal plane.
Zoom lens: A lens that increases or decreases magnification and is usually operated by a foot pedal.

patient and to protect the microscope from damage. Box 25.1 lists common microscope terminology. Refer to Chapter 19 to study microscope draping.

HANDLING THE MICROSCOPE The following guidelines should be observed when the microscope is handled:

1. Before moving the microscope, secure the arms. This prevents them from swinging out and striking the wall or other equipment.
2. The microscope must be balanced before use. This is necessary to ensure that the head of the microscope does not drift up or down. Always consult the manufacturer's instructions for balancing.
3. The microscope must be adjusted to accommodate the surgeon's and assistant's eyesight. Always test the microscope before moving it to the surgical field.
4. Check the brake and other controls to ensure that they are tight before using the microscope.
5. Take special care to ensure that the microscope head control knob is secure before surgery.
6. Check all cords for fraying or loose wires. Light bulbs also should be tested before surgery, and an extra bulb should be kept in the surgical suite.
7. Some microscopes are equipped with an X-Y axis carrier; this must be centered before the microscope is positioned at the field.
8. When moving the microscope, handle it with *both hands* on the vertical column. Moving the microscope by the head can cause it to tip over.
9. Make all adjustments to the vertical oculars before surgery.

CARE OF THE MICROSCOPE

1. The microscope should be damp-dusted before use. Follow the manufacturer's recommendations for use of a disinfectant. Never use detergent or disinfectant on the lenses. They should be cleaned with a lens cleaner or water and wiped with lens paper. Do not use cloth, which leaves lint on the lens.
2. Do not touch the lenses.
3. The scope and all its openings and attachments should be covered at the end of the day to prevent the accumulation of dust.

ROLE OF THE SCRUBBED SURGICAL TECHNOLOGIST

Assisting in eye surgery is a specialty that requires particular skills and techniques. The scrubbed technologist must learn to focus on minute detail, develop steadiness, and communicate clearly with the surgeon. Many eye surgeons hire their own surgical technologist. Ophthalmic technologists perform duties in the eye clinic and in the operating room. They are familiar with eye diseases, diagnostics, and surgical procedures. They may also counsel surgical patients preoperatively and follow their progress through the course of treatment. Many surgical facilities, both outpatient and inpatient, hire ophthalmic surgical technologists.

The following general pointers are intended as an introduction to ophthalmic cases:

- When preparing microsurgical instruments, the ST should check for burrs (rough or jagged spots on sharp instruments). This is done by inspecting the instruments visually under microscope magnification or by running a lint-free microsurgical wipe gently along the edges of the instrument to feel for any sharp edges.
- Instruments are kept clean during each procedure. Only lint-free microsurgical wipes are used on instruments.
- Practice is required to handle and load sutures properly. When a locking needle holder is used, gentle pressure is applied on the shaft. Too much pressure prevents the needle holder from locking. A needle that is too large for the needle holder also may prevent locking.
- To cut suture under a microscope, the ST should place the scissors within the scope's field of vision. Only then should the scissors' tip be positioned at the suture. The scissors are then gently lowered for cutting.
- To cut sutures, the forefinger is placed over the center point on the shank of the scissors. This steadies the instrument and the hand. The point of the scissors is lowered over the suture to cut the ends.
- The ST must keep all instruments in a specific order on the Mayo stand. When returning instruments to the Mayo stand, the ST should place them in their original position and not rearrange them.
- Microsurgery requires dexterity and a steady hand. What appears to the naked eye as a small tremor can be severe under magnification.
- Experienced surgical technologists do not remove their eyes from the microscope to orient an instrument to the surgeon's hand.
- The eye normally produces lubricating fluid that nourishes and protects it from infection and drying. The ST is required

to irrigate the eye periodically during surgery to prevent drying. BSS (commercially supplied in a small squeeze vial) is used for this purpose. During irrigation, the tip of the vial is held over the tissue *but never touches the tissue.*

SURGICAL PROCEDURES

EXCISION OF A CHALAZION

In the excision of a chalazion, nodal tissue arising from a sebaceous gland is excised from the tarsal plate. Chalazion surgery is normally performed in the outpatient setting or clinician's office.

Pathology

A chalazion is an inflammatory benign growth that originates in a sebaceous gland of the eyelid. As in other areas of the body, a sebaceous gland may become impacted, causing inflammation. A chalazion is not infectious, but a granuloma (semisolid tissue) develops, which can enlarge and rupture. Surgery is indicated when conservative treatment fails.

POSITION:	Supine
INCISION:	Conjunctival
PREP AND DRAPING:	Eye
INSTRUMENTS:	Chalazion set including chalazion clamp; fine-toothed forceps; curette; meibomian expression paddle; Beaver knife handle and #67 blade; Westcott scissors
POSSIBLE EXTRAS:	Bipolar ESU; ophthalmic cautery

Technical Points and Discussion

1. ***An incision is made into the tarsal plate.***
   After infiltration with local anesthetic, the surgeon clamps the lid with a chalazion clamp. The lid is everted, and a vertical incision is made through the tarsal plate with a Beaver blade #67. A #11 Bard-Parker blade may also be used.

2. ***The contents of the chalazion are removed with a curette.***
   A curette is used to remove the contents of the chalazion. Bleeding on the edges of the tarsal plate is controlled with the bipolar ESU or eye cautery. A dressing is applied. Patients may be advised to apply ice to the area on the first postoperative day.

DACRYOCYSTORHINOSTOMY

Dacryocystorhinostomy is the creation of a permanent opening in the tear duct for the drainage of tears. The procedure is performed using open technique (discussed here) or endoscopic technique (Fig. 25.9). The procedure is best understood by reviewing the anatomy of the lacrimal system. The procedure is usually performed using the microscope, although some surgeons use surgical loupes. The endoscopic technique is usually performed by an ENT specialist.

Pathology

Dacryocystitis is an inflammation of the lacrimal sac, causing pain, redness, and swelling at the site of the medial canthus. This condition appears as a red mass in the septo-orbital area. Pus or a mucoid material may be seen in the punctum. This condition arises from an obstruction or stricture of the nasolacrimal duct.

Lacrimal sac inflammation and infection usually are seen in adults older than 40 years. Dacryocystorhinostomy surgery reestablishes drainage into the lacrimal duct system by creating a new opening in the nasal sinus to bypass the lacrimal sac.

POSITION:	Supine
INCISION:	Median canthus
PREP AND DRAPING:	Eye prep with head and body drape
INSTRUMENTS AND SUPPLIES:	Lacrimal set; silicone tubes or intubation set; diamond-shaped or spatula miniblade (surgeon's preference); Freer elevator; Gelfoam; fine rongeurs; fine periosteal or Freer elevator
POSSIBLE EXTRAS:	Nasal endoscope; diamond drill

Technical Points and Discussion

1. ***The patient is prepped and draped.***
   The patient is positioned supine, and the head is placed on a head ring or headrest for stability. A local anesthetic (usually 2% Xylocaine with epinephrine) may be infiltrated into the operative site to promote hemostasis. The nasal sinus is packed with gauze impregnated with a topical anesthetic. The skin prep starts at the medial canthus and includes the nose, orbital rim, and cheek.

2. ***A medial canthal incision is made.***
   To begin the procedure, the surgeon makes an incision along the medial canthus of the nose with a #15 blade. Small bleeding vessels are managed with the bipolar ESU. The surgeon uses a Frazier suction during the dissection. The ST should also have numerous cotton-tipped applicators to sponge the wound. A 4-0 suture may be placed in the incision for traction, or small dull rakes can be used for retraction. Stevens tenotomy scissors are used to separate the orbicularis muscle until the periosteum is exposed.

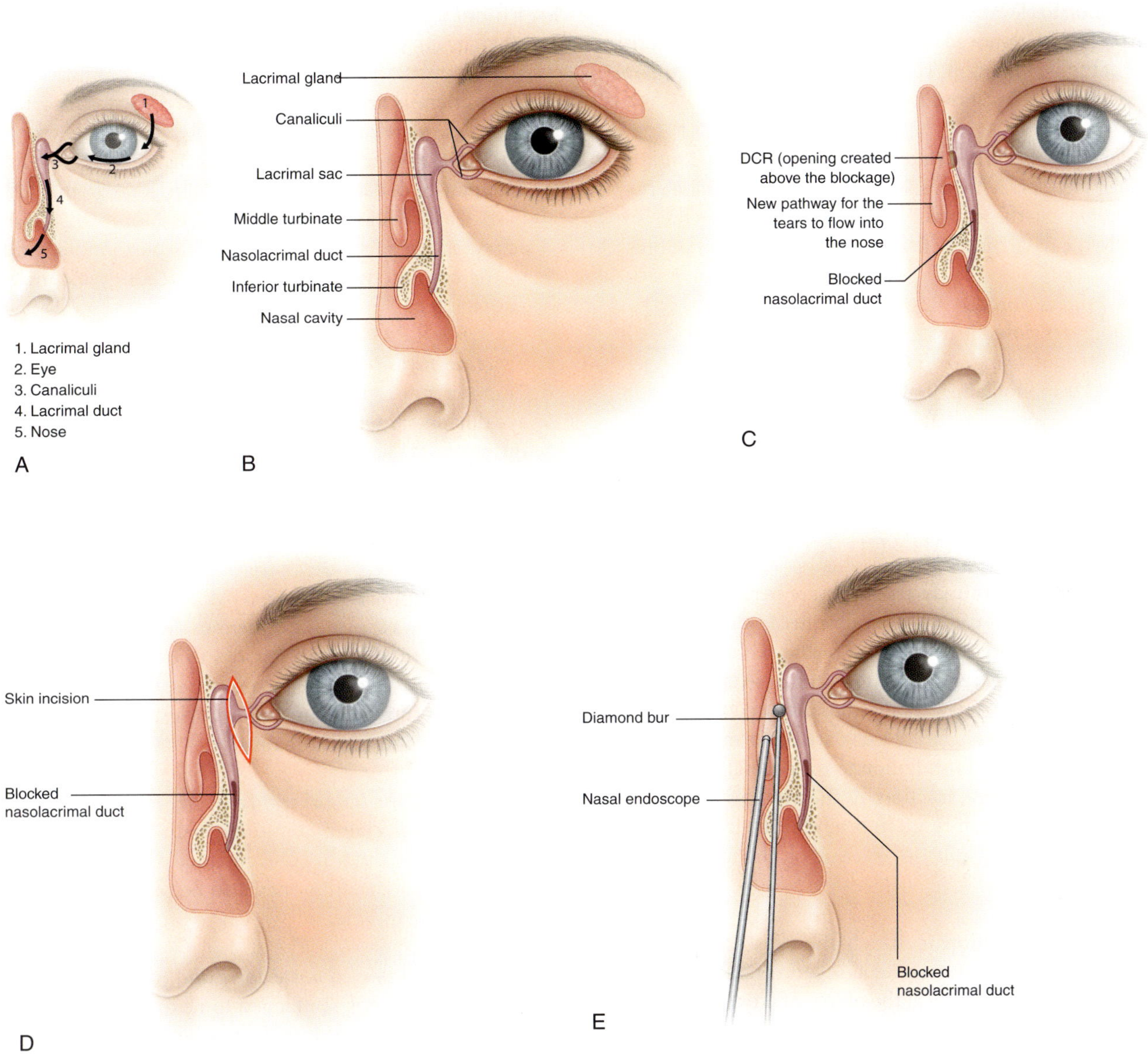

FIG. 25.9 Dacryocystorhinostomy. (A) Normal flow of tears. (B) Anatomy. (C) Surgical objective. (D and E) Comparison of open and endoscopic technique for DCR. (Courtesy Dr. Santiago Ortiz-Perez.)

3. ***An osteotomy is performed in the lacrimal bone.***
The surgeon incises the periosteum and uses a Freer or periosteal elevator to raise the periosteum from the bone. An opening is made in the bone using the periosteal elevator, and the opening is enlarged with a small Kerrison rongeur. The ST will need to remove bits of bone from the tip of the rongeur between bites to keep the tip clean. This can be done using a moist sponge. The opening in the bone exposes the lacrimal sac.

4. ***An incision is made in the lacrimal sac.***
A Bowman lacrimal probe is inserted into the upper punctum and advanced until the tip can be seen pushing on the wall of the lacrimal sac. An incision is made over the probe using an angled crescent blade or the bipolar ESU. The probe is removed and the incision is then extended using Stevens tenotomy scissors. Suction must be immediately available to drain the contents of the lacrimal sac.

5. ***An opening is made in the nasal mucosa.***
The nasal packing is removed for better visualization in the nasal cavity. An opening is made in the nasal mucosa using the tenotomy scissors and bipolar ESU.

6. ***Silicone tubes are inserted into the puncta.***
Silicone lacrimal tubes are now passed through the upper and lower puncta and advanced through the lacrimal sac incision. Ophthalmic antibacterial ointment may be used to lubricate the tubes. An intubation system such as the Guibor tube may be used. This system has one silicone tube with a metal probe attached at each end. The probes are inserted into each punctum and advanced into the lacrimal sac and nasal cavity. A loop of tube remains at the canthus. If a proprietary system is not available, each silicone tube can be fitted over a lacrimal probe and introduced into the canthus. A straight mosquito clamp is used to grasp the probe and tube as it emerges into the nasal cavity. The surgeon may use

a dull hook to elevate the loop slightly to release any tension. The probes are removed and the tubes sutured or tied at the level of the skin incision. The ends of the tube lie in the nasal cavity and will be removed after healing.

7. ***The lacrimal sac is anastomosed to the nasal mucosa.***
A small piece of Gelfoam soaked in thrombin or saline may be inserted into the wound. The lacrimal sac flaps are then sutured to the nasal mucosa flaps using size 6-0 Vicryl sutures.

8. ***The wound is closed.***
The wound is closed in layers, including reattachment of the canthal tendon using size 6-0 Vicryl. Skin is closed with size 5-0 or 6-0 monofilament synthetic suture such as nylon. The silicone tubes are left in place for up to 4 to 8 weeks postoperatively. Patients are advised to use ice to reduce swelling and to keep the head elevated during rest and sleep.

MUSCLE RESECTION AND RECESSION

Muscle resection and **muscle recession** are performed to correct deviation of the eye caused by strabismus. In this procedure, the affected muscles are detached and reattached at the correct location. The procedure requires an eye muscle setup and minor soft tissue instruments. General anesthesia is used for pediatric patients. Routine eye prep and draping are performed. A retrobulbar block may be used in addition to the general anesthetic.

During the procedure, traction on the muscles can cause a vagal response, which can result in bradycardia. If this occurs, the surgeon temporarily releases traction on the muscles.

Pathology

Strabismus is a condition in which the eyes are unable to focus on point because the muscles lack coordination. One eye (the fixing eye) looks directly at the object of attention, but the other eye (the deviating eye) does not.

Two surgical procedures are commonly used to treat strabismus. In lateral rectus resection, a portion of the muscle is excised and the severed end is reattached at the original site of insertion. This limits the drift of the eye. In medial rectus *recession*, the muscle is detached from its insertion, moved posteriorly, and reattached. This releases the eye and allows it to move farther in a lateral position.

A recent innovation in strabismus surgery is the use of adjustable sutures on the muscles. In this technique, a sliding knot is used to secure the muscle. Traction sutures are placed and the ends secured to the patient's face. The adjustable suture can then be used in the clinic to adjust the rotation of the eye under local anesthesia.

POSITION:	Supine with slight elevation of the shoulders
INCISION:	Conjunctiva
PREP AND DRAPING:	Eye
INSTRUMENTS:	Strabismus set

Technical Points and Discussion

RESECTION OF THE LATERAL MUSCLE

1. ***The patient is prepped and draped.***
2. ***The conjunctiva is incised.***
To begin a lateral rectus resection, the surgeon inserts an open-ended eyelid retractor and grasps the limbus with Castroviejo forceps. With tenotomy or Westcott scissors, the surgeon then makes a buttonhole incision in the conjunctiva at the limbus. Bleeding is controlled with cautery.

3. ***Traction sutures are placed.***
Traction sutures are used to help position the operative eye during surgery. A suture of 4-0 silk is passed through the sclera at the 6 and 12 o'clock positions. The ends are held using a small clamp, and the eye is rotated into position to expose the muscle.

4. ***The muscle is measured with calipers.***
A muscle hook is used to separate the attachments between Tenon's capsule and the muscle sheath. An incision is made with tenotomy scissors to expose the tip of the muscle hook. Two Stevens hooks are guided down the lateral rectus muscle, exposing the sclera. A caliper is used to measure and mark the muscle.

5. ***A portion of the lateral rectus muscle is excised.***
The muscle is clamped and cut with tenotomy scissors, and a piece of the muscle is retained as a specimen. Note that muscle shortening may also be performed by taking a tuck in the muscle.

6. ***The muscle is moved posteriorly and reattached.***
The muscle then is reattached to its original site with 6-0 double-arm, nonabsorbable synthetic suture. The conjunctiva can be closed with absorbable suture or left open, depending on the surgeon's preference. Refer to Fig. 25.10 for illustrations on the procedure.

RECESSION OF THE MEDIAL MUSCLE

The procedure for medial rectus recession is identical to that for lateral rectus resection to the point of the conjunctival incision. The surgeon uses tenotomy scissors to undermine the conjunctiva.

1. ***The insertion point is measured and marked.***
Using a previously adjusted caliper, the surgeon then measures the distance from the original insertion point to its new one. The new insertion point is indicated with a surgical marker.

2. ***The muscle is incised.***
Two sutures of 5-0 or 6-0 absorbable material are placed at the end of the muscle but are not tied. A straight mosquito clamp or muscle clamp is placed across the muscle between the sutures and the insertion point. The clamp is allowed to

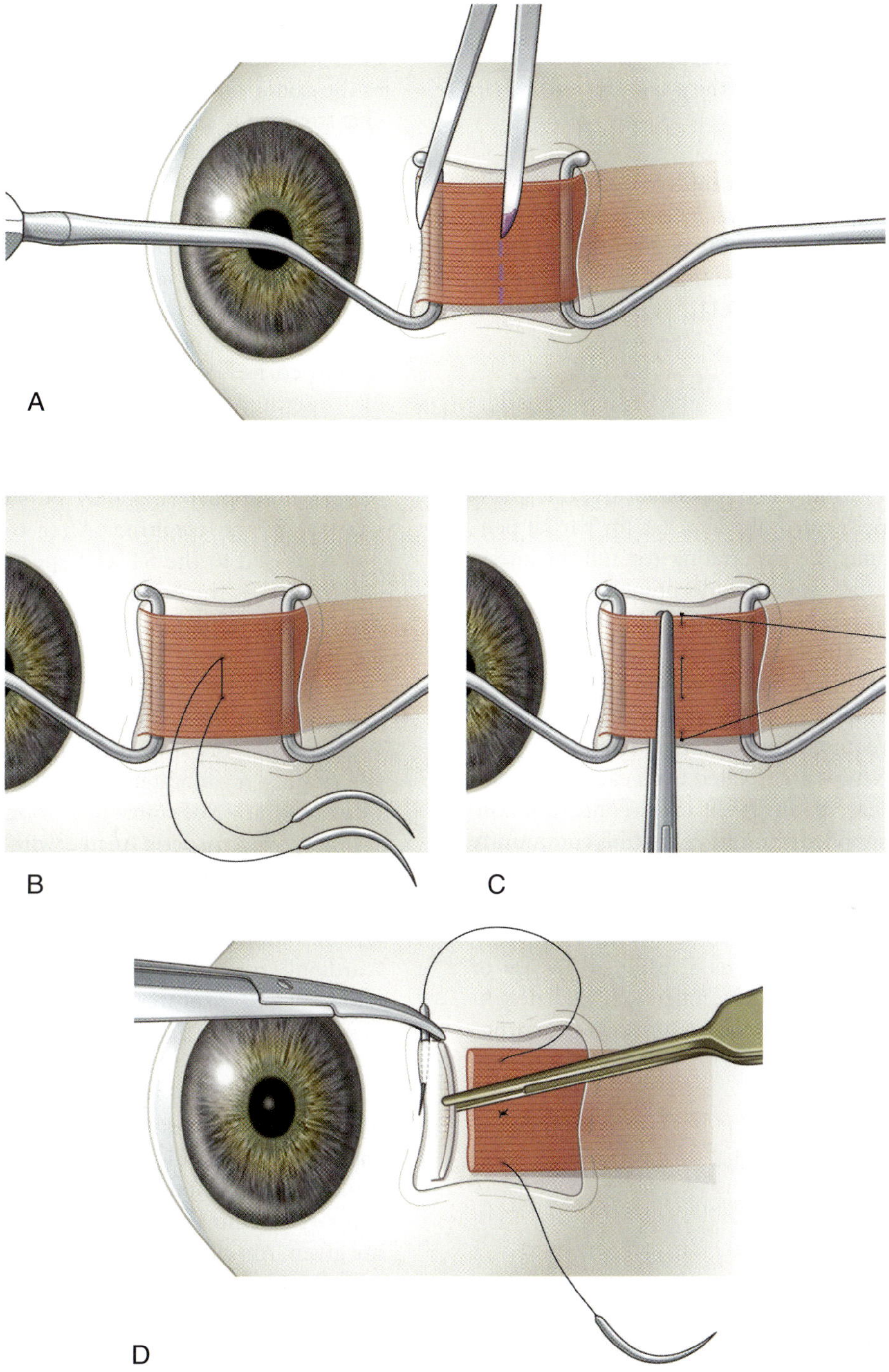

FIG. 25.10 Lateral rectus resection. (A) After making a limbal incision, the surgeon marks the length of the resection by putting ink on the caliper tips. Note position of the muscle hooks. (B) A central knot is placed in the muscle on the ink line. Both arms of the suture are woven through the muscle. (C) A straight mosquito hemostat is used to crush the muscle, which is incised at the crush line. (D) The resected muscle is reattached to the sclera at the original insertion site. (From Spaeth G, Danesh-Mayer H, Goldberg I, Kampik A. *Ophthalmic Surgery Principles and Practice.* 4th ed. Philadelphia: Elsevier; 2012.)

remain on the muscle for up to 3 minutes to provide hemostasis. After the clamp is removed, the surgeon passes a muscle hook under the muscle to elevate it away from the globe. The muscle is then incised with straight iris scissors. At this point, the cautery unit may be needed to control bleeding.

3. ***The muscle is attached to its new location.***
   The ST now passes an empty needle holder and smooth tissue forceps, and the surgeon moves the muscle back to the scribe mark and secures it with the previously placed sutures.

4. ***The conjunctiva is closed.***
The conjunctival incision is closed with 5-0 or 6-0 absorbable sutures swaged to a **spatula needle.** Antibiotic ophthalmic ointment is instilled, and the eye is dressed with a cotton eye pad and rigid shield.

Patients, especially children, who undergo muscle procedures often experience postoperative nausea and vomiting, which are caused by the vagal reflex during surgery. These are treated with antiemetics and are self-limiting. Technical points of the procedure are shown in Fig. 25.11.

PENETRATING KERATOPLASTY (CORNEAL TRANSPLANTATION)

Penetrating **keratoplasty** is full-thickness transplantation of a donor cornea to restore vision. Two types of corneal transplantation are commonly performed: the lamellar (or partial penetrating) keratoplasty and the penetrating (or full-thickness) keratoplasty. In the partial penetrating technique, the anterior chamber is not entered, and one-half to two-thirds of the cornea is transplanted. In the penetrating technique, the anterior chamber is entered, and a full-thickness corneal graft is transplanted.

In full-thickness keratoplasty, a separate instrument table and Mayo setup are required to prepare and transplant the donor tissue. The two setups are isolated from each other, and instruments are not shared to prevent cross-contamination. The donor cornea is supplied through a routine community tissue bank procedure or by the health care facility's bank.

Pathology

The cornea may become damaged as a result of disease or injury. Chemical and thermal burns, infection, and degenerative disease are the most common indications for cornea transplantation.

POSITION:	Supine
INCISION:	Corneal
PREP AND DRAPING:	Eye
INSTRUMENTS:	Corneal transplant set with implant

Technical Points and Discussion

The patient is placed in the supine position with the head stabilized. Before beginning the patient prep, the circulator or ST positions the microscope above the patient, and the surgeon adjusts it to his or her needs. The microscope is then locked into position and rotated out of the field.

1. ***The patient is prepped and draped.***
The eye is prepped in a routine manner. If a regional block anesthetic is to be used, the postauricular area also is prepped. The patient is then draped for an eye procedure.

2. ***The donor cornea is prepared.***
The donor cornea is prepared for transplantation. After determining the size of cornea required, the surgeon places the donor tissue on a silicone block and uses a disposable trephine to incise the cornea. The trephine is a circular cutting instrument that produces a tissue button. The donor trephine is larger than the recipient's cornea. The donor tissue is placed in the surgeon's choice of preservative and protected from contamination or injury.

3. ***The recipient cornea is trephined.***
Several different techniques are used to extract the recipient cornea, including vacuum-operated and manually operated trephines. In addition to the trephine, miniature Westcott or Vannas scissors are also needed to complete the trephination and also to trim the edges. A scleral support ring may be sutured for additional support of the trephine. After trephination, the cornea is passed to the ST as a specimen. Removal of the cornea makes the eye extremely vulnerable to environmental contamination; this phase often is referred to as "open sky."

4. ***The graft is sutured in place.***
A scleral support ring is sutured to the cornea with 6-0 silk sutures. A calibrated marker can then be used to indicate the location of suture sites for closure.
The donor tissue is treated with viscoelastic solution, lifted out of its container with a 0.12-mm forceps, and manipulated onto the recipient's eye. The surgeon uses size 10-0 interrupted nylon sutures to form landmark or "cardinal" sutures in the cornea. After these are placed, additional 10-0 sutures are used to complete the corneal closure (Fig. 25.12).

5. ***Fluid in the anterior chamber is replaced.***
The cardinal sutures may be removed at the end of the case. If needed, sodium hyaluronate can be injected into the anterior chamber to replace lost fluid. The scleral ring support is removed, and antibiotic and steroid injections are given. Antibiotic ointment is applied, and an eye patch with shield is secured with tape.

Full visual recovery after surgery may take up to 1 year. Most patients with successful corneal transplants enjoy good vision for many years. In some cases, the body rejects the transplanted tissue, but this is a rare occurrence. Other risks of corneal transplantation include bleeding, infection of the eye, glaucoma, and swelling of the front of the eye.

EXTRACAPSULAR CATARACT EXTRACTION (PHACOEMULSIFICATION)

Phacoemulsification is the fragmentation of tissue by ultrasonic vibration. This technique is the most common form of cataract removal. The goal of cataract extraction is to remove an opaque lens (cataract) and replace it with an intraocular

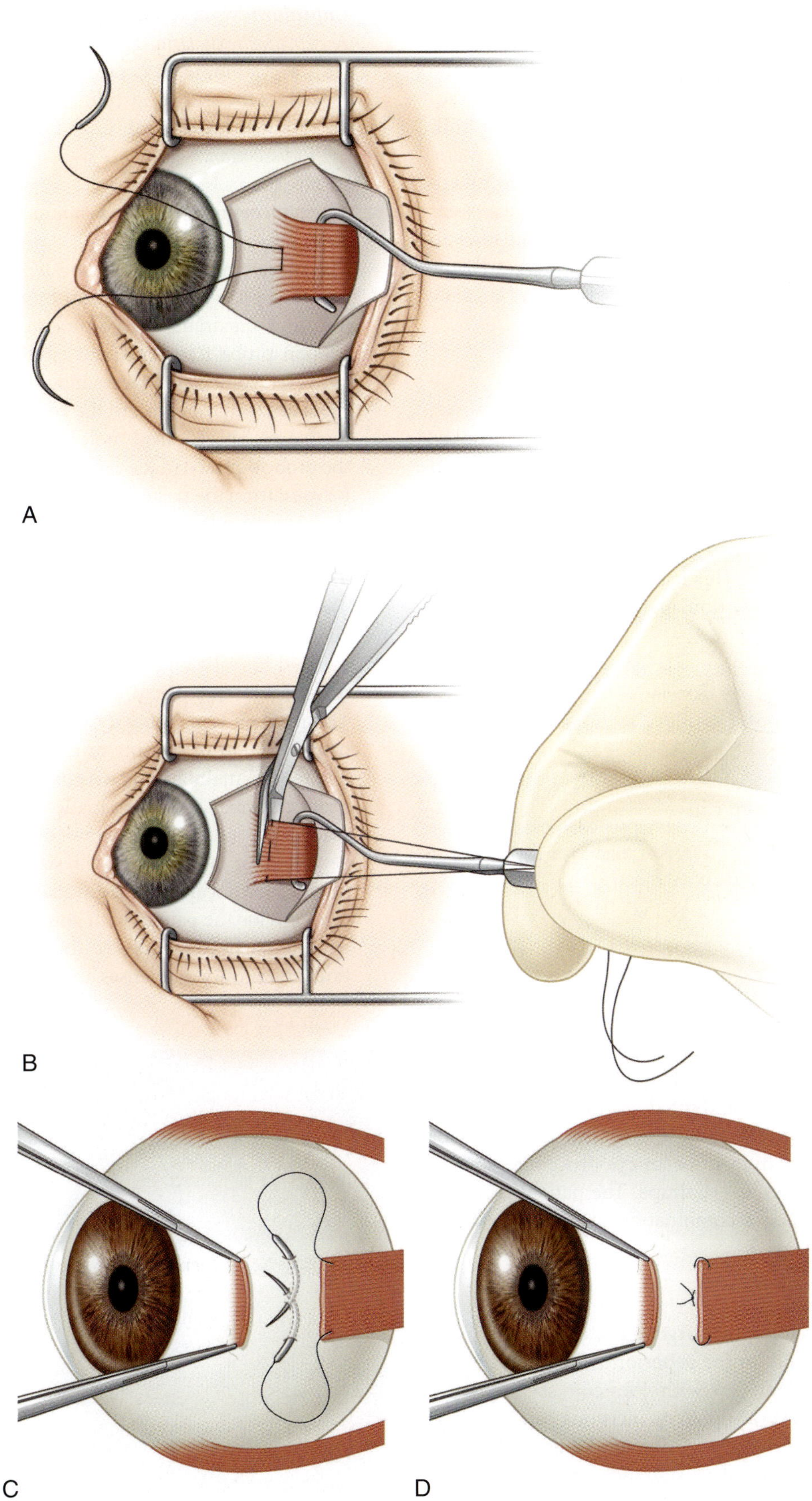

FIG. 25.11 Lateral rectus recession. (A) A security stitch is placed through the muscle at its attachment. (B) The muscle is detached. (C) The suture is passed through the sclera at the correct position. (D) The muscle is reattached. (From Spaeth G, Danesh-Mayer H, Goldberg I, Kampik A. Ophthalmic Surgery Principles and Practice. 4th ed. Philadelphia: Elsevier; 2012.)

lens (IOL) implant to restore vision. Cataract extraction is most often performed using the extracapsular cataract extraction technique. This is removal of the lens only, leaving the lens capsule intact. Historically, extracapsular cataract extraction has been performed with a cryoprobe to remove both the lens and the capsule. This procedure requires enzymatic destruction of the zonules that attach the lens. The intracapsular method has been largely replaced by the extracapsular technique. Current technology allows the phacoemulsifier to be tuned to a frequency that destroys only the target tissue. After the tissue is fragmented and liquefied, it can be safely aspirated.

Pathology

A **cataract** is opacity of the lens. The disease has many causes, including genetic defect, injury, overexposure to ultraviolet light, metabolic disease (e.g., diabetes), and age. Certain drugs, such as corticosteroids and busulfan, are known to cause cataracts. Age-related cataracts are the most common type, because the composition of the lens changes with age and as metabolic changes occur. This leads to progressive loss of transparency and visual distortion, glare, and myopia.

POSITION:	Supine
INCISION:	Anterior chamber
PREP AND DRAPING:	Eye
INSTRUMENTS:	Cataract set with implant supplies, phacoemulsification equipment

Technical Points and Discussion

1. ***The patient is prepped and draped.***
The patient is placed in the supine position with a headrest to immobilize the head. During the prep, several drops of povidone-iodine, diluted according to the surgeon's orders, are instilled into the eye for antibacterial effect. The patient is draped for an eye procedure with a head drape and adhesive eye drape. The patient receives conscious sedation or a combination of topical and regional anesthetics.

2. ***The incision is made.***
To begin the procedure, the surgeon places a traction suture of 3-0 or 4-0 silk in the superior rectus muscle and creates a conjunctival flap with Westcott scissors and toothed forceps. Several different incisions can be used to make the corneal incision. A diamond knife, slit knife, or keratome is used to make a stab incision at the limbus into the cornea. This creates a triangular cut. A second incision is made into the anterior chamber, and a viscoelastic substance such as sodium hyaluronate (Healon) is injected.

3. ***Capsulorhexis and hydrodissection are performed.***
A *capsulorhexis* (incision into the capsule) is performed with a cystotome or capsulorhexis forceps. The surgeon mobilizes the lens by instilling BSS into the eye with a size 26 cannula and a 5-mL Luer-Lok syringe. This is called *hydrodissection.*

4. ***The phacoemulsification probe is used to fragment the cataract.***
The phacoemulsification probe is then introduced. Many surgeons groove the nucleus of the cataract and separate it into four quadrants before proceeding. The phacoemulsification probe fragments and emulsifies most of the lens. However, some small pieces may remain. The surgeon manipulates the probe toward the edges to aspirate the remaining pieces. This is called "polishing the posterior capsule." If the probe is placed in the center, the vitreous may be brought forward from the posterior capsule. This is a complication of the surgery and may necessitate an anterior vitrectomy.

5. ***The intraocular lens is implanted and the wound closed.***
The scleral incision is enlarged, and an IOL is manipulated into the posterior chamber of the capsule. Healon is injected into the chamber and onto the lens. The incision either is closed with 8-0 or 9-0 or 10-0 suture or the incision may self-seal. Many styles of IOLs are available, but the design primarily consists of a central biconvex optic and two tabs to maintain the lens in position. The newest posterior chamber lenses are made of flexible materials, such as silicone and acrylic polymers. This allows the lenses to be folded for insertion and the size of the incision to be reduced. Multifocal optics are available; the goal of this design is to provide the patient with good near and distance vision without the need for glasses. The incision, phacoemulsification, and intraocular lenses are shown in Fig. 25.13.

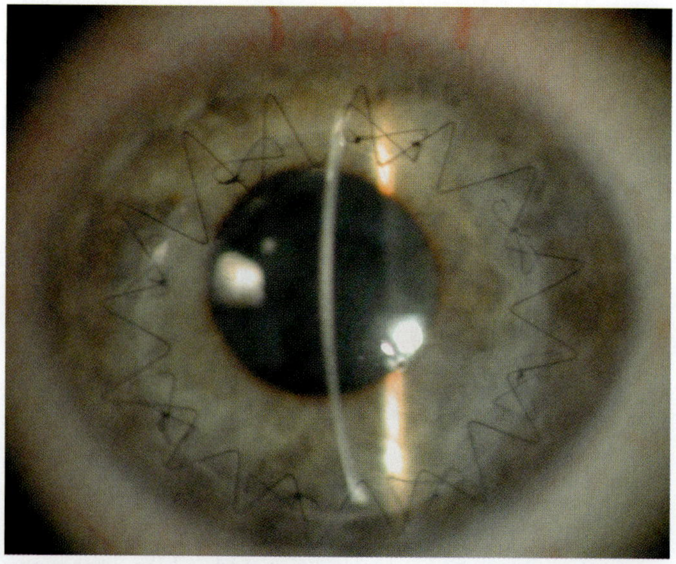

FIG. 25.12 Corneal transplantation. Cornea sutured in place. (From Spaeth G, Danesh-Mayer H, Goldberg I, Kampik A. *Ophthalmic Surgery Principles and Practice.* 4th ed. Philadelphia: Elsevier; 2012.)

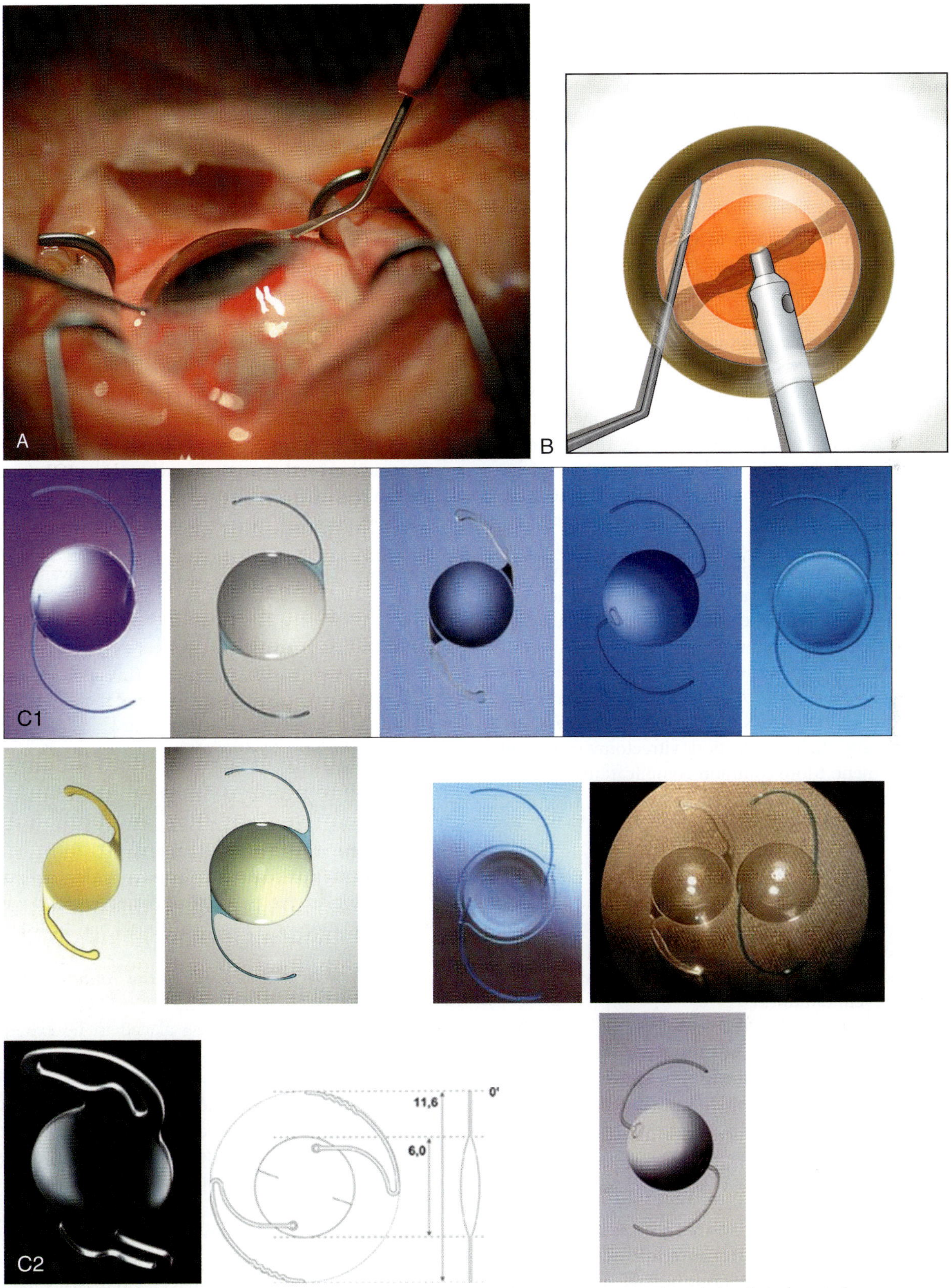

FIG. 25.13 Extracapsular cataract extraction. (A) The phaco incision is made with the slit knife. (B) The lens is obliterated by means of the phaco. (C) Intraocular lenses made of acrylate and silicone. (A and B, From Spaeth G, Danesh-Mayer H, Goldberg I, Kampik A. *Ophthalmic Surgery Principles and Practice.* 4th ed. Philadelphia: Elsevier; 2012. C, From Albert D, Miller J. *Albert and Jakobiec's Principles and Practice of Ophthalmology.* 3rd ed. Philadelphia: Saunders; 2008.)

ANTERIOR VITRECTOMY

An anterior vitrectomy is performed to remove the vitreous from the anterior chamber.

Pathology

An anterior vitrectomy may be performed for a variety of conditions, such as opacity of the anterior segment of the vitreous and loss of vitreous during cataract extraction. This is a complication in which rupture of the posterior capsule allows vitreous to prolapse into the anterior chamber. The phacoemulsification equipment can quickly be adapted to vitrectomy mode. Surgery for removal of vitreous in the anterior chamber is described here.

Technical Points and Discussion

Once the posterior chamber rupture is assessed, the phacoemulsification instrument is stopped and only the irrigation cannula is used. The primary corneal incision may be closed to prevent loss of vitreous. Usually a stab incision is made at the limbus to allow for entry of the vitreous cutter. The irrigation cannula is maintained above the vitreous cutter. A cyclodialysis spatula is used to sweep the vitreous strands posteriorly. The vitreous can also be teased through the incision using a cellulose eye sponge and detached with Westcott scissors. This process is called *manual vitrectomy*. The anterior chamber is reformed with viscoelastic solution. The original incision can then be opened and the IOL inserted. Finally, the conjunctiva is closed using a 10-0 nylon suture.

After the surgery, patients use eye drops for several weeks or longer to allow the surface of the eye to heal. Heavy lifting is avoided for several weeks. Along with the usual complications of surgery, such as infection, vitrectomy can result in retinal detachment. More common complications are high IOP, bleeding in the eye, and recurrent cataracts.

SCLERAL BUCKLING PROCEDURE FOR DETACHED RETINA

Scleral buckling surgery is performed when the sensory layer of the retina becomes separated from the pigment epithelial layer. The surgical goal is to restore the layers to their normal positions and prevent blindness.

Retinal detachment requires immediate repair to prevent the tear from extending. Several techniques are used to repair detached tissue. A common technique is to produce adhesions between the layers with **cryotherapy** (freezing of the tissue) or **diathermy** (mild heat created by a diathermy unit or laser). Neither of these techniques damages the eye, and both create points of scar tissue, although cryotherapy is more common. This is followed by immediate scleral buckling, in which a Silastic band is attached to the sclera. One or more synthetic "buckles" are placed over the band, causing it to indent. This technique puts the tissue in close contact with the retina during healing. An alternative technique is to implant individual Silastic sponges over small tears to bring the retina in contact with the sclera without encircling the entire globe. There are many variations of the techniques used for detached retina. The procedure described here is just one.

Another common technique is to perform a vitrectomy in conjunction with scleral buckling. In this procedure, the vitreous gel is replaced with Healon or gas through a small puncture wound. This method is used to eliminate traction and tearing on the retina. Two puncture sites are made in the sclera to accommodate the microinstruments used to perform cryotherapy or diathermy. The eye remains pressurized throughout the microsurgical procedure. The procedure described here is for scleral buckling and cryotherapy.

Pathology

The vitreous normally adheres to the retina in several locations. A tear in the retina causes sudden painless loss of vision, or "shadowing," which appears as a curtain that descends over the patient's field of vision. Light flashes and "floaters" often accompany the vision loss.

A tear in the retina (called a *rhegmatogenous detachment*) creates a passage for the vitreous to seep between the pigment epithelium and the neural layer of the retina. This seepage separates the layers and may extend the tear. A vitreous tear usually is caused by aging. As the vitreous begins to shrink, this creates traction on the retina. Detachment also may be caused by trauma or diabetes mellitus.

POSITION:	Supine
INCISION:	Conjunctival
PREP AND DRAPING:	Eye
INSTRUMENTS:	Scleral buckling set with diathermy unit or cryo unit

Technical Points and Discussion

1. ***The patient is prepped and draped.***
   The patient is placed in the supine position, prepped, and draped for an eye procedure. A nerve block with conscious sedation or general anesthesia may be used.

2. ***The conjunctiva is incised at the limbus with spring scissors.***
   An open-ended retractor is placed in he eye. Toothed forceps and Westcott scissors are used to make an incision in the sclera and Tenon's capsule. The rectus muscle is then slung with a muscle hook. Traction sutures of size 4-0 silk are placed under each muscle. The traction suture is left long, tagged with a hemostat, and used to retract the globe for access to the posterolateral surface.

3. ***Diathermy or cryotherapy is applied to the area of detachment or tear.***
   Using the diathermy unit, the surgeon makes many small burn marks or "spot welds" over the area of detachment. The diathermy electrode produces a high-frequency electrical current that causes mild burning. If the cryosurgical probe is used, the detached area is treated in the same manner.

4. ***Sutures are placed in the sclera.***
The assistant steadies the eye by holding the traction sutures while the surgeon compresses the globe with cotton-tipped applicators. The sclera then is approximated with fine suture of 4-0 Prolene.

5. ***The buckling components are implanted.***
A double-arm suture of Dacron or other synthetic material is placed in the sclera and secured over the buckling device. This compresses the eye inward at the area of detachment. A Silastic band may be placed 360 degrees around the eye and a scleral buckle sutured into place under the muscles. Sutures are secured to the buckle so that it remains in place. Sutures of 7-0 Vicryl may be used to secure the conjunctiva at the limbus.

6. ***Intravitreal gas may be injected.***
Intravitreous gas injection is the injection of intraocular gas through a handheld syringe. The gas infusion exerts pressure on the retina while subretinal fluid is reabsorbed and scarification takes place. The gases include sulfur hexafluoride (SF_6) and perfluoropropane (C_3F_8).

The scleral buckling procedure is illustrated in Fig. 25.14.

FILTERING PROCEDURES AND TRABECULECTOMY

A *trabeculectomy* is performed to create a channel from which the aqueous humor may drain from the anterior chamber. This procedure is performed for the treatment of glaucoma.

Pathology

Glaucoma is a group of diseases characterized by optic nerve damage and visual field loss. In the past, glaucoma was defined by an IOP above the normal range in association with nerve damage. However, more recent definitions include cases in which IOP is normal. In most types, IOP is elevated and the unrelieved pressure can result in ischemia of the optic nerve, which leads to progressive blindness. The IOP is normally maintained by the aqueous humor, which is secreted by the ciliary epithelium (posterior chamber) and drained between the lens and iris, through the pupil into the anterior chamber. Fluid exits through the trabecular network and the canal of Schlemm. The balance in pressure is maintained by the rate of secretion and drainage. Several pathological conditions can disturb this balance. In nearly all cases of glaucoma, the problem is with drainage rather than overproduction of aqueous humor (Fig. 25.15).

There are many different types of glaucoma. The most common are described below:

- *Primary angle closure glaucoma:* This type of glaucoma accounts for 30% of all cases. The incidence is higher in women. A sudden rise in IOP is caused by total blockage or obstruction of the aqueous humor at the root of the iris (the limbal drainage system). This is considered a medical emergency, because blindness may result if the blockage is not relieved.
- *Primary open angle glaucoma:* This is a chronic disease occurring in both eyes. It develops in the middle years or later. In this condition, the outflow of aqueous humor is obstructed in the trabecular meshwork, which can be caused by different factors.
- *Normal tension glaucoma:* This is a subtype of open angle glaucoma in which IOP is normal. There is retinal damage and visual field loss with migraine and optic disc hemorrhage.
- *Congenital glaucoma:* In congenital glaucoma, the fluid drainage system is abnormal at birth. The infant's eye distends, and corneal haziness occurs. Symptoms include light sensitivity and excessive tearing. Surgery is indicated to prevent blindness.

POSITION:	Supine
INCISION:	Conjunctiva
PREP AND DRAPING:	Eye
INSTRUMENTS:	Trabeculectomy instruments with diathermy unit or cryo unit; shunting device as indicated by the surgeon

Technical Points and Discussion

1. ***The patient is prepped and draped.***
2. ***A conjunctival flap is created.***
To begin the procedure, the surgeon inserts a lid speculum. Size 4-0 traction sutures may be placed in the superior rectus muscle. The conjunctiva is incised at the limbus with toothed forceps and the knife. The Tenon capsule is separated from the sclera with Westcott scissors in the direction of the limbus. This creates a conjunctival flap.

3. ***A scleral flap is created.***
The limbal area is gently scraped with a Beaver blade to remove any blood clots. This technique prevents accidental puncture of the conjunctiva. The sclera is then cauterized in the shape of the flap. The surgeon uses the Beaver blade to make an incision in the sclera, following the outlines of the cautery. Dissection of the scleral flap starts at the apex and extends upward toward the iris.

4. ***A portion of the trabecular meshwork is excised.***
A stab wound is made through the cornea to drain the aqueous humor. This incision is self-sealing and can be used later to reinflate the anterior chamber. If necessary, the scleral flap is retracted, and Vannas scissors are used to excise a portion of the trabecular meshwork.
A complication of the procedure may occur at this point; that is, the iris may spontaneously prolapse into the wound. In such cases, an iridectomy is performed. The surgeon grasps the iris with forceps and removes a portion, taking care not to damage the ciliary body.

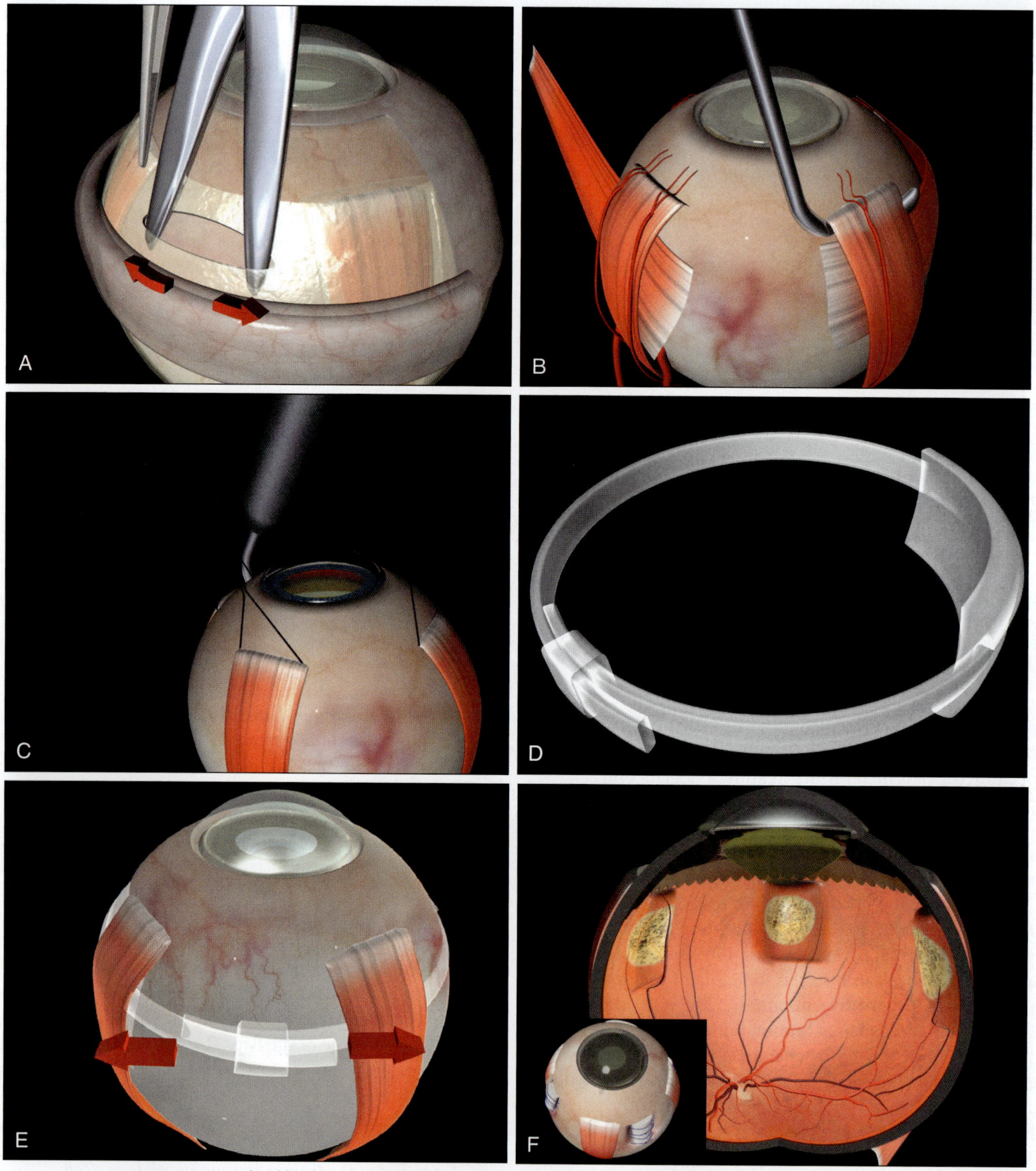

FIG. 25.14 Scleral buckling procedure for retinal detachment. (A) Westcott scissors are used to incise the sclera and Tenon's capsule. (B) A muscle hook is passed behind the rectus muscles. (C) Traction sutures are placed behind each muscle. (D) The Silastic band and buckle. (E) The band is sutured in place. (F) Example of a single sponges used for multiple tears. (From Ryan S, ed. *Retina*. 5th ed. Philadelphia: Elsevier Saunders; 2013.)

5. ***The tissue flaps and incisions are closed.***
In an uncomplicated procedure, BSS is instilled into the anterior chamber to re-inflate it. The scleral flap is closed with 10-0 nylon sutures. The conjunctiva and Tenon's capsule are approximated with 8-0 absorbable suture. BSS is then instilled into the anterior chamber. An eye sponge is placed over the incision site to check for leakage. Subconjunctival antibiotics and steroids are injected, and antibacterial ointments are instilled into the eye.

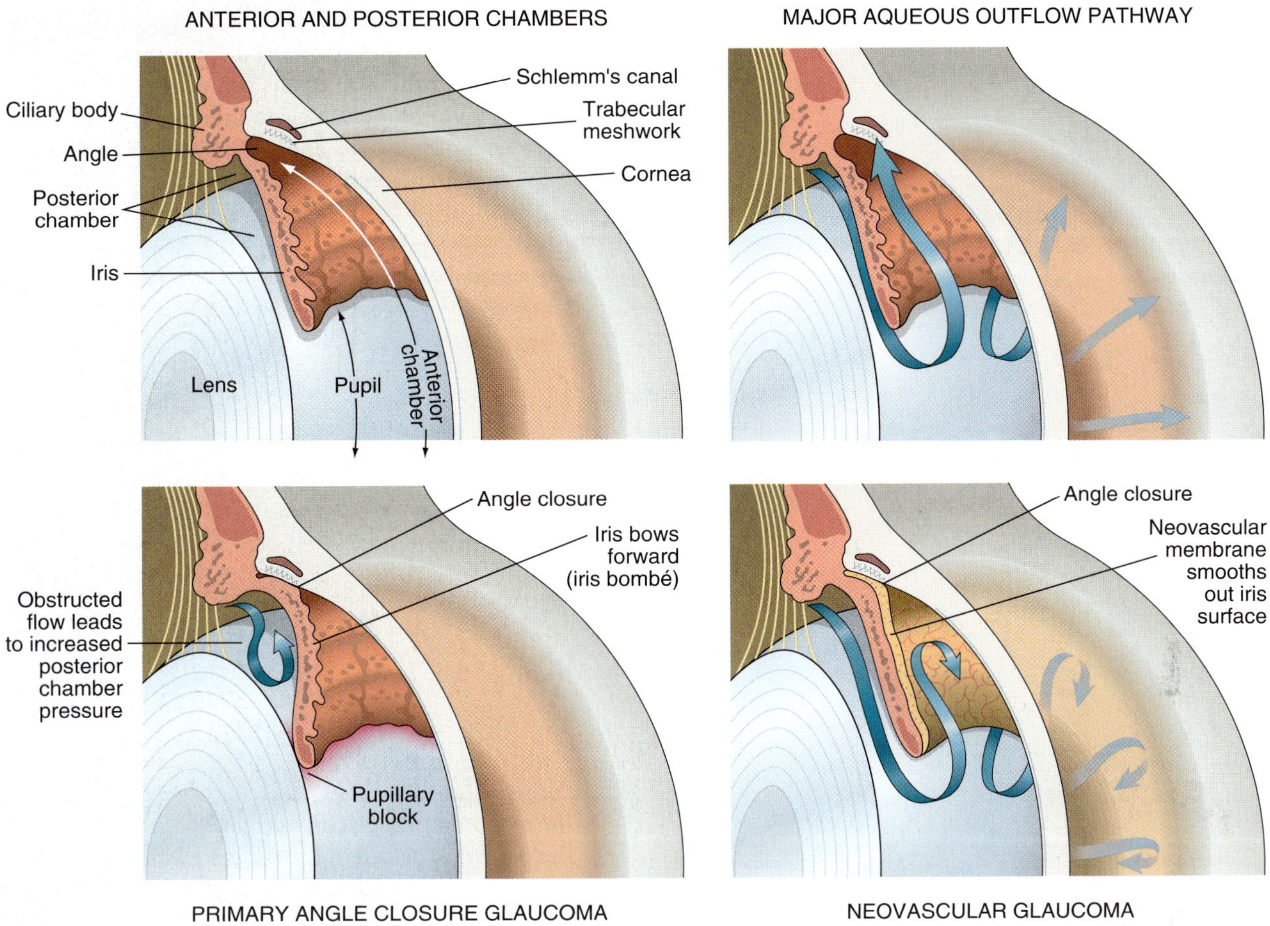

FIG. 25.15 Pathology of glaucoma. *Upper left,* A normal eye, showing the drainage pathway of the aqueous humor. *Lower left,* Primary closure glaucoma, in which the iris is in close contact with the lens. Increased pressure obstructs the trabecular meshwork. *Lower right,* Contraction of the myofibroblasts in the vascular membrane causes the iris to obstruct drainage. (From Kumar V, Abbas A, Fausto N. *Robbins and Cotran Pathologic Basis of Disease.* 7th ed. Philadelphia: WB Saunders; 2004.)

6. ***Adjunctive chemotherapy is performed.***
If the filtering procedure is at risk of failure or if a low IOP is indicated, the surgeon may use a chemotherapeutic agent, such as 5-fluorouracil (5-FU), and mitomycin. If this is the case, a sponge soaked with the agent is placed at the surgical site for approximately 1 minute. After removal of the sponge, the entire field is irrigated with BSS, and the instruments that were exposed to mitomycin are removed from the field. Because of the potential toxicity of the drugs, protocols for their disposal and for instrument decontamination are required in all health care facilities.

The trabeculectomy will fail if a flat bleb does not form in the first few postoperative days. If a bleb leak develops, a bandage contact lens may be inserted and repair may be necessary. Cataract formation may occur as a result of the trabeculectomy, and additional surgery may be required.

The trabeculectomy procedure is illustrated in Fig. 25.16.

REMOVAL OF THE EYE

There are several approaches to eye removal, depending on the pathology. It is important for the surgical technologist to understand the major types for case planning. **Enucleation** is complete removal of the eyeball (globe) while the eye muscles are left intact. **Evisceration** is a similar procedure in which the contents of the eye are removed, but the outer shell of the sclera and the muscle attachments are left intact. **Exenteration** is the most radical of the procedures in which all the structures of the eye socket, including the globe, muscles, fat, and eyelids, are removed. The following describes an enucleation with implant. Procedures for placing an implant after eye removal surgery vary according to the type of defect and desired results.

Evisceration with removal of the cornea and implant procedure is described here.

Pathology

Enucleation is performed to treat intraocular malignancy (e.g., retinoblastoma, melanoma), a penetrating ocular wound, a painful blind eye, or an eye that is blind and painless but disfigured. An artificial prosthesis may be inserted to replace the globe.

Removal of the eye is a psychologically traumatic experience for the patient. Many hospitals now perform this surgery in an outpatient setting. This increases the anxiety and grief experienced by the patient and family, because professional support may not be available immediately after the surgery.

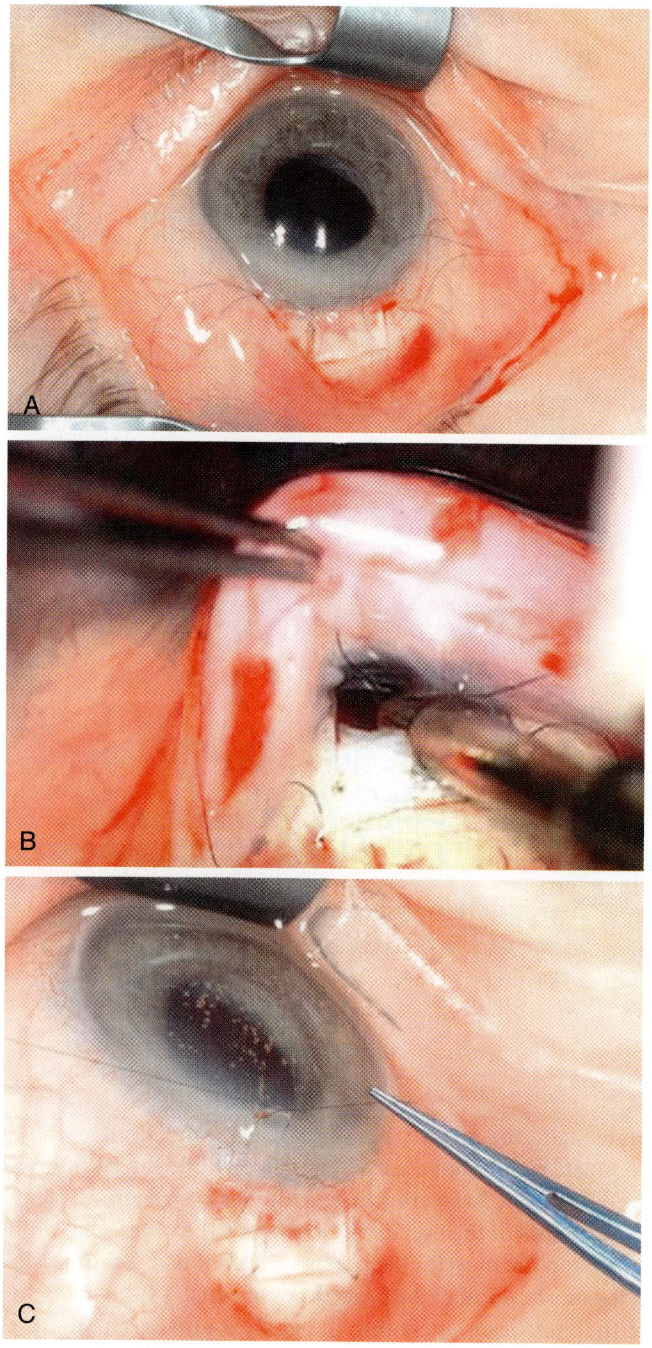

FIG. 25.16 Trabeculectomy (A) Creation of the scleral flap. (B) A block of tissue has been incised at the corneo-scleral junction and is removed here with a punch. (C) The scleral flap is closed (seen here) followed by the conjunctival closure. (From Spaeth G, Danesh-Mayer H, Goldberg I, Kampik A. *Ophthalmic Surgery Principles and Practice*. 4th ed. Philadelphia: Elsevier; 2012.)

Great care must be taken to provide a comforting environment in the operating room. All team members must be sensitive to the psychosocial and emotional effects of losing an eye. General anesthesia is preferred, for obvious psychological reasons. However, hospital protocol may require a regional anesthetic with monitored sedation.

After enucleation or evisceration, a transitional implant is inserted to shape the orbital cavity. This implant is called a *sphere*. A *conformer* is a shield placed over the sphere to cover its surface. The conformer provides support to the eyelids during healing. The conformer and sphere are replaced by an artificial eye after the wound has healed. Orbital implants are designed to allow blood vessels to infiltrate the implant material. Porous polyethylene and hydroxyapatite are the most common implant materials.

The American Society of Ocularists' website provides information on eye prosthetics. The website is available at https://www.ocularist.org/resources_surgical_procedures.asp.

POSITION:	Supine
INCISION:	Conjunctiva
PREP AND DRAPING:	Eye
INSTRUMENTS:	Enucleation or evisceration set; sizers, sphere, and conformer; ESU

Technical Points and Discussion

1. ***The patient is prepped and draped.***
The patient is placed in the supine position and prepared for routine eye surgery, as previously discussed.

2. ***The conjunctiva is incised.***
A retractor is placed in the eye. A circular incision is made as close to the limbus as possible. This conserves as much conjunctiva as possible for closure later in the procedure. The incision is made with a #15 blade or with iris scissors. The surgeon undermines the conjunctiva and Tenon's capsule and prepares to sever the rectus and oblique muscles from the globe.

3. ***The cornea is excised with a Graef knife.***
A Graef knife or scalpel blade placed under the cornea, which is excised. The excision is completed using curved scissors.

4. ***The ocular contents are removed.***
Using the enucleation spoon, the surgeon removes the ocular contents. Any remaining tissue may be removed using a moist gauze sponge. The ST should be prepared to receive the specimen in a small specimen cup or plate.

5. ***Two scleral incisions are made to relieve tension.***
The sclera is incised using straight scissors to continue the dissection and allow the placement of the implant.

6. ***The optic nerve is severed.***
The optic nerve is separated from the remaining sclera using a radiofrequency needle or scalpel. Additional relieving incisions are made.

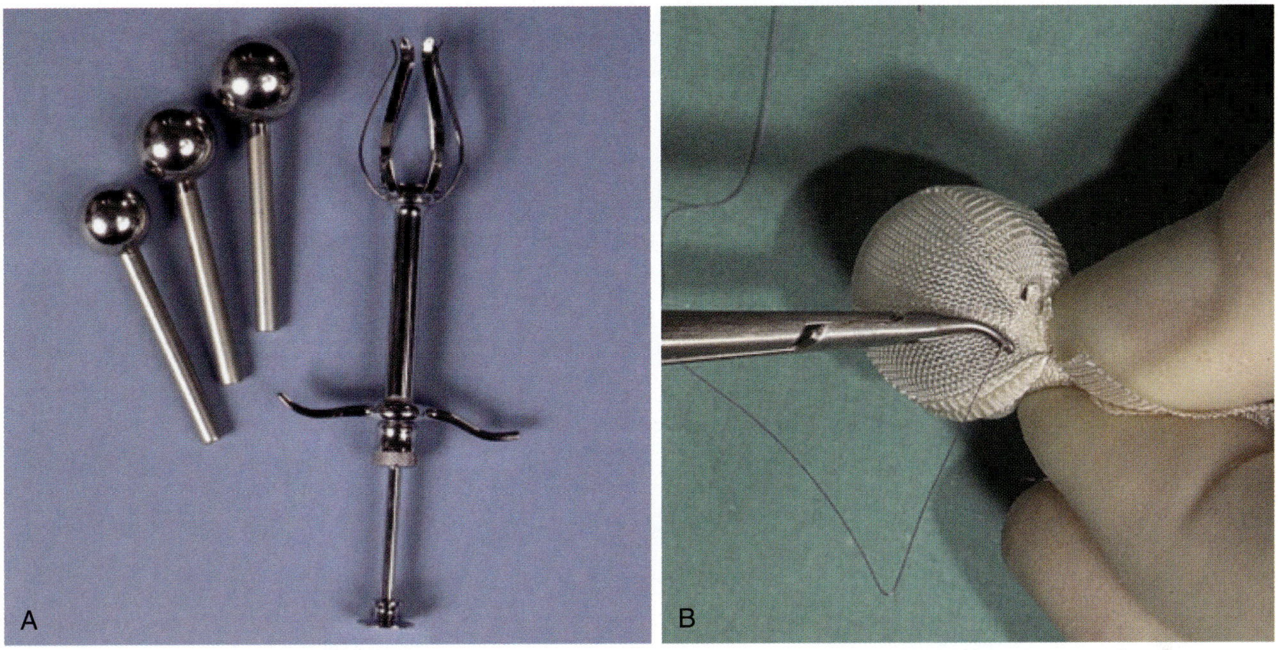

FIG. 25.17 (A) Trial spheres and introducer used during enucleation, evisceration, and exenteration of the eye. (B) The actual sphere implant may be wrapped in synthetic absorbable mesh and secured with sutures as shown before placement. (From Tyers AG, Collin, JRO. *Colour Atlas of Ophthalmic Plastic Surgery*. 4th ed. Elsevier; 2019.)

7. ***An implant sphere is inserted.***
   If any intraocular contents have been extruded into the socket, they must be cleaned out with irrigation solution and a 4 × 4 gauze sponge. Hemostasis is secured with pressure and the bipolar ESU.
   The optic nerve is cut beyond the implant. The technologist should have several sizes of implant spheres and a sphere introducer available from which the surgeon can choose the correct size (Fig. 25.17). Adult sizes usually range from 14 to 22 mm.
   The surgeon selects the implant and conformer, and the sphere is introduced into the orbit. A sphere introducer may be used to place the implant.
8. ***The rectus muscles and Tenon's capsule, as well as conjunctiva are sutured.***
   The rectus muscles are sutured over the sphere with 4-0 or 5-0 absorbable sutures. Next, Tenon's capsule is pulled over the sphere and sutured into place with scleral biting forceps and 4-0 absorbable synthetic suture. A purse-string suture may be used for this step. The conjunctiva is closed with 5-0 sutures.
9. ***The eyelids are sutured together.***
   The conformer may be placed over the sphere. Retraction sutures are removed, and antibiotic ointment is instilled into the eye. The eyelids are then sutured together. The eye is dressed with a soft pad secured with tape. The patient will return for additional surgery to replace the damaged eye with an orbital implant—usually in about 6 weeks, when healing is complete. Fig. 25.18 illustrates the procedure.

REPAIR OF ENTROPION LOWER LID

Entropion is an abnormal inversion of the lower eyelid. The goal of surgery is to restore the eyelid to correct anatomical position by resection. Many different procedures have been devised for correction of entropion and ectropion. In the one described here the retractor muscles are exposed and plicated (folded inwardly) with sutures (Fig. 25.19).

Pathology

An entropion is an inwardly turned eyelid, which causes the eyelashes to rub on the cornea. The condition occurs primarily in older individuals and is caused by weakness and imbalance of eyelid muscles. The condition almost always affects the lower, rather than the upper, eyelids.

POSITION:	Supine
INCISION:	Eyelid
PREP AND DRAPING:	Eye
INSTRUMENTS:	Oculoplastic set
POSSIBLE EXTRAS:	Bipolar cautery

Technical Points and Discussion

1. ***The lid is incised following skin marking.***
   After administration of local anesthetic, a corneal shield is placed in the eye. The incision line is marked with a

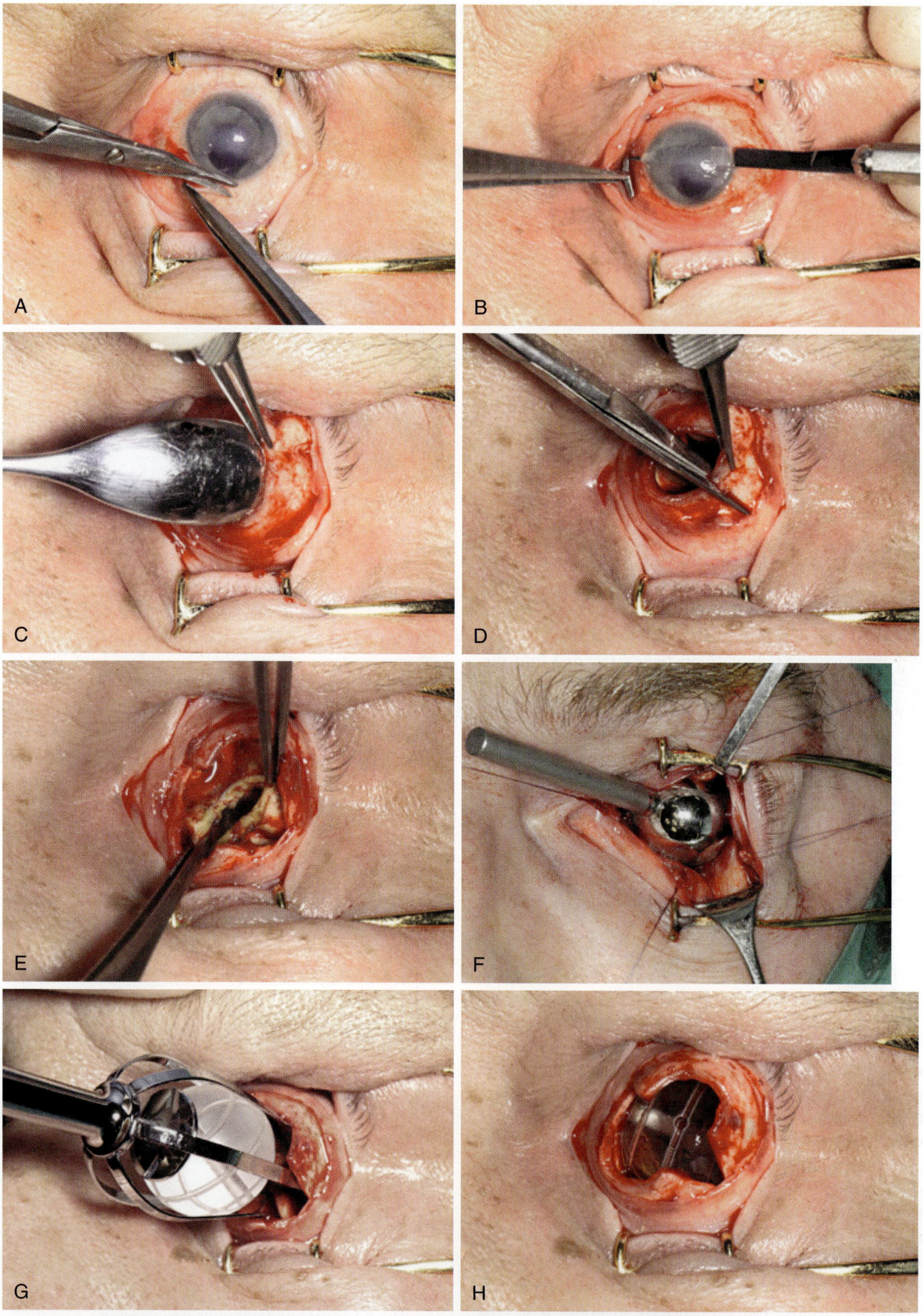

FIG. 25.18 Evisceration. (A) The initial incision is made at the limbus. (B) The cornea is removed. (C) The evisceration spoon is inserted between the uveal tract and the sclera. (D) The ocular contents are removed and a "relieving incision" made in the posterior sclera to accommodate the implant sizer. (E) The optic nerve is separated from the sclera. (F) Sizers and an introducer are used to determine the correct implant size. (G) The correct size implant is placed in position. The implant is put into place with a sphere introducer. (H) The implant in place.

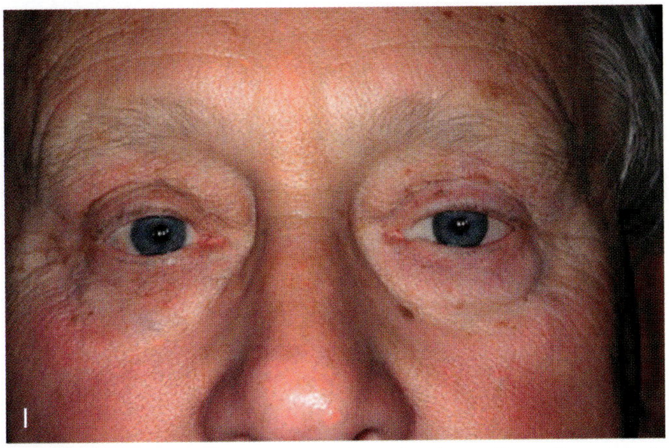

FIG. 25.18 cont'd (I) Three months after surgery with artificial eye. (From Tyers AG, Collin JRO. *Colour Atlas of Ophthalmic Plastic Surgery*. 4th ed. Elsevier; 2019.)

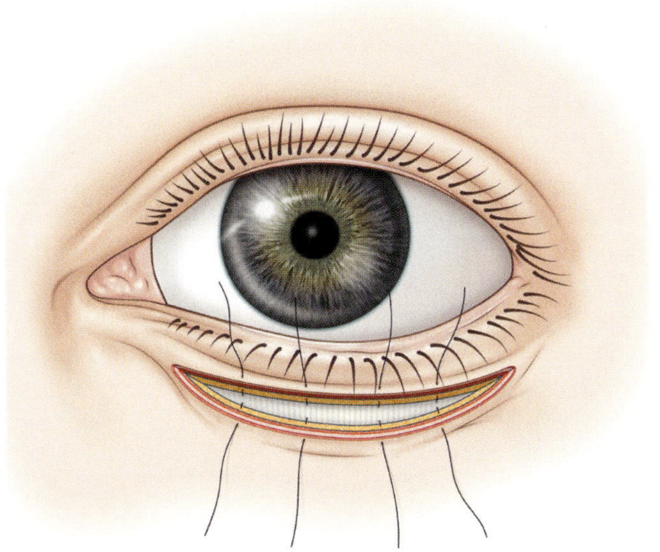

FIG. 25.19 Entropion. An incision is made in the lower lid to expose the retractor muscles. The deep tissue is plicated (folded into sutures) and the wound closed. (From Stein H, Stein R, Freeman M. *The Ophthalmic Assistant*. 9th ed. Philadelphia: Saunders; 2013.)

surgical marker just below the tarsal plate. A horizontal incision is made with a #15 Bard-Parker blade. A lower lid ret retractor is placed. The incision is deepened to until the retractor muscles are exposed. Straight iris scissors or ESU may be used to extend the incision. Small bleeders are controlled with the bipolar ESU or eye cautery unit. During the procedure, the surgical technologist irrigates the incision and blots away excess fluid as necessary.

2. ***The lid is sutured.***
   To perform the plication, the ST should prepare 5-0 or 6-0 Vicryl sutures. The surgeon places the plicating sutures. Tying forceps are used to secure the knots.

3. ***Redundant skin is removed.***
   To complete the repair, the surgeon removes excess skin and muscle tissue from the linear incision using iris scissors or ESU.

4. ***The wound is closed.***
   The wound is closed with size 5-0 or 6-0 nylon or polypropylene sutures. Antibiotic ointment may be applied to the suture line. The eye is dressed with a soft cotton shield and eye protector.

REPAIR OF ECTROPION LOWER LID

Ectropion is drooping of the lower eyelid. This creates an overflow of tears and exposes the conjunctiva, which becomes dry and irritated. The goal of surgical treatment is to restore the eyelid to its normal position. Many approaches to ectropion repair can be used. In the following procedure, a wedge of tissue is removed from the lower tarsal plate, and the excess tissue is excised to tighten the lid.

Pathology

An ectropion is an outwardly turned eyelid. The condition most often is associated with age, although it may also occur congenitally, as a result of scarring, or secondary to facial nerve paralysis (Bell's palsy). Aging may cause the orbicularis muscle to relax. If it is not repaired, the condition may lead to thickening of the mucosal surface on the inside of the eyelid (conjunctiva) and inflammation of the eye itself.

POSITION:	Supine
INCISION:	Lower eyelid
PREP AND DRAPING:	Eye
INSTRUMENTS:	Oculoplastic set
POSSIBLE EXTRAS:	Bipolar ESU

Technical Points and Discussion

1. ***A lateral incision is made below the eye.***
   The surgeon may mark the incision before or after the skin prep. A corneal shield may be placed in the eye.

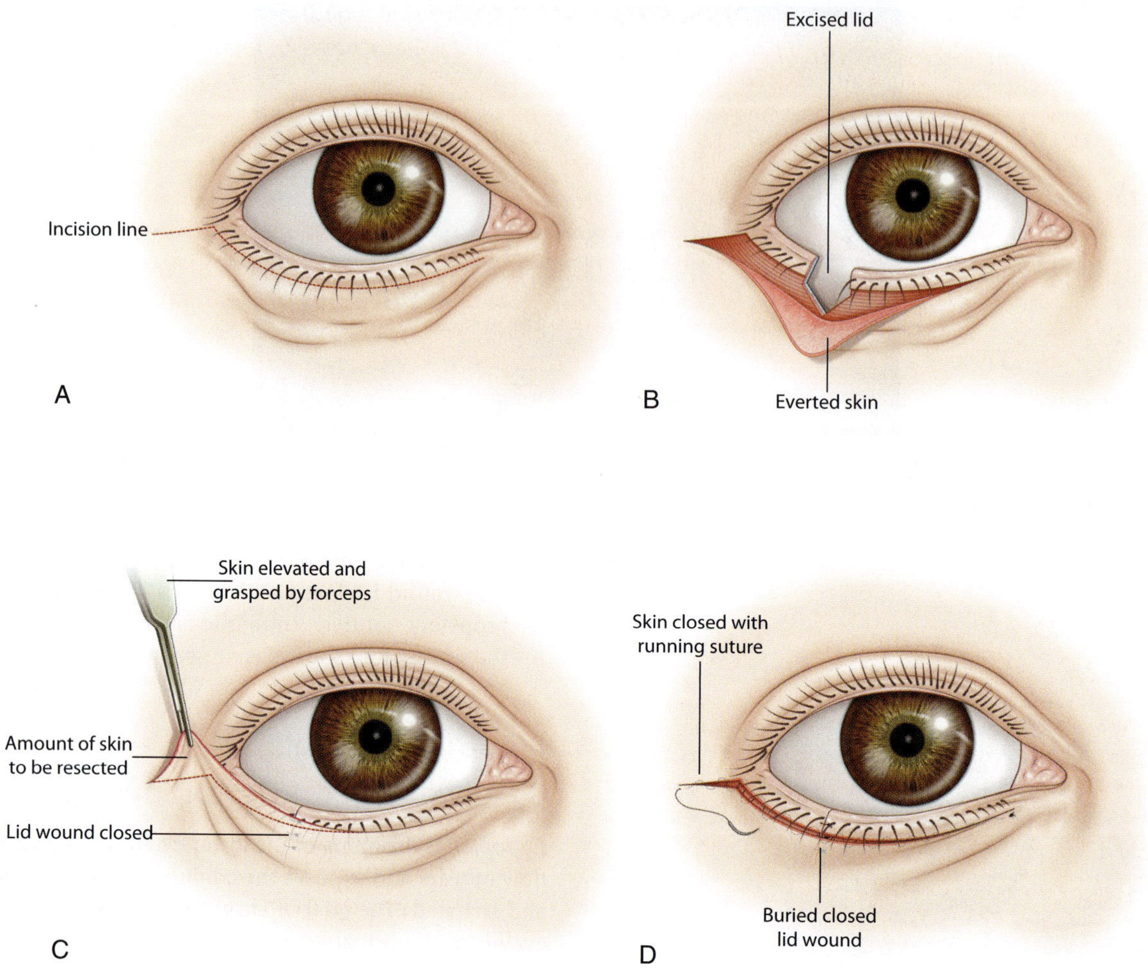

FIG. 25.20 Ectropion. (A) Incision line. (B) The skin is everted and a wedge section is removed from the lower tarsal plate. The wedge edges are approximated to tighten the lid. (C) Redundant skin is removed. (From Stein H, Stein R, Freeman M. *The Ophthalmic Assistant*. 9th ed. Philadelphia: Saunders; 2013.)

The incision is made below the lash line with fine-toothed forceps and a #15 knife blade or straight tenotomy scissors. The surgeon extends the incision using bipolar ESU for coagulation. The ST irrigates the cornea and blots any excess blood or irrigation fluid as necessary.

2. ***A skin flap is raised.***
   Using the ESU and iris scissors, a skin flap is created above and laterally.

3. ***A tissue wedge is excised in the tarsal plate.***
   A full thickness wedge is excised in the lid using straight iris scissors or #11 knife blade. The edges of the tarsal plate are then approximated with size 6-0 silk. The ends are left long.

4. ***The wound is closed.***
   Using size 6-0 Vicryl sutures, the tarsus is closed. Redundant skin is removed with the ESU or straight scissors. Skin is closed with size 6-0 nylon suture. Repair of an ectropion is illustrated in Fig. 25.20.

Related Procedure

Blepharoplasty: Refer to Chapter 28.

PERIORBITAL LACERATIONS

Laceration of the eyelids and margins may result in damage to deeper structures, requiring complex procedures. Specific areas of concern are the lacrimal gland, trochlea, the tear duct system, orbicularis muscles, and the angular artery. These structures lie relatively close to the surface of the skin and can be severely damaged by blunt and sharp injury. This discussion covers laceration of the eyelids.

Preoperative Assessment

Superficial injury to the external structures of the eye can cause a great deal of damage to inner structures because of their close proximity to the surface. Preoperative testing is very important as facial and eye injuries often cause extreme anxiety and fear, which can deter the patient from providing a thorough history. Therefore diagnostic tests are carried out before any closure is attempted. Preoperative diagnostic tests, including imaging of the entire eye, are often carried out to rule out severe injury to the posterior structures. These include intraocular foreign body (IOFB), retinal damage, blowout fracture, iris injury, lens injury, and blunt trauma glaucoma.

Computed tomography defines the soft tissues, infraorbital and intraocular air, foreign bodies, bony orbit, and sinuses. Ultrasound is used to detect retinal detachment, *hyphemia* (bleeding within the interior chamber), and foreign bodies in the anterior chamber. Magnetic resonance imaging (MRI) can detect vegetative material, wooden foreign bodies, and optic nerve laceration.

Patient Prep

Patient preparation for eye laceration surgery includes debridement of the wound, skin antisepsis, and anesthesia. Most superficial injuries can be managed with local infiltration of anesthetic with or without epinephrine. If the injury involves deeper structures such as the lacrimal system or bone, a general anesthetic is used. A routine skin prep is performed using dilute Betadine solution and irrigation of the eye with BSS.

Eyelid Lacerations

Most lacerations of the *upper eyelid* are horizontal. These can be repaired in one or two layers depending upon whether the laceration also includes the tarsal plate. Usually a single layer of size 6-0 nylon or size 7-0 Vicryl rapid suture is used to close vertical lacerations.

Laceration of the lower lid can include damage to the lacrimal structures, namely, the lacrimal canaliculus and nasolacrimal duct. The medial palpebral ligament may also be involved. Injury to these structures may require an endoscopic approach.

Injury to the levator muscle, which controls eyelid movement, is apparent when periorbital fat extrudes from the laceration. Repair of the muscle can be performed using size 5-0 or 6-0 Vicryl.

Intramarginal lid lacerations must be precisely approximated during repair to avoid eversion or inversion of the lower lid. This type of repair can be performed using fine Vicryl sutures.

KEY CONCEPTS

- Knowledge of key anatomical structures of the eye is necessary to understand a surgical procedure.
- Familiarity with diagnostic procedures of the eye contributes to an understanding of the pathology involved and appropriate patient care.
- Most surgical procedures of the eye are performed using the operating microscope, which requires distinct techniques for handling and passing microinstruments.
- Familiarity with common surgical procedures of the eye is necessary for safe handling of instruments and equipment, and for assisting in eye surgery.

REVIEW QUESTIONS

1. What is the rationale for documenting lens implants in the patient's medical record?
2. Why do children experience nausea after strabismus surgery?
3. What methods may the surgical technologist use to keep ophthalmic needles from becoming caught in instruments and drapes?
4. What procedure is used for verification of the correct site and side in ophthalmic surgery? Describe or list the steps of the procedure.
5. Explain the anatomical locations of the anterior and posterior chambers.
6. List the ophthalmic procedures discussed in this chapter that may be performed as emergencies. Explain briefly *why* each example may be an emergency.
7. One of the responsibilities of the surgical technologist during ophthalmic surgery is to frequently irrigate the operative site. Describe the typical appearance of dehydrated eye tissues (e.g., cornea, sclera, and conjunctiva). How should the tissues appear when irrigated frequently?
8. Define *trabeculectomy.*

BIBLIOGRAPHY

Albert D, Miller J. *Albert and Jakobiec's Principles and Practice of Ophthalmology*. 3rd ed. Philadelphia: Saunders; 2008.

Foster CS, Azar DT, Claes HD, eds. *Smolin and Thoft's the Cornea: Scientific Foundations and Clinical Practice*. 4th ed. Philadelphia: Lippincott Williams & Wilkins; 2005.

Riordan-Eva P, Whitcher J. *Vaughan and Asbury's General Ophthalmology*. 17th ed. New York: McGraw-Hill; 2008.

Ryan S. *Retina*. 5th ed. Philadelphia: Elsevier; 2013.

Spaeth G, Danesh-Mayer H, Goldberg I, Kampik A. *Ophthalmic Surgery Principles and Practice*. 4th ed. Philadelphia: Elsevier; 2012.

Stein H, Stein R, Freeman M. *The Ophthalmic Assistant*. 9th ed. Philadelphia: Saunders; 2013.

Tyers AG, Collin JRO. *Colour Atlas of Ophthalmic Plastic Surgery*. 2nd ed. Oxford: Butterworth-Heinemann; 2001.

Tyers AG, Collin JRO. *Colour Atlas of Ophthalmic Plastic Surgery*. 4th ed. Elsevier; 2018.

Yanoff M, Duker J, Augsburger J, et al. *Ophthalmology*. 2nd ed. St Louis: Mosby; 2004.

26 SURGERY OF THE EAR, NOSE, PHARYNX, AND LARYNX

KNOWLEDGE AND SKILLS REVIEW

The following skills and knowledge should be reviewed before you start this chapter:
Surgical pharmacology: Handling black box drugs; use of topical hemostats and hemostatic agents
Minimally invasive and endoscopic surgery: Instruments, equipment, supplies, care in handling

LEARNING OBJECTIVES

After studying this chapter, the reader will be able to:

1. Identify the key anatomical structures of the ear, nose, pharynx, and larynx
2. Discuss key aspects of case planning, including instrumentation, for ear, nose, pharynx, and larynx procedures
3. Describe common procedures of the ear, nose, pharynx, and larynx

TERMINOLOGY

Cerumen: A substance produced by the cerumen glands of the ear (i.e., earwax).
Cholesteatoma: A benign tumor of the middle ear caused by the shedding of keratin.
Effusion: Fluid in the middle ear.
Epistaxis: Bleeding arising from the nasal cavity.
Evert: To turn outward or inside out.
Hypertrophy: Enlargement of an organ or tissue.
Ossicles: The bones of the middle ear that conduct sound (i.e., the malleus, incus, and stapes).
Ototoxic: A substance that can injure the ear.
Packing: A method of applying a dressing to a body cavity. In nasal procedures, ¼- or ½-inch gauze strips are inserted into the nasal cavity to absorb drainage, control bleeding, or expose the mucosa to topical medication. "Packing" a wound may refer to any dressing that is introduced into an anatomical space or cavity.
Papilloma: A benign epithelial tumor characterized by a branching or lobular tumor (also called a papillary tumor).
Paranasal sinuses: Air cells surrounding or on the periphery of the nasal cavities. These are the maxillary, ethmoid, sphenoid, and frontal sinuses.
Paresis: Paralysis of a structure (e.g., vocal cord paresis).
Perforation: A defect in the tympanic membrane caused by trauma or infection.
Phonation: Vibration of the vocal cords during speaking or vocalization.
Polyp: Excessive proliferation of the mucosal epithelium.
Sensorineural hearing loss: Hearing impairment arising from the cochlea, auditory nerve, or central nervous system.
TM: The tympanic membrane.
Transcanal: Surgical access through the external auditory canal (EAC).
Transsphenoidal: Literally, "across or through the sphenoid bone." Surgery of the pituitary gland may be performed by approaching it through the sphenoid bone.
Tympanostomy tube: A tube that is placed in a myringotomy to produce aeration of the middle ear.

SECTION I: THE EAR

Otorhinolaryngology is the medical specialty concerned with the ear, nose, and throat. Surgery of the ear includes procedures of the outer, middle, and inner ear. Procedures are performed using the microscope.

Many patients undergoing ear surgery have a hearing deficit. The perioperative team should adjust their communication methods to accommodate the patient's needs. The patient may state which method is best for communication and which ear has the deficit, and whether written communication is needed.

Some patients with a hearing deficit develop a sense of isolation. The hearing world often is impatient when individuals are unable to communicate quickly and easily. Equality in patient care sometimes requires extra effort for patients with sensorial loss. One of the primary goals of the perioperative protocol is to provide comfort and healing whenever possible. This begins with compassionate patient communication.

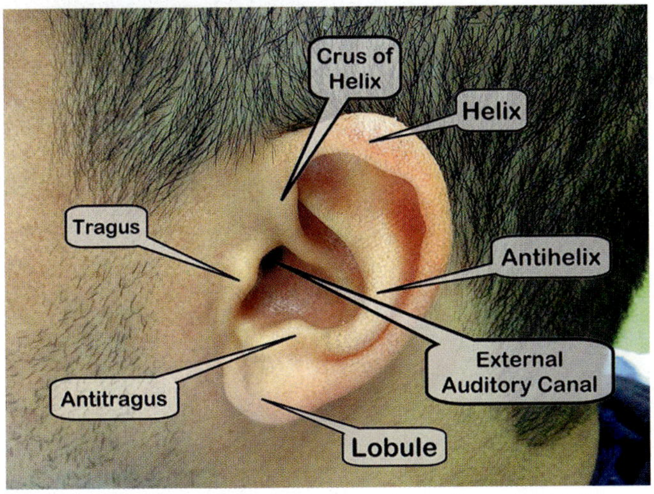

FIG. 26.1 Structures of the external ear. (From Critical ENT skills and procedures in the emergency department. *Emerg Medicine Clin North Am.* 2013;31:1.)

SURGICAL ANATOMY

The anatomy of the ear is divided into three regions: the *external ear,* the *middle ear,* and the *inner ear.*

EXTERNAL EAR

The structures of the external ear include the outer surface of the TM and all structures lateral to it (Fig. 26.1). This includes the *helix, antihelix, tragus, crus of the helix, antitragus, lobule,* and *external auditory canal.* The auricle is a cartilaginous structure covered by skin. Its function is to gather sound waves. The center of the auricle contains the external auditory meatus, which leads to the external auditory canal. The lateral third of the external auditory canal is surrounded with cartilage and is lined with glands that secrete a waxy substance called **cerumen.** The external auditory canal measures approximately 1 inch (2.5 cm) and terminates at the tympanic membrane (**TM**). The TM also serves as a barrier between the external and middle ear.

MIDDLE EAR

The middle ear extends from the TM to the medial wall of the middle ear cleft (Fig. 26.2). It includes the TM, the **ossicles** (i.e., the *malleus, stapes,* and *incus*), the opening to the eustachian tube, the opening of the mastoid cavity, and the intratympanic portion of the facial nerve.

The TM, which is elliptical and conical, aids in the process of hearing by transmitting sound waves to the ossicles, which are just posterior to it. The malleus (hammer bone), the most lateral of the ossicles, is partly embedded in the TM. The incus (anvil) connects the stapes to the malleus. The stapes (stirrup) transmits the vibrations of the TM and the other ossicles to the inner ear via the oval window.

The proximal *eustachian tube* is composed of connective tissue and lined with mucous membrane. It extends into the nasopharynx at its distal end and assists in equalizing pressure between the external environment and the middle ear. It also is a pathway for bacteria to spread from the nasopharynx to the inner ear, causing *otitis media* (middle ear infection).

INNER EAR

The inner ear contains receptors for hearing and balance and is composed of a series of hollow tunnels called *labyrinths.* The inner ear has two separate labyrinth systems. The *bony labyrinth* is formed by the temporal bone and is filled with *perilymph fluid.* Within the bony labyrinth is the *membranous labyrinth.* This structure has three parts: the cochlea, the semicircular canals, and the vestibule.

The spiral-shaped *cochlea* contains the cochlear duct and the organ of hearing, the *organ of Corti.* This organ extends along the length of the membranous labyrinth in the cochlea. It is lined with cilia, which project into the endolymph and receive the sound waves transmitted by the middle ear.

The *semicircular canals* communicate with the middle ear via the oval and round windows. These are located within the temporal bone and contain endolymph fluid. Each of the semicircular canals contains an enlarged space called the *ampulla.* The *crista ampullaris,* located within the ampulla, is responsible for equilibrium of the body in motion (called *dynamic equilibrium*). Fig. 26.3 illustrates the structures of the inner ear.

SOUND TRANSMISSION IN THE EAR

Hearing is the neural interpretation of sound transmission. Sound waves in the air enter the ear and are transmitted to the TM. The membrane vibrates against the malleus, which is attached on the posterior side. This causes vibration in the incus and in the stapes, which is connected to the oval window. From there, sound is transmitted into the perilymph of the cochlea, through the vestibular membrane, to the basilar membrane of the organ of Corti. Nerve transmission occurs from the basilar membrane to the cochlear nerve. This pathway is illustrated in Fig. 26.4.

DIAGNOSTIC PROCEDURES

CLINICAL EXAMINATION OF THE EAR

- The external auditory canal, auricle, mastoid, and surrounding tissues are examined for signs of infection, inflammation, neoplasm, scars, and lesions.
- An *otoscope* is used for the initial examination of the TM. If necessary, any cerumen is removed to allow complete visualization of the TM.
- If further examination of the TM is warranted, microscopic examination may be performed with a 250-mm lens and an ear speculum.
- Nasal and oropharyngeal examinations are performed with a tongue blade and a penlight (or the light from an otoscope) to detect any blockage of the eustachian tube by infection, inflammation, or tumor.
- More in-depth evaluations are performed using computed tomography (CT) or magnetic resonance imaging (MRI).

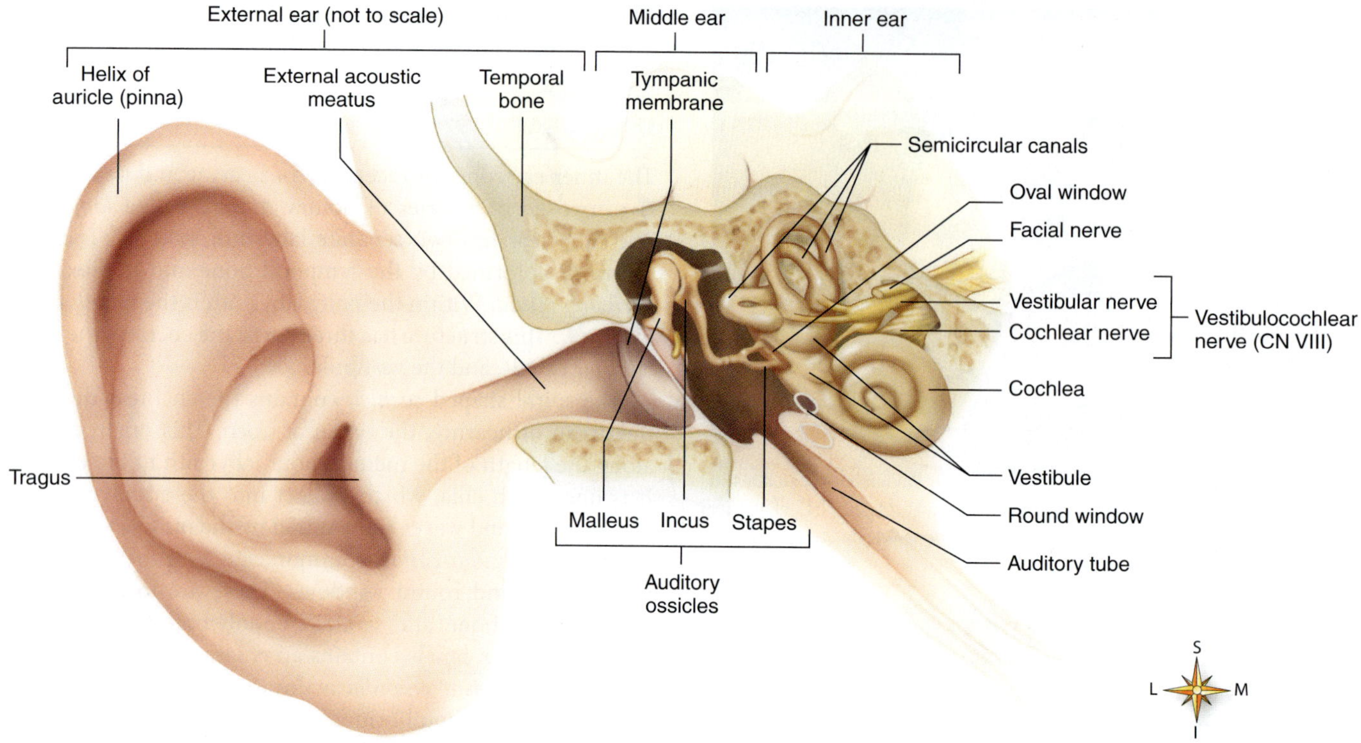

FIG. 26.2 Structures of the middle ear. (From Patton KT, Thibodeau GA, Douglas MM. *Essentials of Anatomy and Physiology—Text and Anatomy and Physiology Online Course*. St Louis: Elsevier-Mosby; 2012.)

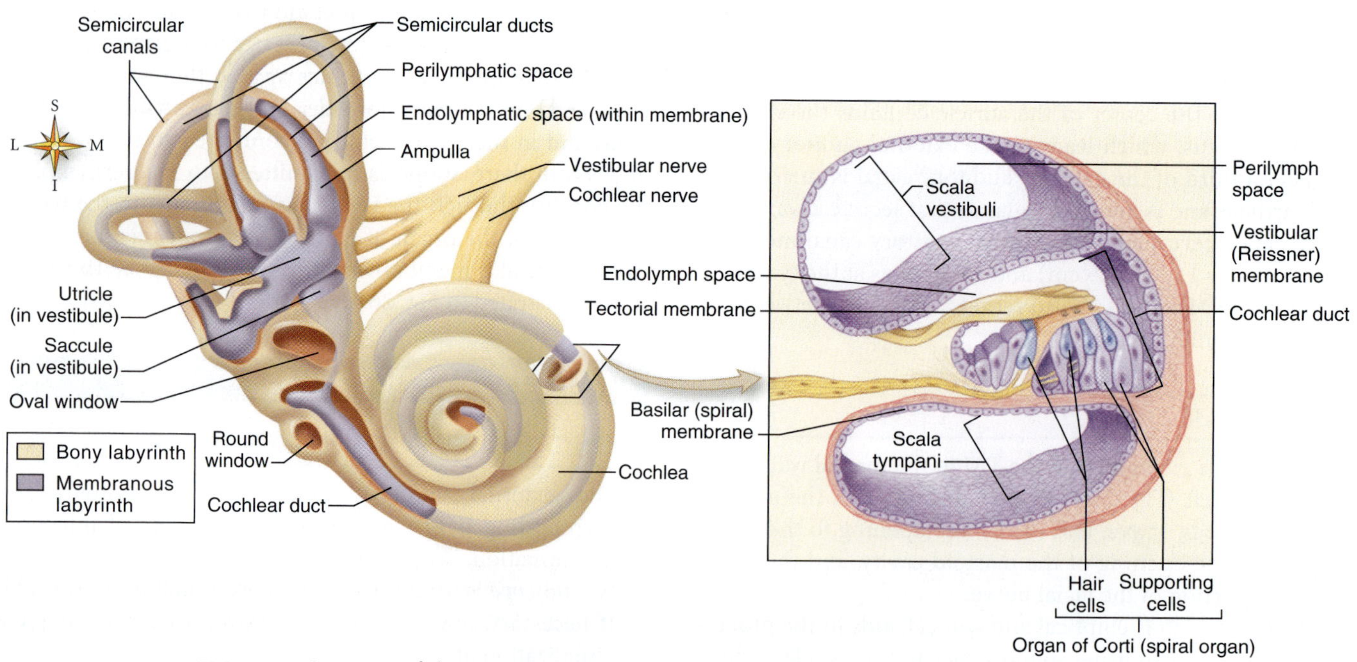

FIG. 26.3 Structures of the inner ear. (From Patton KT, Thibodeau GA, Douglas MM. *Essentials of Anatomy and Physiology—Text and Anatomy and Physiology Online Course*. St Louis: Elsevier; 2012.)

CASE PLANNING

As mentioned previously, many patients undergoing ear surgery have a hearing deficit. Sensitivity to the patient's needs is extremely important because the environment can be frightening, and communication can be difficult. A dry erase board, hand signals, and other methods of communication should be used if necessary.

The results of diagnostic tests should be made available in the operating room during surgery. These include imaging studies and sensory evaluations made in the preoperative period. Table 26.1 lists common diagnostic tests of the ear.

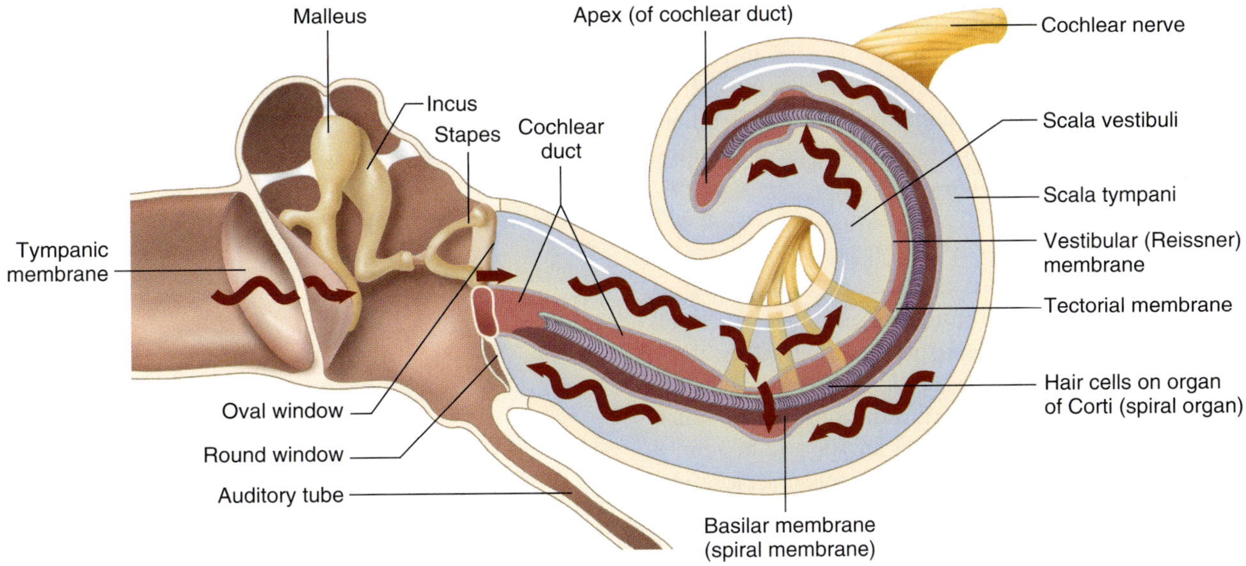

FIG. 26.4 Transmission of sound waves. (From Patton KT, Thibodeau GA, Douglas MM. *Essentials of Anatomy and Physiology—Text and Anatomy and Physiology Online Course.* St Louis: Elsevier; 2012.)

TABLE 26.1 Diagnostic Tests of the Ear

Test	Description
Tuning fork test (Rinne and Weber tests)	Test bone conduction and sensorineural hearing function of cochlea
Audiological testing (hearing test)	Usually conducted by an audiologist; can include air conduction, bone conduction, and speech recognition tests
Electronystagmography (ENG) testing	Tests for nystagmus
Head-positioning tests	Test for benign paroxysmal positional vertigo (BPPV)
Balance testing	Tests stance, gait, and balance for signs of vertigo
Caloric testing	Tests for vertigo and nystagmus; warm or cool water is instilled into the external ear canal to determine whether those conditions are elicited
Auditory brainstem response (ABR)	Usually conducted by an audiologist or neurologist; measures the response of the brainstem to electrical stimulus as it relates to the ear

POSITIONING

Surgical procedures of the ear generally are performed with the patient in the supine position with the head turned. The lateral position may also be used in some cases. Elevation of the head or the table or reverse Trendelenburg position may be used to minimize intraoperative bleeding. A doughnut or horseshoe neurosurgical headrest is used in open (but not in endoscopic) ear surgery to stabilize the head. Special positioning accommodations may be required for a patient with a previous neck injury or other skeletal problems that may cause discomfort during surgery.

PREPPING AND DRAPING

Prepping and draping for ear procedures focus on the ear and postauricular area. A secondary site is prepped for a skin graft. Selected procedures may require the clipping of a small amount of hair in the preauricular region.

Before prepping begins, the circulator verifies that the correct prepping solution is being used. Iodine-based prep solution may be used on the external ear but not on the internal structures. Sensitivity to iodine must be verified in all cases.

IMPORTANT TO KNOW *Chlorhexidine gluconate must never be used in or around the ear. It is* **ototoxic** *and may damage the ear if allowed to drain into the middle ear through the incision or a puncture in the TM.*

A sterile cotton ball is placed in the ear canal to prevent prep solution from entering the canal. The circulator then preps the surgical site, extending to the cheek medially, the occiput laterally, the temporal bone superiorly, and the upper neck inferiorly.

The ear is draped with four towels, which are covered with a fenestrated transparent or U-drape. The drape may be stapled in place. Next, a fenestrated ear drape is used to complete the sterile field.

IRRIGATION

Irrigation is used frequently during surgery to remove blood and tissue debris from the operative field. Because the site is extremely small, even small particles of tissue or blood can obscure the entire field. A suction irrigator provides a fine stream of saline or lactated Ringer solution and removes fluid from the field. The suction irrigator also is used to remove bone fragments and to irrigate the drill tip during bone drilling. The suction irrigator may be combined in one instrument or as separate instruments as illustrated below. a combination suction tip and a smaller irrigator.

INSTRUMENTS

The primary instruments used in ear surgery include a small number of plastic surgery instruments: hook retractors, mosquito forceps, #15 knife, and delicate skin forceps. Ear instruments are designed with a short fulcrum and long shanks, which are extremely delicate. The working tips are short (2 to 5 mm). These include grasping forceps, cup forceps, scissors, picks, elevators, and knives with cutting surfaces of different shapes. Several types of small spring retractors are also used. Various sizes of ear speculums are included in the set. These are designed to fit into the outer ear canal without external support. Ear instruments are maintained in a rack on the instrument table or Mayo stand. They must be arranged so that the tips are easily visible.

Microsurgery instruments are considerably smaller than regular ear instruments. A dedicated light source should be directed over the Mayo stand so that the instruments can be identified. Like all microinstruments, ear instruments must be handled gently and protected from damage. Instruments are illustrated in the Ear Instruments section of the Ear, Nasal, Laryngeal, and Pharyngeal Instruments table.

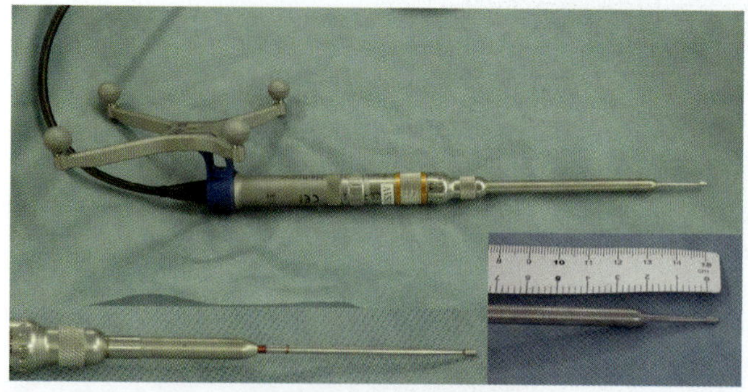

FIG. 26.5 High-speed drill. Midas stealth drill. This particular drill is fitted for navigation-guided drilling. (From Takeshi H, et al. Efficacy of atlantoaxial transarticular screw fixation using navigation-guided drill: technical note. *World Neurosurg.* 2020;134:378–382.)

EQUIPMENT AND SUPPLIES

Power Drill

A high-speed power drill is needed in all ear surgery that involves bone (Fig. 26.5). For example, a drill is used to open the mastoid bone, to enlarge the bony portion of the ear canal, and to drill through the small stapes footplate.

EAR, NASAL, LARYNGEAL, AND PHARYNGEAL INSTRUMENTS

EAR INSTRUMENTS

MYRINGOTOMY KNIFE 6½″	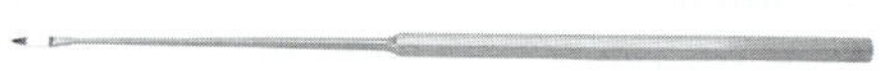 Photo courtesy Aesculap, Inc., Center Valley, PA.
SICKLE KNIFE 5{⅛}″	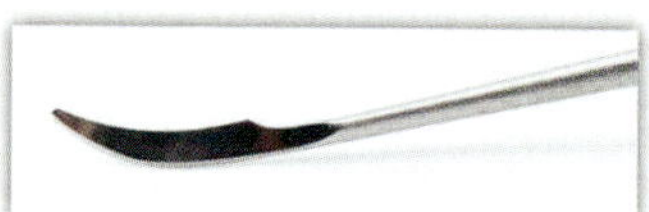 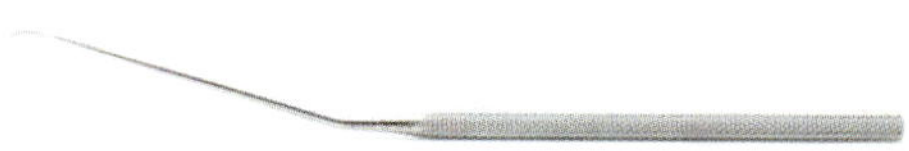 Photo courtesy Aesculap, Inc., Center Valley, PA.
FLAP KNIFE 6{⅝}″	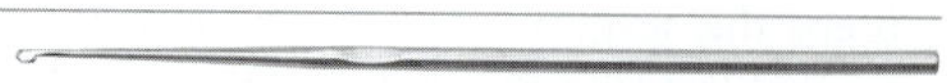 Photo courtesy Aesculap, Inc., Center Valley, PA.
ROSEN KNIFE/ ELEVATOR 6¼″	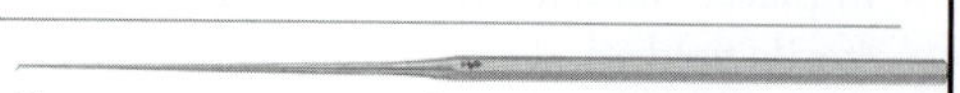 Photo courtesy Aesculap, Inc., Center Valley, PA.
HOUSE KNIFE 6½″	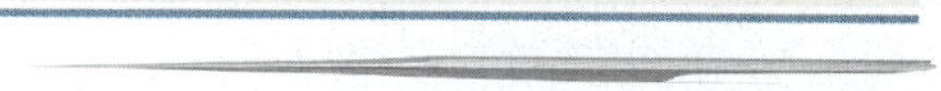 Photo courtesy Aesculap, Inc., Center Valley, PA.
MCCABE CANAL KNIFE 6¼″	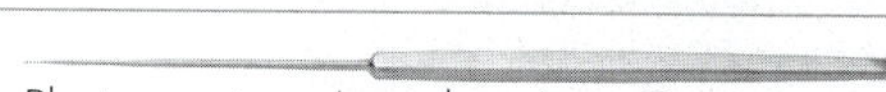 Photo courtesy Aesculap, Inc., Center Valley, PA.
FOOTPLATE KNIFE 6¼″	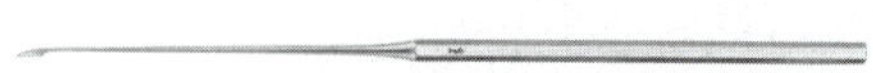 Photo courtesy Aesculap, Inc., Center Valley, PA.
BELLUCCI SCIS 5½″	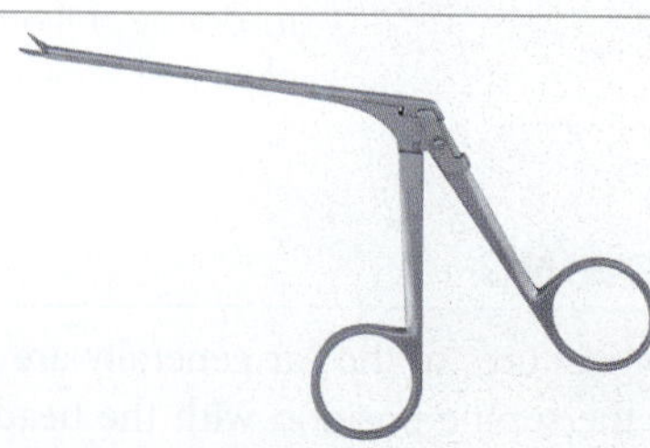 Photo courtesy Symmetry Surgical Inc.

EAR, NASAL, LARYNGEAL, AND PHARYNGEAL INSTRUMENTS—cont'd

ALLIGATOR SCIS 5½″

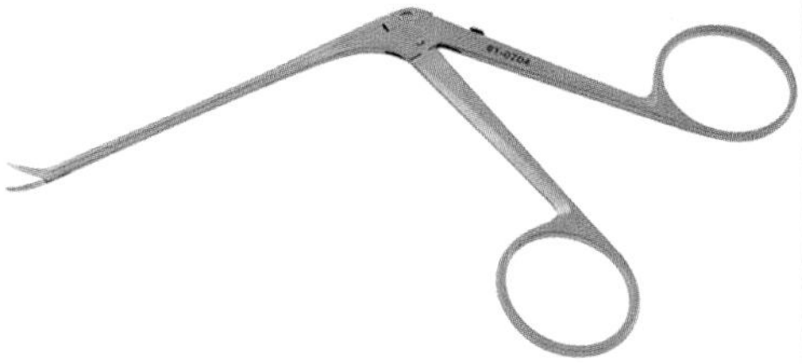

Photo courtesy Symmetry Surgical Inc.

ADSON FCPS BAYONET SERRATED 7″

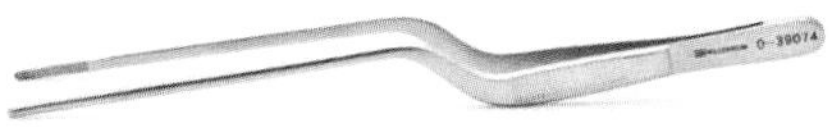

Photo courtesy Millennium Surgical Corp.

MICRO ALLIGATOR FRCP 5½″

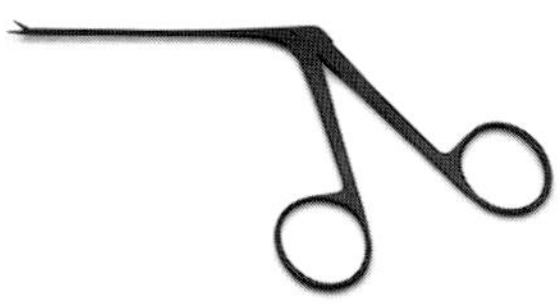

Photo courtesy Millennium Surgical Corp.

HOUSE "GIMMICK" ELEVATOR 6½″

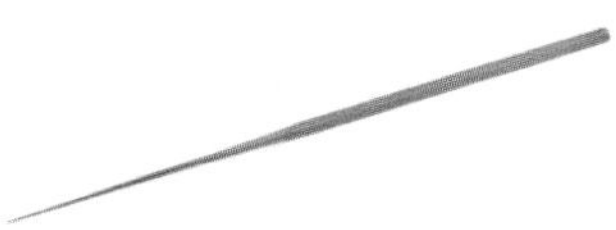

Photo courtesy Symmetry Surgical Inc.

DUCKBILL ELEVATOR 6½″

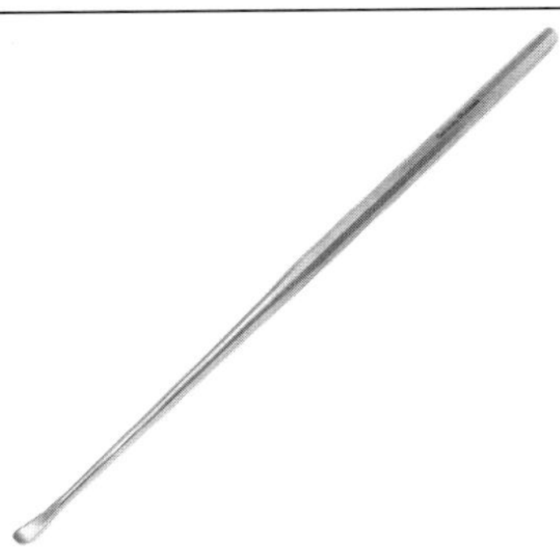

Photo courtesy Symmetry Surgical Inc.

WIET BAYONET SCIS 6½″

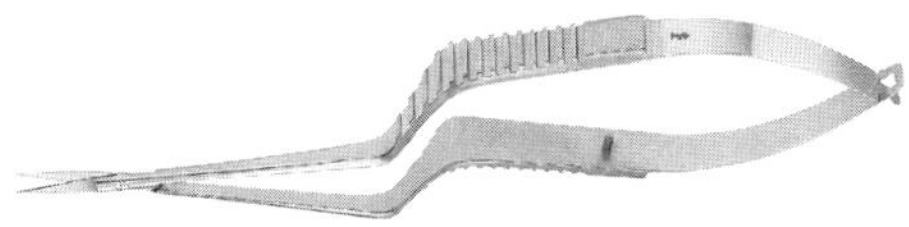

Photo courtesy Aesculap, Inc., Center Valley, PA.

ALLIGATOR FRCP 5½″

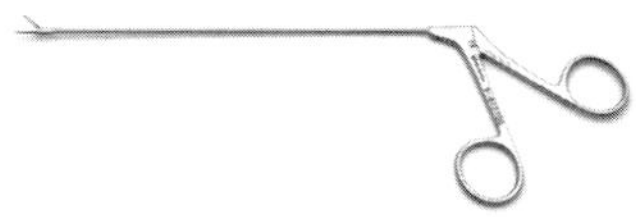

Photo courtesy Millennium Surgical Corp.

CUP FRCP DELICATE 6″

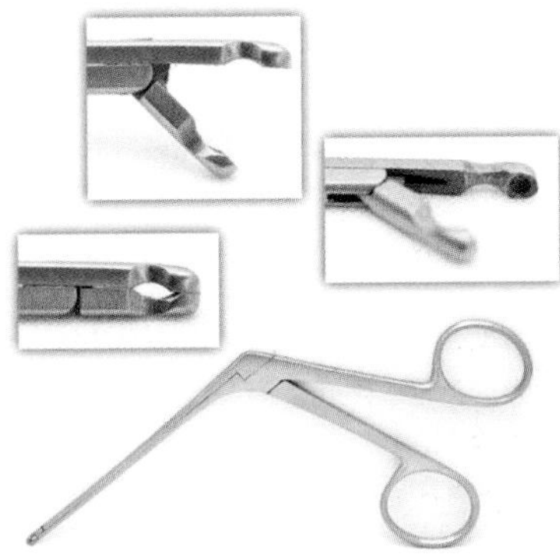

Photo courtesy Aesculap, Inc., Center Valley, PA.

HOUSE ALLIGATOR AND CRIMPER FRCP 5{⅛}″

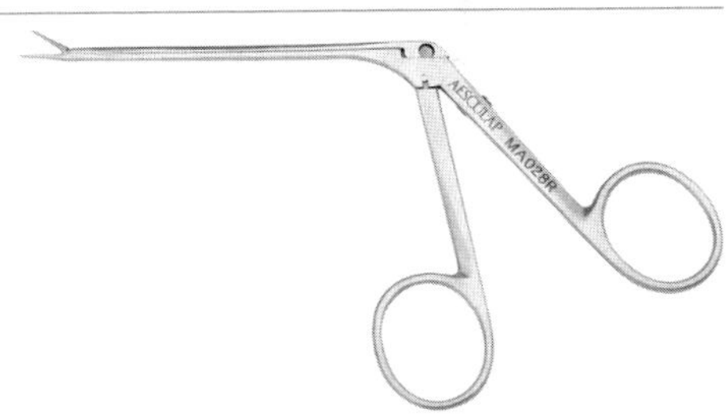

Photo courtesy Aesculap, Inc., Center Valley, PA.

ROSEN PICK 6½″

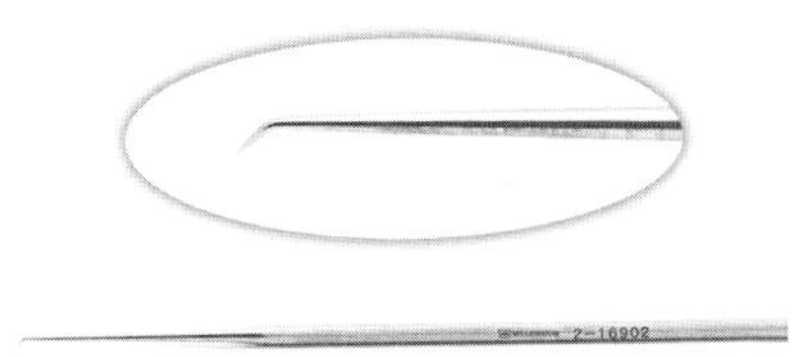

Photo courtesy Millennium Surgical Corp.

EAR, NASAL, LARYNGEAL, AND PHARYNGEAL INSTRUMENTS —cont'd

HOUSE-CRABTREE DISSECTOR PICK "JIMMY"

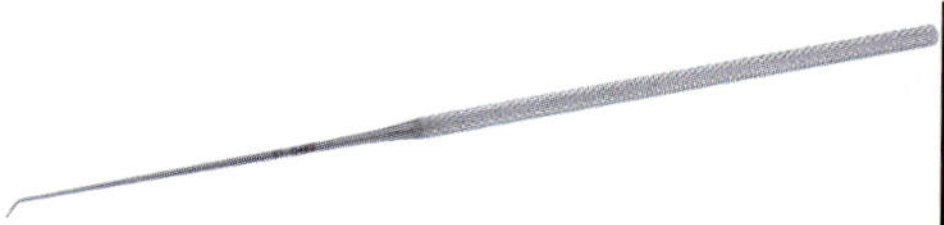

Photo courtesy Symmetry Surgical Inc.

HOUSE STRUT PICK 6½″

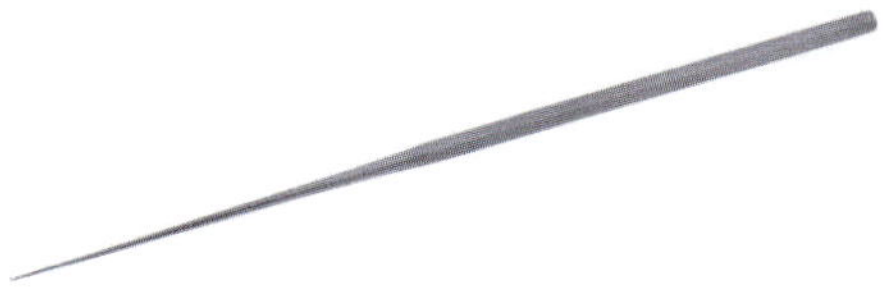

Photo courtesy Symmetry Surgical Inc.

HOUSE CURETTE DOUBLE END CURVED 6″

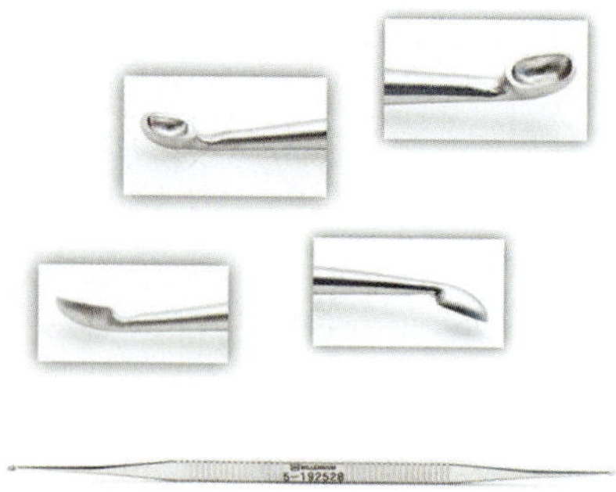

Photo courtesy Symmetry Surgical Inc.

BELLUCCI-WULLSTEIN RETRACTOR 5″

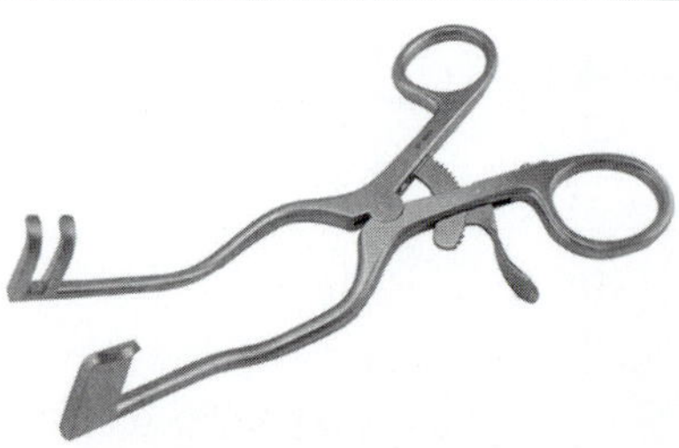

Photo courtesy Symmetry Surgical Inc.

STAPES PICK 90 ° 6″

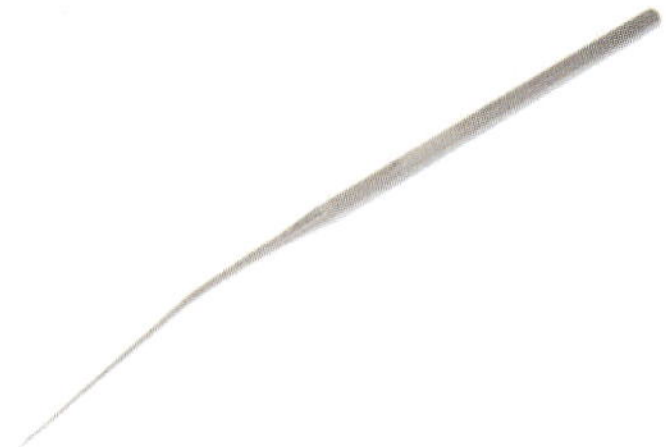

Photo courtesy Symmetry Surgical Inc.

HOUSE CURETTE ANGLED AND STRAIGHT 5½″

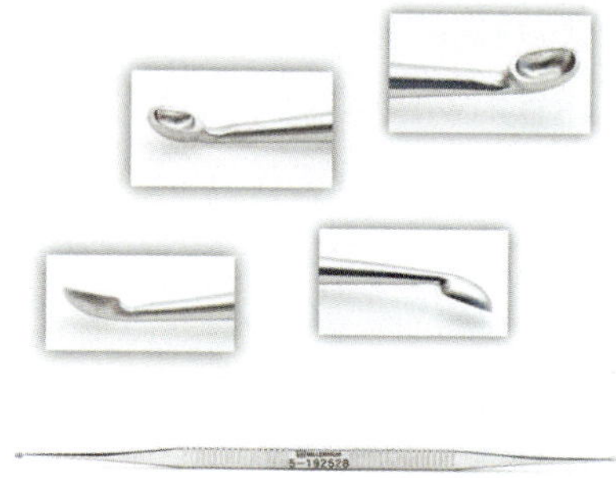

Photo courtesy Millennium Surgical Corp.

HOUSE-SHEEHY KNIFE CURETTE "SMALL WEAPON" 6½″

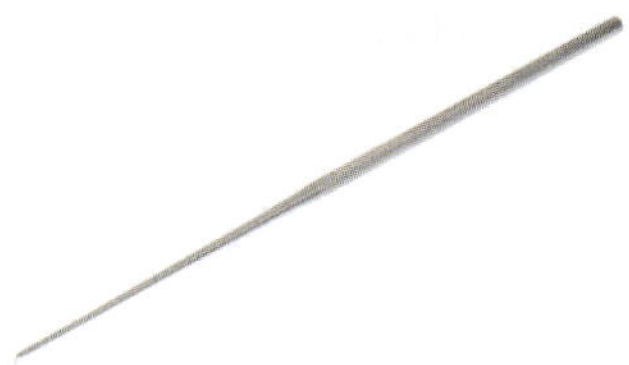

Photo courtesy Symmetry Surgical Inc.

FARRIOR EAR SPECULUM

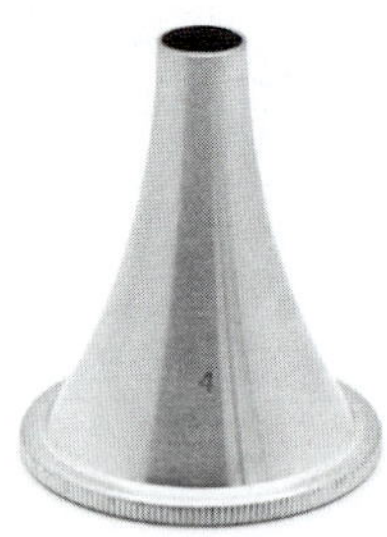

Photo courtesy Millennium Surgical Corp.

FACIA PRESS 7½″

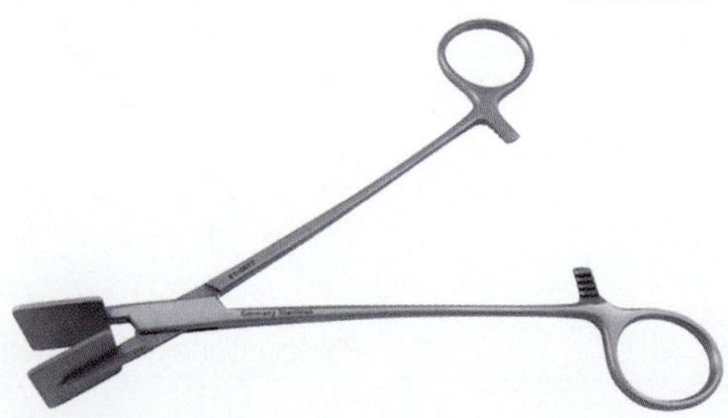

Photo courtesy Symmetry Surgical Inc.

EAR, NASAL, LARYNGEAL, AND PHARYNGEAL INSTRUMENTS—cont'd

BARON SUCTION TUBE 5½″

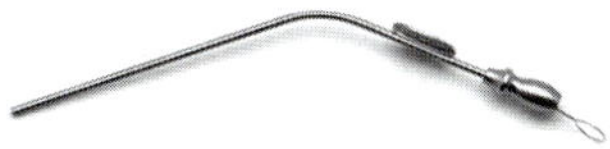

Photo courtesy Millennium Surgical Corp.

NASAL INSTRUMENTS

BALLENGER SWIVEL KNIFE 8″

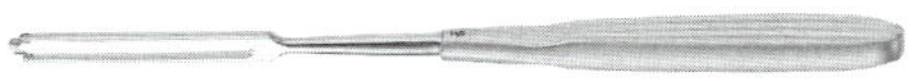

Photo courtesy Aesculap, Inc., Center Valley, PA.

FREER SEPTUM KNIFE 7″

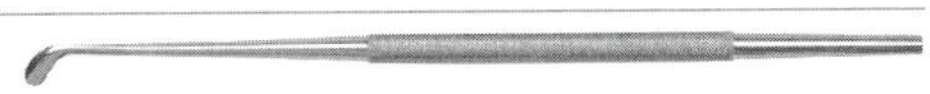

Photo courtesy Aesculap, Inc., Center Valley, PA.

FOMAN DORSAL SCISSORS 5¼″

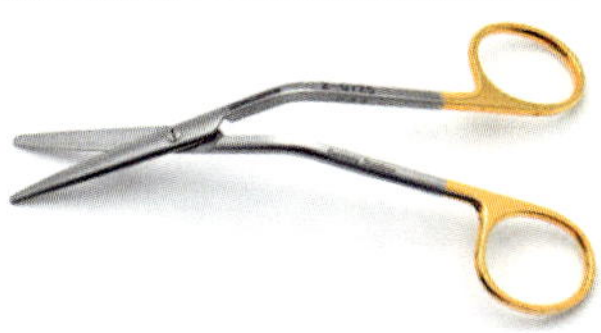

Photo courtesy Millennium Surgical Corp.

BLAKESLEY NASAL FRCP UPBITING 7″

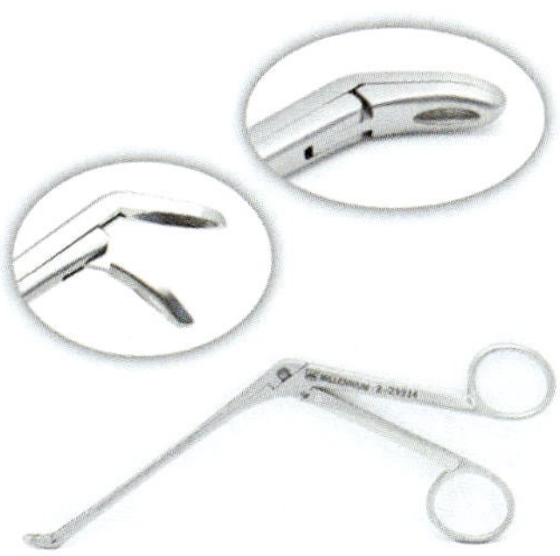

Photo courtesy Millennium Surgical Corp.

JANSEN BAYONET FRCP 6¼″

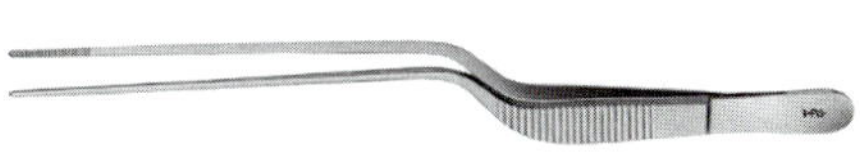

Photo courtesy Aesculap, Inc., Center Valley, PA.

COTTLE NASAL KNIFE 6″

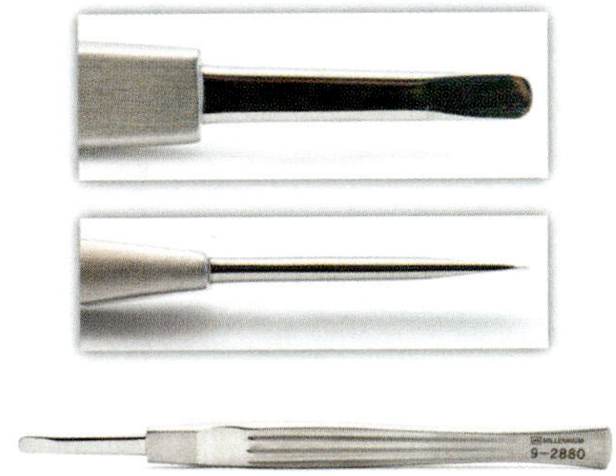

Photo courtesy Millennium Surgical Corp.

BUTTON KNIFE 7″

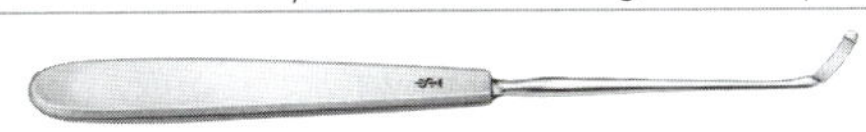

Photo courtesy Aesculap, Inc., Center Valley, PA.

JOSEPHSCISSORS 4½″

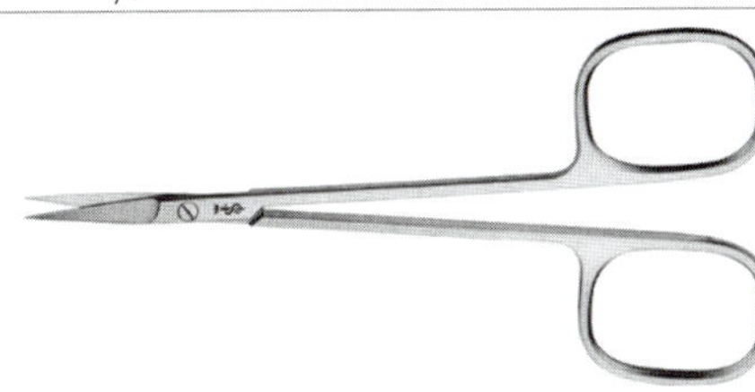

Photo courtesy Aesculap, Inc., Center Valley, PA.

ASCH SEPTUM STRAIGHTEN-ING FRCP 8{¾}″

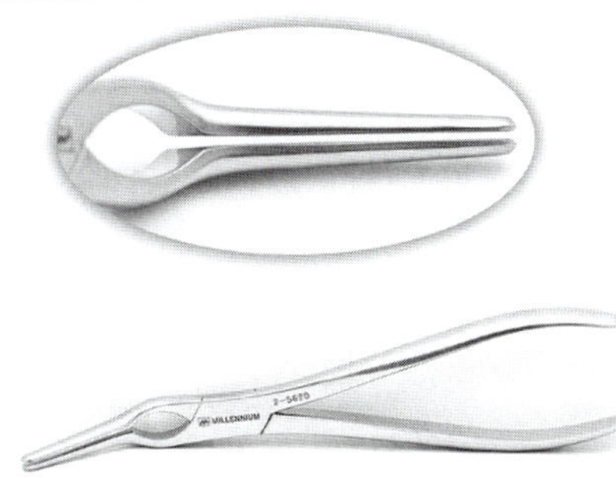

Photo courtesy Millennium Surgical Corp.

WILDE TISSUE FORCEPS

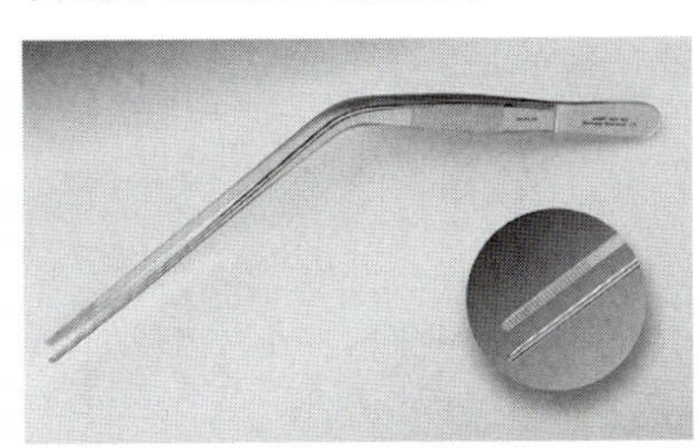

From Nemitz R. *Surgical Instrumentation: An Interactive Approach*, 3rd ed. Elsevier.

EAR, NASAL, LARYNGEAL, AND PHARYNGEAL INSTRUMENTS —cont'd

HARTMANN NASAL DRESSING FRCP 7″

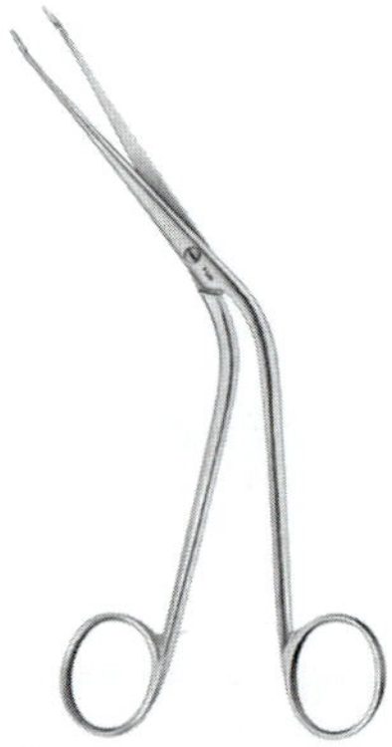

Photo courtesy Aesculap, Inc., Center Valley, PA.

TAKAHASHI RONGEUR 5½″

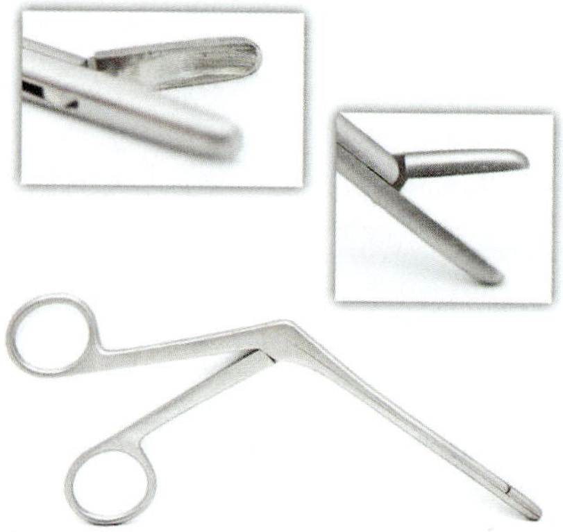

Photo courtesy Millennium Surgical Corp.

NASAL GOUGE

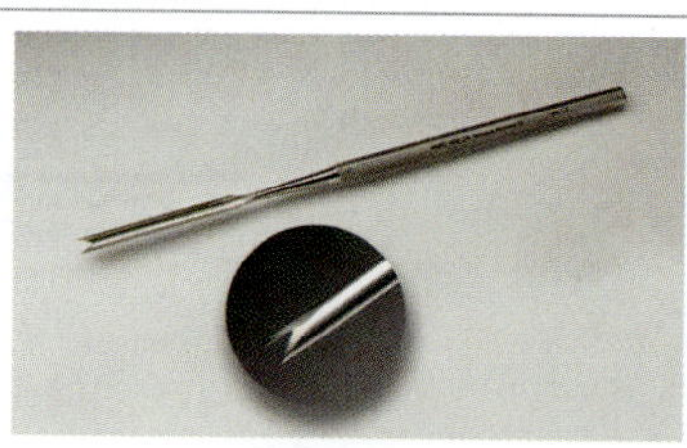

From Nemitz R. *Surgical Instrumentation: An Interactive Approach*, 3rd ed. Elsevier.

FOMAN RASP

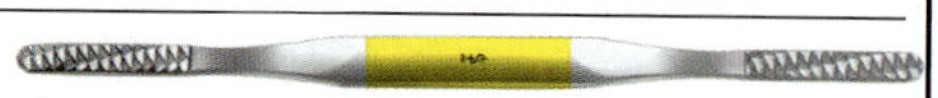

Photo courtesy Aesculap, Inc., Center Valley, PA.

JOSEPH NASAL SAW 6¾″

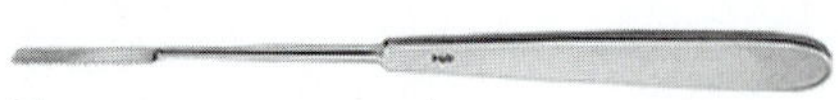

Photo courtesy Aesculap, Inc., Center Valley, PA.

TAKAHASHI FRCP (UPBITING OR DOWNBITING) 5¾″

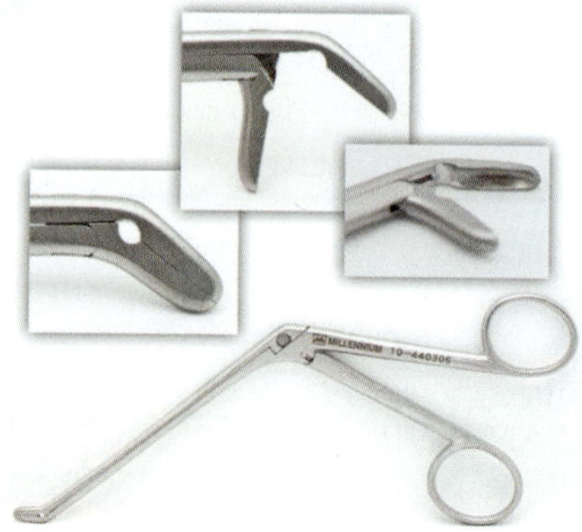

Photo courtesy Millennium Surgical Corp.

LEMPERT BONE RONGEUR 8″

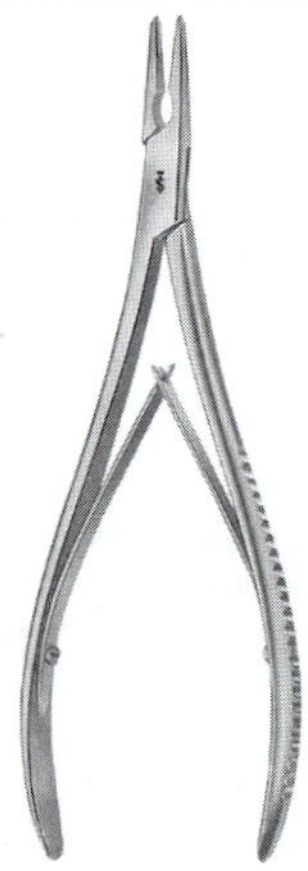

Photo courtesy Aesculap, Inc., Center Valley, PA.

COTTLE SEPTUM CHISEL 7″

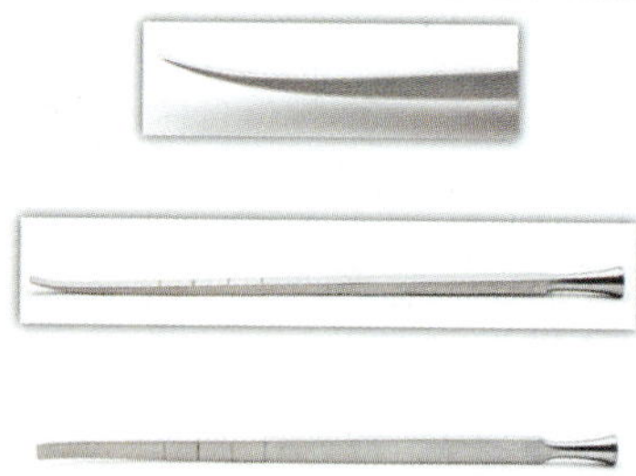

Photo courtesy Millennium Surgical Corp.

LEWIS RASP 7″

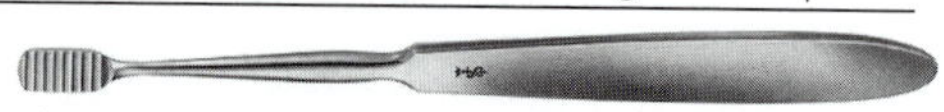

Photo courtesy Aesculap, Inc., Center Valley, PA.

JOSEPH PERIOSTEAL ELEVATOR CU. 6 {⅞}″

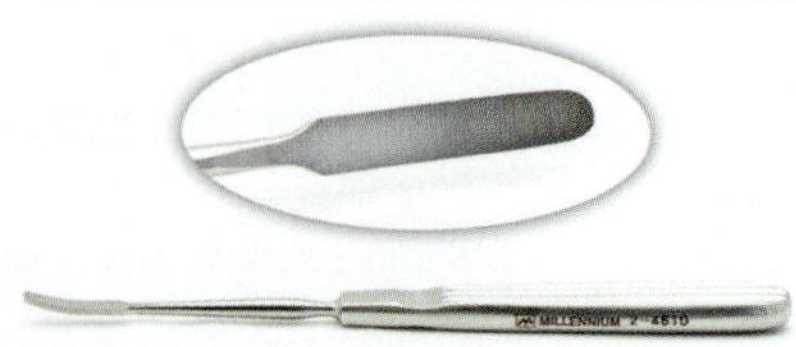

Photo courtesy Millennium Surgical Corp.

EAR, NASAL, LARYNGEAL, AND PHARYNGEAL INSTRUMENTS —cont'd

LEMPERT ELEVATOR 6¾″

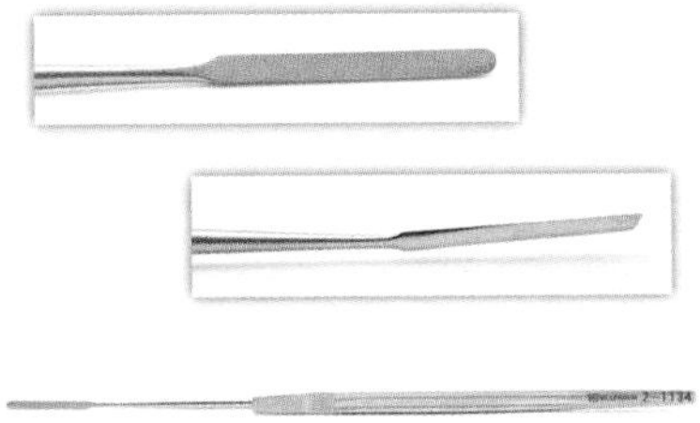

Photo courtesy Millennium Surgical Corp.

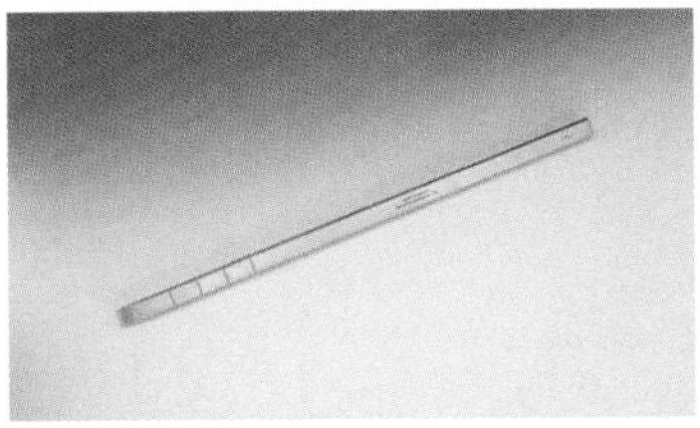

COTTLE CHISEL

From Nemitz R. *Surgical Instrumentation: An Interactive Approach*. 3rd ed. Elsevier.

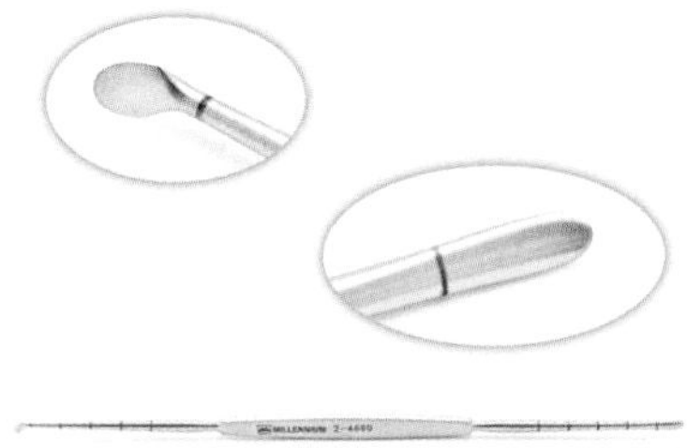

COTTLE SEPTUM ELEVATOR 6¼″

Photo courtesy Millennium Surgical Corp.

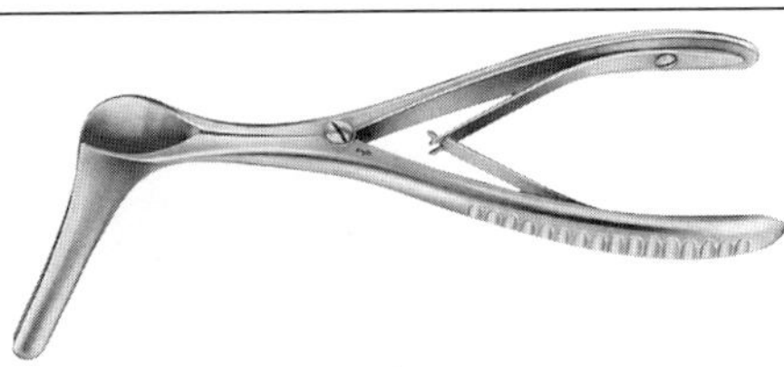

KIILLIAN NASAL SPECULUM 5½″

Photo courtesy Aesculap, Inc., Center Valley, PA.

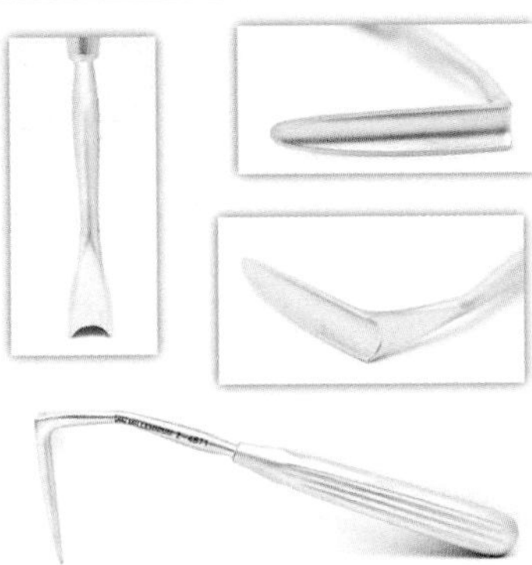

AUFRICHT RETRACTOR 7{⅛}″

Photo courtesy Millennium Surgical Corp.

COTTLE OSTEOTOME

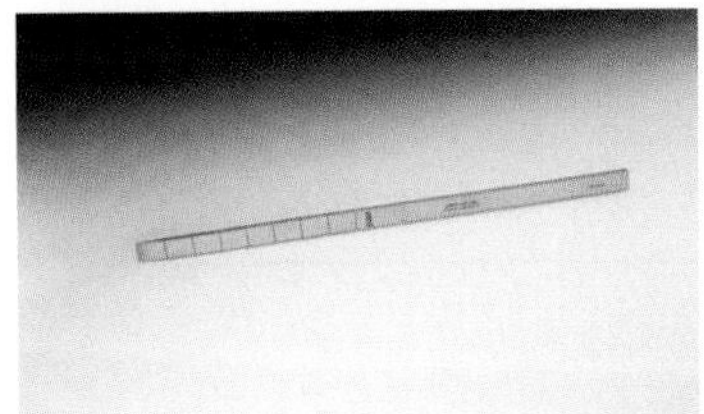

From Nemitz R. *Surgical Instrumentation: An Interactive Approach*. 3rd ed. Elsevier.

JANSEN MIDDLETON RONGEUR

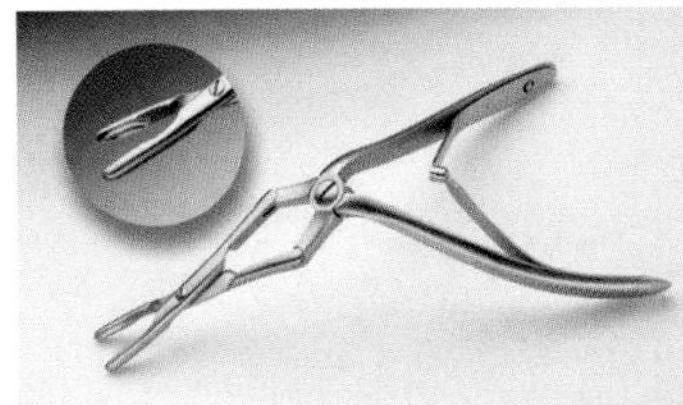

From Nemitz R. *Surgical Instrumentation: An Interactive Approach*. 3rd ed. Elsevier.

COTTLE COLUMELLA CLAMP 4½″

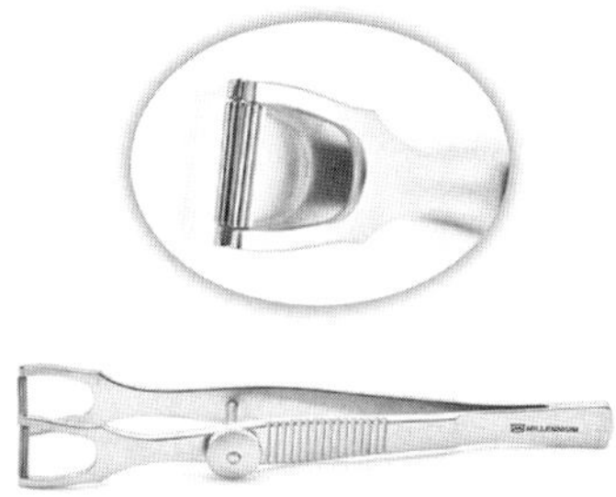

Photo courtesy Millennium Surgical Corp.

COTTLE ALAR RETRACTOR 6¼″

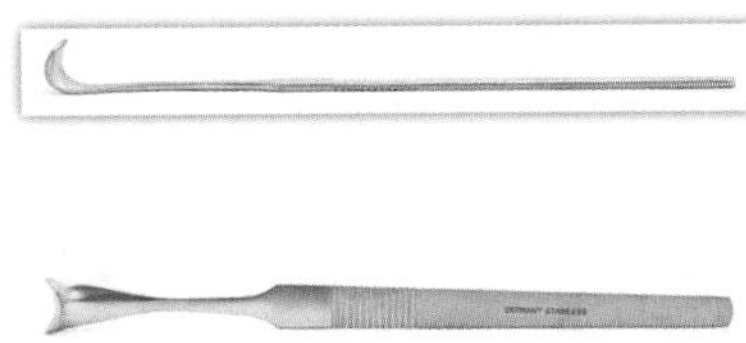

Photo courtesy Millennium Surgical Corp.

COTTLE-JOSEPH DOUBLE HOOK RET 5½″

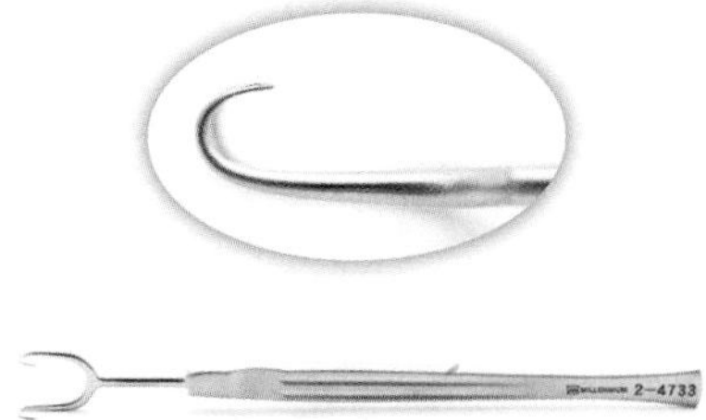

Photo courtesy Millennium Surgical Corp.

EAR, NASAL, LARYNGEAL, AND PHARYNGEAL INSTRUMENTS —cont'd

FOMAN RETRACTOR BLUNT 5¾″

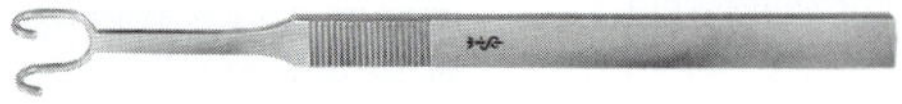

Photo courtesy Aesculap, Inc., Center Valley, PA.

FRAZIER SUCTION TUBE 5¼″

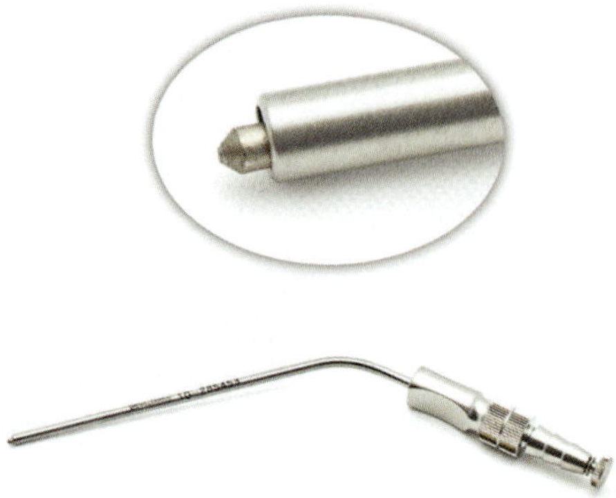

Photo courtesy Millennium Surgical Corp.

COTTON APPLICATOR 7″

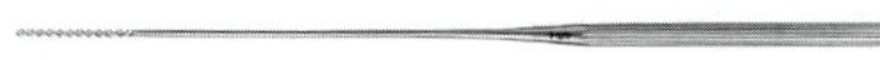

Photo courtesy Aesculap, Inc., Center Valley, PA.

BONE/CARTILAGE CRUSHER 5/8″ × 2¾″

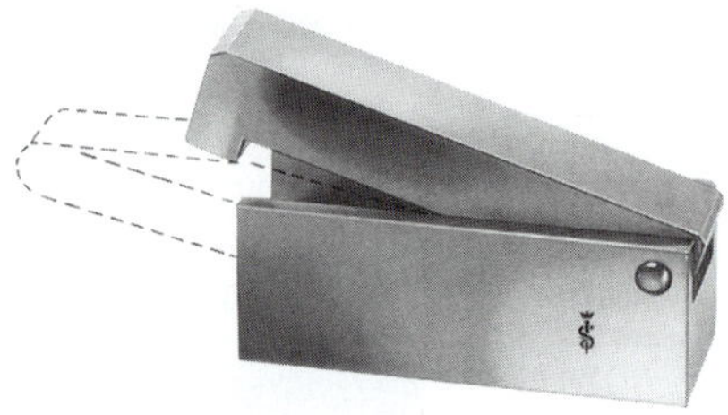

Photo courtesy Aesculap, Inc., Center Valley, PA.

MOUTH AND THROAT INSTRUMENTS

WHITE TONSIL FORCEPS 9½″

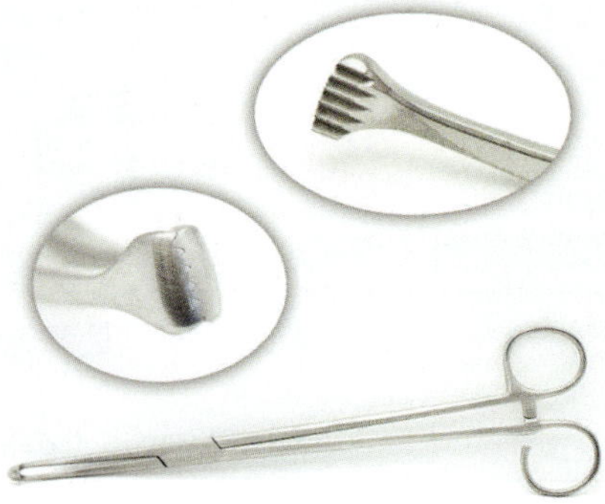

Photo courtesy Millennium Surgical Corp.

FISHER TONSIL KNIFE 8¼″

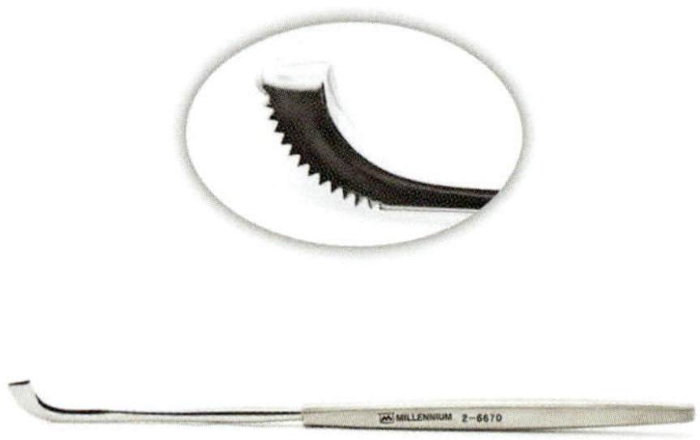

Photo courtesy Millennium Surgical Corp.

SCHNIDT HEMOSTATIC CLAMP 7″

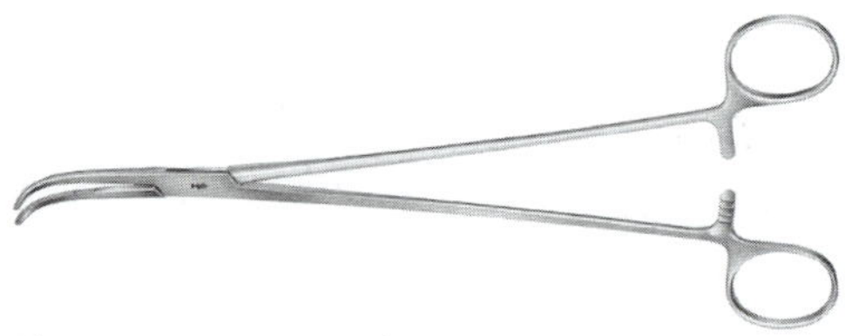

Photo courtesy Aesculap, Inc., Center Valley, PA.

SUCTION COAGULATOR

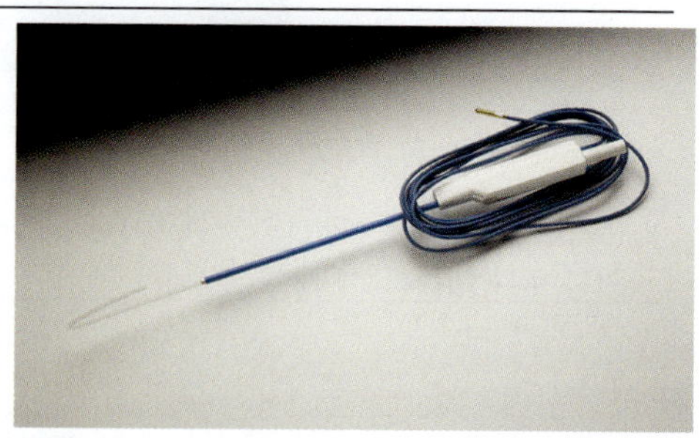

From Nemitz R. *Surgical Instrumentation: An Interactive Approach*. 3rd ed. Elsevier.

EAR, NASAL, LARYNGEAL, AND PHARYNGEAL INSTRUMENTS —cont'd

HURD DISSECTOR & PILLAR RETRACTOR

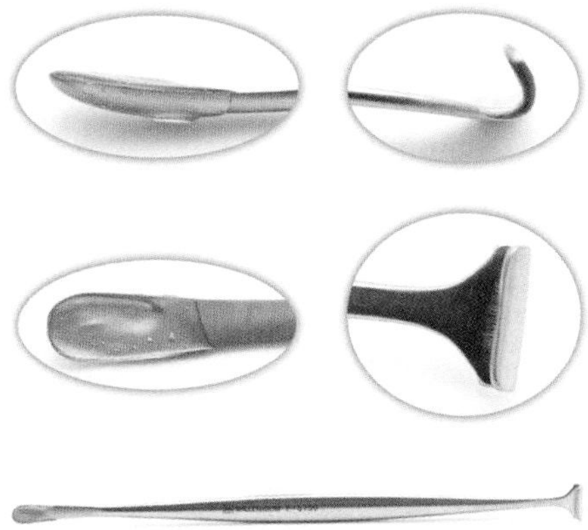

Photo courtesy Millennium Surgical Corp.

BALLENGER SPONGE FORCEPS 7″

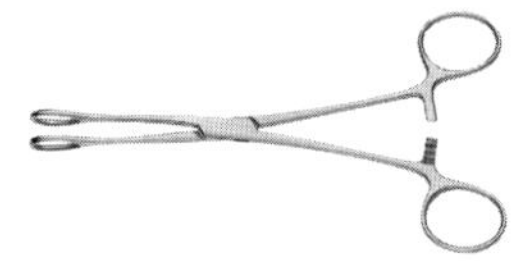

Courtesy of V. Mueller

TONSIL SNARE WITH WIRES

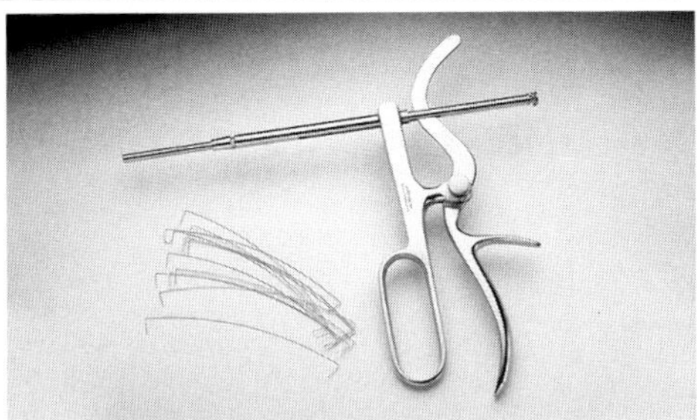

From Nemitz R. *Surgical Instrumentation: An Interactive Approach*. 3rd ed. Elsevier.

ADENOID CURETTES

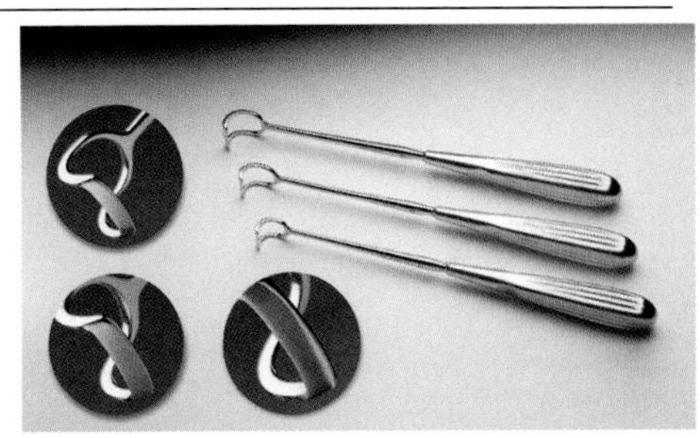

From Nemitz R. *Surgical Instrumentation: An Interactive Approach*. 3rd ed. Elsevier.

JACKSON CUP FRCP ANGLED

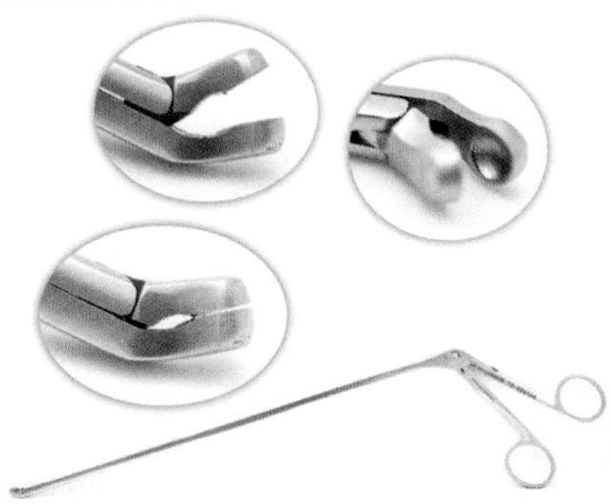

Photo courtesy Millennium Surgical Corp.

JACKSON ALLIGATOR FRCP 50 CM

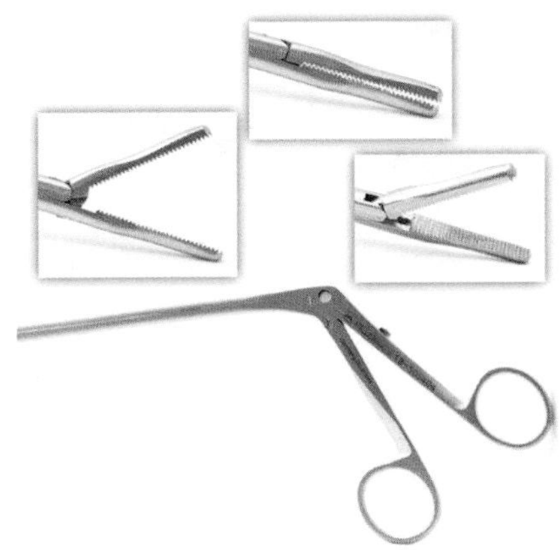

Photo courtesy Millennium Surgical Corp.

EAR, NASAL, LARYNGEAL, AND PHARYNGEAL INSTRUMENTS —cont'd

JACKSON CROSS ACTION FRCP 23 CM

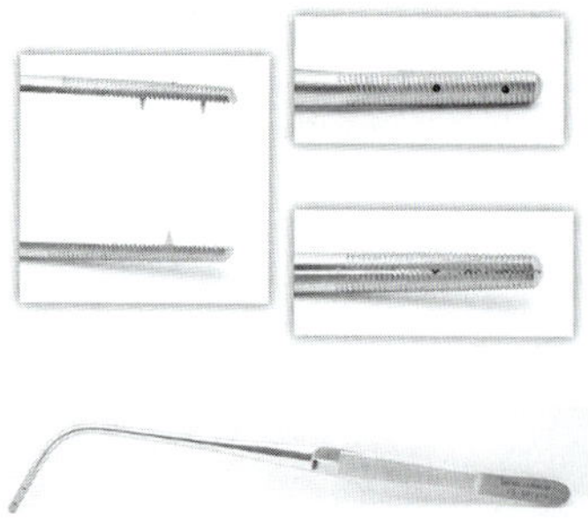

Photo courtesy Millennium Surgical Corp.

FEDER-OSSOFF MICROLARYN SCIS BLUNT

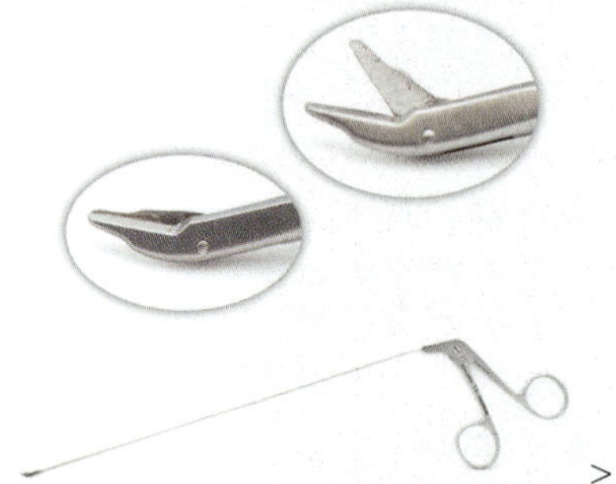

Photo courtesy Millennium Surgical Corp.

JAKO MICRO LARYNGOLOGY SCIS-STRAIGHT

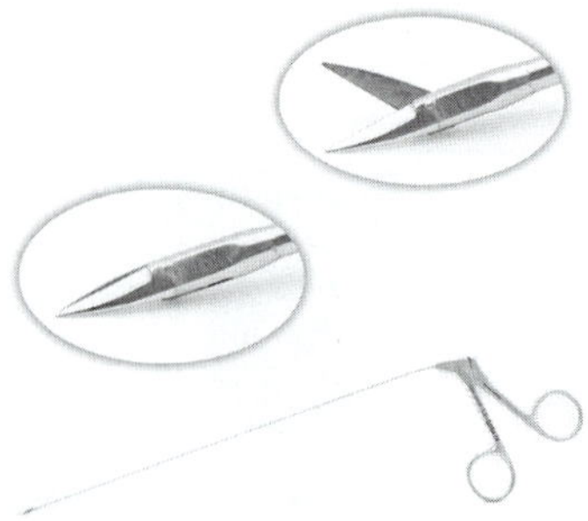

Photo courtesy Millennium Surgical Corp.

PHONO SCIS ANGLED AND STRAIGHT

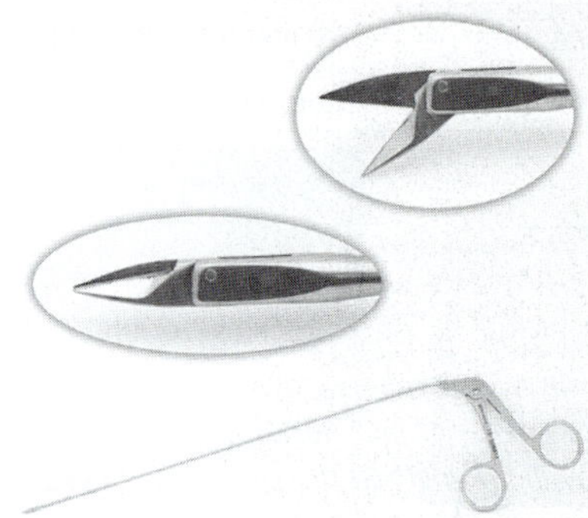

Photo courtesy Millennium Surgical Corp.

LARYNGEAL MIRROR

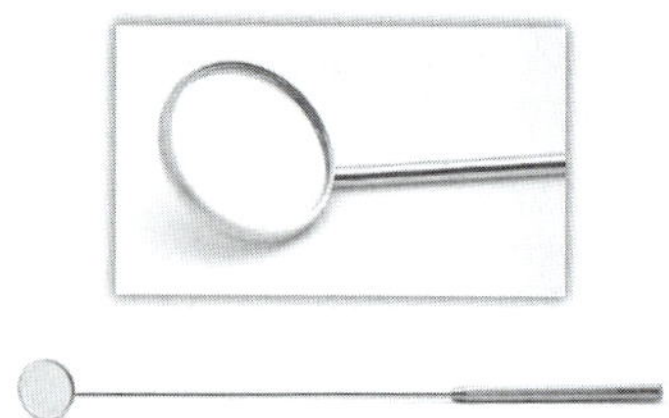

Photo courtesy Millennium Surgical Corp.

All drills are used with small cutting or diamond burrs, which vary in size from 0.5 to 7 mm. The scrub must irrigate the tip of the drill during operation to prevent tissue heating. A suction irrigator or a 3- to 5-mL syringe fitted with an 18-gauge angiography catheter is used for irrigation. If an angiography catheter is used, it is important that only the tip of the Angiocath be visible in the operating field so that the surgeon's vision is not obscured.

Operating Microscope

The operating microscope can be used in all procedures of the middle or inner ear. The standard operating lens for ear surgery has a focal length of 250 mm. However, some surgeons prefer a 200-, 300-, or 400-mm lens. For simple procedures, such as a myringotomy, a small operating microscope on a floor stand may be used. Complex procedures, such as a tympanoplasty or mastoidectomy, require a larger, more mobile operating microscope on a floor stand or ceiling mount. Coarse adjustments are made before surgery, and the microscope is draped within an hour of use. (Chapter 25 presents a complete discussion of the use and care of the operating microscope.)

Sponges

Cotton pledgets, such as those used during neurosurgery, are commonly used in ear procedures. These are pictured in Chapter 19. Square 4 × 4 Raytec sponges should also be available. Even though the operative site may be small, counts are routinely performed for all ear surgeries.

Hemostasis

Absolute hemostasis is necessary during ear surgery; even a small amount of bleeding can fill the operative field. Hemostasis is maintained using vasoconstricting drugs such as topical epinephrine 1:100,000 or injectable lidocaine with epinephrine 1:100,000. The surgical technologist should prepare small (2- to 4-mm) cotton balls soaked in topical solution. Up to 10 cotton balls are prepared and counted before surgery begins. Cotton felt pledgets and gelatin sponges should also be available on the sterile field.

IMPORTANT TO KNOW *Epinephrine must be labeled immediately upon receiving it on the back table. It must be placed in a dedicated area. Strict protocol is followed for verification of the amount and strength before and after it is received on the field and whenever it is passed for use by the surgeon.*

Absorbable gelatin sponge is used alone or in conjunction with vasoconstricting drugs. Oxidized cellulose and microfibrillar collagen may also be used. Refer to Chapter 12 for a complete discussion of hemostatic agents.

Dressings

Two types of dressings are commonly used in ear procedures, the *mastoid* and the *Glasscock*. The mastoid dressing is a bulky gauze dressing applied after complex procedures of the ear, especially those that require drilling of the mastoid. The dressing consists of several fluffed gauze sponges to cover the ear and incision, as well as rolled gauze (Kling or Kerlix), which is wrapped around the patient's head to hold the dressing in place (Fig. 26.6). The Glasscock dressing is prepackaged and includes multiple gauze sponges, which are held in place with a molded plastic shield secured with Velcro straps (Fig. 26.7).

ENDOSCOPIC EAR SURGERY

After the advance of endoscopic sinus surgery, which was introduced in the 1980s, the endoscopic approach to ear surgery was developed and is now commonly used. Endoscopy provides superior visualization of the surgical field and the ability to look around anatomical corners and crevices. As with other surgical specializations, endoscopic ear surgery (EES) often requires a surgical technologist specifically trained in the skills, equipment, instruments, and techniques required.

One of the main differences between EES and microsurgery using the operating microscope is that in EES the surgeon must operate with one hand while holding the endoscope in the other. An endoscope holder is not used because it may cause serious injury to the ear if moved abruptly. Table 26.2 compares the two approaches.

EQUIPMENT

The setup for endoscopic ear surgery includes the standard endoscopic equipment discussed in Chapter 20. These are the imaging system, video monitor, light source and cables, and camera control unit.

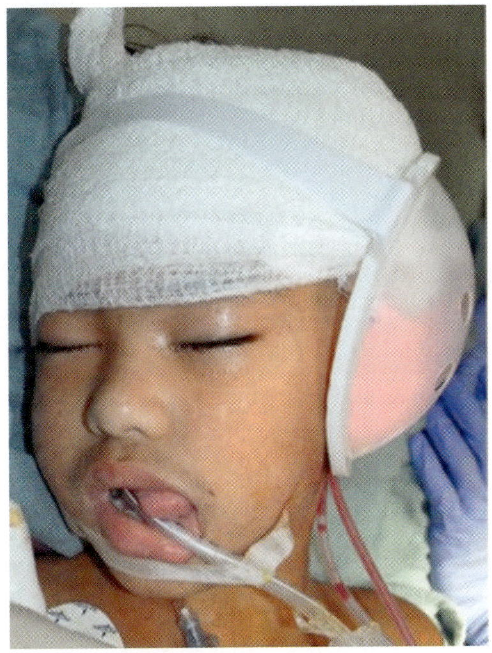

FIG. 26.7 Glasscock dressing. (From Owen S, et al. Alloplastic reconstruction of the microtic ear. *Oper Tech Otolaryngol Head Neck Surg*. 2017;28:2:97–104. doi:10.1016/j.otot.2017.03.007.)

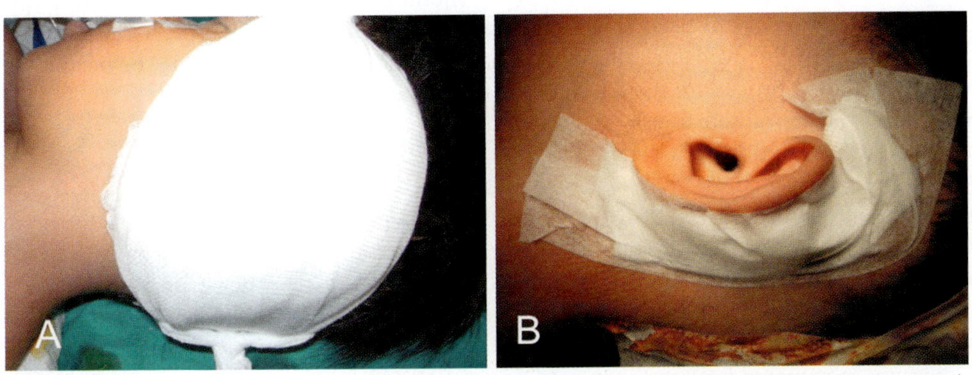

FIG. 26.6 Ear dressings. (A) Mastoid dressing. (B) Simple ear dressing. (From Sheng-Dean L, et al. Mastoid pressure dressing for cochlear implantation—is it necessary? *Internat J Pediatr Otorhinolaryngol*. 2009;73:6:857–860. doi:10.1016/j.ijporl.2009.03.001.)

TABLE 26.2 Basic Differences Between Endoscopic and Microscopic Ear Surgery

	Endoscope	Microscope
Number of hands for dissection	One-handed	Two-handed
Typical surgical approach	Transcanal, postauricular, via the antrum	Transcanal using speculum endaural or postauricular incision
Resolution	High	High
Binocular vision	No	Yes
Field of view	Wide	Narrow
Ability to look around corners	Yes (0–70 degrees)	No
Size of entry needed for visualization	Narrow	Wide

From Kozin ED, et al. Incorporating endoscopic ear surgery into your clinical practice. *Otolaryngol Clin North Am.* 2016; 49:5:1237–1251. https://doi.org/10.1016/j.otc.2016.05.005.

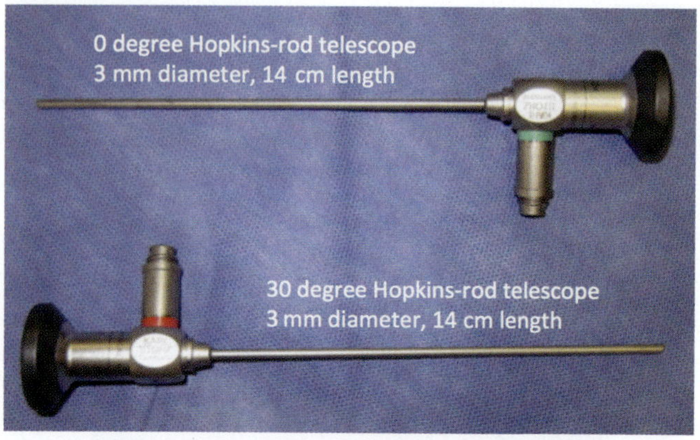

FIG. 26.8 Hopkins telescope used during endoscopic ear surgery. (From Miller KA, et al. 2 principles of endoscopic ear surgery. *Endoscopic Ear Surg.* 2019;52:5:825–845. doi:10.1055/b-0035-121089.)

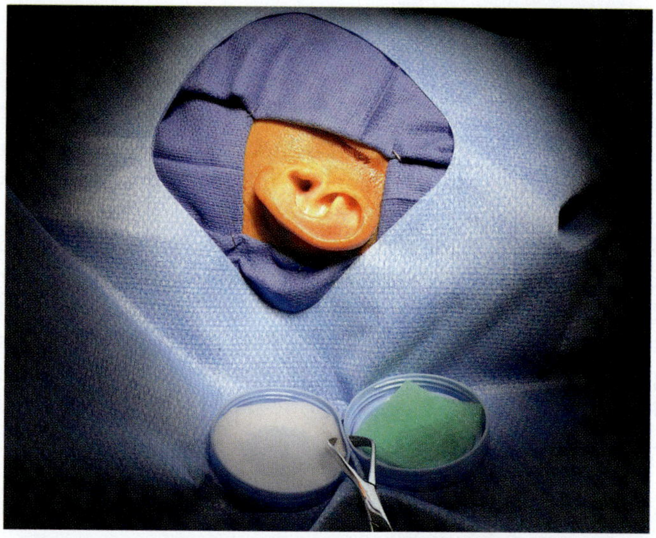

FIG. 26.9 Draped ear with lens cleaner attached. This is a method for maintaining lens cleaner on the sterile field during endoscopic ear surgery. (From Kozin ED, et al. Incorporating endoscopic ear surgery into your clinical practice. *Otolaryngol Clin North Am.* 2016;49:5:1237–1251. doi:10.1016/j.otc.2016.05.005.)

IMPORTANT TO KNOW *The light intensity of the endoscope must not exceed 50% to prevent thermal injury to the external auditory canal and middle ear structures. The light intensity setting must be verified during TIMEOUT before surgery begins (described in Chapter 18).*

The surgeon may use the flexible or rigid telescope. For most cases the 0-degree Hopkins rod lens 2.7-, 3.0-, or 4-mm diameter, 14-cm length telescope is used (Fig. 26.8). A 30-degree telescope should also be available, although it is used less frequently. During the procedure the ST should maintain a *micro wipe* (special material safe to use on lenses) soaked in saline to wipe the lens and keep it clean. This is shown in Fig. 26.9.

Suction is necessary in all procedures (endoscopic and microscopic). Size 5-Fr or 20-Fr otologic (Baron) suction tips are commonly used. These should be attached to flexible tubing as shown in Fig. 26.10. A suction dissector can be used to simultaneously dissect tissue and suction any fluids (Fig. 26.11).

The operating microscope is prepared for standby in case it is needed during the procedure. Complex procedures require ample sterile surfaces to accommodate instruments and supplies.

ROOM SETUP

The surgical technologist should be positioned to provide assistance without blocking the surgeon's view of the video monitor. Fig. 26.12 illustrates several setups for endoscopic ear surgery. The ST must be able to see the video monitor to follow the procedure and anticipate the need for specific instruments and supplies.

ENDOSCOPIC TYMPANOTOMY

Tympanotomy is surgical access to the middle ear through the tympanic membrane. Simple EES is described here as an introduction to other **transcanal** endoscopic procedures, with which the student or newly certified surgical technologist may be required to assist. No pathology is described in this procedure because it is used for any procedure in which endoscopic access through tympanic membrane is required.

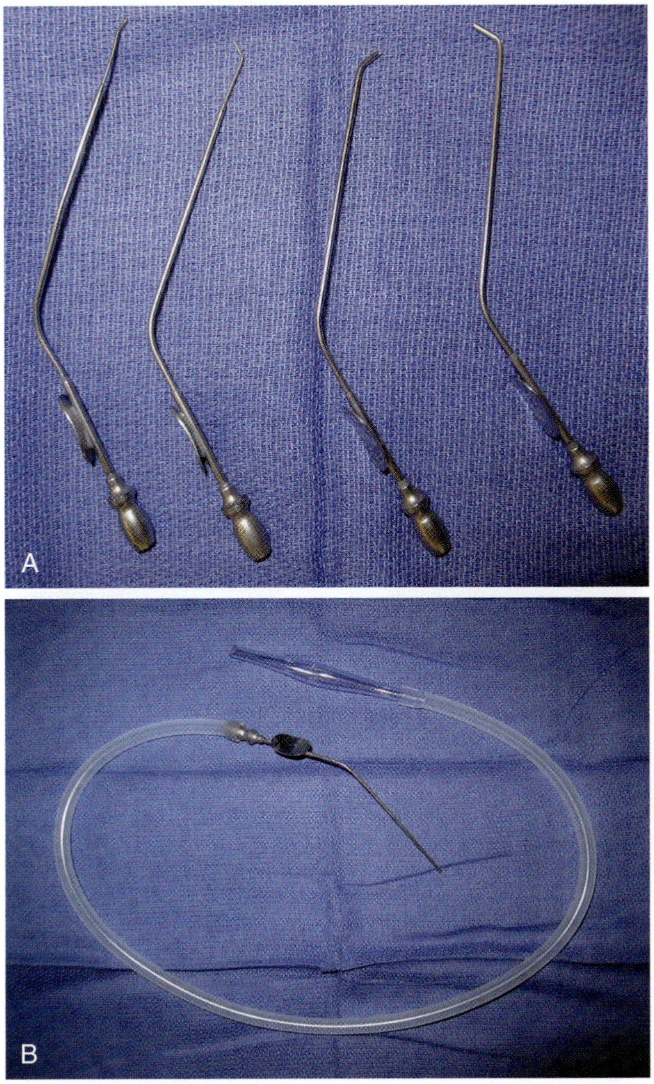

FIG. 26.10 Suction. (A) Suction tubes. (B) Suction attached to flexible tubing. (From Kozin ED, et al. Incorporating endoscopic ear surgery into your clinical practice. *Otolaryngol Clin North Am.* 2016;49:5:1237–1251. doi:10.1016/j.otc.2016.05.005.)

POSITION:	Supine (reverse Trendelenburg with affected ear up may be used to control bleeding)
INCISION:	Tympanic membrane
PREP AND DRAPING:	External and internal ear prep followed by trimming of the external auditory canal hairs. Cerumen is then removed from the EAC using gentle irrigation
INSTRUMENTS:	Otoendoscope; basic microsurgical ear set; specialty ear sets according to the procedure

Technical Points and Discussion

1. ***The patient is prepped and draped.***
The patient is placed in supine position (no headrest) with the head turned to expose the operative ear. The external ear is prepped with 10% povidone-iodine solution. The external auditory canal is flushed with sterile saline until it runs clear. This is followed by close trimming of the hairs in the EAC using curved iris scissors. Using the endoscope for visualization, cerumen is removed from the EAC using sterile saline irrigation, suction, and microcup forceps. The ST should place a Raytec sponge on the field for wiping the tips of the instrument. When the cleansing procedure is complete, the sponge should be removed from the field.

NOTE *Do not use a 4 × 4 Raytec sponge on the endoscope lens because it may cause scratches.*

2. ***The tympanic membrane is incised.***
The patient is placed in reverse Trendelenburg position to aid in hemostasis. Before making the incision, the surgeon injects a small amount of epinephrine in the skin of the EAC. The epinephrine-soaked cotton balls may

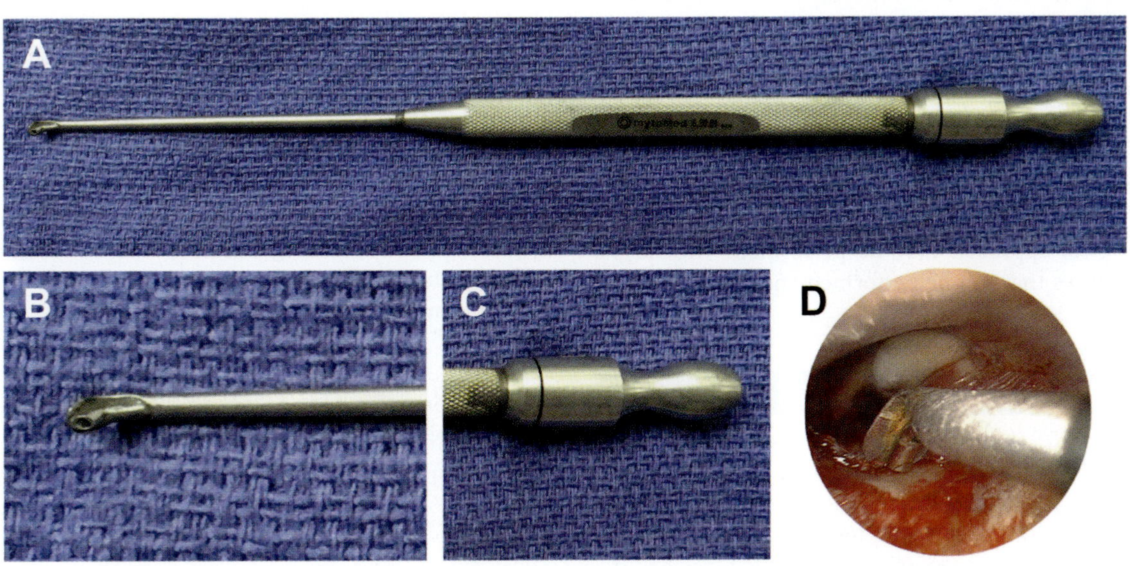

FIG. 26.11 Suction dissector. This instrument combines a Frazier suction tip with a tissue dissector. (From Kozin ED, et al. Incorporating endoscopic ear surgery into your clinical practice. *Otolaryngol Clin North Am.* 2016;49:5:1237–1251. doi:10.1016/j.otc.2016.05.005.)

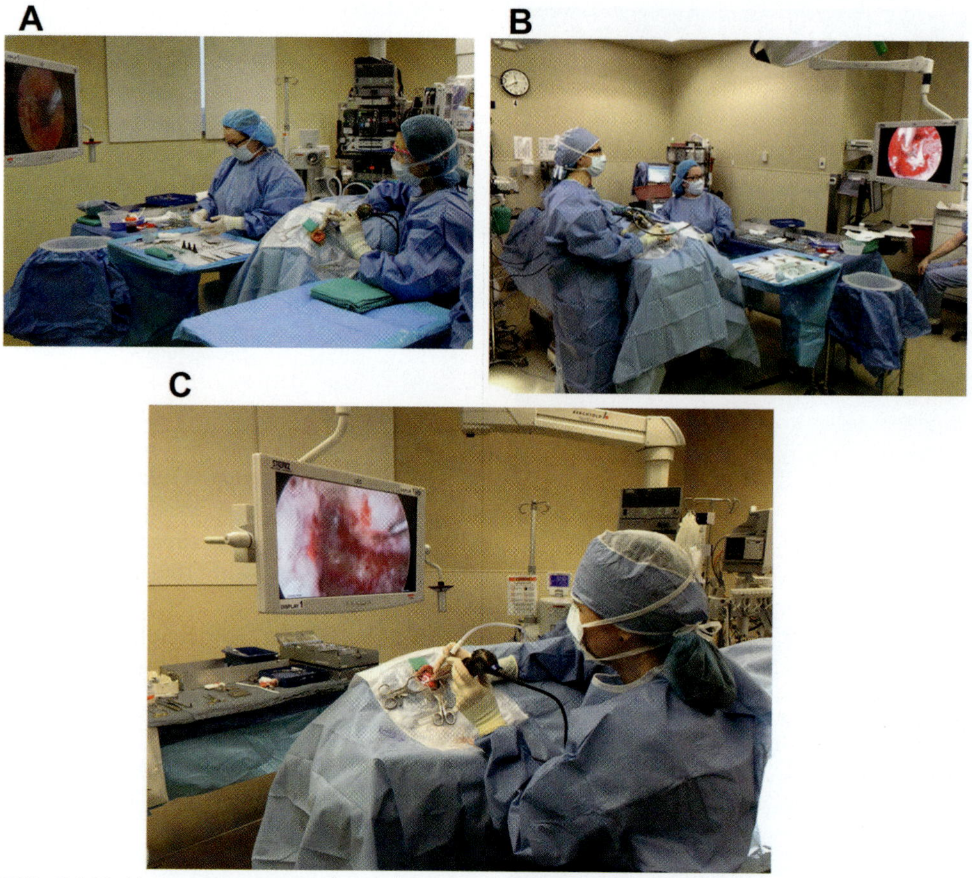

FIG. 26.12 Various room setups for endoscopic ear surgery. Setups should be the result of communication among all members of the surgical team. (From Miller KA, Fina M, Lee DJ. Principles of pediatric endoscopic ear surgery. *Otolaryngol Clin North Am.* 2019;52:5:xix-xx. doi:10.1016/j.otc.2019.06.011.)

now be placed in the EAC, allowing a few minutes for vasoconstriction to take place. He or she then incises the tympanic membrane with the Rosen knife or similar instrument. Suction is required to keep the visual field clear. Several epinephrine-soaked cotton balls are placed at the incision and timed at 1 to 3 minutes. The cotton balls are then suctioned dry and left in place to soak up any blood. They are then replaced with fresh epinephrine sponges (Fig. 26.13). Fig. 26.14 shows the endoscopic view of middle ear structures.

3. *A specific procedure is performed.*
   Endoscopic approach or a combination endoscopic and microsurgical approach may be performed. The surgical procedures that can be performed endoscopically are listed in Box 26.1.

OPEN PROCEDURES OF THE EAR

MYRINGOTOMY

A myringotomy is a surgical opening made in the TM to release fluid from the middle ear. Middle ear **effusion** (presence of fluid) can be treated by making a small incision in the TM (myringotomy). The procedure allows equalization of air pressure between the middle ear and the outside barometric pressure. This allows trapped fluid to drain. To maintain open drainage, a **tympanostomy tube** is placed in the incision. The procedure most often is performed in children. Examples of tympanostomy tubes are shown in Fig. 26.15.

Pathology

Fluid in the middle ear can be caused by inflammation of the mucosa and by eustachian tube dysfunction, in which airflow between the nasopharynx and the middle ear is inadequate; the result is negative pressure in the middle ear and retraction of the TM. Eustachian tube dysfunction can be caused by a congenital anomaly, inflammation of the nasal mucosa, or enlarged adenoids. If left untreated, the effusion may lead to infection, mastoiditis, hearing loss, or perforation.

POSITION:	Supine with affected ear up
INCISION:	Tympanic membrane
PREP AND DRAPING:	The skin prep is usually omitted. Abbreviated ear draping with four towels is used
INSTRUMENTS:	Myringotomy tray and tubes

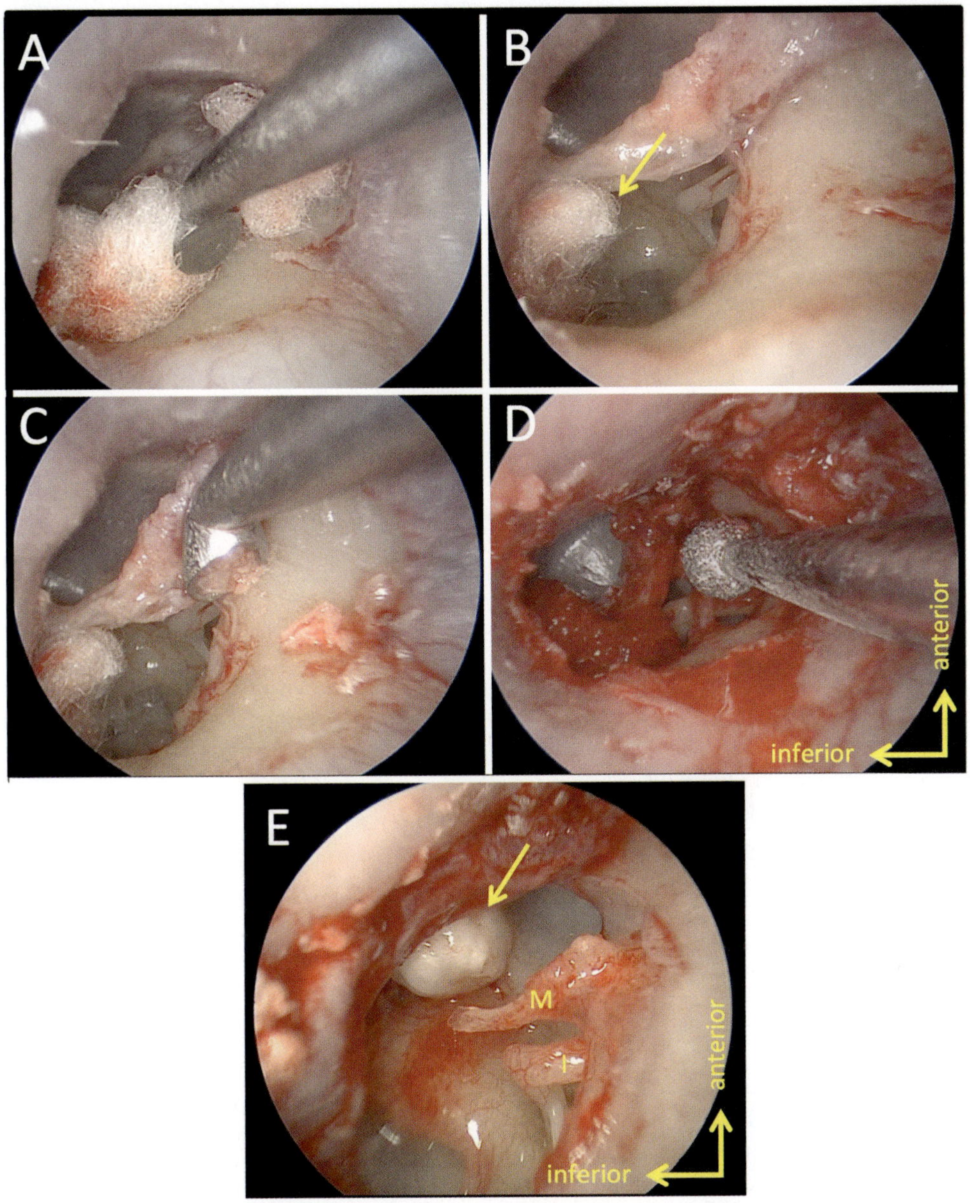

FIG. 26.13 Transcanal endoscopic tympanotomy. (A) Hemostasis using cotton balls soaked in epinephrine solution during elevation with the round knife. (B) Cotton balls used for retraction of the TM. (C and D) The diamond drill and stapes curette are used to remove debris. (E) Exposing the diseased tissue. (From Jan T. Transcanal endoscopic tympanotomy. *Oper Tech Otolaryngol Head Neck Surg*. 2017;28:3.)

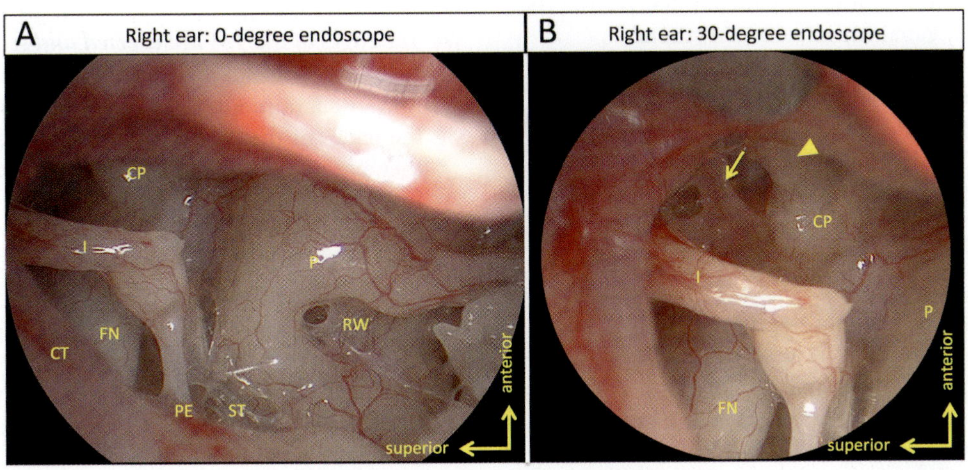

FIG. 26.14 Middle ear structures (endoscopic view). Using the 0-degree scope: *CT*, Chorda tympani; *FN*, facial nerve; *I*, incus; *PE*, pyramidal eminence; *RW*, round window. (From Jan T. Transcanal endoscopic tympanotomy. *Oper Tech Otolaryngol Head Neck Surg*. 2017;28:3.)

BOX 26.1 Indications for Endoscopic Ear Surgery

OUTER EAR
- Cholesteatoma
- Exostosis repair
- Canalplasty
- Debridement and biopsy

MIDDLE EAR
- Myringotomy
- Myringoplasty
- Medial graft tympanoplasty
- Lateral graft tympanoplasty
- Tympanic membrane retraction
- Acquired cholesteatoma
- Congenital cholesteatoma
- Neoplasms of middle ear (e.g., glomus tympanicum)
- Ossiculoplasty

INNER EAR/SKULL BASE
- Intracochlear schwannoma
- Small symptomatic neoplasms of internal auditory canal (IAC) fundus or facial nerve
- Petrous apex cyst
- Perilymph fistula repair (congenital or traumatic) Middle cranial fossa
- Superior canal dehiscence repair
- Posterior fossa/cerebellopontine angle
- Identification of residual schwannoma in IAC fundus
- Localization and plugging of exteriorized air cells during IAC decompression

From Kozin ED, et al. Incorporating endoscopic ear surgery into your clinical practice. *Otolaryngol Clin North Am.* 2016;49:5:1237–1251. https://doi.org/10.1016/j.otc.2016.05.005.

Technical Points and Discussion

1. ***The ear is cleaned of wax and debris.***
The surgeon sits while operating and uses a microscope with a 250-mm lens. The microscope is brought into position as soon as the surgeon is seated. To begin the procedure, the surgeon inserts a Farrior speculum into the external ear canal. The speculum size is determined by the diameter and depth of the ear canal. With the speculum in place, the surgeon removes any wax or debris from the external auditory canal with a cerumen curette.

2. ***A small incision is made in the TM.***
A 2- to 3-mm incision is made in the TM with a myringotomy knife. Fluid behind the TM is suctioned with a small Frazier microsuction (no. 3 or no. 5).

3. ***The tube is inserted.***
The scrub uses alligator forceps to grasp the tube. The surgeon inserts the tube into the myringotomy incision. Next, a Rosen needle is used to seat the tube in the incision. Combinations of antibiotic and steroid drops or antibiotic drops alone are then instilled into the external canal, and the speculum is removed. The external canal is packed with cotton.

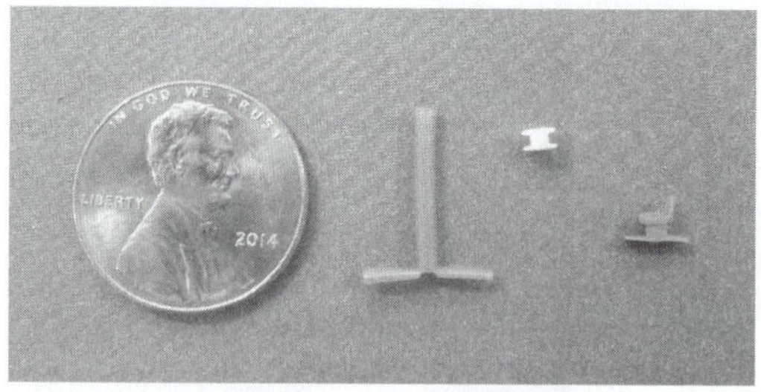

FIG. 26.15 Ventilated tympanostomy tubes. There are many different types of tubes placed within the tympanic membrane to drain the middle ear in chronic otitis media. *Left to right:* T tube, bobbin tube, flanged tube. (From Scholes MA, Ramakrishnan VR. *ENT Secrets*. Philadelphia: Elsevier; 2016.)

MYRINGOPLASTY

A myringoplasty is performed to close a small nonhealing hole in the TM. The procedure is performed without entering the middle ear.

Pathology

Causes of **perforation** of the TM may include a persistent opening after removal of a tympanostomy tube, a blast injury, or a penetrating foreign body in the ear.

POSITION:	Supine with affected ear up
INCISION:	None
PREP AND DRAPING:	External ear
INSTRUMENTS:	Myringoplasty set
POSSIBLE EXTRAS:	Minor plastic set

Technical Points and Discussion

1. ***A speculum is placed in the external canal for microscopic examination.***
The operating microscope is fitted with a 250-mm lens. The microscope usually is not draped for the procedure. To begin the procedure, the surgeon places a Farrior speculum into the external auditory canal.

2. ***The edges of the TM are everted and scored.***
The external canal is cleaned with a cerumen curette and Frazier suction. The surgeon then can **evert** (turn back) the edges of the perforated TM and score them with either a fine Rosen needle or a fine right-angle pick. Several types of patches can be used to close the defect (e.g., gelatin foam, fat graft).

3. ***A fat graft is taken from the ear lobe.***
The surgeon makes a small incision (approximately 5 to 8 mm) on the posterior side of the ear lobe with a #15 blade. Single skin hooks are used to expose the subcutaneous tissue. A small piece of the tissue is excised with a #15 blade and a hemostat or toothed Adson forceps. The graft is placed in a small amount of saline to keep it moist

until the surgeon is ready to implant it. The donor site is closed with 4-0 synthetic absorbable suture.

4. ***The graft is positioned.***
The graft is positioned over the defect in the TM. The external auditory canal is packed with gelatin sponges soaked in a steroid-antibiotic solution, and a Glasscock-style dressing is applied.

TYMPANOPLASTY

A tympanoplasty is the surgical removal of a **cholesteatoma** and mastoid bone, with or without reconstruction. Two methods are commonly used to perform a tympanoplasty. The approach depends on the condition of the TM, the size and position of the perforation, and the surgeon's preference.

In the *underlay* technique, the TM is lifted away and the middle ear is filled with a gelatin sponge to support a graft on the undersurface of the TM perforation. This is used for a small visible perforation with minimal signs of infection.

The *overlay* technique is used for a large perforation, for a severely damaged TM, or for extensive infection. In this procedure, the TM remnants and bony canal skin are removed. The bony canal is enlarged with a drill, and the TM is recreated with a fascia and skin graft (usually from the abdomen, upper arm, or pinna).

Pathology

A tympanoplasty is performed to treat several disorders affecting the TM. These conditions include a nonhealing perforation of the TM, a dysfunction of the eustachian tube that causes retraction of the TM, and a cholesteatoma. In dysfunction of the eustachian tube, inadequate airflow between the nasopharynx and the middle ear causes negative pressure in the middle ear and retraction of the TM. This causes the TM to vibrate incorrectly and can lead to a perforation or cholesteatoma. A cholesteatoma may cause infection, otorrhea, bone destruction, hearing loss, and paralysis of the facial nerve.

POSITION:	Supine
INCISION:	Postauricular; a second incision is made for the skin graft
PREP AND DRAPING:	Ear and skin graft site
INSTRUMENTS:	Tympanoplasty set; graft block

Technical Points and Discussion

1. ***A skin graft is taken.***
If a skin graft from the arm or abdomen is planned, it may be removed before the skin prep and draping. The arm is prepped and draped with towels. The surgeon removes the graft with a sharp, double-edged razor blade (e.g., a Gillette or a Watson) or a Weck skin graft knife. The graft is placed in a small basin and protected from damage or contamination. A small amount of saline is used to keep the graft moist. The donor site is covered or may be dressed. The patient is prepped and draped for the ear procedure.

2. ***A fascia graft is removed.***
The surgeon makes a postauricular (behind the ear) incision and carries it through the temporalis fascia to the mastoid tip. A temporalis fascia graft is harvested with Brown–Adson forceps and a #15 blade. A *fascia press* is used to flatten and shape the graft. A separate sterile table may be set up for this, or the surgeon may use an area of the back table to prepare the graft. The fascia press with the graft on it should be left in the open position unless the surgeon requests otherwise. This allows the graft to dry so that it can be trimmed and placed in the ear later in the procedure.

3. ***The native tympanic membrane is removed or prepared for grafting.***
The microscope is fitted with a 250-mm lens, draped, and moved into position. The TM is exposed with a Gimmick or House knife and removed with Bellucci scissors or knife. If a canaloplasty (reconstruction of the canal) is to be performed, the ear canal is enlarged with a small cutting drill and a small 4 × 5 suction irrigator. This permits better visualization of the middle ear and provides a larger space in which to work.

4. ***The grafts are positioned.***
The middle ear is then prepared to receive the graft. The surgeon trims the fascia to the appropriate size using the fascia press and a #15 blade. The graft is grasped with a smooth alligator forceps and removed from the fascia press. The surgeon reconstructs the middle ear by placing the fascia graft in position with the alligator forceps and a fine Rosen needle. The skin grafts, if taken, are then laid over the fascia graft with alligator forceps and Rosen needle.

5. ***The ear is packed and incision closed.***
The ear is packed with small pledgets of gelatin or collagen sponge to hold the graft in position. The wound is closed in layers with 3-0 absorbable sutures, and the skin is closed with 4-0 absorbable sutures. The ear is dressed with a mastoid dressing.

MASTOIDECTOMY

A mastoidectomy or tympanomastoidectomy is the removal of diseased bone, the mastoid air cells, and the soft tissue lining the air cells of the mastoid. The operating microscope is used during the surgery.

Pathology

The mastoid is composed of many air cells similar to the nasal sinuses. Inadequate flow of air through the sinuses can lead to infection and erosion of the surrounding bone. Cholesteatoma, eustachian tube dysfunction, neoplasm, or congenital malformation of the middle ear may block airflow to the mastoid and cause chronic mastoiditis. An advanced cholesteatoma may spread into the mastoid. In this case, mastoidectomy with tympanoplasty is performed.

POSITION:	Supine
INCISION:	Postauricular; a second incision is made for the skin graft

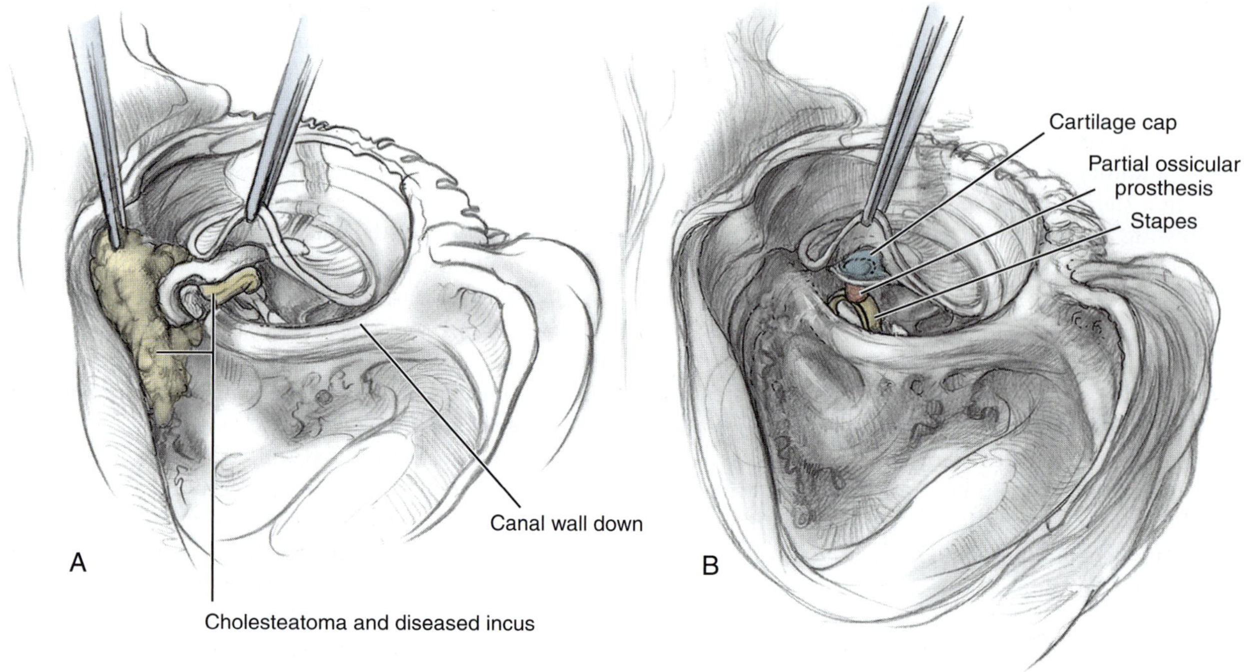

FIG. 26.16 Mastoidectomy. (A) The mastoid air cells are removed and cholesteatoma revealed near the ossicles. (B) In cases where the diseased tissue has invaded the ossicles, an oculoplastic surgery can be performed. (From Brackmann D, Shelton C, Arriaga M. *Otologic Surgery*. 4th ed. Philadelphia: Elsevier; 2016.)

PREP AND DRAPING:	Ear and skin graft site
INSTRUMENTS:	Mastoidectomy set; graft block

Technical Points and Discussion

1. ***The patient is prepped and draped.***
The patient is placed in the supine position, and the arm on the operative side is tucked at the patient's side. General anesthesia is used. A skin graft is taken before the ear prep, as described previously. A 27-gauge needle is used to inject the ear incision site with lidocaine with epinephrine. The patient is then prepped and draped for an ear procedure.

2. ***A postauricular incision is made.***
The surgeon makes a postauricular incision and raises the skin flaps. Once the periosteum has been exposed, the incision is made deeper using a needlepoint electrosurgical unit (ESU). The periosteum is lifted using an elevator. A self-retaining retractor such as a small Weitlaner may be placed at this point.

3. ***A fascia graft is taken.***
A temporalis fascia graft is removed using a knife blade, fine tissue forceps, and scissors. Once it is removed, it is placed in a small basin and prepared. The surgeon may tease out the periphery and smoothen the graft onto a fascia press and allow it to dry on a cutting block. The scrub should keep the graft in a secure location on the back table until it is needed.

4. ***The mastoid bone is drilled.***
The incision is carried to the bone, and the diseased mastoid tissue is excised with a power drill with a large cutting burr. During use of the power drill, the scrub or assistant must provide continuous irrigation and suction to remove bone debris and prevent overheating of the tissues. The surgeon may use a variety of burrs to remove the bone. The microscope is moved into position. Drilling continues to the point where the mastoid bone connects to the middle ear.

5. ***A cholesteatoma is removed.***
A Rosen needle, Gimmick, or picks are used to assess the patency of the mastoid and determine the need for continued drilling. If a cholesteatoma is to be removed, the surgeon uses the Gimmick and Rosen needle. Removal of the ossicles may be necessary if they are diseased.

6. ***The graft is put in place.***
The surgeon prepares the fascia graft by trimming it. A graft block and knife are needed for this step. The surgeon places the fascia graft over the remaining ossicles; this is done as described for a tympanoplasty. The skin graft is placed in position over the fascia. The surgeon then uses a serrated alligator forceps and a Gimmick to pack the mastoid cavity and middle ear with absorbable gelatin matrix sponges that have been soaked in saline solution or a combination steroid-antibiotic. The external auditory canal is also packed with absorbable gelatin matrix, as for the mastoid cavity. The incisions are closed in layers with 3-0 absorbable sutures. The skin is closed with 4-0 absorbable sutures. A mastoid dressing is applied. Refer to Fig. 26.16 for technical highlights of mastoidectomy.

STAPEDECTOMY

A stapedectomy is the reconstruction of the ossicles to restore conduction to the oval window.

Pathology

A stapedectomy, or ossicular reconstruction, is usually performed to treat profound hearing loss related to sclerosis of the stapes. Sound normally is received at the TM, which transmits vibrations through the ossicles and the oval window, which amplifies the sound. If the bony chain is immobile or discontinuous, not only is amplification lost but sound perception can also be severely dampened. The most common cause of ossicle immobility is *otosclerosis* of the stapes. This is abnormal bone growth that locks the stapes into place and prevents it from vibrating and carrying the stimulus. Otosclerosis generally begins at age 30 and progresses with age. After surgery, 90% of patients have a permanent hearing gain, and 1% sustain a permanent hearing loss.

The most common cause of a break in the ossicle chain is a cholesteatoma, which erodes the ossicles. The shape and articulation of the ossicles provide minimal sound amplification (1.7:1). The size ratio between the TM and the oval window provides most of the amplification (17:1). This is important, because a mobile connection between the TM and the oval window can ensure that vibrations are transmitted through the semicircular canal to the inner ear.

POSITION:	Supine
INCISION:	None
PREP AND DRAPING:	Postauricular and auditory canal
INSTRUMENTS:	Stapedectomy set; micro drill; stapes sizers and implant

Technical Points and Discussion

1. ***The auditory canal is injected with lidocaine and epinephrine.***
   The patient is placed in the supine position, and the arm on the operative side is tucked at the patient's side. General anesthesia is used. The external ear canal is injected with a local anesthetic before being prepped. The patient is prepped and draped for an ear procedure.

2. ***The external ear canal is cleared of fluid.***
   The operative microscope with a 250-mm lens is used to examine the middle ear. The external ear canal is irrigated and cleaned with a 7-Fr Frazier suction tip. In this procedure, a speculum holder is used. The surgeon places the speculum in the external canal and attaches it to a universal speculum holder for stabilization. This allows the surgeon to operate with both hands while the speculum is held in the external canal. The surgeon then changes to a 5-Fr Frazier suction tip to clear any fluid from the ear.

3. ***The TM is elevated and stapes superstructure removed.***
   The TM is elevated and the posterior bony ledge is removed with a House knife. With the TM elevated, the surgeon can visualize the ossicular chain. The incudostapedial joint is cut with a joint knife and the stapedial tendon is severed with Bellucci scissors. The stapes superstructure is then fractured with a fine Rosen needle and microcup forceps. Note: The stapes superstructure may be removed using a CO_2 laser.

4. ***A hole is drilled in the stapes footplate.***
   The surgeon then drills a hole in the stapes footplate with the microdrill using a 1-mm cutting burr. A prosthesis sizer is used to measure for the correct implant. The prosthesis is loaded onto a smooth alligator forceps or hook and implanted into the hole in the footplate. A crimper is used to secure the prosthesis.

   The surgeon packs the ear with gelatin sponges soaked in normal saline or steroid antibiotic ointment.

5. ***The TM is put back into position.***
   A Gimmick and a fine Rosen needle are used to replace the TM. The external auditory canal is packed with gelatin sponges soaked in saline or an antibiotic-steroid solution. A Glasscock or mastoid dressing is applied. See Fig. 26.17 for a schematic illustration of the implants.

COCHLEAR IMPLANT

A cochlear implant is used to transmit external sound directly to the eighth cranial nerve. It is used in the treatment of sensorineural deafness. Patients with **sensorineural hearing loss** have functional outer and middle ear structures. However, the cilia, which receive and transmit sound to the ocular nerve and brain, are damaged or absent. The cochlear implant is a device that receives sounds and transmits them as electrical impulses to the brain.

The cochlear implant has two primary components. An electronic processor, which is implanted outside the ear over the temporal bone, captures sound and sends it in digital form to an internal transmitter. The transmitter conveys signals to electrodes, which are implanted into the cochlea. The transmitter takes over the functions of the cochlear cilia. Instead of moving the cilia to transmit sound, the signals are interpreted directly by the acoustic nerve. The patient must learn to interpret the sounds and make sense of their meaning. This requires extensive postoperative rehabilitation and psychological support.

A facial nerve monitor is used to protect the nerve during surgical dissection and implantation of the implants. The monitoring electrodes are placed before the prep and draping.

Pathology

Sensorineural deafness can be congenital or acquired. It has many different causes, including the following:

- Viral or bacterial infection causing damage to the cilia
- Acoustic trauma (caused by loud noise), which results in permanent injury to the cilia

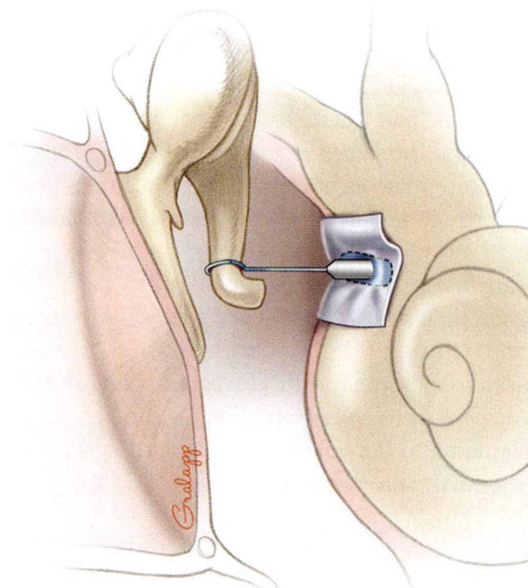

A

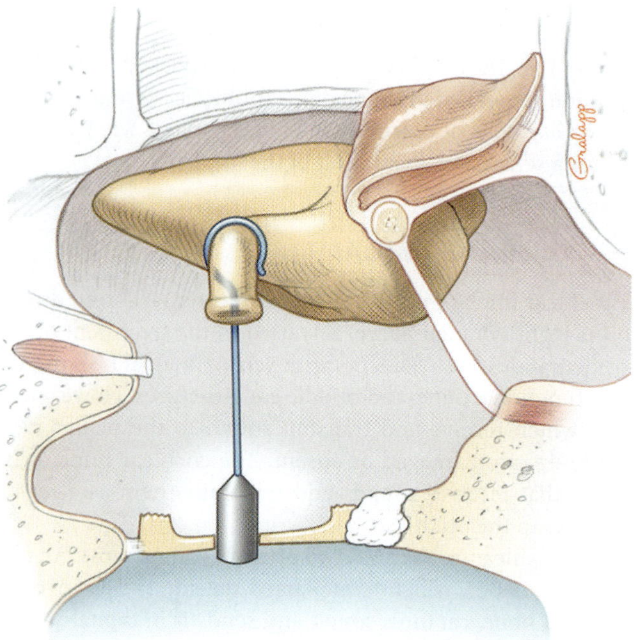

B

FIG. 26.17 Stapedectomy. (A) The prosthesis is inserted between the process of the incus and the tissue graft over the oval window. (B) The prosthesis is inserted through an opening in the stapes footplate to recreate the ossicular chain movement into the labyrinth. (From Cheng H. Stapedectomy versus stapedotomy. *Otolaryngol Clin North Am.* 2018;1:375–392.)

- Tumor of the ocular nerve
- Drugs such as certain antibiotics that cause permanent hearing loss
- Autoimmune disease, stroke, or brain tumor

A cochlear implant provides the perception of sound. However, significant postoperative rehabilitation is required for the patient to turn this into cognitive information. Congenital deafness in the child can be treated with a cochlear implant, but surgery is delayed until the age of 2 years.

POSITION:	Supine
INCISION:	Postauricular and mastoid
PREP AND DRAPING:	External ear, auditory canal, mastoid region
INSTRUMENTS:	Cochlear implant set; minor surgery instruments; ENT drill and burrs; major ear set; bipolar forceps

Technical Points and Discussion

1. ***The patient is prepped and draped.***
The patient is placed in the supine position. The surgeon may clip the hair in the temporal region and outlines the incision with a surgical marking pen. The site is injected with 1% lidocaine with epinephrine 1:100,000. The surgeon implants the electrodes for facial nerve monitoring and connects them to the monitor. The patient then is prepped and draped for an ear procedure.

2. ***The cranium is exposed.***
The surgeon makes a postauricular incision and extends it superiorly using a #15 blade. A skin flap is elevated with a needle-tip ESU and retracted with double-prong skin hooks or wire rakes. The flap is extended deeper to include the muscle. With the flaps elevated, the surgeon places a Beckman-Adson retractor or similar self-retaining retractor under the flaps to expose the cranium.

3. ***A recessed space for the internal receiver is created in the bone.***
The receiver template is placed in position and outlined with the surgical marker or the ESU. The surgeon then drills out the circumscribed area of the temporal bone using a medium cutting burr with irrigation. The template periodically is positioned in the drilled space to ensure a correct fit. A medium diamond burr is used to finish the edges of the temporal bone. Suture tunnel holes are placed, two on each side of the recess. These are used to secure the processor.

4. ***A mastoidectomy is performed.***
The surgeon drills the mastoid with a large cutting burr and suction irrigator, preserving the bony ear canal and the opening of the facial recess. The medial wall of the middle ear is identified.

5. ***The implant set is opened.***
The implant is opened onto the sterile field. Implants are packaged individually and must be opened in a manner that limits or prevents the discharge of static electricity created during opening, because a static charge can interfere with the function of the implant electrodes. The circulator opens the outer package slowly onto the instrument table. The inner (sterile) package may then be submerged in a basin of normal saline and opened below the surface.

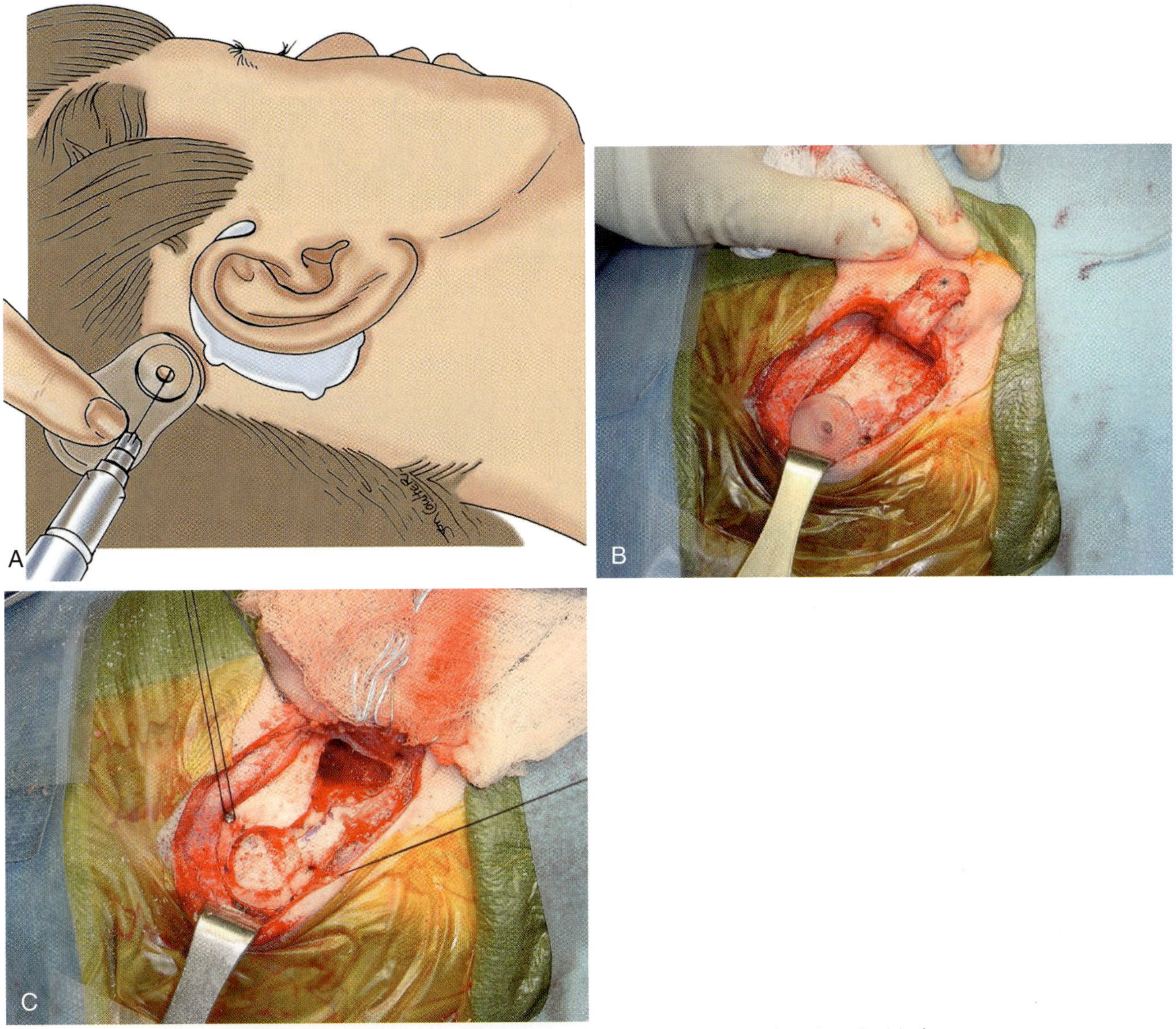

FIG. 26.18 Cochlear implant. (A) A template of the transmitter is sized and marked before surgery. (B) Skin incision and elevation of flaps. (C) The recess is drilled to accommodate the receiver. (D) The device is secured in the bony recess under the temporalis muscle. The electrodes will be placed through the facial recess. (From Meyers E, ed. *Operative Otolaryngology Head and Neck Surgery*. 2nd ed. Philadelphia: Elsevier; 2008.)

6. ***The internal electrodes of the implant are placed into the cochlea via the round window.***
The surgeon places the internal processor into the drilled recess of the temporal bone. The active electrode is passed through the facial recess and round window into the cochlea. This is done using the electrode positioner provided in the implant kit. The active electrode is secured in the round window with a Gimmick or Rosen needle.

7. ***The internal receiver is implanted and secured.***
The surgeon secures the internal processor by placing 2-0 or larger polypropylene suture through the suture holes and tying the knots diagonally across the holes. Bleeding is controlled with the bipolar ESU (monopolar ESU is not used, because it could cause current to be passed through the receiver).

8. ***The incisions are closed.***
With the implant secured, the fascia overlying the cranium is closed with a 2-0 absorbable suture. A 3-0 absorbable suture is used to close the subcutaneous tissue. The skin then is closed with a nonabsorbable suture. A mastoid dressing is placed over the wound.

To allow wound healing, the implant is activated several weeks after surgery. It is activated slowly so that the patient can adjust to the hearing world. Refer to Fig. 26.18 for technical points of the procedure.

An excellent video demonstrating cochlear implant surgery is available at the *Surgeries* website. This is a peer-reviewed, physician-owned company that provides high-quality surgical videos available to students and surgical professionals: https://www.csurgeries.com/video/modified-rambo-transcanal-approach-cochlear-implantation-charge-syndrome/.

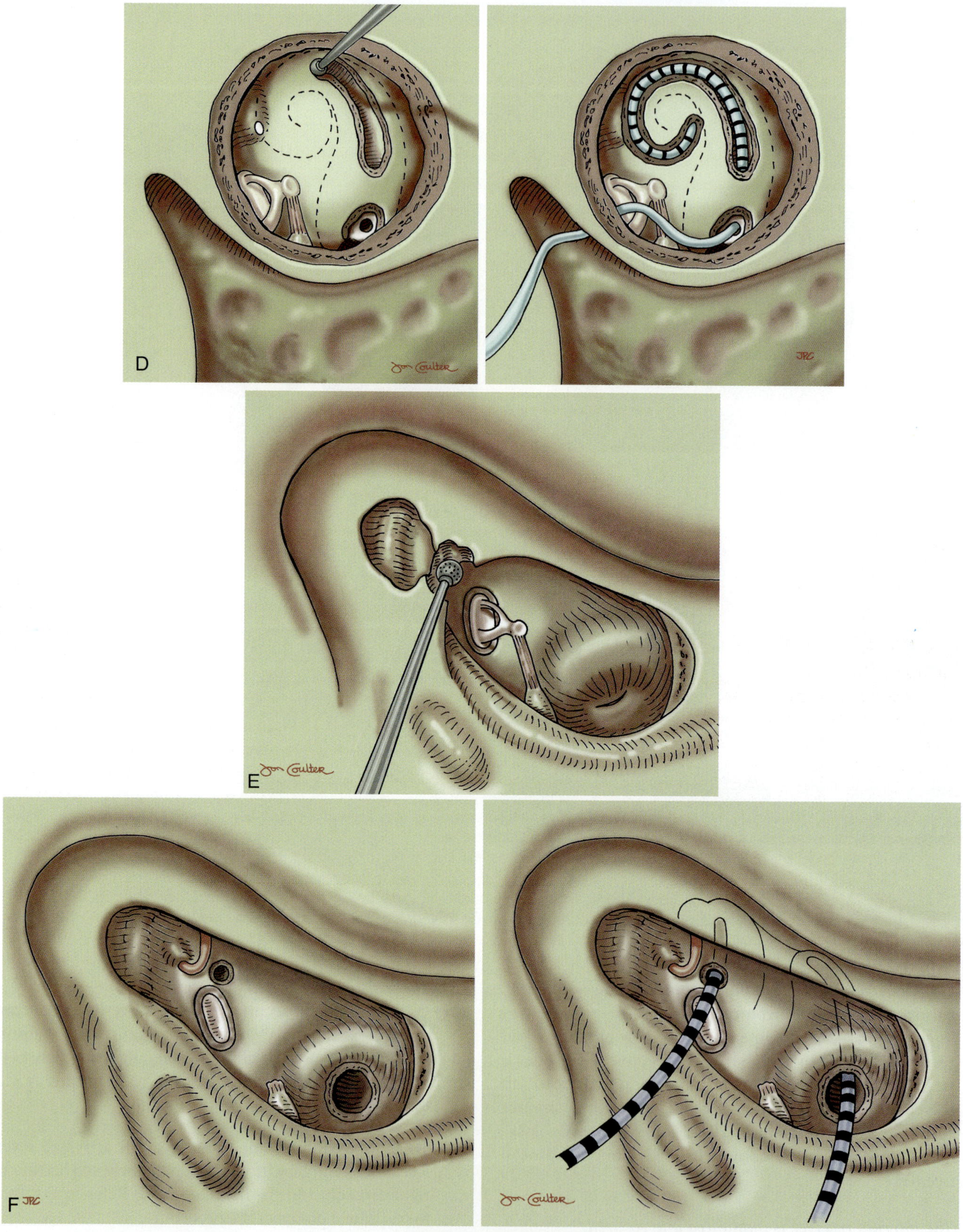

FIG. 26.18, cont'd

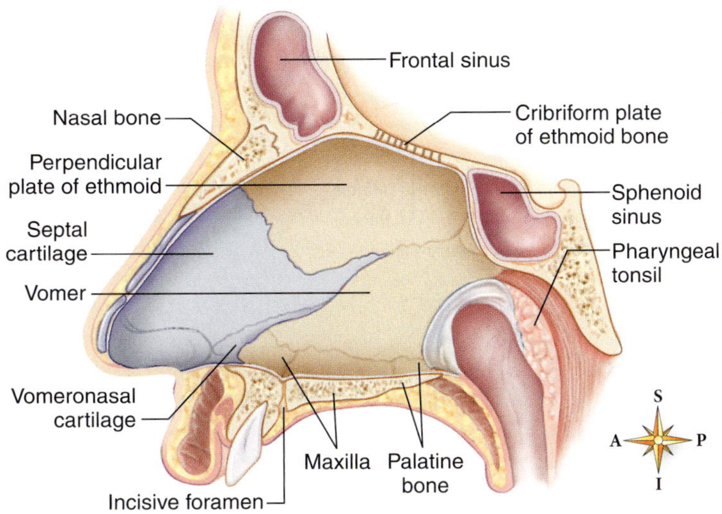

FIG. 26.19 The nasal cavity showing paranasal sinuses and olfactory structures. (From Patton KT, Thibodeau GA, Douglas MM. *Essentials of Anatomy and Physiology—Text and Anatomy and Physiology Online Course*. St Louis: Elsevier; 2012.)

SECTION II: THE NASAL CAVITY, OROPHARYNX, AND LARYNX

Surgery of the nose, oropharynx, and larynx is performed by an otorhinolaryngologist. Most of the structures in these anatomical regions are related to respiration and vocalization, although some share functions with the digestive system. Surgery of lymph and secretory glands in the oropharynx are included in this specialty.

Procedures for pharyngeal and laryngeal tumors may extend into the neck, which contains large blood vessels and nerves that must be protected. Head and neck surgery require meticulous dissection to avoid injury to these vital structures.

SURGICAL ANATOMY

EXTERNAL NOSE

The external nose is formed by two U-shaped, cartilaginous structures called the *lower lateral cartilages,* two rectangular structures called the *upper lateral cartilages,* and two nasal bones. The nares are the flared portions of the lower nose (nostrils). These are lined with skin. Fine hairs in this area filter the air as it enters the nasal cavity. The right and left nostrils are divided by the nasal septum, which is composed of cartilage.

NASAL CAVITY AND SINUSES

The nasal cavity is located over the palatine bone, which is the "floor" of the nose; the "roof" of the nose is formed from the cribriform plate in the ethmoid bone. This is a significant structure, because it separates the nasal cavity from the cranial cavity. Infection or disease arising from the nose may enter the cranial cavity and spread to brain tissue. The nasal cavity has **paranasal sinuses,** or spaces. These are formed by extensions of the ethmoid bone and the frontal, maxillary, and sphenoid bones. The extensions are referred to as the *turbinates* or *nasal conchae.* The sinuses are lined with a highly vascular mucosa. As air passes through the sinuses, it is warmed, humidified, and filtered.

The nasal cavities drain into the superior, inferior, and middle meatus. The nasolacrimal duct drains into the inferior meatus. The posterior aspect of the nasal cavities is the *choana,* which separates them from the nasopharynx. This is an important structure because of the congenital anomaly known as *choanal atresia.* In this condition, infants are born with one or both choanae obstructed, requiring emergency surgery to restore airflow (see Chapter 33).

The paired *maxillary sinuses* are the large sinuses below the ocular orbits. The apices of the tooth roots are found in the floor of these sinuses. The paired frontal sinuses lie behind the lower forehead. The ethmoid sinuses consist of many small air cells in the lateral wall of the nasal cavity between the lateral nasal wall and the turbinates. The sphenoids lie at the posterior superior extent of the nasal cavity. The optic nerves and carotid arteries are within the lateral wall of these sinuses, and the pituitary gland lies behind and above them. Surgery of the pituitary gland may be performed through a **transsphenoidal** approach. The anatomy of the nose and sinuses is shown in Figs. 26.19 and 26.20.

ORAL CAVITY

The oral cavity is divided into two sections, the vestibule and the oral cavity proper. The *vestibule* lies between the inner surfaces of the lips, the buccal mucosa (cheeks), and the lateral aspects of the mandible and maxilla. The oral cavity proper lies within the medial surfaces of the maxillary and mandibular teeth. The roof of the oral cavity proper consists

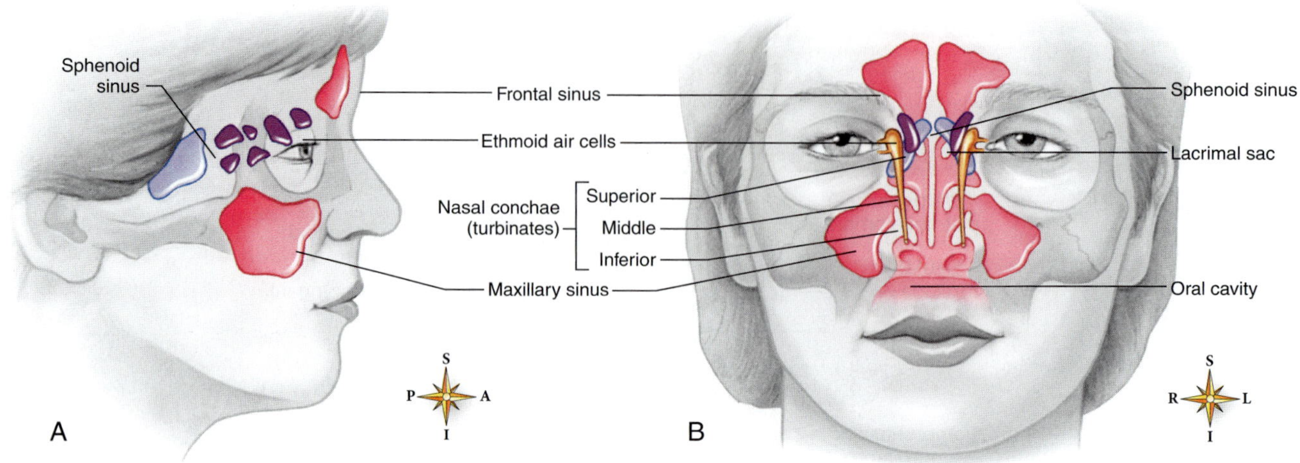

FIG. 26.20 Anatomy of the nasal sinuses. (From Patton KT, Thibodeau GA, Douglas MM. *Essentials of Anatomy and Physiology—Text and Anatomy and Physiology Online Course*. St Louis: Elsevier; 2012.)

of the hard and soft palates, which separate it from the nasal cavity (Fig. 26.21). The soft palate meets in the middle to form the uvula.

The floor of the mouth contains the ducts for the paired submandibular and lingual salivary glands. The tongue is attached in the midline to the floor of the mouth by a membranous structure called the *frenulum*. The tongue is a muscular structure covered by mucous membrane. The surface of the tongue is covered by papillae, or projections that contain taste buds. These are divided by types and regions of the tongue. Various types of papillae and taste buds are capable of separate sensations of taste. The undersurface of the tongue is highly vascular and has large blood vessels. The *sublingual* salivary gland ducts open into each side of the sublingual area. The salivary glands are shown in Fig. 26.22.

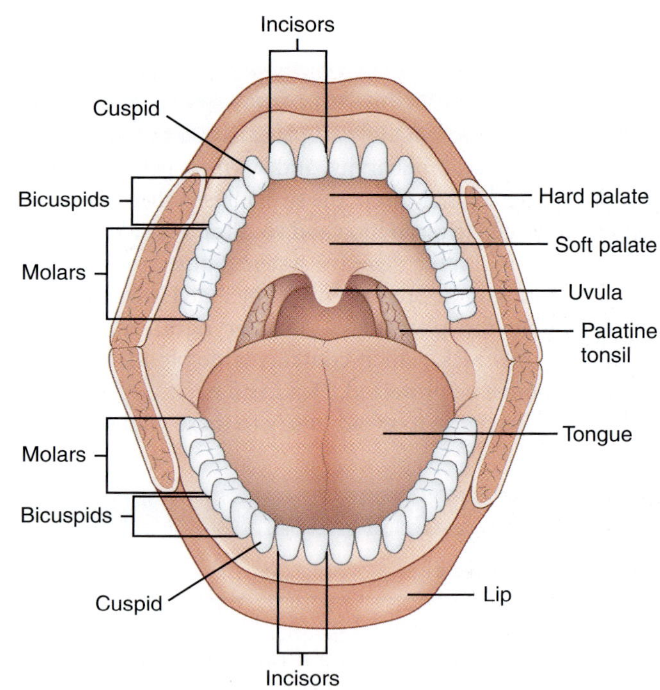

FIG. 26.21 Anatomy of the oral cavity. (From Herlihy B, Maebius NK. *The Human Body in Health and Illness*. 2nd ed. Philadelphia: WB Saunders; 2003.)

PHARYNX

The *pharynx* is a tubular structure extending from the nose to the esophagus. It is separated into three areas: the *nasopharynx, oropharynx,* and *laryngopharynx*. The nasopharynx (Fig. 26.23) extends from the posterior choanae of the nose to the palate. The adenoids lie in the posterosuperior aspect of the nasopharynx, and the eustachian tubes open on each side of the adenoids. The oropharynx extends from the palate to the hyoid bone. The soft palate, tonsils, and posterior third of the tongue (the base of the tongue) lie in the anterior portion of the oropharynx. The *hypopharynx* extends from the hyoid bone to the esophagus.

LARYNX

The larynx is composed of nine segments of cartilage, three paired sets and three unpaired segments. The unpaired cartilages are the cricoid, thyroid, and epiglottis segments; the paired sets are the arytenoids, corniculate, and cuneiform segments.

The larynx is separated into three spaces (Fig. 26.24). The *supraglottis* lies above the true vocal cords and contains the vestibule, false vocal cords, and *epiglottis,* which is composed of cartilage. The *glottis* extends from the true vocal cords to about ½ inch (1 cm) below the free edge of the true vocal cords. The subglottis extends below this position to the inferior edge of the cricoid cartilage. The arytenoid cartilages lie in the posterior larynx and have processes that extend anteriorly (the vocal processes) and that lie within the true vocal cords. The area between the arytenoids is called the *posterior commissure*.

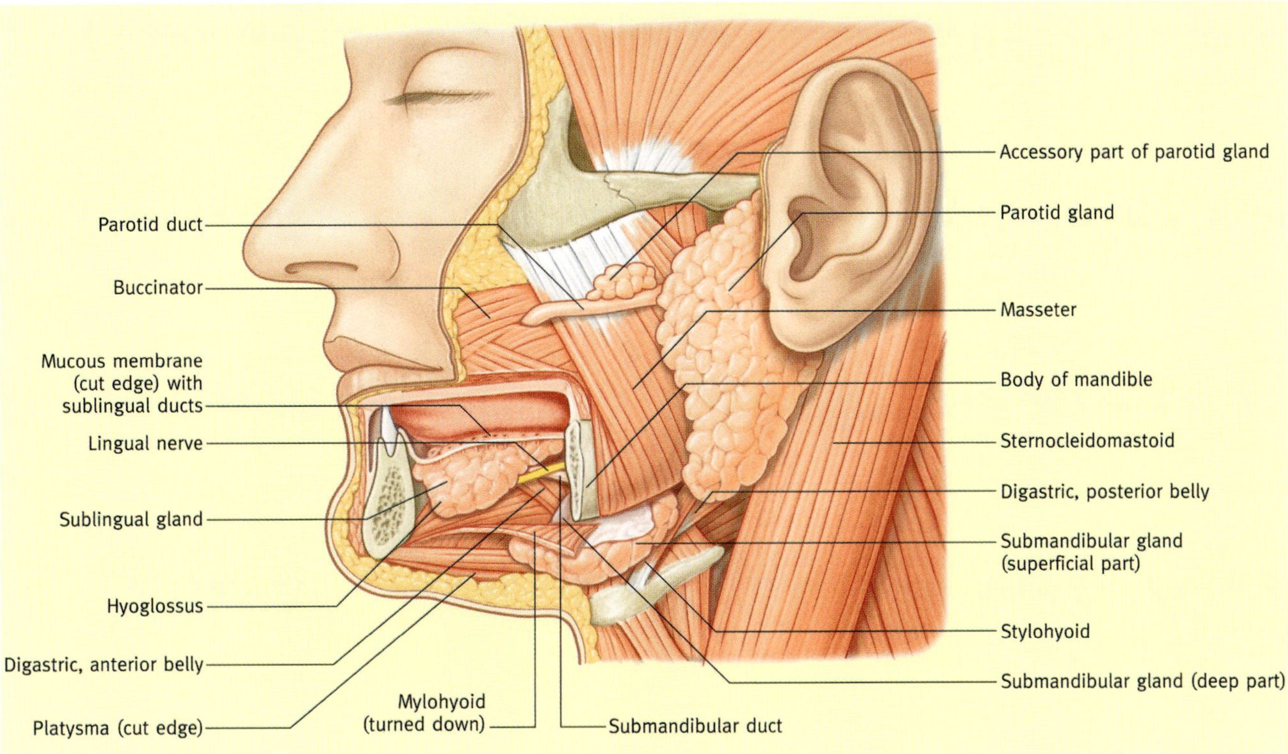

FIG. 26.22 Anatomy of the salivary glands. (From Ellis H. Anatomy of the salivary glands. *Surgery*. 2012;30:11.)

The true vocal cords meet anteriorly at the anterior commissure and connect to the thyroid cartilage. The free edge of the true vocal cords has a loosely covered membrane that vibrates to produce the voice.

The trachea extends from the cricoid to the carina. It is composed of approximately 20 incomplete cartilaginous rings. The cricoid is the only closed ring of the upper airway. The posterior aspect of the trachea is membranous and has no cartilaginous structures.

DIAGNOSTIC TESTS

Diagnostic endoscopy procedures of the upper respiratory tract (larynx and pharynx) are commonly performed for direct visualization of the anatomy. Procedures include sinusoscopy, laryngoscopy, and bronchoscopy. Selected operative procedures such as biopsy and removal of small lesions may also be performed using endoscopic techniques. Pathology specimens are obtained by removing tissue or by cell washing, in which the mucosa is irrigated with saline and cells are collected with a biopsy brush. Fine-needle aspiration and biopsy are also performed before surgical excision.

Imaging studies such as MRI, CT, and ultrasonography are commonly used to confirm or rule out disease or structural abnormalities.

CASE PLANNING

PREPPING AND DRAPING

Patients undergoing nasal procedures generally are prepped from the forehead to the upper neck, including the entire face. Patients having intranasal and endoscopic procedures may not be prepped, because these are considered clean rather than sterile cases. For nasal procedures, the patient is draped with a head drape. A three-quarter sheet is placed under the patient's head. The face then is draped with four towels secured with towel clips, and a split sheet is placed over the patient's body and around the face. If the full face is exposed, the eyes must be protected with eye shields or tape.

Procedures of the pharynx and larynx are approached transorally, and little or no prep is necessary because these are clean procedures. Often these patients are draped with a three-quarter sheet over the chest. A head drape may be applied and the eyes are protected.

EQUIPMENT AND SUPPLIES

Operating Microscope

The operating microscope with a 400-degree lens is used frequently in surgery of the upper airway. The microscope is not draped for procedures of the mouth and throat. While the microscope is in use, the scrub must insert and guide the microinstruments into the laryngoscope, because the surgeon does not turn away from the microscope to receive instruments.

Sponges

Flat cottonoid sponges (patties), and round gauze sponges are commonly used in procedures of the nasal cavities, mouth, and throat. All sponges have strings sewn into them for identification and retrieval to prevent loss and aspiration, which can result in injury or death. All sponges are counted according to routine policy. During nasal procedures the surgeon

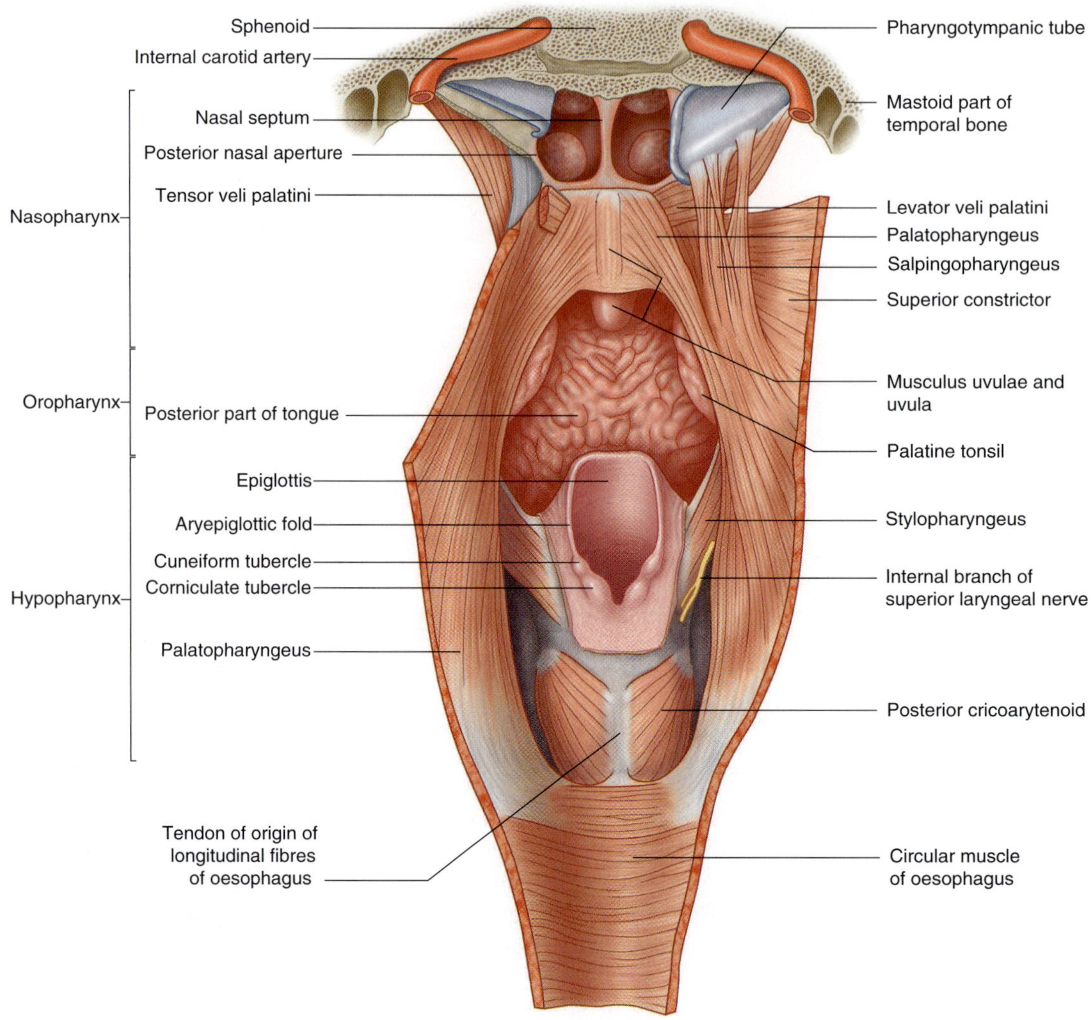

FIG. 26.23 The pharynx. (From Standring S. *Gray's Anatomy*. 41st ed. Philadelphia: Elsevier; 2016.)

may use flat cottonoid sponges soaked with local anesthetic or other agents. Flat cottonoids are illustrated in Chapter 19, Figure 19.4E.

Dressings

No dressings are applied to the mouth and throat after the procedure. A variety of nasal dressings may be used, depending on the procedure. The interior nasal passages may be "splinted" or packed with a continuous ¼- or ½-inch gauze strip. Packing material may be impregnated with a bacteriostatic agent before insertion. Nasal **packing** is the process of placing soft gauze material inside the nose to provide support and absorb fluid.

Nasal packing also helps control bleeding or drainage after septoplasty or rhinoplasty. Exterior nasal splints are used to maintain the shape of the nose in the immediate postoperative period. Several types of external splints are available, made of metal, foam, and fiberglass.

Medications

Medications used for procedures of the nose, mouth, and throat include regional anesthetics, vasoconstrictive agents, and decongestants. A local anesthetic with epinephrine is injected into the nasal mucosa and turbinates for most nasal procedures. Cocaine in solution may be used as a vasoconstrictive agent in the nose or larynx for topical use only. Solutions are administered by infiltration (injection) or may be applied topically with flat cottonoid sponges.

NASAL INSTRUMENTS

Specialty nasal instruments are designed for use on soft tissue and bone. Soft tissue instruments are required for skin, submucosa, and soft connective tissue; bone and cartilage require heavier instruments. In many cases, the complex structure of the nasal cavity requires the surgeon to alternate frequently between these two types of instruments during a surgical procedure. All nasal instruments must be designed to reach deep into the nasal cavities from the outside. Instruments are balanced so that the hinge or fulcrum is much farther from the finger rings than in general surgery instruments. Instrument tips are available in an angled configuration for optimum access. Refer to the Nasal Instruments section of the Ear, Nasal, Laryngeal, and Pharyngeal Instruments table to see common nasal instruments.

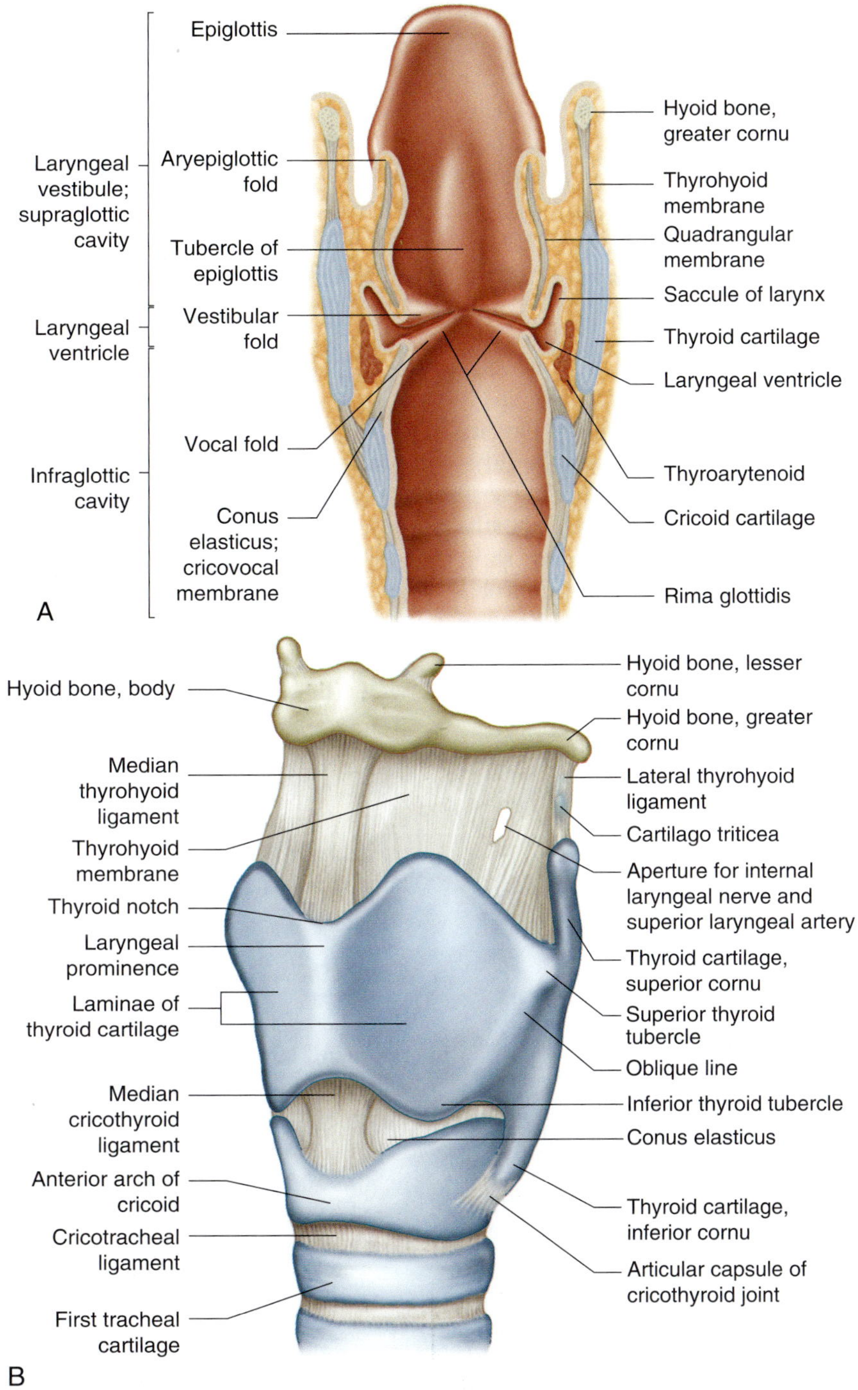

FIG. 26.24 The larynx. (A) The soft tissue structures of the larynx. (B) Bone and cartilage structures. (From Standring S. *Gray's Anatomy*. 38th ed. Edinburgh: Churchill Livingstone; 2004.)

Retractors

A nasal speculum is used for viewing tissue just inside the nares. Fine skin hooks or rakes are used to retract skin tissue in this area. Common retractors include the following:

- Alar retractor
- Fomon retractor
- Aufricht retractor
- Cottle retractor

Knives

Knives must have a delicate tip so that they can be manipulated in the small space of the nasal cavity. A #15 scalpel blade (knife) mounted on a #7 knife handle often is used for skin and submucosal incisions in the naris. The following are used for deeper dissection:

- Ballenger swivel knife
- Button knife

Elevator or Dissector

Elevators are used to lift the periosteum or submucosa from the surface of bone or cartilage. They are available in a wide variety of designs to conform to the complex structure of the nasal cavity. The edge of the elevator is beveled but not sharp. Commonly used elevators include the following:

- Cottle knife or elevator
- Lempert elevator
- Freer elevator

Forceps

Forceps are used for grasping and modeling tissue. The tips of the forceps may be cupped or beveled for cutting or flat and serrated. An example of the cutting type of forceps is the Takahashi ethmoid forceps, which has small, cupped tips. The term *alligator forceps* refers both to the instrument design and to the instrument itself. Alligator forceps have a long shank, short "working" tips, and two hinges, one at the base of the movable tips and one at the fulcrum that opens the tips. The distinction is made clear by the individual surgeon during the procedure. Dressing forceps are bayonet shaped and used to handle nasal packing.

Commonly used tissue forceps include the following:

- Takahashi forceps
- Jackson alligator forceps
- Jackson cup forceps
- Wilde tissue forceps
- Asch septum straightening forceps
- Jansen bayonet forceps

Rongeur

The rongeur is used specifically to cut bone. To provide enough leverage to cut through bone, many rongeurs have two hinges; these are identified as *double-action* rongeurs. A common double-action rongeur is the Jansen-Middleton rongeur shown in the Nasal Instruments section of the Ear, Nasal, Laryngeal, and Pharyngeal Instruments table. The downturned shape is typical of many instruments used in nasal and sinus surgery.

Rongeurs with long shanks are used to reach deep into small spaces, such as the nasal sinus. Some of the rongeurs used in nasal surgery also are used in other specialties, such as neurosurgery. An example is the Kerrison rongeur. Commonly used rongeurs include the following:

- Takahashi rongeur
- Lempert bone rongeur
- Wilde tissue forceps

Gouge, Chisel, and Osteotome

The gouge, chisel, and osteotome are used with a small mallet to model nasal bone. Those used in nasal surgery are smaller and finer than those used in orthopedics. The sharp end of the instrument is angled against the bone and lightly struck with the mallet. This cuts the tissue by increments, producing bone shavings, which are removed with a forceps. The gouge is V-shaped, although the chisel and osteotome are straight. The chisel tip is beveled on both sides, but the osteotome has only one bevel.

Rasp and Saw

A nasal rasp is used to shave bone tissue. The handheld rasp usually is bayonet shaped. Note that the endoscopic shaver or microdebrider is used for the same purpose (discussed later). The bayonet saw is angled (right and left) and used to reduce small defects in bone.

TONSIL AND ADENOID INSTRUMENTS

Tonsil and adenoid instruments include the Crowe-Davis gag and McIvor mouth gag. The tonsil snare was used commonly in the past to remove the tonsils but has been replaced by newer and safer technologies such as ESU ablation or ultrasonic energy. These are discussed in Chapter 15. Adenoid curettes were once very commonly used to remove the adenoids. The mouth gag is placed in the patient's mouth and attached to the edge of the Mayo stand during surgery. Tonsil snares are loaded with short strands of stainless steel wire. The snare is looped around the tonsil and retracted to transect the tonsillar fossa and release the tissue. Basic tonsil and adenoid instruments are shown in the Mouth and Throat Instruments section of the Ear, Nasal, Laryngeal, and Pharyngeal Instruments table. However, these instruments are used less commonly than in the past as new technologies have taken their place.

SHAVER AND DRILLS

The *microdebrider* (Fig. 26.25) is used to excise tissue during nasal and laryngeal surgery. It is a small, powered handpiece with rotating blades. The microdebrider removes small segments of tissue and suctions them, removing blood and debris from the surgical field. Blades are available in a variety of lengths and as straight blades or blades with a 15- or 30-degree bend. A high-speed drill is used to drill bone in the ear and in nasal surgery.

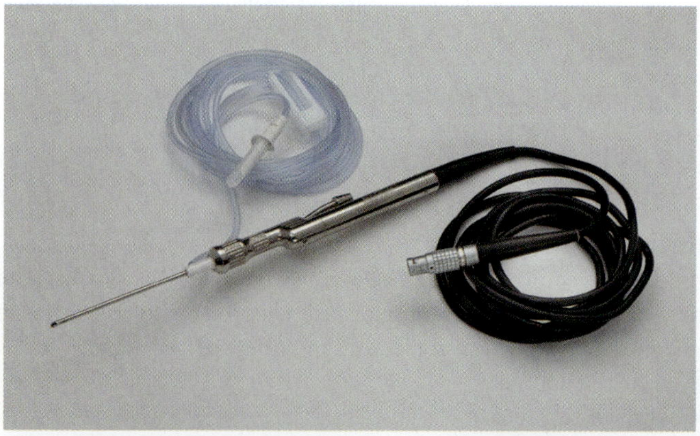

FIG. 26.25 Microdebrider. This instrument is used to remove tissue during sinus surgery. (From Nemitz R. *Surgical instrumentation: an interactive approach*. 3rd ed. St Louis: Elsevier; 2019.)

SINUS SCOPE

The sinus endoscope is used to visualize the sinus passages of the nose and face. The endoscope is available in focal angles of 0, 30, and 70 degrees. The 0-degree scope is used for sinus exploration and evaluation in all procedures. The 30-degree scope is used for maxillary, sphenoid, and ethmoid sinus procedures. The 70-degree scope is used for procedures of the frontal sinus. Refer to Chapter 20 for illustrations of these endoscopes.

SURGICAL PROCEDURES

ENDOSCOPIC SINUS SURGERY

Endoscopic sinus surgery is performed to treat disease of the paranasal sinuses, nasal cavity, and skull base and to improve nasal airflow. Endoscopic techniques are used in the following procedures:

- Polypectomy
- Maxillary antrostomy
- Ethmoidectomy
- Turbinectomy
- Sphenoidectomy

Most endoscopic procedures of the nose are done to treat inflammatory or infectious diseases. A **polyp** is redundant mucosal tissue that prevents airflow and drainage of the paranasal sinus. In rare cases, intranasal neoplasms, **epistaxis** (nasal bleeding), and cerebrospinal fluid leakage may be treated endoscopically.

Patient Preparation

The patient is placed in the supine position with the head stabilized on a doughnut headrest and the arms tucked at the sides. General anesthesia is used. A local anesthetic (usually 1% lidocaine with epinephrine 1:100,000) is injected into the nasal mucosa to provide hemostasis. The surgeon uses a nasal speculum and bayonet forceps to pack the nose with small cottonoids soaked in topical anesthetic or a vasoconstrictor (e.g., cocaine solution, topical adrenaline 1:1000, or Afrin). The patient is prepped and draped for a nasal procedure. The 0-degree sinus endoscope is inserted.

Polypectomy

Under direct visualization with the nasal endoscope, Wilde tissue forceps and microdebrider are commonly used to remove nasal polyps. A #12 Frazier suction device is used to remove the morcellated tissue.

The antrum is enlarged with a microdebrider or a reverse biting forceps. Redundant mucosa and polyps are removed from the maxillary sinus with a microdebrider or Wilde tissue forceps.

Ethmoidectomy

Under direct visualization with a 0-degree endoscope, the surgeon removes (medializes) the middle turbinate up to the midline and bony process of the ethmoid bone. This allows visualization of the middle meatus. The ethmoids are removed with either a microdebrider or a Wilde tissue forceps.

Turbinectomy

Under direct visualization with a 0-degree endoscope, the surgeon displaces the middle turbinate and removes the uncinate, as in the maxillary antrostomy. This allows visualization of the middle meatus. The surgeon changes to a 30- or 70-degree endoscope. Any bony obstruction at the frontal sinus ostium is excised with either Wilde tissue forceps and small bone forceps or with a microdebrider.

Sphenoidectomy

The posterior ethmoids are removed with a microdebrider or Wilde tissue forceps. A 30-degree endoscope is used to view the sphenoid sinus. The ostium is opened with the microdebrider or Wilde tissue forceps. Diseased tissue is removed with Wilde tissue forceps or Takahashi forceps.

Bleeding is controlled with nasal packing saturated with a vasoconstrictive agent. The packing is removed after several minutes and, if necessary, fresh packing saturated with antibiotic ointment is inserted.

CALDWELL-LUC PROCEDURE

A Caldwell-Luc procedure is a technique used to enter the maxillary sinus through an incision made in the gingival-buccal sulcus (the junction of the gum and upper lip). The procedure is commonly performed for drainage of an abscess in the maxillary sinus and surgical removal of granulation tissue that has accumulated as a result of chronic sinus infection. The procedure is illustrated in Fig. 26.26.

Pathology

Access to the maxillary sinus and orbital floor is required for treatment of neoplasms and infection of the orbital cavity.

POSITION:	Supine
INCISION:	Gingival-buccal
PREP AND DRAPING:	Head drape; body sheet
INSTRUMENTS:	Submucosal resection set

Technical Points and Discussion

1. ***The patient is prepped and draped.***
   The patient is placed in the supine position with the head on a doughnut headrest and the arms tucked at the sides. Local anesthesia can be used. Skin prep is omitted for procedures in which an oral approach is used. The patient is draped as for a nasal procedure.

2. ***An incision is made in the gingival-buccal sulcus.***
   The lip is retracted upward with a gauze sponge, and the gingival-buccal sulcus (gum line) is incised with the ESU. The incision is extended from the lateral incisor to the second molar and carried to the periosteum. The mucous membrane is retracted superiorly to expose the periosteum overlying the canine fossa.

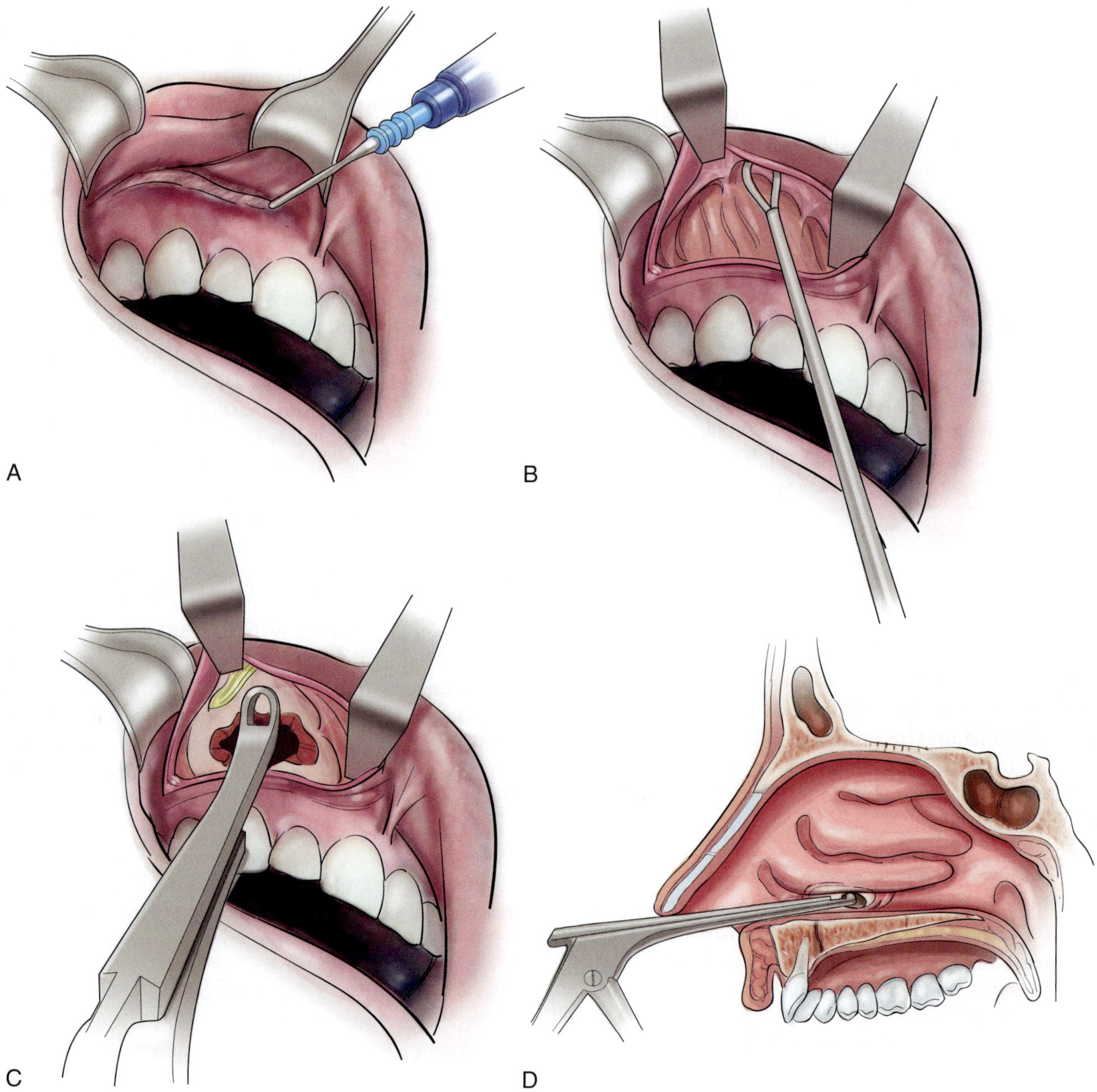

FIG. 26.26 Anterior antrostomy (Caldwell-Luc procedure). (A) An incision is made at junction of the gum and the upper lip. (B) The canine fossa is exposed using a curette. (C) The sinus is opened using a small osteotome and Kerrison rongeur. (D) The antrostomy is performed to make an opening in the inferior turbinate. (From Myers E. *Operative Otolaryngology: Head and Neck Surgery*. St Louis: Elsevier; 2018.)

3. ***The periosteum over the canine fossa is elevated.***
   The periosteum is elevated with a periosteal elevator to the level of the infraorbital nerve. The nerve is identified and preserved.

4. ***The anterior wall of the antrum is opened.***
   Once the periosteum has been removed, the surgeon uses a drill and small cutting burr to enter the maxillary sinus. The opening is enlarged with small Kerrison bone-cutting forceps; this exposes the diseased tissue. Cysts and tumors are removed with small cutting instruments, such as a Wilde tissue forceps or Takahashi forceps. Small bone curettes may also be used. The sinus is irrigated, and small fragments are removed with suction.

5. ***The gingival-buccal incision is closed.***
   The gingival-buccal incision is closed with 3-0 absorbable sutures.

TURBINECTOMY/TURBINATE REDUCTION

Turbinectomy is removal of the bony turbinate to increase airflow through the nose. There are many different techniques used to reduce the inferior turbinate. The goal of all procedures is to restore the function of the turbinate mucosa while reducing its bulk. Turbinectomy may be performed during septoplasty.

Pathology

Nasal airflow may be impaired by chronic engorgement of the inferior turbinate or congenital malformation of the middle turbinate, called *concha bullosa*.

POSITION:	Supine
INCISION:	Intranasal
PREP AND DRAPING:	Head drape and body sheet
INSTRUMENTS:	Septoplasty set shaver, microdebrider

Technical Points and Discussion

1. ***The patient is prepped and draped.***
   The patient is placed in the supine position with the head on a doughnut headrest and the arms tucked at the sides. General or local anesthesia may be used. The patient is prepped and draped for a nasal procedure.

2. ***Local anesthetic and epinephrine are infiltrated into the mucosa.***
   The surgeon begins by infiltrating the turbinate with a local anesthetic with epinephrine. The nose may be temporarily packed with 1/4 or 1/2 wide gauze packing impregnated with a vasoconstrictive agent such as lidocaine with epinephrine. The surgeon then places a nasal speculum in the nose to retract the nostril and expose the turbinates.

3. ***A section of turbinate is removed through a mucosal incision.***
   A #15 blade is used to make an incision into the mucosa at the anterior border of the inferior turbinate. The mucosa is elevated from the underlying bone with a Freer or Cottle elevator. A portion of the bone is removed with a Wilde tissue forceps. The mucosa may be closed with 3-0 chromic suture.

TURBINATE REDUCTION

If a turbinate reduction is planned, a sharp, two-prong bipolar electrode (ESU), sometimes called a *turbinate bipolar,* is inserted into the turbinate and activated for several seconds, causing desiccation of the tissue. The surgeon also may use coblation, which uses radiofrequency energy to desiccate the turbinate. This will result in physical shrinkage of the turbinates, allowing greater flow of air. The nasal cavity is packed as necessary to absorb drainage.

SEPTOPLASTY

A septoplasty is surgical manipulation of the septum to return it to the correct anatomical position or to gain access to the sphenoid sinus for removal of a pituitary tumor.

Pathology

Septal deformity may be caused by trauma, infection, neoplasm, or birth trauma. It may contribute to nasal obstruction, disrupted sleep patterns, headaches, and cosmetic deformities. Septoplasty may be performed with other procedures, such as rhinoplasty or sinus surgery.

POSITION:	Supine
INCISION:	Intranasal/submucosa
PREP AND DRAPING:	Skin prep is omitted. Head drape and body sheet
INSTRUMENTS:	Septoplasty set

Technical Points and Discussion

1. ***The patient is prepped and draped.***
   The patient is placed in the supine position with the head on a doughnut headrest and the arms tucked at the sides. General anesthesia or local anesthesia with monitored intravenous sedation may be used. Before the patient is prepped and draped, the surgeon instills the nose and turbinates with a local anesthetic (1% lidocaine with epinephrine 1:100,000) and using cotton balls soaked in a vasoconstrictive agent (e.g., adrenaline 1:1000, Afrin, or a local anesthetic with epinephrine as described earlier). The patient is then prepped and draped for a nasal procedure.

2. ***The nasal septum is mobilized.***
   The surgeon removes the nasal packs and inserts a nasal speculum. An incision is made in the nasal septum below the obstruction with a #15 blade. Small tenotomy scissors are used to gently dissect the membranous nasal septum and expose the cartilaginous portion of the septum. The septum is raised from the underlying tissue with a Freer or Cottle elevator.

3. ***Deviated tissue is remolded.***
   With the nasal septum free, the surgeon removes the deviated bone with a 4-mm chisel and a small mallet. The fractured portions of the septum are grasped with a Takahashi forceps and removed. The incision is closed with 4-0 chromic suture, and internal nasal splints are positioned bilaterally to stabilize the septum. These are sutured to the membranous septum with 3-0 nonabsorbable suture.

OPEN RHINOPLASTY

Rhinoplasty is remodeling of the nose to improve function or appearance, or both. This is a commonly performed procedure that can be approached two ways—open surgery, explained here, and closed or submucosal resection. In open surgery, the skin and fascia layer of the outer nasal tissues are lifted off the cartilage and bone for direct exposure and remodeling.

Pathology

Alterations in nasal appearance may be due to genetics, ethnicity, and trauma. During the presurgical consultation, the surgeon assesses the patient's expressed desire for a specific outcome. Attention is paid to skin thickness, dorsal height, length, asymmetry, tip definition and shape, and any specific deformities such as a dorsal bump.

POSITION:	Supine
INCISION:	Nasal
PREP AND DRAPING:	Face with head drape
INSTRUMENTS:	Rhinoplasty set, bipolar ESU

Technical Points and Discussion

1. ***The patient is prepped.***
   The patient is placed in the supine position with the arms tucked at the sides. The face is prepped and draped using a head drape and body sheet. Skin markings are then made in the columella, extending intranasally on both sides.

2. ***The columella is incised and the incision carried into the mucosal tissue.***
   A skin incision is made in the thinnest part of the columella with a #15 knife. The surgeon inserts a double-prong, round-tipped skin hook and elevates the dome of the nose. The incision is then carried intranasally along the cartilage border.

3. ***The columnar incision skin flap is developed.***
   The surgeon develops the skin flap over the dome of the nose using curved iris or Stevens tenotomy scissors. As the flap is developed, the skin over the dome of the nose can be lifted completely from the underlying cartilage and nasal bone. An Aufricht nasal retractor is used to lift the skin flap up to the nasal bone.

4. ***The dorsal cartilage is reduced.***
   With the skin flap fully developed, the surgeon reduces the upper nasal cartilage (UNC) using Foman scissors or a #15 blade. The scrub should keep any resulting slivers of tissue in case they are needed later in the procedure. The bony hump is reduced using an osteotome or rasp. This may leave a gap in the two nasal bones, called an *open roof* deformity.

5. ***Bilateral osteotomies are performed.***
   To close the open roof deformity, the nasal bones are broken on each side using a fine osteotome. The bones are then brought together manually by the application of pressure on both sides.

6. ***The nasal tip is modified.***
   The nasal tip is modified, exposing the crural cartilage, and both sides are trimmed using iris scissors. Sutures may also be placed to approximate the two structures, which results in a narrower tip. If sutures are placed, size 5-0 monofilament suture is used. The tip may also be rotated to correct a hook tip using sutures.

7. ***The incisions are closed and dressed.***
   The nasal cavity may be packed using Vaseline gauze or Telfa. Interior splints may be used to support the septum. The mucosal incisions are closed using size 5-0 synthetic absorbable suture. The columellar incision is closed using monofilament synthetic sutures. Steri-Strips and an exterior splint are placed over the nose. Technical points are shown in Fig. 26.27.

   Packing is normally removed within 48 hours. Splints are removed in 4 to 7 days.

An excellent video of a rhinoplasty procedure can be viewed at https://www.csurgeries.com/video/surgical-treatment-nasal-tip-hemangioma-using-open-rhinoplasty-approach/.

TONSILLECTOMY

Tonsillectomy is performed to reduce the frequency of ear, nose, and throat infection. During the procedure, the mouth is held open using a retractor, which is attached to the Mayo stand tray. Until the 1980s, tonsillectomy was performed mainly using "cold" technique, which features sharp dissection. Now a number of different energies can be used for dissection, including radiofrequency, electrodissection, harmonic scalpel, coblation, and laser. The following description covers the basic anatomical progression of the procedure.

Pathology

Tonsillectomy is indicated for several different diseases. Among the most common is chronic infection, **hypertrophy** (enlargement). Recurrent tonsillitis, chronic tonsillitis, or peritonsillar abscess can lead to hypertrophy, causing sleep apnea, and airway obstruction.

POSITION:	Supine with a rolled towel under the shoulders
INCISION:	Peritonsillar
PREP AND DRAPING:	Skin prep is omitted; a head drape and body drape are used
INSTRUMENTS:	Tonsillectomy set

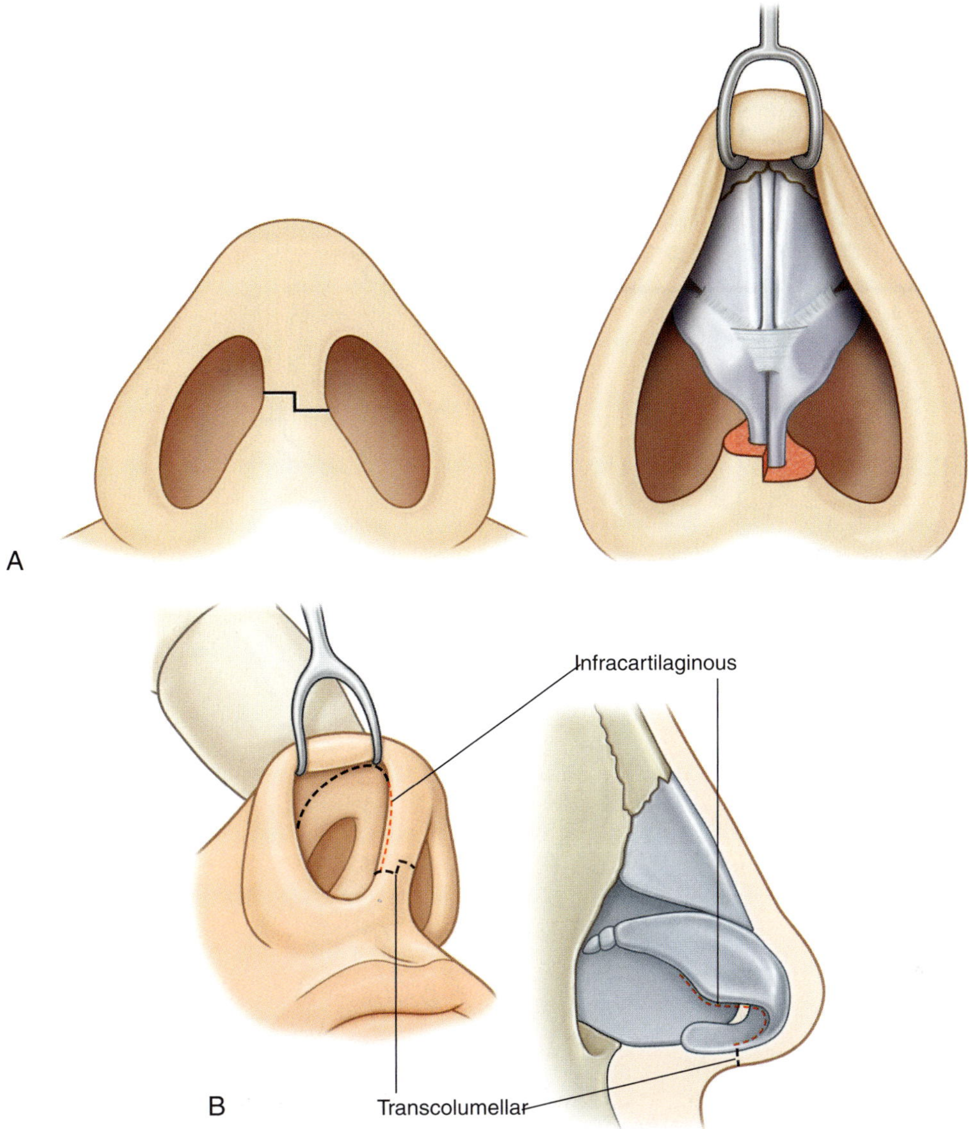

FIG. 26.27 Open rhinoplasty. *Blue shading* indicates cartilage, and bone is shown in *tan*. *Green* indicates grafting material. (A) A midcolumnar incision is made and the hood of the nose retracted upward with a double prong retractor. (B) A separate incision is started inside the naris and connected to the first incision.

Technical Points and Discussion

The patient is placed in the supine position with a doughnut headrest and a shoulder roll, and the arms are tucked at the side. General anesthesia is administered so that the airway can be supported by endotracheal intubation. The patient is rotated 90 degrees to give the surgeon full access to the head.

1. ***The Crowe-Davis or McIvor mouth gag, including tongue blade, is inserted into the mouth and attached to the Mayo stand.***
   A Crowe-Davis or McIvor retractor is inserted into the oral cavity and secured to the edge of the Mayo stand. This is mechanical retraction, not under direct control of the assistant, surgeon, or scrub. After the retractor has been positioned in the mouth, it is attached to the Mayo stand. This holds the jaw open and provides access to the throat.

IMPORTANT TO KNOW *When the retractor has been secured, the Mayo stand must not be moved or jarred, because this can cause injury. During a tonsillectomy, suction must be available at all times.*

2. ***A peritonsillar incision is made.***
   The surgeon grasps the tonsil with a White tonsil forceps or curved Allis clamp and retracts it toward the midline. A peritonsillar incision is made with the ESU or a #12 blade. The initial incision exposes the tonsillar capsule. The tonsil is separated from the underlying muscle and tonsillar fossa (tonsil bed) with an energy device (e.g., electrosurgical, harmonic scalpel) or with Metzenbaum scissors. Bleeders are managed using the device, or they may require clamping and ligation. Note: Some techniques may require the use of a Hurd pillar and tonsil retractor to expose the tonsillar fossa (refer to laryngeal and pharyngeal instruments).

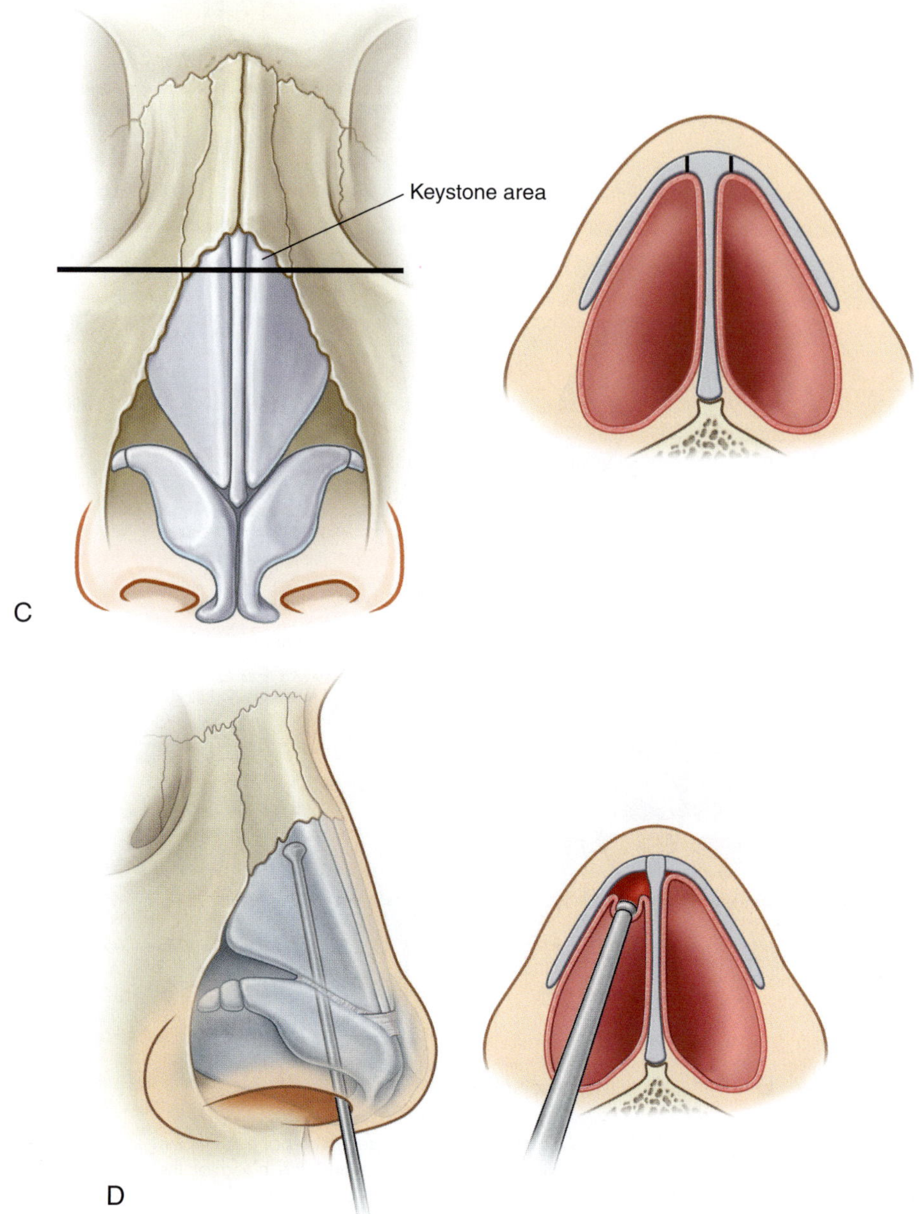

FIG. 26.27, cont'd (C) The nasal skin is elevated from the bone with a Joseph type elevator, and a rasp is used to remove a dorsal hump. (D) The cartilage is dissected away from the mucous tissue layers. The cartilage can then be trimmed with scissors. The tissue is retained for grafting.

3. ***The tonsil pillar is severed.***
   Once the tonsil has been separated from the fossa, only the pillar remains. This is severed using the electrosurgical unit. Throughout the procedure, the assistant uses suction to remove smoke from the oral cavity and to remove blood and oral secretions. The tonsils are kept as separate specimens and identified as right and left.

4. ***Bleeding is controlled.***
   Bleeding from the fossa may be persistent after tonsillectomy. Large vessels are clamped with Schnidt clamps and ligated with 3-0 absorbable suture, or suture ligatures may be used. Tonsil sponges are placed in the tonsil fossa to control bleeding. The oral cavity is irrigated with warm saline, and a final assessment of the operative site is made. The tension of the retractor is then released.

During emergence after tonsillectomy, the patient may experience gagging and "bucking" related to blood and other throat secretions. This can quickly develop into an airway emergency. The scrub should maintain all instruments, including suction, ESU, and retractors, until the patient has been taken to the postanesthesia care unit. Bleeding is a primary concern after a tonsillectomy. Instruments must remain available for immediate use until the patient has been extubated and transported to the postanesthesia care unit, where immediate surgical care is available in case of postoperative bleeding after extubation. See Fig. 26.28 for technical points.

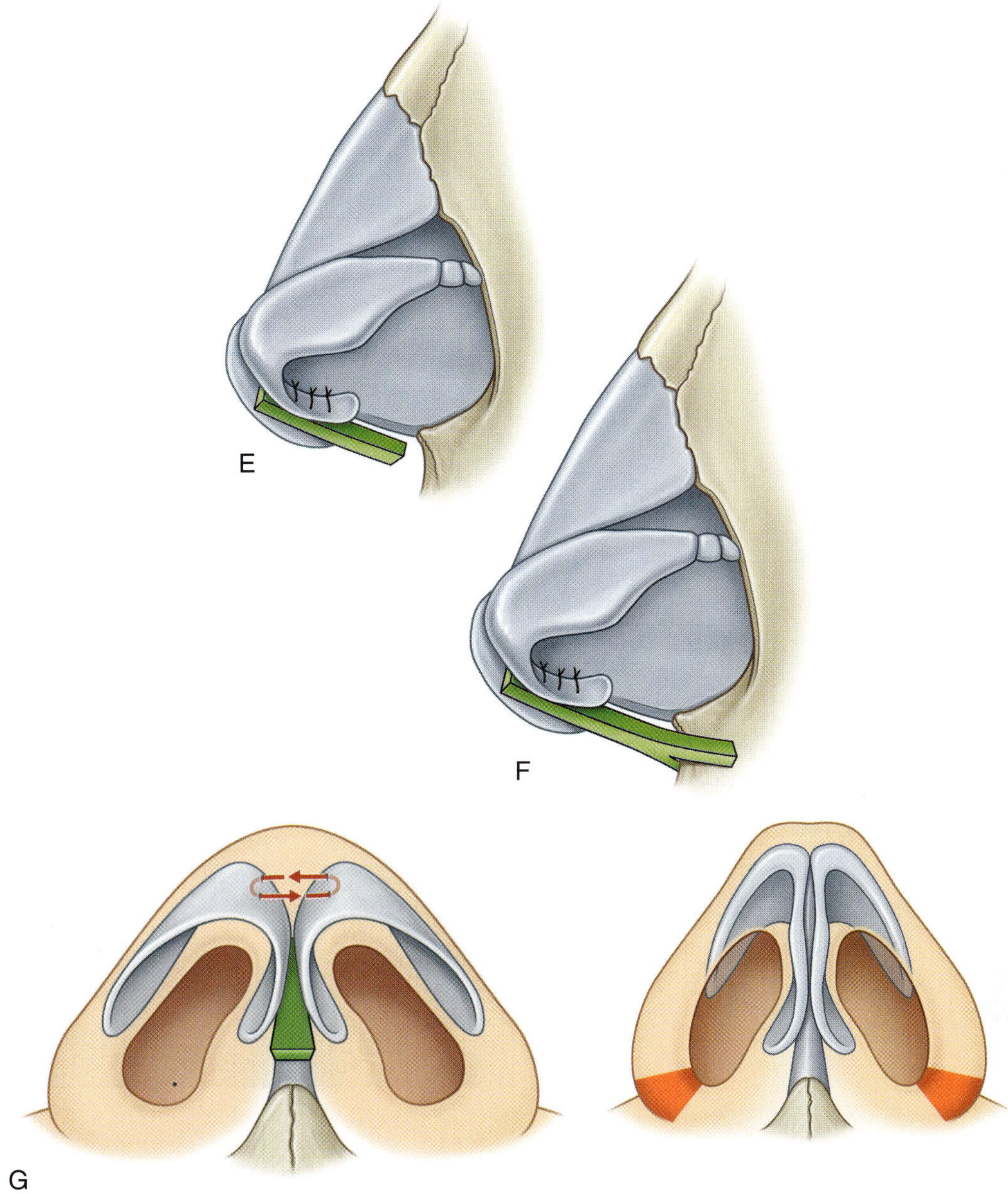

FIG. 26.27, cont'd (E) A columnar strut graft may be used (shown in *green*). (F) The two nasal cartilage tips are sutured together. (G) Wedges (shown in *red*) are removed from the alar to reduce flaring. (From Neligan P, Buck D, eds. *Core Procedures in Plastic Surgery*. St Louis: Elsevier; 2019.)

ADENOIDECTOMY

An adenoidectomy is the surgical removal of the adenoids.

Pathology

The primary reasons for an adenoidectomy are chronic infection and obstruction caused by hypertrophy of the tissue. This often leads to obstruction of the eustachian tube and chronic otitis media. Enlarged adenoids may also contribute to upper airway obstruction, resulting in snoring and sleep apnea. Children are affected more often than adults because the tissue naturally atrophies during adolescence. Adenoidectomy often is performed during tympanostomy and insertion of myringotomy tubes or tonsillectomy. Like tonsillectomy, energy instruments have replaced cold dissection in many cases. However, traditional adenoid curettes are still used by some surgeons.

POSITION:	Supine
INCISION:	None
PREP AND DRAPING:	Skin prep is omitted; a head and body drape are used
INSTRUMENTS:	Tonsillectomy and adenoidectomy set; Robinson catheter size 12 or 14 Fr

Technical Points and Discussion

1. ***The patient is prepped and draped.***
The patient is placed in the supine position, and a doughnut headrest and shoulder roll are used. The arms are tucked at the sides. General anesthesia is administered so that the airway can be supported by endotracheal intubation. The

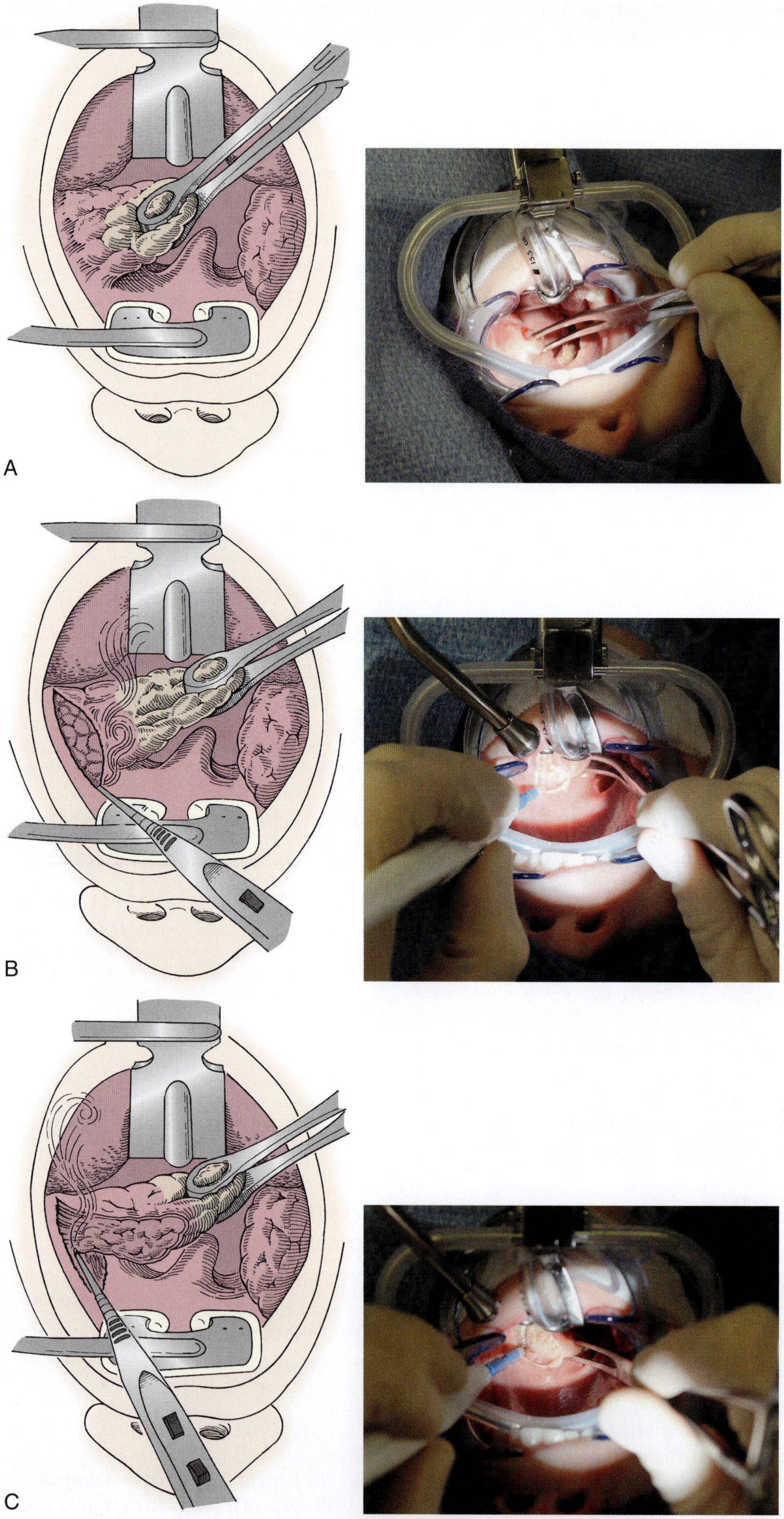

FIG. 26.28 Tonsillectomy. (A) The mouth gag is positioned. (B and C) The tonsil is grasped with forceps or a tenaculum, and the ESU is used to make the peritonsillar incision. A #12 knife blade and Freer elevator may also be used for this step. The ESU can be used to free the tonsil, or a snare may be used. (D and E) The dissection is continued within the tonsil fossa and bleeding vessels coagulated using the ESU. (From Myers E. *Operative Otolaryngology: Head and Neck Surgery*. 8th ed. Philadelphia: Elsevier; 2018.)

patient is draped as for a tonsillectomy. A Crowe-Davis or McIvor retractor is inserted into the oral cavity and secured on the edge of the Mayo stand, as described previously. All precautions regarding the retractor are observed.

2. ***The soft palate is retracted.***
The surgeon retracts the palate using a straight (Robinson) catheter (12 or 14 Fr) inserted through the nose and brought out through the mouth. The ends of the catheter are secured with a clamp. Next, the surgeon uses a dental mirror to inspect the adenoids. Dipping the mirror in antifog solution helps to keep the mirror clear.

3. ***The adenoid tissue is removed.***
If the adenoid tissue is substantial, the surgeon uses an adenoid curette to remove it. The size of the curette depends on the size of the nasopharynx. Adenoid tissue may also be treated with suction ESU. After the tissue has been removed, the oral cavity and nasopharynx are irrigated with an Asepto syringe. The surgeon again uses the mirror to ensure that bleeding has stopped and that all of the adenoid tissue has been removed. Tension is carefully released from the mouth gag, and the catheter and mouth gag are removed. Refer to Fig. 26.29 for patient positioning showing the mouth retractor system and retraction of the soft palate during the procedure.

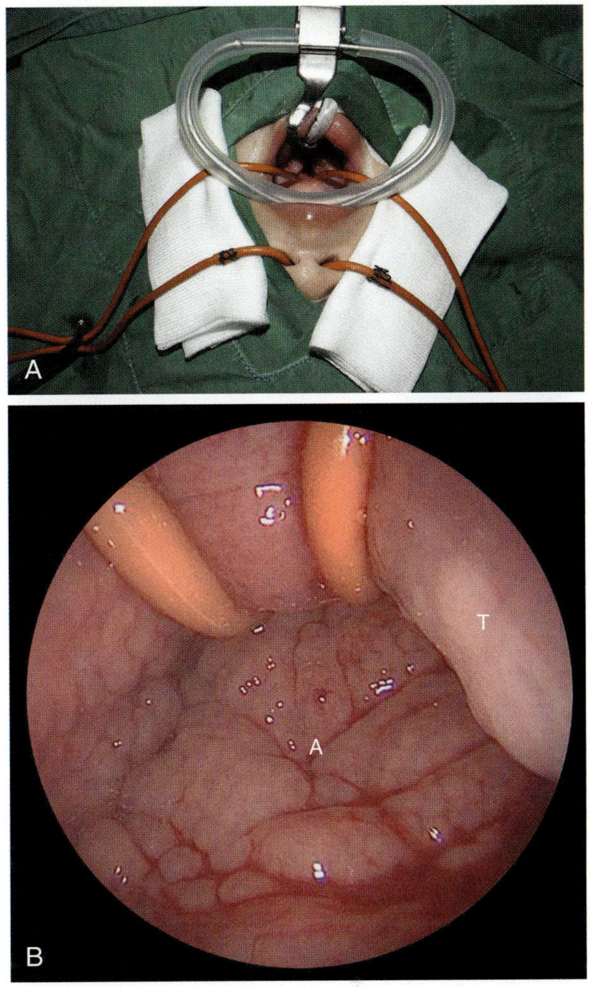

FIG. 26.29 Adenoidectomy. (A) The McIvor mouth gag has been positioned and attached to the Mayo tray. Note that red Robinson catheters are used to retract the soft palate. (B) Combination suction-electrosurgical unit used in adenoidectomy. (From Myers E. *Operative Otolaryngology: Head and Neck Surgery*. 8th ed. Philadelphia: Elsevier; 2018.)

UVULOPALATOPHARYNGOPLASTY

Reconstruction of the uvula and oropharynx, or *uvulopalatopharyngoplasty* (UPP), is performed to reduce and tighten oropharyngeal tissue.

Pathology

Enlarged or redundant oropharyngeal mucosa may collapse on inspiration during the deep stages of sleep as muscles lose tone. This leads to high intrathoracic pressure as air is pulled through the obstruction, causing sleep apnea or interruption of deep sleep. Obstructive sleep apnea can cause a variety of sleep disorders, ranging from sleep deprivation to dangerous pulmonary and cardiovascular complications, including hypertension, cardiac arrhythmias, and neurological dysfunction.

POSITION:	Supine
INCISION:	Oral
PREP AND DRAPING:	Skin prep is omitted. Head and body drapes are used
INSTRUMENTS:	Tonsillectomy and adenoidectomy set; Robinson catheter 12 Fr or 14 Fr; suction-electrosurgical unit

Technical Points and Discussion

1. ***The patient is prepped and draped.***
The patient is positioned as for a tonsillectomy. General anesthesia is used to protect the airway. A tracheotomy setup should be available in case of difficult intubation. The patient then is draped as for a tonsillectomy. Prepping is unnecessary.

2. ***A tonsillectomy is performed.***
A Crowe-Davis or McIvor retractor is inserted and secured to the Mayo stand. The tonsils are removed as necessary, as described previously.

3. ***The uvula and a portion of the soft palate are excised.***
After the tonsillectomy, the uvula is grasped with an Allis clamp and retracted posteriorly. The surgeon excises the redundant soft palate and uvula with the ESU.

4. ***The incision is closed.***
The incision is approximated with 2-0 synthetic absorbable suture. The oropharynx is irrigated, and any residual bleeding is controlled with the ESU. The tension on the retractor then is released. The tonsils and uvula are preserved as separate specimens and labeled appropriately.

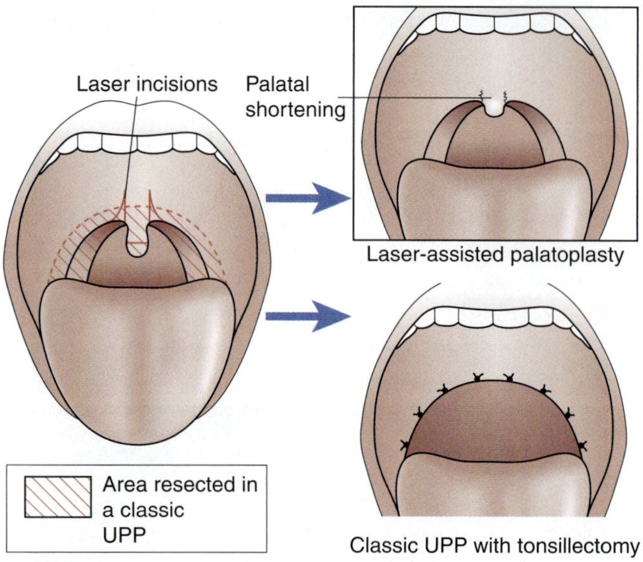

FIG. 26.30 Uvulopalatopharyngoplasty (UPP). Surgical options for shortening the palate in the treatment of upper airway obstruction. (From Dhillon RS, East CA. *Ear, Nose, and Throat and Head and Neck Surgery*. 3rd ed. Edinburgh: Churchill Livingstone; 2006.)

Instruments are kept for immediate use until the patient has been transported to the postanesthesia care unit because of the risk of bleeding after extubation. Selected patients remain in the hospital overnight to ensure that no airway complications arise. Fig. 26.30 shows the incisions and closure.

LARYNGOSCOPY

Laryngoscopy is endoscopic assessment of the larynx. Tissue specimens are removed for pathological examination.

Pathology

Laryngeal lesions include neoplasms, foreign bodies, papilloma, laryngeal polyps, leukoplakia, and laryngeal web. A **papilloma** is a benign proliferative overgrowth of epithelium. Leukoplakia is a benign lesion of the laryngeal epithelium.

Technical Points and Discussion

INDIRECT LARYNGOSCOPY

1. ***The patient is prepped and draped.***
   The patient is placed either in the sitting position or supine with a doughnut headrest. If the patient can cooperate throughout the procedure, no anesthetic is necessary. However, sedation or general anesthesia may be needed. A plain sheet is positioned over the upper body.

2. ***The larynx is assessed using a dental mirror.***
   After examining the mouth, the surgeon retracts the patient's tongue manually with a gauze sponge. The surgeon then positions an examination mirror against the uvula to inspect the larynx, base of the tongue, and pharyngeal wall. The patient may be asked to speak (**phonation**), if possible, so that the surgeon can observe the larynx in motion. The mirror then is removed.

DIRECT LARYNGOSCOPY

1. ***The patient is positioned.***
   General anesthesia is administered. The patient is positioned supine with a shoulder roll. The head is stabilized on a doughnut headrest. The operating table is tilted into reverse Trendelenburg to allow full access to the operative area.

2. ***The rigid laryngoscope is introduced.***
   The surgeon introduces a tooth guard to protect the teeth from injury during the procedure. The rigid laryngoscope is introduced on the right side of the mouth and advanced into the upper airway.

3. ***The laryngoscope is advanced.***
   Oral secretions are suctioned with an open-tip or a velvet-tip laryngeal suction device. The scrub assists by guiding the instruments into the working channel of the laryngoscope and advancing them a short distance into the scope. The surgeon then continues to advance the scope to the level of the larynx and vocal cords. The surgeon also examines the subglottic region and the upper portion of the trachea.

4. ***Biopsies are taken.***
   Any suspicious tissue is biopsied with a long, cupped biopsy forceps. The scrub receives biopsy tissue and ensures that all specimens are kept separate and identified by the exact location and side. *It is extremely important that all tissue be collected from the tips of the biopsy instrument and carefully labeled.*

5. ***Hemostasis is maintained.***
   Bleeding is controlled by applying flat pledgets soaked in a vasoconstrictive agent (e.g., adrenaline, Afrin, or cocaine). The scope is gently withdrawn after all specimens have been removed and bleeding has been controlled. Instruments used in laryngoscopy are shown in Fig. 26.31.

TRACHEOTOMY/TRACHEOSTOMY

A tracheotomy or tracheostomy is performed to provide a patent airway. The procedure may take place in the emergency department, ICU, or operating room.

Pathology

Tracheostomy is indicated for patients who require emergency or elective airway management for prolonged ventilator dependence or acute or chronic upper airway obstruction. Upper airway obstruction may be the result of mechanical obstruction, redundant pharyngeal mucosa (causing sleep apnea), a tumor, foreign body, infection, or secretions. Obstruction also may be caused by congenital, neurological, or traumatic conditions. Such obstructions can include a foreign body in the larynx or hypopharynx, acute laryngotracheal bronchitis in children, laryngeal edema, or some other condition that obstructs the airway.

POSITION:	Supine
INCISION:	Neck
PREP AND DRAPING:	Neck
INSTRUMENTS:	Tracheotomy set with tube and kit

Technical Points and Discussion

1. ***The patient is prepped and draped.***
The patient is placed in the supine position with the head on a doughnut headrest, with the neck hyperextended and the arms tucked at the sides. General anesthesia is used. The patient is prepped and draped for a neck procedure.

2. ***An incision is made over the anterior tracheal wall.***
Using a #15 blade, the surgeon makes an incision to the midline of the neck; the incision may be vertical or horizontal. The skin flaps are elevated with double-prong skin hooks and a #15 blade. With the flaps elevated, the strap muscles are separated in the vertical midline, with a hemostat or the ESU. The isthmus of the thyroid also may be divided to allow visualization of the anterior tracheal wall. A tracheal hook then is placed into the cricoid cartilage to elevate the trachea.

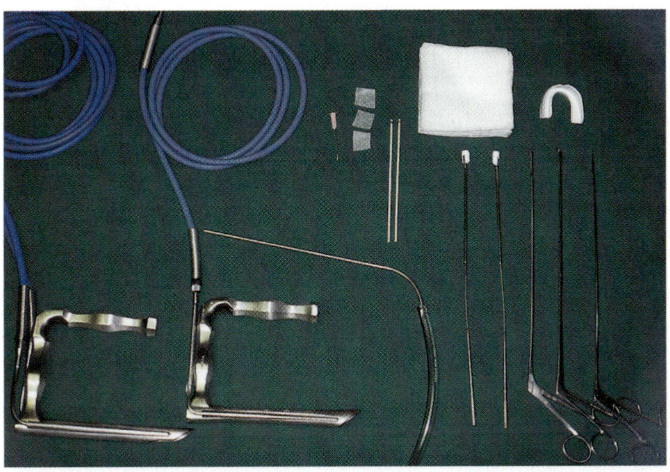

FIG. 26.31 Direct laryngoscopy instruments. *Left to right,* Rigid laryngoscopes, suction tips, sponge carriers, and forceps for biopsy. (From Shah JP, Patel SG. *Head and Neck Surgery and Oncology.* 3rd ed. London: Mosby; 2003.)

3. ***A tracheal incision is made, usually between the third and fourth tracheal rings.***
An incision is made into the trachea between the second and third or third and fourth tracheal rings with a #15 blade. In adults, the tracheal incision is vertical and may include removal of an anterior square of tracheal cartilage. In infants, the tracheal incision is made vertically, and no tracheal cartilage is removed. The inferior edge of the trachea may be anchored to the skin using absorbable sutures, size 3-0.

4. ***The tracheotomy tube is inserted.***
After the tracheal incision is made, the anesthesia provider withdraws the endotracheal (ET) tube to the level just above the tracheal incision. A tracheostomy tube then is placed into the tracheal incision with the obturator in place.

When patient ventilation through the tracheostomy tube has been established, the ET tube is completely removed. Bleeding is controlled with the ESU.

5. ***The tracheostomy tube is secured to the skin.***
The tracheostomy tube may be sutured to the skin with 2-0 nonabsorbable suture (e.g., polypropylene or silk). Drain sponges and tracheostomy ties are then applied. The obturator must be sent along with the patient after surgery. Fig. 26.32 shows an assortment of tracheostomy tubes, and the procedure for tracheostomy is illustrated in Fig. 26.33.

IMPORTANT TO KNOW *The obturator of the tracheostomy tube is kept with the patient as long as the tracheal tube is in place. If the tube becomes dislodged or is traumatically removed, the obturator is needed to replace the tube.*

SECTION III: THE NECK

The neck is extremely complex and highly vascular. It is a critical area of the body as it contains major nerves, blood vessels,

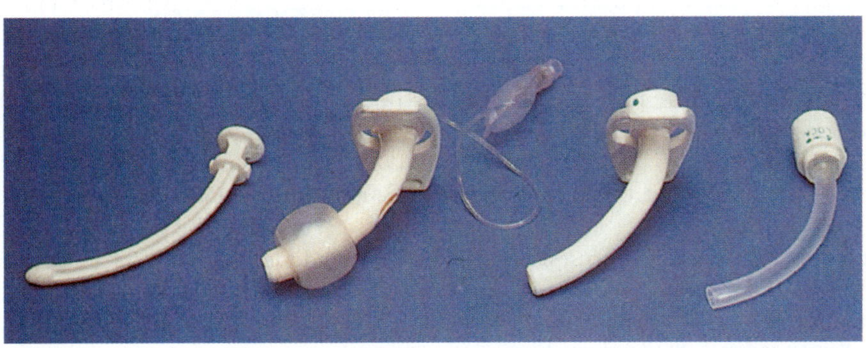

FIG. 26.32 Tracheostomy tubes. *Left to right,* Obturator, cuffed fenestrated outer tube, uncuffed nonfenestrated outer tube, inner tube. (From Dhillon RS, East CA. *Ear, Nose, and Throat and Head and Neck Surgery.* 3rd ed. Edinburgh: Churchill Livingstone; 2006.)

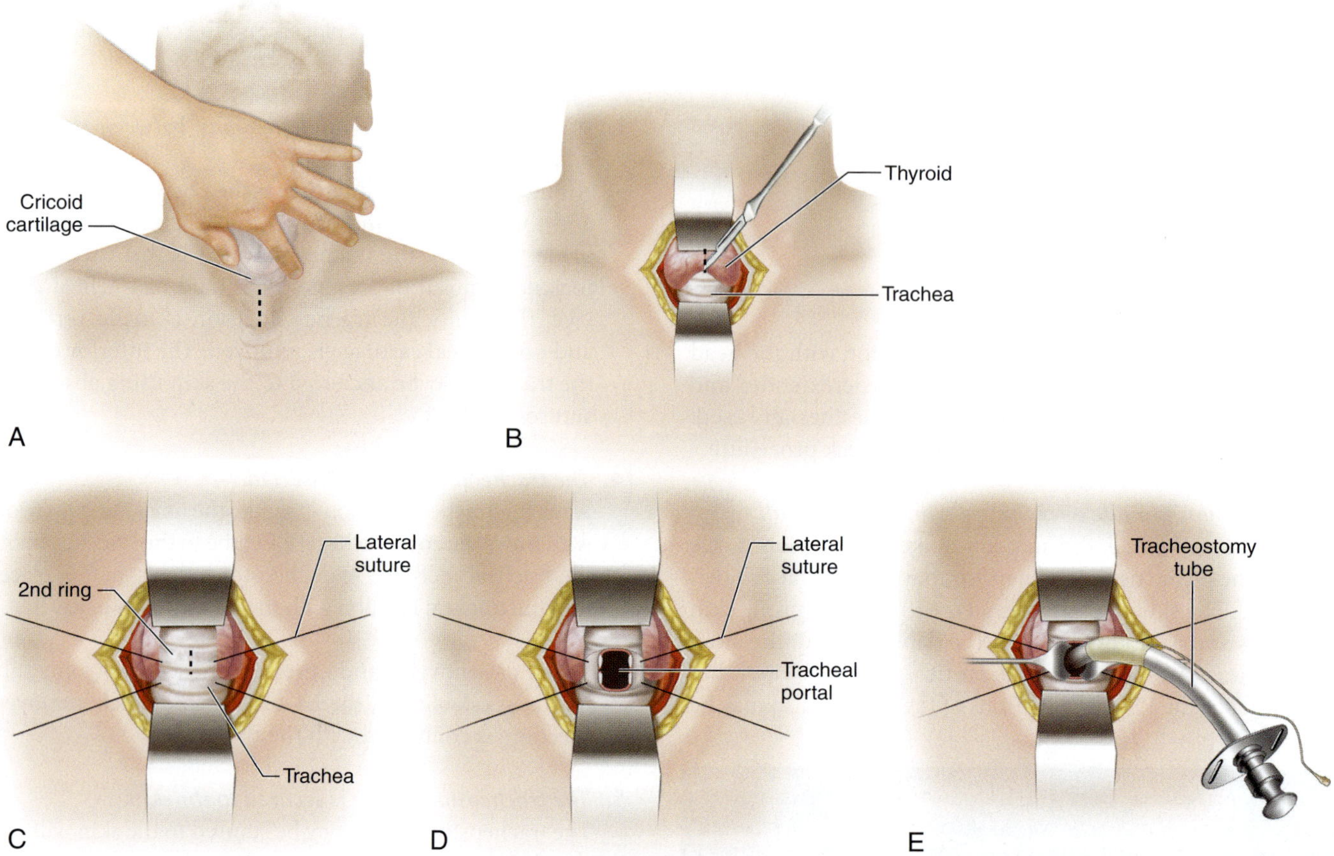

FIG. 26.33 Tracheostomy. (A) A vertical incision is made over the cricothyroid cartilage. (B) The incision is carried deeper by hemostats or ESU. (C) Traction sutures are placed on each side of the exposed trachea. (D) A vertical incision is made across two tracheal rings. (E) A tracheal dilator and hook may be used to insert the tracheal tube. The obturator is removed and the balloon inflated. (From Cioffi W, et al. *Atlas of Trauma Emergency Surgical Techniques. Philadelphia*: Elsevier; 2014.)

the airway, and a significant network of lymph tissue, which drains from the head. Surgical dissection of the region requires advanced technical skills and knowledge of the anatomy. Surgery of the neck most often is performed to remove or debulk tumors arising from the mouth or upper respiratory system and for surgery of the salivary and thyroid glands.

SURGICAL ANATOMY

NERVES, VASCULAR SUPPLY, AND MUSCLES OF THE NECK

Each side of the neck is divided into two large triangles separated by the sternocleidomastoid muscle (SCM), which attaches at the superior end to the mastoid process below the ear and inferiorly to the sternum and clavicle. Below the SCM is the carotid sheath, which contains the carotid artery and its bifurcation, the internal jugular vein, and the vagus nerve.

The spinal accessory nerve (cranial nerve XI) crosses the posterior triangle of the neck behind the SCM. The anterior cervical triangle is located anterior to the SCM. The digastric muscle crosses this triangle. Finally, the submandibular triangle occurs above the digastric muscle. This section contains the submandibular gland and the hypoglossal nerve (cranial nerve XII).

The space below the digastric muscle contains an important structure, the carotid sheath. The larynx, pharynx, thyroid gland, and parathyroid glands lie on the medial side of the carotid sheath.

Cervical lymph nodes are located throughout the anterior neck. The thoracic duct, which connects the body's entire lymphatic system to the vascular system, is located in the left lower neck behind the carotid sheath, where it inserts at the junction of the left internal jugular vein and subclavian vein. Structures of the neck are shown in Fig. 26.34.

SALIVARY GLANDS

There are three pairs of salivary glands: the parotid, submandibular, and sublingual salivary glands. Many minor salivary glands are found throughout the oral cavity and pharynx. The largest of the glands, the parotid gland, is situated over the mandible, anterior to the ear. It extends anteriorly to the masseter muscle. The tail of the parotid gland extends below the mandible into the upper neck. The parotid duct drains into the mouth and the cheek opposite the upper second molar. The facial nerve passes through the gland, where it branches and then exits from the anterior aspect.

The submandibular gland is the second largest salivary gland. It is C-shaped and wraps around the lower (inferior)

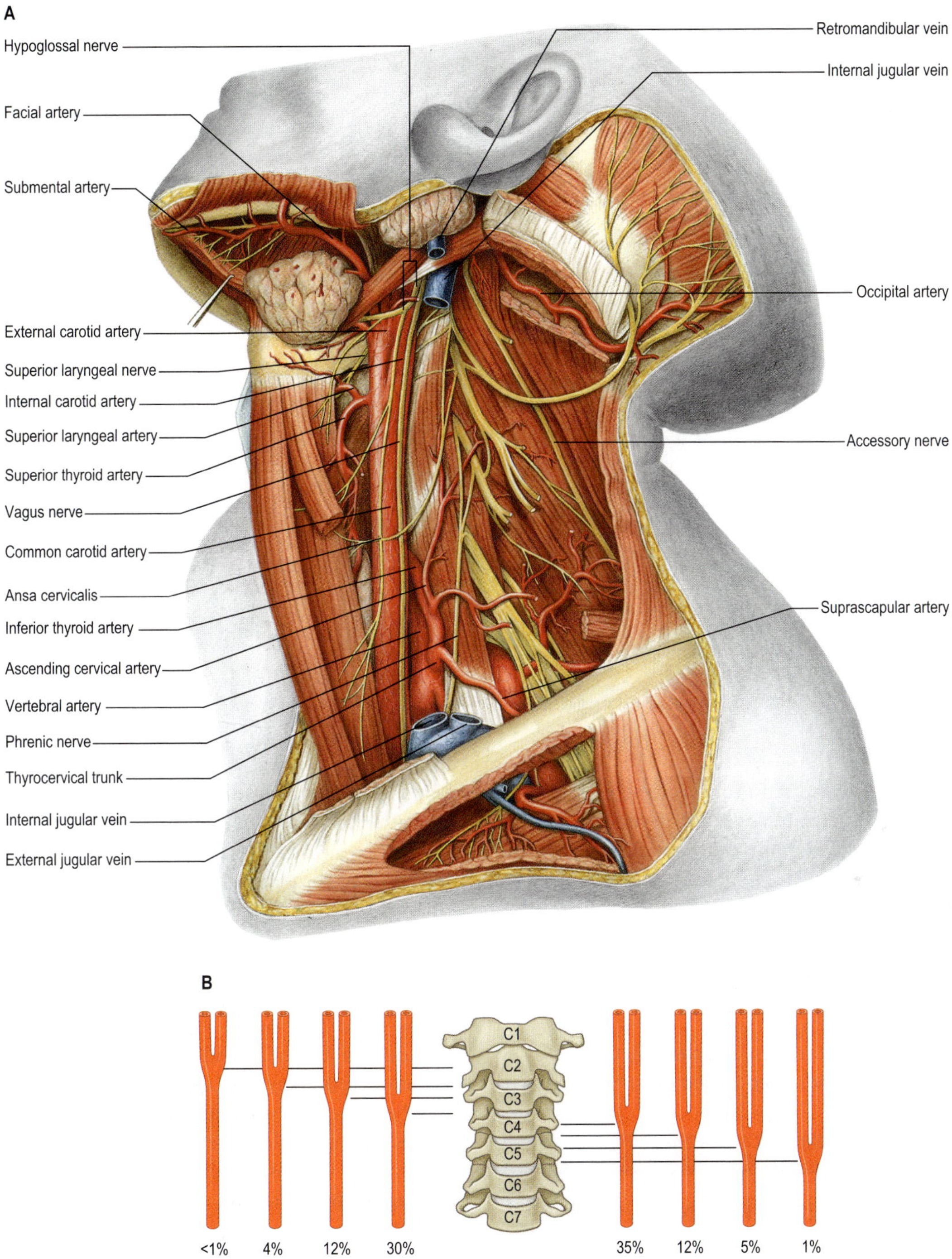

FIG. 26.34 Anatomy of the neck. (From Standring S. *Gray's Anatomy*. 41st ed. St Louis: Elsevier; 2016.)

border of the mandible. The submandibular duct, or Wharton duct, emerges from the deep anterior portion of the gland and drains into the anterior floor of the mouth. A branch of the facial nerve lies within the superficial fascia of the gland. The hypoglossal nerve (cranial nerve XII) and the lingual nerve lie beneath the gland.

The smallest of the salivary glands, the sublingual glands, lie in the floor of the mouth just beneath the mucosa and empty into the oral cavity via multiple small ducts (ducts of Rivinus).

The salivary glands produce saliva, which irrigates the oral cavity and contains enzymes for breaking down simple carbohydrates. Buffers in saliva reduce acidity in the mouth and protect against pathogenic bacteria and demineralization of the teeth. The salivary glands are illustrated in Fig. 26.35.

THYROID GLAND

The thyroid gland is located in the mid-neck and overlies the trachea below the larynx. It has two lobes, which are connected by a central band of thyroid tissue called the *isthmus*. A thin strip of thyroid tissue also projects from the superior edge of the isthmus. The thyroid secretes the

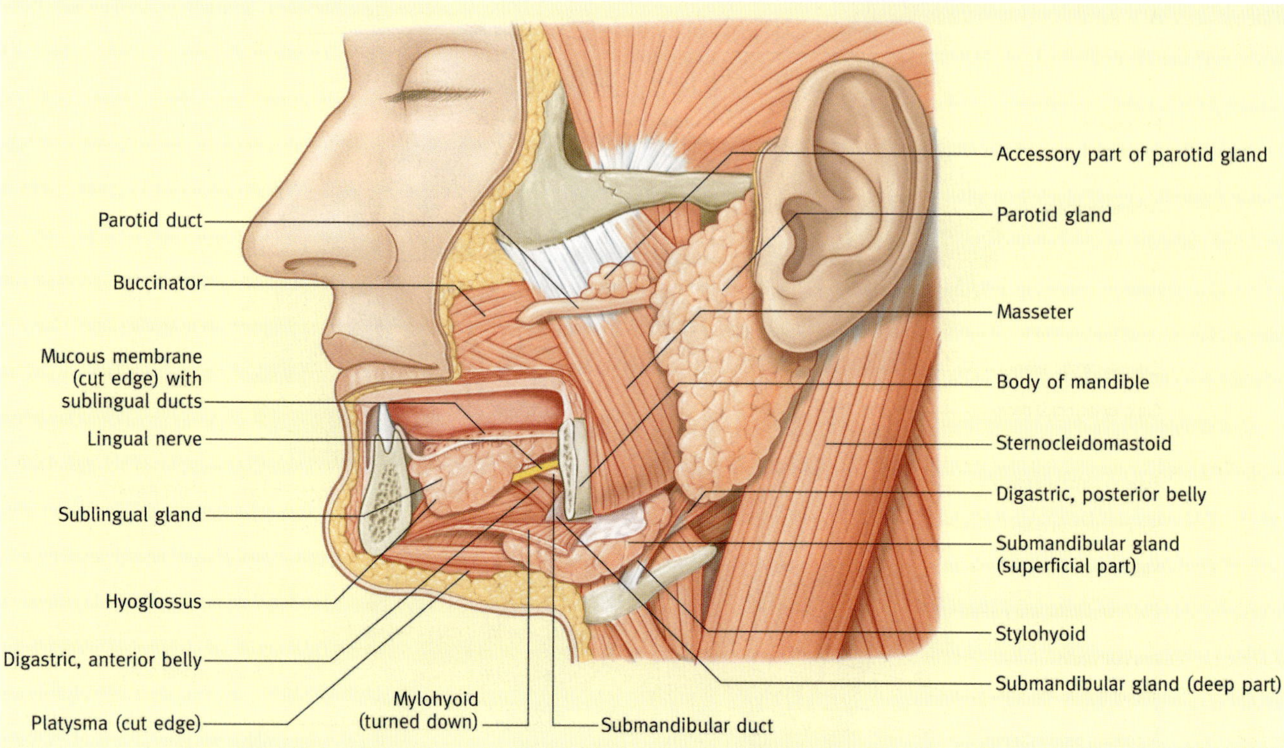

FIG. 26.35 Anatomy of the salivary glands. (From Ellis H. Anatomy of the salivary glands. *Surgery.* 2012;30:1.)

hormones thyroxine (T_4) and triiodothyronine (T_3). These thyroid hormones (THs) are necessary for regulating cell metabolism and growth. Calcitonin, which is also secreted by the thyroid, is necessary for calcium regulation. The parathyroid glands are situated within the lobes of the thyroid. These small glands produce parathyroid hormone (PTH), which influences calcium and phosphate levels in the blood.

NOTE Thyroidectomy *is discussed in Chapter 22, General Surgery, as it is commonly performed by the general surgeon.*

CASE PLANNING

POSITIONING THE PATIENT FOR NECK SURGERY

Procedures of the neck are performed with the patient in the supine position with the head stabilized on a doughnut headrest. The arms are secured at the patient's sides or according to the surgeon and anesthesia provider's preference. The neck may be hyperextended for better access; this is achieved by placing a padded roll at the shoulders. The roll must be carefully positioned to prevent compression of the cervical nerves.

DRAPING

Patients undergoing procedures of the neck are draped to exclude the face and to maintain a sterile field. The surgical site is draped with towels, which are secured with towel clips or skin staples. A clear incise drape commonly is used to cover the towels and operative site. The patient then is draped with a split sheet that surrounds the head. It may be helpful to cover the patient's chest with a towel and place a magnetic drape on top of the towel to prevent instruments from dropping to the floor during surgery.

INSTRUMENTS

General surgical instruments are required for procedures of the head and neck. Additional special instruments are included in tracheal and thyroid sets. These include neck retractors and thyroid grasping clamps. Vascular clamps may be added for radical neck procedures. Numerous vital nerves and large blood vessels in the neck require soft retraction with a Penrose drain or surgical vessel loops. Numerous right-angle clamps are needed during extensive neck dissection.

Neck dissection involves a significant risk of injury to peripheral nerves. A peripheral nerve stimulator or nerve monitoring device often is used to prevent this injury. Thyroid instruments may be used in procedures of the neck. These are shown in the Mouth and Throat Instruments section of the Ear, Nasal, Laryngeal, and Pharyngeal Instruments table.

DRESSINGS

Neck dressings vary according to the procedure. Tracheotomy incisions generally are dressed with drain sponges (4×4 gauze that has been split to include the tracheotomy tube) and tracheal ties. Other procedures of the neck may be dressed with Telfa and Tegaderm or 4×4 sponges and tape. After radical neck procedures, a suction drain may be placed in the wound before closure.

MEDICATIONS

The medications most often used in head and neck surgery are local anesthetics and hemostatic agents. Hemostatic agents such as absorbable gelatin matrix and topical thrombin should be available for extensive neck dissection.

SURGICAL PROCEDURES

PAROTIDECTOMY

A parotidectomy is the surgical removal of the parotid gland.

Pathology

A parotidectomy most often is performed for the treatment of a neoplasm. The facial nerve splits the parotid gland into superficial and deep lobes. Disease most often occurs in the superficial lobe and rarely involves the deep lobe. Involvement of the deep lobe usually indicates malignancy. However, most neoplasms of the parotid gland are benign.

POSITION:	Supine
INCISION:	Facial anterior to ear
PREP AND DRAPING:	As for face and thyroid procedures
INSTRUMENTS:	Major general surgery set, plastic surgery set, vessel loops, vessel clips, monopolar and bipolar ESU
POSSIBLE EXTRAS:	Nerve stimulator

Technical Points and Discussion

1. ***The patient is prepped and draped.***
   The patient is positioned and draped for a neck procedure. General anesthesia is required. However, neuromuscular blocking agents are not used to allow stimulation of the facial nerve for identification.

2. ***A skin incision is made anterior to the ear.***
   The incision begins just anterior to the helix of the ear and extends downward to the tragus. If necessary, the incision can be extended for greater access. The surgeon creates skin flaps by dissecting the subcutaneous layer with Metzenbaum scissors. The skin flaps are retracted with skin hooks or rake retractors.

3. ***The facial nerve is identified.***
   The gland is separated from the SCM and the cartilaginous portion of the external auditory canal with Metzenbaum scissors. The facial nerve trunk then is identified. A nerve stimulator may be required to identify the nerve.

   Dissection is continued along the facial nerve branches, either superiorly or inferiorly, with a mosquito clamp and bipolar ESU or McCabe dissector until the superficial portion of the gland is removed. If the deep lobe of the parotid must be excised, the facial nerve is elevated and retracted with vessel loops. With the facial nerve retracted, the facial nerve branches are elevated off the underlying deep lobe of the parotid gland with a hemostat and bipolar ESU.

   Dissection continues using the same technique to separate the gland from the underlying muscle. Allis clamps are used to grasp the gland and provide countertraction as it is elevated and removed.

4. ***The wound is irrigated and closed.***
   After the gland is removed, the wound is irrigated and a drain is placed. The wound then is closed in layers with absorbable sutures. The skin may be closed with either absorbable or nonabsorbable sutures.

MODIFIED RADICAL NECK DISSECTION

Neck dissection is performed for the removal of a tumor and affected lymph nodes. The traditional radical neck procedure has been almost completely replaced by modifications of the procedure. Three types of neck dissections may be performed, depending on tumor staging. *Radical neck dissection* is the removal of all cervical lymph nodes and surrounding structures, including the spinal accessory nerve, the internal jugular vein, and the SCM. *Modified neck dissection* is the excision of all lymph nodes with the preservation of one or more of the nonlymphatic structures (e.g., spinal accessory nerve, internal jugular vein, or SCM). *Selective neck dissection* is the removal of the upper two-thirds of the cervical lymph nodes and structures with preservation of the neurovascular and musculoskeletal structures.

Pathology

Many head and neck cancers, including malignant tumors of the oral and pharyngeal cavities, cutaneous malignant melanoma, and skin cancer, metastasize to the cervical lymph nodes.

POSITION:	Supine
INCISION:	Neck
PREP AND DRAPING:	Neck and upper thorax
INSTRUMENTS:	Neck dissection instruments, tracheotomy set, vessel loops, vessel clips

Technical Points and Discussion

1. ***The patient is prepped and draped.***
   The patient is placed in the supine position on a doughnut or Mayfield headrest with the affected side of the neck upward. The arms are tucked at the patient's sides, and a

shoulder roll is placed to hyperextend the neck slightly. General anesthesia is used. The patient is prepped, including the face, neck, and chest, and draped for a head and neck procedure.

2. ***The skin is incised and SCM mobilized.***
The skin incision is made with a #15 blade. The incision is extended through the platysma and the ESU. Double-prong skin hooks are used for retraction. Bleeding vessels may be ligated with 2-0 or 3-0 silk ties.

The surgeon mobilizes the SCM using blunt dissection and then retracts it laterally with an Army-Navy retractor. If the SCM is to be sacrificed, it is severed with the ESU. This allows the surgeon to visualize the neurovascular sheath. Dissection continues along the neurovascular sheath to expose the anterior portion of the specimen. This dissection is performed bluntly with hemostats.

3. ***Large veins, arteries, and nerves are identified.***
With the neurovascular sheath exposed, the surgeon identifies the carotid artery, internal jugular vein, and vagus nerve. Silastic vessel loops may be used to provide traction on the structures. The neurovascular sheath is retracted with a Cushing vein retractor. If the internal jugular vein is to be sacrificed, it is double-clamped, transected, and ligated with multiple 2-0 silk ties and 2-0 stick ties.

4. ***The lateral cervical triangle is exposed, and a tracheotomy is performed as needed.***
The surgeon then retracts the SCM anteriorly, exposing the lateral cervical triangle. The subcutaneous tissue is removed with blunt dissection or Metzenbaum scissors. Bleeders are clamped with hemostats and 2-0 silk ties or the ESU. A tracheotomy is performed if necessary. The wound is then irrigated with normal saline. A drain is placed in the wound, and the wound is closed in layers with absorbable suture. Technical points are illustrated in Fig. 26.36.

GLOSSECTOMY

A glossectomy is the removal of the tongue for the treatment of cancer. A partial glossectomy is removal of less than half of the tongue *(hemiglossectomy)*. Simple excision includes primary closure or application of a split-thickness skin graft (STSG) to the anterior tongue. A secondary goal is to ensure that closure of the floor of the mouth prevents a fistula or leakage of saliva from the oral cavity into the neck tissues.

Pathology

The entire neurovascular supply of one side of the tongue passes through the base of the tongue; therefore, if one side of the base of the tongue requires excision, that entire side must be removed. A total glossectomy is the excision of tissue in the anterior two-thirds of the tongue. A pectoralis major myocutaneous (PMC [also called PMMC]) flap or a free flap is constructed to produce a watertight seal. A total glossectomy is almost always combined with a total laryngectomy to treat laryngeal metastasis or problems with aspiration.

POSITION:	Supine with head turned
INCISION:	Neck
PREP AND DRAPING:	Neck
INSTRUMENTS:	Major general surgery set, vascular set, vessel loops, vessel ties, facial fracture instruments, needlepoint and spatula ESU electrodes
POSSIBLE EXTRAS:	Brown dermatome or small disposable dermatome, small power drill, bone plates and screws, power saw with sagittal and reciprocal blades

Technical Points and Discussion: Partial Glossectomy—Primary or STSG Closure

1. ***The patient is prepped and draped.***
The patient is placed in the supine position on a doughnut or Mayfield headrest with the arms tucked at the sides. General anesthesia is used. The patient is prepped and draped for a head and neck procedure.

2. ***A traction suture is placed in the tongue.***
The surgeon grasps the tongue either by using large towel clips at the midline or by suturing the midline with a size 0 silk suture and grasping the ends of the suture with a hemostat. The tongue is pulled anteriorly to expose the affected tissue.

3. ***The tumor is excised and the wound closed.***
The surgeon excises the tumor and a wide margin with the ESU blade or needle tip. The tongue is then closed. If primary closure is possible, the tongue is closed with 3-0 absorbable sutures.

4. ***An STSG is secured over the defect.***
If primary closure is not possible, the defect is closed with an STSG. The graft is sutured into place with 3-0 absorbable suture (refer to Chapter 28).

Technical Points and Discussion: Glossectomy With Mandibulotomy

1. ***The patient is prepped and draped.***
The patient is placed in the supine position on a doughnut or Mayfield headrest with the arms tucked at the sides. General anesthesia is used. Often, a tracheotomy has been performed or will be performed before the glossectomy. The patient is prepped and draped for a head and neck procedure, including the chest in case a PMC flap is needed.

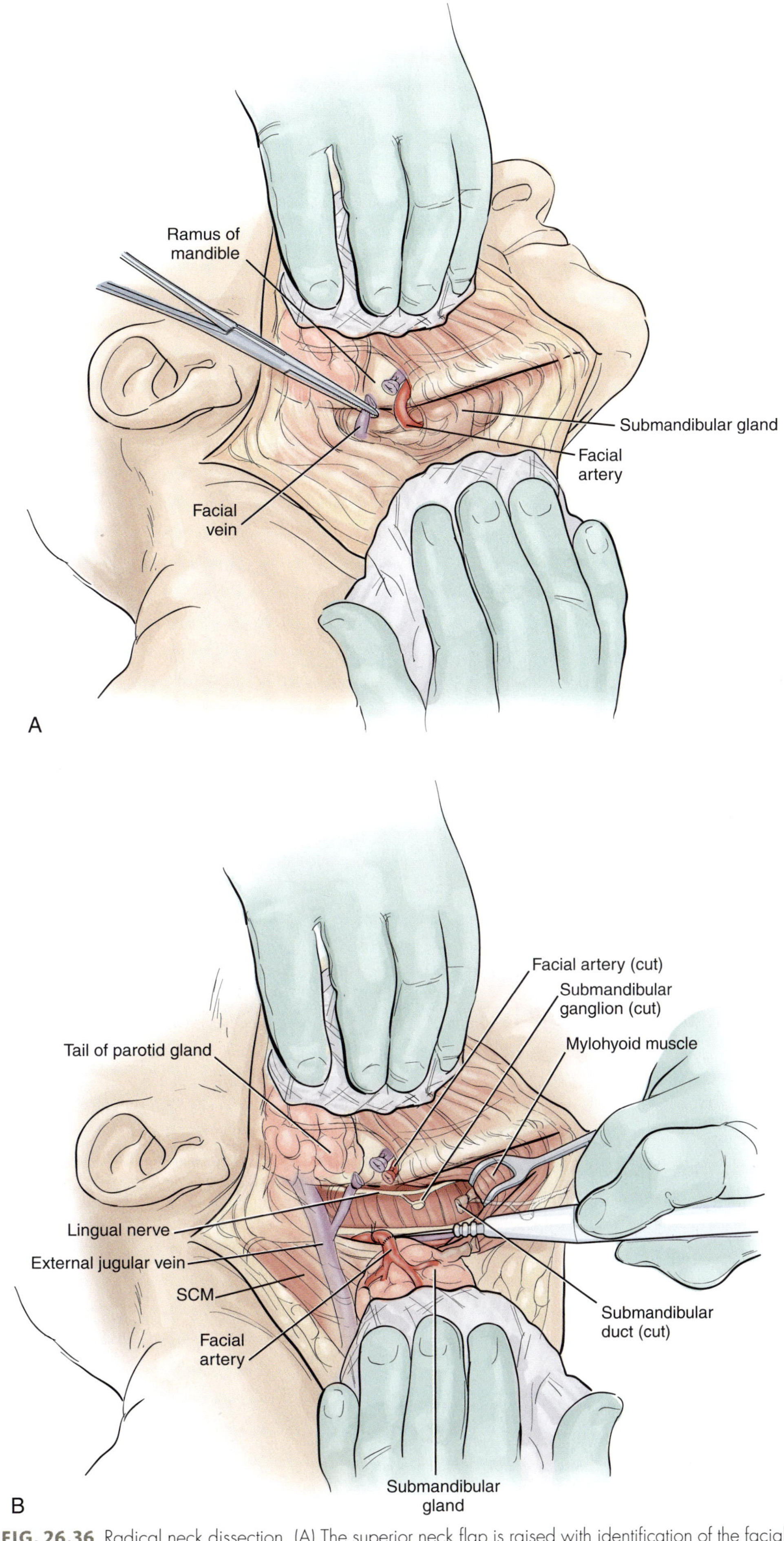

FIG. 26.36 Radical neck dissection. (A) The superior neck flap is raised with identification of the facial artery and vein. (B) The sternocleidomastoid muscle (SCM) is incised along with the tail of the parotid gland.

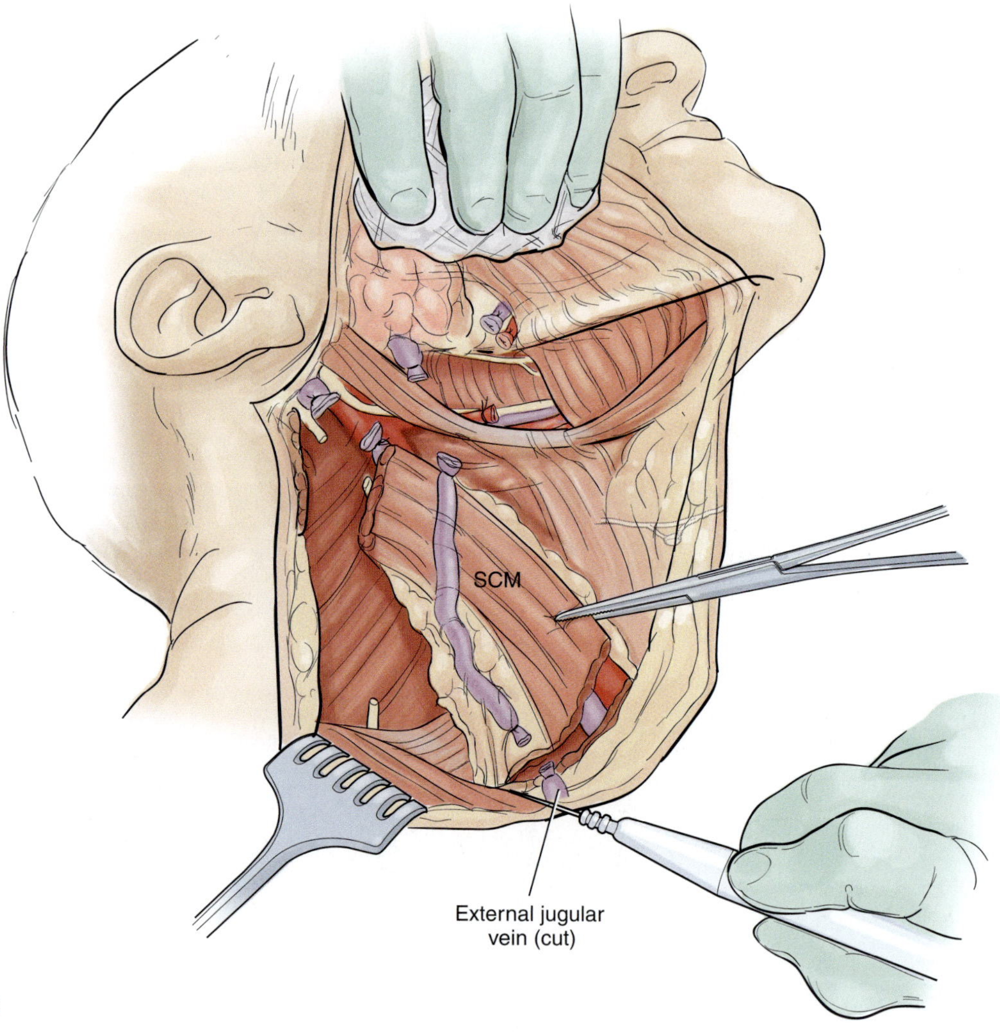

FIG. 26.36, cont'd (C) The external jugular vein is ligated and divided. The omohyoid muscle is severed (shown in D). Note the use of Kocher clamps, which provide traction on the muscle flaps and rake retractors on the wound edges.

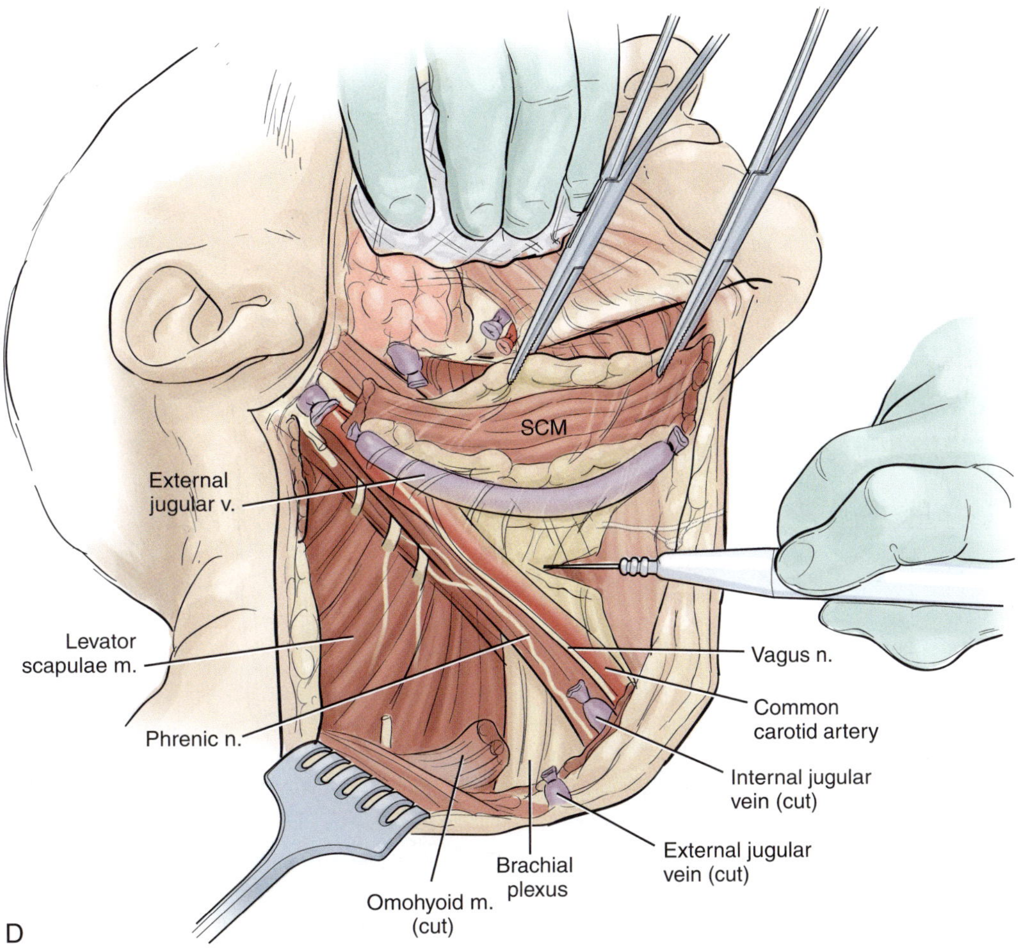

FIG. 26.36, cont'd (D) The completed dissection. (From Khatri V. *Atlas of Advanced Operative Surgery*. Philadelphia: Saunders; 2013.)

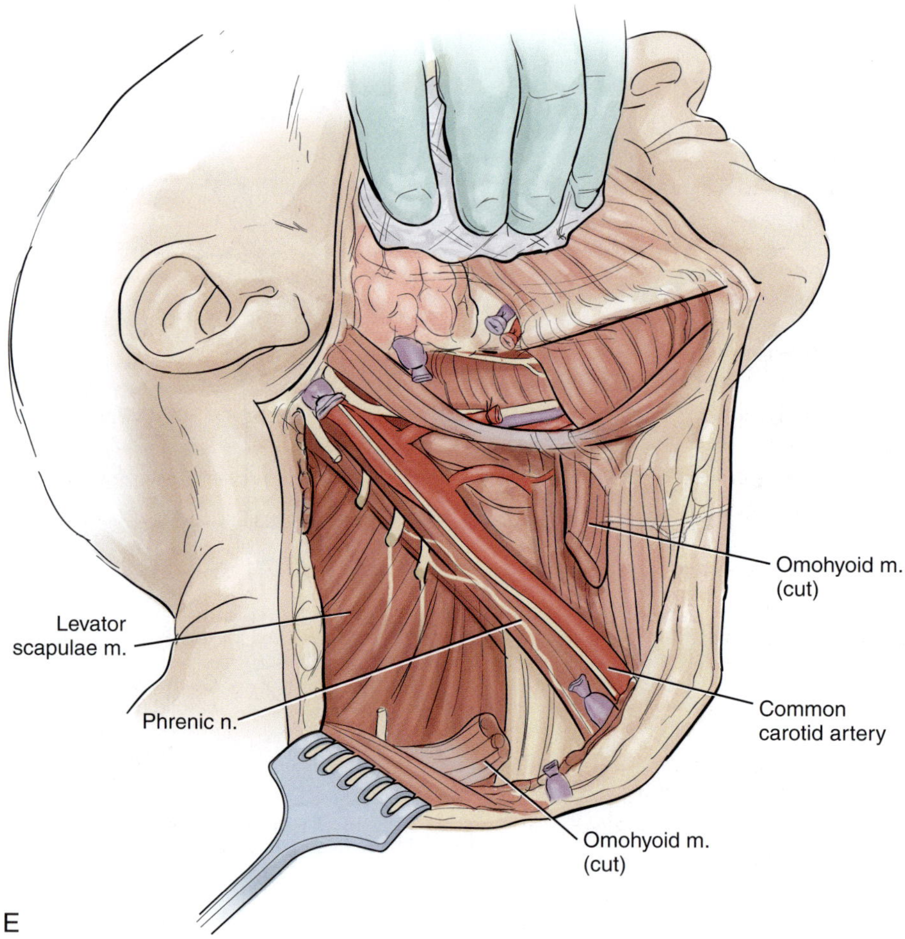

FIG. 26.36, cont'd

2. ***An incision is made at the midline of the lip and extended to the submental region.***
A #15 blade is used to make an incision through the midline lip; the incision is extended to the submental border. Skin flaps are elevated with the ESU. Senn rakes are used for retraction.

3. ***A titanium plate is fitted over the proposed site of division and the mandibular split.***
When the mandibular surface is exposed, a titanium plate is positioned in the region of the planned division. The screw holes are drilled with a small power drill. The plate is secured to the mandible with screws. The surgeon removes the plate after placement and splits the mandible at the midline, using a small power saw with a medium saw blade.

NOTE *If a mandibulectomy is to be performed, segmental resection of the bone may be performed at this stage of the procedure. The top of the mandible may have to be sacrificed, and further resection is performed after verification of tumor margins.*

4. ***The oral floor and body of the tongue are divided.***
In a hemiglossectomy, the anterior part of the oral floor and the body of the tongue are divided at the midline with the ESU. The incision is extended to the tongue base. The affected side of the tongue is then excised with the ESU. The incision is closed primarily or with a skin graft.

5. ***The mandible is reduced and the plate attached.***
The mandible is approximated and internally fixed with the plate. The incision is closed in layers with absorbable suture.

NOTE *For a total glossectomy, the incision is made between the floor of the mouth and the mandible and extended to the base of tongue with the ESU. The tongue is excised from the epiglottis with the ESU. A neck dissection is performed on one or both sides of the neck (see earlier).*

If the incision cannot be closed primarily or with an STSG, a pedicle or free pedicle flap is harvested (see Chapter 28). The flap is sutured into the defect with the skin taking the place of the tongue. The skin is sutured to the remaining mucosa of the floor of the mouth (and to the epiglottic or pharyngeal mucosa if a total laryngectomy was performed in the same procedure). Size 3-0 absorbable suture is used for closure. The mandible is approximated and internally fixed with the titanium plate.

6. ***The lip, oral, and skin incisions are closed.***
The lip incision, oral mucosa, and deep portions of the skin incisions are closed with drains in place using 3-0 absorbable sutures. The skin is closed with fine, nonabsorbable suture. A nasal feeding tube is placed and secured with 2-0 silk suture through the nasal septum.

The patient is transferred to the intensive care unit for airway monitoring. A gastrostomy tube may be inserted to provide nutrition.

LARYNGECTOMY

A laryngectomy is the removal of the larynx, usually with wide excision and tissue grafting. In recent years, conservative laryngectomy has been performed in many cases that would formerly have required radical surgery.

Pathology

A laryngectomy may be performed for the following indications:

- Cancer of the larynx
- Diversion for total separation of the respiratory and digestive tracts
- Major trauma that precludes open reduction and internal fixation

POSITION:	Supine
INCISION:	Neck
PREP AND DRAPING:	Midface to thorax
INSTRUMENTS:	Radical neck set, vascular set, thyroid set, vessel loops, vessel clips
POSSIBLE EXTRAS:	Nerve stimulator

Technical Points and Discussion

1. ***The patient is prepped and draped.***
The patient is placed in the supine position on a doughnut or Mayfield headrest with the arms tucked at the sides. A shoulder roll may be placed to hyperextend the neck. General anesthesia is used. The patient is prepped from the level of the nose to the level of the umbilicus and draped for a head and neck procedure, including the face, neck, and chest.

2. ***A skin incision is made.***
Using a #15 blade, the surgeon begins by making an apron incision, either from mastoid to mastoid (for laryngectomy with neck dissection) or from mid-SCM to mid-SCM (for laryngectomy alone). The flaps are elevated about ½ to 1 inch (1 to 2 cm) above the sternal notch from below and ½ to 1 inch (1 to 2 cm) below the hyoid bone. The flaps generally are secured back with fishhook retractors or suture.

3. ***The larynx and neck structures are exposed.***
The surgeon detaches the strap muscles from the sternum using the ESU or Mayo scissors and retracts them laterally with Army-Navy retractors. This exposes the

carotid sheath, the thyroid, and a portion of the trachea. The carotid sheath is dissected laterally and retracted with a Cushing vein retractor. The thyroid veins may be ligated with hemostat clamps and 2-0 silk ties.

4. ***The thyroid is dissected.***
   The thyroid isthmus is divided, and the lobe on the affected side is mobilized with the ESU or scissors. The thyroid lobe then is dissected free. Scissors are used to remove the fat and lymph tissue from the gland. The inferior thyroid artery is ligated and transected, and the recurrent laryngeal nerve is transected. The dissection of the thyroid continues with blunt dissection to the level of the trachea. The remaining portion of the gland is grasped with a Kocher clamp and divided from the trachea with the ESU.

5. ***The thyroid cartilage is dissected.***
   A cricoid hook is placed in the right side larynx to allow rotation of the larynx and exposure of the constrictor muscles on the thyroid cartilage. These muscles are detached from the cartilage with the ESU. A periosteal elevator then is used to remove the soft tissue from the underside of the thyroid cartilage. The larynx is rotated to the left with a cricoid hook to free the larynx from the remaining muscle and soft tissue of the thyroid. The surgeon then uses Metzenbaum scissors or a hemostat clamp to dissect the thyroid cartilage from the hyoid bone. Any vessels and nerves that are exposed at this point in the dissection are ligated.

6. ***The hyoid bone is exposed.***
   All muscular attachments between the tongue base and hyoid bone are separated with the ESU. With the hyoid bone exposed and free, the surgeon uses heavy Mayo scissors to sever the attachments of the hyoid bone.

7. ***A tracheotomy is performed.***
   A tracheotomy is performed at this point because the surgeon is ready to enter the airway. The surgeon sews the anterior tracheal wall to the posterior skin flap to secure it in place. The ET tube then is removed and the anesthesia circuit is switched to the tracheotomy tube.

8. ***The hypopharynx is incised and the larynx opened.***
   The surgeon uses scissors or the ESU to make an incision into the hypopharynx in the midline over the hyoid bone. The hypopharynx is opened with a hemostat, and the epiglottis is grasped with an Allis clamp and rotated out of the larynx. The lateral pharyngeal walls are incised with heavy Mayo scissors, sparing as much mucosa as possible. The larynx is then opened out.

9. ***The larynx is removed.***
   The tracheal tube is removed, and the posterior membranous trachea is incised with a #15 blade. The trachea is dissected from the anterior esophageal wall with Metzenbaum scissors. The surgeon also transects any fibrous attachments to the larynx at this point. The larynx is removed, and the tracheal tube is replaced.

10. ***The pharyngeal mucosa is closed.***
    With the larynx removed, the pharyngeal mucosa is closed with or without a rotation or free flap (discussed in Chapter 28) in two layers. The first layer is closed with a long 3-0 absorbable suture on a tapered needle, and the second layer is closed with 3-0 absorbable horizontal mattress sutures.

11. ***A stoma is created and the skin closed.***
    With the pharynx closed, the surgeon creates a stoma by attaching the anterior tracheal wall to the inferior skin flap and the posterior tracheal wall to the superior skin flap, using either absorbable or nonabsorbable. The wound is irrigated with normal saline. Drains are placed, and the skin is closed in layers with absorbable suture.

The patient is transferred to the intensive care unit. Chemotherapy and radiation are initiated as soon the wound is sufficiently healed to tolerate them.

Related Procedure

Partial cricoidectomy is subtotal and submucosal resection of the cricoid performed in the treatment or control of chronic aspiration after radical pharyngeal surgery, including removal of the tongue. In this procedure the pharyngeal inlet is enlarged and the laryngeal inlet reduced so that the voice is preserved and aspiration is controlled.

TEMPOROMANDIBULAR JOINT ARTHROPLASTY

The temporomandibular joint (TMJ) connects the mandible to the temporal bone. It enables jaw movement. The *articular disc* is an avascular cushion that glides over and under the bony attachments when the jaw is opened and closed. The disc is continuous and attaches to the muscles anteriorly and ligament posteriorly. Arthroscopy of the joint is performed to diagnose conditions of the joint, which usually involve displacement of the disc.

Pathology

Disc displacement is a forwardly displaced disc that is unable to retract back into normal anatomical position when the jaw is closed. This can result in pain and restricted movement of the mandible.

POSITION:	Supine
INCISION:	Arthroscopic
PREP AND DRAPING:	Face
INSTRUMENTS:	TMJ arthroscopy set with instruments

Technical Points and Discussion

1. ***The trocar points are marked.***
   The mandible is manipulated to identify the puncture points, which are then marked on the skin.

2. ***Local anesthetic with epinephrine is instilled at the site.***
   Lidocaine with epinephrine is used to distend the joint and provide hemostasis. This is done with a 27-gauge, 1½-inch needle.

3. ***A trocar with sheath is inserted.***
   A stab wound is made with a #11 blade, and a sharp trocar and sheath are inserted into the incision. The sharp trocar is then exchanged with a blunt obturator. When the sheath is advanced into position, the obturator is removed and a 30-degree Hopkins telescope is inserted into the sheath (discussed in Chapter 20). The joint may be irrigated to improve visualization of the anatomy.

4. ***Additional trocars are inserted to accommodate instruments.***
   A second incision can be made to accommodate the arthroscopic instruments. The arthroscope may be used with a working sheath, which has an irrigation channel and instrument channel. The working instruments include scissors, forceps, sickle knives, and probes.

5. ***The instruments and fluid are withdrawn and incisions closed.***
   At the conclusion of the procedure, the joint space is decompressed and all instruments removed. The incisions may be closed using fine monofilament skin sutures or Steri-Strips.

KEY CONCEPTS

- Surgical procedures of the ear involve delicate soft and connective tissues but may also require small bone instruments.
- Middle and inner ear instruments are extremely delicate and are best managed by keeping them in their racks during surgery.
- Absorbable gelatin matrix is used frequently during ear surgery for hemostasis and also for packing the bony spaces and graft sites.
- When operating under the microscope, the scrub must pass surgical instruments in correct orientation of their use because the surgeon cannot look away to receive an instrument.
- Surgical procedures of the nose may be performed using open or closed technique. During open technique, the superficial tissues are elevated off the bony and cartilaginous structures. In closed technique, the operation is performed through the submucosa.
- Endoscopy is frequently combined with open techniques of the nasal cavity and sinuses.
- Procedures of the ear and nasal structures require a dry field at all times. The scrub may be required to manage the suction in these delicate procedures.
- Procedures involving the salivary and parotid glands require careful dissection to avoid injury to the facial nerves. These may be isolated during surgery to prevent injury during dissection.
- Procedures of the neck are superficial. However, the anatomy is highly vascular. These procedures require many hemostats and meticulous attention to hemostasis.
- Instruments used during neck surgery, including retractors, are generally very shallow and of short or medium length.

REVIEW QUESTIONS

1. Why is a myringotomy performed?
2. Describe a mastoid dressing.
3. Why is it important to submerge the cochlear implant in normal saline after it is opened onto the sterile field?
4. List three causes of upper airway obstruction that result in the need for a tracheostomy.
5. Why is the obturator of a tracheotomy tube kept with the patient in the recovery period?

BIBLIOGRAPHY

Cioffi W, et al. *Atlas of Trauma Emergency Surgical Techniques*. Philadelphia: Elsevier; 2014.

Jandial R, McCormick P, Black P. *Core Techniques in Operative Neurosurgery*. Philadelphia: Elsevier; 2011.

Khatri V. *Atlas of Advanced Operative Surgery*. Philadelphia: Saunders; 2013.

Myers, E. *Operative Otolaryngology: Head and Neck Surgery*. Elsevier; 2018.

Roberts JR, Custalow CB. *Roberts and Hedges' Clinical Procedures in Emergency Medicine and Acute Care*. Elsevier; 2019.

27 ORAL AND MAXILLOFACIAL SURGERY

LEARNING OBJECTIVES

After studying this chapter, the reader will be able to:

1. Identify key anatomical structures of the face and oral cavity
2. Discuss diagnostic procedures used in the maxillofacial specialty
3. Discuss specific elements of case planning for oral and maxillofacial surgery
4. Discuss pathology of the facial bones and oral cavity
5. List and describe common oral and maxillofacial surgical procedures

TERMINOLOGY

Arch bars: Metal plates wired to the teeth to occlude the jaw during maxillofacial surgery or during healing. Arch bars maintain the patient's normal bite (occlusion).

Bicortical screws: Screws that penetrate both cortical layers and the intervening spongy layer of the bone.

Blowout fracture: A severe fracture of the orbital cavity in which a portion of the globe may extrude outside the cavity.

Dentition: The number, type, and pattern of the teeth.

Le Fort I fracture: A horizontal fracture of the maxilla that causes the hard palate and alveolar process to become separated from the rest of the maxilla. The fracture extends into the lower nasal septum, lateral maxillary sinus, and palatine bones.

Le Fort II fracture: A fracture that extends from the nasal bone to the frontal processes of the maxilla, lacrimal bones, and inferior orbital floor. It may extend into the orbital foramen. Inferiorly, it extends into the anterior maxillary sinus and the pterygoid plates.

Le Fort III fracture: This fracture involves separation of all the facial bones from their cranial base. It includes fracture of the zygoma, maxilla, and nasal bones.

Mastication: Chewing.

Maxillomandibular fixation (MMF): See arch bars.

Occlusion: In maxillofacial surgery, this refers to the patient's bite pattern when the jaw is closed.

Odontectomy: Tooth extraction.

Oromaxillofacial surgery: Surgery involving the bones of the face, primarily for repair of fractures and reconstruction of congenital anomalies.

Subciliary incision: Skin incision made approximately 2 mm inferior to the lower eyelashes.

Transconjunctival incision: Incision made through the conjunctiva.

Oral and maxillofacial **(OMF)** surgery is a specialty that involves diagnosis and treatment of disease, defects, and trauma of the soft tissues and bones of the face and oral cavity. Surgery may involve reconstruction after radical surgery, trauma, congenital deformity, or disease. The face is particularly susceptible to injury in motor vehicle and industrial accidents, high-speed sports, and intentional violence. In recent years there has been a reduction in facial fractures resulting from motor vehicle accidents since the public health campaign to promote the use of seat belts. However, motor vehicle accidents and interpersonal violence continue to be the primary causes of maxillofacial and cranial injury in adults and children.

Maxillofacial injuries can be complex, involving skin, muscle, nerves, and blood vessels. The long-term physiological effects of injury or congenital anomalies can affect speech, **mastication** (chewing), and tooth development. The psychological effects are equally important, because disfigurement often results in social and emotional isolation. Maxillofacial procedures are performed primarily by surgeons specializing in oromaxillofacial, plastic, or otorhinolaryngology surgery.

Surgery for maxillofacial injuries is performed as soon as the patient's general condition permits it. Although usually not considered an emergency surgery, early or immediate repair can provide a better outcome because traumatized tissues become swollen, which may obscure the anatomy.

SURGICAL ANATOMY

BONES OF THE FACE

The bones of the face are divided into three regions: the upper face, the midface, and the lower face.

The *upper face* contains the frontal bone, which forms the forehead and contains portions of the nasal sinuses and the superior margin of the bony orbit.

The *midface* contains the ethmoid, nasal bone, zygoma, and maxillary bones.

The ethmoid bone is a complex structure that contributes to the floor of the cranium and contains numerous sinus cavities. The nasal bone forms the bridge of the nose and articulates with the ethmoid and the maxilla. Fractures of the nasal ethmoid area may injure the lacrimal apparatus, including the ducts and lacrimal glands. The dura is also vulnerable and may require neurological surgery. The zygoma forms the lateral walls and floor of the bony orbit, which houses the eyeball. The zygomatic arch is the cheekbone. Fractures in this area are important because of their association with injury to the eye, especially in displaced fractures. The most common causes of injury are assault, motor vehicle accidents, and sports injuries. The bony orbit is formed by the frontal bone, but it also contains portions of other bones of the face, including the zygoma, maxilla, lacrimal, ethmoid, sphenoid, and palatine bones. The orbital floor is formed by the maxillary sinus. The bilateral maxillae come together to form the upper jaw, the anterior hard palate, and a portion of the orbital cavities.

The *lower face* contains the mandible, which is the only movable bone of the face. It is a U-shaped bone suspended from the temporal bone. The condyles insert into the glenoid fossa of the temporal bones to form the temporomandibular joints. The ramus extends inferiorly from the condyle to the angle, where it joins the body of the mandible and extends anteriorly and medially to join the other half of the mandible. The teeth are embedded in the alveoli of the body of the mandible. Fig. 27.1 shows the bones of the face and cranium. Fig. 27.2 illustrates the skull as viewed from below.

TEETH

The teeth are embedded in the maxilla (top) and mandible (bottom). Each single tooth has distinct tissue layers including outer enamel, soft dentin, and inner vascular pulp. Each tooth socket within the bone is lined with the periodontal ligament, which maintains contact between the tooth's roots and the gum tissue (Fig. 27.3). Humans form two sets of teeth, the temporary (primary) teeth and the permanent teeth as shown in Fig. 27.4.

CLASSIFICATION OF FACIAL FRACTURES

An international standard for the classification of facial fractures is used to address specific complications associated with the fracture's *location* and level of *anatomical alteration*. The system was developed by a French military doctor, René Le Fort, in 1901. The system is still used today. However, a "pure" Le Fort fracture is seldom seen. It is more common to see complex fractures involving two or more Le Fort fractures, including those extending beyond the Le Fort demarcations. The three Le Fort classifications are the following:

- **Le Fort I fracture:** This is a horizontal fracture of the maxilla that causes the hard palate and alveolar process to become separated from the rest of the maxilla. The demarcation extends into the lower nasal septum, lateral maxillary sinus, and palatine bones.
- **Le Fort II fracture:** This type of fracture is pyramidal. It extends from the nasal bone to the frontal processes of the maxilla, lacrimal bones, and inferior orbital floor and may extend into the orbital foramen. Inferiorly, it extends into the anterior maxillary sinus and the pterygoid plates. This type of fracture also is associated with leakage of cerebrospinal fluid (CSF) into the nasal sinuses.
- **Le Fort III fracture:** This fracture involves separation of all the facial bones from their cranial base. It includes fracture of the zygoma, maxilla, and nasal bones. The demarcation line extends through the ethmoid bone and bony orbit, with severe facial flattening and swelling.

Fig. 27.5 shows the Le Fort classification of facial fractures. Potential soft tissue injury is discussed later with the specific fracture site.

INCISIONS OF THE FACE

Access to the fracture site can be made through the injury itself or by incisions. Fig. 27.6 illustrates incisions commonly used in facial fracture.

CASE PLANNING

INSTRUMENTS

Maxillofacial surgery involves both the bones and soft tissue of the head and neck. The instrumentation used for these procedures therefore includes fine orthopedic instruments, implants, and grafting materials, as well as plastic surgery, nasal, and dental instruments. Injury or disease involving the frontal bones may require neurosurgery instruments. Soft tissue injury in facial trauma may require specialty instruments for assessment and repair. Eye injury, including damage to the globe, eye muscles, eyelids, and nasolacrimal system, requires eye and nasal instruments. Muscle and skin repair are common to most facial fracture procedures.

IMPLANTS

Chapter 29 presents a complete discussion of the biomechanical and surgical techniques used in bone trauma and reconstruction, including power drills and techniques for their use. Maxillofacial fracture repair and remodeling systems have been developed by major instrument companies and provide essential instruments needed for the implantation of plates, and mesh used to bridge bone fragments during repair. The primary means of joining the facial bones are miniplates with cortical screws and lag screws.

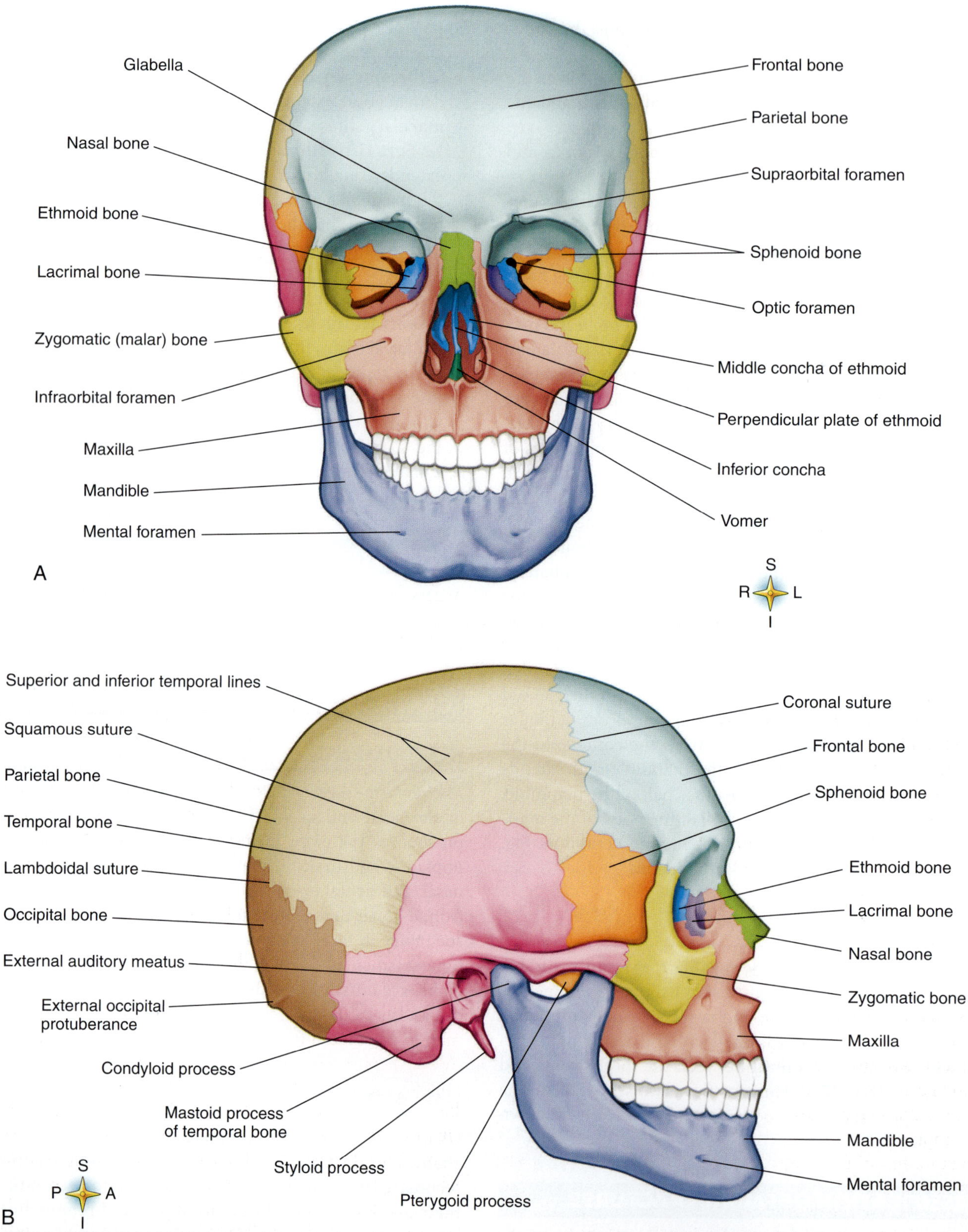

FIG. 27.1 The cranium. (A) Anterior view. (B) Side view. (From Thibodeau GA, Patt KT, eds. *Anthony's Textbook of Anatomy and Physiology*. 17th ed. St Louis: Mosby; 2003.)

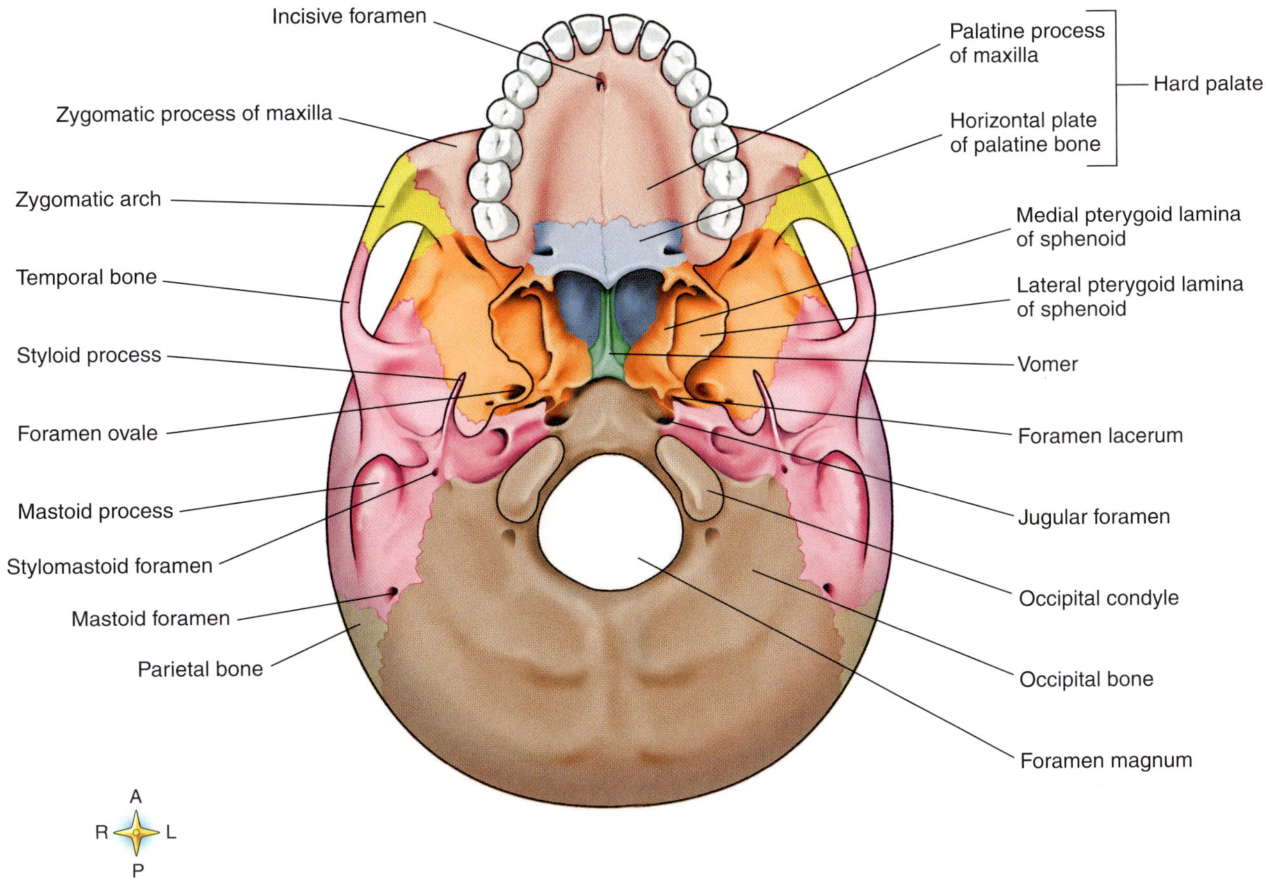

FIG. 27.2 The skull (viewed from below). (From Thibodeau GA, Patton KT, eds. *Anthony's Textbook of Anatomy and Physiology*. 17th ed. St Louis: Mosby; 2003.)

A combination of orthopedic implants is used for complex bone repair and remodeling.

Metal mesh systems are malleable so they can be molded to fit over the contours of facial bone. Small cortical screws or **bicortical screws** are used to implant the titanium or stainless-steel mesh plates, which provide stability during healing. In addition to mesh material and plates, these systems also include plate benders, cutters, forceps, and screwdrivers, which are custom-made to fit the individual manufacturer's system. Many systems are color coded with regard to component size.

The following is the general sequence for implantation of mesh and plates:

1. Assessment of the bone and tissue and planning
2. Selection of hardware to be used
3. Preparation of the hardware, including bending and contouring of the mesh or plate
4. Preparation of graft sites and management of the bone graft or implant
5. Preparation of the surgical site—debridement, remolding, and hemostasis
6. Application of the hardware

The reader is advised to consult Chapter 29 for a complete discussion on orthopedic techniques, including drill terminology and management, types and uses of bone screws, and the instruments required to install them. Surgical implant materials have been specially developed for use in maxillofacial surgery and the repair of defects. *SynPOR* implants, provided by DePuy Synthes, Inc., are manufactured from ultra-high-molecular-weight polyethylene, which has been used for many years for filling defects. A special product for orbital injury incorporates titanium mesh with a SynPOR sheet to support tissue growth.

Resorbable plates are designed like titanium mesh but are slowly absorbed by the body. These are implanted using fixation instruments that are available as a set with the plates. Resorbable plates, mesh, and sheets must be heated to 70°F to be easily molded. A small water bath is draped and used on the surgical field for molding these implants. The implants can be remolded up to 10 times.

PREPPING AND DRAPING

Facial fractures are prepped with dilute povidone-iodine because it has been shown to be the safest and most effective antiseptic for use on the face. Note that hexachlorophene and chlorhexidine are not used on the face because they are ototoxic. The entire face is prepped, from the hairline to the sternal notch, as described in Chapter 17. An endotracheal or nasotracheal tube is usually part of the surgical field and therefore must be included in the prep. The patient is draped with four towels secured with clips to expose the surgical site. A split sheet is then draped over the patient and around the face, with the mouth, nose, and eyes included in the surgical field.

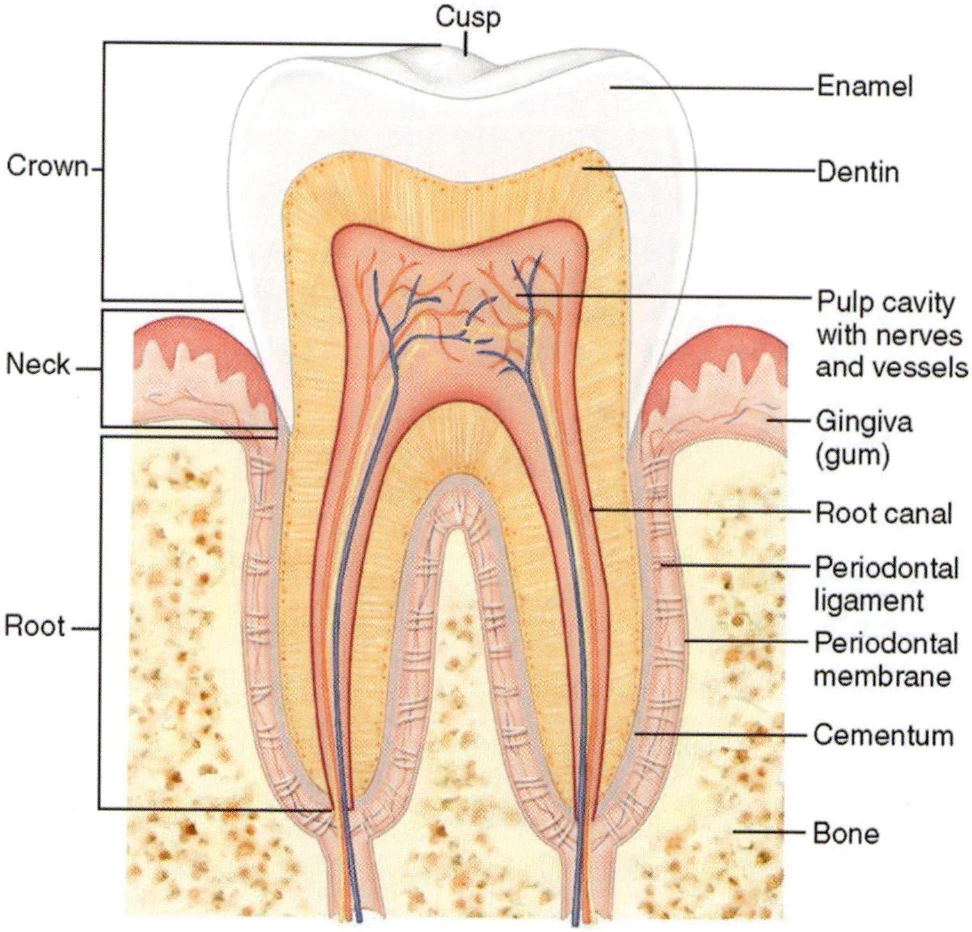

FIG. 27.3 Anatomy of the tooth. See text for details. (From Patton K, et al. *Essentials of Anatomy and Physiology*. St Louis: Elsevier; 2012.)

NOTE *During procedures in which oral and orthopedic (facial bone) techniques are required, the instruments used within the oral cavity (a nonsterile area) must be isolated from the orthopedic setup and procedure, which is sterile.*

SPONGES AND DRESSINGS

Dressings are used to protect the wound and to absorb exudate. Antibiotic ointment may be applied to the incision, and Telfa or other nonadherent dressing may be placed directly over the site. Flat gauze or gauze fluffs may be placed on top of the dressing. Kerlix (rolled) wrap can be used to secure dressings on the head or face. Kerlix is soft and expandable and conforms to the contours of the skull and facial bones.

SURGICAL PROCEDURES

OPEN REDUCTION AND INTERNAL FIXATION: ORBITAL FLOOR FRACTURE

Open reduction and internal fixation (ORIF) of an orbital floor fracture is performed to reduce a fracture of the orbital floor, to prevent entrapment of the extraocular muscles, and to support the orbital contents. In case of injury to the eye, the ST should ask the surgeon which specific sets are required for the repair. These may include an eye muscle, cataract, or enucleation instrument. A fracture resulting in small fragments of bone in the posterior orbit may require optic nerve decompression. Retinal damage may also occur with orbital fracture. If the tissue between the lacrimal punctum and medial canthus is lacerated, there is a strong possibility of damage to the lacrimal system. A stenting procedure is required in the first 72 hours.

Pathology

Orbital floor fractures, or **blowout fractures,** are caused by high-speed blunt force to the globe. Fractures of the orbital floor usually result from the increased orbital pressure caused by the impact on the globe. A portion of the globe may extrude into the nasal sinus (enophthalmos), or the globe can be displaced posteriorly. Entrapment of the eye muscles can result in *diplopia* (double vision). The most common causes of the injury are intentional violence and being struck by a high-velocity object (Fig. 27.7).

POSITION:	Supine
INCISION:	Subciliary or conjunctiva
PREP AND DRAPING:	Eye
INSTRUMENTS:	Ophthalmic; facial fracture set; minor plastic surgery set; facial fracture plates and screws
POSSIBLE EXTRAS:	Eye instruments

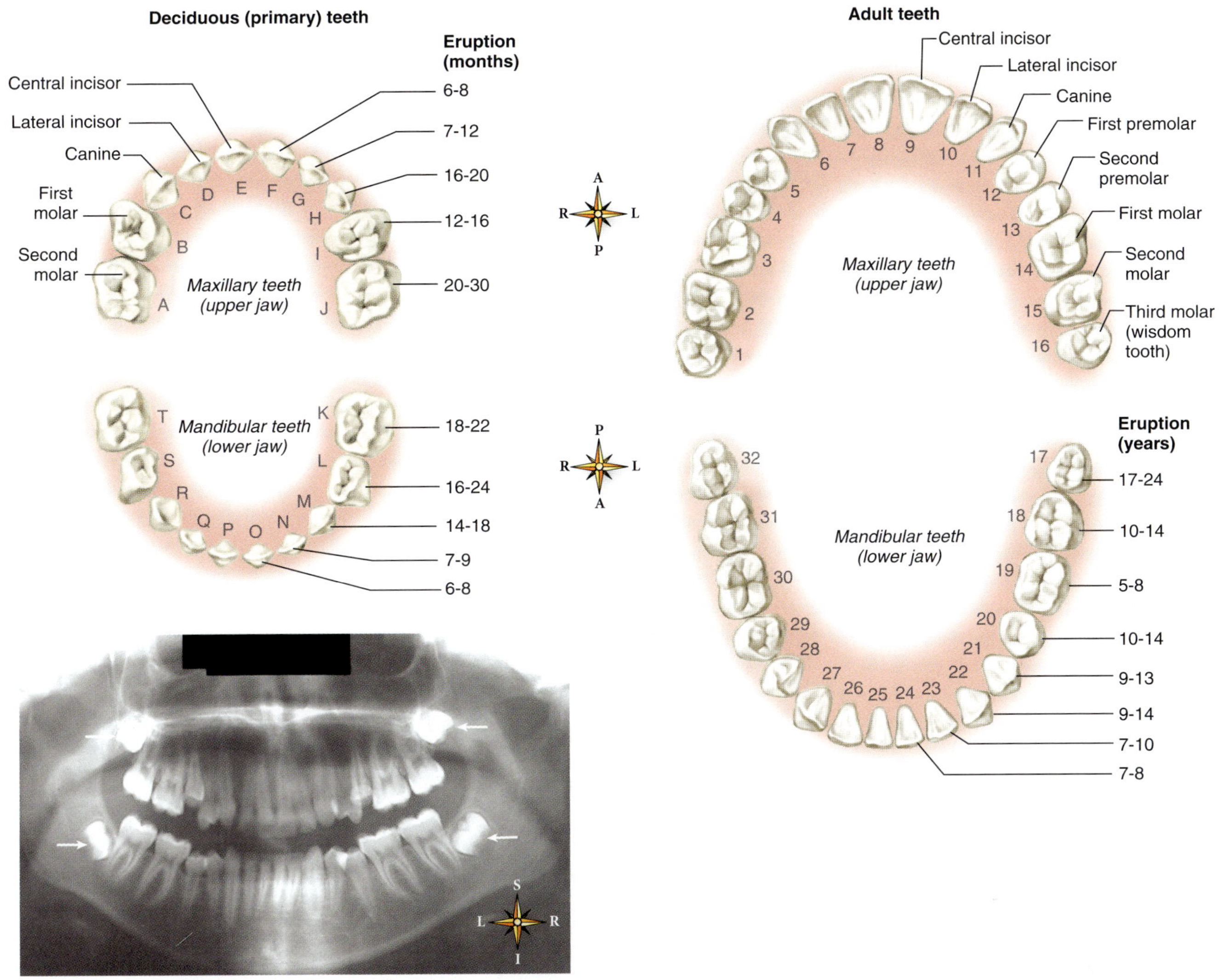

FIG. 27.4 The teeth. Humans form two sets of teeth: the deciduous or primary teeth and the adult permanent teeth. Note the numbering and alphabetic systems used to map out each tooth. The dental x-ray demonstrates the wisdom teeth that have not yet erupted in this individual. (From Patton K, et al. *Essentials of Anatomy and Physiology*. St Louis: Elsevier; 2012.)

Technical Points and Discussion

1. ***The patient is prepped and draped.***
The patient is positioned and prepped as for an eye procedure. General anesthesia is administered. Ophthalmic ointment may be placed in the eyes before the skin prep. The prep is performed carefully to prevent solution from draining into the eyes and ears.

2. ***The orbit is exposed.***
The surgeon begins by placing corneal protectors in the operative eye. Ophthalmic balanced salt solution is instilled into the eye to provide moisture at this stage and as needed throughout the case. The ST may perform this task.

With the cornea protected, the surgeon makes the incision. Either of two incisions can be used. A **subciliary incision** is made 2 mm under the eyelashes with a #15 blade. A **transconjunctival incision** is made in the conjunctiva of the inferior eyelid. The surgeon exposes the orbit by placing small, malleable retractors or brain spatula retractors into the wound and retracting superiorly and inferiorly. The wound is exposed to the level of the orbital rim, and the periosteum is elevated with a Freer or similar elevator. The surgeon then elevates and retracts the orbital contents superiorly with a small malleable retractor.

3. ***The fractures are reduced and repaired.***
After assessment, the surgeon may reconstruct the floor of the orbit using nylon sheeting, polypropylene mesh, Gelfilm, Silastic sheeting, or an orbital floor plate. Typically, a 1-, 1.3-, or 1.5-mm plate or mesh is selected for orbital fractures. The surgeon cuts the selected material to size with plate cutters or scissors (depending on the material) and positions it between the orbital floor and the orbital contents. An orbital floor plate is secured in place with screws in the infraorbital rim.

4. ***The incision is closed.***
With the orbital contents supported, the retractors are removed and the wound is closed. Subciliary incisions are closed with 5-0 absorbable sutures. Transconjunctival incisions are not closed. The surgeon removes the corneal protector after the incisions have been closed. Antibiotic ophthalmic ointment may be placed in the eye and on the incision.

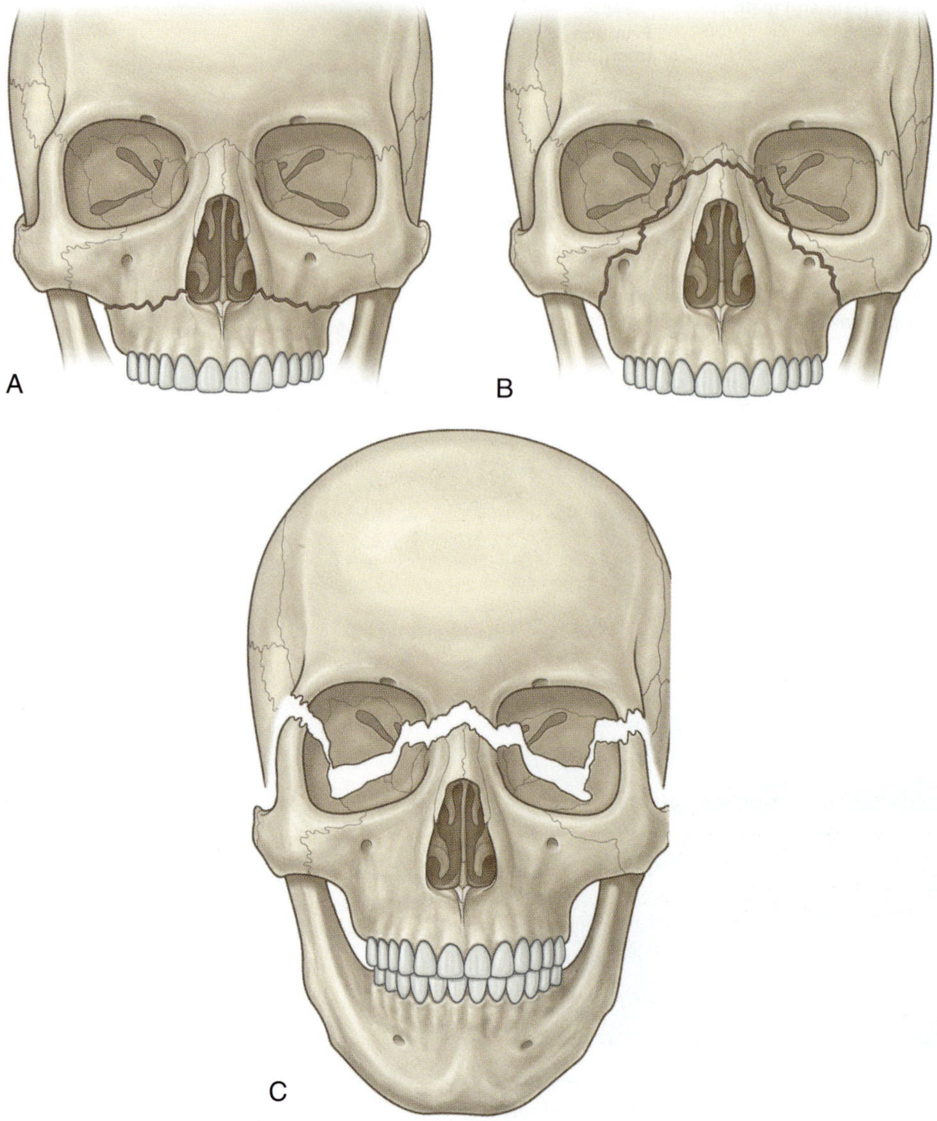

FIG. 27.5 Le Fort classification of facial fractures. (A) Le Fort I—transverse fracture of the maxilla. (B) Le Fort II—pyramidal fracture of the maxilla. The fracture may traverse the nose through the nasal cartilage or bone. It can also separate the zygoma from the maxilla. (C) Le Fort III—The entire facial bone mass is separated from the frontal bone through the zygoma, nasoethmoid, and nasofrontal bone junctions. (From Neligan P, Buck D. *Core Procedures in Plastic Surgery*. Philadelphia: Elsevier; 2014.)

MAXILLOMANDIBULAR FIXATION (APPLICATION OF ARCH BARS)

Maxillomandibular fixation (MMF) is a procedure to wire the jaws in a closed position. The hardware used in this technique is the **arch bar.** This is a malleable stainless steel strap or bar with intermittent smooth hooks. The band is cut to size and fixed to the teeth in the upper and lower jaw using stainless steel suture. The jaw is then closed and wires used to bind the maxilla and mandible together. The purpose of arch bars is to maintain stability of the upper and lower jaws during the procedure or for extended use while a facial fracture heals.

Pathology

Misalignment of the teeth and jaws often accompanies facial fracture. Application of arch bars is a routine procedure in many types of maxillomandibular repairs.

POSITION:	Supine
INCISION:	None
PREP AND DRAPING:	Facial
INSTRUMENTS:	Arch bar set including oral retractors or facial fracture set, stainless steel suture strands, arch bars

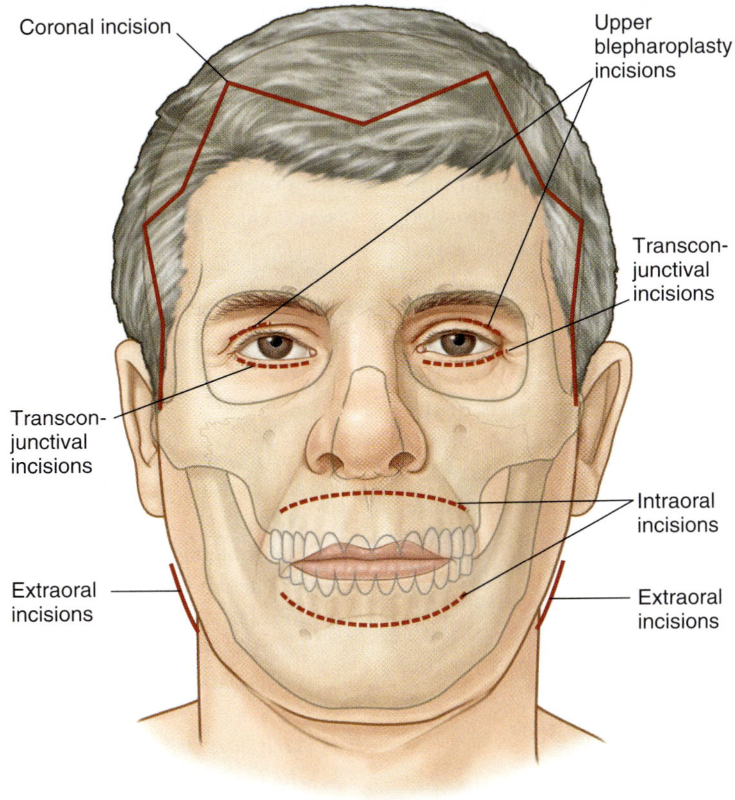

FIG. 27.6 Incisions of the face. Skin incisions are indicated by *solid lines*. The conjunctival incision *(dotted line)* provides access to the orbital floor and anterior maxilla. Intraoral (inside the mouth) incisions are also indicated by a *dotted line*. This is indicated for Le Fort I maxillary and anterior mandible fractures. A lateral incision of the nasal bone provides access to the nasal structures. However, a coronal incision (near the hairline) is preferable. (From Neligan P, Buck D, eds. *Core Procedures in Plastic Surgery*. Philadelphia: Elsevier; 2014.)

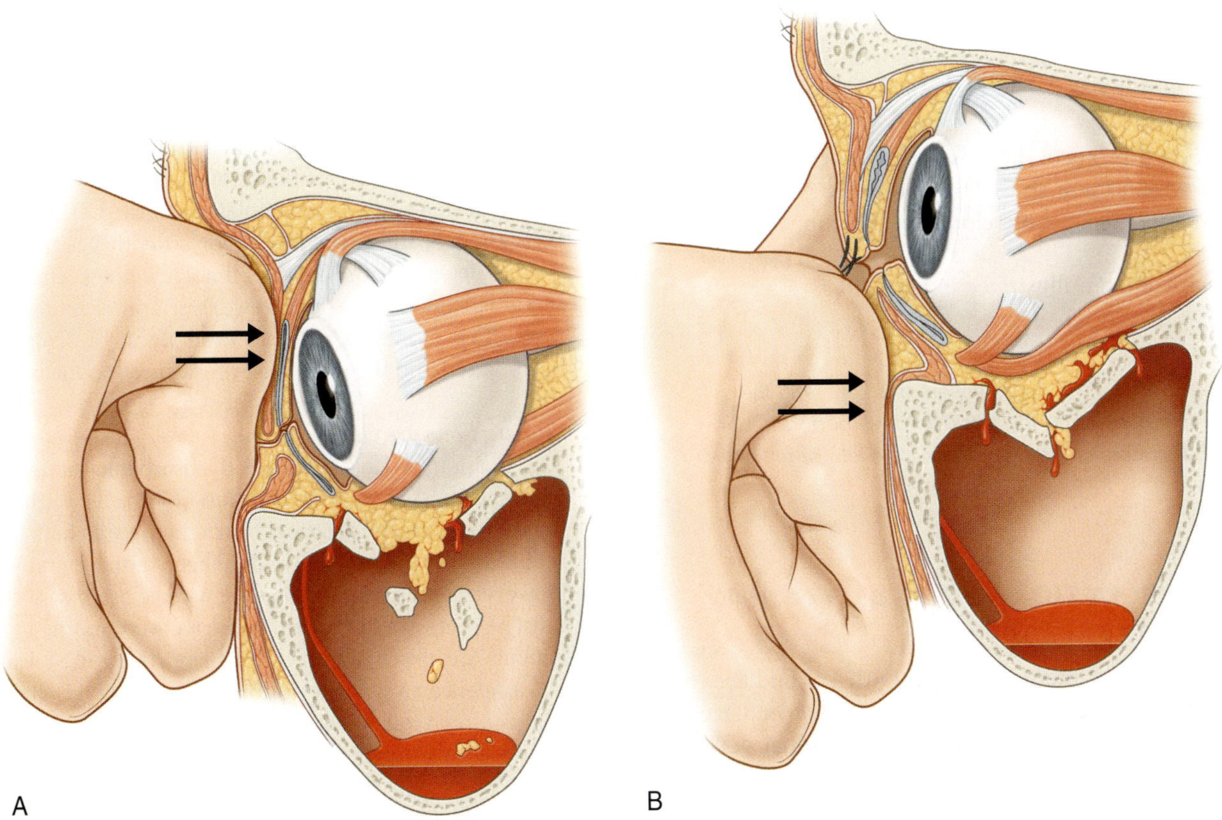

FIG. 27.7 Blowout fracture of the orbit. (A) In this type of fracture, the globe is forced into the orbital wall. (B) Force transmission fracture of the orbital floor. (From Neligan P, Buck D, eds. *Core Procedures in Plastic Surgery*. Philadelphia: Elsevier; 2014.)

Technical Points and Discussion

1. ***Arch bars are wired to the teeth with 24- or 26-gauge wire sutures.***
   The surgeon shapes an arch bar to fit over the patient's upper teeth and gums. The cheek and tongue are retracted by a cheek retractor, intraoral sweetheart or cloverleaf retractor, and the bar is wired into place with 24- or 26-gauge stainless steel suture wires, which are cut into thirds.
   A steel wire mounted on a needle holder is passed to the surgeon. The ST should control the ends of the suture to prevent contamination or injury. A designated clamp may be fixed to the end of the suture for this purpose. The wire is clamped with a Rubio needle holder, threaded between the teeth, wrapped around the bar, and twisted to be tightened. The suture ends are cut with a wire cutter. Three wires are placed on each side of the mouth if there is sufficient space to accommodate them. The procedure is repeated for the lower teeth.

2. ***The jaws are wired together.***
   When the arch bars have been applied to both the upper and lower teeth, the jaw is closed in normal position, and the top and bottom arch bars are approximated with precut lengths of steel suture. Size 24- or 26-gauge stainless steel suture is twisted into a clockwise loop and wrapped around the upper and lower bars with the wire twister. The wire is twisted clockwise until tight against the arch bars and then is cut with a wire cutter. To prevent the suture ends from injuring the soft tissues, a "rosebud" is made in the suture ends by grasping the wire with a hemostat and crimping it inward. The end may be buried in the patient's gingiva.
   Standard protocol dictates that wires be tightened in a clockwise fashion so that any other surgeon knows to remove them in a counterclockwise direction.

Arch bar fixation is illustrated in Fig. 27.8.

IMPORTANT TO KNOW *Wire cutters are kept with the patient at all times during the postoperative period to allow for immediate access to the mouth in the event of an airway emergency.*

OPEN REDUCTION/INTERNAL FIXATION: MIDFACE FRACTURE

Open reduction and internal fixation (ORIF) of midface fractures is performed as follows. Fractures of the midface are reduced (bone fragments are brought into normal position) and fixed in place using metal pins, plates, and bars. The buttressing structures (those under force during dental occlusion) are also reinforced.

Pathology

POSITION:	Supine
INCISION:	Oral
PREP AND DRAPING:	Facial
INSTRUMENTS:	Facial fracture instrument set; power drill and screws; facial fracture plates and screws

Technical Points and Discussion

1. ***The patient is anesthetized, positioned, prepped, and draped.***
   The patient is placed in the supine position on a doughnut or Mayfield headrest with the arms tucked at the sides. General anesthesia is administered through a nasotracheal tube. For extensive trauma, a tracheotomy may be performed first.
   The patient is prepped and draped for a facial procedure.

2. ***Arch bars are applied as required.***
3. ***The fracture is exposed and reduced.***
   The surgeon makes the incision in the upper gingival mucosa on the affected side with a #15 blade. The incision is extended through the mucosa to the level of the maxilla. The surgeon then elevates the periosteum with a Freer or periosteal elevator. The zygoma is reduced with Hohmann retractors or a bone hook, or both.

4. ***The fracture is fixed internally using miniplates and screws.***
   The surgeon selects the size and type of plate to be used. The plates usually are 1.7 or 2 mm. Cortical screws are used to secure the plate to the bone. The plate is held in place with a plate-holding forceps or hemostat. The appropriate drill bit (according to the size of the screw) is loaded onto a small power drill, and the screw holes are drilled. The surgeon then chooses the screw length, or a depth gauge may be used to determine the depth of the screw holes. The correct screw is loaded onto the screwdriver and is screwed into place. This process is repeated until all of the screws have been placed and the plate has been secured to the bone.

5. ***The incisions are closed.***
   The incision is closed with 3-0 absorbable sutures. The wound is dressed with flat and fluffed gauze. A Kerlix wrap is used to secure the dressing. Note that the arch bars may be removed after the fracture(s) have been reduced and plated. However, as always, if the jaws are wired closed, wire cutters must be sent with the patient to the recovery room.
   Patients are closely observed for hemorrhage, CSF leakage, and a patent airway in the postoperative period. Healing usually requires 4 to 8 weeks. Complications include dehiscence of oral lesions, especially when oral hygiene is suboptimal.
   Fig. 27.9 shows a three-dimensional CT of a midface fracture before and after repair.

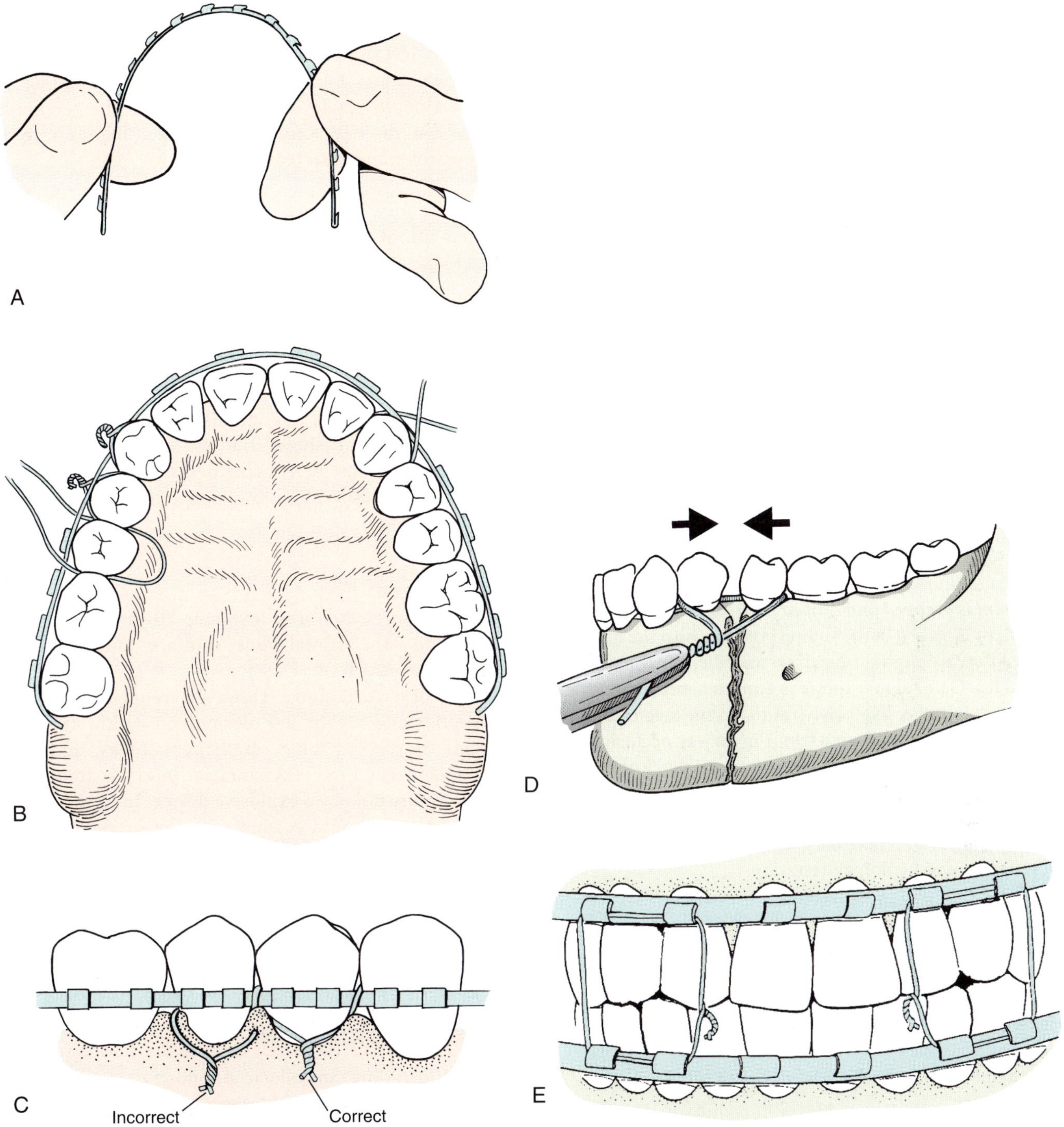

FIG. 27.8 Application of arch bars. (A) A section of arch bar is cut to the correct size and shape of the dentition. (B) The bar is fixed to the teeth with stainless steel wire. (C) The wires are passed between the tooth and the dental papilla. (D) A "bridle wire" is fixed to the bicuspids. (E) Wire loops are placed between the upper and lower arch bars to maintain dental occlusion. (From Meyers E, ed. *Operative Otolaryngology Head and Neck Surgery*. 2nd ed. Philadelphia: Elsevier; 2008.)

OPEN REDUCTION AND INTERNAL FIXATION: MANDIBULAR FRACTURE

In this procedure, the mandibular fracture is repaired and **occlusion** is restored. Miniplates or lag screws may be used in the repair.

Pathology

ORIF of the mandible is performed to treat facial trauma involving the mandible. Intentional trauma and motor vehicle accident are the most common causes of a mandibular fracture.

POSITION:	Supine
INCISION:	Buccal mucosa
PREP AND DRAPING:	Face
INSTRUMENTS:	Facial fracture set; arch bar set; facial fracture plates and screws

Technical Points and Discussion

1. ***The patient is prepped and draped for a facial procedure.***
The patient is placed in the supine position with the head stabilized on a doughnut headrest and the arms tucked at the sides. General anesthesia is administered through a nasotracheal tube. Extensive trauma of the face results in massive swelling and may result in airway occlusion. Therefore a tracheotomy may be performed before the ORIF.
After administration of anesthesia, the surgeon assesses the fractures. If necessary, arch bars may be applied before fracture reduction and fixation.

2. ***A transoral or external incision is made.***
An incision is made in the gingival-buccal mucosa with the electrosurgical unit (ESU) or in the skin over the fracture site with a #10 or #15 blade. If a skin incision is used, Senn retractors are used to retract the skin and subcutaneous tissue. This exposes the mandible and periosteum, which can be elevated with a Freer or other type of periosteal elevator.

3. ***The fracture is exposed and reduced.***
The surgeon reduces the fracture with a small bone clamp. Radiographs or fluoroscopy may be used to evaluate the reduction.

4. ***Miniplates and screws are used to fix the fracture.***
The surgeon selects the plates needed for fixation. The 2.4- and 2.7-mm plates are commonly used. Most mandibular fractures require two plates per fracture: a large plate is used on the inferior side, and a miniplate or tension band device is used on the superior aspect. A small drill bit is fitted to a high-speed drill. The plate is stabilized against the mandible with a plate-holding forceps, and the screw holes are drilled. A drill guide may be used to stabilize the drill bit. If a drill guide is used, a depth gauge is used to measure the required screw length. The appropriate screw is loaded into a screwdriver and inserted.

5. ***The incisions are closed.***
When all of the fractures have been reduced and fixed, the incisions are closed. Transbuccal incisions are closed with 3-0 absorbable sutures, external incisions are closed in layers with 3-0 absorbable sutures, and the skin is closed with 4-0 absorbable sutures. The arch bars may be removed or left in place as needed.
Fig. 27.10 shows a mandibular repair using miniplates. Fig. 27.11 shows the use of a lag screw to approximate the bone fragments. The lag screw draws the two bone fragments together during implantation.

Panfacial Fractures

Panfacial fractures are those involving all three maxillofacial segments—the frontal bone, midface, and mandible. These injuries are treated systematically using the same techniques described above. However, frequently, the surgical wounds and repairs are reexamined within 48 hours to extend the debridement, drain hematomas, and plan further reconstruction. The panfacial injury is frequently caused by a gunshot or an explosive device. In terms of case planning, the ST should consult with the surgeon, if possible, before the case begins, to plan the case and avoid having excess sterile supplies and instruments while having the correct instrument sets available. Fig. 27.12 shows a panfacial injury as a result of a self-inflicted gunshot, including the repair.

TOOTH EXTRACTION

Patients undergoing maxillofacial surgery often require extraction of one or more teeth or extraction may be required as a stand-alone case. A patient requiring general anesthetic or monitored sedation may be operated on in an outpatient clinic. Instruments required for tooth extraction are relatively straightforward. Fig. 27.13 shows a basic extraction tray. Extractors are added according to the patient's age and location of the teeth to be removed.

Pathology

Odontectomy, or tooth extraction, may be performed for a variety of reasons, including damaged or decayed teeth or impaction, which often affects the third molars (wisdom teeth).

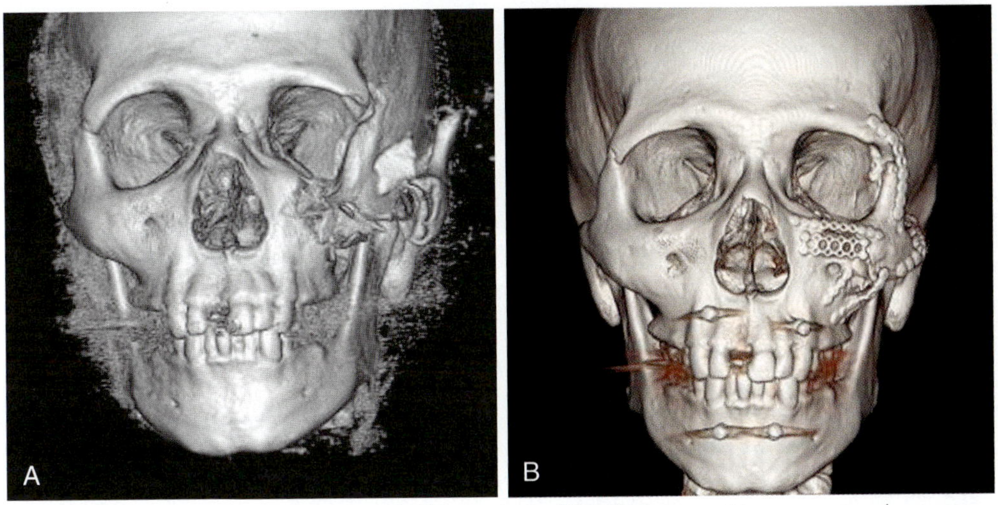

FIG. 27.9 Midface fractures (motor vehicle accident). (A) Before repair. Note extensive damage to the left zygoma and lower orbital rim. (B) Repair of the orbital rim and zygoma maxillary complex with miniplates and screws. (From Meyers E, ed. *Operative Otolaryngology Head and Neck Surgery*. 2nd ed. Philadelphia: Elsevier; 2008.)

POSITION:	Supine
INCISION:	Periodontal
PREP AND DRAPING:	Draping only with head drape and body sheet
INSTRUMENTS:	Dental extraction set

Technical Points and Discussion

1. ***After intubation using a nasotracheal tube, the patient is positioned.***
   The patient is induced and a nasotracheal tube inserted to maintain anesthesia.
   The patient is placed in the supine position with the arms tucked at the sides. The patient is draped to allow adequate access to the mouth.

2. ***An incision is made in the gingiva of the affected tooth.***
   The surgeon reviews imaging studies to ensure that the correct teeth are extracted. A #15 blade is used to make a gingival incision to the level of the bone. A Molt elevator is used to elevate the tissue, including the periosteum, surrounding the tooth.

3. ***The tooth is elevated out of the alveolus, making it mobile.***
   The surgeon then elevates the tooth out of the alveolus with an elevator; this breaks the attachment of the ligament holding the tooth in place, allowing the tooth to become mobile.

4. ***The tooth is extracted using a dental extractor, and the incision is closed.***
   The tooth is extracted with the appropriately sized dental extractor. The size of the extractor varies, depending on the tooth being extracted and the patient's age. If necessary, the incision is closed with absorbable 3-0 sutures (this is usually required with impactions). Dental packs may be placed to prevent postoperative bleeding.

KEY CONCEPTS

- Oral and maxillofacial (OMF) surgery involves surgical repair of fractures and skeletal defects to restore function and aesthetic appearance to the bony and soft tissues of the face.
- OMF trauma procedures are rarely performed as emergencies but are usually repaired within 24 hours of the trauma.
- The face and mouth are highly vascular, which provides some measure of postoperative infection. However, an attempt should be made to separate instruments used in the oral cavity from those used on the facial bones.
- Suction, rather than sponges, is used throughout maxillofacial procedures to maintain a dry field. A Yankauer or smaller round-tipped suction tip is used. Frazier suction tips should also be available.
- Basic instruments required for facial fractures are miniplates and screws, which are available as a commercial

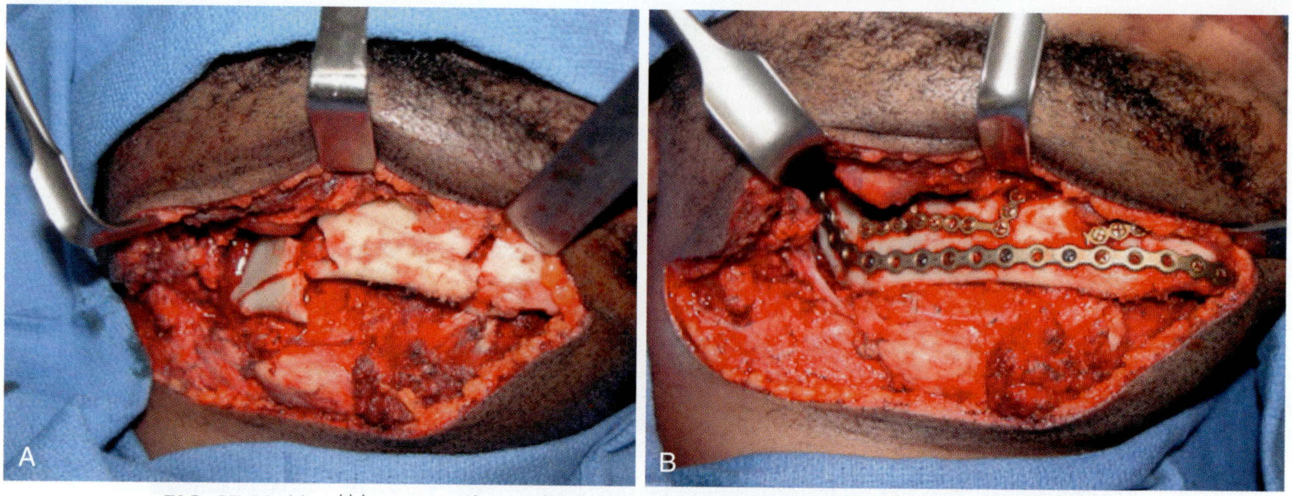

FIG. 27.10 Mandible repair with miniplates. (A) Fracture exposed. (B) Completion. (From Neligan P, Buck D, eds. *Core Procedures in Plastic Surgery*. Philadelphia: Elsevier; 2014.)

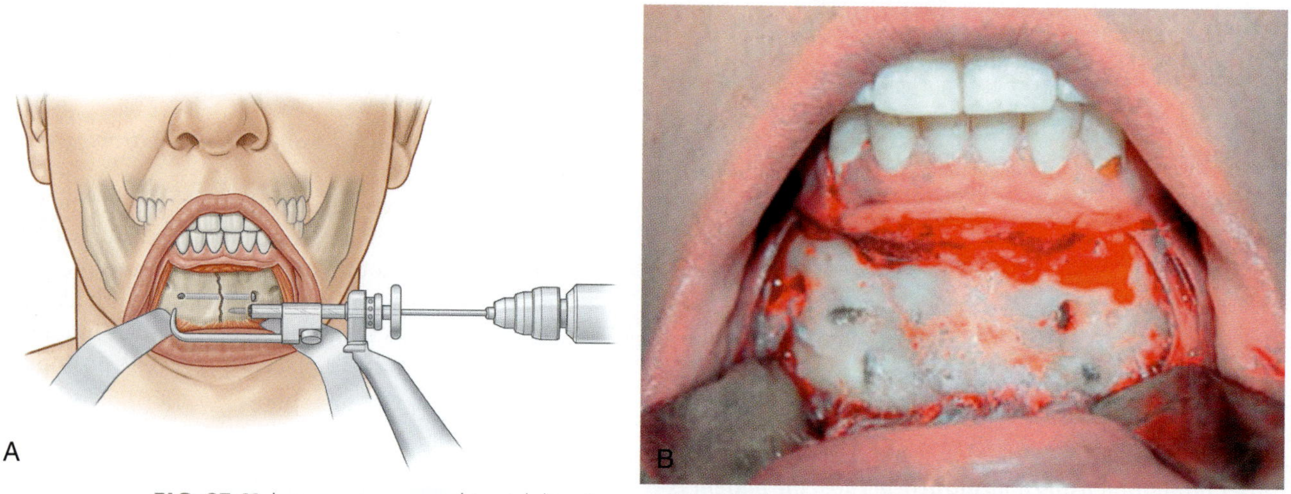

FIG. 27.11 Lag screws are used to stabilize the mandible. (A) The screws are inserted using a high-speed minidrill. (B) Finished repair. (From Neligan P, Buck D, eds. *Core Procedures in Plastic Surgery*. Philadelphia: Elsevier; 2014.)

set along with the instruments required to install them. A basic minifracture and soft tissue set may also be added.

- Facial trauma often involves important soft tissues such as the globe, lacrimal system, nerves, and muscles. Additional instruments may be required for these repairs.
- Management of the patient's airway is a primary concern in facial trauma. A nasotracheal tube is used for fractures involving the maxilla and mandible. A presurgical tracheostomy may be required.
- Maxillofacial patients are positioned supine, with the upper body slightly elevated.
- Insertion of arch bars is used to maintain stability in maxillary and mandibular fractures. The jaws are wired in the closed position. This requires that wire cutters be sent with the patient to the recovery room in case of airway emergency.

REVIEW QUESTIONS

1. Why are arch bars used during open reduction and internal fixation of facial fractures?
2. How should stainless steel sutures be handled? (Review Chapter 22 if necessary.) Expand your answer to include care of sharp ends and preparation.
3. What type of facial fracture may result in leakage of cerebrospinal fluid?
4. What causes a CSF leak?
5. What basic instruments are needed for arch bars?
6. Explain how a depth gauge is used to implant screws (refer to Chapter 29).
7. Why is it important to repair facial fractures as soon as the patient is stable?
8. What causes the orbital rim to rupture in a blowout fracture?

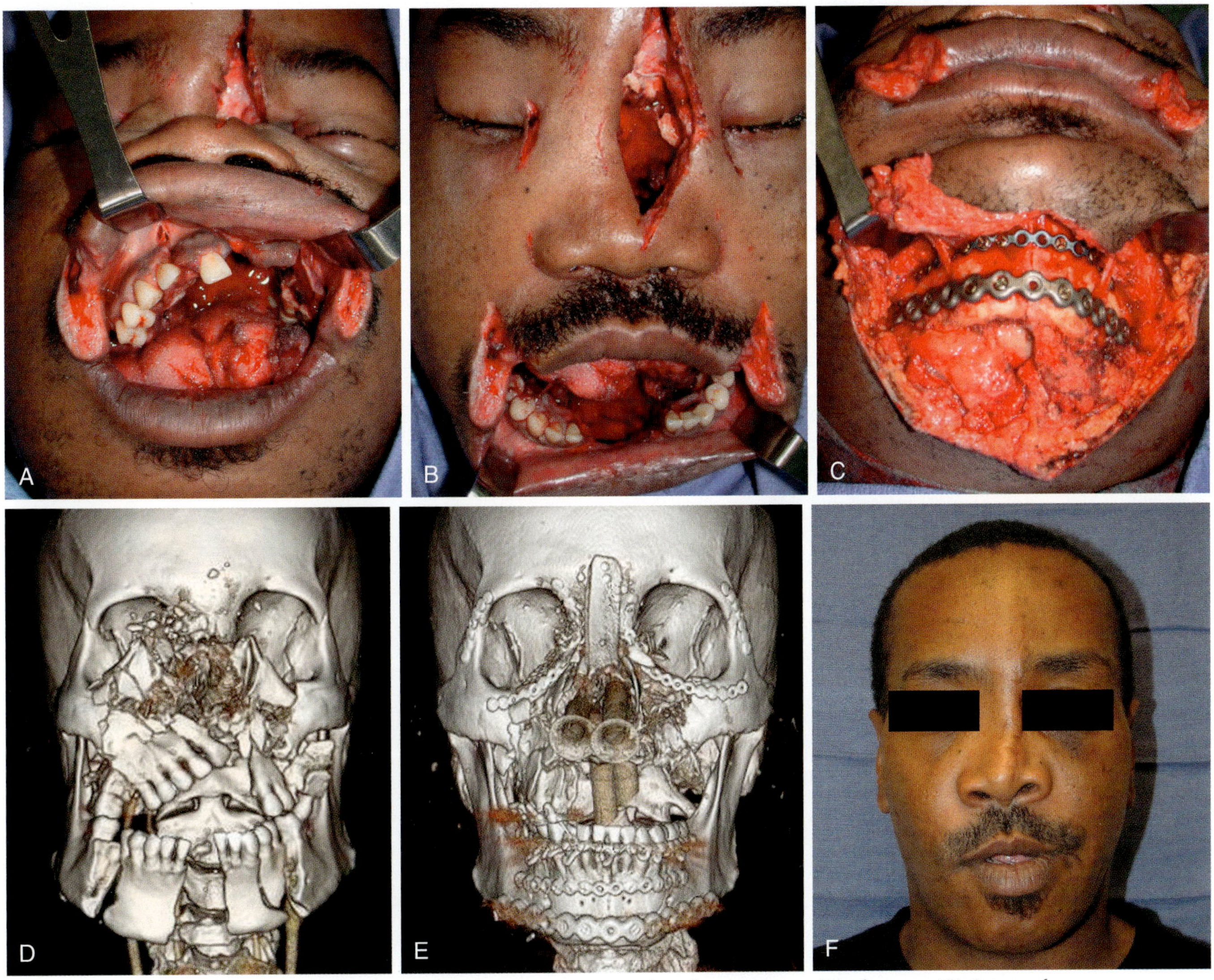

FIG. 27.12 Panfacial injury. (A and B) Demonstration of midface and mandible fractures. (C) Repair of the mandible with miniplates. (D) Three-dimensional CT demonstrating the extent of injury. (E) CT after repair. (F) Final outcome. (From Neligan P, Buck D, eds. *Core Procedures in Plastic Surgery*. Philadelphia: Elsevier; 2014.)

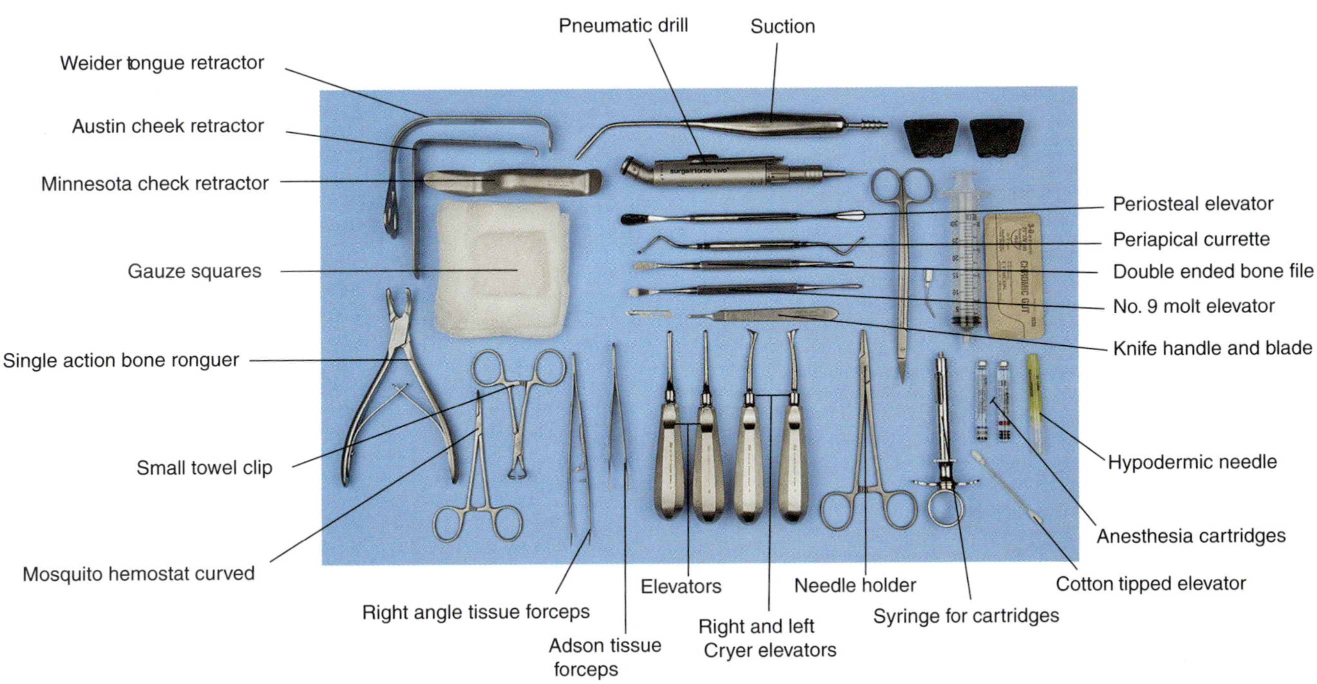

FIG. 27.13 Basic extraction tray. (From Hupp J. *Contemporary Oral and Maxillofacial Surgery*. Philadelphia: Elsevier; 2019.)

BIBLIOGRAPHY

Flint PW, Haughey BH, Lund VJ, Niparko JK, eds. *Cummings Otolaryngology: Head and Neck Surgery*. 5th ed. Philadelphia: Mosby; 2010.

Marks SC, ed. *Nasal and Sinus Surgery*. Philadelphia: WB Saunders; 2000.

Meyers E, ed. *Operative Otolaryngology Head and Neck Surgery*. 2nd ed. Philadelphia: Elsevier; 2008.

Neligan P, Buck D, eds. *Core Procedures in Plastic Surgery*. Philadelphia: Elsevier; 2014.

Thibodeau GA, Patt KT, eds. *Anthony's Textbook of Anatomy and Physiology*. 17th ed. St Louis: Mosby; 2003.

Weerda H, ed. *Reconstructive Facial Plastic Surgery: A Problem-Solving Manual*. New York: Thieme; 2001.

PLASTIC AND RECONSTRUCTIVE SURGERY 28

KNOWLEDGE AND SKILLS REVIEW

The following skills and knowledge should be reviewed before you start this chapter:
Procedure for frozen section specimens (Chapter 19)
Intraoperative management of grafts and implants (Chapter 18)

LEARNING OBJECTIVES

After studying this chapter, the reader will be able to:

1. Identify key anatomical features of the integumentary system
2. Discuss specific elements of case planning for plastic and reconstructive surgery
3. Discuss grafting techniques used in plastic and reconstructive surgery
4. Explain the principles of flap, transverse rectus abdominis myocutaneous (TRAM), and deep inferior epigastric perforator (DIEP) grafts

TERMINOLOGY

Aesthetic surgery: Surgery that is performed to improve appearance but not necessarily function.

Allograft: A tissue graft in which the donor and recipient are of the same species.

Autograft: The surgical transplantation of tissue from one part of the body to another in the same individual.

Biological graft: Grafts derived from live tissue, either human or animal.

Biosynthetic graft: A type of graft or implant material made of synthetic absorbable material.

Composite graft: A biological graft composed of different types of tissues such as skin and muscle.

Debridement: The surgical removal of devitalized tissue, debris, and infectious material from a wound.

Dermatome: A medical device used to remove single-thickness skin grafts.

Eschar: Thick, nonelastic, blackened tissue that forms over a full-thickness injury (usually third-degree burn or gangrenous wound).

Fasciotomy: Longitudinal incisions made in the fascia to release severe swelling or stricture, in compartment syndrome.

Full-thickness skin graft (FTSG): A skin graft composed of the epidermis and dermis.

Hypertrophic scar: A raised scar characterized by excess collagen.

Keloid: Excess scar tissue occurring in dark-skinned individuals. The scar may become bulbous and usually does not reduce over time.

Mohs micrographic surgery (MMS): A procedure in which a malignant tissue mass is removed and cut into quadrants before frozen section. These quadrants are used to map the tumor and determine the malignant margins.

Plication: Folding of tissue and securing it in place surgically.

Porcine: Derived from pig tissue.

Ptosis: Drooping or sagging of any anatomical structure.

Rule of nines: A method of estimating the percentage of burned tissue which relates to the patient's prognosis.

Split-thickness (or partial-thickness) skin graft (STSG): A skin graft that consists of the epidermis and a portion of the papillary dermis.

Synthetic grafts: Grafts derived from synthetic material compatible with body tissue. Synthetic grafts may be soft, semisolid, or liquid.

Undermine: A surgical technique in which a plane of tissue is created or an existing tissue plane is lifted, such as skin from the fascia.

Xenograft: A graft made up of tissue taken from one species and grafted into another species (e.g., a porcine graft implanted into human tissue).

The surgical objectives of plastic and reconstructive surgery are the following:

- To restore function lost because of trauma, disease, or a congenital anomaly
- To produce a physical outcome that is aesthetically acceptable to the patient within the individual's cultural and social environment

Plastic and reconstructive surgery involve the treatment of defects and anatomical abnormalities that are present at birth or acquired through disease or injury. Restoration of form and function is the primary goal of treatment. Plastic and reconstructive surgery crosses nearly all subspecialties and varies from simple procedures to extremely complex and technically demanding operations.

Aesthetic surgery, also called *cosmetic surgery*, is performed to improve an individual's appearance but does not necessarily address function.

An individual's personal, professional, and social goals are deeply connected with society's standards of acceptable appearance. In Western culture, body image is highly influenced by pressure to appear youthful (i.e., smooth, wrinkle-free skin; a slim body; and high definition of secondary sexual characteristics). Many plastic and reconstructive procedures are specifically intended to provide these changes. The basis of surgery is to fulfill a fundamental need for social acceptability. Individuals who have been disfigured by trauma, a congenital defect, or disease may experience a level of self-consciousness that prevents them from achieving a fulfilling life. For these patients, plastic surgery offers a path to integration into and acceptance by their social culture.

Whether the patient arrives in surgery for an elective or a nonelective procedure, special psychological needs must be met. Patients usually benefit from an honest, straightforward manner and should receive emotional support throughout the perioperative period.

SURGICAL ANATOMY

INTEGUMENTARY SYSTEM (SKIN)

The skin, or integumentary system, performs numerous vital functions:

- Protects underlying tissues and organs
- Excretes organic waste and stores nutrients
- Excretes water and dissipates heat as a means of thermoregulation
- Contains sensory nerves that inform the individual about the environment

Epidermis

The epidermis is the outer layer of the skin. The primary tissue cells of the epidermis are the keratinocytes. Five distinct epidermal layers represent various developmental stages of the keratinocyte:

- The *stratum corneum* is the most superficial layer. It is relatively transparent and composed of dead keratinocytes that are filled with a protein called *keratin.* The stratum corneum is thicker on areas of the body that are weight bearing or exposed to friction, such as the hands and feet.
- The *stratum lucidum* is composed of dead or dying cells that are flattened and densely packed. This layer is extremely thin (approximately five cells thick). It may be absent on areas of the body with thin skin.
- The *stratum granulosum* is several cells thick and produces keratin.
- The *stratum spinosum* contains undifferentiated cells that become specialized as they migrate to the skin surface.
- The *stratum germinativum*, also called the *stratum basale*, is the deepest layer of the epidermis attached to the dermis. The cells in this layer undergo mitosis, producing daughter keratinocytes that migrate through the layers of the epidermis. The melanocytes also are found in this layer; these cells are responsible for the production of melanin, a substance that gives rise to skin pigmentation.

Dermis

The dermis lies between the epidermis and the subcutaneous fatty layer. It provides nourishment and innervation to the epidermis. The blood vessels of the dermis are responsible for oxygenation of the tissue and thermoregulation. A large portion of the vascular plexus in the dermis bypasses the capillaries through an arteriovenous network in which small arteries flow directly into venules. This allows the vessels to dilate and constrict as the environmental temperature rises and falls. The dermis has numerous sensory receptors (i.e., for pain, touch, heat, cold, and pressure), which inform the brain about environmental change or danger.

Skin Appendages

Skin contains several specialized structures called *appendages*, such as hair, sweat, and oil glands, which have protective functions.

HAIR Hair is a protective structure that covers most areas of the body, except the palms and soles of the feet. Each hair is surrounded by a follicle located in the dermis. The follicle consists of the hair itself, a sebaceous gland, muscle, and sometimes an apocrine (sweat) gland. The hair shaft, the visible portion of the hair, varies in size, shape, and color. The *sebaceous glands* discharge a waxy, oily secretion called *sebum* into the hair follicles and acts as a lubricant. The hair muscle (arrector pili muscle) aids thermoregulation of the body by contracting in a cold environment; this reduces the surface area of the skin and prevents heat loss.

SWEAT GLANDS Two types of *sweat glands* are found in the human body. The *apocrine sweat glands* arise from the dermis and are located mainly in the axilla and groin. They open out into the hair follicles. The oily secretion has no odor unless it comes in contact with bacteria. The *eccrine glands* secrete sweat over the surface of the body through small tubules. Sweat helps regulate the body temperature by cooling it through evaporation.

As mentioned, sebaceous glands produce sebum, a combination of wax, lipids, cholesterol, and triglycerides. These glands are distributed over the entire body, except on the palms and the soles of the feet. Their functions are to lubricate the skin and hair and to prevent evaporation in a cold environment. The sebaceous glands are responsive to hormonal influence, and their size is proportional to the amount of sebum produced. A cross-section of skin showing the layers is shown in Fig. 28.1.

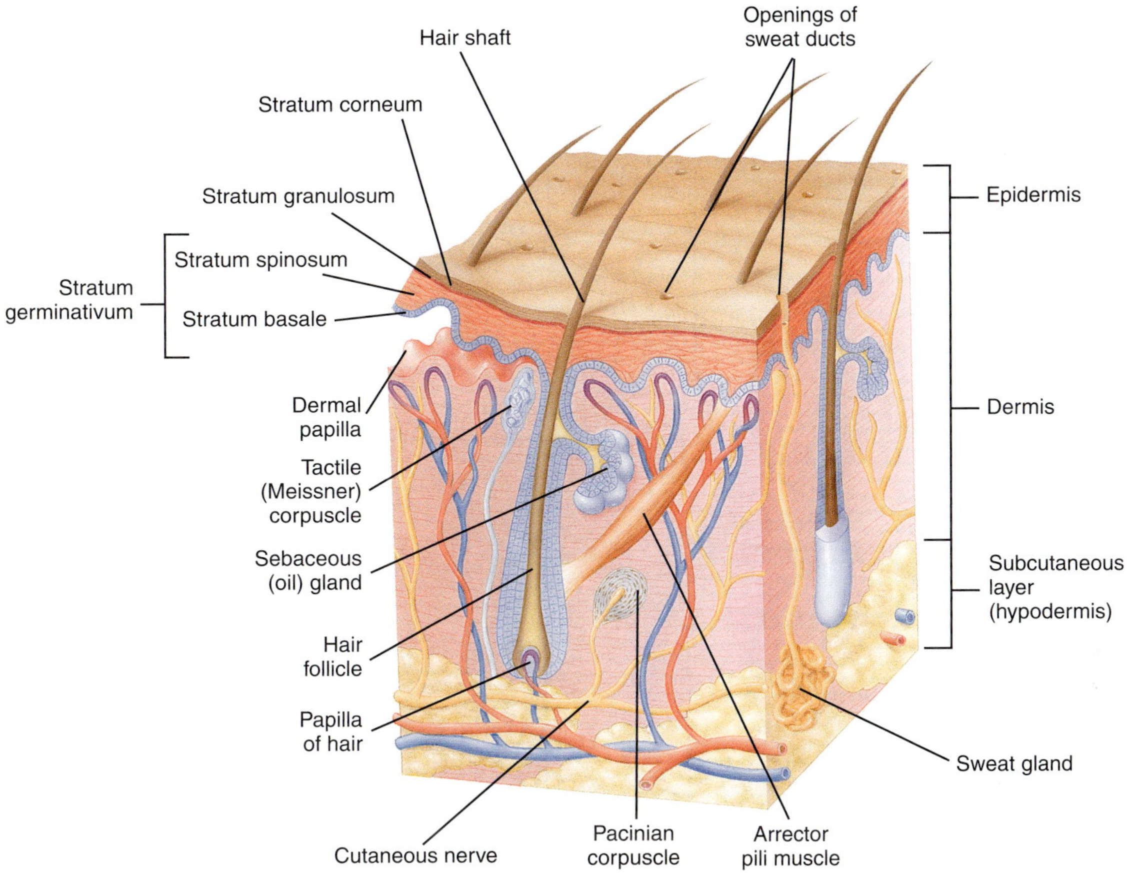

FIG. 28.1 The skin, including the dermis and epidermis. (From Thibodeau GA, Patton KT, eds. *Anthony's Textbook of Anatomy and Physiology*. 17th ed. St Louis: Mosby; 2003.)

ANATOMY OF THE FACE

Many aesthetic surgical procedures are performed on the face. The soft tissues of the face include skin, fat (adipose tissue), muscle, fascia, and ligaments (Fig. 28.2). The subcutaneous fatty tissue is separated into deep and superficial layers by a tissue plane called the *superficial musculoaponeurotic system* (commonly called the SMAS). The fat of the superficial layer is composed of lobes, which are deposited unevenly over the surface of the face and integrated within the fibrous tissue of the SMAS. The fat is very dense in the cheek and neck region. The deep fat layer, under the SMAS, is thinner and divided by fibrous bands. The ligaments of the face support the soft tissue and attach it to the bone.

CASE PLANNING

PREPPING AND DRAPING

Povidone-iodine is used to prep the skin for surgical procedures. However, the specific dilution of this prep solution is ordered by the surgeon. Regardless of the prep solution used, care must be taken not to allow the prep solution to drain into the eyes or ears. For a complete discussion of an eye prep, refer to Chapter 25.

Draping routines in plastic and reconstructive surgery follow the general techniques described in Chapter 17. Extra draping towels, plain sheets, and adhesive drapes should be available for complex draping routines. For procedures involving the face, most surgeons use a head drape. This prevents the hair from falling into the field and allows the surgeon to visualize the entire face during the procedure. Hair that may interfere with the operative site can be pulled back into multiple sections and held with elastic bands. Fenestrated or split sheets are used for draping a limb. Whenever large amounts of solution are required, such as during debridement, an impervious pocket drape should be used to collect and isolate runoff. Multiple draping sites are commonly required during plastic and reconstructive surgery.

INSTRUMENTS

Plastic surgery instruments include a variety of devices for cutting, sculpting, retracting, and grasping tissue. Superficial procedures of the dermis require short instruments (5-inch to 7-inch). Shallow retractors including skin hooks, rakes, and self-retaining spring retractors are included in the basic plastic surgery set. Procedures that involve deep tissues such as muscles, the body wall, and breast tissue require deeper retractors such as those used in general surgery. Specialized retractors for elevating the body wall are required during abdominoplasty. Lighted retractors such as the one shown in Fig. 28.3 are also used in plastic and reconstructive procedures.

Sharp dissection is performed with very fine, sharp scissors and toothed tissue forceps. Many other kinds of delicate

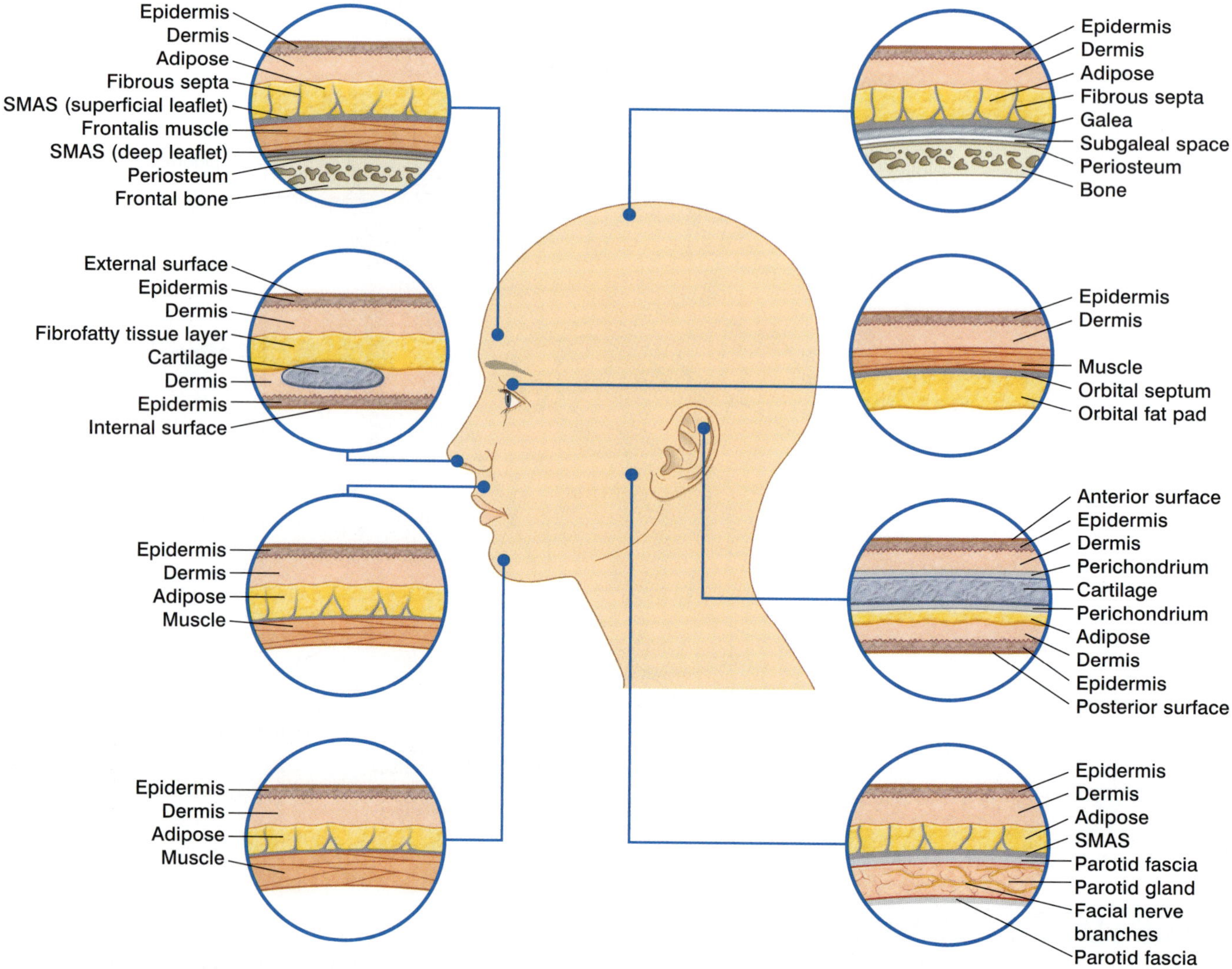

FIG. 28.2 Tissue layers of the face. (From Robinson J, Hanke C, eds. *Surgery of the Skin: Procedural Dermatology*. 3rd ed. Philadelphia: Saunders Elsevier; 2015.)

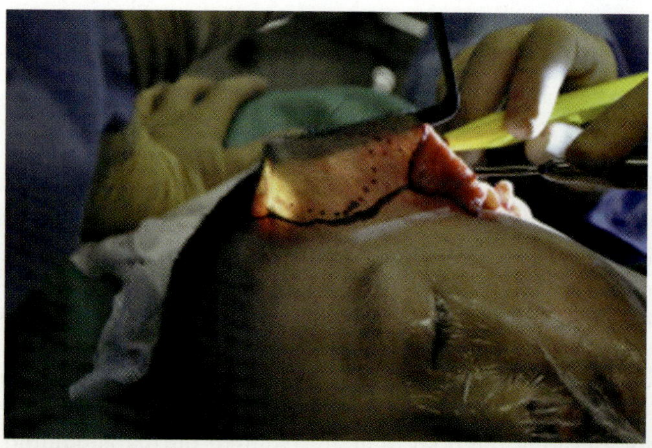

FIG. 28.3 Lighted retractor—frequently used in plastic and reconstructive surgery. (From Stephan S, Reinisch J. Auricular reconstruction using porous polyethylene implant technique. *Facial Plast Surg Clin North Am* 2018;26(1):69–85. https://doi.org/10.1016/j.fsc.2017.09.009.)

scissors are available, and most plastic surgeons have one or two favorites, which the surgical technologist should have available.

Toothed forceps are used for grasping skin. Adson or fine single-toothed forceps are used for procedures that do not require magnification. Hemostats are not used on the skin but are required for superficial blood vessels or for tagging suture. Fine mosquito forceps are commonly used.

Reconstruction procedures may require fine orthopedic instruments, including small bone clamps, toothed tissue forceps, and small Kocher clamps. Rasps, small osteotomes, and fine curettes also should be available during procedures involving bone tissue. Curved and straight Mayo scissors are needed for trimming cartilage and soft implants. Many facilities develop custom-made sets for specific procedures, often based upon their surgeons' preferences and techniques. Basic plastic instruments are shown in the Plastic Surgery Instruments table.

PLASTIC SURGERY INSTRUMENTS

Par Scissors Sharp 5¾″

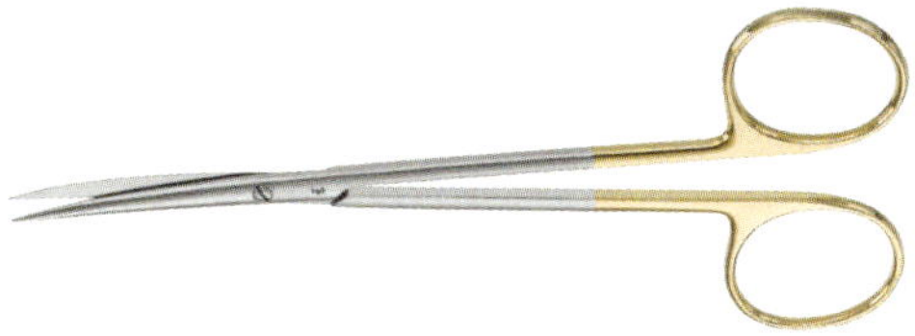

Photo courtesy Aesculap, Inc., Center Valley, PA.

Strabismus SCIS 4½″

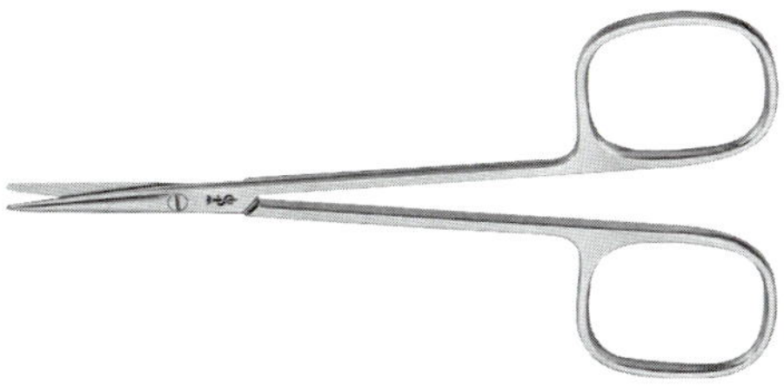

Photo courtesy Aesculap, Inc., Center Valley, PA.

Supercut scissors 5½″

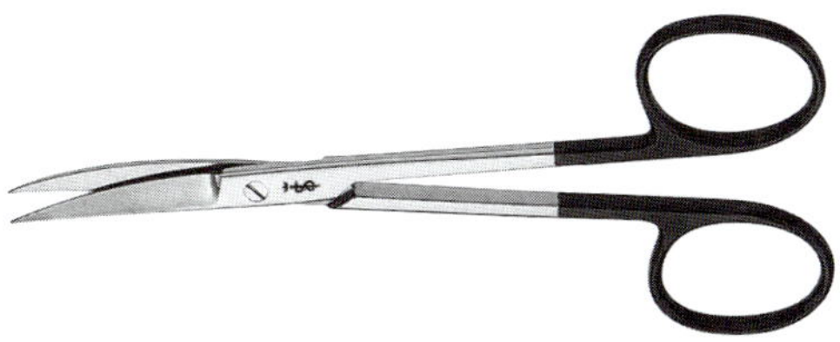

Photo courtesy Aesculap, Inc., Center Valley, PA.

Suture SCIS 4¾″

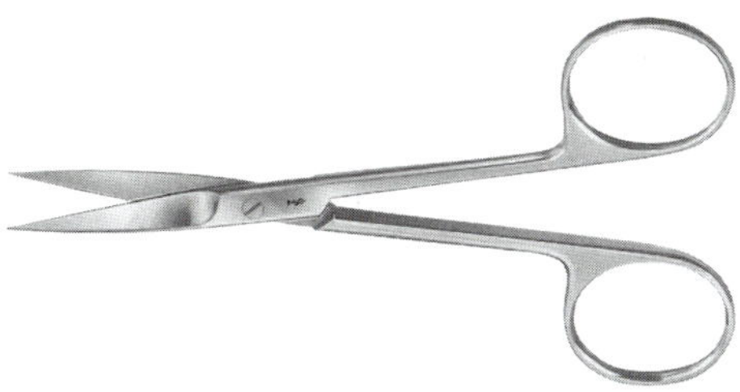

Photo courtesy Aesculap, Inc., Center Valley, PA.

Fraser-Kelly FRCP 5½″

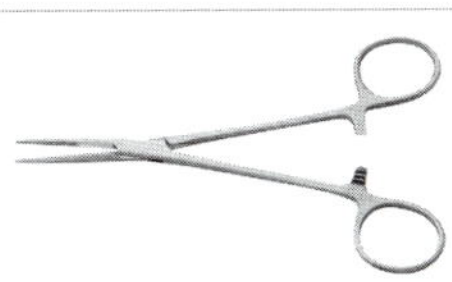

Courtesy and copyright Becton, Dickinson and Company.

Mosquito FRCP Cu. 5″

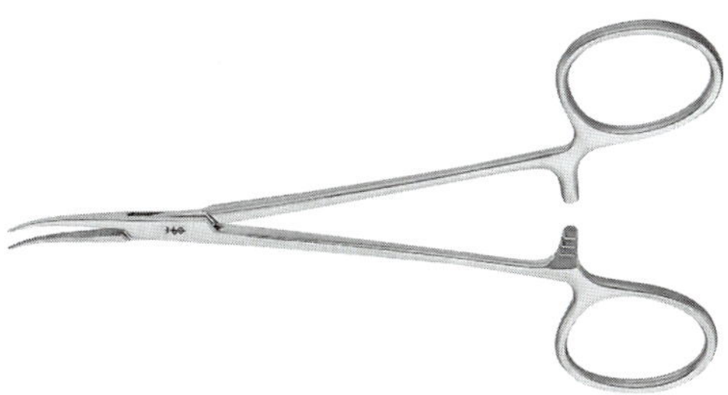

Photo courtesy Aesculap, Inc., Center Valley, PA.

Kaye Facelift SCIS 7½″

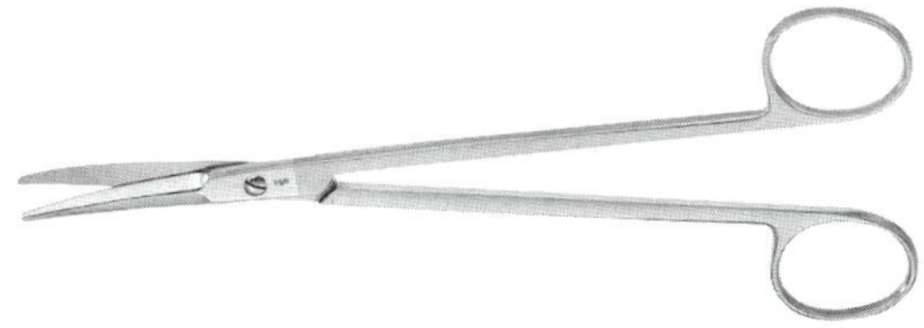

Photo courtesy Aesculap, Inc., Center Valley, PA.

Metzenbaum SCIS St. 5¾″

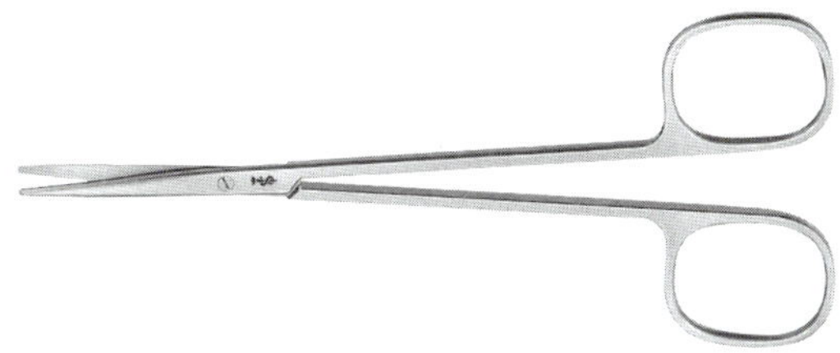

Photo courtesy Aesculap, Inc., Center Valley, PA.

Straight Dissecting SCIS

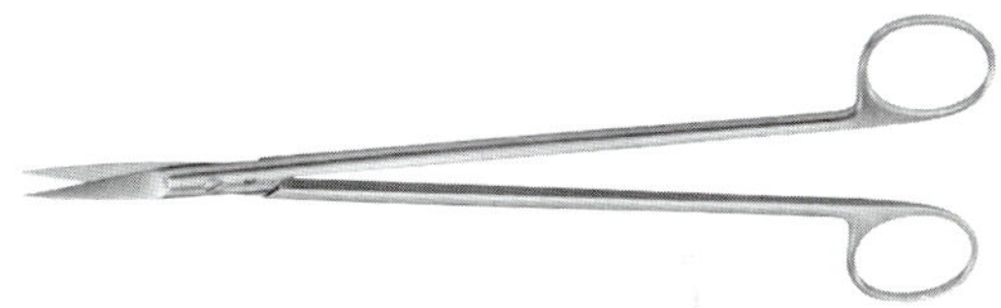

Photo courtesy Aesculap, Inc., Center Valley, PA.

Kelly FRCP St. 5½″

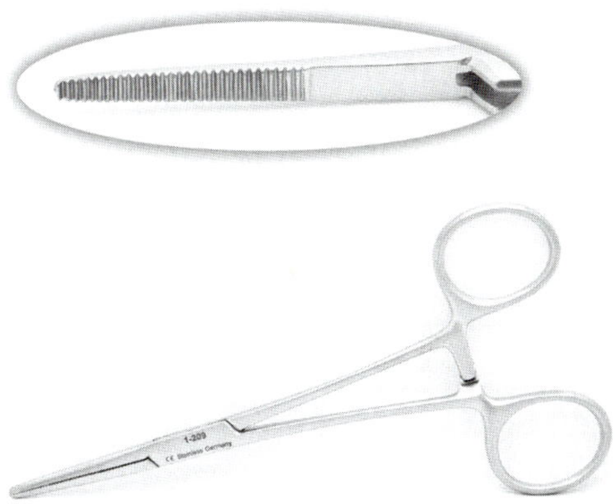

Photo courtesy Millennium Surgical Corp.

Kocher CLMP 5½″

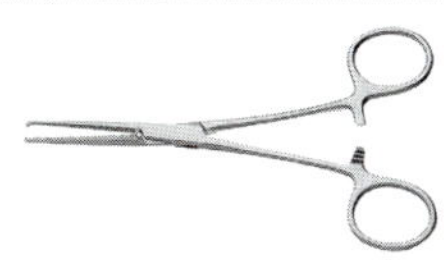

Courtesy and copyright Becton, Dickinson and Company.

Hartman Mosquito CLMP 5″

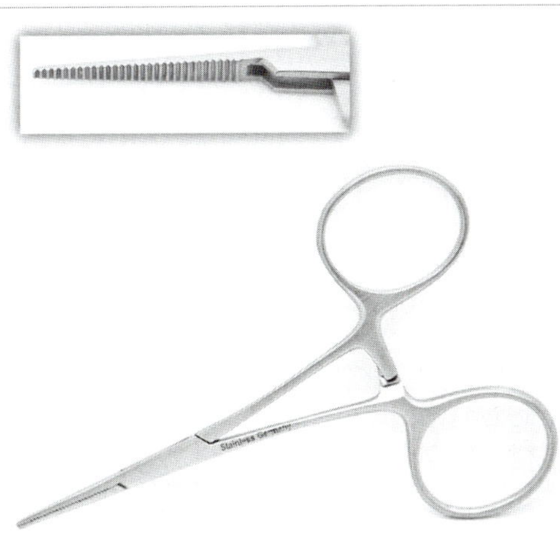

Photo courtesy Millennium Surgical Corp.

Continued

PLASTIC SURGERY INSTRUMENTS —cont'd

Watson Skin Graft Knife

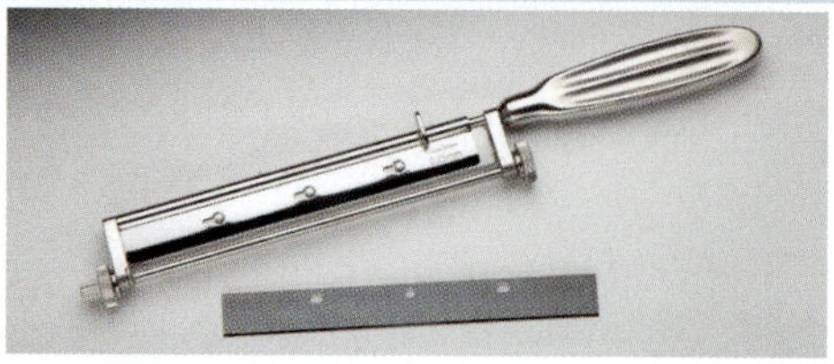

From Nemitz. *Surgical Instrumentation: An Interactive Approach*. 3rd ed. St. Louis: Elsevier; 2019.

Graefe Tissue FRCP 4½″

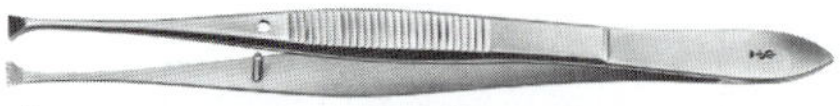

Photo courtesy Aesculap, Inc., Center Valley, PA.

Gerald FRCP 1 × 2 teeth 5½″

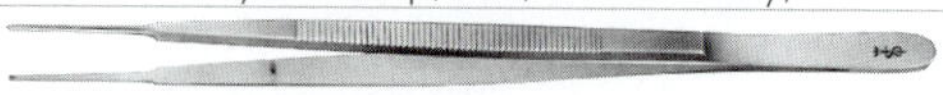

Photo courtesy Aesculap, Inc., Center Valley, PA.

Jewelers forceps cu tips 4⅜″

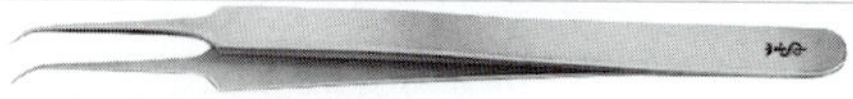

Photo courtesy Aesculap, Inc., Center Valley, PA.

Liposuction Cannula

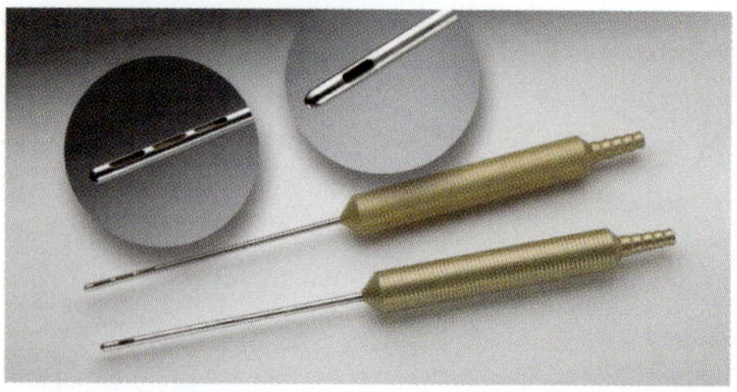

From Nemitz. *Surgical Instrumentation: An Interactive Approach*. 3rd ed. St. Louis: Elsevier; 2019.

Allis tissue FRCP 5½″

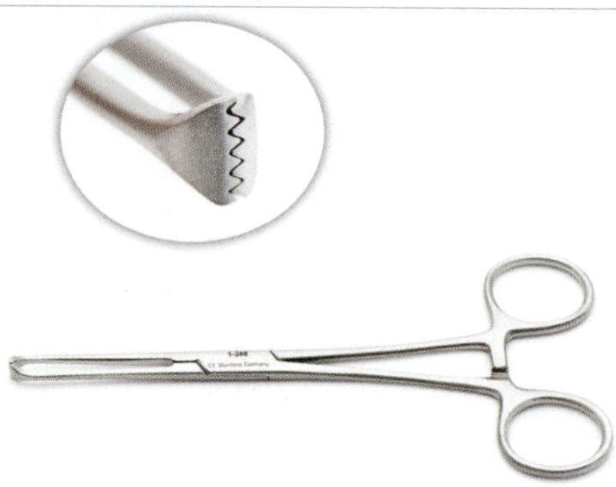

Photo courtesy Millennium Surgical Corp.

Skin hook 7½″

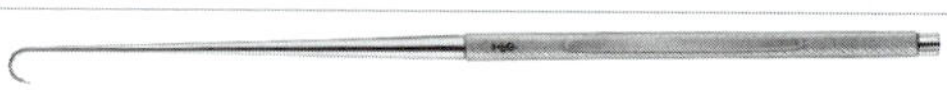

Skin hook 2 Prong 5½″

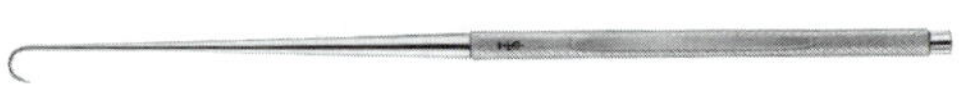

Photo courtesy Aesculap, Inc., Center Valley, PA.

Ball Hook Retractor {5/12}″

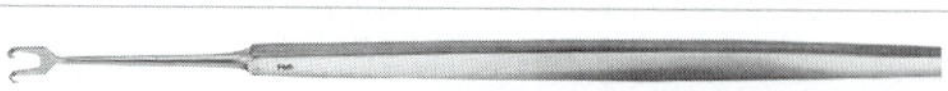

Photo courtesy Aesculap, Inc., Center Valley, PA.

Senn Retractor 6¾″

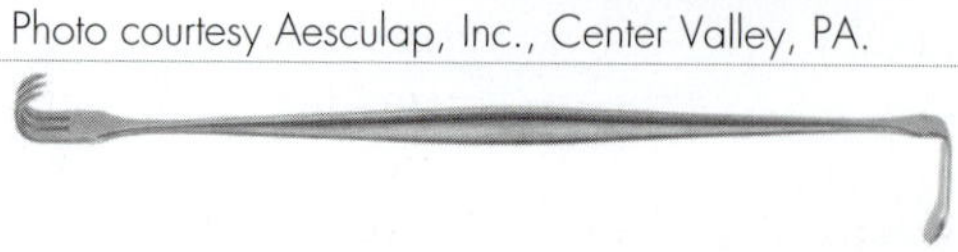

Courtesy and copyright Becton, Dickinson and Company.

Weitlaner Retractor 4⅜″

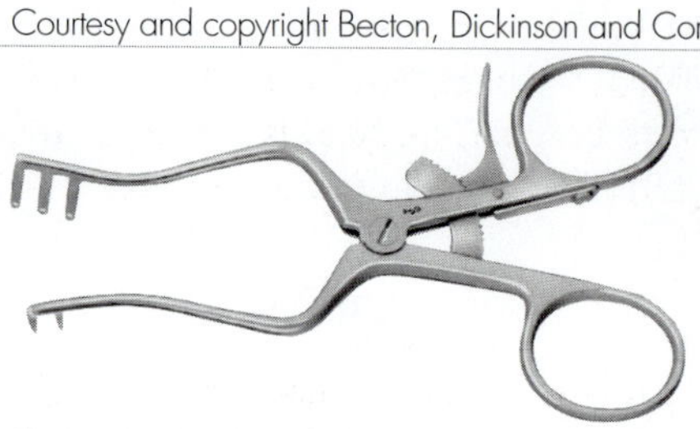

Photo courtesy Aesculap, Inc., Center Valley, PA.

Adson FRCP Smooth 4½″

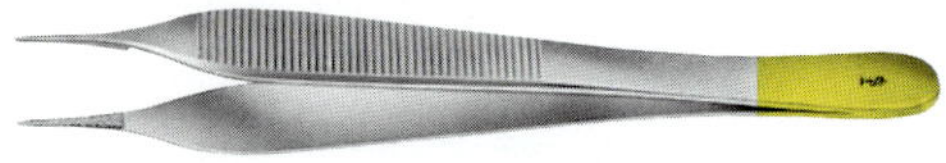

Photo courtesy Aesculap, Inc., Center Valley, PA.

Brown Tissue FRCP 4½″

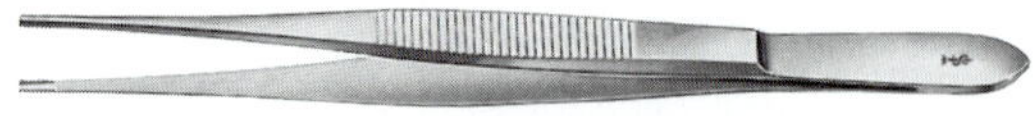

Photo courtesy Aesculap, Inc., Center Valley, PA.

Jewelers FRCP 5¼″

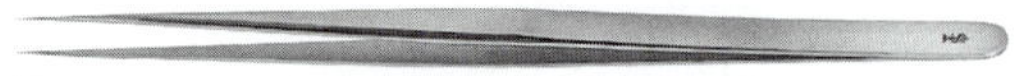

Photo courtesy Aesculap, Inc., Center Valley, PA.

Micro Lazar suture forceps 6″

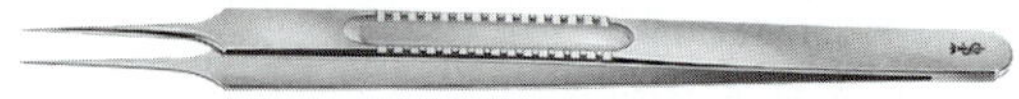

Photo courtesy Aesculap, Inc., Center Valley, PA.

Tissue forceps 1 × 2 teeth 4½″

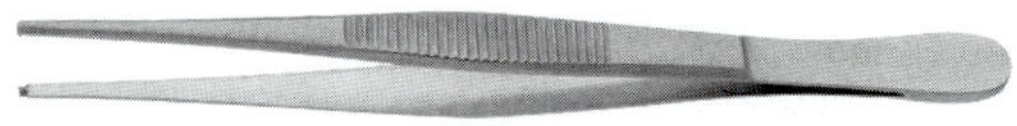

Courtesy and copyright Becton, Dickinson and Company.

Delicate Kocher 5″

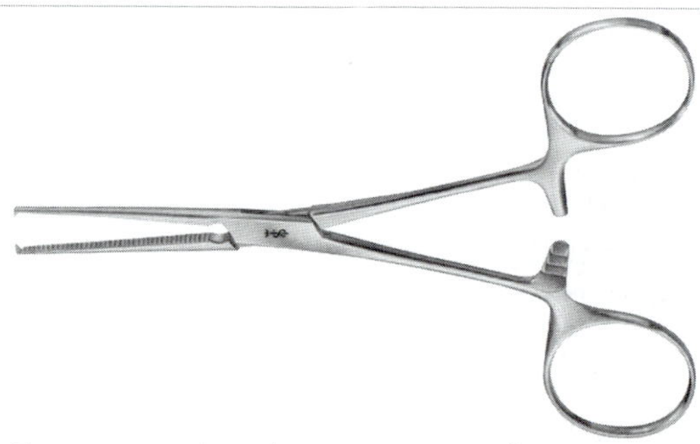

Photo courtesy Aesculap, Inc., Center Valley, PA.

Vein retractor 7½″

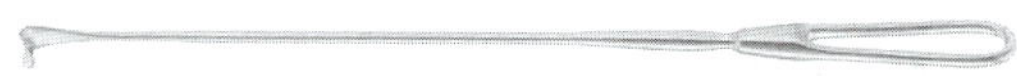

Photo courtesy Aesculap, Inc., Center Valley, PA.

Graefe Skin Hook 5½″

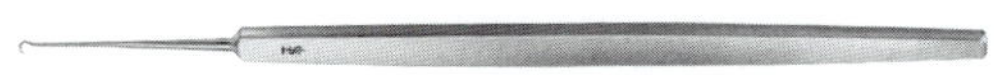

Photo courtesy Aesculap, Inc., Center Valley, PA.

Graefe Nerve/ vessel Hook 6″

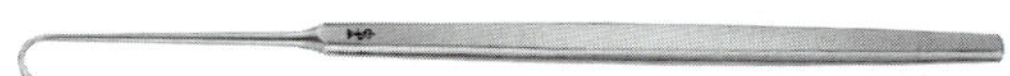

Photo courtesy Aesculap, Inc., Center Valley, PA.

Breast Retractor 12½″

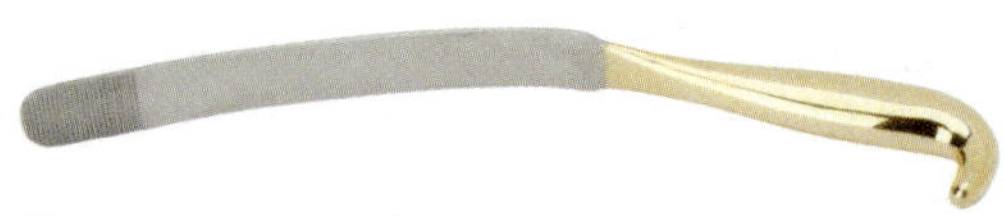

Photo courtesy Aesculap, Inc., Center Valley, PA.

Frazier Suction Cannula 3½″

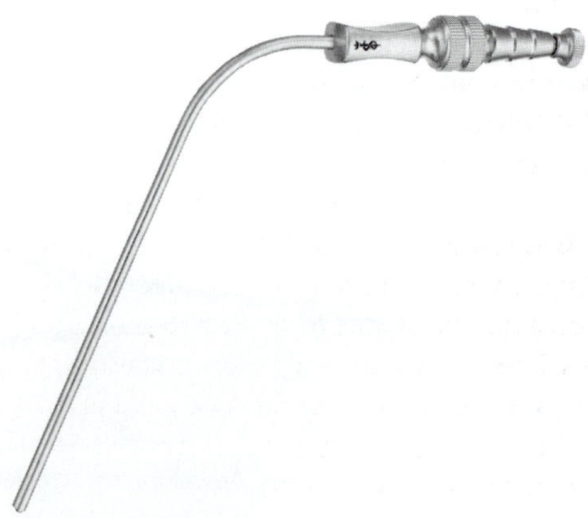

Photo courtesy Aesculap, Inc., Center Valley, PA.

PLASTIC SURGERY INSTRUMENTS —cont'd

Rosen Suction Cannula ½″

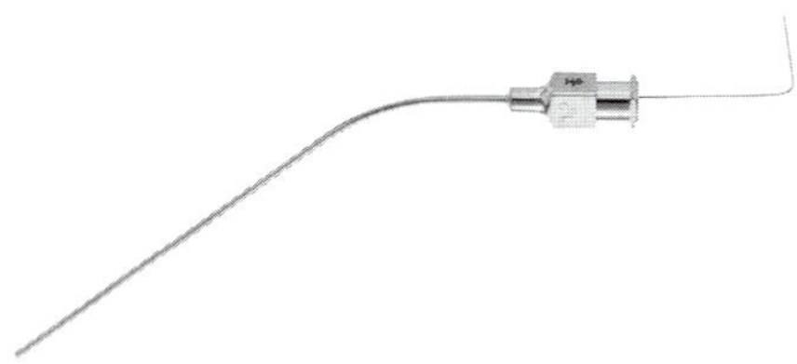

Photo courtesy Aesculap, Inc., Center Valley, PA.

Lempert Bone Rongeur 6½″

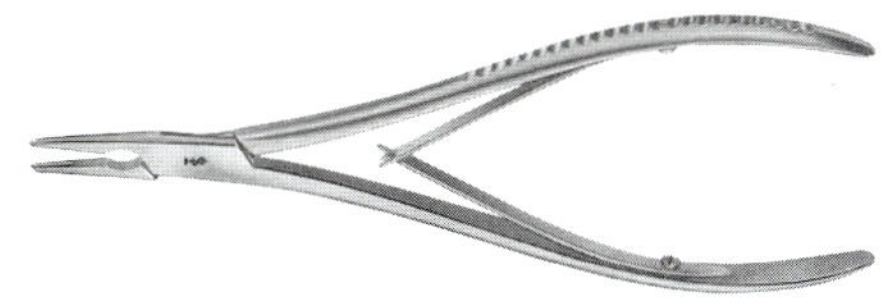

Photo courtesy Aesculap, Inc., Center Valley, PA.

SCIS scissors; FRCP forceps; Cu curved; St straight; CLMP clamp;

Bone-Cutting Instruments

Plastic and reconstructive surgery may require powered orthopedic instruments for the following techniques:

- To model bone tissue with a rotating burr or cutter
- To create anchor holes for screws or pins
- To cut through bone with an oscillating or reciprocal saw blade

Power drills are available in a wide variety of sizes and designs. The ST is responsible for proper assembly and safe management of these instruments. Refer to Chapter 29 for more information.

SURGICAL PROCEDURES

SURGICAL MANAGEMENT OF BURNS

Burns are caused by heat, flame, scalding (liquid), electrical current, radiation, or chemicals. Hospitals that contain a burn ICU also have surgical facilities to provide complete care to the burn patient. Management of burns is a specialization that requires specific advanced training of all staff. Severely burned patients frequently require extensive plastic or reconstructive surgery.

Classification of Burns

The current system for classifying burns established by the American Burn Association, http://www.ameriburn.org, describes the depth of tissue injury:

- **Superficial partial-thickness first-degree:** Only the outer layer of the epidermis is injured. The skin is red or pink, dry, and painful to touch.
- **Partial-thickness second-degree:** The epidermis and various degrees of the dermis are injured. The skin is blistered, red, and moist. The burn is very sensitive to environmental exposure and touch.
- **Full-thickness second-degree:** The epidermis and full dermis are injured. These burns are characterized by a white, smooth, shiny surface with dry blisters and edema.
- **Full-thickness third-degree:** The skin, subcutaneous tissue, muscle, and bone are burned. The third-degree burn is centered in an area of second-degree injury. The skin may be white, brown, or black with a waxy appearance. There is no pain because nerves have been destroyed. Third-degree burns develop **eschar,** which is devitalized nonelastic tissue that adheres to the wound site.

Extensive second- and third-degree burns can result in fluid and electrolyte imbalance, infection, inadequate nutrition, respiratory deficit, and vascular damage. Circumferential

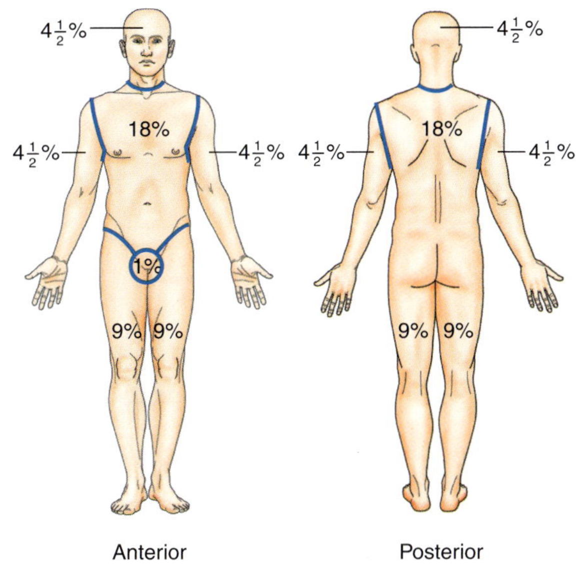

FIG. 28.4 Rule of nines for estimating body surface area burned. Burned areas are calculated according to the anatomical area. Greater than 15% affected area relates to a high probability of burn shock. (From Garden OJ, Parks RW. *Principles and Practice of Surgery*. Edinburgh: Elsevier; 2018.)

eschar (thick charred tissue resulting from a burn) has a tourniquet effect on the affected body part and thus can extensively damage underlying muscle, bone, and vascular tissue. In this case, an **escharotomy** or **fasciotomy** (multiple incisions through the eschar or fascia) is performed to release the stricture.

Estimating Surface Area of Burns

Estimating the percent of body surface area that has been burned is important for emergency treatment such as fluid resuscitation and for predicting levels of morbidity and mortality. Patients with greater than 15% surface area burned (adults) are likely to develop hypovolemic shock. In children, the same risk occurs when 10% of total body surface area is burned. There are two systems commonly used to determine surface area of burns. The **Rule of Nines** (Fig. 28.4) is used in *adults only*. In this system areas of the body are assigned fractions or multiples of 9% of total body surface area. The **Brower and Lund** system (Fig. 28.5) is used for children as it accounts for developmental differences in surface area by age.

DEBRIDEMENT OF BURNS

Debridement is the removal of nonviable tissue from a nonhealing or traumatic wound. Burn wounds require

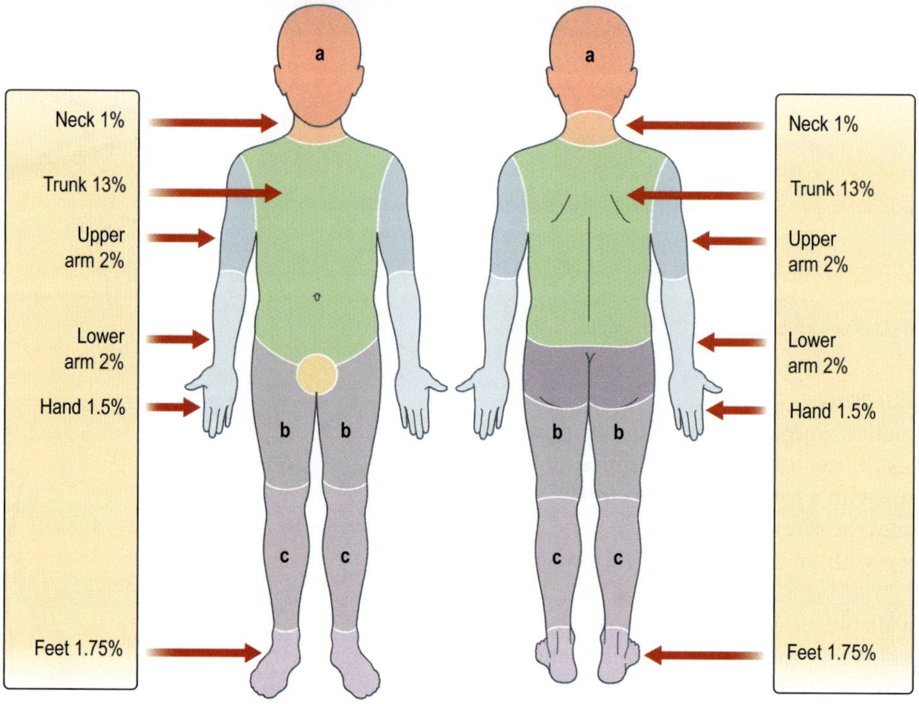

Body part	0 yr	1 yr	5 yr	10 yr	15 yr	Age
	relative % of body surface area					
a = 1/2 of head	91/2	81/2	61/2	51/2	41/2	
b = 1/2 of thigh	23/4	31/4	4	41/4	41/2	
c = 1/2 of lower leg	21/2	21/2	23/4	3	31/4	

FIG. 28.5 Browder and Lund method of estimating body surface area burned in children. (From Lee R, Teven CM, Neligan P. *Plastic Surgery: Volume 4: Lower Extremity, Trunk, and Burns*. 2018.)

repeated debridement to remove dying and dead tissue so that healing can continue.

Pathology

Debridement may be necessary for any type of contaminated or complex traumatic wound. Tissue damage from burns continues after the event. This is related to disrupted physiological processes in and around the burn. Burn patients are also susceptible to fluid volume and electrolyte abnormalities, which contribute to tissue sloughing and infection.

POSITION:	According to the location of the wound(s)
INCISION:	The wound site
PREP AND DRAPING:	The sites are prepared separately
INSTRUMENTS AND SUPPLIES:	Minor plastic surgery set including fine scissors and fine Adson and Brown forceps; saline irrigation at body temperature; bulb syringes
POSSIBLE EXTRAS:	Protective dressings according to the surgeon's preferences

Technical Points and Discussion

Preparation of the burn patient requires extensive thermoregulation and physiological monitoring. The temperature in the operating room is raised to reduce the risk of hypothermia.

1. ***The patient is positioned and prepped.***
The patient is positioned to allow for adequate exposure of the burn. General anesthesia is used. The patient is prepped with povidone-iodine and draped with towels and three-quarter sheets. A pneumatic tourniquet may be used for burns of the extremities.

2. ***Nonviable skin is removed.***
The surgeon begins by removing all nonviable skin with scissors and a #10 or #20 knife blade. A Braithwaite or Watson knife (see later) may also be used. The tissue is removed until only a viable layer remains. The ST should have a small basin available to receive the specimens. The surgeon may irrigate the wound with saline at room temperature.

3. ***Hemostasis is maintained.***
Lap sponges soaked in a solution of sterile saline and topical epinephrine are applied to control bleeding. The

concentration most often used is 1000 mL of normal saline, with 4 mL of topical epinephrine (1:1000) added according to the surgeon's orders.

4. ***An allograft or nonadherent and padded protective dressing are applied.***
When hemostasis has been achieved, an allograft may be applied. The graft is stapled over the debrided burns to create a layer of protection until autografting can be performed (usually several days after the initial debridement). Nonadherent dressings (e.g., Xeroform) and fluffs are applied. The extremities are wrapped with compression bandages.

SKIN GRAFTS

An introduction to tissue grafts was presented in Chapter 18. The technical details of skin grafting are presented here.

A graft is tissue taken from a distant site on the patient, from another individual, or animal and used to replace tissue lost from disease or injury. A graft can also be manufactured (synthetic material). Skin grafting is a common procedure in plastic surgery. The ST must be familiar with the type of graft planned for a particular surgery. This information determines the preoperative preparation; the instruments, equipment, and supplies used; and the procedural steps of the surgery.

CLASSIFICATION OF SKIN GRAFTS

Split-thickness skin graft (STSG): Contains epidermis and papillary dermis, which is a highly bioactive portion of the dermis

Full-thickness skin graft (FTSG): Contains the complete dermis and epidermis

Fig. 28.6 illustrates the difference between a split-thickness and a full-thickness skin graft.

MATERIALS USED FOR SKIN GRAFTS

Three categories of materials are used in skin grafting:

- **Biological:** Derived from living tissue
- **Synthetic:** Derived from manufactured materials
- **Biosynthetic:** Absorbed by the body or enhances healing but is not derived from biological tissue

TYPES OF BIOLOGICAL GRAFTS

The ST should become familiar with terms used to describe implants and grafting techniques in these categories:

- **Allograft:** A graft transferred from one individual to another. An allograft, also called *homograft*, is harvested from donors and preserved by the tissue bank until needed. Skin, bone, and cartilage are commonly used allografts. Once the allograft has been implanted, it is incorporated into the patient's tissues and eventually absorbed.

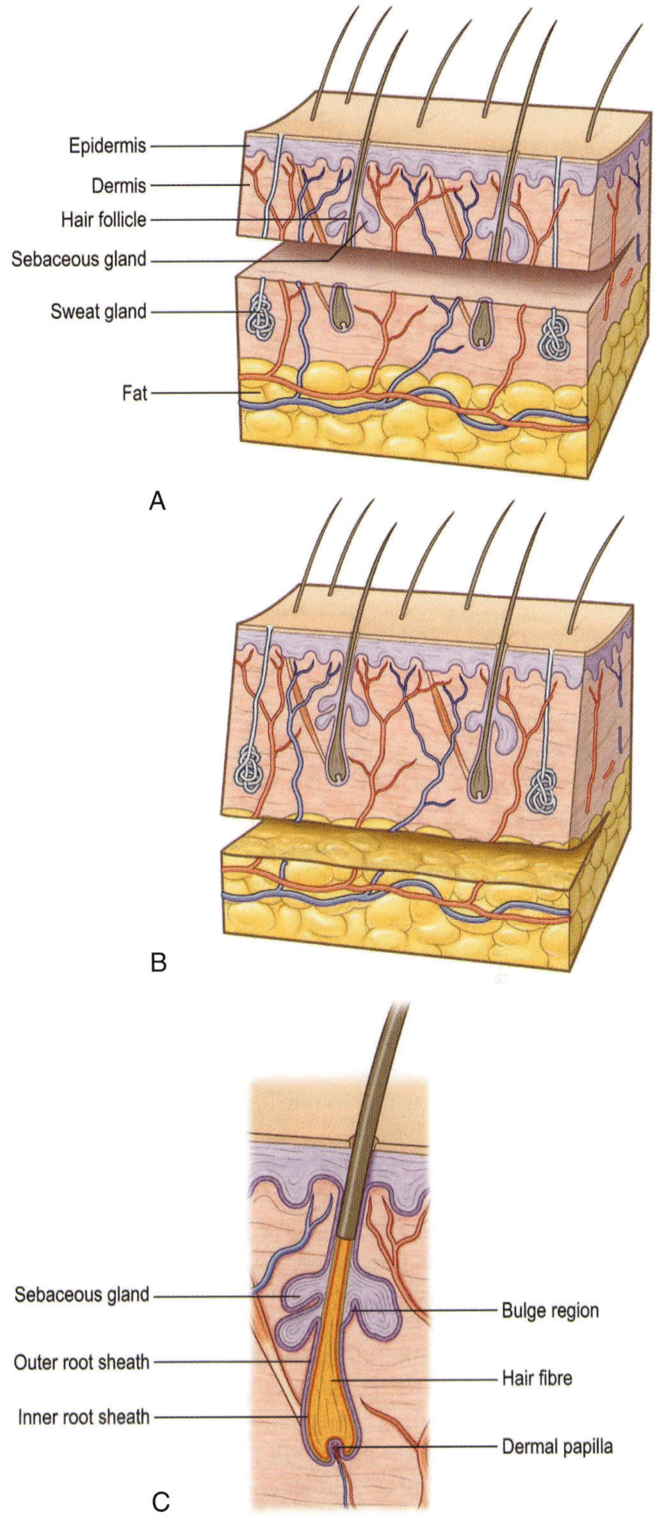

FIG. 28.6 Skin grafts. These illustrations demonstrate the appendages and tissue layers of skin grafts. (A) Split thickness. (B) Full thickness. (From Velasco J, Ballo R, Hood K, Jolley J, Rinewalt D, Veenstra B, eds. *Essential Surgical Procedures*. Philadelphia: Elsevier; 2016.)

- **Autograft:** A biological graft taken from one area of the body and transplanted to another area in the same patient. Commonly used tissues are skin, bone, cartilage, and fat.
- **Composite graft:** A biological graft consisting of more than one tissue type (e.g., skin, blood vessels, nerves, fascia).

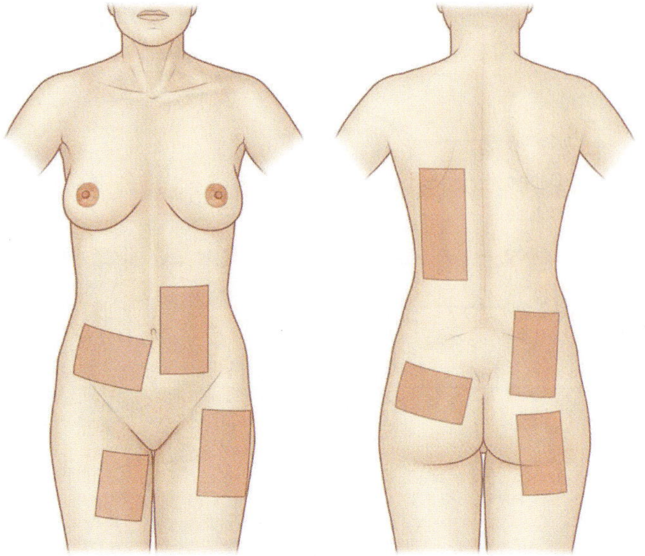

FIG. 28.7 Split-thickness skin graft donor sites. (From Velasco J, Ballo R, Hood K, et al, eds. *Essential Surgical Procedures*. Philadelphia: Elsevier; 2016.)

Composite grafts are classified according to the method of transplantation (described with the surgical procedures later in this chapter).

- **Xenograft:** A graft made up of tissue taken from one species that is grafted into another species (e.g., **porcine** [pig], bovine [cow] skin grafted into a patient).

SPLIT-THICKNESS SKIN GRAFT

A split-thickness skin graft (STSG) is used to replace skin that has been lost as a result of trauma or disease. The STSG can be harvested using a dermatome or graft knife. Very small grafts can be taken using a #15 knife blade. Fig. 28.7 illustrates potential STSG sites. These areas are fleshy and broad.

Special Equipment

DERMATOME Skin grafting is a common technique in plastic and reconstructive surgery. Grafts taken from the patient's own body are used to extend the edges of a wound or to cover an area in which skin has been lost to trauma or disease. A large split-thickness graft is removed with a **dermatome.**

The hand-held oscillating dermatome may be powered by compressed air or electricity. The most commonly used models are the Brown, Padgett, and Zimmer dermatomes. A handheld, battery-operated dermatome can be used for very small grafts. The knife dermatome with detachable blade is used for debridement and for harvesting grafts. Fig. 28.8 illustrates these dermatomes.

The oscillating dermatome has a flat blade housed within an adjustable head. The instrument head is placed over the lubricated graft site and advanced forward. The ST should prepare the dermatome in advance of the procedure, although some surgeons prefer to have this responsibility. The dermatome set includes blade guards, a screwdriver, and a disposable blade. The ST must make sure the blade knife and guards are properly assembled and the correct blades for that instrument are mounted. This is a critical process, because if incorrectly installed, the blade guard and knife can work loose and injure the donor site or tear the graft. The Brown dermatome requires a new blade for each use. The blade and guard are inserted into the head of the instrument and secured with screws.

The Reese *drum dermatome* (Fig. 28.9) requires skin adhesive, which is applied to the donor site in the shape and size of the graft required. The edge of the donor site is fixed to the drum, which elevates the skin while an oscillating blade separates the skin from the underlying tissue.

GRAFT MESHER An STSG is usually modified before implantation in the recipient site. The graft is "aerated" by transforming it from a solid sheet of skin to a mesh configuration. This is done with a graft mesher. The graft is placed on a flexible *carrier plate* and carefully fed into the mesher, which cuts small, diamond-shaped holes in the skin (shown later).

IMPORTANT TO KNOW *The ratio of skin to aerated spaces is marked on the carrier plate. The surgical technologist must ensure that the required plate, as determined by the surgeon, is used during meshing. Aeration prevents blood and serum from accumulating under the graft during healing and also increases the surface area of the graft.*

Pathology

Skin is necessary for the protection and nourishment of underlying tissues. Minor injuries or defects can regenerate sufficient skin to create a scar. Large defects require a skin graft to protect underlying tissues from infection and injury.

POSITION:	According to the location of the graft site
INCISION:	Two sites are prepared—the donor and recipient sites
PREP AND DRAPING:	The sites are prepared separately
INSTRUMENTS AND SUPPLIES:	Minor plastic surgery set including fine scissors and fine Adson and Brown forceps, mineral oil, dermatome
POSSIBLE EXTRAS:	Tongue blade

Technical Points and Discussion

1. ***The patient is prepped and draped.***
The patient is positioned for exposure of the donor site (i.e., supine position for the lower extremities and trunk, prone position for the buttocks and back). The donor and recipient sites are prepped and draped separately. Some surgeons use a clear prep product such as chlorhexidine gluconate with isopropyl alcohol (ChloraPrep) rather than Betadine on the donor site. The donor site is selected from a fleshy area of the body. Typical sites are shown later.

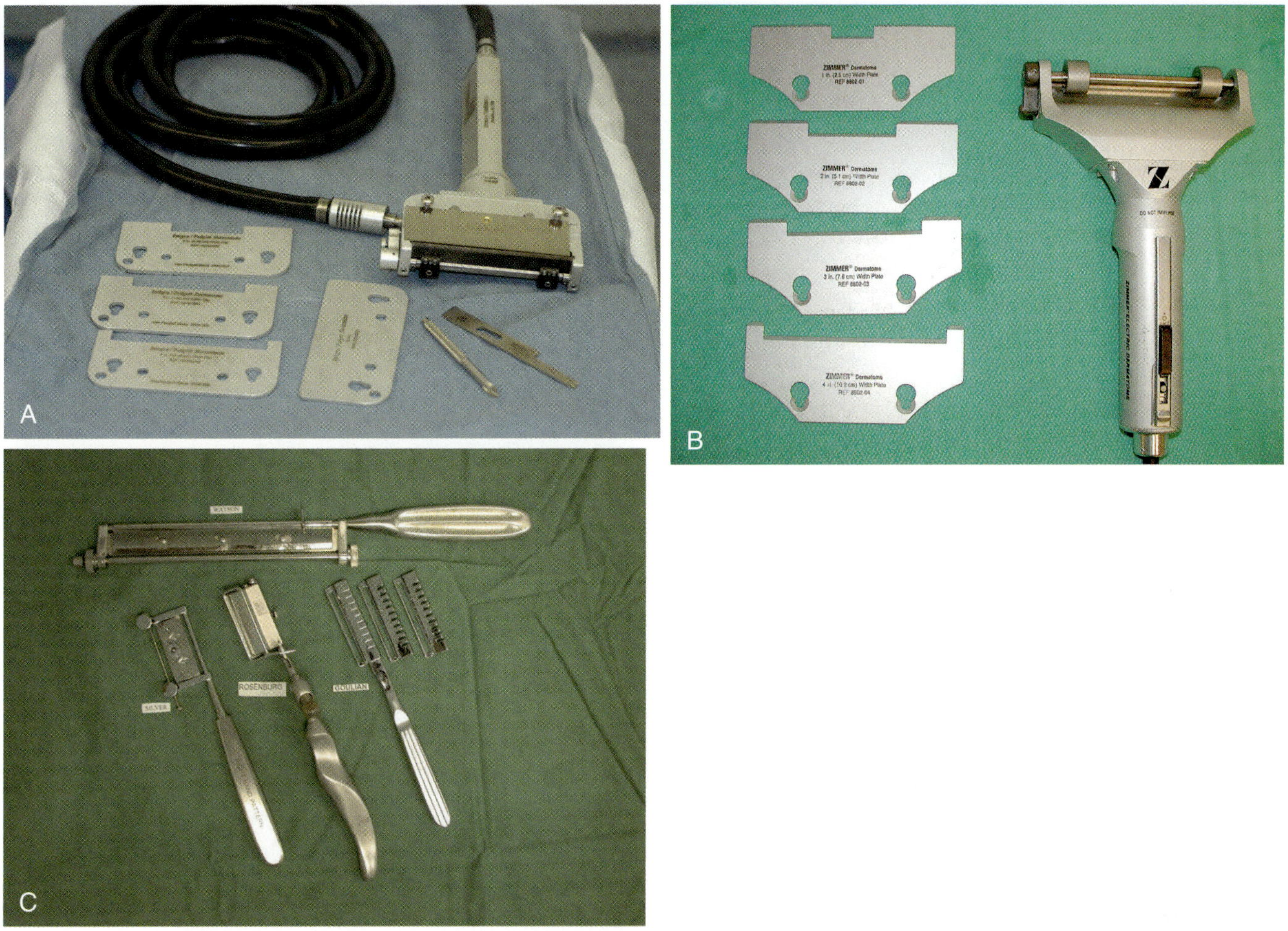

FIG. 28.8 Dermatomes. (A) Padgett dermatome. (B) Zimmer dermatome with blades. (C) Hand-guided knife dermatomes used mainly for debridement. (A, From Wolf S, Hotchkiss W, Pederson W. *Green's Operative Hand Surgery*. 17th ed. Elsevier; 2017. B, From Tyers AG, Collin JRO. *Colour Atlas of Ophthalmic Plastic Surgery*. Elsevier; 2018. C, From Herndon D. *Total Burn Care*. 5th ed. Edinburgh: Elsevier; 2018.)

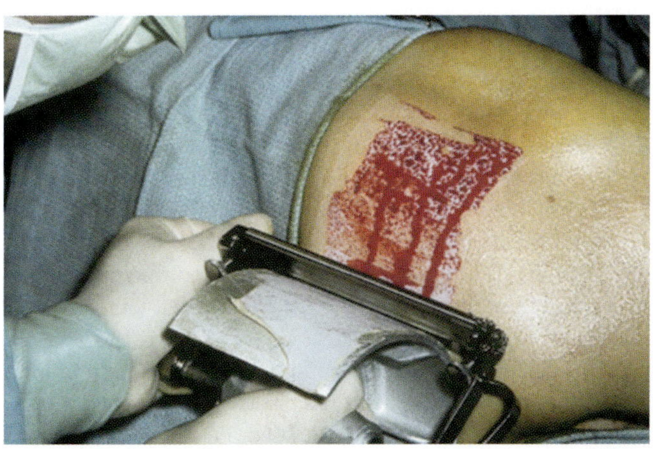

FIG. 28.9 Taking a graft with the Reese drum dermatome. The Reese dermatome is used with skin glue, which is painted on the skin. The drum is rolled over the area, which causes it to adhere to the drum while the oscillating blade releases the skin. (From Baggish MS, Karram MM. *Atlas of Pelvic Anatomy and Gynecologic Surgery*. Philadelphia: Elsevier; 2016.)

2. ***The recipient site is prepared.***
   If the graft recipient site was created in the same surgery as the skin-grafting procedure, the recipient site will be ready for graft placement. However, if grafting takes place as a separate procedure as a step in the healing process, the site must be prepared. This is done by debridement of the area. This is necessary to ensure that all devitalized tissue has been removed and healthy vascularized tissue remains. The recipient site can be covered with a surgical towel or moist sponges while the graft is prepared.

3. ***The donor site is prepared (Brown, Padgett, Zimmer dermatomes).***
   The surgeon may mark the donor site before the graft is taken. To maintain hemostasis the graft site may be infiltrated with epinephrine diluted with injectable saline. The ST should have 10-cc syringes available fitted with Luer-Lok needles, size 25 or 28 × 2 inches.

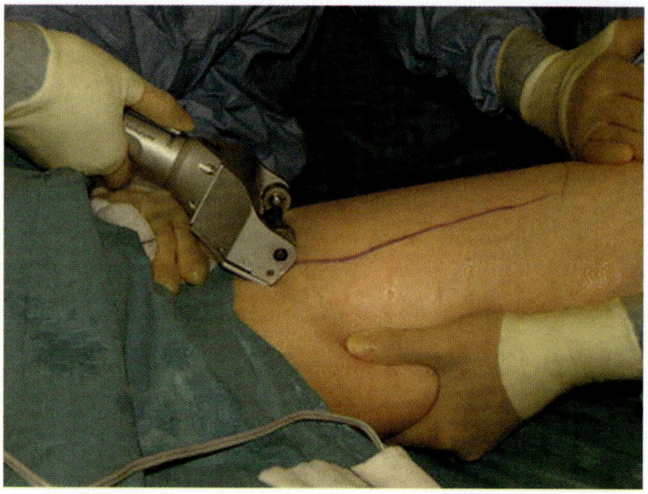

FIG. 28.10 Taking a split-thickness graft with an oscillating dermatome (Padgett or Zimmer). The surgical technologist places tension on the graft site manually or with a wooden tongue blade. The surgeon advances the dermatome. (From Velasco J, Ballo R, Hood K, Jolly J, eds. *Essential Surgical Procedures*. Edinburgh: Elsevier; 2016.)

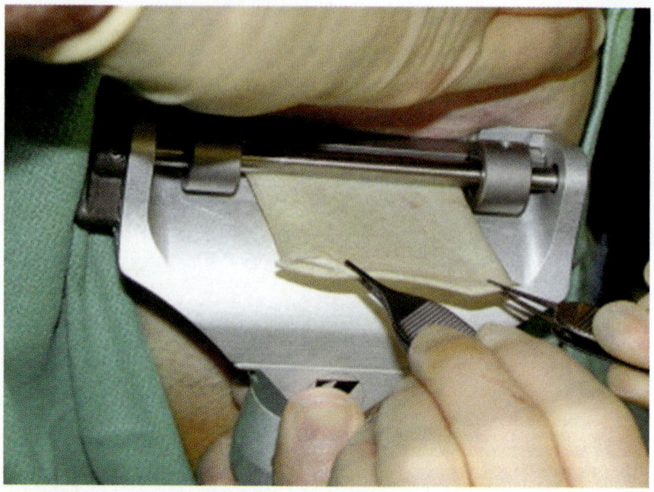

FIG. 28.11 As the graft emerges from the back of the dermatome, the surgical technologist or assistant must elevate the skin to protect it from damage. (From Robinson JK, Hanke C, Seigel D, et al. *Surgery of the Skin: Procedural Dermatology*. London: Elsevier Saunders; 2015.)

Mineral oil is applied to the graft site to reduce friction as the blade glides over the skin.

4. ***The graft is harvested.***
The dermatome should always be handed to the surgeon with the depth gauge set at 0. This allows the surgeon to select the depth setting for the blade, usually 0.012 to 0.015. To assist the surgeon in taking the graft, the assistant or ST pulls the donor skin taut using either 4 × 4 gauze sponges or tongue blades. The surgeon positions the dermatome at the donor site and advances it forward. The graft emerges from the back of the instrument as the dermatome is advanced across the skin.

The assistant grasps and elevates the graft with fine Adson or Brown tissue forceps as it emerges from the blade. The surgical technologist may be asked to perform this task. When sufficient skin has been removed, the dermatome is angled upward; this severs the graft. If it is not released, the graft can be separated from the donor bed with fine scissors such as sharp iris scissors. The scrub immediately places the graft in a small basin to protect it from contamination and injury. Alternatively, the surgeon may transfer the graft immediately to a *carrier* plate for meshing (see next section).

The graft should be kept moist but not wet and should be covered with Telfa or gauze, according to facility protocol. The donor site is covered with a sponge soaked in saline or a solution of saline and topical epinephrine (1:1000) to aid in hemostasis. These steps are shown in Figs. 28.10 and 28.11.

5. ***The graft is meshed using a graft mesher.***
The skin is placed on a plastic carrier plate with fine-toothed forceps, spreading it evenly over the surface with the exterior side facing upward. The plate is inserted into the mesher, which is hand operated. The carrier plate and graft emerge from the instrument as the handle is operated. The ST may be required to operate the mesher while the surgeon holds the carrier plate in alignment (Fig. 28.12).

6. ***The graft is secured over the recipient site.***
The surgeon gently transfers the graft to the recipient site and spreads it. Excess tissue is trimmed with curved iris scissors The graft is attached to the skin surrounding the defect with staples or interrupted sutures size 3-0 or 4-0. If the graft is implanted onto an exposed area of the body, such as the hands or face, it is sutured in place. On areas that are not exposed, such as the abdomen or back, the graft may be stapled.

7. ***The recipient site is dressed.***
There are numerous ways to dress the recipient site. The recipient site is first covered with non-adherent Vaseline gauze or Xeroform gauze.

8. ***A stent is constructed.***
To maintain contact between the skin graft and the tissue bed below it, a bolster is secured over the graft with sutures. This technique is referred to as a *stent* or a *tie-over* dressing. To begin the technique, the surgeon places numerous sutures around the edge of the graft. The ends are left long. The bolster may be constructed of surgical cotton moistened with saline, a commercially prepared foam material, or moldable silicone can be used. With the bolster in place, the long sutures are drawn over the top and tied (Fig. 28.13). The bolster is then covered with fluffed or flat gauze. If the site is on a limb, it may be further protected with rolled gauze.

9. ***The donor site is dressed.***
The donor site is dressed using Xeroform gauze and flat dressings, or it can be covered with a synthetic dressing such as *OpSite* or *Suprathel*.

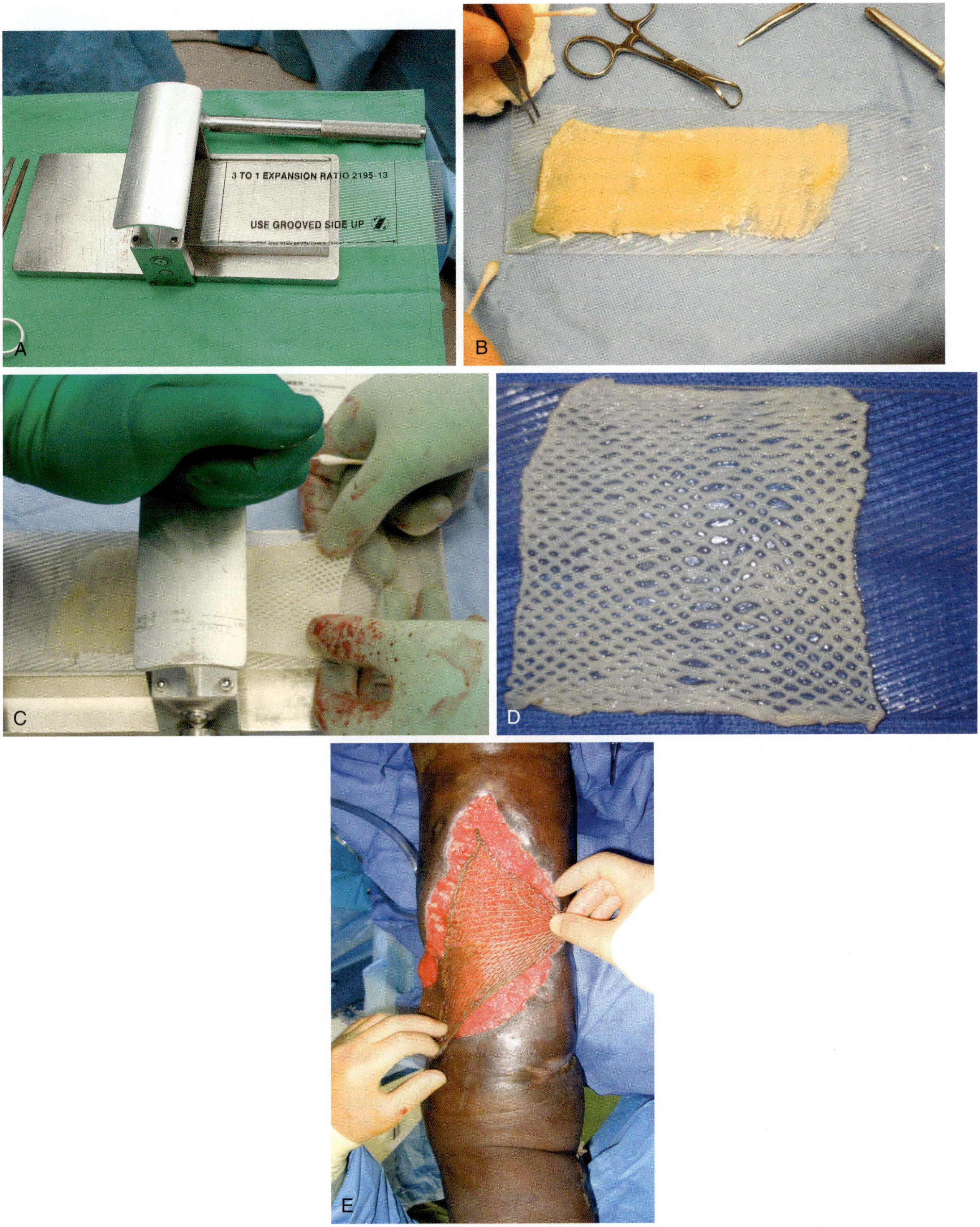

FIG. 28.12 Meshing the graft. (A) Graft mesher with carrier plate. This device is used to aerate the graft, increasing its surface area and improving contact between the graft and the recipient site. Note the ratio of skin to aerations printed on the plate. (B) Fitting the graft to the carrier plate. (C) The carrier plate and graft are fed into the graft mesher. The surgical technologist operates the mesher while the surgeon keeps the carrier plate in alignment. (D) The aerated graft. (E) The graft is fitted over the recipient site. (A, From Robinson JK, Hanke C, Seigel D, et al. *Surgery of the Skin: Procedural Dermatology*. London: Elsevier Saunders; 2015. E, From Dockery G, Crawford M, eds. *Lower Extremity Soft Tissue and Cutaneous Plastic Surgery*. 2nd ed. Philadelphia: Elsevier; 2012.)

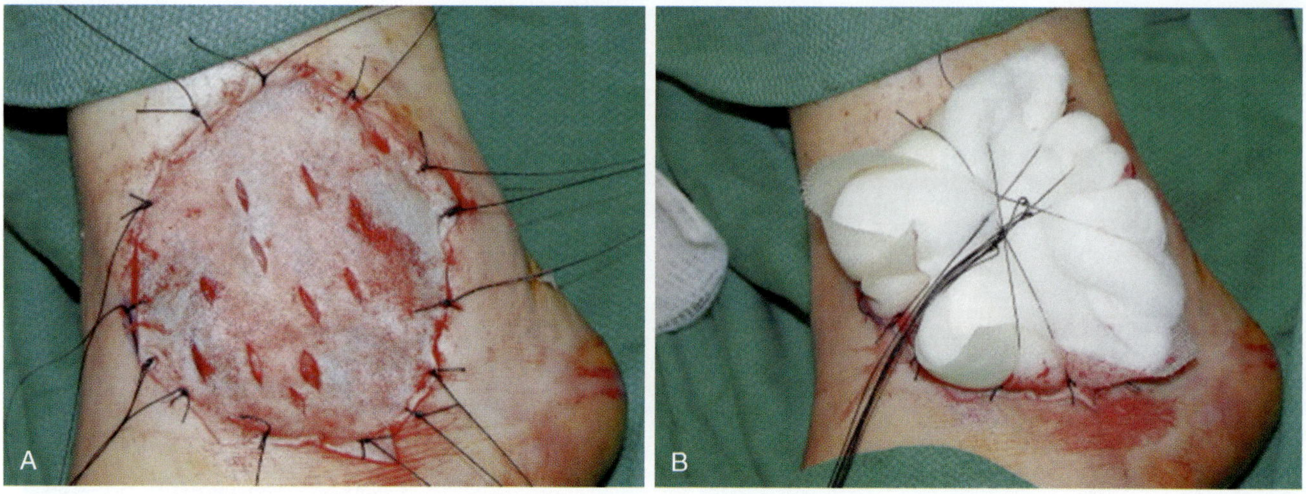

FIG. 28.13 Creating a stent. (A) Sutures are used to attach the graft to the recipient site. The ends are left long. (B) A layer of non-adherent (Vaseline) gauze is placed over the graft. This is topped with surgical cotton or other moldable material. The long sutures are brought over the top of the dressing and tied in place. (From Robinson JK, Hanke C, Seigel D, et al. *Surgery of the Skin: Procedural Dermatology*. 3rd ed. London: Elsevier Saunders; 2015.)

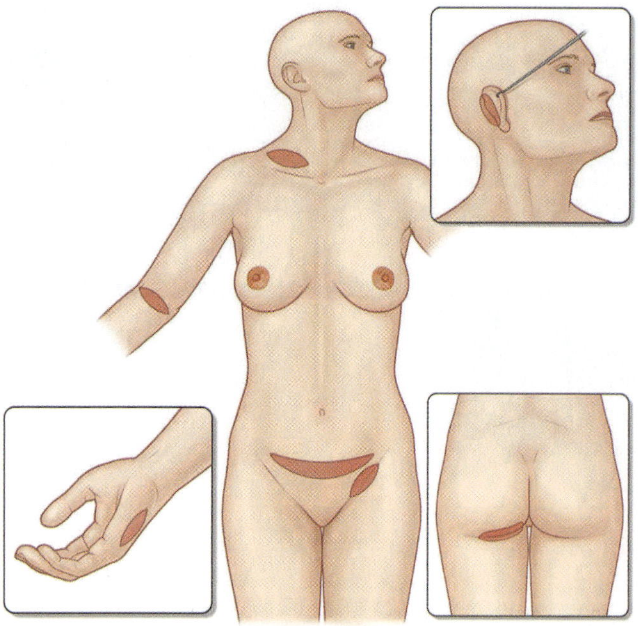

FIG. 28.14 Full-thickness skin graft. Potential graft sites. (From Velasco J, Ballo R, Hood K, et al, eds. *Essential Surgical Procedures*. Philadelphia: Elsevier; 2016.)

FULL-THICKNESS SKIN GRAFT

A full-thickness skin graft (FTSG) is composed of both dermis and epidermis. It is used to cover a deep defect created by surgical removal of a lesion, trauma, or disease.

An FTSG is usually harvested using the knife and sharp scissors. The donor site is selected in areas of the body that have somewhat loose skin. These include the subclavicular area, groin, lower abdomen, and clavicle as shown in Fig. 28.14. Grafts taken from these areas can be closed directly with sutures after the graft has been removed.

Pathology

Areas of the body that have lost both the dermis and epidermis require a graft that can bring blood supply to the area. The dermis contains the cell components that promote normal healing.

POSITION:	According to the location of the recipient and donor sites
INCISION:	As above
PREP AND DRAPING:	Skin prep for the donor site is cleansed with dilute Betadine. Draping according to the donor and recipient sites
INSTRUMENTS:	Minor plastic surgery set, bipolar ESU

Technical Points and Discussion

1. ***The recipient site is prepared.***
The recipient site of the graft must be prepared for the graft to become integrated into the new site. Removal of a lesion at the time of grafting includes this preparation. The site must be free of all devitalized tissue and may require further dissection to expose its vascularity.

2. ***The donor graft is taken.***
The donor site is prepped in routine fashion and draped at the same time as the recipient site. A template is sometimes made using available materials such as a glove wrapper. The template is placed over the recipient site and sized accordingly using a marking pen. The template is then placed over the donor site and its outline drawn with a skin marker. The surgeon uses a #15 blade, tissue scissors (e.g., iris, Stevens, and Metzenbaum), and Adson or other fine-tissue forceps to take the graft. Use of the ESU is limited as this creates debris

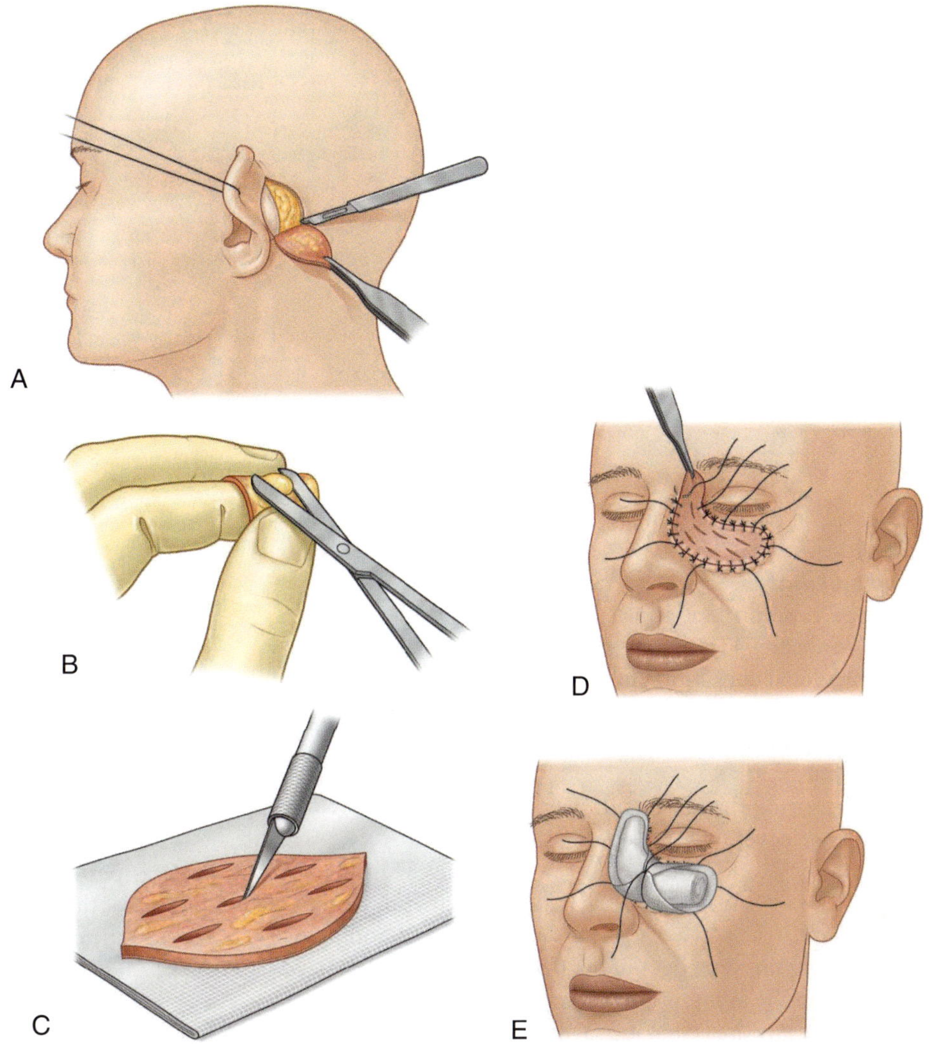

FIG. 28.15 Full-thickness skin graft technique. (A) Harvesting the graft. (B) Trimming fat from the graft. (C) Scoring the graft using a silastic plate and #11 knife. (D) The graft is sutured in place. (E) A stent is constructed over the graft. (From Velasco J, Ballo R, Hood K, et al, eds. *Essential Surgical Procedures*. Philadelphia: Elsevier; 2016.)

that can slow recipient site healing. The graft is immediately placed in a small basin and kept moist using Telfa moistened with saline.

3. ***The graft is prepared.***
   All subcutaneous tissue is removed from the graft. The surgeon does this using Stevens or curved iris scissors. The graft is implanted quickly to maintain its viability.

4. ***The graft is sutured to the donor site.***
   The graft can be sutured to the donor site using interrupted sutures of size 5-0 or 4-0 synthetic absorbable suture. One or more tacking sutures may be placed in the middle of the graft to maintain contact with the donor bed. After all sutures have been placed, the site is dressed using petrolatum or Xeroform gauze, flat gauze, and fluffed gauze. A pressure dressing is usually not required. Technical points are illustrated in Fig. 28.15.

FLAP GRAFT

Pedicle grafts provide coverage and vascularization to a soft tissue defect. A pedicle graft (also called a *flap graft*) is raised from the donor site but not immediately severed free. This distinguishes the flap graft from a *free graft,* in which the entire graft is raised (excised) and transferred to the recipient site. The pedicle graft donor site tissue is partly severed, and the flap is brought into contact with the recipient site. The graft is sutured in place to cover the defect and the donor site covered with a split thickness skin graft. During the healing process, the graft tissue infiltrates and develops over the recipient wound. When healing is complete, the flap is released. Pedicle grafts are classified as near or distant. A near graft is created in adjacent tissue (e.g., from the palm for use on the finger). Distant grafts are created from the trunk or other areas for use on a limb.

An advancement flap (see the following section) is raised from the tissues in the immediate area of the defect. Rotational flaps are semicircular and require some degree of turning to reach and cover the recipient tissue defect.

Pedicle flaps contain good blood supply from vessels that infiltrate the recipient site during healing.

Pathology

This type of graft is used when the recipient site requires skin and deeper tissue layers to fill a large tissue defect resulting from radical surgery, disease, or trauma.

POSITION:	According to the site
PREP AND DRAPING:	According to the site
INSTRUMENTS:	General surgery, plastic set

Technical Points and Discussion

ADVANCEMENT FLAP

1. ***The patient is prepped and draped.***
The patient is placed in a position that allows access to both the defect and the donor site. Depending on the size of the defect, general or regional anesthesia may be used.

2. ***The incision lines of the flap are measured and drawn on the skin.***
The surgeon begins by measuring the defect and the proposed flap to ensure complete coverage. The incision lines are drawn on the skin.

3. ***The recipient site is debrided.***
The surgeon cleans any rough, uneven edges of the defect with a #15 blade and scissors. It is important to expose only viable tissue and remove any areas that are ragged or nonvascular.

4. ***The flap is elevated and positioned.***
Next, the donor site is incised. The flap is elevated with the knife or tenotomy scissors. Retraction is applied with double-prong skin hooks. When the flap has been raised sufficiently, it is advanced into position over the recipient site. The surgeon does this by simply approximating the edges of the skin flap to cover the defect; 3-0 or 4-0 absorbable sutures are used for deep tissue, and 5-0 or 6-0 nonabsorbable sutures are used for the skin.

5. ***The donor site is closed.***
Exposed tissue of the donor site is covered with an STSG. A bulky protective dressing is applied.

These techniques are illustrated in Fig. 28.16.

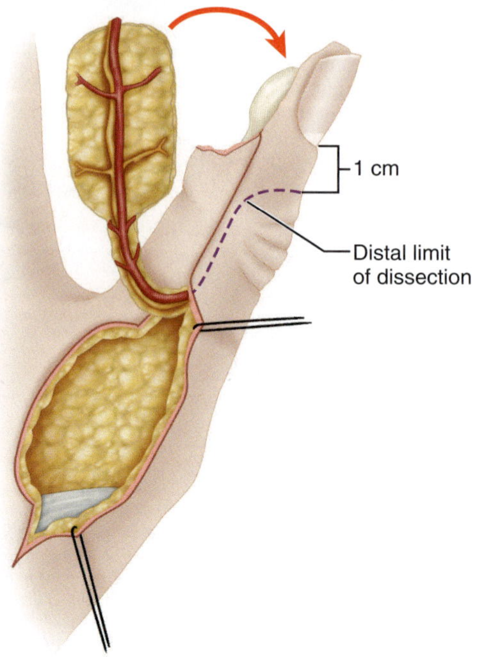

FIG. 28.16 Flap (rotational) graft. A flap of tissue with its blood supply is raised from an adjoining area and sutured to the fingertip. The flap remains attached to its original location until the new site has healed. The donor site is covered with a split-thickness skin graft. (From Canale S, Beaty J, eds. *Campbell's Operative Orthopaedics*. 12th ed. Philadelphia: Mosby; 2013.)

MOHS MICROGRAPHIC SURGERY

Mohs micrographic surgery (MMS) is a technique of excising a malignant skin lesion by systematic removal of the margins and immediate microscopic examination. Wound margins found to contain malignant cells are removed until the site is clear of malignancy. MMS is performed in conjunction with frozen section technique so that the results of the microscopic evaluation can be obtained quickly and wider excision performed as needed. Fig. 28.17 illustrates the concept of MMS.

Pathology

Malignant lesions of the skin may be caused by excessive exposure to ultraviolet light (sun or artificial) in combination with genetic susceptibility. The most common types of skin lesions are basal cell carcinoma, squamous cell carcinoma, and malignant melanoma. Of these, malignant melanoma is the lesion of most concern.

POSITION:	According to the location of the lesion
INCISION:	Follows the periphery of the lesion
PREP AND DRAPING:	According to the location of the lesion
INSTRUMENTS:	Minor plastic surgery set, bipolar ESU
ADDITIONAL SUPPLIES:	Skin markers; multiple specimen containers; Telfa strips

Technical Points and Discussion

1. ***The patient is prepped and draped to expose the lesion.***
The patient is positioned to allow maximum exposure to the diseased tissue. Surgery of the face requires stabilization of the head using a gel doughnut pad or similar device. Dilute povidone iodine may be used to prep the skin.

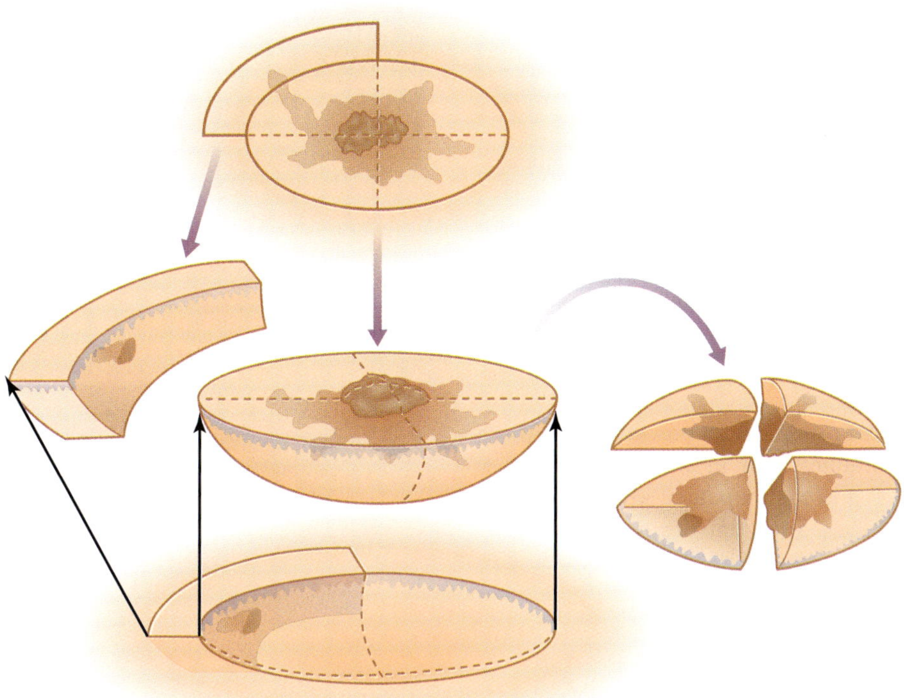

B

FIG. 28.17 Mohs micrographic surgery for removing a malignant skin lesion. (A) The technique is based on sectional removal of tissue, immediate microscopic examination. (B) This is repeated until no further malignancy is detected in the specimens. (From Usatine R, Phenninger J, Stulbert D, Small R. *Dermatologic and Cosmetic Procedures in Office Practice*. Philadelphia: Saunders; 2012.)

2. ***The surgeon marks the periphery of the lesion and orientation marks with ink.***
Mohs surgery requires meticulous orientation marks to demonstrate areas of remaining malignancy once the specimen has been removed. This is necessary to ensure that only diseased tissue is removed.

Individual surgeons have specific preferences for a method of marking the tissue. A routine gentian violet skin marker can be used; many surgeons prefer dyes such as methylene blue or carmen red. These can be applied with a wooden cotton-tipped applicator that is broken in half. The cotton portion is discarded, and the broken tip used like a quill pen. Another method is to mark the periphery of the lesion and cut small hash marks across the line. These cuts are strategically placed to represent a clock face orientation. Other orientation methods include sutures placed at strategic points in the specimen. The surgical technologist should consult the surgeon's preference card to plan the case and supplies needed.

An additional method used for orientation is to place one or more dye marks corresponding to anatomical locations (lateral, medial, superior, inferior) outside the lesion periphery. These would match up to the marks in the lesion itself.

3. ***The lesion is excised.***
Lesions are usually removed using a #15 knife blade. The assistant or ST may use double- or single-prong skin hooks to retract the skin edges during excision. The ESU is generally not used when frozen section is planned because super-heating the tissue distorts it and may lead to a misdiagnosis.

4. ***The surgical technologist receives the specimen.***
The scrubbed surgical technologist should receive the specimen in a clear Petri dish or shallow specimen container. All specimens must be kept separate. The ST is responsible for ensuring that marks or other means of orientation are maintained while the specimen is handled on the sterile field. Specimens received during surgery should be kept separated, identified, and placed carefully on a Telfa pad moistened with saline. Normally, specimens for frozen section are passed off the field immediately.

NOTE *A complete discussion on the management of surgical specimens can be found in Chapter 19.*

5. ***The pathologist receives the specimen and preforms a frozen section. She or he reports the results back to the surgeon.***

6. ***According to report, additional areas of malignancy are excised using the orientation marks for guidance.***
The surgeon repeats the excision in the areas of malignant tissue. These are again referred to the pathologist for

frozen section. This step is repeated until the margins of the lesion are free of malignant cells.

7. ***The wound is closed primarily or a skin graft is harvested to cover the defect.***
Deep excision of a lesion may require a split-thickness graft. If the wound can be closed with sutures, fine nylon or polypropylene, size 4-0 or 5-0 may be used.

The techniques described are illustrated in Fig. 28.18.

SCAR REVISION

Scar revision is performed to remodel a previous scar. There are many different techniques used in scar revision. Laser therapy is commonly used in the outpatient setting. Surgical revision aims to remove the old scar and create a new pattern that is less noticeable. A Z-plasty or W-plasty is used in this case. When healed, these configurations are less noticeable than a straight-line scar.

IMPORTANT TO KNOW *Scar revision involving the removal of tissue deeper than skin requires more complex techniques. Incisional hernia repair and release of burn contracture involving subcutaneous tissues are examples.*

Pathology

Scar formation is a normal phase of healing. Clean surgical wounds usually heal with minimal scarring, especially when little or no tension is put on the wounds. However, infection or excess tension on a wound may result in a scar that appears ragged, misshapen, or undulating. Scars resulting from traumatic injury are particularly prone to uneven scar formation. A **hypertrophic scar** is one that develops excess tissue and may be red or raised. This type of scar generally heals after 6 months and may resolve over a period of years. However, **keloid** scars, which often develop in dark-skinned individuals, continue to form at the wound site and may become bulbous and unsightly. Keloids also can invade nearby tissue. This type of scar is difficult to treat and usually does not resolve naturally. Scars that develop over skin grafts may have excessive bulk, or the graft may have buckled during healing, giving it a quilt-like appearance.

Discussion

The surgeon begins by marking the planned revision including the lines of incision and location of skin flaps. A zigzag incision is made on one side of the scar and a straight incision on the other side with a #15 blade and Adson toothed forceps. Fine skin hooks may be used to provide traction on the scar during excision. The next step is to **undermine** the surrounding tissue with Metzenbaum or curved iris scissors to release the scar. Undermining involves separation of the skin from deeper tissues. The wound edges are closed with 4-0 or 5-0 absorbable synthetic sutures and dressed with Telfa and flat gauze. Fig. 28.19 shows a Z-plasty correction.

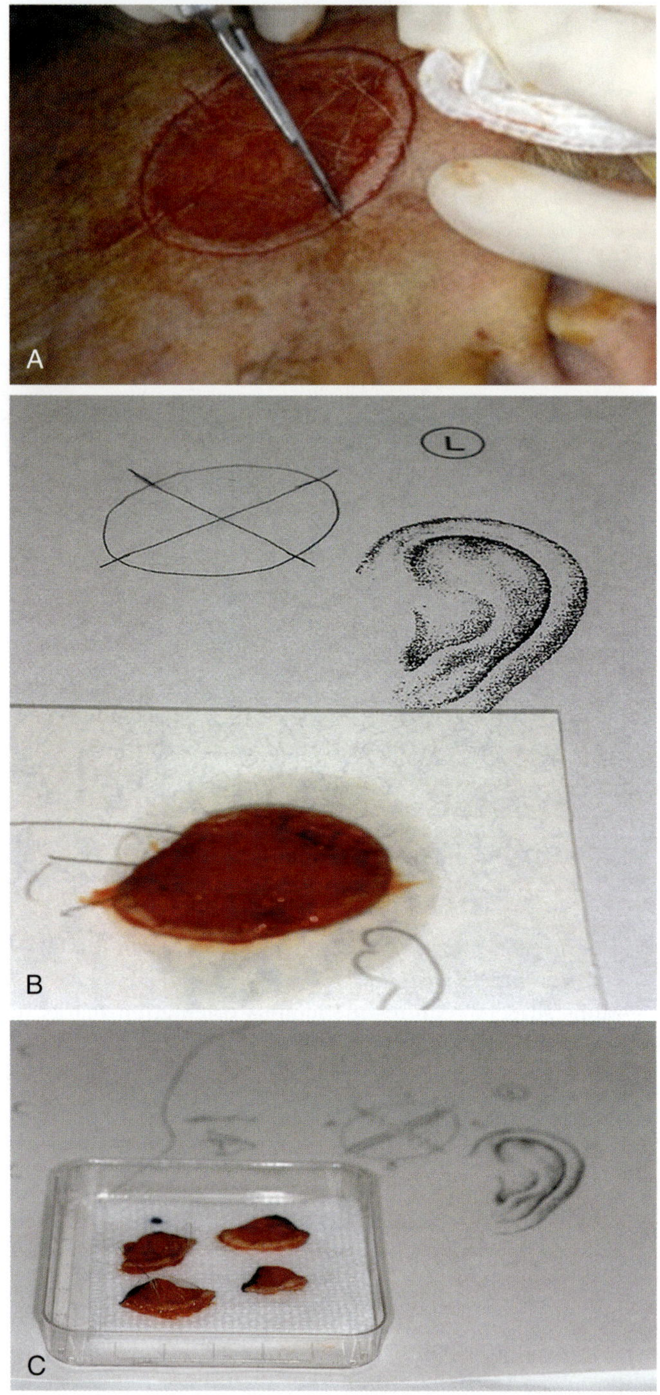

FIG. 28.18 Mohs micrographic surgery. (A) The periphery of the lesion has been drawn. Hash marks are made with the knife across the primary incision line to orient the specimen to its anatomical location. (B) The intact specimen is placed on a sheet of paper with its anatomical location marked. (C) Successive sections of the specimen are oriented in their relation to the ink dot in the left corner of the gauze. The dot is oriented to the drawing. (From Benedetto PX, Poblete-Lopez C. Mohs micrographic surgery technique. *Dermatol Clin.* 2011;29[2]:141–151. https://doi.org/10.1016/j.det.2011.02.002.)

BLEPHAROPLASTY

Blepharoplasty is resection of the eyelid to improve vision of the upper visual fields. There are many different techniques used to achieve the surgical goal. These include simple skin

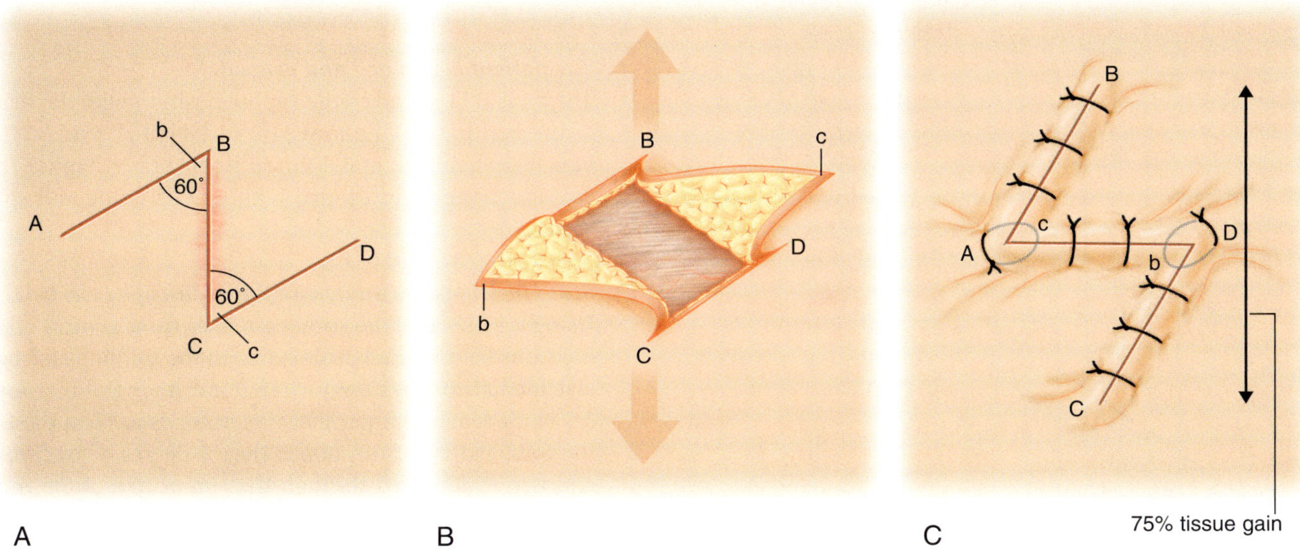

FIG. 28.19 Simple Z-plasty scar revision. This technique provides greater flexibility of the available skin and provides a cosmetically appealing result. This technique is also used for severe scar constriction such as that caused by burns. (From Robinson J, Hanke C, eds. *Surgery of the Skin, Procedural Dermatology*. 3rd ed. Philadelphia: Saunders; 2015.)

excision, removal of fat, repositioning of muscle, and canthopexy (suspension of the lateral canthus). The instrumentation used for these approaches is the same. A combination skin blepharoplasty and fat removal are described here.

Pathology

With advancing age, the eyelids lose elasticity and tone and may droop over the eye, interfering with vision. The procedure also may be performed for cosmetic purposes.

POSITION:	Supine
INCISION:	Eyelids
PREP AND DRAPING:	Eye
INSTRUMENTS:	Minor plastic set including fine scissors and forceps, corneal shields, bipolar ESU
POSSIBLE EXTRAS:	Cotton-tipped applicators

Technical Points and Discussion

1. ***The patient is prepped.***
   With the patient sitting, the surgeon marks the incision lines before the surgery. The patient is placed in the supine position with the head on a doughnut headrest and the arms tucked at the sides. A local anesthetic is instilled into the lid using a 30-gauge, 1½-inch needle. The patient is prepped and draped with a head drape and split sheet. Corneal shields are inserted to protect the cornea from injury during the procedure.

UPPER LID BLEPHAROPLASTY

2. ***The skin is incised and subcutaneous tissue removed.***
   The incision is made with a #15 blade. Dull rakes are used to retract the skin and expose the subcutaneous tissue. Depending on the amount, the fatty tissue may be excised with tenotomy scissors. A needlepoint bipolar ESU is used to control bleeding in the fatty tissue. If excess muscle also is present, it is removed with curved iris scissors. The incision is closed with size 6-0 nonabsorbable subcuticular suture and several interrupted sutures to reinforce the primary suture Line. The ends of this suture are left long for easy removal. A simple blepharoplasty is illustrated in Fig. 28.20.

LOWER LID BLEPHAROPLASTY: SUBCILIARY APPROACH

3. ***The skin and orbicularis muscle are incised.***
   Using a #15 blade, the surgeon makes the incision in the subciliary region, 2 to 3 mm below the lower lash line. The lower lid skin is elevated upward and outward so that the amount to be removed can be determined. The skin is excised with a #15 blade. To gain access to the infraorbital fat pads, the surgeon makes an incision into the orbicularis muscle. Double-prong skin hooks are used to retract the skin. The excess fat is removed with iris scissors.

4. ***The muscle is reattached and incisions closed.***
   The orbicularis oculi muscle is reattached to the periosteum at the lateral orbital rim with clear, nonabsorbable sutures. This prevents the lower lid from drooping after blepharoplasty. The incisions are closed as described previously.

BROW LIFT: ENDOSCOPIC TECHNIQUE

Brow lift procedures are done to lift the supportive structures of the brow and alleviate drooping of skin, muscle, and fascia. Numerous approaches can be used for a brow lift. These include the coronal approach (behind the hairline), the pretrichial approach (at the hairline), or the direct approach (at the level of the brow itself). An endoscopic technique is discussed

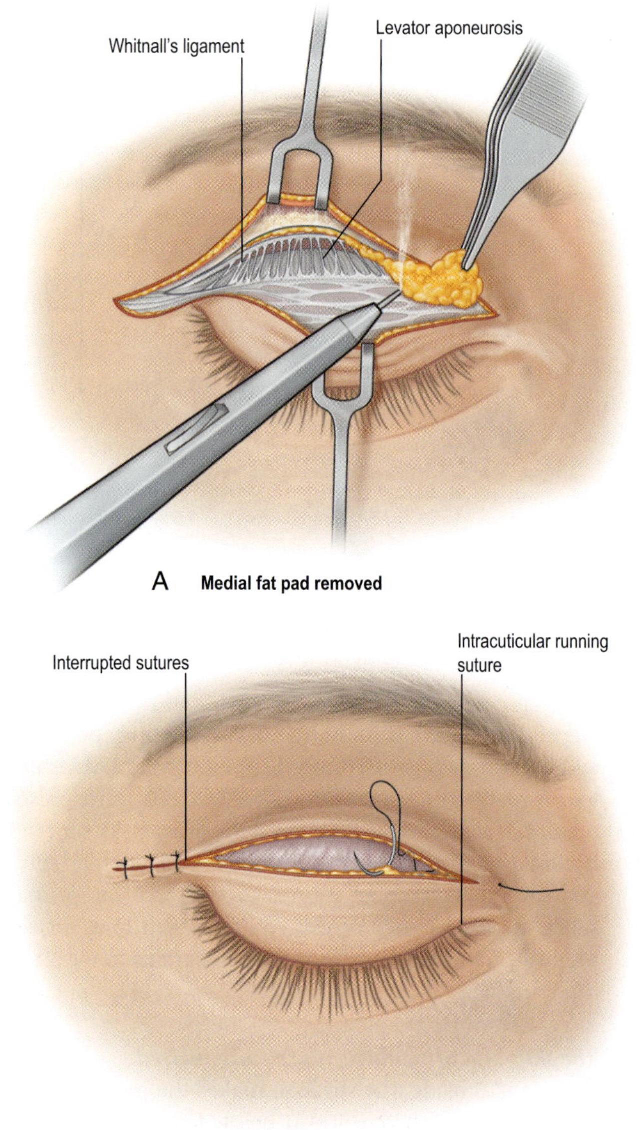

FIG. 28.20 Simple blepharoplasty. (A) Fat pad is removed. (B) Sutures are placed. (From Neligan P, Buck D, eds. *Core Procedures in Plastic Surgery*. Philadelphia: Elsevier; 2014.)

here. Some surgeons use an Endotine fixator to reattach the scalp to the bony cranium. This is a tissue-tacking device that places tacks made of synthetic absorbable polymer.

Pathology

The soft tissues of the brow may droop with age and deepen the furrows over the eyes. This may also lead to eyebrow **ptosis** (pronounced *toh-sis*) and upper lid "hooding" of the eye.

POSITION:	Supine
INCISION:	Bicoronal
PREP AND DRAPING:	Face and head, exposing the coronal area excluding nose and mouth
INSTRUMENTS:	Endobrow set; endoscope 30-degree, 4- or 5-mm; ESU; power drill
POSSIBLE EXTRAS:	Endotine fixators

Technical Points and Discussion

1. ***The patient is prepped and draped.***
The patient is placed in the supine position with the head of the bed raised. The arms are tucked at the sides. The hair is pulled back and secured with rubber bands. The face is prepped and draped with a head drape and split sheet.

2. ***Scalp incisions are made and the endoscope inserted.***
Using a #10 blade, the surgeon makes three central scalp incisions behind the hairline, one in the midline and two just medial to the superior temporal line. The incisions are extended, and a periosteal elevator is used to dissect the forehead flap from bone. The 30-degree 4- or 5-mm endoscope is passed through the rim of one of the incisions. Undermining is continued to a point approximately 0.8 inch (2 cm) above the supraorbital rim.

3. ***The temporal and frontal fascia is elevated.***
Next, a straight periosteal elevator is used to elevate the temporal fascia with the endoscope in place. The two temporal dissections are connected with a straight periosteal elevator and the 30-degree endoscope. The surgeon elevates the frontal fascia to the level of the supraorbital rim.

4. ***The lateral brow is fixed.***
When the periosteum has been mobilized, the surgeon elevates and fixes the lateral brow. (The medial brow usually is not fixed, because if it is elevated too much, the brow looks unnatural.)

The surgeon may fix tissue by drilling into the bone and passing absorbable sutures through the holes and soft tissue. The incision is closed with staples. A head dressing consisting of Kerlix fluffs and rolled gauze is applied.

RHYTIDECTOMY

Redundant and sagging supportive tissue of the face is reduced or modified to provide a more aesthetic appearance. There are many different rhytidectomy techniques. The objective is to release the subcutaneous connective tissues of the face, including the superficial muscular aponeurotic system (SMAS), so that it can be retracted and reattached to tighten the tissues. The connective tissues are accessed through several incisions. Local anesthetic with epinephrine is instilled for hemostasis. The procedure described here demonstrates the basic techniques for rhytidectomy. Other procedures, such as liposuction of the neck and mentoplasty, may be performed at the same time.

Pathology

The aging process and gravity affect the skin and the structures that lie beneath it. This results in hollow infraorbital regions, nasolabial folds, jowls, and excess skin below the chin. Certain environmental factors contribute to laxity and wrinkling of the skin. Wrinkles are a normal product of aging. However, **photo damage** occurs with extended, excessive exposure to

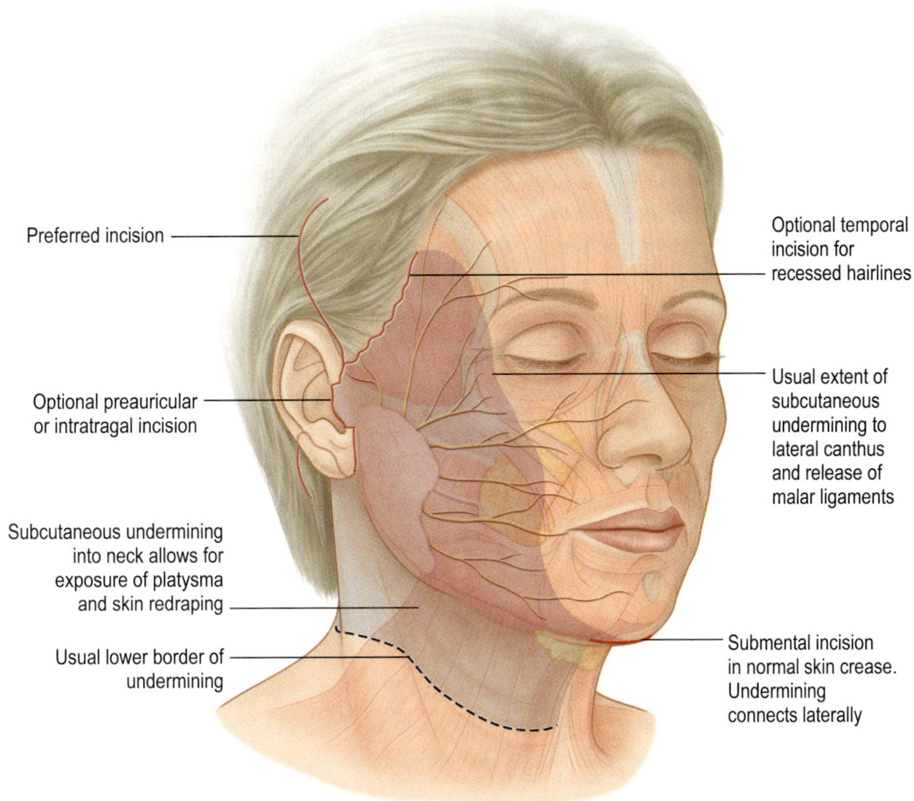

FIG. 28.21 Subcutaneous rhytidectomy. Incision lines and areas of undermining are shown. (From Neligan P, Buck D, eds. *Core Procedures in Plastic Surgery*. Philadelphia: Elsevier; 2014.)

ultraviolet light. Smoking also causes extreme wrinkling of the skin.

POSITION:	Supine
INCISION:	Periauricular
PREP AND DRAPING:	Face exposing the frontal scalp
INSTRUMENTS:	Rhytidectomy, bipolar ESU
POSSIBLE EXTRAS:	Lighted facial retractor

Technical Points and Discussion

1. ***The patient is prepped and draped.***
The patient is placed in the supine position with the head stabilized on a doughnut or Mayfield headrest and the head of the bed raised. The surgeon marks the skin with a skin marker before the prep is performed. The patient is prepped and draped for a face procedure.

   The surgeon injects the excisional areas with local anesthetic containing epinephrine as a vasoconstrictor to provide hemostasis. A fine-gauge spinal needle and 10-mL syringe are used for the injection.

2. ***Skin incisions are made.***
Skin incisions are made with a #15 blade, and double-prong skin hooks are used for retraction. The dissection continues with rhytidectomy scissors. The bipolar ESU is used to control small bleeders. The surgeon may use a fiber-optic retractor to aid exposure during dissection. At this point, the surgeon may overlap the underlying fascial attachment with 2-0 or 3-0 absorbable suture.

3. ***The skin is trimmed.***
Excess skin is excised with Metzenbaum scissors, and the subdermal layer is closed with 3-0, 4-0, and 5-0 absorbable sutures. A small Penrose drain may be placed during closure. The skin is closed with a combination of staples and 5-0 absorbable or nonabsorbable sutures. A head dressing is placed to support the incisions. Gauze sponges with an Ace wrap or a fascioplasty splint are commonly used to dress the wound. Fig. 28.21 illustrates the incision lines and areas of undermining for a subcutaneous facelift.

MENTOPLASTY

Mentoplasty is one of many different facial augmentation procedures in which synthetic implants are used. Surgery to place a chin implant is called *mentoplasty*. Many different materials are used as implants, including silicone, acrylic polymers, polyethylene, Gore-Tex, and mesh. Several types of subdermal and subcutaneous injectable filler materials are available. These include Dermalogen, AlloDerm, Restylane, collagen, and liquid silicone. An autograft (fat, bone, or cartilage) may also be used. The type of implant chosen depends on the

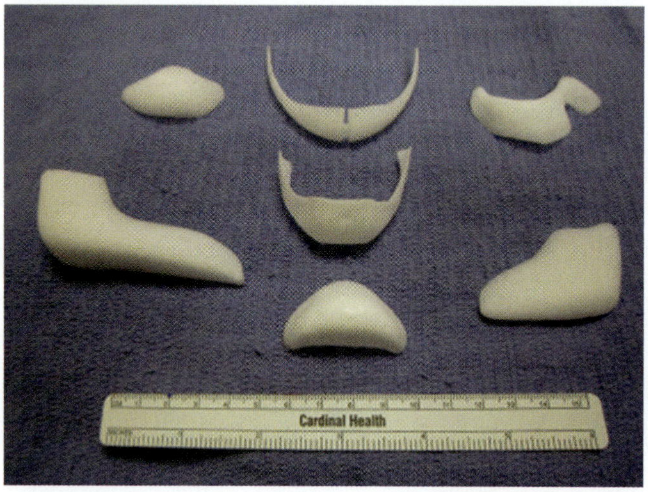

FIG. 28.22 Facial augmentation implants made of high-density polyethylene. (From Gurtner G, Neligan P. *Plastic Surgery: Principles*. 4th ed. vol 1. London: Elsevier; 2018; Gurtner G, Neligan P. *Plastic Surgery: Aesthetic*. 4th ed. vol 2. London: Elsevier; 2018.)

surgeon's preference and the type of defect to be filled. Fig. 28.22 illustrates various facial augmentation implants.

Pathology

Facial augmentation corrects malformation or loss of facial tissue caused by congenital anomaly, trauma, or radical surgery in which bone and other connective tissue was removed. Patients may also seek augmentation for aesthetic reasons in the absence of deformity.

POSITION:	Supine
INCISION:	Chin
PREP AND DRAPING:	Face
INSTRUMENTS:	Minor plastic set, minor orthopedic set

Technical Points and Discussion

1. ***The patient is prepped and draped.***
The patient is placed on the operating table in the modified sitting position with the arms tucked at the sides. General anesthesia may be used or local anesthetic is instilled into the region of the mental nerve, the incision line, and the surrounding soft tissue. Draping fully exposes the face to allow the surgeon to assess the projection given by the implant. A head drape and a split sheet are commonly used.

2. ***A skin incision is made and extended into deep tissue.***
A 10- to 15-mm incision is made vertically in the midline on the chin with a #15 blade. The incision extends through the subcutaneous fat and muscle to the layer of the periosteum. The assistant retracts the skin flaps with double-prong skin hooks. Bleeders are controlled with ESU. The periosteum is incised with a #15 blade.

3. ***The implant is placed and the wound closed.***
Next, the surgeon elevates the periosteum with a periosteal elevator (e.g., Joseph elevator). The implant is eased into position; the periosteum is elevated with a Senn retractor during implantation. Absorbable sutures may be placed in the distal end of the implant and periosteum to prevent the implant from shifting.

The wound is closed in two layers. The periosteum is closed with interrupted 3-0 absorbable sutures, and the skin is closed with 6-0 nonabsorbable suture or a 5-0 fast-absorbing suture. Gauze dressings are applied.

MALAR AUGMENTATION

Malar augmentation is an operative procedure to increase the height of the cheekbone for aesthetic improvement. Numerous methods are used to augment the malar region. These include injection of biosynthetic materials and silicone implants. In the following procedure, a polyethylene implant is used.

POSITION:	Supine
INCISION:	Oral
PREP AND DRAPING:	Face with head drape
INSTRUMENTS:	Minor plastic set with cheek retractors, bipolar ESU

Technical Points and Discussion

1. ***A buccal incision is made.***
An intraoral incision is made at the junction of the gum and soft tissue of the upper lip using a #15 knife or needle-point ESU. The incision is carried into deep connective tissues using the ESU, blunt dissection, or scissors. Angled retractors are placed in the wound to hold back the upper lip.

2. ***A pocket is created in the malar space.***
Dissection continues laterally, and a tissue pocket is created over the cheekbone. Narrow periosteal elevators are used to raise the tissue over the bone. Malar implant sizers are now used to select the correct implant. The correct implant is then inserted into the pocket. Some surgeons place a pullout suture into the implant and tissue to hold it in place. This is removed within the first few days postoperatively. Small microscrews may also be used to keep the implant from sliding during healing.

3. ***The incision is closed.***
The incision is closed in layers using synthetic absorbable suture.

OTOPLASTY

Otoplasty is surgical modification of the external ear. Surgery in children is planned before a child enters school or at 5 years

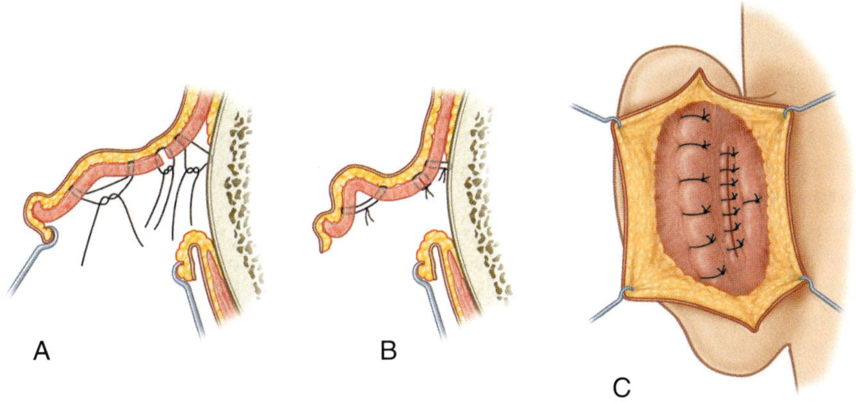

FIG. 28.23 Otoplasty for prominent ears. (A and B) The concha is resected and two suture lines placed. (C) Completed repair. (From Neligan P, Buck D, eds. *Core Procedures in Plastic Surgery*. Philadelphia: Elsevier; 2014.)

of age. The adult patient may undergo otoplasty at any time. The procedure can be performed under local anesthesia with sedation. Two separate procedures are illustrated here: the first for prominent ears and the second for correct of Stahl's ear (see subsequent figures). Surgery to modify or construct the external ear often requires tissue or **synthetic grafts** to create the scaffolding, which is covered with a skin graft. Split- and full-thickness grafts may be necessary to accomplish the surgical goals.

Pathology

Otoplasty is performed to correct a congenital malformation of the external ear or to recreate an ear destroyed by trauma or disease.

POSITION:	Supine
INCISION:	Postauricular
PREP AND DRAPING:	Ear
INSTRUMENTS:	Minor plastic surgery set; cartilage rasp (ear)
POSSIBLE EXTRAS:	Size 27- or 28-gauge hypodermic needles

Technical Points and Discussion

1. ***The patient is prepped.***
   The patient is placed in the supine position with the head of the table raised. A doughnut headrest is used to stabilize the patient's head and allow access to the posterior ear. If the procedure is bilateral, the patient is prepped and draped to allow access to both ears. The incisions are marked in the postauricular area. An ellipse of skin is usually removed.

2. ***The skin incision is made following the lines marked and carried to the cartilage.***
   The postauricular skin is injected with local anesthetic with epinephrine. With the ear held forward, an incision is made in the postauricular skin with a #15 blade to expose the cartilage. Double-prong skin hooks are placed at the incision, which is completed following the elliptical pattern. This exposes the cartilage of the ear and also the fascia overlying the mastoid. The skin edges are undermined using curved iris scissors. Bleeders are managed using the needlepoint ESU.

3. ***Sutures are placed through the mastoid fascia and attached to the posterior cartilage.***
   Several monofilament nonabsorbable sutures are placed in the mastoid fascia and then into but not through the posterior cartilage of the conchal bowl.

4. ***The helical fold is reduced.***
   A small skin incision is made in the anterior helix and a Freer elevator inserted along the cartilage at the helical fold. This creates a tissue plane for insertion of a rasp. The rasp is inserted into the tunnel created by the Freer elevator and passed over the helical cartilage several times. This reduces it and allows it to bend more easily. To keep the ear in the new position closer to the head, the surgeon may pass two or three hypodermic needles, size 28-gauge, through the helical fold.

5. ***Sutures are placed in the cartilage on the posterior side.***
   Synthetic absorbable sutures size 5-0 are placed at the posterior cartilage. The sutures previously placed through the mastoid fascia are now secured. Finally, the skin is closed using synthetic monofilament sutures size 4-0 or 5-0. This is shown in Fig. 28.23.

   The reconstructed ear is reinforced with ointment-impregnated cotton balls and a mastoid dressing.

CORRECTION OF STAHL'S EAR

Stahl's ear is the pointed appearance of the normally rounded crus of the ear. The technique used here is similar to the previous procedure. Fig. 28.24 illustrates the procedure and outcome.

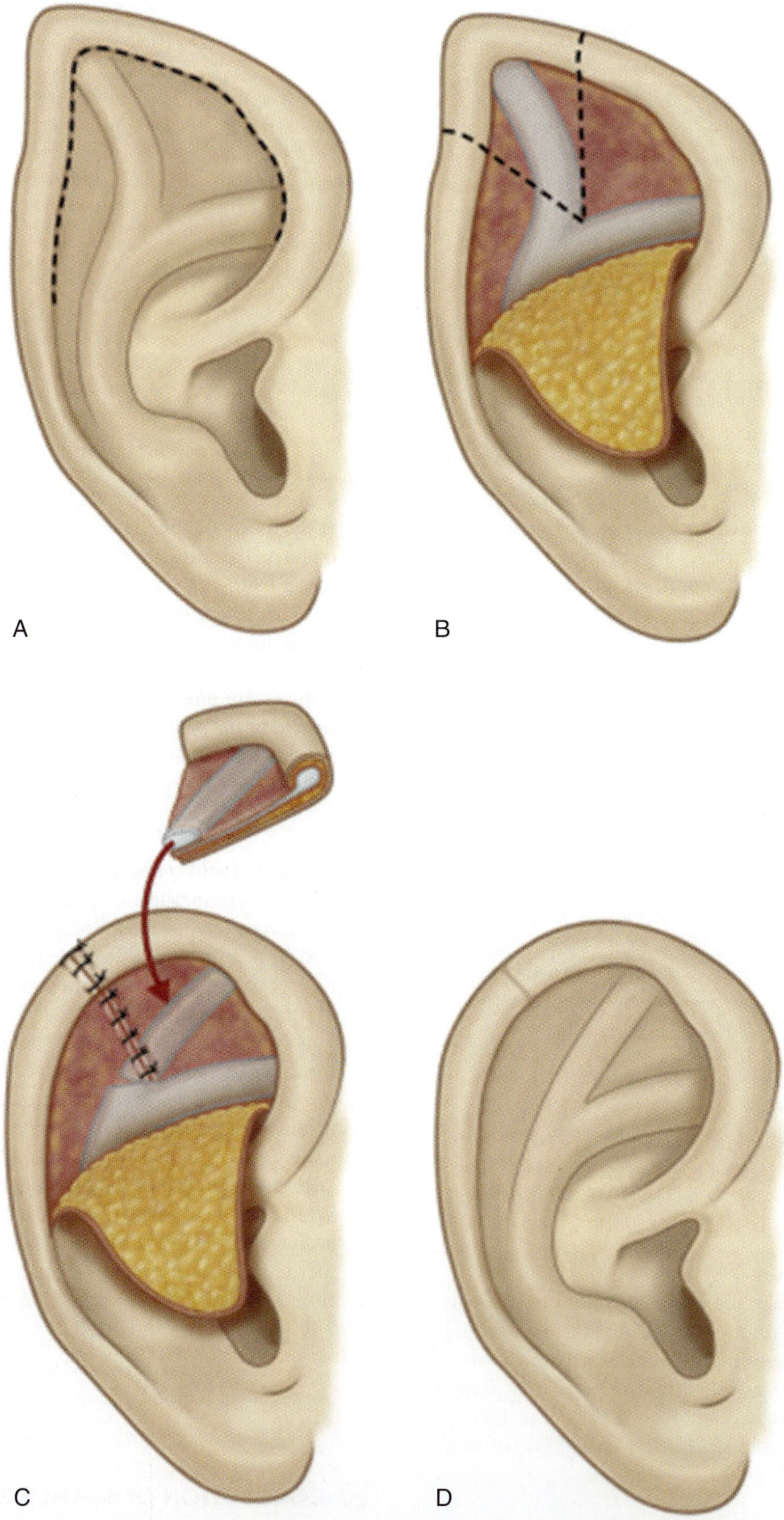

FIG. 28.24 Otoplasty for Stahl's ear. (A) The skin incision is made inside the helical rim. (B) The crus is excised. (C) The cartilage is approximated and the specimen is used as an only graft to reconstruct the crus. (D) Final result. (From Gurtner G, Neligan P. *Plastic Surgery: Principles*. 4th ed. vol 1. London: Elsevier; 2018; Gurtner G, Neligan P. *Plastic Surgery: Aesthetic*. 4th ed. vol 2. London: Elsevier; 2018.)

AUGMENTATION MAMMOPLASTY

Simple breast augmentation is performed to increase the size and improve the shape of the breast or to create a new breast after mastectomy. This is commonly performed using breast implants or with transplanted tissue. The implants are constructed with a silicone outer layer and a saline or silicone inner space. Sometimes a tissue expander is used to create space for the implant. The expander is inflated with sterile saline after fitting it into the tissue pocket. The following is a description of the simple insertion of breast implants.

POSITION:	Supine or modified Fowler
INCISION:	Breast
PREP AND DRAPING:	Prep extends from neck to umbilicus. Drape as for thoracic procedure. Thorax
INSTRUMENTS:	Mammoplasty set or general surgery set with breast retractors, breast tissue expander, and implant

Technical Points and Discussion

POSTMASTECTOMY RECONSTRUCTION

1. ***The patient is prepped and draped.***
The patient is placed in the supine or modified Fowler position, prepped, and draped for a breast procedure, including the sternal notch and xiphoid process. This allows the surgeon to use midline anatomical marks that have not been altered by previous surgeries.

2. ***A pocket is created under the pectoralis major muscle.***
A #15 blade is used to make an incision in the axillary region, around the lower half of the areola and nipple, or in the inframammary fold. Hemostasis is maintained with the ESU.

   The surgeon creates a pocket in the musculofascial tissue of the pectoralis major. This is done with a blunt hemostat or with gentle digital separation of the tissue.

3. ***A tissue expander is inserted.***
A tissue expander is inserted into the pocket and filled in 60-mL increments. The ST must record the amount of fluid used in the expander, because the same amount will be used if an expandable implant is used. Once the pocket has been expanded, the permanent implant is inserted.

4. ***The incision is closed.***
The incision is closed with 3-0 and 4-0 absorbable suture. The skin is closed with a subcuticular suture.

REDUCTION MAMMOPLASTY WITH MASTOPEXY AND NIPPLE RECONSTRUCTION

Mammoplasty with mastopexy involves removal of excess breast tissue and reconstruction (mammoplasty) to provide an aesthetic appearance. The breast attachment is lifted (mastopexy) and the nipple reconstructed. Many different techniques are used to perform breast reduction and lifting. The selection of any one procedure depends on the surgeon's training and on the specific needs of the patient. Preoperative preparation of the patient takes place in the surgeon's clinic. The procedure is planned using computer modeling and calibration. The incisions are clearly marked with a skin marker. The procedure here describes a free nipple graft.

Pathology

Combination mammoplasty and mastopexy may be performed for cosmetic or medical reasons. Macromastia (excessively large breasts) is related to the weight and size of the breast. The increased forward weight can cause cervical and thoracic pain. Patients also may suffer socially and psychologically. Macromastia in males is referred to as *gynecomastia*.

POSITION:	Semi-Fowler
INCISION:	Breast
PREP AND DRAPING:	Thorax with bilateral exposure to the breasts
INSTRUMENTS:	Major general surgery set, breast retractors
POSSIBLE EXTRAS:	Doppler ultrasound

Technical Points and Discussion

1. ***The patient is prepped and draped.***
The patient is positioned in the semi-Fowler position so that the position of the breasts can be observed during the procedure. The patient is prepped and draped for a breast procedure as previously described.

2. ***An incision is made around the areola and extended in a wide triangle to the inframammary line.***
The surgeon begins by making a circular incision using a #15 blade around the areola, with the breast held in extension. Next, the surgeon makes a triangular or anchor-shaped incision with the apex at the nipple margin and the base along the inframammary fold. The skin is undermined with Adson toothed forceps or Metzenbaum scissors.

3. ***Glandular and connective tissue is excised.***
The breast is then manually retracted superiorly, and the glandular and loose connective tissue excised. This step is performed with the ESU and Metzenbaum scissors. Any tissue removed is passed off the field and may be weighed. This is done to ensure that approximately the same amount of tissue is removed from each breast.

4. ***The inframammary and triangular incisions are closed.***
The surgeon approximates the breast tissue at the midline by bringing the sides of the triangle together and suturing them with absorbable 3-0 suture on a curved

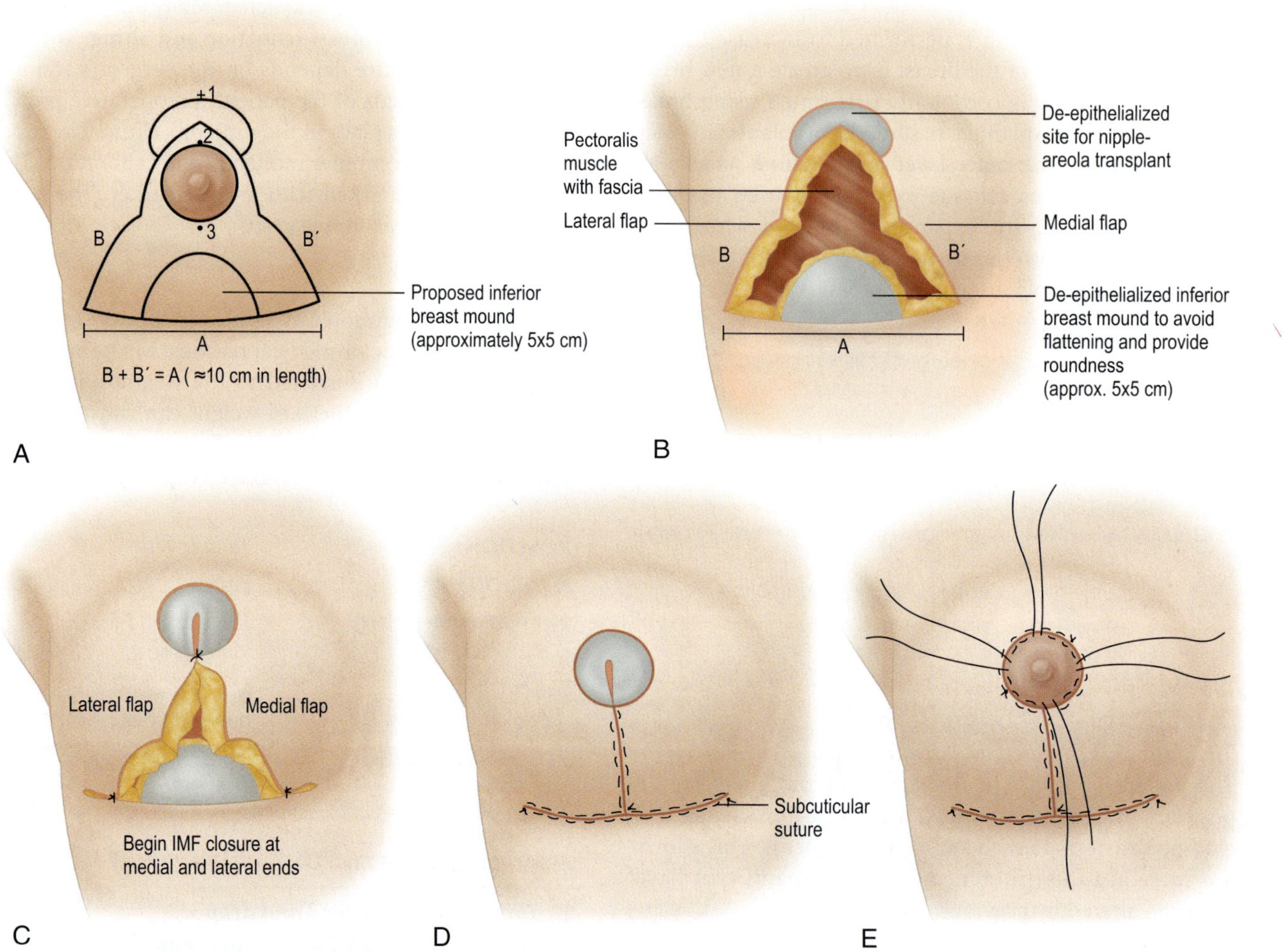

FIG. 28.25 Reduction mammoplasty/mastopexy with free nipple graft. (A) Surgical plan. (B) Resection of breast tissue. (C) Initial sutures. (D and E) Closure before and after the graft is sutured. (From Neligan P, Buck D, eds. *Core Procedures in Plastic Surgery*. Philadelphia: Elsevier; 2014.)

needle. Any excess skin at the inframammary incision is trimmed with Metzenbaum scissors or a #15 blade. The incision is closed with 3-0 absorbable suture. Both skin incisions are then closed with 4-0 subcuticular suture.

5. ***The nipple is transposed.***
   The surgeon uses a nipple marker to make a circular incision at the apex of the triangular incision. The tissue is excised with a #15 blade. This creates a new position for the areola and nipple, which are pulled through the incision line and sutured in place with nonabsorbable or synthetic absorbable subcuticular suture size 5-0. Gauze fluffs and supportive dressings are then applied. Technical points are illustrated in Fig. 28.25.

TRANSVERSE RECTUS ABDOMINIS MYOCUTANEOUS FLAP

A transverse rectus abdominis myocutaneous (TRAM) flap procedure is performed to reconstruct the breast without the use of implants. In this procedure, a pedicle graft including fatty tissue, muscle, and skin is transposed from the lower abdominal area to the mastectomy site through a tunnel in the abdominal wall. The flap is transferred while retaining its blood flow from the abdominal vessels. The procedure can be performed at the same time as the mastectomy or at a later date. In the following procedure, the breast is reconstructed at a later date.

Pathology

Mastectomy is performed for the treatment of breast cancer. Details of the pathology are described in Chapter 22.

POSITION:	Supine
INCISION:	Transverse pelvic, breast
PREP AND DRAPING:	A combined prep and draping procedure are carried out on the lower abdomen and chest wall. A Foley catheter is placed and sequential compression device applied to the patient's legs.

INSTRUMENTS AND SUPPLIES:	Major laparotomy instruments with breast retractors, table-attached retraction system, extra right-angle and long curved hemostatic clamps, vessel loops, vascular graft tunneler, vessel clips
POSSIBLE EXTRAS:	Doppler ultrasound

Technical Points and Discussion

1. ***The patient is prepped and draped.***
The patient is placed in the supine position and prepped from the neck to the pubis. Draping exposes the abdomen and the breasts.

2. ***The mastectomy scar is excised and the incision carried to the chest wall.***
The surgeon grasps the mastectomy scar with Adson toothed forceps or Allis clamps and excises it with a #15 blade. After any bleeders are controlled, the incision is covered with a moist lap tape or surgical towel.

3. ***A lower abdominal incision is made.***
An elliptical incision including the umbilicus is made in the lower abdomen. The incision is carried deeper to the rectus sheath. Richardson and Deaver retractors may be used to retract the incisional walls. A table-attached retractor system may also be used to maintain traction on the upper edge of the incision throughout the procedure.

4. ***The tissue flap is separated from its attachments.***
To bring the tissue flap into the chest wall and reconstruction of the breast, the tissue flap must be separated from its attachments in the abdomen. The deep epigastric vein and artery are clamped using right-angle or curved hemostats, then divided. The rectus muscle is detached from the pubic bone. The muscle may be grasped with Allis clamps and the pubic attachment incised with Metzenbaum scissors and ESU.

5. ***The rectus sheath is separated from the rectus muscle.***
The rectus sheath is separated from the muscle. This is accomplished using blunt and sharp dissection.

6. ***The tissue flap is brought into the chest wall.***
The first step in bringing the tissue flap up to the reconstruction site is creation of a tunnel in the fascia of the abdominal and chest wall. This is usually done digitally. The tissue flap can be brought through the tunnel by inserting a grasping clamp through the tunnel from top to bottom and then pulling the graft carefully back through. The vascular supply to the graft is maintained by the superior epigastric vessels.

7. ***The breast reconstruction is performed.***
Once the pedicle flap is brought through the incision at the mastectomy site, it can be trimmed to create a new breast. The surgeon may use the knife or scissors to size the flap graft.

   The flap is attached to the mastectomy site using a combination of staples and absorbable sutures. Attachments are made in the pectoral fascia and skin. The skin is closed using size 3-0 and 4-0 Monocryl. Two suction drains are placed in the chest wall on each side of the new breast.

8. ***The abdominal incision is closed.***
The surgeon closes the abdomen in layers. The rectus sheath is approximated with 2-0 absorbable synthetic suture. The skin is closed with staples or an absorbable subcuticular suture. Synthetic mesh may be used to reinforce the closure (described in Chapter 22). Technical points are illustrated in Fig. 28.26.

MICROVASCULAR DEEP INFERIOR EPIGASTRIC PERFORATOR GRAFT

The deep inferior epigastric perforator (DIEP) procedure is a method of transplanting a free graft from the abdomen to the chest wall to reconstruct a breast after mastectomy. The procedure uses microvascular anastomosis techniques. Whereas the blood supply of the TRAM flap graft is carried from the recipient site to the donor site, the *microvascular free flap* obtains its blood supply from the recipient site. The techniques involved in microvascular free graft surgery are similar regardless of the location of the graft donor site and recipient site, and the DIEP graft is just one of many different kinds. In cases where nerves and connective tissue structures are also transplanted, microsurgical techniques are also used to join the donor and recipient structures. Replantation procedures such as attachment of a severed limb use such techniques. Other procedures in which microvascular techniques are used include free flaps that cover deformities resulting from radical cancer surgery of the breast, face, head, and neck. This procedure may be performed at the time of mastectomy or at a later date. Microvascular technique is used to create the anastomosis between the epigastric perforators and the internal mammary vessels. This allows breast reconstruction with ample vascularization and decreased risk of graft necrosis. Two surgical teams are often used: one for the chest wall and the other for the pelvic dissection and graft harvesting. Before surgery, the surgeon uses a duplex Doppler and computerized tomography (CT) to detect and measure the pelvic perforators where they emerge through the fascia and muscle. Their location is then marked on the skin using a surgical pen. The pelvic elliptical incision lines and other landmarks are also marked preoperatively.

Pathology

Refer to Chapter 22 for a discussion on the incidence and surgical options available to breast cancer patients who require radical or tissue-sparing mastectomy.

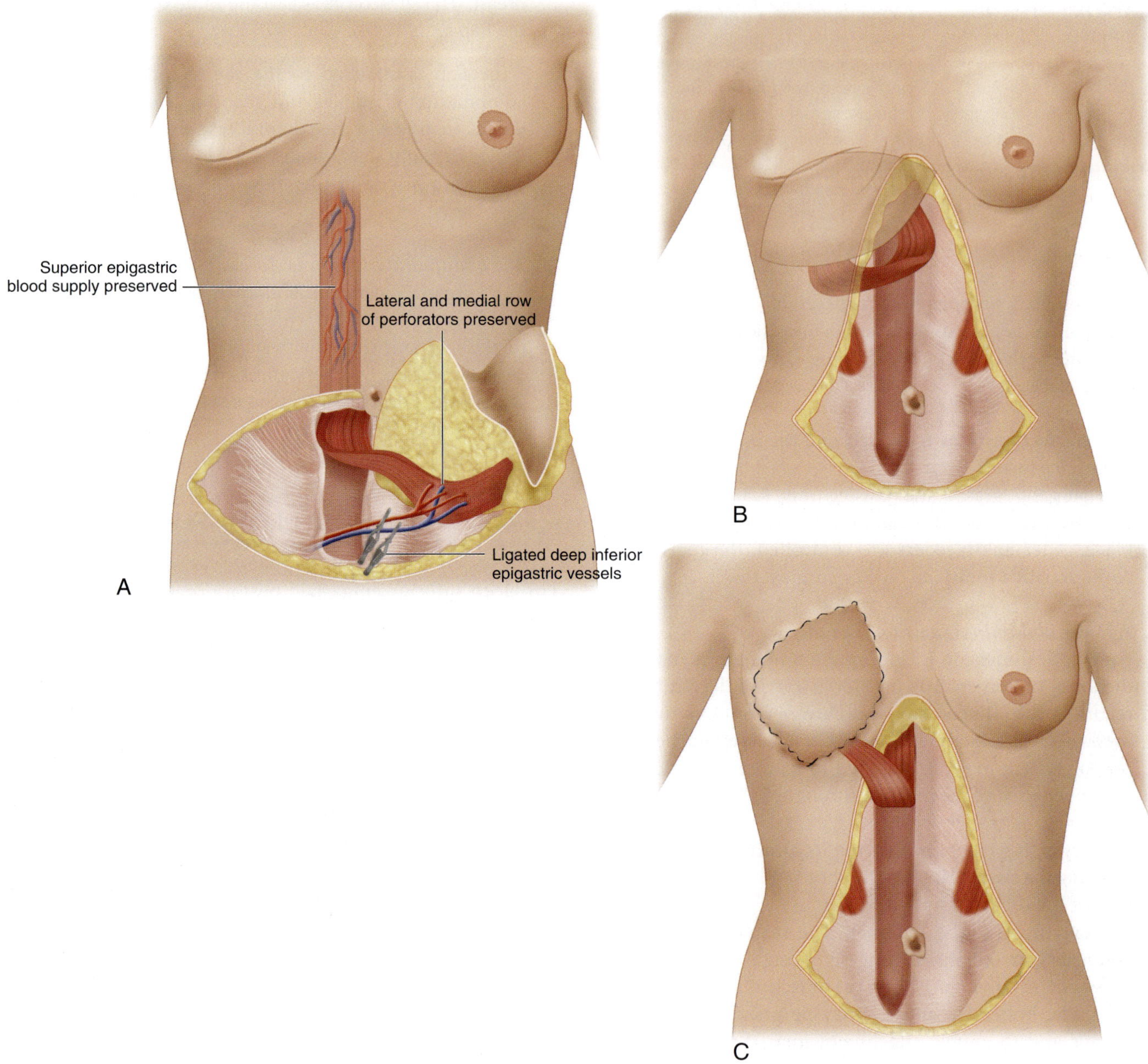

FIG. 28.26 Transverse rectus abdominis myocutaneous (TRAM) flap breast reconstruction. (A) The TRAM flap is released from the pelvic wall. (B) A subcutaneous tunnel is made, and the flap is transposed into the mastectomy defect. (C) The flap is sutured to form the breast mound. (From Klimberg V, Townsend C, Evers M, eds. *Atlas of Breast Surgical Techniques.* Philadelphia: Saunders; 2012.)

POSITION:	Supine
INCISION:	Transverse pelvic; mastectomy site
PREP AND DRAPING:	A combined prep and draping procedure are carried out on the lower abdomen and chest wall. A Foley catheter is placed and sequential compression device applied to the patient's legs
INSTRUMENTS AND SUPPLIES:	Major laparotomy instruments with chest wall retractors; extra right-angle and curved hemostatic clamps: vessel loops; vessel clips; *Micromat*; microvascular instruments; microvascular clamps and venous couplers; Freer elevator, Cobb elevator; double action rongeur; monopolar and bipolar ESU; sterile Doppler ultrasound
POSSIBLE EXTRAS:	Loupe magnifiers for each surgeon or operating microscope

Technical Points and Discussion

1. ***The patient is prepped and draped.***
The patient is placed in supine position and prepped from the neck to the pubis. Draping exposes the abdomen and the thorax.

PREPARATION OF THE DONOR SITE

2. ***An elliptical incision is made in the lower pelvis.***
Using a #10 or #20 knife blade, the surgeon incises the skin following skin markings made previously.

3. ***The abdominal flap is raised and the perforators identified.***
The incision is carried to the anterior fascia and exterior oblique muscles using the monopolar ESU. The tissue flap is raised from one corner of the ellipse using the monopolar ESU. A sterile Doppler is used to guide the dissection and prevent damaging the perforator vessels. As the perforators are approached, the surgeon may use the bipolar ESU for hemostasis. Rake or medium Richardson retractors may be used for exposure. The perforators that will be used for the flap are then carefully dissected through an incision in the anterior rectus fascia and muscle to their origin at the external iliac vessels. Dural hooks such as those used in neurosurgery are used to retract the muscle fibers. The ST should also have vessel clips and microvascular clamps available during the dissection. Irrigation should be available throughout to prevent the vessels from drying. Tenotomy scissors may be used for fine tissue dissection of the perforators including a small cuff of fascia around each vessel. Vessels that are *not* to be included in the flap are clamped with *Acland* microsurgical occluding clamps (shown in the illustrations following). The flap is then assessed for adequate perfusion. If the perfusion is inadequate, a different set of perforators are selected.

NOTE *If all attempts to demonstrate perfusion fail, the procedure may be converted to a TRAM flap as described previously.*

Once the vessels have been isolated, a vessel loop is placed around each.

4. ***Preparation of the mastectomy site: a partial rib resection is performed.***
If two teams are available to operate simultaneously on both the recipient (mastectomy) site and the abdominal portion, the donor flap can be immediately transferred to the chest wall. However, if the reconstruction is delayed, deep scar tissue is scored to allow the flap to be introduced aesthetically without tension. To begin the procedure on the recipient site Weitlaner or Gelpi retractors are placed in the chest wall incision. The internal mammary vessels, which are used for the microvascular anastomosis, are accessed by removing a portion of the third rib. The surgeon divides the pectoralis major fibers and anterior perichondrium, which lies over the costal cartilage using the ESU. A Cobb or Freer elevator may then be used to elevate the anterior perichondrium. A portion of the costal cartilage is removed using a double-action rongeur, exposing the posterior perichondrium with the mammary vessels lying just under it. The ESU is used to carefully incise the perichondrium. Using a Freer elevator and Adson forceps, the surgeon gently clears the perichondrium from the vessels.

5. ***The mammary vessels are isolated.***
The ST should now have microvascular instruments immediately available. Micro forceps, scissors, and an elevator are used to isolate ("skeletonize") the veins from the surrounding tissue. Once this is done, a flat neurosurgical sponge soaked with a vasodilating agent such as papaverine, verapamil, or lidocaine is placed over the vessels to reverse any spasm.

6. ***The donor flap is released.***
Once the donor vessels have been isolated and the recipient vessels prepared, the flap may be released. A marking suture of 5-0 Prolene may be used to identify the skin site over the perforator for Doppler assessment after transfer. The size and weight of the flap is then assessed. The entire flap or only a portion may be released according to the dimensions of the mastectomy defect. The vascular bundles with their perforators are then clamped, ligated with vessel clips, and released. Heparinized saline is used to flush the artery and prevent clotting.

7. ***The microsurgical anastomosis is performed.***
If the operating microscope is used, it is placed in position at this time.

The graft is oriented correctly to prevent torsion, and several temporary tacking sutures are placed through the chest wall. A background patch of colored silicone (*MicroMat*) is placed behind the vessels to provide contrast during the anastomoses. The microsurgical anastomoses of veins and arteries are then performed using size 9-0 nylon suture. Alternatively, the veins may be joined using venous microvascular coupling devices. These consist of two collars, which are fitted to the ends of the two veins. The collars are then fitted together and crimped, forming an end-to-end anastomosis. However, the arterial anastomoses are always sutured by hand. The 11th intercostal nerve may also be anastomosed using size 11-0 nylon suture. When all vessel anastomoses have been completed, the clamps or clips are removed and perfusion assessed. Several small, loose fat grafts may be placed around the vessels to help prevent them from rotating.

8. ***The DIEP flap is set into the mastectomy site.***
Up to this point the free DIEP flap has been positioned in correct orientation to the mastectomy site and vessels but not securely attached to the chest wall. Now the surgeon shapes the flap and removes a margin of skin from the periphery so that the edges can be embedded into the mastectomy defect. The skin margins of the flap are removed with Mayo scissors and toothed Adson forceps. The flap is then set into the mastectomy defect and sutured in place. A narrow Deaver retractor is used to elevate the edge of the defect. Interrupted sutures of size 3-0 Vicryl are placed through the edges of the flap, where they meet the subcutaneous chest tissue. Skin is closed using clear Prolene sutures, size 4-0. A colored Prolene marking suture, size 5-0 is inserted over the site of the anastomosis for Doppler testing postoperatively.

9. ***The abdominal wound is closed.***
The abdominal incision is closed in layers. The fascia defect is sutured with size 0 non-absorbable suture such as

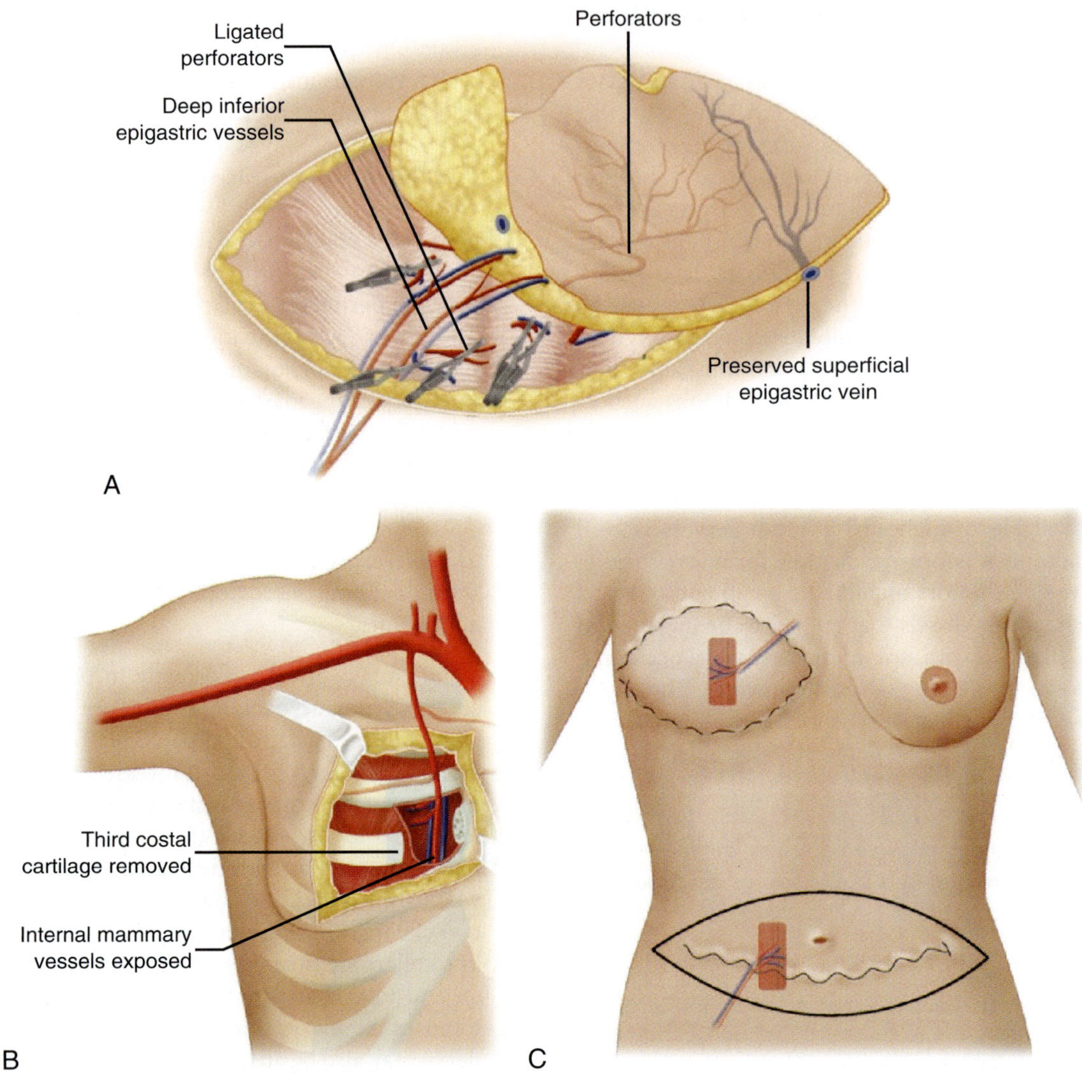

FIG. 28.27 DIEP free graft. (A) The donor graft is harvested from the lower abdomen. Microvascular clamps are seen on the vascular structures. (B) The mammary vessels are prepared for anastomosis. (C) The DIEP graft is implanted in the mastectomy site. (From Klimberg V, Townsend C, Evers M. *Atlas of Breast Surgical Techniques*. Philadelphia: Saunders; 2012.)

Prolene. Interrupted sutures are placed first, followed by a running suture. Any remaining portion of abdominal flap may be removed and an abdominoplasty performed. Size 2-0 Vicryl suture is used to close Scarpa's fascia. The umbilicus is positioned and secured during closure. Two suction drains are placed and skin approximated with size 3-0 Monocryl subcuticular or interrupted sutures. The recipient site wound is dressed with Telfa, gauze fluffs, and flat gauze. The abdominal wound is dressed with nonstick gauze, an abdominal pad, and tape. Patients recover in the intensive care unit overnight followed by 5 or more days in the surgical ward. The procedure for a DIEP graft is shown in Fig. 28.27.

NIPPLE RECONSTRUCTION

After a TRAM flap or DIEP reconstruction, the nipple and areola may be reconstructed to create a more natural appearance. A common approach to nipple reconstruction is the *skate flap*. In this procedure, a small flap of existing skin and fatty tissue of the reconstructed breast is elevated. The incision is shaped as three elliptical extensions or wings arising from a central point. The skin is incised using a #15 blade following skin markings made before surgery. The incisions are carried into the fatty tissue to release tension on the skin. A needlepoint ESU is used to control small bleeders. The three flaps are then used to form a skin projection and sutured in place using size 5-0 Vicryl. The skin forming the base of the new nipple is approximated using interrupted Vicryl sutures. The nipple may be tattooed to provide color contrast at the time of reconstruction or at a later date (Fig. 28.28).

LIPOSUCTION

Liposuction is performed to remove excess deep fat. High-vacuum suction, a rigid cannula, and a large-bore suction tube (at least ⅜ inch [0.9 cm] in diameter) are used in the

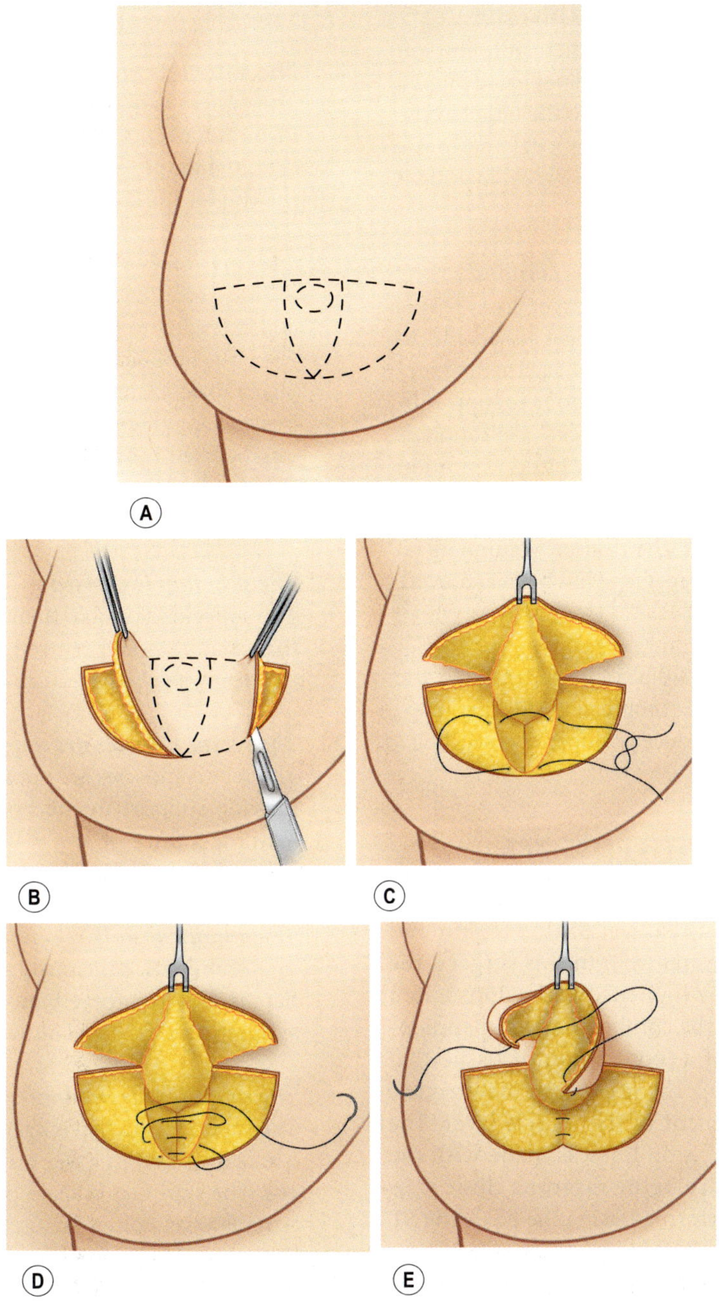

FIG. 28.28 Nipple reconstruction using the skate flap. (A) The flap design. (B) The wings are elevated. (C) The central portion is elevated. (D) The lateral wings and core are demonstrated. (E) The lateral wings are wrapped around the core of adipose tissue. The flap is closed. The skin may be tattooed at a later date. (From Nahabedian M, Neligan P. *Plastic Surgery, Volume 5: The Breast*. 4th ed. Elsevier; 2018.)

procedure. This is performed to remove excess fat from the body—usually in the abdomen, neck, and upper arms.

POSITION:	For abdominal liposuction—supine
INCISION:	Multiple small incisions in the target tissue
PREP AND DRAPING:	Abdominal or according to other areas to be treated
INSTRUMENTS:	Liposuction cannulas and instruments

Technical Points and Discussion

1. ***The patient is prepped and draped.***
The patient is placed in the supine position with the arms at a 90-degree angle to the body (for liposuction of the abdomen). Depending on the extent of the procedure, either general anesthesia or local anesthesia with intravenous sedation is used. The patient is prepped and draped with towels and three-quarter sheets to allow exposure of all the sites to be treated.

2. ***Local anesthetic is injected into the operative site.*** The surgeon begins by injecting an anesthetic into the soft tissue. A large volume of lidocaine and epinephrine diluted in lactated Ringer solution is injected into the targeted tissue until it is taut. The injection provides local anesthesia and hemostasis and expands the operative area, making it easier to insert the liposuction cannula.

3. ***Cannulas are inserted through multiple incisions.*** Multiple incisions are made into each target area. This is done to provide easier access to the target tissue and to prevent depressions around the access sites. The liposuction cannula is connected to the large-bore suction tubing and high-vacuum suction. Superficial aspiration is performed with a 2- or 3-mm cannula. Deep aspiration requires a 4- or 5-mm cannula.

   Aspiration is continued until the desired volume of fat has been removed or the desired shape has been achieved.

4. ***The wounds are closed.*** The incisions are closed with 3-0 absorbable suture. If the extremities have been treated, a compression stocking is applied to provide support and reduce postoperative swelling.

ABDOMINOPLASTY WITH POSSIBLE PANNICULECTOMY

Abdominoplasty is the surgical removal of excess skin and adipose tissue from the abdominal wall. In this surgery, the abdominal muscles may also be tightened and a liposuction performed. The procedure may be combined with a panniculectomy, which is reduction of a loose apron of tissue that arises from the lower abdomen. The procedure may require the use of mesh for reinforcement of the muscle layer. The surgical plan, including the incision lines, is made with the patient standing. This takes place in the surgeon's clinic.

Much of the dissection is performed using the ESU. The ST should periodically remove the buildup of charred tissue on the instrument tip to prevent superheating.

Pathology

Abdominoplasty usually is performed as a cosmetic procedure, but it also can be performed for medical reasons. After significant weight loss, the skin of the abdomen hangs flaccid and can interfere with normal body movement. In some cases, the redundant skin can hang to the level of the knees. This "apron" makes movement and activities of daily living very difficult.

POSITION:	Supine
INCISION:	Low transverse abdominal from one iliac crest to the other
PREP AND DRAPING:	Abdominal
INSTRUMENTS:	Laparotomy set with long instruments, a table-attached self-retaining retractor, large Deaver retractors

Technical Points and Discussion

1. ***The patient is prepped and draped.*** The patient is placed under general anesthesia and placed in the semi-Fowler position to reduce tension on the abdominal tissue. The patient is prepped from the nipples to the thighs and draped for an abdominal procedure.

2. ***The incision is made and the tissue edges elevated.*** A transverse, U-shaped incision is made in the abdomen and extended to the fascia. Skin flaps are elevated with the ESU. The umbilicus is excised and left in its natural position. Sharp towel clamps are placed in the upper margin of the incision for traction. As the procedure continues, a table-attached self-retraining retractor may be needed to elevate the upper skin flap. The skin flap is further elevated to the level of the xiphoid process and the inferior sternal borders.

3. ***The skin flap is excised.*** The superior skin flap then is pulled inferiorly to measure the amount to be removed. This tissue is then excised using heavy sharp dissection scissors.

4. ***The rectus muscles are approximated.*** The rectus muscles are approximated to tighten them and provide support to the body wall. This is done using a running suture of size 3-0 polydioxanone (PDS) or another absorbable synthetic suture.

5. ***The umbilical stalk is reinforced.*** The umbilicus, previously separated from the abdominal flap, is now reinforced and secured using size 4-0 or 3-0 synthetic absorbable suture.

6. ***The umbilicus is implanted into the flap.*** The superior skin flap is again placed over the abdomen and a hole incised with a #15 blade to accommodate the umbilicus. The skin flap is again pulled down over the abdomen. Several towel clamps are used to approximate the upper and lower flaps. A Kocher clamp is used to grasp the umbilicus and bring its edges to the level of the abdominal skin. It is sutured to the abdominal wall using size 3-0 absorbable sutures.

7. ***The abdominal wall incision is closed.*** Before the wound is closed, the patient may be placed in the semi-Fowler position, and, one or two drains are placed. These may be suction drains or gravity drains, depending on the amount of tissue removed.

   The abdominal wound is closed in two layers with absorbable suture. The skin is closed using staples. Dressings are applied, and the patient is maintained in the semi-Fowler position to prevent tension on the suture line. An abdominal binder may be applied.

Abdominoplasty procedure is demonstrated on the following website: https://www.youtube.com/watch?v=0o_424ckxW0.

KEY CONCEPTS

- *Plastic and reconstructive surgery* involves the treatment of congenital defects and anatomical abnormalities caused by disease and injury. Restoration of form and function is the primary goal of treatment.
- *Aesthetic surgery*, also called *cosmetic surgery*, is performed to improve the appearance but does not necessarily address function.
- Most cosmetic surgery involves only the skin; therefore the instruments are short and have fine tips.
- Reconstruction procedures may require fine orthopedic instruments, including small bone clamps, toothed tissue forceps, and small Kocher clamps. Rasps, small osteotomes, and fine curettes should also be available during procedures involving bone tissue.
- The dermatome is used to remove split-thickness skin grafts. The Brown-type dermatome is the most commonly used.
- Dressings in plastic and reconstructive surgery provide wound protection and physical support to remodeled structures. Complex reconstructive procedures require a variety of materials and techniques. Dressing routines in these procedures are exact and are considered a critical step in the procedure.
- Grafting is the surgical implantation of biological or manufactured material into an area of the body.
- A split-thickness skin graft (STSG) contains only the dermis, whereas a full-thickness skin graft (FTSG) contains both dermis and epidermis. A composite graft is one that contains two or more types of tissue.
- An implant is a synthetic, natural, or biosynthetic substance used to fill in or replace an anatomical structure.
- For diseased or traumatized tissue to heal, all devitalized or infected areas must be removed. The process of removing the diseased, damaged, or infected tissue is called *debridement*.
- During *Mohs surgery*, a malignant skin lesion is removed and cut into quadrants before frozen section. These quadrants are used to map the tumor and determine the exact location of malignant margins. Further excision is performed until the specimen is clear of all malignancy.
- Burns are classified according to the depth of tissue injury.
- In a superficial partial-thickness first-degree burn, only the outer layer of the epidermis is injured. The skin is red or pink, dry, and painful to touch.
- A partial-thickness second-degree burn is one in which the epidermis and various degrees of the dermis are injured. The skin is blistered, red, and moist. The burn is very sensitive to environmental exposure and touch.
- In a full-thickness second-degree burn, the epidermis and full dermis are injured. These burns are characterized by a white, smooth, shiny surface with dry blisters and edema.
- Proper assembly of the dermatome blade and head is critical to prevent skin tissue from tearing during the procedure.
- The skin graft mesher is used to perforate a skin graft. This increases its surface area and prevents serum from accumulating under the graft once it is in place.
- In a full-thickness third-degree burn, the subcutaneous tissue, muscle, and bone are burned. The third-degree burn is centered in an area of second-degree injury. The skin may be white, brown, or black, and appears waxy. There is no pain because nerves have been destroyed.
- Third-degree burns develop *eschar*, which is devitalized, nonelastic tissue that adheres to the wound site.
- Mineral oil is applied to the donor skin graft site to reduce the friction between the skin and dermatome blade.
- A stent is a special dressing applied over a skin graft. The dressing provides continuous pressure on the site to keep the graft in contact with the wound during healing.
- A pedicle graft is a composite graft in which a flap of tissue is partially released from one area of the body and attached to the wound site. When healing is complete, the flap is released and the donor site defect is closed primarily with sutures.
- Blepharoplasty resection of the eyelid is done to improve vision of the upper visual fields.
- Brow lift procedures are done to lift the supportive structures of the brow and alleviate drooping of skin, muscle, and fascia.
- The normal aging process and certain environmental factors such as smoking and exposure to excessive ultraviolet light contribute to sagging and wrinkling of the skin. Rhytidectomy is performed to remodel the skin and underlying tissue.
- Facial augmentation is performed to give normal contours to the chin or cheek. This is achieved by inserting a molded implant into the affected area.
- Otoplasty is performed to correct a congenital malformation of the external ear or to re-create an ear destroyed by trauma. Procedures for otoplasty often involve multiple surgeries. These procedures are somewhat complex and many approaches can be used, depending on the pathological condition and the patient's needs.
- Augmentation mammoplasty is performed to increase the size and improve the shape of the breast. The procedure is performed in post-mastectomy patients and those desiring larger breasts for aesthetic reasons.
- Reduction mammoplasty may be performed for cosmetic or medical reasons. Macromastia (excessively large breasts) is related to the weight and size of the breast. The increased forward weight can cause cervical and thoracic pain.
- A transverse rectus abdominis myocutaneous (TRAM) flap procedure is performed to augment the breast without the use of implants. In this procedure, a flap is raised from the abdomen and transferred to the chest wall as a pedicle graft.
- Panniculectomy (abdominoplasty) is performed for cosmetic reduction of abdominal fat. An "apron" of tissue is removed in severe cases to improve the patient's quality of life.
- A deep inferior epigastric perforator flap is a microvascular free graft obtained from the pelvis and used to reconstruct the breast after mastectomy.

REVIEW QUESTIONS

1. What are the three classifications of burns? Describe them.
2. When is debridement necessary for the treatment of burns?
3. What is compartment syndrome?
4. Differentiate full-thickness from split-thickness skin grafts.
5. Explain the purpose of a flap graft.
6. What is a biosynthetic material?

BIBLIOGRAPHY

Aston SJ, Beasley RW, Thorne CHM, eds. *Grabb and Smith's Plastic Surgery*. 5th ed. Philadelphia: Lippincott-Raven; 1997.

Baggish MS, Karram MM. *Atlas of Pelvic Anatomy and Gynecologic Surgery*. Philadelphia, PA: Elsevier; 2016.

Benedetto PX, Poblete-Lopez C. Mohs Micrographic surgery technique. *Dermatol Clin*. 2011;29(2):141–151. https://doi.org/10.1016/j.det.2011.02.002.

Canale S, Beaty J, eds. *Campbell's Operative Orthopaedics*. 12th ed. Philadelphia: Mosby; 2013.

Cummings C, Flint P, Haughey B, et al., eds. *Cummings Otolaryngology—Head and Neck Surgery*. Philadelphia: Mosby; 2005.

Dockery G, Crawford M, eds. *Lower Extremity Soft Tissue and Cutaneous Plastic Surgery*. 2nd ed. Philadelphia: Elsevier; 2012.

Garden OJ, Parks RW. *Principles and Practice of Surgery*. Edinburgh: Elsevier; 2018.

Hall-Findlay E, Evans G, eds. *Aesthetic and Reconstructive Surgery of the Breast*. Philadelphia: Elsevier Saunders; 2012.

Herndon DN. *Total Burn Care*. Edinburgh: Elsevier; 2018.

Klimberg V, Townsend C, Evers M, eds. *Atlas of Breast Surgical Techniques*. Philadelphia: Saunders; 2012.

Neligan P, Buck D, eds. *Core Procedures in Plastic Surgery*. Philadelphia: Elsevier; 2014.

Robinson J, Hanke C, eds. *Surgery of the Skin, Procedural Dermatology*. 3rd ed. Philadelphia: Saunders; 2015.

Robinson JK, Hanke C, Seigel D, Fratilla A, Bhatia A. *Surgery of the Skin Procedural Dermatology*. London: Elsevier Saunders; 2015.

Tyers AG, Collin JRO, eds. *Colour Atlas of Ophthalmic Plastic Surgery*. 2nd ed. Oxford: Butterworth-Heinemann; 2001.

Usatine R, Pfenninger J, Stulberg D, Small R. *Dermatologic and Cosmetic Procedures in Office Practice*. Saunders; 2012.

Velasco J, Ballo R, Hood K, Jolly J, eds. *Essential Surgical Procedures*. Edinburgh: Elsevier; 2016.

ORTHOPEDIC SURGERY 29

LEARNING OBJECTIVES

After studying this chapter, the reader will be able to:

1. Identify major bones of the body
2. Discuss specific types of instruments used in orthopedic surgery
3. Explain the uses of common orthopedic implants and hardware
4. Discuss basic techniques used in fracture reduction and fixation

TERMINOLOGY

Alloys: Metal that is composed of a mixture of pure metals.

Aponeurosis: A tendinous sheet that separates muscles or attaches a muscle to bone.

Arthrodesis: Surgical fusion of a joint.

Bioactive material: One that brings about a specific biological response at the interface of the material and the tissue.

Biocompatibility: A term that describes a material that is compatible with the tissue (i.e., causes no toxic or inflammatory effect).

Biomechanics: The relationship between movement and biological or anatomical structures.

Broaches: Fin-shaped rasps used to enlarge the medullary canal for the insertion of an implant.

Cannulated: A device having a hollow core; for example, an instrument with a central channel that can be fitted over a guidewire or pin.

Casting: A method of immobilizing a limb by the application of rigid or semi-rigid material along the length of the limb. A cast can be fully or partially circumferential.

Closed reduction: Alignment of bone fragments into anatomical position by manipulation or traction of the limb.

Comminuted: A fracture in which there are multiple bone fragments.

Compartment syndrome: Extreme tissue swelling within a closed compartment of the body or closed external device such as a cast. Edematous tissue can exceed the capacity of the space it is held in, causing sufficient pressure to cause tissue necrosis.

Compression: Mechanical force in which a structure is compacted or pressed together. A compression injury (e.g., compression fracture) results when bone or other tissue is compacted.

Cruciate: Cross shaped.

Dislocation: Displacement of a joint from its normal anatomical position.

Distraction: A mechanical process in which a structure is elongated. Distraction can be used to suspend a limb (and thereby stretch the soft tissue and bones) during surgery. A distraction injury is caused by the pulling apart or stretching of tissue (the opposite of a compression injury).

External fixation: A method of maintaining bone fragments in anatomical position from outside the body. A cast is an example of an external fixation device.

Internal fixation: Surgical repair of a fracture by implanting a device such as a metal plate, rod, or nail that holds the bone fragments in correct position during healing.

Open reduction: Surgical access (through an incision) to bring bone fragments into anatomical alignment.

Orthopedic system: A specific (usually patented) set of instruments and implants used for an orthopedic technique.

Press-fit: To impact or press a joint implant into position. Press-fitted implants do not require bone cement.

Ream: To enlarge a preexisting hole, depression, or channel, such as the medullary canal.

Reduction: The process of manipulating bone fragments to restore anatomical position.

Replantation: Surgical attachment of a limb (e.g. hand, fingers, arm) after traumatic amputation.

Tap: A spiral path drilled through the bone before inserting a screw.

Traction: A mechanical method of applying pulling force to a fractured bone in order to bring the fragments into alignment.

Orthopedic surgery is a specialization of the body's connective tissues. These tissues are the framework of the body, with a supporting and binding function. Surgery is performed to treat or correct injuries, congenital anomalies, and diseases of the bone, joints, ligaments, tendons, or muscle. Most orthopedic procedures focus on restoring bone and joint function that has been lost or reduced because of traumatic injury or disease. Alleviating pain is also a primary goal of surgical intervention. This chapter is presented according to the anatomical location of the pathology and surgery and encompasses bone and soft tissue repair.

Proficiency in orthopedic techniques relies heavily on a thorough understanding of the instrumentation and implants used for repair and reconstruction. Orthopedic techniques and **biomechanics** share many of the principles and language used in carpentry and engineering. Many procedures rely on the use of a proprietary **orthopedic system** developed and manufactured for sale or rent by a company or organization. This type of system contains patented surgical instruments and devices designed for use in a specific surgical technique. This means that the surgical team, including the surgical technologist, must learn the way a system works and the devices required for that procedure. Most manufacturers' system components are not interchangeable with those of another manufacturer.

Although a daunting number of systems are available and in development, the biomechanical principles of orthopedics remain constant. Surgical approaches (systems, procedural technique, and technology) to orthopedic injury and disease may seem complex, but they follow a basic pattern based on the mechanical and physiological aspects of bone structure. This chapter explains the basic generic techniques and mechanics and introduces common approaches while pointing out the possibility for variation. The key to developing advanced skills is to learn basic principles and apply them to complex systems.

SURGICAL ANATOMY

BONES AND THEIR STRUCTURE

The skeleton (Fig. 29.1) provides structural support to the soft tissues of the body. The individual bones of the body are divided into two groups called the *axial skeleton* and the *appendicular skeleton*.

The axial skeleton is composed of the cranium and facial bones, the bones of the ear, the spinal column, sternum, and ribs.

The cranium has eight bones that are connected by tough connective tissue called *sutures*. The brain is encased within the cranium, which includes the floor of the skull, and the sphenoid bone. At birth, the cranial bones are loosely fused. In the prenatal period, the sutures are wide and soft, which allows the head to mold as it passes through the mother's pelvis during birth. The *fontanels* are areas where the joint space is particularly wide. These occur in the posterior skull at the junction of the parietal and occipital bones and in the anterior skull between the parietal and frontal bones. The posterior fontanel usually closes by 8 weeks of age and the anterior fontanel between 3 and 18 months of age. The cranium is discussed in more detail in Chapter 34.

The *facial bones* are more complex and form the structure of the nasal sinus, orbit of the eye, and jaw. Only the *mandible* (lower jaw) is freely moveable. The *zygoma* and *orbital rim* are common sites of fracture in sports and motor vehicle accidents. The facial bones are discussed in detail in Chapter 27.

The *vertebral column* consists of 24 individual vertebrae: 7 *cervical*, 12 *thoracic*, and 5 *lumbar*. In adults, the *sacrum* is composed of five vertebrae that are fused. The *coccyx* is formed by the fusion of four or five vertebrae. The vertebra are discussed in detail in Chapter 34.

The *sternum* forms the anterior chest wall and is composed of three sections: the *manubrium*, the *body*, and the *xiphoid process*.

Twelve pairs of ribs connect to their corresponding vertebrae. Ribs 1 through 8 attach to the sternum and are connected by costal cartilage. Ribs 11 and 12 are "floating" ribs (i.e., they are not attached anteriorly).

The *appendicular skeleton* is composed of the upper extremities, pelvic girdle, and the lower extremities.

The shoulder includes the *scapula* and *clavicle*. The long bone of the upper arm is the *humerus*. It articulates proximally with the *glenoid fossa*. The *ulna* and *radius* form the forearm, and the *carpal* and *metacarpal* bones form the hand and wrist.

The pelvis consists of the *ilium, ischium,* and *pubis*. The *femur*, or thigh bone, is the longest bone of the body. The *patella* is located between the femur and the lower leg. The lower leg bones are the *tibia* and *fibula*. The bones of the foot are anatomically divided into three groups: the posterior foot contains seven *tarsal* bones. The mid-foot contains five *metatarsal* bones, and the toes contain the *phalanges*.

BONE TISSUE

Bone tissue is classified into two types:

- *Cortical bone,* which is also known as *compact bone,* is the denser of the two types. It is found in the shaft of long bones, at the ends of joints, and in vertebrae, where it surrounds the softer cancellous bone. The structure of cortical bone is highly structured in concentric circles and canals, which contain blood vessels, nerves, and lymph vessels.
- *Cancellous* bone (also called *spongy* or *trabecular* bone) is softer than cortical bone found at the ends of the long bones, within the ribs, flat bones of the cranium, the scapula, and other smaller flat bones of the body. Cancellous bone is less dense than cortical bone and has no geometric structure. Instead, the structure resembles a sponge, and the spaces are filled with red or yellow *marrow*, a soft connective tissue. Red marrow, which produces blood cells, is found in the center of certain long bones, in the vertebrae, and in pelvic bones. Important components of the immune system originate as precursor cells in the marrow. These include lymphocytes, monocytes, and macrophages.

BONE MEMBRANES

Bones are covered with a tough, bi-layered membrane called *periosteum*. The function of the periosteum is to protect the bone surface and provide attachment for tendons. It also contains osteoblasts. These are the bone's growth cells; they provide a source of development and repair in the same way that tree bark functions.

NOTE *The periosteum is an important tissue in orthopedic surgery. It must be scraped from the bone before cutting or remodeling. This is done with a periosteal elevator.*

The *endosteum* lines the inner channels of long bones. It also fills the *interstitial spaces* (i.e., the spaces between cells) of cancellous bone, as well as the Haversian canals. The endosteum initiates bone growth and provides nutritional substances to bones.

BONE STRUCTURE AND SHAPE

Long bones are characterized by a middle shaft, called the *diaphysis*, and the two ends, called the *epiphyses* (singular, epiphysis). Long bones include the bones of the legs, arms, and digits (i.e., the fingers and toes). The shaft is mostly composed of a compact bone and has a hollow center. The transition between the diaphysis and epiphysis is not readily apparent except during development, when the region is filled with cartilage. This developmental tissue is called the *epiphyseal plate* or *metaphysis*. It is significant in fracture pathology because a break in this area may delay growth of the bone in a child. The hollow cavity inside a mature long bone is called the *medullary*

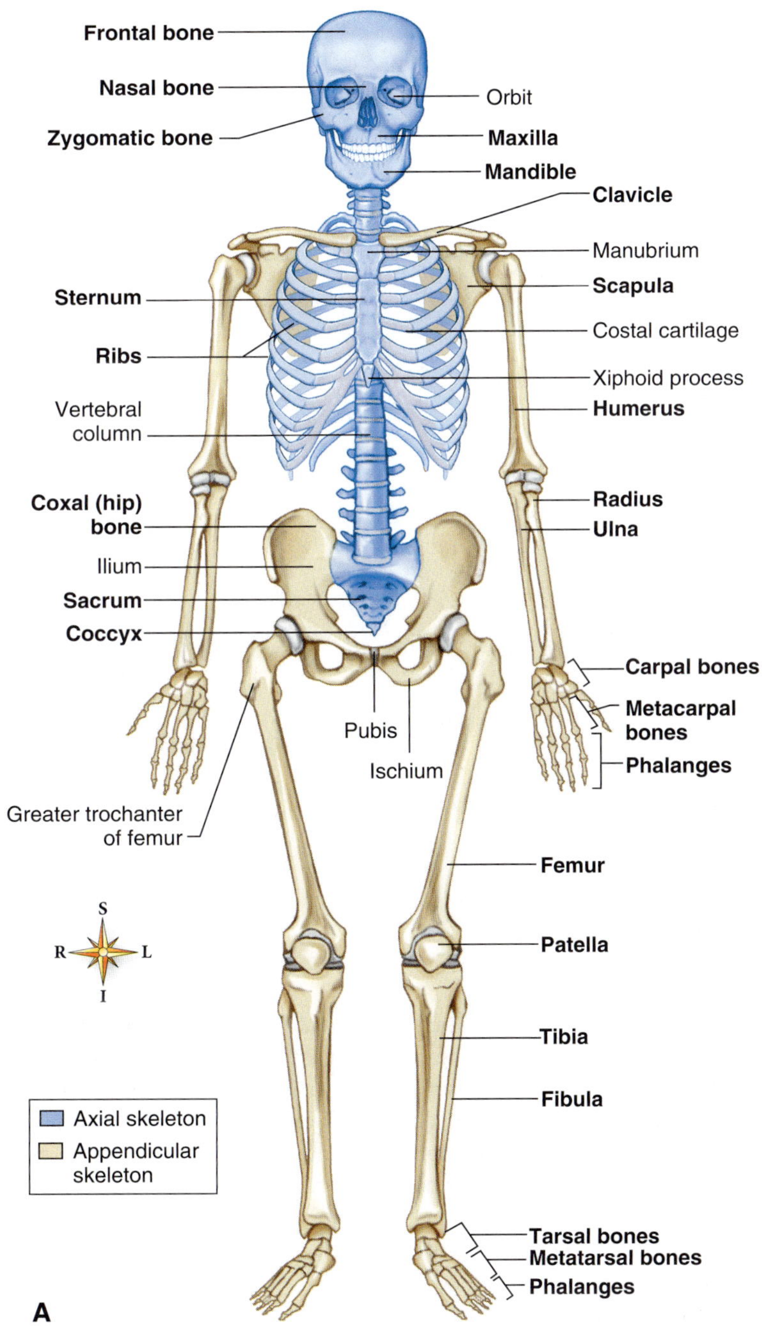

FIG. 29.1 Axial and appendicular skeleton. (A) Anterior view.

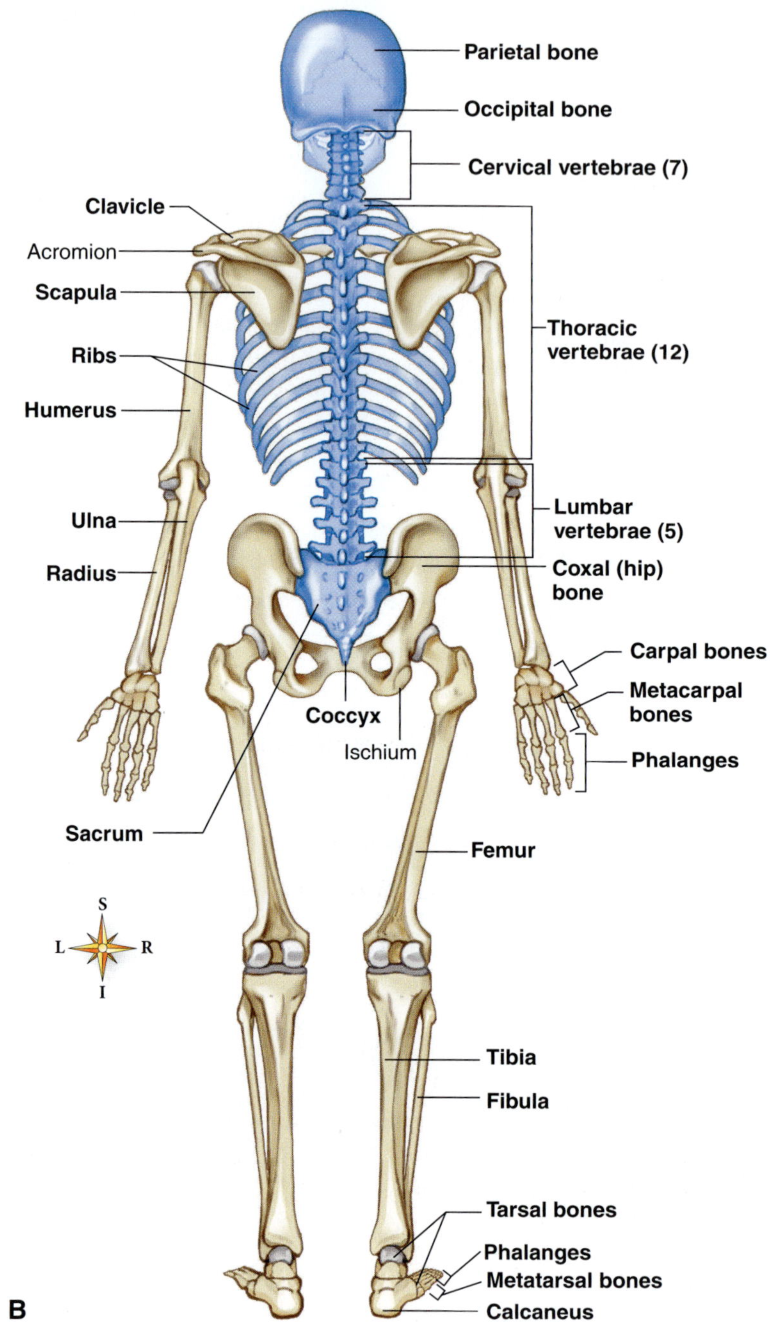

FIG. 29.1, cont'd (B) Posterior view. Patton K, Thibodeau G, Essentials of anatomy and physiology. 1st ed. St Louis: Elsevier; 2012.

canal. The epiphyses are wider and have bony outcroppings and protrusions where the ligaments are attached. The epiphyses, which are composed of cancellous bone, form the joints, which are covered with cartilage, a resilient connective tissue that increases the strength of the joint and reduces friction between the bones. Fig. 29.2 illustrates the structure of a long bone and its membranes.

Bones can be classified by their shape. The *short* bones are those of the wrist and ankle. *Irregular* bones include the vertebrae, spine, and face. A few irregularly shaped bones occur singly; these are referred to as *sesamoid bones*. The patella is an example of a sesamoid bone.

Flat bones are usually thin compared to other types of bones. In adults, the inner cancellous layer of the flat bones contains red marrow. (In other types of bones, red marrow converts to yellow marrow during childhood and persists into adulthood.) The ribs, cranial bones, scapula, and sternum are examples of flat bones.

LANDMARKS

Bones have many different irregularities called *landmarks*. These function as areas of attachment for tendons and ligaments or provide a passageway for nerves and blood vessels. They appear as

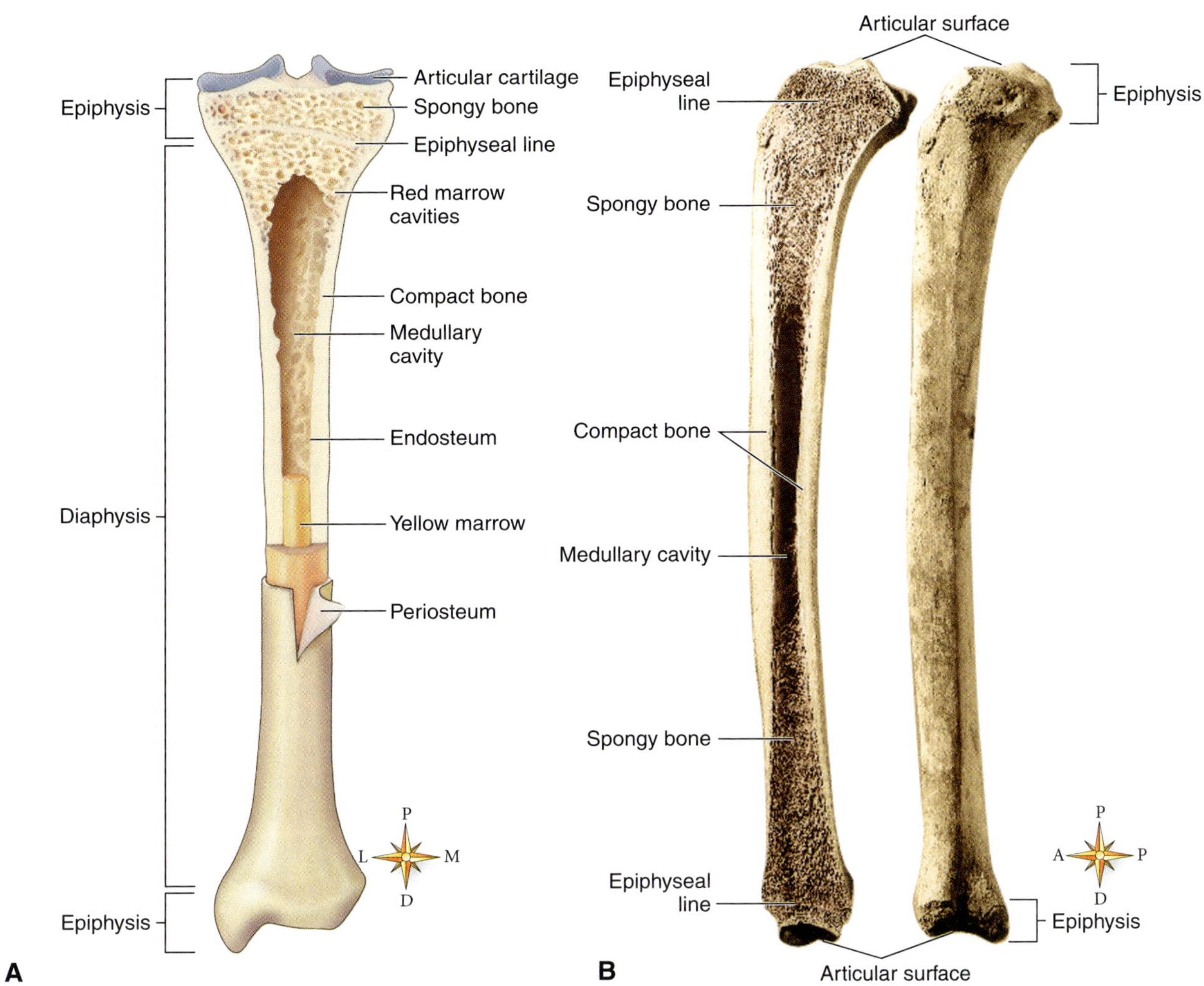

FIG. 29.2 (A) Frontal section of a long bone (tibia). (B) Sagittal section. (From Thibodeau G, Patton K. *Essentials of Anatomy and Physiology*. St Louis: Mosby; 2012.)

raised projections, bumps, ridges, channels, and tunnels. Some common types of landmarks are listed in Box 29.1. The body has many hundreds of bone landmarks. Differentiating the different types of landmarks is less important than recognizing them as identifiers of significant or common anatomical sites. Specific landmarks are referred to in surgical procedures to clarify the technique. For example, "An osteotomy was performed in the femoral neck." This means that the neck of the femur was incised or cut. Another example of an important landmark is the *iliac crest*, which is a common site for harvesting a bone graft.

JOINTS

The articular system (joints) includes the areas of the body where two bones meet and some degree of movement occurs. The movement may be small, as in the ossicles of the ear, or large, as in the hip joint.

Classification

Joints are classified according to the degree of movement they allow and by the shape of the articulating surfaces. Joint classifications are as follows:

BOX 29.1	Common Landmarks of Bone
Condyle	A knuckle-shaped portion of bone generally found in association with a joint
Crest	A ridge of bone (e.g., iliac crest)
Foramen	A rounded orifice in a bone (e.g., olfactory foramen); usually a passageway for blood vessels or nerves
Fossa	A depression in a bone (e.g., iliac fossa)
Neck	A narrow bridge of bone between two other structures (e.g., neck of the femur, neck of the humerus)
Process	A projection of bone (e.g., coracoid process)
Sinus	A cavity within a bone (e.g., nasal sinus)
Spine	A sharp, narrow projection (e.g., spinous process)
Sulcus	A groove in a bone
Tubercle	A small rounded projection (e.g., deltoid tubercle)
Tuberosity	A large rounded projection (e.g., ischial tuberosity)

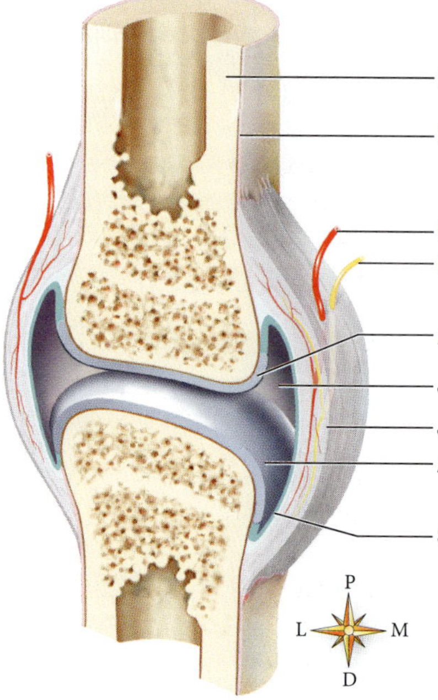

FIG. 29.3 Synovial joint structure. (From Thibodeau G, Patton K. *Essentials of Anatomy and Physiology*. St Louis: Mosby; 2012.)

- ***Synarthrosis:*** A joint with limited movement or fixed articular surfaces, such as between the bones of the cranium.
- ***Amphiarthrosis (cartilaginous joint):*** A joint in which the bones are connected by cartilage and only slightly moveable. The symphysis joints are included in this category (e.g., symphysis pubis).
- ***Diarthrosis:*** A joint that is freely moveable, such as the hip or shoulder.
- ***Synovial Joints*** A synovial joint is composed of articulating bone ends and connective tissues that surround them (Fig. 29.3).

The joint capsule surrounds the joint and contains nerves and blood vessels. The capsule is lined with a synovial membrane, which produces a viscous fluid that lubricates and nourishes the joint. The synovial fluid flows out of the joint capsule when it is injured or incised. The articular surfaces of the bones in the joint are covered with cartilage, which aids smooth gliding of one bone surface over the other. The space inside the joint capsule is called the joint cavity. During endoscopic joint surgery (arthroscopy), the telescope and instruments are inserted into the joint cavity through the capsule.

Joint Mobility

The flexibility of the joints is the basis of body movement. When a joint becomes diseased or is injured, movement becomes difficult or impossible because of mechanical restrictions or pain.

Joint movement is carefully described in medicine. In surgery, movement terminology often is used during the assessment of a joint. Terms are also used to direct patient positioning. In both cases, the surgeon may ask other team members to move a limb in a certain direction or in a spatial orientation. For example, the surgeon may request "more internal rotation" or "increased abduction." Specific terminology is used because less precise terms may cause confusion, resulting in injury to the patient.

Anatomically, a joint moves within its normal range of motion. Each moveable joint of the body is classified according to specific anatomical movements (e.g., pivot joint and ball-and-socket joint). The important point is that joints must be manipulated *only within their normal range of motion* to prevent injury. (Chapter 16 reviews terms and presents illustrations related to joint movement.) The types of moveable joints are as follows:

- *Hinge joint:* A joint that has rocker and cradle components, which allow extension and flexion only (e.g., the elbow).
- *Saddle joint:* A joint in which the two components have a complementary convex–concave shape, and the bones slide over each other. The body has only one saddle joint, which is in the thumb. This joint allows flexion, extension, *abduction*, and *adduction*.
- *Gliding joint:* A joint in which relatively flat surfaces of bone slide over each other (e.g., the vertebrae, movement of which allows the spine to flex).
- *Ball-and-socket joint:* A joint with a spherical component and a concave component. Movement occurs in several planes, making this joint the most freely moveable type (e.g., the hip and humerus). Ball-and-socket joints allow flexion, extension, abduction, adduction, rotation, and circumduction.
- *Pivot joint:* A joint composed of a bony protuberance and an open collar component (e.g., the first and second vertebrae of the neck). This type of joint allows rotation.
- *Condyloid joint:* A joint in which a small protrusion (condyle) slides within a slightly elliptical component (e.g., the carpal bones of the wrist). Condyloid joints allow flexion, extension, abduction, and adduction.

TENDONS, LIGAMENTS, AND MUSCLES

Tendons, ligaments, fascia, and muscle are the primary soft connective structures encountered in orthopedic surgery.

Tendons can take the form of a fibrous cord or a sheet of connective tissue called an **aponeurosis.** *Ligaments* attach bones to each other, providing flexibility and strength to the skeletal structure. When attached to the cartilage, they stabilize the joint and limit movements that may injure it. Neither tendons nor ligaments have significant blood supply.

Striated muscle, also commonly called *skeletal muscle*, facilitates movement of the skeletal system. It is composed of fibers that are bound together by sheaths of fascia. Each group of fibers and its associated sheath are bound together to form one muscle. Striated muscle is under voluntary control and makes up most of the body's muscle tissue. The primary functions of muscle are to provide skeletal movement, support the body's posture, and to maintain body heat through anaerobic metabolism. Muscle groups are attached to bone by tendons at two fixed points to allow skeletal movement. These points are called the *origin* and *insertion* of the muscle.

PATHOLOGY OF SOFT CONNECTIVE TISSUES AND JOINTS

The most common pathology of tendons, ligaments, and muscles is injury related to trauma, overuse, and certain autoimmune diseases such as rheumatoid arthritis, scleroderma, and lupus.

Surgery to restore function to damaged tendons, ligaments, and muscles usually requires reattachment, or anastomosis. Tendon, ligament, and muscle repair is commonly performed using non-absorbable sutures and suture-anchor systems.

The stability of a joint relies on the health of the soft connective tissues that support the bones and enable movement. Tendons and ligaments are frequently involved in joint surgery. In some cases, they required transposition (moving from one attachment point to another), modification such as shortening removal of damaged segments, or the use of tissue grafts. Joint pathology is frequently related to advancing age, previous trauma, or infection. The autoimmune diseases that can cause inflammation, damage, and pain also affect joint function. *Osteoarthritis* is the most common cause of arthritis and is usually a result of advancing age and previous trauma to the joints. It is a degenerative process that results in pain and loss of function and can occur in any joint. Joint surgery for full or partial repair and replacement is called *arthroplasty*.

ORTHOPEDIC PATHOLOGY

The following basic terms are used to discuss orthopedic pathology:

Fracture: Break of continuity in bone because of trauma or disease

Rupture: Torn or detached tendon, ligament, or muscle. Although frequently a sudden event related to trauma, it can also take place slowly when the tissue is exposed to sharp bony growths (spicules) or bone fragments

Avulsion: Partial or complete tearing away of tissue from its normal attachment (e.g., bone, tendon, muscle, or ligament). This term may also apply to a specific body structure (e.g., ear, hand, finger)

Overuse injury: Damage and disease of soft connective tissues caused by repetitive motion or repetitive stress

FRACTURES

Fractures occur as a result of trauma or disease and represent the majority of pathology requiring orthopedic surgery. Traumatic bone injury may be complicated by soft tissue injury, with critical damage to nerves and blood vessels. Motor vehicle accidents, pedestrian versus vehicle, sports injuries, and interpersonal violence are the primary causes of fractures.

Fracture Classification

Fractures are classified to enable communication among health care professionals. Several classification systems are used. Classification is important to the surgical technologist because it provides information needed for the preparation of the appropriate instrumentation, positioning, and surgical approach. Systems of classification vary according to the type of criteria they use:

- *Name of the bone and location:* The distinguishing features are the name of the bone (e.g., tibia, femur, third phalanx) and the anatomical area (distal or proximal). For example, a fracture may be located in the distal tibia or the proximal humerus.
- *Pattern of fracture:* Fractures may be described by the pattern of the break. This helps identify the forces involved and the methods required for repair.
- *Level of comminution:* This is the extent of fragmentation. For example, a severely comminuted fracture is one that has many fragments. Mild comminution describes a fracture with few fragments. A highly comminuted fracture requires a longer surgical time and complex instrumentation.
- *Displacement:* This factor describes whether the bone fragments are in anatomical alignment. A nondisplaced fracture is one in which the bone fragments are in alignment.
- *Pathological origin:* A pathological fracture can occur with normal load. It is caused by any disease that weakens the structure and composition of the bone.

Fracture Patterns

Fracture patterns can be associated with the impact and environment that caused them (Fig. 29.4). Common fracture patterns include the following:

- *Transverse:* Fracture line that is perpendicular to the long axis of the bone
- *Oblique:* Type of transverse fracture that occurs at an angle
- *Spiral:* Fracture of the long bone that occurs in a spiral pattern as the result of twisting or torsion on the bone
- *Impacted:* Fracture in which bone fragments are driven into each other or into another bone
- *Comminuted:* Fracture with two or more pieces
- *Open:* Fracture in which the fractured end penetrates the skin
- *Greenstick:* Fracture of immature bone that is soft and less brittle than mature bone. The fracture is incomplete or the impact results in severe bending and bruising
- *Depressed:* Cranial fracture in which the fragments are displaced inwardly
- *Pathological fracture:* Fracture resulting from disease such as osteoporosis, which is caused by calcium deficiency

Fracture Repair

REDUCTION For a fracture to heal, the bones must be brought into anatomical alignment. This is called **reduction** (of the bone fragments). Mechanical or manual reduction of the bone fragments is performed with the patient under anesthesia. Reduction is a physical (kinetic) process and may require the mechanical advantage of a traction device that pulls the injured bones into alignment. After injury, severe tissue swelling can make reduction more difficult, requiring mechanical aid. If the fracture is minor, manual reduction may be adequate. Two types of reduction are as follows:

- ***Open reduction (OR):*** Performed using a surgical incision
- ***Closed reduction (CR):*** Performed by the manipulation of the bone or with an external traction device that pulls the

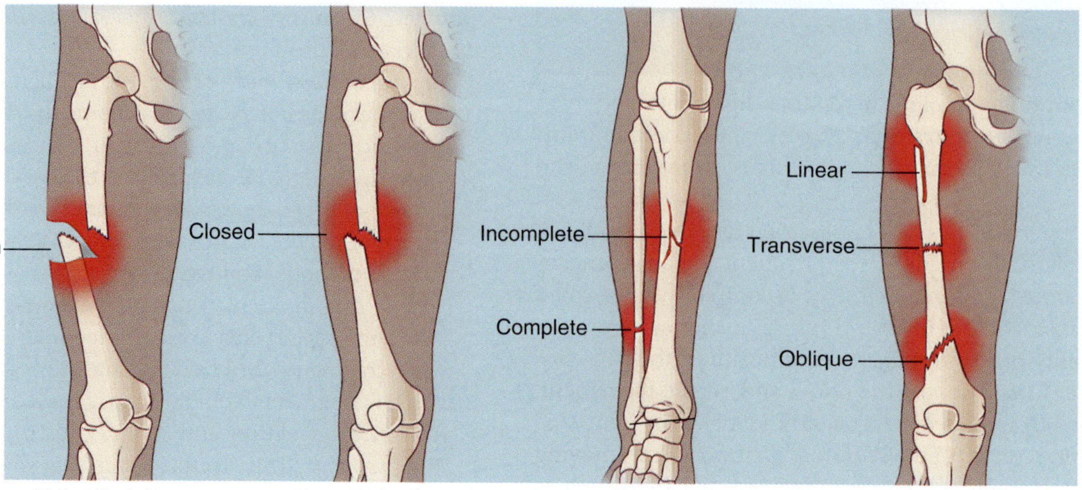

FIG. 29.4 Fracture types. (From Thibodeau G, Patton K, eds. *Anthony's Textbook of Anatomy and Physiology*. 17th ed. St Louis: Mosby; 2003.)

bone fragments into position; no incision is made in the skin

FIXATION After reduction, the bone fragments must be stabilized and protected from shifting out of alignment. This is called fixation. Fixation is the mechanical or structural method used to hold bone fragments in anatomical position during healing. Much of the orthopedic surgery focuses on various methods of fixation. The two main types of fixation are the following:

- ***Internal fixation (IF):*** Requires surgery to insert or implant a device that holds the bone fragments in place. Metal plates, rods, pins, and screws are examples of internal fixation devices.
- ***External fixation (EF):*** Is a means of stabilizing bone fragments from outside the body. A cast is an example of an external fixation device. Other devices, including external frames and cages, are also used. Pins or wires may be inserted through the skin and into the bone to support the external fixation device.

Surgical repair of fractures are specifically described according to the type of reduction and repair. The surgical options are as follows:

- ***Closed reduction and external fixation (CREF):*** The fracture is reduced manually or with a traction device. Except for casting and other types of noninvasive splinting, an external fixation device requires the insertion of wires, pins, or other devices to support the external structure. Some devices can be inserted transcutaneously (through the skin). A very small incision is made in the skin, and the pin or wire is drilled into the deeper tissue and bone.
- ***Open reduction external fixation (OREF):*** The fracture is exposed surgically; fixation is applied externally as described for CREF.
- ***Closed reduction internal fixation (CRIF):*** The fracture is reduced without surgical exposure; fixation is externally applied.
- ***Open reduction and internal fixation (ORIF):*** This procedure requires open surgery to expose the bone and reduce the fracture. Internal orthopedic implants are used to achieve fixation.

TIMING AND URGENCY OF SURGICAL TREATMENT

Surgical procedures for orthopedic injury are classified by the level of urgency:

1. ***Emergency***: Emergency procedures must be performed *as soon as possible* to prevent infection, neurological damage, amputation, and possible death. Injuries include open fractures, dislocation of a major joint, fracture with deep penetrating or macerated wounds, spinal injury, fracture or dislocation that impairs blood supply, and fractures with compartment syndrome (severe internal swelling and pressure that compromises blood supply to tissues).
2. ***Urgent:*** Urgent procedures are required within *24 to 72 hours* after the injury. These include debridement or repeat debridement of open fractures, limb stabilization in cases of multiple trauma, hip fracture, and unstable fracture and or dislocation.
3. ***Elective:*** Elective surgery after trauma can be delayed from *3 to 4 days* or, in some cases, several weeks. Injuries of this type include fracture or joint injury that has been stabilized but requires surgery to provide a better outcome.

PHYSIOLOGY OF BONE HEALING

Bone healing takes place through a complex physiological process that resembles soft tissue repair. However, the process is slower. Return of full function may take 6 months or longer, especially in weight-bearing bones. The three phases of bone healing are the inflammatory, reparative, and remodeling phases. These are described in Fig. 29.5. Bone healing, like all tissue healing, is affected by the health of the individual.

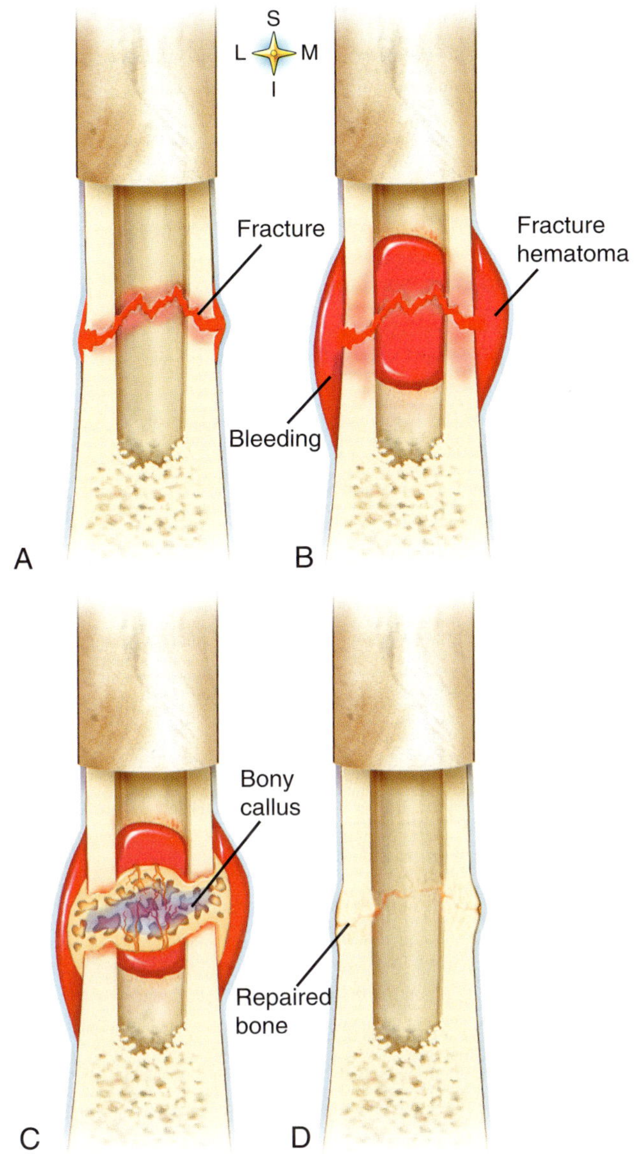

FIG. 29.5 Process of bone healing. (A) Fracture site. (B) Inflammatory phase. Blood accumulates at the fracture site, and fibroblasts create a network of granulation tissue. (C) Reparative phase with formation of callus (bone cells and cartilage), which fills the space between the bone fragments. (D) Remodeling phase in which the bone matrix is replaced by compact bone cells and excess callus is absorbed. (From Thibodeau G, Patton K, eds. *Anatomy and Physiology*. 6th ed. St Louis: Mosby; 2007.)

ORTHOPEDIC CASE PLANNING

Effective case planning for an orthopedic procedure requires specific knowledge, which can be complex:

1. What is the planned surgical approach (e.g., anterior, posterior, lateral)?
2. What position will be used, and what table is required (e.g., fracture table, hand table)?
3. What positioning accessories and table attachments are required?
4. What instrument sets are needed including joint arthroplasty? These should have been scheduled ahead of time.
5. Are implants required? What type and size? This information should have been checked at the time the surgery was scheduled.
6. Are power instruments needed? Which ones? Are the correct attachments available (e.g., drill bits, saw blades, burrs, reamers, motorized shaver)?
7. What imaging equipment is required (e.g., fluoroscopy, O-arm, C-arm)?
8. Will there be a need for cement, topical hemostatic agents, tissue glues, special irrigation solutions, bone grafting supplies, bone substitute?
9. If *arthroscopy* (minimally invasive surgery) is scheduled, are the instruments and components available? What type of joint irrigation and distension fluids are required? What size irrigation tubing is needed?
10. What specific energy devices are needed (e.g., ESU, laser, radiofrequency)?
11. What sutures and suture devices and anchors are required?

PATIENT POSITIONING

Positioning for orthopedic surgery varies according to the anatomical location requiring access and any physical limitations of the individual patient (Table 29.1). Positioning for multiple operative sites such as the primary operative site and an additional site for harvesting a graft should enable exposure to both without re-positioning during the procedure.

The standard operating table with accessories can be used for most orthopedic procedures. A fracture (distraction) table is preferred for hip procedures (Fig. 29.6). This table supports the operative leg while providing open access to the femur. An anti-skid device is used to prevent the patient from sliding on the table. The open design of the table also allows safe and rapid positioning of the C-arm fluoroscope. Features of the orthopedic table include the following:

- Jointed (articulated) components to hold the leg in traction
- Open design of the lower portion to allow positioning of the C-arm
- Translucent support surfaces

NOTE *Refer to Chapter 16 for additional photos and positioning details using the fracture table.*

Many standard operating tables can be converted to allow femoral or lower extremity surgery by removing the foot section and replacing it with adjustable leg suspension devices. The Fowler position can be created for shoulder surgery by adjusting the articulated sections of the table and replacing the normal headboard with an open-design head stabilizer. It is important to give adequate time to make these modifications before the patient arrives in surgery. Table accessories can be heavy; therefore adequate personnel should be available for assembly.

Standard positioning devices used in other surgical specialties are also used in orthopedic procedures with some additions. Sometimes is it necessary to suspend or apply traction to a limb. In these cases, a **distraction** system is used. This is a system that pulls the fractured limb along the long axis of the bone to maintain alignment and elevates it for operative exposure. Fig. 29.7 illustrates the use of a suspension system for the arm during arthroscopic surgery of the wrist.

TABLE 29.1 Positions for Surgical Exposure in Orthopedic Surgery

Anatomical Area	Position	Special Features*
Shoulder and humerus	Beach chair (modified Fowler position)	Head may be stabilized with a Mayfield headrest or similar attachment.
		Upper body is flexed 45 to 60 degrees.
		Operative shoulder is slightly over the table edge.
		Non-operative shoulder is padded at the scapula.
		Vertical footboard may be required.
Forearm and elbow	Supine with hand table extension	Operative arm is extended on a hand table at no greater than 90 degrees of abduction.
	Supine or semi-lateral with "over chest" extension	Operative arm is abducted and elevated over the thorax with the elbow flexed.
		Stabilizers are used to maintain the semi-lateral position (table supports, foam wedges, beanbag).
Wrist and hand	Supine with hand table extension	Operative arm is extended on a hand table at no greater than 90 degrees of abduction.
		Pad or "bump" is placed under the wrist for stabilization; a surgical hand holder may also be used.
	Supine with hand suspended in sterile distractor	Separate sterile accessories are required for the distractor.
Pelvis	Supine	Precautions are taken to protect nerves and blood vessels.
	Prone	Lower extremities may be held in traction.
		Precautions are taken for respiratory clearance.
		Lower table section may be removed.
Hip and femur	Supine using standard operating table	No special accessories are required.
	Supine using fracture table	Operative leg is in traction or distraction.
		Non-operative leg is positioned in a well leg holder to provide clearance for C-arm fluoroscopy or is extended in a boot as accessory.
		Perineal stop (post) requires substantial padding.
		Allows complete clearance above and below lower extremities.
	Lateral	Stabilizers are used to maintain the lateral position (table supports or peg board stabilizer).
Knee and lower leg	Supine	Operative knee is supported in variable degrees of flexion using an alvarado knee positioner**.
		Operative leg may be suspended over the table edge for intraoperative manipulation.
Ankle and foot	Supine	Supine or prone position is used with the operative leg in free position or elevated on padding.

*Normal precautions to protect nerves, vessels, and respiratory clearance are observed for all positions.
**https://www.youtube.com/watch?v=JRxnuXQvnFU

HEMOSTASIS

Pneumatic Tourniquet

The pneumatic tourniquet provides a bloodless operative site by blocking the flow of blood. The components of the tourniquet are the cuff, regulator, and tubing. An appropriately sized cuff must be selected according to the patient's size. The tourniquet cuff is placed proximal to the surgical site before the patient is prepped. Webril bandaging material is wrapped over the tourniquet site carefully to reduce any folds or pinching in the skin. The cuff then is secured over the padding. The regulator is adjusted for the correct pressure but not activated. After the surgical prep and draping, a latex bandage (Esmarch bandage) is used to exsanguinate the limb. This device is introduced in Chapter 13 during the discussion of an intravenous regional anesthesia (Bier block). The bandage is applied in a proximal direction, causing blood to flow out of the limb. The tourniquet is then inflated.

IMPORTANT TO KNOW *Application and monitoring of the pneumatic tourniquet is performed by qualified surgical personnel only, usually the anesthesia provider and registered perioperative nurse who have been trained in the use of the pneumatic tourniquet. Improper use of the pneumatic tourniquet, including failure to perform a preoperative patient risk assessment, inadequate or incorrect preparation of the*

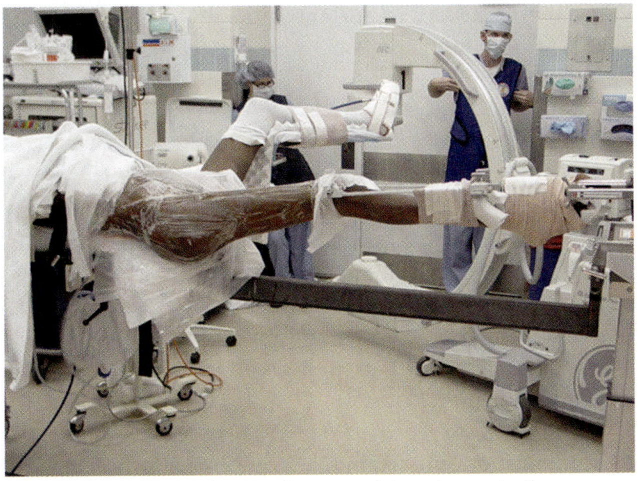

FIG. 29.6 Fracture table. The fracture table reduces the fracture using traction while providing excellent exposure to the surgical site. The table and accessories require detailed training to prevent injury. (From Browner B. *Skeletal Trauma: Basic Science Management and Reconstruction*. 6th ed. Philadelphia: Elsevier; 2020.)

limb with padding, incorrect pressure settings, tourniquet time, and improper placement of the tourniquet on the limb is associated with nerve, vessel damage, and circulatory emboli and may lead to severe patient injury.

Hemostatic Agents

During surgery, a moldable preparation called *bone putty* (Ostene) is pressed into bleeding areas to control oozing. Beeswax combinations (bone wax) traditionally have been used for this purpose, but these have been largely replaced with more effective and safer materials. Other hemostatic agents, such as topical thrombin, are used in peripheral tissues during microsurgery of the hand.

ORTHOPEDIC SUTURES

INFECTION CONTROL

Orthopedic surgery is performed with particular attention to the risk of airborne and droplet contamination. Postoperative infection after joint replacement (arthroplasty) can result in the destruction of the joint, with no recourse for further treatment. Osteomyelitis after any orthopedic surgery can result in long-term disability.

Orthopedic procedures are commonly performed in operating suites with laminar airflow or "super clean" air capability. A laminar airflow system moves air in linear patterns, entering at one wall and exiting at another. Super clean air is created with fresh air exchanges that occur at a rate of more than 300 changes per minute. Laminar airflow and filtering systems used to create super clean air significantly reduce the number of airborne organisms.

IMPORTANT TO KNOW *Refer to Chapter 9 for surgical guidelines necessary during the use of laminar airflow.*

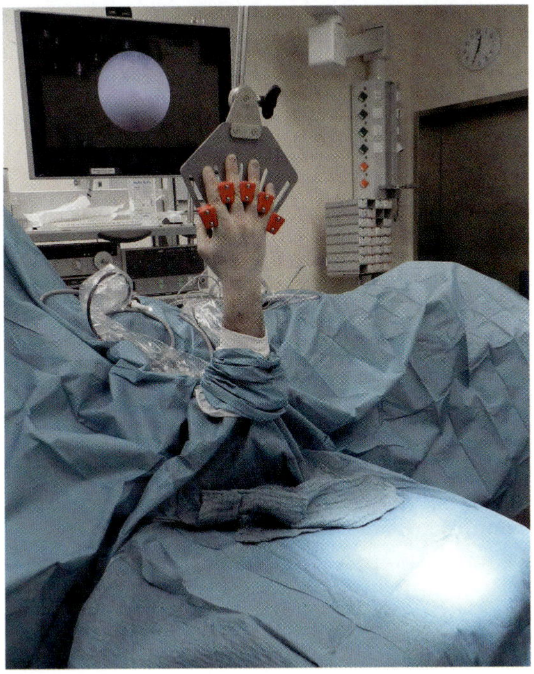

FIG. 29.7 Arm suspension (detraction) device. This device provides traction of the arm and wrist. (From Baur E. Arthroscopic-assisted partial wrist arthrodesis. *Hand Clin.* 2017;33[4]:735–753.)

Another method used to reduce the risk of surgical site infection during joint replacement procedures is the use of a sterile surgical helmet system (SSHS). The helmet system creates a closed air environment around the surgical team member and prevents its release at the surgical site. Refer to Chapter 9 for a discussion on the use of SSHS and regulatory requirements for infection control.

DRESSINGS

Surgical dressings are used to protect the incision from contamination and injury. The orthopedic dressing frequently provides support, as well as protection. Plaster of paris (POP) and resin casts are examples of external support. Many other types of soft or semi-rigid support systems are used on the limbs. Orthopedic appliances such as combined Velcro and hard plastic splints, foot boots, and other postoperative support systems are usually fitted to the patient by a trained physiotherapist shortly after the operative procedure. However, the surgical *dressing* is applied in the operating room at the close of surgery. The surgical technologist should become familiar with dressing combinations used by surgeons at her or his facility. Some of the most common materials are as follows:

- *Gauze "fluffs"* are made with Kerlix or plain gauze squares that are pulled apart from the center to make them fluffy rather than flat. These are used to provide cushioning in small areas such as between the fingers or toes.
- *Thick cotton wrap* is used to provide support to a limb.
- *Cotton wadding* is molded to the contours of the affected area for padding and support, commonly used in hand and foot dressings.

- *Ace-type stretchable fabric bandages* are used to wrap a limb, usually on top of cotton wrap, to provide extra support and mild **compression.**
- A *Coban-type dressing* is a common roller bandage with superior stretching and self-sticking capability. This type of material does not offer as much support as the Ace type of fabric bandage but conforms more easily to the shape of the limb.
- *Stockinet* is commonly used under splits and casts. It is a stretchable, tube-shaped fabric that is fitted over the limb and folded over at the top to form a smooth, padded edge.

CASTING

Casting is a method of external fixation in which a limb is immobilized by applying plaster or synthetic resin. Acute or open fractures are not treated with a cast because of the high risk of complications, such as compartment syndrome and infection. Surgical technologists who are required to learn casting techniques are best trained by orthopedic surgeons in their facility. The role is usually that of an orthopedic technician, who has completed training in the techniques required, including the medical aspects of the role.

Casts differ by location and medical objectives. A cylinder cast is a simple wrap along the length of the limb to immobilize a fracture. A spica cast is used in pediatrics to immobilize hip fractures or deformities. The spica cast covers the trunk and one or both limbs. Casting splints sometimes are applied longitudinally over the arm or wrist to provide rigid support after surgery. The splints do not cover the surgical incision or encase the limb.

Casting materials include plaster and polyurethane resin. Plaster is used less commonly than resins, which are stronger and resistant to breakdown by moisture. Resin casts are also more manageable for the patient because of their light weight. Casting materials are available in 2- to 6-inch (5- to 15-cm) widths.

Before a cast is applied, the limb is wrapped with padding. Two types of padding are commonly used. A stockinet is first applied to the limb. This is followed with felted (batted) cotton Webril. Rolled Webril is applied from the distal to proximal end of the limb. At least two layers of Webril are needed. Extra padding is needed for bony prominences.

Rolls of cast material are immersed in cold water before use. During application, the limb is lightly supported by the assistant. Plaster hardens within 30 minutes but requires 24 to 48 hours to set completely. Resin casts dry in 15 to 30 minutes. The single largest patient risk associated with casting is **compartment syndrome.** This is edema (swelling) of tissue within a closed compartment of the body (such as the cranium) or inside an external cast. When pressure on the tissues exceeds the space in the compartment, a tourniquet effect takes place, preventing the flow of blood to the tissues. In orthopedics this can lead to necrosis of the entire limb and eventual amputation if circulation is not restored. Safeguards to prevent this include using splints rather than cylindrical casting and judicious use of cotton Webril, which can be constricting when improperly applied. Naturally, postoperative swelling must be taken into account when a cast is applied directly after surgery. Careful monitoring of the limb and postoperative instructions to the patient are very important in the detection of compartment syndrome in the postoperative period.

ORTHOPEDIC POWER EQUIPMENT

Power equipment is used in orthopedic surgery to cut, drill, and remodel bone. The surgical technologist should be familiar with the safety and mechanical features of power equipment. The most important points are as follows:

- Safety features of the equipment and power source
- How to connect the power equipment to the power source
- Types of accessories and their function
- How to attach accessories
- Assisting the surgeon during the use of the equipment
- Cleaning and reprocessing the equipment

Power equipment used in surgery uses compressed nitrogen or compressed medical air (pneumatic energy). The force exerted through the hose and instrument is very powerful and can cause serious injury. A complete discussion of gas cylinder and regulator safety can be found in Chapter 7. The following are general safety precautions for the use of pneumatic instruments:

1. Inspect the instrument and hose before use. Make sure the instrument is properly assembled.
2. Place the instrument in the safe position (i.e., with the safety catch "on") before attaching accessories or the power hose.
3. Make sure that accessories are attached correctly, using guards where applicable. A drill or saw attachment that is incorrectly seated can be propelled from the handpiece with extreme force and may cause serious injury.
4. Inspect accessories before attaching them. Never attach a bent drill tip or other accessory because it can wobble and become disengaged from the handpiece. Never use a cracked or chipped cutting accessory.
5. Put the safety catch "on" before passing it to the surgeon.
6. Test the pressure before using the instrument. Ensure that the pressure does not exceed the level recommended by the manufacturer.
7. Always "bleed" the air hose before detaching the handpiece. With the compressed gas tank valve turned off, activate the instrument to remove any remaining gas from the hose.
8. Follow the manufacturer's guidelines for decontamination and sterilization.
9. To prevent tissue injury, continually irrigate the tip of the instrument while in use. Power instruments generate heat as a result of friction between the tissue and tip. The temperature can be high enough to destroy tissue in the vicinity of the tip.

DRILL

A drill is used whenever torque (rotational energy) is required.

An orthopedic drill is similar to a carpenter's drill. The drill has two main components, the head and handle. Attachments for the drill are inserted at the drill head. Many different kinds of attachments are available. The surgical technologist must be familiar with the specific functions and handling of surgical drills (Fig. 29.8).

Drill Attachments and Accessory Devices

The following are the most commonly used drill attachments and accessories:

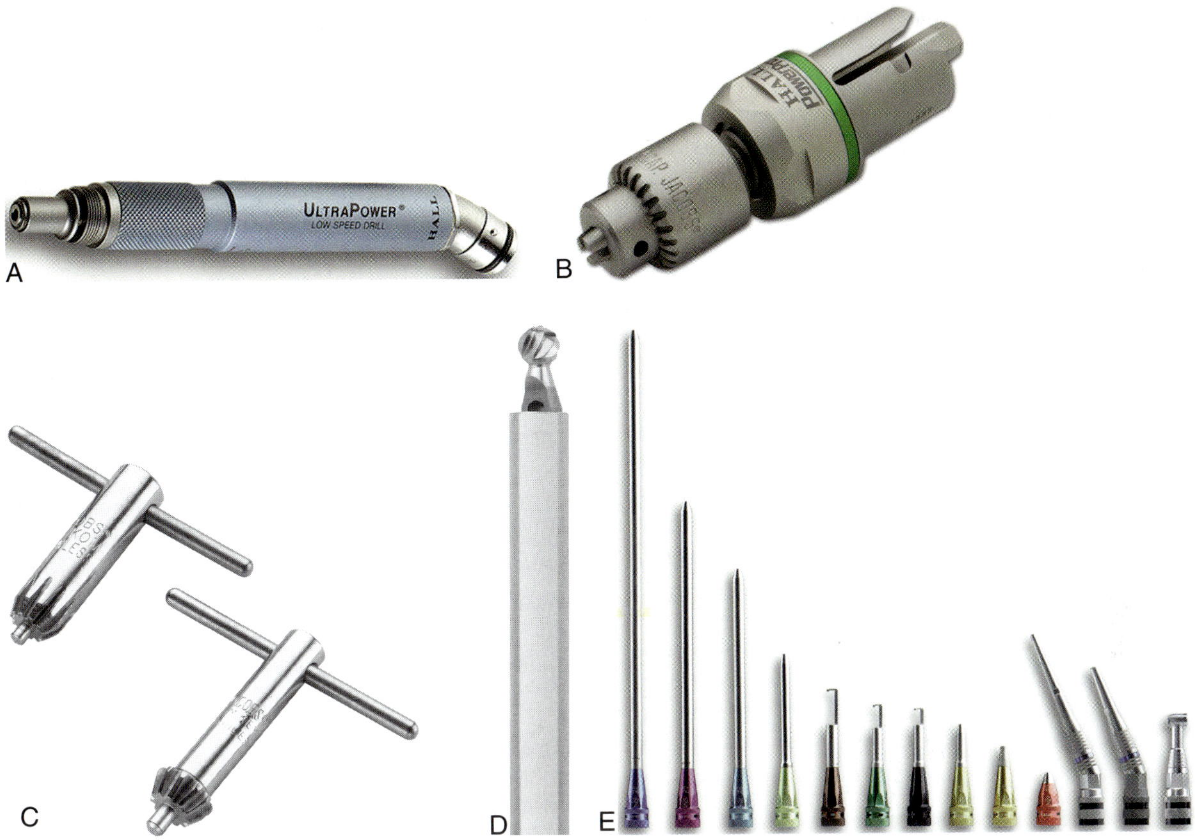

FIG. 29.8 Orthopedic drill and accessories. (A) Pneumatic low-speed drill. (B) Jacob chuck. (C) Jacob chuck keys. (D) Diamond burr. (E) Drill tips. (C, D, and E, Courtesy Zimmer, Warsaw, IN.)

- *Burr:* A round, conical, or tapered tip used for making narrow holes or for smoothing very small areas. Burrs are made from stainless steel, titanium, or diamond.
- *Chuck:* The chuck is attached to the drill head and receives attachments such as reamers, burrs, drill bits, or other rotational cutting tips, which fit into the central hole of the chuck. A chuck key is used to open and close the chuck's jaws, which are shaped like a cloverleaf. Most types of chucks are tightened and loosened manually.
- *Depth gauge:* A small calibrated rod used to measure the depth of a drilled or reamed hole in bone.
- *Drill bit:* A pin with wide cutting threads that is used to make a smooth-sided hole in the bone. Flutes (phalanges) in the drill bit allow cut bone to escape from the thread channels. Drill bits are supplied singly or in standard sizes in a metal rack.
- *Drill guide (drill sleeve):* An instrument inserted near or at the screw hole to correctly aim the angle of a screw, pin, nail, or wire as it enters the bone. The drill guide may be a single instrument or part of an assembly. Although many designs are available, the function is the same for all types.
- *Reamer:* A rod-shaped or chisel-pointed cutter used to **ream,** or clear, the medullary canal. A rounded or cup-shaped reamer is used for dishing surfaces such as the acetabulum. Reaming is used to prepare the bone for an implant. A reamer may be attached to a power drill or used manually.
- *Shaver:* A type of burr used mainly on cartilage for shaping and removing tissue such as the meniscus.
- *Tap:* An instrument similar to a screw that is used to cut threads in the bone. The tap corresponds to the diameter of the screw, its shape, and the pitch. Pre-tapping prevents bone from becoming embedded in threads of the screw as it is inserted. However, some screws are self-tapping.

SAWS

Power saws are used to cut bone in a precise direction and angle. The saw blades generally are fine toothed and vibrate or oscillate rapidly. This produces a smooth cut with little bone loss. Orthopedic saws are identified mainly by the movement of the blade. The name of the saw is also the category of the blade that the device uses:

- *Reciprocating saw:* The blade moves "in and out" of the handpiece along the axis of the handpiece.
- *Sagittal saw:* The blade is fixed at a right angle (90 degrees) to the handpiece and oscillates in the perpendicular axis.
- *Oscillating saw:* The blade is mounted along the same axis as the handle and moves "back and forth."

Each type of blade is available in many shapes, which are identified by the length of the blade shaft and type and the width of the blade edge.

ORTHOPEDIC INSTRUMENTS

Many orthopedic instruments have been designed for use with a specific system. These specialized instruments are classified by type (e.g., impactor) and system (e.g., Sirus tibial nail).

Generic instruments, which are not associated with a specific system, are classified by type and sometimes more specifically by anatomical region (e.g., hip, knee). Surgical technologists should be familiar with the standard instruments used in their facility. Commonly used orthopedic instruments are shown below (see Orthopedic Instruments.)

RETRACTORS AND BONE-HOLDING CLAMPS

Because bone does not yield to retraction the way soft tissue does, the surgeon most often retracts the surrounding tissue away from the bone or uses a bone-holding clamp or hook to grasp a bone for manipulation. Certain types of bone retractors (e.g., Blount and Bennett retractors) are designed to be used as levers against the bone, to shift its position. Soft tissue retractors are designed for a specific anatomical location, such as the shoulder, and some general surgery retractors (e.g., Army-Navy and Weitlaner retractors) are also used in orthopedic surgery.

RONGEURS AND BONE CUTTERS

Rongeurs and bone cutters are used for trimming and modeling bone and cartilage. Double-action instruments have two hinges for increased force at the tips (from increased leverage). Cutting edges may be cupped, anvil tip, or double bladed.

CHISELS, OSTEOTOMES, GOUGES, AND CURETTES

Chisels, gouges, and osteotomes are used with a mallet to model bone or to remove bone for a graft. Each has a specific type of cutting tip. Instruments in this group usually are supplied in graduated sizes and secured in a metal rack.

- *Chisel:* Beveled (sloped) on one side only
- *Osteotome:* Beveled on both sides
- *Gouge:* V- or U-shaped chisel

A curette is used without a mallet. It has a cup-shaped cutting edge and is used for scooping out bone and other dense tissue.

ELEVATORS AND RASPS

A periosteal elevator (or simply, elevator) is used in nearly every open orthopedic procedure. Although it has many uses, its main function is to remove the periosteum (the tough outer membrane of the bone) from the bone surface. This is necessary to cut or saw through bone tissue because the periosteum tends to shred or tear on contact with a rongeur or cutting instruments, preventing a clean cut. Many sizes and types of elevators are available. The most common are the smooth-tip joker elevator and the larger, square-tip key elevator. A bone rasp is used to model and shape bone or to roughen the bone surface.

MEASURING DEVICES

Measuring devices commonly used in orthopedic procedures include the protractor, caliper, screw depth gauge, and ordinary ruler. Computerized mapping has replaced some but not all of the measuring techniques previously used in joint replacement surgery.

ORTHOPEDIC INSTRUMENTS

Wire Cutter 5½″

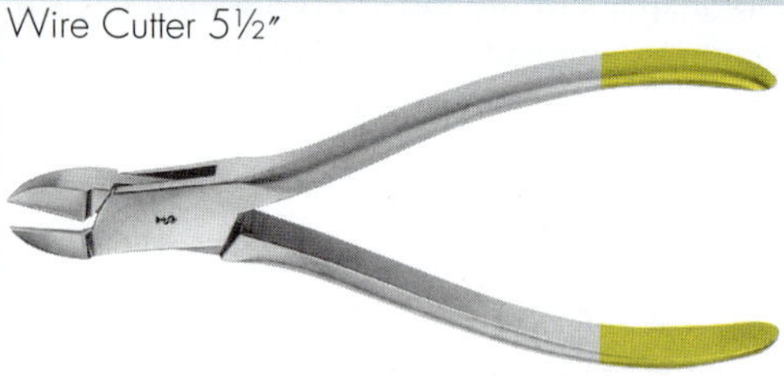

Photo courtesy Aesculap, Inc., Center Valley, PA.

Straight Dissecting Scissors 5″

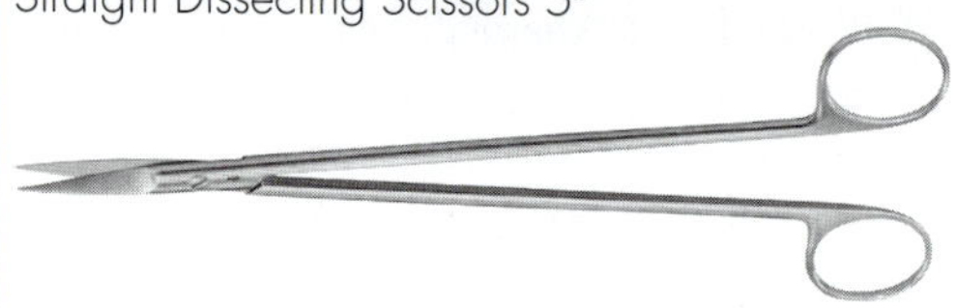

Photo courtesy Aesculap, Inc., Center Valley, PA.

Bone Curette 7″

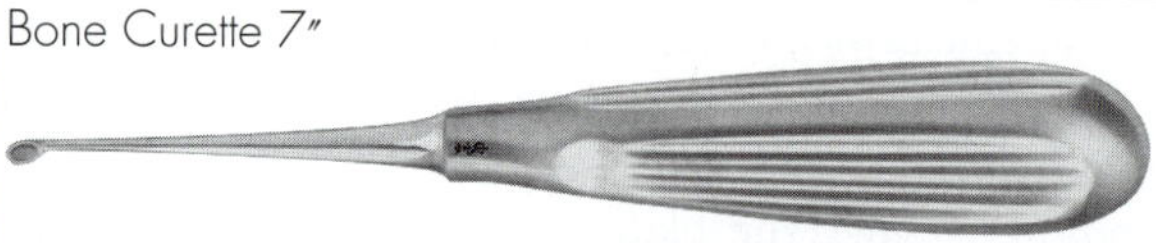

Photo courtesy Aesculap, Inc., Center Valley, PA.

Cobb Elevator 11″

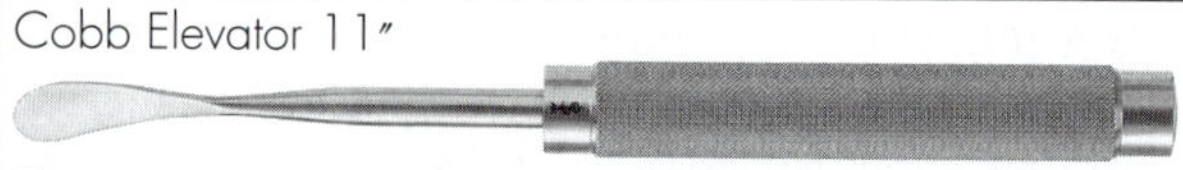

Photo courtesy Aesculap, Inc., Center Valley, PA.

Gouge 8″

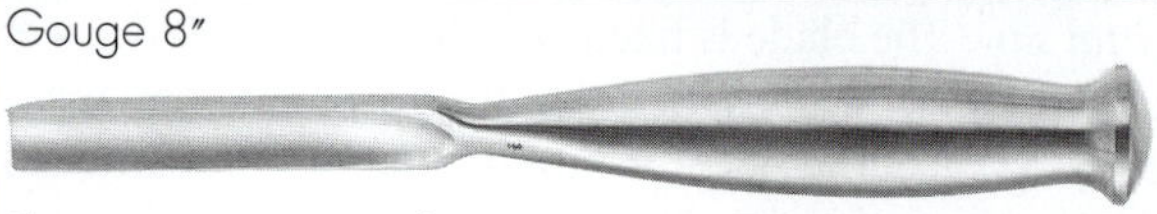

Photo courtesy Aesculap, Inc., Center Valley, PA.

Lambotte Osteotome 9¾″

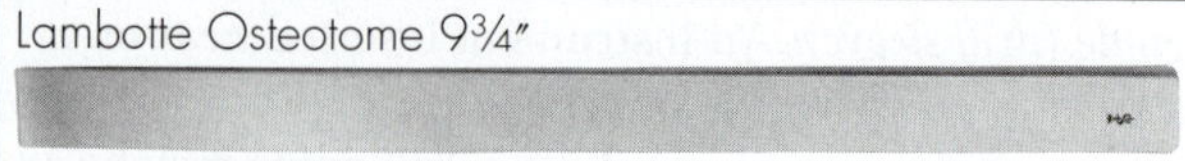

Photo courtesy Aesculap, Inc., Center Valley, PA.

Mallet 7½″

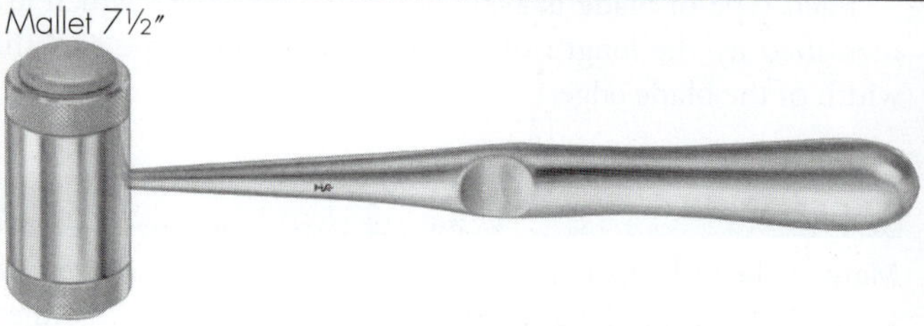

Photo courtesy Aesculap, Inc., Center Valley, PA.

Putti Bone File 10¾″

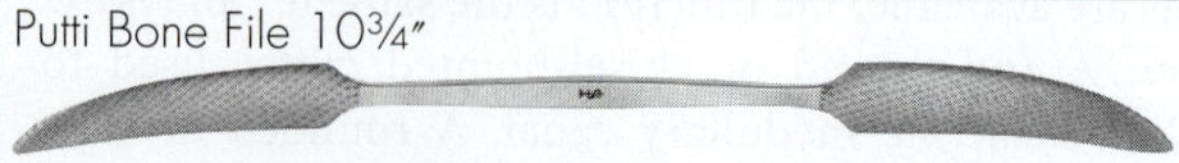

Photo courtesy Aesculap, Inc., Center Valley, PA.

Leksell Double-Action Rongeur 9¾″

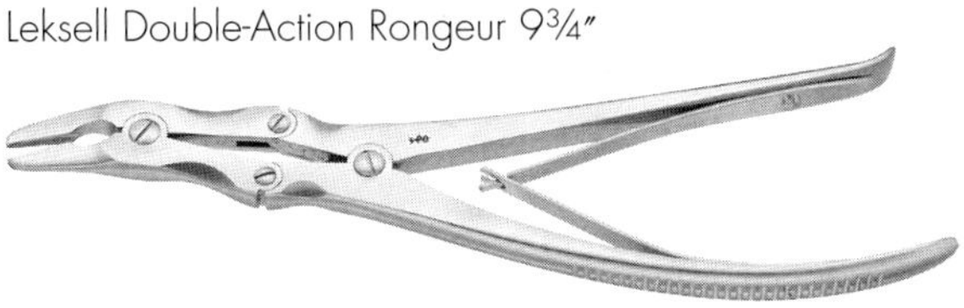

Photo courtesy Aesculap, Inc., Center Valley, PA.

Martin Cartilage Clamp 8″

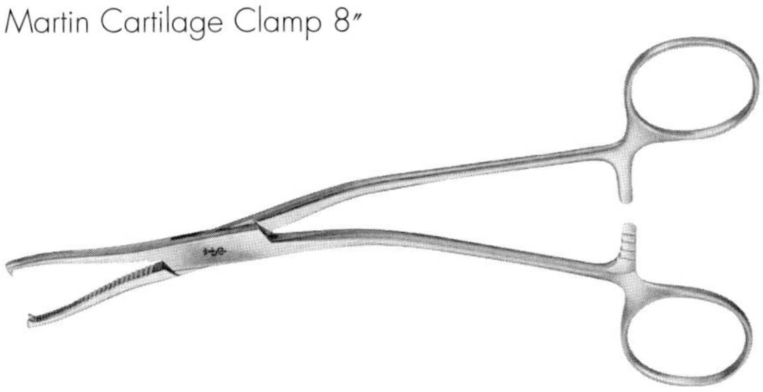

Photo courtesy Aesculap, Inc., Center Valley, PA.

Smilli Meniscus Knife 6¾″

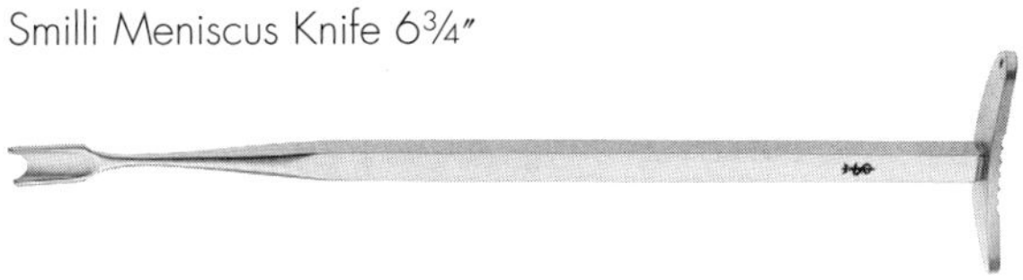

Photo courtesy Aesculap, Inc., Center Valley, PA.

Volkman Retractor

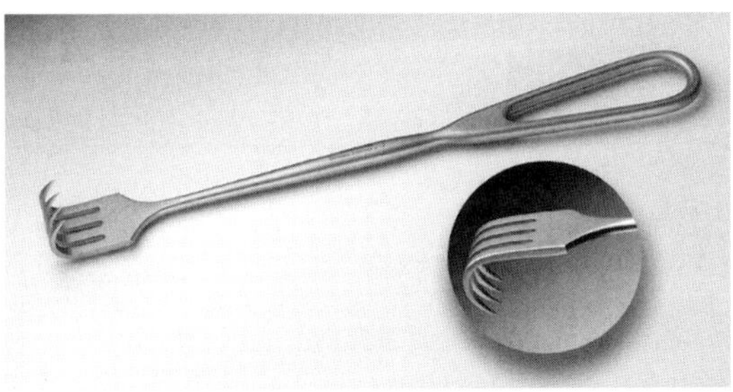

From Nemitz. *Surgical Instrumentation: An Interactive Approach.* 3rd ed. St. Louis: Elsevier; 2019.

Lewin Bone Clamp

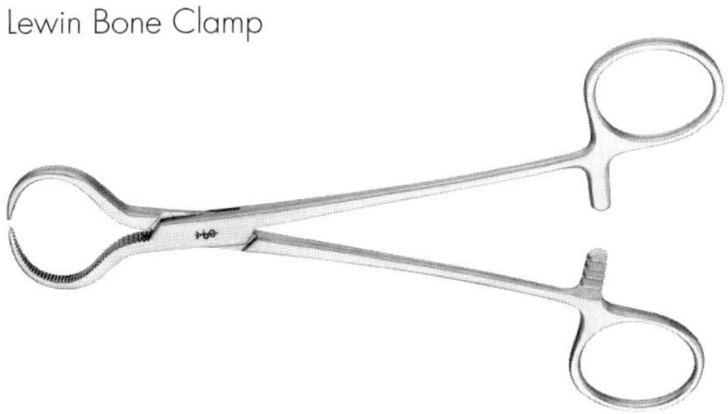

Photo courtesy Aesculap, Inc., Center Valley, PA.

Pelvic Reduction Forceps 9{⅞}″

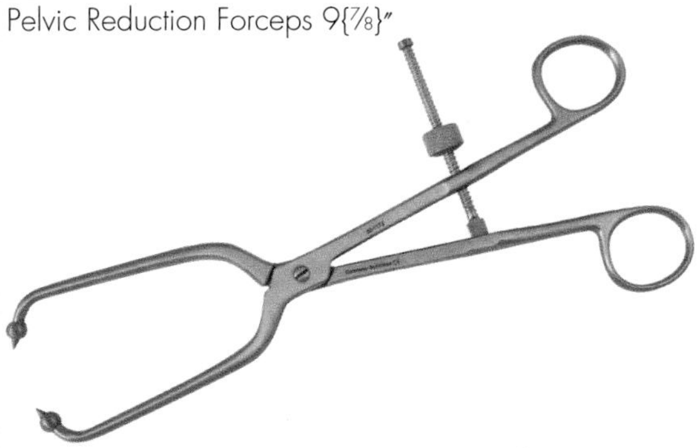

Photo courtesy Aesculap, Inc., Center Valley, PA.

Liston Single Action Bone Cutting Forceps

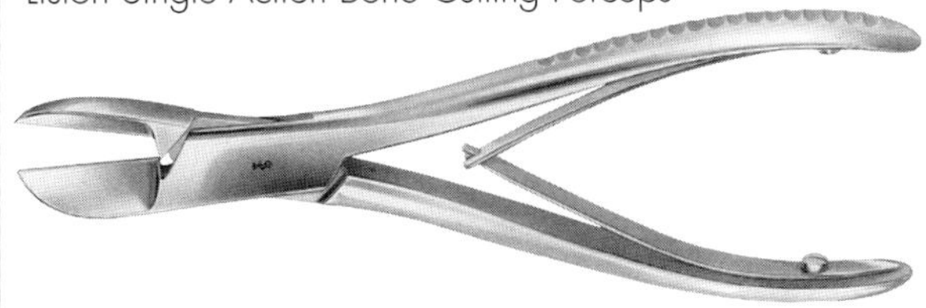

Photo courtesy Aesculap, Inc., Center Valley, PA.

Key Periosteal Elevator 7″

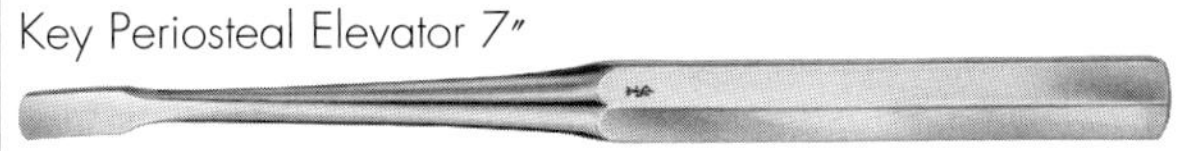

Photo courtesy Aesculap, Inc., Center Valley, PA.

Bolt and Nail Cutter 18½″

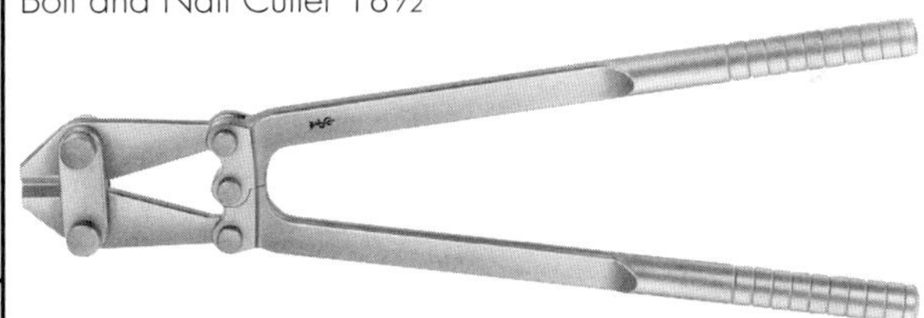

Photo courtesy Aesculap, Inc., Center Valley, PA.

Lowmann Bone Clamp

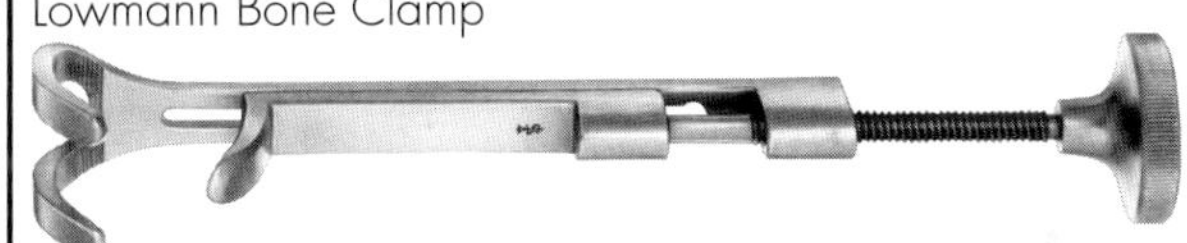

Photo courtesy Aesculap, Inc., Center Valley, PA.

Langenbeck Bone Holding Forceps

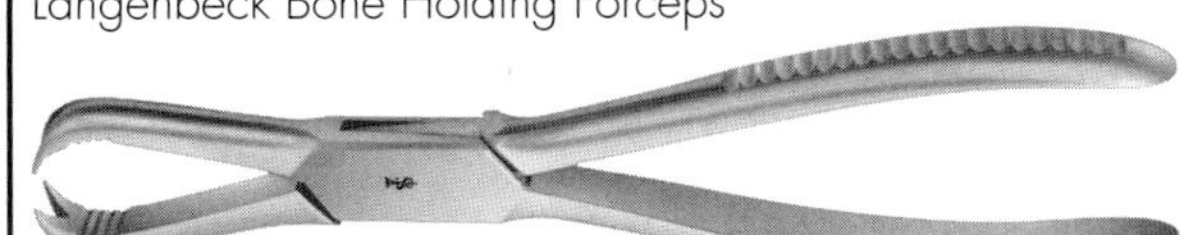

Photo courtesy Aesculap, Inc., Center Valley, PA.

Doane Knee Retractor

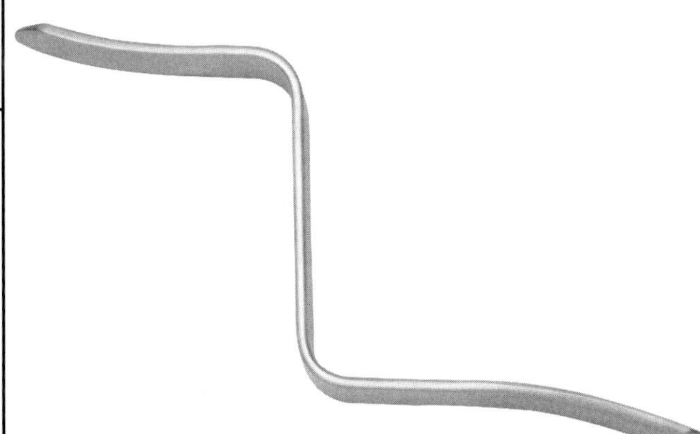

Photo courtesy Aesculap, Inc., Center Valley, PA.

Blount Knee Retractor 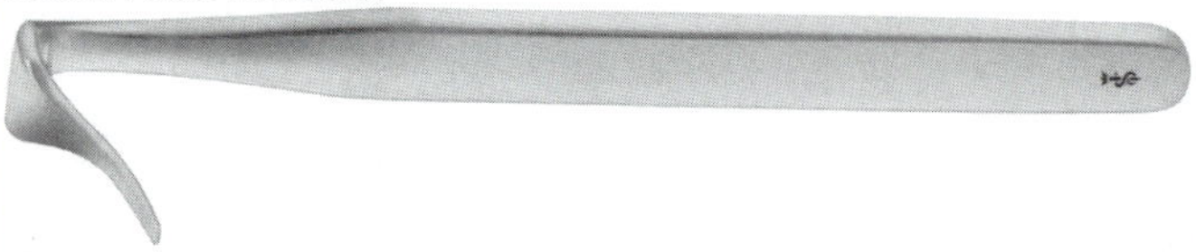 Photo courtesy Aesculap, Inc., Center Valley, PA.	Hibbs spinal retractor 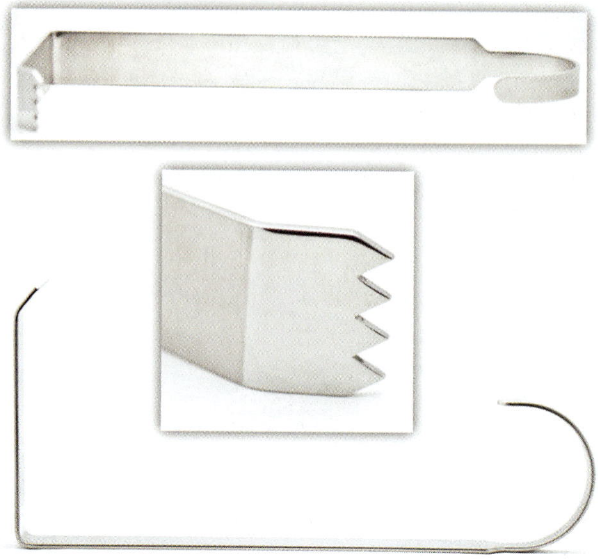 Photo courtesy Aesculap, Inc., Center Valley, PA.
Bennett Retractor 9¼″ 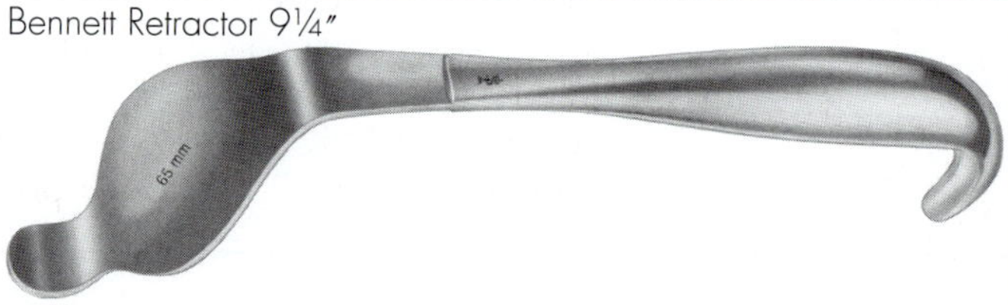 Photo courtesy Aesculap, Inc., Center Valley, PA.	

ORTHOPEDIC IMPLANTS

Orthopedic implants or *hardware* are the devices used to attach or fix bone and other connective tissue (joint replacement implants are discussed separately). Many hundreds of different implants are available for orthopedic repair. However, a relatively simple classification system (i.e., implant type and use) is used for them. The manufacture and use of orthopedic hardware are regulated to protect the public. The U.S. Food and Drug Administration (FDA) requires strict documentation and tracking of implant devices.

Surgical facilities maintain an inventory or supply of sterile implants for surgical cases routinely performed in that facility. A database of all implants is maintained for regulatory purposes and restocking. A surgical technologist (team leader or orthopedic specialist) may be designated to maintain implant inventories and implement the documentation and supply system.

IMPLANT MATERIALS

Metals are commonly used in the manufacture of implants because metal can withstand the load required of the bone. Current research is aimed at creating new metal **alloys** (made from a mixture of different metals) that are highly biocompatible and inert. Stainless steel remains the alloy most commonly used for implants. However, titanium is also used because of its light weight and strength.

Bioactive Implants

Materials that are bioactive cause a biological response in tissue at the interface with the implant. Bioactive coatings and substances used in the manufacturing of orthopedic implants can result in improved bone support during healing. Specific coatings can also provide an anti-infective environment during healing. *Bioresistance* is another desirable quality of implant material. Particular materials that make up an implant may make it resistant to infectious agents. **Biocompatibility** means that the implant is compatible with the tissue and does not cause tissue reaction. This includes a possible allergic reaction or other immune response. A material that is *inert* does not react with other nonorganic or biological substances. This quality is also critical because metals, in particular, can interact at the molecular level, creating ions that are harmful to the body. Reactions can also lead to corrosion or oxidation of the implant, leading to weakness or breakdown. For these reasons, it is important for the surgeon to make sure that devices composed of different metals are not implanted near each other in the body.

DOCUMENTATION

All implants stored in the operating room must be documented on a database for tracking, retrieving, and stock replacement. When an implant is used, specific information about the implant is recorded in the patient's record. This includes but is not limited to the following:

- Date and name of the facility
- Type of implant and size (where applicable)
- Location of implant in the body
- Name of the surgeon
- Manufacturer's identification number, including the batch, lot, and serial numbers

Implant Log

The facility keeps information about each implant in a permanent log. This can be an electronic database or a written log. The FDA requires the following information:

- Name and address of the surgical facility
- Manufacturer's identification information
- Implant serial number, lot number, batch number, and any other identifying information (e.g., size, type)
- Patient's identification details
- Surgeon's identification details
- Implant expiration date (if applicable)

IMPLANT STERILIZATION

Many implants, including joint components, are supplied by the manufacturer individually in sterile packages. Plates, screws, pins, and rods are not wrapped individually but supplied in sterile sets, from which the appropriate size is selected during surgery. Joint and other specialty implants that are sterilized and packaged by the manufacturer are opened onto the sterile field only after the exact size and type have been determined. This reduces environmental exposure during surgery, as well as the need for an excessive implant inventory.

Implants must not be processed using immediate-use steam sterilization (IUSS) except in extreme emergency. The Association for the Advancement of Medical Instrumentation (AAMI) is an accredited agency for setting safety standards in health care. In its most recent update on the sterilization of implants, it recommends that if an emergency situation makes IUSS unavoidable, a biological monitoring device must be used, along with a chemical indicator. The implant must not be used until the biological indicator provides a negative result.

The patient's permanent operative record must reflect the details of the sterilization process and the outcome of the biological and chemical indicators. The sterilizer log (computer printout), which includes all sterilization parameters achieved when the implant was flashed, must be included in the patient's chart. The AAMI provides yearly updates of accepted sterilization practices through its *Standards Registry*. Standard *ST79* provides current practices regarding steam sterilization for implants and should be consulted yearly for updated information.

SCREWS

The orthopedic screw is among the most commonly used orthopedic implants. Screws are supplied in different types, sizes, shapes, and designs. They are made of titanium, stainless steel, or bioabsorbable material. The function of a screw is to fix an orthopedic implant such as a plate to a bone or fix bone to bone, or bone fragments or bone to soft connective tissue.

The parts of a screw are as follows:

- *Head:* The flat or conical part of the screw. The recess of the screw may be hexagonal, a straight slot, or *cruciform* (cross-shaped). This is important to selecting the correct screwdriver.
- *Shaft:* The long section of the screw. The outside of the threads (thread diameter) determines the screw's numerical diameter. This measurement is important because the ST selects the correct drill bit size to match the screw size (non–self-tapping screws only) to be used.
- *Threads:* The spiral-shaped ridges along the screw shaft. The threads on most screws are asymmetrical (i.e., flat on the top and rounded underneath). This provides a wide surface for placing the screw into the bone. Some screws are only partially threaded.
- *Tip:* The tip of the screw may be blunt, corkscrew, or trocar shaped. The shape determines whether it requires a predrilled hole.

Types of Screws

When assisting in orthopedic procedures requiring the use of screws, the surgical technologist must be able to differentiate among the different types and understand the nomenclature used to describe the size required by the surgeon. Size is measured in millimeters (mm) diameter and length.

Screws are classified according to the type and function:

- *Cancellous:* Used on cancellous bone
- *Cortical:* Small diameter and decreased pitch; used in cortical bone to fix a plate. Fig. 29.9A shows a comparison of the cancellous and cortical screw, which the surgical technologist must be able to differentiate. Fig. 29.9B illustrates the basic design of orthopedic screws
- *Lag:* Exerts compression on bone fragments, either directly or with a plate (Fig. 29.10)
- *Locking:* Used with a special plate that has threaded holes to secure the screw head to the plate
- *Cannulated:* A screw with a hollow core. The hollow center allows the screw to be fitted over a prepositioned guidewire to ensure precise placement (Fig. 29.11)
- *Fixation*: Used to exert pressure between the bone and the plate or washer
- Self-tapping: Has flutes at the tip that cut a passage for the threads as the screw is inserted
- *Non–self-tapping:* Requires a pre-drilled pilot hole
- *Compression:* The compression screw was originally designed to be used with a plate for repair of fracture of the femoral neck

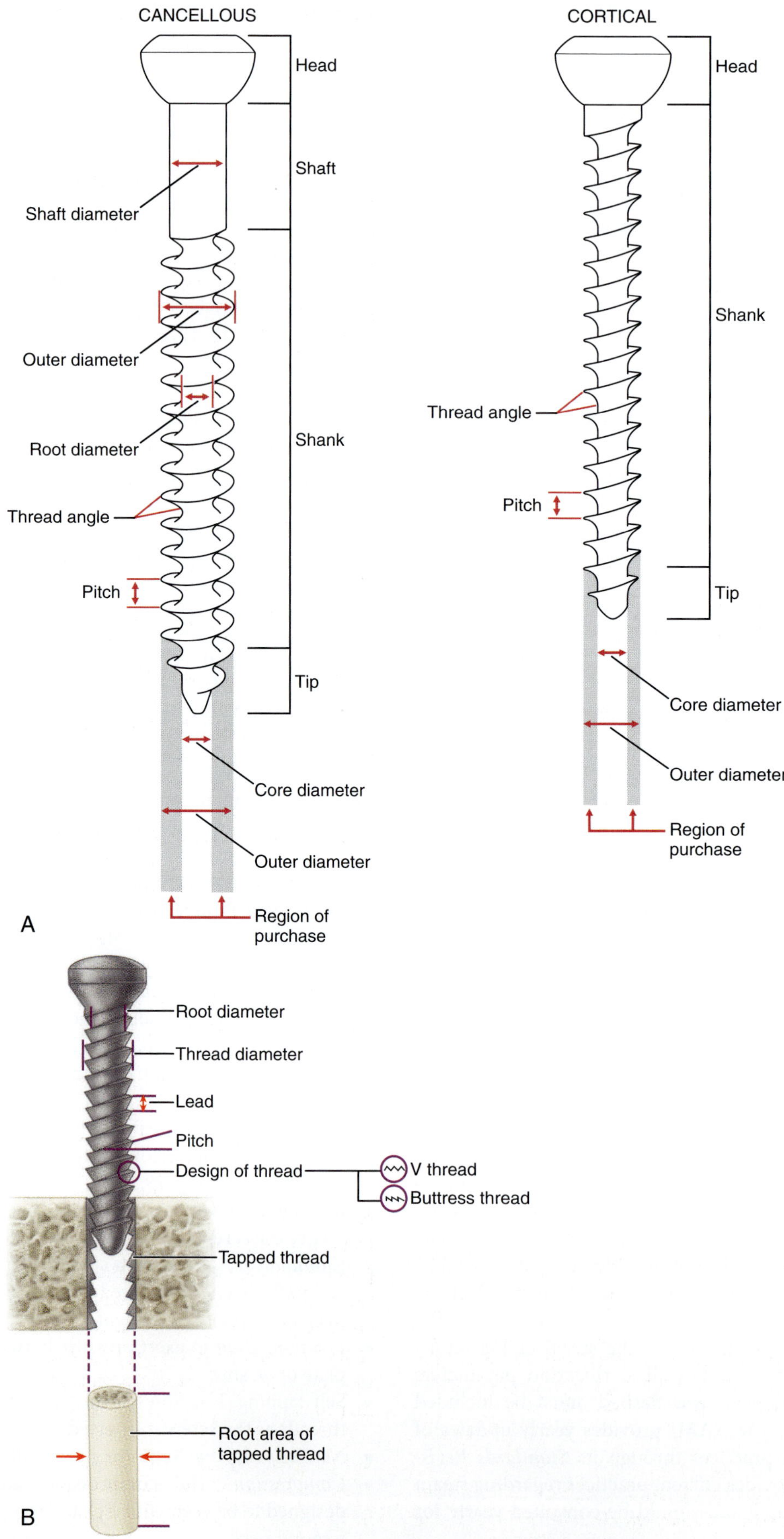

FIG. 29.9 (A) Comparison of cortical and cancellous screws. (B) Design of orthopedic screws. (A, From Browner B. *Skeletal Trauma: Basic Science Management and Reconstruction*. 6th ed. Philadelphia: Elsevier; 2020. B, From Canale T, Beaty J, Azar F. *Campbell's Core Orthopedic Procedures*. Philadelphia: Elsevier; 2016.)

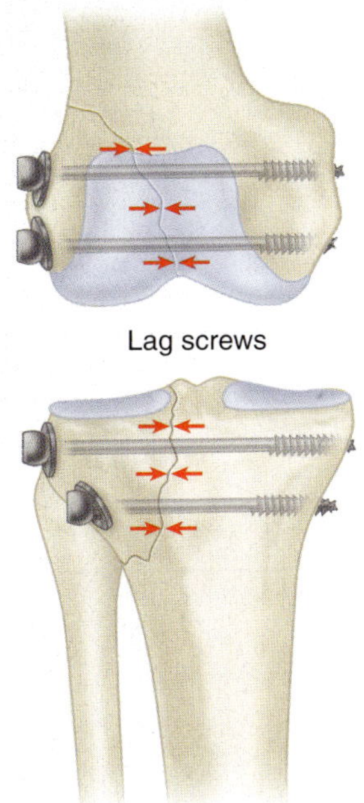

FIG. 29.10 Lag screw, may be used with or without a washer. This type of screw provides compression of the bone fragments by drawing the far one into the near one. Note that the near end is smooth. (From Canale T, Beaty J, Azar F. *Campbell's Core Orthopedic Procedures*. Philadelphia: Elsevier; 2016.)

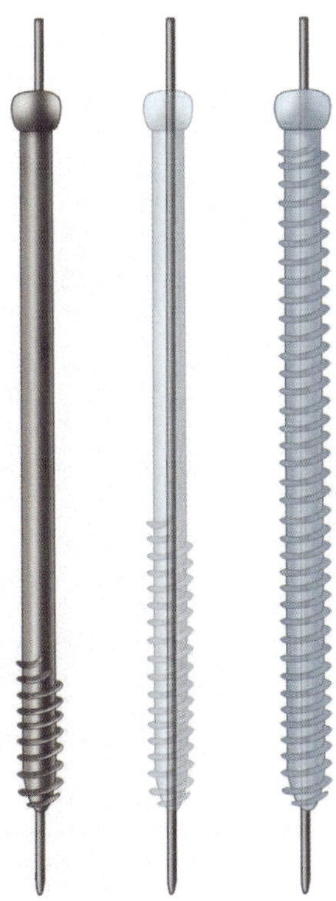

FIG. 29.11 Cannulated screw. This screw is hollow so that it can be fitted over a guide wire for proper placement. (From Canale T, Beaty J, Azar F. *Campbell's Core Orthopedic Procedures*. Philadelphia: Elsevier; 2016.)

Placement of Screws

Unless a screw is *self-tapping*, it requires the use of a power drill and **tap,** also called a *drill bit*, which creates a pilot hole to accommodate the screw. The depth of the hole is measured using a *depth gauge*. A *drill guide* attaches to the bone and maintains the correct angle of the tap during drilling. The screw is seated using a handheld screwdriver. If the screw is cannulated, it is drilled over a pre-placed guidewire. Fig. 29.12 illustrates the instruments required for screw placement.

PLATES

Plates provide stability and support during healing. Plates are made of titanium or stainless steel and are available in a matte or polished finish. Plates are fixed to the bone using screws. Plates can be straight, contoured, or beveled to fit smoothly over bone and joint surfaces. The screw holes can be smooth sided, threaded, oblique, or straight.

Functions of various plating systems are as follows:

- Protect and neutralize the fracture
- Span the fracture
- Provide compression
- Reduce the fracture (bring the bone fragments together)
- Buttress (support) structures or fragments

Reconstruction Plate

A reconstruction plate may be bent to fit the contours of the bone surface. First, an aluminum template is fitted over the bone to duplicate its contour. The template is then taken to the back table, and the implant plate is shaped with a plate press or plate benders. More delicate reconstruction plates may be shaped and cut to size by hand. This type of plate is used commonly in pelvic fractures and in cranial and facial trauma (Fig. 29.13).

Locking Plate

A locking plate has threaded screw holes that lock the screws into the plate. This prevents the screws from rocking, which loosens them or causes them to back out.

Dynamic Compression Plate

A dynamic compression plate has screw holes that are inclined (sloped) and offset. This design feature provides reduction and compression of the fragments. Anchor screws are inserted into one fragment. As the screws are tightened, the plate slides along the bone, drawing the two bone fragments together (Fig. 29.14). The term *dynamic* refers to the compression of bone fragments produced by the natural load exerted on the bones by the body itself.

A low-contact dynamic compression plate is designed to reduce contact between the plate and the bone. The plate sits just above the surface of the bone, secured by screws. This prevents direct pressure on the periosteal vascular supply and may enhance healing. Another type of plate is used to reduce contact with the periosteum is the wave plate, which is contoured to intermittently curve away from the bone. This type of plate is used in fractures that have failed to heal by other methods.

Tension Band Plate

A tension band plate provides a mechanical advantage in the fixation of the long bones. Asymmetrical loading occurs in all long bones; that is, more weight is carried on the concave side of the long axis of the bone. A partial fracture on the convex side tends to widen under load. The tension band plate is

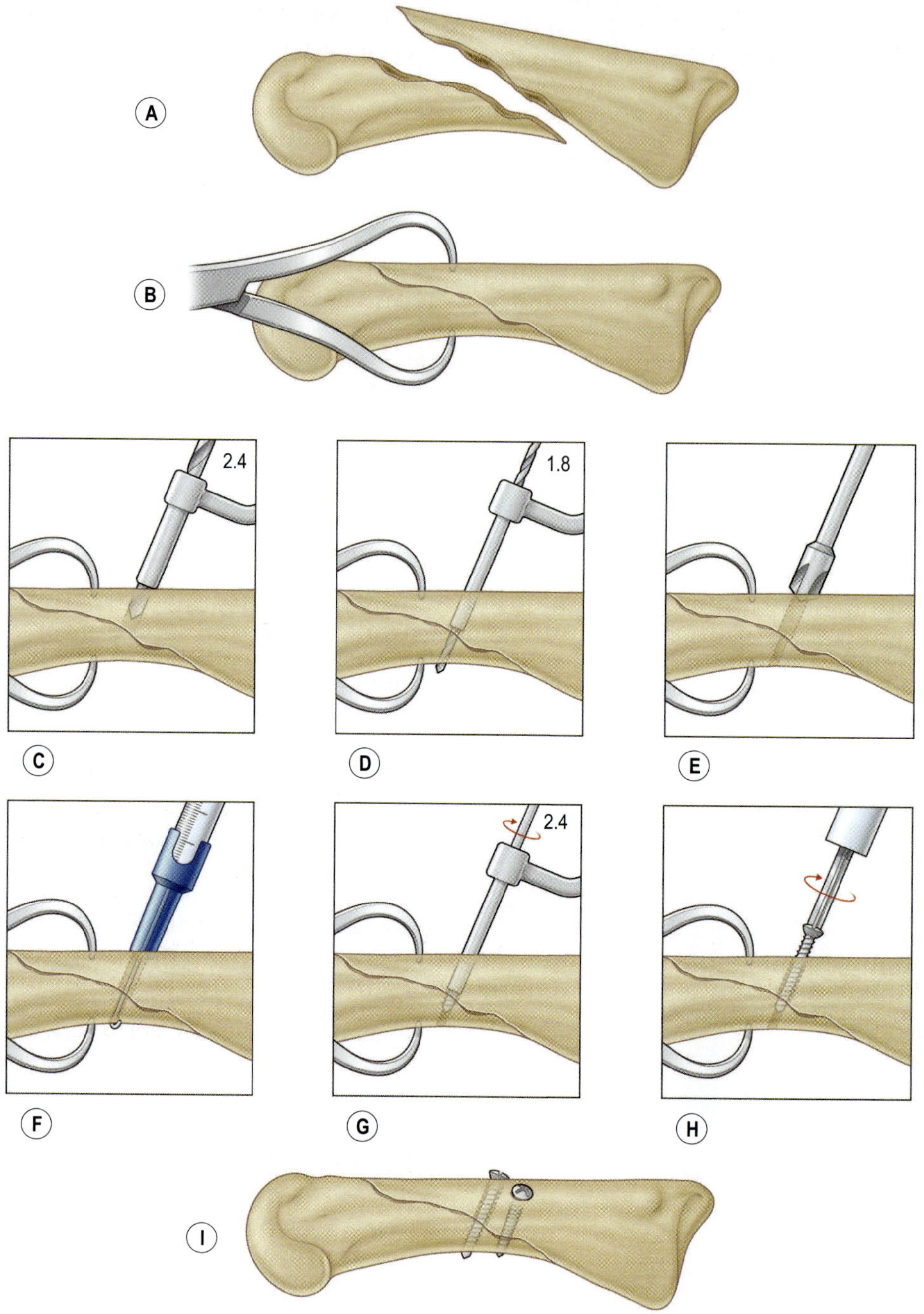

FIG. 29.12 Instruments used to set a screw. This illustration shows lag screw insertion. The instruments are the same for most types of orthopedic screws. (A and B) A bone clamp is used to approximate the bone fragments. (C and D) Sequential drill bits are used with the drill guide to form the pilot holes for the screws. (E) A countersink enables the screw head to be seated into bone. (F) A depth gauge is inserted to determine the length of the hole needed for the screw. (G) A tap sleeve protects the adjacent soft tissues (for non–self-tapping screws). (H) A 2.4-mm screw is inserted. (I) A second screw is set in a different plane. (From Chang J. *Plastic Surgery: Hand and Upper Extremity*. vol 6. 4th ed. Elsevier; 2018.)

placed on the convex or gap side of the fracture to counteract the load and prevent the gap from widening (Fig. 29.15).

Buttress Plate

A buttress is a supporting structure that prevents an adjoining object or structure from collapsing. An example of common buttressing is a lean-to shed. The structure supporting the roof at its highest point is a buttress. The supporting structure is "pushing" on the roof to support it at an angle. In orthopedics, a buttress plate is used to give added strength or to "prop" one structure against another.

Condylar Plate

A condylar plate is often used in conjunction with compression screws for the fixation of fractures of the *condyle* (the rounded end of a long bone). The end of the plate is contoured to fit over the surface of a condyle, and compression lag screws are inserted through the fracture fragments (Fig. 29.16).

Intertrochanteric Nail and Plate Combination

Fractures that occur across the trochanter of the hip often require stabilization from a side plate, which is implanted at the proximal end of the femur. An older prototype of this device is the Jewett nail. Although the Jewett nail is still occasionally used, it has been largely replaced by more efficient systems, such as the dynamic hip screw and the dynamic compression–sliding hip screw. This implant has two primary pieces: a lag screw, which is inserted into the trochanter, and a locking plate, which is inserted over the screw and extends along the proximal femur (Fig. 29.17). During healing, the plate-nail combination shifts the load from the trochanter (normal loading) to the long axis of the femur, removing excess pressure from the trochanter.

NOTE *Refer to Repair of Intertrochanteric Fracture (Figure 29.34) later in this chapter.*

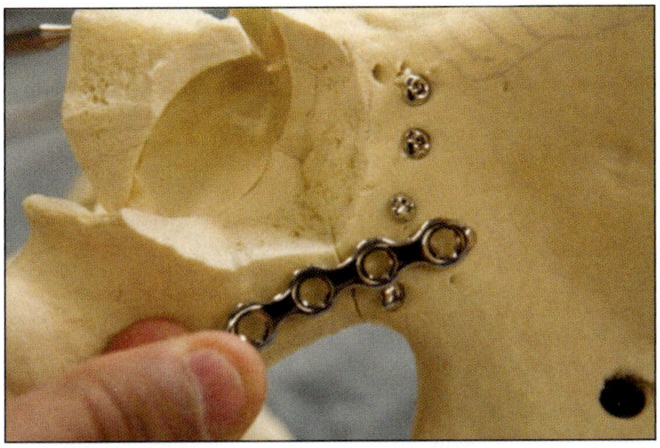

FIG. 29.13 Reconstruction plate. This type of plate is commonly used in the reconstruction of contoured bones, where the load is not extreme. (From Schemitsch E, McKee M, eds. *Operative Techniques: Orthopedic Trauma Surgery*. Philadelphia: Saunders; 2010.)

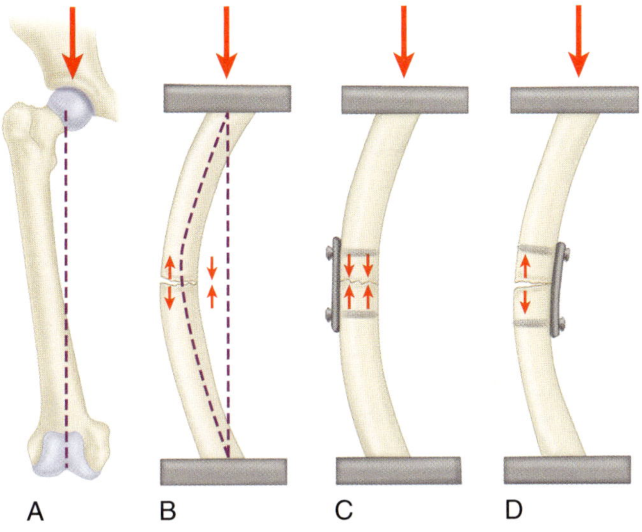

FIG. 29.15 Principles of tension band plate. (A and B) Long bones may be subject to peripheral loading. (C) A plate is applied to the A plate is fixed to the convex side of the bone to counteract tension and provide internal fixation. (D) The plate fixed to the concave side does not provide traction and induces stress in the plate, which results in fracture. (From Canale T, Beaty J, Azar F. *Campbell's Core Orthopedic Procedures*. Philadelphia: Elsevier; 2016.)

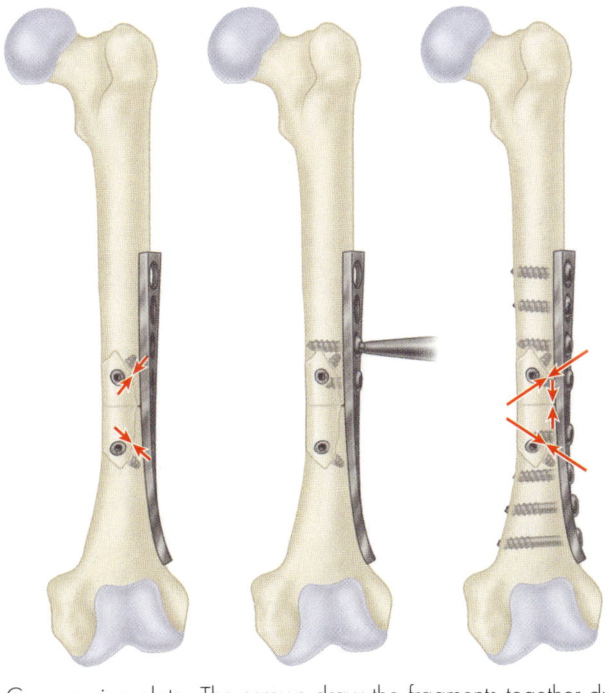

FIG. 29.14 Compression plate. The screws draw the fragments together during fixation. (From Canale S, Beaty J, eds. *Campbell's Operative Orthopaedics*. 12th ed. Philadelphia: Mosby; 2013.)

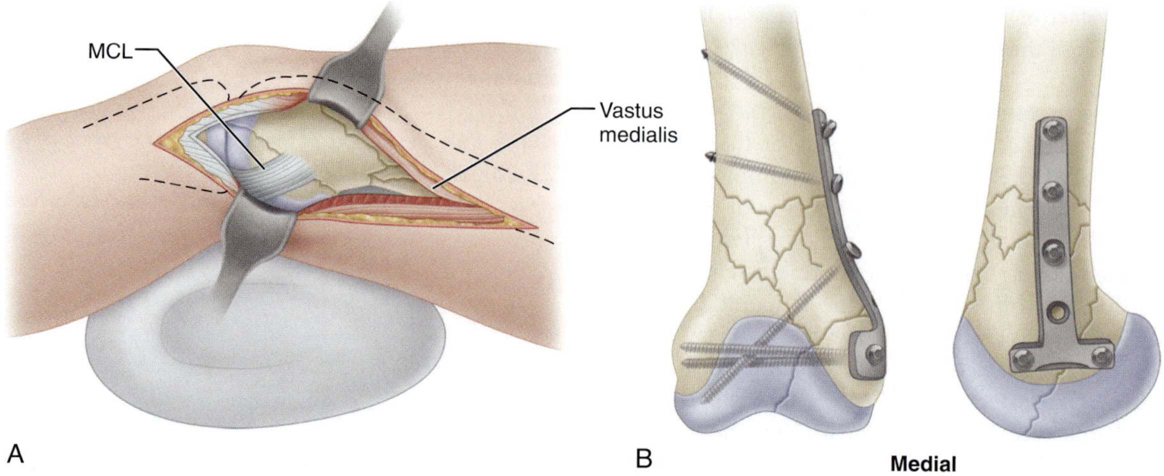

FIG. 29.16 Condylar plate. (A) Exposure of the condyle. (B) This plate fits over the contours of a condyle and is secured with compression screws (two views shown). (From Canale T, Beaty J, Azar F. *Campbell's Core Orthopedic Procedures*. Philadelphia: Elsevier; 2016.)

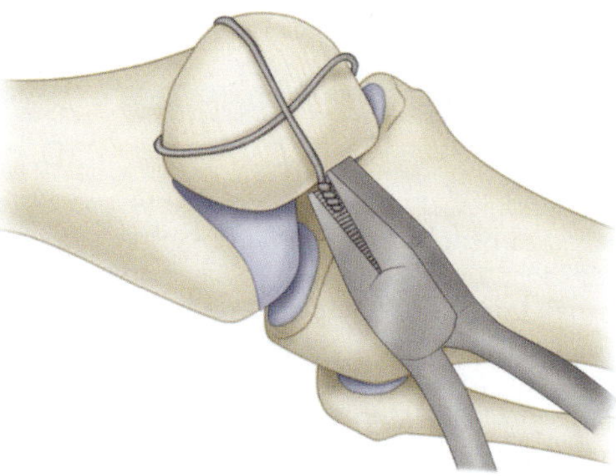

FIG. 29.17 Tension band wire fixation. Stainless steel wire is used to provide fixation in the fractured patella. (From Azar F. *Campbell's Operative Orthopaedics*. 13th ed. Philadelphia: Elsevier; 2017.)

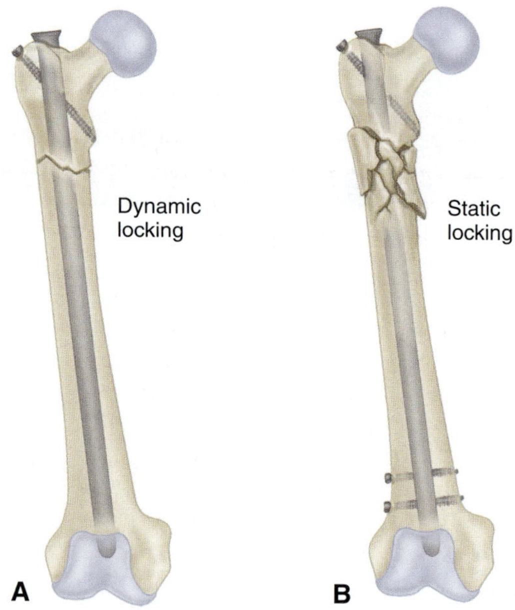

FIG. 29.18 Intramedullary femoral nail. (A) The dynamic nail controls bending and prevents rotation. (B) The static nail is more load bearing. (From Canale S, Beaty J, eds. *Campbell's Operative Orthopaedics*. 12th ed. Philadelphia: Mosby; 2013.)

INTRAMEDULLARY NAIL OR ROD

An intramedullary (IM) nail is a thick rod inserted into the medullary canal of long bones to provide structural support from inside the bone. This device is used for the fractures of long bones, such as the femur, tibia, and humerus. IM nails are made of titanium and stainless steel. They are supplied as slotted, cannulated (hollow), or solid. Nails are inserted by reaming the intramedullary canal or by impacting the nail through the marrow tissue to seat it. The *Ender nail* and *Rush rod* are older-style nails that are used in multiples and impacted with a mallet. Modern IM systems include the nail itself plus two or more transverse locking bolts, which increase contact with the bone and provide structural support. Locking bolts are placed at the proximal and distal ends of the nail and prevent it from drifting or backing out of the medullary canal. They also provide rotational support. Fig. 29.18 shows a femoral nail with locking screws.

WIRES AND CABLES

Flexible wire and cable are used in a variety of techniques to approximate bone and soft tissue and for stabilization. Wire most often is used to reduce small bone fragments. This is done by drilling holes in the fragments, inserting a wire through the holes, and drawing the fragments together. The wires are then twisted, and the resulting knot is buried in the adjacent soft tissue or flattened against the bone. Wire or cable is also used in cerclage (encircling) reduction to provide added strength to another type of implant, such as an IM nail. Cables are closed at their ends with a cable clamp.

KIRSCHNER WIRES AND STEINMANN PINS

Kirschner wires (K-wires) and Steinmann pins are thick wires that are inserted with a drill. The wires have a sharp, diamond-shaped point that penetrates the bone and soft tissue. They are inserted directly into tissue with a drill. They are extremely sharp and can easily puncture gloves and drapes. They should be handled with caution. After insertion, the surgeon cuts the excess wire with cutters. All pieces are retrieved from the surgical field and placed in a magnetic container to prevent injury or loss in the wound.

The main advantages of K-wires and Steinmann pins are their size and ease of insertion. They cause little trauma to bone and can be easily withdrawn. They commonly are used for the following purposes:

- As a guidewire for cannulated screws and instruments
- To provide temporary or final stabilization for a fracture
- As an intramedullary device to span a fracture in a small bone (e.g., the digits)
- To position multiple fragments of a comminuted fracture
- As a template for cannulated nails
- As a component of traction devices

MODULAR ROD AND PIN FIXATION

Modular rod and pin fixation is used for external stabilization of a fracture. The system is very flexible and can be used for fractures of the long bones and pelvis and to distract (separate) bone in which loss has occurred as a result of trauma or disease. The external framework maintains alignment with expansion of the limb to create space for new bone growth.

The basic design is based on external metal rods, which act as a superstructure to the bone. The rods are held in place with bolts and pins, which are inserted through the bone to support the outer framework. The modular system can be used as a unilateral frame (a single rod attached by internally placed pins) or a modular frame or cage constructed with multiple rods and pins, which are inserted into the bone fragments and connected with clamps (Fig. 29.19). Many types of pins do not require predrilling and are inserted with a power drill. This type of traction is commonly used in patients with severe open trauma.

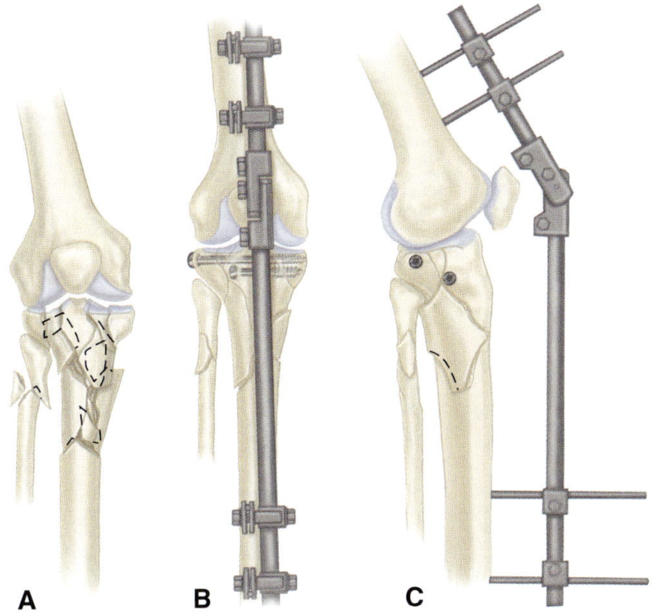

FIG. 29.19 Rod and pin external fixation. This system is used in fractures where there is extensive soft tissue damage—often as a temporary measure in polytrauma cases. (A) Comminuted fracture of the tibia. (B and C) Joint reconstruction using lag screw and external frame. (From Canale S, Beaty J, eds. *Campbell's Operative Orthopaedics.* 12th ed. Philadelphia: Mosby; 2013.)

SUTURE AND SUTURE DEVICES

Sutures are used in orthopedic surgery to repair soft connective tissue, for attaching tendon to bone, and for routine closure of tissue planes. Non-absorbable materials are used for repair to reduce any possible tissue reaction and also to provide superior strength during healing. The following suture materials are commonly used:

- Braided polyester (e.g., Fiberwire, Ticron)
- Caprolactam (e.g., Caprosyn, Supramid)
- Polydioxanone
- Braided polypropylene
- Stainless steel
- Polytetrafluoroethylene (PTFE)

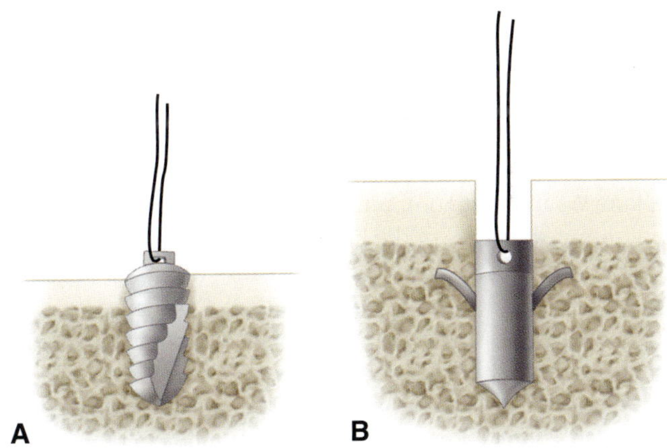

FIG. 29.20 Suture anchor. This device is used to attach soft tissue to bone. (A) The anchor is drilled into the bone, and sutures are used to attach soft tissue. (B) Hook device with suture attached. (From Canale S, Beaty J, eds. *Campbell's Operative Orthopaedics.* 12th ed. Philadelphia: Mosby; 2013.)

A variety of ***anchoring devices*** have been developed in the past decade. These include biosynthetic tacks, screws, biosynthetic cord, and patching material. Companies that manufacture the systems also provide special insertion instruments to accompany their product. As with many orthopedic systems, the ST should take advantage of in-service and online educational materials designed for the surgical technologist. Anchoring devices are made of materials such as polyetheretherketone (PEEK) or methylmethacrylate. A non-absorbable cord is attached to the anchor (Fig. 29.20).

Orthopedic buttons, another type of suture anchor, are used with stainless steel suture to fix the suture in place

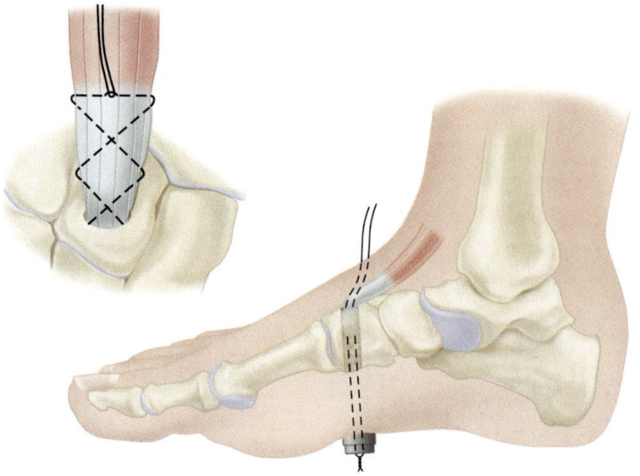

FIG. 29.21 Button. This technique combines suture repair with an orthopedic button. Suture strands are brought out through the skin and attached to a button, which prevents them from retraction during healing. (From Azar F. *Campbell's Operative Orthopaedics*. 13th ed. Philadelphia: Elsevier; 2017.)

during healing. The repair is performed and the suture material brought out through the skin and attached to the button until healing is complete (Fig. 29.21).

JOINT REPLACEMENT IMPLANTS

Joint implants are metal or synthetic components used to replace the diseased or injured tissue. This type of surgery is referred to as *arthroplasty*. The load placed on a joint requires that the implant meet criteria to prevent degradation of the implant. As implant components slide over each other in the joint, minute particles of the implant materials can be released into the joint cavity. These particles cause a cellular reaction that leads to the destruction of bone tissue. Different types of implant materials are designed to help overcome this problem through greater resistance to wear. No implant material or design is suitable for all patients. The selection is based on the patient's bone type, age, activity level, and general health.

ARTHROPLASTY MATERIALS

Metals

Metal alloys are used in the manufacture of joint implants. The metals and alloys most commonly used are the following:

- Cobalt-chromium-molybdenum
- Titanium-aluminum-vanadium
- Pure titanium
- Tantalum

Metal-on-metal components were the first type to be used in joint replacement. Some researchers have returned to this design, using more advanced metallurgy. However, metal can release ions into the body, causing toxicity. This type of a system is not used in patients with kidney disease or in women of childbearing age.

Polyethylene is a highly durable, low-friction plastic in the form of ultra-high molecular weight, highly cross-linked polyethylene (UHMWPE). This is a modified form of polyethylene made through a process of irradiation. Although very strong, highly cross-linked polyethylene breaks down through wear and delamination (separation of layers). UHMWPE components are commonly used in joint replacement procedures.

Ceramic materials were developed in orthopedic technology to increase resistance to wear. This type of a component is mainly limited to hip replacement. Three types of ceramic materials are currently used: alumina, zirconium, and oxidized zirconium. Ceramic materials have been used for the manufacture of femoral heads for several decades. Ceramic-on-polyethylene, ceramic-on-ceramic, and ceramic-on-metal implants are currently available. The advantages of ceramic are that it is very hard, it can be highly polished, and it remains resistant to scratching. The greatest disadvantage is that the material is brittle and can fracture or shatter.

Coatings may be applied to implants to enhance healing and resist wear. Metal fibers or "beads" are applied to the surface of the implant to create microscopic pores that accept bone cement during implantation. In **press-fit** implants, bone tissue infiltrates the pores during healing. Metal coatings are used or the original surface material may be altered by infusing it with gas or exposing it to nitrogen ions.

DESIGN STRUCTURE

The structure and surface of a joint implant are extremely important to the safety and function of the joint postoperatively. Joint stability is achieved by the basic design and surface coating.

Modular components are now used in most joint replacement systems. These are joint systems that contain several parts. Modular components can be manufactured from different materials or the same material and assembled inside the patient. An inventory of modular components allows surgical facilities to maintain a variety of sizes of components within a single system. Nonmodular systems may provide greater longevity because they have fewer components.

Joint implants may be cemented in place with bone cement or they may be press-fitted by impaction. The choice of cemented or press-fit design depends on the bone quality and the patient's age, health, and desired level of activity.

BONE CEMENT

Implants used in arthroplasty (joint replacement) may be cemented in place with polymethylmethacrylate (PMMA). Bone cement is an interface or a grout (rather than glue) between the joint implant and tissue. It is formed by mixing two components, PMMA powder and a liquid monomer of methylmethacrylate. When dry, the cement forms strong radiopaque filler. Bone cement is supplied plain or with an antibiotic additive that is released into the bone.

Bone cement is prepared during surgery to a doughy consistency. It is instilled into the joint manually or with a cement gun. After mixing, it hardens within 15 minutes. During mixing, the two components create an exothermic (heat-releasing) reaction.

PMMA is a hazardous chemical and must be handled according to regulations established by the National Institute for Occupational Safety and Health (NIOSH) and the hospital's policies and protocols. Exposure to PMMA vapor is an occupational risk, and use of the cement is associated with toxic and cardiovascular events in patients.

Occupational Risk

Vapor released when the dry and liquid components of PMMA are mixed is known to cause serious eye damage and respiratory tract and skin irritation. An allergic reaction may also occur. The effects of vapor inhalation are cumulative and are associated with kidney and liver damage. Inhalation may also cause neurological symptoms and pregnancy complications.

> More information on occupational risk is available on the NIOSH website at http://www.cdc.gov/niosh/data.

Patient Risks

Patient risks associated with PMMA include toxicity and vascular events. Acute toxicity causes sudden cardiovascular complications and possible cardiac arrest. Increased intramedullary pressure may force marrow tissue into the circulation, resulting in embolism. Bone cement implantation syndrome includes life-threatening hypotension, pulmonary edema, and cardiogenic shock. These hazards can be reduced by the use of good surgical technique, such as low-pressure pulse lavage to clear the medullary canal before the cement and implant are inserted.

Safety Precautions

The cement is supplied to the sterile field in its two components, as a dry powder and a liquid solvent. These are combined and mixed in a closed container specially designed for use with PMMA. The bone cement mixer is fitted with a vacuum tube that shunts vapor away from the surgical field. They then are dissipated through a charcoal filter. The vacuum system also removes air pockets, which destabilize the cement. Surgical technologists can become familiar with the operation and assembly of bone cement mixers used in their facility.

Preparing Bone Cement

The manufacturer's instructions for mixing bone cement should always be consulted before the process is started. Cement is injected into a prepared joint with a cement gun. Some mixers have a cartridge that is transferred directly to the cement gun after mixing. General preparation includes the following steps:

1. Assemble the mixing apparatus according to the manufacturer's specifications. Attach one end of the vacuum tubing to the mixer. The circulator receives the other end and attaches it to a vacuum pump, which is operated with compressed nitrogen.
2. Pour the powdered and liquid cement components into the mixer.
3. Secure the lid of the mixer. Rotate the lid handle to mix the components.
4. Continue to mix the cement until it reaches a doughy consistency. At this stage, it is removed from the mixer and molded to shape. When it is no longer sticky, it is ready for use.
5. If a cartridge mixer is used, remove the cartridge from the mixer and transfer it immediately to the cement gun.
6. Change sterile gloves when the cement no longer requires handling.
7. Discard any unused cement according to hospital policy. *Do not handle unused cement.*

BONE GRAFTS AND BONE SUBSTITUTES

Bone transplantation is usually performed using a segment of the patient's own bone (autograft) or cadaver bone (allograft). Cadaver bone is reprocessed to remove minerals and protein and then is freeze dried. Bone is stored in the hospital bone bank and supplied in a sterile form.

The most common anatomical areas used for autograft donor bone are the iliac crest and tibia. Grafts are usually taken using an osteotome and mallet. The graft site is prepped separately. If it is not closed promptly after the graft is out, the surgical technologist should keep the site covered and protected with sterile towels or a small drape. Bone graft tissue is covered with moist saline sponges or in antibiotic solution and kept on the back table in a basin until needed. Do not soak a bone implant unless requested by the surgeon. Never use water to moisten bone implants because this causes cellular damage.

BONE GRAFT HARVESTING

A bone graft may be harvested directly from the iliac crest, tibia, or rib. The most common site is the iliac crest. In this case the bone is exposed through a linear incision and the graft removed using a chisel. This produces slices of bone, which can be further shaped with a small bone rongeur.

A newer method, which has shown to be superior, is with the use of the reamer irrigator aspirator (RIA) device (Fig. 29.22). The RIA works by reaming, irrigating, and aspirating the contents of the medullary canal of the donor bone. A ball tip guidewire is inserted into the medullary canal, and the RIA instrument is inserted over it under fluoroscopic guidance. The reamer and irrigation system are activated to collect the intramedullary contents. The RIA removes excess fluid from the collection chamber and the remaining material collected. The surgeon may add antibiotic or other substances to increase the volume of the graft before implanting it at the recipient site (Fig. 29.23). The system must be used according to the guidance of the manufacturer. Individual systems vary, so it is important to follow the recommendations closely because the design of the RIA device and accessories are complex.

BONE GRAFT SUBSTITUTES

Bone graft substitutes are commonly used to repair and reconstruct bone. A shortage of graft materials and interest in **bioactive materials** has led to the development of new graft substitutes:

- Ceramic: Composites of calcium phosphate, calcium sulfate, and bioactive glass (paste, chips, granules)

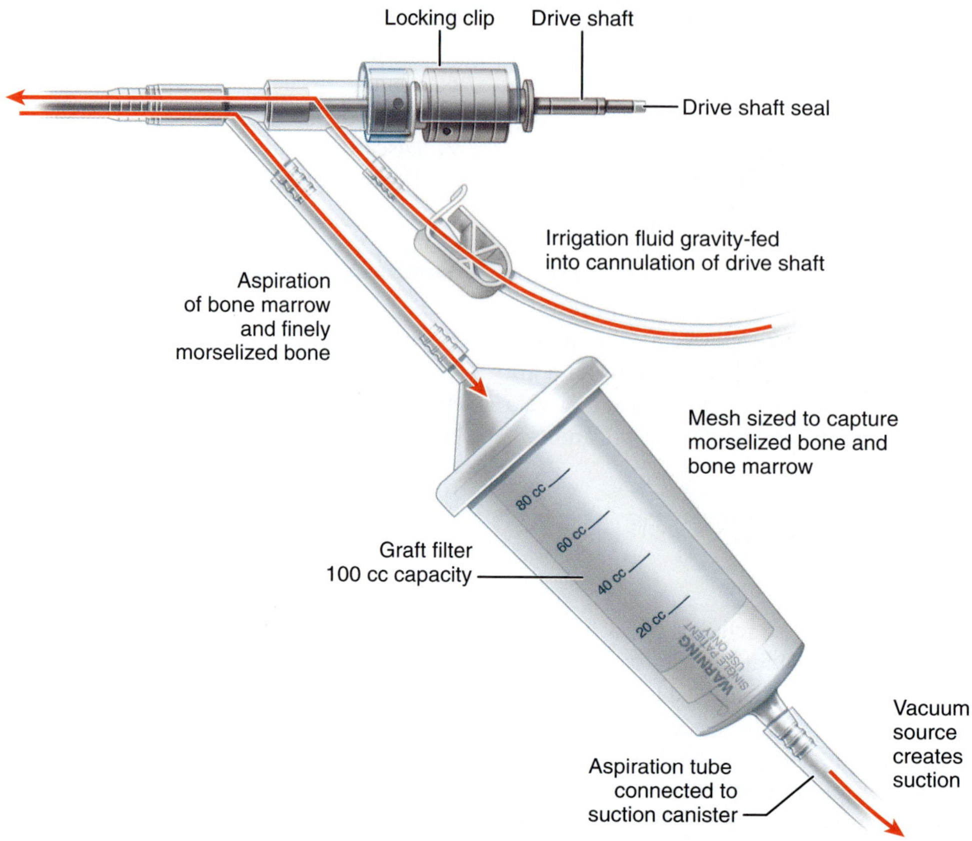

FIG. 29.22 Reamer irrigator aspirator (RIA). This device is used for harvesting medullary canal tissue for autografting. The device and technique require training according to the manufacturer's detailed instructions. (From Azar F. *Campbell's Operative Orthopaedics*. 13th ed. Philadelphia: Elsevier; 2017.)

- Polymer: Cross-linked collagen-based or hydroxyapatite-coated, resin-based
- Bone graft substitutes are supplied in the following forms:
  - Injectable paste
  - Block form
  - Granules
  - Putty
  - Chips

TRACTION

Traction is a mechanical method of applying a pulling force or elongation to fractured bone. Traction is used to do the following:

- Prevent injury to soft tissues, especially blood vessels and nerves near the fracture site
- Align bone after a fracture or **dislocation**
- Prevent movement of a fractured limb
- Reduce pain in acute orthopedic trauma patients before surgical repair
- Reduce muscle spasm in orthopedic injuries

Traction is used much less often in modern orthopedics than it was in the past. Advances in orthopedic implant surgery and techniques have replaced long-term traction as a primary method of treatment except in certain circumstances. The two types of traction are as follows:

- *Skin traction* requires taping a traction system to the skin. It generally is used only as a temporary measure (e.g., Buck traction). Skin traction is seldom used in adults. Modern external traction frames provide temporary traction for emergency use.
- *Skeletal traction* requires surgical insertion of metal pins or rods through the bone distal to the fracture. The pins are attached to a traction device that applies force or is drawn by a weighted pulley.

ARTHROSCOPIC SURGERY

Arthroscopic surgery is a minimally invasive surgery (MIS) of the joints. This technique is used for diagnostic procedures and for repair and reconstruction of soft tissue. Most open soft tissue procedures of the joints can be performed arthroscopically.

Before studying the minimally invasive techniques presented in this chapter, the reader should review Chapter 20. The principles are the same; only the instrumentation, patient preparation, and specific operative techniques are different.

INSTRUMENTS

Many orthopedic MIS instruments resemble those used in open procedures. In addition to the instruments described

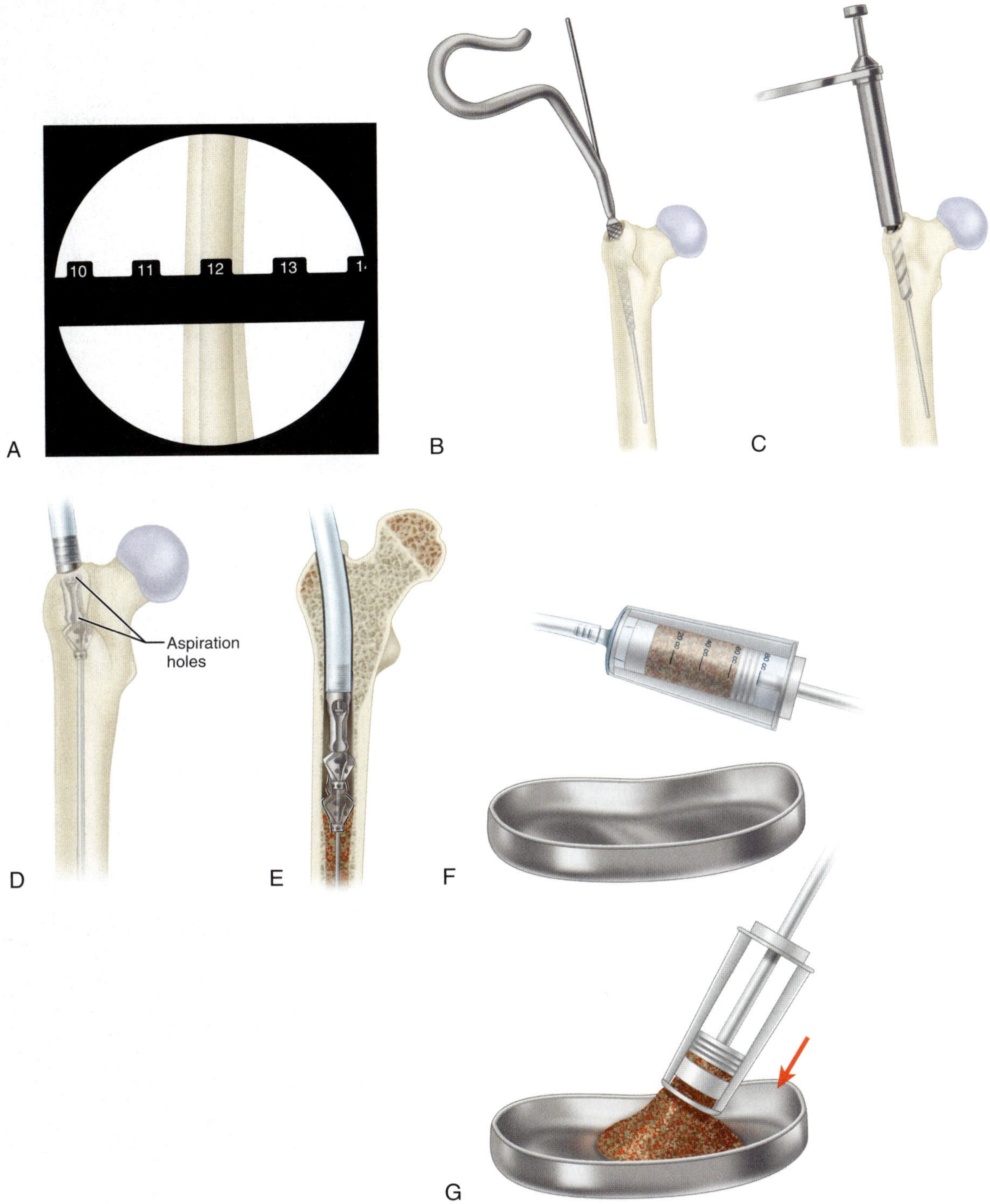

FIG. 29.23 RIA technique for harvesting femoral or tibial bone graft. (A) Confirmation of the reaming diameter. (B and C) Access to and reaming of medullary canal. (D) Insertion of reamer. (E) Reaming the canal. (F) Removing the graft material. (G) Graft material pushed out of inner filter. (From Azar, F. *Campbell's Operative Orthopaedics*. 13th ed. Philadelphia: Elsevier; 2017.)

below, a number of sophisticated devices are available for passing sutures through bone and cartilage.

Basic arthroscopy instruments include 30- and 70-degree arthroscopes, probe, knives, a motorized meniscus cutter and shaver, and radiofrequency ligation/cutting instruments. A variety of instruments are shown in Orthopedic Instruments.

Scissors

Arthroscopic scissors are available in diameters of 3 to 4 mm and may be straight or hook-tipped. The hook tip pulls the tissue into the instrument as it cuts. Right- and left-curved scissors and angled scissors are useful in cutting meniscus.

Basket Forceps

Biopsy punch or basket forceps are very commonly used. The open base allows tissue to drop from the instrument so that it does not have to be withdrawn for cleaning, as in open surgery. Basket forceps are hooked or straight; these are available in 30-, 45-, and 90-degree angles.

Suction Punch

This instrument is used to take small bits of meniscus and other connective tissue while suctioning fragments out of the joint through a channel in the instrument.

Probe

The probe is the most commonly used instrument in arthroscopic surgery. It is used to evaluate tissue and structures by touch and to retract structures in the joint during exploration. It allows the surgeon to feel the texture and density of joint structures and identify tears and tissue debris. The tip is round and right angled.

Grasping Forceps

Grasping instruments are used to maintain traction on tissue during cutting with the knife or scissors. It is also used to pick up loose bodies of cartilage and other tissue. Grasping instruments often are designed with a ratchet system to close the jaws over tissue. The tips may be serrated or contain teeth at the tip. Double- and single-action forceps are available.

Knife Blades

Knife blades for use inside the joint are available in a variety of configurations: straight, curved, hooked, or retrograde. The blades have magnetic properties so that if the tip breaks off during surgery, it can be retrieved more easily. Knife blades are inserted into the cannula sheath or through a retractable sheath system that protects the tissue until it enters the field of vision.

Shaving Instruments

A motorized shaver is used to smooth joint surfaces and remove redundant tissue. The instrument head contains a cylindrical blade, which rotates as it cuts tissue. The rotating cannula is set within a hollow sheath with windows. Suction is introduced through the cylinder that draws the tissue into contact with the tissue fragments and cuts them. The tissue fragments are suctioned out of the joint and into a tissue trap. Tips are available in a variety of sizes. The system is operated by a foot pedal, which allows the instrument to work at variable speed.

IMPORTANT TO KNOW *When the motorized shaver is in use, the outflow channel of the arthroscope must be closed to avoid oversuction and to prevent pulling contaminated irrigation fluid back into the joint.*

JOINT DISTENTION

Joint distention with saline or lactated Ringer solution is necessary for arthroscopy of the shoulder and knee. Fluid is instilled into the joint through one port and exits through another. Inflow tubing and outflow tubing are required to maintain continuous flushing of the joint.

As with other forms of MIS, expansion of the operative field from within allows greater visibility of the structures. Free-flowing solution keeps the operative field free of tissue debris and blood, which can obscure the endoscopic image transmitted to the monitor.

Fluid distention also acts as a *tamponade* (pressure to control bleeding). This is particularly important in rotator cuff surgery, in which bleeding can be brisk. In knee surgery, the synovial capsule may be inflamed, which can contribute to capillary bleeding. When tamponade is required, the inflow of fluid must be adjusted to keep up with the outflow. The circulator is responsible for making adjustments in the pump system (or gravity system) as necessary.

SURGICAL PROCEDURES

SHOULDER

The shoulder is composed of three main bones: the scapula, clavicle, and humerus. The head of the humerus fits into the glenoid socket of the scapula; this forms the glenohumeral joint. The socket is surrounded by a rim of cartilage called the *labrum,* which helps stabilize the head of the humerus. The labrum also attaches to several ligaments, which further support the joint.

The clavicle moves in coordination with the humerus and is a primary site of sports injury. Clavicular joints include the following:

- *Acromioclavicular (AC) joint:* Clavicle to acromion
- *Sternoclavicular (SC) joint:* Clavicle to sternum

The shoulder is a mechanically unstable structure. It is suspended from the skeleton by soft tissue and is mobile in all directions. The head of the humerus technically is a ball-and-socket joint, but the glenoid socket, which holds the head of the humerus, is shallow. As mentioned earlier, the labrum encircles the rim of the glenoid. The labrum is a cartilaginous structure similar to the meniscus in the knee. It increases the amount of contact between the humeral head and the glenoid, but joint stability relies on the ligaments, muscles, and tendons. The muscles that attach the humerus to the glenoid socket are jointly called the *rotator cuff.* These muscles also add to the stability of the joint; however, they can be torn as a result of sports injury or other traumatic stress.

The shoulder joint is shown in Fig. 29.24. Inside the joint capsule is a layer of connective tissue that is thickened at three points; these are the *glenohumeral ligaments.* When these soft tissues fail because of injury or repetitive stress, shoulder dislocation can occur. Recurrent dislocation requires surgical treatment in most cases.

POSITIONING AND SURGICAL EXPOSURE

Two positions are commonly used for shoulder surgery: lateral decubitus and beach chair. The affected arm may be unsecured so that it can be moved through different positions during the procedure, or it may be suspended using a

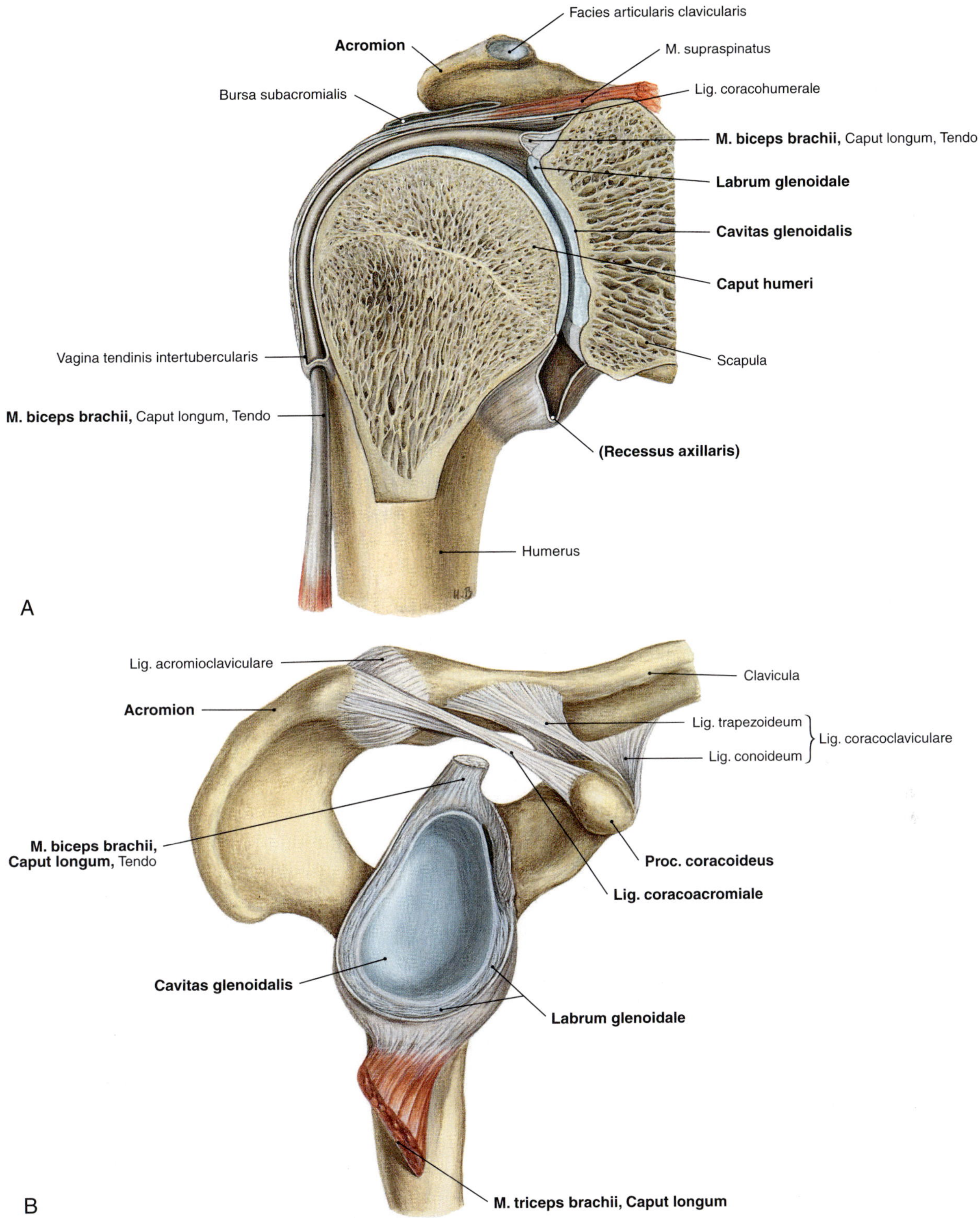

FIG. 29.24 Shoulder joint anatomy. (A) Section of the shoulder in the scapular plane. (B) Ventral and lateral view. (From Paulsen F. *Sobotta Atlas of Human Anatomy*. Vol 1. 15th ed. Munich, Germany: Elsevier GmbH; 2013.)

distractor system. The skin prep includes the chin, neck, thorax, shoulder, and arm; however, the lower arm is enclosed in sterile drapes so that only the shoulder and upper arm are exposed.

There are many different incisions used to access the shoulder for repair. Shoulder access may be anterior, or an anterior approach is used for many types of shoulder procedures. Another common approach is directly over the deltoid at the acromion. The posterior approach is used less commonly.

BANKART PROCEDURE (OPEN)

In the Bankart procedure, the glenoid rim is reattached to the joint capsule with a biosynthetic or other anchoring device or with heavy sutures. There are many different proprietary systems available for repair of a Bankart lesion. The principle in any system is to reattach the labrum to the glenoid rim. Each type of system used for the repair includes the tools and materials required for that system. These may include screws, biodegradable tacks, and sutures. The exact technique used to install these systems is specific to the system. Most require holes to be drilled in the glenoid rim, through which the suture is passed.

Pathology

An important cause of recurrent glenohumeral dislocation is the tearing or separation of the labrum (the rim of the glenoid capsule) from the joint capsule. The glenoid capsule is concave and normally cups the humeral head with support from the labrum and ligaments. However, the glenoid becomes shallow when the labrum and ligaments are torn away. Without support, the humeral head is forced out of the glenoid.

POSITION:	Beach chair
INCISION:	Anterolateral or anterior shoulder
PREP AND DRAPING:	Chin to waist, affected arm and axilla (prepped last), and anterior and posterior shoulder. Standard shoulder draping is used
INSTRUMENTS:	Major orthopedic; shoulder instruments; tacking device and accessories

Technical Points and Discussion

1. ***The patient is prepped and draped.***
The patient is placed in the beach chair position. A pad is placed under the scapula to lift the shoulder and bring the scapula forward. The shoulder and arm are prepped and draped, and the arm is left free for intraoperative manipulation.

2. ***An anterolateral or anterior incision is made and extended to the joint.***
An anterior or anterolateral incision is made near the axillary crease. The incision is carried into deep tissue using sharp dissection with Metzenbaum scissors and the electrosurgical unit (ESU). Rake retractors are used superficially to expose the muscles. As the incision is extended, deep handheld or self-retaining retractors are used to expose the joint. When the muscles have been exposed, the conjoined tendon is dissected free and retracted.

3. ***The joint capsule is incised and prepared.***
The capsule is divided and the glenoid rim is elevated with a retractor such as a ring retractor. The glenoid is prepared for the anchoring devices. In some cases, the tear may require remodeling with small rongeurs. An osteotome or rasp is used to score the glenoid rim and produce a raw surface on the bone (to expose the capillary blood supply and initiate bone healing) to which the capsule will be attached.

4. ***The capsule is attached to the glenoid.***
The capsule is attached with biosynthetic bone anchors, staples, or heavy sutures. If anchors are used, the ST should have several anchors available. For a thick bone, a pilot hole may be required. Size 0 or 2-0 Mersilene sutures are used in the traditional method of repair.

5. ***The joint capsule and wound are closed.***
After inspecting the repair, the surgeon uses the long suture ends to close the joint capsule. The shoulder then is manipulated into all ranges of motion to test the repair. The wound is irrigated and closed with continuous or running sutures. A simple dressing is applied, and the shoulder is placed in a soft immobilizer.

Technical points of the procedures are shown in Fig. 29.25.

After an open procedure for shoulder instability, dislocation can recur in 30% to 60% of cases. The patient may return to some activity within several months. Physical therapy is required to strengthen the rotator cuff muscles. Healing usually is complete within 6 months.

ARTHROSCOPIC MODIFIED BANKART PROCEDURE

POSITION:	Beach chair or lateral decubitus
INCISION:	Arthroscopic ports
PREP AND DRAPING:	Chin to waist, affected arm and axilla, and anterior and posterior shoulder. Standard shoulder draping is used
INSTRUMENTS:	30-degree and 70-degree arthroscope; arthroscopic shoulder instruments; tissue shaver; anchor suture system; drill

Technical Points and Discussion

1. ***The patient is positioned, prepped, and draped.***
The patient is placed in beach chair or lateral position and prepped for a shoulder procedure. After draping, the operative arm may be placed in a distractor. The surgeon draws the locations of the arthroscopic portals with the surgical marker.

2. ***Arthroscopic ports are placed.***
In this procedure three arthroscopic ports are used. The posterior port is the main entry point. It is used for the insertion of the arthroscope and guides the placement of other ports. To establish the posterior port, an 18-gauge

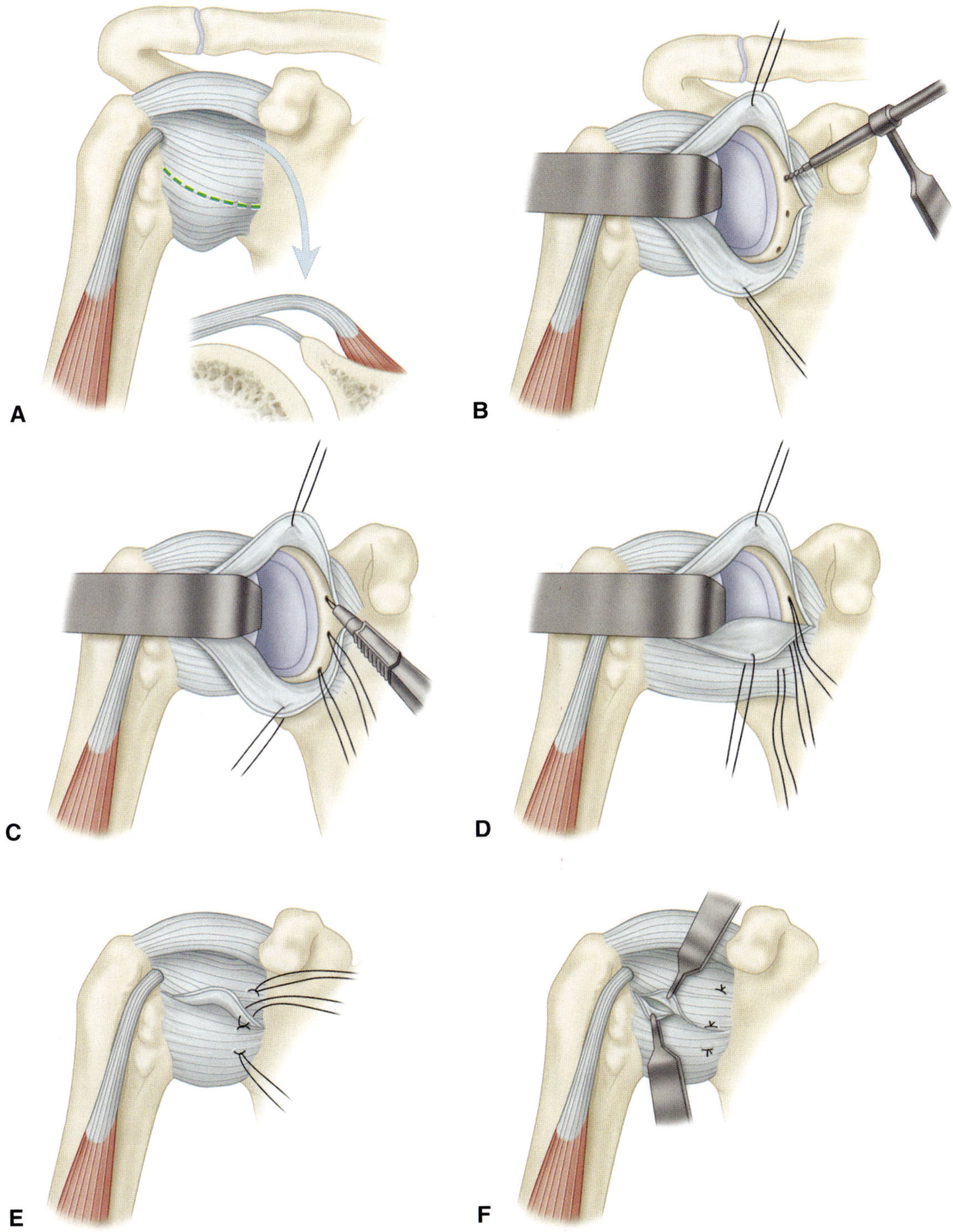

FIG. 29.25 Open Bankart procedure for recurrent dislocation. (A) The capsular incision is made. A stay suture is placed to identify the attachment of the glenoid. (B) Drill holes are made in the scapular neck adjacent to the glenoid surface. A Hohmann retractor is in place. (C) Suture anchors are placed in each drill hole. The sutures are pulled to set the anchor. (D) The capsule is approximated. An Allis clamp is used here to hold traction on the capsule while the sutures are tied. (E) Suture anchors are used to secure and tighten the superior flap. (F) Final capsule imbrication with interrupted non-absorbable sutures. (From Canale S, Beaty J, eds. *Campbell's Operative Orthopaedics.* 12th ed. Philadelphia: Elsevier; 2013.)

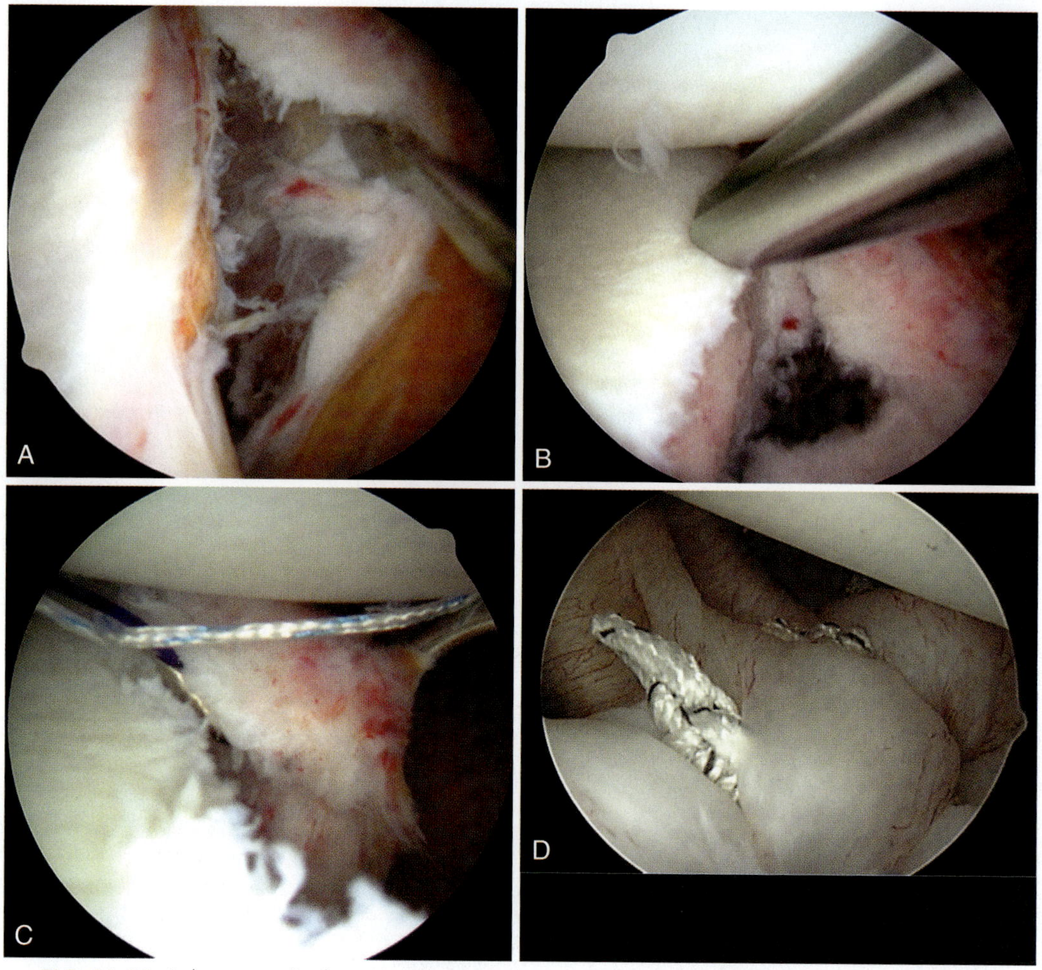

FIG. 29.26 Arthroscopic Bankart procedure. (A) The capsule and labral complex freed. (B) An anchor is inserted on the edge of the glenoid. (C) A 1-cm bite of suture is taken and then passed distal to the anchor. (D) Knots are tied to create a soft tissue bumper. (From Azar F. *Campbell's Operative Orthopaedics.* 13th ed. Philadelphia: Elsevier; 2017.)

spinal needle is directed into the joint space. When it is in place, 30 to 40 mL of saline is injected. After the skin incision is selected for the first portal, local anesthetic with epinephrine is injected for hemostasis. An incision is made with a #11 blade. A trocar and cannula is then passed from the back to the front of the shoulder until the trocar tents the skin on the anterior side. An incision is made over this trocar, and a cannula is passed over its tip. As the trocar is withdrawn, it carries the new cannula with it for proper placement. The arthroscope with fiberoptic light and fluid inflow tubing is then inserted into the posterior cannula. A third cannula may be inserted in the same way.

3. ***The joint is explored and assessed.***
The surgeon performs a complete arthroscopy of the joint to determine the extent of injury.

4. ***The glenoid surface is prepared.***
A rasp, shaver, or burr is used to debride the glenoid below the labrum to create a fresh bleeding surface, which enables healing.

5. ***Anchor sutures are placed.***
The anterior working cannula is now replaced with a threaded 8.5 cannula. This cannula is used to pass the drill, drill guide, and other instruments required for the repair. In this procedure, small-size suture anchors and loop sutures of PEEK are passed between the labrum and glenoid using a hooked suture carrier. The carrier can be used to directly pass the sutures, and a grasper is used to pull the ends out through the cannula. A drill is inserted, and a "socket" is created in the glenoid. The sutures are passed through an anchor, which is fixed in the glenoid along with the sutures. Three anchors are usually sufficient to reattach the labrum to the glenoid.

6. ***The wound is irrigated and closed.***
The wound is irrigated with saline, and the cannulas are withdrawn. The incisions are closed with subcuticular non-absorbable sutures. Flat gauze dressings are applied. Placement of suture anchors is shown in Fig. 29.26.

The patient is fitted for a sling immobilizer after surgery. Physical therapy is performed starting at week.

Related Procedure: Arthroscopic Acromioplasty

Arthroscopic acromioplasty is the removal of bony spurs from the undersurface of the acromion. Spurs can lead to impingement and swelling of the supraspinatus tendon, causing swelling and pain. The inflammation may also cause weakness in the muscles of the rotator cuff. Acromioplasty is performed as a stand-alone procedure or during surgery for other repairs. A posterior approach is most commonly used. Spurs are reduced using a cartilage shaver.

ROTATOR CUFF REPAIR

In this procedure, the tendons of the rotator cuff are attached to the humerus with sutures or anchor-suturing devices. Small bony outgrowths may also be removed to prevent impingement on the rotator cuff (**acromioplasty**).

An open or arthroscopic approach can be used.

Pathology

The rotator cuff is composed of four tendons that attach to the humerus. Each tendon is continuous with a muscle that originates at the scapula. The muscles are the *supraspinatus, subscapularis, infraspinatus,* and *teres minor.* One or more tendons may be damaged by traumatic injury or as a result of recurrent shoulder dislocation. A rotator cuff tear usually occurs where the supraspinatus tendon inserts into the humerus. The injury can be superficial or can involve the entire tendon. Degenerative conditions, in which the tissue is weakened because of past injury or previous surgery, can also result in tearing.

POSITION:	Beach chair or lateral decubitus
INCISION:	Anterior shoulder
PREP AND DRAPING:	Chin to waist and anterior and posterior shoulder and arm. The shoulder is draped free using standard techniques
INSTRUMENTS:	Major orthopedic set; shoulder set; small drill and bits
POSSIBLE EXTRAS:	Suture anchor system; collagen or biosynthetic mesh

Technical Points and Discussion

1. ***The patient is positioned, prepped, and draped.***
The patient is prepared for a shoulder procedure with the arm draped free.

2. ***The incision is made.***
A vertical anterior skin incision is made with a #10 knife and carried through the deltoid muscle using a needle-point ESU. Rake retractors are used on the wound edges.

3. ***The deltoid and coracoacromial ligament are divided.***
Using a deep #10 knife the surgeon incises the aponeurosis of the deltoid and coracoacromial ligament. The deltoid attachment is also severed from the clavicle and acromion using the spatula tip ESU. The ST should have ample lap sponges available.

4. ***The bursa is incised.***
The incision is carried to the joint capsule with the ESU and Metzenbaum scissors. A self-retaining retractor (e.g., Gelpi or Beckman retractor) is used to expose the rotator cuff tendons and muscles.

5. ***The acromion is prepared.***
If sutures are used to repair the tear, the acromion must be prepared. If acromioplasty is required after the resection of the joint capsule, it may be necessary for the surgeon to perform an osteotomy at the superior acromion and incise the anterior acromion. The cut surfaces are remodeled to remove any spurs or other rough spots on the bone. This technique can also be applied in arthroscopic surgery. Several small holes are made in the surface of the humerus with an awl or drill.

6. ***Sutures or an anchoring device are passed through the bone and tendon.***
Braided polyester sutures are passed through the bone and the tendon; two lines of sutures may be placed. The suture ends are left long and tagged with hemostats. This step is repeated until all sutures are in place. The arm is raised and the shoulder is adducted to reduce tension on the suture line. The sutures are then tied. Biosynthetic or collagen material is secured over the repair site to strengthen the tissue. If anchor screws are used for the repair, pilot holes are drilled before insertion of three or more anchors. The anchor is implanted, and the sutures are drawn through the edge of the tendon and then tied. If the deltoid muscle was severed, it is reattached to the acromion with several heavy sutures passed through drill holes. The wound is irrigated with antibiotic solution, and bleeding is controlled with the ESU.

7. ***The wound is closed.***
The incision is closed with 2-0 and 3-0 absorbable suture. The subcutaneous tissue is closed with 4-0 absorbable suture and Steri-Strips. The incision is covered with 4 × 4 gauze and a bulky dressing and is immobilized with a sling or shoulder immobilizer. A repair using collagen patch material is illustrated in Fig. 29.27.

TOTAL SHOULDER ARTHROPLASTY

In total shoulder arthroplasty, the humeral head and glenoid capsule are replaced with artificial components to restore function and relieve pain. In hemiarthroplasty, only the humeral component is used. A total joint system includes both the humeral and glenoid components. The stem portion may be press-fit or cemented. The glenoid component is replaced with a pegged cup, usually constructed of polyethylene.

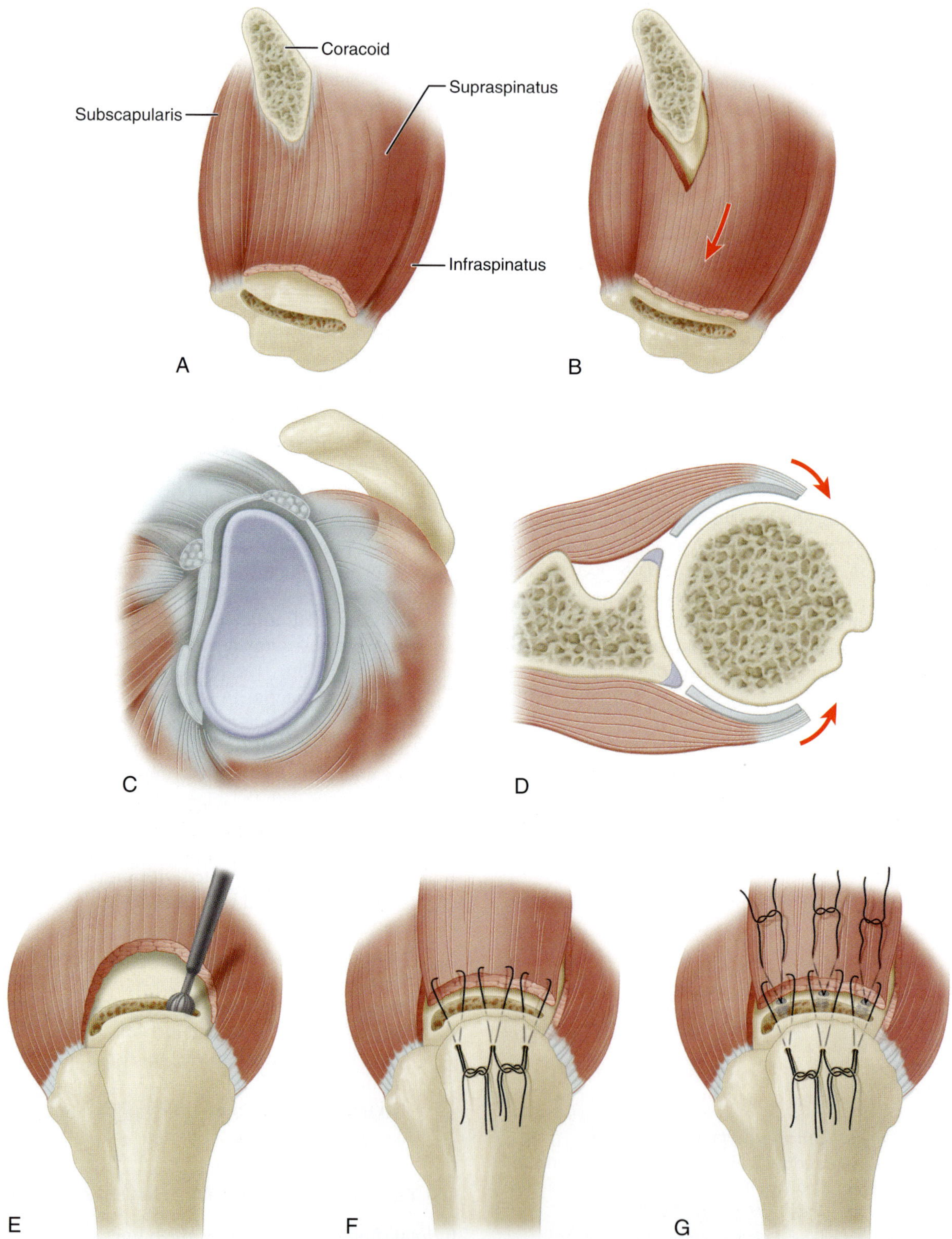

FIG. 29.27 Rotator cuff repair. (A and B) The cuff is mobilized by releasing the soft tissues. (C and D) The capsule is incised at its attachment at the glenoid labrum. (E) An osteotome is used to create a trough. (F) Suture holes are drilled 2 to 3 cm from the trough. (G) Suture anchors are inserted proximal to the trough margin. (From Azar F. *Campbell's Operative Orthopaedics*. 13th ed. Philadelphia: Elsevier; 2017.)

In preparation for shoulder arthroplasty, the surgical technologist should have all the components and sizers needed for the selected system. A major orthopedic set and shoulder instruments are added, and ample table room should be provided to accommodate the instrument trays. A pneumatic oscillating saw is needed to perform the osteotomy. Reamers are required for the medullary canalization of the humerus. **Broaches** (fin-shaped rasps that closely match the contour of the medullary implant) that fit the specific system implant are also needed for canalization. If a cemented prosthesis is planned, provisions should be made for these components (e.g., mixer, tubing). A magnetic instrument pad should be used to prevent instruments placed on the surgical field from falling. The ESU and suction are used continuously during the procedure, and holsters should be provided for these on the field.

An excellent video demonstrating total shoulder arthroplasty can be viewed at https://www.youtube.com/watch?v=3VTiMjDYdAs.

Pathology

The indications for shoulder arthroplasty are persistent pain that is not relieved by more conservative surgery and inability to perform activities of daily living because of loss of function. Osteoarthritis is the primary cause of these symptoms. Rheumatoid arthritis, traumatic arthritis, and shoulder instability related to rotator cuff disease are less commonly indicated for joint replacement.

POSITION:	Fowler or beach chair; sequential compression device needed
INCISION:	Anterior shoulder
PREP AND DRAPING:	Chin to waist, including the affected arm, posterior shoulder, and axilla. Standard shoulder drapes are used
INSTRUMENTS:	Shoulder arthroplasty set; high-speed drill; oscillating saw; shoulder replacement system
POSSIBLE EXTRAS:	Instruments and supplies for rotator cuff repair

Technical Points and Discussion

1. ***The patient is positioned, prepped, and draped.***
The patient is placed in beach chair position with the affected shoulder exposed anteriorly and posteriorly. The affected arm is left free for manipulation during the procedure. The shoulder and upper body are prepped widely.

2. ***The entry incision is made.***
An anterior (deltopectoral) approach is most commonly used for the procedure. The deltoid muscle is mobilized. The incision is carried to the joint capsule, which is incised to allow the humerus to be released from the glenoid fossa. Slotted or Darrach retractors or elevators may be used to dislocate the humerus. Hohmann retractors are used to support the position of the humeral head. Heavy non-absorbable sutures are placed in the rotator cuff. The ends are left long to be used in closure at the end of the procedure.

3. ***The humeral head is dislocated.***
After anatomical landmarks are identified, the humeral head is dislocated from the joint.

4. ***The humeral head is reamed.***
The center point of the humeral head is identified and an entry hole made to accommodate a reamer. A round reamer is used to create and enlarge the hole.

5. ***The humeral head is severed.***
A resection guide is put in place with a cutting block, and the humerus is severed using an oscillating saw. Irrigation with a bulb syringe will be needed during cutting. Any osteophytes (bone spurs) are removed with a rongeur. The ST should place the humeral head in the protected area of the back table, where it is kept moist.

6. ***The medullary canal is prepared.***
The medullary canal is prepared for reaming by delivering the humerus out of the incision. A pilot hole is made in the cancellous bone with a small reamer, and increasingly larger reamers (8 to 12 mm) are used to enter the medullary canal. An osteotome is used to remove a "fin" of bone to fit the shape of the prosthesis. When the cancellous bone has been penetrated, modular broaches are used to form a space for the humeral stem. When the last modular rasp has been used, it is left in place. Preliminary trial of humeral heads is carried out over the modular rasp. The trial head is removed, but the modular rasp left in place.

7. ***The glenoid fossa is prepared.***
The glenoid rim often must be trimmed and osteophytes and other bony growths removed. The fossa can be lowered (the rim taken down) with rongeurs or by reaming the fossa with a high-speed burr or cup-shaped reamers.

8. ***The glenoid is reamed and pin holes are drilled.***
Two types of glenoid prostheses are commonly used: a pegged and a keeled design. Holes must be drilled to accommodate a pegged component. Pegged systems provide a drill guide for the exact placement of the holes.

NOTE *A pegged system is shown in the accompanying figures.*

A centering pin is used to start the glenoid hole. The hole is then carefully enlarged using a circular disc-shaped reamer. After bone debris is removed from the surgical wound, individual peg holes are drilled to accommodate the pins of the glenoid component. This is done using a peripheral drill guide.

9. ***The trial glenoid is placed.***
The glenoid trial is put in place to ensure that the drill holes are set correctly and that the rim of the implant matches the edge of the real glenoid.

10. ***The glenoid component is cemented in place.***
The ST should have irrigation and suction available to remove debris from the peg holes. All bits of bone are removed from the pin holes. Bone cement is required to set the glenoid component. The ST must time the preparation of the cement correctly to have it ready when needed. The surgeon may request additives to the cement or a commercially prepared formulation can be used. The cement is injected into the peg holes and a compactor used to remove air spaces in the cement columns. The glenoid component is then placed. The ST should have a small elevator ready to clear cement that has extruded from the component.

11. ***The humeral stem is impacted in place.***
After the wound is irrigated, it is cleared of all debris. The ST should have fresh sponges up on the field. Following these steps, the humeral stem can be impacted.

12. ***The humeral head is trialed and selected.***
The final humeral head trials are used to determine the correct size. The joint capsule tissue may require adjustment to ensure the correct amount of tension is created around the implants. The humeral head is then placed and the shoulder reduced. Before the final closure, the joint is assessed for mobility.

13. ***The wound is closed.***
The incision is closed in layers. The subscapularis sutures are secured, and the rotator cuff is closed with synthetic non-absorbable sutures. The superficial layers are closed with absorbable synthetic sutures. A suction drain may be placed before closure. The wound is dressed with Kerlix fluffs and an abdominal pad. A shoulder brace is applied for stability. Fig. 29.28 shows technical points of the procedure.

FOREARM

The forearm includes two bones: the radius and ulna (see Fig. 29.1). Fractures of the forearm may occur during sports, industrial accident, or motor vehicle accident. The forearm bones are critical to pronation and supination, and their relationship is sometimes referred to as a *functional joint*. Surgical treatment is indicated in nearly all "both-bone" fractures in the adult. Fixation using plates is a common technique.

OPEN REDUCTION INTERNAL FIXATION OF FOREARM FRACTURES

Fractures of the mid-radius and ulna are usually repaired using a dynamic compression plate. Closed reduction using a cast for external fixation is applied only to children. Closed reduction with external fixation is used only as a temporary measure in unstable poly trauma patients with multiple traumatic injuries or fractures that are highly contaminated. A dynamic compression plate repair of the radius with fluoroscopy is presented here (refer to earlier section on plates for reference). If both the ulna and the radius are fractured, both incisions are made at the start of the case. The dynamic compression plate contains slotted holes. When the first screw is fixed, it is left in a neutral position in the slot. As subsequent screws are applied, the plate moves along the bone and fracture, bringing the two segments together.

POSITION:	Supine with the affected arm placed on an arm table
INCISION:	Volar (inner) surface of the forearm
PREP AND DRAPING:	The arm and a wide area of the axilla and chest are prepped. Standard arm draping is used
INSTRUMENTS:	Small fragment set; 3.5-mm dynamic compression plates; sharp and blunt reduction forceps

Technical Points and Discussion

1. ***The patient is positioned, prepped, and draped.***
The patient is placed in supine position with the anterior side of the affected arm up on a translucent hand table. A pneumatic tourniquet is applied to the upper arm. The arm and hand are prepped. The hand is excluded from the draping exposure. The surgeon marks the incision line on the skin. An Esmarch bandage is used to exsanguinate the arm, and the tourniquet is inflated.
2. ***The entry incision is made.***
The skin incision is made using a #10 blade. The incision is carried to deep tissue layers using the deep knife, Metzenbaum scissors, and ESU. Rake retractors are used to expose the deep anatomy until the level of the radius. At this level, the ST should provide two Beckman retractors. The fracture site is examined.
3. ***The dynamic compression plate is prepared.***
The surgeon selects the correct length and configuration plate to be used. This is done by comparing the x-ray of the non-injured arm. The radius is bowed. Therefore the plate must be contoured using the plate benders, which are included in the compression plate set. The number of bicortical screws required is determined.
4. ***The fracture is reduced.***
The fractured ends of the bone must be brought into alignment (reduced) before fixation with the plate. This is done using two bone-holding forceps—one at each end

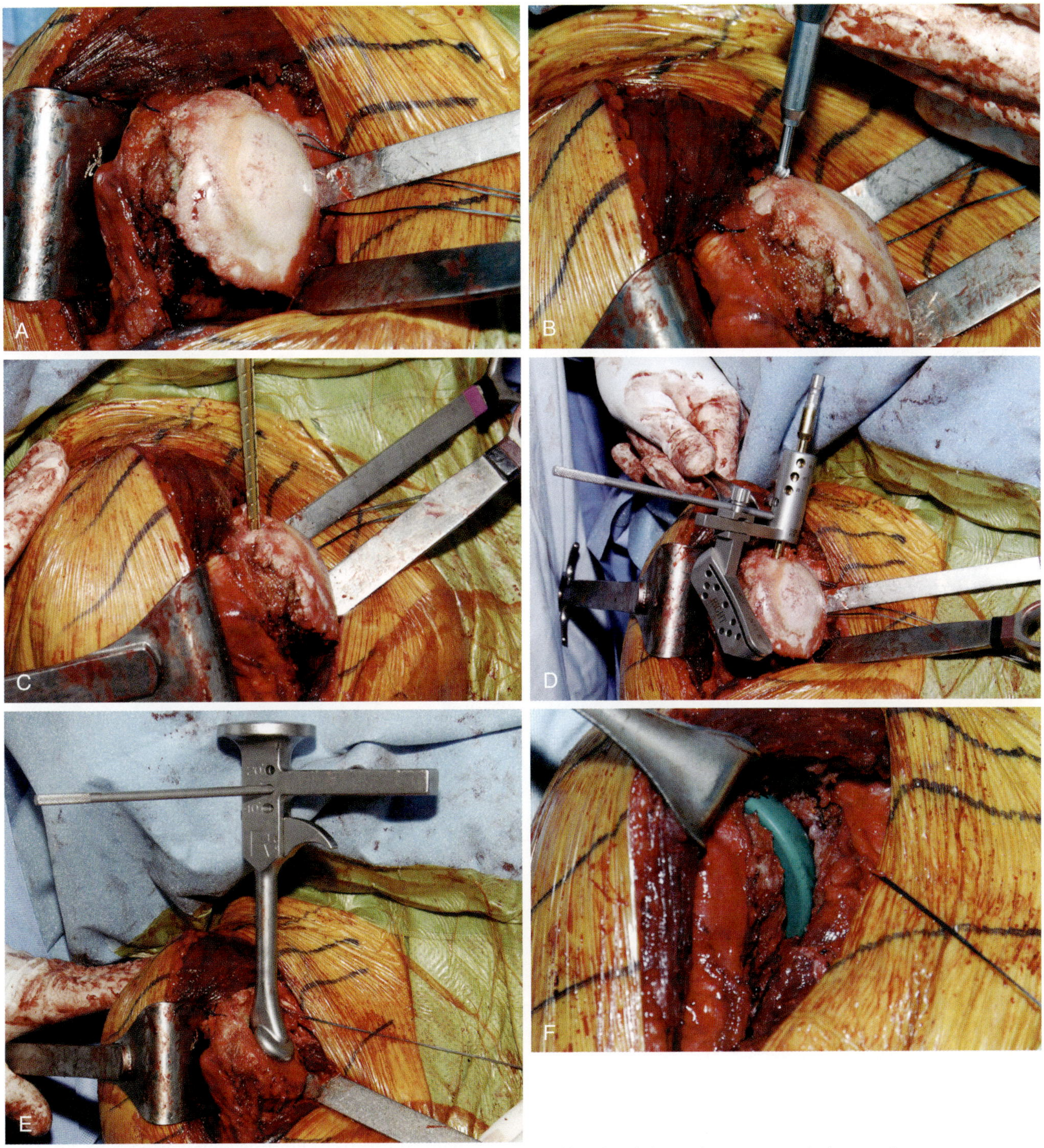

FIG. 29.28 Total shoulder arthroplasty. (A) The humeral head is dislocated. (B) An entry hole is made. (C) Reamers are used to prepare the medullary canal. (D and E) A resection guide and cutting block is placed and the humeral head removed. The angle of the cut is confirmed. (F) A trial humeral stem is placed.

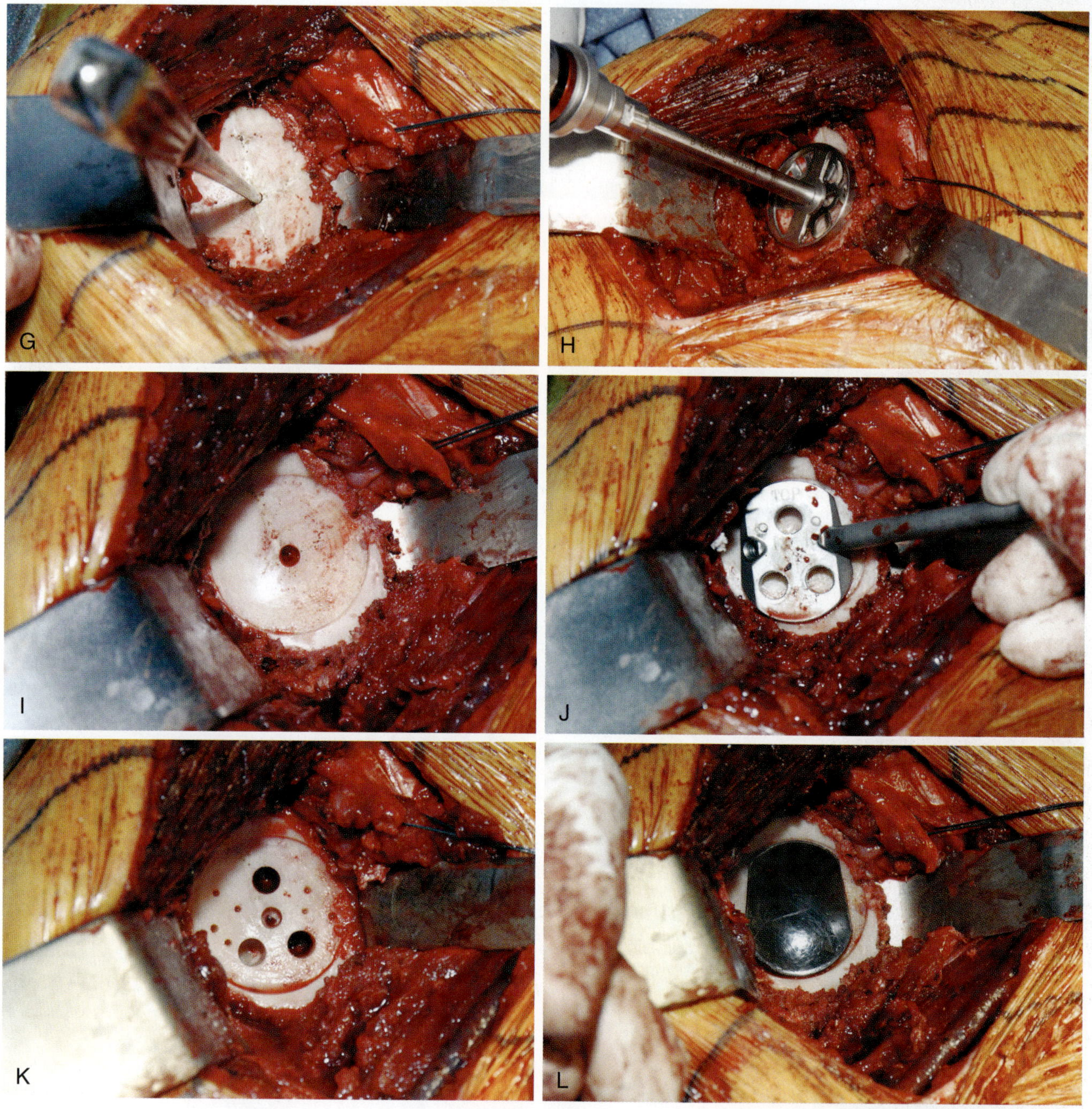

FIG. 29.28, cont'd (G) A trial humeral head is placed. (H) Center hole of the glenoid is made. (I) A peripheral drill guide is used to drill the glenoid peg holes. (J) The trial glenoid component is placed. (K) The final glenoid component. (L) The final humeral head is impacted in place and the shoulder joint reduced. (From Lee D, Neviaser J. *Operative Techniques: Shoulder and Elbow Surgery*. 2nd ed. Philadelphia: Elsevier; 2019.)

of the fracture. Blunt forceps are commonly used here. A small S curve bone lever may be needed to achieve reduction.

5. ***The bicortical screws are implanted in the plate.***

The screw holes are drilled using a drill guide to correctly angle the drill bit. The bent plate is fixed to the bone, and the first screw is inserted using a screwdriver. The screw is left in neutral position. Reduction forceps are placed in the opposite fragment to maintain the reduced position against the plate. The second screw is inserted on the opposite fragment. This screw is tightened, and this compresses the two fragments into anatomical position. Additional screws are placed in neutral position. Fluoroscopy is used to verify the positions of the screws and plate, and the forearm rotation is checked manually.

6. ***The wound is closed.***

The wound is irrigated and closed in layers using synthetic absorbable suture. Skin is closed with staples or interrupted synthetic sutures size 4-0. A flat dressing is placed over the wound.

Fig. 29.29 shows the application of a dynamic compression plate.

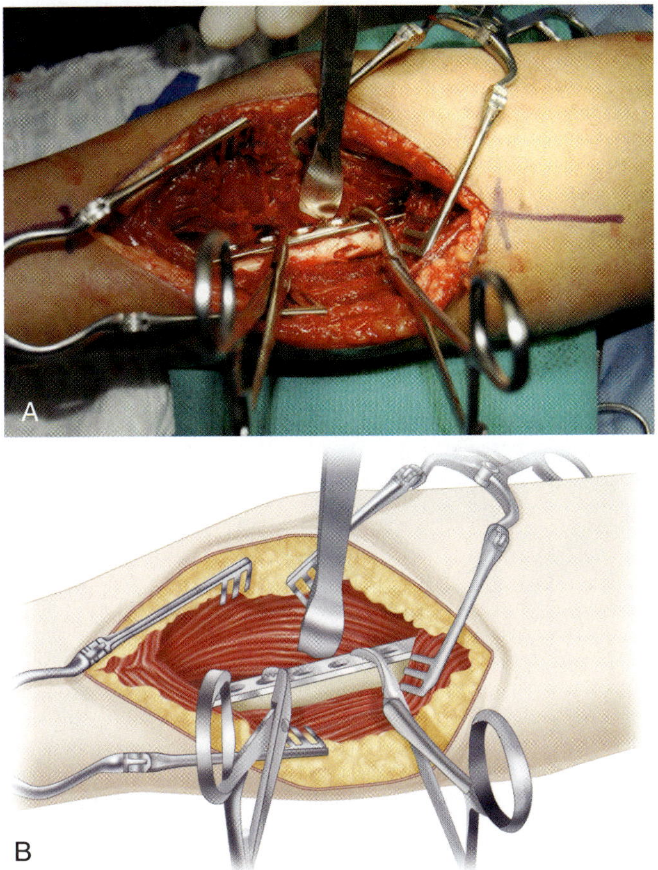

FIG. 29.29 Forearm fracture using dynamic compression plate. (A) The fracture has been reduced and held temporarily by clamps. Note the use of Beckman retractors. (B) Illustration of plate in place. (From Schemitsch E, McKee M. *Operative Techniques: Orthopaedic Trauma Surgery*. Philadelphia: Elsevier; 2020.)

EXTERNAL FIXATION OF THE RADIAL SHAFT

External fixation of the radius mid-shaft is performed as a temporary repair of severe open fractures or those with severe soft tissue injury. A unilateral modular rod and pin system is used (review earlier section on modular external fixation). The components of the system are as follows:

- Threaded self-drilling/self-tapping pins
- Pin-to-bar clamps
- Bars
- Bar-to-bar clamps

IMPORTANT TO KNOW *All commercially available rod and pin systems are designed to be used according to the manufacturer's specific technique. The surgical technologist must be familiar with the system instruments and implants and the surgical technique required.*

POSITION:	Supine with affected arm on hand table
INCISION:	Over fracture or through existing wound
PREP AND DRAPING:	Arm with hand excluded
INSTRUMENTS:	Modular pin and rod system; drill; minor orthopedic set

Technical Points and Discussion

1. ***The patient is positioned, prepped, and draped.***
The patient is placed in supine position with the affected arm on a translucent hand table. The hand is excluded from the draping exposure.
2. ***The incisions are made.***
The pin sites are determined, and small stab incisions are made over each site. The deep tissues are divided bluntly using Langenbeck or similar small retractors until the bone is reached.
3. ***The pins inserted.***
The drill sleeve and trocar are inserted and advanced to the bone. The trocar is then withdrawn. A pilot hole is drilled into the bone using the appropriate size drill bit. A depth gauge is used to measure the hole. The pin is then inserted manually or using a drill. This step is repeated for each pin. Fluoroscopy is used to determine the depth of the pin in the bone.
4. ***The rod system is assembled.***
The rod system is loosely assembled by connecting the pins with the bar using appropriate pin-to-bar clamps. The fracture is reduced by placing traction on the bar and manipulating the bone fragments into place. This position is maintained by the assistant while the clamps are tightened. The completed reduction is verified on fluoroscopy. Pin sites are not sutured. Xeroform gauze strips are wrapped around the base of each pin, where it contacts the skin.

Technical points of the procedure are illustrated in Fig. 29.30.

WRIST AND HAND

Wrist and hand surgery is a specialty that combines orthopedics, vascular surgery, and neurosurgery. Microsurgical techniques are commonly used for **replantation** of the hand and for repair of nerves, blood vessels, tendons, and ligaments after trauma. Technological advances in instrumentation within the past 15 years have greatly improved recovery after complex hand trauma and soft tissue diseases such as fascia contraction and nerve entrapment. Innovative joint replacement procedures are now common for the treatment of joint diseases, such as degenerative and rheumatoid arthritis.

Hand surgery and many forearm procedures are performed using a hand table. The surgeon and assistant (or surgical technologist) are seated facing each other. The surgical technologist may have a major role in assisting during hand procedures. This includes not only providing irrigation and retraction but also stabilizing the hand as shown in Fig. 29.31. Important to know: the surgeon and assistant (or surgical technologist) operate while seated at the hand table, the top surface of the hand table is the only sterile at table level.

The sterile field is extended to the draped surface of the table, never below it. The arm and hand are prepped using standard techniques. The hand may require scrubbing to remove dirt, especially from under the fingernails. Trauma cases involving shards of glass, metal, wood, or other foreign objects that are embedded in soft tissue require more complex *debridement*. This usually is performed outside the operating room, often in the emergency department. Industrial accidents may result in tissue injection of oil and other chemicals, which also require extensive debridement.

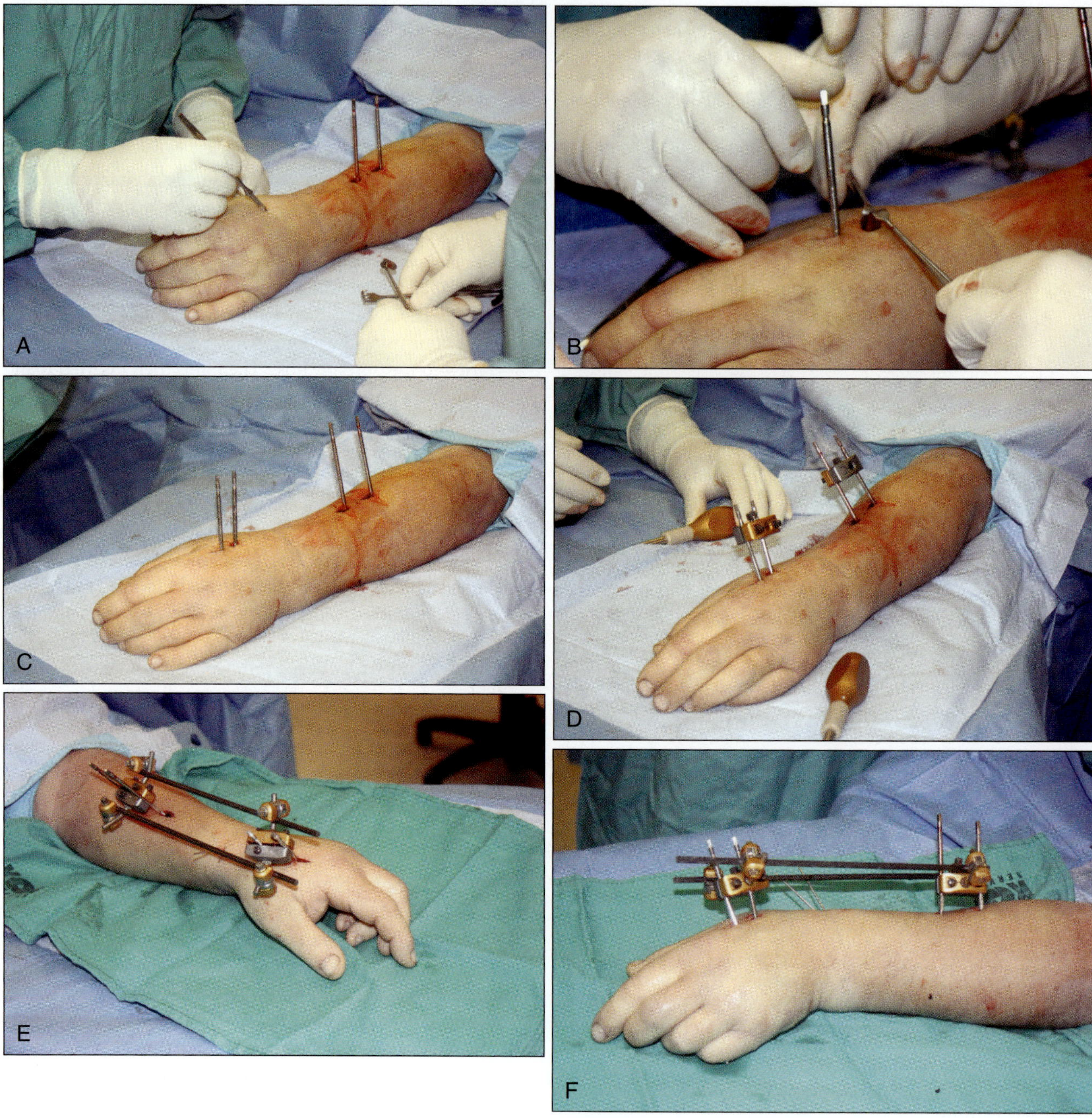

FIG. 29.30 External fixator. (A) A #15 knife is used to make stab incisions. In this repair, four pins will be placed. (B) Pin placement. (C) Completion of all pins. (D) Clamps are placed over the pins. (E and F) Rod assembly is completed. (From Schemitsch E, McKee M, eds. *Operative Techniques: Orthopedic Trauma Surgery*. Philadelphia: Saunders; 2010.)

A regional or local anesthetic is used for many hand procedures. A combination of lidocaine and a long-acting local anesthetic (e.g., bupivacaine) is commonly used. Vasoconstrictive agents (e.g., epinephrine) are not used because they can cause damage to delicate vessels and nerves. A pneumatic tourniquet is used for all hand cases.

Short plastic surgery instruments are used for all hand procedures. Delicate orthopedic instruments are required for joint and trauma surgery involving bone. A small drill and fine Steinmann pins or K-wires are commonly used for internal fixation. Reconstruction procedures require small vascular clamps and short right-angle clamps. The bipolar ESU with a fine-needle point and bipolar forceps are used to prevent lateral heating of adjacent tissues. Silastic vessel loops are used to retract tendons and ligaments. The surgeon may use magnifying loupes or operating microscope during surgery.

Delicate tendons, ligaments, nerves, and blood vessels are critical for the precise movement of the hand. These tissues must be kept moist during surgery. The surgical technologist assisting in hand procedures irrigates the surgical wound with saline. A small bulb syringe or standard syringe fitted with an irrigation tip may be used. Low-pressure suction with fine-angled suction tips is used to prevent injury to the tissue. Neurosurgical patties and small gauze sponges dipped in saline are also required.

In reconstructive hand surgery, sutures are required for tendon, nerve, and ligament repair. These tissues must heal with as

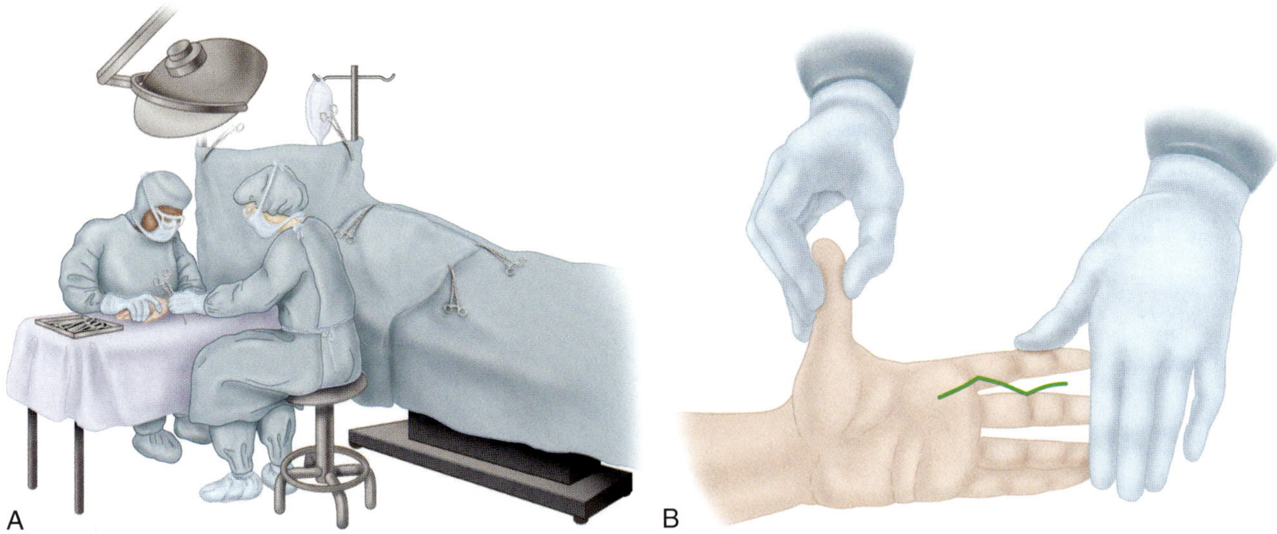

FIG. 29.31 Hand surgery is performed using a hand table. The surgeon and assistant sit across from each other.

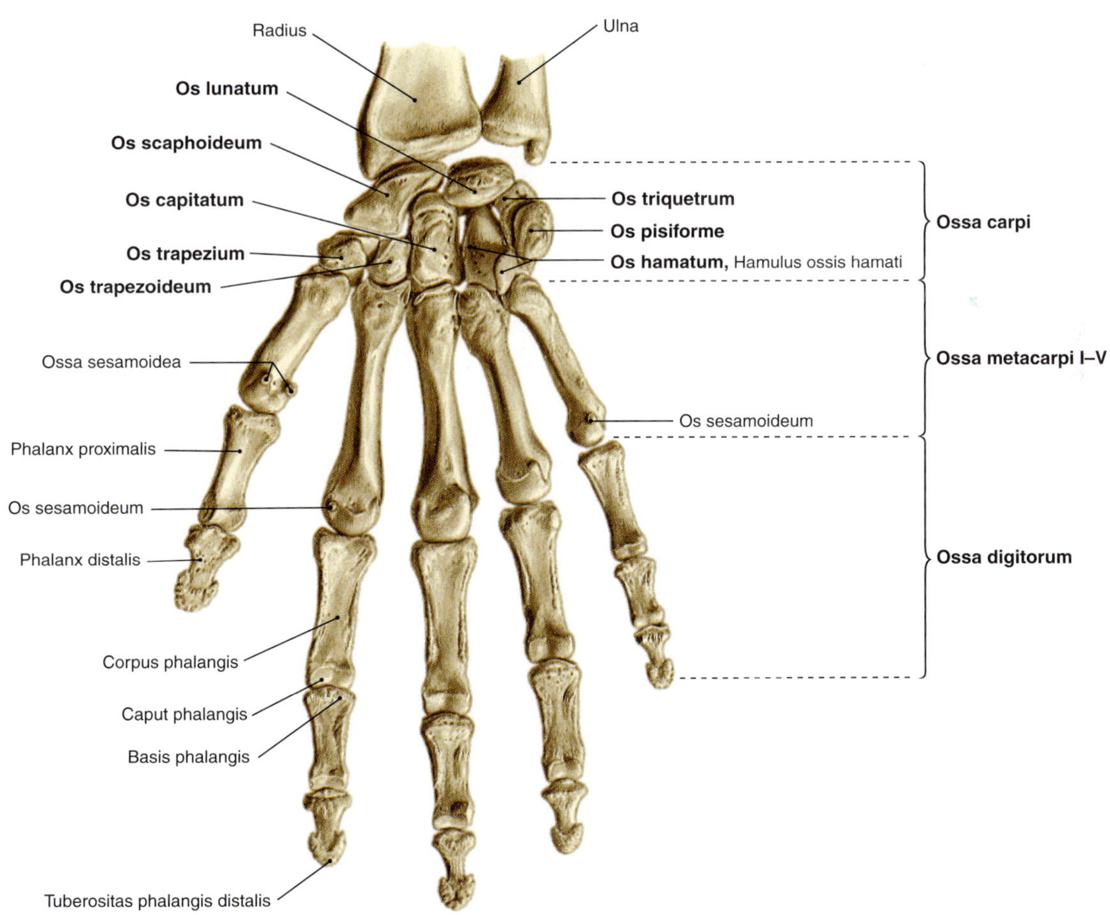

FIG. 29.32 Bones of the wrist and hand. (From Paulsen F. *Sobotta Atlas of Human Anatomy*. Vol 1. 15th ed. Munich, Germany: Elsevier GmbH; 2013.)

little scar formation as possible to preserve function. Inert suture materials, such as 6-0 and 7-0 polypropylene stainless steel, and polyester are commonly used. A fine ⅜ cutting curve is commonly used. Vascular sutures are required for trauma, reconstruction, and replantation, also called *reimplantation* (reattachment of a digit or a portion of the hand). Double-arm sutures are used for the anastomosis of vessels, tendons, and nerves.

NOTE *Procedures of the hand involving nerve repair are located in Chapter 34, Neurosurgery.*

Bones of the wrist and hand are shown in Fig. 29.32. Tendon sheaths of the hand are shown in Fig. 29.33.

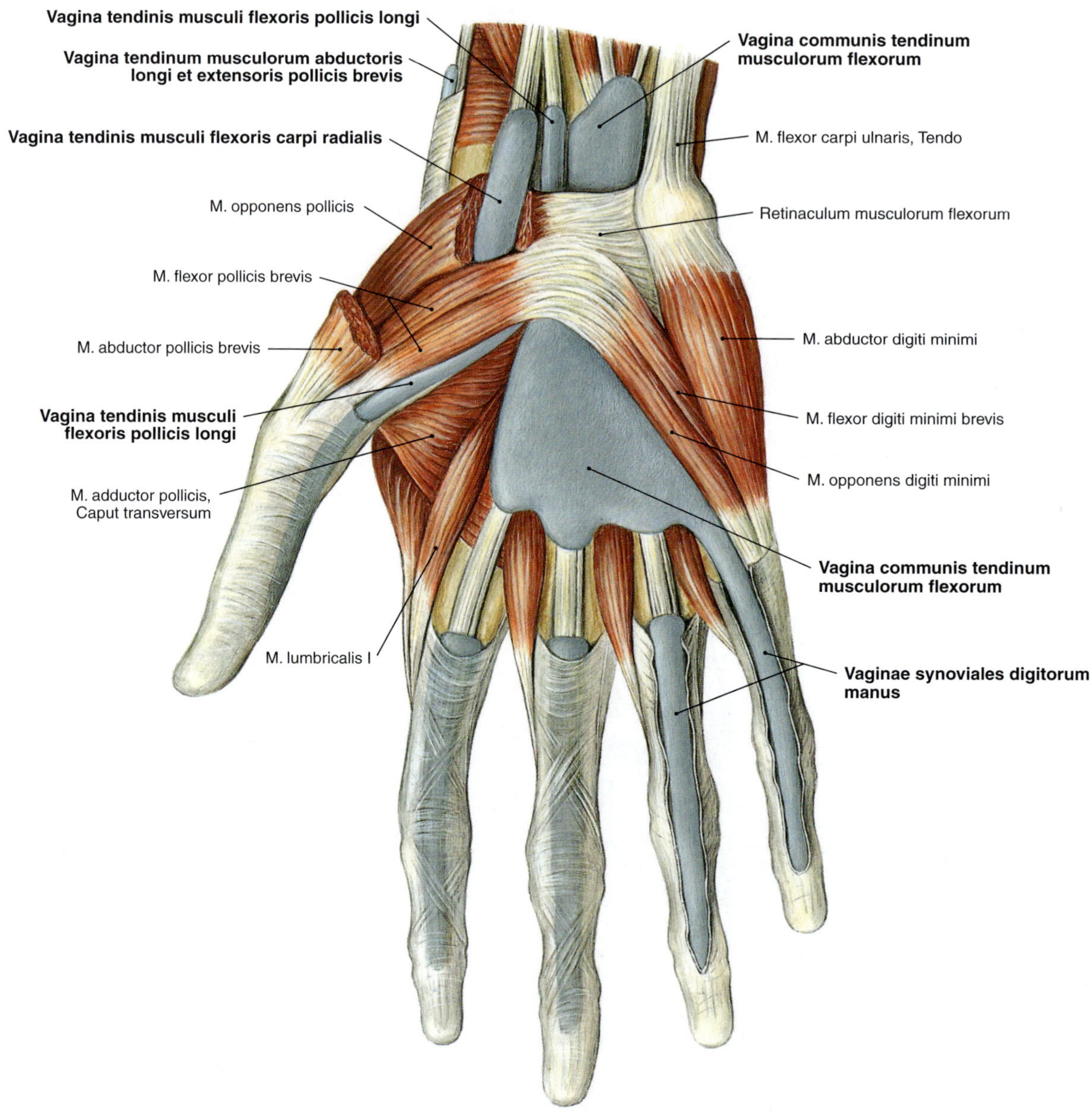

FIG. 29.33 Tendon sheaths of the hand. (From Paulsen F. *Sobotta Atlas of Human Anatomy*. Vol 1. 15th ed. Munich, Germany: Elsevier GmbH; 2013.)

OPEN REDUCTION AND INTERNAL FIXATION OF THE WRIST

Pathology

The scaphoid is the most common site of a wrist fracture because of its vulnerable location. A common cause of fracture is a fall when the wrists are flexed to break the impact. Simple nondisplaced fractures are treated with casting. Open reduction and internal fixation are required for a displaced or unstable fracture. One or more cannulated screws are used for the fixation of the scaphoid. The Herbert cannulated screw, the Synthes 3.0 cannulated screw, and the AO screw are surgical options. The procedure is done under fluoroscopic guidance.

POSITION:	Supine with affected arm on hand table; pneumatic tourniquet
INCISION:	Anterior longitudinal wrist
PREP AND DRAPING:	Forearm and hand; possible iliac crest for bone graft
INSTRUMENTS:	Hand instrument set; drill; K-wires; Herbert cannulation screw system; vessel loops
POSSIBLE EXTRAS:	Instruments for iliac bone graft

Technical Points and Discussion

1. ***The patient is positioned, prepped, and draped.***
The patient is placed in the supine position with the operative arm on a hand table. A tourniquet is applied, and the hand and arm are prepped and draped in a routine manner.
A rolled towel may be placed under the wrist to stabilize it or the hand may be placed in a distractor.

2. ***The entry incision is made.***
The surgeon makes a small incision over the scaphoid bone and inserts two rake retractors to expose the flexor carpi muscle. This is divided with a curved hemostat and scissors. The tendon sheath is incised, and the flexor tendon is isolated and refracted using a vessel loop. Depending on the approach, a branch of the radial artery may be encountered. This is divided and ligated with 3-0 or 4-0 non-absorbable suture. The joint capsule is then incised to expose the scaphoid bone. A small Weitlaner retractor is placed in the wound, and Hohmann small bone elevators are used to expose the fractured bone.

3. ***K-wires are placed through each section of the fractured bone.***
Using a small drill, the surgeon places K-wires through each pole of the fractured bone. These are used to manipulate the fragments and reduce the fracture.

4. ***The screw hole is drilled into the bone.***
The fracture is reduced under fluoroscopy to ensure correct alignment. For the placement of a cannulated screw, a threaded guidewire is inserted over the fracture site. A drill sleeve may be used to direct the wire at the correct angle. The screw hole may be pre-drilled with a small power drill and cannulated drill bit. A space for the threaded washer is also created.

5. ***The screw assembly is inserted.***
The washer is inserted with the cannulated driver. A measuring device similar to a drill tap is inserted over the guidewire to measure the depth of the pre-drilled hole and washer. The screw is threaded over the guidewire and tightened with a screwdriver. The guidewire is removed by using the power drill in a reverse mode.

6. ***The wound is closed.***
The wound is irrigated and closed in layers. The capsule is closed with a 4-0 synthetic absorbable suture. Skin and subcutaneous tissue are closed with 4-0 non-absorbable sutures. The wound is dressed with flat gauze. A plaster cast is usually applied over the wrist and arm.

RELEASE OF DUPUYTREN CONTRACTURE

Constricted palmar fascia is incised and released to restore mobility to the hand and fingers. A Bier block or general anesthetic may be used.

Pathology

A Dupuytren contracture is a condition in which the fascia of the palm or fingers contracts. The disorder has a strong familial component, and the deformity progresses rapidly.

POSITION:	Supine with affected arm on hand table
INCISION:	Palmar
PREP AND DRAPING:	Hand and arm prep and draping; pneumatic tourniquet
INSTRUMENTS:	Hand set

Technical Points and Discussion

1. ***The patient is positioned, prepped, and draped.***
The patient is placed in the supine position with the operative arm on an arm board. A pneumatic tourniquet is placed. The hand and lower arm are prepped and draped.

2. ***The contracture is released.***
The surgeon uses a #15 blade or Beaver blade to make the incision on the ulnar side of the palmar fascia, as well as the apex of the fascia. Tenotomy scissors and fine forceps or fasciotome are used to dissect the tissue and expose the tendons. After the tendons have been freed and the fingers can be moved without impingement, the tourniquet is released and the wound is checked for hemostasis and then irrigated. The skin is closed with interrupted non-absorbable sutures. A bulky compression dressing using gauze fluffs is applied.

HIP

As the number of people over the age of 60 years continues to increase in the United States, the number of hip surgeries has also increased. Falls continue to be a major contributor to hip fracture in older people. However, an increasing number of younger people are presented in surgery for hip fractures related to high-impact vehicle accidents.

Positioning for hip surgery is aided by the use of a fracture table (discussed earlier in the chapter), which places the affected leg in boot traction while allowing circumferential access to the hip for operative techniques and also for C-arm fluoroscopy (refer to Chapter 16 for additional photos). When the standard operating table is used, the patient can be placed in supine or lateral position. Fractures of the hip include the trochanter, femoral neck, femoral head, and acetabulum. The technique used in treatment depends on the degree of complexity, age of the patient, and level of activity expected after recovery. A combination of plates, heavy screws, and rods are commonly used in treatment. Hemiarthroplasty and total arthroplasty of the hip are now commonly performed with many new advances in materials and methods to provide short recovery times and a long-lasting repair.

FEMORAL NECK FRACTURE

A number of options are available for the surgical treatment of a fracture of the femoral neck (located across the trochanter or the neck itself). These include the following:

- Trochanteric fracture: Compression screw and plate system
- Femoral neck fracture: Dynamic compression screws
- Displaced fracture: Arthroplasty

A procedure using a compression screw and sliding plate is discussed here. C-arm fluoroscopy and an image intensifier are used intermittently during the procedure.

Pathology

The femoral neck is a common site of injury in a fall. The fracture may occur alone or may be accompanied by a fracture of the femur.

POSITION:	Fracture table supine with affected leg in traction; both legs in abduction
INCISION:	Lateral hip
PREP AND DRAPING:	Waist to ankle. Standard hip draping with impervious drapes and Ioban adhesive drape
INSTRUMENTS:	Major orthopedic set; drill, K-wires, Steinmann pins, plate system

Technical Points and Discussion

1. ***The patient is positioned, prepped, and draped.***
A general anesthetic is administered, and the patient is placed in position for traction using a fracture table (refer to Chapter 6 for a complete discussion of the fracture table). The fracture is reduced using boot traction, and the position is verified on fluoroscopy.

2. ***The entry incision is made.***
A lateral or posterolateral incision is used for the surgical treatment of a hip fracture. Rake retractors are placed in the wound, and the ESU is used to divide the subcutaneous tissue and fascia. The muscle is then divided and retracted. Richardson, Army-Navy, Hibbs, or Deaver retractors may be used for deep retraction.

3. ***A guide pin is inserted.***
A guide pin is inserted to establish the correct angle for the trochanter compression screw and plate. A Steinmann (guide) pin and drill are used for this purpose. The guide pin remains in place during most of the procedure, and cannulated instruments are inserted over it. For the insertion of the guide pin, a 6.4-mm drill bit is used to make a pilot hole in line with the femoral neck. An angle guide is used to obtain the correct angle of the guide pin. The pin is then drilled following the angle of the guide and viewed under fluoroscopy.

4. ***A cannulated reamer is fitted over the pin.***
Next, the depth of the guide pin is determined with a cannulated depth gauge. An appropriately sized reamer is used to drill over the guide pin according to the depth gauge measurement. This is the starter channel, or *tap.* A long reamer designed for lag screw insertion is calibrated for the channel, which then is reamed to the appropriate depth. The reamer is cannulated and fits over the guidewire during this process.

5. ***The pin angle is verified with a trial plate.***
The angle of the pin may be checked using a trial plate. The size should be verified with the surgeon before the sterile implant is opened. The ST may receive the plate from the circulator at this time.

6. ***The lag screw and plate are inserted.***
The lag screw is inserted with or without pre-tapping. A calibrated tap drill (reamer) is used as necessary, and the reading is taken from the back of the tap. The surgeon then determines the correct size for the lag screw. The plate component is fitted into the lag screw inserter, and the T-handle and lag screw are inserted into the assembly. The assembled unit is placed over the guide pin and into the prepared channel. The surgeon advances the lag screw and plate barrel. The guide pin is removed, and the traction is released.

7. ***The side plate is installed.***
The ST should prepare a drill, drill guide, and drill bit for attaching the side plate to the femur. The surgeon then drills the holes and measures them with a depth gauge. The ST selects the correct size of screw and passes it with the screwdriver. When the side screws have been placed, an impactor may be used to secure the plate barrel. A compression screw is inserted into the tube and tightened by hand. This brings the femoral neck fragments into contact. The compression screw is then removed.

8. ***The wound is closed.***
The wound is irrigated and checked for bleeders. A suction or gravity drain may be placed in the wound before closure. The muscle is closed with 2-0 or 3-0 interrupted absorbable synthetic sutures. The fascia is closed with the running suture of the same material. Subcutaneous tissue is closed with 3-0 absorbable sutures, and the skin is approximated with staples. A compression dressing consisting of flat gauze and an abdominal pad is placed over the incision. A triangular pad is placed between the legs to splint them and keep the hip abducted.

The patient is usually able to begin weight bearing within 24 hours after surgery. Patients are discharged as soon as they can walk over a level surface, climb several steps, and get into and out of bed.

Technical points of the procedure are shown in Fig. 29.34.

TOTAL HIP ARTHROPLASTY

The goal of hip arthroplasty is to replace diseased components of the hip joint, including the acetabulum, trochanter, and ball of the femur, with one or more artificial implants. Many surgical approaches can be used for hip arthroplasty. Aside from variations in the implant design, the main technical differences important to the surgical technologist are as follows:

- One or both components of the hip joint may be replaced.
- The implants may be cemented or press-fitted.
- One or two incisions may be used for the surgical approach.

The surgical options are chosen on the basis of the patient's *physiological* age and desired level of activity after surgery, the condition of the bone, and the surgeon's specific training. The following procedure is based on a traditional approach to non-cemented hip arthroplasty as a basis for

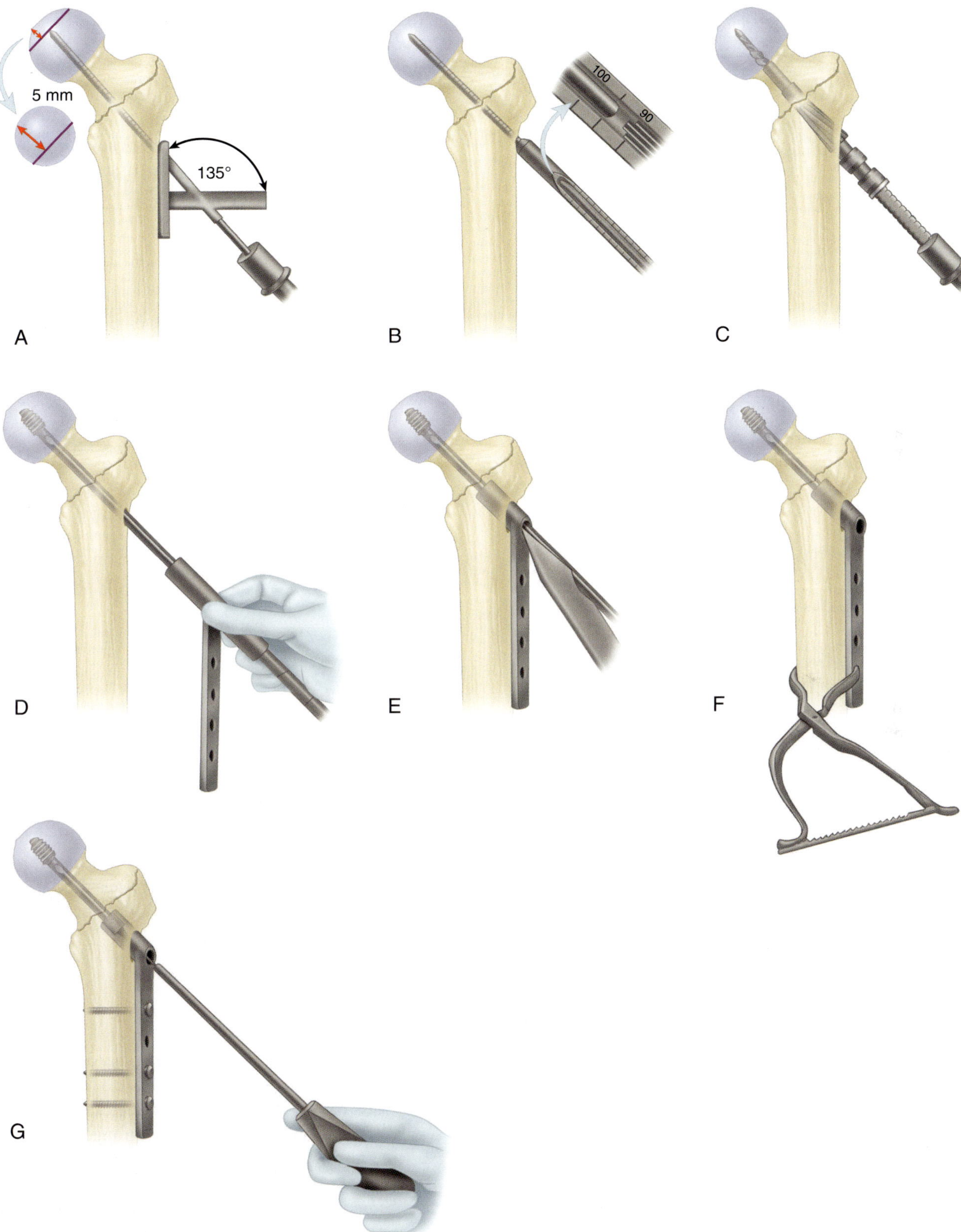

FIG. 29.34 Repair of intertrochanteric fracture. (A) A pin is inserted through the femur using a guide. (B) A depth gauge is placed anteriorly along the femoral neck to measure depth. (C) A reamer is used to place the hole for the nail. (D) The lag screw is inserted with the plate to the correct depth. (E) The side plate is advanced to make contact with the bone. (F) A plate or bone clamp is used to secure the plate. (G) Bicortical screws are used to fix the plate. (From Canale S, Beaty J, eds. *Campbell's Operative Orthopaedics*. 12th ed. Philadelphia: Mosby; 2013.)

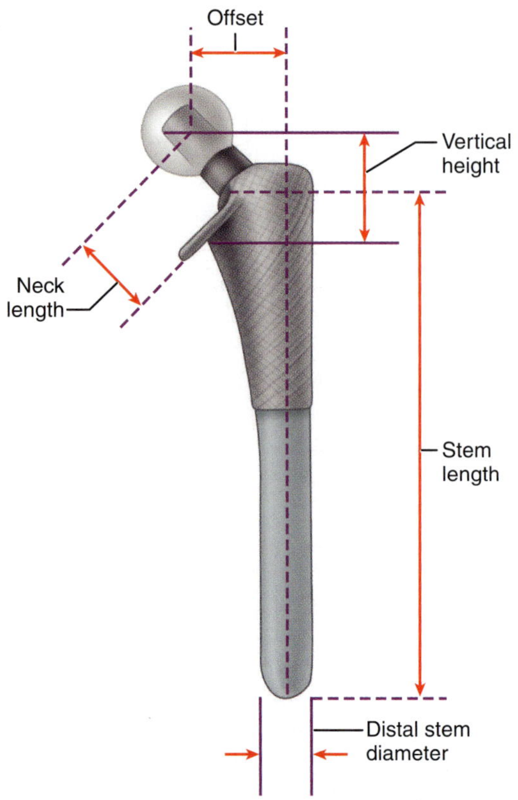

FIG. 29.35 Modern femoral hip component. (From Azar F. *Campbell's Operative Orthopaedics*. 13th ed. Philadelphia: Elsevier; 2017.)

more specific training required by a surgical facility and its surgeons. A posterolateral approach to the femur is used. As with all orthopedic systems, it is very important that the instruments specific to that system are used. Each system has its own training manuals, which instruct the user on the use of the instruments.

Hip Components

Modular implant systems for hip arthroplasty include the following components:

- *Femoral component:* Includes the stem, neck, and head. The neck is usually adjustable for angle (called the *offset*) and length. The femoral component may be press-fitted or cemented.
- *Acetabular components:* Includes an acetabular liner, which is seated into the prepared acetabulum, and a shell, which fits into the liner. The outside of the shell may be spiked or smooth, or it may have drill holes for screws.

There are many different types and styles of hip arthroplasty components. Like all other orthopedic systems, each manufacturer offers a variety of components and instrumentation required for their implantation. Nearly all systems are modular—that is, the parts that make up the joint component can be selected to meet the specific anatomical and medical needs of the patient. Fig. 29.35 illustrates the features of the femoral component.

Pathology

Hip arthroplasty is performed to treat a number of arthritic conditions:

- *Osteoarthritis:* Results in the loss of cartilage and eventual erosion of bone. The disease is usually associated with the aging process.
- *Osteonecrosis:* Death of bone and marrow tissue, usually related to trauma or disease
- *Acetabular fracture:* Hip trauma, commonly associated with falls and motor vehicle accidents
- *Femoral neck fracture:* Commonly associated with falls
- *Avascular necrosis:* Death of bone tissue related to the interruption of blood supply to the hip

POSITION:	Lateral or supine
INCISION:	Anterolateral
PREP AND DRAPING:	Waist to knee prep. Standard hip draping including a pouch drape for fluid runoff
INSTRUMENTS:	Major orthopedic set with hip instruments; bone hooks; bone clamps; chisels; osteotomes; drill and drill bits; hip replacement components including sizers, bone-cutting instruments, measuring devices, impactor, screwdrivers; broaches
POSSIBLE EXTRAS:	Bone cement and mixing apparatus with exhaust system

Technical Points and Discussion

1. ***The patient is positioned, prepped, and draped.***
The patient is placed in the lateral position using a bean bag positioner. The skin is prepped from the waist to the foot. Draping exposes the hip and thigh. The foot is not exposed but is wrapped in sterile towels so that the hip and leg can be manipulated during the procedure. The lower leg may be draped with impervious tube stockinet. An incise drape impregnated with iodophor antiseptic is used to cover the operative site.

2. ***The entry incision is made.***
A posterolateral incision is made using a #10 knife. The ESU is used to deepen the incision. Initially, medium Richardson or similar retractors are placed in the wound edges. The subcutaneous tissue and fascia lata are divided along with the fascia covering of the gluteus maximum. The ST should have ample dry lap sponges and suction available during this part of the procedure. The edges of the fascia are dissected bluntly. At this stage, moist lap sponges may be sutured to the edge of the fascia to collect bits of cement and tissue debris during the procedure. A Charnley or other self-retaining retractor can be inserted at this level. Dissection is continued to expose underlying muscle.
At this level the surgeon may request size 2-0 nonabsorbent tag sutures to place in the tendons for identification later in the procedure. As dissection continues,

blunt cobra or Hohmann retractors may be required. The capsule is divided and retracted. The patient's leg length may be measured at this point. The teres ligament ruptures during avulsion. However, if it does not, it must be severed to release the femoral head.

3. ***The hip is dislocated.***
The hip is then dislocated by flexing, adducting, and internally rotating the hip. A bone hook is placed under the femoral neck to lift the head out of the acetabulum. Once the hip is dislocated, the femur can be delivered into the wound. A broad flat retractor is required for this.

NOTE *If the hip cannot be dislocated, the femoral neck is divided with an oscillating saw and the femoral head removed.*

5. ***The femoral neck is divided.***
The next step is the osteotomy (bone cut), in which the femoral head is removed. First, the surgeon marks the osteotomy site using the ESU or osteotome. The ST should prepare a narrow-width oscillating or reciprocating blade and power saw and bulb syringe irrigation. The saw is then used to divide the femoral neck. The assistant irrigates the cutting site during the osteotomy.
The ST receives the femoral head, which is set aside on the back table and preserved with moist saline sponges. The ST should stand close to the operating table when receiving the specimen to prevent it from dropping to the floor. The humeral head may be required for bone grafting later in the procedure.

6. ***The acetabulum is prepared for the implant.***
To prepare the acetabulum for the implant, the surgeon passes a curved clamp within the sheath of the psoas muscle. A large bone hook is used to retract the femur. The capsule is then divided. Additional cobra or Hohmann retractors are needed for exposure.
The surgeon trims any loose tissue or (bony spurs) from the rim of the joint. An osteotome, knife, and curette are used to remove the tissue.
The surgeon then dishes out the surface of the acetabulum using power-operated reamers in graduated sizes. Irrigation fluid should be available for the surgeon's assistant. The ST should clean excess tissue from the reamers and broaches between uses. A basin of sterile water should be available for this.

7. ***The acetabular component is inserted.***
Before the acetabular component is inserted, it may be necessary to prepare the bone for fixation devices required for a specific component. This is done following the manufacturer's specifications. The acetabulum component is attached to the positioning rod that is included in the system. The size of the component is the same as the size of the last reamer used.
The acetabular component is impacted by hand using a mallet or slap hammer. The area is irrigated to remove any tissue debris. Finally, the polyethylene liner is inserted according to the system design and specifications.

8. ***The femoral medullary space is reamed.***
To prepare the femoral side of the joint, the surgeon creates an intramedullary space in the femur to accept the femoral stem. The exact depth of the space may be determined before surgery by comparing the radiograph with a transparent template. The surgeon may measure the femur again before reaming. A hand awl or "cookie cutter" is used to start the opening for the femoral canal. This is followed by broaches or power reamers. The broach is impacted into the canal with a mallet or slap hammer and guide, which is fitted over the broach. Broaches are used in successively larger sizes. Immersing the rasps in a basin of water is helpful for removing tissue debris from the instruments after each use. A precision reamer is sometimes used to plane the end surface of the femur. If this is required, the broach handle is removed and the planer attached.

9. ***A trial femoral head is inserted.***
In the next phase of the procedure, a trial femoral head is tested for fit. In most systems, the trial head is fitted onto the broach. The hip is then reduced and assessed. The hip is dislocated, and the femoral component and neck are implanted. If a broach is still in place, it is removed.

10. ***The femoral component is inserted.***
Before the femoral component is inserted, the medullary canal is irrigated to remove any loose debris. The component is then gently impacted with the device provided in the system.
The femoral head component is seated using a plastic-capped impactor. The hip is then reduced.

11. ***The wound is closed.***
The wound is thoroughly irrigated, and bleeders are checked. A closed suction drainage system can be placed at this point. The capsule is closed using heavy non-absorbable sutures placed using the holes previously made in the trochanter. in the of the trochanter. The tagged tendons are reattached, and any large muscles that were divided are repaired with interrupted sutures of the surgeon's choice of size and material. The fascia is closed using interrupted synthetic sutures. The subcutaneous layer can be closed with interrupted absorbable sutures and the skin closed with staples or other sutures of the surgeon's choice. A flat dressing with abdominal pad is placed over the wound and the drain secured to the skin with a non-absorbable

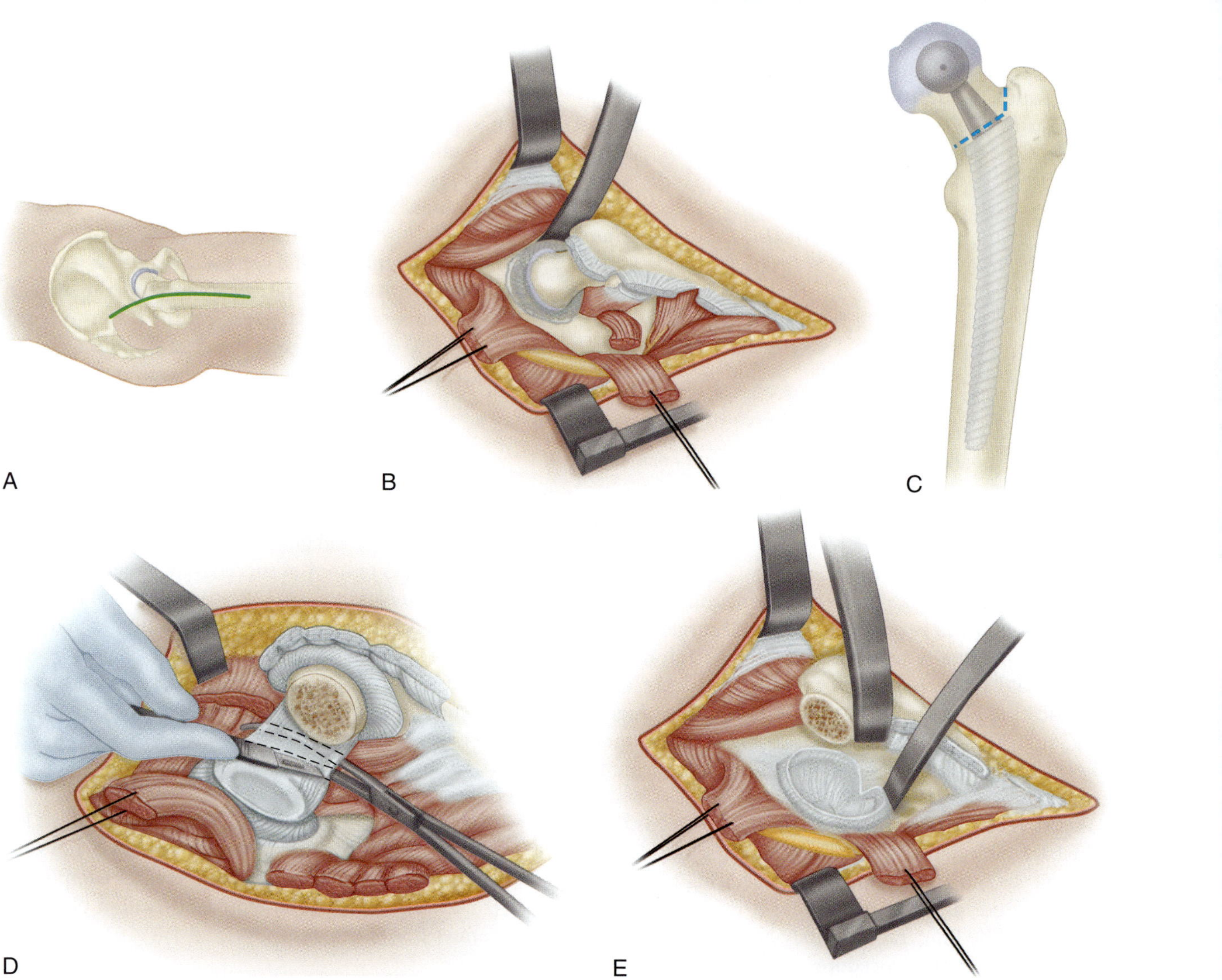

FIG. 29.36 Incisions for total hip arthroplasty. (A) Posterolateral skin incision. (B) Dissection in soft tissue completed. (C) Femoral neck osteotomy (cut). (D) Anterior capsule divided. (E) Femur is retracted for access to acetabulum. (From Azar F. *Campbell's Operative Orthopaedics*. 13th ed. Philadelphia: Elsevier; 2017.)

suture. Important technical points are shown in Figs. 29.36 and 29.37.

Patients are closely monitored for hemorrhage and embolism after arthroplasty. Deep vein thrombosis or a fat embolism may occur in the immediate postoperative period or weeks after surgery. Patients are encouraged to begin walking within 24 hours of surgery.

FRACTURE OF THE PELVIS

An unstable pelvic fracture can be life threatening and is treated as soon as possible after the trauma. The mortality rate for pelvic fractures can approach 35% in open fractures. The high mortality rate is associated with uncontrollable retroperitoneal hemorrhage and other life-threatening injuries.

Patients arrive in surgery with a rigid or soft pelvic binder in place to limit the movement of fractured bones, which can extend the injuries. A simple stabilizing surgery using an external pelvic clamp is the preferred method so that soft tissue injuries such as bladder rupture can be attended to first. More complex procedures are performed after the patient is stabilized. All assessment scans must be available during surgery. These may include CT scans, MRI scans, contrast angiogram, and cystogram. If the patient arrives in traction, weights are attached to the operating table until reduction is secured.

The surgical technologist and circulating nurse are informed about instrumentation for internal or external fixation. However, the decision may be changed during surgery. This procedure involves an anterior repair using a reconstruction plate. Fig. 29.38 illustrates important technical points of the procedure.

Open reduction is the preferred method of repair of an unstable fracture. A number of surgical options for fixation are available on the basis of the location of the fracture:

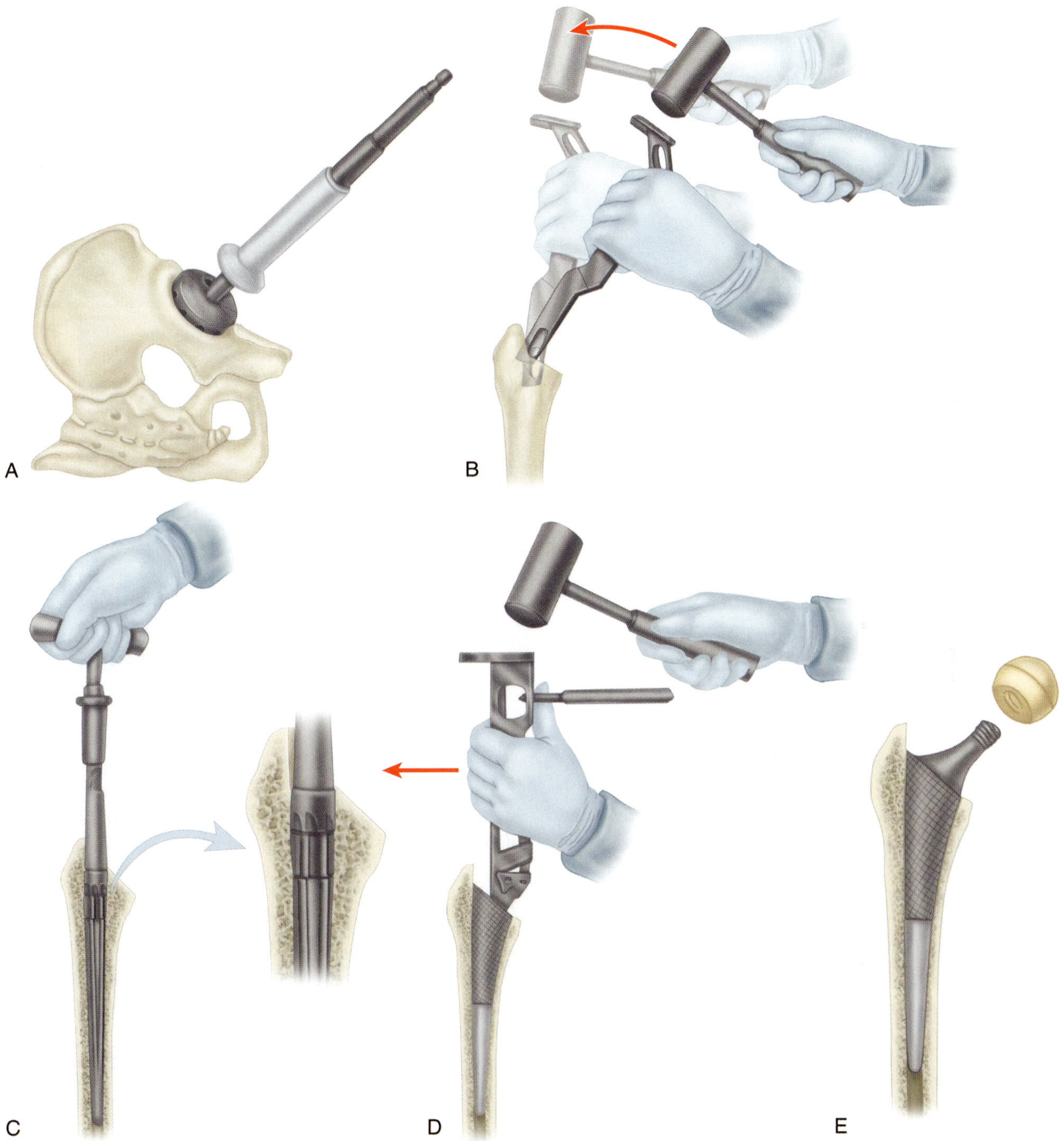

FIG. 29.37 Key technical points in total hip arthroplasty (non-cemented). Refer to text for discussions. (A) Reaming the acetabulum. (B) Broaching the acetabulum. (C) Reaming the femoral canal. (D) Broaching the femoral canal. (E) Assembly of trial head and femoral neck segments. (From Azar F. *Campbell's Operative Orthopaedics*. 13th ed. Philadelphia: Elsevier; 2017.)

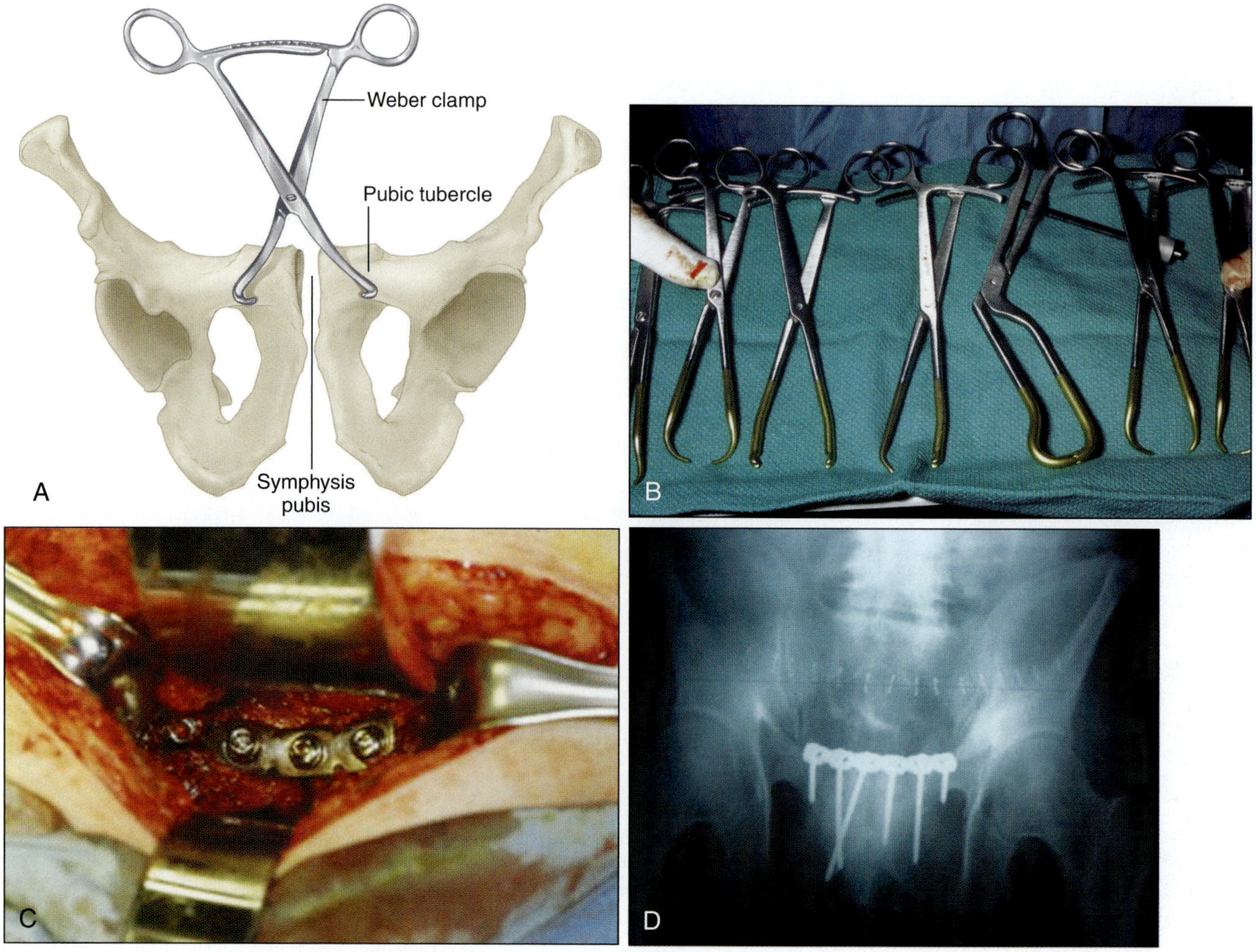

FIG. 29.38 Internal fixation of anterior pelvic fracture. (A) A Weber clamp is used to maintain the reduction of the symphysis. (B) Assortment of Weber clamps used for pelvic fractures. (C) Fixation of the fracture using a reconstruction plate. (D) X-ray of repair. (From Schemitsch E, McKee M, eds. *Operative Techniques: Orthopedic Trauma Surgery*. Philadelphia: Saunders; 2010.)

- Fracture of the ilium is fixed internally with lag screws and fragment plates.
- Surgical options for the fracture of the pubic rami are percutaneous pins or internally placed screws.
- Sacral fracture is treated with plates, screws, or rods. External fixation with a rod and pin system may also be used.
- Fracture of the symphysis pubis can be repaired using one or more reconstruction plates.
- A definitive procedure such as the following one described is performed after the patient has been stabilized in an external fixation device. Refer to Chapter 35 for a discussion on the stabilization of trauma patients.

Pathology

Fractures of the pelvis are often the result of a high-impact trauma and frequently are accompanied by significant injury to the genitalia, intra-abdominal, urological, and neurovascular structures.

A type B fracture of the symphysis *(open book)* is presented here. In this injury, the symphysis is split resulting in rotation instability and deformity and may include fracture of the sacroiliac joint. This can result in an opening out of the pelvis, hence the name *open book fracture*.

POSITION:	Supine with legs in internal rotation
INCISION:	Pfannenstiel
PREP AND DRAPING:	Lower margin of rib cage to base of pubis; Foley catheter; laparotomy draping
INSTRUMENTS:	Major orthopedic including pelvic clamps; curved or dynamic compression plate set; drill; laparotomy set
POSSIBLE EXTRAS:	Intestinal instruments; genitourinary instruments

Technical Points and Discussion

1. ***The patient is position, prepped, and draped.***
   The patient is placed in supine position on the operating table with both legs in internal rotation. A Foley catheter

is necessary, although in most cases this will have been inserted previously. The skin prep extends from the lower margins of the rib cage to the base of the pubis. Draping follows a laparotomy technique.

2. ***The entry incision is made.***
A long Pfannenstiel (lower vertical) incision is made just above the symphysis pubis using a #10 or #20 knife. The incision is extended deeper using the ESU to the level of the rectus sheath.

Right-angle retractors can be placed at this level. The linea alba is incised lengthwise, exposing the space of Retzius, which is developed using blunt dissection. The bladder is protected using a ribbon retractor and moist lap tapes. The rectus abdominis muscle is retracted, and the insertion into the pubic body is elevated with a periosteal or Cobb elevator.

3. ***The fracture is reduced.***
To reduce the anterior fracture, a Weber clamp is placed, inserted into both pubic tubercles. It may be necessary to insert 4.5-mm screws into each pubic body. Both screws are grasped in the jaws of a pelvic reduction clamp. As the jaws are closed, the two pubic bodies are drawn together. The clamp is also used to manipulate and reduce any external rotation displacement. Reduction is confirmed on fluoroscopy.

4. ***The fracture is fixated.***
A contoured, four- to six-hole 3.5-mm reconstruction plate is used to fixate the fracture. The plate is placed over one pubic ramus. An appropriate size drill bit and sleeve are used to drill the first medial hole. The hole is measured using a depth gauge. The second medial hole is drilled on the opposite side of the fracture using the same technique. Screws are inserted using a handheld screwdriver. Locking screws may be required. The repair is checked on fluoroscopy. If necessary, a posterior repair is made using a single sacroiliac screw.

5. ***The wound is closed.***
Before the wound is closed, a suction drain (Jackson-Pratt or Hemovac) is placed in the retropubic space. The rectus abdominis muscle is repaired with interrupted non-absorbable sutures of size 0. The subcutaneous layer is closed with interrupted absorbable synthetic sutures. The skin is closed with interrupted nylon or Prolene sutures, or skin staples may be used. The wound is dressed using bulky gauze.

Depending on the extent of soft tissue and organ trauma, the patient is only partially mobile for approximately 6 weeks. Postoperative complications include embolism, infection, and chronic pain.

INTRAMEDULLARY FEMORAL NAILING

A femoral shaft fracture can be repaired with an intramedullary femoral nail. A femoral nail is a rigid rod that is seated in the medullary canal and held in position with locking screws placed at a 90-degree angle to the nail. The procedure can be done using open (incision) or closed (no incision) technique. Antegrade (insertion of the nail at the proximal end of the bone) or retrograde (insertion of the nail at the distal end of the bone) can be used. Closed antegrade intramedullary nailing is presented here.

Pathology

The femoral shaft fracture is among the most common injuries of the leg. The intramedullary technique for repairing a femoral fracture may be used for a comminuted fracture or a proximal and distal fracture.

POSITION:	Supine with knee flexed at 30 degrees or held in abduction
INCISION:	Lateral hip
PREP AND DRAPING:	Waist to knee prep; standard hip draping
INSTRUMENTS:	Major orthopedic set; hip retractors, drill, Steinmann pin set, femoral nailing system

Technical Points and Discussion

1. ***The patient is positioned, prepped, and draped.***
The patient is placed in the supine position on the fracture table with the affected hip flexed 15 to 30 degrees. Traction is applied using the traction boot. The position is verified on fluoroscopy. The prep includes the knee, hip, thigh, buttock, and trunk, including the axilla. Draping is standard, using a large U-drape that extends to the knee.

2. ***The entry incision is made.***
An incision is made over the trochanter and carried through the subcutaneous, fascial, and muscle layers. Richardson or large rake retractors can be used to expose the trochanter. The fracture may be reduced by manual manipulation or by using a bone hook.

3. ***A guidewire is inserted.***
An awl may be used to form the entry points in the medullary canal. A threaded guidewire is inserted into the trochanter and verified by fluoroscopy. The guidewire is then advanced.

4. ***The medullary canal is prepared for reaming.***
To prepare for medullary reaming, a cannula (metal sleeve) and bushing are placed over the guidewire. The cannula is advanced over the guidewire until it is seated. A cannulated reamer is inserted over the pin to the trochanter. The guidewire is then replaced with a ball tip wire, which is manipulated into the canal beyond the fracture site. A cannulated nail length gauge is used to measure the depth of the canal. Fluoroscopy is used to assess the position and depth.

5. ***The medullary canal is reamed.***
Graduated intramedullary reamers are used to increase the space for nail insertion. The technologist should have several reamers of incremental sizes ready for this part of the procedure; sizes 8 to 17 mm in 0.5-mm increments should be available. The first reamer is an 8-mm end-cutting reamer.

6. ***The intramedullary nail is inserted.***
When the medullary canal has been prepared, the correct nail is selected and prepared on the back table. An interlocking nail guide is used to align the cross-screw position in the nail. A driver and slap hammer attachment are used to drive the nail into the canal while the nail guide maintains the correct position. The nail is driven into the medullary canal, and the driver is disengaged. Nail caps, if used, are inserted by hand at this time with a nail cap inserter.

7. ***The screws are placed.***
A screw guide with protective bushing is inserted into the targeting device, and the proximal screw holes are drilled. A depth gauge is used to measure the holes, and the appropriately sized screws are placed through the bone and nail by hand. A freehand targeting device is used to locate the distal screw hole using fluoroscopy. The targeting device is positioned over the distal nail hole, and a combination trocar-drill is used to penetrate the bone through the targeting device. The position is confirmed with fluoroscopy. An incision is made over the trocar, and the nail hole is located with a hemostat. The trocar is centered in the nail hole, and the hole is completed. A depth gauge is used to measure the drill hole, and the appropriate-size screw is inserted and hand-tightened.

8. ***The wound is closed.***
The position of the nail and screws is assessed, and the wound is irrigated. All tissue debris is removed from the wound and any potential bleeders are checked with the ESU. The wound is closed with interrupted absorbable synthetic sutures and skin staples. A flat dressing is placed over the incision.

NOTE *The techniques used in this procedure closely follow those used in intramedullary nailing, which is discussed later in this chapter.*

Related Procedure: Repair of a Supracondylar Fracture

Distal femoral fractures may be repaired using a lag screw–plate combination. The techniques described previously are used for this procedure. The patient is placed in the supine position with the operative flank raised slightly for better exposure of the distal femur.

KNEE

The knee is the most complicated joint of the body. It is vulnerable to a variety of injuries, which are caused mainly by sports and motor vehicle accidents. The knee is the largest joint, and it carries a great deal of body weight, especially when in motion. It also has the longest mechanical levers of the body. Pathogenic conditions in the knee are often very disabling because of the weight-bearing function of the joint. The joint is divided into separate compartments, which are created by the structures contained within it. However, no separate fibrous capsule binds the joint together. The ligaments and tendons surround the two joints that make up the knee: the tibiofemoral joint and the patellofemoral joint. The patella forms a part of the knee joint on the anterior side. The *menisci* (single—meniscus) separate the femoral and tibial condyles and provide shock absorption (Fig. 29.39).

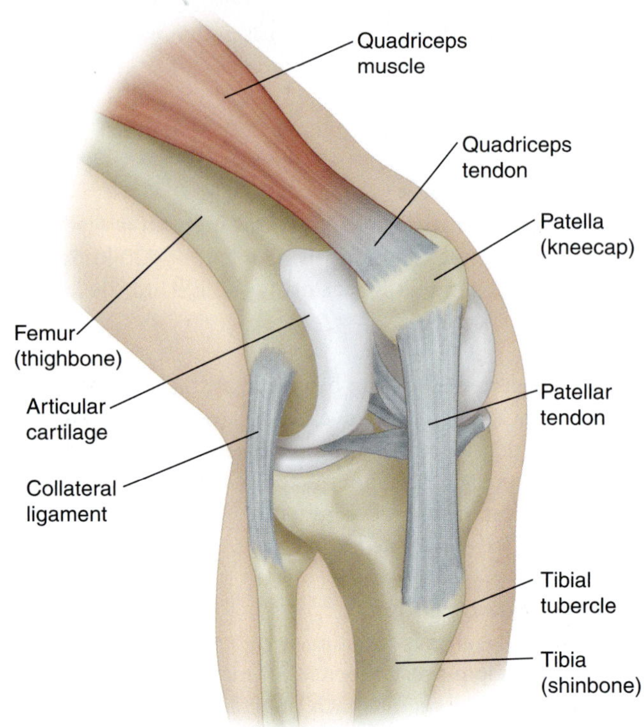

FIG. 29.39 Anatomy of the knee. (From Schemitsch E, McKee M. *Operative Techniques: Orthopaedic Trauma Surgery.* Philadelphia: Elsevier; 2020.)

Many procedures of the knee are approached endoscopically. The open technique is most often used with a parapatellar, medial, lateral, or posterior approach.

KNEE ARTHROSCOPY

Knee arthroscopy is a common technique for assessing and correcting problems arising from injury and disease. Diagnostic arthroscopy can take place just before a definitive procedure or as a stand-alone operation. The procedure may be performed under local anesthesia with sedation. General anesthesia is used for more complex procedures.

IRRIGATION

Lactated Ringer solution is used in the irrigation system to extend the knee spaces and to flush debris from the wound.

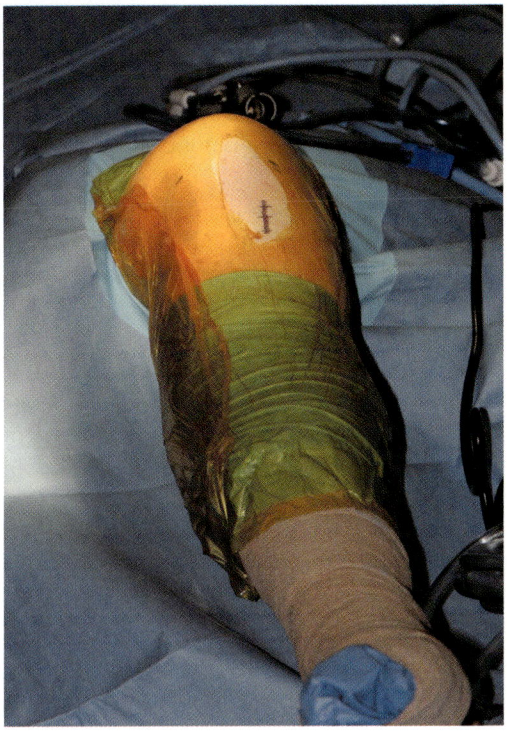

FIG. 29.40 Knee arthroscopy draping. (From Azar F. *Campbell's Operative Orthopaedics*. 13th ed. Philadelphia: Elsevier; 2017.)

The inflow may be directed through the scope or through a separate dedicated cannula. Irrigation fluid is suspended and pulled through a pump or allowed to feed by gravity. Five-liter bags of solution are placed 3 to 4 feet above the joint. The basic steps of knee arthroscopy are presented here.

POSITION:	Supine. The operative leg may rest on a leg holder or may be placed off the lateral edge of the operating table
INCISION:	Port sites
PREP AND DRAPING:	Prep mid-thigh to mid-ankle; draping for knee exposure with lower leg excluded with secure drapes
INSTRUMENTS:	Knee arthroscopy set including cutdown instruments; surgeon's choice of trocars and cannulas; a 4-mm 30-degree scope

Technical Points and Discussion

1. ***The patient is positioned, prepped, and draped.***

The patient is placed in supine position. The operative leg may be placed in leg support or positioned off the lateral side of the table. A third option is to lower the bottom table break and allow both legs to dangle over the edge. This provides the greatest flexibility for moving the joint through various positions during the surgery. The surgeon may mark the port sites in the skin. A pneumatic tourniquet is placed at the upper thigh. For short diagnostic procedures the tourniquet may not be necessary. The operative leg is prepped from the mid-thigh to ankle and draped using routine orthopedic procedure with split sheets, body drape, and impervious Ioban at the operative site. The foot and lower leg is wrapped in sterile towels and covered with a stockinet and adhesive drape (Fig. 29.40).

2. ***The ports are placed.***

A stab incision is made with a #11 blade lateral to the patella and just above the joint line, allowing an inflow cannula to be inserted into the knee joint without damaging the cartilage.

When the knee has been infiltrated with fluid, a second incision is made medially, and a sharp trocar and sheath are inserted into the knee joint. The trocar is then removed and replaced with a blunt trocar. The knee is irrigated, any fluid is removed, and a 30-degree scope is inserted.

An 18-gauge spinal needle is inserted into the knee joint under direct visualization to determine the placement of a third incision. This incision creates an opposite portal for the insertion of the probe and operative instruments. The exact location of this incision depends on the type of surgery to be performed. During complex procedures in which the cannulas are exchanged frequently, a "switching stick" is inserted within the cannula to hold its place while another cannula is placed.

3. ***The knee is explored.***

A systematic assessment of the knee joint is carried out during diagnostic or preoperative arthroscopy. This requires the manipulation of the knee through many different positions to open up the spaces. A probe is often used to palpate the tissues.

4. ***A definitive procedure is performed.***

If arthroscopy is the basis of a definitive procedure, it is started soon after the evaluation of the joint. At the close of the procedure, the trocars are removed and individual port sites are closed and dressed.

ARTHROSCOPIC MENISCECTOMY

The meniscus is a horseshoe-shaped cartilage that distributes load across the joint and creates stability. A tear in the meniscus is the most common knee injury. The medial meniscus is injured more often than the lateral meniscus. Meniscectomy may be partial or complete. Complete meniscectomy leaves the medial rim of the structure to share load bearing and stabilize the knee.

When the meniscus is in view, the surgeon locates the tear with a probe. The attachment of the meniscus is divided with a hook knife. A motorized shaver is used to remove frayed edges from the cartilage. Complete removal, if required, is performed with meniscus knives and scissors.

CRUCIATE LIGAMENT REPAIR

The goal of surgery is to repair a torn anterior **cruciate** ligament (ACL) and restore the stability of the joint. A graft is taken from the central portion of the patellar tendon to replace the torn ACL. Other graft sites include the hamstring or quadriceps tendon. The graft is secured by passing it through tunnels made in the tibia and femur and attached with sutures or biosynthetic interference screws, which prevent the graft from being pulled out of the tunnels.

Pathology

The ACL stabilizes the knee in the anterior-posterior position, preventing buckling of the knee. It crosses the center of the knee joint, attaching to the femur superiorly and the tibia inferiorly. ACL tears usually occur during a twisting motion of the leg, often during sports or other strenuous activity.

POSITION:	Supine; the foot of the table may be lowered
INCISION:	Patellar
PREP AND DRAPING:	Knee
INSTRUMENTS:	Knee set; ACL system instruments, including cannulated burrs, guidewires, and attachment devices (e.g., interference screws); microsagittal saw; motorized arthroscopy shaver; minor soft tissue set with right-angle retractors

Technical Points and Discussion

1. ***The patient is positioned, prepped, and draped.***
The patient is placed in supine position on the operating table with the operative knee flexed over the lower table break, which is flexed downward. A pneumatic tourniquet is positioned on the upper thigh. The affected leg is prepped from the foot to mid-thigh. The knee is draped in a routine fashion.

2. ***Diagnostic arthroscopy is performed.***

3. ***The entry incision is made.***
An anterior incision is made over the patellar tendon using a #10 knife. Subcutaneous tissue is divided with the ESU. Small rake retractors are used at the wound edges. Metzenbaum scissors are then used to separate the paratenon, which lies directly over the tendon. This exposes the patellar tendon. Army-Navy retractors should be available to expose the joint.

4. ***The graft is removed from the central patellar tendon.***
A disposable double-bladed knife or #15 knife blade is used to notch out a section of tendon, which remains attached to the patella at the upper pole and the tibia at the lower pole. An oscillating saw is then used to cut through the bone at each end of the graft. A 0.25-inch (0.63-cm) osteotome is used to divide the bone plugs at each end. This produces a strip of tendon with small bone plugs attached at each end. The ST should have a small basin to receive the graft, which is moved to the back table for preparation. The graft should be kept in a basin with lactated Ringer solution and antibiotic.

5. ***The graft is prepared.***
The bone ends are trimmed with a small, single-action rongeur. The ST must preserve any bone chips in a basin with a small amount of saline because they may be replaced in the wound when the graft is placed. The surgeon passes the graft through a 10-mm sizer tube to try the graft and ensure that it fits. The bone plugs are trimmed as necessary. The surgeon then makes a small hole in each bone plug using a small drill and a fine drill bit. Size 1 non-absorbable sutures are passed through each hole, and the ends are left long and tagged with hemostats. The surgeon then uses a surgical pen to mark the graft at the bone-tendon margin. These marks are used to align the graft in the joint during insertion. The graft is ready for insertion. It is preserved in the specimen basin until the surgeon is ready to insert it.

   The surgeon irrigates the wound and closes the remaining patellar tendon with 2-0 absorbable suture. Skin closure is delayed until the end of the procedure.

6. ***ACL remnants are removed.***
A motorized shaver or rongeurs are used to remove the damaged ACL tissue. A torn meniscus may be removed at this stage.

7. ***The graft tunnel is prepared.***
To prepare the joint for the graft, a drill guide is used to position the tunnel that will receive the graft. A guidewire is drilled into the tibia. A tunnel is then drilled over the guidewire with a cannulated reamer or burr. This step is repeated on the femoral side. A calibrated aiming device may be used to locate the exact angle of the tunnels before drilling. An eyed pin is drilled through the bone tunnels and brought out through the skin.

8. ***The graft is implanted.***
The ST should bring the graft to the field when directed by the surgeon. The preplaced sutures are threaded through the eye of the pin and pulled through the tunnel at both ends. Biosynthetic interference screws are placed in the tunnel against the bone plugs to provide a tighter fit. A small guidewire is placed first, and the screws are placed over the wire. The screws are seated with a screwdriver. The preplaced sutures are then removed.

9. ***The wound is closed.***
The wounds are closed with synthetic absorbable sutures. The wound is dressed with gauze, and a leg brace is applied.
Fig. 29.41 illustrates the technical points of the procedure.

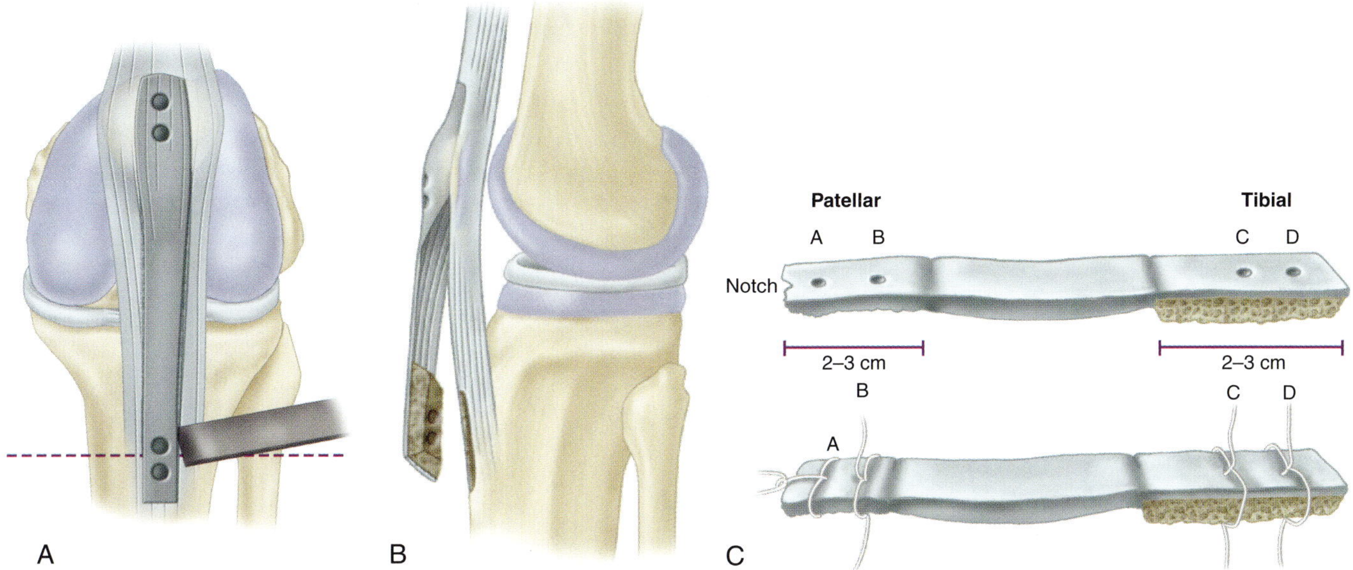

FIG. 29.41 Anterior cruciate ligament repair. (A) Release of the graft. (B) Graft freed from the tibial tuberosity. (C) Preparation of the graft.

The patient remains on crutches for 2 to 3 weeks using a leg brace. Physical therapy is initiated within the first week of recovery. The total recovery period is 4 to 6 months. The patient usually is able to return to normal activities after a successful repair.

Related Procedure: Repair of a Torn Lateral Collateral Ligament

A torn lateral collateral ligament can be repaired using the techniques described for the repair of the ACL. A patellar tendon graft is used to replace the damaged collateral ligament. With a less severe injury, the ligament may be reattached with biosynthetic screws, staples, or sutures of heavy Dacron.

TOTAL KNEE ARTHROPLASTY

The knee has three cartilaginous surfaces: the patella, tibia, and femur. Any or all three surfaces may be involved in a joint disease. In unicompartmental total knee arthroplasty (TKA), the medial or lateral surfaces of the femur and tibia are replaced. In total knee replacement, all three components are replaced. Unicompartmental replacement often requires total knee replacement later in the patient's life and is suitable for patients with intact supporting structures.

Knee replacement is a complex procedure. Many systems are available and are continually being refined. In particular, the unicompartmental approach has been under intense development. Electronic systems that aid the precise alignment of the joint components are now used in some facilities. An alternative is the custom-made cutting block, which is made before surgery using the patient's MRI scans to develop precise cutting guides. Use of these systems requires instructions by the manufacturer.

Components of the total knee implant are as follows:

- A metal femoral component inserted over the distal femur
- A tibial base plate and a metal tray that is placed in the proximal tibia and a polyethylene patellar component. The components may be implanted with bone cement or may be press fitted

A hinged implant contains two polyethylene and chrome bearings, which provide flexion-extension and axial rotation. This design is used in patients with significant ligament insufficiency, flexion-extension mismatch, and neuromuscular diseases.

The procedure presented here includes basic techniques for TKA and does not attempt to describe specific joint systems and techniques specified by the manufacturer of a specific system.

Pathology

Three common forms of arthritis affect the knee: osteoarthritis, rheumatoid arthritis, and post-traumatic arthritis. Inflammation and degeneration of the joint surfaces result in pain and loss of function. Osteoarthritis is the most common indication for arthroplasty.

POSITION:	Supine using a leg support or total knee replacement positioner
INCISION:	Midline patellar
PREP AND DRAPING:	Foot to mid-thigh prep with a routine knee draping technique
INSTRUMENTS:	Total knee system instrument set; major orthopedic set with knee instruments; chisels and osteotomes; double-action rongeurs; bone cement mixing system

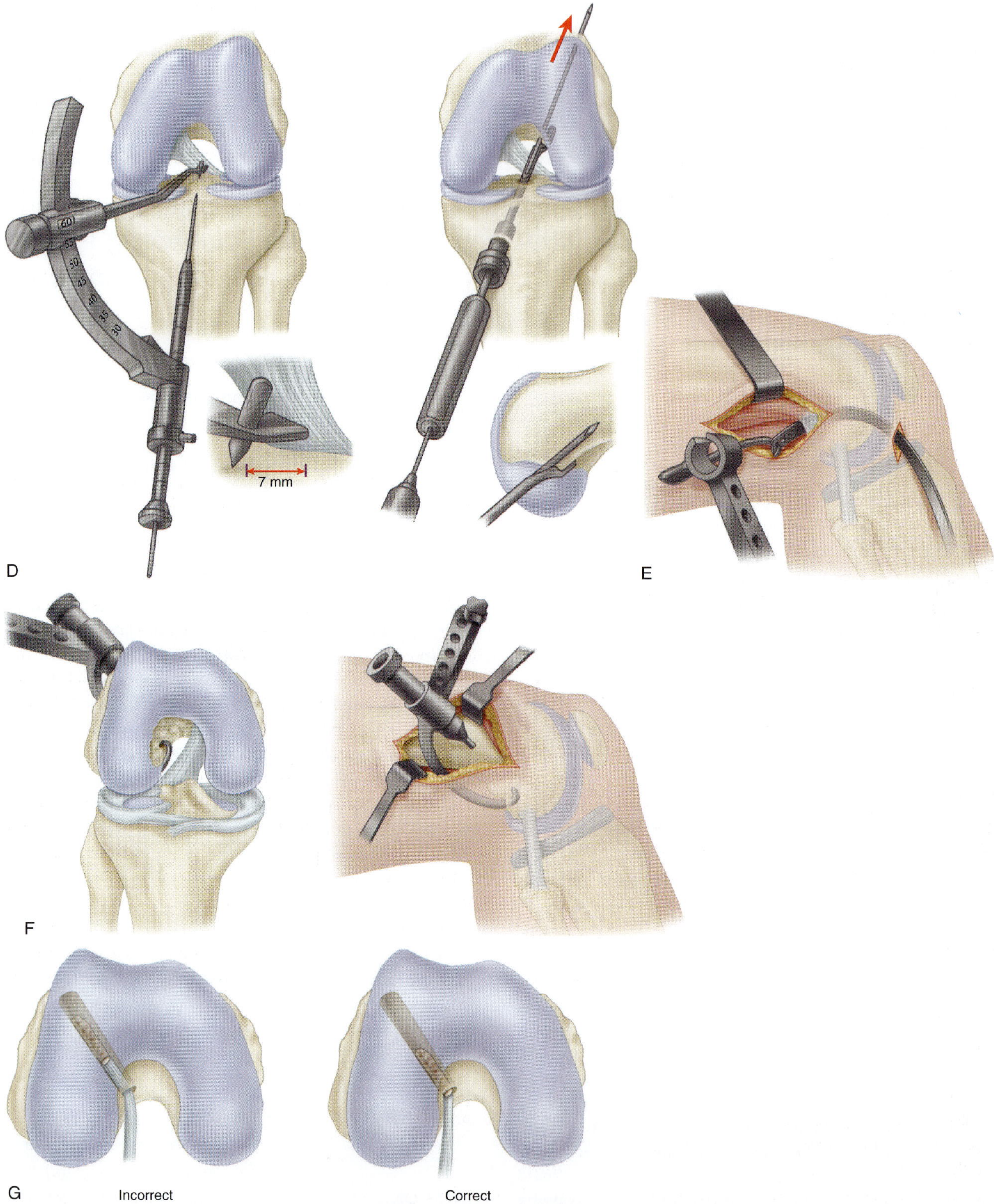

FIG. 29.41, cont'd (D) Use of tibial drill guide for measuring the tunnel. (E) The rear entry guide is fixed to the eye of the passer to bring the graft through the tunnel. (F) The guide is engaged, and the screw is positioned. (G) The screw is placed. (From Azar F. *Campbell's Operative Orthopaedics*. 13th ed. Philadelphia: Elsevier; 2017.)

Technical Points and Discussion

1. ***The patient is position, prepped, and draped.***
   The patient is placed in supine position with the knee positioned over the lower table break or in a leg positioner. The skin prep extends from the foot to mid-thigh. The incision line and boundaries of the patella are marked before the Ioban adhesive drape is applied. The leg is draped as described for a knee procedure. The leg is then attached to a flat leg holder. The leg is exsanguinated and tourniquet inflated.

2. ***The entry incision is made.***
   A curved midline patellar incision is made using a #10 or #20 knife with the knee in flexion. The incision is extended to deep tissues using a deep knife. Wide rake retractors are needed to pull back the tissue flaps. The capsule is incised using a #10 or #15 deep knife. A periosteal elevator may be used to lift the capsule and medial collateral ligament off the tibia. The knee is then extended, and the patella everted. A small Richardson retractor and deep rakes are used at this level. The anterior cruciate ligament and anterior horns of the menisci are removed using a deep knife. The fat pad is also removed at this time. Heavy Kocher forceps are required along with the deep knife. Blount knee retractors may be used.

3. ***The femoral canal is entered.***
   A drill is used to enter the femoral canal. A large Frazier suction is needed at this point. The canal is irrigated and suctioned to remove fat.

4. ***The femur is prepared.***
   An intramedullary cutting guide and jig are placed over the canal. The distal femoral cuts are made using a wide oscillating saw under irrigation with an Asepto syringe. The ST should retrieve all bone fragments and keep them in a moist condition on the back table. An osteotome is used to remove the posterior condyles. The menisci may be removed at this time using the knife and Kocher clamp. Preparation of the femur is completed with anterior and posterior chamfer (rounding off) of the previously cut surfaces.

5. ***The proximal tibia is prepared.***
   A tibial jig and alignment rod are used to obtain the correct cutting angle. The proximal tibia cut is made using the oscillating saw and irrigation. The cut is levered away from the knee using an osteotome. The cut tissue is then released from the tibia using the deep knife and Kocher clamp. A Hohmann retractor is used to lever the tibia forward. A tibial template can then be used to size the tibia. The alignment is checked with an alignment rod. A bone punch is used to prepare the medullary canal for the tibial steam. Osteophytes are removed using a double-action rongeur. The flexion and extension gaps are assessed using spacer blocks. The soft tissues are balanced by trimming those tissues under tension using a #15 blade on a #7 handle.

6. ***The components are implanted.***
   The trial components are put into place, and the alignment is checked again using the alignment rod. The patella may be trimmed and measured at this point. A trial patella is placed and marked. The trial tibia base plate is placed, and a punch is driven into the bone. The cut bone surfaces are irrigated with pulse lavage and dried. The ST should prepare the bone cement. When it is ready, all components are cemented into place. Excess cement is trimmed. The femoral component is impacted using a mallet. Any cement that was extruded is removed. The cement is allowed to cure. Hemostasis is then maintained. The joint is again checked for cement fragments. The knee is irrigated, and the polyethylene component is levered into place.

7. ***The wound is closed.***
   A suction drain is placed, and the knee is closed in layers using synthetic absorbable sutures. The skin is closed with an absorbable subcuticular stitch. An occlusive dressing is placed over the incision, followed by a support bandage.

INTRAMEDULLARY NAILING (TIBIA)

In this procedure an intramedullary rod (nail) is inserted into the tibia for fixation and stabilization of a fracture.

The selection of an IM nail for a fracture of the tibia is based on the type and severity of the fracture, the patient's age, and the surgeon's preference. Two types of IM nails are commonly used: the cannulated nail and the solid nail. Although called "nails," these devices are rod implants that are impacted into the intramedullary space along the parallel axis. Stabilizing screws may be placed at the proximal and/or distal ends to prevent the nail from slipping. The nail may be inserted without the preparation of the medullary canal, or the canal may be reamed before the insertion of the nail.

C-arm fluoroscopy is used intraoperatively. The C-arm is adjusted before the skin prep to ensure full exposure of the operative site. A pneumatic tourniquet may be used to maintain hemostasis.

Pathology

Fractures of the tibia are commonly the result of a high-velocity impact caused by a motor vehicle accident or sports trauma.

POSITION:	Supine using standard operating table or fraction table
INCISION:	Proximal tibia
PREP AND DRAPING:	Lower leg to above the knee
INSTRUMENTS:	Major orthopedic set; tibial nail system with accessory instruments; knee instruments; power drill; general surgery set

Technical Points and Discussion

1. ***The patient is positioned, prepped, and draped.***
The patient is placed in the supine position on the standard operating table with the thigh supported over a padded bolster or similar device. If the traction table is used, the thigh is elevated over a padded crossbar. The foot is placed in traction using a skeletal nail.

2. ***The entry incision is made.***
The surgeon makes an incision over the patellar tendon using a #10 knife blade. The ST should have retractors, and the ESU should be immediately available.

3. ***A threaded-tip guidewire is inserted under fluoroscopic guidance.*** The ST should prepare a threaded guidewire, drill, and soft tissue sleeve. With the sleeve in place, the surgeon advances the guidewire through the trochanter while imaging the entry to ensure proper placement. The position of the guidewire is verified before inserting the intramedullary reamer.

4. ***The entry point is created.***
With the initial guidewire in place, an entry site is made using a cannulated entry reamer with a soft tissue sleeve in place. A ball tip guide pin is inserted into the tibial space and advanced across the bone fragments.

5. ***The tibial canal is reamed.***
The tibial canal can be cleared using several different techniques. A cannulated reamer with power drill can be placed over the guide pin and the canal cleared for nail insertion. When a power reamer is used, the ST should collect and contain bits of tissue that are created in the reaming process. If reamers are not used, the surgeon may use sizers to determine the correct nail size.

6. ***The nail size is determined and appropriate nail inserted.***
After the canal has been reamed, the hand assembly is removed and medullary tube is inserted over the reamer. The reamer is then removed and may be replaced with a ball tip guide rod, which is used to guide the IM nail into position.
The selected nail implant is then inserted. At each step, the position of the guidewires is verified, and the hollow medullary tubes are used to protect the tissue of the endosteum while drilling takes place. The medullary tube and guidewires are removed only when the IM nail is in place. Note that no guidewire is used for solid nails.
Depending on the system and the manufacturer, a number of methods can be used to insert the nail. A hollow nail can be grasped with a targeting device or guide, which keeps the nail straight and angled correctly as it is inserted over the guidewire. The nail is inserted manually with a twisting or oscillating movement. A metal driver may be used to seat the nail. The position of the implant is verified fluoroscopically, and the guidewire is removed.

7. ***The locking pins are placed.***
Locking pins are inserted. These fit into the nail at a right angle through the proximal and distal ends of the nail. To line up the entry point of the locking bolts with the nail, a targeting guide or similar right-angle aiming device is used. The IM guidewire is removed, and the targeting device is attached. The skin is incised over the site for the locking bolts, and the tissue is dissected to bone. The drill holes are then made through the tissue protector. Screw length is determined with a depth gauge. The locking screws are inserted and tightened manually with a screwdriver. End caps may be inserted over each locking pin. This prevents the ingrowth of bone tissue.

8. ***The wound is closed.***
After the final repair is checked using fluoroscopy, the wound is irrigated and closed in layers. The patellar tendon and paratenon are approximated with interrupted sutures size 0 or 2-0. Skin is closed using an absorbable synthetic subcuticular suture or skin staples. The wound is dressed with a flat dressing, fluff gauze, and a compression bandage.
Technical points are shown in Fig. 29.42.

ABOVE-KNEE AMPUTATION (AKA)

Leg amputation is classified according to the level of the amputation and whether the limb is ischemic (lacking blood supply) or non-ischemic (blood supply is intact). In a non-ischemic limb, the muscle must be stabilized by myoplasty or *myodesis* (fixing the muscle to the bone) to provide a strong stump with sufficient power for adduction. However, this is not possible in an ischemic leg because the vascular supply may be further compromised. Muscle stabilization is performed on the ischemic limb.

Pathology

The most common indication for amputation is ischemia caused by diabetes mellitus primary vascular disease. The number of amputations for other causes, including trauma, infection, or tumors, has decreased in the United States as a result of improved medical technology and the enforcement of occupational safety guidelines. The level of the amputation is important for the healing of the wound and for fitting prosthesis. The lowest level possible is selected.

POSITION:	Supine using a leg holder
INCISION:	Midfemoral circumferential
PREP AND DRAPING:	Waist to ankle prep. Draping for midfemoral exposure with the leg draped free. The foot and groin are excluded from the draping

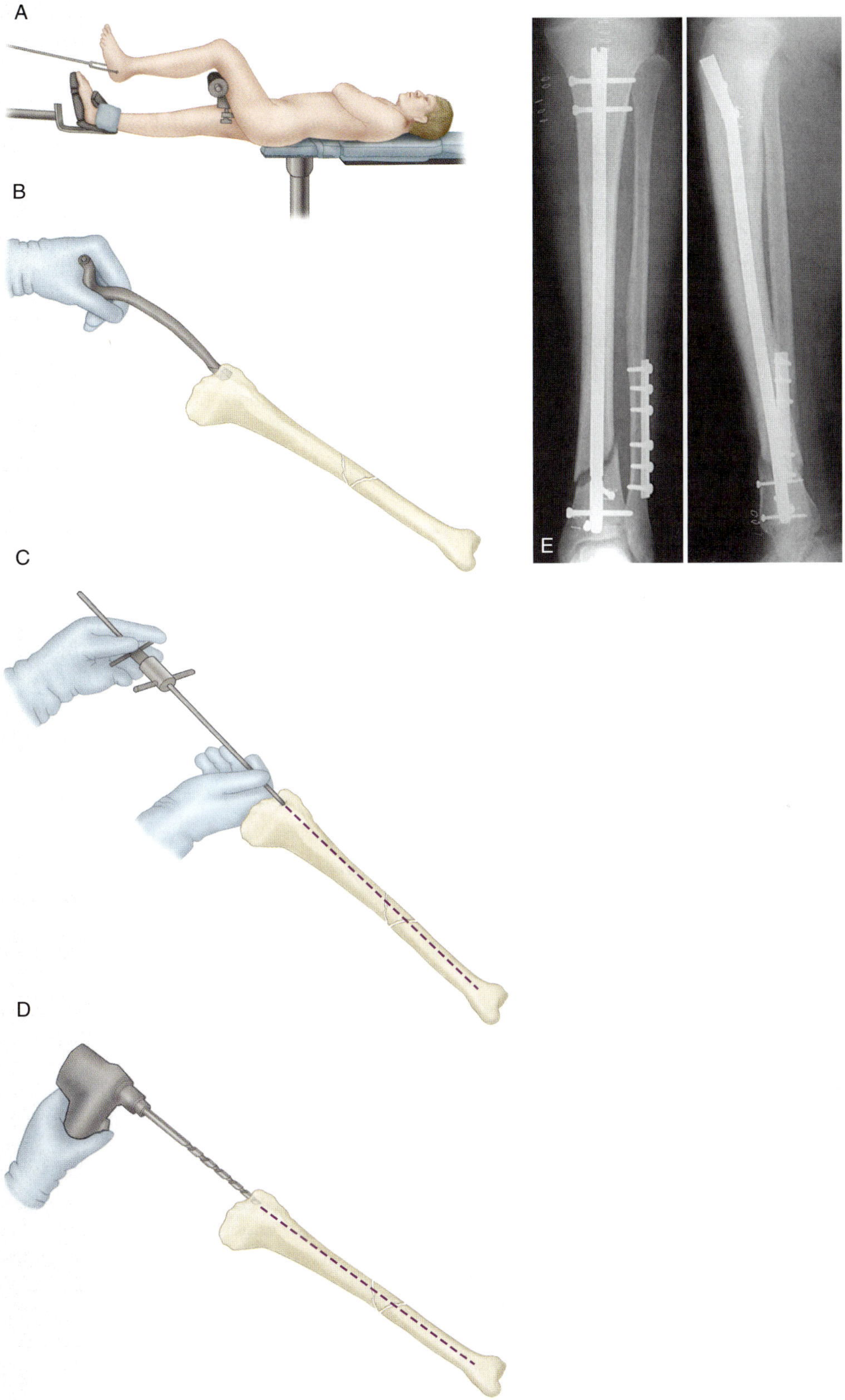

FIG. 29.42 Intramedullary tibial nail. (A) Patient position using a fracture table. (B) An awl is used to open the medullary canal. (C) A ball tip guide rod is inserted under image intensification. (D) Graduated cannulated reamers, which fit over the guide rod, are used to clear the medullary canal. (E) X-ray of completed repair. (From Azar, F. *Campbell's Operative Orthopaedics* (13th ed.). Philadelphia: Elsevier; 2017.)

INSTRUMENTS:	Lower limb amputation set including Gigli saw, amputation knives, and rasps

Technical Points and Discussion

1. ***The patient is positioned, prepped, and draped.***
The patient is placed in supine position. A leg holder may be used. A pneumatic tourniquet is placed at the upper thigh. The surgeon outlines the proposed tissue flaps on the patient's skin. The prep extends from the waist to the ankle. The leg is draped for a midfemoral incision with the lower leg wrapped in impervious drapes followed by an adhesive drape.

2. ***The tissue flaps are developed.***
The incision starts with the anterior tissue flap using a #20 knife. A curved line is followed. The posterior flap is made using the same pattern. The incisions are extended through the subcutaneous tissue and fascia. Rake retractors are inserted. The quadriceps muscle is divided. Small bleeders are managed with the ESU. The femoral artery and vein are ligated with a non-absorbable suture and divided.

3. ***The femur is cut and shaped.***
The femur is exposed, and the periosteum is incised circumferentially using a deep knife. The bone is cut using a Gigli saw or an amputation saw. The posterior muscles are then divided, and the ends are allowed to retract. The leg is removed. The ST may maintain the limb on the back table or immediately pass it to the circulator, who receives it in a plastic bag. A rasp is then used to smooth the cut edges of the femur.

   The cutaneous nerves are sectioned so that they retract well away from the cut edge of the muscle. The wound is then irrigated to remove all bone dust.

4. ***The muscles are attached to the bone.***
With use of a small drill bit, several holes are placed near the lower edge of the femur. The abductor and hamstring muscle are sutured to the bone using absorbable or non-absorbable sutures. The tourniquet is released at the point, and hemostasis is attained.

   The quadriceps flap is extended over the end of the cut femur. The fascia layer is sutured to the posterior thigh fascia.

5. ***The wound is closed.***
A Hemovac suction drain is placed in the wound under the muscle. The ends are brought out through the skin. The subcutaneous layer and skin are closed with absorbable synthetic suture. The wound is dressed using a flat dressing and rolled gauze, followed by a light compression dressing.

   Technical points of the procedure are illustrated in Fig. 29.43.

BELOW-KNEE AMPUTATION

Below-knee amputation (BKA) techniques are similar to transfemoral amputation. The flap design and attachment of muscles are extremely important to the rehabilitation of the patients and their ability to bear weight on the stump. The exact technique varies somewhat between the ischemic limb and the non-ischemic leg. In the non-ischemic limb, myoplasty is performed, which is the attachment of divided muscle groups to the bone. In this technique, the muscle groups are sutured to the opposing muscles or fascia.

Pathology

Amputation may result from trauma, vascular insufficiency, congenital anomaly, tumor, or infection.

POSITION:	Supine. A triangular leg rest may be used. A pneumatic tourniquet is positioned over the upper leg
INCISION:	Lower limb, circumferential
PREP AND DRAPING:	Lower limb with the foot is excluded
INSTRUMENTS:	Lower limb amputation set; bone saws; large rake retractors; drill

Technical Points and Discussion

1. ***The patient is positioned, prepped, and draped.***
The patient is placed in prone position. A triangular leg rest may be used to flex the knee and allow access to the full circumference of the limb. The surgeon marks the skin incisions and length of the stump on the patient's skin.

   The skin prep extends from the ankle to mid-thigh. Draping follows routine exposure to the lower leg with the foot wrapped and excluded using an impervious drape secured by an adhesive drape.

2. ***The entry incision is made.***
Using a #10 or #20 knife, the surgeon makes the anterior incision following the skin flap marking. The incision is carried to the posterior side. Using a deep knife, the surgeon deepens the posterior incision through the fascia. Rake or right-angle retractors may be placed to expose the tibia. This deep incision is carried anteriorly. The level of bone transection is marked.

3. ***The anterior muscles are divided.***
The superficial peroneal nerve is identified and pulled distally using a clamp. It is then divided and allowed to retract away from the end of the stump. The anterior muscles are divided using a deep knife or ESU. The tibial vessels and peroneal nerve are identified, ligated, and divided using a ligature of size 2-0 or 3-0 non-absorbable suture.

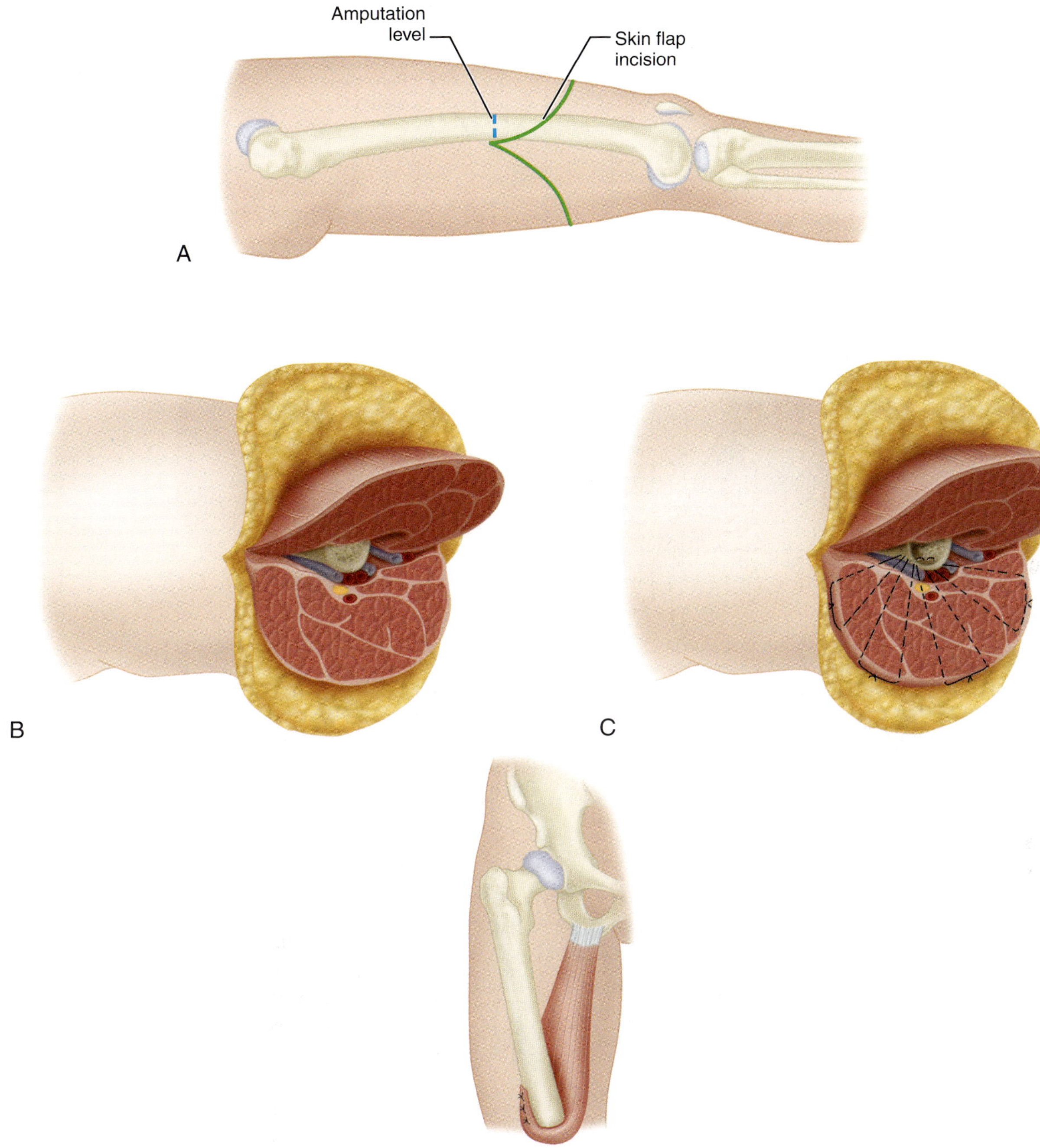

FIG. 29.43 Above-knee amputation. (A) Incision and bone level. (B) Myofascial flap. (C) Muscles attached to the femur through holes drilled in bone. (From Canale S, Beaty J, eds. *Campbell's Operative Orthopaedics*. 12th ed. Philadelphia: Mosby; 2013.)

4. ***The bones and posterior muscles are divided.***
The tibia and fibula are divided using a Gigli or amputation saw. The posterior muscles are divided using a deep knife. The posterior tibia, peroneal vessels, and tibial nerve are now exposed. Each is doubly ligated using size 2-0 suture and divided. The gastrocnemius-soleus muscles are beveled using a large amputation knife. The bone ends are rounded with a rasp. The wound is now irrigated.

5. ***The wound is closed.***
The tourniquet is released, and all bleeding is controlled with the ESU or suture ties. The muscle flap is brought over the ends of the bones and sutured to the deep fascia and periosteum on the anterior side. Size 3-0 or 2-0 non-absorbable suture is used. A suction drain is placed under the muscle flap and brought out through the skin. The skin flaps are brought together and secured using size 3-0 non-absorbable sutures. The skin is closed with size 3-0 or 4-0 subcuticular absorbable synthetic suture. The wound is dressed with bulky gauze and an elastic compression bandage.

Technical points are illustrated in Fig. 29.44.

The patient is rehabilitated as soon as possible after surgery. A rigid dressing may be used to protect the stump and control postoperative edema. Weight bearing is

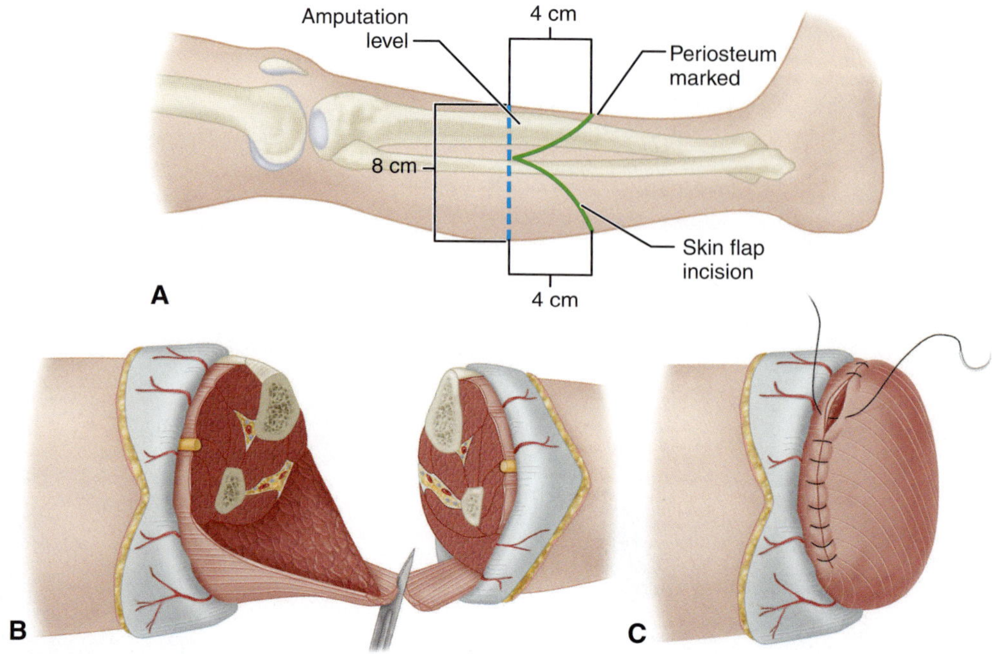

FIG. 29.44 Below-knee amputation. (A) Amputation and flap design. (B) Posterior myofascial flap. (C) Suturing the myofascial flap to the periosteum. (From Canale S, Beaty J, eds. *Campbell's Operative Orthopaedics*. 12th ed. Philadelphia: Mosby; 2013.)

limited at first, using the parallel bars or walker. The patient may be fitted with a temporary prosthesis in the early weeks of rehabilitation.

FOOT

Fracture and sprain of the foot and distal tibia are common sport injuries. Motor vehicle accidents also contribute to the total number of foot injuries. Other injuries can be caused by walking over uneven ground, trips, and falls.

The foot and ankle are complex structures bearing the entire weight of the body. The foot contains 26 bones in three regions. The many tendons of the foot provide great flexibility to the joints. In the ankle, the articulation is between the lower tibia, malleoli, and talus. This joint provides flexion of the ankle. The subtalar joint between the talus and calcaneus allows inversion and eversion of the ankle (Fig. 29.45).

REPAIR OF THE ACHILLES TENDON

Surgical repair of a ruptured Achilles tendon is the "gold standard" for active individuals. The procedure may involve grafting and application of biosynthetic scaffolds for the infiltration of normal tissue during healing.

Pathology

A ruptured tendon is one that is shredded and torn and partially avulsed but not completely severed. Rupture commonly occurs in active sports, especially those involving jumping, such as tennis, basketball, gymnastics, and volleyball. A low-level injury may occur in other activities, such as cycling.

POSITION:	Prone
INCISION:	Along the long axis of the Achilles tendon
PREP AND DRAPING:	Mid-thigh to foot; standard foot draping
INSTRUMENTS:	Minor orthopedic set including tendon instruments—tendon stripper and fascia needle; polyethylene block for trimming the graft

Technical Points and Discussion

1. ***The patient is positioned, prepped, and draped.***
   The patient is placed in prone position. The lower legs should rest on an elevated pad. A pneumatic tourniquet is placed at the upper thigh. The skin prep extends from the mid-thigh to the foot. Draping should provide open access to the foot and ankle.

2. ***The entry incision is made.***
   A posteromedial incision is made off center along the axis of the tendon. The incision is carried to the subcutaneous tissue and the tendon sheath. Sharp rake retractors may be placed at this level. This exposes the fascia (paratenon), which is incised to expose the tendon.

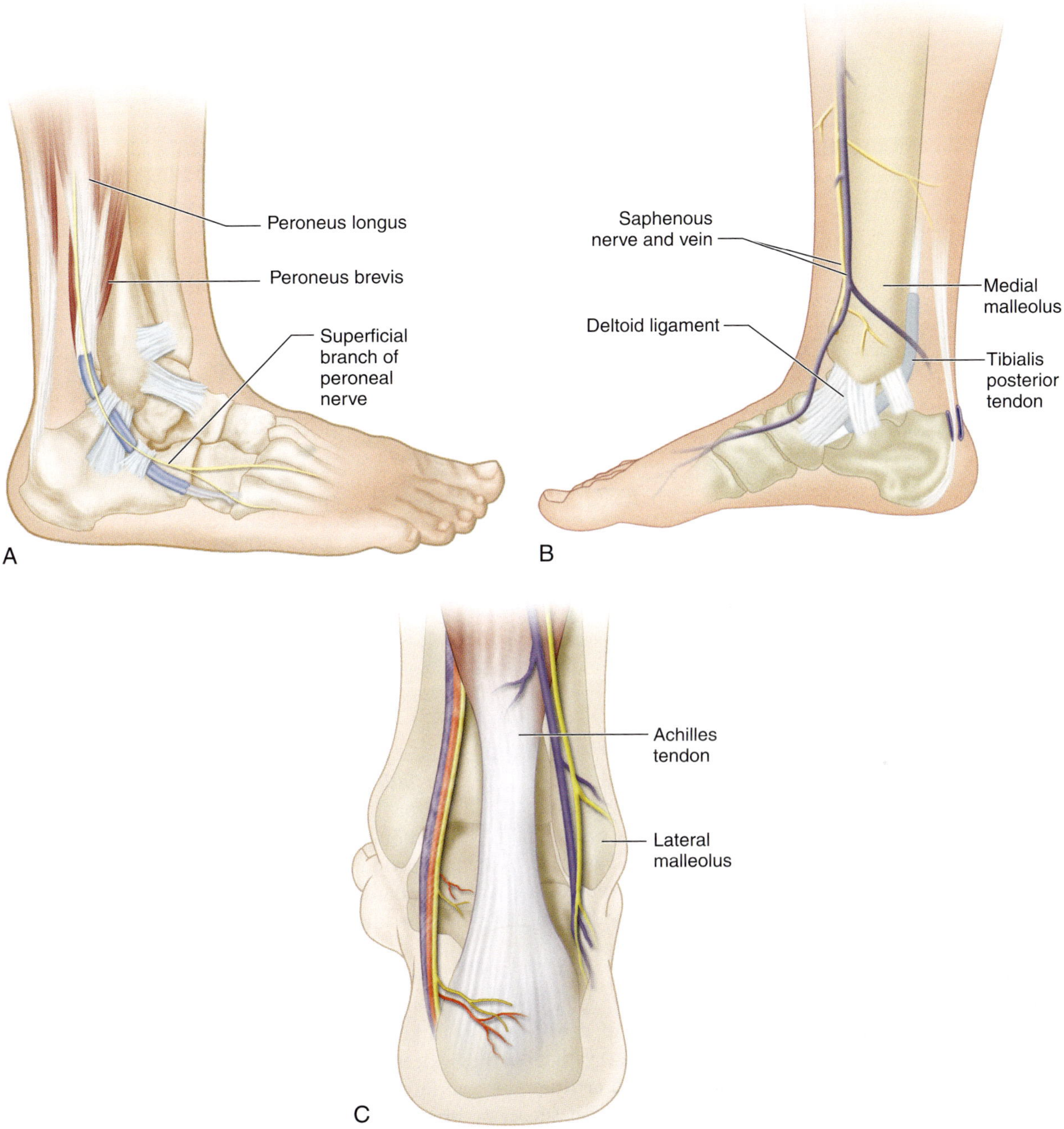

FIG. 29.45 Anatomy of the foot. (A) Lateral view. (B) Medial view. (C) Posterior view. (From Schemitsch E, McKee M, eds. *Operative Techniques: Orthopedic Trauma Surgery*. Philadelphia: Saunders; 2010.)

3. ***The tendon is approximated.***
The ruptured ends of the tendon are secured using #1 non-absorbable suture of the surgeon's choice of material. The knee and foot are flexed, and the sutures are tied.

4. ***A tendon graft may be placed.***
A plantaris tendon graft may be harvested using a tendon stripper. The ST should place the graft on the back table and keep it moist with saline. The edges of the torn tendon are trimmed using Metzenbaum scissors and approximated with size 2-0 absorbable sutures. The tendon graft is threaded on a fascia needle. The graft is then sutured to the anterior and posterior tendon. Size 2-0 absorbable synthetic sutures are then used to secure the graft to the Achilles tendon. The distal tendon graft can be spread out and tacked over the repair.

5. ***The wound is closed.***
The wound is irrigated and closed in layers. The fascia sheath and subcutaneous layer are closed with size 2-0 absorbable sutures. The skin is closed using interrupted non-absorbable sutures. A flat dressing is applied to the wound, followed by a short leg cast.

Technical points are shown in Fig. 29.46.

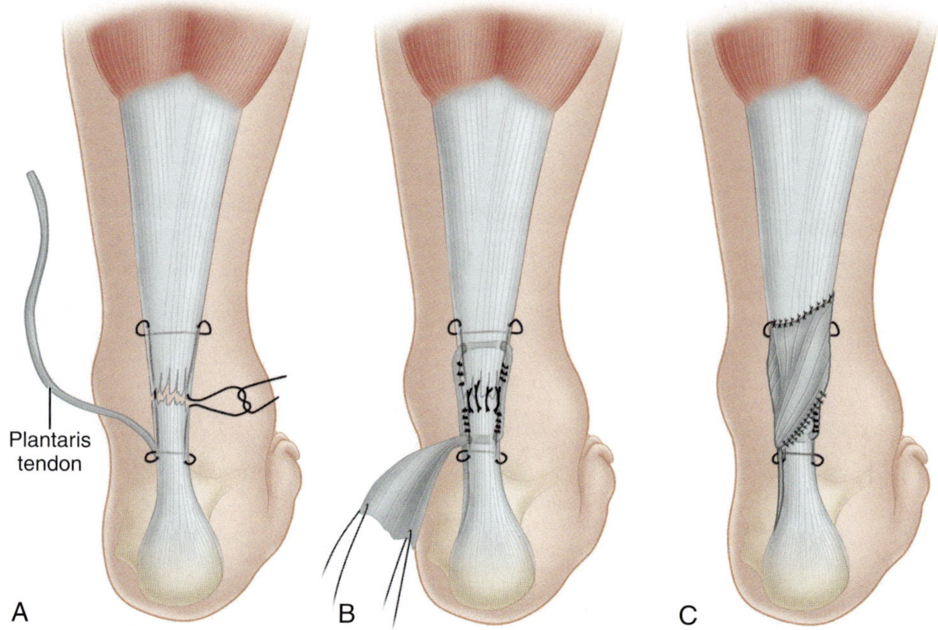

FIG. 29.46 Repair of Achilles tendon. (A) The ruptured ends are approximated using heavy nonabsorbable suture. (B) The frayed edges of the tendon are repaired. (C) The graft is opened out and tacked over the repair. (From Canale S, Beaty J, eds. *Campbell's Operative Orthopaedics*. 12th ed. Philadelphia: Mosby; 2013.)

TRIPLE ARTHRODESIS

Triple **arthrodesis** is the fusion of the talocalcaneal, talonavicular, and calcaneocuboid joints. This is performed by removing the cartilage from each joint. Bone grafts or biosynthetic graft material is used to replace the cartilage and enable the joints to fuse. The surgical goal is to prevent the movement of these joints and thereby prevent pain and joint instability.

Pathology

Triple arthrodesis is performed to treat a number of painful, chronic joint diseases that are not helped by conservative therapy. These include congenital defects, rheumatoid arthritis, post-traumatic arthritis, and neuromuscular disease. These conditions cause deformity and pain in the joints.

POSITION:	Supine
INCISION:	Ankle—two incisions (description follows)
PREP AND DRAPING:	Knee to foot; iliac crest if a bone graft is needed. Standard lower leg draping
INSTRUMENTS:	Foot and ankle set including lamina spreader, bone saw, drill, K-wires, burrs. Include a cannulated screw system and medium size osteotomes and curettes

Technical Points and Discussion

1. ***The patient is positioned, prepped, and draped.***
The patient is placed in supine position. A pneumatic tourniquet is place at the upper thigh. The foot and leg are prepped to the knee. The foot and ankle are draped using a standard technique. The surgeon outlines the incisions with a skin marker.

2. ***The entry incision is made and tendons dissected.***
An anterior or anterolateral incision is made using a #15 knife. The incision is carried deeper using the ESU or deep knife. Small right-angle retractors can be placed at this point. The extensor digitorum brevis and hallucis brevis tendon insertions are dissected using a deep knife. The dissection is carried along the extensor digitorum brevis to expose the calcaneocuboid joint.

3. ***The calcaneocuboid joint is debrided.***
A Gelpi retractor, rake, or lamina spreader can be inserted in the incision. All surfaces of the joint are debrided using a curette and osteotome. Several holes are now drilled on each side of the joint.

4. ***The subtalar joint is debrided.***
The subtalar joint is identified, and the ligaments are removed. A Hohmann retractor is placed in the wound to lift the peroneal tendons providing better exposure. The joint is debrided using a curette or osteotome. Holes may be drilled to provide increased space for debridement if required. The bony surfaces are removed using small osteotomes.

5. ***The talonavicular joint is exposed and debrided.***
An anteromedial incision is made to expose the talonavicular joint. Branches of the saphenous vein are ligated or managed with the ESU. A full-thickness flap is raised to expose the deep surfaces of the joint. These are debrided using a curved osteotome and curette. A double-action rongeur may be used to trim the talus so that it can rest in anatomical position in the navicular. A right-angle retractor such as a US or small Richardson retractor is placed in the wound to expose the lateral talonavicular joint. The surfaces are debrided as explained earlier.

6. ***The talonavicular joint is fixed.***
A large, partially threaded cancellous screw size 6.5 or 7.0 mm is used to fix the talonavicular joint. A guidewire (K-wire size 0.062) is first drilled across the arthrodesis site, and the position is checked using fluoroscopy. The drill hole is made, and the screw is inserted. An additional screw may be required.

7. ***The calcaneocuboid joint is fixed.***
A separate incision is made at the base of the fourth and fifth metatarsals. A guidewire is passed into the cuboid and across the joint to the calcaneus. A screw hole is drilled and tapped over the guidewire. The guidewire is removed.

8. ***Gaps are filled with bone graft.***
Before all gaps are closed in the arthrodesis, sites are filled with bone grafts. The tuberosity of the calcaneus or iliac crest can be used.

9. ***The wounds are closed.***
The tourniquet is released, and the wound is irrigated. All bleeders are controlled with the ESU. A Hemovac or Jackson-Pratt suction tube is placed in the wound, which is then closed in layers. Absorbable synthetic sutures are used to close the subcutaneous layers. Synthetic non-absorbable sutures are used on skin. A large compression dressing is applied to the ankle, and a short-leg cast or splint is applied.

Patients use a wheelchair for 4 to 6 weeks. After 3 weeks, the sutures are removed. The cast is removed after 12 weeks.

BUNIONECTOMY (MODIFIED MCBRIDE PROCEDURE)

In a bunionectomy, an enlarged metatarsal head (hallux valgus) is reduced or removed. The goal of surgery is to alleviate pain and increase patient mobility.

Pathology

Hallux valgus is a deformity of the first metatarsal head and is associated with various structural anomalies of the entire toe. Poorly fitting shoes contribute to the pathology. An enlarged metatarsal head is painful and often limits the patient's mobility.

POSITION:	Supine
INCISION:	Over the hallux joint
PREP AND DRAPING:	Knee to foot prep. The foot is draped free
INSTRUMENTS:	Small bone fragment set; oscillating saw (narrow blade); drill; K-wires

Technical Points and Discussion

1. ***The patient is positioned, prepped, and draped.***
The patient is placed in the supine position. Regional anesthesia is administered, and a pneumatic tourniquet is applied. Standard draping for the foot is used.

2. ***The entry incision is made.***
An incision is made in the medial side of the metatarsal shaft and extended through the fascia using a #15 knife. Double hook or Senn retractors are placed in the wound. Any superficial bleeders are controlled using a needle point ESU. The incision is then carried to the deep metatarsal space.

3. ***Soft tissues are released.***
The conjoined tendon is exposed and incised using the deep #15 knife. The lateral joint capsule is released along with the extensor tendon. The periosteum and medial joint capsule are incised. This exposes the bunion.

4. ***The bony prominence is removed.***
With use of a sagittal saw, the medial bony prominence is removed. Bone may be removed from the side and top of the metatarsal. The sides of the osteotomy are smoothed using the saw.

The tip of the saw blade must be irrigated during the procedure. Any redundant capsule tissue is trimmed using the deep knife and fine tissue forceps.

5. ***The wound is closed.***
The joint capsule and periosteum are closed using absorbable synthetic sutures, size 4-0. Skin is closed using interrupted nylon sutures. The wound is dressed with a flat dressing and gauze fluffs.

KEY CONCEPTS

- Instruments used in orthopedic surgery perform the same functions as their counterparts in soft tissue (e.g., grasping, cutting, viewing).
- Infection control in orthopedic surgery is a critical issue that is addressed using laminar air flow in the operating room, helmet systems for team members, and particular attention to skin preparation.

- Many different types of orthopedic implants and hardware are used in bone repair and reconstruction. Basic techniques are common to most types, although it is important to follow individual manufacturers' recommendations for specific techniques.
- Orthopedic technology has borrowed many terms from carpentry. It is important to learn the meaning of these terms to enhance communication with the orthopedic team.
- Implants require special handling on the field in sterilization. An implant must never be flash sterilized unless absolutely necessary. A biological indicator must be included in every sterilization batch.
- Bone grafts, cements, and bioactive materials are commonly used in orthopedic surgery. Bioactive and synthetic substitutes have been developed to address the shortage of banked bone.
- PMMA bone cement carries health risks while unset. Mixing must be done using a closed device with suction to vent the fumes through a charcoal filter.
- Arthroscopic surgery is based on techniques used in other minimally invasive specialties, including joint distention using intermittent irrigation, which is gravity or pump controlled.
- Positioning for orthopedic surgery can require up to 20 minutes, which should be considered during case planning.
- Draping techniques used in orthopedic procedures can be complex. Most procedures involving the upper and lower limbs require the use of split sheets or U-drapes and occlusive adherent plastic drapes impregnated with iodophor.
- Whenever power instruments that cut bone are in use, such as drills, reamers, and saws, the tip of the instrument must be continuously irrigated to prevent the buildup of heat and prevent excess friction. Irrigation can be delivered using a bulb syringe or Asepto syringe (see Chapter 12).
- When disconnecting power instruments from compressed gas, bleed the instrument first. This is done by turning off the gas source and then activating the instrument. This depressurizes the system and enables a safe disconnect.
- When a limb is draped, it may be necessary to drape it "free." This means that the limb is placed through the drape aperture or split drapes are used to allow unrestricted movement of the limb during surgery.
- In arm and lower leg surgery, the hand or foot may be "excluded" from the access. This means that the hand or foot is enclosed using impervious drapes covered by an adherent plastic drape.
- Dressings used to protect the incision are often bulky or rigid to provide support to the repair. These techniques are best learned by watching others and participating in the technique.

REVIEW QUESTIONS

1. Define the following important terms in your own words for surgical technique in orthopedics:
   - Internal fixation
   - External fixation
   - Open reduction
   - Closed reduction
2. Give an example of a specific orthopedic procedure for each of the four techniques listed in question 1.
3. What techniques and specific instruments must be used to insert simple bone screws that are not self-tapping?
4. Describe the sterilization requirements for orthopedic implants.
5. What is a lag screw? How does it work?
6. What special equipment is used to mix bone cement? Why is this equipment necessary?
7. Define *torque*.
8. What is meant by the term *cannulated* as it applies to orthopedic hardware?
9. What are the most important reasons for the immediate stabilization of a fracture?
10. What is biosynthetic graft material?

REFERENCE

Association for the Advancement of Medical Instrumentation. *ANSI/AAMI ST79:2017 Comprehensive Guide to Steam Sterilization and Sterility Assurance in Health Care Facilities*. Arlington, Va: AAMI; 2017.

BIBLIOGRAPHY

Baur E. Arthroscopic-assisted partial wrist arthrodesis. *Hand Clin*. 2017;33(4):735-753.

Browner B. *Skeletal Trauma Basic Science Management and Reconstruction*. 6th ed. Elsevier; 2020.

Browner B, Jupiter J, Krettek C, Anderson P. *Skeletal Trauma: Basic Science, Management, and Reconstruction*. 6th ed. Philadelphia: Elsevier; 2020.

Canale T, Beaty J, Azar F. *Campbell's Core Orthopaedic Procedures*. Philadelphia: Elsevier; 2016.

Kollimorgen R, Ellis T, Lewis B, Harris J. Achieving post-free distraction in hip arthroscopy with a pink pad patient positioning device using standard hip distraction tables. *Arthrosc Tech*. 2019;8(4):e363-e368.

Lee D, Neviaser J. *Operative Techniques: Shoulder and Elbow Surgery*. 2nd ed. Philadelphia: Elsevier; 2019.

Miller M, Hart J, MacKnight J. *Essential Orthopaedics*. 2nd ed. Philadelphia: Elsevier; 2020.

Paulsen F. *Sobotta Atlas of Human Anatomy*. Vol 1. 15th ed. Munich, Germany: Elsevier GmbH; 2013.

Schemitsch E, McKee M. *Operative Techniques: Orthopaedic Trauma Surgery*. Philadelphia: Elsevier; 2020.

Young A, Sonnabend A. *Operative Techniques: Shoulder and Elbow Surgery*. Philadelphia: Elsevier; 2019.

VASCULAR AND MICROVASCULAR SURGERY 30

LEARNING OBJECTIVES

After studying this chapter, the reader will be able to:

1. Identify key anatomical features of the peripheral vascular system
2. Discuss diagnostic procedures of the vascular system
3. Discuss specific elements of case planning in vascular surgery
4. Describe surgical techniques used in vascular and microvascular surgery
5. Discuss vascular pathology
6. List and describe common vascular procedures

TERMINOLOGY

Aneurysm: Ballooning of an artery as a result of weakening of the arterial wall. It may be caused by atherosclerosis, infection, or an anatomical defect in the vascular system.

Angioplasty: Restoration of blood flow to a blocked artery using endovascular techniques.

Arteriosclerosis: A disease characterized by thickening, hardening, and loss of elasticity of the arterial wall.

Arteriotomy: An incision made in an artery.

Atherosclerosis: The most common form of arteriosclerosis, which causes plaque to form on the inner surface of an artery.

Bifurcation: The Y-shape of an artery or graft.

Doppler duplex ultrasonography: A type of ultrasonography that produces a visual image of blood flow.

Embolus: A moving substance in the vascular system. An embolus may consist of air, a blood clot, atherosclerotic plaque, or fat.

Endarterectomy: The surgical removal of plaque from inside an artery.

Endovascular: Refers to the interior of a blood vessel.

Hemodialysis: A process in which blood is shunted out of the body and passed through a complex set of filters for the treatment of severe renal disease and as an emergency procedure in cases of acute poisoning.

Hemodynamic: Referring to the pressure, flow, and resistance in the cardiovascular system.

Hybrid operating room: A specially equipped operating room designed to perform endovascular and open surgical procedures.

In situ: In the natural position or normal place, without disturbing or invading surrounding tissues.

Infarction: A blockage in an artery that may lead to tissue ischemia and tissue death.

Intimal hyperplasia: A thickening of the innermost layer of a vessel as a result of long-term central line placement, graft placement, or other interventions that stimulate the overgrowth of intima.

Intravascular ultrasound: A diagnostic tool in which a transducer is introduced into an artery, and ultrasound is used to translate the physical characteristics of the lumen into a visible image.

Ischemia: The decrease in or absence of blood supply to a localized area, usually related to vascular obstruction.

Lumen: The inside of a hollow structure, such as a blood vessel.

Microsurgery: Surgery performed using microscopic techniques, instrument and imaging technology in a variety of different surgical specialties.

Percutaneous: Literally, "through the skin." In a percutaneous approach in surgery, an incision is not made; rather, a catheter or other device is introduced through a puncture site.

Stent: A tubular device placed inside a vessel to provide support and to prevent stricture.

Thrombus: Any organic or nonorganic material blocking an artery; generally refers to a blood clot or atherosclerotic plaque but also includes fat or air.

Umbilical tapes: Lengths of cotton mesh tape used to loop around a blood vessel for retraction. See *vessel loop.*

Venous stasis: Pooling of blood in the veins caused by inactivity or disease. Stasis can cause distention of the veins.

Vessel loop: A device used to retract a vessel during surgery. A length of thin Silastic tubing or cotton tape (umbilical tape) is passed around the vessel. The ends can be threaded through a bolster (a ⅛- to ¼-inch [0.3- to 0.6-cm] length of rubber or Silastic tubing) to secure the loop against the blood vessel.

Peripheral vascular surgery is a specialty of the arteries, veins, and lymphatic vessels lying outside the immediate area of the heart. Vascular procedures are performed to treat disease, injury, and congenital malformation. Like many other surgical specialties, many vascular procedures that have been traditionally performed as open surgeries are now performed using endoscopic and **endovascular** techniques which are performed with instruments that enter the blood vessel. Depending on the procedure, they may be performed in the interventional radiology clinic or **hybrid operating room** to have access to advanced imaging technology while providing the instruments and supplies required in case of an emergency. This chapter provides information on the technology and procedural techniques commonly used in vascular procedures. It also discusses the techniques required for **microvascular surgery.** This is surgery performed using the operating microscope or surgical loupes. The technique can be applied not only to vascular procedures but also across many other surgical specialties, including replantation procedures after traumatic amputation of a limb or digit, plastic and reconstructive surgery, trauma surgery, urology, neurosurgery, and genitourinary surgery.

PATHOLOGY OF THE ARTERIAL SYSTEM

An important source of vascular disease is **arteriosclerosis, atherosclerosis,** or thromboembolic disease. Surgical intervention for these diseases includes open and minimally invasive procedures. Many conditions that required open surgery in the past may now be performed using endovascular techniques, with far less trauma and a more rapid recovery. Sophisticated diagnostic technology has contributed to early diagnosis and a decrease in the number of open surgical procedures.

Vascular access for **hemodialysis** is another function of vascular surgery. Patients with end-stage renal disease who require hemodialysis also require surgery to create a vessel suitable for puncture by the large-bore needles (typically 15 to 17 gauge) used to carry the blood to and from the dialysis machine. For urgent hemodialysis access, a double-lumen dialysis catheter can be inserted and used immediately.

Trauma to arteries is commonly treated using vascular surgery techniques. Gunshot and stab wounds can often be repaired by patching or bypassing the damaged vessel. Deceleration injury, caused by a sudden stop from high speeds common in motor vehicle accidents, can cause a **dissection** (splitting of the layers of the aortic wall). If treated in time, these injuries can often be repaired using open or endovascular techniques.

Reconstruction and grafting procedures often require temporary clamping of large vessels or those that contribute the main blood supply to vital organs. Timing is important to minimize the risk of **ischemia** (loss of blood supply) to tissue during selected grafting procedures. Some procedures require temporary occlusion of major blood vessels. During these minutes when blood flow is stopped, the surgical technologist must be particularly attentive to the field and technical requirements. Complex vascular surgery requires a high degree of knowledge and a well-organized instrument table.

PATHOLOGY OF THE VENOUS SYSTEM

Venous blood returns to the heart from the extremities aided by the contraction of skeletal muscles. The intraluminal valves of the veins prevent blood from returning by gravity to the extremities. Valve incompetency or chronic inactivity may cause stasis of venous blood and distention in the veins. In primary varicose veins, the superficial saphenous veins are affected. Secondary varicose veins originate from the deep saphenous vein.

SURGICAL ANATOMY

The peripheral vascular system is a complex network of vessels, which carry blood cell components and nutrients (including oxygen) to all parts of the body and remove the waste products of metabolism. The major structures of this system are the arteries, veins, and capillaries.

STRUCTURE OF BLOOD VESSELS

All blood vessels except the capillaries are composed of three main layers or walls. From the outside to the inside, they are as follows:

- The *tunica externa* (also called the *adventitia*), which is composed of connective tissue, protects the vessel from injury and provides structural strength.
- The *tunica media*, which is composed of inner layers of smooth muscle bounded by connective tissue
- The *tunica intima,* which secretes substances that cause vasodilation or constriction and those that prevent platelet aggregation in the vessel

The structure of arteries and veins is shown in Fig. 30.1.

ARTERIES

The *arteries* carry oxygenated blood from the heart to the rest of the body. The only exception is the *pulmonary arteries,* which carry deoxygenated blood from the heart to the lungs. Arteries and the smaller arterioles have distinct characteristics that enable them to transport a large volume of blood under pressure. Arteries of the heart, also called *elastic arteries,* are capable of stretching without injury. These vessels can withstand the pressure of blood being pumped by the heart muscle. The *muscular* arteries carry blood to specific organs. These are much smaller than the great vessels of the heart but have a thick muscular layer. The arteries are thick walled and highly elastic and contain mostly smooth muscles.

The elastic nature of arteries allows them to contract during *systole* (ventricular contraction) and relax during *diastole* (the resting phase of the heart) to maintain vascular pressure. Arteries dilate and contract to accommodate the metabolic needs of the body. For example, inflammation causes the expansion of arteries and the release of blood through arterioles; this increases blood supply to injured or infected tissue. Vasodilation lowers the body temperature because it exposes the blood to surface cooling provided by the evaporation of sweat from the skin. Peripheral vasoconstriction occurs during shock and

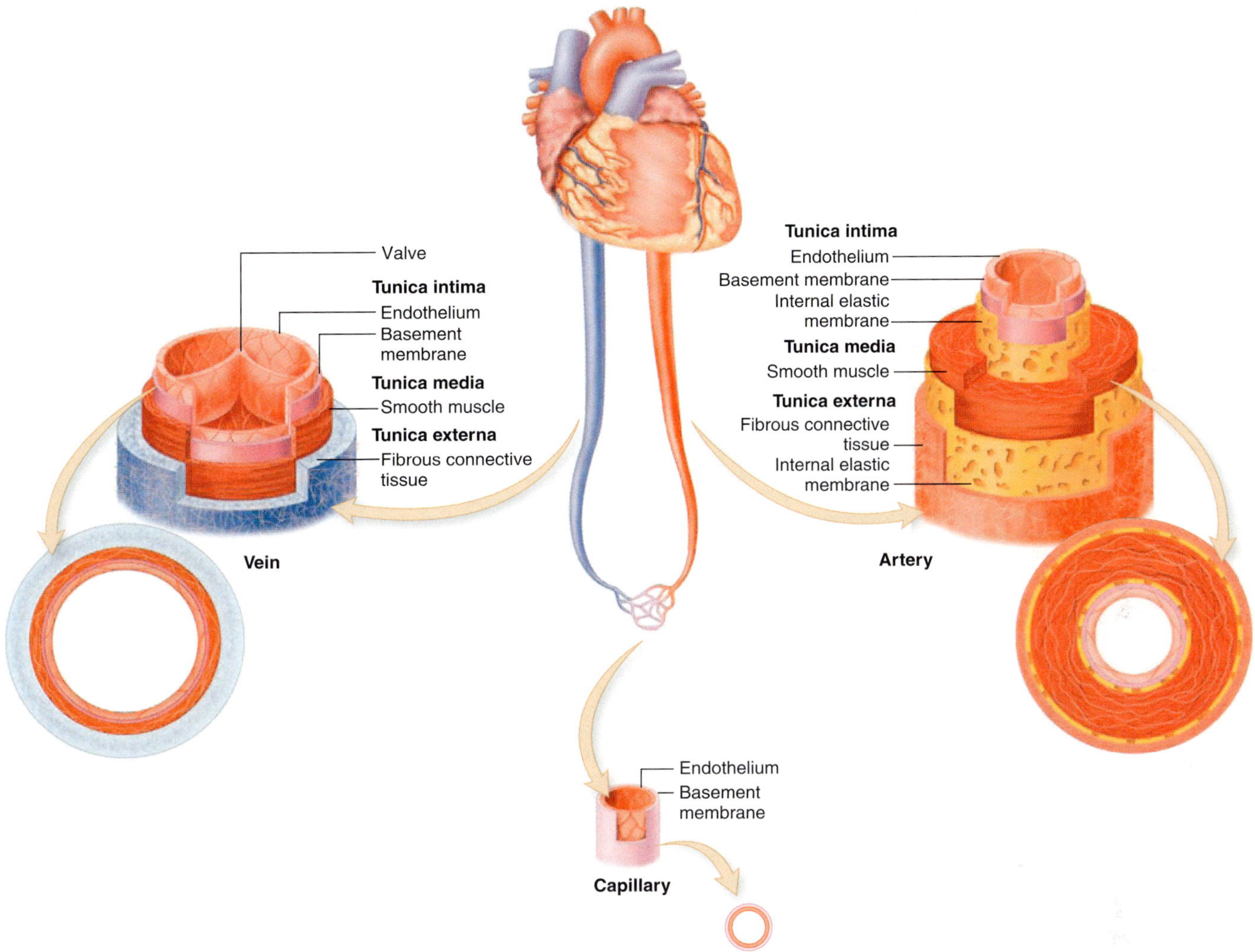

FIG. 30.1 The structure and tissue layers of veins and arteries. Note that the muscle layer of arteries is much thicker than that of the veins. (From Patton KT, Thibodeau GA, Douglas MM. *Essentials of Anatomy and Physiology—Text and Anatomy and Physiology Online Course.* St Louis: Elsevier-Mosby; 2012.)

when the body's core temperature is subnormal; this concentrates the greatest volume of blood in the heart and brain and prevents further cooling at the surface of the body.

ARTERIOLES AND CAPILLARIES

Arteries branch into arterioles, which transition into capillaries, where oxygen is released into tissues. Arterioles provide vascular resistance, regulating the flow of blood into organs and tissues.

The *capillaries* are microscopic vessels that function as the transition and exchange mechanism for oxygen and other substances between the vessel walls and tissue cells. Capillaries are composed of endothelial cells and have no muscle fibers. Precapillary sphincters control the flow of oxygenated blood into the capillary. The walls of the capillary are one cell thick and allow selected substances, including oxygen, to diffuse through the capillary membrane into the tissue. The microcirculation of the capillary system is illustrated in Fig. 30.2.

Some tissues, such as the liver and spleen, have a rich supply of capillary networks. Because of this, these tissues bleed easily and profusely when injured. Capillary bleeding is managed using topical thrombin or tissue sealants. Refer to Chapter 12 for a complete discussion of these substances.

VEINS

The venous system carries blood back to the heart from the peripheral tissues. After passing through the capillary network, blood enters the venules, which transition into increasingly larger branches of veins that run roughly parallel to the arteries on their way to the heart.

Veins are thin walled, which allows them to expand. They function as vessels for transporting blood and also as storage units for blood. Like arteries, larger veins contain muscle fibers that allow them to constrict. However, unlike arteries, veins have valves that open only one way, preventing blood from backing up.

Blood is not pumped through the veins; rather, it is milked toward the heart by contractions in skeletal muscles in the peripheral system (Fig. 30.3) and by intraabdominal and intrathoracic pressure in the trunk of the body. Malfunction of the veins' one-way valves results in **venous stasis** or pooling, which can cause the veins to dilate abnormally (called a *varicosity*). A number of physiological functions prevent blood from clotting in the vessels. Movement is among the most important. Stasis and pooling can cause thrombosis or blood clots in peripheral or cardiac circulation.

Box 30.1 presents important differences between arteries and veins.

CIRCULATORY PATHWAYS

The circulatory system is divided into two main pathways: the systemic system and the pulmonary system as shown in Fig. 30.4. These systems function simultaneously. The heart acts as a pump for both systems.

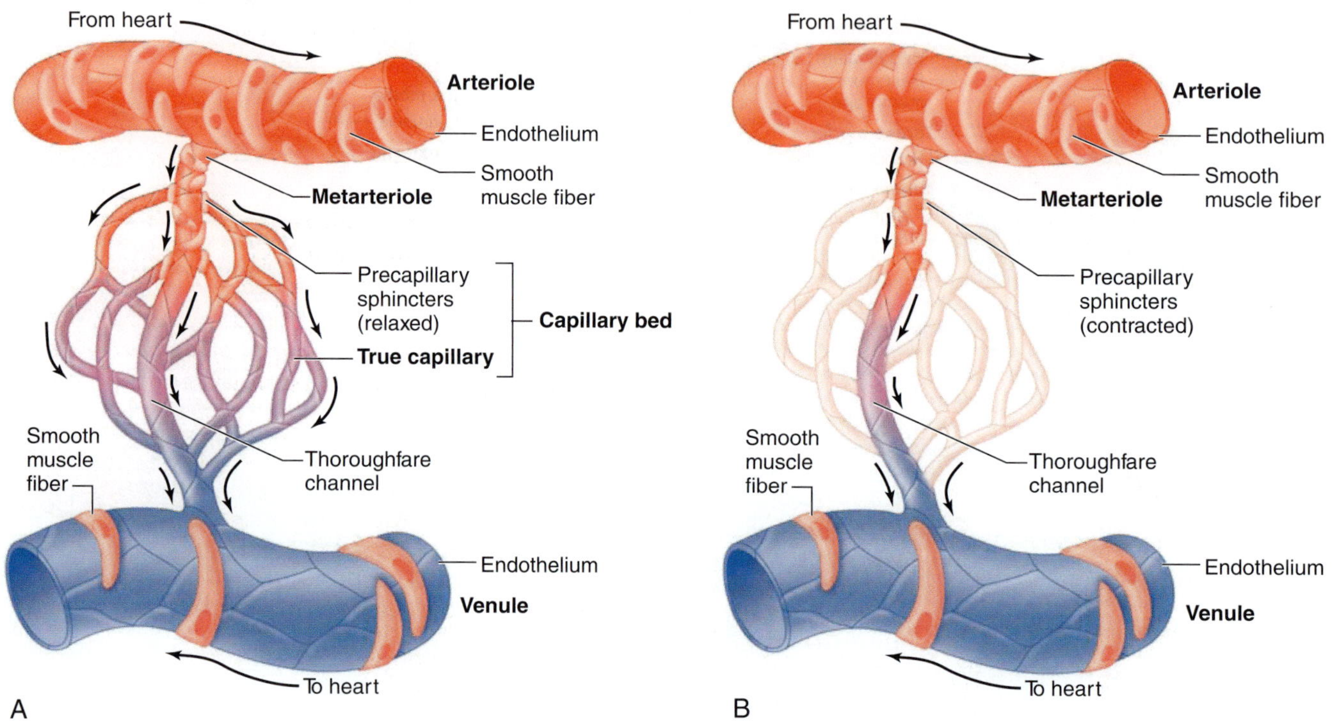

FIG. 30.2 Microcirculation in the capillary system. (A) Precapillary sphincters relaxed—blood flows through the capillary bed. (B) Precapillary sphincters contracted—blood flows through larger arterioles only. (From Patton KT, Thibodeau GA, Douglas MM. *Essentials of Anatomy and Physiology—Text and Anatomy and Physiology Online Course*. St Louis: Elsevier-Mosby; 2012.)

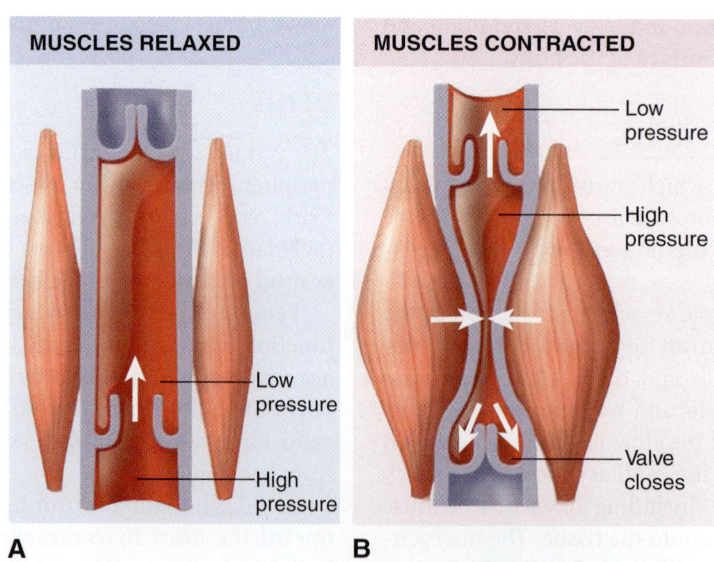

FIG. 30.3 Skeletal muscle "pump." One-way valves in the veins prevent blood from backing up. Blood in the extremities is milked toward the heart by skeletal muscle contraction. (From Patton KT, Thibodeau GA, Douglas MM. *Essentials of Anatomy and Physiology—Text and Anatomy and Physiology Online Course*. St Louis: Elsevier-Mosby; 2012.)

BOX 30.1 Comparison of Arteries and Veins

ARTERIES
- Thick walls
- Elastic
- Blood moves through arteries by the pumping action of the heart
- No internal valves
- Loss of function can lead to tissue injury or death
- When severed, spurt blood (because of pumping action of the heart)
- Blood loss can be rapid and severe
- Arterial pressure is higher than venous pressure

VEINS
- Thin walls
- Less elastic than arteries
- Blood moves through veins by the contraction of skeletal muscles
- Internal valves prevent backflow
- Loss of function not as medically significant as with arteries
- When severed, tend to bleed slowly
- Tend to be closer to the skin surface than arteries

SYSTEMIC CIRCULATION

The systemic circulatory path carries blood to all organs and tissues of the body *except the lungs* and then returns it to the heart. The circuit from the heart to the organs and tissues includes the arteries, arterioles, and capillaries. It is here, at the capillaries where nutritive substances including oxygen are exchanged for carbon dioxide and other waste products. The deoxygenated blood begins its path from capillary to venule, to the systemic veins and back to the heart, which pumps it into the pulmonary circuit.

PULMONARY CIRCULATION

The pulmonary circuit moves blood to the lungs and back to the heart. After the deoxygenated blood has entered the heart from the two vena cavae, it flows into the right atrium and then into the right ventricle to be pumped into the pulmonary arteries and into the lungs.

IMPORTANT TO KNOW *The pulmonary arteries are the only arteries of the body that carry deoxygenated blood.*

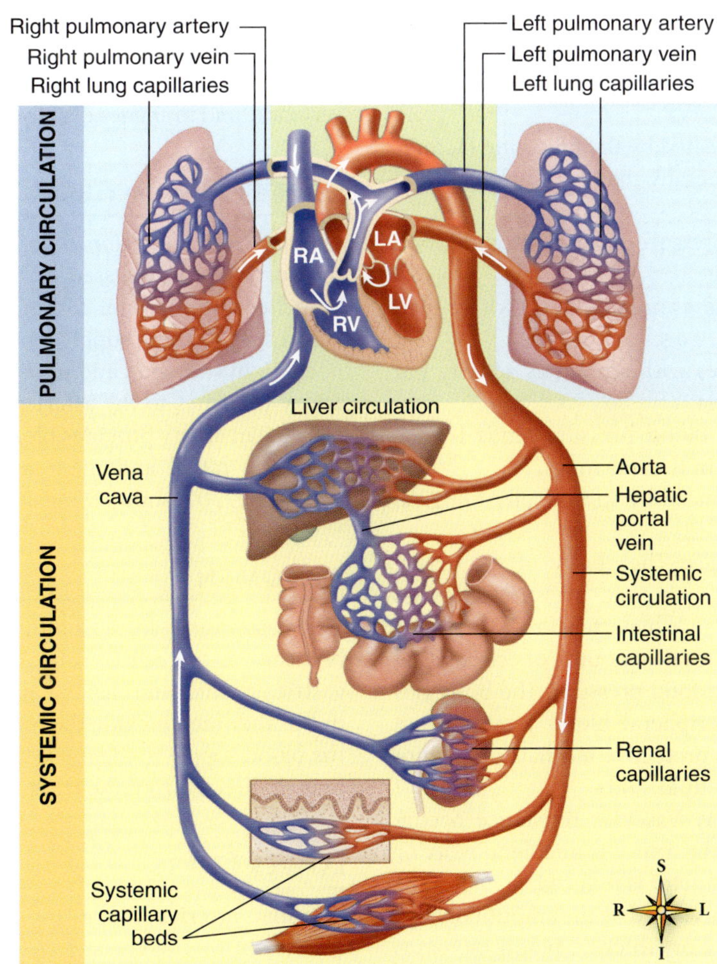

FIG. 30.4 Cardiac and systemic circulation. (From Patton KT, Thibodeau GA, Douglas MM. *Essentials of Anatomy and Physiology—Text and Anatomy and Physiology Online Course.* St Louis: Elsevier-Mosby; 2012.)

Carbon dioxide in the deoxygenated blood is exchanged for oxygen in the capillaries of the alveoli in the lungs. The newly oxygenated blood is then transported into the venules and pulmonary veins. From there it enters the left atrium of the heart.

BLOOD PRESSURE

Blood pressure is the force exerted on the arterial wall by the pumping action of the heart. The *systolic pressure,* the higher pressure, occurs during the contraction of the ventricles (systole). The lower pressure, the *diastolic pressure,* occurs during the relaxation phase of the cardiac cycle (diastole).

Regulation of blood pressure is influenced by chemicals released by the autonomic nervous system in response to injury, body position, temperature, pain, and emotion. The complex hormonal regulation of arterial pressure, which is called the *renin-angiotensin-aldosterone system,* is influenced by fluid volume and other factors.

A decrease in blood pressure *(hypotension)* can be caused by hypovolemia (a precipitous drop in blood or fluid volume), fluid shifts between the spaces in the body, shock, or infection.

Hypertension, or abnormally high blood pressure, often is caused by cardiovascular disease, such as arteriosclerosis, but it also occurs with chronic renal failure and hypermetabolic conditions (e.g., malignant hyperthermia and hyperaldosteronism).

Normal blood pressure is affected by the following factors:

- *Gender:* Adult females generally have a higher blood pressure than males.
- *Age:* A gradual rise in blood pressure occurs from childhood to adulthood.
- *Weight:* Blood pressure is higher in individuals with a high body mass index, regardless of age.
- *Exercise:* Blood pressure rises with strenuous activity but returns to baseline level at rest.
- *Diurnal (daily) fluctuation:* Blood pressure tends to rise during the day and is lowest in the mornings.

Blood pressure is also influenced by specific physiological parameters:

- *Elasticity of the arterial walls:* The ability of the artery to expand and relax affects systemic pressure. Arteries stiffened by atherosclerosis cause hypertension.
- *Total blood volume:* The total amount of circulating blood has a direct effect on blood pressure. The body has mechanisms to constrict peripheral blood vessels when volume is low. However, this protective mechanism cannot overcome large blood loss or fluid shifts.
- *Peripheral vascular resistance:* Vascular resistance occurs when the muscular layer of the artery is unable to relax or arteries are stiff and their diameter is reduced.
- *Blood viscosity:* Viscosity is measured by the amount of fluid in the blood. Lower viscosity or "thicker" blood increases blood pressure.

MAJOR ARTERIES

The largest artery of the body is the aorta. It emerges from the heart in an arch at the left ventricle and curves downward to descend through the thoracic cavity, passing behind the heart but in front of the spinal column. As it enters the abdomen, it passes through the diaphragm behind the retroperitoneum space. The aorta terminates at the pelvic **bifurcation** (splitting into a Y), which forms iliac arteries.

THORACIC CAVITY

The aorta arises from the left ventricle of the heart to form an arch (the *aortic arch*). Three major arteries arise from the top of the arch: the *brachiocephalic* artery, the *left common carotid* artery, and the *left subclavian* artery. Beyond these branches, the aortic arch curves downward and is called the thoracic *descending aorta.* It passes through the diaphragm and leaves the thoracic cavity and enters the abdominal cavity. It is called the *abdominal aorta* at this level. There are many branches of the aorta at all levels.

HEAD

The *brachiocephalic artery* gives rise to the *right common carotid artery,* which branches to form the *external carotid artery* and the arteries of the brain (Fig. 30.5). The vertebral artery, which branches from the *brachiocephalic artery,* follows the cervical vertebrae and branches distally to the arteries of the head.

UPPER EXTREMITIES

The arteries of the upper body begin at the three vessels of the aortic arch discussed earlier. The brachiocephalic artery branches into the right common carotid and the right subclavian arteries. These supply blood to the right side of the head, neck, right shoulder, and upper arm. The left common carotid artery branches to the arteries of the neck and head. The left subclavian artery provides blood to the left shoulder and right arm. The radial and ulnar arteries arise from the brachial artery. Fig. 30.6 shows the major arteries of the body.

ABDOMEN

The descending aorta continues through the abdomen and branches to the celiac trunk, a network that gives rise to the gastric, splenic, and hepatic arteries. Other significant arteries in the abdomen include the mesenteric arteries, which provide the blood supply to the intestines, and the renal arteries, which branch directly from the aorta and supply blood to the kidneys.

LOWER LIMBS

The iliac arteries divide into the internal and external iliac arteries in the pelvis, and the external iliac artery converges into the femoral artery in the groin. Traveling distally, the

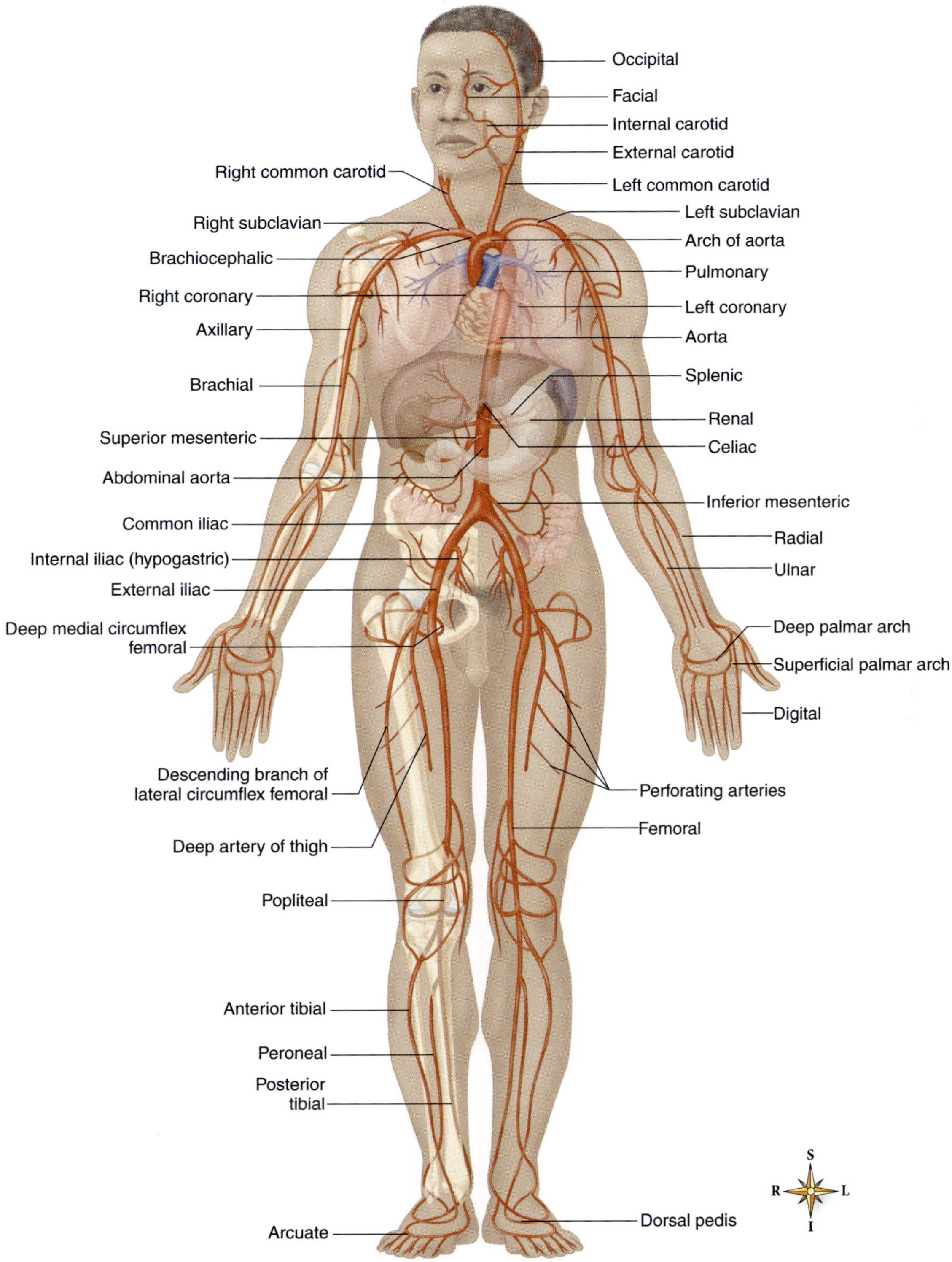

FIG. 30.5 Major arteries of the body. (From Patton KT, Thibodeau GA, Douglas MM. *Essentials of Anatomy and Physiology—Text and Anatomy and Physiology Online Course*. St Louis: Elsevier-Mosby; 2012.)

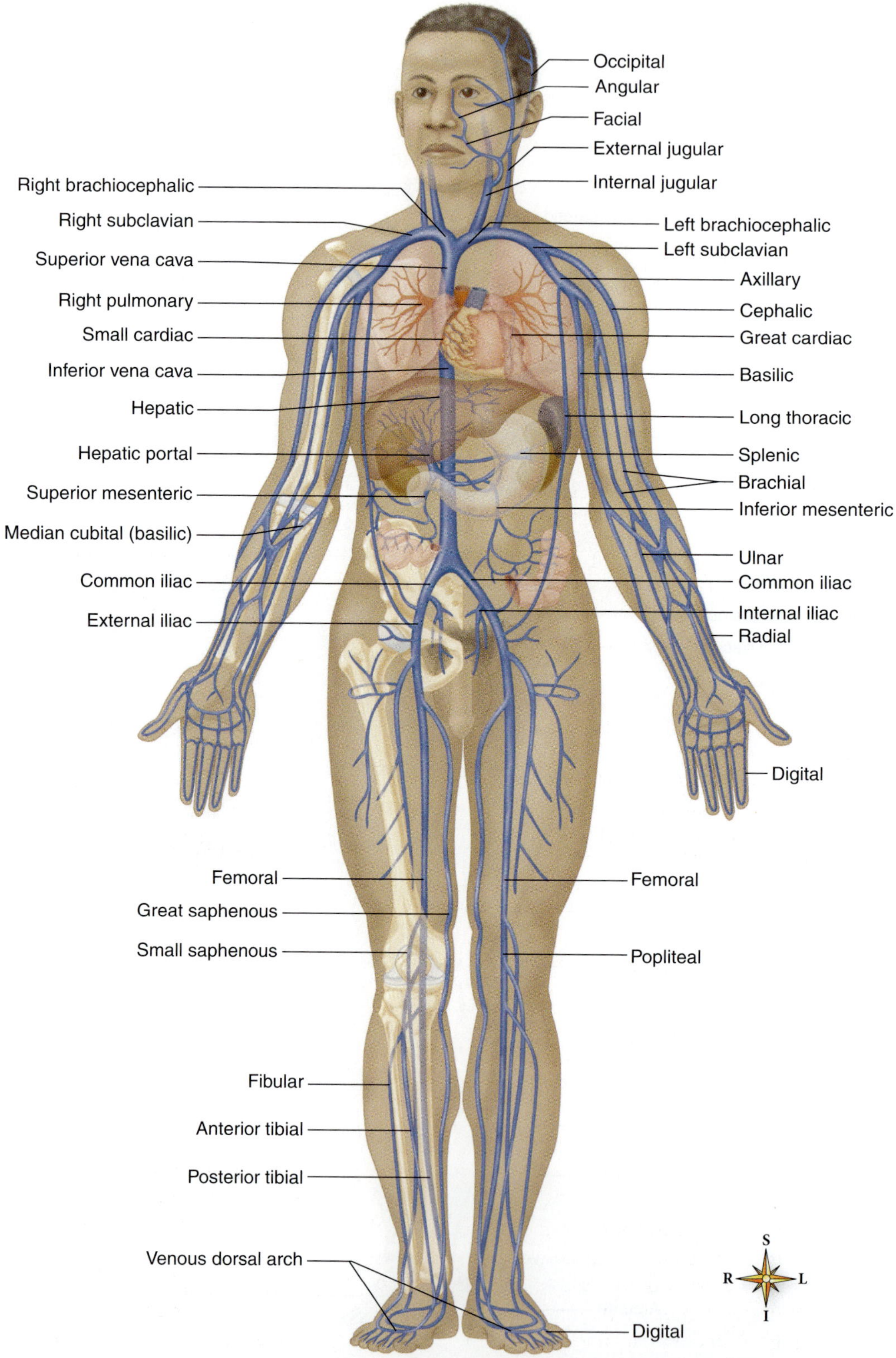

FIG. 30.6 Major veins of the body. (From Patton KT, Thibodeau GA, Douglas MM. *Essentials of Anatomy and Physiology—Text and Anatomy and Physiology Online Course*. St Louis: Elsevier-Mosby; 2012.)

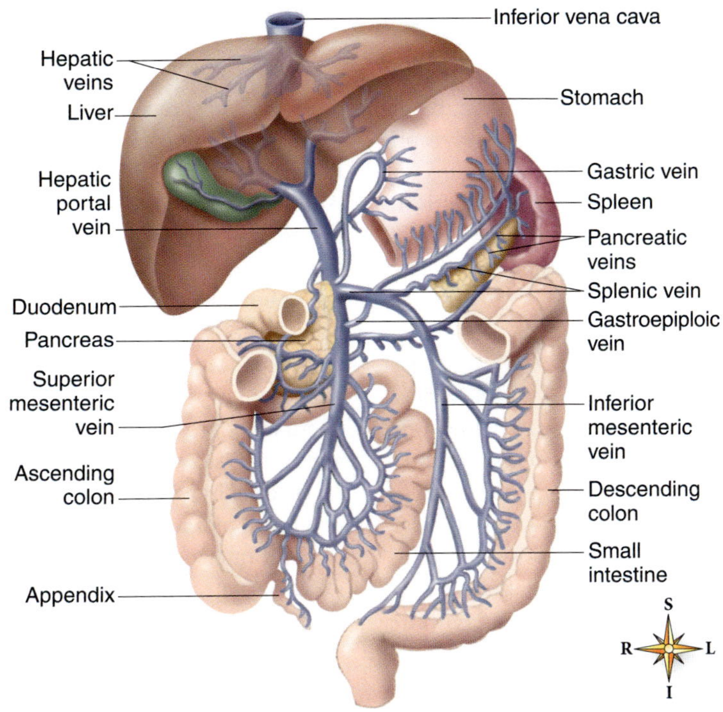

FIG. 30.7 Hepatic portal circulation. In this system veins are located between two capillary beds. The hepatic *portal* vein collects blood from the abdominal viscera and shunts it to the liver. The hepatic vein returns the blood to the inferior vena cava.

femoral artery communicates with the popliteal artery in the knee area. The popliteal artery branches into the anterior tibial, peroneal, and posterior tibial arteries. The dorsal pedis emerges from the anterior tibial artery and then further divides into smaller arteries of the foot and phalanges.

MAJOR VEINS

The largest vein of the body is the vena cava, which is divided into *inferior* and *superior* segments. The venae cavae communicate with the heart through the right atrium. The superior vena cava receives deoxygenated blood from the head, neck, and upper extremities, and the inferior vena cava receives blood from the lower body and extremities. The major veins are illustrated in Fig. 30.6.

PORTAL CIRCULATION

The hepatic portal circulation is unique in structure and function. The superior mesenteric and splenic veins converge to form the portal vein. This large vessel carries nutrients from the digestive system into the liver and supplies about 60% of that organ's oxygen requirements. The hepatic veins carry blood out of the liver to the vena cava. However, a pressure difference between the hepatic and portal veins allows the liver to store approximately 450 mL of blood. This can be released back into the systemic circulation as needed.

Microscopic sinuses (sinusoids) in the liver, which are lined with epithelium, filter and remove bacteria, toxins, and cell remnants from the blood. The blood then is shunted back into the hepatic veins and into the vena cava (Fig. 30.7). Because of the structure of the liver and sinusoids, fibrotic diseases of the liver, such as cirrhosis and hepatitis, can prevent the flow of venous blood out of the sinusoids. Blood backs up into the veins of the digestive system, causing varicosities and rupture of the vessels.

LYMPHATIC SYSTEM

The lymphatic system is composed of ducts (vessels), regional lymph nodes, and lymph (fluid). Lymph tissue such as the tonsils, adenoids, and Peyer's patches, in the large intestine, are important surveillance tissues that help to mediate the immune system. Lymph contributes to the formation of plasma, the liquid portion of blood, which is derived from intercellular components. Lymph vessels follow the anatomical pattern of arteries and veins. Like veins, lymph vessels contain valves that prevent reverse flow. The complex lymph system drains into two primary collection ducts. The right lymphatic duct drains lymph from the head, neck, thorax, and right arm. Lymph from the right lymphatic duct enters the subclavian vein. The second collecting system is the thoracic duct, which receives lymph from other parts of the body and drains into the left subclavian vein. Occlusion of these ducts (e.g., during radical surgery) results in lymphedema or swelling of the lymph vessels. Certain diseases and tumors also cause blockage of the lymph system.

Lymph nodes are located at intervals along the lymph ducts. Nodes are composed of lymphatic tissue that collects and filters fluid from the system. They also produce lymphocytes (white blood cells). Nodes occur in groups or chains in collection areas. For example, the axillary nodes drain lymph from the breasts. Lymph from the pelvic organs drains to nodes in the inguinal area. During lymph node dissection, specific nodes are removed and assessed according to the organ suspected of cancer to determine whether metastasis has occurred.

VASCULAR DISEASE

There are many different types of vascular disease. However, *atherosclerosis* is the most common pathology requiring surgery. This is an obstructive arterial disease that causes stiffening and loss of elasticity of the artery wall. In peripheral atherosclerosis, fatty plaque and calcium are deposited on the tunica intima, causing stenosis and poor circulation. Areas of plaque are most dense near arterial bifurcations. Circulatory obstruction in the lower limbs leads to intermittent *claudication* (severe pain related to obstructed arterial flow) and ischemia. Dry gangrene may develop in untreated severe obstruction. In addition to causing reduced blood flow to vital organs and tissues, atherosclerosis can also result in embolism when fragments of the plaque are released into the bloodstream. This can result in brain attack (stroke). Atherosclerosis is the primary cause of high blood pressure. *Thrombophlebitis* affects the superficial veins of the legs. In this condition, painful clots form as a result of venous stasis often related to inactivity. *Deep vein thrombosis* is the presence of one or more clots in the deep veins of the leg.

IMPORTANT TO KNOW *The difference between a thrombus and an embolus is that a thrombus is stationary in the vessel, whereas an embolism moves through the circulatory system until it reaches a location that is too small for it to pass through.*

An **aneurysm** is a portion of an artery that has increased in size by greater than 50% of the normal diameter. Aneurysms may occur as a result of infection, disease, or trauma. An aneurysm can potentially occur in any part of the body but is most frequent in areas where the artery branches into two tributaries, such as the iliac bifurcations of the aorta. As the aneurysm expands, it can eventually and catastrophically burst. There are three structural forms of aneurysms: saccular, fusiform, and dissecting (Fig. 30.8). Abdominal aortic aneurysm is discussed in this chapter. Thoracic and cardiac aneurysms are covered in their respective chapters. Cerebral aneurysm is covered in Chapter 34.

Intimal hyperplasia is a thickening of the tunica intima layer as a result of long-term central line placement, graft placement, or other interventions that irritate the intima. Intimal hyperplasia can occur in both arteries and veins. In arteries, symptoms similar to those of atherosclerosis often result; in veins, poor venous return, swelling, and tissue breakdown can occur.

DIAGNOSTIC PROCEDURES

Diagnosis of peripheral vascular disease is based first on the patient's history, the physical examination findings, and the results of routine blood tests. More specific studies may be performed on the basis of the findings of these tests and the patient's signs and symptoms.

ARTERIAL PLETHYSMOGRAPHY

A pulse volume recorder is used to measure the arterial pulse waveform during systole. For this test, three blood pressure cuffs are placed on the leg and inflated to 65 mm Hg. Each cuff reading produces a waveform, which is compared with the

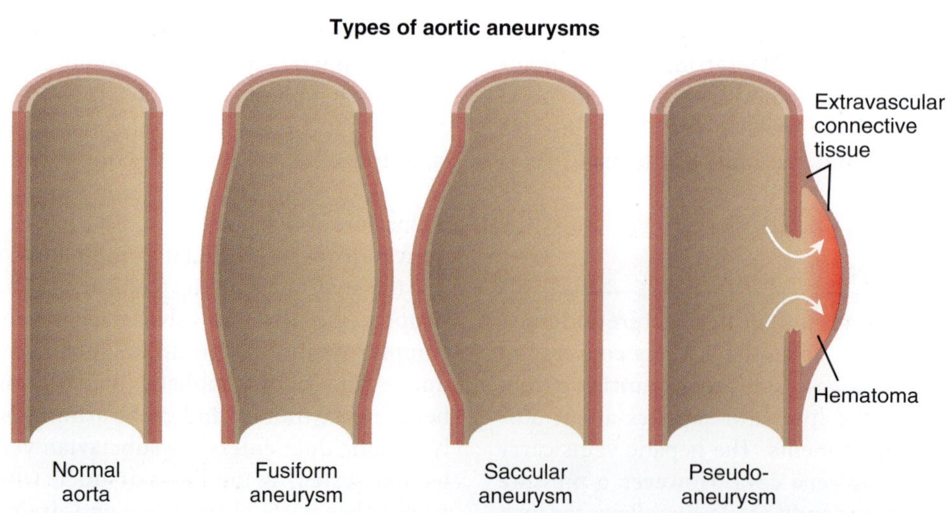

FIG. 30.8 Structural types of aortic aneurysms. The fusiform is the most common. It bulges outward symmetrically. The saccular aneurysm protrudes from one wall only. The pseudo-aneurysm is characterized by a hematoma that arises from the vessel wall. The dissecting aneurysm (not shown) results from a tear in the innermost tissue layer of the vessel (intima), which gives rise to splitting of the arterial wall. (From Solomon S, Wu J, Gillam L. *Essential Echocardiography: Companion to Braunwald's Heart Disease*. Philadelphia: Elsevier; 2019.)

waveforms from the other two cuffs. A reduced wave in one area may indicate reduced blood flow at that point.

DOPPLER SCANNING

Doppler scanning intensifies the sounds made by blood flowing through a vessel. The pitch, rhythm, and quality of the sound reflect pressure, volume, and flow rate. The tip of the Doppler probe is placed over a pulse point or other area that requires evaluation. The high-frequency sound waves generated by the probe are reflected back to a data recorder. Intraoperative Doppler scanning is performed with a sterile probe. **Doppler duplex ultrasonography** combines Doppler scanning with ultrasound to produce visual images of the vessel. Decreased blood flow, strictures, thrombi, turbulence (swirling motion of blood characteristic at a stricture), and other abnormalities are displayed on a monitor in real time and can be preserved for permanent documentation.

ARTERIOGRAPHY AND ANGIOGRAPHY

Angiography refers to imaging of arteries or veins. This is done as an intraoperative, diagnostic, or interventional procedure to delineate the lumen and interior surface of the arteries.

Angiography to obtain a diagnosis before surgery is commonly performed in the interventional radiology department's *angiography suite*. This is a specific department of the hospital or health care facility. The angiography suite is staffed by radiologists, certified radiology technologists trained in interventional angiography techniques, nurses, and anesthesiologists. The surgical technologist may have an opportunity to work in this setting; however, the angiography technologist is usually the professional who assists. Angiography performed as a step in a surgical procedure is similar.

During angiography a contrast medium is injected into the artery under fluoroscopy or computed tomography. Complex studies that provide three-dimensional images and time flow data are commonly used in diagnosis. *Multidetector computed tomography angiography* has taken the place of conventional angiography for diagnostic studies of the arterial system. Interventional arteriography is performed in conjunction with the insertion of stents, angioplasty balloons, and other devices.

INTRAVASCULAR ULTRASONOGRAPHY

Intravascular ultrasound is used in both peripheral and coronary surgery to map the **lumen** of a vessel. A rotating flexible catheter carrying a transducer is introduced into the vessel. Ultrasonic energy is generated and interpreted by the transducer. The lumen of the vessel can be mapped (including density, accumulation of atherosclerotic plaque, and wall thickness), and a visual image can be produced. Because the catheter is able to rotate, intravascular ultrasound produces a 360-degree image.

VASCULAR INSTRUMENTS

Vascular surgery is performed with general surgical and vascular instruments. Other instruments are added according to the regional anatomy. All vascular procedures require right-angle (Mixter type) clamps, tonsil (Schnidt) clamps, and Kelly, Crile, and mosquito forceps. General dissecting scissors and general surgery forceps are also used on nonvascular tissue. Common vascular instruments are shown in the Vascular Instruments table.

VASCULAR INSTRUMENTS

METZENBAUM SCIS DELICATE 5¾″	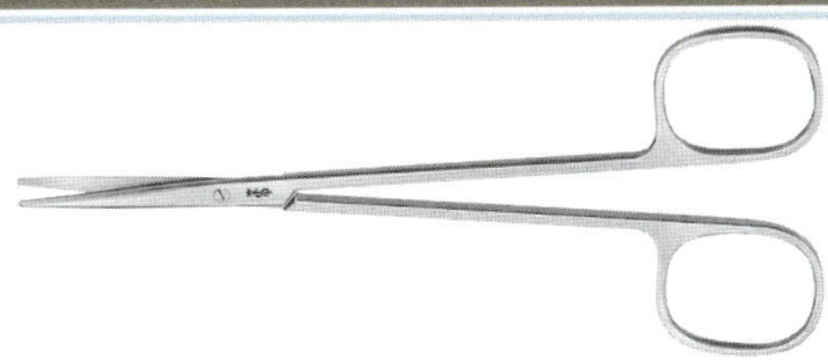 Photo courtesy Aesculup, Inc., Center Valley, PA.	STRAIGHT DISSECTING SCIS 7½″	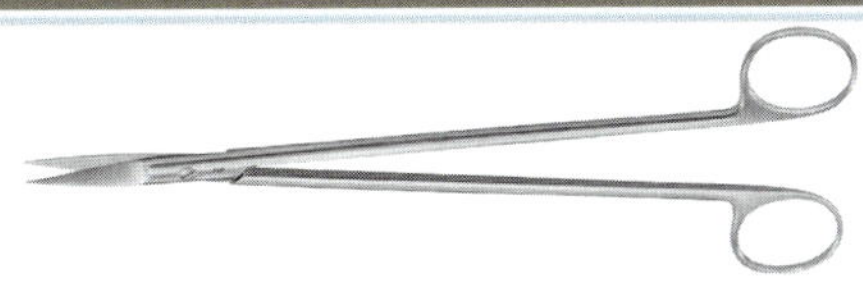 Photo courtesy Aesculup, Inc., Center Valley, PA.
POTTS-DEMARTEL SCIS 8½″	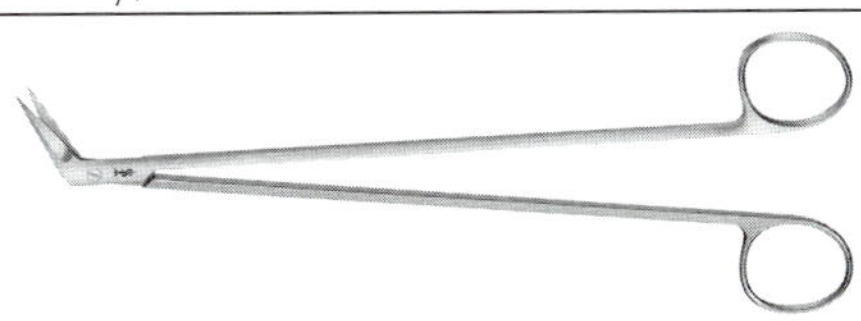 Photo courtesy Aesculup, Inc., Center Valley, PA.	DEBAKEY DIETH TISSUE FCPS	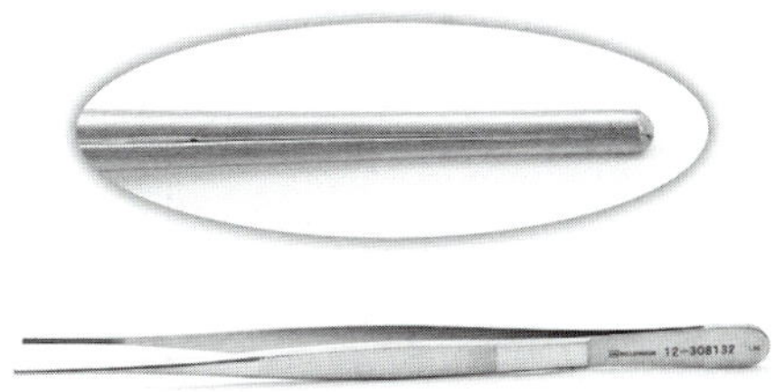 Millennium Surgical Corp.
DEBAKEY ATRAUMATIC TISSUE FCPS 6″	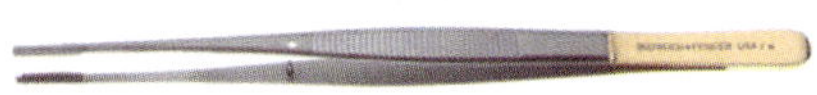 Millennium Surgical Corp.	CUSHING ANGLE FCPS 7″	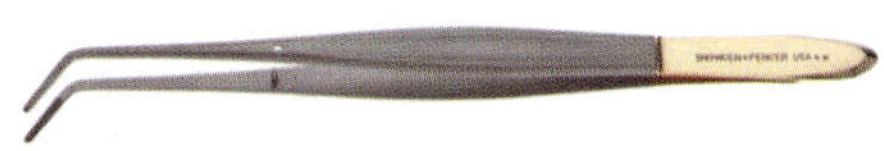 Courtesy and copyright Becton, Dickinson and Company.

VASCULAR INSTRUMENTS —cont'd

JAVID CLAMP 7″

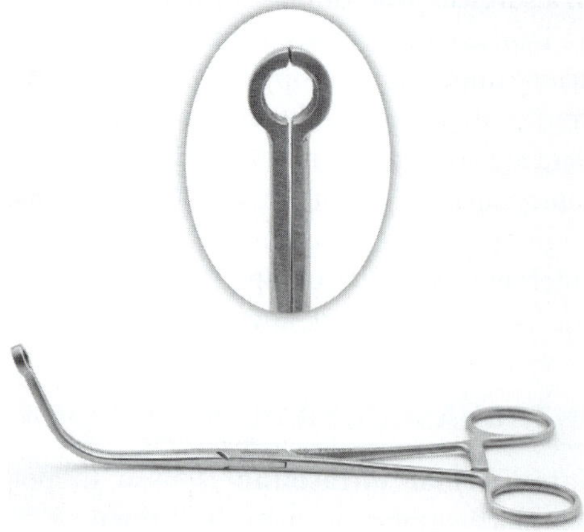

Millennium Surgical Corp.

COOLEY PERIPHERAL CLAMP 7″

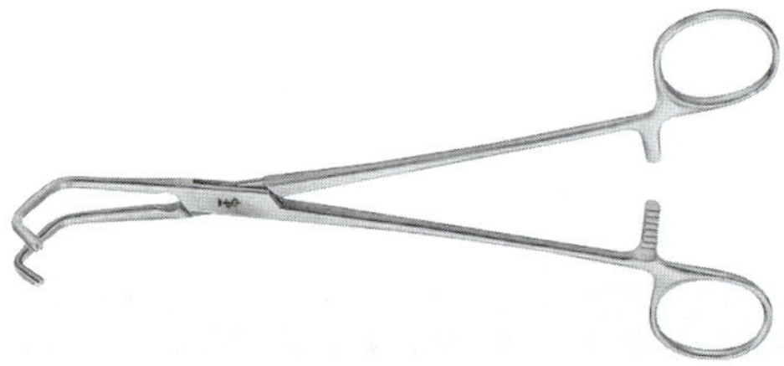

Photo courtesy Aesculup, Inc., Center Valley, PA.

Penfield 4 Dissector 8″

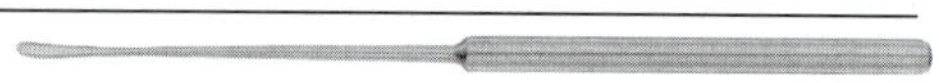

Photo courtesy Aesculup, Inc., Center Valley, PA.

DEBAKEY ATRAUMATIC VENA CAVA CLAMP 8″

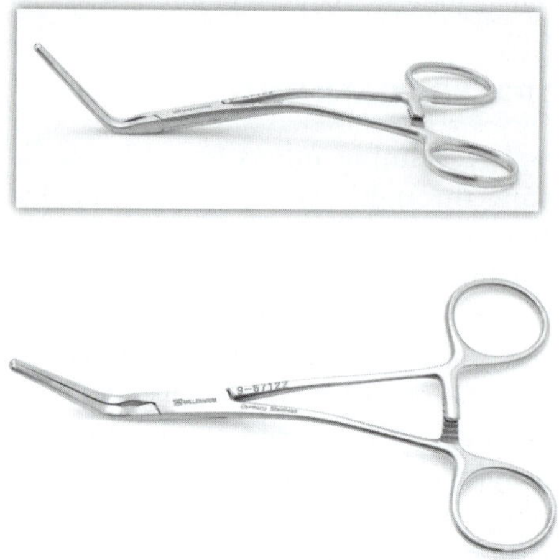

Photo courtesy Aesculup, Inc., Center Valley, PA.

DERRA ANASTOMOSIS CLAMP 6½″

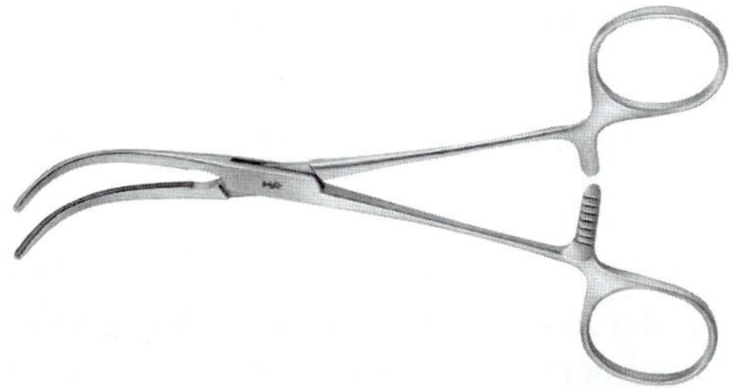

Millennium Surgical Corp.

GLOVER BULLDOG CLAMP

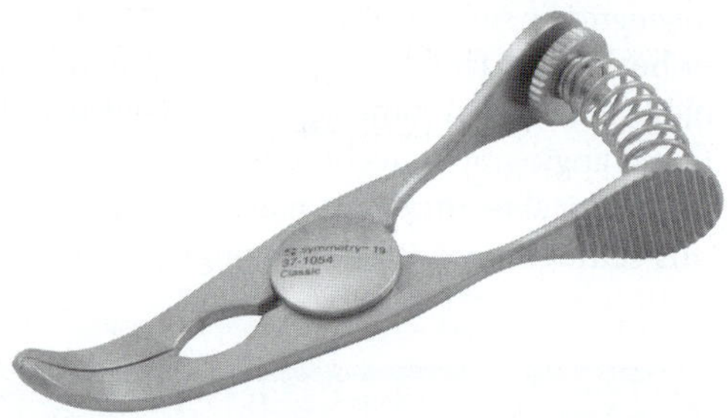

Courtesy and copyright Becton, Dickinson and Company.

OLIVE TIP IRRIGATION NEEDLE

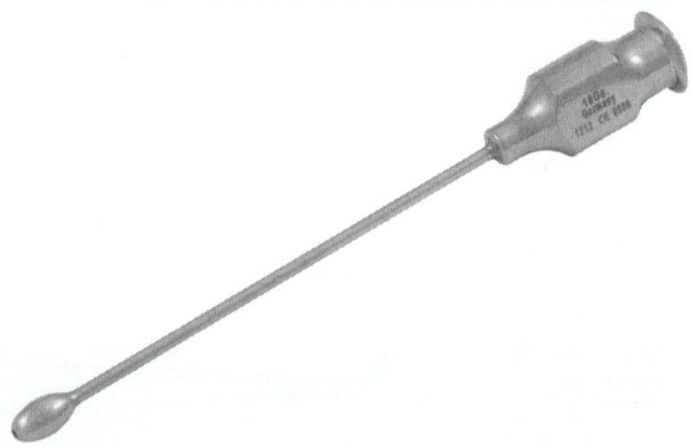

Copyright Symmetry Surgical Inc.; photo courtesy of Symmetry Surgical Inc.

VASCULAR INSTRUMENTS —cont'd

CASTROVIEJO MICRO NEEDLE HOLDER 4¾″ (size 7-0 suture and smaller)

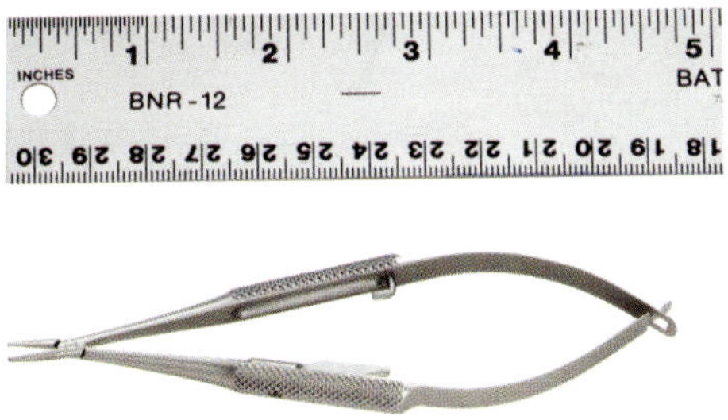

MICRO NEEDLE HOLDER (size 5-0 suture and smaller) 4¾″

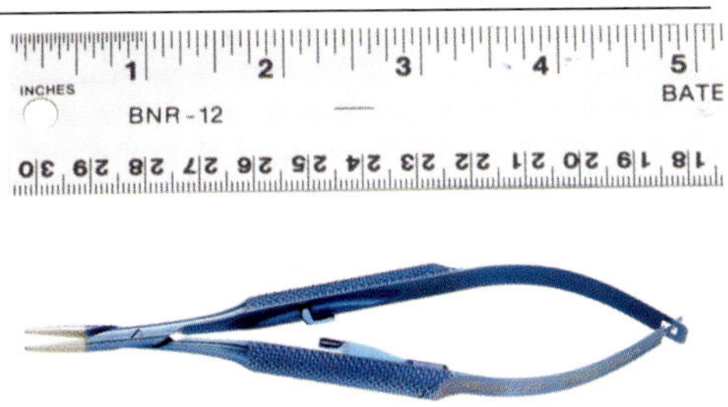

MICRO SUTURE TYING FORCEPS ANGLED 5½″

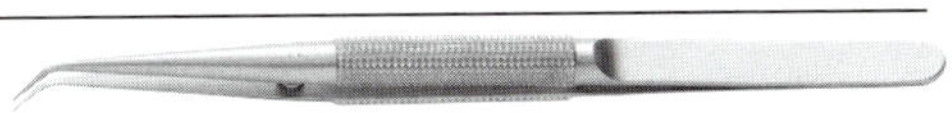

CASTROVIEJO MICRO SCISSORS (1 blade with bead) 4⅛″

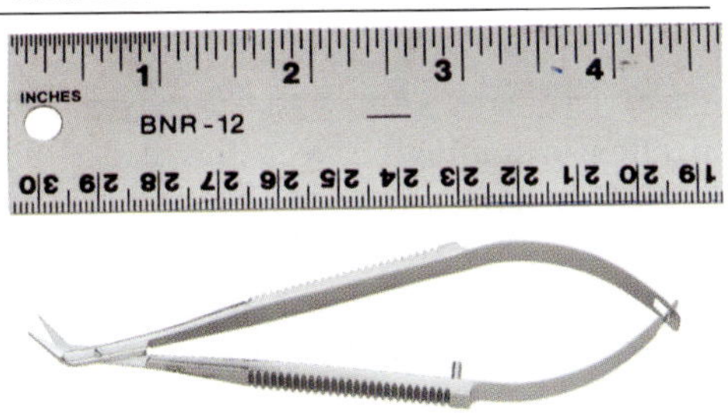

JACOBSON MICRO SCISSORS STRAIGHT BLADES 6″

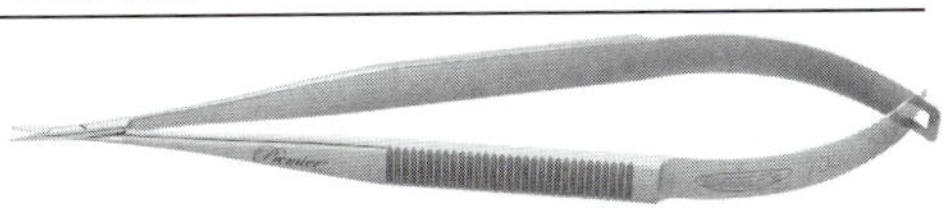

TITANIUM RICHARDS MICRO NEEDLE HOLDER 6¾″ (size 6-0 suture and smaller)

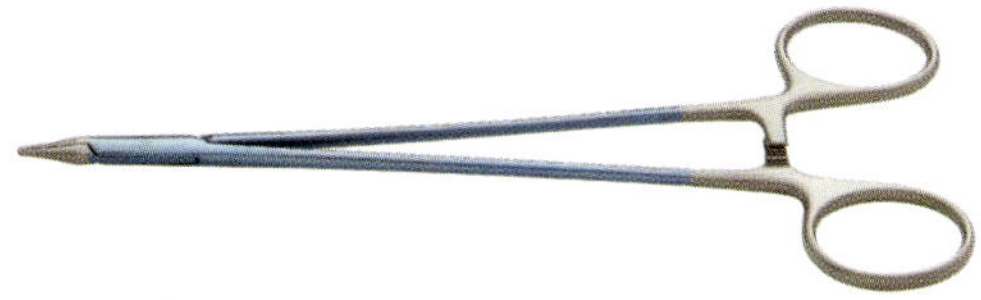

JEWELERS FORCEPS 4½″

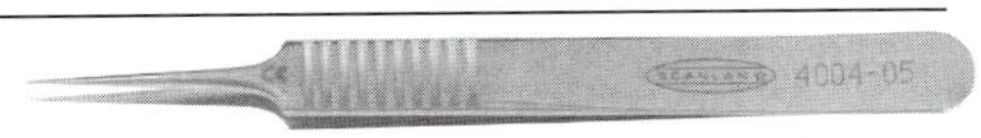

MICRO SUTURE TYING FORCEPS 6″

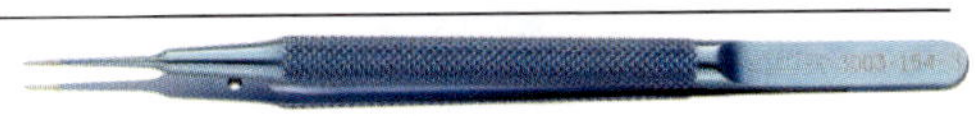

CASTROVIEJO MICRO SCISSORS CURVED BLADES 5½″

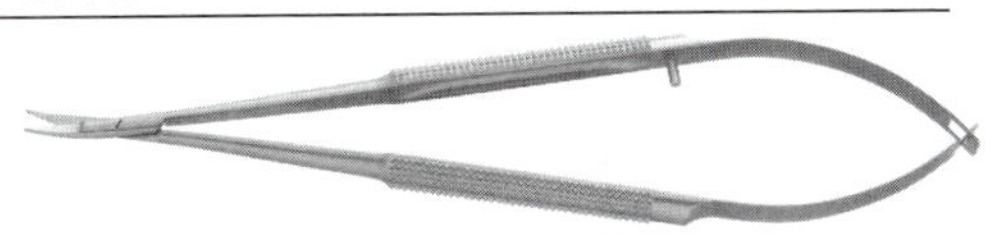

IRIS-EYE SCISSORS 4″

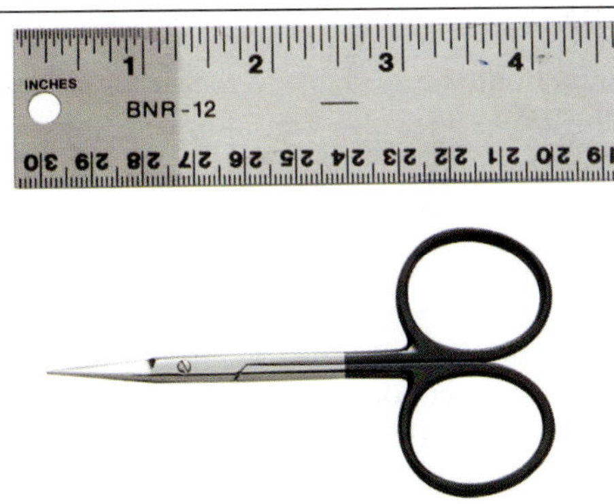

VASCULAR INSTRUMENTS—cont'd

STEVENS TENOTOMY SCISSORS 4⅝″

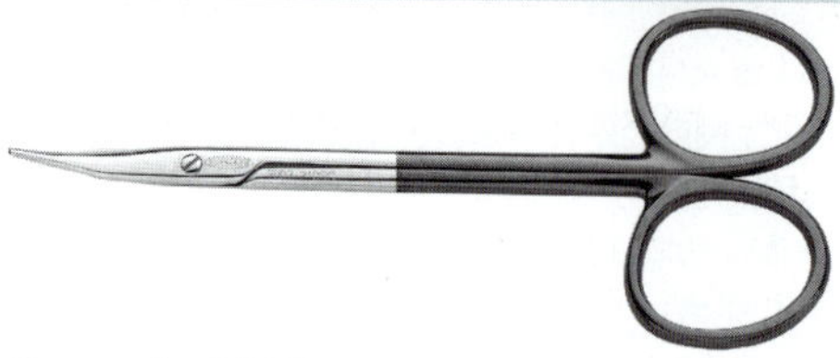

Copyright 2019; Image courtesy Scanlan International, http://www.scanlaninternational.com

BABY METZENBAUM SCISSORS 4¾″

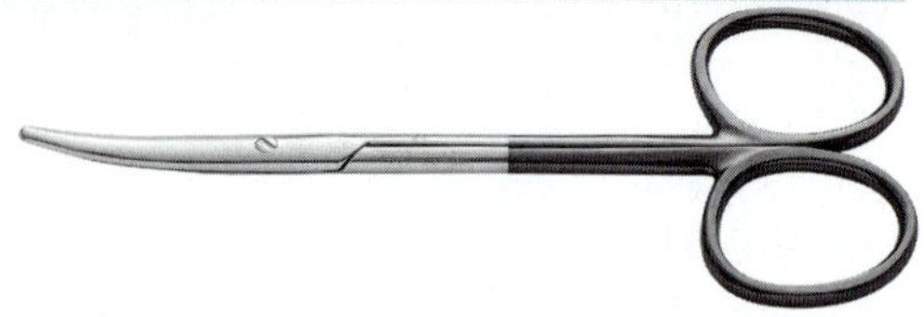

Copyright 2019; Image courtesy Scanlan International, http://www.scanlaninternational.com

RAGNELL DISSECTION SCISSORS 6″

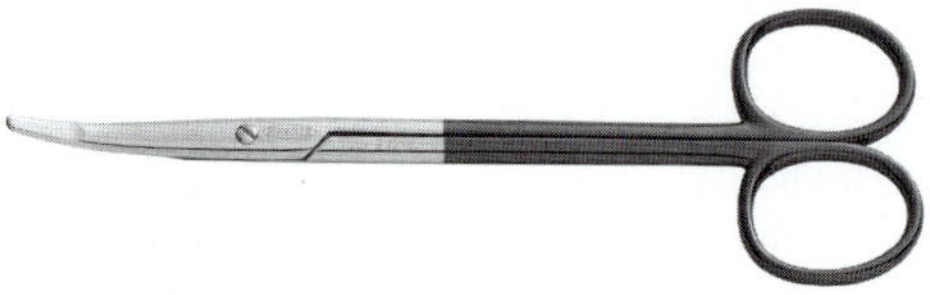

Copyright 2019; Image courtesy Scanlan International, http://www.scanlaninternational.com

VASCULAR MOSQUITO FORCEPS 4½″

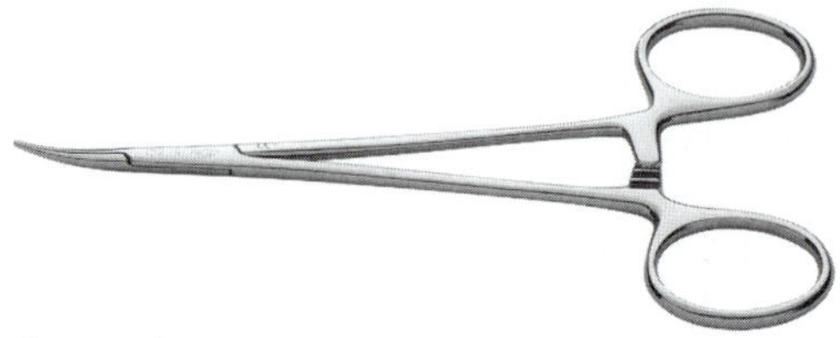

Copyright 2019; Image courtesy Scanlan International, http://www.scanlaninternational.com

FOGARTY CLAMP WITH JAW INSERTS

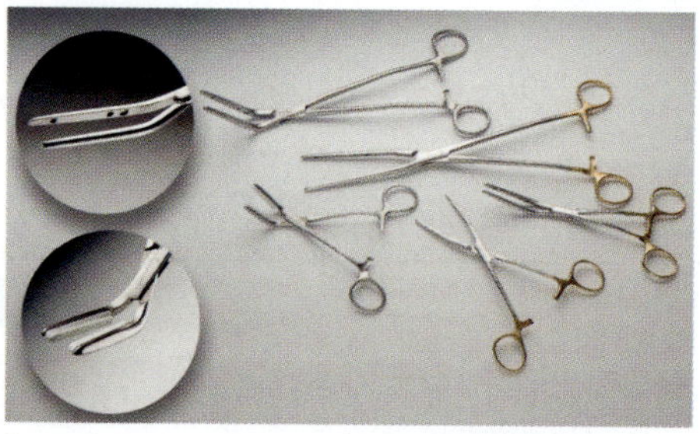

From Nemitz. *Surgical Instrumentation: An Interactive Approach*. 3rd ed. St. Louis: Elsevier; 2019.

IMPORTANT TO KNOW *The nomenclature used to differentiate vascular instruments often contains the name of the inventor(s) (e.g., Potts, Satinsky, DeBakey, Potts-Smith, Satinsky-DeBakey) followed by the type of instrument and finally the generic description. Examples include Potts coarctation clamp, Satinsky vena cava clamp, DeBakey tangential occlusion clamp, Potts-Smith scissors, DeBakey forceps.*

It is common for surgeons to specify exactly which instruments should be available in the sterile setup of a specific procedure. This provides continuity during the procedure and decreases the possibility of the wrong instruments, especially during critical stages during the procedure.

CLAMPS

Vascular clamps are specifically designed to occlude large blood vessels without damaging them. Their jaws contain finely serrated inserts that grip the tissue but do not crush or damage the surface of the vessel, even when fully closed. Clamps are available in a wide variety of shapes and sizes to fit around a vessel as it lies in normal anatomical position. Peripheral vascular clamps are smaller than those used in cardiac surgery. Hundreds of types of vascular clamps are available.

SCISSORS

Vascular scissors are extremely delicate. It is very important that the blades are well maintained to prevent tissue from buckling or folding between the blades. Scissors are sharply pointed or have a rounded probe tip. The most commonly used vessel dissection scissors are Potts (angled) and De Martel (straight) scissors. Fine Metzenbaum scissors are also used in vascular dissection. Vascular scissors must never be used to cut any materials such as suture or grafts because this can dull or cause misalignment of the blades.

FORCEPS

Vascular forceps (pickups) have very fine serrations at the tips to allow a secure grip on veins and arteries without injuring the tissue.

Surgeons generally do not ask for a specific type of vascular forceps during surgery. They assume that their personal preference is on record and have been placed on the instrument table. Vascular forceps are always passed to the surgeon when it is apparent they will be used to grasp a blood vessel or other delicate tissue. Plain general surgical forceps are not suitable for use on vascular tissue because they do not have the precision or gripping ability of vascular forceps. Toothed forceps are never used on blood vessels because they can puncture the walls of the vessel.

RETRACTORS

There are few vascular-specific retractors except small vein retractors, which are also used in general surgery. Nonpenetrating shallow retractors are commonly used during superficial vascular surgery. A blunt-tip Weitlaner (self-retracting) or spring retractor should be available for shallow retraction. Handheld retractors include the Senn retractor, vein retractor, and shallow Richardson retractor. Skin hooks may be occasionally needed. Extreme care is taken with any sharp retractors because of the delicate nature of vessels and surrounding structures.

For deeper surgery, general surgery retractors are used (e.g., Deaver, Richardson, and Army-Navy retractors). An Omni-Tract self-retaining retractor can be used for procedures of the abdominal arteries. Smaller self-retaining retractors are used to expose the below-knee popliteal and anterior tibial artery during procedures in this area.

SUCTION

Small suction tips, such as the Frazier, are commonly used in most vascular procedures. The suction pressure should be lowered for use on the actual vessels. Frazier suction tips are available in a wide variety of French (Fr) sizes, and the size used depends on the tissue. During surgery, suction tips must be kept clear of blood and tissue debris by suctioning a small amount of water through the tip. Larger suction tips are used according to the regional anatomy. General surgical tips, such as the Poole (vented) or Yankauer suction tip, are used in abdominal vascular surgery.

A dry surgical site is critical in vascular surgery, and suction must be available at all times. Because vascular suction tips (e.g., the smaller Frazier tip) clog easily, two should be immediately available: one on the field and another held in reserve. This allows the clogged tip to be flushed or cleared with a metal stylet while the other is used.

Large vessels, such as the abdominal aorta, require larger suction tips. Two suctions may be necessary to maintain a dry field. In general, suction is used more often than sponges to maintain a dry operative field.

TUNNELER

A tunneler is used to burrow a channel through connective tissue to make space for a tubular vascular graft. Occasionally during surgery, the graft anastomosis sites are surgically exposed but located some distance apart. The tunneler is inserted into one site and pushed through the subcutaneous tissue to the other wound site. This creates a path for the graft, which can then be pulled through in preparation for anastomosis.

CASE PLANNING

SUTURES

Vascular sutures range in size from 3-0 to 12-0. Cutting and taper needles used for anastomosis have a ⅜-inch or ½-inch curve. Synthetic monofilament or coated suture is preferred over plain braided suture because it is nonreactive and prevents endovascular clotting and emboli.

Vascular suture materials include polyester (Mersilene), polypropylene (Prolene), nylon, polyhexafluoropropylene (Pronova), Gore-Tex, and silk. Suture-needle combinations are very delicate and require careful handling. Only fine-tipped needle holders should be used. Cardiovascular (CV) sutures are available as single needles or double-arm needles.

The CV needle is grasped in the usual position behind the swage, and the suture is gently withdrawn from the package. When passing a double-arm suture, mount one needle on the needle holder and place a small hemostat fitted with jaw covers on the other needle. Instrument jaw covers are short lengths of Silastic tubing, which are fitted over the tips of an instrument to cushion the grip and prevent damage to the suture. Note that there are regional differences in the term *jaw cover.* Jaw cover is the generic name for "suture boot" and "booty." Surgipaw is a trademarked name, and in some health care facilities the jaw cover is called a "paw."

IMPORTANT TO KNOW *During surgery, do not remove a loaded needle holder from the field unless you are certain it is free and clear of the anastomosis. Double-arm sutures are used in tandem, and removing one may drag the other out of the tissue.*

Vascular sutures may also be loaded with felt pledgets (small squares of felted material) attached to the suture (Fig. 30.9). The pledget prevents the suture material from cutting through the arterial wall. These are available in pre-cut sizes.

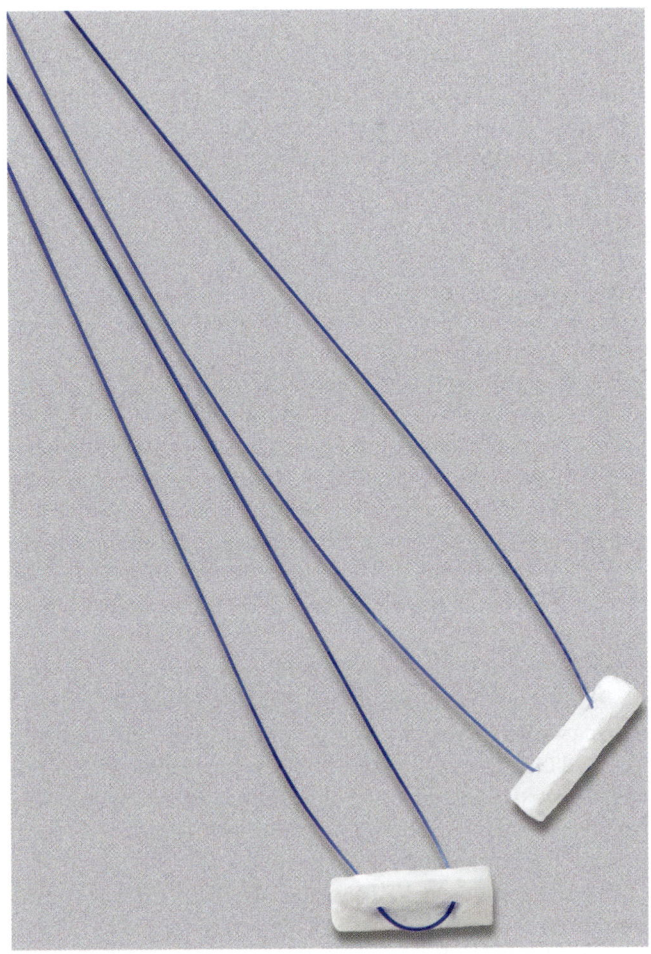

FIG. 30.9 Suture pledget. These are used to prevent sutures from cutting through delicate tissues. (Courtesy Medtronic. All rights reserved. Used with the permission of Medtronic.)

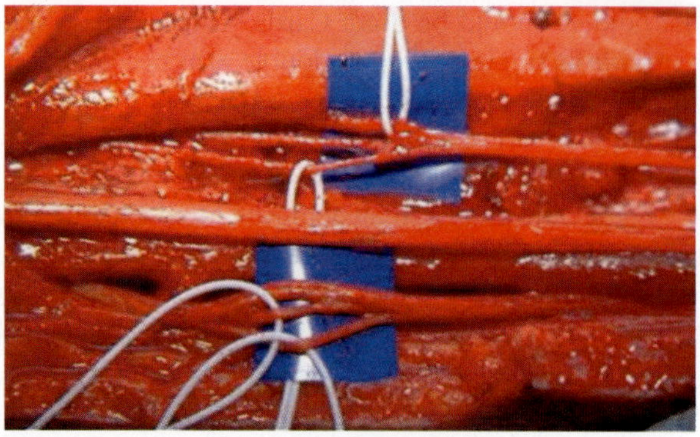

FIG. 30.10 Vessel loops. Silastic bands are commonly used to mobilize and provide traction on blood vessels. Blue visibility aid is also shown. (From Cioffi W, et al, eds. *Atlas of Trauma/Emergency Surgical Techniques*. Philadelphia: Saunders; 2014.)

EXPOSURE AND CONTROL OF BLOOD VESSELS

During vascular surgery, blood vessels are mobilized and prepared for incision and entry. Retraction is performed with a **vessel loop.** Several types of loops are available. The most common is a thin length of Silastic material, which is carried around the vessel with a right-angle clamp. The ends of the vessel loop are clamped together with a hemostat as shown in Fig. 30.10. **Umbilical tapes** are made of cotton that come prepackaged for use for retraction of vessels. A Rummel tourniquet consists of an umbilical tape that is passed around a blood vessel. The free ends of the tape are threaded through a (bolster) silastic or Robnel tubing. The tubing is then tightened against the vessel by pulling on the umbilical tape providing a tourniquet effect. It is secured with a hemostat (Fig. 30.11).

VASCULAR GRAFTS

Vascular grafts are used to replace a blood vessel, to patch a vessel, or to provide dialysis access. Synthetic grafts are made of Dacron, polyester, or polytetrafluoroethylene (PTFE). Some types are impregnated with antibacterial substances to decrease the risk of postoperative infection. Sources of biological materials are banked human umbilical cord, bovine carotid artery, and autograft (usually from the saphenous vein). Grafts may be straight or bifurcated (Y-shaped). The length is measured in centimeters, and the diameter reflects the outside diameter in millimeters.

Synthetic grafts require no special preparation except trimming. Patch grafts are cut into elliptical sections and sutured in place with a double-arm suture. Bovine grafts are soaked in normal saline as per the manufacturer's instructions. All prepared grafts are intended for use as directed by the manufacturer. Harvested vein should be kept moist while the surgeon prepares the anastomosis sites.

Vascular grafts are extremely expensive. They must not be distributed on the surgical field until the surgeon is ready to insert them and has verbally requested the size required. All manufactured grafts are identified by size, lot, and identification number, which must be recorded on the patient's operative record.

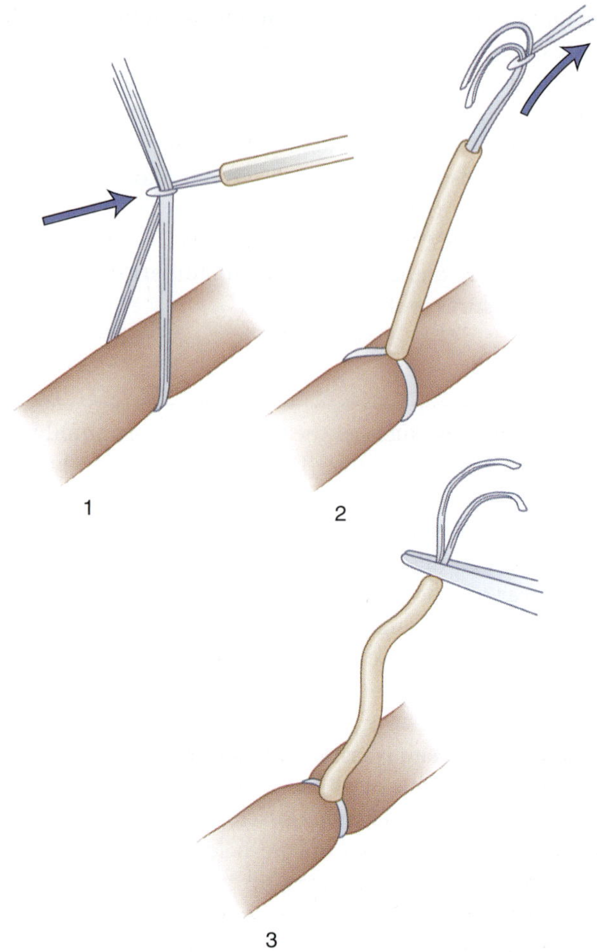

FIG. 30.11 Rummel tourniquet. The tourniquet is constructed of an umbilical tape secured with a length of latex tubing. These are frequently used in cardiovascular surgery. (From Ouriel K, Rutherford R, eds. *Atlas of Vascular Surgery: Operative Procedures*. Philadelphia: WB Saunders; 1998.)

DRUGS

Vascular surgery requires a number of important and high-alert intraoperative drugs. Safety protocols for the distribution and labeling must be followed. These protocols are discussed in detail in Chapter 12. Specific drugs are used to prevent blood from clotting at the operative site (anticoagulation) or to enhance coagulation. Other drugs can be used intraoperatively to dilate vessels, prevent vasospasm, and irrigate vessel lumens.

Anticoagulation

During vascular surgery, heparinized saline solution is used to prevent coagulation in the area of the operative vessels. This prevents thrombi from forming at the surgical site and reduces the risk of embolus. Systemic heparin may be administered just before an artery is clamped when preparing for **arteriotomy** (incision into the operative artery). Heparinized saline is prepared by the pharmacist or circulating nurse. He or she receives both heparin and *intravenous saline*, which are mixed in a ratio according to the surgeon's orders. For use on the field, the solution is drawn up with a 20- or 30-mL syringe fitted with a tapered irrigation tip. Systemic heparin is reversed with protamine sulfate, which is administered by the anesthesia care provider. Dextran-40 is an antithrombotic. It is often administered intravenously (IV) to patients after bypass or endarterectomy procedures but can also be used in a diluted form as an irrigation on the field during these procedures.

Coagulation

Hemostasis is maintained at anastomosis sites with collagen or fibrin products, such as microfibrillar collagen hemostat (Gelfoam, Avitene) or topical thrombin. Topical thrombin is a dry powder that is reconstituted with intravenous saline. Topical hemostatic collagen materials are used on anastomosis sites and capillary beds. Small squares (1 cm) of Gelfoam may be soaked in topical thrombin before use. Surgicel may also be placed on the site of the anastomosis.

NOTE *It is critically important that all medications on the field be clearly marked as soon as they are received.*

Vasodilation

Papaverine is a drug that relaxes smooth muscle of the vascular wall, which results in dilation and increased blood flow. It is sometimes injected into autologous vein grafts during bypass procedures to counteract vasoconstriction that occurs during vein harvest.

Prevention of Vasospasm

Vasospasm can occur during vascular surgery, resulting in constriction of the blood vessels at the operative field. The surgeon may use a topical agent such as papaverine, lidocaine, or verapamil. The selected drug is used to moisten a gauze sponge, which is then placed over the vessel.

TECHNIQUES IN VASCULAR SURGERY

ENDARTERECTOMY

Many vascular procedures require removal of atherosclerotic plaque from the inside of an artery (**endarterectomy**). Plaque is a rubbery substance that adheres to the tunica intima, causing stenosis or occlusion. Plaque may also be hard, or *calcified*, or a combination of soft and calcified plaque may be present. When the surgeon removes the plaque, there is a risk it will break apart, causing an embolus, especially when clamps are removed to test blood flow. Endarterectomy requires meticulous technique and fine instruments. Plaque can be removed in one piece (Fig. 30.12). The surgeon may use a Penfield or Freer elevator to separate the plaque from the intima layer of the vessel while applying gentle traction. An alternative technique is to transect the artery at its bifurcation and remove the plaque circumferentially. The artery may be closed using the technique shown in Fig. 30.13.

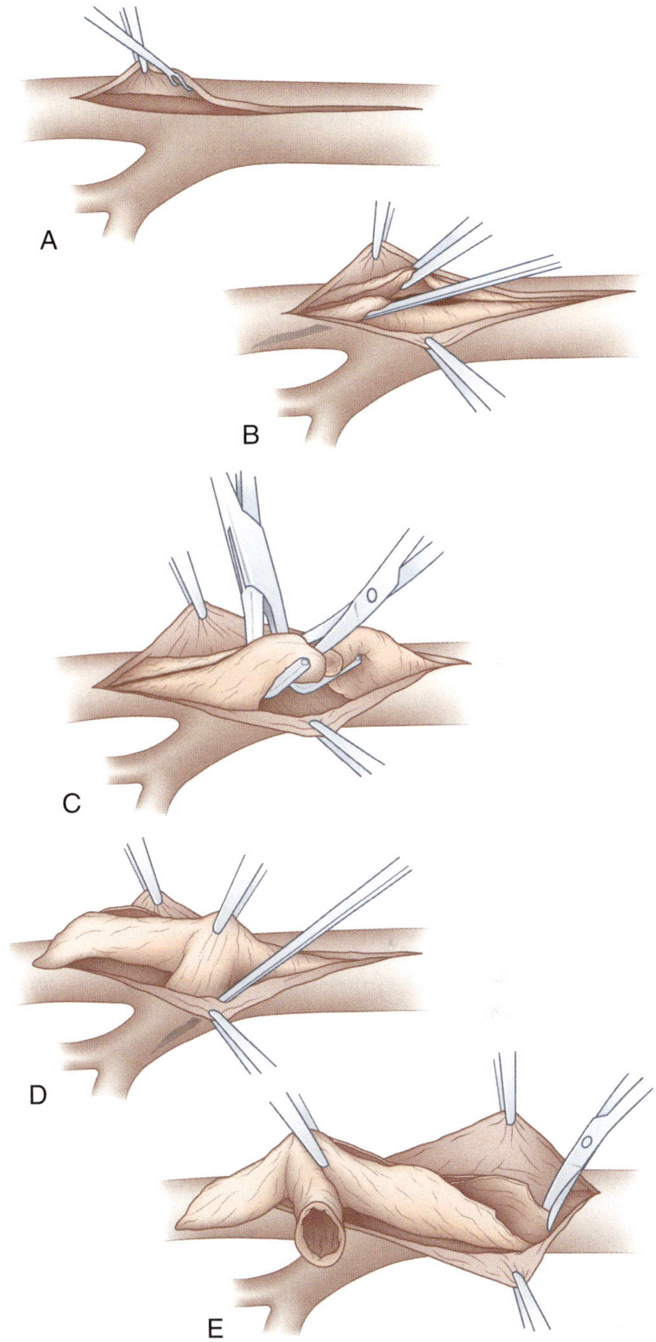

FIG. 30.12 Endarterectomy technique. (A) An arteriotomy is performed. (B) A plane is created between the vessel wall and plaque. (C) The plaque is divided over a right-angle clamp. (D) The plaque is mobilized distally. (E) The proximal end of the plaque is trimmed. (From Ouriel K, Rutherford R, eds. *Atlas of Vascular Surgery: Operative Procedures*. Philadelphia: WB Saunders; 1998.)

VESSEL ANASTOMOSIS

Blood vessel anastomosis is performed using end-to-end, end-to-side, or side-to-side technique. Longitudinal or circumferential incisions in the blood vessel are closed with a double-arm suture. Traction sutures are often placed at one or both ends of the incision. Figs. 30.14 and 30.15 illustrate the techniques.

GRAFT TUNNELING

Vascular grafts must often be tunneled through subcutaneous tissue or other layers to connect one vessel to another. Two techniques are used. The surgeon may use the fingers to separate the tissue digitally or a graft tunneler (discussed previously) can be used. The tunneler is a long metal shaft with blunt tips that is pushed manually through the tissue. As the tunneler is advanced, it creates a tubular space through which the graft can be threaded. The surgeon usually performs this step by inserting a long clamp (e.g., a Péan clamp) into the tunnel and grasping the graft from the entry site. If the tunnel is short, the surgeon can pass it easily. Longer grafts may require an intermediate incision in the skin and subcutaneous tissue.

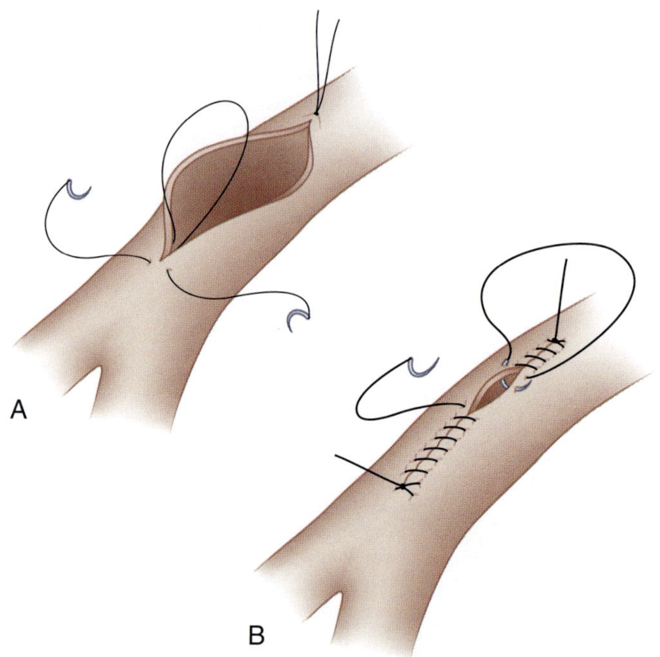

FIG. 30.13 Suturing technique for closing a longitudinal arteriotomy. (A) Double-arm suture is placed at each end. (B) Continuous sutures are placed to provide a sealed closure. (From Ouriel K, Rutherford R, eds. *Atlas of Vascular Surgery: Operative Procedures*. Philadelphia: WB Saunders; 1998.)

ENDOVASCULAR TECHNIQUES

Endovascular surgery is performed within the blood vessels. To understand advanced techniques in which the surgical technologist is required to assist, a basic understanding of the principles involved is helpful. A series of devices are inserted into the blood vessel in a prescribed sequence. Some of the devices are used to simply "hold a place" for the insertion of those that are used to achieve a surgical objective such as dilating a vessel, removing an embolus, or providing support to the wall of a blood vessel.

There are two basic methods used to access a blood vessel. In *open endovascular access,* an incision is made over the access point. The vessel is mobilized, and the devices are inserted directly into the blood vessel under direct vision. In ***percutaneous*** *access*, there is no incision. Instead, an 18-gauge needle is inserted into the target vessel using ultrasound guidance. The first device is inserted through the needle. A guidewire is then inserted into the needle, which is then removed. An access sheath is inserted over the guidewire. Finally, catheters and stents used to perform the surgical objective are inserted into the sheath.

The basic technical requirements include the following:

- Access to the point of entry to the vascular system
- Appropriate level of anesthesia and physiological monitoring
- A method of visualizing and thereby guiding the blood vessels and devices

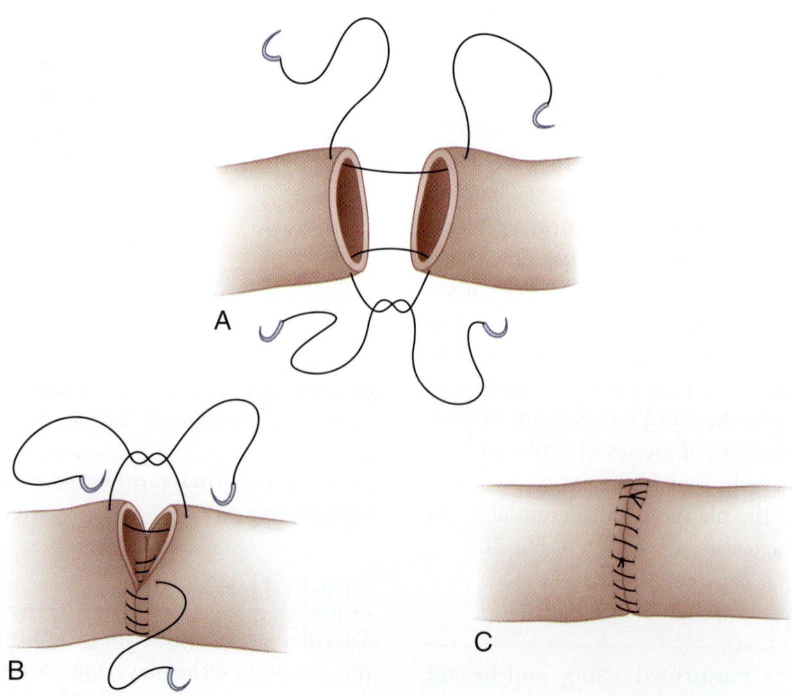

FIG. 30.14 End-to-end anastomosis. (A) Two double-arm sutures are placed in opposite locations. (B) Continuous sutures are placed circumferentially. (C) Completed closure. (From Ouriel K, Rutherford R, eds. *Atlas of Vascular Surgery: Operative Procedures*. Philadelphia: WB Saunders; 1998.)

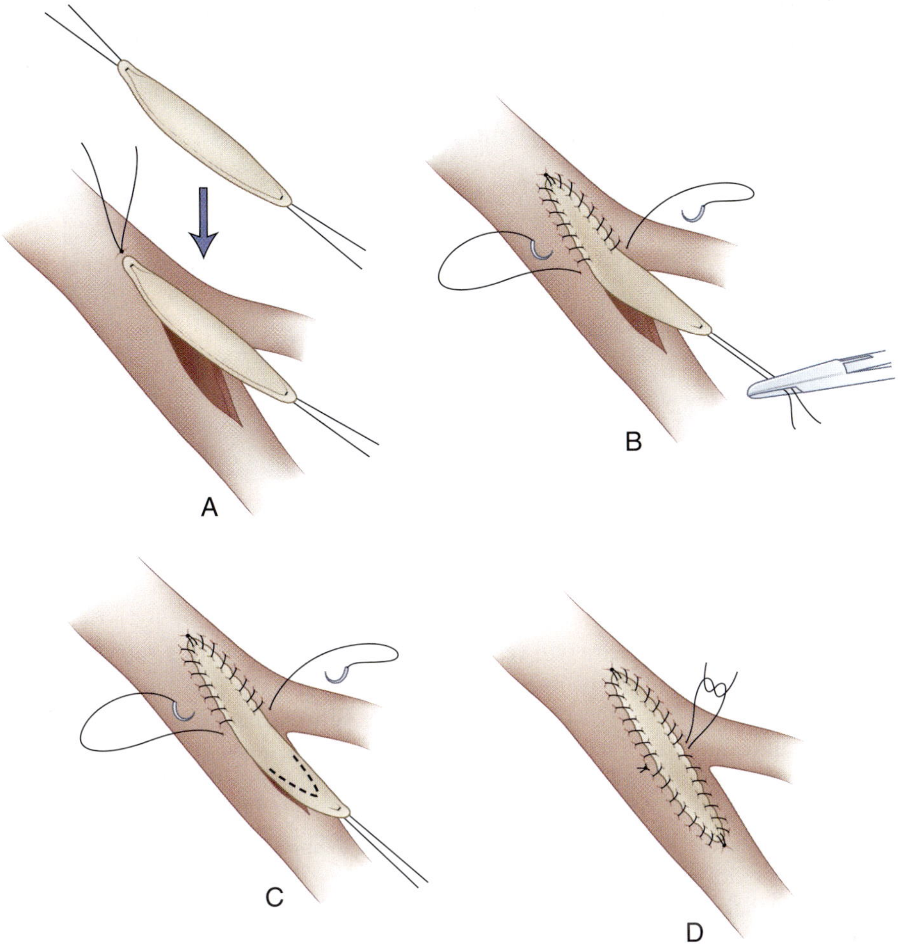

FIG. 30.15 Technique for placing a patch graft. (A) Traction sutures are placed at each end of the graft. (B) Sutures are applied at both sides of the graft. (C) The graft may be trimmed as needed *(dotted line)*. (D) Completed graft. (From Ouriel K, Rutherford R, eds. *Atlas of Vascular Surgery: Operative Procedures*. Philadelphia: WB Saunders; 1998.)

- A technique for introducing and manipulating endovascular devices

ACCESS

Access to the vascular system is either *retrograde* (against the flow of blood) or *antegrade* (in the same direction as blood flow). The access site may not be the actual vessel in which the pathology lies. Instead, the access vessel is selected for its size and condition, taking into consideration any medical condition that would prevent the use of a particular vessel such as scarring or atherosclerosis at the access point. The surgical position is selected on the basis of the access point.

The most common arterial access point used in endovascular procedures is the common femoral artery. However, the brachial and axillary arteries are also used. Venous access is obtained using the internal jugular, common femoral, brachial, and popliteal veins.

ANESTHESIA

Most patients undergoing percutaneous endovascular procedures require only short-acting intravenous sedatives and infiltration of local anesthetic at the access. However, patients who are highly anxious may be given a general anesthetic. Physiological monitoring is very important during the procedure regardless of the type of anesthetic used. Many vascular patients have a history of cardiac, vascular, or kidney disease, which can complicate their risk factors during the procedure.

IMAGING

Fluoroscopy is used during percutaneous endovascular procedures. Ultrasound is also used to define the tissue planes in reference to the entry needle during access. Once access is secured, fluoroscopy is used to guide the various devices inside the vascular system. Angiography is also used in conjunction with fluoroscopy.

Guidewires

Once direct or percutaneous access to the blood vessel is secured, a *guidewire* is inserted into the vessel and acts as a pilot for all subsequent devices. Guidewires also hold the place in the vessel while different catheters and other devices are exchanged. Guidewires come in a variety of lengths, from 50 to 260 cm, to accommodate smaller peripheral procedures

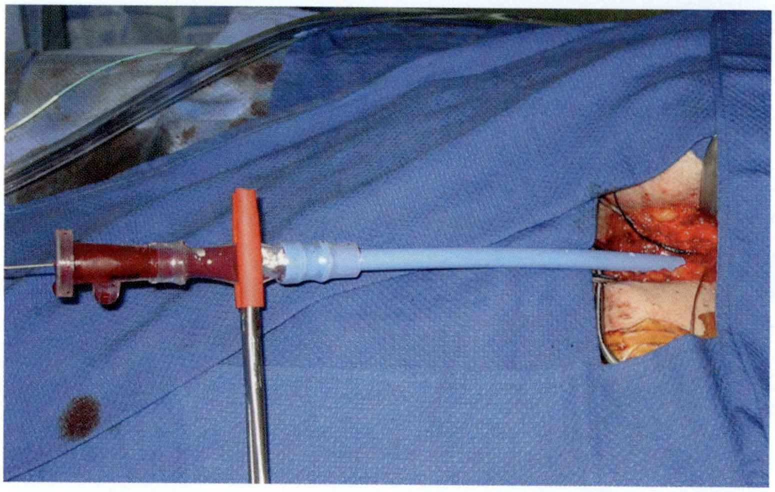

FIG. 30.16 Access sheath. This device is used during endovascular procedures, when it is inserted over a guidewire to protect the vessels walls from injury. It also acts as a conduit for catheters and stents used during the procedure. (From Cioffi W, et al, eds. *Atlas of Trauma Emergency Surgical Techniques.* Philadelphia: Saunders; 2014.)

up to larger aorta repairs. The diameter of the wire will typically be 0.014, 0.018, or 0.035 inch. Catheter lumen sizes correspond to these wire diameters.

Guidewires are made from stainless steel or a more flexible metal alloy known as Nitinol. The tips of the wires vary; some are stiff and rigid, some are J-curved, and some have floppy, flexible tips to protect delicate vessel walls. Great care must be taken to keep wires wet and free of clot and debris. A moistened Raytec sponge should be available to wipe wires down before and after each insertion. Handling longer wires can be a challenge, and several devices are available to keep the wires from falling out of the sterile field. A skilled surgical technologist is adept at re-wrapping the wires quickly and safely after each use.

Access Sheath

An access sheath is a tube that is introduced directly into the blood vessel over the guidewire. The sheath is a *protective device* that prevents the vessel walls from injury as other endovascular devices are inserted through it in a sequence. It also serves as the delivery system for these other devices (e.g., catheters, stents). If a larger sheath is needed during the procedure, a guidewire is inserted to maintain access to the vessel, while the small sheath is removed and a larger one replaced over the wire using the same method. The sheath remains in place until the completion of the procedure.

Access sheaths are made of Teflon-coated polyvinyl chloride (PVC). They contain an introducer/dilator, a port on the side for flushing with heparinized saline, and a stopcock for hemostasis. Sheaths vary in size from 4 to 24 Fr, depending on the vessel being treated and the devices used. To avoid tearing delicate vessel walls, the ST should flush the sheath with heparinized saline before passing it to the surgeon for insertion. At the end of the case, the sheath will be removed by the surgeon while an assistant holds pressure distal to the insertion site. For venous sheaths, pressure is held on the insertion site for a minimum of 10 minutes to stop bleeding. For arterial sheaths, the surgeon will close the insertion site with a 5-0 to 7-0 vascular suture. Percutaneous closure devices are also available that insert a purse-string suture around the insertion site, which is tightened after sheath removal. Fig. 30.16 shows an access sheath in the femoral artery.

NOTE *Whenever a wire, catheter, or sheath is introduced into or removed from a vessel, the lumen should be flushed and the outside wiped down with a moist gauze sponge. This prevents the formation of thrombus that could be introduced into the bloodstream upon the insertion of the device.*

Catheters

Most endovascular procedures use a variety of catheters to accomplish different tasks. All endovascular catheters have a lumen through which a guidewire can be passed or through which contrast medium can be injected. *Sizing catheters* have radiopaque markings in centimeter increments to assist in measuring the length of a vessel under fluoroscopy. *Directional catheters* have specially shaped tips to assist in guiding a wire into the correct vessel at a bifurcation. *Exchange catheters* are used to hold the place in a vessel while the surgeon exchanges one wire for another. *Balloon catheters* (Fig. 30.17) have an inner lumen and are surrounded by a balloon that is filled with contrast medium (or a mixture of heparinized saline and contrast medium) for visualization under fluoroscopy.

Stent expansion balloons are inflated to expand stents to fit snugly in the lumen of an artery. *Angioplasty balloons* are used to treat stenosis in veins or enlarge an arterial lumen that is restricted by plaque. The balloons are typically inflated and then held open for several seconds to several minutes using an *insufflation device* or manual pressure on the syringe of contrast. Intravascular ultrasound, discussed in the Diagnostic Procedures section of this chapter, is delivered into the artery on a catheter. One endovascular procedure may require several different catheters throughout the procedure.

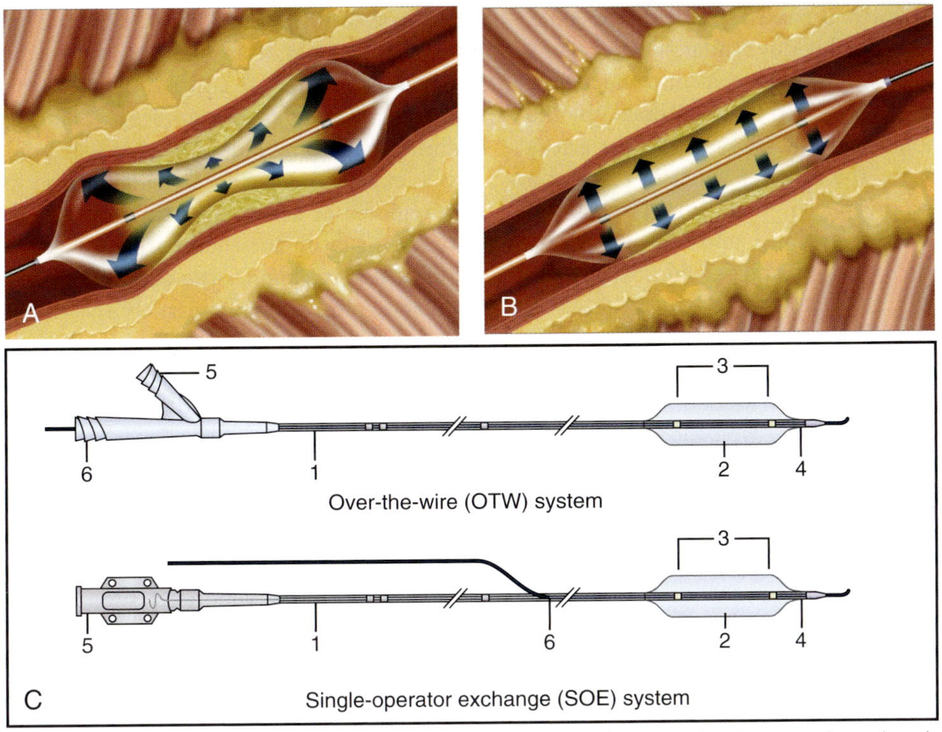

FIG. 30.17 Balloon catheters. Coaxial *over-the-guidewire* catheter *(top)* and monorail rapid exchange catheter *(bottom)*. *1*, Catheter shaft; *2*, balloon; *3*, marker; *4*, tapered tip; *5*, inflation port; *6*, guidewire exit port. (From Cronenwett JL, Johnston KW, eds. *Rutherford's Vascular Surgery*. 7th ed. Philadelphia: Saunders; 2010.)

Endovascular Stent

An endovascular **stent** is a tubular mesh implant that fits against the wall of an artery. The stent thus provides a physical barrier between the atherosclerotic plaque and the vessel lumen. It also holds the vessel open so that blood can flow freely without platelet aggregation. Covered stents, also known as *stent grafts*, are used to reinforce aneurysmal artery walls and create a smooth path for blood flow while walling off the aneurysm sac. Stents are made of stainless steel, titanium, or Nitinol. Stent grafts may be constructed as a metal mesh covered in expanded polytetrafluoroethylene (ePTFE) or woven polyester.

Stents are implanted permanently. Three common types of stents are the balloon stent, the self-expanding mesh stent, and the covered stent (stent graft).

The *balloon stent* is a fine catheter with a balloon tip. A mesh stent is fixed over the balloon, and when the balloon is expanded, the mesh stent is pushed into position against the vessel wall. The *self-expanding stent* opens to provide a similar effect. A stent graft is self-expanding to a point and is then pressed against the arterial wall using a balloon catheter to ensure a snug fit with no leaks.

Fig. 30.18 illustrates different types of stents.

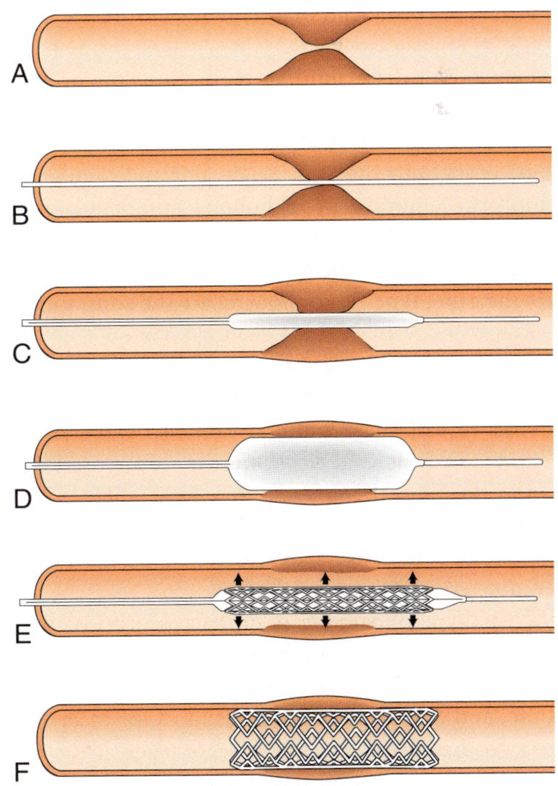

FIG. 30.18 Percutaneous angioplasty. (A) Stenosis of the artery. (B) Insertion of a guidewire. (C) A balloon catheter is inserted over the guidewire. (D) The balloon is inflated. (E) A mesh stent is inserted over the guidewire. (F) The stent is inflated, and the guidewire is removed. (From Garden O, et al. *Principles and Practice of Surgery*. 6th ed. Edinburgh: Churchill Livingstone; 2012.)

ENDOVASCULAR PROCEDURES

ANGIOPLASTY

Angioplasty is the insertion of an arterial balloon catheter into an artery to establish patency and normal blood flow. A large-bore needle is inserted into the vessel distal to the area of stenosis. A flexible guidewire is passed through the needle, which is withdrawn, and a small endovascular sheath (4 to 8 Fr) is inserted. Contrast medium is injected into the artery, and the area of stricture is marked on films produced by the data recorder. The balloon catheter is inserted into the artery to the level of the stricture. The catheter is left in place at a specific pressure and for a specific length of time. The balloon catheter is filled with contrast medium, and both the vessel walls and catheter balloon are observed using fluoroscopy.

NOTE *An insufflation device is used to inflate the angioplasty balloon to the exact pressure (measured in standard atmospheric units, or atm). This device is loaded with 10 to 20 mL of contrast solution and connected to the balloon catheter. The ST should take care to remove all air from the insufflator, tubing, and balloon before inflating because trapped air will distort the fluoroscopic image and may cause an air embolus if the balloon were to rupture.*

CENTRAL VENOUS LINE

The central venous catheter, known commonly as a *central line*, was introduced in Chapter 12 as a method of administering IV drugs, solutions, and parenteral nutrients and for blood draws in patients who require long- or medium-term therapy. Central line catheters are constructed of PVC, Teflon, polyurethane, or Silastic (silicone elastomer blend). The main line of the device is a soft tube with an insertion end that remains in the vein and a distal end that remains outside the body. The distal end may have two or three extensions (lumens), which are designated for drug, fluid, or blood infusion, or for blood withdrawal. The catheter is inserted into the superior vena cava near the right atrium through a percutaneous (through the skin) entry into the subclavian, internal jugular, or less commonly the femoral vein. Although a number of companies manufacture and distribute central venous catheters under their own brand name, the generic names remain in use and identify the exact type. The following are the common generic types:

- *Tunneled catheter:* A portion of the catheter is embedded or "tunneled" in the subcutaneous tissue. There is an insertion site and an exit site. Common tunneled catheters are the Hickman, Broviac, and Groshong. These are used for long-term intravenous therapy and may have single or multiple lumens.
- *Non-tunneled catheter:* This catheter is used for short- or medium-term intravenous therapy.
- *Port:* This type of catheter has an access port or reservoir, which is implanted under the skin.

Central lines, like other medical devices, have evolved over time, and complexity and procedures for insertion have changed. In the past, central lines were place at the patient's bedside and often required repeated sticks with a large-bore needle or an incision (called a *cutdown*) to expose the vein directly. This resulted in high infection rates and limited success rates. Modern central line placement is performed using a strict aseptic technique, in the interventional radiology department or in the operating room using guided fluoroscopy technique or ultrasound to pinpoint the exact entry site and correct placement of the catheter in the vena cava.

Two techniques are commonly used for central line placement, *tunneled* and *non-tunneled* (Seldinger method). Both techniques require wide skin prep using chlorhexidine, draping to expose the sternoclavicular region including the chin, and regional or general anesthesia with routine physiological monitoring by an anesthesia provider.

Tunneling technique: The entry vein (subclavian or inferior jugular) is punctured percutaneously with a syringe and *introducer needle* supplied in the catheter insertion kit. With the needle held in position, the syringe is removed, and a *guidewire* is placed into the needle, which is then removed. Some central line kits contain a catheter that can be placed over the needle. The guidewire is advanced to the inferior vena cava, and the distal end of the catheter is threaded over the guidewire. An exit site for the distal end of the catheter is selected a few inches below the insertion site, and a plastic *tunneler* is inserted near the venotomy site. This is advanced subcutaneously to the exit site, where a small stab wound is made with a scalpel over the tip of the tunneler. The catheter is then pulled through the tunnel to emerge through the stab wound. The catheter is flushed, checked for placement, and sutured in place.

Seldinger technique: The entry vein is punctured with an introducer needle. A guidewire is threaded through the needle, which is then withdrawn, leaving the guidewire in place. The catheter is threaded over the guidewire for exact placement. The guidewire is removed, the catheter is flushed, and sutured in place.

INTRAOPERATIVE ANGIOGRAPHY

Preoperative angiography (arteriography) is the injection of contrast medium into a selected artery and its branches to determine the exact location of strictures, occlusion, or malformation. During surgery, intraoperative angiography is used in conjunction with angioplasty and other procedures to allow the surgeon to see the position of the stricture and to place the catheter in the correct location. It is also used during the placement of endovascular stent grafts and after bypass procedures to verify the new bypass' effectiveness. Intraoperative angiography is performed with intravascular ultrasound and fluoroscopy because it allows the surgeon to see obstructions or emboli distal and proximal to the operative area. All team members must wear a lead apron during a procedure involving fluoroscopy.

In this procedure, the contrast medium is injected directly into the operative artery, and the interior configuration of the vessel and its branches are observed by fluoroscopy. The contrast medium is flushed through the vessel with sterile intravenous saline at the completion of the procedure. Repeat injections and data recording may be required to clarify an image. The diameter of a vessel can also be measured with some types of imaging equipment. This assists the surgeon in sizing for a balloon catheter or stent.

The C-arm should be draped just before the procedure and moved slightly out of the field.

POSITION:	According to the location of the entry vessel; usually supine
INCISION:	According to the location of the entry vessel
PREP AND DRAPING:	According to the location of the entry vessel(s)
INSTRUMENTS:	Minor plastic surgery set; minor peripheral vascular set; vessel loops; hemostat jaw covers; small self-retaining retractor
EXTRAS:	Doppler; see later

Supplies

- Two or more 30- or 60-mL syringes
- Arterial needle
- One or more IV catheter extension tube(s)
- 3-way stopcock
- Contrast medium as specified by the surgeon
- Angiocath or IV catheter for injection of the contrast medium
- Intravenous saline
- Intravenous heparin according to the surgeon's order

Technical Points and Discussion

1. ***The circulator distributes the contrast medium to the scrubbed surgical technologist.***
The circulator distributes the contrast medium to the ST, who draws it up into two syringes. A solution of 60% Renografin is frequently used. A third syringe of IV saline is prepared to flush the contrast medium from the arteries when fluoroscopy or radiography has been completed. One end of the angiography needle is attached to IV extension tubing and the other end to a 3-way stopcock, which is attached to a syringe of dye. All air bubbles must be removed from the tubing to ensure that air is not introduced into the artery. A Kelly or Mayo hemostat is placed across the tubing to prevent air from backing into it. The stopcock is secured in the closed position. The procedure and photos for setting up the devices with contrast medium can be found in Chapter 12.

2. ***A sterile field is prepared for imaging.***
In preparation for fluoroscopy, metal instruments should be moved out of the immediate operative site. Fluoroscopy is the most common imaging process used intraoperatively. However, if standard x-rays are to be taken, the ST receives the cassette in a cassette pouch. A deep fold is made in the edge of the sterile cassette cover, making a wide sterile cuff. After the cassette has been dropped inside, the edges of the pouch are turned up and secured. The cassette is placed under the limb, the radiography machine is positioned, and films are taken. The cassette and cover are removed from the field.

3. ***The surgeon injects the contrast medium into the artery, and images are recorded during injection.***
The surgeon may choose one of the several techniques to inject the contrast medium:
   - If the arteriotomy (incision in the artery) has already been sutured, an angiography needle is inserted between the sutures.
   - A catheter can be inserted into the vessel and secured with a suture tie.
   - If a sheath is already present in the vessel, the surgeon will inject contrast through the stopcock and tubing attached to the sheath.

   After the procedure, the contrast medium is flushed from the artery with sterile saline.

INSERTION OF A VENA CAVA FILTER

A vena cava filter is a metal, umbrella-shaped filter inserted into the inferior vena cava to prevent emboli from entering the pulmonary system. The filter can be temporary or permanent.

Insertion of a vena cava filter is commonly performed in the catheter lab or operating room using fluoroscopy. New filter devices can be inserted at the patient's bedside in the intensive care unit (ICU).

The vena cava filter is inserted by percutaneous needle insertion. The procedure requires a guidewire and filter introducer. The filter, which resembles an umbrella without fabric, is made of titanium, stainless steel, or Nitinol. When the filter is deployed, it opens out to the edges of the vessel.

Pathology

Pulmonary emboli occur when one or more thrombi move from the venous system into the pulmonary vascular system. The vena cava filter is a method of capturing and preventing further movement of emboli. Candidates for the surgery include the following:

- Patients who have a venous thrombus but cannot tolerate anticoagulant therapy; these include patients who have had recent surgery or have a history of hemorrhagic stroke
- Patients who have had a massive pulmonary embolism and survived but for whom a subsequent embolism would be fatal
- Patients with chronic or venous thromboemboli in spite of anticoagulant therapy
- Patients at high risk for pulmonary embolism

POSITION:	Supine
INCISION:	Groin
PREP AND DRAPING:	Groin
INSTRUMENTS:	Minor plastic surgery set; minor peripheral vascular set; vessel loops; hemostat jaw covers (booties); small self-retaining retractor
EXTRAS:	Doppler

Technical Points and Discussion

1. ***The patient is positioned and prepped.***
The patient is placed in the supine position on the fluoroscopy or radiology table. The operative site is prepped with povidone-iodine solution, and the area is draped in the usual manner. Local anesthesia with or without sedation is administered.

2. ***The femoral, inferior jugular, or subclavian veins are accessed percutaneously.***
The surgeon or radiologist begins the procedure by inserting a large-bore needle into the femoral, inferior jugular, or subclavian vein. A guidewire is inserted through the needle, and the needle is withdrawn.

3. ***A filter introducer and flexible guidewire is inserted.***
With the aid of fluoroscopy, the introducer is passed over the guidewire, and the filter is ejected from the tip. The final position of the filter is confirmed under fluoroscopy. The introducer and guidewire are withdrawn, and pressure is applied to the puncture site for 10 to 15 minutes.

4. ***A pressure dressing is applied to the insertion site.***
The patient must remain in the flat supine position for at least 4 hours after the procedure to prevent postoperative hemorrhage. Many vena cava filters can be removed at a later date if deemed necessary. Retrievable filters feature a small hook at the top. By placing a sheath (8 to 15 Fr) in the inferior jugular or subclavian vein superior to the filter, the surgeon can thread a snare over a guidewire, grab the top of the filter, and gently pull upward. The filter will then collapse upon itself as it enters the sheath, much like an umbrella. After the filter is removed, an intraoperative angiogram is taken to confirm that the vena cava did not sustain damage during the removal. The sheath is withdrawn, and pressure is held for 10 to 15 minutes before a pressure dressing is applied.

ENDOVASCULAR ANEURYSM REPAIR (EVAR)

In this procedure, an abdominal aortic aneurysm is surgically managed using an expanding stent deployed from the femoral artery either by percutaneous or open technique. The design of most endovascular stents is sectional. That is, the main body of the stent is separate from the graft limbs, which form the bifurcated Y. The stent segments are deployed through a device that places the proximal end of the stent, expands it, and opens it by the manipulation of the controls at the head of the device.

The exact technique used depends on the graft system. However, patient preparation is the same for all proprietary systems. The patient is prepped in supine position to include the possibility of conversion to an open procedure. The percutaneous approach uses the guidewire and stent method previously described. Open procedures require an incision of the femoral artery and may include retroperitoneal access through an abdominal incision. Fig. 30.19 illustrates the procedure.

OPEN VASCULAR PROCEDURES

VASCULAR ACCESS FOR RENAL HEMODIALYSIS

Patients with severe renal disease require frequent hemodialysis. This treatment requires long-term access to the patient's vascular system. An anastomosis between the arterial and venous systems is created surgically to produce this access. Two techniques usually are used to create vascular access: an arteriovenous shunt or an arteriovenous (AV) fistula.

Pathology

Severe renal disease results in electrolyte imbalance and uremia (nitrogenous wastes in the blood). When the kidneys' filtering ability drops below 5%, hemodialysis is necessary for survival. During extracorporeal *hemodialysis,* the patient's blood is shunted outside the body through an artery. The blood is pumped through a series of filters to remove the waste products and excess electrolytes that normally would be filtered by the kidneys. The blood is then returned to the body through a vein.

POSITION:	Supine with operative arm placed on operative arm board
INCISION:	Arm—exact site depends on dialysis access vessels
PREP AND DRAPING:	May include the hand, arm, chest, and axilla
INSTRUMENTS:	Minor plastic surgery set; peripheral vascular set; vessel loops; mosquito hemostat jaw covers (booties); small self-retaining retractor; vascular graft according to surgeon's preference
POSSIBLE EXTRAS:	Magnifying loupes

Technical Points and Discussion

ARTERIOVENOUS SHUNT

1. ***The patient is prepped and draped.***
The patient is placed in the supine position with the arm extended on a large arm board. The arm is prepped and draped free. A local anesthetic is usually administered.

2. ***The cephalic vein is mobilized.***
A skin incision is made over the cephalic vein and carried through the fascial layer with a curved hemostat and tenotomy or plastic surgery scissors. The vein is identified and mobilized circumferentially. A vessel loop is placed around the vein, and a small bulldog or similar vascular clamp is placed over the proximal end of the vessel.

3. ***The cephalic vein is divided and ligated; the radial artery is mobilized.***
The vein is transected, and the distal end is ligated with size 2-0 silk or polypropylene suture. The radial artery is identified and mobilized. Two small vessel loops or small

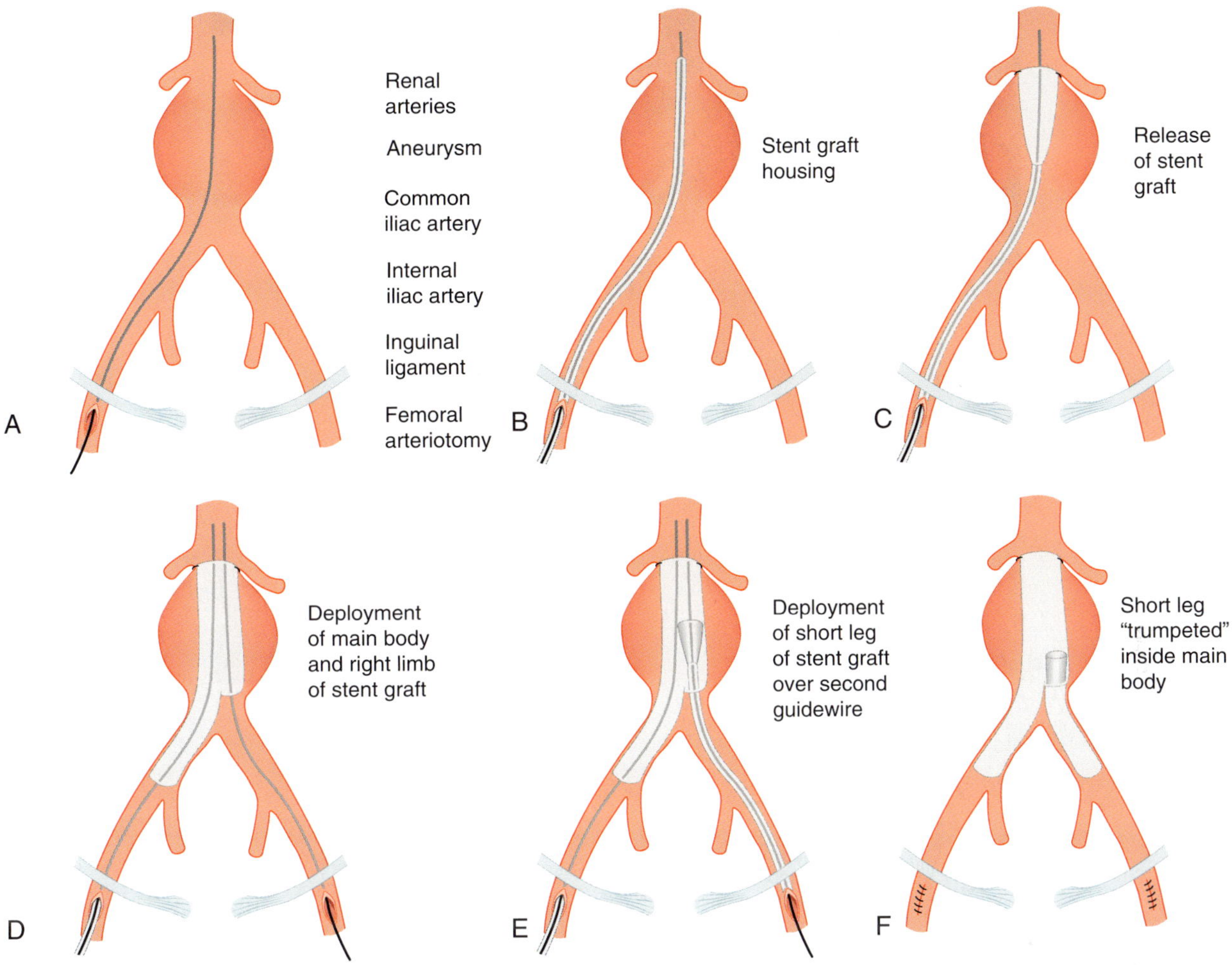

FIG. 30.19 Endovascular aneurysm repair (EVAR) using a wire stent. (A) A guidewire is passed through the aneurysm through the right common femoral artery. (B) A catheter containing the stent graft is passed over the guidewire and into position in the aneurysm. (C) The outer cover of the catheter is removed, allowing the proximal end to remain open. (D) The rest of the graft is removed, allowing the deployment of the main body and right limb of the stent graft in the common iliac artery. (E) A second guidewire is passed through the short limb of the stent graft. (F) Deployment is complete, and the aneurysm sac is excluded from the circulation. (From Garden O, et al. *Principles and Practice of Surgery*. 6th ed. Edinburgh: Churchill Livingstone; 2012.)

vascular clamps are placed on either side of the proposed anastomosis site.

4. ***An arteriotomy is performed.***
A small arteriotomy is performed to accommodate the graft. A graft tunneler may be used to insert the graft into the subcutaneous fat just under the skin of the forearm. The ends of the graft are brought in close approximation to both vessels.

5. ***The graft is prepared, and anastomosis is performed.***
The graft is trimmed, if necessary, and sutured in place with 6-0 or 7-0 polypropylene suture. The venous anastomosis is created using an end-to-end technique and the arterial anastomosis using an end-to-side technique. The incisions are closed in layers and dressed with Telfa and dry gauze.

Brachiocephalic Arteriovenous Fistula

An *arteriovenous (AV) fistula* is a direct anastomosis between an artery and a vein. The site is selected for patency and accessibility. After routine prep and draping of the area, an incision is made over the vessels. The vessels are mobilized with sharp dissection and prepared as for an arteriovenous shunt. An end-to-side anastomosis is performed using a 6-0 or 7-0 polypropylene suture. The wound is closed in layers and dressed with Telfa and dry gauze. The anastomosis is shown in Fig. 30.20.

Weeks or months may be required for complete recovery of the AV fistula before it can be used for dialysis. Postoperative complications include infection, thrombosis, and a condition known as *steal syndrome*. This occurs when the fistula or shunt directs too much blood away from the hand, distal to the anastomosis. The new shunt or fistula is "stealing" blood from the hand and can cause ischemia. The treatment for this condition is ligation of the fistula or removal/revision of the graft.

THROMBECTOMY

Thrombectomy is the removal of a stationary clot in an artery. This restores circulation and prevents the development of

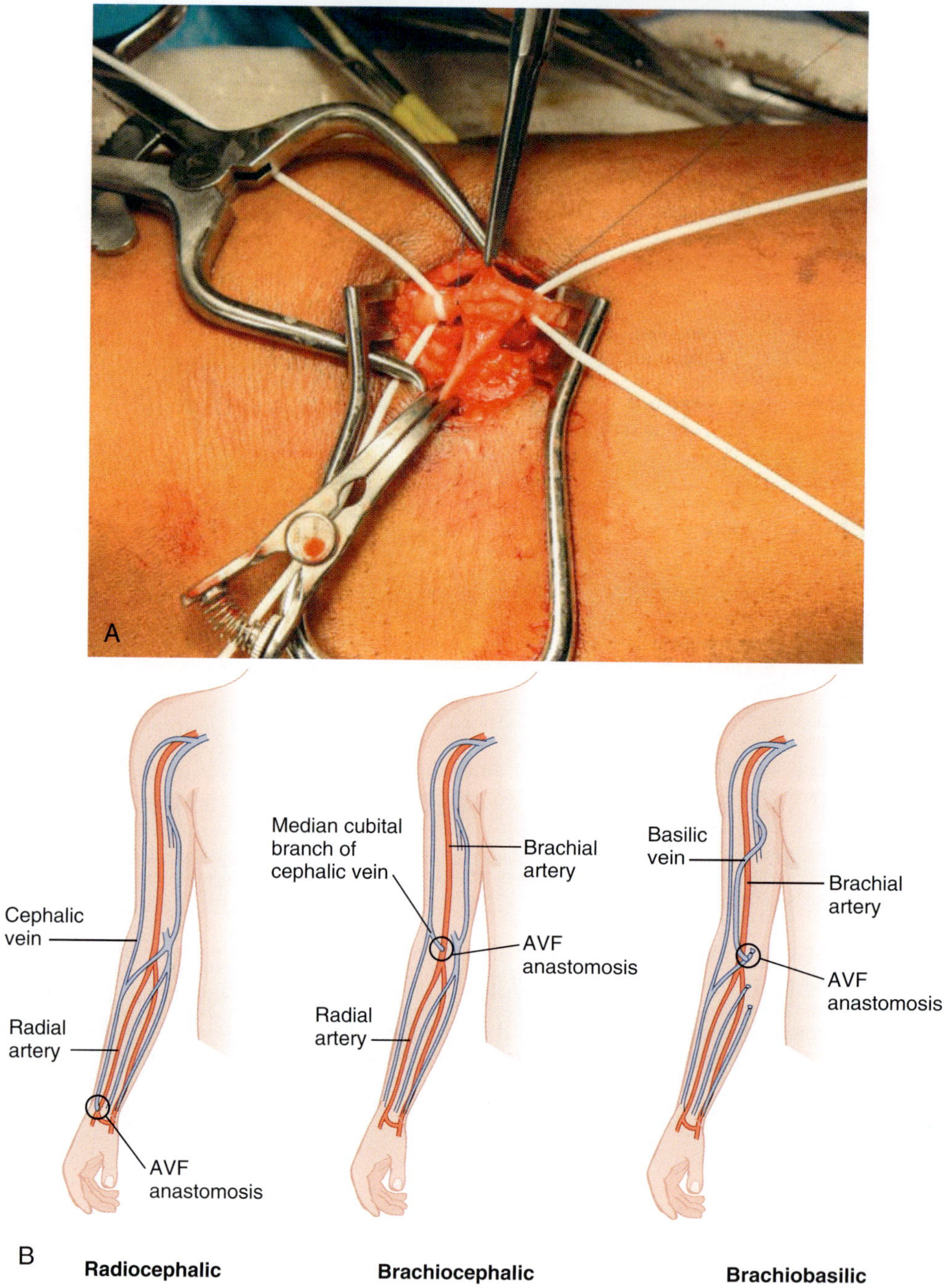

FIG. 30.20 Arteriovenous fistula for renal dialysis access. (A) The brachial artery and cephalic vein are isolated and exposed. Note the use of Silastic vessel loops for traction and bulldog clamp at the 7 o'clock position. (B) Locations of AV fistulas for dialysis access. (From Chaikof E, Cambria R, eds. *Atlas of Vascular Surgery and Endovascular Therapy Anatomy and Technique*. Philadelphia: Elsevier; 2014.)

emboli. Thrombectomy is commonly performed with an embolectomy catheter. Patient preparation depends on the location of the thrombus as determined by angiograms, duplex Doppler ultrasonography, and magnetic resonance imaging. Thrombi from the lower extremities are often removed from the groin. Mesenteric thrombi may require an abdominal approach (laparotomy) but are often accessible using a femoral approach. The following discussion presents the techniques of thrombectomy, beginning with isolation of the vessel and use of the embolectomy catheter. Surgical incisions and closures are found in chapters associated with particular anatomical areas.

Pathology

A **thrombus** is a stationary clot in the arterial or venous system. A thrombus that breaks away from the vessel wall is called an **embolus.** As an embolus travels through increasingly smaller vessels of the vascular system, it may lodge in the heart, brain, kidney, mesentery, or other vital organ. This causes vascular obstruction (**infarction**), leading to tissue death. Thrombectomy therefore can be a life-saving procedure. Common causes of thrombi are as follows:

- Atherosclerosis
- Surgery, especially when large blood vessels are exposed to air and clots form at the surgical site.
- Orthopedic trauma, especially of the hip or other large bone
- Pulmonary emboli (those that lodge in the lung) usually originate in the venous system of the lower extremities

POSITION:	Supine or according to the location of the clot
INCISION:	According to the location of the thrombus
PREP AND DRAPING:	According to the location of the thrombus
INSTRUMENTS:	Laparotomy or general set; vascular set; vessel irrigation tips; vascular suction (e.g., Frazier tips); 30- and 60-mL syringes; heparinized saline; embolectomy catheters should be available but not opened until needed
POSSIBLE EXTRAS:	Topical hemostatic agents

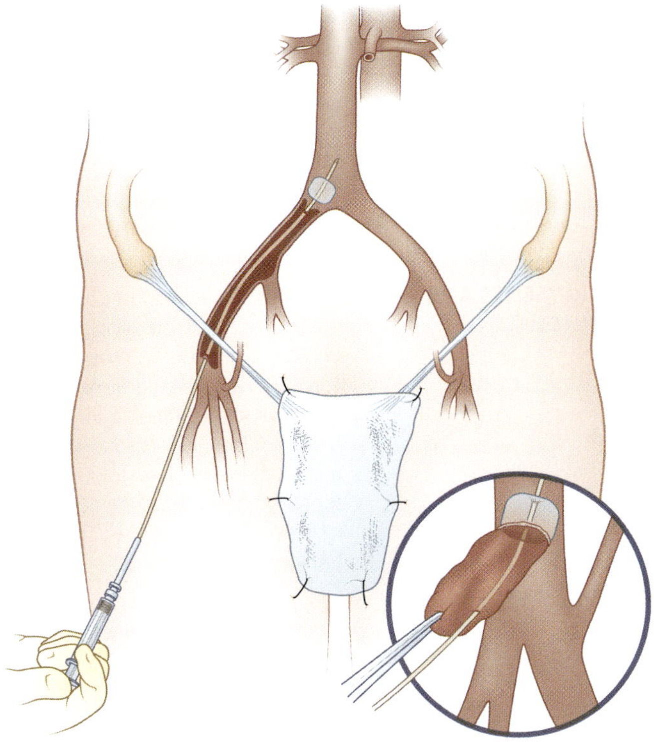

FIG. 30.21 Open thrombectomy. A thrombectomy catheter is inserted through a femoral venotomy and advanced past the thrombus. The balloon is inflated, and the catheter is carefully withdrawn, pulling the thrombus with it. (From Ouriel K, Rutherford R, eds. *Atlas of Vascular Surgery: Operative Procedures*. Philadelphia: WB Saunders; 1998.)

Technical Points and Discussion

1. ***The patient is positioned, prepped, and draped according to the location of the thrombus.***
The patient is placed in the supine position for abdominal, lower extremity, and upper extremity surgery. A general or regional anesthetic is used. The surgical site is prepped in normal fashion.

2. ***The target vessel is mobilized.***
After surgical exposure of the target vessel, the surgeon places several vessel loops around the vessel and its nearby tributaries. This allows the manipulation of the vessel and traction as needed.

3. ***An arteriotomy is performed.***
The surgeon clamps the vessel distal to the thrombus. A vascular clamp is selected to fit the configuration of the vessel and its position in the wound. An arteriotomy is made with a #11 scalpel blade. Suction is applied at the arteriotomy site. Heparin is administered, and the vessel is clamped distal to the thrombus.

4. ***Thrombectomy is performed.***
The prepared embolectomy catheter is carefully threaded into the vessel, past the site of the thrombus. The balloon is inflated, and the catheter is withdrawn (Fig. 30.21).This pulls the thrombus back through the vessel. Angioscopy and intraoperative Doppler duplex ultrasonography may be performed. The thrombus should be retained as a specimen.

Arteriotomy is closed, followed by wound closure. Arteriotomy is closed with 6-0 or 7-0 non-absorbable vascular suture. The wound is closed in layers according to the incision site.

CAROTID ENDARTERECTOMY

Carotid endarterectomy is the surgical removal of atherosclerotic plaque from the carotid artery. Plaque is removed through an open incision in the artery. This reestablishes the flow of oxygenated blood to the brain.

During carotid endarterectomy, the surgeon may temporarily occlude or bypass the carotid artery while removing plaque. The instruments and Mayo table must be kept neat and organized to ensure maximum efficiency during the procedure. All essential instruments, catheters, and vascular clamps must be prepared and in view. Attention to the surgical wound is important throughout the procedure.

Carotid endarterectomy may be performed using either a general or regional anesthesia. When a regional anesthetic is used, the patient will respond to simple neurological tests, such as hand strength tests or speaking. An electroencephalogram (EEG) is commonly used to measure the brain's electrical activity during the procedure. Electrical activity is affected by oxygen supply to the tissue, a component of carotid surgery.

Pathology

Partial obstruction of the carotid artery forms at the bifurcation of the common carotid artery with the internal and external carotid branches. The obstruction causes restricted arterial blood flow to the brain, which may result in neurological symptoms. These may advance from transient ischemic attack to major brain accident. Patients with complete blockage of the carotid artery are generally not considered for carotid endarterectomy.

POSITION:	Supine with head turned away from the operative site. The neck may be slightly hyperextended.
INCISION:	Lateral neck
PREP AND DRAPING:	As for thyroidectomy
INSTRUMENTS AND SUPPLIES:	Vascular set; selected right-angle vascular clamps (surgeon's choice); right-angle clamps; Freer elevator; Penfield elevators; vessel loops; Rummel tourniquets; hemostat jaw covers (booties); umbilical tapes or vessel loops for retraction; topical hemostatic materials (e.g., Surgicel, Gelfoam, Avitene)
POSSIBLE EXTRAS:	Internal carotid shunt; ring shunt clamp (e.g., Javid clamp); contrast media; C-arm; Doppler ultrasound

Technical Points and Discussion

1. ***The patient is positioned, prepped, and draped.***
The patient is placed in the supine position, and the head is turned away from the affected side. A small gel roll or pad may be placed under the shoulders to hyperextend the neck. If EEG monitoring will be used, electrodes are placed. The skin prep extends from the chin to the axillary line. Draping is similar to that for thyroidectomy.

2. ***An incision is made on the anterior border of the sternocleidomastoid muscle.***
The surgeon begins the procedure by incising the neck along the anterior border of the sternocleidomastoid muscle. The incision is carried deeper with the vascular forceps, electrosurgical unit (ESU), Metzenbaum scissors, and sponge dissectors to the level of the common, internal, and external carotid arteries. The ST should have a variety of retractors available, including dull Weitlaner, dull rakes, and Army-Navy retractors.

3. ***The common, external, and internal carotid arteries are mobilized and controlled with vessel loops.***
The common, external, and internal carotid arteries are mobilized with fine vascular tissue forceps and Metzenbaum scissors. The bifurcation itself is not mobilized fully. Vessel loops are placed around each of the three arteries. Small hemostats are used to clamp the ends of the loops. Small sections of tubing or Rummel tourniquets may also be used.

4. ***The internal, common, and external carotid arteries are clamped.***
Before the surgeon makes the arterial incision, the anesthesia care provider administers systemic heparin to the patient. This prevents clotting and reduces the risk of emboli. The carotid sinus may be injected with 1% lidocaine to prevent bradycardia and hypotension associated with manipulation of the carotid body.

Before the carotid artery is incised, the ST should have a number of instruments ready: a #11 scalpel blade, Potts and De Martel scissors, and neurosurgical elevators (Penfield or similar), a Freer elevator, and straight hemostats. Wide-tip atraumatic suction is also needed. The surgeon indicates the preferred vascular clamps.

5. ***An arteriotomy is made into the common carotid artery and extended upward.***
To begin the endarterectomy, the surgeon clamps the internal, common, and external carotid arteries. The surgeon then notifies the anesthesia care provider and circulator that the arteries have been clamped. The length of time the artery is occluded is timed. The EEG is closely monitored until the clamps are released. The surgeon makes a small incision into the common carotid artery with the #11 scalpel blade. The incision is extended with Potts or De Martel scissors. Arterial plaque is identified as a thick, yellow, rubbery material that adheres to the lumen (intimal layer) of the artery.

6. ***An intraluminal shunt may be put in place to provide continuous cerebral blood flow.***
To provide continuous blood flow to the cerebrum while plaque is removed, the surgeon may insert a flexible internal shunt into the internal and common carotid arteries. Many types of shunts are available. The ST must flush the shunt with heparinized saline before passing it to the surgeon. Use of a shunt during the procedure is shown in Fig. 30.22.

If a shunt is to be used, it is inserted at this point. A shunt ring clamp such as the *Javid clamp* and vessel tourniquets are used to maneuver and hold the shunt in place. The previously placed cross-clamps may be released once the shunt is in place.

7. ***Atherosclerotic plaque is dissected from the vessel wall.***
The surgeon grasps the edge of the plaque with vascular forceps or a straight hemostat and lifts it gently from the intima. Penfield or Freer elevators are used to create a dissection plane between the plaque and the lumen wall. The ST may have a small basin ready on the field to collect the plaque fragments. The arterial plaque and lumen of the artery are flushed with heparinized saline. During dissection, the plaque is passed to the ST as a specimen or placed in a small basin. The arterial lumen is flushed with heparinized saline solution.

8. ***A patch graft is sutured over the arteriotomy.***

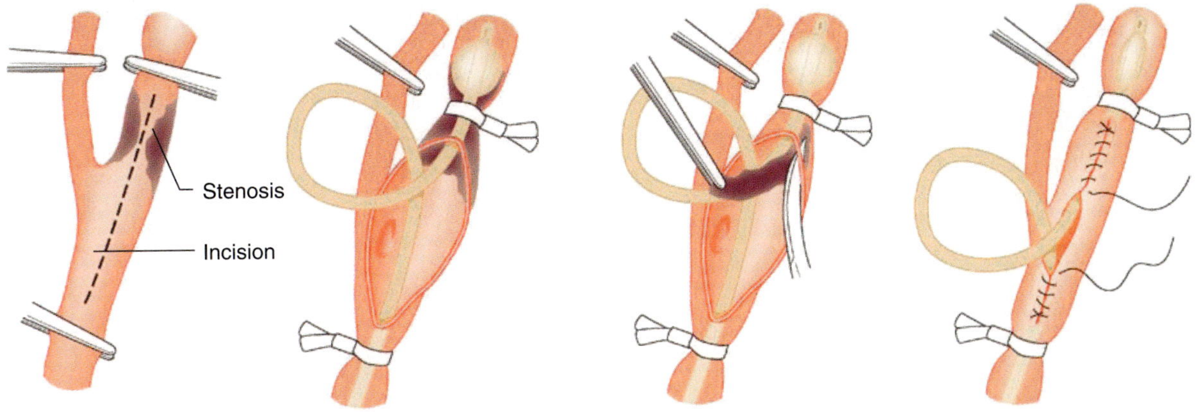

FIG. 30.22 Use of the Javid shunt during endarterectomy. The arteriotomy is performed, and the shunt is inserted, allowing partial blood flow during the removal of plaque. (From Garden O, et al. *Principles and Practice of Surgery*. 6th ed. Edinburgh: Churchill Livingstone; 2012.)

At this point, a patch graft may be placed over the arteriotomy. Graft materials include PTFE, vein, or Dacron. The surgeon will determine what material is to be used and shapes the graft using suture scissors. The graft is sutured over the arterial defect using interrupted polypropylene sutures, size 6-0 or 7-0. If a shunt was used, it is removed just before the arterial incision is completely closed. The ring clamp holding the shunt is released from the internal carotid artery, and the shunt removed. The arterial clamps are removed sequentially (e.g., external, common, and internal).

9. ***The graft is checked for leaks, and additional sutures are placed as needed.***
The ST should have topical hemostatic agents of the surgeon's choice available. Gelfoam, Surgicel, and Avitene are commonly used. The suture line is observed for leaks and blood flow confirmed with Doppler. Any leaks are repaired with additional sutures and controlled with topical hemostatic agents.

C-arm fluoroscopy may be used at this time to check the patency of the vessel superior to the surgical site. Doppler and intravascular ultrasound may also be used. All bleeders are controlled with the ESU, and the neck incision is irrigated with warm saline. The deep layers of the arterial incision are closed with 3-0 synthetic absorbable sutures. The skin is closed with 4-0 nylon or other synthetic, non-absorbable material. The wound is covered with a gauze dressing. The procedure for carotid endarterectomy is shown in Fig. 30.23.

Patients may be taken to the neurosurgical ICU after the procedure and observed closely for neurological deficit, hemorrhage, and respiratory complications.

ABDOMINAL AORTIC ANEURYSM (OPEN)

An abdominal aortic *aneurysm* is a condition in which a section of the abdominal aorta wall weakens and bulges. The surgical goal is to implant a graft extending from the aorta to both iliac arteries. This restores circulation to the lower extremities and pelvis.

Repair of an aortic aneurysm may be scheduled (elective) or an emergency procedure.

Pathology

A peripheral aortic aneurysm can occur at any location in the artery. However, the most common location is below the renal arteries extending into the bifurcation of the common iliac arteries or just above it. If the disease remains undiagnosed, the walls of the aorta become increasingly stretched and finally rupture. A *dissecting aneurysm* is one in which blood seeps between the layers of the vessel, causing it to tear and split. Atherosclerosis and degeneration of the muscular layer of the vessel are the most common causes of aortic aneurysm. Although the aneurysm may not extend into the iliac arteries, a bifurcated graft is often used in the repair.

POSITION:	Supine
INCISION:	Abdominal midline
PREP AND DRAPING:	Laparotomy
INSTRUMENTS:	Major laparotomy set including long laparotomy instruments; Deaver retractors; Thompson, Bookwalter, or Omni-Tract self-retaining retractor; Beckman retractor; major vascular set; vessel loops; umbilical tapes; suture bumpers; long Penrose drain for retraction; aortic graft; topical hemostatic materials; IV saline and heparin; topical thrombin
POSSIBLE EXTRAS:	Blood recovery system (e.g., Cellsaver or Haemonetics system)

Technical Points and Discussion

1. ***The patient is positioned and prepped.***

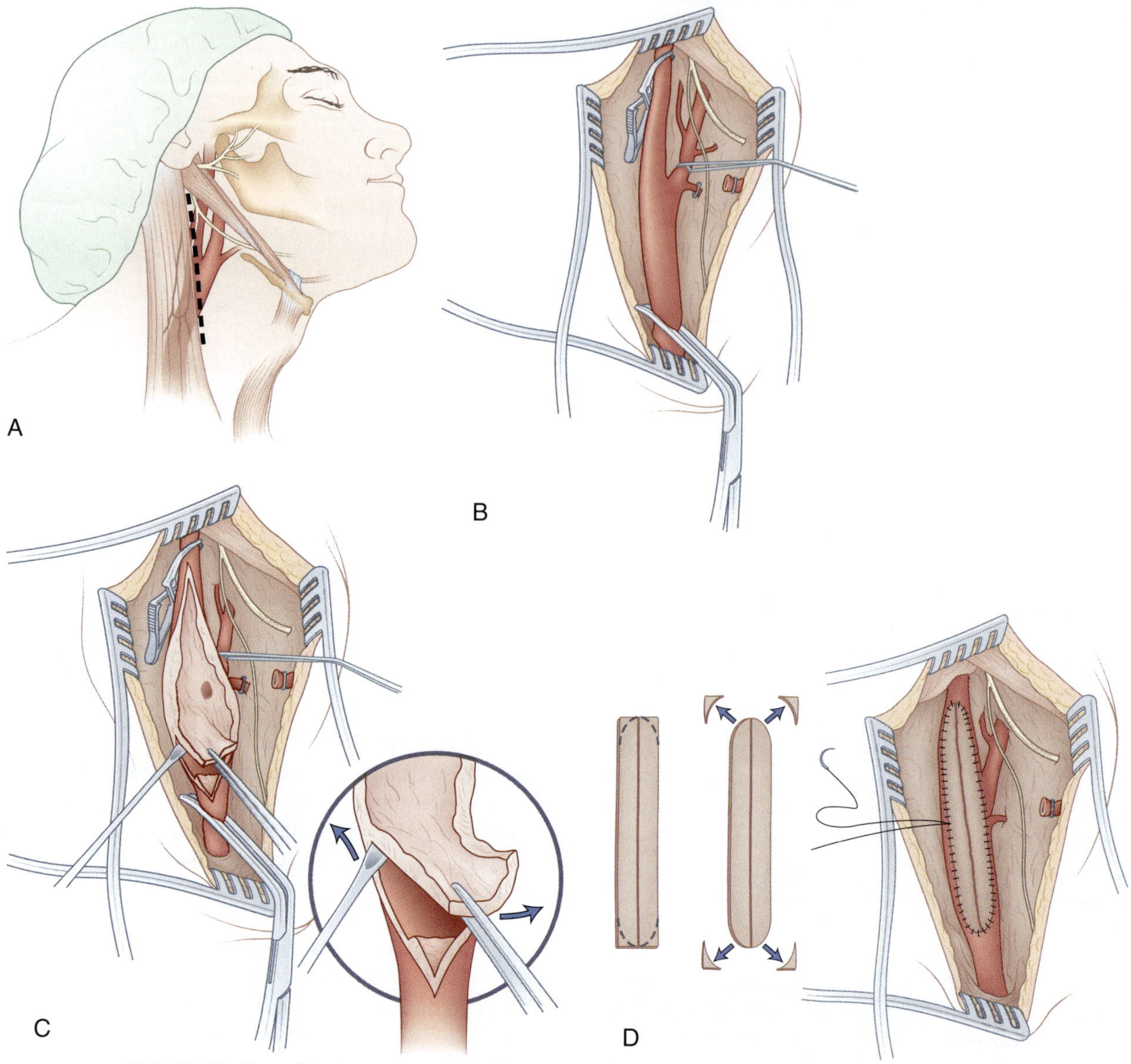

FIG. 30.23 Carotid endarterectomy. (A) The incision is made parallel to the sternocleidomastoid muscle. (B) The internal jugular vein is mobilized, and the carotid vessels are exposed. (C) An arteriotomy is performed and plaque is extracted from the vessel. (D) Closure with a patch graft. (From Ouriel K, Rutherford R, eds. *Atlas of Vascular Surgery: Operative Procedures*. Philadelphia: WB Saunders; 1998.)

The patient is placed in the supine position, prepped, and draped for a midline incision extending from the xiphoid to the pubis. A Foley catheter is inserted before the skin prep.

2. ***The abdomen is entered.***
The surgeon enters the abdomen through a long midline incision. The transverse colon is moved aside and packed with moist lap sponges. The bowel may be contained in a bowel bag or moist lap tapes for protection. A self-retaining retractor fixed to the table or standard Balfour retractor is placed in the abdomen.

3. ***The retroperitoneal space is entered.***
The retroperitoneum and fatty tissue are incised over the aorta using the long Metzenbaum scissors and ESU. Depending on the size of the patient, a long electrode tip may be needed for the ESU.

4. ***The abdominal aorta is partially mobilized.***
With use of both sharp and blunt dissection, the aorta is partially mobilized. DeBakey forceps and long Metzenbaum scissors may be used. The ST should also have several sponge sticks and small sponge dissectors prepared. A vessel loop may be placed around the aorta. If the vena cava is damaged in this stage, it is immediately repaired using a size 4-0 or 5-0 vascular suture. The neck of the aneurysm is clamped.

5. ***The common iliac arteries are exposed.***
Dissection of the distal aorta is performed at the level of the iliac arteries. These are mobilized using mainly blunt dissection. The lumbar arteries that

enter the aorta from the posterior side may be occluded with size 2-0 or 5-0 Prolene or braided polyester sutures. The iliac arteries are clamped using Fogarty clamps.

6. ***The aneurysm is incised and opened.***
   If a risk of excessive bleeding exists in spite of cross clamping the aorta, a Foley catheter with 30 mL balloon may be prepared for use as an intraluminal tamponade in the aorta. Extra aortic clamps, suction, and mounted sutures should be prepared. A basin is used to collect large clots and atherosclerotic debris. Before the aneurysm sac is opened, the patient is heparinized and the common iliac arteries are clamped using DeBakey or similar right-angle vascular clamps. The proximal aorta is cross-clamped using the surgeon's preference for Crafoord coarctation or Satinsky, Potts, or Cooley aortic clamp.

   A longitudinal incision is made in the aneurysm using the ESU or #15 knife blade. Smaller lateral (T-shaped) incisions are made at each end of the long incision. This provides greater access to the cavity.

7. ***Blood clots and plaque are removed from the aneurysm sac.***
   The ST should place a basin on the field as blood clots and atherosclerotic plaque are removed piecemeal from the aneurysm cavity. The surgeon uses vascular forceps to grasp the plaque and separate it from the wall of the aorta. Bleeding arising from the lumbar arteries, which perforate the aorta, is controlled by ligation using Prolene vascular suture. If the iliac arteries are to be grafted, each is opened and irrigated with heparinized saline. The aneurysm sac is not removed but is opened out, and the graft is positioned between the leaves of the sac.

8. ***A graft is implanted in the aorta.***
   A tube graft or bifurcated graft specified by the surgeon is prepared. The ST should pass the graft in a basin along with straight Mayo scissors to the surgeon. A collagen-impregnated Dacron graft is commonly used. The distal ends of a bifurcated graft are anastomosed with a double-arm suture size 3-0 or 4-0 Prolene or polyester vascular suture. The suture lines may be tested by irrigating the graft with saline or slight release of the cross clamps.

   The graft is sutured to the aorta and aneurysm using a double-arm vascular suture of size 3-0 Prolene. Leaks are repaired with 3-0 Prolene figure-of-eight sutures. Suture pledgets may be required for the closure. If the anastomosis was tested using blood (by releasing the cross clamp), blood is removed from the graft. A topical hemostatic agent may be used on the suture lines. At this time the patient's pedal pulses are checked using the Doppler.

9. ***The aneurysm wall is sutured over the graft.***
   After bleeding is controlled, the aneurysm wall is jacketed around the graft and closed with a size 3-0 Prolene running suture.

10. ***The retroperitoneal space is closed.***
    After the wound is irrigated and all tissue and plaque debris removed, the retroperitoneum is closed using a running synthetic absorbable suture size 3-0. The abdomen is closed as a single layer with polydioxanone surgical (PDS) suture or in multiple tissue layers. Skin is closed with staples and dressed with flat gauze. Technical points of the procedure are illustrated in Fig. 30.24.

AORTOBIFEMORAL BYPASS

An aortobifemoral bypass is performed to treat aortoiliac occlusive disease. A bifurcated graft is implanted between the aorta and the femoral arteries to bypass the iliac arteries and restore circulation. Bilateral tunnels are made in the tissue between the aorta and the femoral arteries. The bifurcated limbs of the graft are brought through the tunnels and anastomosed to the arteries.

Pathology

The iliac artery is a common site of atherosclerosis. An aortobifemoral bypass is performed instead of an endarterectomy or aortoiliac bypass because it produces increased patency and can be performed in patients with extensive calcification of the arteries.

POSITION:	Supine
INCISION:	Midline
PREP AND DRAPING:	The prep area extends from the axillary line to the mid-thighs. Both legs are draped circumferentially, and the genitalia are covered with a towel and barrier drape. A Foley catheter is inserted before the skin prep.
INSTRUMENTS:	Major laparotomy set; Beckman retractors; major vascular set; vessel loops; umbilical tapes; suture bumpers; vessel clips; topical hemostatic materials; IV saline and heparin; topical thrombin; suture pledgets; surgeon's choice of graft
POSSIBLE EXTRAS:	Long Penrose drains; straight Robinson catheter

Technical Points and Discussion

1. ***A laparotomy is performed through a long midline incision, and the aorta is exposed.***
   A midline abdominal incision is made and carried to the aorta, as described in the previous procedure. The proximal portion of the aorta is dissected to the renal veins using sharp and blunt dissection. The

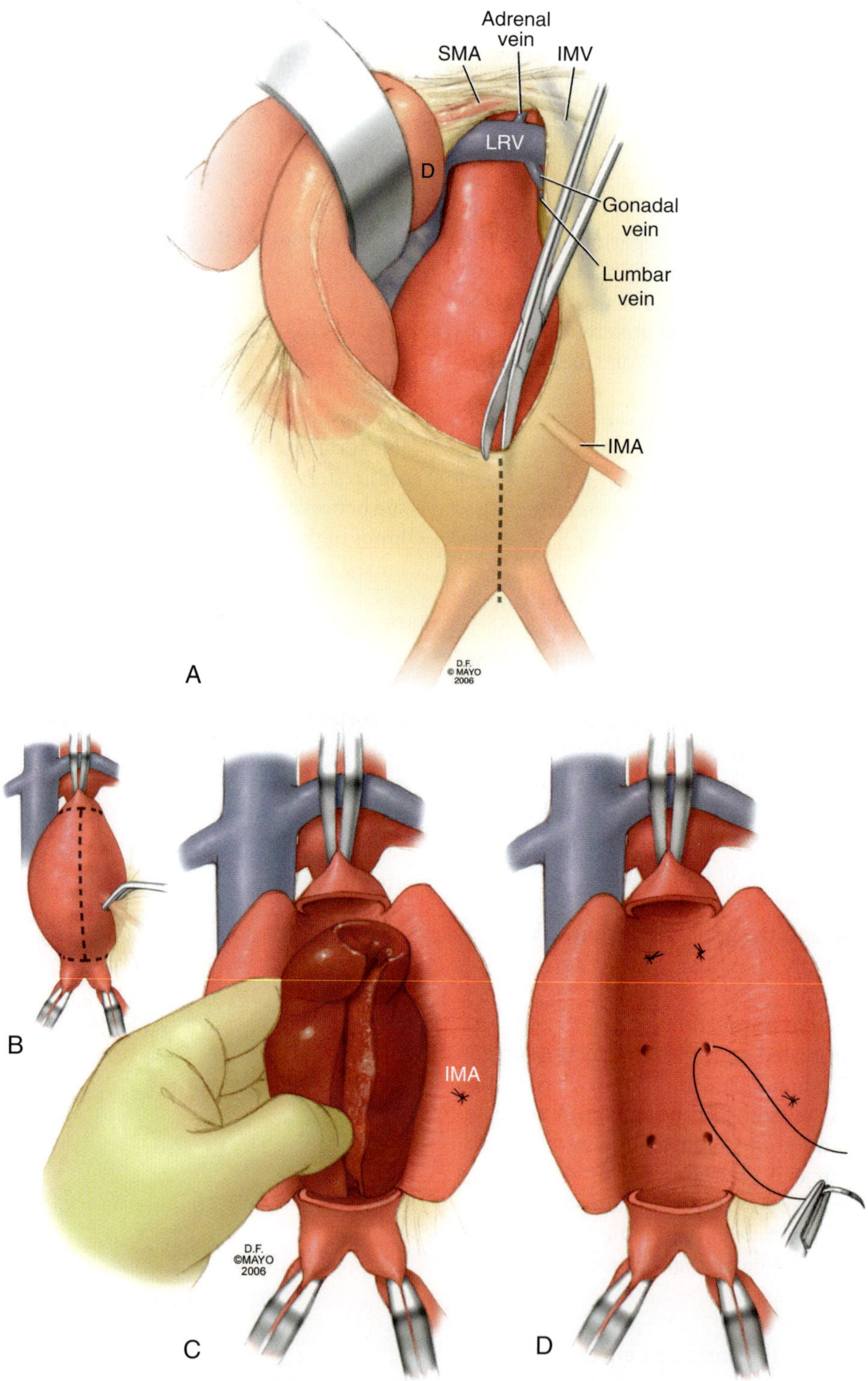

FIG. 30.24 Abdominal aortic aneurysm with graft insertion. (A) The retroperitoneum is incised. (B) Proposed incision in aorta. Aneurysm is exposed. (C) The leaves of the sac are opened; blood clots and plaque are removed. (D) Here the communicating lumbar arteries are oversewn.

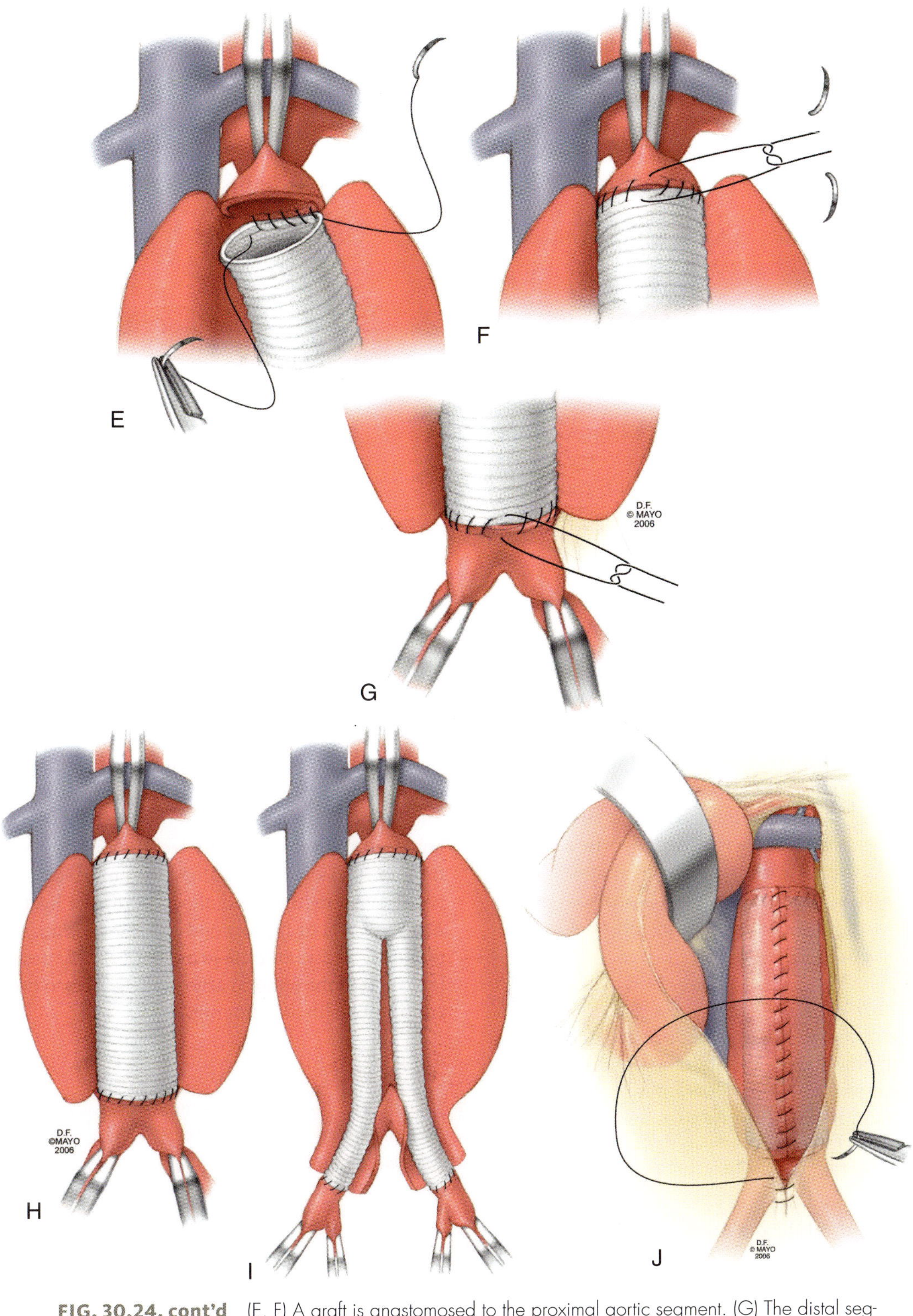

FIG. 30.24, cont'd (E, F) A graft is anastomosed to the proximal aortic segment. (G) The distal segment is anastomosed. (H) A bifurcated graft may also be used. (I) Completed anatomosis. (J) Closing the aorta over the graft. (From Townsend CM, Beauchamp EM, Mattox K. *Sabiston Textbook of Surgery*. Philadelphia: Elsevier; 2017.)

duodenum is mobilized to expose the renal vein. Vessel loops should be available. The distal aorta is then exposed.

2. ***The femoral arteries are exposed.***
   Bilateral groin incisions are made using a knife. Dissection is performed with Metzenbaum scissors, sponge dissectors, and the ESU. A Weitlaner or similar self-retaining retractors are used superficially, and Richardson retractors are used for deeper hand retraction. The larger arteries (common, superficial, and profunda) are dissected out, and vessels loops are applied as needed for traction and protection. After the femoral vessels have been exposed, the incisions may be covered with sterile towels.

3. ***The graft tunnels are constructed.***
   Bilateral tunnels are made from the groin on both sides to the bifurcation of the aorta. The surgeon may construct the tunnels using gentle digital dissection or may use a Pèan clamp or graft tunneler. Long Penrose drains or Robinson catheters may be inserted into the tunnels using a Pèan clamp to enable passage of the graft limbs. The ends of the drains or catheters are tagged with hemostats to prevent them from backing out of the tunnels.

4. ***The distal aorta is clamped and divided.***
   The patient is heparinized and the aorta is clamped using the surgeon's preferred vascular clamp. The aorta is then divided. Lumbar branches may be ligated at this time. The distal aorta is oversewn using a size 3-0 vascular suture. Suture pledgets may be required.

5. ***End-to-end anastomosis is performed on the aorta.***
   Before implanting the graft, the surgeon trims it using straight Mayo scissors. If there is atherosclerotic plaque at the cuff of the proximal aorta, this may be removed using vascular forceps and scissors. The graft is anastomosed to the proximal aorta using a double-arm suture of size 3-0 Prolene or polyester.

6. ***The wounds are closed.***
   The groin incisions are closed using size 2-0 and 3-0 absorbable synthetic sutures. The abdomen is closed with a single running suture of size 1 PDS suture or in multiple tissue layers. Skin is closed with staples and dressed with flat gauze. Fig. 30.25 shows the completed graft. Patients recover in the ICU or surgical unit. Doppler testing is performed throughout the first 48 hours of postoperative recovery to ensure that the peripheral circulation remains intact.

NOTE *A technically similar procedure is the femorofemoral bypass shown in Fig. 30.26. This figure demonstrates the technique of tunneling through the superficial tissue layers. This type of tunneling is different from a tunneling procedure used in endovascular procedures.*

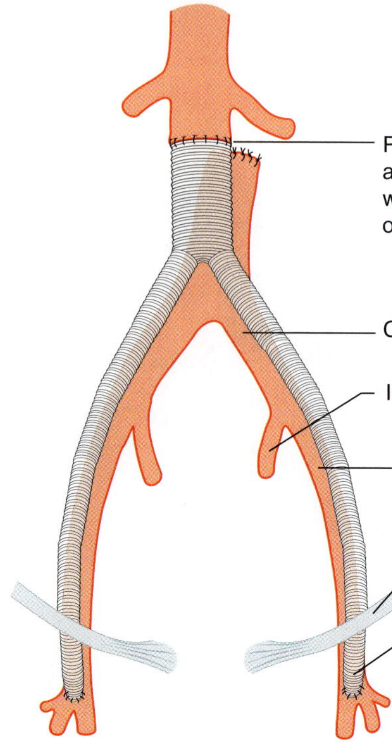

FIG. 30.25 Aortobifemoral bypass. A graft is implanted between the aorta and the femoral arteries to bypass the iliac arteries and restore circulation. (From Garden O, Bradbury A, Forsythe J, Parks R, eds. *Principles and Practice of Surgery*. 6th ed. Edinburgh: Churchill Livingstone; 2012.)

IN SITU SAPHENOUS FEMOROPOPLITEAL BYPASS

In situ saphenous vein bypass is a surgical alternative to the use of a synthetic graft to bypass a diseased femoral artery. The saphenous vein is not removed but is left in its normal anatomical position. In the technique described here, a continuous incision is made along the entire saphenous vein. This is the safest method and allows complete ligation of tributaries. The distal or narrow end of the vein is anastomosed to the popliteal artery, and the proximal vein is anastomosed to the large end of the femoral artery. The goal is to produce vascular continuity with an autograft.

POSITION:	Supine
INCISION:	Midline and groin
PREP AND DRAPING:	The prep area extends from the umbilicus to both groins to both legs, including the ankles and feet. Both legs are draped circumferentially, and the genitalia are covered with a towel and barrier drape. A Foley catheter is inserted before the skin prep.
INSTRUMENTS:	Major laparotomy set; Beckman retractors; major vascular set; vessel loops; umbilical tapes; suture bumpers; hemostat jaw covers (booties), vessel clips; topical hemostatic materials; IV saline and heparin; topical thrombin; suture pledgets; surgeon's choice of graft

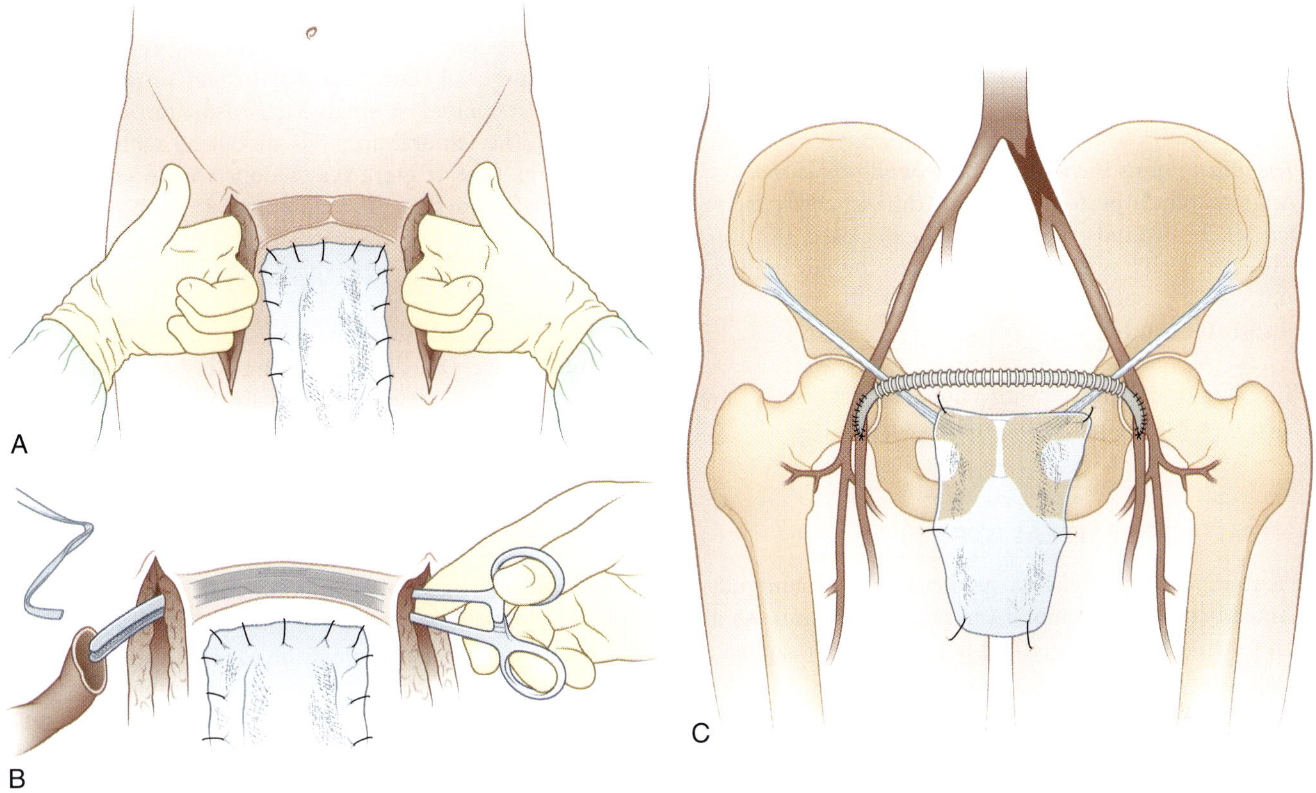

FIG. 30.26 Femorofemoral bypass. (A) A suprapubic tunnel is created digitally. (B) The midline fascia is pierced with a long clamp, which grasps a Penrose drain or umbilical tape to facilitate the delivery of the graft without kinks or twists. (C) Bilateral end-to-side anastomoses are constructed; each anastomosis is run onto the profunda femoris artery if the superficial femoral arteries are occluded. (From Ouriel K, Rutherford R, eds. *Atlas of Vascular Surgery: Operative Procedures.* Philadelphia: WB Saunders; 1998.)

POSSIBLE EXTRAS: Long Penrose drains, straight Robinson catheter

Technical Points and Discussion

1. ***The patient is prepped and draped.***
The patient is placed in supine position. The operative leg, lower abdomen, and groin are prepped and draped with the operative leg and groin exposed. The incision site and pedal pulse points are marked on the skin.

2. ***An incision is made, and the saphenous vein is mobilized.***
The medial aspect of the thigh is incised from above the ankle to the groin, following the saphenous vein. The incision is carried deeper with dissecting scissors and the ESU. This exposes the saphenous vein, which is partly or completely mobilized. Vessel loops are placed around the vein for traction.

3. ***The branches of the vein are mobilized.***
Branches of the vein are sequentially clamped with mosquito forceps and clipped or ligated with size 3-0 silk. They are then divided from the vein. The distal and proximal ends of the saphenous vein are clamped and divided.

4. ***Internal venous valves are obliterated.***
Before the anastomoses are performed between the saphenous vein and femoral and popliteal arteries, the valves must be incised so that arterial blood can flow through them easily. Several techniques are used. The angioscope is passed through the lumen of the vein, and a system is used to sever the valves and remove tributaries. This avoids extensive dissection of the vein. An alternative method is to incise the first two valves under direct vision with valve scissors and then to use a valvulotome, with or without the angioscope, to release the others.

5. ***The anastomosis is performed.***
Anastomoses are created between the saphenous vein and the femoral artery. The vein is trimmed to a bevel and a small incision is made in the femoral artery with Potts scissors or a #11 scalpel blade. An end-to-side anastomosis is formed with 6-0 or 7-0 non-absorbable sutures with a double- or single-arm needle. The profunda femoris can also be used for anastomosis. The distal anastomosis is made using the same technique.

6. ***Tributaries to the vein are occluded.***
Next, the small tributaries that branch from the saphenous vein must be occluded. These are located with Doppler ultrasound unless the vein is completely exposed. The surgeon applies digital pressure over the vein while observing the Doppler wave. Increased flow indicates an

area of arteriovenous fistula (a vascular connection between the arterial circulation and the venous flow). These areas are exposed and each individual tributary is clipped or ligated and incised.

7. ***The anastomosis is checked, and wounds are closed.*** Angiography is performed at this time to check for patency. The wounds are irrigated and closed in layers, with absorbable synthetic sutures used for subcutaneous and fascial tissue. The skin is closed with clips or nonabsorbable suture.

   The wounds are dressed with a nonadherent dressing and then with gauze squares and roller gauze.

FEMOROPOPLITEAL BYPASS

In a femoropopliteal bypass, a synthetic graft or autograft is implanted between the femoral and popliteal arteries. As discussed previously, in situ grafting uses the greater saphenous vein as a shunt.

Pathology

Femoropopliteal bypass is indicated for atherosclerosis of the femoral artery.

POSITION:	Supine
INCISION:	Groin and leg
PREP AND DRAPING:	The prep area extends from the axillary line or umbilicus to the mid-thighs. Both legs are draped circumferentially, and the genitalia are covered with a towel and barrier drape. A Foley catheter is inserted before the skin prep.
INSTRUMENTS:	Major laparotomy set; Beckman retractor; major vascular set; vessel loops; umbilical tapes; instrument jaw protectors; vessel clips; topical hemostatic materials; IV saline and heparin; topical thrombin; suture pledgets; surgeon's choice of graft

Technical Points and Discussion

1. ***The patient is prepped and draped.*** The patient is placed in the supine position, prepped, and draped with the affected leg and groin exposed. The incision site and pedal pulse points are marked on the skin.

2. ***The femoral artery is exposed and mobilized.*** An incision is made on the medial side of the thigh, below the groin. Dissection is performed with the scalpel, Metzenbaum scissors, sponge dissectors, and the ESU. A Weitlaner or other small self-retaining retractor is used for superficial retraction. For deeper retraction, Army-Navy retractors or small Richardson retractors may be used. The femoral artery is mobilized with careful dissection. One or more vessel loops are placed around the artery for traction and manipulation.

3. ***The popliteal artery is exposed and mobilized.*** A second vertical incision is made on the medial side of the knee below the patella. The subcutaneous, fascial, and muscle layers are dissected with both sharp and blunt dissection. A self-retaining retractor is used to expose the popliteal space. The popliteal artery is mobilized with sponge dissectors and scissors. A vessel loop is placed around the artery. Angiography may be done at this time to verify that the popliteal artery is patent.

4. ***The graft is measured and tunneled.*** The surgeon chooses the appropriately sized graft. The greater saphenous vein may be used instead of a synthetic graft. The procedure for harvesting a saphenous graft is discussed in Chapter 32. A tunnel is made in the subcutaneous tissue, and the graft is carried from the upper to the lower wound. The graft is then drawn back into the popliteal space.

5. ***The graft is anastomosed.*** To perform the anastomosis, the surgeon first places a vascular clamp across the femoral artery. A small incision is made in the artery with a #11 scalpel blade followed by vascular scissors. Using running sutures of 5-0 or 6-0 polypropylene, the surgeon creates the anastomosis between the femoral artery and graft.

   The popliteal anastomosis is created in the same manner as the femoral anastomosis. During both anastomoses, the ST should have heparinized saline solution available for the irrigation of the arterial sites. Hemostatic agents are used to check bleeding at the anastomosis and additional sutures are placed if needed.

6. ***Circulation is verified, and the wounds are closed.*** Angiography may be done at this time, and the patency of the arterial system is monitored with the Doppler or intravascular ultrasound. The wound is irrigated and closed in layers. The popliteal space is closed with 2-0 or 3-0 interrupted absorbable synthetic sutures. The skin is commonly closed with staples or nylon sutures. The groin incision is closed in layers and dressed with gauze squares.

   A femoropopliteal bypass is illustrated in Fig. 30.27.

During the immediate postoperative period, the patient's pedal pulses are monitored carefully. Possible complications include blockage of the graft and infection. Patients may experience some numbness of the lower leg. Swelling of the operative leg is common after surgery.

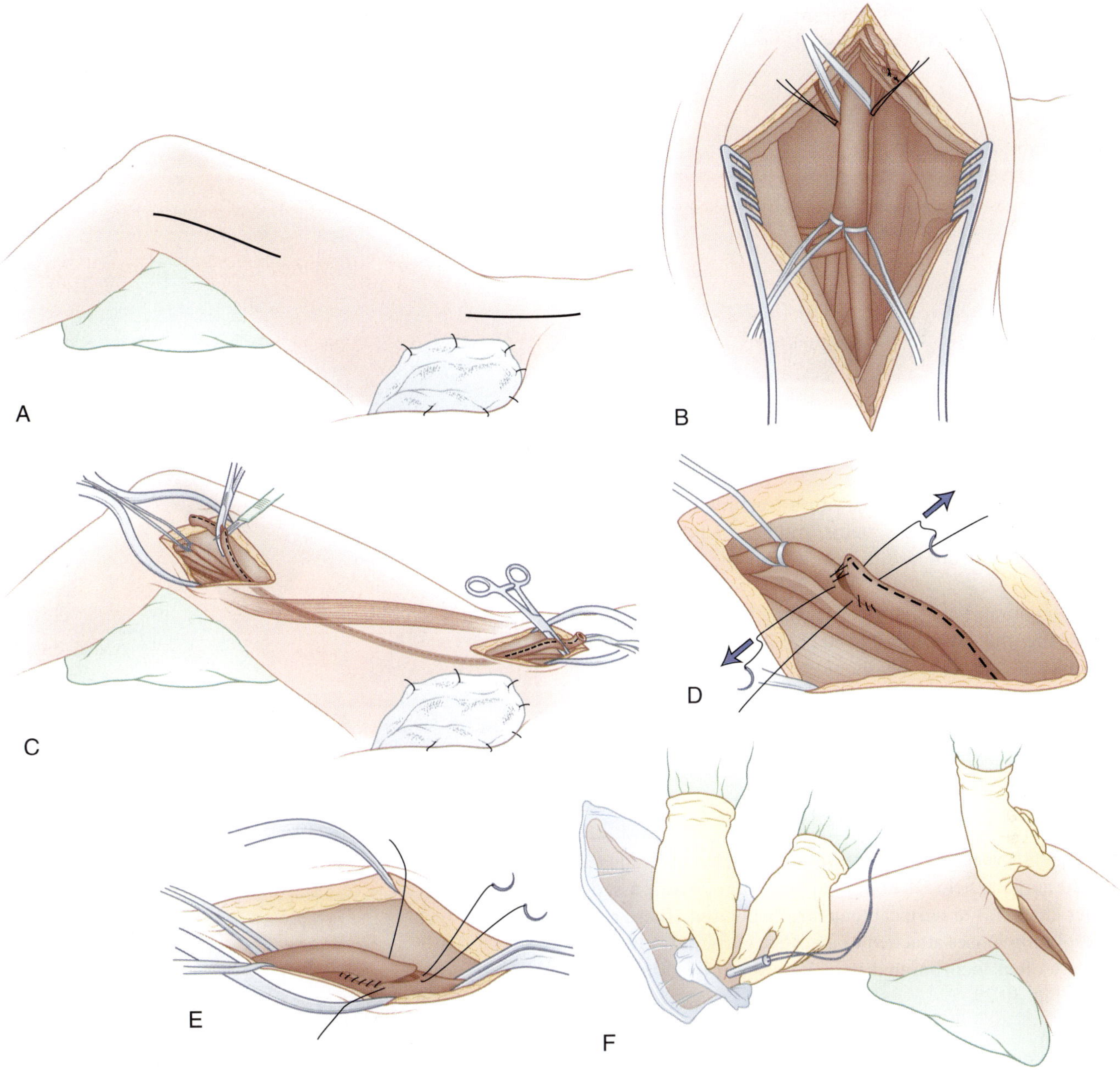

FIG. 30.27 Femoropopliteal bypass. (A) A femoral incision is made at the level of the inguinal ligament. A popliteal incision is made on the medial side of the distal thigh. (B) The common femoral, superficial femoral, and profunda femoris arteries are exposed in the groin. (C) A curved hemostat and the knife blade are used to bevel the graft for the anastomoses. (D) Completion of the popliteal anastomosis. (E) The proximal anastomosis is completed with a two-suture technique. (F) Doppler ultrasound is used to assess the hemodynamic result intraoperatively. (From Ouriel K, Rutherford R, eds. *Atlas of Vascular Surgery: Operative Procedures*. Philadelphia: WB Saunders; 1998.)

MICROVASCULAR SURGERY

Microsurgery refers to any surgical procedure that requires magnification. Examples of microsurgical procedures include microneural (nerves), microlymphatic (lymphatic vessels), and microtubular (performed on the small delicate tubules) of the reproductive and genitourinary systems. Microvascular procedures involve very small (approximately 1 mm in diameter) blood vessels. The techniques required for most microsurgical procedures, including microvascular, are similar.

Case planning for microvascular procedures requires specific considerations for room preparation patient position and draping, the surgeon's preferences for magnification, instruments, irrigation solutions, surgical drugs and adhesives, and special supplies.

ROOM PREPARATION AND TEAM POSITION

Microvascular surgery can be performed in a standard operating room with accommodation for equipment including

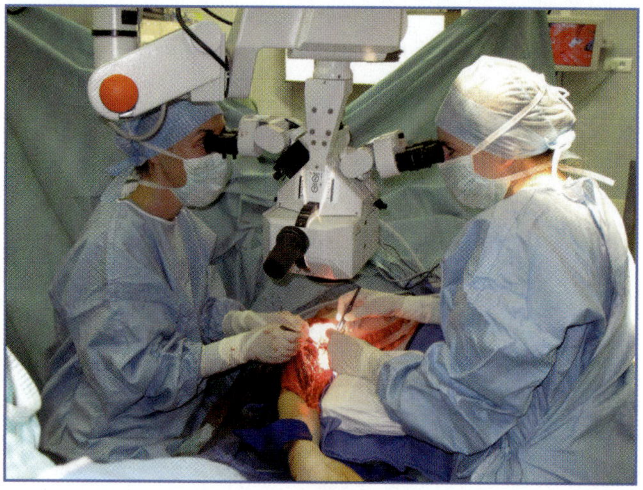

FIG. 30.28 Microsurgical team. (From Merle M, Dautel G. *Emergency Surgery of the Hand*. 4th ed. Philadelphia: Elsevier; 2017.)

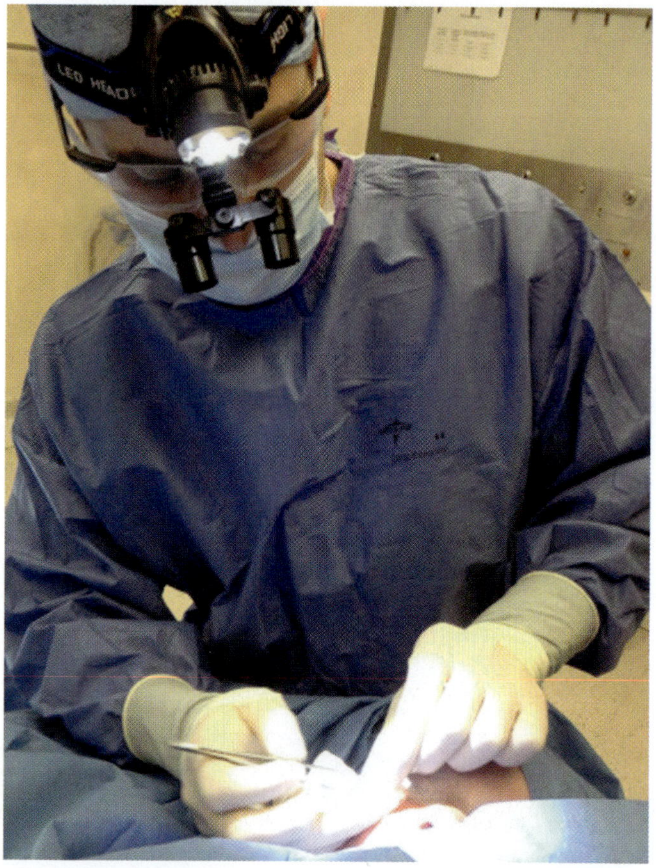

FIG. 30.29 Surgical loupes for use in microsurgery. Shown here are loupes combined with a surgical headlight. (From Miranda BH, et al. Building the headlight: An illuminating experience. *J Plastic Reconstr Aesthet Surg*. 2014;67[8]:1158–1160. https://doi.org/10.1016/j.bjps.2014.03.011.)

the operating microscope fitted with a teaching head (dual-head microscope), imaging systems, and hand table (used for hand and arm procedures) sitting stools for the surgeon and assistant.

The surgeon and assistant may operate while standing or seated during microsurgery (Fig. 30.28). If they are to remain seated, fully adjustable stools should be available. The procedures are often tedious and require wrist and arm supports to prevent hand and arm fatigue. The surgical technologist may stand next to the surgeon's assistant.

MAGNIFICATION OF THE SURGICAL FIELD

Microsurgical procedures, by definition, require magnification of the surgical field. The operating microscope (discussed in earlier chapters) or surgical loupes may be used. These are high-resolution lenses attached to an eyeglass frame and lens. Loupes are often incorporated into the surgical head light as shown in Fig. 30.29.

MICROVASCULAR INSTRUMENTS

Instruments used in microvascular surgery are constructed for maximum control over the instrument and tissues. They are extremely delicate and easily ruined by improper handling. Instruments should be contained in a protected tray with slots to keep them separated during transport and sterilization (Fig. 30.30). This type of tray can also be used on the instrument table. When not in use, tip guards should be used to protect the instruments (Fig. 30.31).

Titanium is used in the manufacturing of high-quality microsurgical instruments. The metal is lightweight and helps prevent the instruments from becoming magnetized.

Scissors

Scissors used in microsurgery are spring loaded to prevent hand fatigue and enable precise mechanical action with minimal movement of the surgeon's hand. Tissue scissors have slightly curved blades and rounded tips. Sharp, straight bladed

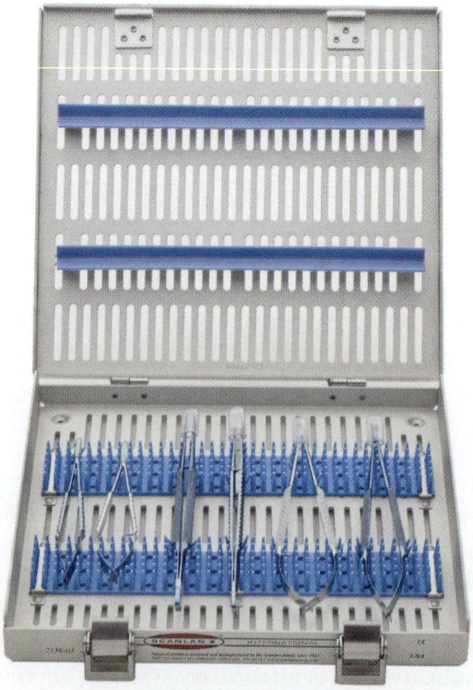

FIG. 30.30 Instrument tray for microsurgical instruments. (Copyright 2019; image courtesy Scanlan International, www.scanlaninternational.com.)

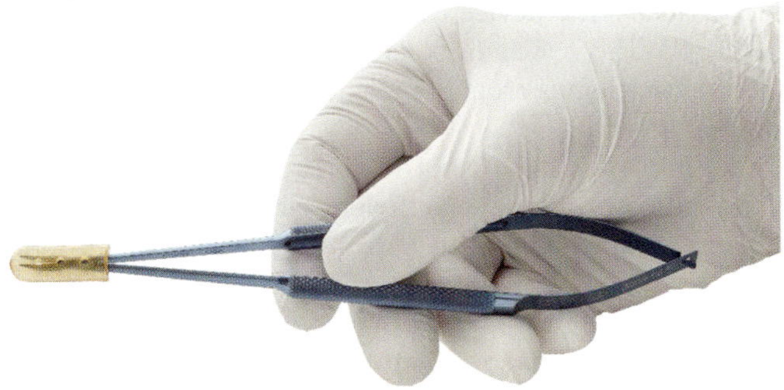

FIG. 30.31 Instrument tip guards for microsurgical instruments. (Copyright 2019; image courtesy Scanlan International, www.scanlaninternational.com.)

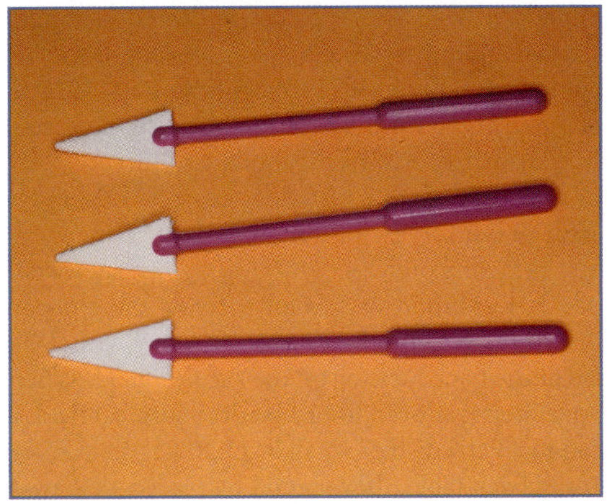

FIG. 30.32 Cellulose sponges used in microvascular surgery. (Copyright 2019; image courtesy Scanlan International, www.scanlaninternational.com.)

scissors are used to separate arterial layers and to cut microsurgical sutures.

Needle Holders

Needle holders may be locking or non-locking, straight or curved. Most types are spring loaded. These are held like a pencil and should be passed to the surgeon so that the instrument is oriented in this position with the handle resting between the surgeon's thumb and its web. When passing a suture loaded in a non-locking needle holder, remember to keep gentle pressure on the handles to avoid dropping the needle. (Detailed instruction on passing sutures can be found in Chapter 19.)

Monofilament non-absorbable nylon or polypropylene suture, size 8-0 to 12-0, is preferred by most surgeons. Microvascular needles are available in ⅜ and ½ curve shapes with taper or spatulated tips. Sutures are placed with the aid of tying or jewelers forceps.

Irrigation and Suction

The surgical technologist or surgeon's assistant is responsible for ensuring that the microvascular site is kept moist during the procedure. Ringer's lactate or heparinized saline are used according to the surgeon's preference. An ophthalmic irrigation tip (olive-tip or similar design) or 24-gauge angiocath can be fitted to a syringe for this purpose.

Suction during microvascular surgery can be problematic. Even with low suction pressure, vessels can be damaged. (Some surgeons therefore prefer to apply the suction tip over a moistened hydrocellulose sponge.) Eye spears of the same material are used to absorb small amounts of blood from the operative site (Fig. 30.32).

Microvascular Clamps

Disposal microvascular clamps are preferred by most surgeons because reusable clamps can lose their gripping pressure (Fig. 30.33). Clamps are available in different shapes and pressures, which are calibrated according to the size of the vessel.

IMPORTANT TO KNOW *Microsurgical clamps for arteries are different from those used on veins. Look for an A or a V engraved on the clamp to select the correct one. Some manufacturers' clamps are color coded for venous and arterial use.*

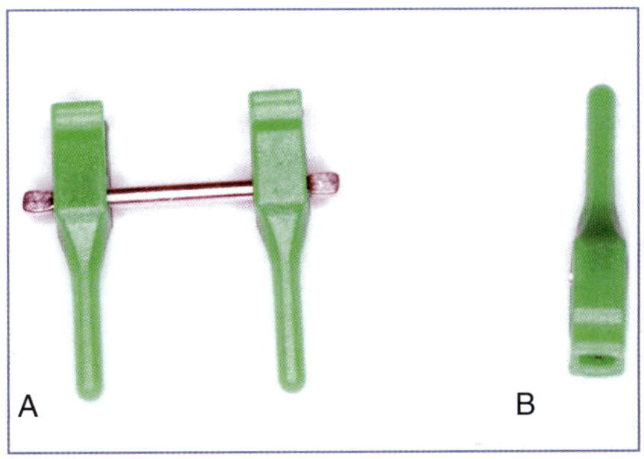

FIG. 30.33 Disposable microvascular clamps. (Courtesy AROSurgical, Newport Beach, CA.) (A) Double vein clamp. (B) Single vein clamp.

Clamps are differentiated according to the size of the vessel to be occluded. The surgeon will request the size and type required. Metal clamps may also be used.

Bipolar ESU

The bipolar ESU is used in microvascular surgery to coagulate small bleeders. The preferred bipolar instrument is the jewelers forceps because of its very fine tips, which minimize the amount of heat dispersed to nearby tissues. Bipolar microvascular scissors are also available for the same purpose.

Visibility Aids

During microvascular and other types of microsurgery, visibility background materials are used to reduce glare and to provide color contrast between the anatomical structures (vessels, nerves, etc.) and the surrounding tissue. Colored silicone patches are positioned under the structures to provide this contrast. An example is shown in Fig. 30.34.

Care of Transplant Tissues

The surgical technologist is responsible for the care of transplant tissues used during microvascular surgery. These include vessels that have been harvested for implantation and free skin flaps that have been harvested from one area of the body for implantation in another. It is particularly important that the tissues are kept moist with normal saline (not water) until the surgeon is ready to perform the implantation.

After the tissue is harvested, it may be covered with a papaverine or lidocaine solution-soaked gauze sponge according to the surgeon's preference. The surgeon may wish to trim the tissue or test blood vessels for patency using heparinized saline or other solution. Free tissue (flaps or vessels) can be prepared at the back table or on the surgical field. Whenever a tissue specimen is moved to or from the surgical field, it must be placed in a Petri dish or small basin. If harvested tissues are kept on the back table, they should be placed well away from the edge.

Microvascular Anastomosis

ANASTOMOSIS DEVICES A number of devices and systems have been developed to aid in microvascular anastomoses. The most commonly used device is the approximator clamp shown in Fig. 30.35. The device consists of two clamps joined by a metal rod. The vessels to be anastomosed are cross-clamped and the two clamps brought together using a hemostat (artery forceps) for suturing.

The *microvascular anastomotic coupler system* (Fig. 30.36) consists of two polyethylene rings fitted with a series of stainless steel pins. Rings are available in many different sizes. The two vessel ends are threaded through the rings, which are brought together by the device. This everts the ends of the vessels so that the intimal layers of the vessels are in contact with each other. Closing the instrument interlocks the pins in place. The rings remain as permanent implants (Fig. 30.37).

SUTURING TECHNIQUES Microvascular anastomosis follows the same general techniques described previously for open vascular surgery. The end-to-end and end-to-side methods are commonly used. The vessels are isolated, trimmed as required, and finally joined by sutures or staples. Figs. 30.38 through 30.40 illustrate these techniques.

Microvascular stapling instruments are also available for vessel anastomosis. These are configured like other surgical

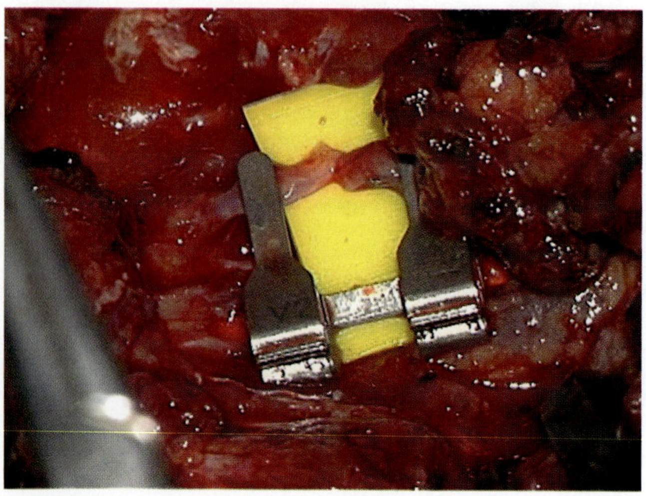

FIG. 30.34 Visibility aids in microvascular surgery. (From Lee L, Karp NS. *Atlas of Reconstructive Breast Surgery*. Edinburgh: Saunders; 2019.)

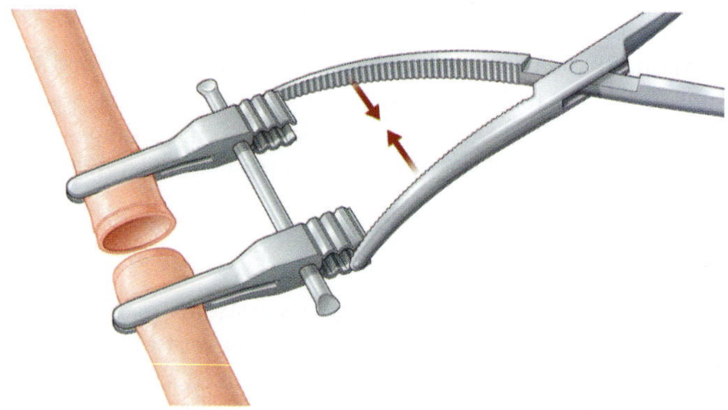

FIG. 30.35 Approximator clamp used to bring vessel ends together for anastomosis. (From Gurtner G, Neligan P. *Plastic Surgery: Principles*. 4th ed. Vol 1. London: Elsevier; 2018.)

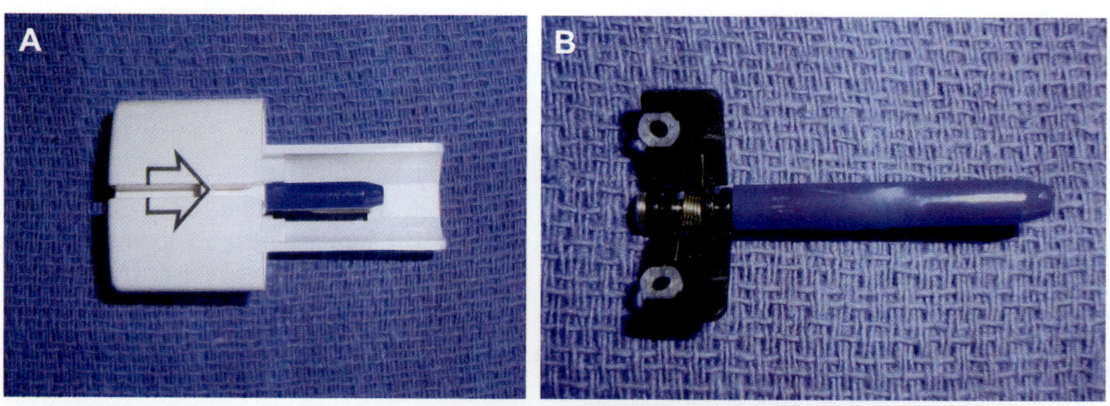

FIG. 30.36 Microvascular anastomotic coupler used to form an end-to-end anastomosis between two arteries. (A) Device as shown before removal from packaging. (B) Coupler with packaging removed. The couplers are color coded for size. This example is a size 1.5 mm. (From Technology in microvascular surgery. *Oral Maxillofacial Facial Surg Clin.* 2010;22:1.)

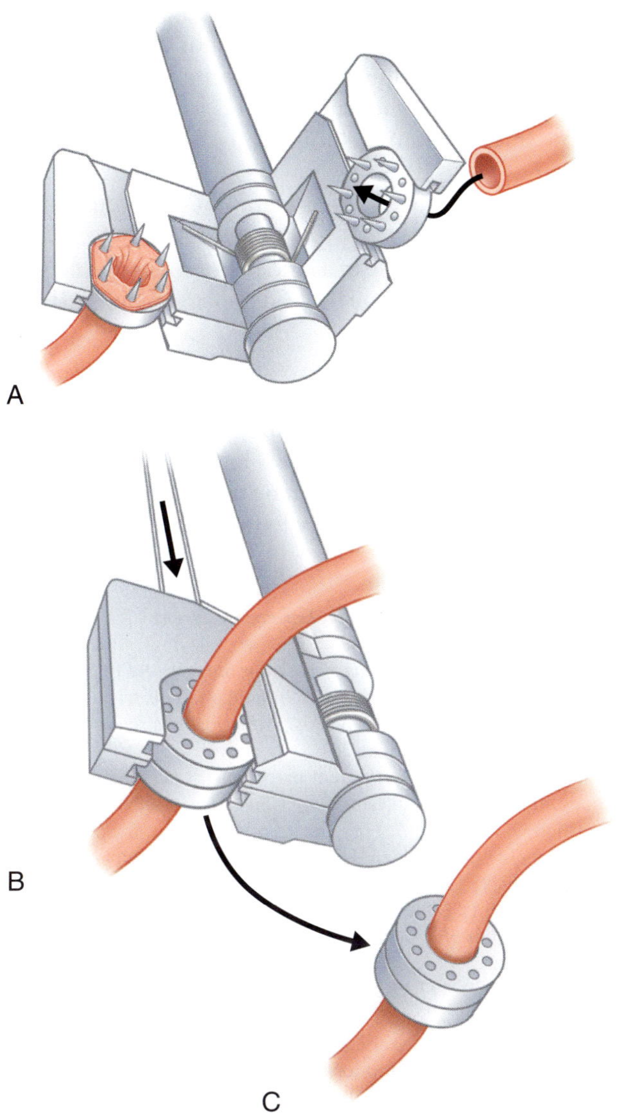

FIG. 30.37 Mechanics of the microvascular anastomotic coupler. (A) The vessel is threaded through the silastic ring on both sides. The ends are everted and impaled over the sharp metal pins. (B) The coupler device is closed and each set of pins is seated into the opposite ring. This brings the intimal layers together. (C) The anastomosed vessel is removed from the device. The rings remain in place as a permanent implant. (From Wei F, Mardini S. *Flaps and Reconstructive Surgery*. 2nd ed. Edinburgh: Elsevier; 2017.)

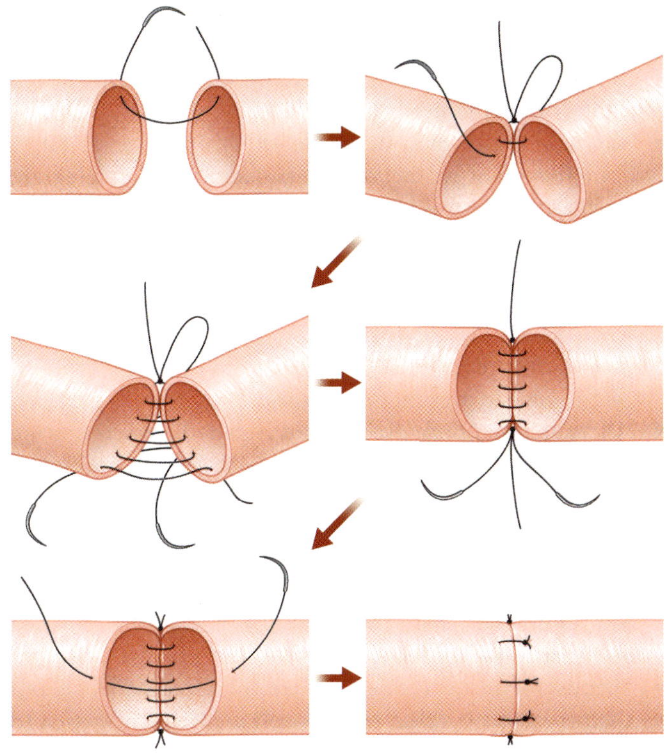

FIG. 30.38 End-to-end vessel anastomosis using interrupted sutures. (From Gurtner G, Neligan P. *Plastic Surgery: Principles*. 4th ed. Vol 1. London: Elsevier; 2018.)

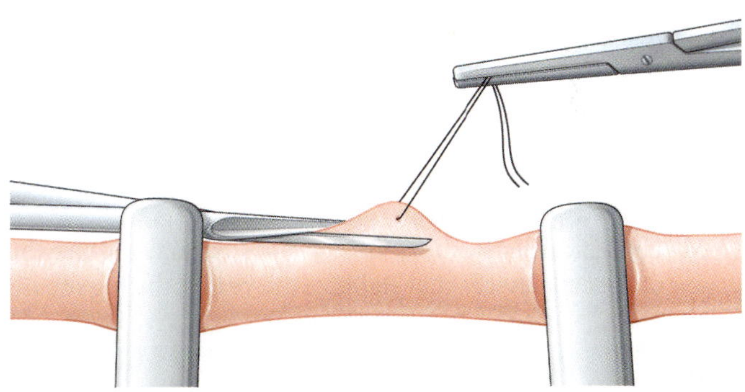

FIG. 30.39 End-to-side anastomosis. Preparation of the vessel (arteriotomy). (From Gurtner G, Neligan P. *Plastic Surgery: Principles*. 4th ed. Vol 1. London: Elsevier; 2018.)

staplers in a disposable format. Refer to Chapter 11 for information on surgical staplers.

KEY CONCEPTS

- Vascular procedures are frequently performed to reestablish blood flow in an obstructed vessel. The bifurcation of the vessel is the most common area of obstruction resulting from atherosclerotic disease.
- Vascular surgery uses specific techniques, including endarterectomy, vessel anastomosis, and the use of vascular grafts.

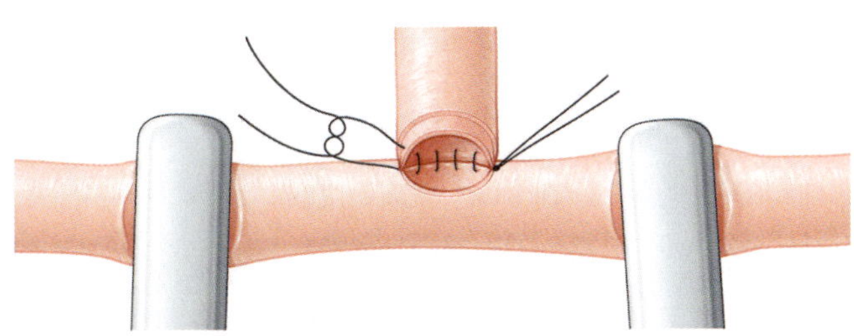

FIG. 30.40 Completion of anastomosis. (From Gurtner G, Neligan P. *Plastic Surgery: Principles*. 4th ed. Vol 1. London: Elsevier; 2018.)

- During endovascular procedures, the ST may be responsible for controlling the ends of guidewires, stents, and catheters. This requires focused response to prevent the devices from falling out of the sterile field.
- Vascular grafts may be made of synthetic material, a combination of synthetic and biomaterials, or an allograft. Each type of graft is inserted using specific techniques.
- Grafts must be handled as little as possible before insertion and protected on the back table.
- During vascular surgery, intravenous heparin is distributed to the ST. This is a high-risk drug, which must be labeled as soon as it is received and isolated from other medications on the table to prevent drug errors.
- All saline solution used to flush blood vessels during vascular surgery must be *intravenous saline*. Topical saline normally used for irrigation of tissues is never injected into a blood vessel.
- Vascular sutures are composed of synthetic material in very small sizes. The end-to-end anastomosis requires a double-arm suture, whereas a linear repair is normally performed with a single-arm suture.
- Hemostatic agents such as Gelfoam, oxidized cellulose, and tissue sealants (CoSeal and Tisseel) are frequently used to control bleeding at anastomosis sites.
- Arteriotomy (incision of an artery) is performed first with a #11 or #15 knife blade and then extended using Potts scissors.
- Microsurgery is performed under the operating microscope or using magnifying loupes worn like eyeglasses.
- Microvascular procedures are performed in many different specialties. Technological advances in optics, sutures, and microinstrumentation have advanced the surgeon's ability in replantation of limbs, transplantation of tissue flaps after cancer surgery, and restoration of nerve function.
- Microsurgical instruments are extremely delicate and must be handled with care at all times.
- Microsurgical anastomosis of blood vessels may require the use of special devices that stabilize the vessels during repair.

REVIEW QUESTIONS

1. Define a vascular *stent.*
2. Why is it important to try and remove sclerotic plaque from an artery in one piece?
3. Why are double-arm needles used for arterial anastomosis?
4. What is the difference between a thrombus and an embolus?
5. What is the effect of venous stasis on the veins?
6. A Freer elevator or a Penfield elevator is used to remove atherosclerotic plaque from an artery. In what other surgical specialties are these instruments used?
7. How should a Rummel tourniquet be passed to the surgeon?
8. What size suture may be used on the aorta during aneurysm repair?
9. Describe the purpose of a guidewire.
10. What instruments may be used to perform an endarterectomy?
11. What drug is used topically to prevent vasospasm during microvascular surgery?
12. How should the ST pass a microvascular spring-loaded needle holder (locking and non-locking)?
13. What suction techniques can be used during microvascular surgery to prevent injury to the tissues?

REFERENCES

1. Cioffi W, et al. *Atlas of Trauma Emergency Surgical Techniques.* Philadelphia: Elsevier; 2014.
2. Chaikof E, Cambria R. *Atlas of Vascular Surgery and Endovascular Therapy Anatomy and Technique.* Philadelphia: Elsevier; 2014.
3. Cronenwett JL, Johnston KW, eds. *Rutherford's Vascular Surgery.* 7th ed. Philadelphia: Saunders; 2010.
4. Eliason JL, Clouse DW. Current management of infrarenal abdominal aortic aneurysms. *Surg Clin N Am.* 2007;87(5).
5. Garden O, Bradbury A, Forsythe J, Parks R, eds. *Principles and Practice of Surgery.* 5th ed. Edinburgh: Churchill Livingstone; 2007.
6. Gurtner, G., & Neligan, P. (2018). *Plastic Surgery:* VOL 1: Principles (4th ed., Vol. 1). London: Elsevier.
7. Khatri V. *Atlas of Advanced Operative Surgery.* Philadelphia: Saunders; 2013.
8. Lee L, Karp NS. *ATLAS of Reconstructive Breast Surgery.* Edinburgh: Saunders; 2019.
9. Kouchoukos N, Blackstone E, Hanley F, Kirklin J. *Cardiac Surgery.* 4th ed. Philadelphia: Saunders; 2013.
10. Merle M, Dautel G. *Emergency Surgery of the Hand.* 4th ed. Philadelphia, PA: Elsevier; 2017.
11. Miller R, et al. *Miller's Anesthesia.* 8th ed. Philadelphia: Saunders; 2012.
12. Moore W. *Vascular and Endovascular Surgery: A Comprehensive Review.* 8th ed. Philadelphia: Elsevier; 2013.
13. Patton KT, Thibodeau GA, Douglas MM. *Essentials of Anatomy and Physiology - Text and Anatomy and Physiology Online Course.* St Louis, MO: Elsevier-Mosby; 2012.
14. Porth CM, ed. *Pathophysiology: Concepts of Altered Health States.* 7th ed. Philadelphia: Lippincott Williams & Wilkins; 2004.
15. Tinkham MR. The endovascular approach to abdominal aortic aneurysm repair. *AORN J.* 2009;89:289.
16. Wei F, Mardini S. *Flaps and Reconstructive Surgery.* 2nd ed. Edinburgh: Elsevier; 2017.

THORACIC AND PULMONARY SURGERY

31

LEARNING OBJECTIVES

After studying this chapter, the reader will be able to:

1. Identify key anatomical features of the respiratory structures in the thoracic cavity
2. Describe diagnostic procedures of the respiratory system
3. Discuss pathology of the respiratory system
4. Discuss specific elements of case planning in surgery of the thoracic cavity and respiratory system
5. List and describe common thoracic procedures of the respiratory system

TERMINOLOGY

Arterial blood gases (ABGs): A blood test that determines carbon dioxide, oxygen saturation, and pH of the blood.

Bleb: Area of overdistention in lung tissue.

Closed chest drainage: A system of removing air or fluid from the thoracic cavity and restoring negative pressure so that the lungs can expand after thoracic surgery or penetrating trauma to the chest wall.

Diffusion (oxygen): The movement of oxygen from the alveoli and into the bloodstream.

Dyspnea: Difficulty breathing.

Empyema: A pus-filled area of the lung.

Expiration: The act of breathing out (exhalation).

Hemothorax: The presence of blood in the thoracic cavity or between the pleural sac and lungs, usually caused by trauma.

Hypoxia: Lower-than-normal oxygen level.

Inspiration: The act of taking a breath (inhalation).

Perfusion (oxygen): The distribution of oxygen to tissues.

Pneumothorax: Air in the chest cavity, which prevents the lungs from expanding and may displace the mediastinal structures.

Pulmonary function tests (PFTs): Tests performed to measure the function and strength of the pulmonary system.

Ventilation: The process of moving air into and out of the lungs during inhalation and exhalation.

Thoracic and pulmonary surgery includes procedures of the respiratory system and thoracic cavity, excluding those that involve the heart and cardiac vessels. Thoracic procedures within the specialty involve the lungs, bronchi, and peripheral bronchial system. Surgery involving other organs located within the thoracic cavity, such as the esophagus and thymus, may be performed by a thoracic surgeon or by a general surgeon with the assistance of a thoracic specialist. This often depends on whether the surgery involves pulmonary structures.

Surgery of the lungs and other pulmonary structures in the thoracic cavity is frequently preceded by the endoscopic assessment of the respiratory structures. Tissue biopsy is performed through the flexible or rigid bronchoscope. Open or video-assisted thoracic surgery may then be used to perform a specific procedure. Interventional procedures such as foreign body removal, biopsy, and removal of small tumors can be performed through the flexible endoscope, or the rigid bronchoscope, which has a larger diameter than the flexible scope.

Maintaining lung inflation is an important procedural consideration in thoracic surgery. The thoracic cavity is under *negative pressure*. Under normal circumstances, the lungs expand freely within a vacuum in the chest cavity. An incision, tear, or puncture of the chest wall allows atmospheric air to rush into the thorax. This results in immediate collapse of the lungs. During *thoracotomy* (open chest surgery), the lungs are inflated with the use of a mechanical respirator managed by the anesthesia provider (AP). In the immediate postsurgical phase and healing phase, the normally negative pressure within the thoracic cavity is maintained with a closed drainage system, which removes air and fluid to allow lung expansion (described later in the chapter).

NOTE *The following procedures involving the upper respiratory system or chest wall are located in specialty chapters:*
Chapter 33 Pediatric Surgery
- *Correction of pectus excavatum*
- *Repair of cleft lip and palate*

Chapter 26 Surgery of the Ear, Nose, Pharynx, and Larynx
- *Turbinectomy*
- *Septoplasty*
- *Tonsillectomy*
- *Adenoidectomy*
- *Uvulopalatopharyngoplasty*
- *Laryngoscopy*
- *Tracheotomy/tracheostomy*
- *Laryngectomy*
- *Radical neck dissection*

SURGICAL ANATOMY

The respiratory system is divided into two parts: upper and lower. The upper tract includes the nose, nasal cavities, mouth, pharynx, and larynx. The lower tract includes the trachea, bronchi, bronchioles, and lungs. The function of the respiratory system is to maintain a steady intake of oxygen from the air and eliminate carbon dioxide from the blood. Oxygen is necessary for life, whereas carbon dioxide is a waste product of normal metabolism.

Three processes are involved in respiratory function:

- **Ventilation:** The breathing process; it involves contraction of the diaphragm and accessory muscles and expansion of the ribs to pull air into the lungs
- **Diffusion (oxygen):** The transfer of oxygen from the alveoli in the lungs to the bloodstream
- **Perfusion (oxygen):** The movement and absorption of oxygen molecules into body tissues, also called *oxygenation*

UPPER RESPIRATORY TRACT

The nose is composed of cartilage and bone covered by skin. The external nose flares to form the nares. The internal nose is lined with mucous membrane and is highly vascular. It is divided by the nasal septum, which is composed of cartilage and bone. Nasal hair in the anterior nasal cavity help filter the air as it enters the upper respiratory tract. Olfactory nerves, which are responsible for the sense of smell, are located in the superior nasal airway and septum.

The nasal sinuses are bilateral structures, each composed of three tiers of bony projections called the *conchae* or *turbinates*. These projections are the superior, medial, and inferior meati (sing., *meatus*). The projections form spaces called the *paranasal sinuses*. Each of these is named after the bone above it (i.e., the maxillary, ethmoid, frontal, and sphenoid bones). The nasal passages are lined with mucous membrane, which warms and humidifies air as it enters the body.

PHARYNX

The pharynx lies behind the oral cavity and communicates with the nasal cavities. It is subdivided into three sections: the oropharynx, nasopharynx, and laryngopharynx or larynx. The oropharynx lies immediately below the mouth. The nasopharynx communicates with the nasal cavities. Two important structures are located in the nasopharynx: the eustachian tube, which drains from the middle ear, and the pharyngeal tonsils (adenoids). The palatine tonsils, the structures commonly referred to as "the tonsils," are located in the oropharynx.

LARYNX

The larynx connects the trachea with the oropharynx. The anatomy of this region is complex and is best understood by studying illustrations of this anatomy. The larynx is a wide, circular cavity formed by cartilage. It contains the vocal cords and prevents food and other foreign bodies from entering the trachea.

The epiglottis is a cartilaginous structure that functions as a flap to close off the entrance to the trachea during swallowing. The epiglottis is also under voluntary control and is closed when a person holds his or her breath. During defecation, the glottis is voluntarily closed and the intraabdominal muscles are contracted. This is referred to as the *Valsalva maneuver.* This action also causes a momentary decrease in intrathoracic pressure and an increased heart rate. The epiglottis often is confused with the uvula, which is the visible projection of epithelial tissue extending from the soft palate of the mouth.

The larynx is divided into bilateral sections by paired folds of tissue, which are the extensions of the epithelial lining of the laryngeal cavity. The upper folds are called the *vestibular folds*. The lower folds form the vocal cords, which produce speech. The space between the folds is the glottis, which is the entrance to the trachea.

Two other important cartilaginous structures in the larynx are the thyroid cartilage and the arytenoid cartilage. The thyroid cartilage is a large "shield" of tissue that forms the anterior wall and protects the larynx from injury. This structure is larger in men than in women. The horn-shaped arytenoids extend superiorly and support the vocal cords. Fig. 31.1 illustrates the upper respiratory system.

TRACHEA

The trachea begins at the larynx and branches into two main airways, the right and left primary bronchi and bronchial tree. The trachea is a semi-rigid tube mainly composed of C-shaped cartilaginous rings. The cricoid cartilage is the only completely closed ring in the structure.

BRONCHI

The trachea branches into the right and left primary bronchi at the carina. Because the right bronchus is straighter than the left, inhaled foreign material is more likely to enter the right lung. As the bronchi enter the lung segments, they branch into smaller and smaller divisions, or bronchioles, forming a tree-like structure. Cartilaginous rings support the primary bronchi. However, as the branches become smaller, the walls are formed by cartilage plates until the level of the bronchioles, where there is no cartilage. The bronchioles are composed of smooth muscle lined with epithelium.

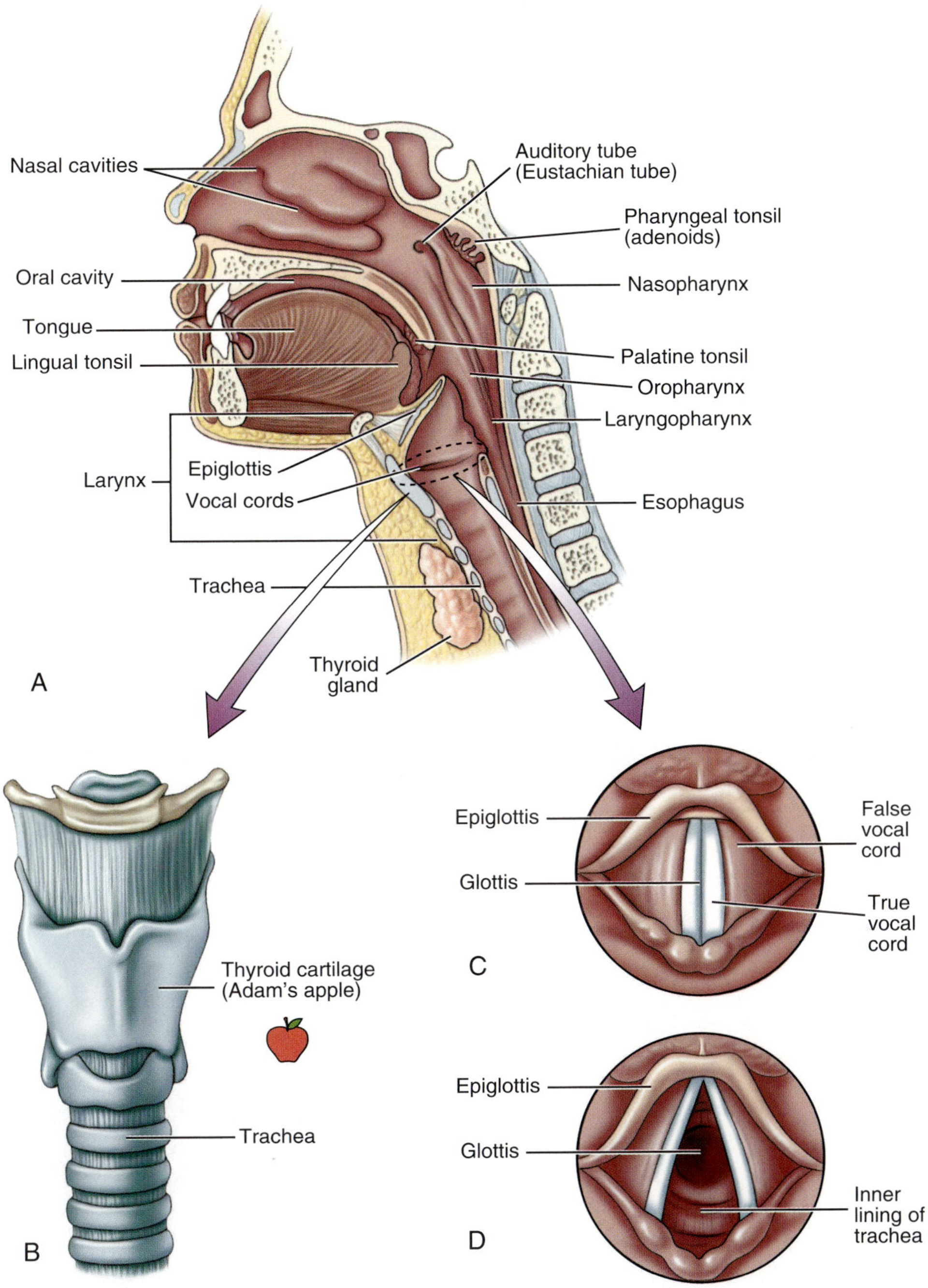

FIG. 31.1 (A) Upper respiratory system. (B) Larynx, showing the thyroid cartilage. (C) Vocal cords and closed glottis. (D) Open glottis. (From Herlihy B, Maebius NK, eds. *The Human Body in Health and Illness*. 2nd ed. Philadelphia: WB Saunders; 2003.)

LUNGS

The lung is divided into anatomical regions. The right lung has three lobes, and the left lung has two lobes. Each lung is composed of smaller segments, called *bronchopulmonary segments,* which contain branches of the main bronchi. The hilum (notch) of each lung is located on the medial side. Large blood vessels and primary bronchi enter the lung at the hilum. The apex of the lung is located at the upper portion and extends just above the clavicle.

The bronchioles terminate in small ducts, alveolar sacs, and individual alveoli. Each alveolus exchanges incoming oxygen molecules with carbon dioxide molecules from the blood.

The lungs are separated in the thoracic cavity by the mediastinum. This space contains the heart, large vessels, bronchi, trachea, esophagus, and thymus gland, which produces hormones necessary for immune function. Each lung is enclosed in a pleural cavity and covered by a double membrane, the pleural sac. The outer membrane forms the parietal pleura, which lines the thoracic cavity and outer mediastinal walls. The inner or visceral pleura cover the lungs. A small amount of pleural fluid is secreted into the pleural space between the two membranes. *Pleuritis* is the inflammation of the pleural membranes. An increase in fluid (e.g., serous fluid, pus, or blood) is called a *pleural effusion*. The pleural space is called a *potential space* because during respiration, the space increases

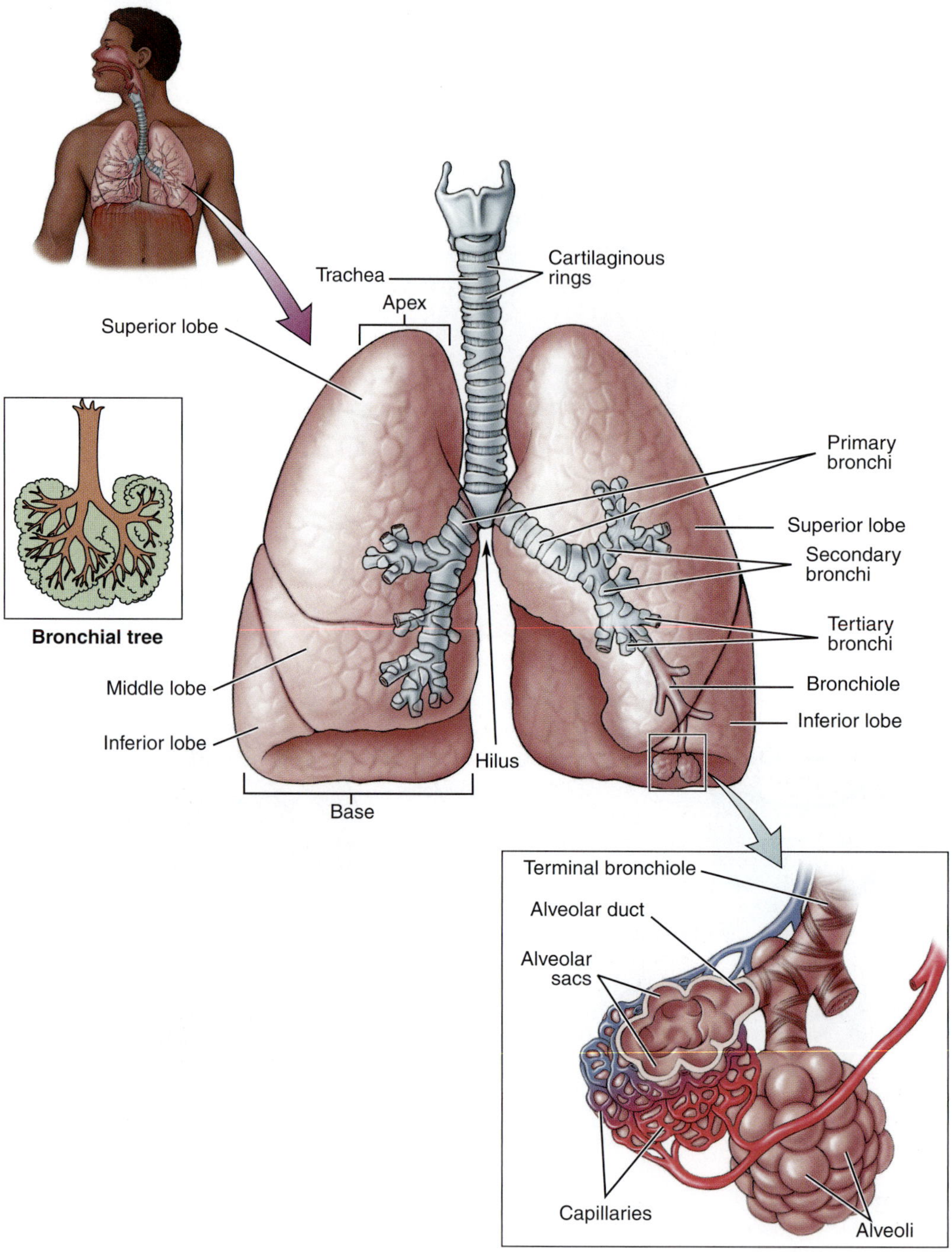

FIG. 31.2 The lungs and bronchial tree. (From Herlihy B, Maebius NK, eds. *The Human Body in Health and Illness*. 2nd ed. Philadelphia: WB Saunders; 2003.)

or decreases as the lungs fill with air. In pleural effusion, the lungs cannot expand fully.

The pleural space normally maintains negative pressure in relation to atmospheric air and the alveoli. If the chest wall and pleural space are opened, such as during trauma or surgery, air rushes in and collapses the lungs. Fig. 31.2 illustrates the lungs and bronchial tree.

MECHANISM OF BREATHING

Breathing is a complex physiological and mechanical process controlled by the autonomic nervous system but also under voluntary control. The thoracic cavity is a closed space. The diaphragm is continuous with the parietal pleural membrane. Recall that the pressure between the two pleural membranes is negative, whereas air pressure in the trachea, bronchi, bronchioles, and alveoli is equal to atmospheric pressure outside the body. When the diaphragm contracts during inhalation, the potential space between the two pleural membranes decreases, and air is pulled into the airways and lungs. When the diaphragm relaxes during exhalation, air flows passively out of the lungs (Fig. 31.3).

A number of important factors affect breathing:

1. An intact pleural membrane is needed to maintain the negative pressure in the pleural space (keep in mind the analogy to the vacuum-sealed package that is created by removing air from the inside—a hole in the package allows air to rush in).

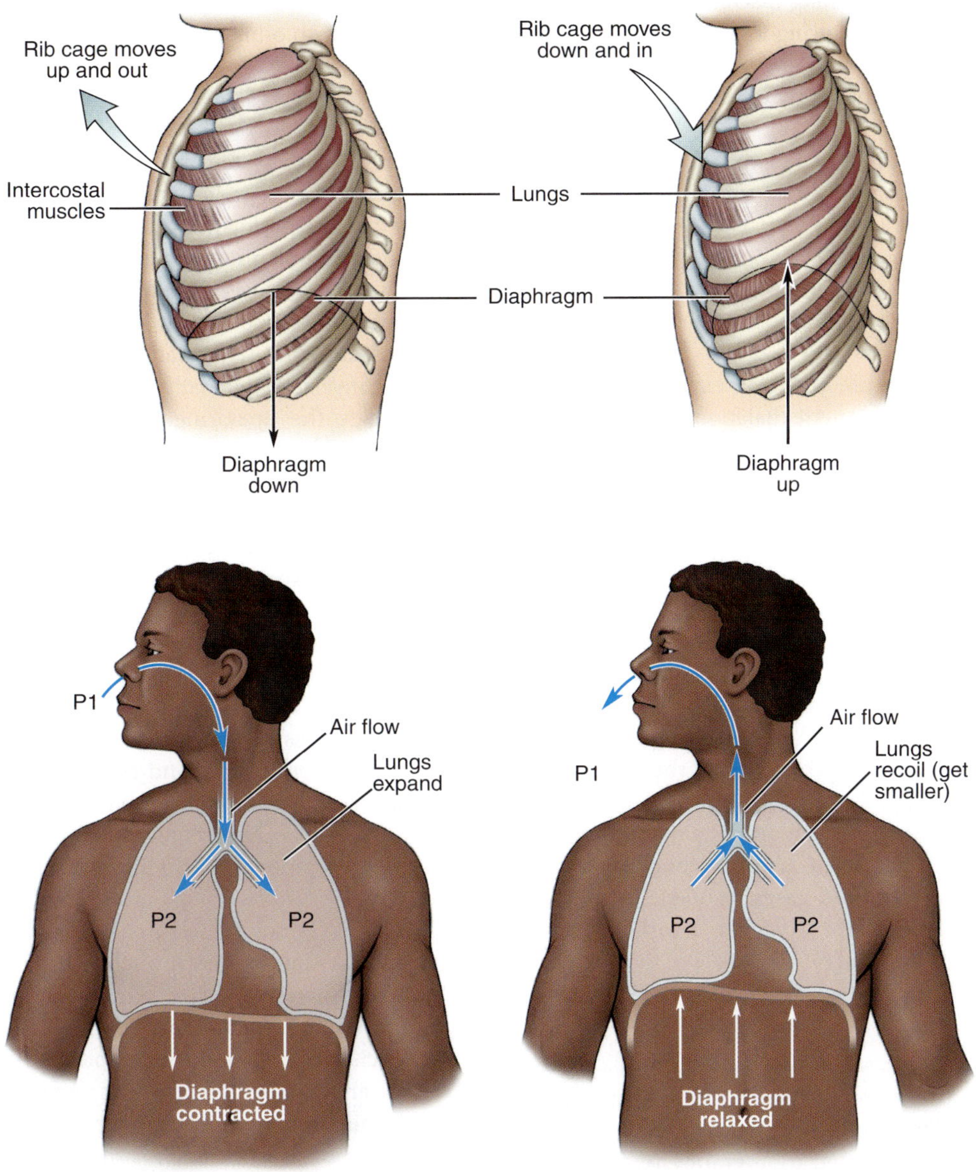

FIG. 31.3 Mechanism of breathing. (From Herlihy B, Maebius NK, eds. *The Human Body in Health and Illness*. 2nd ed. Philadelphia: WB Saunders; 2003.)

2. Penetrating trauma to the chest cavity causes air to rush in and collapses the lungs. Air (**pneumothorax**), blood (**hemothorax**), or exudate in the pleural space displaces and compresses the lungs. This prevents their expansion and, if severe enough, may result in full collapse of the lung.
3. The alveoli must have sufficient elasticity to expand and fill with air. Diseases that constrict the alveoli, such as emphysema, cause loss of alveolar elasticity. The result is inability to exchange oxygen with carbon dioxide.
4. An intact central nervous system is required to initiate transmission to the phrenic nerve, which controls the diaphragm. For example, barbiturate drugs can depress the central nervous system to the level at which breathing stops.
5. The chest cavity must be able to expand freely. An example of pathological restriction is eschar from extensive third-degree burns.

DIAGNOSTIC TESTS

Diagnostic tests for the respiratory system assess the function of the lungs, thoracic space, and bronchial system. Terms related to the medical assessment of respiration:

- *Apnea:* Cessation of respiration
- *Dyspnea:* Difficulty or painful respiration
- *Hyperventilation:* Abnormally fast rate of respiration
- *Hyperpnea:* Excessively deep respiration
- *Cyanosis:* Bluish tint to skin seen in patients with poor oxygenation
- *Hyperventilation:* Abnormally rapid rate of respiration

PULMONARY FUNCTION

Pulmonary function tests (PFTs) are a specific group of procedures that measure lung function. These noninvasive tests are performed with a complex breathing machine, which measures the parameters digitally. The following tests are included in this group:

- *Tidal volume:* The amount of air exhaled during normal respiration
- *Minute volume:* The amount of air exhaled per minute
- *Vital capacity:* The total volume of air exhaled after maximum **inspiration**
- *Functional residual capacity:* The volume of air remaining in the lungs after exhalation
- *Total lung capacity:* The total amount of air in the lungs when fully inflated
- *Forced vital capacity:* The amount of air expelled in the first, second, and third seconds after exhalation
- *Peak expiratory rate:* The maximum amount of air expelled in forced **expiration**

LABORATORY TESTS

A complete blood count (CBC), including white blood cell differential, is performed as a basic screening tool for surgical patients. More specific laboratory tests, such as those for tumor markers, are performed according to the suspected pathological condition. Culture and sensitivity tests may be performed on exudate collected from the respiratory tract.

Among the most important blood tests for pulmonary function is the determination of arterial blood gas values, commonly called **arterial blood gases (ABGs).** In this test, the arterial blood is assessed for oxygen and carbon dioxide levels and pH (acid–base balance).

IMAGING STUDIES

Imaging studies of the pulmonary and thoracic structures include radiographs, magnetic resonance imaging (MRI), ultrasound scans, and computed tomography (CT). Radiographs are used to screen patients for tuberculosis and other fibrotic diseases. Fluid and air in the pleural space, tumors, and anatomical deformities are also detected on radiographs. MRI and CT scans are used for more definitive analysis of masses.

Pulmonary angiography is performed when CT scans are inconclusive for the diagnosis of pulmonary embolism. During angiography, the blood vessels of the lungs are injected with a contrast medium, and fluoroscopy or CT is used to detect any abnormalities.

Endoscopic procedures (discussed later in the chapter) are performed to obtain biopsy specimens of cells, fluid, and tissue. Visual examination of the respiratory tract by endoscopy, along with other diagnostic tools, assists in diagnosis.

CASE PLANNING

Most respiratory system procedures (80% to 90%) are now performed using video-assisted thoracic surgery (VATS), which can be performed without painful muscle-splitting incisions. Case planning is dependent on what approach and technique will be used. However, even when VATS surgery is planned, instruments and supplies for an open procedure must be immediately available so that the procedure can be quickly converted. Normally, these supplies are kept in reserve just outside the operating room suite, unless the surgeon requests that they are opened in advance.

INSTRUMENTS

Open thoracic surgery of the respiratory structures requires the following instruments:

- General surgery instruments, including long instruments (shanks must be at least 9 inches [22.5 cm] for most adult patients)
- Chest wall instruments, including self-retaining chest, rib, and scapula retractors and rib approximators. Orthopedic rongeurs, periosteal elevators, and rib-stripping instruments are also required for some procedures.
- Lung instruments, including atraumatic tissue-grasping clamps
- Bronchus clamps, which are large, right-angle clamps used to occlude the primary bronchi. The jaws of the clamps are stippled for greater grip on the cartilaginous tissue.
- Surgical stapling instruments, which are commonly used in thoracic surgery (both open and endoscopic procedures). These are used in lung resection and for the occlusion of the bronchial stem after resection.
- Vascular clamps (needed for some lung procedures)

IMPORTANT TO KNOW *With the patient in a lateral position, it is necessary to position a magnetic instrument pad over the top drape to serve as a neutral zone and to retain any instruments that are placed on the drape. Side pockets attached to the drape are also useful to keep instruments on the field.*

Refer to the Thoracic Instruments table to review instruments commonly used in thoracic procedures. Instruments used in VATS are also included in this group. Cardiac-specific instruments are shown in Chapter 32.

OPEN THORACIC SURGERY INSTRUMENTS

STRAIGHT DISSECTING SCIS 7 ½″

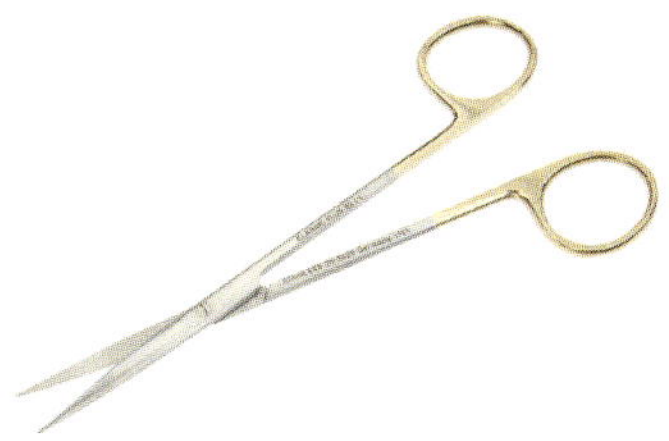

Courtesy and copyright Becton, Dickinson and Company.

MIXTER THORACIC FRCP 9″

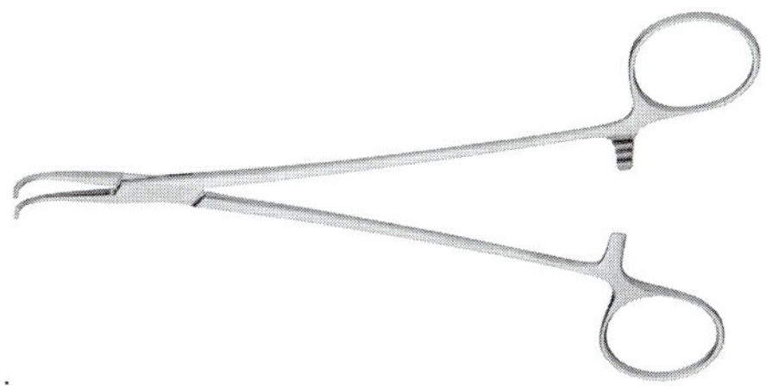

Courtesy and copyright Becton, Dickinson and Company

MIXTER FRCP FINE TIP 9″

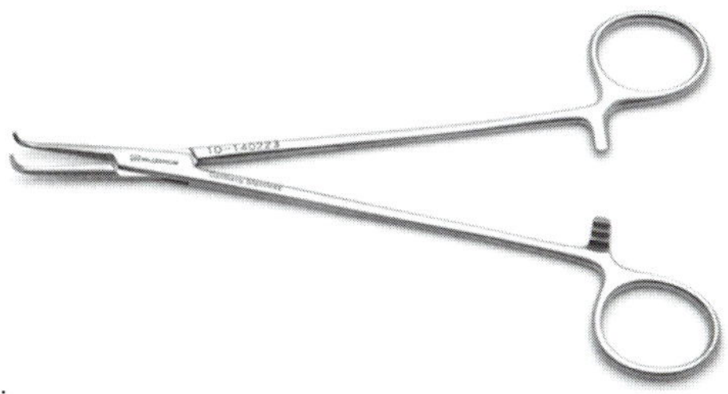

Millennium Surgical Corp.

SAROT BRONCHUS CLAMP

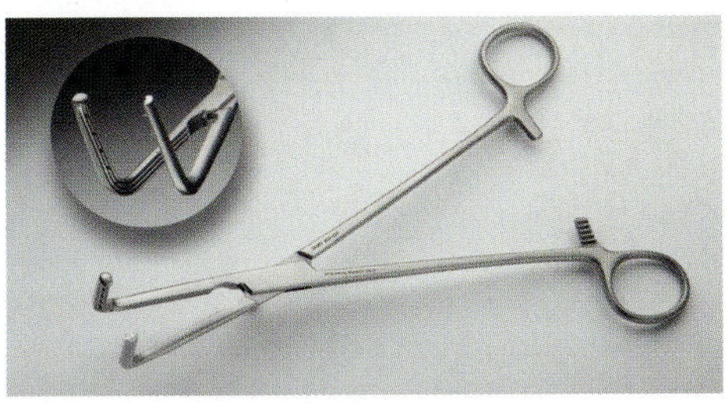

From Nemitz. *Surgical Instrumentation: An Interactive Approach*. 3rd ed. St. Louis: Elsevier; 2019.

STILLE-LUER BONE CUTTER 9″

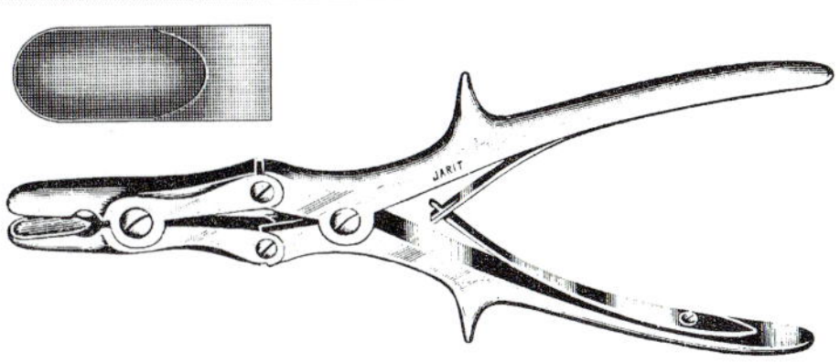

Courtesy Jarit Surgical Instruments, Hawthorne, NY.

GEMINI MIXTER FRCP FULL CURVE 8″

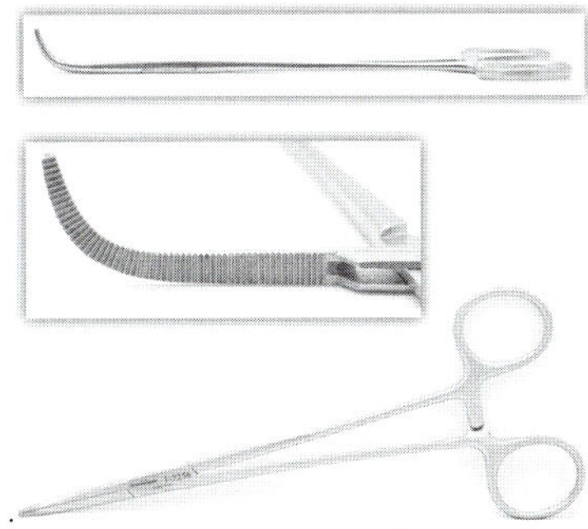

Millennium Surgical Corp.

RIGHT-ANGLE MIXTER 9″

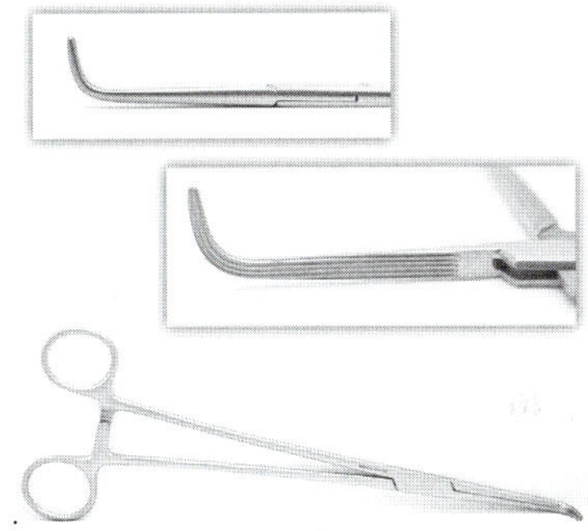

Millennium Surgical Corp.

DUVALL LUNG GRASPING FRCP 7¾″

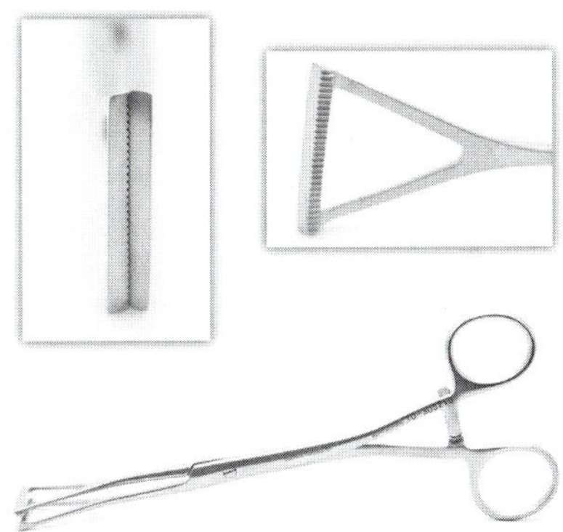

Millennium Surgical Corp.

BETHUNE RIB SHEARS 13½″

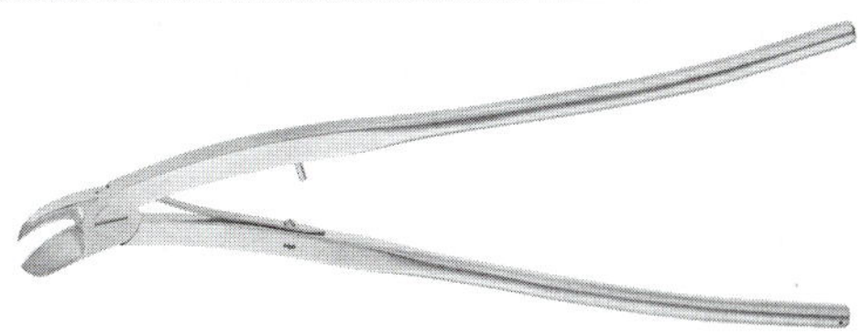

Photo courtesy Aesculap, Inc., Center Valley, PA.

MATSON RIB STRIPPER 8¾″

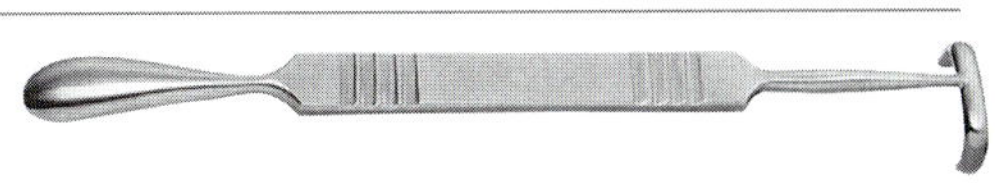

Courtesy and copyright Becton, Dickinson and Company.

OPEN THORACIC SURGERY INSTRUMENTS—cont'd

BAILEY RIB CONTRACTOR 8″

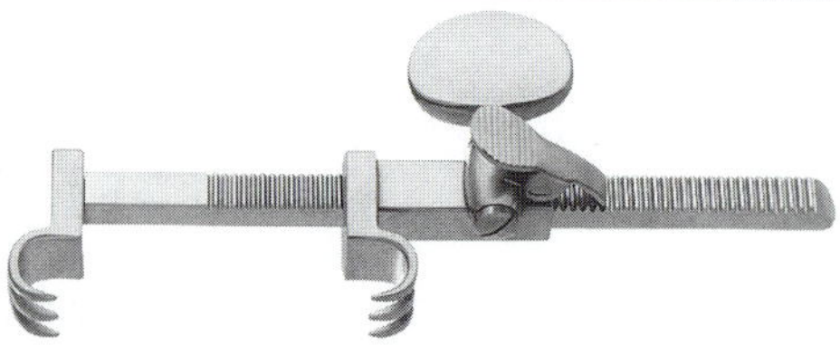

Courtesy and copyright Becton, Dickinson and Company.

SEMB LUNG RETRACTOR 10″

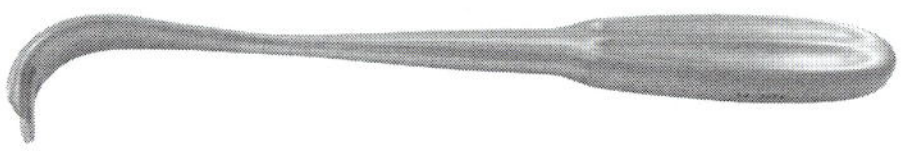

Copyright 2016 Symmetry Surgical, Inc.; photo courtesy Symmetry Surgical, Inc.

DOYEN RIB RASPATORIES

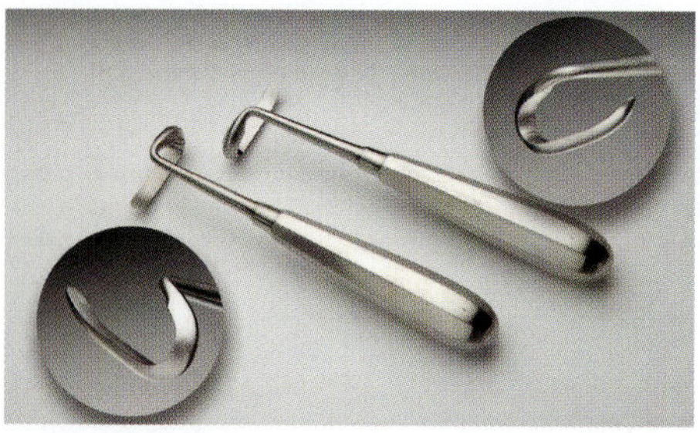

From Nemitz. *Surgical Instrumentation: An Interactive Approach*. 3rd ed. St. Louis: Elsevier; 2019.

FINOCHIETTO RETRACTOR 7 7/8″

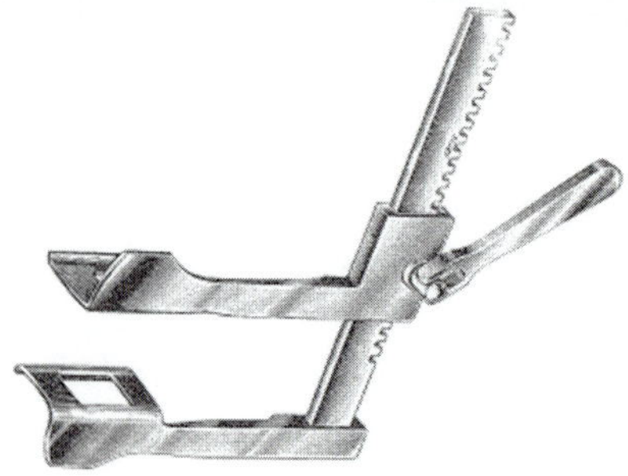

Courtesy Jarit Surgical Instruments, Hawthorne, NY.

RYDER NEEDLE HOLDER

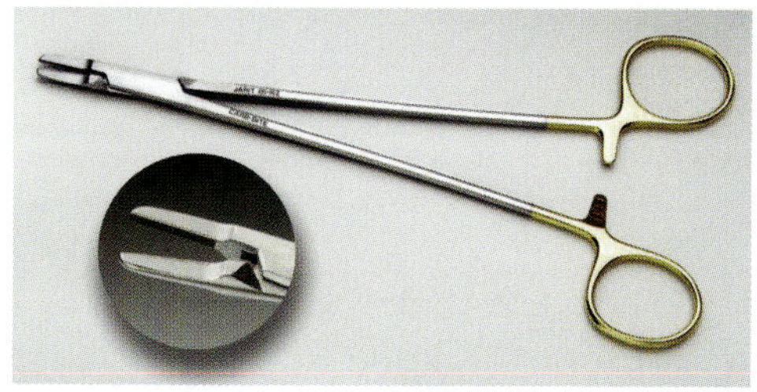

From Nemitz. *Surgical Instrumentation: An Interactive Approach*. 3rd ed. St. Louis: Elsevier; 2019.

SAROT CLASSIC PLUS NEEDLE HOLDER 7″, 10″

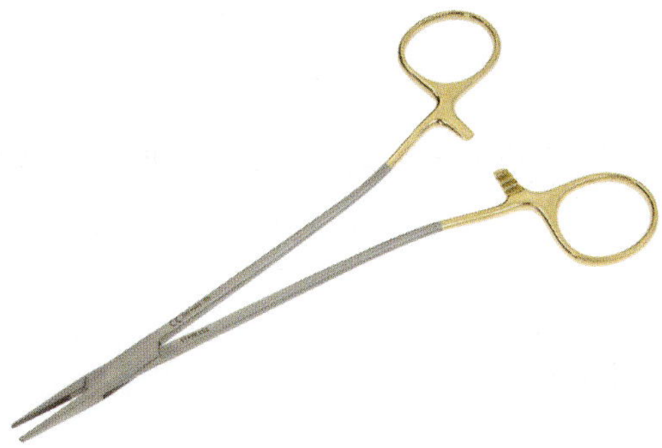

Copyright 2016 Symmetry Surgical, Inc.; photo courtesy Symmetry Surgical, Inc.

VIDEO-ASSISTED THORACIC SURGERY (VATS) INSTRUMENTS

ROCCO NODULE CLAMP 13¼″

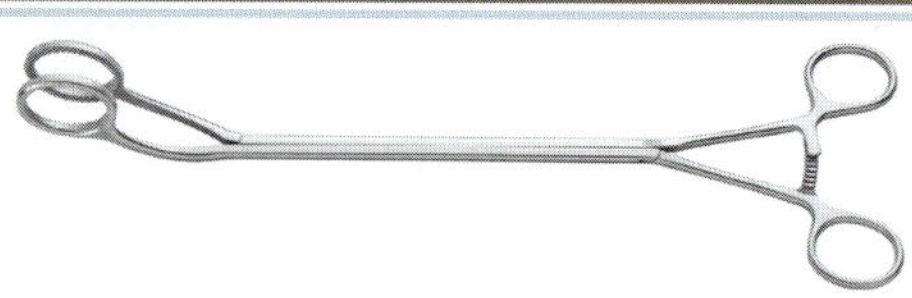

Courtesy Scanlan International, Inc.

FOERSTER LUNG-GRASPING CLAMP 13¼″

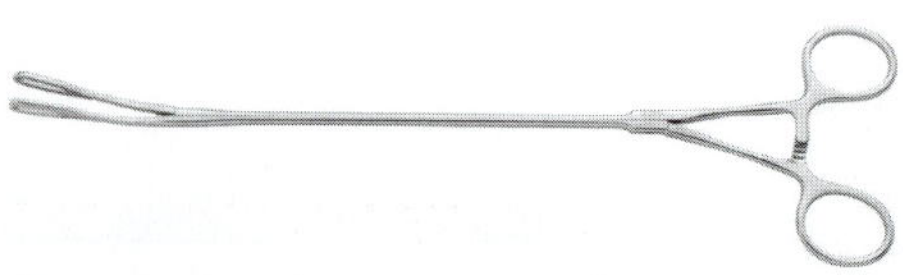

Courtesy Scanlan International, Inc.

NODE GRASPING CLAMP 13″ 1

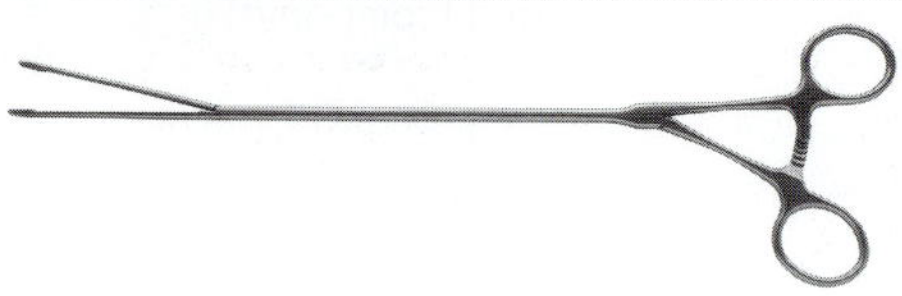

Courtesy Scanlan International, Inc.

GONZALEZ-RIVAS LUNG-GRASPING CLAMP 9¾″

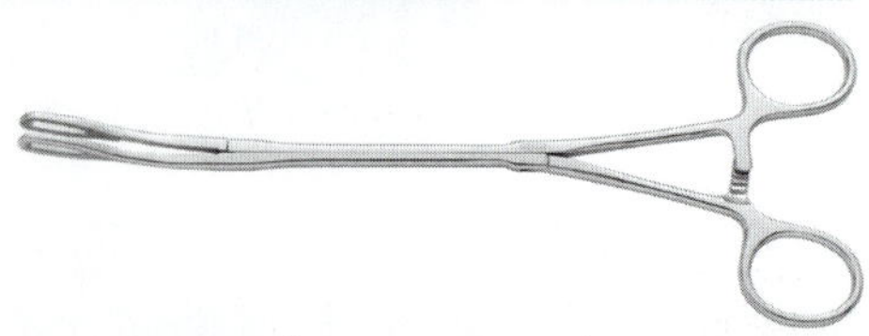

Courtesy Scanlan International, Inc.

DUVAL LUNG-GRASPING CLAMP CURVED LEFT 13½″

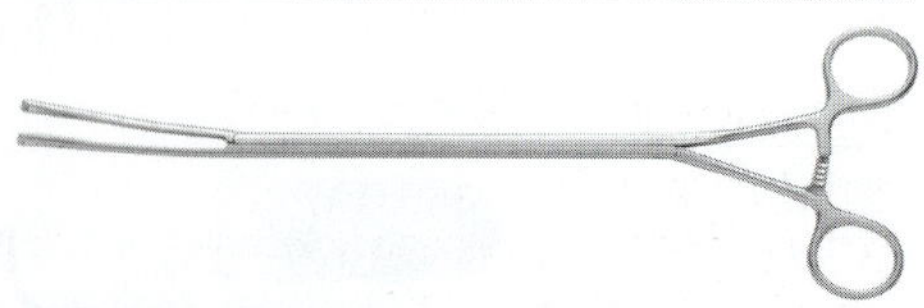

Courtesy Scanlan International, Inc.

KHAN DECORTICATION GRASPER 13¼″ 2

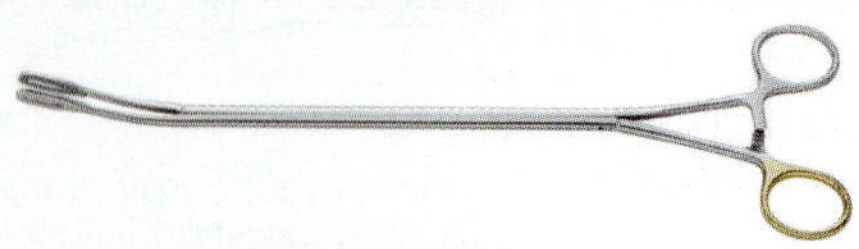

Courtesy Scanlan International, Inc.

VIDEO-ASSISTED THORACIC SURGERY (VATS) INSTRUMENTS—cont'd

GONZALEZ-RIVAS DISSECTOR 13⅓″ 3

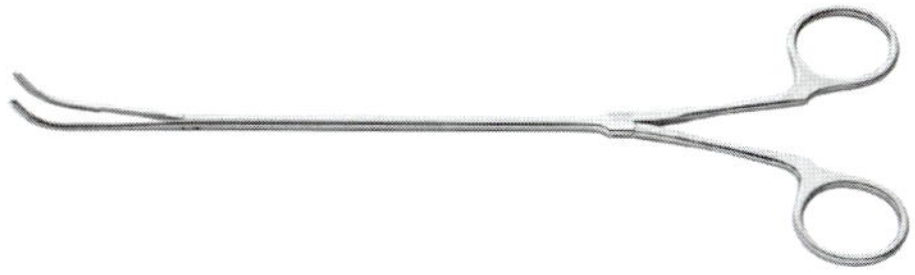

Courtesy Scanlan International, Inc.

GENING J SPH SNAKE DISSECTOR 13⅓ 1/3″ 4

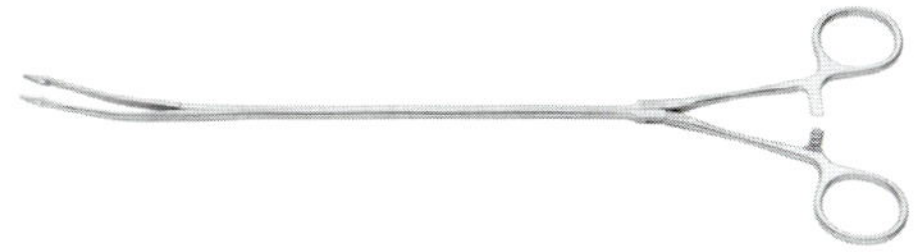

Courtesy Scanlan International, Inc

DENNIS DISSECTOR 13¼″ 5 >

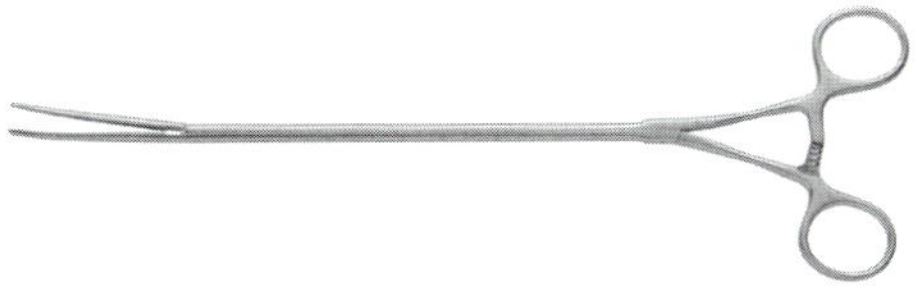

Courtesy Scanlan International, Inc.

DEBAKEY COOLEY CLAMP 13½″ 6

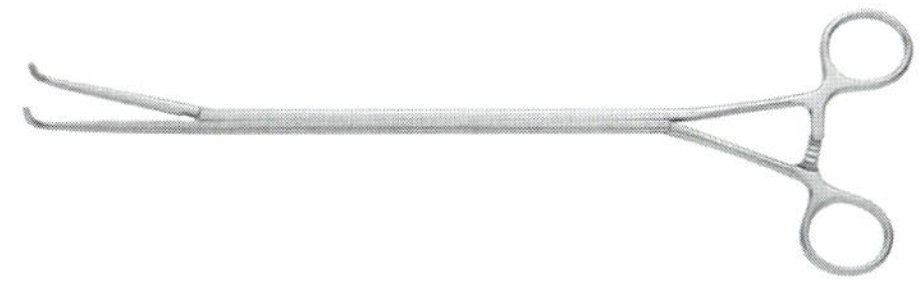

Courtesy Scanlan International, Inc.

HARKEN CLAMP 11½ 7

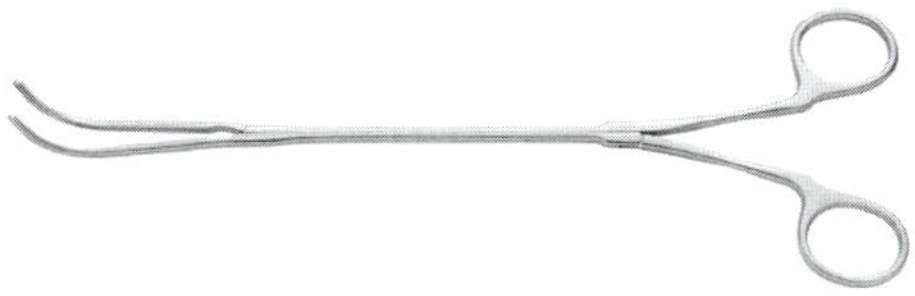

Courtesy Scanlan International, Inc.

ALLIS FORCEPS 11½″ 8

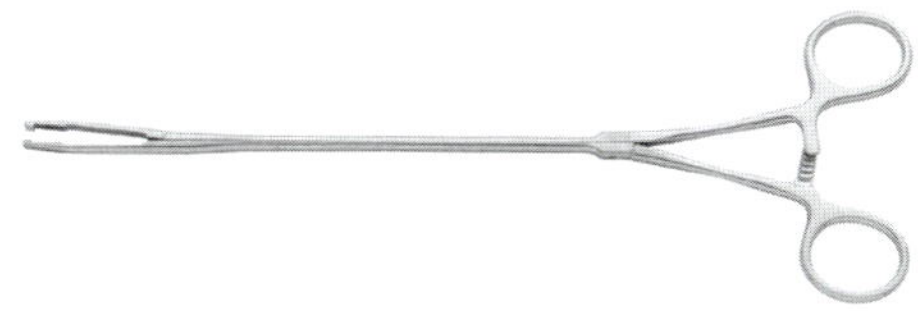

Courtesy Scanlan International, Inc.

CHITWOOD DEBAKEY CLAMP 10⅜″ 9

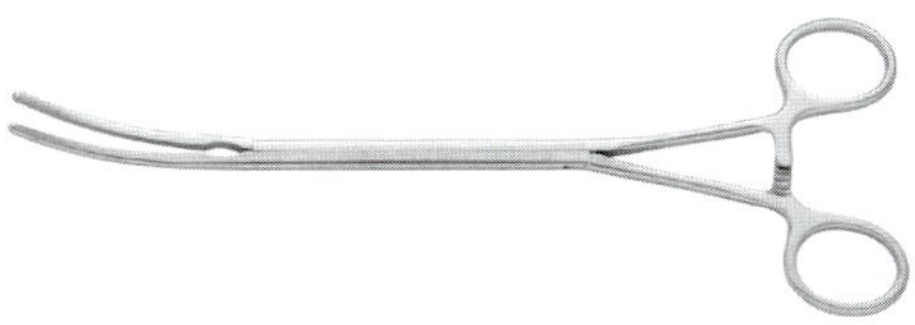

Courtesy Scanlan International, Inc.

CHITWOOD DISSECTING SCISSORS 10½″

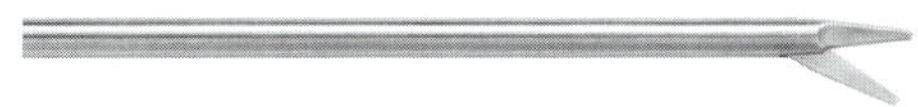

Courtesy Scanlan International, Inc.

METZENBAUM SCISSORS 11½″

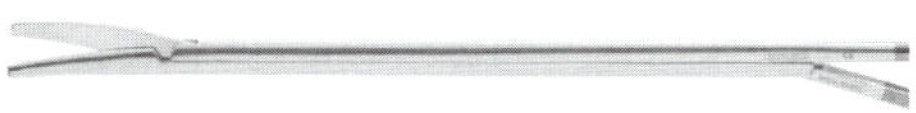

Courtesy Scanlan International, Inc.

GONZALEZ-RIVAS FORCEPS 12¾″

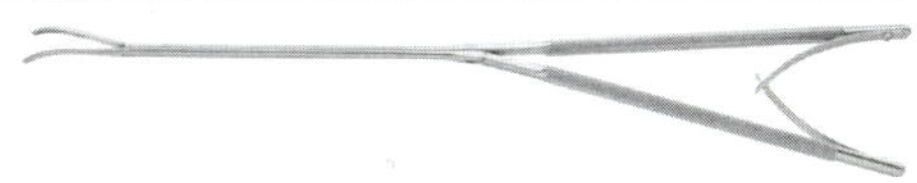

Courtesy Scanlan International,

AXIAL HANDLE FORCEPS 14½″

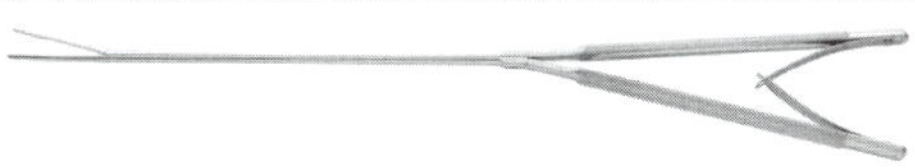

Courtesy Scanlan International,Inc.

ROCCO ADVENTITIA ELEVATOR 12¾″

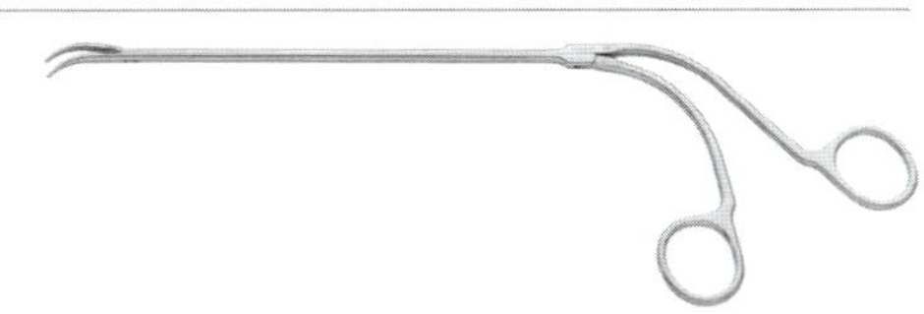

Courtesy Scanlan International,

RING HANDLE NEEDLE HOLDER 17½″

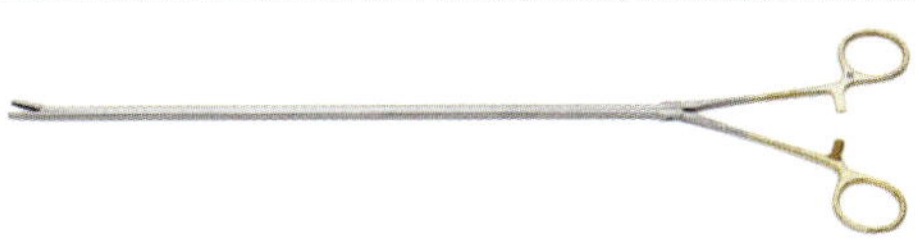

Courtesy Scanlan International, Inc.

RING HANDLE NEEDLE HOLDER 14⅜″

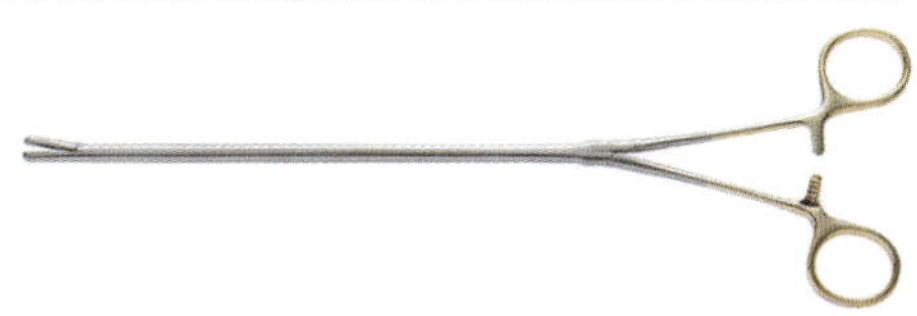

Courtesy Scanlan International, Inc.

AXIAL HANDLE NEEDLE HOLDERS 14⅜″

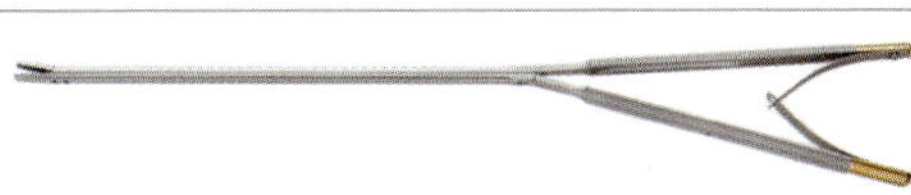

Courtesy Scanlan International, Inc.

GONZALEZ-RIVAS KNOT PUSHER 14¾″

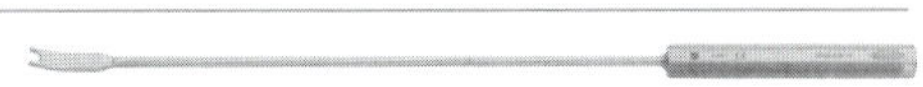

Courtesy Scanlan International, Inc.

CHITWOOD KNOT PUSHER MINI "TRAP MODEL" 13⅝″

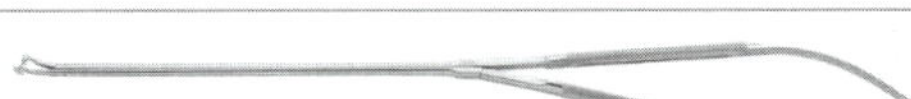

Courtesy Scanlan International, Inc.

CHITWOOD SUPER CUT SUTURE CUTTER 13″

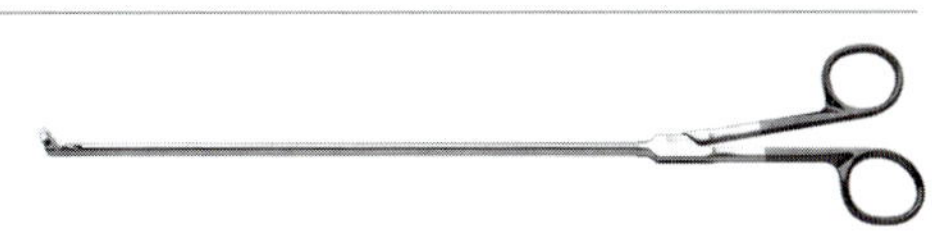

Courtesy Scanlan International, Inc.

WOLF SUCTION INSTRUMENT 14¼″

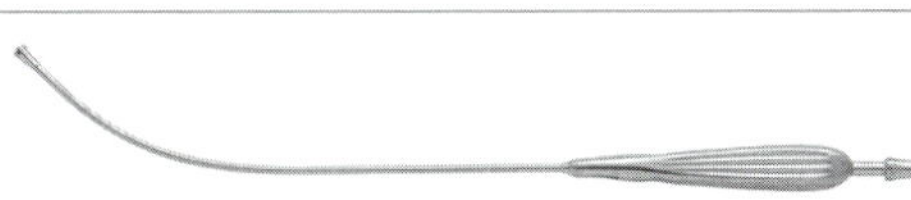

Courtesy Scanlan International, Inc.

D'AMICO SUCTION INSTRUMENT 17¾″

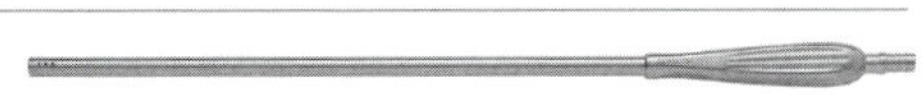

Courtesy Scanlan International, Inc.

VIDEO-ASSISTED THORACIC SURGERY (VATS) INSTRUMENTS—cont'd

DENNIS RIB CUTTER 13½″	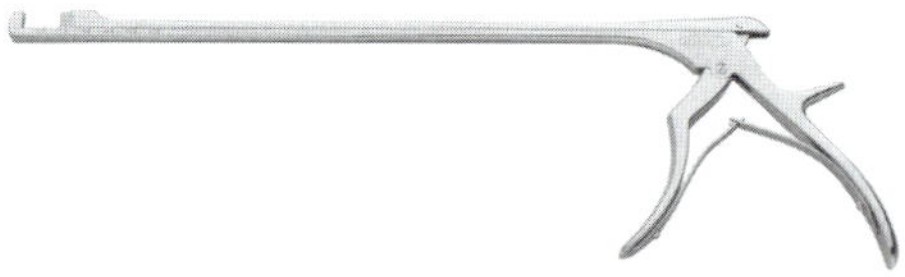 Courtesy Scanlan International, Inc.
CHITWOOD SUTURE PULLER 11½″	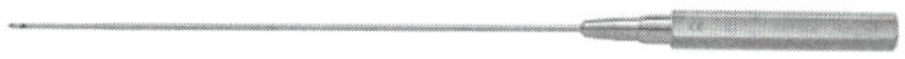 Courtesy Scanlan International, Inc.
AXIAL HANDLE FORCEPS	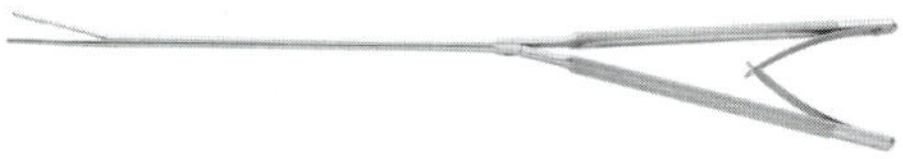 Courtesy Scanlan International, Inc.
RING HANDLE NEEDLE HOLDER	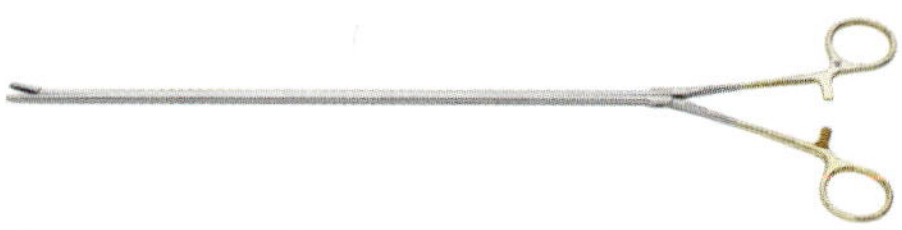 Courtesy Scanlan International, Inc.
CHITWOOD KNOT PUSHER MINI TRAP MODEL	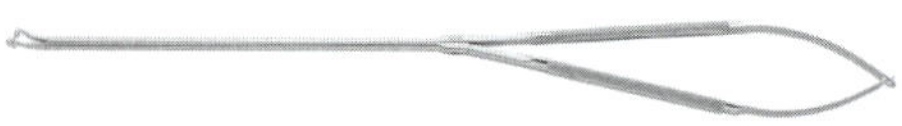 Courtesy Scanlan International, Inc.
STERN CHEST TUBE PASSER 9¾″	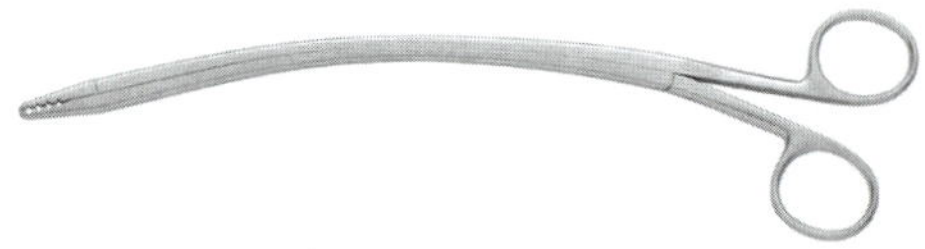 Courtesy Scanlan International, Inc.
GONZALEZ-RIVAS KNOT PUSHER	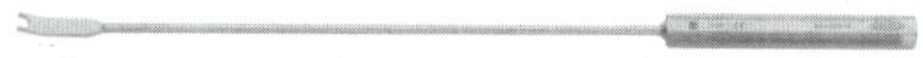 Courtesy Scanlan International, Inc.
ROCCO ADVENTITIA ELEVATOR (FORCEPS)	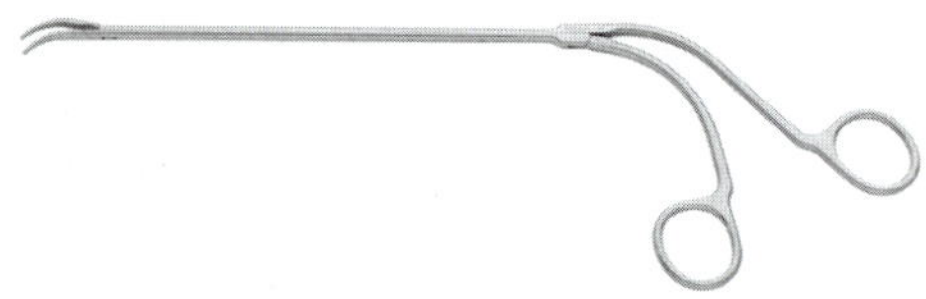 Courtesy Scanlan International, Inc.
AXIAL HANDLE NEEDLE HOLDERS	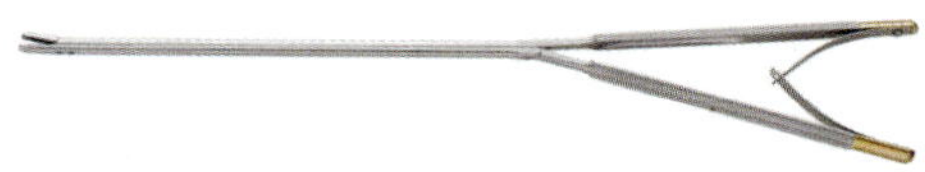 Courtesy Scanlan International, Inc.
CHITWOOD SUPER CUT SUTURE CUTTER	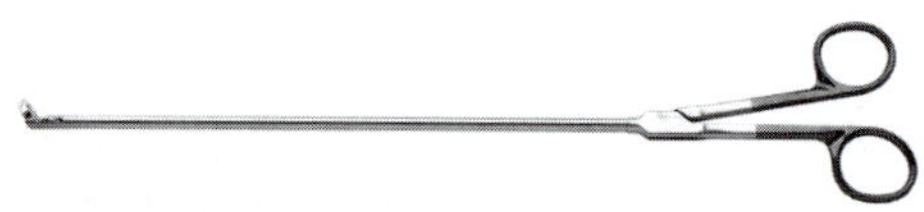 Courtesy Scanlan International, Inc.

DRUGS AND SOLUTIONS

Hemostatic agents are commonly used in thoracic surgery to control capillary bleeding from the lung surface and for coagulation at the site of anastomosis of the large vessels. Gelfoam soaked in thrombin and oxidized cellulose or absorbable collagen should be available according to the surgeon's preference. Bone sealant (Ostene) may also be required to seal the cut edges of a rib or sternum. Fibrin sealant is used to prevent the escape of air from a lung or bronchial anastomosis. Refer to Chapter 12 for discussions on the pharmacology and preparation of these materials.

PREPPING AND DRAPING

The incisions most commonly used in pulmonary surgery are the posterolateral and anterolateral thoracotomy, with the patient in the lateral position (see Chapter 16). The skin prep may extend from the neck to the iliac crest. Minimum draping includes a body sheet, towels for squaring the incision, an incise drape, and a fenestrated thoracotomy drape.

CLOSED CHEST DRAINAGE

As explained above, negative pressure in the thoracic cavity is lost when the chest wall and pleura are opened or punctured. This occurs during trauma, disease, and thoracic surgery. For the lungs to expand, negative pressure must be restored. This is achieved with **closed chest drainage,** also called *closed underwater drainage* (Fig. 31.4).

One or more chest tubes are inserted through the body wall and into the pleural space. The distal end of the tubes is connected to a set of chambers. The first container drains blood, fluid, and air from the thoracic cavity. The second container is partly filled with water to prevent air from entering the system from the distal end. The system works by gravity or active suction. As long as the sealed chambers remain below the level of the patient's chest, fluid and air drain from the thoracic cavity. However, if the drainage system is raised, fluid flows back into the chest cavity and can collapse the lungs or heart.

NOTE *The prototype for disposable (single-use) closed chest drainage systems was the Pleur-evac (Teleflex Medical, Research Triangle Park, NC), which was introduced in 1967. The term Pleur-evac is often used as a generic term for all closed chest drainage systems, although other companies manufacture similar devices.*

During closure, a chest tube is placed in one or more locations in the thoracic cavity. If two tubes are required (in one or both pleura), they can be joined with a Y-connector and attached to the drainage system.

A patient with a chest drainage system must be moved carefully to avoid the disruption of the chest tubes. If a chest tube becomes dislodged from the thoracic cavity, the proper emergency response is to prevent air from entering the wound. Sterile petroleum gauze is kept with the patient at all times for this purpose. In the event a drainage tube comes out, the gauze

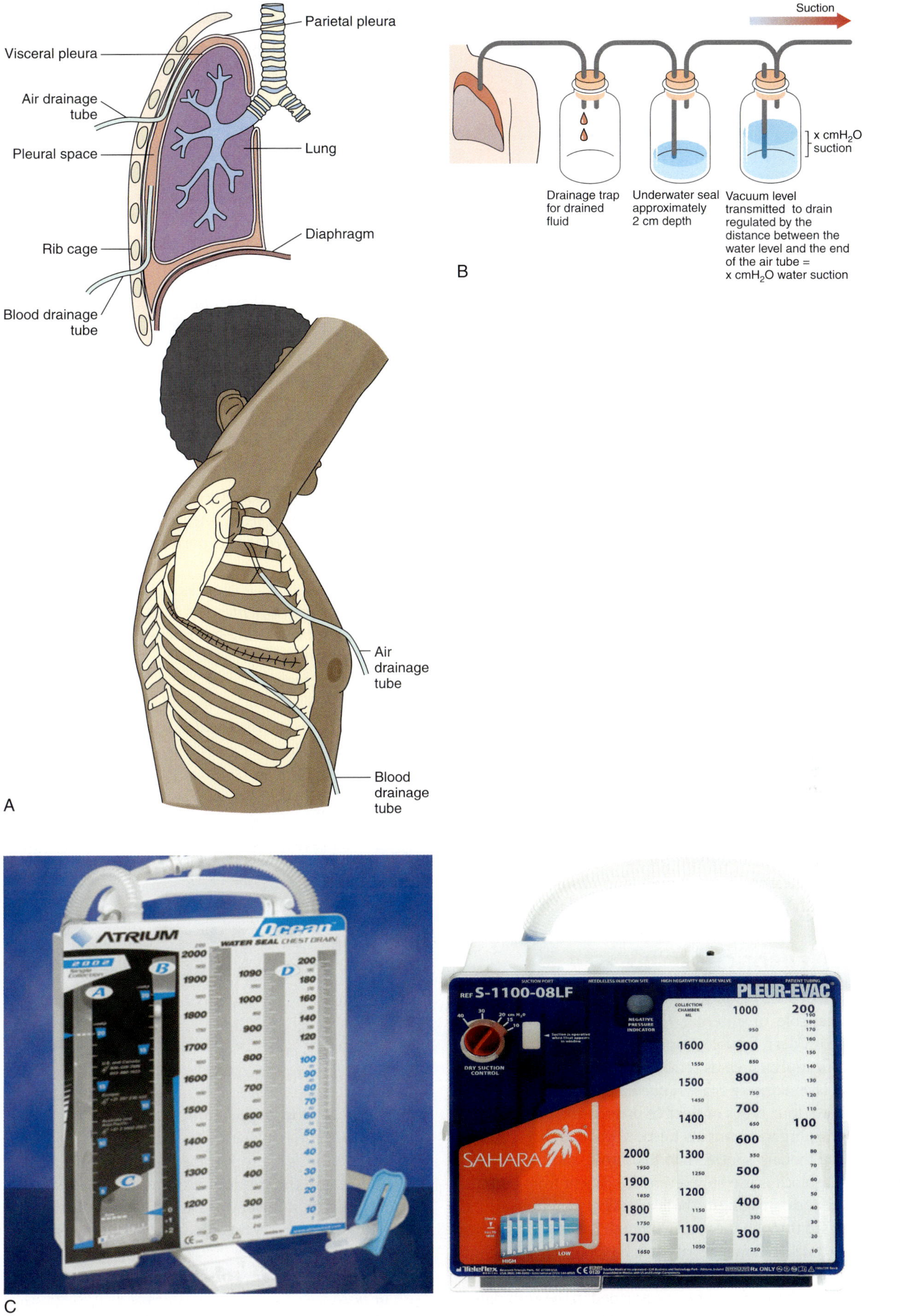

FIG. 31.4 Closed chest drainage system. (A) Chest tubes are placed in the pleural space. (B) Mechanics of closed chest drainage. (C) Modern chest drainage systems, which operate on the 3-bottle drainage concept. (A, From Potter, P, Perry A, Stockert P, Hall A, eds. *Fundamentals of Nursing*. 8th ed. St Louis: Mosby; 2013. B, From Cassivi SD, Deschamps C, Pastis NJ. Chest tube insertion and management. *Clin Respir Med.* 2012;862–868. https://doi.org/10.1016/b978-1-4557-0792-8.00072-6. C, From Boujaoude Z, Shersher D. *Critical Care Medicine: Principles of Diagnosis and Management in the Adult.* 5th ed. Philadelphia: Elsevier; 2019.)

is immediately placed over the wound to prevent air from filling the thorax and deflating the lung. The three-chamber unit is always kept upright and never raised to the level of the chest because this causes fluid to flow back into the chest cavity.

Students sometimes have difficulty understanding how an underwater chest drainage device works. This knowledge is critical to setting up the system and preventing patient injury related to errors. To view a video on the theory of the "three-bottle system," refer to the following website: https://www.youtube.com/watch?v=AtkkqlCrUpE. Note that once you understand the principles, you can proceed to the manufacturer's instructions for setup of the chest drainage system used in your facility. An advance understanding of the science involved in the system greatly increases your ability to set it up correctly.

SURGICAL PROCEDURES

INSERTION OF CHEST TUBES

To provide closed chest drainage, chest tubes must be surgically inserted. In the case of a surgical procedure involving thoracotomy, the tubes are inserted just before the chest is closed to establish negative pressure after endotracheal extubation. After a spontaneous or traumatic air leak or a surgical procedure in which the right or left pleural cavity is opened, negative pressure must be restored to allow the lungs to expand. The surgeon achieves this by making an opening into the affected pleural cavity through a small thoracic incision. One or more chest tubes are inserted and connected to a water-seal chest drainage system to remove air, blood, and exudate from the thoracic or pericardial cavity. Suction is applied.

Chest tubes are made of heavy Silastic or polyvinyl chloride tubing that has numerous perforations at the proximal end. Chest tubes may be placed in one or more locations. They are sutured to the chest wall with heavy, non-absorbable sutures and dressed with petroleum gauze, fluffed, and flat gauze.

FLEXIBLE BRONCHOSCOPY

Flexible bronchoscopy is performed with a slender fiber-optic endoscope capable of entering the primary and peripheral bronchi. The modern flexible scope may also be used for interventional procedures such as retrieval of a foreign body, cryosurgery, and laser surgery. Sizes range from 2.8 mm to 5.9 mm. Fig. 31.5 shows four types of flexible bronchoscopes. Fig. 31.6 illustrates grasping instruments for removal of a foreign body.

A local anesthetic is sprayed into the throat, and the patient is sedated. A bite block is used to prevent the patient from biting on the endoscope and damaging it. The flexible fiber-optic tube is lubricated and passed through the patient's mouth or nose. Unlike rigid bronchoscopy, which allows the patient to be ventilated through the tube, the patient must breathe around the flexible endoscope.

Flexible bronchoscopy is often performed in the ambulatory surgery facility, or in a designated department of the hospital facility. It is common for the surgeon to perform both flexible and rigid bronchoscopy during the same procedure. Rigid bronchoscopy (described later) requires general anesthesia.

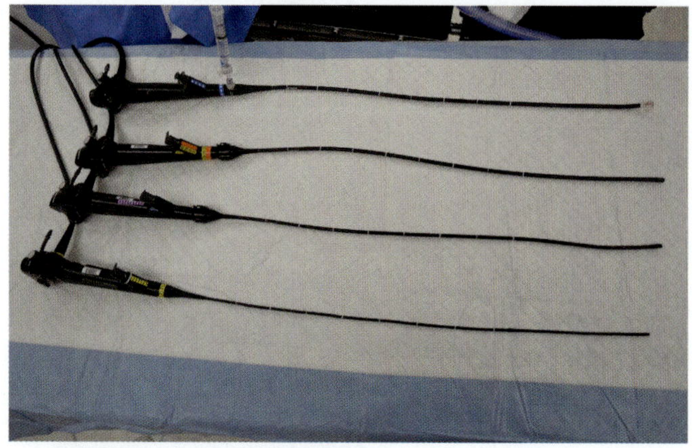

FIG. 31.5 Flexible bronchoscopy. Four types of flexible bronchoscopes top to bottom: endobronchial ultrasound bronchoscope, therapeutic bronchoscope, regular adult bronchoscope, pediatric bronchoscope. (From Myers E, Snyderman C. *Operative Otolaryngology*. 3rd ed. Philadelphia: Elsevier; 2018.)

The instruments should be set up on separate tables to facilitate the changeover from one system to the other.

Instruments needed to perform specific tasks include the following:

1. *Suction*
2. *Grasping instruments*
3. *Baskets for retrieving specimens*
4. *Optical forceps*
5. *Irrigation system*
6. *Laser fiber*
7. *Biopsy instruments: needles, brushes, forceps*
8. *Sponge carrier*
9. *Specimen containers, slides, fixatives*

POSITION:	Semi-Fowler
INCISION:	None
PREP AND DRAPING:	Body drape and towel for eye protection, bite block
INSTRUMENTS:	Flexible bronchoscopes; biopsy forceps; cytology brush; suction catheters; 10-mL syringes with slip tip; collection tubes; Lukens tissue trap; suction
POSSIBLE EXTRAS:	Microscope slides; tissue fixative

Technical Points and Discussion

1. ***The patient is prepped and draped.***
   The patient is placed in a sitting position. There is no prep, although a top drape is used to protect the patient and secure the instruments and leads. The eyes are protected with a towel or head drape. The throat is sprayed with local anesthetic before the scope is inserted.

2. ***The bronchoscope is inserted through the patient's mouth or nose.***
   The surgeon inserts the bronchoscope and advances the endoscope through the trachea and bronchial tree. When cancer is suspected or known, the healthy lung is examined first to avoid seeding it with cancer cells.

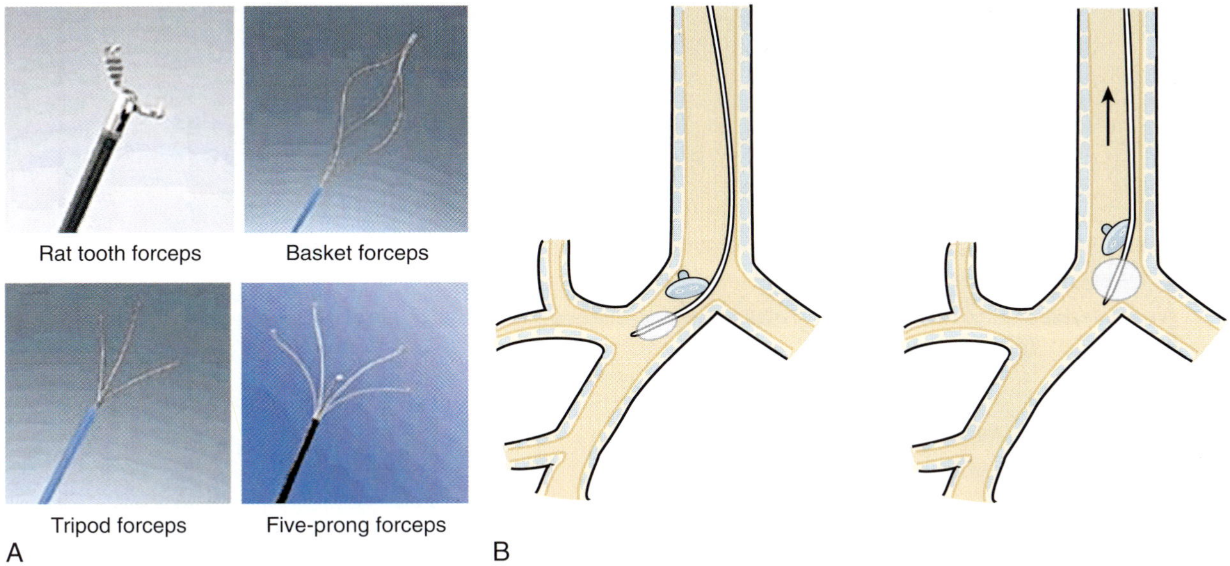

FIG. 31.6 (A) Instruments for removing foreign body. (B) Balloon catheter used to extract foreign body using backward pull. (From Broaddus VC, Mason RJ. *Murray & Nadel's Textbook of Respiratory Medicine*. Philadelphia: Elsevier Saunders; 2016.)

3. ***Cytology or biopsy specimens are taken.***
   The surgeon obtains cytology samples by inserting a small brush through the operating channel. The technologist must make sure the instrument is long enough to extend outside the tip of the scope. After the brush is removed, the scrub dips it in a specimen container holding a small amount of saline. Alternatively, the brush may be gently wiped on a microscope slide, which is immediately placed in a fixative. This process may be repeated several times. In some cases, the tip of the cytology brush may be cut from the wire and placed in the container.

   Biopsy forceps may be used to obtain small tissue samples. These forceps must be handled carefully because the specimens are very small and easily lost. After the forceps are withdrawn from the scope, the sample should be placed immediately in a specimen container or on a Telfa pad. A hypodermic needle is helpful for removing bits of tissue from the biopsy forceps. A suction cannula is used to remove secretions. These are trapped in the Lukens specimen trap, just as in rigid bronchoscopy. After all specimens have been obtained, the scope is withdrawn.

Innovations in tumor-ablating devices have increased the use of flexible bronchoscopy for tissue debridement. The *microdebrider* used commonly in sinus surgery has been modified for use in flexible bronchoscopy. Cryotherapy and argon laser are also used for interventional procedures. These modalities are discussed in Chapter 15.

NAVIGATIONAL BRONCHOSCOPY

Navigational bronchoscopy is performed during flexible bronchoscopy (described above). Navigational refers to a method that can be used to accurately identify the location of suspicious lymph nodes. *Electromagnetic navigational bronchoscopy* (ENB) requires the use of navigational software. The patient is placed on a board that generates an electromagnetic field. Electromagnetic sensors are placed strategically on the patient's thorax. Bronchoscopy is then initiated using a location guide threaded into the working channel of the bronchoscope. A sensing probe located at the tip of the guide can move in three directions as it moves through the electromagnetic field while being tracked by the computer system. A virtual map is aligned with the patient's anatomy derived from CT scanning displayed on the monitor. The bronchoscope is then positioned in the suspicious area of the lung, as the surgeon views the computer monitor. When the target area is reached, the working channel is locked into position. At this point the guide is removed and biopsies taken as described earlier. This procedure is shown in Fig. 31.7.

Endobronchial ultrasound (EBUS) with needle biopsy is another navigational procedure used during bronchoscopy. In this procedure a radial probe is inserted into the working channel of the bronchoscope and used to identify the mediastinal and hilar lymph nodes (Fig. 31.8). An ultrasound puncture bronchoscope can be used to assist in identification of the suspicious node. A needle biopsy is taken for confirmation of the diagnosis.

RIGID BRONCHOSCOPY

Rigid bronchoscopy is an endoscopic procedure performed for assessment and interventions of the of the trachea and bronchi. Rigid bronchoscopy is required when large-bore instruments are required.

> The following website provides general instruction on how to assemble the rigid bronchoscope: http://www.karlstorznetwork1.com/videos/karl-storz-quick-reference-guide-to-rigid-bronchoscopy. An additional video, which highlights the parts of the Karl Storz bronchoscope and their function, is available at https://www.broadcastmed.com/otolaryngology/5562/videos/karl-storz-rigid-bronchoscopy-in-service.

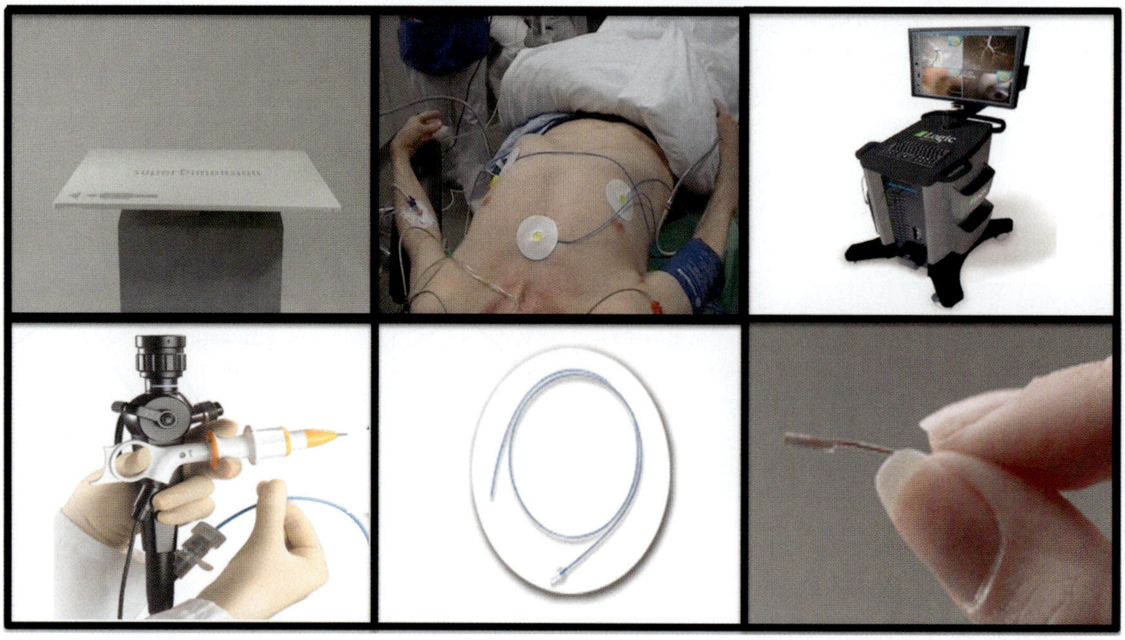

FIG. 31.7 Electromagnetic navigational bronchoscopy. *Clockwise from top left:* Procedure table with location board that generates the electromagnetic field. Patient sensors that enable tracking. Procedure cart with location processor, cables, and computer software. Location guide with probe being inserted into the working channel. Probe. Probe tip. (From Madariaga ML, Lanuti M. Sampling of suspicious solitary pulmonary nodules: electromagnetic navigational bronchoscopy and video-assisted thoracoscopic surgery. *Semin Roentgenol*. 2017;52[3]:178–184. https://doi.org/10.1053/j.ro.2017.06.003.)

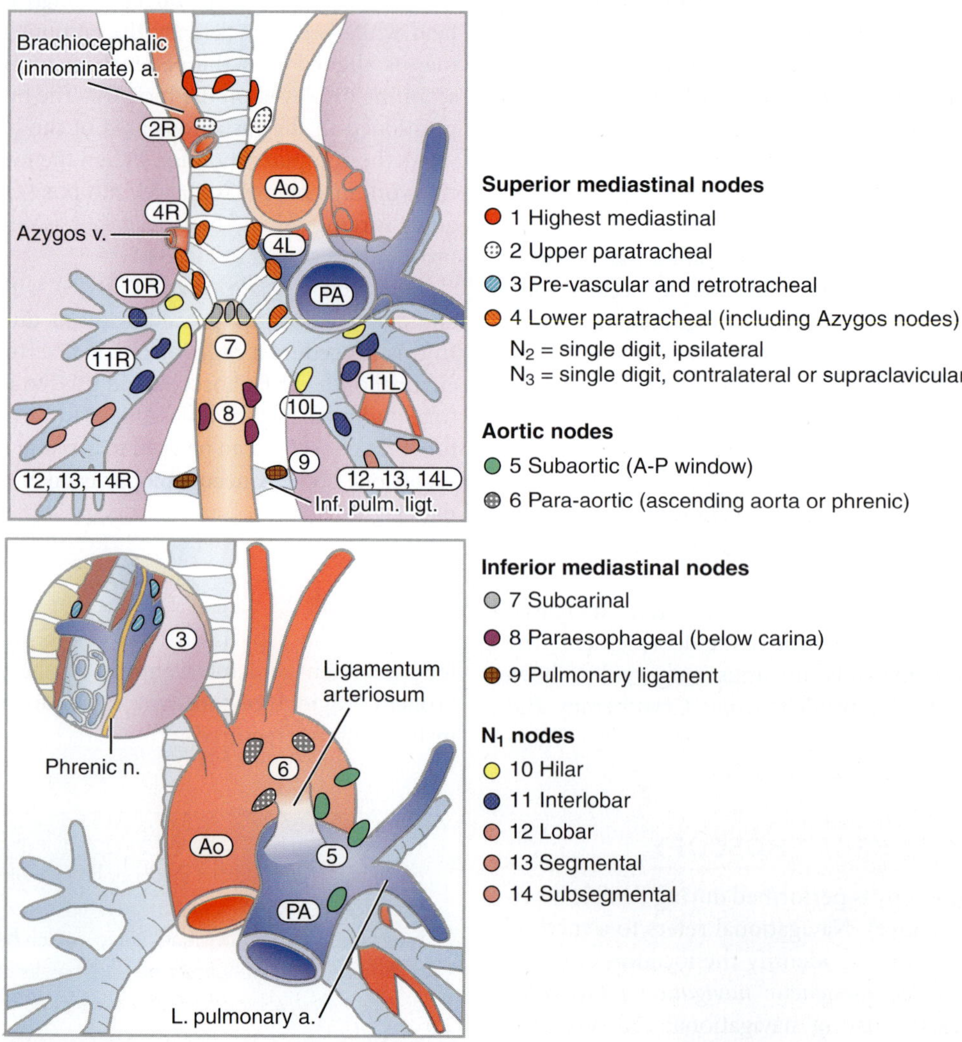

FIG. 31.8 Stations used to identify lymph nodes for staging lung cancer. (From Broaddus C, et al. *Murray and Nadel's Textbook of Respiratory Medicine*. 6th ed. Philadelphia: Saunders; 2016.)

Rigid bronchoscopy is performed under general anesthesia. The ventilation circuit of the anesthesia machine is attached to the bronchoscope for intermittent ventilation and administration of anesthetic.

Role of the Surgical Technologist

Interventional bronchoscopy is a specialty that requires the surgical technologist to have hands-on training on the equipment, techniques used, and management of the bronchoscopy supplies. Like other types of minimally invasive specialties, this requires not only an initial orientation to the procedures and technology but also detailed care and use of the instruments.

Before surgery, the bronchoscope, imaging system, and supplies must be assembled and set up according to the specific intervention and facility policy. During surgery the ST directly assists the surgeon. The ST guides instruments into the side channel of the bronchoscope and withdraws them under the direct supervision of the surgeon. The ST also assists in collecting, identifying, and managing specimens as they are withdrawn (see techniques described for flexible bronchoscopy). Identification and source of each specimen is verified in coordination with the circulating nurse and surgeon.

Instruments and Equipment

The basic components of the rigid bronchoscope are the *outer sheath;* the *bridge,* which accommodates the fiber-optic endoscope; and the fiber-optic endoscope (Figs. 31.9 and 31.10). A complete imaging system, which is common to minimally invasive devices, is also required (refer to Chapter 20). Additional instruments are needed to perform interventional procedures. *Basic* instruments include the following:

- Airway adapter
- Suction
- Graspers
- Baskets
- Biopsy forceps

Rigid Bronchoscopy Instruments

A basic bronchoscopy setup includes the following:

- Rigid bronchoscope of appropriate size
- Optical telescope and bridge
- Light carrier
- Suction and suction catheter guide
- ESU
- Graspers
- Biopsy forceps

Basic bronchoscopy instruments are shown in Fig. 31.11.

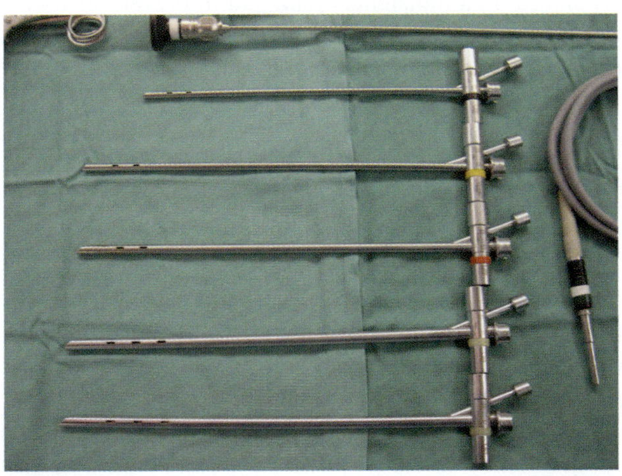

FIG. 31.9 Rigid bronchoscopy. Rigid bronchoscopes of different sizes. (From Hagberg CA, Artime CA, Aziz MF, Benumof JL. *Hagberg and Benumof's Airway Management.* 4th ed. Philadelphia: Elsevier; 2018.)

Team Positions

The surgeon stands at the patient's head to maintain alignment with the patient's upper airway. The surgical technologist is positioned next to the surgeon or at the patient's chest level. The team must be able to view the flat-screen monitor during the procedure (Fig. 31.12).

Pathology

The effects of diseases of the bronchi are visible with the aid of endoscopy. Rigid bronchoscopy is used for the following interventions:

- Laser and cryo treatment
- Foreign body extraction

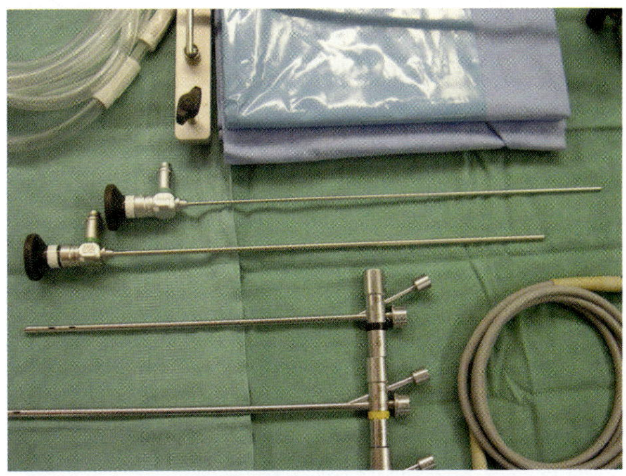

FIG. 31.10 Rigid bronchoscopy optical telescopes. (From Hagberg CA, Artime CA, Aziz MF, Benumof JL. *Hagberg and Benumof's Airway Management.* 4th ed. Philadelphia: Elsevier; 2018.)

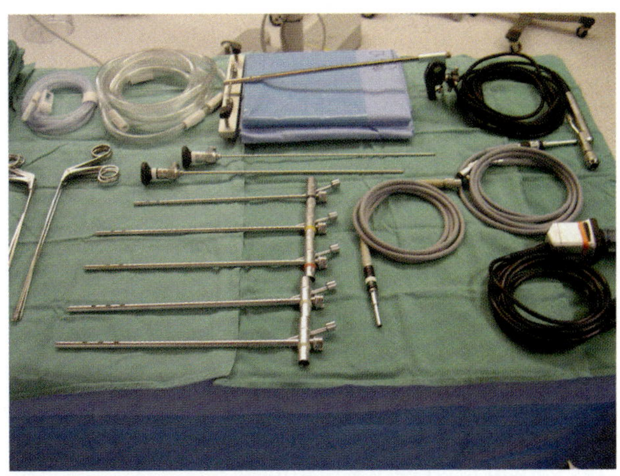

FIG. 31.11 Rigid bronchoscopy. Simple setup, including bronchoscopes, telescopes, suction tubing, grasping instruments, and power cables. (From Hagberg CA, Artime CA, Aziz MF, Benumof JL. *Hagberg and Benumof's Airway Management.* 4th ed. Philadelphia: Elsevier; 2018.)

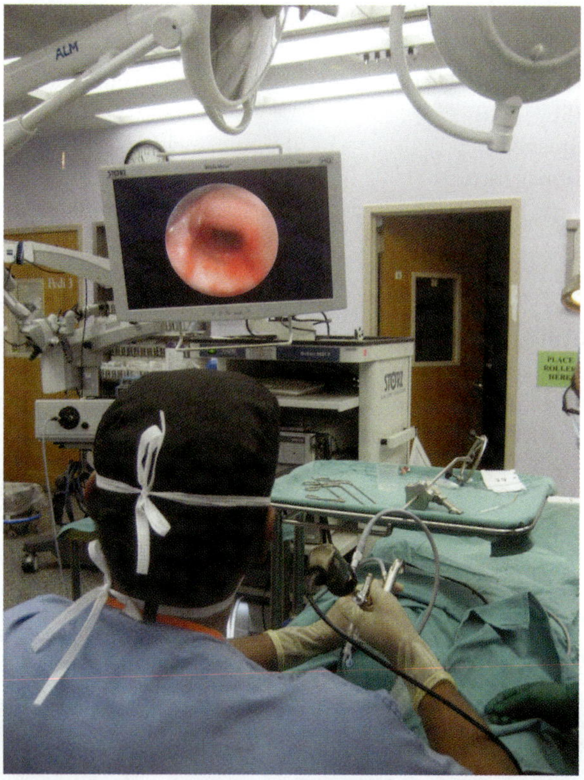

FIG. 31.12 Rigid bronchoscopy. Team positions. Note position of the Mayo over the patient. The ST normally stands at the patient's side with access to the Mayo and within view of the flat screen. (From Hagberg CA, Artime CA, Aziz MF, Benumof JL. *Hagberg and Benumof's Airway Management.* 4th ed. Philadelphia: Elsevier; 2018.)

- Dilation of stenosis
- Intraluminal (inside the airway) tumor debulking
- Placement of an airway stent

The following website demonstrates assembly of Karl Storz rigid bronchoscopes: http://www.karlstorznetwork1.com/search?q=Bronchoscopy. Note that this video does not replace hands-on in-service instruction on the rigid bronchoscope.

POSITION:	Supine
INCISION:	None
PREP AND DRAPING:	Skin prep is omitted; draping includes a body sheet, and towel or eye shield is used to protect the eyes from injury
INSTRUMENTS:	Rigid bronchoscope and its accessories; tooth guard; basic bronchoscopy instruments (as above)

Technical Points and Discussion

1. ***The patient is prepped and draped.***
   The patient is placed in the supine position with the neck slightly hyperextended. A body drape and head drape are applied. An eyepiece adapter should be placed over the scope to protect the surgeon from contamination by the patient's body fluids. A tooth guard is placed in the patient's mouth to prevent injury to the teeth.

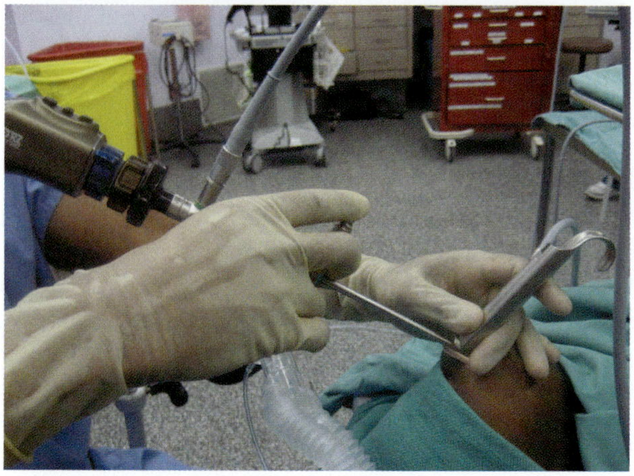

FIG. 31.13 Rigid bronchoscopy. Advancing the bronchoscope. (From Hagberg CA, Artime CA, Aziz MF, Benumof JL. *Hagberg and Benumof's Airway Management.* 4th ed. Philadelphia: Elsevier; 2018.)

2. ***The bronchoscope is inserted into the trachea and slowly advanced (Fig. 31.13).***
   The surgeon inserts the rigid scope into the trachea. Side channels on the bronchoscope allow for the insertion of irrigation and suction devices and other instruments. The ST may be asked to assist by guiding the instruments into the side channels as directed by the surgeon.

3. ***Interventional procedures, such as tissue biopsy or extraction of a foreign body, are performed.***
   If sputum or fluid samples are to be taken, suction tubing adapted with a Lukens trap is attached to the tubing. Cells are washed free from the bronchus and retrieved with the suction cannula attached to a Lukens trap. This small vial collects solutions as they are suctioned. The trap must be held upright to avoid losing the specimen. The surgeon performs bronchial lavage by injecting saline into the side channel.

Biopsy tissue is removed with cup forceps. The scrub is responsible for removing the tissue from the forceps. The sample is placed on a moistened Telfa pad to prevent its loss. The tissue must be handled gently when removed from the forceps so that it is not crushed because this may distort the pathology.

Foreign bodies are retrieved with a basket similar to that used to remove kidney stones. The basket instrument is threaded into the side channel. Grasping forceps may also be used to retrieve a foreign body.

At the close of the procedure, before the scope is withdrawn, the surgeon suctions the patient free of all secretions. The scope is then withdrawn.

An important complication of rigid bronchoscopy is injury to the tracheobronchial structures, which may occur if the patient moves during the procedure. The autonomic gag reflex may cause the patient to arch and cough, even during heavy sedation or light general anesthesia. A local anesthetic is sprayed into the trachea before the endoscope is inserted to help prevent bucking during the procedure.

Complications include possible injury to the bronchial tree and lung tissue. Additional complications include the laceration of blood vessels near the bronchial tissue and infection.

MEDIASTINOSCOPY

Mediastinoscopy is endoscopic examination of the mediastinum through an incision. Thymus and lymph node biopsies are performed to establish a diagnosis. A rigid mediastinoscope is a stainless steel endoscope inserted through a small incision at the suprasternal notch. Mediastinoscopy has been largely replaced by EBUS.

Pathology

Mediastinoscopy is performed for diagnostic or interventional surgery. The thymus gland, which is located in the mediastinal space in children, regresses in adulthood. Biopsy of the thymus gland and regional lymph nodes within the mediastinal space is performed to determine or rule out a cancer diagnosis.

POSITION:	Supine with neck hyperextended
INCISION:	Upper thoracic
PREP AND DRAPING:	Thyroid
INSTRUMENTS:	Mediastinal set

Technical Points and Discussion

1. ***The patient is prepped and draped.***
The patient is placed in the supine position with the neck hyperextended. The patient is prepped and draped for a thoracic incision. The procedure is performed using general anesthesia. The surgeon may stand at the patient's head or side.

2. ***The incision is made.***
A small incision is made over the suprasternal notch with a #10 knife blade. The incision is carried through the subcutaneous and muscle layers, commonly with Metzenbaum scissors and tissue forceps. The fascial layer on the anterior surface of the trachea is identified. The surgeon clamps small veins with mosquito hemostats and ligates them with fine silk ties. The ESU is used for smaller bleeders. The surgeon uses blunt finger dissection to make a plane between the tissues into the superior mediastinum. The scope is then inserted into this tissue plane and carefully advanced.

3. ***Lymph node biopsy is performed.***
Lymph node biopsy is performed routinely during the procedure. A biopsy needle attached to a metal stylet is used to pierce the target node and aspirate the contents. The technologist attaches a syringe to the stylet before handing it to the surgeon. This procedure is done to verify that the specimen is nodal tissue. When this is confirmed, the surgeon uses cup biopsy forceps to obtain a pathology specimen. The technologist removes the tissue from the forceps and places it in a specimen container or on a Telfa pad moistened with saline.

4. ***The wound is closed.***
After specimens have been obtained, the surgeon dries the wound and checks for bleeding. The ESU and hemostatic agents (e.g., absorbable gelatin sponge) may be used to control bleeding. The surgeon then withdraws the scope and closes the incision with synthetic absorbable sutures and skin staples.

VIDEO-ASSISTED THORACIC SURGERY (VATS)

Video-assisted thoracic surgery (VATS) is minimally invasive surgery of the thoracic cavity. This technique is similar to other types of minimally invasive procedures in which cannulas are inserted through the body wall and used to receive a rigid scope and instruments. This technique is different from bronchoscopy surgery, in which a flexible or rigid scope is inserted through the airway via the trachea. The term *video-assisted thoracic surgery* or *VATS* was coined at a time when minimally invasive endoscopic surgery was in its early development. At that time, video display from the endoscope to a monitor was a relatively new technology. VATS has now been developed to the extent that it has replaced most open procedures of the respiratory system.

To view a VATS procedure including instrumentation, see the following video: *VATS Right Middle Lobe Lobectomy in the Setting of Oligometastatic Lung Cancer,* available at https://www.youtube.com/watch?v=tGDP75MXEZ4.

VIDEO-ASSISTED THORACIC SURGERY (VATS)

It is important to distinguish the difference between thoracoscopy or pleuroscopy) and video-assisted thoracic surgery (VATS). Different textbooks and authors use the term *thoracoscopy* without making a clear distinction between thoracoscopy and video-assisted thoracic surgery. The differences are noted below:

- Thoracoscopy is a minimally invasive procedure that can be performed under local anesthetic and conscious sedation. VATS is invasive surgery performed under general anesthesia.
- Thoracoscopy is performed through a *flexible or semi-rigid fiber-optic endoscope* with a narrow working channel. VATS is performed through multiple ports or one large port using a rigid scope and modified (long) thoracotomy instruments.
- Thoracoscopy is performed mainly for assessment and minor procedures of the pleura. VATS technique is a surgical procedure which requires a full surgical team. The surgical goals are the same as those performed through open thoracotomy.

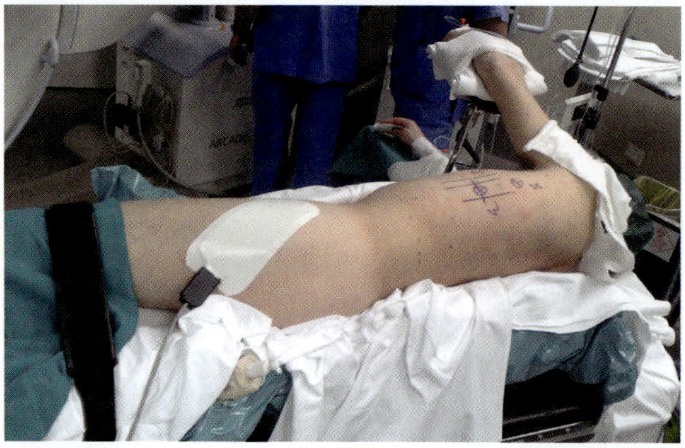

FIG. 31.14 Video-assisted thoracic surgery. Patient in lateral position. Note the extensive markings to indicate the location of important landmarks, and position of the electrosurgical return electrode pad. (From Longo UG, Papapietro N. Thoracoscopy for minimally invasive thoracic spine surgery. *Orthop Clin North Am.* 2009;40[4]:459–464.)

PATIENT PREPARATION

The patient is placed in the lateral position with the operative side up. The operative side arm is brought above the chest so that it does not block access to the operative site. It may be positioned on an overhead arm board or secured in a cradle. The downside arm rests on an arm board (Fig. 31.14). Positioning must be meticulous because there are risks to the cervical vertebrae, brachial plexus, and ulnar nerves.

A general anesthetic is administered through a double-lumen endotracheal tube. The double lumen allows the operative lung to collapse while the anesthetic and oxygen are administered to the opposite lung.

The patient is prepped from the neck to the iliac crest and from bedside to bedside. The exposed shoulder and arm may also be prepped, and the arm is placed on an overhead cradle.

Before starting surgery, the surgeon marks key locations on the skin, including the scapula, and port positions, which are measured to ensure access to the target tissues.

PORTS

Ports to accommodate the video thoracoscope and instruments are placed according to the procedure. Three or four individual ports are usually required. The ports are positioned in a "baseball diamond" pattern. This prevents instruments from crossing over within the thoracic cavity (Fig. 31.15). A single-port or "uniport" approach may also be used. In this technique a single large port is placed in the subxiphoid area or lateral thoracic wall to accommodate the instruments (Fig. 31.16).

INSTRUMENTS AND SETUP

VATS in an adult requires a 5-mm or 10-mm lens in sizes 0 and 30 degrees. The scope, camera, and light source are managed as for all minimally invasive endoscopic procedures (see Chapter 20). VATS instruments contain two fulcrums rather than just one. This allows the instruments to be opened within the small spaces of the ports without placing pressure on peripheral tissues. This is especially important for avoiding contact with the major nerves of the thoracic cavity.

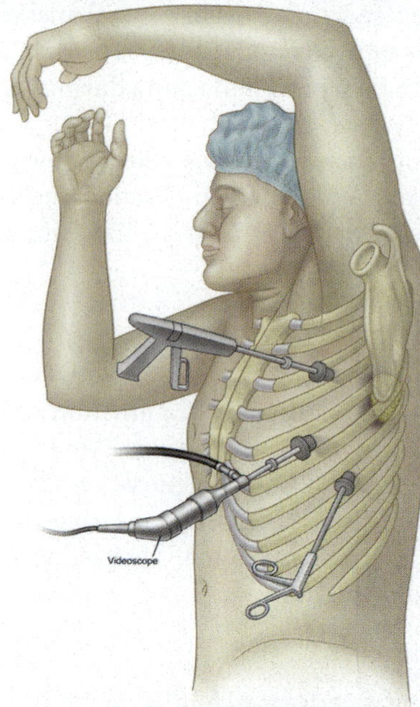

FIG. 31.15 Video-assisted thoracic surgery. Location of ports for mediastinal surgery. (From Ng CS, Yim AP. Technical advances in mediastinal surgery: videothoracoscopic approach to posterior mediastinal tumors. *Thorac Surg Clin.* 2010;20[2]:297–309. https://doi.org/10.1016/j.thorsurg.2010.02.003.)

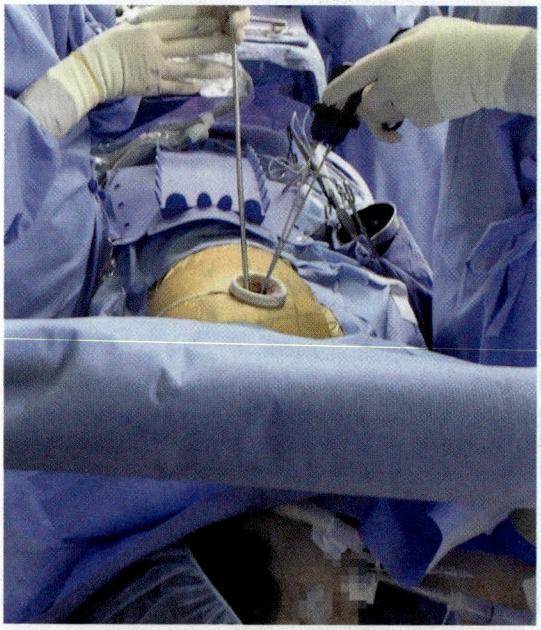

FIG. 31.16 Video-assisted thoracic surgery. Single port large enough to accommodate several instruments. The larger port requires a minithoracotomy incision. Some procedures use more than one uni-port plus single ports strategically placed. Note the Mayo positioned over the patient's legs *(top of photo)*, magnetic pad and pockets in drape *(top right)*. (From Kim HK, Han KN. Uniportal video-assisted thoracoscopic surgery segmentectomy. *Thorac Surg Clin.* 2017;27[4]:387–398. https://doi.org/10.1016/j.thorsurg.2017.06.007.)

VATS is frequently performed in conjunction with diagnostic procedures such as rigid and flexible bronchoscopy. Each stage of these multiple procedures must be set up separately. Sterility is maintained at all times. However, most facilities require that each setup be handled as a separate procedure without cross-over. Once the diagnostic portion of the procedure is complete, the instrument table should be covered and moved out of the immediate surgical field. This requires careful case planning ahead of the procedures to ensure that all needed equipment and instruments can be dedicated to the individual procedures.

Since the VATS procedure can be used for many different procedures of the thoracic cavity, specific instrumentation for a procedure depends on the surgery to be performed. System-specific instruments include those for the respiratory system, spine, and upper gastrointestinal tract.

Familiarity with VATS procedures and their instrumentation must be acquired with experience and study. Most thoracic instruments used in open thoracotomy have been modified for use in VATS procedures (see VATS Instruments table).

TEAM POSITIONS

In most VATS procedures with the patient in lateral position with the operative side up, the surgeon and assistant stand *at the patient's anterior side.* This is different from open thoracotomy, in which the surgeons are positioned at the patient's dorsal side. Both the surgeon and assistant surgeon remain side by side. The scrubbed surgical technologist stands on the posterior side at the level of the patient's legs (Fig. 31.17).

VATS LUNG BIOPSY

In this procedure lung tissue is removed for pathological assessment.

POSITION:	Lateral
INCISION:	Mini-thoracotomy and/or multiple entry ports for the VATS instruments and camera
PREP AND DRAPING:	Lateral thoracotomy
INSTRUMENTS:	VATS imaging system, biopsy instruments, resection instruments
POSSIBLE EXTRAS:	Linear endo stapler

Technical Points and Discussion

1. ***The patient is prepped and draped, and the cannulas are inserted.***
   The patient is placed in the lateral position and prepped and draped for a thoracostomy. A 2-cm skin incision is made between the ribs to accommodate the first cannula. Size 10- or 12-mm trocars are used. A 10-mm thoracic telescope is introduced.

2. ***A small section of the lung is removed.***
   A wedge resection is a large tissue biopsy or the removal of a small peripheral lesion. These are commonly removed with the linear surgical stapler.

Small sponge forceps are inserted through one of the instrument ports, and a 30-mm endoscopic linear stapler is introduced through a separate port. The biopsy specimen is removed with the stapling device, which divides the lung and closes the cut portion. Additional specimens, including lymph node samples, may also be removed.

3. ***The edges of the divided lung tissue are assessed for bleeding and air leakage.***
   The surgeon carefully inspects the suture line for air leaks by filling the chest cavity with warm saline solution. The ACP then inflates the lung, and the surgeon observes the suture line for bubbles. The surgeon or assistant applies pressure to the site, and additional sutures or tissue sealant is placed as needed.

4. ***The wounds are closed.***
   The instruments are withdrawn, and a chest tube is inserted into the lower incision and secured with heavy silk. The wounds are sutured with synthetic absorbable suture and skin staples. Steri-Strips may also be used to close the skin.

NOTE *If a small open incision is necessary for biopsy, the procedure is performed as described with the linear stapler. A chest tube is inserted, and the wound is closed with synthetic absorbable sutures and skin staples.*

Related Procedure

Pleuroscopy, endoscopic surgery of the thorax, may be performed in place of VATS for diagnostic purposes and some surgical interventions. During this procedure, a flexible fiberoptic endoscope is inserted through a single incision in the chest wall. Talc pleurodesis is a procedure commonly performed using the pleuroscope. During this procedure, talc is applied to the pleural space to create adhesions and prevent recurrent spontaneous pneumothorax. The talc is introduced through the endoscopic working channel using an atomizer.

ACUTE PULMONARY THROMBOEMBOLECTOMY

In this procedure, thrombi of the pulmonary vessel(s) are removed through a mid-sternotomy incision. The procedure is carried out using cardiopulmonary bypass (CPB), which is discussed in detail in Chapter 32, Cardiac Surgery.

Pathology

Pulmonary thromboembolic disease is caused by the remnants of emboli that have arisen from the deep veins of the lower extremities (called *deep venous thrombosis*). These remnants adhere to the walls of the pulmonary arteries. Eventually, this substance converts to connective and elastic tissue, in which acute pulmonary embolectomy is performed in patients with life-threatening circulatory insufficiency related to an embolism. In an acute situation only, the visible emboli are removed, and endarterectomy is not attempted.

POSITION:	Supine
INCISION:	Thoracotomy
PREP AND DRAPING:	Thoracotomy; Foley catheter
INSTRUMENTS:	Thoracic instruments; open heart instruments; linear endo stapler; vessel clips; bipolar ESU; embolectomy catheters; closed chest drainage system

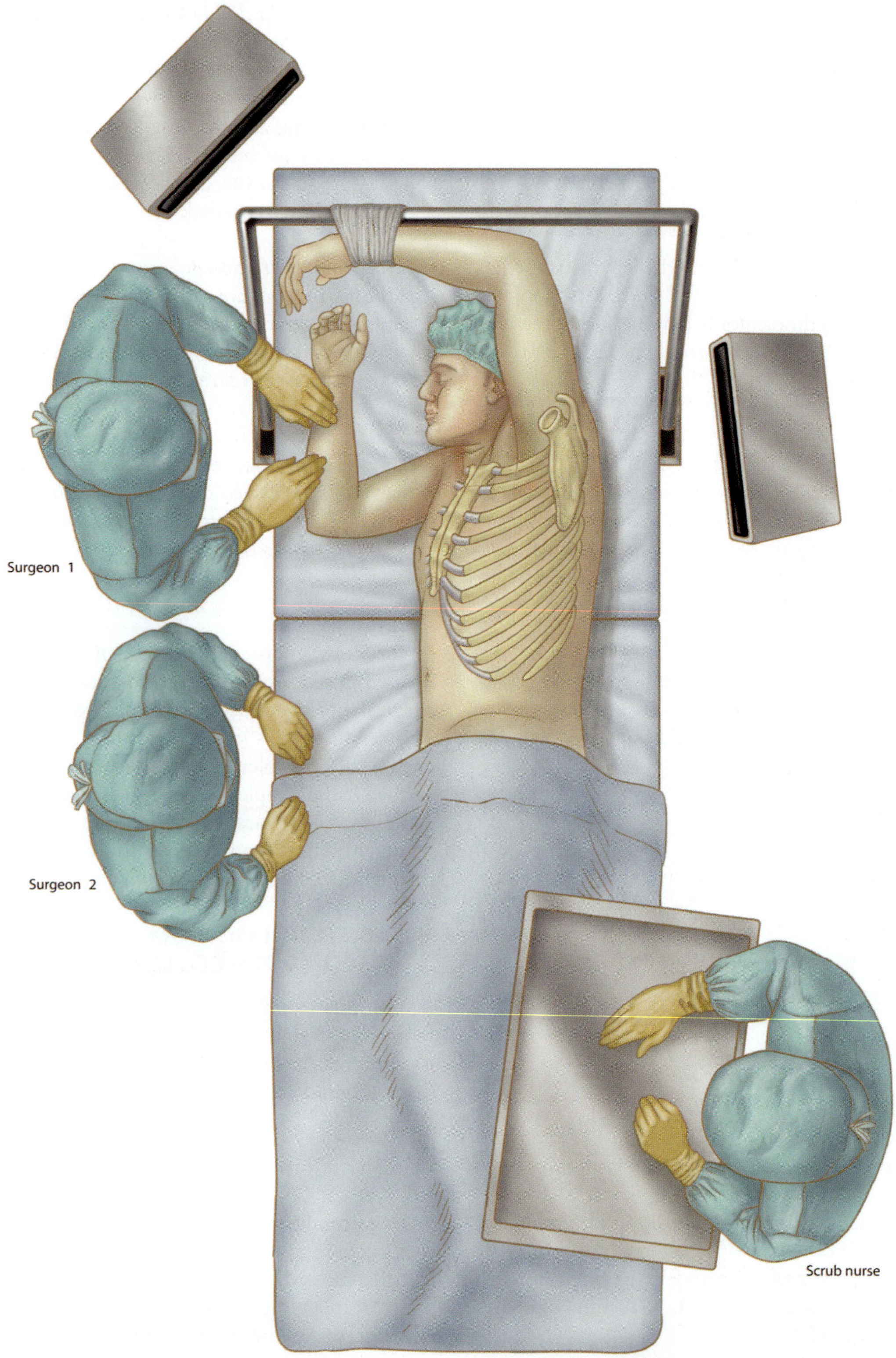

FIG. 31.17 VATS team positions. Whereas in open thoracotomy the surgeons face the patient's dorsal side, in VATS procedures they are positioned on the anterior side, facing the pathology. The surgical technologist may need to position the Mayo closer to the surgeons. (From Ng CS, Yim AP. Technical advances in mediastinal surgery: videothoracoscopic approach to posterior mediastinal tumors. *Thorac Surg Clin*. 2010;20[2]:297–309.)

Technical Points and Discussion

1. ***The patient is prepped and draped.***
The patient is anesthetized and placed in supine position, prepped, and draped for a midline thoracotomy incision.

2. ***A median sternotomy incision is made.***
A midline sternotomy incision is made, and a sternal retractor such as a Finochietto is positioned in the incision. Cardiopulmonary bypass is initiated. Cardiac arrest is not usually performed, and the heart remains warm during the procedure.

3. ***The mid-pulmonary artery is isolated.***
The scrub should have Rommel tourniquets prepared. These are placed around the superior and inferior vena cavae. Two polypropylene sutures are then placed in the mid-pulmonary artery and used for traction.

4. ***An arteriotomy is performed.***
The surgeon makes an incision in the pulmonary trunk between the preplaced sutures using a #11 knife blade and angled Potts scissors. Suction should be immediately available. Visible emboli are removed using vascular forceps. A balloon catheter may also be used to remove emboli. The incisions may then be extended to remove additional emboli. The scrub should remove emboli from the field and retain them as specimens. A pediatric bronchoscope or sinuscope may be used to explore the pulmonary branches for additional emboli.

5. ***The pleural spaces are entered and the lungs compressed to eject small clots.***
The surgeon enters the pleural spaces to manually compress the lungs. This is done to milk clots from the distal vessels, where they can be removed with suction.

6. ***The arteriotomy is closed.***
After the wound is flushed, the arteriotomy is closed using size 6-0 polypropylene suture. The patient is then weaned from bypass. Some surgeons may insert a vena cava filter to prevent further pulmonary emboli. This procedure is described in Chapter 30.

The wound is then closed in layers, and chest tubes are placed. Patients may be transported to the intensive care unit (ICU) for recovery.

LUNG VOLUME REDUCTION SURGERY (LVRS): OPEN TECHNIQUE

In lung volume reduction surgery (LVRS), portions of the lung severely affected by chronic pulmonary emphysema are removed to improve pulmonary function. Segmental resection is performed using linear cutting staples. In this procedure the staple lines are re-enforced using Gore-Tex strips or biological glue (see Chapter 12 for a discussion on tissue adhesives). This is done to prevent the stapled tissue from tearing when the lung is reinflated. A bilateral resection is described here. Although most LVRS procedures can be managed using VATS technique, the surgical technologist should acquire knowledge on access through the sternum. The median sternotomy incision described in the following section provides access to the mediastinum, upper lobes of the lung, and is used in cardiac procedures.

Pathology

Chronic pulmonary emphysema is marked by the loss of elasticity and destruction of lung tissue, usually related to chronic cigarette smoking. The disease is characterized by the stiffening of the tissue and inability to empty the alveoli, which results in abnormal enlargement of the lungs. Gas exchange is severely impaired, and the result is **dyspnea** (difficulty breathing) and **hypoxia.** Areas of overinflation, or **blebs,** develop in the most severely affected tissue. Segmental removal of diseased lung tissue improves pulmonary function and tidal volume in particular.

POSITION:	Supine
INCISION:	Median sternotomy
PREP AND DRAPING:	Midline sternotomy
INSTRUMENTS:	Thoracotomy instruments; sternal saw, linear staplers; gastrointestinal clamps; bovine pericardium graft, PTFE or similar material; vessel clips; bipolar ESU
POSSIBLE EXTRAS:	Tracheostomy instruments

Technical Points and Discussion

1. ***The patient is prepped and draped.***
The patient is placed in supine position, prepped, and draped for a midline sternal incision for bilateral lung access.

2. ***A median sternotomy incision is made to expose the sternum, which is divided using a sternal saw.***
Soft tissues are divided using the monopolar ESU. A sternum retractor is placed in the wound.

3. ***To inspect the lung, the anesthesia care provider deflates the first lung.***
Adhesions are dissected with Metzenbaum scissors, right angle clamps, and the ESU.

4. ***Lung clamps are used to grasp and seal the portion of the lung to be excised.***
The surgeon uses Duval lung forceps or other atraumatic forceps or a gastrointestinal clamp is used to isolate areas that are to be transected.

5. ***A GIA stapler is placed across the lung tissue, which is then severed and stapled.***
A leak-proof seal is achieved by placing polytetrafluoroethylene (PTFE), Gore-Tex strips, or biological glue on the edges of the resection.

The lung is inflated and the pleural cavity filled with saline to check for leakage. If no leaks are detected, the transection procedure is carried out on the second lung.

6. ***Chest tubes are inserted, and the wound is closed.*** Chest drains are inserted and attached to a sealed chest drainage unit. The sternum is closed using stainless steel wire, size 5. The fascia and linea alba are sutured with running sutures of absorbable synthetic material. Skin is closed according to the surgeon's preference. The patient may be transferred to the postanesthesia care unit or the intensive care unit.

Refer to Fig. 31.18 for technical highlights of the procedure.

Related Procedure: Lung Volume Reduction Surgery VATS

LVRS is performed as an open procedure (as described earlier) or using the VATS technique. The two procedures are very similar: both use linear staples and re-enforcement of the staple lines with synthetic patching materials.

THORACOTOMY

Thoracotomy is the general term for *open surgery* of the thoracic cavity. The procedure for opening and closing the chest is generally the same for any thoracotomy. Thoracic emergencies involving open or penetrating wounds with severe hemorrhage may require the thoracotomy to be performed in the emergency department. In these cases, the patient is rushed to the operating room as soon as hemostasis is controlled. Refer to Chapter 35 for a more detailed description of emergency thoracotomy.

Pathology

Thoracotomy may be performed for any condition that requires access to the thoracic cavity.

POSITION:	Supine or lateral
INCISION:	Midline thoracotomy or anterolateral

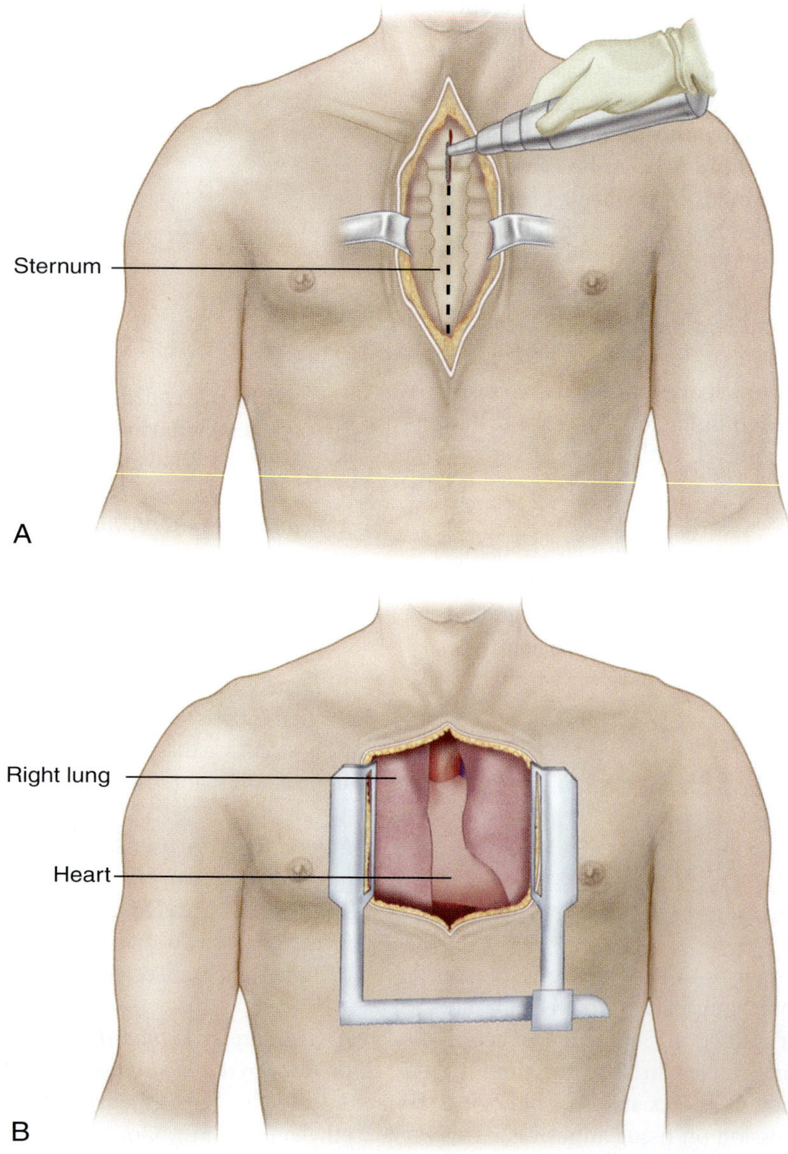

FIG. 31.18 Lung volume reduction surgery (LVRS): open technique. (A) A mid-sternal incision is made to access both lungs. (B) Sternal retractor in place.

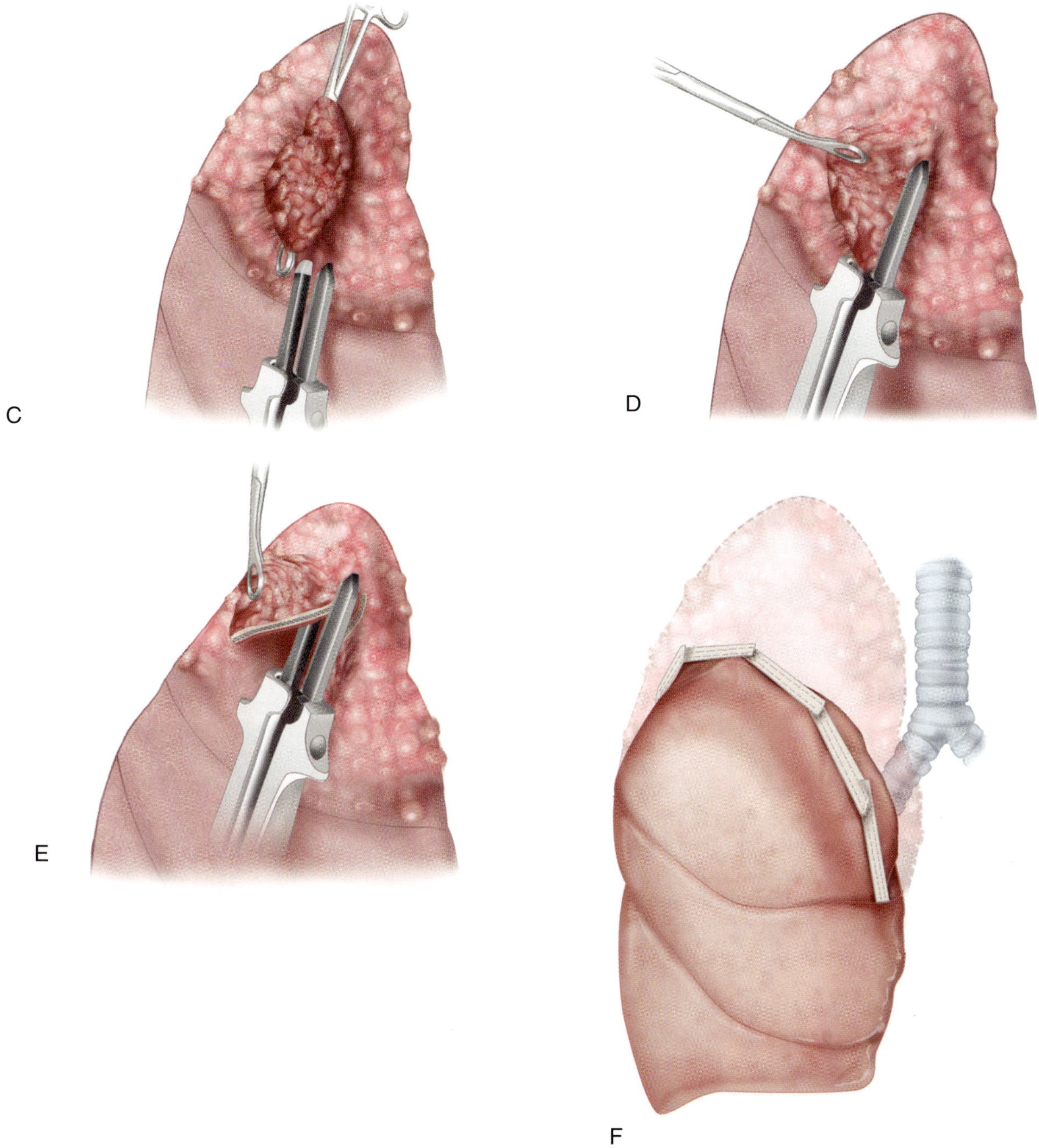

FIG. 31.18, cont'd (C) The affected lung tissue is clamped using an atraumatic intestinal clamp. (D) The GIA stapler is placed across the tissue and fired. (E) Resection continues using the GIA. (F) The staple lines are re-enforced using PTFE, Gore-Tex, and biologic adhesive. (B and F, From Zwischenberger JB, Townsend CM, Evers BM. *Atlas of Thoracic Surgical Techniques E-Book: A Volume in the Surgical Techniques Atlas Series*. Saunders; 2010.)

PREP AND DRAPING:	Thoracotomy
INSTRUMENTS:	Major thoracotomy set; long ESU electrode; Deaver retractors; malleable ribbon retractors; scapular retractor; vascular forceps; rib instruments; long Penrose drain for traction; Silastic vessel loops; umbilical tapes
POSSIBLE EXTRAS:	Bronchus clamps; deep vascular clamps

Technical Points and Discussion

1. ***The patient is prepped and draped.***
The patient is placed in the lateral position, prepped, and draped for a lateral thoracotomy.

2. ***The incision is made and carried to deep tissue.***
An anterolateral incision is made. Subcutaneous and muscle layers are then divided with the knife or ESU. Bleeders are coagulated or clamped and ligated with silk ties.

The surgeon inserts a scapular retractor beneath the shoulder muscles and elevates the scapula. An intercostal incision is made with the knife or ESU.

3. ***A rib may be removed.***
Occasionally, a rib must be removed. If this is necessary, the surgeon incises the periosteum along its anterior surface. A periosteal elevator or rib rasp is used to strip the periosteum from the rib. The surgeon severs the rib from its attachment at the spine and sternum using Bethune or similar rib shears. The entire rib is removed. The surgeon then trims the sharp edges of the remaining rib end using Sauerbruch rib shears or a rongeur.

4. ***Retractors are placed, and surgery is continued.***
The edges of the wound are covered with laparotomy sponges to protect them from bruising. A self-retaining retractor is placed in the wound and opened slowly. Surgery then continues as planned.

Closure

After chest tubes have been inserted and instruments have been removed, the surgeon places pericostal sutures (e.g., size 1 or 2 absorbable suture) around the two ribs and tags the suture ends with a hemostat. Alternatively, the surgeon may drill small holes through the ribs and bring the suture through these holes. Four to six sutures are usually required. A rib approximator (e.g., the Bailey approximator) is used to bring the ribs together. The pericostal sutures are tied securely while the approximator is in place.

A size 0 continuous absorbable suture may be used to approximate the periosteum between the two ribs. The surgeon then closes the muscles with a size 0 continuous or interrupted non-absorbable suture. Subcutaneous tissue is closed with 3-0 absorbable sutures. The skin is closed with staples, 4-0 non-absorbable interrupted suture, or a 4-0 absorbable subcuticular stitch. Chest tubes are connected to the sealed drainage system, and the wound is dressed with absorbent pads and tape. A local anesthetic infusion catheter (such as ON-Q) may be inserted in the chest wall, or a cryoablation device may be used to freeze intercostal nerves for pain management postoperatively.

LOBECTOMY: VATS

Lobectomy is the removal of a portion of a lung to prevent the spread of cancer or to treat a benign tumor. Lobectomy may be performed as a VATS procedure or as an open procedure. The principles and anatomical divisions are the same for open and closed procedures.

Pathology

A lobectomy is most often performed to in the treatment of lung cancer, but it may be indicated in other conditions such as cysts, localized infection, or trauma to a portion of the lung.

POSITION:	Lateral
INCISION:	Posterolateral thoracotomy
PREP AND DRAPING:	Thoracotomy
INSTRUMENTS:	Major thoracotomy set, major general surgery set; bronchus instruments; deep vascular clamps and forceps
POSSIBLE EXTRAS:	Silastic vessel loops: umbilical tapes; vessel clips, linear stapling instruments; fibrin tissue adhesive

Technical Points and Discussion

1. ***The patient is prepped and draped.***
The patient is placed in the lateral position, prepped, and draped for a thoracotomy incision.

2. ***A thoracotomy is performed.***
A posterolateral thoracotomy is performed. The surgeon examines the entire lung and mediastinum closely to make certain no evidence of disease exists beyond that previously diagnosed.

3. ***The hilum of the lobe is identified, and individual arteries and veins are divided.***
The lobe is retracted with lung-grasping forceps, and the pleura is incised. The pulmonary artery and vein are dissected free at the hilum. Sponge dissectors and right-angle clamps are used to help separate the vessels from the connective tissue at the hilum.

Silastic vascular loops may be used to retract the bronchus and large vessels. Smaller vessels are mobilized with scissors, clamped with right-angle clamps, and ligated with size 2-0 silk ties.

4. ***The bronchus is mobilized and separated from the hilum.*** The bronchus is occluded with a bronchus clamp. Suction is very important while the bronchus is open to prevent blood or fluid from draining into the opposite lung. The scrub may be needed to manage the suction while the surgeons transect and suture the bronchus. Interrupted sutures of 3-0 silk, 4-0 synthetic absorbable suture, or a linear stapler are used to occlude the proximal bronchus, which is divided with the knife.

5. ***The lobe is removed, and the bronchial stump is closed.*** When all vessels and the bronchus have been occluded, the lobe can be removed. The bronchial stump is covered with the pleura and sutured with interrupted 3-0 polyethylene sutures.

6. ***The wound is irrigated and closed.*** The wound is irrigated, and the lung is inflated to check for leaks. A chest tube is inserted, and the wound is closed in layers.

Several technical points for VATS lobectomy are illustrated in Fig. 31.19.

OPEN PNEUMONECTOMY

Pneumonectomy is the removal of the entire lung.

Pathology

Removal of a lung reduces the size of a tumor that may be impinging on vital structures. Debulking is also a palliative measure to slow the progression of cancer. Other indications for lobectomy include extensive or chronic abscess or bronchiectasis (chronic dilation of the bronchi) caused by infection, pulmonary obstruction, or tuberculosis.

POSITION:	Lateral
INCISION:	Thoracotomy
PREP AND DRAPING:	Thoracotomy
INSTRUMENTS:	Major thoracotomy set; major general surgery set; bronchus instruments; deep vascular clamps and forceps; Silastic vessel loops; umbilical tapes; vessel clips; long spatula ESU electrode
POSSIBLE EXTRAS:	Linear stapling instruments

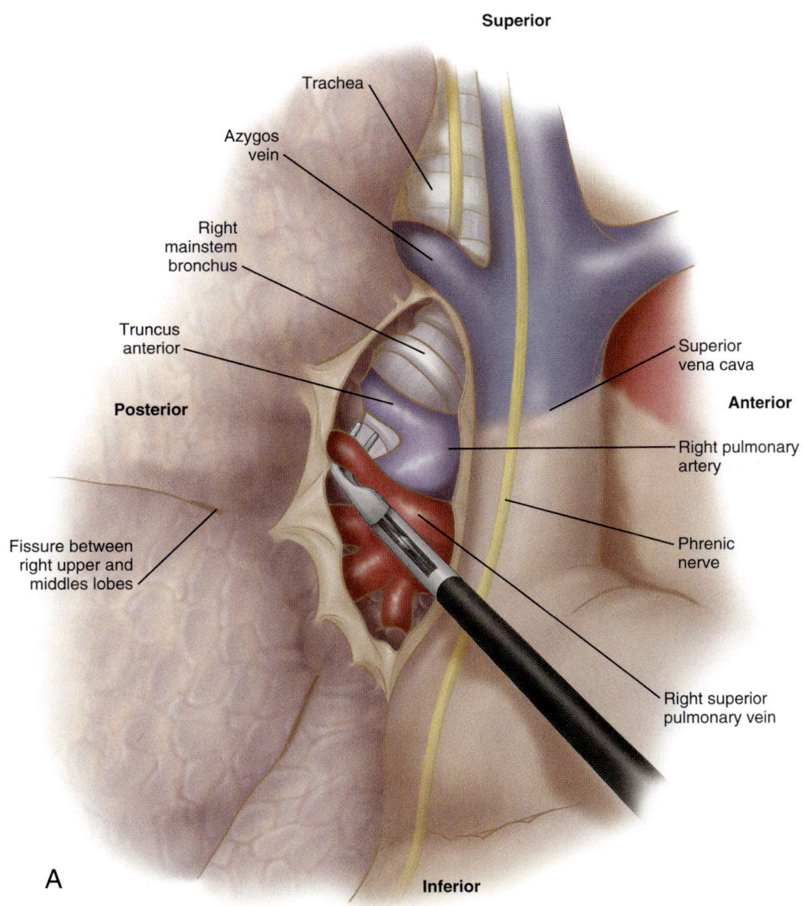

FIG. 31.19 Lobectomy (VATS). (A) The anterior hilum is exposed and the right superior pulmonary vein is dissected using right angle clamp.

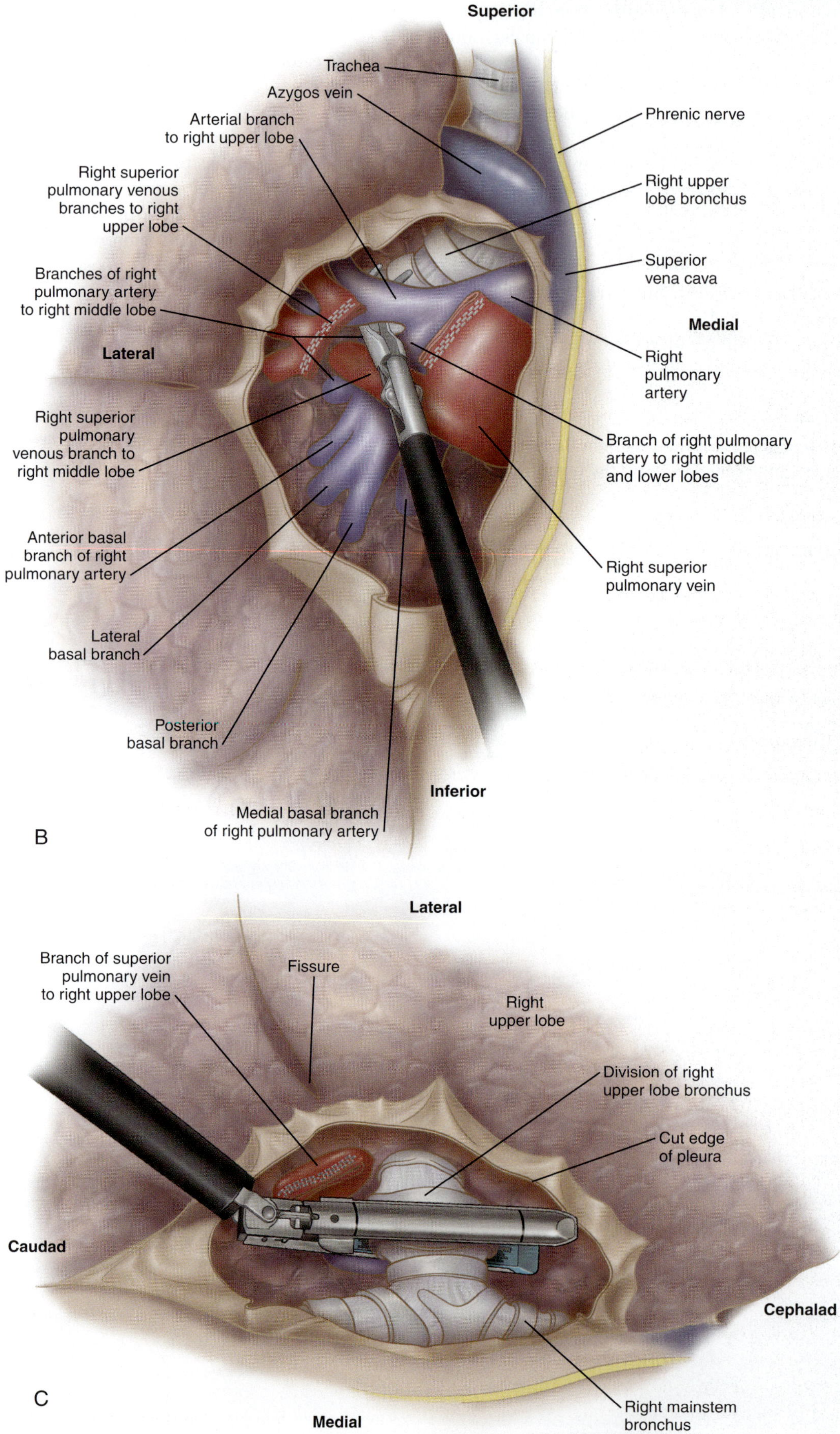

FIG. 31.19, cont'd (B) The pulmonary vein has been divided and sealed with linear staples. The pulmonary artery is dissected. (C) The bronchus is divided and sealed. (From Frantizides C, Carlson M. *Video Atlas of Advanced Minimally Invasive Surgery*. Philadelphia: Elsevier Saunders; 2013.)

Technical Points and Discussion

1. ***A thoracotomy is performed.***
   The patient is placed in the lateral position, and thoracotomy is performed. The entire lung and surrounding tissues are examined closely to evaluate the extent of the disease. The lung is retracted with nonmalleable or malleable retractors or Duval lung forceps to expose the mediastinal pleura. The pleura is incised with scissors and smooth tissue forceps. Blunt dissection along the edge of the parietal pleura is performed with sponge dissectors. Dissection is carried to the hilum.

2. ***The major vessels are divided (i.e., bronchus, pulmonary artery, and superior and inferior pulmonary veins).***
   The major structures connected to the lung are isolated, including the bronchus, pulmonary artery, and pulmonary vein. The pulmonary artery and vein are carefully separated, clamped with right-angle vascular clamps, and divided. Heavy silk sutures are used to ligate the vessels. The vagus, recurrent laryngeal (left side only), and phrenic nerves are retracted with vessel loops or moist umbilical tapes.

The pulmonary artery is clamped, divided, and ligated. The surgeon may oversew the cut edges of the artery with a fine suture, such as 4-0 or 5-0 silk or polypropylene. The superior and inferior veins are ligated and divided in similar fashion. Ligation clips may be used for smaller vessels.

3. ***The bronchus is divided and closed.***
   The bronchus is commonly occluded with a Sarot clamp and divided with the knife. The lung can then be removed from the wound. The open end of the bronchus is closed with interrupted sutures (e.g., 3-0 polypropylene sutures) or the stapler. The bronchus is divided, and the lung is removed from the wound. Surgical staples with a cutting blade may also be used to divide and seal the bronchus.

4. ***The wound is closed.***
   The wound is irrigated with warm saline, and any leaks are identified and repaired with sutures. The pleura is sutured over the bronchus. Chest tubes may be inserted and brought out through stab wounds adjacent to the incision. These are secured with heavy silk sutures. The upper mediastinal pleura is closed with absorbable suture, and the wound is closed in layers.

DECORTICATION OF THE LUNG

Decortication of the lung is the surgical removal of fibrous tissue overlying the lung.

Pathology

Chronic inflammation, infection (**empyema** or tuberculosis), or a lung tumor causes the formation of exudate in the pleural space. Because of effusion or tumor, fibrin deposits form, and the parietal pleura can adhere to the chest wall and prevent the lungs from inflating. The fibrous tissue is referred to as a *peel*. Removal of the peel or affected pleura aids the treatment of chronic infection and eases restriction of the pleura. Pleurectomy (removal of the pleura) is performed to treat pleural cancer, such as mesothelioma.

POSITION:	Lateral
INCISION:	Posterolateral
PREP AND DRAPING:	Thoracotomy
INSTRUMENTS:	Major thoracotomy set; major general surgery set; bronchus instruments; deep vascular clamps and forceps; Silastic vessel loops; umbilical tapes; vessel clips; long spatula ESU electrode
POSSIBLE EXTRAS:	Linear stapling instruments; curettes

Technical Points and Discussion

1. ***A thoracotomy incision is made in the fifth intercostal space.***
   After the thoracic incision has been made, the subcutaneous tissue and muscle are dissected with scissors and ESU. A rib spreader is inserted to expose the affected portion of the lung. A portion of the fifth or sixth rib may be resected with rib shears. Multiple adhesions are usually present. These are removed with careful dissection.

2. ***The fibrous tissue is removed.***
   Empyema or other fluid is drained and cultured. The ACP expands the lung intermittently to demonstrate areas requiring additional decortication. The peel is then carefully dissected using sponge dissectors.

3. ***Chest tubes are inserted, and the wound is closed.***
   After sufficient dissection and removal of the fibrous membrane, drainage tubes are inserted and the incision is closed.

LUNG TRANSPLANTATION

Transplantation of one or both lungs is performed to remove a diseased lung and replace it with a donor lung. Single-lung transplantation is increasingly being used as a way to maximize the allocation of donor lungs. If both lungs are diseased, bilateral transplantation is indicated. Living donor transplantation involves removal of the donor's lower lobes only. Procurement of lung tissue (and other organs) is a very precise procedure that requires knowledge of protocols and procedures, as well as problem-solving abilities.

Pathology

Single- or double-lung transplantation is indicated for patients with restrictive lung disease, emphysema, pulmonary hypertension, and other noninfectious end-stage pulmonary diseases.

Technical Points

LUNG DONOR

1. *The donor is prepped from chin to knees.*
2. *A median sternotomy is performed.*
3. *A sternal (or rib) retractor is inserted.*
4. *The pleura is opened longitudinally, and the pericardium is divided.*
5. *Umbilical tapes are placed around the aorta and the superior and inferior venae cavae.*
6. *Pleural adhesions are divided and the proximal pulmonary arteries are dissected.*
7. *The superior vena cava is ligated with heavy silk ties.*
8. *The aortic arch is dissected free, and the ligamentum arteriosum (the remnant ductus arteriosus) is divided.*
9. *The pulmonary artery is encircled with an umbilical tape and separated from the ascending aorta.*
10. *Cardioplegia solution is infused through the proximal aorta into the heart via the coronary arteries; pulmoplegia (perfusion) solution is infused into the pulmonary organs.*
11. *Cardiac veins and arteries are separated, and the heart is removed and placed in a cold preservative solution.*
12. *The pulmonary arteries are separated from the mediastinum.*
13. *The trachea is dissected free.*
14. *The lungs are inflated and then stapled and removed.*
15. *The lungs are placed in a cold preservative solution.*

LUNG RECIPIENT

1. *The patient is placed in the lateral position with the operative side up. The individual is prepped from chin to knees.*
2. *A thoracotomy incision is made, and a retractor is inserted.*
3. *If the recipient's right lung is to be removed, the pulmonary vein, pulmonary artery, and azygos vein are isolated and divided.*
4. *If the recipient's left lung is to be removed, the ligamentum arteriosum is divided.*
5. *The lung to be removed is collapsed, and the proximal pulmonary artery is occluded. If hemodynamic instability is a factor, a femoro-femoral bypass may be performed.*
6. *The lung is removed.*
7. *The pulmonary veins are divided, and branches of the pulmonary artery are separated.*
8. *The bronchus is divided, and the diseased lung is removed.*
9. *The bronchus-to-bronchus anastomosis is performed with 3-0 absorbable suture.*
10. *The pulmonary artery-to-pulmonary artery anastomosis is performed with running 4-0 polypropylene suture.*
11. *The recipient pulmonary veins are attached to the donor atrial cuff with running 4-0 polypropylene suture.*
12. *The new lung is inflated and inspected.*
13. *Chest tubes are inserted, and hemostasis is achieved.*
14. *The chest is closed.*
15. *Bronchoscopy may be performed to suction secretions and confirm an intact anastomosis.*

   Advanced-level techniques used during the procedure include shortening the donor bronchial stump, wrapping the anastomosis with omentum or an intercostal muscle pedicle, and performing an intussuscepting (e.g., telescoping) bronchial anastomosis technique.

KEY CONCEPTS

- Thoracic surgery focuses on the structures of the respiratory system, especially the trachea, bronchi, and lungs.
- Thoracic surgery is performed with specialty instruments, including atraumatic lung clamps, rib instruments, and bronchial clamps. Surgical stapling instruments are used frequently for lung resection. Long general surgery instruments are often required for the adult patient.
- The thoracic cavity is normally under negative pressure. When the chest wall is punctured or opened, air rushes into the chest cavity and collapses the lungs.
- Negative pressure in the chest cavity is restored after surgery with a closed chest drainage system.
- Bronchoscopy involves endoscopic examination of the respiratory structures. Rigid and flexible bronchoscopes are used. The rigid bronchoscope is used most often for interventional procedures.
- The most common incision used in thoracic surgery is the posterolateral, performed with the patient in the lateral position.
- Video-assisted thoracic surgery is minimally invasive surgery performed with a trocar-cannula system and telescope. The techniques are similar to laparoscopy.
- Pulmonary diseases that may require surgery include structural anomalies, cancer of the respiratory tissues, benign mass, diseases related to environmental toxins, and the effects of long-term infection. Circulatory diseases such as arteriosclerosis may also affect the lungs.
- Lung volume reduction surgery is performed to remove lung tissue that has lost elasticity because of emphysema.
- The surgical technologist must understand the dynamics of breathing and the concept of negative pressure in the thoracic cavity. This is critical to responding to emergency surgery and emergency situations that arise during thoracic surgery.
- Video-assisted thoracic surgery (VATS) is not a simplification of open thoracic surgery. These procedures require the same instruments used in open thoracotomy with modifications in the fulcrum. The primary difference between open thoracotomy and VATS is in its "muscle-sparing" approach.
- All procedures performed with the patient in lateral position require the use of a magnetic instrument pad and side pockets in the drape to prevent instruments from falling to the floor during surgery.
- Chest tubes are needed to evacuate fluid (including blood) and air from the pleural space after trauma and surgery in which negative pressure has been lost.

- Flexible bronchoscopy is used for assessment of the bronchial tree and minor procedures of the pleura.
- Rigid bronchoscopy is used when large-bore instruments are required for a procedure.
- All bronchoscopic procedures are performed using sterile instruments. This is to prevent cross-infection between patients.
- Staging for lung cancer involves identification of the station of each lymph node specimen. The surgical technologist must understand the terminology of this system to ensure that no errors are made in identification of a specimen.
- The surgical technologist coordinates closely with the circulating nurse in the management of specimens.
- During assessment procedures, methylene blue dye is injected into tissue suspected of malignancy. This allows the surgeon to identify the area during surgery, which follows the assessment.
- Flexible bronchoscopy is referred to as *medical bronchoscopy* to distinguish it from video-assisted thoracic surgery.
- Rigid bronchoscopy can be performed for procedures of the major airways because its large-bore channels can accommodate instruments.
- Before VATS procedure begins, the surgeon may measure the distance between the port sites and mark the lines on the patient's skin. This is to prevent instruments in different ports from clashing during surgery.
- Tissue glue is commonly used to seal bronchial anastomoses and lung resection lines.
- The most common incisions used in thoracic surgery are the anterolateral, posterolateral, and midline sternotomy.

REVIEW QUESTIONS

1. Explain the process of breathing, including the influence of negative pressure in the thoracic cavity.
2. Why must a closed chest drainage unit be kept lower than the patient's body?
3. What are the differences among lobectomy and pneumonectomy?
4. What is the difference between thoracotomy and thoracostomy?
5. Explain pneumothorax and why it occurs.
6. What is the purpose of debulking a tumor?
7. What instruments are needed to perform a rib resection?

BIBLIOGRAPHY

Broaddus VC, Mason RJ. *Murray & Nadel's Textbook of Respiratory Medicine*. Philadelphia: Elsevier Saunders; 2016.

Cassivi SD, Deschamps C, Pastis NJ. Chest tube insertion and management. *Clin Resp Med*. 2012:862–868. https://doi.org/10.1016/b978-1-4557-0792-.

Cameron J, Cameron A, eds. *Current Surgical Therapy*. 11th ed. Philadelphia: Saunders; 2014.

Christie S. Electromagnetic navigation bronchoscopy for identifying lung nodules for thoracoscopic resection. *AORN*. 2014;99(6):750–763.

Gonzalez-Rivas D, Sihoe AD. Important technical details during uniportal video-assisted thoracoscopic major resections. *Thorac Surg Clin*. 2017;27(4):357–372. https://doi.org/10.1016/j.thorsurg.2017.06.004.

Hagberg CA, Artime CA, Aziz MF, Benumof JL. *Hagberg and Benumof's Airway Management*. 5th ed. Philadelphia, PA: Elsevier; 2018.

Hervé D. Rigid bronchoscopy. *Clin Chest Med*. 2013;34(3):427–435.

Khatri V, ed. *Atlas of Advanced Operative Surgery*. Philadelphia: Saunders; 2013.

Kim HK, Han KN. Uniportal video-assisted thoracoscopic surgery segmentectomy. *Thorac Surg Clin*. 2017;27(4):387–398. https://doi.org/10.1016/j.thorsurg.2017.06.007.

Longo UG, Papapietro N. Thoracoscopy for minimally invasive thoracic spine surgery. *Orthop Clin North Am*. 2009;40(4):459–464.

Madariaga ML, Lanuti M. Sampling of suspicious solitary pulmonary nodules: electromagnetic navigational bronchoscopy and video-assisted thoracoscopic surgery. *Sem Roentgenol*. 2017;52(3):178–184. https://doi.org/10.1053/j.ro.2017.06.003.

Marino KA, Sullivan JL, Weksler B. Electromagnetic navigation bronchoscopy for identifying lung nodules for thoracoscopic resection. *Ann Thorac Sur*. 2016;102(2):454–457. https://doi.org/10.1016/j.athoracsur.2016.03.010.

Ng CS, Yim AP. Technical advances in mediastinal surgery: videothoracoscopic approach to posterior mediastinal tumors. *Thorac Surg Clin*. 2010;20(2):297–309. https://doi.org/10.1016/j.thorsurg.2010.02.003.

Salvin S.H. Ng MD, Anthony P.C. Yim MA,

Sellke F, del Nido P, Swanson S, eds. *Sabiston and Spencer Surgery of the Chest*. 9th ed. Philadelphia: Elsevier; 2016.

Sellke F, Ruel M, eds. *Atlas of Cardiac Surgical Techniques*. Philadelphia: Saunders; 2010.

Suda T. Uniportal subxiphoid video-assisted thoracoscopic thymectomy. *Asvide*. 2016;3:287–287. https://doi.org/10.21037/asvide.2016.287.

Valasco JM. *Essential surgical Procedures*. Elsevier; 2016.

Zwischenberger JB, Townsend CM, Evers BM. *Atlas of Thoracic Surgical Techniques E-Book: A Volume in the Surgical Techniques Atlas Series*. Saunders; 2010.

32 CARDIAC SURGERY

LEARNING OBJECTIVES

After studying this chapter, the reader will be able to:

1. Identify key anatomical features of the heart and great vessels
2. Describe diagnostic procedures commonly used in cardiac medicine
3. Describe specific elements of case planning for cardiac surgery
4. Discuss cardiac pathology
5. Define the primary surgical goals for common cardiac procedures
6. Discuss what instrument sets may be used for common cardiac procedures

TERMINOLOGY

Aneurysm: A weakness in the arterial wall resulting in ballooning of the artery and possible rupture.

Aortotomy: Incision into the aorta.

Apex: The lower left tip of the left ventricle of the heart.

Arrhythmia: An abnormal heartbeat (also called *dysrhythmia*).

Arteriosclerosis: Disease of the arteries characterized by the loss of elasticity and hardening of the arterial walls.

Atherosclerosis: A disease characterized by the buildup of cholesterol deposits in the arterial lining.

Bicaval cannulation: The use of two (single-stage) venous cannulas. One is placed in the superior vena cava, the other in the inferior vena cava. They are connected to the venous return line via a Y-connector.

Bradycardia: A slow heart rate (usually a heart rate under 60 beats per minute in an adult).

Cardiac cycle: A complete heartbeat, from the beginning of one heartbeat to the beginning of the next.

Cardioplegia: Intentional stoppage of all cardiac activity during cardiac surgery.

Cardiopulmonary bypass machine: Medical equipment that provides bypass circulatory support to the heart and lungs.

Coarctation: A congenital narrowing or stricture in the aorta.

Conduit: A channel through which fluid can pass.

Congenital: A condition present at birth.

Cross-clamp: A clamp placed across a blood vessel to occlude it.

Diastole: The phase of the cardiac cycle when the heart muscle relaxes to allow the chambers to fill with blood.

Endovascular repair: Endoscopic surgery of the vascular system.

Femoral cannula: A type of vascular catheter used for intravenous and intraarterial femoral access during on-pump cardiac surgery.

Fibrillation: Uncoordinated muscular activity in the heart muscle, which results in a "quivering" rather than pumping action.

Infarction: Necrosis of tissue related to decreased blood flow to the tissue.

Ischemia: Inadequate blood supply to a localized area related to blockage of vessels leading to that area.

Node: In cardiac anatomy, a group of specialized nerve cells that transmit electrical impulses that stimulate cardiac contractions.

Off-pump procedure: An open-heart procedure without the use of cardiopulmonary bypass (i.e., "the pump").

Pacemaker: A device that helps control abnormal heart rhythms.

Shunt: To bypass a structure or carry fluid from one anatomical location to another.

Stenosis: The narrowing of a hollow structure such as a blood vessel or duct.

Sternotomy: An incision made into the sternum.

Systole: The heart muscle contracts to allow blood to be pumped into the aorta.

Tachycardia: A fast heart rate (usually over 120 beats per minute in the adult).

Thoracoabdominal aortic aneurysm: An aneurysm of the aorta extending from the chest to the abdomen.

Thoracotomy: An incision made into the thoracic cavity.

Type A aortic dissection: A tear in the inner lining of the aorta that begins at the ascending aorta and may extend into femoral arteries.

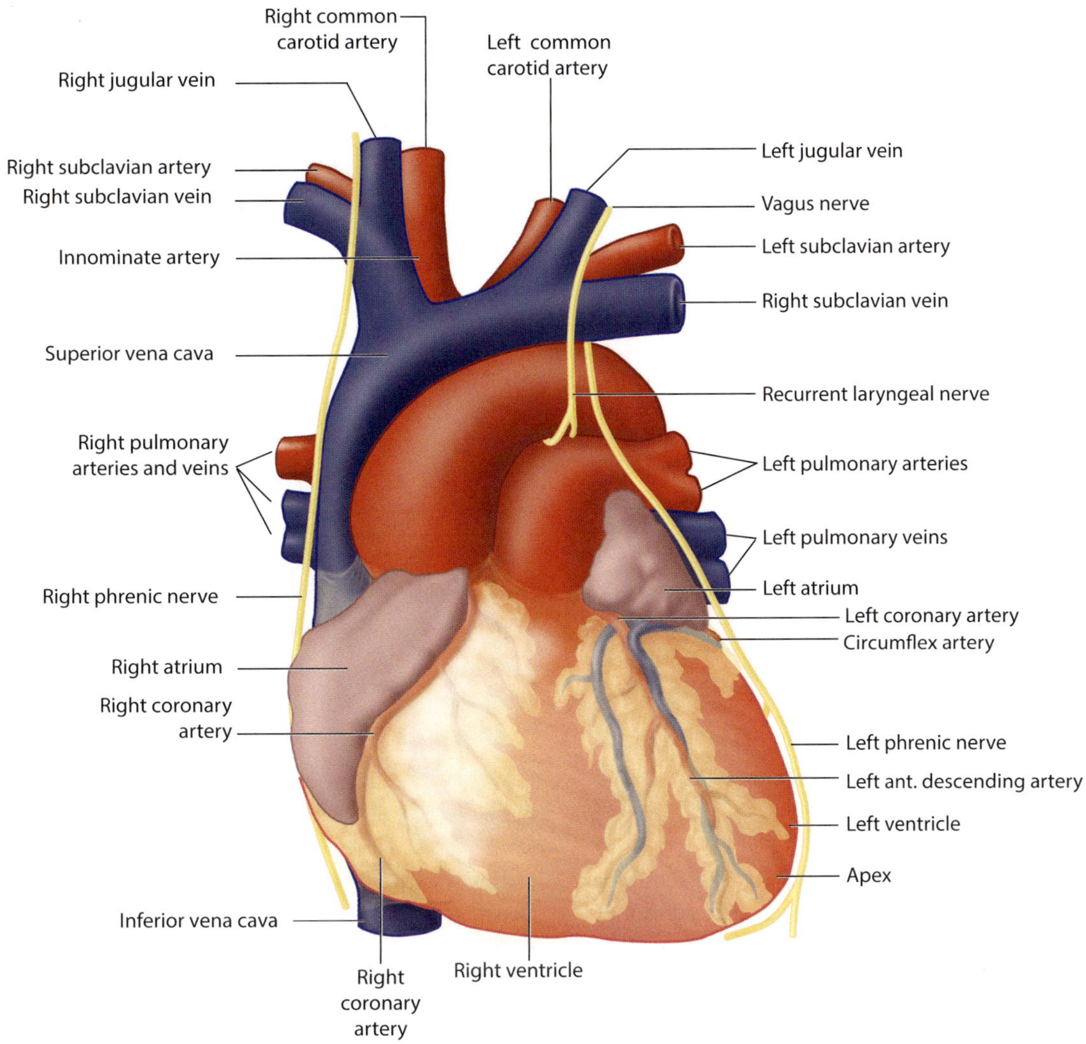

FIG. 32.1 The heart and great vessels. (From Cioffi W, et al. *Atlas of Trauma Emergency Surgical Techniques*. Philadelphia: Elsevier; 2014.)

Cardiac surgery encompasses procedures of the heart and associated great vessels performed to treat acquired or **congenital** disease. Open techniques and minimally invasive endoscopic procedures are used. The techniques used in cardiac surgery build on those used in thoracic, general, and vascular procedures. However, cardiac procedures are generally more complex and require equipment not used in other specialties. The surgical technologist may become a specialist in cardiac surgery after training in general, peripheral vascular, and thoracic surgery. This specialty requires a thorough understanding of cardiothoracic anatomy and cardiac function, as well as the ability to work in a complex surgical environment with multiple technologies.

SURGICAL ANATOMY

The thoracic cavity contains the heart and its great vessels, the lungs and their associated respiratory structures, the mediastinum, and a portion of the esophagus.

HEART

The heart is a muscular organ that contains four chambers. The two upper chambers are the right atrium and the left atrium; the two lower chambers are the right ventricle and the left ventricle (Fig. 32.1). The heart lies within a closed cavity called the *mediastinum*, between the two lungs, posterior to (behind) the sternum. Most of the heart lies to the left of the midline.

The heart is enclosed by a double-layered membrane called the *pericardium*. Pericardial fluid between the outer parietal and inner visceral pericardium lubricates the layers and prevents friction. Three tissue layers make up the heart wall: the outer *epicardium*, middle *myocardium*, and *inner endocardium*. Myocardium is a specialized muscle tissue (cardiac muscle) capable of generating electrical impulses, which cause the heart to contract.

Heart Valves

The valves of the heart maintain unidirectional blood flow. The atria are separated from the ventricles by the atrioventricular (AV) valves. The tricuspid valve lies on the right side, and the bicuspid (mitral) valve lies on the left side. The leaflets of the valves open as blood is pumped and close when the pressure on the other side of the valve exceeds the entry pressure. The AV valve leaflets are attached to the papillary muscle of the ventricles by connective tissue called *chordae tendineae*.

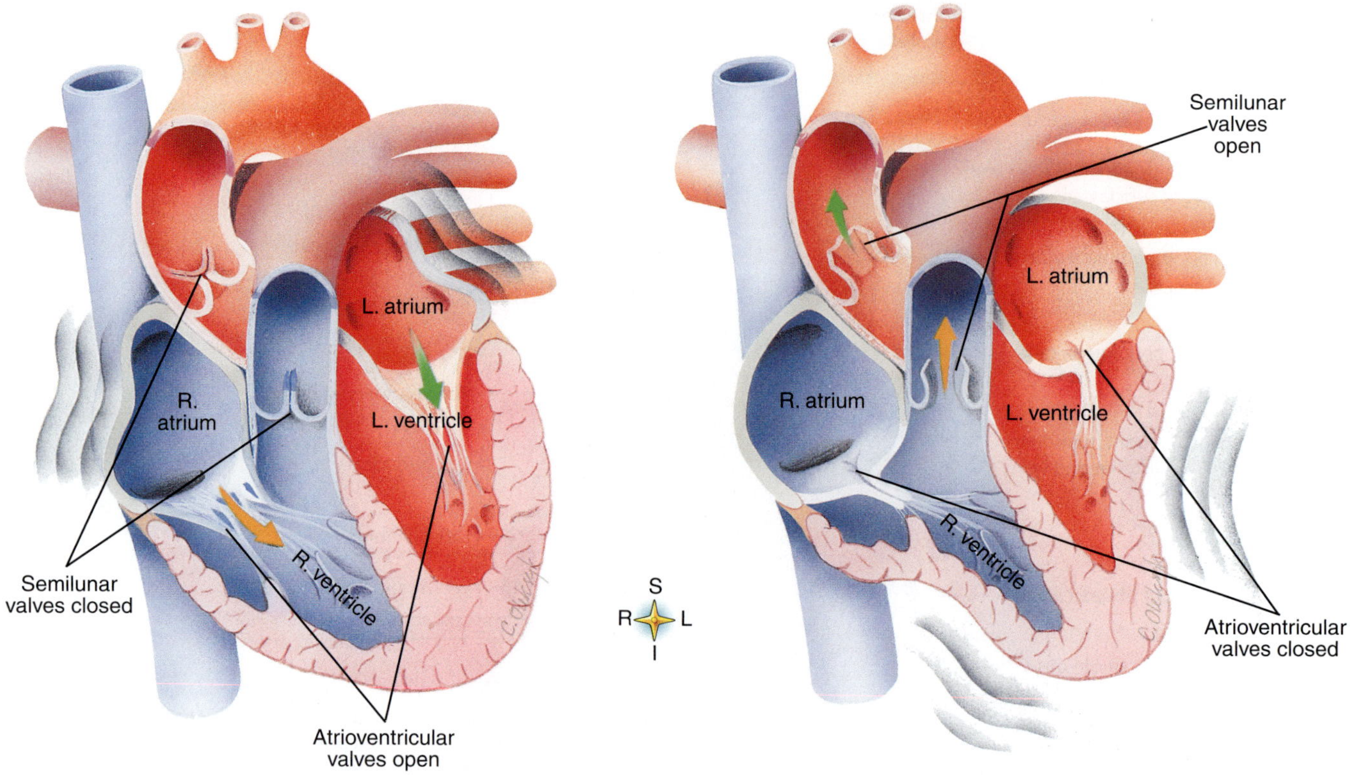

FIG. 32.2 Chambers and valves of the heart. *L.,* Left; *R.,* right. (From Patton KT, Thibodeau GA. *The Human Body in Health & Disease.* 6th ed. St Louis: Elsevier; 2014.)

The large vessels of the heart also have valves. The semilunar valves connect the ventricles to the large vessels. The pulmonary valve connects the right ventricle with the pulmonary artery. The left aortic valve connects the left ventricle to the aorta.

CARDIAC CYCLE

The pumping action of the heart from one beat to the next is called the **cardiac cycle.** The cycle occurs in two phases, systole and diastole. During **systole,** the ventricles contract; in **diastole,** they relax and fill with blood. The cycle is fully defined by the electrical impulses that occur in specific areas of the heart, the muscular activity, and the flow of blood through the chambers and vessels. The heart's four chambers are divided by a septum (Fig. 32.2). Deoxygenated blood enters the right atrium through the vena cava. The right atrium contracts and sends the blood through the tricuspid valve into the right ventricle. As the right ventricle becomes full, the tricuspid valve closes. The right ventricle then pumps blood through the pulmonic valve into the pulmonary artery and lungs, where carbon dioxide is replaced with oxygen. The pulmonary veins carry the oxygenated blood from the lungs to the left atrium. As the atrium contracts, the mitral valve opens, allowing blood to enter the left ventricle. The left ventricle is the strongest pump of the heart. It sends the blood out of the left ventricle to the aortic arch and on to the rest of the body. The heart's own blood supply is delivered by the coronary artery circulation (Fig. 32.3).

CONDUCTION SYSTEM

The electrical conduction system contains a network of specialized cells, which generate electrical activity along conduction pathways. These cells, which are found in several areas of the heart, transmit nerve signals that cause the heart muscle to contract in a coordinated way. A group of these specialized cells is called a **node.**

The sinoatrial (SA) node initiates the cardiac cycle and is sometimes called the heart's pacemaker. Impulses travel from the SA node to the AV node in the interatrial septum. From the AV node, they travel to the bundle of His at the AV junction. Conduction continues through the right and left bundle branches, ventricular walls, and Purkinje fibers. Disease or interference in the conduction system results in uncoordinated electrical activity in the cardiac muscle and may cause ineffective contractions. The conduction system is illustrated in Fig. 32.4.

DIAGNOSTIC PROCEDURES

Before surgery, the patient undergoes diagnostic studies to identify pathological conditions or anomalies. Many of these studies are performed in the interventional radiology department. Cardiac function tests may require sophisticated imaging techniques, injection of radionuclide, and physical stress tests.

Routine laboratory tests are performed to identify abnormalities of the blood, urine, cardiac enzymes, and waste products, which may indicate myocardial damage. Common tests are listed in Box 32.1.

CARDIAC CATHETERIZATION

Cardiac catheterization is an interventional radiology procedure that involves the insertion of a cardiac catheter into

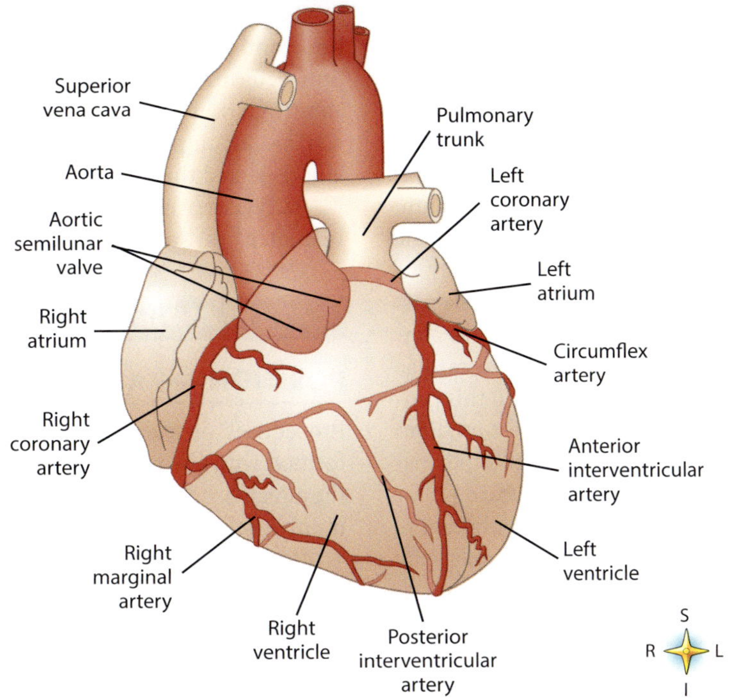

FIG. 32.3 Coronary arteries that supply blood to the heart tissue. (From Patton KT, Thibodeau GA. *The Human Body in Health & Disease*. 6th ed. St Louis: Elsevier; 2014.)

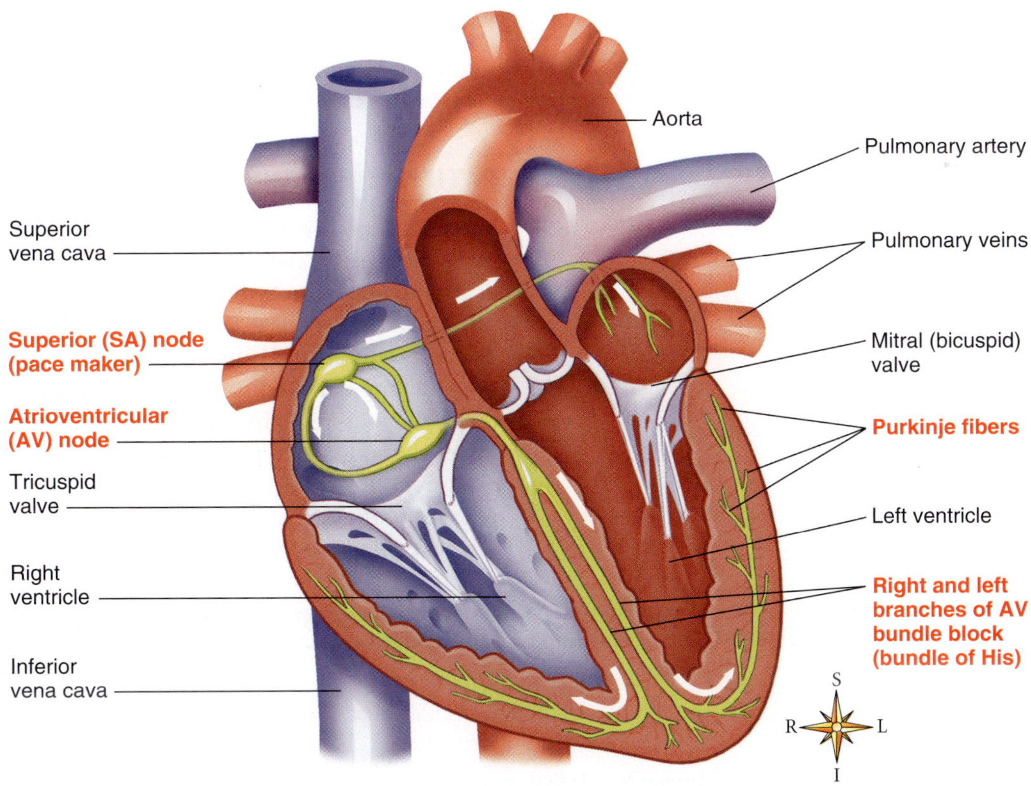

FIG. 32.4 Conduction system of the heart. (From Patton KT, Thibodeau GA. *The Human Body in Health & Disease*. 6th ed. St Louis: Elsevier; 2014.)

the heart chambers and large vessels via a peripheral artery or vein. Specific tests are then performed inside the heart and vessels, such as intravascular ultrasonography, angiography (including coronary artery imaging), and endocardial biopsy.

Left heart catheterization is often performed to assess the coronary arteries, systemic vascular resistance, aortic and mitral valve function, and left ventricular pressure. These tests are performed through a percutaneous puncture of the femoral, radial, or brachial artery, with catheterization through these vessels.

Right heart catheterization is performed to assess the right atrium and ventricle and the pulmonary artery. Pulmonary artery occlusion pressure (PAOP) is a significant test that determines cardiac volume and output. Valve function may also be tested through right heart catheterization. In this procedure, a catheter is inserted percutaneously through the femoral, subclavian, or internal jugular vein; advanced into the right atrium; and then advanced farther, into the pulmonary artery, via the tricuspid valve, right ventricle, and pulmonary valve.

Cardiac imaging has become increasingly complex in the past 10 years. In addition to standard angiography, in which a contrast medium is injected to obtain real-time images of the cardiac system, digital subtraction angiography is also used. In this process, only the vessels and chambers in which contrast medium is injected are shown on the fluoroscopic image. All other tissues are masked or subtracted. Aortic imaging is performed for the assessment of **coarctation** of the aorta, valve regurgitation, congenital anomalies, and **aneurysm.** Ventricular angiography demonstrates the movement of blood through the valves and can be used to measure the ejection fraction (the amount of blood pumped from the ventricles) and end-systolic and end-diastolic volumes. Cardiac imaging data are shown in Table 32.1.

Intravascular ultrasound is performed with an end catheter transducer (catheter fitted with a transducer at its end), which can be advanced into the lumen of the blood vessel to determine the rate of blood flow.

BOX 32.1 Cardiac Diagnostic Tests

Resting electrocardiogram (ECG)
Exercise ECG (stress test)
Chest radiography
Echocardiogram
Radionucleotide scanning
Computed tomography (CT) scan
Positron emission tomography (PET) scan with or without stress test
Magnetic resonance imaging (MRI) and magnetic resonance angiography (MRA)
Pulmonary function tests
Aortography
Electrophysiology
Cardiac catheterization
Endomyocardial biopsy
Mediastinoscopy

Oxygen saturation can be measured at various points in the heart and large vessels during catheterization. This information determines whether blood is being shunted (taking an abnormal route).

Cardiac output is measured by calculating the amount of blood ejected through the heart per minute.

Cardiac muscle biopsy is performed to detect tissue rejection after heart transplantation.

CASE PLANNING

POSITIONING AND INCISIONS

Procedures of the heart and associated structures are performed with the patient in the supine or lateral position with the affected side up. The following are the incisions most commonly used in open cardiac surgery:

- *Median* **sternotomy** *(supine):* A partial or full midline incision is made through the sternum.
- *Anterolateral, posterolateral:* This is a modification of the lateral position in which the patient is supine with soft padding under the hip and shoulder of the affected side. This rolls the thorax slightly upward. The shoulder of the affected side then is abducted, and the arm is suspended safely on an overhead table brace (see Chapter 16).
- *Mini-***thoracotomy** *(supine):* The 2-inch (5-cm) right or left mini-thoracotomy is made between the ribs for access during minimally invasive and robotic procedures.

(See **Table 32.2** for thoracic incisions.)

PATIENT PREP

Many cardiac procedures require a skin prep that extends beyond the incisional area. This is because access to peripheral veins and arteries may be needed for cannulation or excision during cardiac surgery. For example, during coronary bypass graft procedures, a full anterior body prep and peripheral limb prep are implemented so that the surgeon can have access to the saphenous veins in the legs and the axillary veins of the upper thorax. Whenever the legs are prepped, a safe method of suspending the legs must be used. This may involve the suspension of the legs or bilateral leg rests. Access to the femoral artery requires a complete groin prep.

TABLE 32.1 Angiographic Data

Angiographic Data	Findings
Coronary arteries	Anatomy/function of the coronary vascular bed, distal coronary flow, atrioventricular fistula, atherosclerosis, anomalous origin of coronary arteries
Ventriculography	Anatomy/function of ventricles and associated structures, left ventricular aneurysm, congenital abnormalities, valvular stenosis/regurgitation, shunts
Valvular angiography	Intact mitral/tricuspid complex, valvular incompetence/stenosis/regurgitation
Pulmonary angiography	Pulmonary embolism, congenital abnormalities
Aortography	Patency of aortic branches; normal mobility, competence, and anatomy of aortic valve; aneurysms (saccular, fusiform); origin of aortic dissection; shunts or anomalous connections; congenital defects or obstructions

Modified from Pagana KD, Pagana TJ, eds. *Mosby's Diagnostic and Laboratory Test Reference.* 7th ed. St Louis: Mosby; 2005.

INSTRUMENTS AND EQUIPMENT

Cardiac surgery requires a general surgery set augmented with cardiac instruments, general thoracic instruments (including stapling devices), and lung instruments, depending on the procedure. Specific instruments for coronary artery, valve, aneurysm, chest wall, and lung surgery may be added. Instrumentation can be complex, requiring experience and advanced organizational skills to anticipate the steps of a procedure. Cardiac-specific instruments are illustrated in the Cardiac Instruments table. Refer also to Chapter 31 to review thoracic instruments.

CARDIAC INSTRUMENTS

POTTS SMITH SCISSORS 8¼″, 12″

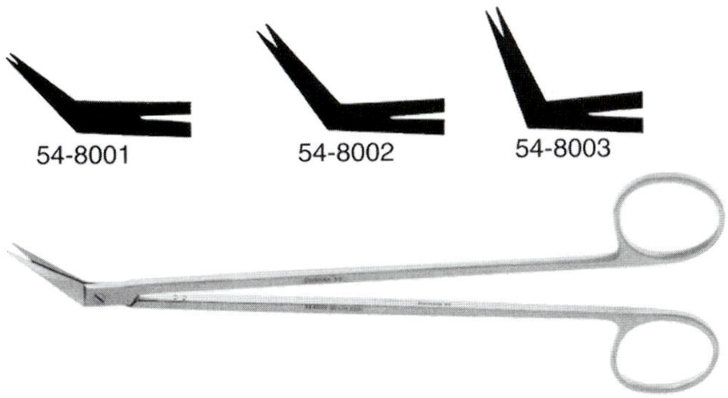

Copyright 2016 Symmetry Surgical, Inc.; photo courtesy Symmetry Surgical, Inc.

DIETHRICH CORONARY ARTERY SCISSORS (ANGLED 25° TO 125°) 7°

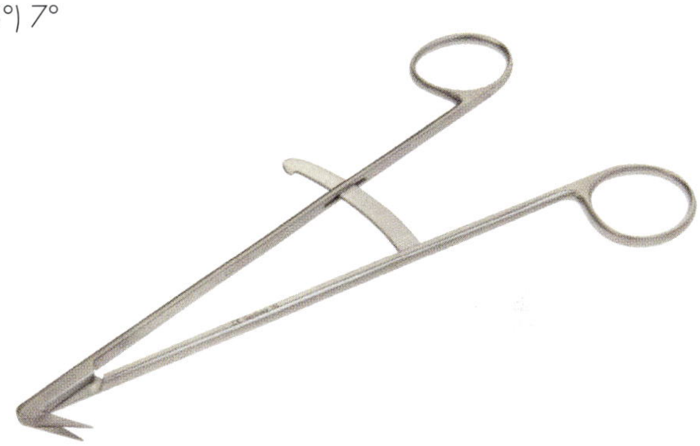

Copyright 2016 Symmetry Surgical, Inc.; photo courtesy Symmetry Surgical, Inc.

METZENBAUM CLASSIC PLUS DISSECTING SCIS 9″

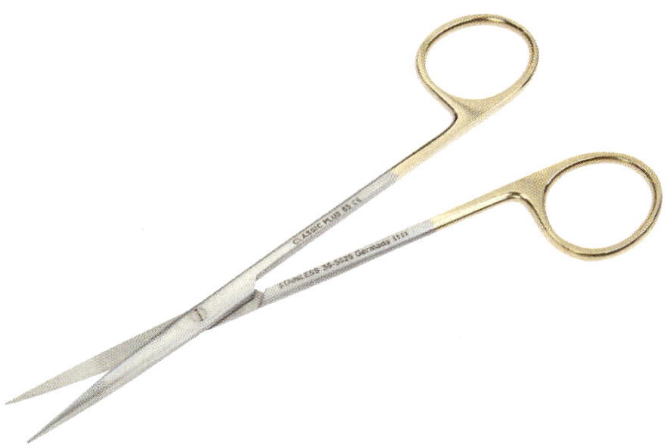

Copyright 2016 Symmetry Surgical, Inc.; photo courtesy Symmetry Surgical, Inc.

GERALD FORCEPS 1 × 2 TEETH 5½″

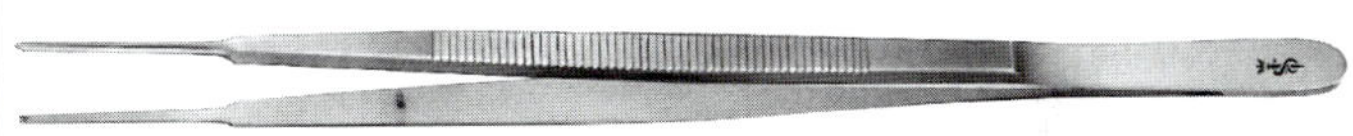

Photo courtesy Aesculap Inc., Center Valley, PA.

COOLEY PEDIATRIC ANASTOMOSIS CLMP 7″

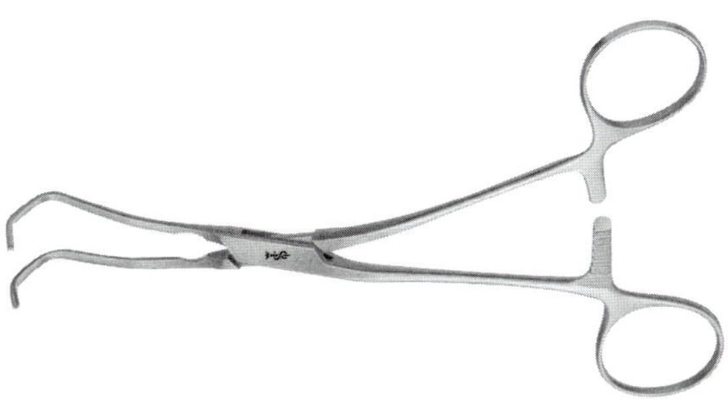

Photo courtesy Aesculap Inc., Center Valley, PA.

DEBAKEY ATRAU VENA CAVA CLMP 8″

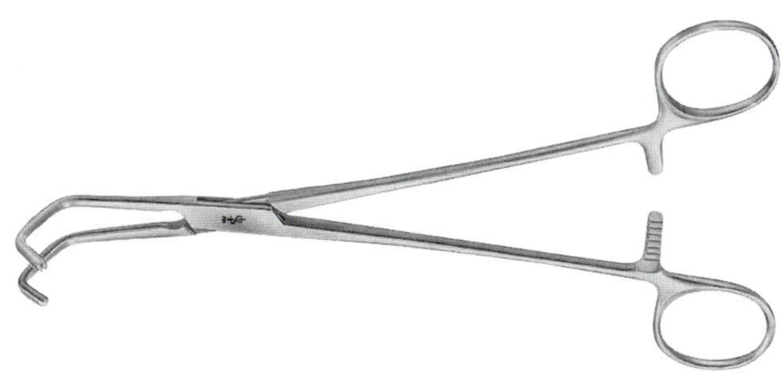

Photo courtesy Aesculap Inc., Center Valley, PA.

CARDIAC INSTRUMENTS—cont'd

DEBAKEY PATENT DUCTUS CLMP 6¼″

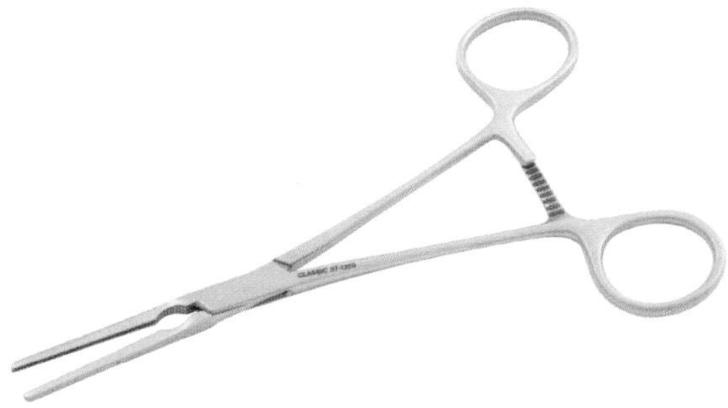

Copyright 2016 Symmetry Surgical, Inc.; photo courtesy Symmetry Surgical, Inc.

DERRA VENA CAVA CLMP 10″

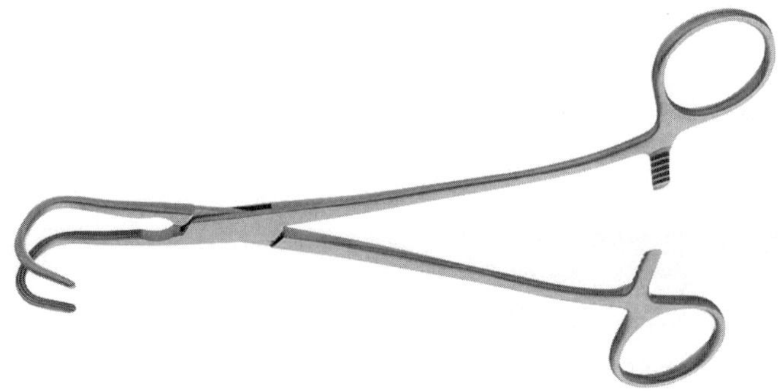

Courtesy and copyright Becton, Dickinson and Company.

GLOVER CLMP CURVED 8½″

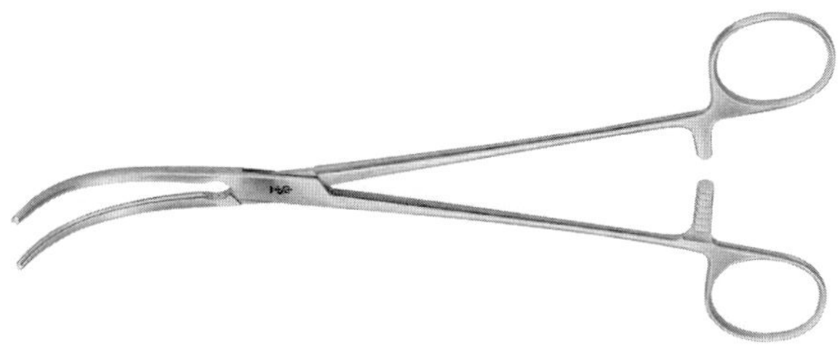

Photo courtesy Aesculap Inc., Center Valley, PA.

SATINSKY TANGENTIAL CLMP 9½″

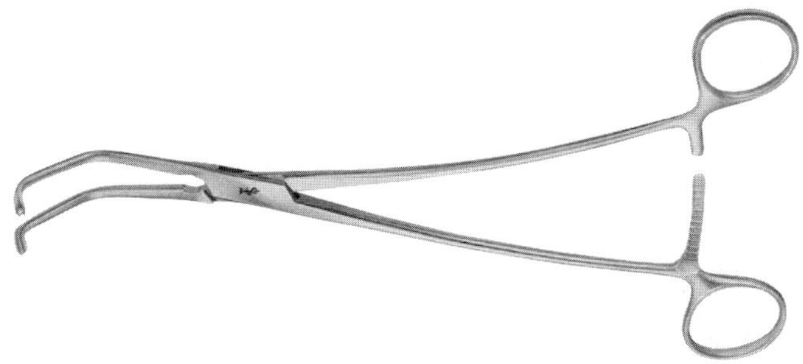

Photo courtesy Aesculap Inc., Center Valley, PA.

DEBAKEY MULTI PURPOSE CLMP 30°

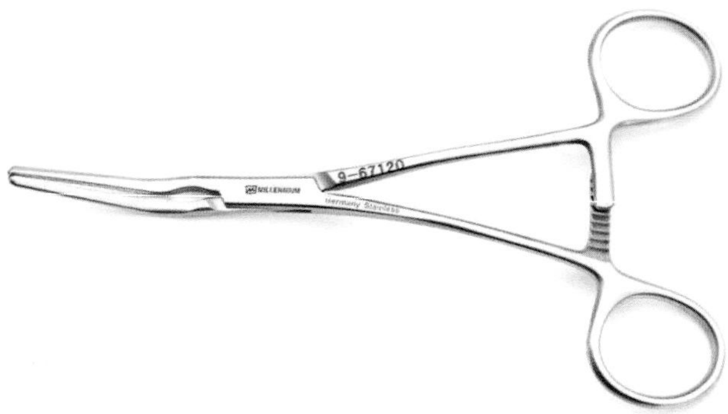

Millennium Surgical Corp.

GLOVER COARCTATION CLMP 10½″

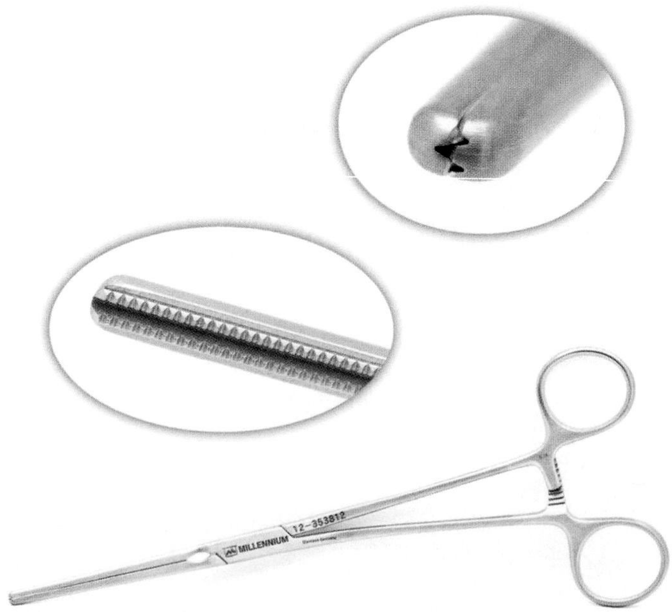

Millennium Surgical Corp.

LEITZ CLAMP 8″

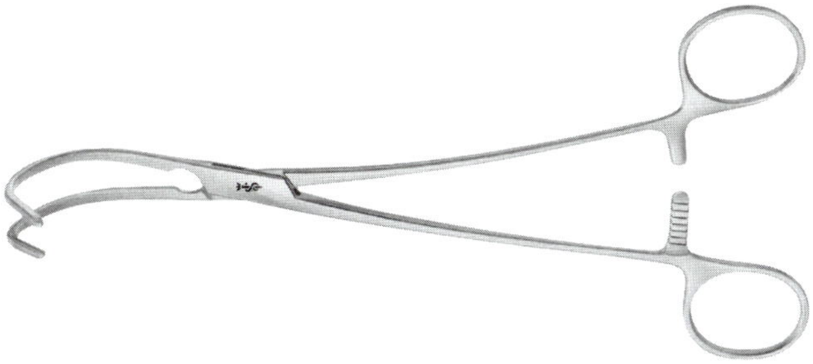

Photo courtesy Aesculap Inc., Center Valley, PA.

DEBAKEY AORTIC ANEUR ISM CLAMP 10½″

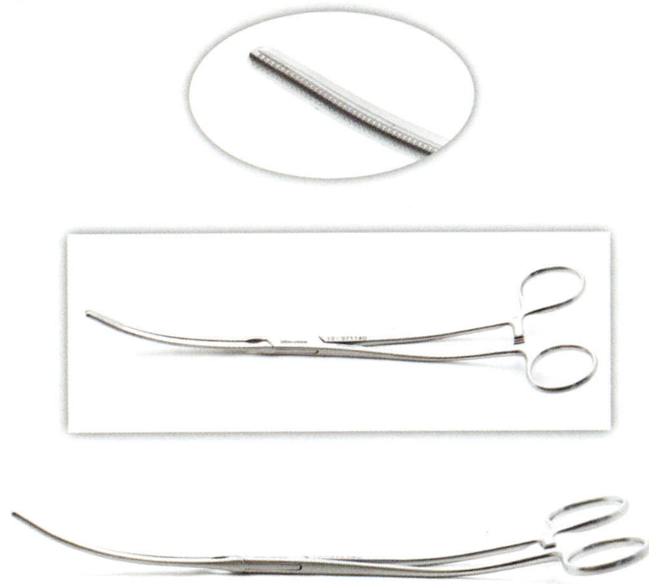

Millennium Surgical Corp.

ALLISON LUNG RETRACTOR

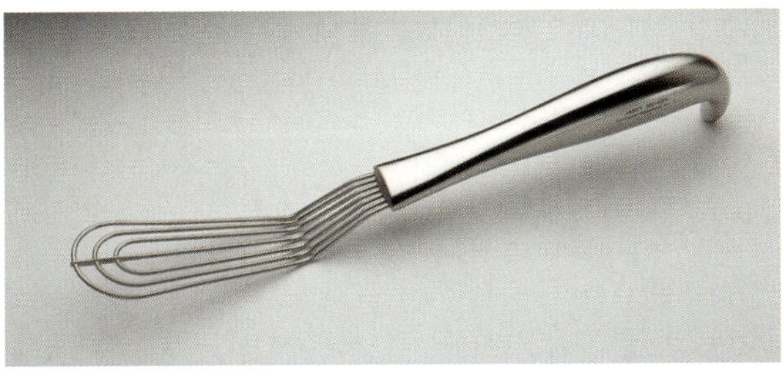

From Nemitz. *Surgical Instrumentation: An Interactive Approach.* 3rd ed. St. Louis: Elsevier; 2019.

MAYO.HEGAR NEEDLE HOLDER 8½″

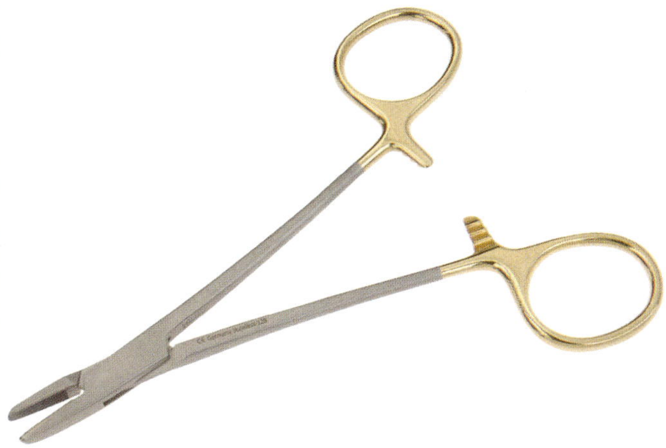

Copyright 2016 Symmetry Surgical, Inc.; photo courtesy Symmetry Surgical, Inc.

DAVIDSON SCAPULA RETRACTOR

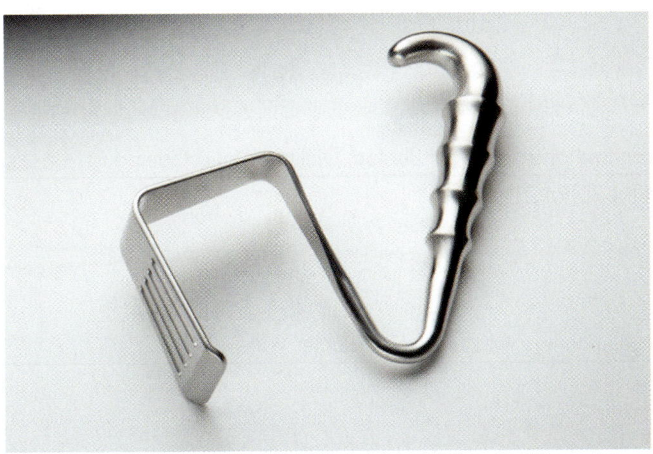

From Nemitz. *Surgical Instrumentation: An Interactive Approach.* 3rd ed. St. Louis: Elsevier; 2019.

FARABEUF RASP

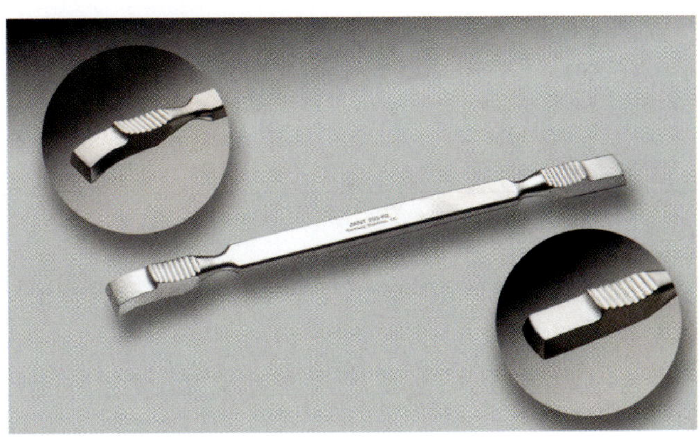

From Nemitz. *Surgical Instrumentation: An Interactive Approach.* 3rd ed. St. Louis: Elsevier; 2019.

CARDIAC INSTRUMENTS—cont'd

STERNAL WIRE TWISTERS 6¼″

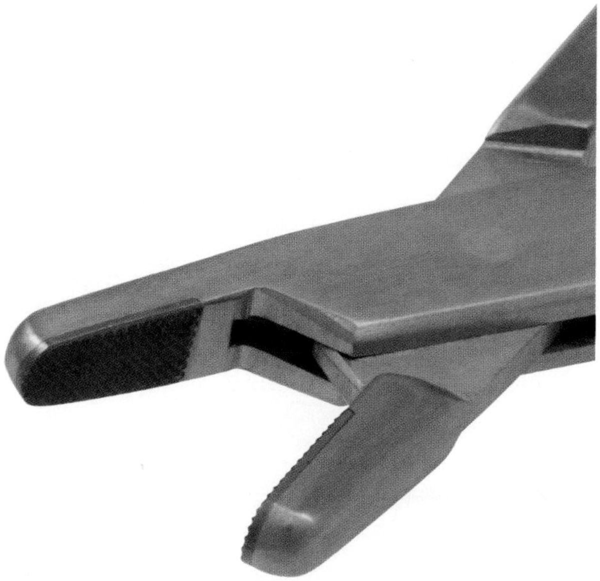

DEBAKEY DILATORS 7½″

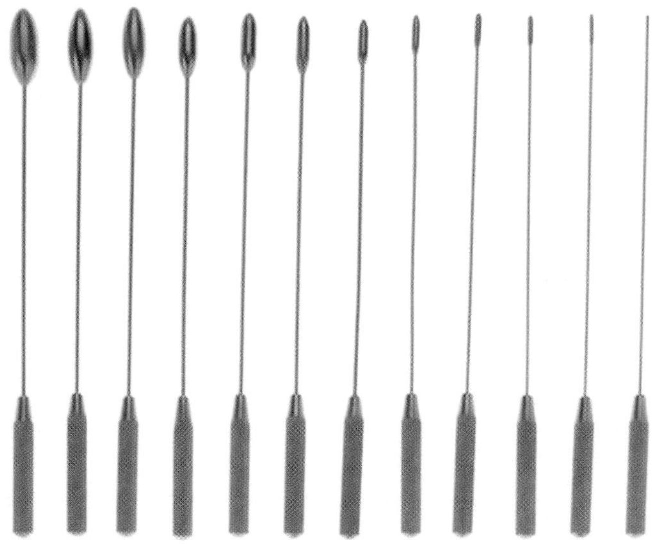

AORTA PUNCH 8½″

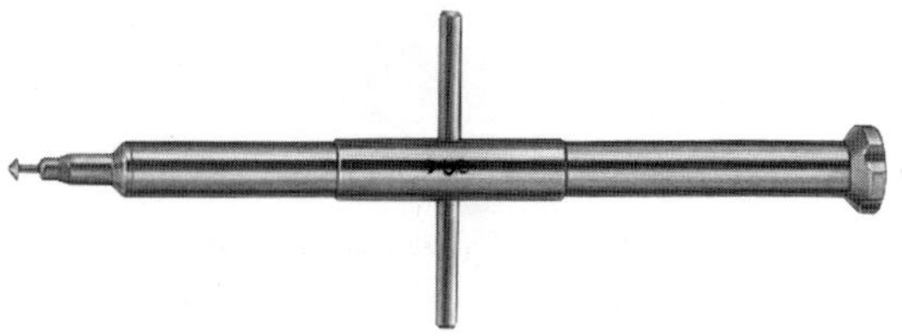

Photo courtesy Aesculap Inc., Center Valley, PA.

FINOCHIETTO RETRACTOR 7⅞″

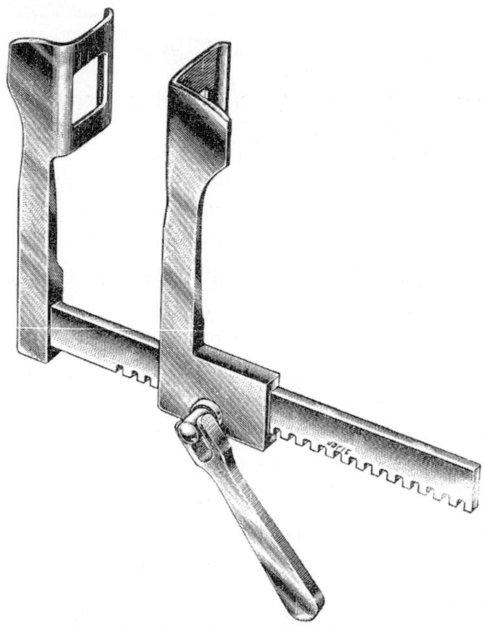

ROCHESTER ATRIAL SEPTUM RETRACTOR 5½″

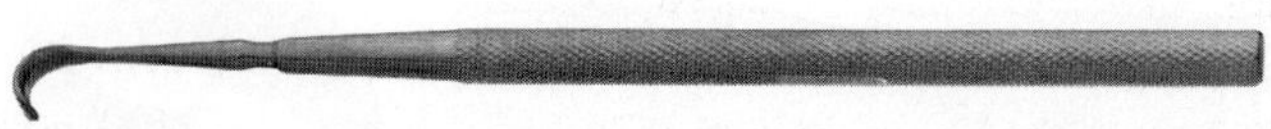

VEIN RETRACTOR 14″

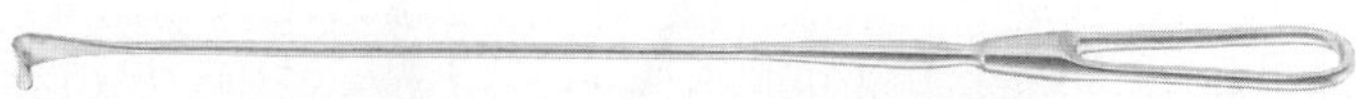

Photo courtesy Aesculap Inc., Center Valley, PA.

CARDIAC INSTRUMENTS—cont'd

ATRIUM RETRACTOR 10¾″

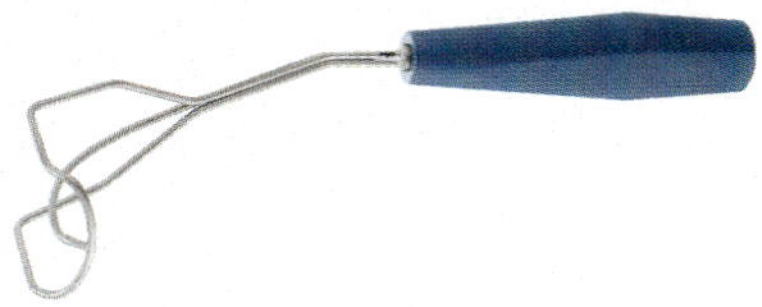

Photo courtesy Aesculap Inc., Center Valley, PA.

WEITLANER RETRACTOR 4⅜″

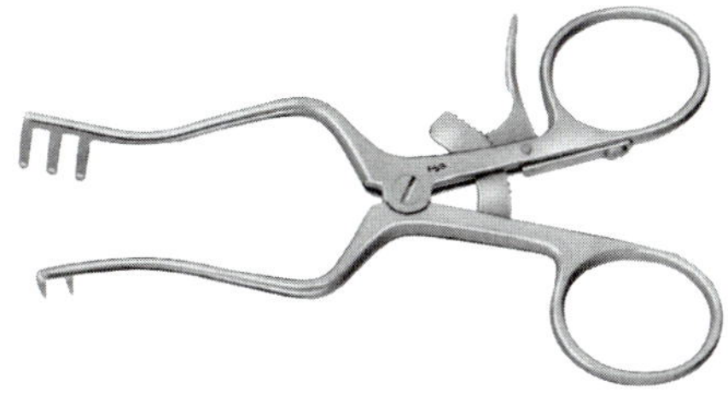

Photo courtesy Aesculap Inc., Center Valley, PA.

PARSONNET EPICARDIAL RETRACTOR

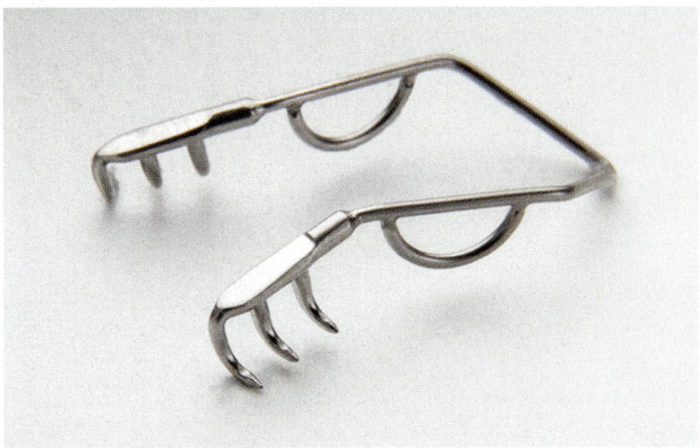

From Nemitz. *Surgical Instrumentation: An Interactive Approach.* 3rd ed. St. Louis: Elsevier; 2019.

The *Rumel tourniquet,* commonly used in cardiovascular surgery, is a short length of synthetic tubing either commercially prepared or cut from a straight (Robinson) urinary catheter. The tourniquet is threaded over cannulation sutures to help hold them in place. The Rumel tourniquet is also used when large vessels are occluded or isolated with a vessel loop or umbilical tape (a length of cotton is passed under a vessel for retraction). A stylet, such as that from a Rumel tourniquet, is used to snare the strands of suture or tape and bring them through the lumen of the tubing. The tubing is tightened against the cannula or vessel by pulling on the strands, which are held using a hemostat placed at the upper end.

A standard open-heart instrument set contains instruments for most procedures. Additional items can be added according to the procedure.

Coronary artery instruments are extremely delicate. They include scissors, forceps, and needle holders, which are similar to routine vascular instruments.

Minimally invasive coronary procedures require longer instruments with the same precision tips. In off-pump coronary anastomosis, a flexible suction tip coronary stabilizing device can be positioned on either side of the coronary artery to minimize cardiac movement. *Valve instruments* include special retractors to expose the valve, suture holders, and accessories for the valve prosthesis. These include sizers and holders.

Instrument and Equipment Management

Among the skills required for participation in a cardiac team is the ability to organize and maintain instrument and equipment tables. Many facilities require a standard setup for the surgical technologist. It is usually necessary to maintain at least two back tables and three Mayo stands. These are set up with specific purpose and design for the scrub to know at any moment where specific instruments are and to provide specific spaces for the preparation of supplies. The cardiac operating room is crowded with physiological monitoring and anesthesia equipment, **cardiopulmonary bypass machine,** instrument tables, solution basins, and electrosurgery equipment. This means that space needed for the surgical instruments must be planned and conserved. Surgical technologists wishing to specialize in cardiac surgery will have ample opportunity to work with mentors whose techniques and wisdom will guide the learning process.

Vessel and Patch Grafts

Many types of grafts are available in assorted sizes; the two most common types are knitted and woven grafts. Knitted grafts are soft and porous. They are preferred for small artery anastomosis or for very fragile vessels. Woven grafts are used for large artery replacement because their tight weave prevents loss of blood through the graft.

Grafts are available as straight or bifurcated tubes made of Teflon, Dacron, or polytetrafluoroethylene (PTFE). To prevent waste and expense, only the appropriate size of graft, as determined by using graft sizers during the procedure, should be opened. As with all implants, the type, size, and serial number of the graft are recorded on the patient's operative record by the circulating nurse.

Patch grafts, made of Teflon (or PTFE), are used to strengthen a suture line or to close a defect (an abnormal opening in the tissue). Patches are cut to size as needed. Teflon felt material in the form of small pledgets is used along

TABLE 32.2 Thoracic Incisions

Incision	Position of Patient	Indications	Special Patient Needs
Median sternotomy: Incision down the center of the sternum	Supine	Most adult cardiac procedures except those on branch pulmonary arteries, distal transverse aortic arch, and descending thoracic aorta; OPCAB	Padding for the hands, elbows, feet, back of head, and dependent bony prominences
Mini-sternotomy: Partial upper or lower sternal incision starting either from the sternal notch or the xiphoid process and extending to the midportion of the sternum; lower end sternal splitting (LESS)	Supine	MAS, on-CPB or off-CPB procedures	Same as for a median sternotomy
Para-sternotomy: Resection of the right or left costal cartilages (from the second to the fifth cartilage, depending on the surgical target)	Supine; a small roll may be placed under the affected side	Left: MAS CABG Right: MAS CABG, valve procedures	Same as for a median sternotomy; risk of postoperative chest wall instability
Anterolateral thoracotomy: Curvilinear incision along the subpectoral groove to the axillary line	Supine with a pad or pillow under the operative site; arm on the affected side is supported in a sling or overarm board; the arm on the unaffected side may be tucked along the side	MAS, MIDCAB, trauma to the anterior pericardium and left ventricle; repeat sternotomy	Padding for extremities; pad or other device to elevate the affected side; arm board or sling for the arm on the affected side
Left anterior small thoracotomy (LAST), right anterior mini-thoracotomy: Curvilinear incision along the subpectoral groove, right or left side	Supine with a small roll under the affected side	Left: MAS, MIDCAB Right: MAS valve procedures or CABG	Same as anterolateral thoracotomy
Lateral thoracotomy: Curvilinear incision along the costochondral junction anteriorly to the posterior border of the scapula	Placed on the side with the arms extended and the axilla and head supported; the knees and legs are protected	Lung biopsies; first rib resection; lobectomy	Arm board, overarm board, axillary roll, padding for extremities, padding between the legs; sandbags, straps, wide tape, or other devices to support the torso
Posterolateral thoracotomy: Curvilinear incision from the subpectoral crease below the nipple, extended laterally and posteriorly along the ribs almost to the posterior midline below the scapula (the location of the intercostal incision depends on the surgical site); used less often with the availability of VATS techniques	Lateral with the arms extended and the axilla and head supported; the knees and legs are protected	First rib resection; lobectomy	Similar to needs for a lateral thoracotomy
Trans-sternal bilateral anterior thoracotomy (clamshell): Sub-mammary incision extending from one anterior axillary line to the other across the sternum at the fourth interspace	Supine	Lung transplantation; emergency access to the heart when a sternal saw is not available	Same as median sternotomy; requires the transection of left and right IMA
Subxiphoid incision: Vertical midline incision from over the xiphoid process to about 4 inches (10 cm) inferiorly (the lower portion of the sternum may be divided to improve exposure)	Supine	Pericardial drainage, pericardial biopsy, attachment of pacemaker electrodes, MAS	Same as median sternotomy
Thoracoabdominal incision: Low curvilinear incision on the left side, extended to the anterior midline, and continued vertically down the abdomen	Anterior thoracotomy with the chest at a 45-degree angle to the table; abdomen supine	Thoracoabdominal aneurysm	Same as anterolateral thoracotomy

CABG, Coronary artery bypass grafting; *CPB*, cardiopulmonary bypass; *IMA*, internal mammary artery; *MAS*, minimal access surgery; *MIDCAB*, minimal access direct coronary artery bypass; *OPCAB*, off-pump coronary artery bypass; *VATS*, video-assisted thoracoscopic surgery.

Modified from Rothrock JC, ed. *Alexander's Care of the Patient in Surgery*. 13th ed. St Louis: Mosby; 2007; Waldhausen JA, Pierce WS, Campbell DB, eds. *Surgery of the Chest. 6th ed.* St Louis: Mosby; 1996; Zipes DP, Libby P, Bonow RO, Braunwald E, eds. *Braunwald's Heart Disease*. 7th ed. Philadelphia: Saunders; 2005.

the suture line to reinforce the anastomosis. To prepare these, the scrub should place a mosquito clamp in the middle of the pledget and pass a suture through the pledget on both sides of the mosquito clamps, or the clamp and pledget are passed to the surgeon for suture attachment.

Prosthetic Valves

A full set of prosthetic heart valves and their sizers, handles, and holders are required for valve replacement. As the surgical technologist you should be familiar with the different types of valves and accessory equipment. Valves are extremely expensive and should be handled as little as possible. The scrub and the circulator must verify the type, size, and identification number of the valve. The circulator records the valve identification information on the patient's operative record. There are many different heart valves produced by a number of different companies internationally. The basic types are mechanical and biological. Biological valves are stored in a glutaraldehyde solution, which must be removed by rinsing the valve according to the manufacturer's specifications.

Pacemaker

A **pacemaker** is a device that produces electrical impulses that stimulate the heart muscle. This process is called *pacing the heart*. Pacing batteries may be temporary (external) or permanent (internal). Temporary electrodes are implanted on the surface of the heart at the time of cardiac surgery. Two types of permanent electrodes are used, endocardial (transvenous) electrodes and epicardial electrodes. An endocardial electrode is inserted into a vein and advanced into the right ventricle under fluoroscopy. An epicardial electrode is sutured directly to the heart on the atrium, ventricle, or both (see procedure later).

Defibrillator

Defibrillator paddles are required to convert **fibrillation** (ineffectual quivering of the ventricles) into a functional rhythm. Internal defibrillator paddles are kept readily available on the sterile field. When needed, such as during ventricular fibrillation, the surgeon places a paddle on each side of the heart and instructs the circulator to set the charge on the defibrillator. The application of electricity to the heart shocks the cells, converting the rhythm back to normal. When the defibrillator is in use, all personnel must stand clear of the patient to avoid receiving an electric shock.

Disposable, adhesive defibrillator pads may be used during repeat sternotomy or minimally invasive procedures.

Cardiopulmonary Bypass Machine and Cannulas

The cardiopulmonary bypass (CPB) machine takes the place of the heart and lungs during open heart surgery. Blood that is returning to the heart is diverted through the pump-oxygenator and then returns to arterial circulation in the body (shown later in CPB procedure).

The surgical technologist should be familiar with the basic function and operation of the pump. This includes the size of the pump lines and how they connect to the patient. The scrub should also know which lines infuse blood and which remove blood, as well as the types of cannulas. The order of cannulation for a standard bypass procedure is aortic, venous, transatrial cardioplegia cannula (retrograde), right superior pulmonary vein vent (LV vent), then antegrade. Femoral arterial and venous cannulas may be used depending on the type of surgery or if the patient's ascending aorta cannot be cannulated.

- *Aortic cannula:* May have a straight or an angled tip to direct the blood toward the descending thoracic aorta. This cannula carries oxygenated (arterial) blood.
- *Venous cannula:* Straight-ended with multiple holes in the distal tip. This type of cannula is used to **shunt** blood from the heart. A two-stage venous cannula also has openings in the midportion of the catheter.
- *Transatrial cannula (retrograde):* Placed into the coronary sinus to deliver cardioplegia to protect the back of the heart. Some are self-inflated; others require the use of a 3-cc syringe.
- *Right superior pulmonary vent catheter (LV vent):* Also used to decompress the left ventricle and remove intracardiac air.
- *Coronary antegrade perfusion cannula:* Has a cuff near its tip to prevent the cannula from being inserted too far into the coronary arteries. A 14-gauge angiocatheter may also be used. It is used to infuse cardioplegic solution directly into the heart.
- *Femoral arterial cannula:* Also carries oxygenated (arterial) blood, is tapered to match the size of the artery, and has a beveled end to allow easier insertion.

Cardioplegic Solution

Cardioplegia is the intentional interruption of the heart's pumping action. A cardioplegic solution contains various additives, the most important being potassium chloride. The solution may be cooled or warmed for administration.

A cardioplegic solution is administered by two methods. In antegrade cardioplegic infusion (after the aortic **cross-clamp** has been applied), an antegrade cannula is placed in the aorta (the aortic "root"). The cardioplegic solution is infused into the aorta. It then flows into the right and left coronary openings and into the coronary circulation. In retrograde cardioplegic infusion, a catheter is placed in the coronary sinus of the right atrium and into the great cardiac vein. The cardioplegic solution is then infused into the coronary venous system.

SURGICAL PROCEDURES

MEDIAN STERNOTOMY

A median sternotomy is a midline incision used for surgical procedures of the heart and large vessels in the thoracic cavity. The following discusses the steps for opening and closing the chest only.

POSITION:	Supine
INCISION:	Median sternotomy
PREP AND DRAPING:	Thoracic
INSTRUMENTS:	Major thoracic set, sternal saw, sternal retractor

Technical Points and Discussion

OPENING THE CHEST

1. ***The patient is prepped and draped.***
The patient is placed in supine position, prepped, and draped for a sternal midline incision.

2. ***The incision is made through soft tissues, and the xiphoid is divided.***
The surgeon makes a midline incision from the sternal notch to approximately 2 inches below the xiphoid. The subcutaneous tissue and linea alba (the fascial layer distal to the xiphoid) are divided with the knife or ESU. The surgeon digitally separates the underlying tissue from the sternal notch and xiphoid. The xiphoid is then divided on the midline with curved Mayo scissors.

3. ***The sternum is divided.***
A sternal saw is placed in the center of the xiphoid or sternal notch, and the sternum is divided. Army-Navy retractors are used to elevate the sternal edge as the periosteum bleeding is controlled using the ESU. Bone wax may be applied to prevent bleeding from the marrow.

4. ***The heart is exposed.***
The surgeon may or may not place a moist laparotomy sponge over the edges of the sternum before the placement of the sternal retractor. The sternal retractor is opened to expose the pericardium. This provides maximum exposure of the heart and ascending aorta.
The surgeon elevates the pericardium with vascular forceps or a clamp to prevent injury to the heart. The pericardium is then incised using the ESU or scissors to expose the heart and ascending aorta.

5. ***If CPB is planned, the heart and aorta are cannulated.***
If the procedure requires bypass, traction sutures may be placed through the edges of the pericardium and sewn to the periosteum. The heart and aorta are then cannulated for CPB. If an **off-pump procedure** is to be performed (i.e., CPB is not needed), cannulation is not required. However, the scrub should be prepared to institute bypass if the patient's condition deteriorates. A median sternotomy is illustrated in Fig. 32.5.

CLOSING THE STERNOTOMY INCISION

Sternotomy Closure

6. ***Chest tubes are positioned.***
Before the chest is closed, two chest drainage tubes are placed in the wound.

7. ***Wires are placed through the sternum, or a sternal plating system may be used.***
After the surgical procedure, drainage catheters are inserted to remove blood, fluid, and air from the pericardium and the pleural spaces (if they have been entered). Temporary pacing wires are placed on the epicardial surface of the heart. The surgeon places six to eight wire sutures through each sternal edge. The size of the wire ranges from 4 to 7. When passing stainless steel sutures, the scrub holds the free ends of the wire to control the ends and protect them from contamination. A wire twister is needed to secure the sutures, which are cut using wire-cutting scissors and buried in the sternum using a heavy straight clamp.

8. ***The sternal edges are approximated.***
The sternal holes are checked for any bleeding. The surgeon tightens the wires and twists each one to bring the sternal edges together. The surgeon uses a wire twister to make a final twist, burying the ends in the periosteum. The surgeon approximates the fascia and periosteum with interrupted sutures, such as size 0 polyester sutures.

CARDIOPULMONARY BYPASS

CPB diverts blood away from the heart and lungs so that surgery can be performed. An increasing number of cardiac procedures are performed without the use of CPB. However, many types of surgery, such as valve replacement, heart transplant, and aneurysm repair, do require bypass.

CPB may be total or partial. The surgeon performs total bypass by tightening umbilical tapes around the venae cavae and cannulas. This forces all blood returning to the right side of the heart into the cannula and pump. It also prevents air from entering the venous line and obstructing the flow of blood to the pump when the right side of the heart is open. Total bypass is also used for procedures such as mitral valve replacement, repair of septal defects, resection of a left ventricular aneurysm, and heart transplant. In partial bypass, blood can escape around the cannula and enter the heart. Partial bypass is often used during aortic valve replacement. It is also used to support a patient in emergencies such as cardiac arrest or a ruptured aneurysm. Fig. 32.6 illustrates a typical bypass circuit.

A median sternotomy incision is used to expose the heart. Access to the circulatory system is performed by inserting cannulas into the venae cavae and ascending aorta. The cannulas are attached to pump tubing. Fig. 32.7 shows an arterial and venous cannula.

In both types of bypass, blood returns to the pump through the cannula by gravity drainage and is pumped back into the circulation by a roller head (or a centrifugal pump) on the bypass machine. When the right side of the heart is open and the patient is on bypass, the risk exists that air will enter the venous line. This can cause an "air lock" (a large amount of air in the venous line), which may obstruct the flow of blood to the pump. The vacuum created by the pump draws the air away from the heart and into the pump.

The surgical technologist must always watch for the presence of air in the heart or pump lines and alert the surgeon immediately if air is noticed. Air must be removed to prevent an air embolus. This can be done by manipulating the venous line.

The cannulation sites are selected according to the patient's pathology and the ability to access preferred anatomical sites.

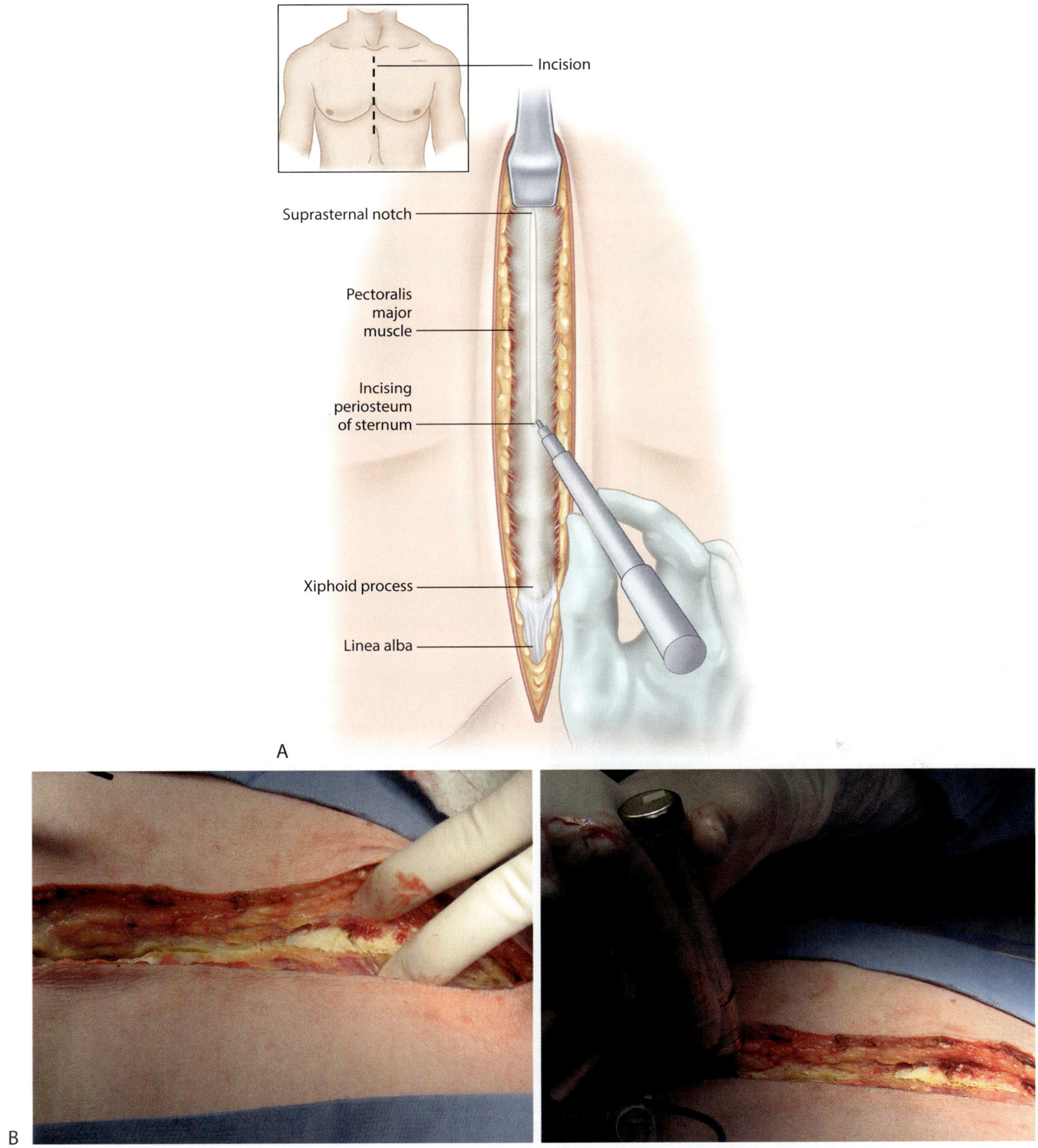

FIG. 32.5 Median sternotomy. (A) Incision. (B) Carrying the incision to the sternum and sternotomy using a powered sternal saw. (From Selke F, Ruel M, eds. *Atlas of Cardiac Surgical Techniques.* Philadelphia: Saunders; 2010.)

Several definitions are important to learn in preparing to assist in surgery requiring CPB:

- *Venous cannulation* pulls blood from the venous circulation. A number of devices are used in CPB by the perfusionist to draw the blood out of the heart. However, the venous cannula is the starting point. Venous cannulation usually takes place through the right atrium.
- *Atrial cannulation* is the means by which blood is returned to the heart during CPB via the atrial cannula. The most common site is the ascending aorta. However, the femoral artery is also used, especially in patients with severe atherosclerotic disease.
- *Cardiotomy blood* is collected directly from the wound cavity using a suction device. The blood is transferred to

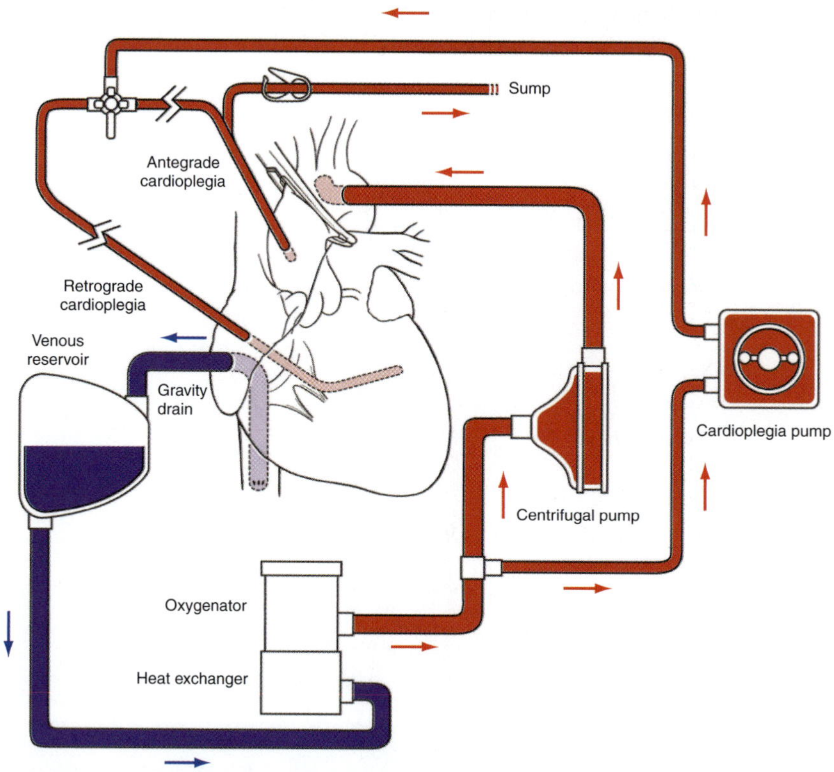

FIG. 32.6 Cardiopulmonary bypass circuit. (From Townsend C, Beauchamp B, Evers B, Mattox K, eds. *Sabiston Textbook of Surgery: The Biological Basis of Modern Surgical Practice*. 19th ed. Philadelphia: Elsevier; 2012.)

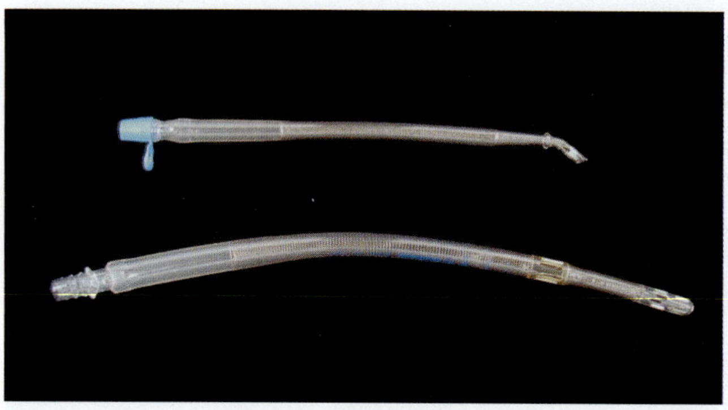

FIG. 32.7 Cardiac cannulas. Top: Aortic cannula. Bottom: Venous cannula. (From Townsend C, Beauchamp B, Evers B, Mattox K, eds. *Sabiston Textbook of Surgery: The Biological Basis of Modern Surgical Practice*. 19th ed. Philadelphia: Elsevier; 2012.)

a cardiotomy reservoir, which removes particulate matter and defoams the blood before shunting into the system.

- *Cardiac venting* refers to the active aspiration of blood from the heart during CPB. This creates a bloodless field and prevents the distension of the cardiac chamber. Cardiac venting through a cannula can be sited in the pulmonary artery, pulmonary vein, left atrium, left ventricle, and the ascending aorta.

POSITION:	Supine or lateral
INCISION:	Thoracic
PREP AND DRAPING:	Thoracic
INSTRUMENTS:	Open heart set

CANNULATION TECHNIQUES IN CARDIOPULMONARY BYPASS

Cannulation is performed in a specific order (according to which sites are used) unless the surgeon specifies otherwise. The order is as follows:

1. Arterial
2. Venous
3. Retrograde
4. LV vent or PA vent
5. Antegrade

The technique for cannulation is similar for each cannulation site. Transesophageal echocardiography (TEE) may be used to guide and confirm cannulation.

Ascending Aorta

1. Two purse-string sutures are placed on the anterior portion of the ascending aorta using a braided polyester or polypropylene suture with or without pledgets. The ends are pulled through a Rumel tourniquet and secured with a hemostat or Kelly clamp. The aortic adventitia is dissected for easier cannulation.
2. An **aortotomy** is made between the purse-strings with a #11 blade. The surgeon blocks the hole digitally.
3. The tip of the aortic cannula is inserted into the opening on the ascending aorta and positioned. The assistant holds the cannula in place as the surgeon tightens the Rumel tourniquets on both sides of the cannula. The tourniquets and cannula are then secured with a heavy #2 silk tie.

4. The cannula is filled with blood to prevent air from being infused in the heart, clamped with a tubing clamp, connected to the arterial perfusion line and unclamped.
   This technique is shown in Fig. 32.8A.

Right Atrial Appendage (Venous)

1. A Cooley spoon clamp is placed across the right atrial appendage and held in place by the assistant.
2. A purse-string suture is placed through the right atrial appendage and above the clamp. The ends are pulled through a Rumel tourniquet and secured with a hemostat or Kelly.
3. The tip of the appendage is then excised by the surgeon using Metzenbaum scissors or #11 or #12 blade. The edges of appendage are held open with forceps while the two-stage venous cannula is being inserted.
4. The assistant removes the clamp, tightens the Rumel tourniquet, and then secures both the Rumel tourniquet and venous cannula with a #2 silk tie.
5. The venous cannula is filled with blood in the same manner as was the aortic cannula. A tubing clamp is placed on the end of the cannula before being connected to the venous line of the CPB machine.

Retrograde

1. The assistant gently presses on the heart with a warm moist laparotomy sponge as the surgeon places a purse-string at the retrograde cannulation site using polyester suture. The ends are pulled through a Rumel tourniquet and secured with a hemostat or Kelly clamp.
2. A stab incision is made using #11 blade and then dilated with a Schnidt tonsil clamp.
3. The retrograde cannula is inserted under TEE guidance to ensure it is in the coronary sinus. Once placement has been confirmed, the stylet is removed, and the tourniquet and cannula are secured in place with a #2 heavy silk tie.
4. The cannula is attached to the cardioplegia line for delivery of retrograde cardioplegia.

The technique for this cannulation is shown in Fig. 32.8B.

Right Superior Pulmonary Vein (Left Ventricular Vent)

1. The assistant retracts the right atrium to expose the right superior pulmonary vein as the surgeon places a purse-string suture. A tourniquet is placed over the suture ends, which are secured with a hemostat.
2. The surgeon makes a stab incision in the vein with a #11 knife blade, dilates the incision with a Schnidt tonsil clamp, and inserts the cannula into the vein. The cannula is manipulated into the left atrium, across the mitral valve, and into the left ventricle.
3. The tourniquet is snugged down and secured with a heavy #2 silk tie. The cannula is then connected to the pump suction line.

Antegrade

1. A 5-0 or 4-0 polypropylene purse-string is placed into the ascending aorta with or without pledgets. The suture ends are passed through a Rumel tourniquet and secured with a hemostat or Kelly.

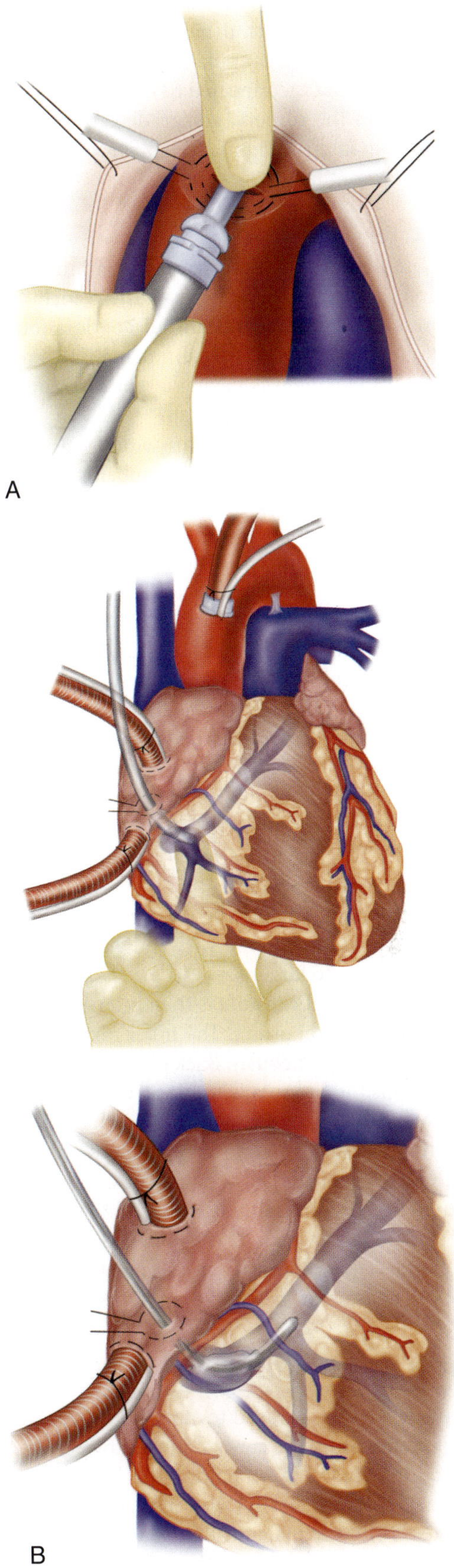

FIG. 32.8 Cannulation for cardiopulmonary bypass. (A) Ascending aorta cannulation. A double row of purse string sutures is placed, and the cannula is advanced into the middle. (B) Retrograde cannulation. (From Selke F, Ruel M, eds. *Atlas of Cardiac Surgical Techniques*. Philadelphia: Saunders; 2010.)

2. The tip of the antegrade cannula is used to puncture the aorta for placement. The tourniquet is snared down and secured to the antegrade cannula with a heavy #2 silk tie. The end of the cannula is connected to the cardioplegia line.
3. Depending on the surgery, antegrade cardioplegia can be given directly into the right and left coronary artery using a handheld cannula.

Femoral Artery and Vein

Femoral cannulation is typically used in minimally invasive cardiac surgeries that require bypass. These include **type A aortic dissections, thoracoabdominal aortic aneurysm,** or if the ascending aorta cannot be cannulated. In some cases, it may be used if the patient is having a repeat sternotomy, and the heart is adherent to the chest wall.

1. An incision is made in the groin with a #10 knife blade. Fascial layers are divided with Metzenbaum scissors.
2. A self-retaining Weitlaner retractor is used to help gain exposure of the common femoral artery and vein.
3. The vessels are mobilized using a right-angle clamp and encircled with either an umbilical tape or vessel loop and tagged with a hemostat.
4. A polypropylene purse-string is placed on the anterior surface of the femoral artery and vein and secured with a Rumel tourniquet and hemostat.
5. Using the introducer needle that comes with the kit, the surgeon inserts the needle into the common femoral artery until there is back bleeding from the needle.
6. A guidewire is then inserted through the needle and threaded up the femoral artery. The needle is removed (leaving the wire in place).
7. The artery is dilated using the dilators from the kit. Each dilator is threaded over the wire individually (beginning with the smallest to largest).
8. The arterial **femoral cannula** is then inserted over the wire and into the femoral artery. The inner obturator and wire are removed simultaneously. Back bleeding from the femoral artery fills the cannula with blood to prevent air embolus.
9. The femoral cannula is connected to the perfusion arterial line. The Rumel tourniquet is tightened, and a heavy #2 silk tie is used to secure the cannula in place (may also be secured to the patient's thigh with a heavy braided or nylon suture). The femoral vein is cannulated in a similar fashion using TEE guidance to ensure proper placement of the cannula tip.

INFUSION OF A CARDIOPLEGIC SOLUTION

A cardioplegic solution is used to stop the heart; this reduces the energy required by the cardiac muscle by eliminating the energy requirements of contraction. The process of infusing a cardioplegic solution into the coronary arteries protects the cardiac muscle from damage while the aorta is occluded and the blood supply is interrupted. The solution may be infused directly into the coronary artery using a handheld cardioplegia cannula or retrogradely into the coronary sinus. A cardioplegic solution can be infused indirectly into the aortic root just above the aortic valve.

Decannulation

The left ventricular catheter is usually removed from the ventricle before bypass is discontinued. The catheter is occluded with a tube-occluding clamp, and the silk suture and tourniquet are removed. The catheter is withdrawn, and the suture is tied securely. Additional sutures (often on pledgets) may be used for hemostasis. Decannulation of the venae cavae and aorta uses the same technique after the bypass has been discontinued.

Femoral Artery and Vein

At the conclusion of the bypass, the surgeon occludes the femoral vein cannula. The assistant releases the cannula from the drapes and other attachments on the field. The surgeon then withdraws the cannula and occludes the vein with a vascular clamp. The venotomy is closed with a continuous suture of 5-0 or 6-0 polypropylene. All clamps are removed, and the artery is decannulated with the same technique.

Bleeding or hemorrhage can occur in the postoperative period if cannulation sites have not been closed securely, if heparin has not been adequately reversed with protamine, if dissection of the cannulated blood vessel occurs, or if surrounding tissue has been damaged. Atelectasis may persist because of lung deflation during bypass. Temporary cognitive, sensory, and perceptual changes may occur as a result of the effects of extracorporeal circulation.

CORONARY ARTERY BYPASS GRAFTING (CABG)

Coronary artery bypass (CAB) of a narrow segment of one or more coronary arteries is performed to improve circulation to the heart. A saphenous vein autograft is commonly used. The procedure is commonly known by its acronym, CABG, for coronary artery bypass grafting.

Pathology

The inner and outer walls of the heart may be affected by coronary artery disease (CAD). CAD is caused by the buildup of cholesterol deposits in the arterial lining, a condition called **atherosclerosis.** This can affect any artery. A closely related disease is **arteriosclerosis,** which is loss of elasticity in and hardening of the arteries. Arteriosclerosis is often the result of diet and other environmental causes. When the flow of coronary blood is reduced, the myocardial cells are deprived of oxygen and other nutrients. This in turn can produce a weakening of the heart muscle or a myocardial **infarction,** resulting in tissue death.

POSITION:	Supine
INCISION:	Median sternotomy
PREP AND DRAPING:	Xiphoid to pubis; bilateral legs and feet; feet may be excluded to the ankles; groin is excluded; Foley catheter
INSTRUMENTS:	Major cardiac set; coronary artery set; vascular set; vessel loops; vessel clips; Rumel tourniquets

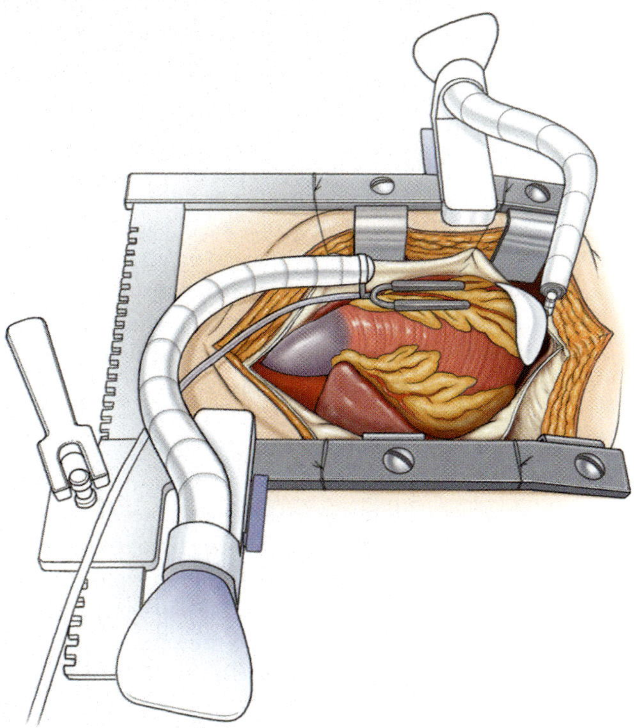

FIG. 32.9 Heart stabilizer. This device is used to decrease cardiac movement during beating-heart procedures. (From Townsend C, Beauchamp B, Evers B, Mattox K, eds. *Sabiston Textbook of Surgery: The Biological Basis of Modern Surgical Practice.* 19th ed. Philadelphia: Elsevier; 2012.)

Technical Points and Discussion

The surgeon performs a median sternotomy and cannulates for CPB. An increasing number of coronary bypass procedures are performed without CPB. In patients with very complex disease involving several vessels, bypass is required as described here. However, the procedure can be done on the beating heart. In this case, a vacuum-assisted stabilizer is required (Fig. 32.9). The device is attached to the sternal retractor, and it minimizes the movement of the heart during surgery.

1. **A segment of the saphenous vein is removed.**
   The assistant removes the greater saphenous vein from the leg, or the left or right radial artery may be harvested for use as a free graft. The harvested vein is placed in a small basin with heparinized blood solution to keep the graft moist. See the Saphenous Vein Graft procedure later in this chapter.

2. **The internal mammary artery is prepared.**
   The internal mammary artery (IMA) takedown is performed by elevating the sternal edge with an IMA retractor (Rultract) that attaches to the side of the bed. In most cases, the left internal mammary artery (LIMA) is used. The right internal mammary artery (RIMA) or both internal mammary arteries (BIMA) may also be used for bypassing the coronary arteries. Coronary forceps and ESU or harmonic scalpel are used to dissect and free the IMA from the chest wall. Bleeding from small branches is controlled with vessel clips. Papaverine is applied topically to the IMA. The distal end is detached by using medium clips, scissors, and a bulldog clamp. The IMA is covered with a surgical sponge soaked with papaverine and tucked away in the chest. The proximal end is left intact to allow blood from the subclavian artery to supply the IMA. The LIMA is used to bypass the left anterior descending (LAD) artery.

3. **The diseased coronary artery is opened, and the graft is sutured in place.**
   After CPB has been instituted (if used), the surgeon identifies the segment of the coronary artery to which the bypass graft will be anastomosed. Excess epicardial fat is removed from the arteriotomy site with a #64 Beaver blade or a #15 blade. The surgeon then occludes the ascending aorta and inserts the indwelling catheter for the infusion of the cardioplegic solution and venting of air. Next, the coronary artery is opened with a #11 knife blade (or Beaver blade), and the incision is extended with Potts coronary scissors. A Garrett coronary dilator may be inserted into the lumen of the artery to assess its size. The surgeon bevels the free end of the vein with tenotomy or fine Metzenbaum scissors. The vein is then sutured to the coronary artery with continuous or interrupted sutures of 7-0 polypropylene. This is referred to as a *distal anastomosis.* When the anastomosis is complete, the assistant inflates the vein with cardioplegic solution to test for leaks and to determine the diameter and length of the graft when it is filled.

4. **Venous and other free grafts are anastomosed to the ascending aorta.**
   The surgeon performs all other anastomoses using the same technique. Size 6-0 or 8-0 polypropylene may be used for the anastomosis. The aorta then is unclamped, and the indwelling catheter is removed. A portion of the aorta is occluded with a vascular clamp (e.g., Lambert-Kay clamp). A #11 knife blade and aortic punch are used to create a hole in the occluded portion.

   The surgeon inflates the vein to make sure it is not twisted and does not have any leaks and to determine the length needed to reach the aorta. The vein is then cut to the appropriate length, and the end is beveled with scissors. The anastomosis is performed between the vein and the hole in the aorta. This is referred to as the *proximal anastomosis.* The surgeon completes each anastomosis and removes the clamp from the aorta. When the procedures are performed off-pump, a small horseshoe retractor is positioned over the coronary arteriotomy to minimize cardiac movement during the distal anastomosis. The proximal aortic anastomosis is performed with the partial occlusion of the aorta. In some patients, both distal and proximal anastomoses are created with the aorta cross-clamped. Air is evacuated from the vein grafts with a 25- or 27-gauge needle. The surgeon inspects each anastomosis for leaks, and any found are repaired before the bypass is discontinued.

5. **CPB is discontinued, and decannulation is performed.** The cannulas are removed, and a pacemaker electrode may be sutured to the heart. Metal rings or radiopaque material may be placed around each vein graft on the aorta. These mark the veins in the event cardiac catheterization is performed in the postoperative period. The wound can then be closed. Harvesting the IMA, distal anastomosis, and completed anastomosis are shown in Fig. 32.10.

Complications of CABG include hemorrhage, atrial and/or ventricular **arrhythmias,** stroke, infection, and cardiac **ischemia.** CABG grafts may also clot, causing a myocardial infarction.

SAPHENOUS VEIN GRAFT

The greater saphenous vein is removed to provide an autograft for peripheral or coronary artery bypass. The goal is to remove the vein yet retain its structural and physiological soundness. A common problem during vein harvesting arises from the practice of one surgeon harvesting the vein while the rest of the team prepares the implant site (e.g., during CAB). In this case, the two overhead operating lights are dedicated to the top of the surgical field, leaving no direct light for the saphenous vein harvest. A third light or headlight should be available to provide lighting on the leg.

Pathology

An autograft is an ideal graft for arterial bypass. The greater saphenous vein has been used more successfully than other materials for small-diameter arterial bypass. It is readily accessible, and its connective tissue layer thickens with increased pressure. This makes it strong and able to withstand high arterial pressure.

POSITION:	Supine
INCISION:	As for CABG
PREP AND DRAPING:	As for CABG
INSTRUMENTS:	Minor vascular set; general surgery set

Technical Points and Discussion

1. ***The groin and inner aspect of the leg are incised over the saphenous vein.*** The knee is flexed to gain access to the medial aspect of the leg. To begin the surgery, the surgeon makes a long incision directly over the saphenous vein from the groin to the point of removal, usually below the knee. The groin incision is made parallel to the upper thigh crease, directly over the saphenous vein. Bleeders are coagulated with the ESU or ligated with 3-0 silk sutures. A dull Weitlaner retractor may be placed in the wound.

2. ***Branches of the vein are clamped, ligated, and divided.*** Branches of the vein are clamped and ligated with silk or clipped and divided. The vein is ligated with heavy silk sutures and divided with scissors.

3. ***The vein is mobilized and removed.*** The surgeon performs the distal excision by first clamping tributaries and ligating them. The vein is carefully dissected along its length to avoid creating wide tissue flaps on each side. The scrub or assistant must keep the vein and incision moist during the surgery. Frequent irrigation with saline solution is necessary. Some surgeons inject papaverine or lidocaine into the subcutaneous tissue to prevent vein spasm.

   The surgeon places Silastic vessel loops around the vein for retraction rather than using forceps, which can damage the vessel. When all tributaries have been divided, the vein is removed and placed in a basin.

Preparation of the Vein

The scrub attaches a blunt-tipped irrigation needle to a 30-mL syringe. The needle is inserted into the tip of the vein and secured with a heavy silk tie. Saline is used to irrigate the vein during the repair. If ordered, heparinized papaverine may be used. The surgeon injects solution into the vein and occludes the branches with size 3-0 silk ties. The vein must be kept moist at all times.

After preparation, the graft is maintained in a moist saline environment until needed. The vein may also be placed in a basin with heparinized papaverine and normal saline solution. This is called a "vein bath." The vein must be carefully monitored and protected at all times.

The leg incision is closed with Vicryl interrupted sutures size 3-0. The skin is closed with staples or monofilament synthetic suture. Harvesting of a saphenous vein is illustrated in Fig. 32.11.

MINIMALLY INVASIVE DIRECT CORONARY ARTERY BYPASS (MIDCAB)

The minimally invasive direct coronary artery bypass (MIDCAB) technique for coronary artery bypass uses an autograft of the left internal mammary artery (LMA) to make the anastomosis with the LAD coronary artery. This is an off-pump procedure performed on the beating heart. Specialized equipment has been developed to facilitate the procedure. An off-pump stabilization system is used to enable surgery on the beating heart.

Pathology

The MIDCAB procedure is performed for essentially the same pathology described for a CABG. However, the minimally invasive procedure is selected for patients with single-vessel disease.

POSITION:	Supine with the left chest elevated
INCISION:	Left anterolateral thoracotomy
PREP AND DRAPING:	Thoracic
INSTRUMENTS:	Off-pump MIDCAB instrument set including heart stabilizer; cardiac set

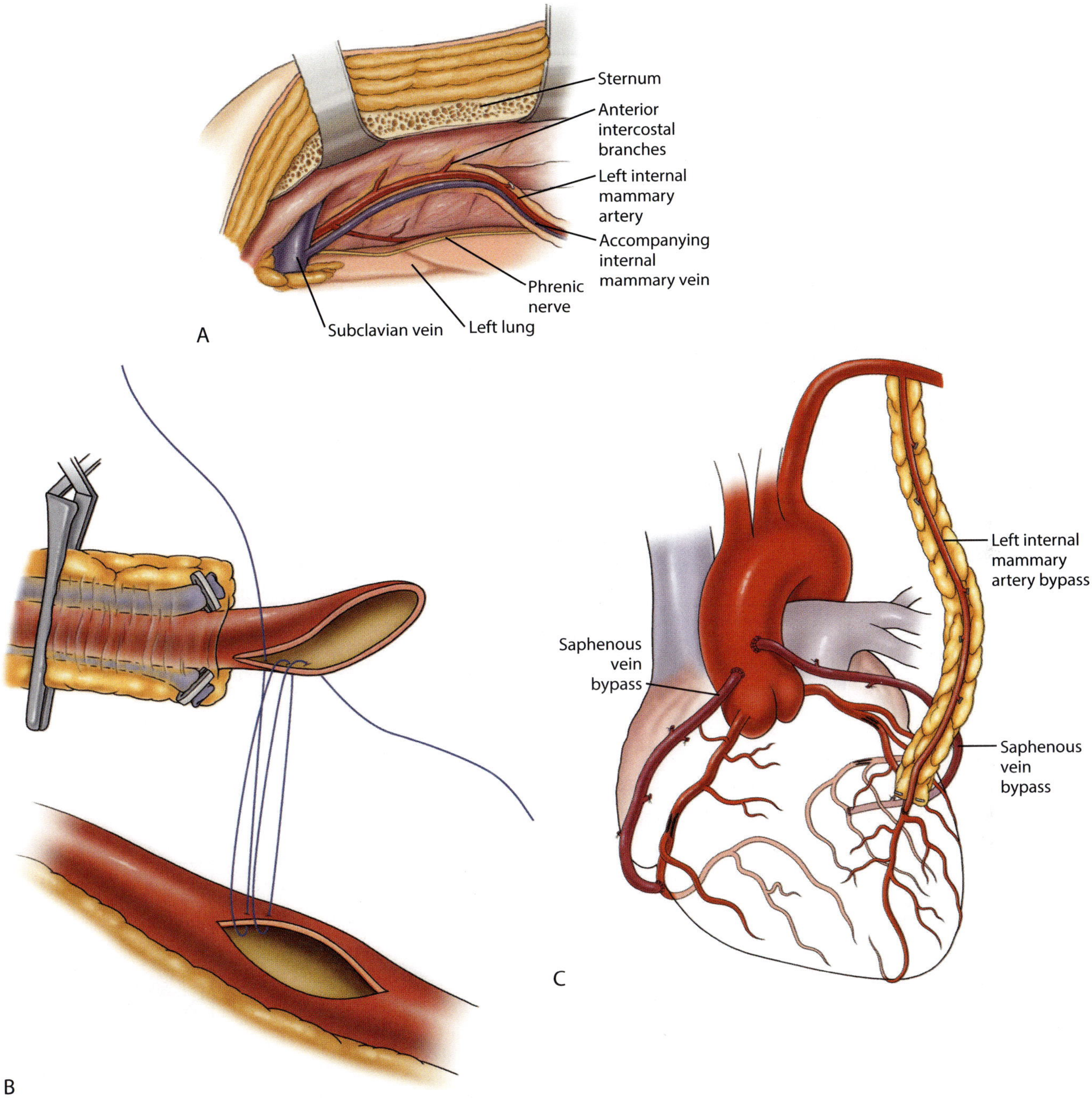

FIG. 32.10 Coronary artery bypass grafting (CABG). (A) Harvesting (takedown) of the internal mammary artery. The artery is dissected from the chest wall as a pedicle including the vein and connective tissue around it. (B) The distal anastomosis technique. A 5-mm arteriotomy is made in the coronary artery to be bypassed. The distal end of the internal mammary artery is spatulated to fit. Prolene sutures are used to form the anastomosis. (C) A three-vessel coronary artery bypass. (From Townsend C, Beauchamp B, Evers B, Mattox K, eds. *Sabiston Textbook of Surgery: The Biological Basis of Modern Surgical Practice*. 19th ed. Philadelphia: Elsevier; 2012.)

Technical Points and Discussion

1. ***The patient is prepped and draped.***
The patient is placed in supine position with the left chest elevated using gel positioners. These may be placed under the left scapula and buttock. The fourth intercostal space is marked. The patient is prepped and draped for a wide thoracotomy. Some surgeons also prep the legs for saphenous autograft in case the LIMA graft cannot be used.

2. ***A left anterolateral thoracotomy incision is made.***
A 10-cm incision is made under the nipple in the fourth intercostal space. The incision is carried through the subcutaneous fat using the ESU. The pectoris muscle is then incised down to the fourth rib. A self-retaining retractor such as a mastoid, Weitlaner, or Beckman retractor can be placed at this point. The intercostal space is incised using the ESU.

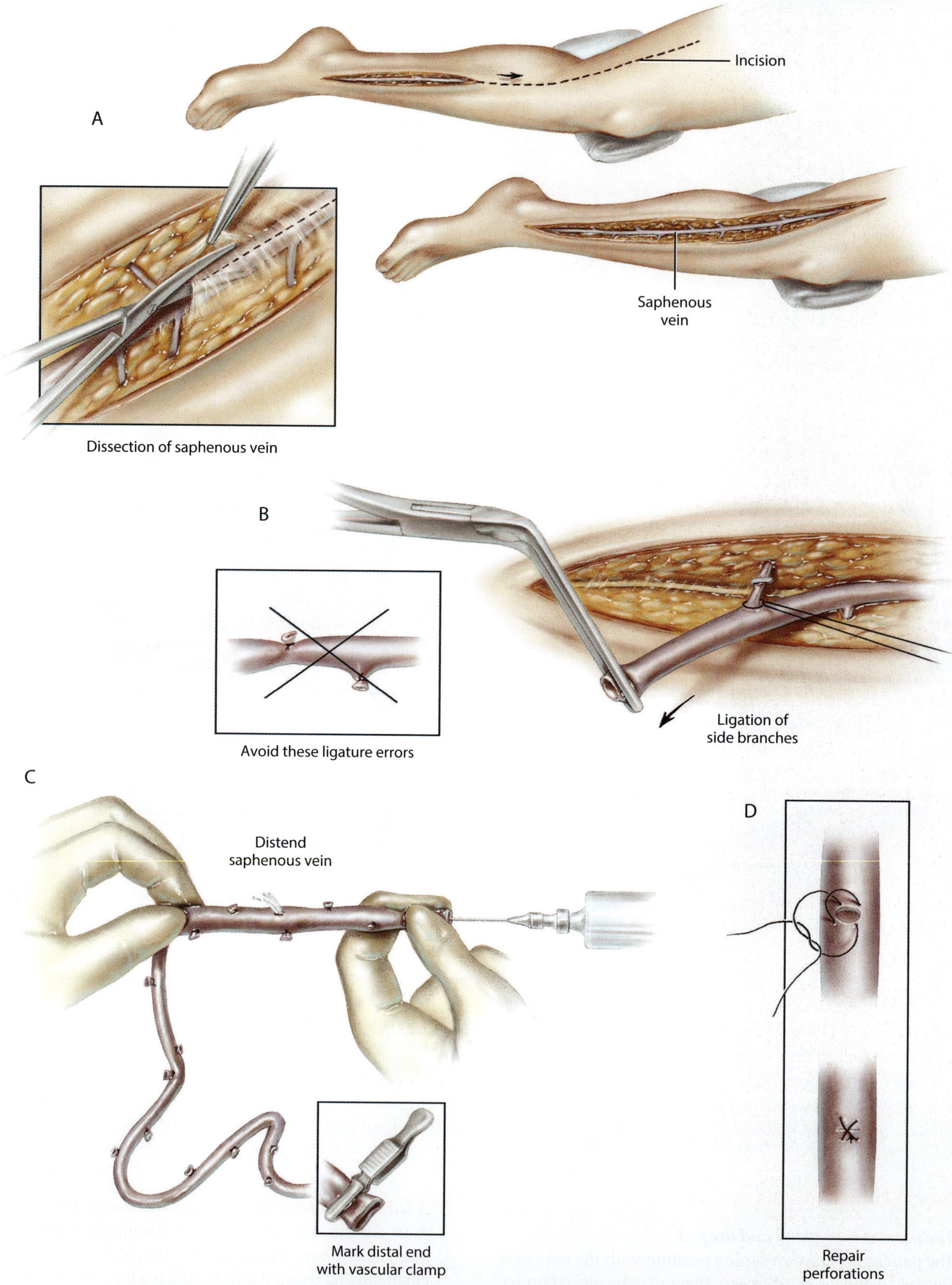

FIG. 32.11 Saphenous autograft. The saphenous vein is commonly harvested to replace a diseased coronary artery and for other bypass procedures. (A) External rotation of the hip exposes the line of incision. (B and C) The saphenous vein and artery are exposed. Tributaries are clamped, tied, and divided. (D) The vein has been removed and is tested for leaks, which are clamped and ligated. (From Doty D, Doty J. *Cardiac Surgery Operative Technique*. 2nd ed. Philadelphia: Saunders; 2012.)

3. ***The pleural space is entered.***
The pleural space is now entered, and the incision is carried toward the sternal edge. A larger retractor is needed at this point. Many different retractors and stabilizers have been specifically designed for the MIDCAB procedure. Examples of such retractors are the retractor system (and the TAVI-MIDCAB retraction system at https://pdfs.semanticscholar.org/bf68/f4d9b402f55933fde1d25e1c8400b60fd048.pdf). The retractor is put in position in the fourth space and opened. The antero-intercostal membrane is incised.

4. ***The LIMA is harvested.***
The LIMA is identified and mobilized. Vessel loops may be used for traction. Tributaries are identified along the length of the vessel. These are clipped and ligated. The mammary artery is then harvested with its pedicle.

5. ***The anastomosis is performed.***
The pericardium is incised to expose the target area of the anastomosis. A heart stabilizer is attached to the retractor. The anastomosis can now be performed. The surgeon places two suture loops of size 5-0 polypropylene around the coronary artery. The heart stabilizer is adjusted and locked. The coronary artery is opened, and the suture loops are tightened to provide hemostasis. The anastomosis is then carried out using a running suture of size 7-0 or 8-0 polypropylene. The LIMA pedicle is tacked to the pericardium with several sutures. The loop sutures are removed.

6. ***The anastomosis is checked, and hemostasis is secured.***
The surgeon checks the anastomosis to ensure that there is no leakage. The wound is irrigated and closed in layers.

RESECTION OF A LEFT VENTRICULAR ANEURYSM

Resection of a left ventricular aneurysm reduces the risk of rupture and embolism.

Pathology

An aneurysm of the left ventricle is most often caused by a reduced blood supply from an infarcted coronary artery.

POSITION:	Supine
INCISION:	Median sternotomy
PREP AND DRAPING:	Chin to mid-thigh
INSTRUMENTS:	Major cardiac set

Technical Points and Discussion

1. ***A median sternotomy is performed and CPB established.***
2. ***The ventricle is incised and assessed.***
A median sternotomy is performed and bypass is initiated. The surgeon cross-clamps the ascending aorta. The ventricle is incised with the long knife, and the incision is extended with curved Mayo scissors. Allis clamps may be applied to the edges of the aneurysm for traction. The surgeon assesses the mitral valve and removes any clots with forceps or suction. The scrub should keep the instruments clean to prevent clots from entering the bloodstream.

3. ***The aneurysm is dissected, and the graft is placed.***
The aneurysm tissue is excised with curved Mayo scissors, and a Dacron patch is inserted to repair the ventricle. An alternate technique is to resect the aneurysm tissue and bring the edges of the ventricle together with suture of size 0 polypropylene or polyester. Strips of Teflon felt or pledgets are incorporated with the suture. A second or third row of sutures is placed through the ventricular edges for a more secure closure. The surgeon decompresses the ventricle using the sump catheter from the CPB machine. The catheter is removed before the final suture is placed. The **apex** of the ventricle may be aspirated with a 18-gauge needle.

4. ***The wound is closed.***
The wound is prepared for closure as previously described, and the incision is closed. Resection of a left ventricular aneurysm is illustrated in Fig. 32.12.

AORTIC VALVE REPLACEMENT

The aortic valve maintains one-way blood flow from the left ventricle to the aorta. The valve is replaced when it has lost function because of disease.

Pathology

Common causes of valve insufficiency are endocarditis, congenital anomalies, and calcification. A leaking valve allows blood to leak back into the left ventricle instead of going through the aorta. The left ventricle eventually fails as a result of increased cardiac work.

Calcification of the valves can also occur. The valve leaflets may become stiff because of calcification or other thickening. This can reduce the opening of the valve to a small slit. The ventricle must work harder to pump a sufficient amount of blood through the narrowed orifice of the stenotic valve. This can lead to ventricular failure and insufficient blood flow to the brain, coronary arteries, and other organs.

POSITION:	Supine
INCISION:	Median sternotomy
PREP AND DRAPING:	Chin to mid-thigh
INSTRUMENTS:	Open heart set; valve set; and selected prosthesis

Technical Points and Discussion

1. ***A median sternotomy and CPB are performed with a two-stage venous cannulation.***

   The surgeon performs a median sternotomy and cannulates for CPB.

2. ***Cardioplegic solution is infused.***

   A retrograde cardioplegic catheter is inserted into the coronary sinus. The ascending aorta is occluded, and the cardioplegic solution is infused. The route through which the cardioplegic solution is delivered depends on the valve pathology. If aortic stenosis is present, the cardioplegic solution is initially infused through the aortic root. After the aorta is opened, subsequent cardioplegic infusions are given through the retrograde catheter. If aortic insufficiency is present, the solution infused into the aortic root preferentially flows into the left ventricle. Fluid in the ventricular chamber distends and damages the ventricular wall. In these situations, retrograde cardioplegic solution is infused. Direct coronary perfusion is rarely needed.

3. ***The valve site is prepared.***

   The surgeon opens the aorta with a transverse incision or, occasionally, a vertical incision. The valve cusps are incised with forceps and scissors or a #11 blade on a long knife handle. If the valve leaflets are extensively calcified, the surgeon may debride the calcium with rongeurs. The technologist should keep the instruments clean with a damp sponge to prevent calcium particles and other materials from dropping back into the wound, where they may cause an embolus.

   The annulus is measured with aortic valve sizers. Different types of valve prostheses have their own unique sizers. The scrub obtains the correct size of prosthesis from the circulating nurse.

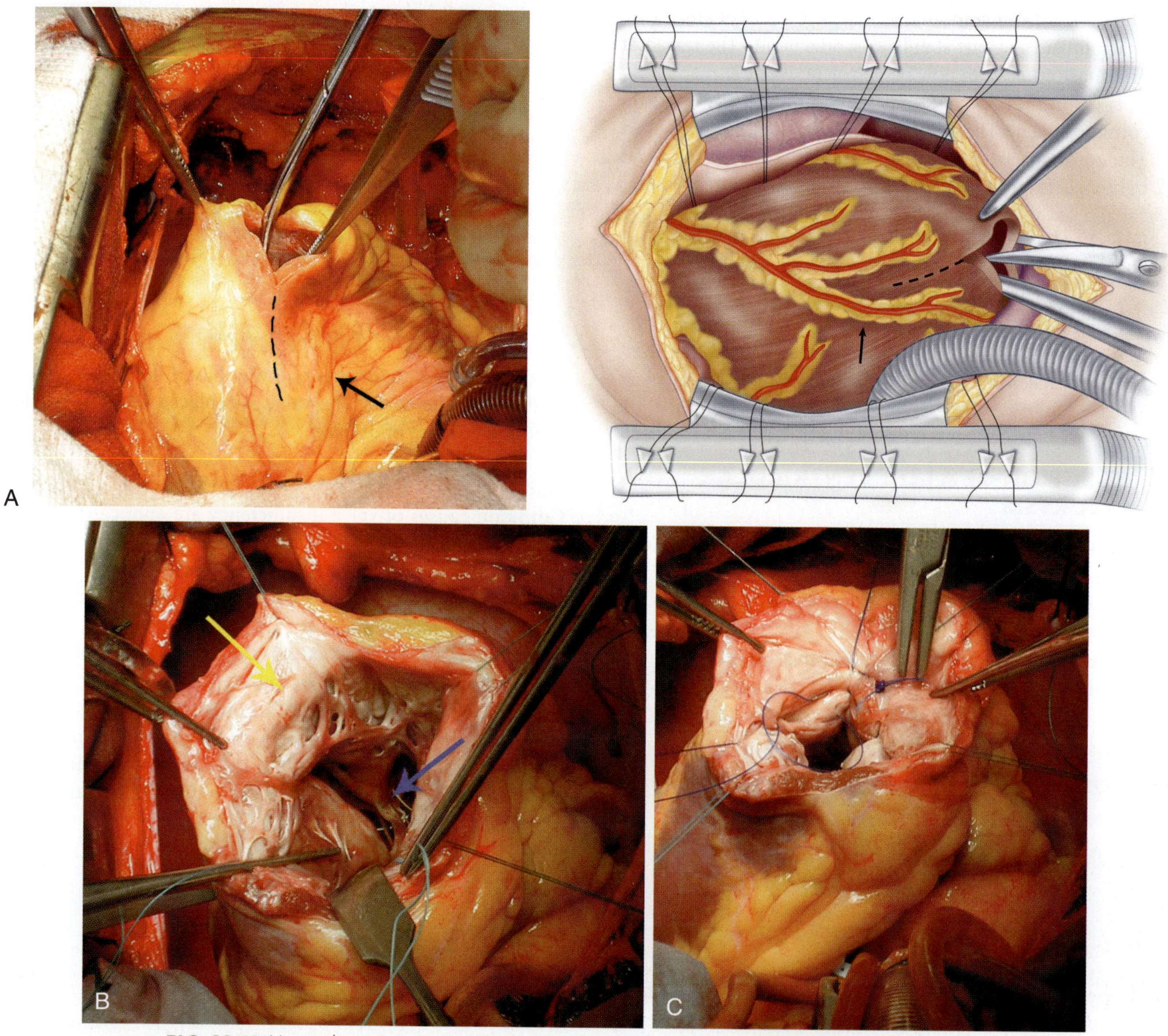

FIG. 32.12 Ventricular aneurysm. (A) The ventricle is opened. (B) Traction sutures are placed, and the cavity is cleared of thrombus material. The scarred area is pointed out with a *yellow arrow*. The *blue arrow* shows the papillary muscles. (C) A circular suture line is placed on the border of the scarred and normal myocardium. Size 2-0 polypropylene is used here.

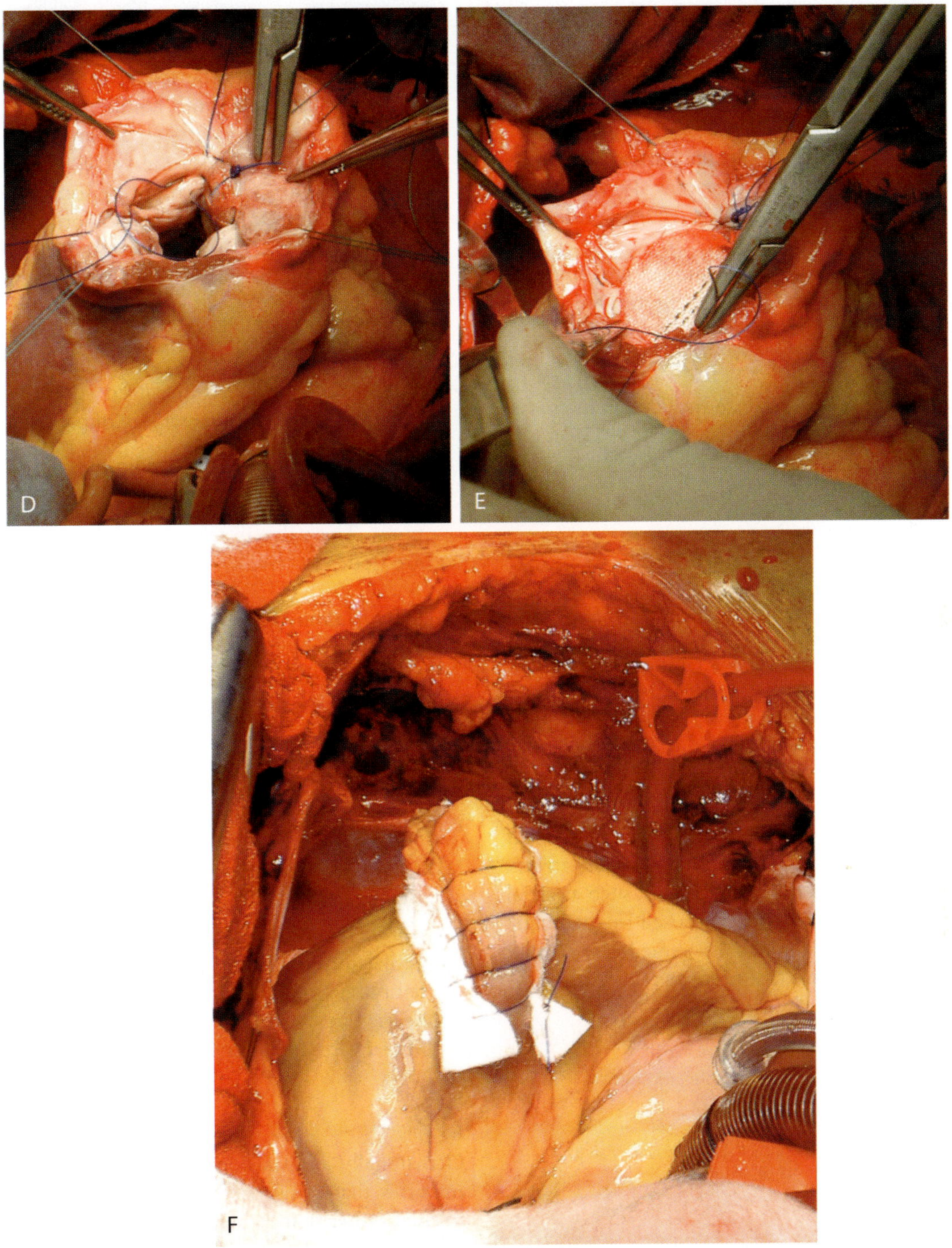

FIG. 32.12, cont'd (D) A Dacron patch is used to cover the opening. (E) The ventriculotomy is closed in two layers. (F) Teflon strips may be used to reinforce the closure as shown here. (From Selke F, Ruel M, eds. *Atlas of Cardiac Surgical Techniques*. Philadelphia: Saunders; 2010.)

4. ***A prosthetic valve is implanted.***
   The surgeon places interrupted sutures of size 2-0 or 3-0 polypropylene through the annulus of the *prosthetic sewing ring.* Interrupted sutures in the aortic valve may be inserted in three series, corresponding to the three cusps of the valve. The distal suture ends are tagged or placed in a suture holder. When biological valves are used, they must be rinsed to remove the glutaraldehyde storage solution; the valve must be kept moist with saline before it is implanted. If the leaflets become dry, the prosthesis can be damaged.

5. ***The valve is sutured in place, and the aortic incision is closed.***
   The surgeon seats the valve in position and ties all sutures. The aortotomy is closed with two polypropylene sutures

size 3-0 placed at each side. Before tying the sutures, the surgeon allows air to escape from the suture line. The surgeon may oversew the initial closure to ensure hemostasis.

6. ***Bypass is discontinued, and the is wound closed.***
The aortic clamp is removed, and the aortic vent line is turned on to aspirate air. The surgeon may also elevate the left ventricular apex and insert an 18-gauge needle into the chamber to allow air to escape.
Bypass is discontinued, and the cannulas are removed. Temporary pacemaker electrodes may be sutured to the heart. Chest tubes are inserted, and the wound is closed in layers.

Complications of the procedure include hemorrhage, atrial and/or ventricular arrhythmias, stroke, infection, ischemia, and death. Additional complications include valve failure or malfunction.

MITRAL VALVE REPAIR AND REPLACEMENT

In mitral valve repair and replacement, a diseased mitral valve is replaced to open a constricted valve (**stenosis**) or to prevent blood from regurgitating into the left atrium. The valve is repaired with an annuloplasty (or other reparative techniques). If the valve is severely damaged, it is replaced.

Pathology

The mitral valve is situated between the left atrium and left ventricle. Over time, a stenotic valve causes the left atrium to become dilated and can lead to arrhythmias, such as atrial fibrillation. Mitral valve disease may be caused by rheumatic heart disease, dilation of the annulus, ischemic heart disease, trauma, or changes in the tissue that produce regurgitation.

POSITION:	Supine
INCISION:	Median sternotomy
PREP AND DRAPING:	Chin to pubis prep
INSTRUMENTS:	Major cardiac set; valve instruments

Technical Points and Discussion

MITRAL VALVE REPLACEMENT

1. ***A median sternotomy is performed, and CPB is initiated.***
A median sternotomy is performed. The aorta is cannulated in the usual fashion. Both venae cavae are cannulated, and umbilical tapes are placed around them secured with a Rumel in preparation for total CPB. A retrograde cannula is inserted into the coronary sinus. The ascending aorta is occluded, and a cardioplegic solution is infused through the aortic root and into the coronary arteries.

2. ***Left atriotomy is performed, and the mitral valve is excised.***
The surgeon opens the left atrium with a #11 or #15 blade on the long knife handle, extends the incision with scissors, and inserts an atrial retractor, which the assistant uses to expose the valve. The surgeon grasps the valve with a valve hook or long Allis clamp and excises the cusps with valve scissors or the knife. The chordae tendineae and papillary muscles of the anterior leaflet are cut; the posterior leaflet chordae are often left intact.

3. ***A prosthetic valve is sutured in place.***
The annulus is then measured so that the technologist can obtain the correct size of prosthetic valve from the circulator. The surgeon places the sutures through the annulus and the prosthetic sewing ring using the same technique as described for aortic valve replacement. The valve is seated in position, and the sutures are tied.

4. ***The atriotomy is closed, and the aorta is unclamped.***
The atriotomy is closed with continuous 3-0 polypropylene suture. Before tying the sutures, the surgeon temporarily releases the vena cava tourniquets and allows the heart to fill with blood. The blood is allowed to spill out of the heart to remove air bubbles. The surgeon then ties the sutures securely. The aortic clamp is removed, and the aorta is aspirated with a vent catheter to ensure that no air remains in the heart.

5. ***Chest tubes and pacing wires are inserted, and the wound is closed.***
CPB is discontinued, and the cannulas are removed. A temporary pacemaker electrode may be sutured to the heart. Chest tubes are inserted, and the wound is closed. Mitral valve replacement is illustrated in Fig. 32.13.

Mitral Commissurotomy

Occasionally, a mitral commissurotomy (opening of the commissures that bring the cusps of the valve together) is performed rather than valve replacement. This technique can be used to relieve stenosis when the valve leaflets are sufficiently flexible to allow it. The procedure is performed during bypass. The surgeon incises the commissures with a knife or breaks them apart with a mitral valve dilator (e.g., Gerbode or Tubbs dilator) to separate the cusps. The atrium is then closed as described for mitral valve replacement.

Mitral Ring Annuloplasty

A dilated mitral valve annulus can be repaired by the placement of an annuloplasty ring in the annulus to allow the valve leaflets to come together more efficiently. Sutures are placed in the annulus and the annuloplasty ring and are tied. This procedure reduces the annular orifice, allowing the valve leaflets to close properly.

Related Procedure

TRICUSPID VALVE REPLACEMENT OR REPAIR

In replacement procedures, the tricuspid valve is excised and replaced with a prosthetic valve through a right atriotomy. Total CPB is required. Tricuspid ring annuloplasty (similar to mitral valve annuloplasty) is often preferred over replacement.

RESECTION OF AN ANEURYSM OF THE ASCENDING AORTA

An aneurysm or dissection of the ascending aorta can rupture or prevent the aortic valve leaflets from closing properly. The goal of resection of an aneurysm of the ascending aorta is to repair the aneurysm and restore function to the valve.

Pathology

An aortic aneurysm is a potentially life-threatening condition in which the walls of the aorta (or any other vessel or heart chamber) balloon out because of cardiovascular disease. Aneurysms can be classified as saccular or fusiform. A *saccular aneurysm* is the ballooning out of a localized area in the artery. A *fusiform aneurysm* involves the entire circumference of the artery. Arteriosclerosis and atherosclerosis both contribute to these conditions. As the disease progresses, the walls of the aorta become increasingly stiff and blocked by fatty deposits. The walls of the segment *distal to* the blockage (in the direction of blood flow) become weak and distended. Finally, the ballooning vessel begins to delaminate (the intimal layer separates), and blood is forced between the layers, resulting in rupture. This delamination is called *dissection,* and the aneurysm then is referred to as a *dissecting aneurysm.*

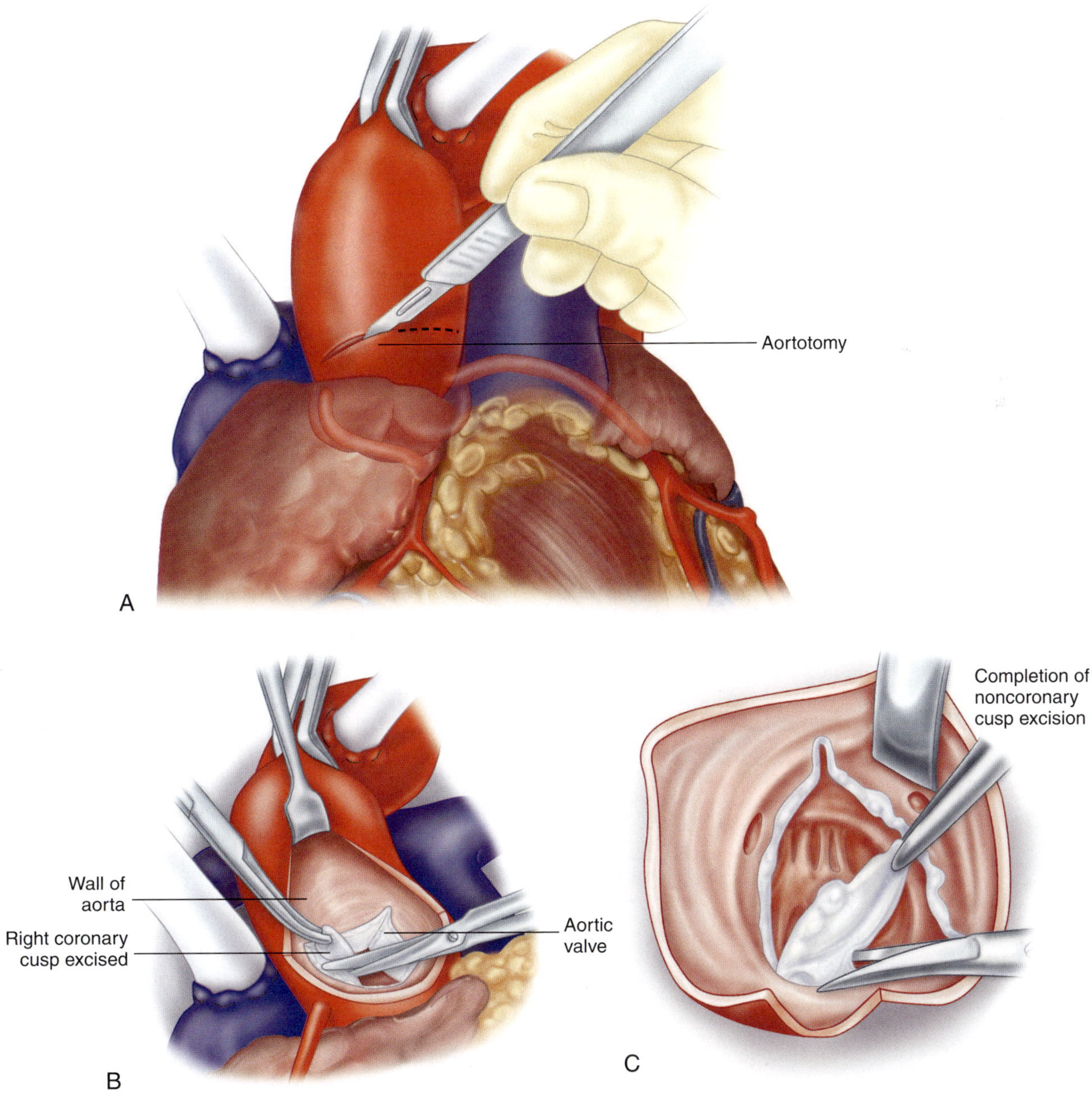

FIG. 32.13 Mitral valve replacement. (A) An aortotomy is made using a #15 knife blade. (B) The valve is exposed, and the annulus is cleared of calcified debris. The commissure is divided from the aortic wall, and the coronary cusp is excised. (C) The left coronary cusp is removed. Resection of the valve continues with the excision of the noncoronary cusp.

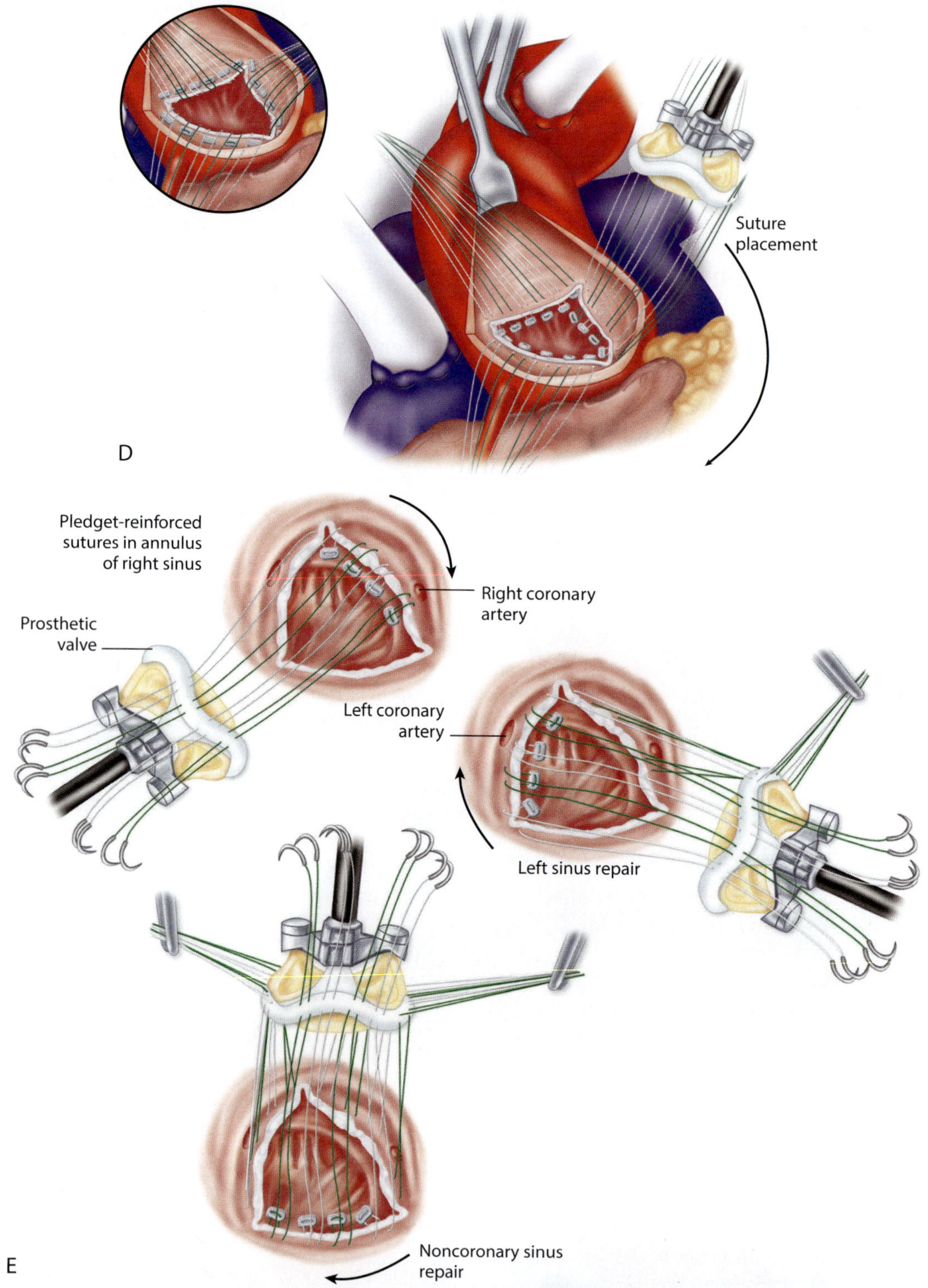

FIG. 32.13, cont'd (D) Attachment of the prosthetic valve. Multiple pledgeted 3-0 Dacron sutures are placed. Here sutures are alternated by color to simplify identification of the pairs. (E) Overhead view of sutures that have been passed through the prosthesis sewing ring.

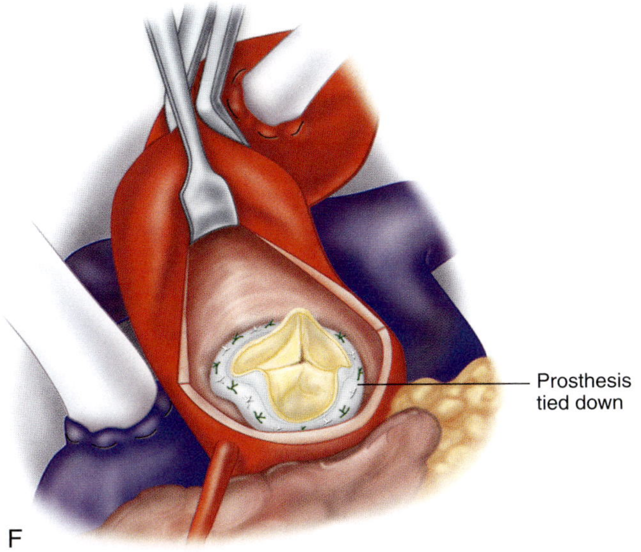

FIG. 32.13, cont'd (F) Completed valve in place. (From Selke F, Ruel M, eds. *Atlas of Cardiac Surgical Techniques*. Philadelphia: Saunders; 2010.)

POSITION:	Supine
INCISION:	Median sternotomy
PREP AND DRAPING:	Chin to mid-thigh
INSTRUMENTS:	Major cardiac set

Technical Points and Discussion

1. ***A median sternotomy is performed.***
2. ***The femoral artery is isolated and cannulated.***
   If there is a risk that the aorta may rupture, the femoral artery and vein are isolated for cannulation.
3. ***The aorta is occluded and aneurysm opened.***
   The surgeon occludes the aorta distal to the aneurysm. The surgeon's preference for aortic cross clamp will be noted on the surgeon's preference card. The aneurysm is opened with scissors, and all clots and debris are removed using tissue forceps and suction. The scrub should have a basin available to receive the debris. If the aorta is dissected, the location of the aortic tear is identified.
4. ***Retrograde cardioplegic solution is infused (the coronary arteries rarely are directly perfused).***
   Retrograde cardioplegic solution is administered through the coronary sinus. The surgeon examines the aortic valve to determine the extent of injury and to replace it if necessary. The technologist should have valve instruments available on the setup tray to prevent delay. Valve suture should be ready for immediate opening if needed.
5. ***A prosthetic graft is anastomosed to the proximal and distal aorta, and the aorta is unclamped.***
   The surgeon obtains the appropriate size of graft from the scrub and performs the proximal anastomosis with a continuous suture of 3-0 polypropylene. When the anastomosis is complete, the surgeon occludes the graft with a vascular clamp and temporarily releases the aortic clamp to test the suture line. Additional sutures are placed as needed. Teflon felt pledgets are used to reinforce the suture line.
   The surgeon cuts the graft to an appropriate length and performs the distal anastomosis. Before tying the suture, the surgeon temporarily releases the aortic clamp to fill the graft and flush out air and clots. The right superior pulmonary vein vent catheter is then removed.
6. ***CPB is discontinued, and the cannulas are removed.***
   After CPB has been discontinued, the cannulas are removed. The surgeon may cover the graft with aneurysm tissue. The assistant closes the groin incision while the surgeon inserts chest tubes and closes the sternotomy.

The surgeon must occasionally replace both the aorta and aortic valve. Special composite graft-valve prostheses are available for these procedures. If the coronary opening is obscured by the composite graft, the surgeon must re-implant the coronary opening or create bypass grafts that attach proximally to the aortic graft. Coronary bypass instruments should be available for this procedure.

Postoperative complications include hemorrhage, stroke, infection, and death. Graft anastomoses may require repair if persistent bleeding arises. Neurological deficit or paralysis may be a complication of surgery on the descending thoracic aorta.

RESECTION OF AN ANEURYSM OF THE AORTIC ARCH

An aneurysm or dissection of the aortic arch can impair blood flow to the brain and the upper body because of the frequent involvement of the aortic branches (i.e., the brachiocephalic artery, left carotid artery, and left subclavian artery). The goal of resection of an aortic arch aneurysm is to repair the aneurysm and restore adequate blood flow to the aorta and its branches.

An aneurysm that extends or is limited to the aortic arch may require resection and anastomosis of both the aorta and its branching arch vessels using a graft. The femoral vein and artery are cannulated as for aneurysms of the ascending aorta. In some cases, the branch vessels cannot be clamped because of their location or because of their involvement in the aneurysm. In these cases, the surgeon may elect to turn off the pump for the period required to anastomose the arch vessels. Once the anastomoses are complete, the pump is started again and the remainder of the procedure is performed under bypass. Fig. 32.14 illustrates the graft replacement of an aortic arch.

RESECTION OF AN ANEURYSM OF THE DESCENDING THORACIC AORTA

The goal of surgical repair of an aneurysm of the descending thoracic aorta is to prevent rupture and life-threatening hemorrhage.

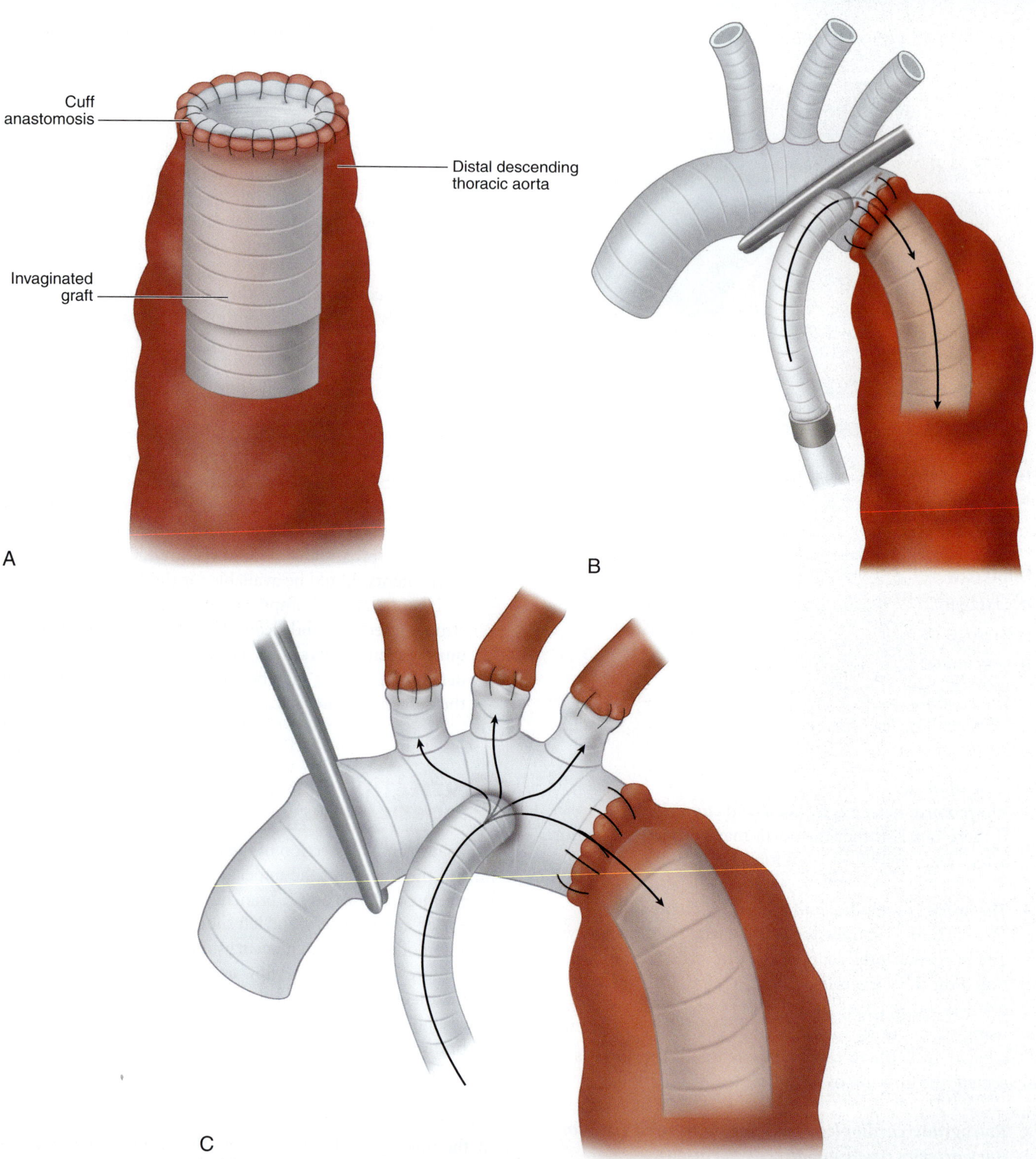

FIG. 32.14 Aneurysm of the aortic arch. (A) A branched graft is inserted into the distal descending thoracic aorta. The cuff anastomosis is performed using 3-0 polypropylene suture. Surgical adhesive may be applied to seal the needle holes. (B and C) The anastomosis continues with the common carotid and innominate arteries. (From Selke F, Ruel M, eds. *Atlas of Cardiac Surgical Techniques*. Philadelphia: Saunders; 2010.)

POSITION:	Right lateral
INCISION:	Left posterolateral thoracotomy
PREP AND DRAPING:	Chin to thigh
INSTRUMENTS:	Major cardiac set

Technical Points and Discussion

1. ***A thoracotomy is performed.***
   A left thoracotomy is performed. After the chest has been opened and the retractors placed, the surgeon retracts the edges of the pleura with 2-0 silk sutures.

2. ***The aneurysm or dissection is mobilized from the surrounding tissue.***
The surgeon begins to free the aneurysm from the surrounding tissue. Femoral vein–femoral artery CPB may be used to perfuse the kidneys and the rest of the lower body. If bypass is not used, speed is essential at this time because there is no flow to the lower body. The scrub must be alert and avoid unnecessary movements and loss of time while handling instruments.

3. ***Vascular occluding clamps are applied to the aorta, and the aneurysm or dissection is resected.***
The surgeon occludes the aorta proximal and distal to the aneurysm. The knife is then used to make a longitudinal incision into the aneurysm, and the incision is extended with scissors. The outer layer of the aneurysm is preserved and retracted with 2-0 or 3-0 silk sutures. These flaps are used later in the procedure to cover the grafts and prevent them from adhering to the lung.
The surgeon removes all debris and blood clots inside the aneurysm using suction and tissue forceps. The technologist should have a small basin to receive loose debris and blood clots and a moist sponge to wipe debris from the instruments.

4. ***The intercostal arteries are ligated.***
The surgeon ligates the intercostal vessels along the posterior wall of the aneurysm with polyester sutures. Identifying the origin of these vessels may be difficult. To aid identification, the surgeon may irrigate the area with warm saline solution and look for bleeding points, indicating an open vessel. When hemostasis is secured, the graft is anastomosed to the aorta.

5. ***The proximal anastomosis is performed.***
The surgeon transects the aorta immediately above and below the aneurysm and removes the middle segment. A graft is then implanted to replace the diseased segment. The surgeon performs the proximal anastomosis with continuous suture of 3-0 or 4-0 polypropylene or polyester.

6. ***The graft is checked for leaks.***
A straight vascular clamp may be placed across the graft while the surgeon releases the proximal aortic clamp briefly to check for leaks. The surgeon reapplies the aortic clamp, removes the graft clamp, and places any additional sutures needed to control leakage. Teflon pledgets may be used to bolster the sutures.

7. ***The distal anastomosis is performed.***
After completing the proximal anastomosis, the surgeon trims the graft to the appropriate length and performs the distal anastomosis. Before the suture is tied, the graft is flushed to clear it of clots and debris. The suture is then tied and all clamps are removed, restoring blood flow to the lower body.

8. ***The graft is covered with aneurysm tissue and the wound is closed.***
If CPB has been used, it is discontinued at this stage, and the cannulas are removed. To complete the procedure, the surgeon covers the graft with remaining aneurysm tissue (if it has not been excised) using absorbable continuous or interrupted 2-0 or 3-0 suture. The mediastinal pleura is closed, chest tubes are inserted, and the wound is closed in layers.

ENDOVASCULAR REPAIR OF A THORACIC ANEURYSM

Endovascular repair of a descending thoracic aneurysm is now frequently used for the treatment of descending thoracic aortic aneurysm (DTAA). Several different devices are currently used. These include the TAG Device (Gore), Talent (Medtronic), and Zenith TX2 (Cook Medical). Others are under investigation at this time. The surgical approach may be through an incision into the femoral artery, or percutaneous insertion (without incision) may be possible. As in the endovascular repair of abdominal aneurysm, a wire stent graft is deployed through the femoral artery and positioned at the level of the aneurysm. This is done under fluoroscopy and intraoperative angiography, using the opposite groin for the entry of angiocatheters. Technical points of the procedure are illustrated in Fig. 32.15.

Pathology

Endovascular repair of descending aortic aneurysms is performed on patients with fusiform-type aneurysms, which are at least double the normal size of the aorta. Computed tomography angiography is used to measure and evaluate the extent of disease to determine whether the patient is suitable for endovascular repair.

POSITION:	Supine
INCISION:	Groin
PREP AND DRAPING:	Lower abdominal, groin
INSTRUMENTS:	Endovascular aneurysm set

Technical Points and Discussion

1. ***The femoral artery is cannulated.***
A transverse incision is made in the groin. The femoral artery is exposed and mobilized. An 18-gauge needle is inserted into the femoral artery, and a flexible guidewire such as a 0.035-inch Bentson wire is threaded into the thoracic portion of the aorta. The needle is removed. Because the guidewires may be more than 6 feet long, the surgical technologist should take precautions to avoid contaminating the wire by anchoring the distal end of the wire with wet, sterile towels or another weighted sterile object.

2. ***The femoral artery is dilated.***
Dilators of increasing size are inserted over the guidewire; each dilator is inserted and removed in succession and

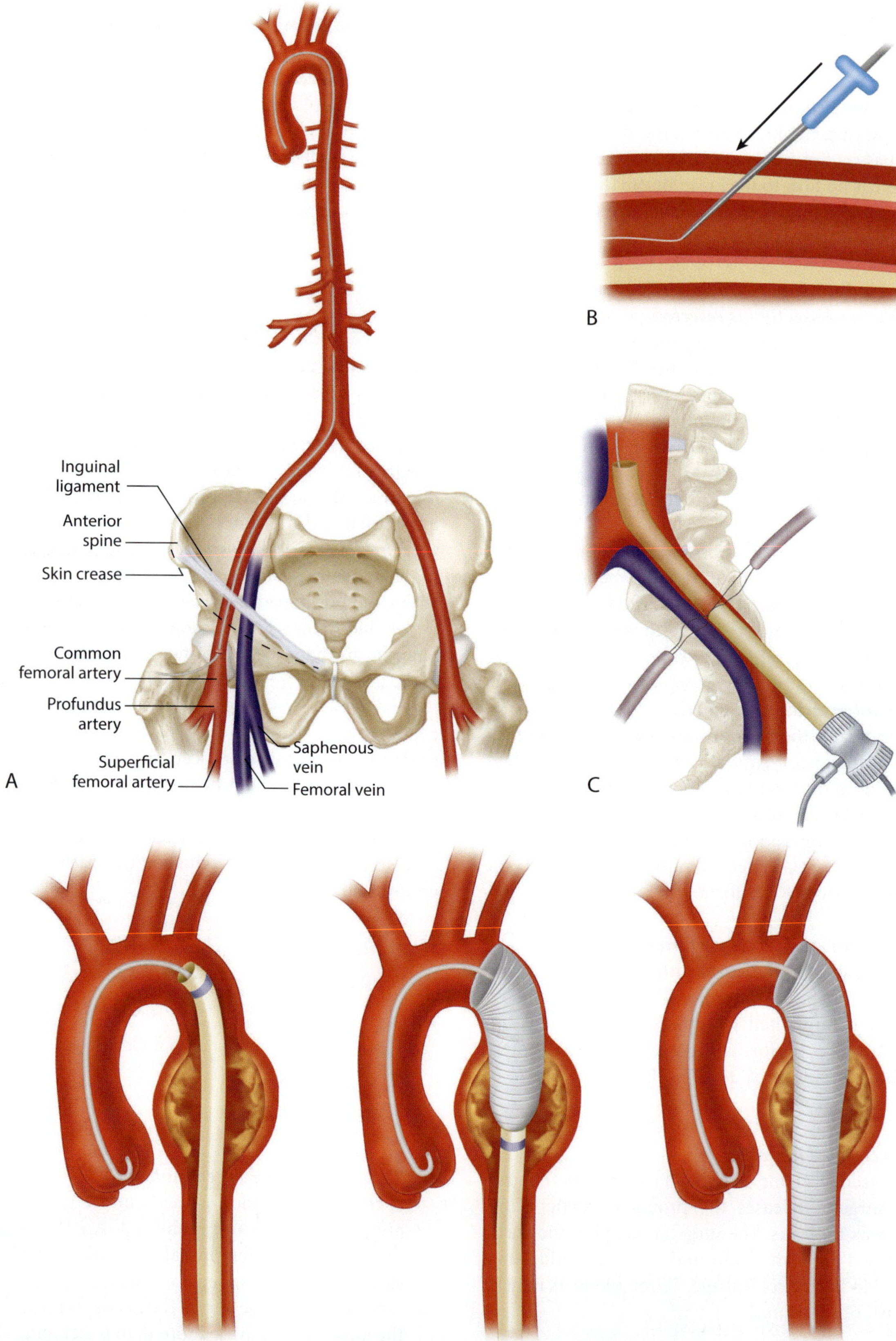

FIG. 32.15 Endovascular aortic aneurysm. (A and B) The femoral artery is exposed, and an 18-gauge needle and guidewire are used to enter the artery. (C) A guide catheter is inserted over the guidewire. An introducer sheath is introduced over a pigtail catheter, the graft is introduced through the sheath, and the sheath is withdrawn, leaving the graft in place. (From Selke F, Ruel M, eds. *Atlas of Cardiac Surgical Techniques*. Philadelphia: Saunders; 2010.)

replaced with a larger guidewire to enlarge the femoral artery.

3. ***The opposite femoral artery is cannulated.***
   An angiographic catheter is inserted into the patient's opposite femoral artery to visualize the interior of the aorta, to perform intraoperative angiograms, and to guide and verify the placement of the deployed stent.

4. ***The arch vessels are identified and measured.***
   The surgeon uses fluoroscopy to identify the location of the arch vessels and to identify normal proximal and distal aortic tissue into which the endovascular stent graft will be secured. Intravascular ultrasound may be used to measure internal diameters and to note anatomical angles that can affect placement of the device(s). More than one device may be deployed when there is an extensive lesion. The guidewire may be exchanged several times to arrive at a suitable one for entry into the aortic arch.

5. ***The endograft is deployed.***
   The endograft is deployed in the aorta using the appropriate introducer sheath if necessary. Intraoperative arteriogram is used to confirm the location of the aneurysm for the exact placement of the graft. When the target area is confirmed, the endograft is positioned and opened in the aorta. The surgeon confirms the proper placement of the endostent(s), and the absence of endoleaks. If hemostasis is not achieved, the surgeon may reposition the graft or replace the existing graft with another stent. If there is acute hemorrhage that cannot be repaired endoscopically, the technologist should be prepared for open surgery to complete the repair.

6. ***The wounds are closed.***
   The wounds are closed using size 2-0 and 3-0 synthetic absorbable sutures. Skin is closed with interrupted nylon sutures or subcuticular Vicryl size 4-0 or 3-0. The wounds are dressed with flat gauze and tape.

   Recovery from an endovascular repair is considerably shorter than recovery from an open thoracotomy. Possible complications include bleeding and migration of the device, requiring adjustment and/or insertion of another device.

INSERTION OF AN ARTIFICIAL CARDIAC PACEMAKER

An artificial pacemaker is implanted in the body to correct cardiac arrhythmia caused by a disease of the conduction system. A *pulse generator* provides electrical impulses through the device's cardiac leads, which are implanted in the conductive tissue of the heart.

A pacemaker may be implanted in the cardiac catheterization suite or in the perioperative period. Postsurgically, a pacemaker can be implanted via the transvenous route (a temporary pacer is used until it is replaced by a permanent pacing system).

A pacemaker may be implanted temporarily, such as during cardiac procedures, or the implantation may be permanent. Three approaches are used for permanent implantation: the transvenous, epicardial, and subxiphoid approaches. The transvenous and subxiphoid procedures, which do not require a thoracotomy, are commonly performed with the patient under local anesthesia with monitored anesthesia care. When the transvenous approach is used, the electrodes are placed with the aid of fluoroscopy.

Pathology

Cardiac arrhythmia is an abnormal pattern of conductivity in the heart. Healthy individuals may have an arrhythmia. However, when the heart's conduction mechanism is affected by disease, certain arrhythmias can be life threatening. Arrhythmias are named by type and origin. Some common arrhythmias are as follows:

- *Ventricular* ***tachycardia:*** A heart rate over 120 beats per minute
- *Atrial flutter:* A heart rate of 240 to 350 beats per minute in an adult
- *Ventricular fibrillation:* Chaotic, disorganized stimulation of one or both ventricles that does not pump the blood
- *Atrial fibrillation:* Chaotic, disorganized stimulation of one or both atria that prevents atrial contraction (which normally fills the ventricle with blood)
- ***Bradycardia:*** A heart rate below 40 to 60 beats per minute

Conduction disease can arise from ischemic heart disease, which can be caused by atherosclerosis, infection, or congenital defects.

TEMPORARY PACEMAKER

POSITION:	Supine
INCISION:	Median sternotomy
PREP AND DRAPING:	Thoracic
INSTRUMENTS:	Cardiac instrument set

Technical Points and Discussion

1. ***A median sternotomy is performed.***

2. ***An electrode is sutured to the right atrium and/or the right ventricle or can be inserted transvenously.***
   A right or left subclavian venotomy is performed, and the electrode is advanced into the right atrium, through the tricuspid valve, and into the right ventricle, where it is placed in the right ventricular apex. The pulse generator is then placed within the superficial tissues of the chest wall. An atrial electrode may also be placed in the atrial appendage for dual-chamber (atrial and ventricular) pacing.

   Temporary pacemaker leads are implanted before CPB is discontinued because the field is more accessible with the lungs deflated (as occurs on bypass). Another reason the leads are implanted before the bypass is discontinued is that if touching the heart during lead attachment causes an arrhythmia, perfusion to the body is not compromised.

The surgeon sutures the metal wire electrode to the heart with 5-0 silk. Only the tip of the electrode is exposed; the remaining section is insulated.

3. ***The free end of the electrode is brought through the skin and secured with a suture.***
The scrub prepares the electrode on a needle holder before or after the bypass is discontinued. The assistant cuts the needle off the electrode after the surgeon places it through the myocardium. The surgeon then secures the electrode with 5-0 silk sutures. The surgeon brings the opposite end of the electrode through the skin and secures it with 2-0 silk sutures. The electrode is connected to an alligator cable and pacemaker generator. The anesthesia care provider can then pace the heart as necessary.

INSERTION OF PERMANENT PACEMAKER (SUBCLAVICULAR)

POSITION:	Supine
INCISION:	Subclavian
PREP AND DRAPING:	Thoracic; axillary; the neck is included for jugular access as needed
INSTRUMENTS:	Minor general surgery set; US retractors; Deaver retractors

Technical Points and Discussion

1. ***The patient is prepped and draped.***
The patient is placed in supine position, prepped, and draped for a subclavicular incision.

2. ***A guidewire is positioned in the right atrium.***
Venous access is gained into the subclavian, internal jugular, or axillary vein using an 18-gauge access needle. A guidewire is threaded over the needle and advanced into the right atrium under fluoroscopy. The needle is withdrawn, leaving only the guidewire.

3. ***A pocket is formed in the subclavicular subcutaneous tissue.***
An incision is made in the skin at the proposed implantation site with blunt dissection and scissors.

4. ***The ventricular lead is placed at the right ventricular apex.***
A sheath and dilator are inserted over the guidewire. The guidewire and dilator are then removed leaving only the sheath. A rigid stylet is advanced inside the center of the pacemaker lead, and the lead-stylet assembly is advanced to the heart chamber.

5. ***The leads are secured to the endocardium.***
The position of the lead is verified, and it is fixed to the pericardium either with a helical screw or other mechanism according to the type of pacemaker set. The screw is inserted using the torque device, which comes with the set. The lead stylet is removed.

6. ***The lead is tested and sutured in place.***
The pacing and sensing levels and impedances are measured using a pacing analyzer. Pacing is performed. The proximal end of the lead is sutured to the muscle tissue.
If a second lead is required, it is introduced through a separate sheath into the atrium.

7. ***The pulse generator is positioned.***
The surgeon irrigates the tissue pocket using antimicrobial solution. The pulse generator is then connected to the leads and positioned in the pocket. Non-absorbable sutures such as Dacron are used to secure the pulse generator. The incision is closed in layers using size 3-0 or 2-0 Vicryl. Skin is closed with Steri-Strips or subcuticular absorbable suture. A flat dressing is applied.

Heart Failure

Surgical techniques to support a failing heart are available for temporary, long-term, or permanent support. When mechanical devices cannot reverse the decline of heart function, cardiac transplantation may be required.

INSERTION OF AN INTRAAORTIC BALLOON PUMP (IABP)

An intraaortic balloon pump (IABP) is a device that increases the supply of oxygen to the heart. When the ventricle contracts, the balloon deflates, creating a vacuum that lowers the pressure in the aorta. When the ventricle relaxes, the balloon inflates, increasing the volume of blood into the coronary arteries and distal organ. This produces additional blood flow to the brain, kidneys, and other organs.

An intraaortic balloon catheter reduces the workload of the heart after myocardial infarction or in patients who cannot be taken off bypass. The device is inserted into the descending thoracic aorta in a retrograde direction via the femoral artery. The device itself is available in a kit that includes all the accessories needed for implantation. The procedure is done under local anesthesia or at the close of cardiac surgery.

Pathology

Myocardial infarction is caused by the obstruction of the coronary artery and results in death of cardiac tissue. An intraaortic balloon catheter reduces the workload of a damaged heart after myocardial infarction. This also reduces the oxygen requirements of heart tissue and compensates for the loss of coronary artery function.

POSITION:	Supine
INCISION:	Groin
PREP AND DRAPING:	Groin
INSTRUMENTS:	Minor general surgery; balloon pump kit and accessories including dilators, sheaths, and guidewires

Technical Points

1. *The patient is placed in the supine position and prepped for a groin incision.*
2. *An introducer needle is used to puncture the femoral artery. A guidewire is placed into the needle.*
3. *The needle is removed leaving the guidewire in place.*
4. *A dilator is threaded over the guidewire to enlarge the artery.*
5. *A small incision is made into the femoral artery.*
6. *A sheath with dilator is advanced. The dilator is removed leaving the sheath.*
7. *Air is removed from the IABP using a one-way valve and syringe.*
8. *The IABP is inserted into the artery over the guidewire into the sheath.*
9. *The device is advanced into the descending thoracic aorta.*
10. *The mechanical ends of the IABP are passed off the field and connected to the machine by the perfusionist.*

IMPLANTATION OF A LEFT VENTRICULAR ASSIST DEVICE

A left ventricular assist device (LVAD) is used in three scenarios. One is to act as a bridge for patients awaiting heart transplantation; another is *destination therapy* in patients who cannot receive a transplant. The LVAD may also be used to wean patients off CPB. The LVAD maintains perfusion through a pump system. Power is provided by pneumatic, electrical, or battery-powered pumps. Right ventricular assist devices are also available.

The implantable LVAD pump is connected to inflow and outflow cannulas, which are implanted in the left ventricle and aorta. There are many different pump manufacturers and several methods used to implant them. A general approach is presented here. The surgical technologist will need to study the types of pumps used at his or her facility. This includes pump preparation and the use of implant accessories. The basic components of the LVAD are the pump, an outflow **conduit**—a large collar and tube that shunts blood out of the ventricle, an inflow conduit or graft that receives blood from the pump, and the power line that is implanted in the body and exits to connect to power source. A common technique for the implantation of the LVAD is to perform implantation during CPB with the heart beating.

POSITION:	Supine
INCISION:	Median sternotomy extended to umbilicus
PREP AND DRAPING:	Abdomen and thorax
INSTRUMENTS:	Cardiac set with LVAD kit and accessories

Technical Points

1. *The patient is prepped and draped for a midline/median sternotomy.*
2. *A midline abdominal incision is made.*
3. *A tissue pocket is made in the right upper quadrant to accommodate the LVAD. A smaller pocket is made opposite (on the left side).*
4. *A sternotomy is performed.*
5. *The LVAD model is placed in the tissue pocket to determine the correct size.*
6. *The apex of the left ventricle is cored using the coring knife component of the set.*
7. *Approximately 20 size 2-0 polyester horizontal mattress sutures are placed around the circumference of the apical core. A felt strip may be placed around the edge to provide cushioning for the sutures.*
8. *Sutures are passed through the inflow conduit (tube) and secured.*
9. *The inner ring of the inflow conduit is removed, and the LVAD is inserted into the left ventricle. Additional 2-0 sutures may be used for hemostasis. Cable ties are secured around the neck of the conduit.*
10. *A Dacron graft is brought into the wound and extended to check for correct length. A bend relief is inserted connecting the LVAD and the graft. This prevents the grafts from crimping after implantation.*
11. *A side clamping aortic clamp is positioned over the aorta.*
12. *A linear incision is made in the aorta, and an end-to-side anastomosis is performed between the aorta and Dacron graft. The aortic clamp is released, and the anastomosis is checked for leakage.*
13. *The pump is positioned in the tissue pocket.*
14. *A percutaneous tube containing the electric cable is tunneled through the abdominal wall through a stab incision.*
15. *The LVAD is connected to the outflow graft.*
16. *The LVAD is initiated while CPB is withdrawn.*

Several different types of LVAD are illustrated in Fig. 32.16.

HEART TRANSPLANTATION

The goal of heart transplantation is to replace a diseased heart with a healthy donor heart. Heart transplantation is undertaken by a specially trained transplant team.

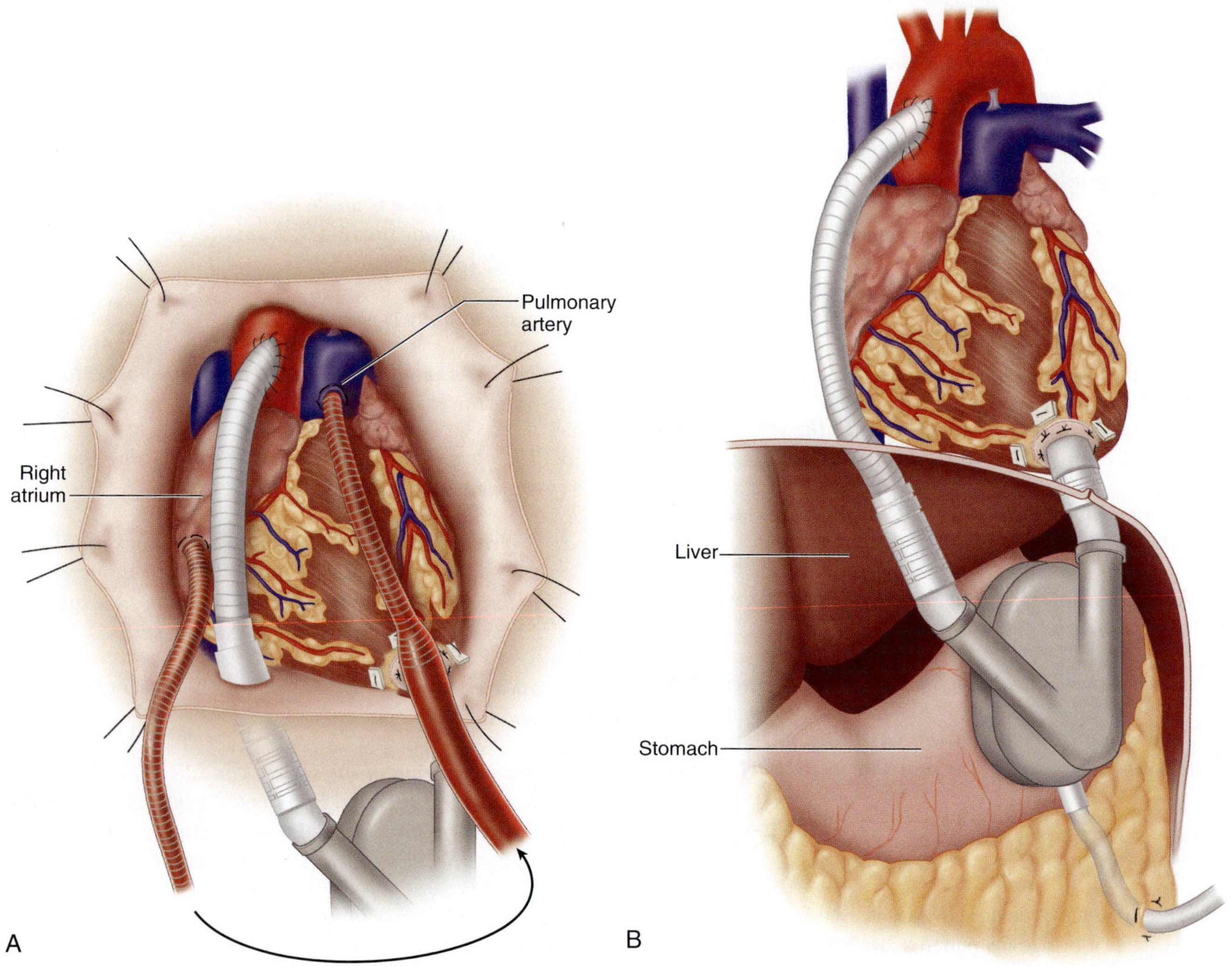

FIG. 32.16 Assistive ventricular devices. (A) Levitronix CentriMag (Levitronix LLC). (B) HeartMate SVE (Thoratec Corp.). (From Doty D, Doty J. *Cardiac Surgery Operative Technique*. 2nd ed. Philadelphia: Saunders; 2012.)

A modification of the orthotopic implantation technique has been developed that reduces some of the cardiac rhythm problems that can occur after transplantation. End-to-end anastomoses between the superior vena cava and the inferior vena cava are performed rather than the traditional atrial-to-atrial anastomoses. A cuff of the recipient left atrium is sewn to the donor left atrium; pulmonary artery and aorta anastomoses are performed in the usual manner. A pulmonary pressure monitoring line may be inserted before the patient leaves the operating room.

Complications of heart transplantation include rejection and infection. Transplant anastomoses may require repair if persistent bleeding develops. Rhythm changes may occur if retained conduction tissue from both the native and donor hearts is present.

Myocardial biopsies are required after surgery to detect possible rejection. Postoperatively, the transplant patient is placed on lifelong therapy with immunosuppressive medications to prevent the rejection of the donor heart. Endomyocardial biopsies are taken regularly to monitor for rejection. Patients who have undergone cardiac surgery are commonly transported to a cardiovascular intensive care unit (CVICU) for the intensive monitoring of blood pressure, heart rate, cardiac rhythm, chest tube drainage, and temperature.

The endotracheal tube may be removed within a few hours after arrival in the CVICU, or it may remain in place until the patient is able to breathe independently. The patient's neurological, renal, pulmonary, and pain status are also closely observed and treated as necessary. Complications can include hemorrhage, prolonged ventilation, renal failure, infection, cardiac arrest, stroke, and death. Patients are often discharged from the hospital within 5 to 7 days unless complications develop. Technical points are illustrated in Fig. 32.17.

Pathology

Heart transplantation may be performed in suitable patients with end-stage cardiac disease. Patients suitable for heart transplantation include those with the following:

- Coronary artery disease
- Congenital heart disease
- Valve disease
- Rejection of a previously transplanted heart

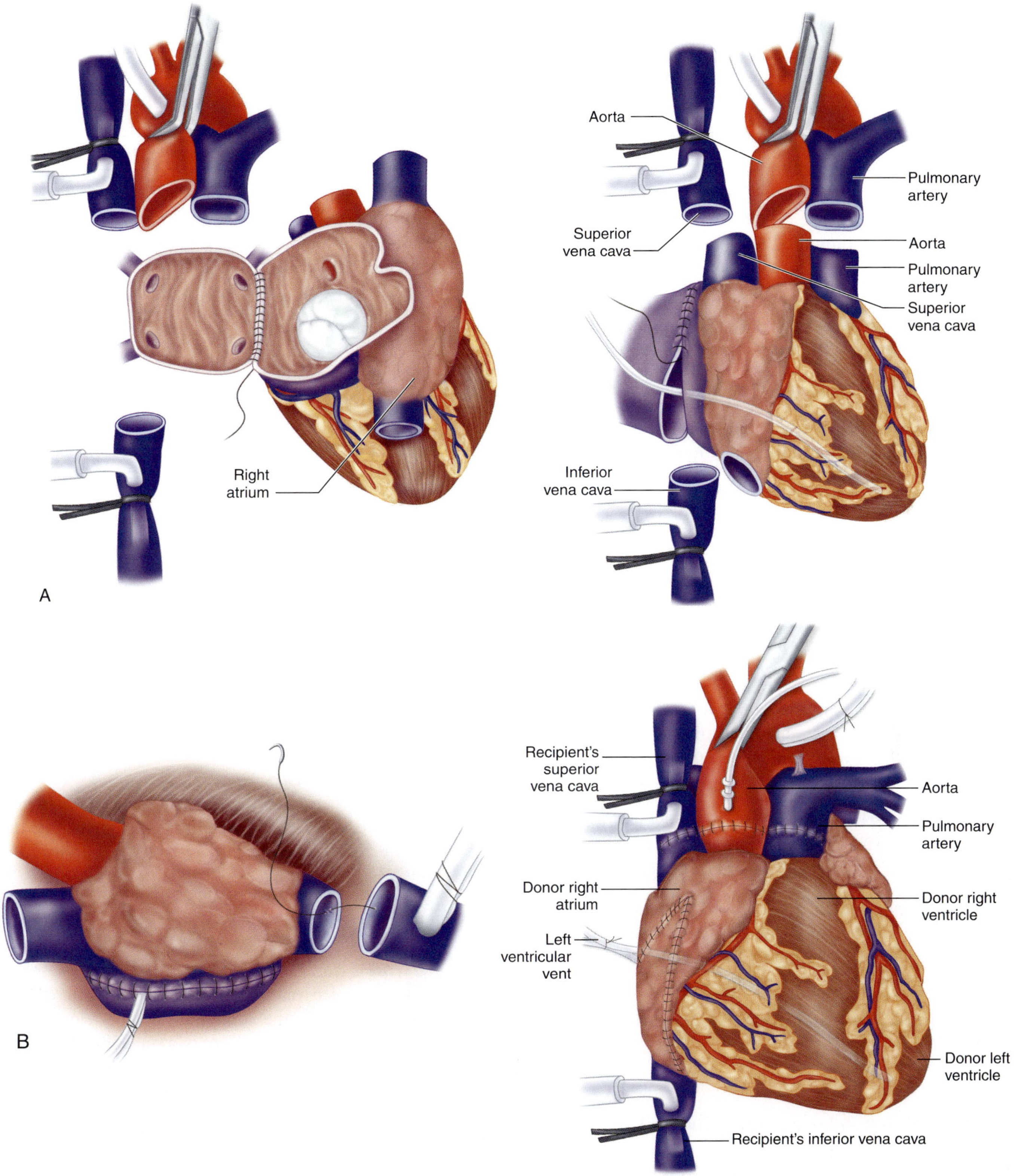

FIG. 32.17 Heart transplantation. (A) Left atrium anastomosis of the donor heart. (B) Anastomosis of the vena cava. (From Selke F, Ruel M, eds. *Atlas of Cardiac Surgical Techniques*. Philadelphia: Saunders; 2010.)

Technical Points

NATIVE HEART EXCISION

1. ***The patient is placed in the supine position and prepped from chin to knees.***
2. ***A median sternotomy incision is made to expose the heart and great vessels.***
3. ***Heparin is administered.***
4. **Bicaval cannulation *for CPB is performed.***
5. ***Caval tapes are placed around each vena cava.***
6. ***The patient is cooled, the aorta is cross-clamped, and the caval tapes are tightened around the venae cavae.***
7. ***The pulmonary trunk and aorta are divided.***
8. ***The atria are incised to leave intact the posterior portions of the right and left atrial walls and the interatrial septum.***
9. ***The recipient's native heart is excised.***

DONOR HEART IMPLANTATION

1. ***The donor heart is removed from the transport container and placed in a basin on the back table.***
2. ***The surgeon inspects the heart and trims the atrial walls and great vessels in preparation for the anastomoses.***
3. ***The donor heart is placed in the pericardial cavity and aligned with the remnant interatrial septum and the right and left atrial wall remnants of the recipient's heart.***
4. ***The donor left atrial wall is anastomosed with running 3-0 polypropylene suture (suture size and type may vary according to the surgeon's preference) (Fig. 32.17A).***
5. ***The inferior vena cava (IVC) and superior vena cava (SVC) are anastomosed with running 3-0 polypropylene suture, followed by pulmonary artery anastomosis with 4-0 polypropylene suture (see Fig. 32.17B).***
6. ***The aorta is anastomosed with 3-0 or 5-0 running polypropylene suture.***
7. ***Air is removed from the heart.***
8. ***Chest drainage tubes and epicardial pacing wires are inserted.***
9. ***The chest incision is closed.***

PEDIATRIC CARDIAC PROCEDURES

CLOSURE OF A PATENT DUCTUS ARTERIOSUS

Surgical closure of a *patent ductus arteriosus* (PDA) is performed to prevent arterial blood from recirculating through the pulmonary circulation. The ductus may be approached by an open incision or by the endoscopic route.

Pathology

The ductus arteriosus is a normal anatomical opening in the fetal heart. During fetal development, blood is pumped from the right ventricle into the systemic circulation via the ductus, which connects the pulmonary artery and descending thoracic aorta. At birth, the lungs expand and the ductus closes spontaneously within a short time. If the ductus fails to close, arterial blood returns to the lungs, putting an added burden on the lungs and heart. The heart becomes enlarged and may fail. The ductus is closed surgically to correct this defect, usually during infancy.

POSITION:	Lateral
INCISION:	Left thoracotomy
PREP AND DRAPING:	Thoracic
INSTRUMENTS:	Cardiac set

Technical Points and Discussion

1. ***The patient is prepped and draped.***
   Surgical repair of a PDA may be performed by minimally invasive surgery. An open procedure is described here.
2. ***A left thoracotomy is performed.***
   To begin the repair, the surgeon places a traction suture through the edges of the pleura usually with 3-0 silk suture. The ends are tagged with a hemostat. The assistant retracts the pleura with the suture.
3. ***The ductus is isolated.***
   The surgeon then carefully dissects the aorta and pulmonary artery with fine dissecting scissors to expose the ductus. A heavy silk suture may be passed around the ductus.
   The surgeon continues the dissection until the ductus is fully isolated.
4. ***The ductus is closed.***
   Straight or angled vascular clamps are placed across the ductus, one close to the aorta and the other close to the pulmonary artery. In a newborn or a small infant, the surgeon may simply tie the ductus with size 0 silk because the ductus is small and may not allow the placement of the vascular clamps. Vascular clips may also be used.
   In other situations, the surgeon may divide and oversew the cut edges. The surgeon cuts halfway through the ductus with Potts scissors or a knife. A 5-0 or 6-0 polypropylene suture is used to begin the closure of the ductus on the aortic side. The surgeon continues to incise the ductus and continues the suture to close the defect on the aortic side. The vascular clamp is then slowly released. Additional sutures are placed if needed. The end of the ductus closest to the pulmonary artery is sutured in the same manner. A topical hemostatic agent can be used to control bleeding at the anastomosis.

5. ***A chest tube is inserted, and the chest is closed.***
The mediastinal pleura is closed with a continuous suture of 3-0 or 4-0 silk or chromic gut. An appropriate-size chest tube is inserted, and the wound is closed in layers.

CORRECTION OF A COARCTATION OF THE THORACIC AORTA

Correction of a coarctation of the thoracic aorta is performed to restore blood flow to the lower body and reduce cardiac workload.

Pathology

Coarctation of the thoracic aorta is a congenital stenosis that usually occurs near the junction of the fetal ductus arteriosus and the aorta. Severe narrowing obstructs the normal flow of blood through the thoracic aorta and to the lower body. The heart becomes enlarged as a result of the increased work required to pump blood through a stricture. The lower body may be underdeveloped as a result of the defect.

POSITION:	Lateral
INCISION:	Posterolateral thoracotomy
PREP AND DRAPING:	Thoracic
INSTRUMENTS:	Cardiac set

Technical Points and Discussion

1. ***The patient is placed in the lateral position, prepped, and draped for a thoracotomy.***
2. ***A thoracotomy is performed.***
The thoracic cavity is entered through a posterolateral thoracotomy. A moist laparotomy sponge is placed over the lung, which is retracted by the assistant.

3. ***The mediastinal pleura is incised.***
The surgeon incises the mediastinal pleura and places 3-0 or 4-0 silk traction sutures in the edges. This exposes the aorta. Moist umbilical tape is placed around the aorta for mobilization and retraction.

4. ***The ligamentum arteriosum is ligated and divided.***
The intercostal arteries are mobilized. Fine dissecting scissors are used to dissect the aorta in the area of the coarctation.
The surgeon ligates and divides the ductus (a ductus that has closed naturally is called the *ligamentum arteriosum*) to free the aorta and prevent bleeding from the ductus or ligamentum if it is still patent. Additional sutures of 4-0 silk are placed in the ductus if needed.

5. ***The aorta is occluded proximal and distal to the coarctation.***
The surgeon occludes the aorta proximal and distal to the coarctation with straight or angled vascular clamps. The arteries that supply the diseased segment are also ligated. Bulldog clamps may be placed on vessels that lie between the diseased segment and the cross clamps of the aorta.

6. ***The aorta is transected, and the stricture is removed.***
The two ends of the aorta are anastomosed with 5-0 or 6-0 continuous suture. Interrupted sutures are often used in pediatric patients to allow growth. (In adults, 3-0 or 4-0 polypropylene suture is used.) If the two limbs of the aorta cannot be brought together easily (often the case in adults), a synthetic tube graft may be inserted, or a proximal portion of the left subclavian artery may be used to form a patch. In this technique, a part of the artery wall is rotated and anastomosed to the resected coarctation. The distal artery is then ligated.

7. ***The aorta is unclamped.***
All clamps are removed from the aorta and intercostal arteries. Blood flow to the lower body is restored. The surgeon inspects all suture lines for hemostasis, and additional sutures are placed as needed. A topical hemostatic agent may be applied to control bleeding.

8. ***The wound is closed.***
The mediastinal pleura is closed with 3-0 or 4-0 suture. A chest tube is inserted, and the wound is closed in layers.

TOTAL CORRECTION OF TETRALOGY OF FALLOT

Tetralogy of Fallot is a combination of congenital defects that include pulmonary stenosis, ventricular septal defect, right ventricular hypertrophy, and dextroposition (displacement) of the aorta. Surgical repair is performed to restore normal blood flow. Repair of each defect is discussed separately below.

Pathology

Tetralogy of Fallot causes reduced pulmonary blood flow and right-to-left shunting (from the right ventricle to the left ventricle) of blood. This shunting mixes deoxygenated blood with oxygenated blood, and the mixture is pumped into the systemic circulation. The right ventricle becomes hypertrophied (enlarged) because of the work needed to pump the blood through the obstructed pulmonary system. The patient is cyanotic and increased oxygen demand results in reduced pulmonary blood flow. If delayed repair is necessary, a systemic-pulmonary shunt may be performed to increase blood flow to the lungs. This shunt improves oxygenation and allows the baby to develop to a stage at which total correction is possible.

POSITION:	Supine
INCISION:	Median sternotomy
PREP AND DRAPING:	Thoracic
INSTRUMENTS:	Pediatric open-heart set

Technical Points and Discussion

1. ***The patient is prepped and draped.***
The patient is prepped and draped for a median sternotomy.

2. ***A median sternotomy is performed and bypass is initiated.***
After the chest has been opened, bypass is initiated. Cardioplegia is then performed as described previously.

3. ***A right ventriculotomy is performed.***
The surgeon performs the right ventriculotomy with a knife and Metzenbaum scissors. Retractors are inserted, and a portion of the infundibular muscle is excised.
A pulmonary valvulotomy is then performed, and the ventricular septal defect is closed as described below. After air is evacuated from the left ventricle, the clamp is removed from the aorta.

4. ***The ventricular septal defect is closed, and the right ventricle is closed with a patch.***
The surgeon closes the ventricle with a continuous suture of 4-0 polypropylene. A patch of woven Dacron or Teflon is used to enlarge the right ventricular outflow tract (the area beneath the pulmonary valve). The pulmonary artery may also be enlarged with a patch, using a smaller size suture.

The pulmonary artery pressure and right ventricular pressure are measured to determine whether the surgery was successful. If the results indicate that additional surgery is required, additional surgical supplies are needed.

5. ***Bypass is discontinued.***
If the surgery is successful, bypass is discontinued, and the wound is prepared for closure as described previously. Chest tubes are inserted, and the wound is closed. Complete repair of tetralogy of Fallot is illustrated in Fig. 32.18.

CORRECTION OF PULMONARY VALVE STENOSIS

Valvulotomy is performed to release fused valve leaflets and restore circulation from the right ventricle to the lungs.

Pathology

Pulmonary valve stenosis is usually a congenital anomaly in which the pulmonary valve is narrowed. Pulmonary stenosis may also occur proximal or distal to the valve. Severe stenosis may require emergency treatment.

POSITION:	Supine
INCISION:	Median sternotomy
PREP AND DRAPING:	Thoracic
INSTRUMENTS:	Cardiac set

Technical Points and Discussion

1. ***The patient is prepped and draped.***
The patient is placed in supine position, prepped, and draped for a median sternotomy.

2. ***CPB is initiated through a median sternotomy.***
The surgeon enters the chest through a median sternotomy. The pericardial sac is incised with scissors, and the incision is extended downward to the diaphragm and upward to the innominate vein. Cannulas of the correct size are obtained and bypass is initiated.
An umbilical tape is placed on the aorta and a purse-string suture of 4-0 polypropylene or polyester is placed. The assistant brings the ends of the suture through a bolster (a short vinyl or Silastic tube that holds the suture ends together) and holds the suture with a hemostat.

3. ***The pulmonary artery is opened, and the fused leaflets are separated.***
To begin the repair, the surgeon isolates the vena cava with umbilical tape, and a tourniquet is placed as previously described. The pulmonary artery above the valve is opened with scissors. The aorta may be temporarily occluded to create a drier field. The fused leaflets are separated with a knife, Metzenbaum scissors, or Potts scissors. The surgeon closes the pulmonary artery with 5-0 continuous suture of polypropylene. If the pulmonary artery is stenotic, a patch graft may be inserted to enlarge the artery.

4. ***CPB is withdrawn, chest tubes are placed, and the wound is closed.***

CLOSURE OF AN ATRIAL SEPTAL DEFECT

An atrial septal defect is a congenital anomaly in which a hole in the interatrial septum allows blood from the left atrium to flow into the right atrium. The goal of surgery is to close the defect and reduce excessive blood flow to the pulmonary system.

Pathology

Blood normally flows from the left atrium into the left ventricle before entering the systemic circulation. An atrial septal defect causes the blood to shunt from the left atrium to the right atrium. This creates increased pressure on the right ventricle and lungs, causing the heart to enlarge and eventually fail. An atrial septal defect is usually closed during childhood. However, some patients reach adulthood before developing symptoms that require surgical repair.

POSITION:	Supine
INCISION:	Median sternotomy
PREP AND DRAPING:	Thoracic
INSTRUMENTS:	Cardiac set
POSSIBLE EXTRAS:	Patch graft

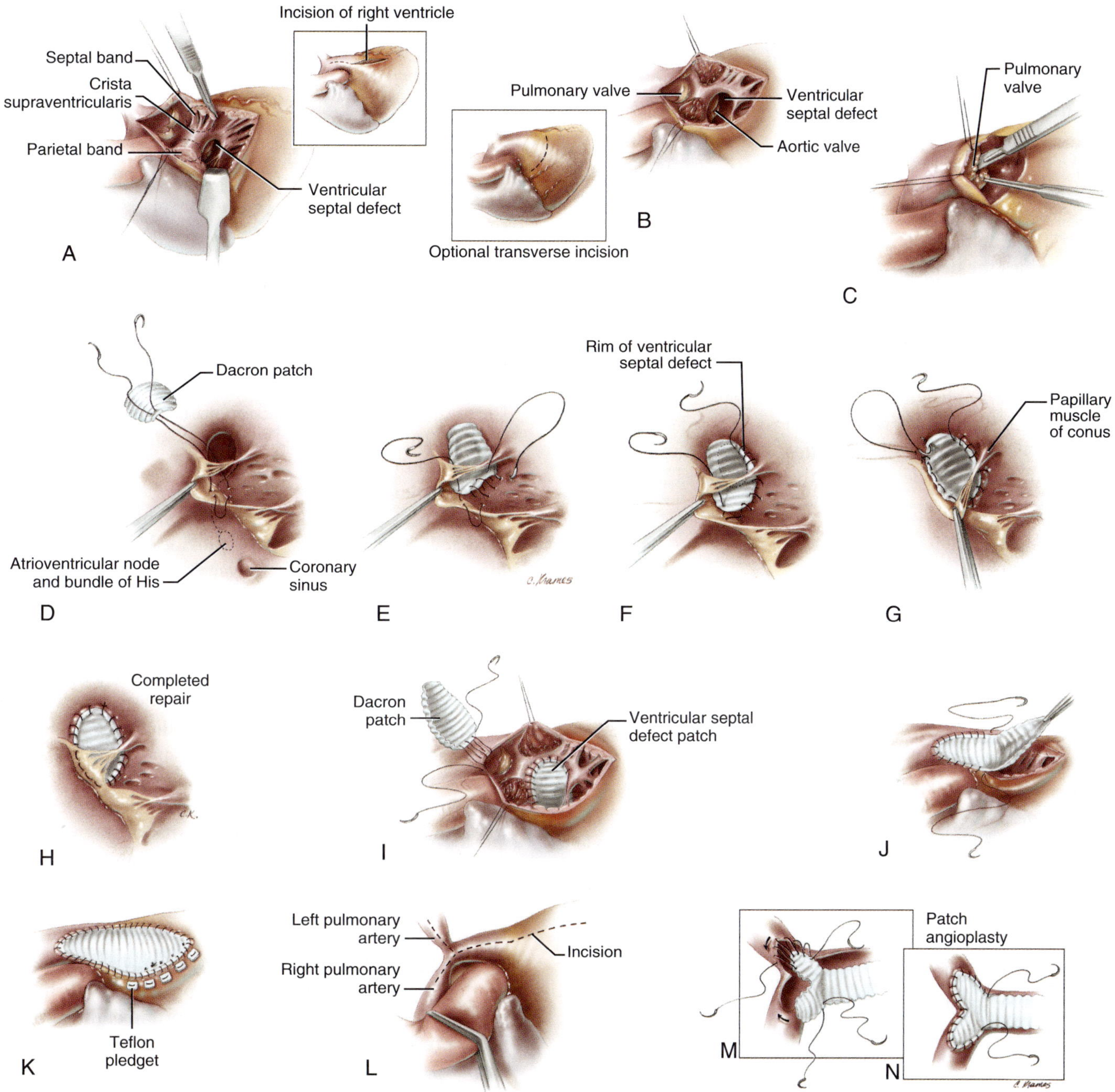

FIG. 32.18 Repair of tetralogy of Fallot. (A) A ventriculotomy incision is made using a #11 knife blade. The incision is carried to the annulus of the pulmonary valve, and a valvotomy is performed. (B) Traction sutures are placed at the annulus of the pulmonary valve, the apex of the ventricular incision, and at the base of the apex muscle band. (C) Optional transverse approach. (D) The septal leaflet of the tricuspid valve is retracted with forceps. A patch graft of woven Dacron is created and secured to the rim of the defect with size 4-0 polypropylene sutures. (E) Several additional sutures are placed in the ventricular septum. (F) Suturing continues around the rim of the defect. (G) A continuous horizontal mattress suture is placed through the base of the defect. (H) The suture line is continued along the ventricular muscle. The repair is completed by tying the two ends of the double arm suture. (I) If the incision was extended across the pulmonary annulus, the pulmonary annulus and arteriotomy are closed using a Dacron or polytetrafluoroethylene (PTFE) graft secured with a running suture of size 4-0 polypropylene. (J) The suture is continued to the annulus of the pulmonary valve. (K) An alternative approach is used when pressure in the right ventricle is expected to rise after the repair. Teflon pledgets are used to increase the strength of the closure. (L) If the right and left branches of the pulmonary artery are hypoplastic, the incision may be carried into the pulmonary arteries to widen the outflow. (M) A Dacron patch is used to reconstruct the vessels. (N) The suture is continued along the edges of the annulus of the pulmonary valve and completed at the ventriculotomy. (From Doty D, Doty J. *Cardiac Surgery Operative Technique*. 2nd ed. Philadelphia: Saunders; 2012.)

Technical Points and Discussion

1. ***The patient is prepped and draped for a median sternotomy.***
   The sternotomy is performed and bypass is initiated.

2. ***An atriotomy is performed.***
   The surgeon may fibrillate the heart and occlude the aorta before performing a right atriotomy. A Richardson (pediatric) retractor is placed in the wound, and the surgeon examines the defect. Additional supplies may be needed, depending on this assessment.

3. ***The defect is repaired.***
   The surgeon may repair the defect with a primary closure or by inserting a patch or pericardial graft. Large defects require a patch graft, which is cut to size and sutured in place with polypropylene sutures. Air is removed from the left side of the heart before the final sutures are placed and tied.

4. ***The wound is closed.***
   Bypass is discontinued, and the wound is prepared for closure. The incision is closed in layers.

CLOSURE OF A VENTRICULAR SEPTAL DEFECT

A ventricular septal defect is the incomplete closure of the septum between the right and left ventricle, which normally occurs during fetal life. This causes increased pulmonary pressure by allowing blood from the left ventricle to flow into the right ventricle and to the lungs, leading to congestive heart failure after birth. The septal defect is repaired to restore normal cardiac circulation.

Pathology

A ventricular septal defect is a hole in the intraventricular septum. It can occur in a variety of locations. Increased pressure in the left ventricle causes blood to flow through the defect into the area of lower pressure, the right ventricle.

Technical Points and Discussion

1. ***The patient is prepped and draped.***
   The patient is prepped and draped for a median sternotomy.
   The surgeon performs a median sternotomy and cannulates for total CPB.

2. ***The aorta is occluded, and a cardioplegic solution is infused into the coronary arteries.***
   The surgeon occludes the aorta with a pediatric vascular clamp and infuses a retrograde cardioplegic solution through the coronary sinus.

3. ***Ventriculotomy is performed, and the defect is closed.***
   A right ventriculotomy is performed with the knife or Metzenbaum scissors. The surgeon may place sutures through the edges of the ventricle for traction.
   The defect is assessed, and a Dacron or pericardial patch graft is sutured into place using size 4-0 or 5-0 polypropylene. Teflon pledgets may be used to reinforce the suture line. Air is removed from the left ventricle before final closure.

4. ***The ventricle is closed, followed by wound closure.***
   After removing the aortic clamp, the surgeon closes the ventricle with continuous suture. Bypass is discontinued, and the cannulas are removed. A temporary pacemaker lead may be sutured to the right ventricle and right atrium. Chest tubes are inserted, and the wound is closed.

KEY CONCEPTS

- The midline sternotomy incision primarily is used for heart surgery. This requires access through soft tissues and the bony sternum.
- Access to the heart for repeat procedures may be complicated by excessive scarring and may require a different incision.
- Cardiac instrumentation may be divided into sets that are appropriate for the specific surgery being performed, such as open heart, valve procedures, and aneurysm.
- The scrub should be prepared for conversion from an endovascular to open surgery in each case.
- Cardiopulmonary bypass is managed by a CPB perfusionist. However, the scrub has specific roles in assisting with the placement of the cannulas and decannulation.
- Some cardiac cases may be performed on the beating heart. In these procedures, a cardiac stabilizer is used.
- The bypass cannulas are inserted into anatomical sites according to the technical requirements of the procedure and the patient's condition. The actual technique used is very similar across all sites.
- The greater saphenous vein is used as an autograft for many bypass procedures. Harvesting the vein is usually performed by a surgical assistant. A separate Mayo tray and dedicated lighting should be available for this procedure, which takes place at the same time as the cardiac portion of the surgery.
- Valve prostheses should be handled as little as possible. Each prosthesis has a unique sizing obturator.
- Vascular sutures are often double armed. The most common suture used on cardiac and vessel tissue is Dacron, polyester, and polypropylene. Size 3-0 is commonly used on the larger vessels, whereas size 6-0 and 5-0 are used on smaller ones.
- Endovascular procedures are becoming commonplace in cardiac surgery. To become proficient, the scrub will need to become familiar with various techniques such as the Seldinger technique along with the types of guidewires, catheters, and access sheaths.
- Cardiac surgery is complex not because of the technical difficulty but more because of the many different types and configurations of equipment required. The best way to become proficient as a cardiac assistant is through practice and study. Many good resources are available from manufacturer's websites and also through in-service training.

REVIEW QUESTIONS

1. Why are multiple prep sites often required in cardiac surgery?
2. What are the specific characteristics of cardiac clamps that differentiate them from other types of clamps?
3. Several techniques are used to isolate and manipulate blood vessels during cardiac surgery. Describe at least two.
4. What is the purpose of suture pledgets?
5. What instruments are needed to divide the sternum?
6. What is the atrial appendage?
7. What technique is often used in valve surgery to help the surgeon identify pairs of sutures between the valve and the annulus?
8. List all the drugs and solutions (and their basic action) likely to be needed and managed by the surgical technologist during open heart surgery. Be sure to include hemostatic agents and tissue adhesives.
9. During cardiopulmonary bypass, the heart may be deliberately stopped. What technique is used to stop the heart? What technique is used to start it again?
10. What are the basic indications for implanting a left ventricular assist device?

BIBLIOGRAPHY

Cameron J, Cameron A, eds. *Current Surgical Therapy*. 11th ed. Philadelphia: Saunders; 2014.

Carabello BA. Aortic stenosis: two steps forward, one step back. *Circulation*. 2007;115:2799.

Cohn LH, ed. *Cardiac Surgery in the Adult*. New York: McGraw-Hill; 2008.

Denholm B. Clinical issues: implant documentation. *AORN Journal*. 2008;87:433.

Doty D, Doty J, eds. *Cardiac Surgery Operative Technique*. 2nd ed. Philadelphia: Saunders; 2012.

Fedak PWM, McCarthy PM, Bonow RO. Evolving concepts and technologies in mitral valve repair (review). *Circulation*. 2008;l117:963.

Haywood PAR, Buxton BF. Contemporary graft patency: 5-year observational data from a randomized trial of conduits. *Ann Thorac Surg*. 2007;84:795.

Khatri V, ed. *Atlas of Advanced Operative Surgery*. Philadelphia: Saunders; 2013.

Kouchoukos N, Blackstone E, Hanley F, Kirklin J, eds. *Cardiac Surgery*. 4th ed. Philadelphia: Saunders; 2013.

Levy MN, Pappano A, eds. *Cardiovascular Physiology*. 9th ed. St Louis: Mosby; 2007.

Miller R, et al., eds. *Miller's anesthesia*. 8th ed. Philadelphia: Saunders; 2012.

Pelter MM. Electrocardiography: normal electrocardiogram. In: Moser DK, Riegel B, eds. *Cardiac Nursing: A Companion to Braunwald's Heart Disease*. St Louis: Saunders; 2008.

Rubertone JA. Anatomy of the cardiovascular system. In: Moser DK, Riegel B, eds. *Cardiac Nursing: A Companion to Braunwald's Heart Disease*. St Louis: Saunders; 2008.

Sellke F, del Nido P, Swanson S. *Sabiston and Spencer Surgery of the Chest*. 9th ed. Philadelphia: Elsevier; 2016.

Sellke F, del Nido P, Swanson S, eds. *Sabiston and Spencer Surgery of the Chest*. 9th ed. Philadelphia: Elsevier; 2016.

Sellke F, Ruel M. *Atlas of Cardiac Surgical Techniques*. Philadelphia: Saunders; 2010.

Thompson J, Bertling G. Endovascular leaks: perioperative nursing implications. *AORN Journal*. 2009;89:839.

Townsend C, Beauchamp B, Evers B, Mattox K, eds. *Sabiston Textbook of Surgery: The Biological Basis of Modern Surgical Practice*. 19th ed. Philadelphia: Elsevier; 2012.

Velasco J, Ballo R, Hood K, Jolley J, Rinewalt D, Veenstra B, eds. *Essential Surgical Procedures*. Philadelphia: Elsevier; 2016.

Wagner GS. *Marriott's Practical Electrocardiography*. 11th ed. Philadelphia: Lippincott Williams & Wilkins; 2008.

33 PEDIATRIC SURGERY

LEARNING OBJECTIVES

After studying this chapter, the reader will be able to:

1. Identify key physiological and anatomical features in pediatric surgery
2. Discuss pediatric pathology with respect to surgery
3. Discuss key elements of case planning for pediatric surgery
4. Describe psychosocial care of the pediatric patient
5. Discuss risk reduction techniques in pediatric surgery
6. List and describe common pediatric surgical procedures

TERMINOLOGY

Acquired abnormality: A physiological or anatomical defect that develops in fetal life as a result of environmental factors.

Bolus: A compact substance (e.g., undigested food, fecal material) that occurs normally in the digestive tract.

Child life specialist: A trained professional who specializes in the psychosocial care of and communication with pediatric patients and their families.

Choana: The communicating passageways between the nasal fossae and pharynx.

Coarctation: Narrowing of the passageway of a blood vessel, such as coarctation of the aorta.

Congenital: A condition or an anomaly that develops during fetal life.

Ductus arteriosus: A normal fetal structure that allows blood to bypass circulation to the lungs. If this structure remains open after birth, it is called a patent ductus arteriosus.

Embryonic life: The first 8 weeks of gestational development.

Exstrophy: The eversion or turning out of an organ.

Fetus: Gestational life after 8 weeks.

Genetic abnormality: A birth anomaly that is inherited.

Homeostasis: The balance of physiological processes that maintain life.

Isolette: An infant-size "bed" that is environmentally controlled and equipped with monitoring devices.

Magical thinking: A psychological process in which a person attributes intention and will to inanimate objects. Magical thinking may also describe a patient's belief that an event will happen because he or she wills it or wishes it. This is a normal developmental stage of toddlers.

Mutagenic substance: A chemical or other agent that causes permanent change in the cell's genetic material.

Nephroblastoma: Pediatric cancer of the kidney, also known as Wilms tumor.

Neural tube defect: A congenital abnormality resulting from failure of the neural tube to close in embryonic development.

Omphalocele: A protrusion of abdominal contents through a congenital defect at the umbilicus.

Pyloric stenosis: A congenital narrowing of the pylorus.

Teratogen: A chemical or agent that can injure the fetus or cause birth defects.

Pediatric surgery is a multidisciplinary field that encompasses many surgical specialties. Most procedures can be classified in one of three groups:

- Surgery for treatment of **congenital** anomalies
- Procedures for treatment of diseases
- Trauma surgery

Innovative techniques in fetal surgery are also being developed and refined as a separate specialty of pediatric medicine.

Pediatrics as a specialty includes care of a child from neonate to late adolescence. However, because many surgical procedures are an integral part of the child's growth and development, the patient is often followed into adulthood.

Pediatric surgery includes a variety of pathologies, which are not restricted to one body system. However, many pediatric surgeons specialize in a particular system or area of medicine, such as pediatric cardiology or maxillofacial or trauma surgery.

An important dynamic of pediatric surgery is the family's experience in the perioperative process. The family and patient cannot be separated in this specialty, and they require equal consideration in communication and psychosocial care.

The purpose of this chapter is to provide an overview of the physiological and psychological needs of the pediatric patient and to present *common* procedures. Procedures that are performed in both adult and pediatric patients are presented in that specialty chapter (e.g., hernia surgery is presented in Chapter 22 because it is performed on adults and children, whereas *omphalocele*, which is also an embryonic abdominal wall defect, is presented in this chapter). The procedures included in this chapter are performed most often in pediatric patients only.

Refer to specialty chapters to review the surgical anatomy associated with each procedure presented in this chapter. Important physiological and psychosocial considerations are provided to highlight special needs of pediatric patients in the perioperative environment. Note that pediatric heart procedures are discussed in Chapter 32.

PHYSIOLOGICAL AND ANATOMICAL CONSIDERATIONS

The body's mechanisms for maintaining **homeostasis** (physiological balance) in a pediatric patient are different from those in an adult in many ways. Some of these differences create increased risks for the pediatric surgical patient.

THERMOREGULATION

All patients are at risk for hypothermia during surgery. However, pediatric patients, especially infants and neonates, are particularly vulnerable to hypothermia and hyperthermia. Important facts to remember are the following:

- Physiological mechanisms that normally regulate temperature in an adult are absent or undeveloped in an infant. Infants and children tend to lose more heat than they generate.
- Infants' relatively large skin surface area and low body weight can contribute to rapid lowering of the core temperature.
- Children and infants have extensive peripheral circulation, which contributes to relatively rapid cooling.
- Infants lack adequate insulation (fatty tissue) to maintain the core temperature in a cold environment.
- Infants and children show a wide range in temperature variation compared with adults.

Hypothermia

Environmental factors are an important cause of hypothermia in pediatric patients:

- Loss of body heat can occur through conduction when the patient's skin comes in contact with cold surfaces (e.g., a cold operating table or transport crib).
- Heat loss by radiation occurs as the patient's own body heat is given up to cold air in the operating room. Heat loss by radiation is intensified when body tissues are exposed during open procedures.
- Prep solutions contribute to hypothermia in two ways. Water absorbs heat from the body much more rapidly than air. Consequently, cool prep solutions lower the body temperature by both conduction and evaporation.
- Wet linens, drapes, and bedclothes are a source of body cooling during the perioperative period.
- Anesthetics can have a profound hypothermic effect in children. This is an added burden to the physiological stress of poor thermoregulation.

MECHANISMS OF HYPOTHERMIA Hypothermia can result in a chain of physiological events that place the pediatric patient at risk for cardiac problems, apnea, and hypoglycemia. Pediatric patients, especially infants, have little metabolic tolerance for cold. They have little reserve fat, and blood vessels are close to the skin, causing rapid heat loss. Approximately 60% to 75% of body heat is lost through radiation of body heat to the air. As the core temperature begins to drop, metabolism slows (approximately 50% at 82.4°F [28°C]). Heart rate and stroke volume decrease and systemic blood pressure falls. A drop in circulating blood and respiratory rate causes a decrease of up to 6% in normal oxygen intake. In a pediatric patient, this can be critical.

Shivering, a compensatory reaction to cold, normally occurs with hypothermia in adults. However, infants lack this mechanism. When an infant is cold, brown fat, found only in infants, is metabolized, using up oxygen and glucose. The result is hypoxemia and hypoglycemia. Electrolyte balance is disturbed, leading to loss of intravascular fluids in the skin. The effects of these physiological events can be rapid and severe. Cardiac arrhythmias, leading to arrest, may occur.

Hyperthermia

Environmental hyperthermia is less of a risk to pediatric surgical patients than hypothermia. However, elevated core temperatures can occur with the misuse of warming devices. Hyperthermia can also be induced in the perioperative period by excessive covering. Waterproof drapes trap heat and may contribute to hyperthermia.

Physiological hyperthermia, such as malignant hyperthermia, is a greater risk in pediatric patients than in adult patients. (Chapter 13 presents a complete discussion of malignant hyperthermia, its causes, and the emergency response.)

PERIOPERATIVE INTERVENTIONS TO MAINTAIN NORMOTHERMIA

Steps to maintain the pediatric patient's temperature are implemented throughout the perioperative period. If the patient becomes chilled, it may be difficult to reestablish warmth, which requires the use of active warming methods.

Transport and Prewarming

Interventions to maintain the patient's temperature begin during transport to the surgical department. Infants and children may become chilled during transport; therefore personnel must make sure that adequate blankets are available *before transport*. Neonates may arrive in a heated **Isolette** (an infant-size transport unit that is environmentally controlled and equipped with monitoring devices). Infants and neonates should wear a head covering at all times. On arrival in the operating room, the patient is taken to a preheated holding area. A period of *prewarming* may be advisable in the holding area of the operating room. The patient is covered with a warm air blanket or placed on a warm air mattress for prewarming.

Intraoperative Warming

During surgery, several methods are used to maintain the core temperature.

- The operating room is prewarmed before the patient arrives. The anesthesia care provider (ACP) and surgeon agree on the correct temperature for preparation of the patient.
- A warm air blanket may remain in use during the procedure. Upper- and lower-body mattresses are available for this purpose.
- A water-filled blanket may be used underneath the patient during surgery. Warm or cool water can be used to treat hyperthermia or to prevent hypothermia. Water blankets are programmable to maintain a constant temperature and have alarms in case flow is occluded or preset temperatures change.
- Overhead heating panels are used during the preoperative prep or whenever supplemental warming is needed. These are commonly used in neonatal and infant care in the surgical environment. A safe distance on the basis of light aperture and intensity is established by the manufacturer. These parameters must be followed precisely, and the patient must be continuously monitored to prevent injury. Dehydration is a risk when overhead heating is used.
- A solution warmer is used during surgical procedures to maintain the correct temperature of irrigation solutions. Intravenous (IV) solutions are also prewarmed before administration.
- Surgical sponges are moistened with warm saline before use.

Monitoring

Pediatric biophysical monitoring uses many of the same techniques as in adult care. Esophageal and rectal probes assess the precise core body temperature. For short procedures, external measuring devices (axillary probes) are used.

FLUID BALANCE

Fluid balance (maintaining the correct amounts and types of fluids in body spaces) is an important goal in the care of pediatric patients. Infants and children can become rapidly dehydrated. Before surgery begins, an IV line is inserted to maintain access to the circulatory system. Renal output is measured carefully and, if needed, tests can be done for specific electrolyte balance at any time. The high ratio of surface area to body volume in young children and infants contributes to an increased risk for acid-base imbalance in the blood. Arterial blood gas determinations can rapidly detect acid-base imbalance.

Certain surgical procedures, such as those of the gastrointestinal system, increase the risk for dehydration and electrolyte shifts. The ACP maintains constant monitoring to ensure that electrolyte imbalance is quickly brought under control.

HEMOSTASIS

Hemostasis is a critical element in pediatric surgery. Infants and children have little blood reserve and cannot tolerate persistent bleeding. All members of the surgical team are jointly responsible for monitoring blood loss as efficiently and accurately as possible. The scrubbed technologist must report the cumulative amount of irrigation fluid used during surgery so that this can be subtracted from the amount of fluid in each suction canister. Used sponges are maintained carefully, according to facility protocol, and weighed to determine blood loss.

The ST should have appropriate clamps, suture, and hemostatic materials and agents available according to the requirements of the procedure. The importance of the ST's role during critical moments of hemorrhage cannot be overstated. The ST should plan for such emergencies before surgery and mentally rehearse the steps needed to act quickly and correctly. Consulting with the surgeon on specific instruments and supplies *before surgery* reinforces preparation.

RESPIRATORY SYSTEM AND AIRWAY

An important anatomical difference between the adult and pediatric respiratory systems is the structure of the airway. Failure to manage a pediatric patient's airway is among the leading causes of death in medical and traumatic emergency. The following are some of the important features of the pediatric airway:

- The tongue is large in proportion to the oral cavity.
- Infants less than 8 weeks of age are *obligate nose breathers*; this means that they can only breathe through the nose; obstruction of the nasal passages may cause severe respiratory compromise.
- In infants and children, the trachea is much shorter and smaller than in adults.
- The airway is more delicate and less rigid than that of an adult.

- The thoracic wall is weak and unstable in children. The costal and suprasternal muscles are prominent during airway obstruction or lung disease (e.g., pneumonia).
- Lung residual capacity is much lower in children than in adults. This contributes to much more rapid hypoxia if the airway is lost.

PATHOLOGY

During early **embryonic life,** organ systems develop from one of three cellular layers: the endoderm, the ectoderm, or the mesoderm. Each layer gives rise to a specific set of organs through a complex process. Disturbances during the critical stages of germ cell differentiation and organ development can result in errors or defects in a structure or organ system.

Much of pediatric surgery is performed to correct structural defects that develop during fetal life; such a defect is called a *congenital or* **genetic abnormality.** The cause of the abnormality may be genetic (inherited) or acquired. An **acquired abnormality** is the result of one or more *environmental agents* or conditions to which the **fetus** is exposed. The most vulnerable period in fetal life is the first 60 days. This is a period of rapid cellular and tissue differentiation.

An environmental agent (a chemical or drug) that injures the embryo or fetus is called a **teratogen.** Examples of teratogens are environmental mercury and alcohol. Certain drugs are also known to cause severe developmental defects.

A **mutagenic substance** causes gene mutation, a chemical change in the genetic structure. Mutation can cause retardation, skeletal deformity, or microcephaly (severely diminished brain development). Gamma radiation (x-rays) is both mutagenic and teratogenic.

The maternal diet is an important source of congenital birth defects. For example, lack of folic acid in the mother's diet causes specific spinal cord **(neural tube) defects,** such as spina bifida and anencephaly (absence of a cranial vault). A low-protein diet results in poor fetal development.

Certain *infection agents* are also known be teratogenic. The following infectious microorganisms cause significant congenital abnormalities (listed in parentheses):

- *Toxoplasma gondii* (cerebral calcifications, microcephaly, heart defects)
- Rubella virus—the causative agent of measles (cataract, glaucoma, deafness, heart defects, retinal defects)
- Cytomegalovirus (hydrocephalus, deafness)
- Herpes virus (microcephaly, microphthalmia, retinal defect)
- Varicella-zoster virus—the causative agent of chickenpox (muscle atrophy, mental retardation)
- *Treponema pallidum*—the causative agent of syphilis (hydrocephalus, deafness, bone defects)

Table 33.1 presents important congenital and inherited abnormalities.

PSYCHOSOCIAL CARE OF THE PEDIATRIC PATIENT

Psychosocial care of the pediatric patient in the perioperative environment is a process that involves the child, his or her caretakers, and perioperative staff. The goal of psychosocial care is to help patients and caretakers develop strategies that support them through the perioperative experience. The child's developmental stage, emotional state, and social support system are considered in planning for a safe, smooth surgical outcome. Planning for surgery usually includes a preoperative visit or counseling session involving the patient, the caretakers, and **child life specialist,** who is trained in providing age-appropriate counseling to children about to undergo surgery and who can explain the perioperative procedures. This helps reduce anxiety and allows the patient and caretakers to ask questions before surgery. One of the most important goals of preoperative planning is to provide education. Allowing the child to ask questions in an informal setting demystifies the fearful aspects of surgery and engenders trust.

It is important for all staff members to understand the basic developmental stages *and their significance in the perioperative setting.* The greatest fears of young children undergoing surgery are the following:

1. Fear of the unknown
2. Fear of separation from the primary caregivers
3. Fear of mutilation

Children appreciate supportive, positive statements about their perioperative experience. Trust in caregivers begins with honest but careful descriptions of what will happen to them. Certain words and phrases are avoided (Box 33.1) so that the patient does not develop a sense of fear or dread.

DEVELOPMENTAL STAGES OF THE CHILD

Traditionally, childhood development is divided into age categories in which children display distinct social and cognitive characteristics. The following categories are described in the *Journal of the American Academy of Pediatrics.*

Refer to https://www.cdc.gov/ncbddd/childdevelopment/positiveparenting/index.html.

Infants: Neonatal Period Through 12 Months

Between birth and 1 year, children begin to develop trust in others. They require tactile comfort and are unable to tolerate sudden environmental changes. Loud noises may cause anxiety and fear. Between 7 months and 1 year, the child begins to fear separation from the parent or caregiver and usually has a strong mistrust of strangers. Transitional objects, such as a soft toy or blanket, are very comforting at this stage of development, and some facilities allow these to be brought into the surgical environment (they are labeled and returned to the parent or guardian for safekeeping). Parents may be allowed into the operating room during induction and may be present in the postanesthesia care unit (PACU), depending on the facility's policy.

Toddlers: 13 Months to 2 Years

Toddlers begin to become autonomous, and although very active, they have a short attention span. They understand more than they can express and require concrete explanations of their environment. They cope with stress best with a favorite toy or stuffed animal. It is usually best to be truthful with the toddler while avoiding details of the procedure.

TABLE 33.1 Congenital and Genetic Abnormalities

Condition	Description	Considerations
Anencephaly	Congenital anomaly in which large parts of the brain fail to develop; occurs in 3 of 10,000 births.	Neonates with this lethal neural tube defect do not survive.
Atrial septal defect	Congenital cardiac defect in which a hole in the interatrial septum allows blood from the left atrium to flow into the right atrium.	Surgical repair may be necessary to close the defect.
Branchial cleft cysts and clefts	These are embryonic remnants or slits in the neck region that persist as cysts or fistulas after birth. They may not be diagnosed unless they interfere with structural function or become infected.	Surgical removal may be necessary.
Chest wall deformities	Two common chest wall deformities are *pectus excavatum* (PE) and *pectus carinatum* (PC). In PE the sternum is concave and may impinge on thoracic structures. In PC the sternum protrudes.	Surgical reconstruction is performed for cosmetic purposes or to relieve pressure on thoracic structures. See Repair of Pectus Excavatum.
Choanal atresia	Choanal atresia is a congenital anomaly characterized by a stricture or blockage of the passage between the nasal sinus and the pharyngonasal airways. Bilateral choanal atresia (both sides of the nasal passage are blocked) is a neonatal emergency; immediate treatment is required to maintain oxygen perfusion in the newborn.	Surgical repair is performed at birth in emergency cases. Endoscopic surgery and splinting of airways may be performed in nonemergency cases.
Cleft lip or palate	Partial or complete division of the lip or palate prevents the infant from suckling effectively. The defect occurs in about 1 in 700 live births.	Surgical reconstruction is performed in stages beginning at about 12 weeks of age. See Repair of a Cleft Lip and Repair of a Cleft Palate.
Coarctation of the aorta	Congenital narrowing of the thoracic aorta that restricts blood flow to the lower body.	Surgical treatment is necessary to restore circulation.
Esophageal atresia	Complete or partial absence of the esophagus. The defect is associated with tracheoesophageal fistula (see Tracheoesophageal Fistula Entry).	Surgical reconstruction of the esophagus is necessary for nutritional intake.
Gastroschisis	An abdominal wall defect in which the viscera form outside the body. In this defect there is no sac surrounding the viscera. The cause is unknown.	Immediate surgical repair is required to preserve the viscera.
Hirschsprung disease (megacolon)	Congenital absence of ganglion cells, which control the relaxation and contraction that occur in peristalsis of the bowel. This causes chronic bowel obstruction.	Surgery is performed to remove the diseased bowel.
Infantile hypertrophic pyloric stenosis (IHPS)	Also called *pyloric stenosis;* a congenital anomaly in which the longitudinal and circular muscles of the gastric pylorus are thickened. This results in obstruction at the pylorus.	Surgical treatment is performed to release the thickened bands of muscle and release the stricture.
Omphalocele	A type of abdominal wall deformity in which the viscera develop outside the body, contained within a peritoneal sac.	Surgery is performed as soon as possible after birth to conserve the tissues involved.
Patent ductus arteriosus	The ductus arteriosus is a fetal heart structure that shunts blood from the right ventricle into the systemic circulation. The ductus normally closes shortly after birth. A persistent or patent ductus arteriosus may result in heart failure.	Surgical repair is necessary to close a patient ductus arteriosus.
Pulmonary valve stenosis	Congenital cardiac defect in which the pulmonary valve leaflets are fused, restricting circulation of blood from the right ventricle to the lungs.	Surgical repair is necessary to restore circulation.
Spina bifida	A congenital anomaly that includes several types of neural tube defects, including incomplete closure of the bony spinal column around the spinal cord. The deformity often causes lower extremity paralysis and loss of bladder and bowel function. Spina bifida is associated with folic acid deficiency during pregnancy.	Surgical repair to close the superficial tissue layers is possible. However, nerve damage is not reversible.

TABLE 33.1 Congenital and Genetic Abnormalities—cont'd

Condition	Description	Considerations
Syndactyly	Webbing of the fingers or toes as a result of incomplete separation of the digits in embryonic life.	See Correction of Syndactyly.
Tetralogy of Fallot	A combination of congenital defects. The anomalies include pulmonary stenosis, ventricular septal defect, right ventricular hypertrophy, and transposition of the aorta.	Treatment is surgical repair of the defects.
Tracheoesophageal fistula	A fistula connecting the esophagus with the trachea. The defect results in aspiration of liquid and food particles into the trachea.	The defect is surgically closed to prevent aspiration.
Ventricular septal defect	Congenital cardiac defect in which blood from the left ventricle flows into the right ventricle and lungs, leading to congestive heart failure.	Surgical repair is necessary to close the defect.
Wilms tumor (nephroblastoma)	The most common primary renal malignancy of children. The tumor can become very large and spread from the abdomen to the lungs.	Surgical en bloc resection is performed when possible. The kidney, ureter, and adrenal gland are removed. More extensive dissection and resection may be required.

BOX 33.1 Terms to Avoid (and Substitutes) in Caring for Pediatric Patients

Avoid	Substitute
Bad, no good	Good, good job!
Gas	Breeze, air
Stick, poke	Pinch
Strap in	Put on the safety belt
Stink	Smells funny
Feels strange	Feels funny
Cold water	Feels cool
Put to sleep	Nap

Preschoolers: 3 to 5 Years

Children in this age group have a strong fear of the unknown and exhibit **magical thinking,** in which ordinary or inanimate objects have intentions (harmful or benevolent). When communicating with the preschooler, health care professionals should give simple explanations and should avoid words that imply harm or injury. Children in this age group are not able to reason fully. Explanations that are simple but factual are best.

Middle Childhood: 6 to 11 Years

Children in the early and middle school years use concrete reasoning (immediate experience) rather than complex abstract thinking; they are curious about objects and events in their environment. Children in this group fear harm and pain but are able to comprehend simple explanations of cause and effect. Patients in this age group can be comforted by knowing what to expect. All children have a need for privacy; however, children in this age group have a heightened sense of invasion when exposed.

Early Adolescence: 12 to 14 Years

Patients between 12 and 18 years of age are able to project the significance of current events into the future. They understand the consequences of their illness but often focus on the social rather than the physical aspects. Among their greatest concerns are separation from their peers (including rejection by peers) and loss of mobility. A change in body image caused by a perceived disfigurement can be very disturbing. Disruption of their normal routines, especially those that contribute to socialization, is also upsetting. Fear of exposure and loss of privacy are extremely important in this age group, especially in middle adolescence.

Adolescents often reject or are mistrustful of care by strangers and need to demonstrate personal independence. This aspect of development increases their stoicism, and they may refuse to take pain medication or to report pain, even when it is severe. Patients in this age group often find it difficult to admit fear, but they usually are grateful for straightforward, "no-nonsense" explanations of what is happening in their environment and why.

Late Adolescence: 15 to 17 Years

Teenagers at this age are developing strong independence from their parents but now appreciate the concept of caring for others. They may strongly resent confinement related to illness and highly value time spent with their peers. They are able to understand illness and the clinical environment and appreciate concrete explanations.

CASE PLANNING

ANESTHESIA

Many procedures that otherwise could be carried out with regional anesthesia or monitored sedation are performed in the pediatric patient with general anesthesia. This is partly because general anesthesia allows the anesthesia care provider to secure the airway and maintain full respiratory control during the

TABLE 33.2 Common Preoperative Medications Used in Pediatric Surgery

Agent/Drug	Route	Comments
H_2 blocker (ranitidine, famotidine)	Oral, intravenous (IV)	Prevents gastrin-stimulated acid secretion
Ketamine	Intramuscular injection	Produces anesthesia within 3 minutes
	Oral	May be combined with midazolam for mask induction
Lidocaine 2.5% and prilocaine 2.5% (EMLA cream)	Topical	Applied to the skin before insertion of an IV cannula to reduce the pain of insertion
Methohexital (Brevital)	Rectal	Produces sleep within about 10 minutes
Metoclopramide (Reglan)	Oral or IV	Antiemetic
Midazolam (Versed)	Oral	May be administered by the parent
	Intranasal	Produces peak effect in 30 minutes
	Sublingual	May prolong anesthesia recovery
	Rectal	Causes anterograde amnesia after 10 minutes
Oral transmucosal fentanyl citrate	Oral transmucosal	May be used in lollipop form for pain relief in short procedures

procedure. General anesthesia is also necessary because children are unable to cooperate during regional anesthesia.

The differences between adult and pediatric anesthesia are primarily related to physiological and anatomical variations between the two populations. Important considerations in learning about pediatric anesthesia are the following:

1. Anesthesia (and surgery) involves the entire family, not just the patient.
2. Children are much more sensitive to small variations in drug doses than are adults.
3. IV fluids are commonly administered with microdrip tubing and a burette chamber and fluid pump. This provides accurate measurement of fluids.
4. Pediatric patients often are induced and maintained with inhalation anesthesia by mask or by laryngeal or endotracheal tube. Inhalation anesthetics are taken up quickly by the brain, allowing for rapid induction.
5. IV access is usually obtained after induction to avoid patient struggling and anxiety.
6. Oral intake is restricted preoperatively in pediatric patients to reduce the risk for aspiration during anesthesia. As a general rule, clear liquids are withheld for 2 hours before surgery and breast milk for 4 hours. Solid food is withheld for 6 hours before surgery.[1]
7. Children are unable to cooperate fully during procedures that could otherwise be performed under regional anesthesia and therefore require a general anesthetic more often.

Preparation for Anesthesia

Pediatric patients are assessed and prepared for anesthesia by methods similar to those used for adults. However, the psychological preparation must take into consideration the child's more extreme fears, especially the trauma of separation and fear of not waking up. Whenever possible, the family is prepared for the experience of anesthesia at least 4 days before surgery. Age-appropriate preparation may include familiarizing the child with anesthesia devices, surgical attire, and other objects that can cause anxiety. A brief review of preoperative preparation as it applies to pediatric patients is presented here:

1. A preoperative history is taken, including current health status, chronic and acute conditions, history of past diseases, and previous surgery.
2. The patient's current medications, anesthesia history, and allergies are recorded.
3. A review of systems is performed (i.e., routine physical assessment of each system).
4. The results of routine laboratory tests are reviewed.
5. Additional tests are requested as needed.
6. The preoperative medication and induction method are discussed with the family.
7. Special considerations for children are taken into account (e.g., loose or missing teeth, cardiac defects, croup, history of apnea, recent respiratory infection).

Preoperative Medication and Induction

Pediatric patients may be given an anxiolytic (anxiety-reducing) medication before surgery. However, this practice varies from institution to institution and among anesthesia care providers. Preoperative sedation may delay recovery from anesthesia, and the method of administration (injection or a bitter-tasting oral medication) may increase anxiety in the child. Other drawbacks include an increased risk for falls and adverse physiological events, such as respiratory depression. If preoperative medication is required, several drugs are available (Table 33.2).

INDUCTION Allowing one or both parents to be present during induction is now an accepted practice in many health care facilities. This has proved to reduce the need for preoperative medication in many pediatric patients. Parents who are not fearful themselves may stay with the patient from the time of arrival in the surgical department through the entire induction process. Patients older than 4 years are the best candidates for parental presence during induction. Infants and young children may be induced in the parent's or nurse's arms. The method of induction depends on the following conditions:

- The child's age
- Whether there is IV access
- The presence of a parent
- The preference and skill of the anesthesia care provider
- The American Society of Anesthesiologists (ASA) case classification (see Chapter 13)

Anesthesia may be induced by a combination of methods or by a single method:

- Mask inhalation
- Intramuscular injection
- Rectal administration
- Oral administration
- IV administration

If the child already has an IV line, IV induction with thiopental or propofol (Diprivan) is often administered for rapid, safe induction. Inhalation induction is easily performed with a cooperative child. The child can be asked to try on a mask and is praised for compliance. Even if the child refuses the mask, it can be held below the face. As soon as the child becomes sleepy, the mask can be fitted over the face. A child who arrives asleep may be administered an anesthetic through this "blow-by" method and quickly induced during sleep.

ANESTHESIA MAINTENANCE After induction or just before, the precordial stethoscope, pulse oximeter, and cardiac electrodes are placed. IV access is secured when the child is unconscious. Inhalation anesthesia is maintained through an endotracheal tube. Continuous inhalation anesthesia by mask can be used for short procedures (lasting less than 1 hour). Intraoperative monitoring is carried out as in adults and includes a minimum of electrocardiography, pulse oximetry, respiratory function, and blood pressure.

EMERGENCE AND RECOVERY When anesthetic agents are withdrawn or reversed, the patient experiences increased physiological stress from pain and other strong stimuli. The child's response during emergence from anesthesia depends on whether opioids, sedatives, or benzodiazepines were given. These can prolong emergence but also contribute to a smoother recovery. Patients who have had a routine surgical procedure without complications may remain in the operating room until the airway reflexes are intact and the endotracheal tube is removed. If the patient is to be transported to the intensive care unit, the endotracheal tube may be left in place and the patient maintained on ventilation. After the patient is admitted to the PACU, parents usually are permitted to remain with the child for comfort and reassurance.

The most common postanesthesia complications in pediatric patients are postoperative nausea and vomiting, which occur in 40% to 50% of children. Other, less common, events include respiratory depression and delirium during emergence. (Chapter 13 presents a complete discussion of postanesthesia complications.)

SAFETY OF THE PEDIATRIC PATIENT

Pediatric specialization involves the same domains of safety required in surgery of the adult. The surgical technologist maintains a safe environment in collaboration with other members of the perioperative team. Pediatric patients *are particularly vulnerable* to risks related to their age, size, and stage of development. The student should review environmental risks that apply to all patients, which are covered in previous chapters. Specific risks and concerns are described in Table 33.3.

Safe Handling of Drugs

Because of their small size and undeveloped organ systems, pediatric patients are at high risk for adverse events from medications. The surgical technologist participates in the medication process while in the scrubbed role. Pediatric medications are prescribed according to the child's weight in kilograms, and the correct dose must be verified by the surgeon, circulating registered nurse, and surgical technologist. Cumulative amounts of drugs, such as local anesthetics and vasoconstriction agents, given throughout the procedure must be recorded and tracked *in real time* to prevent an overdose. All safety precautions discussed in Chapter 12 apply to the pediatric patient, with special emphasis on the potential risks for errors made in measuring, dispensing, and documentation.

TRANSPORT OF THE PEDIATRIC PATIENT

Neonates and infants are usually transported to the operating room in a heated Isolette. Occasionally, a neonate may be carried to the operating room by a parent. Young children may walk to the surgical department (for outpatient cases) and are placed on a gurney in the holding area for transportation to the operating room. Any patient on a monitoring device or those with an artificial airway in place must be transported by a registered nurse and one other person. Transporting an inpatient toddler can present challenges because of this age group's innate curiosity and agility. The hospital crib is equipped with side and bottom pads, and a flexible top may be used over the crib. During transport, a child may attempt to climb over the crib or stretcher rails. Furthermore, it is critical to ensure that the child does not extend a limb through the rails.

POSITIONING THE PATIENT

The principles of safe patient positioning apply to pediatric patients as well as adults. Although the principles are the same for adults and children, it is important to use appropriate-size padding to fit the pediatric patient. Gel and foam pads are appropriate for infants and children, whose delicate skin must be protected from shearing and pressure injury at all times. When creating a surgical position, the surgical technologist must keep in mind that a child's joints are extremely flexible. Care must be taken to move the patient's body within the normal range of motion and to consider anatomical restrictions related to injury or congenital defect. Adhesive tape should not be used when positioning children, because it can cause severe skin injury. Instead, soft Velcro straps designed for use with foam pads and supports should be used.

ELECTROSURGERY

All types of electrosurgical units (ESUs) are used in pediatric procedures, including monopolar and bipolar (high-frequency

TABLE 33.3 Risks in the Perioperative Care of Pediatric Patients

Domain of Care	Specific Risk	Precautions/Prevention	Rationale
Electrosurgery	Burns	• Use a pediatric-size patient return electrode (PRE) according to the manufacturer's specifications. • Never cut a PRE.	A PRE must be the correct size to properly disperse electricity flowing from the active electrode through the patient's body.
Patient transport	Falls	• Never turn your attention away from the patient during transport. • Do not abandon the patient *for any reason*. • Make sure that crib rails are secure.	Children (especially toddlers) are curious and extremely active. A child can quickly climb over the top of a crib or over stretcher rails.
• Skin prep	• Chemical burn • Hypothermia	• Prep solutions may be diluted to prevent skin burns. • Follow the surgeon's orders for solution strength. • Use warmed solutions to prevent loss of body heat.	Infants and toddlers have very delicate skin. About 60% to 75% of body heat is lost through radiation. Additional cooling by evaporation can rapidly cause hypothermia.
• Positioning	• Skeletal injury	• Follow all the usual precautions for positioning the patient. • Pay careful attention to moving the patient's body within the normal range of motion. • Provide ample padding over skin, nerves, and blood vessels.	Children's joints are very flexible but fragile. Limbs and joints may be overstretched, causing injury because of the patient's small stature and apparent flexibility.
Surgical technique	Injury to body tissue	• Do not put any pressure on the patient's body (e.g., from heavy instruments, tension from power cords, or leaning over the patient during surgery).	Bruising and other injury can result from weight or pressure, not directly observed because drapes hide the patient's body. Pressure on the thorax may result in respiratory compromise.

or radiofrequency) units. The safety principles for adult electrosurgery are the same for pediatric patients. The primary differences are the size of the active electrodes and the patient return electrodes (PREs). Active electrodes are selected according to the tissue and location in the body. Special pediatric-size PREs are used on children according to the child's weight. The parameters for size are established by the manufacturer of the electrode and must be followed. A PRE must *never* be cut or trimmed, because this can result in patient injury. (Chapter 15 presents a complete discussion of electrosurgery hazards for adults and pediatric patients.)

INSTRUMENTS

Pediatric instrument sets are assembled for a specialty such as cardiac, genitourinary, or gastrointestinal surgery. The instruments themselves may be smaller in all dimensions, or only the tips (working ends) may be smaller. For example, adult microsurgical instruments and those used in eye surgery often are used in pediatric plastic and genitourinary procedures. Fine scissors, needle holders, forceps, and calipers are found across these specialties. Pediatric instruments used in general surgery include a greater number of mosquito forceps (to replace Kelly and Crile clamps) and short Babcock and Allis clamps. Plastic shods (short lengths of plastic or silastic tubing) should be available to place over the tips of fine hemostats and should be available for all tag clamps. Smaller retractors (e.g., narrow Deaver, small Richardson, and "baby Balfour" retractors) are suited to children older than toddlers. Smaller self-retaining retractors are useful in pediatric general surgery, such as the small Weitlaner and various small spring retractors from thyroid and vascular surgery.

Minimally invasive techniques use very small trocars and endoscopes, which are designed in proportion to an infant's or a child's body size. The instruments themselves are shorter and have finer tips than the adult-size versions.

NOTE *Instrument sets mentioned in the procedures should all be available in sizes appropriate to infants through adolescents.*

SPONGES

Sponges used in open pediatric procedures often are smaller than those used in adult procedures. This includes radiopaque lap and gauze sponges. Dissecting sponges must be mounted on a clamp, as in adult surgery; however, smaller, shorter clamps are used. For example, short ring forceps (sponge clamps) are used for gauze sponges. Mayo clamps, rather than long Péan clamps, are used for sponge dissectors. The guidelines and protocols for using only radiopaque sponges in the body cavity apply in pediatric surgery, just as in adult surgery.

SUTURES

Pediatric sutures are naturally smaller to meet the needs of more delicate tissues. In general, suture materials more often are absorbable than synthetic, except in cardiac, orthopedic, and reconstructive surgery. Nylon, Prolene, and other monofilament sutures are commonly used for skin and other connective tissues because they are the least reactive and rarely tear when pulled through tissue. The size of sutures depends on the patient's age and the tissue involved. Skin most often is closed with subcuticular sutures and colloidal skin adhesive.

SURGICAL PROCEDURES

REPAIR OF A CLEFT LIP

Repair of a cleft lip involves the closure of a cleft defect in the lip.

Pathology

The *philtrum* (the groove that extends from the upper lip to the nose) is formed during embryonic development by the joining of the median nasal processes. The lateral portions of the upper lip are formed by the maxillary processes. These formations occur during the first 8 weeks of development. Interruption of normal development and closure of these structures may result in a cleft lip. The cleft may be complete or incomplete and unilateral or bilateral. Bilateral cleft lip is often associated with clefts of the soft palate. An infant with a cleft lip is referred to a surgeon immediately after birth. The cleft is repaired in stages, and the initial repair is performed at 10 to 12 weeks of age. Repair of cleft lip can be complex, especially during the preoperative planning phase in which many precise measurements of each anatomical landmark must be taken.

POSITION:	Supine
INCISION:	Face
PREP AND DRAPING:	Face
INSTRUMENTS:	Plastic set; cleft lip and palate instruments
POSSIBLE EXTRAS:	Bipolar ESU

Technical Points and Discussion

1. ***The patient is prepped and draped.***
The patient is placed in the supine position with the head on a doughnut headrest and the arms at the sides. Before the prep, the surgeon draws the anatomical landmarks and the planned incisions on the skin with a surgical marker. If local anesthetic is to be used, it is injected at this time. The patient is prepped with povidone-iodine solution and then draped for a head-and-neck procedure.

2. ***The incisions are made.***
The incision is made with a #15 blade along the vermilion border toward the cleft-side midline. Double- or single-prong skin hooks are used for retraction. The mucosa is separated off the orbicularis oris muscle with a #15 knife or tenotomy scissors. The surgeon then detaches the medial lip from the maxilla by incising the cleft at the top of the labial sulcus. This releases the medial lip.

3. ***Z-plasty flaps are created.***
A Z-plasty incision is made through the skin, muscle, and mucosa with a #11 or #15 blade. Hemostasis is maintained with the ESU. The procedure is repeated on the lateral portion of the cleft. When the dissection has been completed and the Z-plasty flaps have been created, the wound is ready to be closed.

4. ***The wound is closed.***
The mucosa is closed with interrupted absorbable sutures size 5-0 or 6-0. The muscle then is closed with subcuticular absorbable sutures through the tips of the Z-plasty flaps. The vermilion border is closed with a subcuticular suture. The skin is then closed with absorbable suture (Fig. 33.1).

REPAIR OF A CLEFT PALATE

Repair of a cleft palate involves closure of the palate to restore normal function.

Pathology

In the development of the midface, the palate arises from the joining of the medial nasal prominences on each side of the oral cavity to the maxillary prominence. Failure of these structures to join results in a cleft palate. The extent of the cleft can be complete or incomplete, depending on the level of fusion that occurred during embryonic development. Although cleft palate is sometimes seen in conjunction with cleft lip, they are separate malformations and are rarely related to one another. Infants with this condition are referred to a surgeon shortly after birth. However, the defects usually are not repaired until the infant is 11 to 12 months old, to avoid interference with facial growth.

Before surgical repair of the palate, the infant may require myringotomy with tube placement, because cleft palate often is associated with chronic ear infection and partial deafness. The infant also may be fitted with a palatal prosthesis to allow for easier feeding until the time of repair.

POSITION:	Supine
INCISION:	Palate; lip; nose
PREP AND DRAPING:	The skin prep may be omitted. Head drape and body drape are used.
INSTRUMENTS:	Cleft palate set; pediatric plastic set
POSSIBLE EXTRAS:	Needlepoint ESU

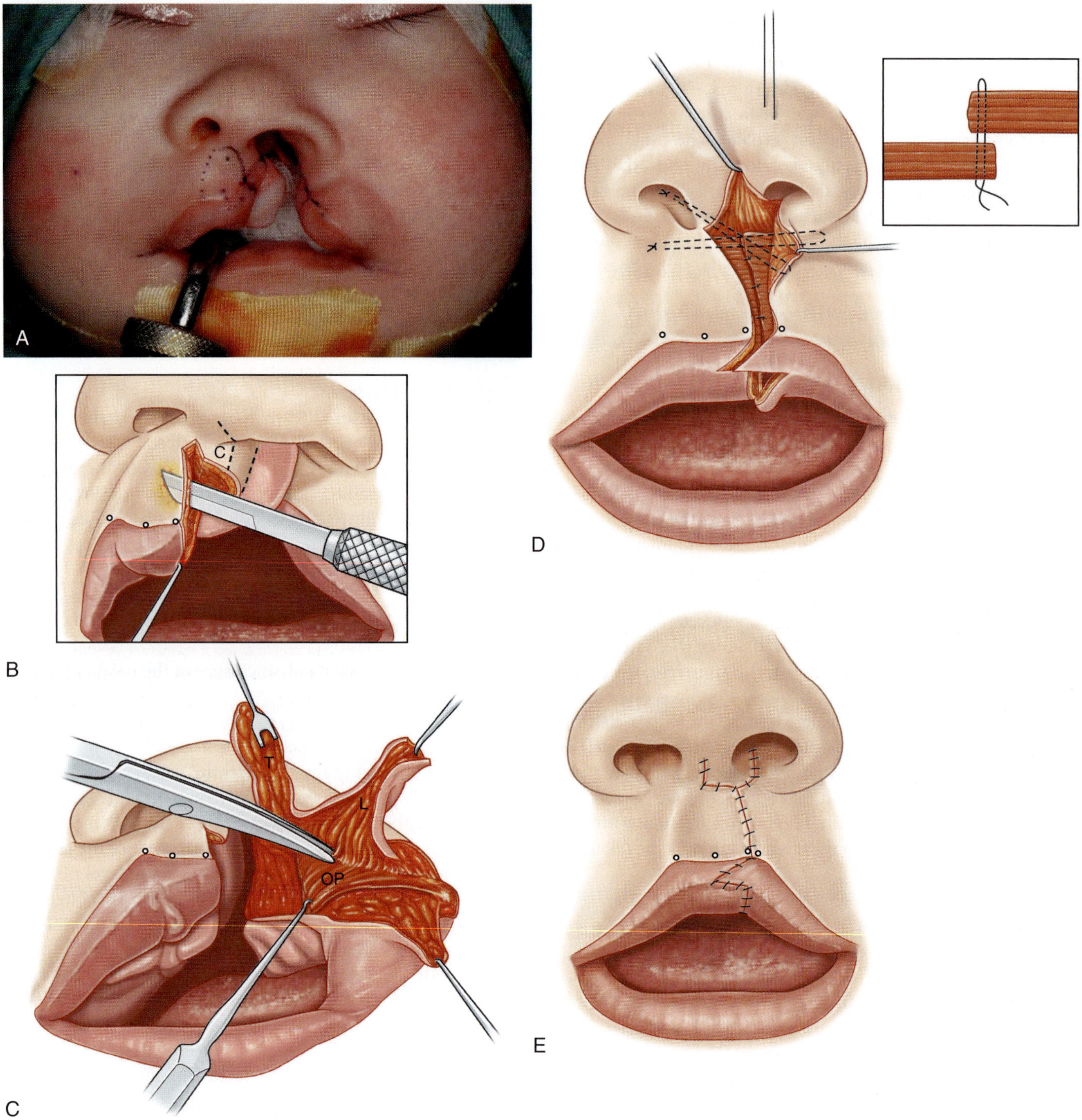

FIG. 33.1 Complex bilateral cleft lip and palate. (A) Proposed incision lines. (B) One flap is raised and rotated medially. (C) The completed dissection with an elevated turbinate. (D) Orbicularis muscle closure. *Inset:* Overlapping the lateral muscle on the medial muscle. (E) Completed closure. (From Neligan P, Buck D, eds. *Core Procedures in Plastic Surgery*. Philadelphia: Elsevier; 2014.)

Technical Points and Discussion

1. ***The patient is prepped and draped.***
The patient is placed in the supine position with the head on a doughnut headrest and with a shoulder roll to hyperextend the head. The surgeon may insert the cleft palate mouth gag, or Dingman mouth gag, before the prep. The palate is injected with a local anesthetic with epinephrine. This injection is given before the prep so that the hemostatic effects of the epinephrine have time to begin working before the initial incision. The patient is then prepped with povidone-iodine soap and paint. If the mouth gag is already in place, it also must be prepped.

   The surgeon first suspends the mouth gag from the Mayo stand. Once the gag is attached, the scrub must avoid jarring the Mayo stand because this can injure the patient.

2. ***Incisions are made in the palate and the muscle.***
The surgeon makes the initial incisions along the borders of the mucosa with a #15 blade. The incisions are extended through the oral mucosa, muscle, and nasal mucosa with a cleft palate blade (#6910 Beaver blade). After making the incisions, the surgeon elevates the nasal mucosa off the underlying muscle with the cleft palate blade and a Freer or Cottle elevator.

3. ***The flaps are prepared.***
This step is performed on both sides of the cleft. Next, the surgeon separates the oral mucosa from the overlying muscle. This step is performed in the same fashion as in the nasal mucosa. This creates three layers for closure.

4. ***The incisions are closed.***
After the mucosa has been elevated to the most lateral edges, the incisions are closed. The nasal mucosa is closed first with 4-0 absorbable suture on a 6-inch (15 cm) Crile-Wood needle holder and DeBakey forceps. The muscle is closed with 4-0 absorbable suture. The oral mucosa is closed with 4-0 or 5-0 absorbable suture. After closing the palate, the surgeon examines the wound and releases any areas under tension. The wound is then irrigated, and the mouth gag is removed.
Infants can begin to take liquids by sippy cup shortly after surgery. Any feeding method that involves sucking (bottles, straws, cups with valves) is not used because this can disrupt the repair. Some surgeons require their postoperative patients to wear arm restraints for several weeks. This prevents the infant from putting anything in the mouth, which may disturb the repair. Fig. 33.2 illustrates the procedure.

CHOANAL ATRESIA

The **choana** is the passageway between the posterior nasal opening and the larynx. Surgery for this defect involves puncture and removal of the tissue and placement of a stent to ensure that the airway remains open during healing. A choanal **atresia** is congenital blockage of this opening resulting from a bony or membranous plate. Infants are obligate nose-breathers, and if the condition is bilateral (both sides of the nasal sinuses are affected), the procedure is an emergency. A pediatric sinuscope is used for the visualization of the obstruction and use of a tissue-shaver and small rongeur to remove the obstruction.

CORRECTION OF ESOPHAGEAL ATRESIA AND TRACHEOESOPHAGEAL FISTULA

The goal of surgical repair of esophageal atresia (EA) is to restore continuity of the esophagus. In repair of a tracheoesophageal fistula (TEF), an abnormal opening between the trachea and the esophagus is closed to prevent the flow of food and saliva from the esophagus to the lungs.

Pathology

EA (the absence or closure of a normal anatomical orifice) is a nongenetic defect in which the esophagus is interrupted. The upper or proximal portion terminates in a blind pouch that does not communicate with the distal esophagus. Numerous variations of the anomaly can be seen, often including a TEF. A TEF is a direct passageway or duct between the esophagus and the trachea.

EA prevents the normal passage of food and saliva to the stomach. A TEF between the proximal esophageal segment and the trachea causes aspiration of saliva and milk into the trachea and lungs; a TEF in the distal esophageal segment causes gastric secretions to flow into the lungs. EA may exist as a single anomaly or, more commonly, with TEF.

EA/TEF is associated with several other birth defects, some of which are lethal. These include the following:

- Imperforate anus
- Ventricular and atrial septal defect
- Tetralogy of Fallot
- Limb deformities
- Neural tube defect

In addition to these and other anomalies, the fetus with EA/TEF is prevented from swallowing amniotic fluid, a source of nutrition in fetal life. This results in low neonatal birth weight and size.

Surgical options for the correction of EA/TEF depend on the type and severity of the defect. Staged or delayed repair may be necessary if other life-threatening conditions (e.g., cardiac defects) take precedence or to allow normal growth and elongation of the esophagus. A colon graft may be used to elongate the esophagus, although primary closure is preferred when possible. Primary repair (anastomosis of the two esophageal segments) is performed when the two segments can be brought together and the infant's general physiological condition is good. An isolated TEF without EA can be repaired through a cervical approach. Primary closure of EA is described here.

POSITION:	Thoracotomy
INCISION:	Posterolateral thoracotomy
PREP AND DRAPING:	Thoracotomy
INSTRUMENTS:	Thoracic set; general surgery set; Finochietto retractor; vessel loops; monopolar ESU; bipolar ESU

Technical Points and Discussion

1. ***The patient is prepped and draped.***
The infant is placed in the thoracotomy position with the head of the operating table slightly elevated. The prep extends from the neck to the iliac crest and includes the anterior and posterior chest.

2. ***A posterolateral thoracotomy is performed.***
The knife is used to make a transverse, posterolateral thoracotomy incision, and the ESU is used to extend it into the latissimus muscles. Rake retractors can be used to retract the skin and subcutaneous layers while the muscle and fascia are divided. The scapula is retracted and the

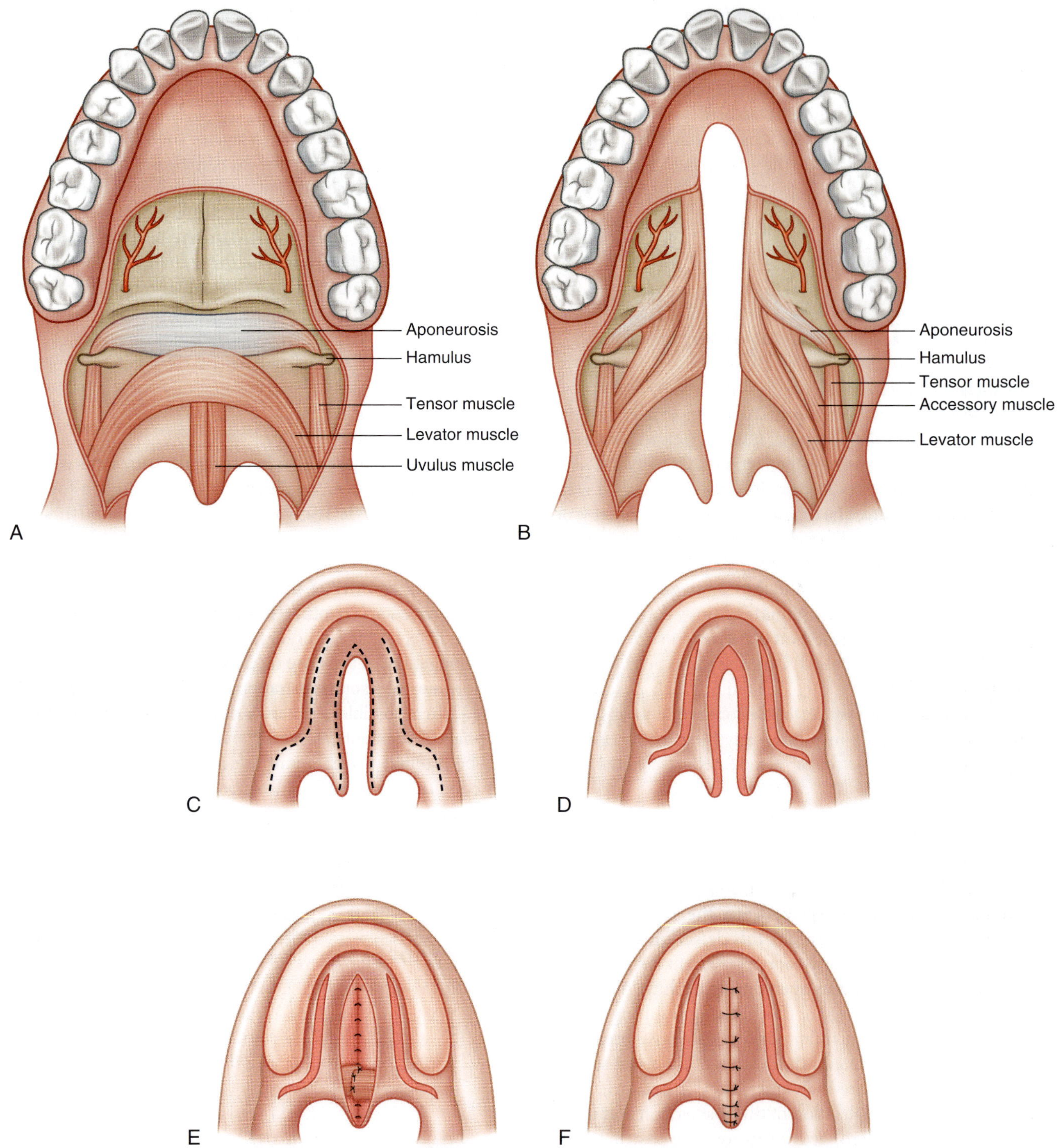

FIG. 33.2 Cleft palate. (A) Normal anatomy. (B) Cleft palate. Note the derangement of muscles. (C) Lines of incision. (D) Opening the palate along the incision lines. (E) Suturing the deep layer and muscle. (F) Final closure leaving the peripheral incision open to close by second intention. (From Neligan P, Buck D, eds. *Core Procedures in Plastic Surgery*. Philadelphia: Elsevier; 2014.)

chest cavity is entered by incising the intercostal muscles. The ESU is used to divide the muscles. This exposes the pleura, which is dissected from the chest wall with small sponge dissectors. A Finochietto retractor is placed in the wound, and pleural dissection continues to expose the azygos vein. This is clamped, ligated with 4-0 silk suture, and divided.

3. ***The TEF is identified and excised.***
The esophageal defect is assessed. The anesthesia care provider advances the preplaced Replogle tube (nasogastric decompression tube). This demonstrates the blind proximal esophageal pouch. The TEF is located and encircled with a Silastic vessel loop. The fistula is then excised with fine dissecting scissors.

4. ***The trachea is closed.***
The tracheal opening is closed with interrupted sutures of 4-0 or 5-0 absorbable synthetic. The surgeon tests the closure with warm saline irrigation solution. Bleeders are controlled with the ESU.

5. ***The proximal and distal esophageal pouches are mobilized.***
The proximal and distal esophageal segments are grasped with Babcock clamps, and the anastomosis site is examined. The esophageal pouches are mobilized by a sharp and blunt dissection.

6. ***An end-to-end or end-to-side anastomosis is performed.***
The surgeon excises the proximal pouch with fine dissecting scissors and smooth forceps. The distal portion, which is larger, is also excised to fit the proximal segment. An end-to-end anastomosis may be planned, or the proximal segment may be implanted in a circular incision made in the distal portion of the esophagus. The Replogle tube is advanced across the anastomosis site, and traction sutures are placed through the esophageal segments. Absorbable 5-0 or 6-0 synthetic suture is used to create a single-layer anastomosis. Surgical alternatives include a double-layer closure and variations in the anastomosis to prevent tension on the esophagus. The Replogle tube may be left in place or withdrawn.

7. ***The wound is irrigated and closed.***
The wound is irrigated with warm saline, and bleeders are controlled with the ESU. A small chest tube may be placed in the extrapleural space. The wound then is closed in layers with absorbable synthetic sutures.
Care of the infant immediately after surgery focuses mainly on the airway. Pharyngeal secretions are suctioned frequently for the first few days until the infant is able to swallow. The chest tubes are securely maintained and the incision sites are monitored for leakage or blockage. Oral feeding begins 2 to 6 days after surgery, after contrast studies have shown that the anastomosis is secure. Complications include infection, recurrent TEF, and leakage of the anastomosis.

PYLOROMYOTOMY

Pyloromyotomy is surgery to correct infantile hypertrophic pyloric stenosis, or simply **pyloric stenosis,** a thickening of the pylorus that results in stricture at the gastric outlet. The goal of surgery is to release the pyloric muscle fibers by incising them. This relaxes the gastric opening and allows food to pass normally out of the stomach into the intestine. Ramstedt pyloromyotomy is commonly performed for the treatment of pyloric stenosis. Either an open or a minimally invasive technique may be used. The laparoscopic procedure is described here.

Pathology

Pyloric stenosis is a congenital anomaly involving the longitudinal and circular muscle fibers of the gastric outlet. The pylorus (or gastric outlet) of the stomach is enlarged and edematous, causing food to be regurgitated almost immediately after intake. This leads to dehydration and failure to thrive. The condition is about four times more common in male children. In the following procedure, the muscle of the hypertrophic pylorus is split, and the mucosa is left intact.

POSITION:	Supine
INCISION:	Laparoscopic
PREP AND DRAPING:	Laparotomy
INSTRUMENTS:	Laparoscopic pyloromyotomy

Technical Points and Discussion

1. ***The patient is prepped and draped.***
The infant is placed in the supine position. Most surgeons place the infant in transverse position on the operating table. The surgeon operates at the feet allowing the anesthesia provider access to the airway. A small roll may be placed at the level of the pylorus to elevate it. The chest and abdomen are prepped with an iodophor-povidone solution and draped for a laparotomy.

2. ***A 5-mm umbilical incision is made.***
The umbilical ring may be opened and a 5-mm or 3-mm trocar inserted. The abdomen is then inflated. A 2-mm stab incision is made through the abdominal wall using a No. 11 blade. A pyloric grasper is inserted and is used to steady the pylorus. An additional stab incision is made on the left side.

3. ***The pylorus is brought out through the incision.***
A beaver knife with a 2-mm banana blade is inserted and used to perform the pyloromyotomy.

4. ***The pyloromyotomy is deepened.***
A pyloric spreader is used to extend and deepen the pyloric incision. The incision is complete when the mucosa becomes visible. The grasper and spreader are then removed. Two blunt graspers are used to hold the edges of the myotomy and demonstrate mobility. Before closing the wounds a grasper is used to occlude the duodenum.

5. ***The stomach is checked for leaks.***
The anesthesiologist uses a bulb syringe and orogastric tube to inflate the stomach. The myotomy is closely observed for any leaks. The omentum is placed in the myotomy.

6. ***The umbilical incision is closed.***
An umbilical suture of 3-0 absorbable material is placed in the fascia to prevent an umbilical hernia. The wound is dressed with adhesive strips.

REPAIR OF AN OMPHALOCELE

An **omphalocele** is a congenital anomaly in which the abdominal viscera develop outside the body, contained within a peritoneal sac. The goal of surgery is to replace the contents of the abdomen in phases until the abdominal wall can be closed.

Surgical options for repair of an omphalocele depend on the size of the defect. Small defects (less than 0.8 inch [2 cm]) can be reduced in one step. In such cases, a primary abdominal closure is performed soon after birth. If the sac is ruptured, emergency surgery is required.

Larger defects require multiple-stage procedures in which portions of the viscera are replaced in the abdominal cavity over a period of days or weeks. To prevent hypothermia, infection, and dehydration, a Silastic, Dacron-reinforced silo is sutured to the abdominal wall. The silo is reduced gradually, over a period of days, while the infant is in intensive care. When the omphalocele has been sufficiently reduced, the infant is taken to the operating room for complete closure of the abdominal wall. If the contents cannot be reduced completely, skin closure alone is performed. This results in a large abdominal wall hernia, which may be repaired later in childhood.

Pathology

An omphalocele is covered by a clear sac or membrane composed of peritoneum and amnion. The size of the omphalocele can range from very small, containing only a small portion of the intestine, to extremely large *(giant omphalocele),* including the intestine and other abdominal viscera, such as the liver and spleen. The anomaly is associated with genetic defects, including trisomies 13, 18, and 21 in 30% of cases. Cardiac, musculoskeletal, and genitourinary defects are also associated with omphalocele.

Gastroschisis is similar to an omphalocele, except that no peritoneal sac or membrane covers the abdominal viscera. Surgical treatment for gastroschisis is similar to that for an omphalocele, involving the use of a Silastic silo and phased reduction. The absence of a peritoneal covering over the viscera may require immediate treatment to protect the tissues.

POSITION:	Supine
INCISION:	Supine
PREP AND DRAPING:	Laparotomy
INSTRUMENTS:	Laparotomy
POSSIBLE EXTRAS:	Biological mesh; Silastic sheeting

Technical Points and Discussion

Shortly after birth, the omphalocele is protected with moist sponges or plastic wrap and the infant prepared for surgery. General anesthesia is induced and the abdomen, umbilical cord, and sac are prepped and draped. A Foley catheter is inserted. Great care is taken not to rupture the sac.

PRIMARY CLOSURE

1. ***The sac is excised.***
   The surgeon grasps the sac using a mosquito clamp or fine forceps. The sac is then entered by means of the knife and fine Metzenbaum scissors. The abdomen is explored.

2. ***The umbilical artery and vein are ligated.***
   The umbilical artery and vein are identified. These are clamped and ligated with size 3-0 silk.

3. ***The skin is undermined.***
   To provide space for reducing the omphalocele, the skin is undermined on both sides of the abdomen. This is done with Metz scissors.

4. ***The omphalocele is reduced and the abdomen closed.***
   When enough space has been created to accommodate the viscera, it is reduced into the abdomen. The fascia is closed transversely with interrupted sutures of size 3-0 silk or synthetic absorbable material. A prosthetic mesh bridge may be necessary to cover the defect. Biological material such as AlloDerm and LifeCell can be used. Gore-Tex may also be used to form the bridge. The material is attached to the fascia with interrupted non-absorbable synthetic sutures. A purse-string suture may be used to close the skin.

STAGED CLOSURE

The patient is prepped as in primary closure. A silo may be used for a ruptured or very large omphalocele. The silo material (usually Silastic sheeting) is attached to the abdominal wall with non-absorbable sutures. A non-absorbable traction suture is placed at the highest part of the silo so it can be suspended during healing. This allows the viscera to reduce by gravity over a period of days or weeks.

Fig. 33.3 illustrates both techniques of management for an omphalocele. Fig. 33.4 illustrates the repair of a gastroschisis.

REPAIR OF BLADDER EXSTROPHY/EPISPADIAS

The surgical goal of reconstruction is to restore the normal functions of the lower urinary tract.

Pathology

Bladder **exstrophy**/epispadias is a complex set of congenital anomalies involving the lower genitourinary tract and skeletal system. The anomalies arise from the same developmental defect, which occurs in the first trimester of fetal life. The anomalies associated with the defect are as follows:

- Bladder exstrophy (the anterior bladder wall is exposed on the outside of the body through an abdominal wall defect)
- Epispadias (the urethra is fully exposed or terminates on the dorsum of the penis)
- Shortening of the penis, which also demonstrates chordee (bands of tissue that cause an upward curvature)
- Opening out of the glans and absence of the dorsal foreskin
- Anterior displacement of the vagina and anus
- Exposure of the bladder neck
- Possible presence of an omphalocele
- Divergence of the rectus muscles and widening of the pubic symphysis

Technical Points and Discussion

Reconstruction usually is performed in three stages, although this varies with the individual patient and with the surgical strategy chosen by the surgeon:

- *First stage:* Closure of the bladder and abdomen (24 to 48 hours of life)
- *Second stage:* Repair of epispadias (2 to 3 years old)
- *Third stage:* Achieving urinary continence (4 to 5 years old)

Repair of an exstrophic bladder in the male is described here.

The following are important technical points of the complex repair.

1. ***The patient is placed in the supine position.***
   A wide area is prepped, including the entire body anteriorly and posteriorly below the level of the nipple so that turning is possible, and the area is draped.
2. ***Traction sutures of 5-0 Prolene are placed in the glans penis, and ureteral catheters are secured in each ureteral orifice.***
3. ***The surgeon incises and completely dissects the periphery of the bladder and urethral plate (endodermal tissue lining the urethral groove).***
4. ***The incision is extended distally to the area where the ejaculatory ducts join the urethra, on both sides.***
5. ***The umbilical cord is excised and an umbilicoplasty is performed during or after the initial procedure.***
6. ***Skin flaps may be created if any question exists about the urethral length.***

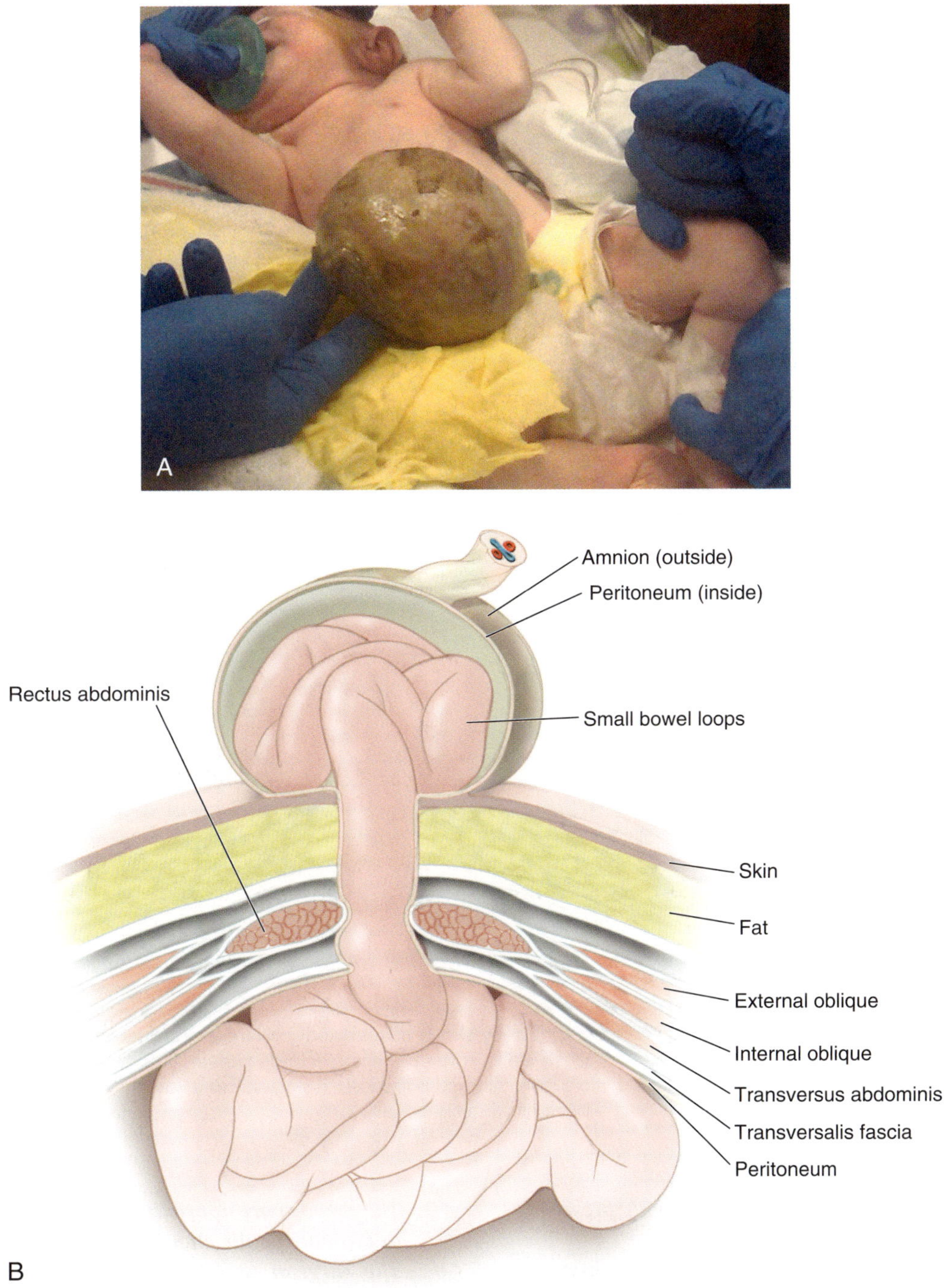

FIG. 33.3 Omphalocele. (A) Large omphalocele in the newborn. (B) Schematic illustration of an omphalocele.

Continued

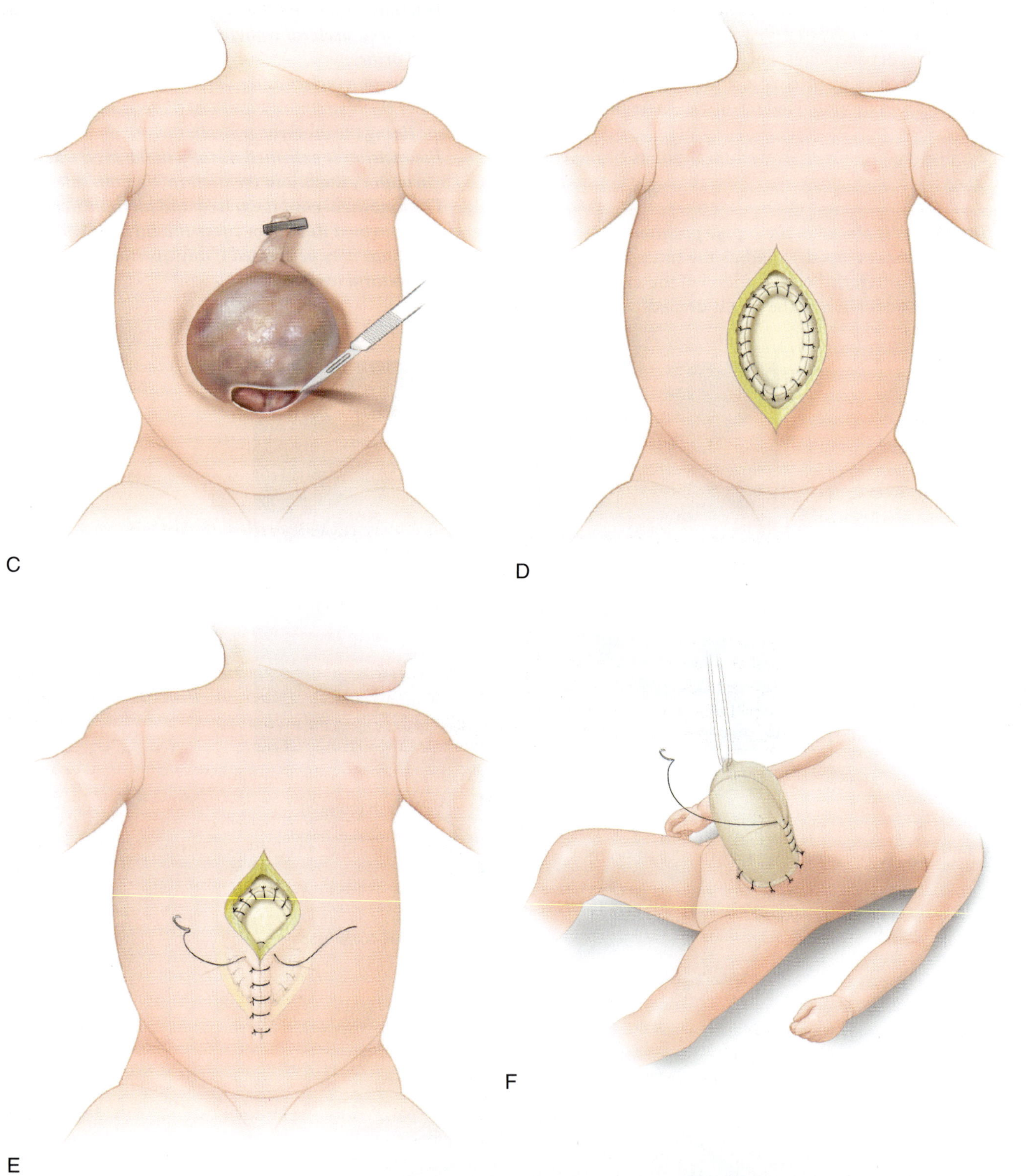

FIG. 33.3, cont'd (C) The sac is incised. (D) The skin is undermined, and the omphalocele reduced into the abdomen. A bridging mesh graft is used to cover the defect. (E) Skin closure. (F) Silo technique. The omphalocele remains contained in a Silastic silo and is reduced in stages. (From Rosen M, ed. *Atlas of Abdominal Wall Reconstruction*. Philadelphia: Saunders; 2012.)

7. ***The bladder is completely mobilized, with preservation of its blood supply.***
8. ***Inversion of the bladder plate and approximation of the corpora are the first stage of epispadias repair.***
9. ***The corpora are approximated carefully in the midline to promote penile elongation.***
10. ***The surgeon approximates the skin at the urethral plate inferiorly.***

11. ***The urethral plate is made tubular and ureteral catheters are placed bilaterally and brought out on each side of the bladder.***
12. ***After two-layer closure of the bladder and urethral plate, the bladder is reduced into the pelvis and fixed with suture.***
13. ***Sutures are placed to approximate the pubic halves. The drainage tubes are brought out superiorly, and the fascia, subcutaneous tissue, and skin are approximated.***

Fig. 33.5 illustrates the technical points of bladder exstrophy and epispadias repair.

ORCHIOPEXY FOR AN UNDESCENDED TESTICLE

The goal of surgery for a congenital undescended testicle is to restore the testicle to its normal position in the scrotum. The procedure is sometimes called an *orchiopexy;* however, this term actually refers only to the surgical attachment of the testicle to the scrotal wall. Orchiopexy is performed for a variety of conditions, including surgical attachment for the prevention and treatment of testicular torsion.

Pathology

During normal fetal life, the testicles are retained within the abdomen. Just before birth, the testicles should descend into the scrotum. Occasionally one or both testicles fail to descend into the scrotum. This can result in sterility because of the testicles' exposure to the increased temperature in the abdominal cavity.

POSITION:	Supine
INCISION:	Inguinal or testicular
PREP AND DRAPING:	Inguinal and scrotal
INSTRUMENTS:	Minor general surgery set; needlepoint ESU

Technical Points and Discussion

1. ***The patient is prepped and draped.***
   The patient is placed in the supine position, prepped, and draped with the inguinal, groin, and scrotal areas on the affected side exposed.
2. ***The surgeon enters and explores the inguinal region.***
   The surgeon makes an incision over the external ring, as for a hernia repair. The incision is carried into the deep inguinal tissues with sharp dissection. Small bleeders are coagulated with the ESU or clamped with mosquito hemostats and ligated with fine absorbable sutures.
3. ***The spermatic cord is mobilized.***
   The spermatic cord is identified and dissected with blunt and sharp dissection. The cord is dissected high in the internal ring to create sufficient slack to bring the testicle into the scrotum.
4. ***A tunnel is made through the inguinal canal into the scrotum.***
   The surgeon uses blunt dissection (e.g., Mayo or sponge forceps, or digital separation of the tissue) to create a tunnel for the testicle. A clamp is advanced through the external oblique fascia, and the tissue is manually separated, forming a pocket in the scrotum.
5. ***The testicle is brought through the tunnel and secured with sutures.***
   The testicle is brought through the tunnel, and the scrotum is incised to expose the scrotal septum. Several 3-0 or 4-0 absorbable sutures are placed through the septum and testicle, securing the testicle in place.
6. ***The inguinal layers are closed.***
   The inguinal layers are closed with size 3-0 or 4-0 Vicryl. Skin is closed with tissue adhesive and Steri-Strips or a subcuticular suture of synthetic absorbable suture, size 4-0 or 5-0.

REPAIR OF PECTUS EXCAVATUM

Pectus excavatum, or funnel chest, is a nongenetic defect of the chest wall marked by overgrowth of the costal cartilages, a sunken appearance in the anterior chest, and a restricted sternum. The goal of surgery is to reconstruct the chest wall to restore normal inspiratory function and improve body image. Surgery for pectus excavatum is frequently performed during adolescence, when the defect can worsen. It involves the implantation of one or more curved bar prostheses into the chest wall. The bars push the chest wall outward. The prosthesis is removed after several years. The procedure is performed using a minimally invasive technique.

Pathology

Pectus excavatum is a congenital defect in the sternum resulting in a longitudinal groove. Children born with the acquired defect may have mild to moderate paradoxical movement of the sternum with inhalation. Children may experience shortness of breath. Although not all cases require repair, shortness of breath and tiring can be corrected with surgery, which also improves body image.

POSITION:	Supine
INCISION:	Thoracic
PREP AND DRAPING:	Thoracic
INSTRUMENTS:	5-mm thoracoscope; pectus excavatum set with prosthesis, bender, fixation plate, and accessories; minor general surgery set; umbilical tape

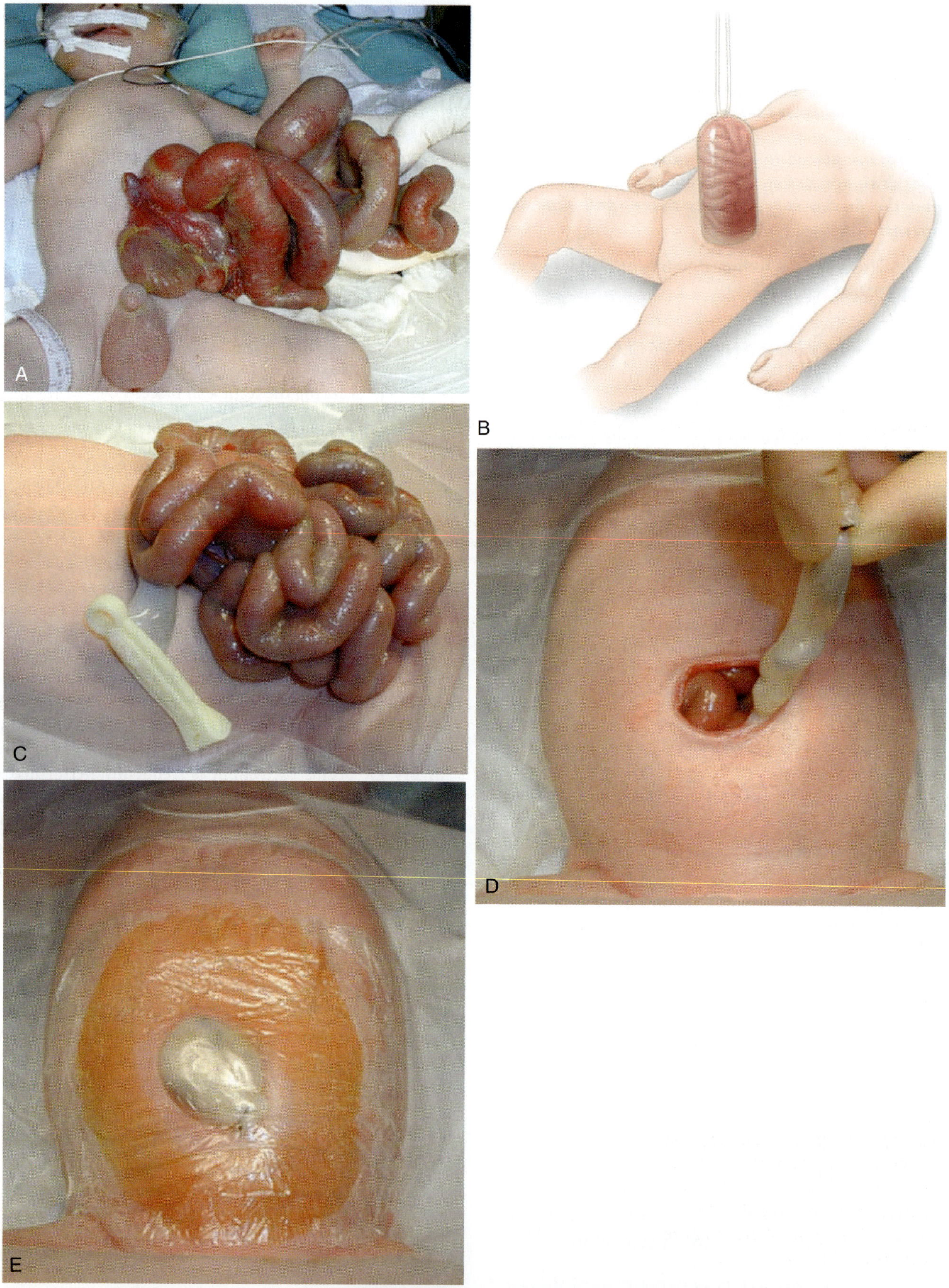

FIG. 33.4 Gastroschisis. (A) Large gastroschisis in newborn. (B) Silo technique. (C) A sutureless technique involves replacing the bowel in the abdomen as far as possible, covering the defect with Silastic sheeting, and allowing gravity to reduce the defect over a period of days. (D) The umbilical cord is coiled over the top of the viscera before the Silastic sheet and Tegaderm are applied. (E) Protective coverings are in place. (From Rosen M, ed. *Atlas of Abdominal Wall Reconstruction*. Philadelphia: Saunders; 2012.)

Technical Points and Discussion

1. ***The patient is prepped and draped.***
The patient is placed in the supine position with both arms extended to 90 degrees; general anesthesia is administered; a thoracic skin prep and draping are performed. The defect is then measured and the skin marked for bar insertion sites. The bar may be sized externally at this point.

2. ***A thoracoscopy is performed.***
A small stab wound is made in the lateral chest wall below the bar insertion sites. A 5-mm blunt trocar is inserted, followed by the thoracoscope. Insufflation of the chest cavity is usually not necessary.

3. ***Two 0.8-inch (2-cm) incisions are made in the midaxillary line following the skin marks.***
Incisions are made with a #11 blade and Metz scissors. A pocket is then created in the subcutaneous tissue to accommodate the bar introducer.

4. ***The pectus bar is prepared by means of a plate bender.***
The pectus bar is now shaped to conform to the depth and curvature of the defect. This is done by means of the plate bender, which is part of the pectus set.

5. ***A bar introducer is inserted.***
Under thoracoscopic visualization, a curved introducer is inserted through one of the incisions and a tunnel is made. The inserted introducer is slowly advanced under the sternum to the opposite incision.
A moistened umbilical tape is threaded through the tip of the introducer and tied snugly. The introducer is then pulled back out of the tunnel, bringing the umbilical tape with it.

6. ***The prosthesis is inserted.***
The preshaped bar is now attached to the umbilical tape and pulled back through the tunnel made by the introducer. The bar is introduced with the convex side facing posteriorly.

7. ***The bar is flipped (inverted).***
When the bar is in place, it is flipped over by means of the pectus inverter. An evaluation can now be made to determine the need for a second bar.

8. ***A bar stabilizer and suture are placed.***
To keep the bar from migrating, a bar stabilizer is inserted into the wound and sutured to the bar with size 3 wire or size 0 non-absorbable suture. The holes in the bar and stabilizer are then sutured to the chest wall muscle. This is done with a figure-of-eight suture size 0 absorbable attached to a right-angle needle.

9. ***The wounds are closed.***
The wound is checked for bleeding and to ensure that the bar is stabilized. The thoracoscope is withdrawn, and the wounds are closed with synthetic absorbable sutures and flat dressings or Steri-Strips. Technical points are illustrated in Fig. 33.6.

As the child emerges from anesthesia, the PACU team ensures that the patient remains in the supine position to prevent the bar from being dislodged. Patients are kept in the hospital for at least 3 to 4 days for pain control and to ensure that the bar is stable. Epidural catheterization for continuous pain control is used in selected patients. Limited activity may be resumed 6 weeks after surgery.

RADICAL NEPHRECTOMY: WILMS TUMOR

The goal of surgical treatment of Wilms tumor is excision of the kidney without trauma to the specimen, which may result in seeding cancerous cells. In some cases, a partial nephrectomy may be performed; however, most cases are advanced at the time of diagnosis, requiring a more aggressive surgical approach. An open approach is usually preferred because it allows for exploration of the perirenal tissues.

The patient presenting for nephrectomy is usually between the ages of 2 and 5 years. A period of illness may have preceded the surgery, or a nonpainful mass may have been diagnosed without other medical consequences. Cancer surgery in all families is emotionally difficult for the patient and family but is often intensified in the pediatric population. Support to the family is necessary throughout the perioperative period.

Pathology

Wilms tumor (**nephroblastoma**) is the most common malignancy of the kidney in children. However, the disease itself is rare. The tumor is responsible for 6% to 7% of all childhood cancers. Most cases are identified in children younger than 5 years. The disease can present in one or both kidneys and is more frequently encountered in females. Early diagnosis and absence of bilateral disease are indications of a successful outcome.

POSITION:	Supine with elevation of the operative flank
INCISION:	Abdominal
PREP AND DRAPING:	Abdominal/flank
INSTRUMENTS:	Kidney set; laparotomy set; Deaver retractors; vascular set; vessel loops; narrow Penrose drain; plastic clamp shods
POSSIBLE EXTRAS:	Gelfoam; topical thrombin; vessel clips

Technical Points and Discussion

1. ***The patient is prepped and draped.***
The patient is placed in the supine position with a small gel pad under the operative flank for elevation and improved exposure.

2. ***The abdomen is entered and the peritoneal reflection mobilized.***
An abdominal incision (lateral or subcostal) is made to enter the abdominal cavity. (Normally a flank incision is not used for this procedure.) After the incision is extended as necessary, a self-retaining retractor may be positioned. The surgeon may gently explore the abdomen, including the liver, inferior vena cava, and periaortic area, for any signs of metastasis.

The scrub should have sponge sticks and a small Deaver retractor available. The surgeon will palpate the renal vein as it emerges from the vena cava to establish a landmark and to check for any thrombosis related to the tumor.

For access to the retroperitoneum, the peritoneal reflection of the colon is identified and mobilized. The ureter is identified and mobilized with a wide Silastic vessel loop or narrow Penrose drain. This allows the ureter to be retracted during dissection.

3. ***The ureter and renal vessels are ligated.***
The perirenal fascia is dissected, and the renal artery, vein, and accessory vessels are dissected, clamped, and ligated or clipped. The ureter can then be ligated with fine absorbable sutures (including one or more suture ligatures) and divided. The kidney and adrenal gland are carefully extracted to prevent seeding of cancer cells, with the Gerota fascia intact. Note that ligatures on pedicle structures may be left long and tagged with mosquito forceps until closure to ensure that hemostasis is secure.

4. ***Lymph nodes are removed.***
Before the wound is closed, several lymph nodes are removed for pathological analysis. However, extensive nodal dissection is not usually performed. Ligatures are now checked to ensure that there is no leakage, and any bleeding is controlled with the ESU. The wound may then be gently irrigated with warm saline and closed in layers. A flat gauze dressing or subcuticular skin closure with Dermabond is used.

Immediate postsurgical complications include small bowel obstruction, hemorrhage, vascular complications, and wound infection. In the postoperative period, patients undergo radiation and chemotherapy according to the postoperative findings (staging). Lifelong care is necessary because Wilms tumor can recur after several years.

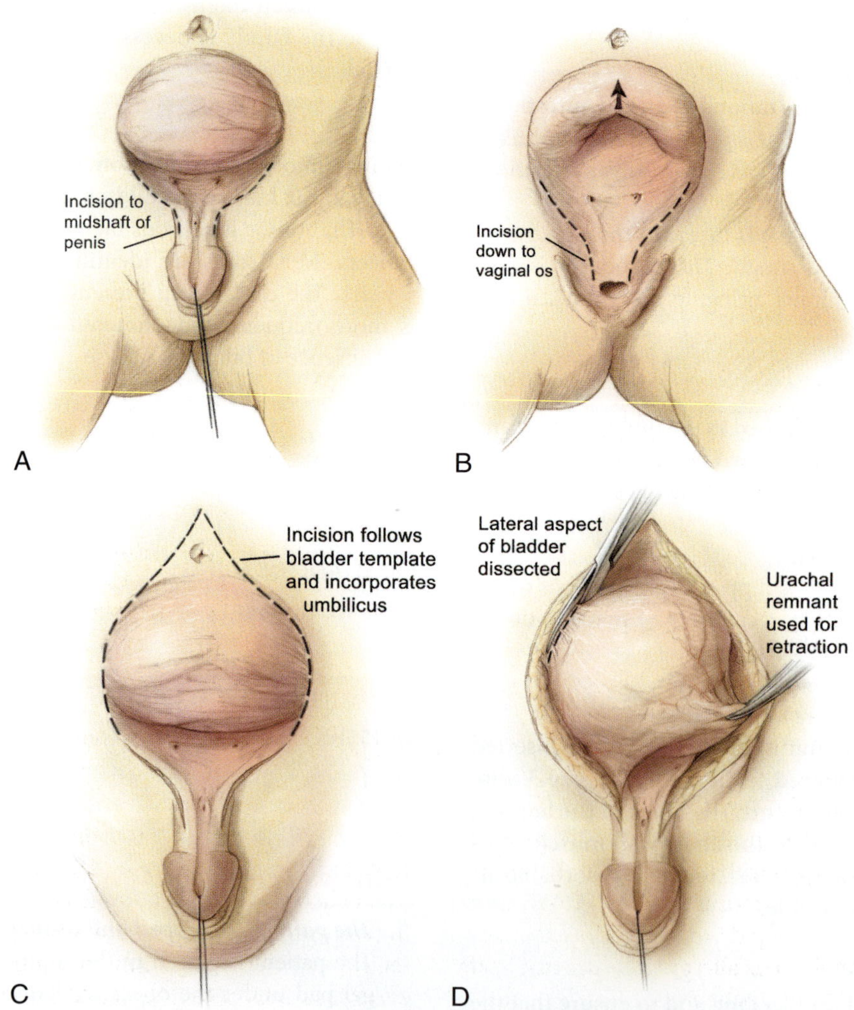

FIG. 33.5 Bladder exstrophy and epispadias. (A) The bladder plate is dissected from the abdominal wall. (B) Incision in the female. (C and D) Continuation of the incision.

Continued

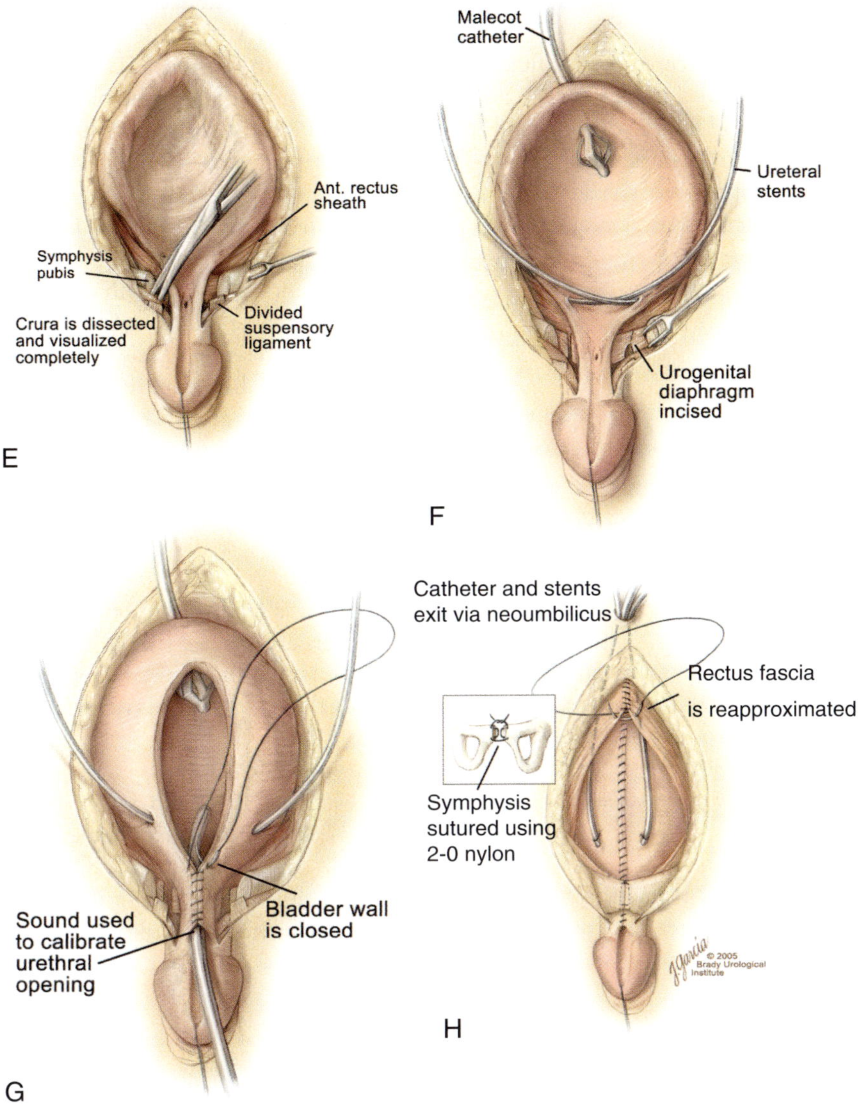

FIG. 33.5, cont'd (E) Dissection of muscles from the symphysis pubis. (F) Stents are placed in the bladder to maintain drainage. (G) A sound is placed in the urethra and closure begins. (H) The symphysis, bladder, and rectus fascia are closed. (From Wein AJ, ed. *Campbell-Walsh Urology*. 9th ed. Philadelphia: WB Saunders; 2007.)

REPAIR OF A MYELOMENINGOCELE

The surgical goal of repair of a myelomeningocele is to close a dural and cutaneous defect and preserve neural function. Immediate surgical repair is essential if the defect is leaking cerebrospinal fluid (CSF); otherwise, the procedure is performed within 48 hours of birth to prevent infection. Infants with a myelomeningocele often undergo many surgical procedures to address the primary defect and associated birth defects. Consequently, latex sensitization often develops in these patients. Many institutions that routinely treat infants with a myelomeningocele use a latex-free protocol to minimize exposure and reduce sensitization. The surgical technologist should be familiar with the facility's policies and procedures for latex allergy to ensure that a safe environment is maintained for the patient.

Infants with a myelomeningocele are more vulnerable to hypothermia because of the exposure of their skin and neural structures to the ambient room temperature. The scrub must ensure that the solutions used during the procedure are warm. Because of the delicate nature of this procedure and the patient's size, small, fine instruments are used.

Pathology

Spina bifida is a birth defect associated with incomplete closure of a section of the vertebral column. Spina bifida may occur at any point in the vertebral column but is most common in the lumbar and sacral spine. The defect may be small (spina bifida occulta) and not cause any neurological deficit for the infant, or it may cause herniation of the meninges and leakage of CSF (meningocele). The most significant form of spina bifida causes the spinal cord, meninges, and nerve roots to herniate through the skin. The structures generally are contained within a cyst or sac-like enclosure. The neural tissue in the myelomeningocele is abnormal, and even with repair the patient still has some degree of neurological deficit, such as paralysis or loss of sensation below the level of the defect. A myelomeningocele often is accompanied by birth defects such as heart and urinary system problems, which may complicate the infant's care.

Hydrocephalus (excessive accumulation of cerebrospinal fluid within the ventricles of the brain) is discussed in Chapter 34. It often is associated with a myelomeningocele. If the hydrocephalus is significant, the surgeon may elect to place a ventricular shunt at the time of myelomeningocele repair. If the hydrocephalus is less of a concern, the surgeon may postpone the shunt placement to allow the infant to recover from the primary surgery.

POSITION:	Prone
INCISION:	Back
PREP AND DRAPING:	Back
INSTRUMENTS:	Neuro set; plastic set; neuro patties; bipolar ESU

Technical Points and Discussion

1. ***The patient is prepped and draped.***
   The infant is positioned prone on the operating table with the use of small chest and hip rolls. The skin is prepped and a procedure drape positioned over the back. If the neural sac is intact, the surgeon decompresses it with a 20-gauge needle and syringe. The fluid is sent for culture and analysis.

2. ***The incision is made around the defect.***
   The surgeon begins the procedure by making a circumferential incision around the defect and placode (an area of thickened tissue over the defect) with a #15 blade on a #3 knife handle. The scrub should be prepared with bipolar ESU and moist 4 × 4 sponges to assist the surgeon with hemostasis. The incision is carried through the subcutaneous tissue until the fascia or dura is visualized.

3. ***The tissue around the defect is explored and dissected free.***
   The surgeon uses Metzenbaum scissors to remove the tissue over the exposed spinal cord and dissects the tissues along the side of the cord to reach the dura. The scrub should be prepared with the bipolar ESU and moistened cottonoids, as necessary, for hemostasis during the dissection. Metzenbaum scissors are used to separate the dura from the fascia, and the dura is closed over the spinal cord with 4-0 braided nylon or silk suture.

4. ***The fascia is separated from the muscle and closed.***
   The fascia is dissected from the muscle layer with Metzenbaum scissors and a #11 blade, as necessary. The fascial layer is closed over the dura with non-absorbable suture.

5. ***The wound is closed.***
   The wound is irrigated with warm saline. The muscle layer is closed with absorbable synthetic sutures. If the defect is small, the surgeon may be able to approximate the skin edges easily; larger defects may require Z-plasty or flap closure with interrupted sutures of synthetic

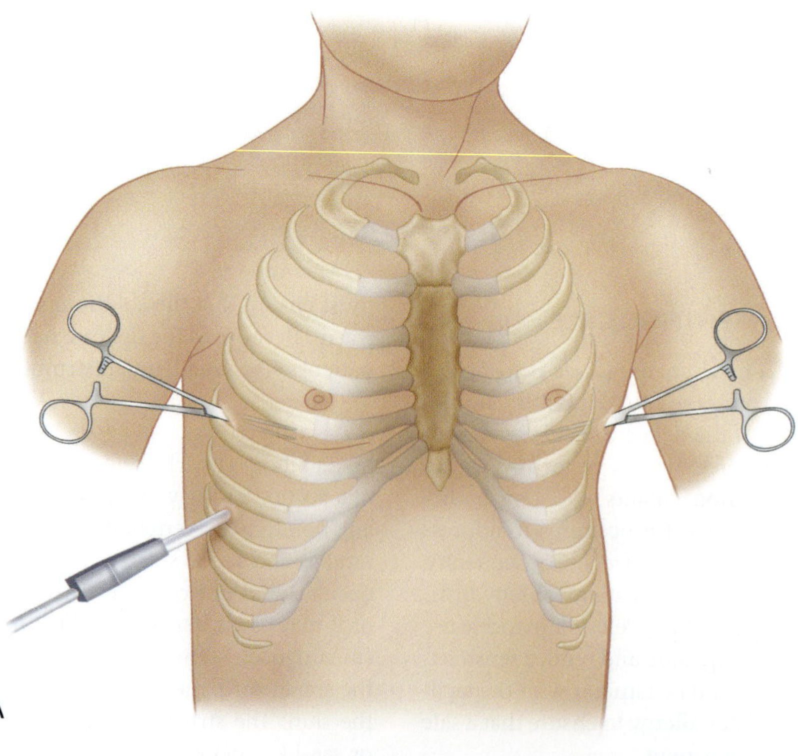

A

FIG. 33.6 Pectus excavatum. (A) Under thoracoscopy, a pocket is made in the subcutaneous tissue behind the sternum.

Continued

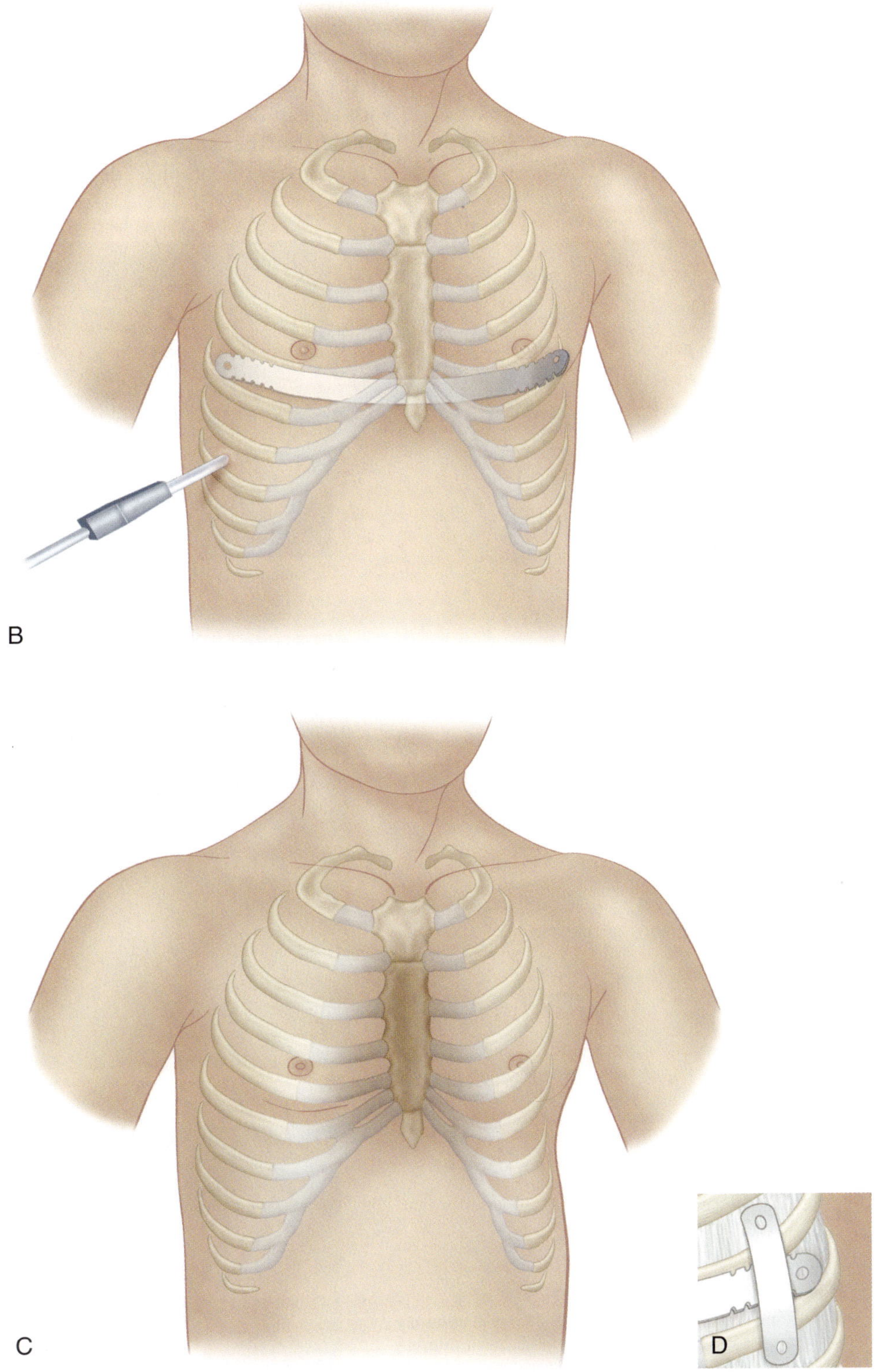

FIG. 33.6, cont'd (B) The bar is pulled into the pocket using an introducer. (C and D) The bar is secured with stabilizer plates at each end. (From Chung DH, Chen MK, eds. *Atlas of Pediatric Surgical Techniques*. Philadelphia: Elsevier Saunders; 2010.)

non-absorbable material. Technical points for the procedure are illustrated in Fig. 33.7.

CORRECTION OF SYNDACTYLY

Surgery is performed to separate the fingers and/or toes, which are joined at birth.

Pathology

During weeks 6 and 8 of gestation, the paddle-shaped hands and feet normally differentiate into separate fingers and toes. Syndactyly results when this separation fails to occur. It is the most common malformation of the limbs and is associated with at least 28 other specific syndromes, occurring in 1 per 2000 births. The cause is unknown. The condition is classified as incomplete or complete, depending on whether the fingers

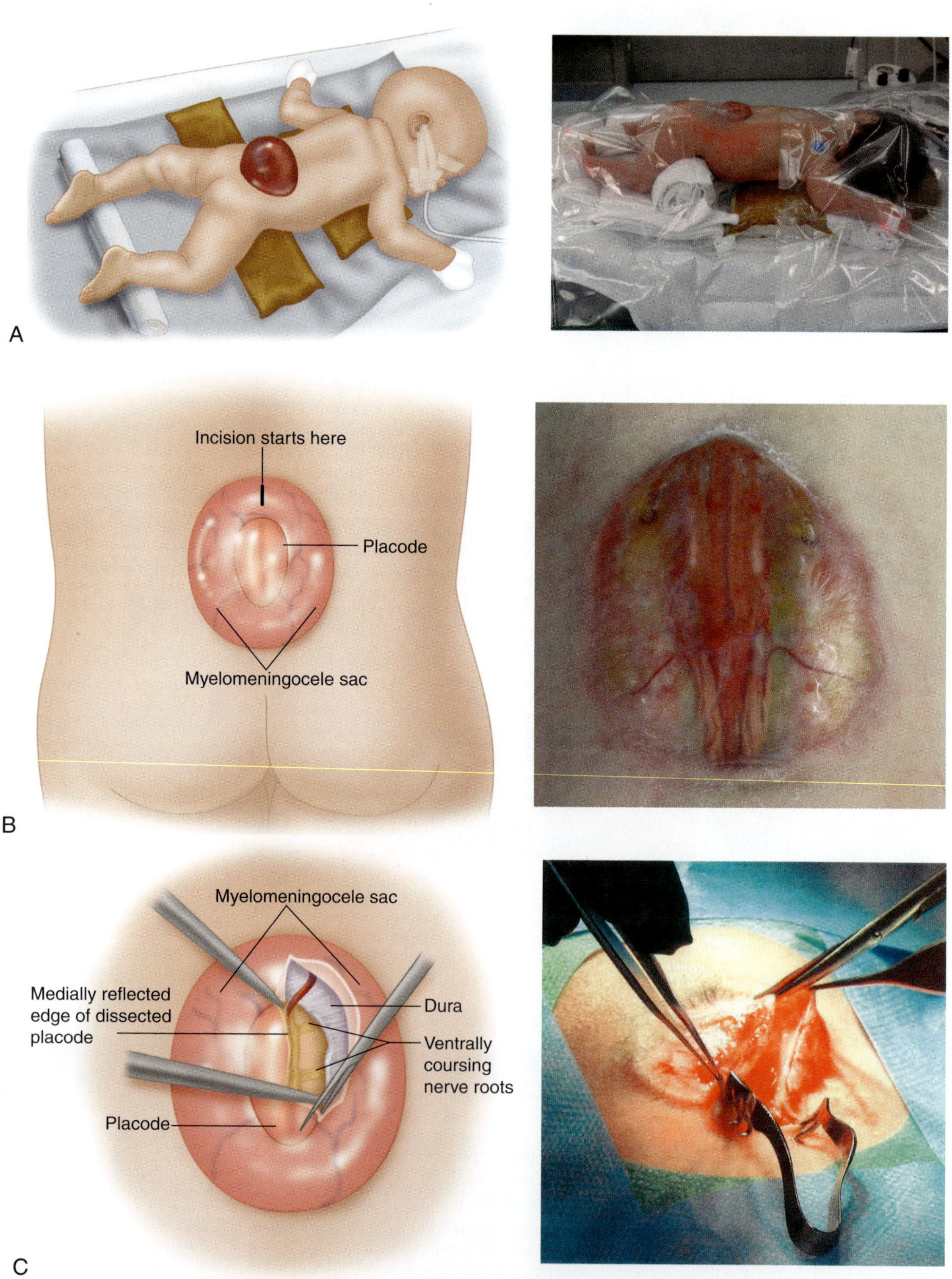

FIG. 33.7 Myelomeningocele. (A) Positioning the patient. (B) The incision is made at the perimeter of the sac and placode (a thickened area of tissue overlying the myelomeningocele). (C) Dissection is carried out circumferentially.

Continued

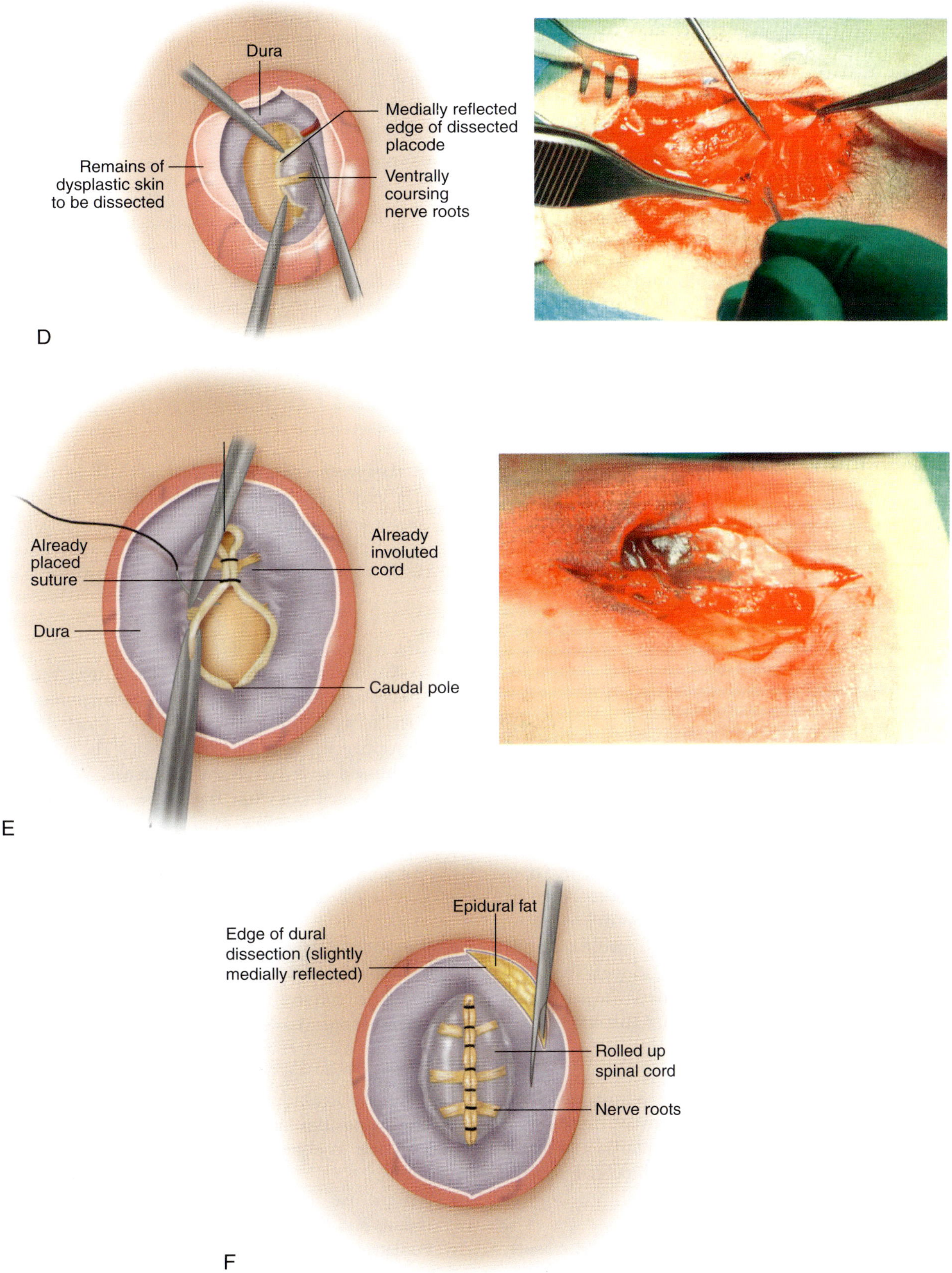

FIG. 33.7, cont'd (D) The edges of the placode are released. (E) The shape of the cord is maintained, and closure is started. (F) The dura is closed.

Continued

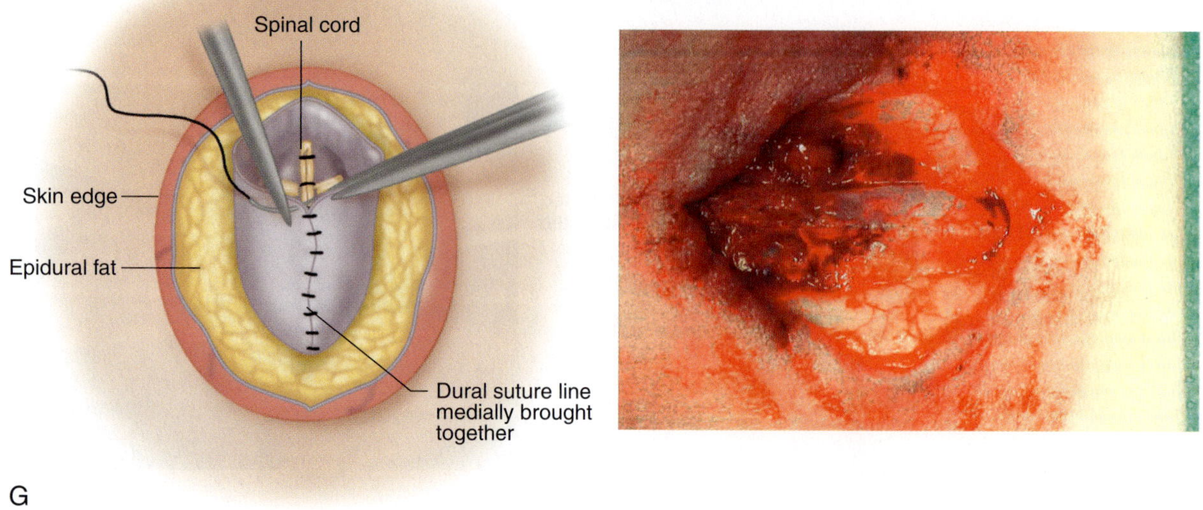

FIG. 33.7, cont'd (G) Closure completed. (From Jandial R, McCormick P, Black P, eds. *Core Techniques in Operative Neurosurgery.* Philadelphia: Elsevier; 2011.)

are joined from the base (web) to the tip. In complex syndactyly, bone and soft tissue are shared by two fingers, whereas in simple syndactyly, only superficial tissues and skin are involved. Surgery is performed before the child reaches school age. The surgical plan for syndactyly is shown in Fig. 33.8.

Technical Points and Discussion

1. ***The patient is prepped and draped.***
   The patient is placed in the supine position with the operative arm on a hand board. General anesthesia is induced. A tourniquet is applied, and the arm is prepped from the elbow to the hand. If a skin graft is required, the donor site is prepped and draped separately.

2. ***A skin graft is taken.***
   To begin the procedure, the surgeon plans the incisions and draws them on the hand. If a graft is to be taken, this is done first. The groin is a common donor site. A small amount of skin is removed from the groin crease by means of the freehand method and a scalpel. The scrub should keep the graft moist until needed. The site is covered with a towel to protect it from contamination.

3. ***Skin flaps are raised.***
   The skin incisions are made with a #15 knife and plastic surgery forceps. A Z-shaped or modified Z-incision is used. The tourniquet is released momentarily, and bleeders are controlled with a needlepoint bipolar ESU. The tourniquet can then be reinflated.

4. ***The web space is reconstructed with a primary Z-closure on one side.***
   The triangular flaps are closed on one finger with anchor sutures of 5-0 nylon and interrupted sutures to complete the repair.

5. ***A skin graft is sutured in place.***
   The graft is positioned over the denuded area of the other finger and trimmed as needed. Tenotomy scissors or iris scissors may be used for this. The graft is sutured in placed with 4-0 or 5-0 interrupted nylon or absorbable synthetic sutures.

6. ***The wounds are dressed.***
   A Xeroform dressing can be placed over the graft site, and a stent dressing can be used to maintain close contact between the graft and finger. (Stent dressings are described in detail in Chapter 28.) The opposite finger is dressed with Xeroform and gauze. Webril is applied around each site while the fingers are widely separated. Many surgeons apply a hard cast to maintain the repair during healing. Figs. 33.8 and 33.9 illustrate the technical points.

KEY CONCEPTS

- Pediatric surgical procedures are performed mainly to correct congenital defects, treat diseases, and address trauma.
- A parent may accompany the child into the operating room for induction. An infant or small child may be held by the parent during induction.
- During positioning, the pediatric patient requires the same attention to potential nerve, vessel, and skeletal injury as adults.
- Always use the appropriate size positioning device for infants and children.
- Pediatric instrument sets are often identified according to the procedure or specialty.
- Prepping solution used on infants and small children may require weaker strength than that used on adults. This is because of the risk for skin irritation and burns.

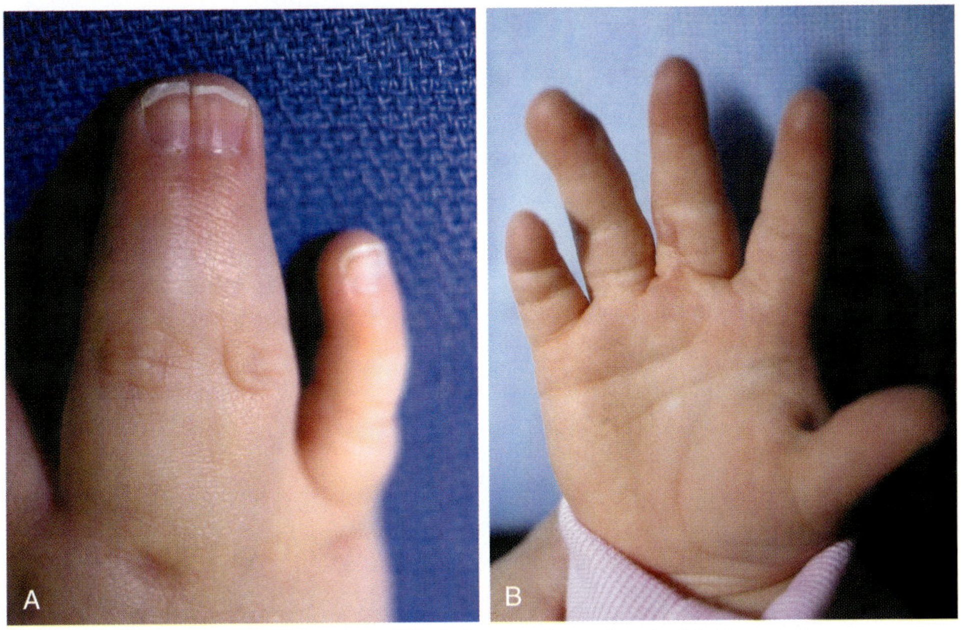

FIG. 33.8 Syndactyly. (A) Complete simple syndactyly. (B) After repair.

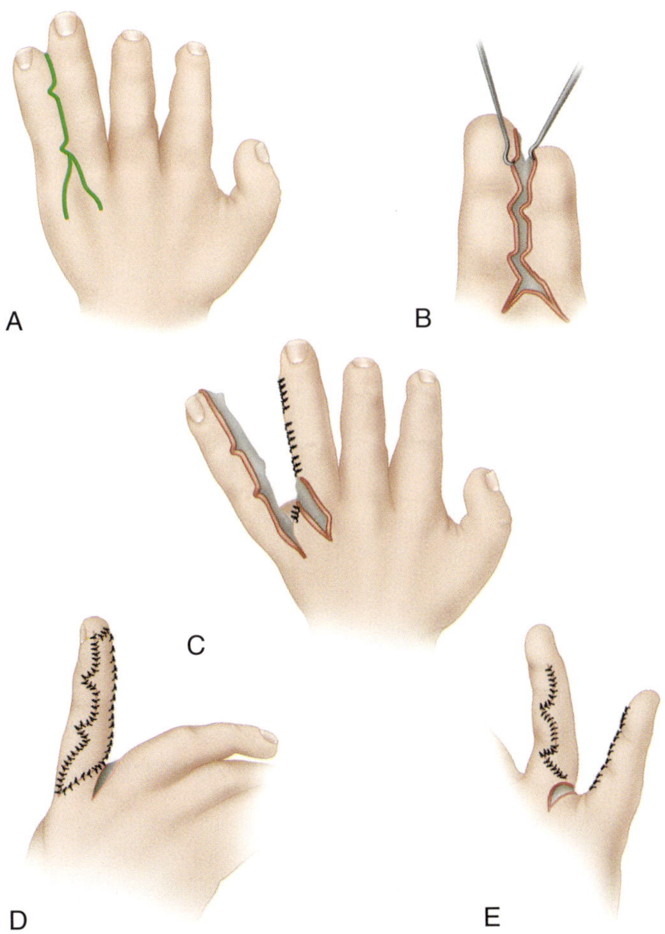

FIG. 33.9 Syndactyly surgical technique. (A and B) Proposed incision lines. Irregular flaps will be created to provide greater coverage. (C) The flaps are raised and the web space reconstructed. (D and E) The flaps are closed on one finger, and a full-thickness skin graft is used for the remaining defect. (From Canale S, Beaty J, eds. *Campbell's Operative Orthopaedics*. 12th ed. Philadelphia: Mosby; 2013.)

REVIEW QUESTIONS

1. What are the disadvantages of administering a preoperative anxiolytic to a pediatric patient?
2. List at least five reasons infants are at risk for hypothermia.
3. Explain magical thinking and how this affects a toddler's view of the perioperative environment.
4. Explain the difference between an omphalocele and gastroschisis.
5. List at least six reasons pediatric patients should not be considered "small adults." Give examples from your knowledge of pediatric physiology.
6. What are the specific risks associated with transporting a pediatric patient?
7. What are the risks to tissue that is left exposed to the environment in conditions such as omphalocele and spina bifida?

REFERENCE

1. American Society of Anesthesiologists. Practice guidelines for preoperative fasting and the use of pharmacologic agents to reduce the risk of pulmonary aspiration: application to healthy patients undergoing elective procedures—a report by the American Society of Anesthesiologists Task Force on preoperative fasting. *Anesthesiology*. 1999;90:3.

BIBLIOGRAPHY

Association of periOperative Registered Nurses (AORN). Pediatric medication safety. *AORN J*. 2006;83:1.

Busen N. Perioperative preparation of the adolescent surgical patient. *AORN J*. 2001;73:2.

Canale S, Beaty J, eds. *Campbell's Operative Orthopedics*. 12th ed. Philadelphia: Mosby; 2013.

Cartwright CC, Jimenez DF, Barone CM, et al. Endoscopic strip craniectomy: a minimally invasive treatment for early correction of craniosynostosis. *J Neurosci Nurs*. 2003;35:3.

Dreger V, Tremback T. Management of preoperative anxiety in children. *AORN J*. 2006;84:5.

Gearhart J, Rink R, Mouriquand P, eds. *Pediatric Urology*. 2nd ed. Philadelphia: Saunders; 2010.
Golden L, Pagala M, Sukhavasi S, et al. Giving toys to children reduces their anxiety about receiving premedication for surgery. *Anesth Analg*. 2006;102:1070.
Hommertzheim R, Steinke E. Malignant hyperthermia: the perioperative nurse's role. *AORN J*. 2006;83:1.
Ingoe R, Lange P. The Ladd's procedure for correction of intestinal malrotation with volvulus in children. *AORN J*. 2007;85:2.
Meyers E, ed. *Operative Otolaryngology Head and Neck Surgery*. 2nd ed. Philadelphia: Elsevier; 2008.
Miller R, et al., eds. *Miller's Anesthesia*. 8th ed. Philadelphia: Saunders; 2012.
Neligan P, Buck D, eds. *Core Procedures in Plastic Surgery*. Philadelphia: Elsevier; 2014.
Phippen ML, Papanier Wells M, eds. *Patient Care During Operative and Invasive Procedures*. Philadelphia: WB Saunders; 2000.
Swoveland B, Medvick C, Thompson G. The Nuss procedure for pectus excavatum correction. *AORN J*. 2001;74:6.
Touloukian RJ, Smith EI. Disorders of rotation and fixation. In: O'Neill JA, Rowe MI, eds. *Pediatric Surgery*. 5th ed. Vol 2. St. Louis: Mosby; 1998.
Viitanen H, Paivi A, Viitanen M, et al. Premedication with midazolam delays recovery after ambulatory sevoflurane anesthesia in children. *Anesth Analg*. 2000;90:498.

NEUROSURGERY 34

LEARNING OBJECTIVES

After studying this chapter, the reader will be able to:

1. Identify key anatomical features of the nervous system
2. Describe the basic physiology of the autonomic nervous system
3. Describe basic diagnostic procedures of the nervous system
4. List and describe common surgical procedures of the nervous system

TERMINOLOGY

Aneurysm: Dilation or ballooning of an artery wall as a result of injury, disease, or a congenital condition.

Arteriovenous malformation (AVM): A collection of blood vessels with abnormal communication between the arteries and veins. It may be the result of injury, infection, or a congenital condition.

Astrocytes: Cells that support the nerve cells (neurons) of the brain and spinal cord by providing nutrients and insulation.

Bone flap: A section of bone removed from the skull during craniotomy procedures.

Craniectomy: Removal of a section of the cranium for treatment of intracranial pressure. A cranioplasty is performed at a later time, once the condition is stabilized.

Cranioplasty: Reconstruction of a portion of the cranium lost as a result of disease or trauma.

Craniotomy: Surgical opening into the cranial cavity.

Embolization: A technique used to occlude a blood vessel. Various materials, including platinum coils and microscopic plastic particles, are injected into the vessel under fluoroscopy control to stop active bleeding or prevent bleeding.

Intracranial pressure (ICP): The pressure within the skull exerted by the brain tissue, blood, and cerebrospinal fluid.

Spondylosis: Narrowing of the spinal canal. The condition can create chronic pain, especially in the areas where the spinal nerves exit the cord.

Stereotactic: A computerized method of locating a point in space or in tissue, by the use of coordinates in three dimensions. During stereotactic surgery, the precise location of a tumor or other tissue can be identified from outside the body. The tissue can then be targeted for destruction.

Neurosurgery is a specialization of the brain, spine, and peripheral nerves. Access to the brain and spinal anatomy often requires penetration or removal of bony tissue. Therefore many procedures require both soft tissue and orthopedic instruments. Unlike most other tissues of the body, nervous tissue does not regenerate after trauma or disease. Many neurosurgical procedures are performed to restore function to other systems and alleviate pain, for tumor removal, and for the treatment of trauma or disease that is life threatening or that greatly reduces the patient's quality of life. Like other specialties, neurosurgical technology has advanced quickly in the past decade. Digital technology has created new techniques in neuroendoscopy, microsurgery, biomodeling, and navigation of the nervous system. This chapter is an introduction to neurosurgical techniques that are the basis of more advanced practice for the surgical technologist.

SURGICAL ANATOMY

The nervous system is a communication center for the body. It receives, processes, and interprets information from the environment. It then coordinates appropriate sensory and motor responses. The nervous system is divided structurally into two parts: the *central nervous system (CNS),* which includes the brain and spinal cord, and the peripheral nervous system (PNS), which includes the cranial and spinal nerves and their branches.

CELLS OF THE NERVOUS SYSTEM

Neurons

The neuron is the primary cell type of the nervous system and is located throughout the body. It transmits information to other neurons, muscle, and glandular tissue. The neuron has three main parts: the body (or soma), the axon, and the dendrites (Fig. 34.1).

- The *soma* acts as the sending and receiving area for nerve impulses and is the energy center for the cell.
- The *axon* carries nerve impulses away (efferent) from the cell.
- The *dendrites* carry nerve impulses toward (afferent) the cell.

Neuroglia and Schwann Cells

Neuroglia and Schwann cells provide support to the neurons. Brain and spinal cord tissue are composed primarily of neuroglia. **Astrocytes**, the most common type of neuroglia, fill the spaces among the neurons. Oligodendrocytes form myelin, the fatty sheath that provides insulation for the dendrites. Microglia are specialized immune cells that remove cellular debris. Ependymal cells line the brain ventricles and are involved in the production of cerebrospinal fluid (CSF). Schwann cells are found in the PNS. Their main functions are the production of myelin and the removal of cellular debris.

CENTRAL NERVOUS SYSTEM

Skull (Cranium)

The skull covers and protects the brain. It is composed of bony plates that are connected by a thin membrane called a *suture*. The major bones of the skull (Fig. 34.2) are as follows:

- One *frontal bone,* which provides structure for the forehead and orbits
- Two *parietal* bones on either side of the skull, which provide structure for the sides and roof of the cranium
- Two *temporal* bones on either side of the skull, which contribute to the structure for the sides of the cranium
- One occipital bone, which provides structure to the back of the skull and a portion of the floor of the cranium

The skull is covered by the multilayered scalp, which is composed of skin and highly vascular subcutaneous tissue. The *pericranium* is the periosteal layer of the skull bones. The pericranium is covered by muscle and the galea, a tough, fibrous tissue sheet. The skin of the scalp is very thick and highly vascular and contains numerous hair follicles.

Meninges

Directly beneath the skull lie the three protective coverings of the brain, the meninges. The outermost layer, the dura mater, is composed of very dense, fibrous tissue. The middle layer is the arachnoid mater. The arachnoid mater is a very delicate, serous membrane that has the appearance of a spiderweb. Beneath the arachnoid mater is the subarachnoid space, which is filled with CSF. The pia mater is the layer closest to the brain. This is a vascular membrane that contains portions of areolar connective tissue. This membrane dips down into the various crevices and convolutions of the brain. The layers of the scalp, superficial brain, and associated structures are illustrated in Fig. 34.3.

Brain

The brain is divided into three main sections: the cerebrum, cerebellum, and brainstem. Each of these sections is further subdivided (Fig. 34.4).

CEREBRUM The cerebrum, or forebrain, controls all motor activity and sensory impulses. It is divided into halves, the right and left cerebral hemispheres. Each hemisphere is subdivided into four lobes:

- The *frontal lobe* is responsible for thought and behavior.
- The *temporal lobe* controls memory, the senses, language, and emotions.
- The *parietal lobe* primarily controls language.
- The *occipital lobe* controls vision.

The cerebrum is the largest part of the brain, accounting for almost 88% of the total weight of the organ. The surface of the cerebrum is convoluted, with small bulges that occur throughout. These bulges are called *gyri* (sing., gyrus). Between the bulges are shallow indentations, called *sulci* (sing., sulcus). Larger, deeper furrows in this area are known as *fissures.*

The outer tissue layer of the cerebrum is known as the *cerebral cortex.* This layer is composed of gray matter and is divided into lobes, which are named for the bones that lie over them. The gray matter is composed of nerve cells and blood vessels.

CEREBELLUM The cerebellum, or hindbrain, lies under the posterior cerebrum and is the second largest area of the brain (Fig. 34.5A). Like the cerebrum, it is covered by a cortex composed of gray matter and is divided into lobes by fissures. The cerebellar lobes are the anterior, posterior, and flocculonodular lobes. The anterior and posterior lobes help control coordination and movement. The flocculonodular lobe helps control equilibrium. Coordination between the cerebrum and cerebellum is necessary for the "planning" and execution of movement. The sensory information provided by the cerebrum guides the coordinated movement of muscles and balance.

BRAINSTEM The brainstem is composed of three sections: the medulla oblongata, midbrain, and pons (Fig. 34.5B). The medulla oblongata is a continuous connection between the spinal cord and the pons. It is made up primarily of gray matter and closely resembles the spinal cord in internal structure except that it is much thicker. Lines of white matter are interspersed within the gray matter, and all impulses into and out of the spinal cord are located here. The medulla is responsible for vital functions such as control of the circulatory system, respiration, and heart rate.

The midbrain is situated between the forebrain and the hindbrain. The major structures of the midbrain are the thalamus, hypothalamus, pituitary gland, and pineal gland. The pituitary gland is composed of two sections, anterior and posterior, which coordinate with the hypothalamus to synthesize and secrete many vital hormones that are responsible for cell activity and physiological processes in the body. These essential hormones that are targeted include the growth hormone, thyroid-stimulating hormone, adrenocorticotropic hormone, prolactin, luteinizing hormone, and oxytocin. The pineal gland lies posterior to the pituitary and secretes melatonin, which regulates periods of wakefulness and sleep (circadian rhythm) through a feedback mechanism from the retina. On the ventral side of the midbrain are two masses of white matter called the *cerebral peduncles.* White matter contains millions of myelinated

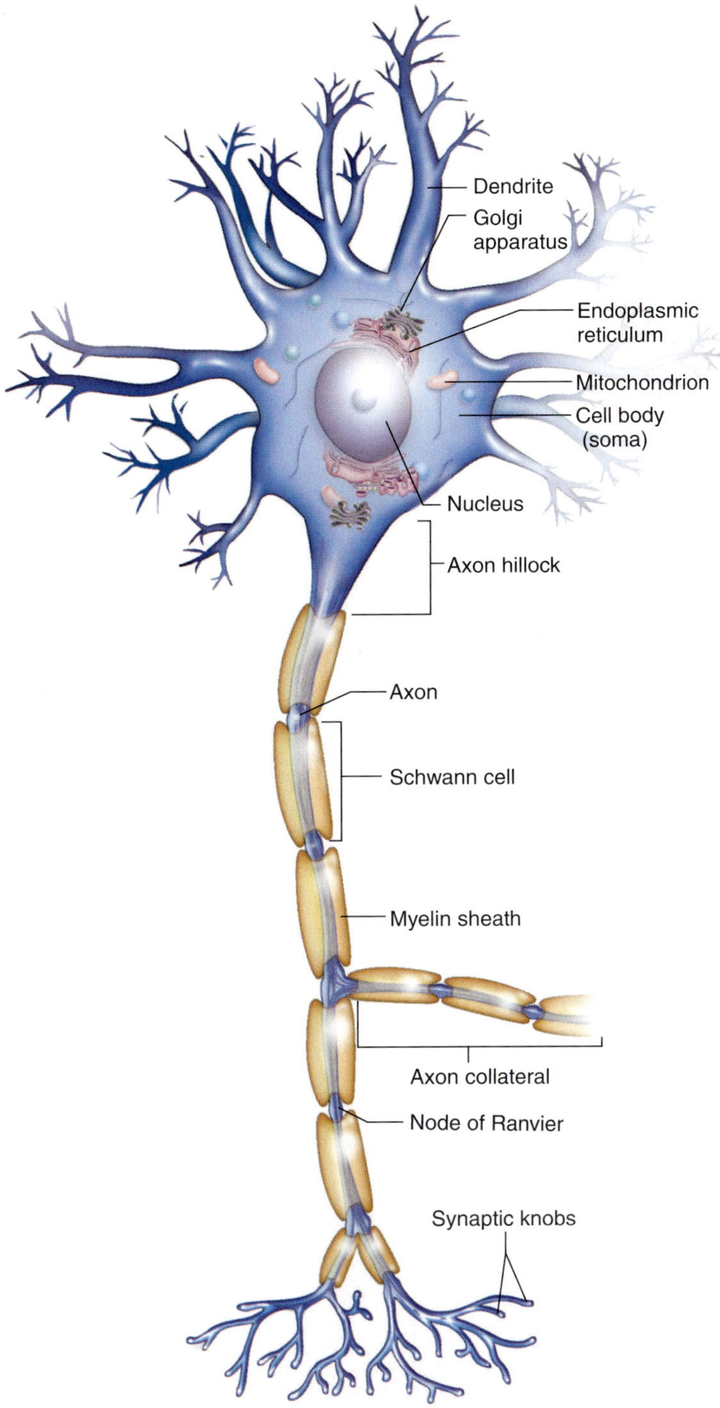

FIG. 34.1 Structure of the neuron. Note the three main sections: the cell body, dendrites, and axon. The myelinated sheath of some neurons affects the speed of nerve transmission. (From Standring S. *Gray's Anatomy*. 41st ed. Elsevier; 2016.)

nerve fibers that carry impulses among the neurons. On the dorsal side are four rounded tissue masses called the *corpora quadrigemina*. This section is responsible for relaying auditory and visual impulses.

The pons lies between the midbrain and the medulla, in front of the cerebellum. It consists mainly of white matter and serves as a relay between the medulla and the cerebral peduncles. The fifth, sixth, seventh, and eighth cranial nerves originate in this portion of the hindbrain.

VENTRICULAR SYSTEM

The ventricles are four cavities that are found between the various sections within the brain. They are filled with CSF, which bathes and nourishes the brain. Two lateral ventricles occupy the two halves of the cerebrum. These are connected by the interventricular foramen, which leads to the third ventricle. This ventricle opens into a narrow path, called the *cerebral aqueduct*, which leads directly into the fourth ventricle, lying

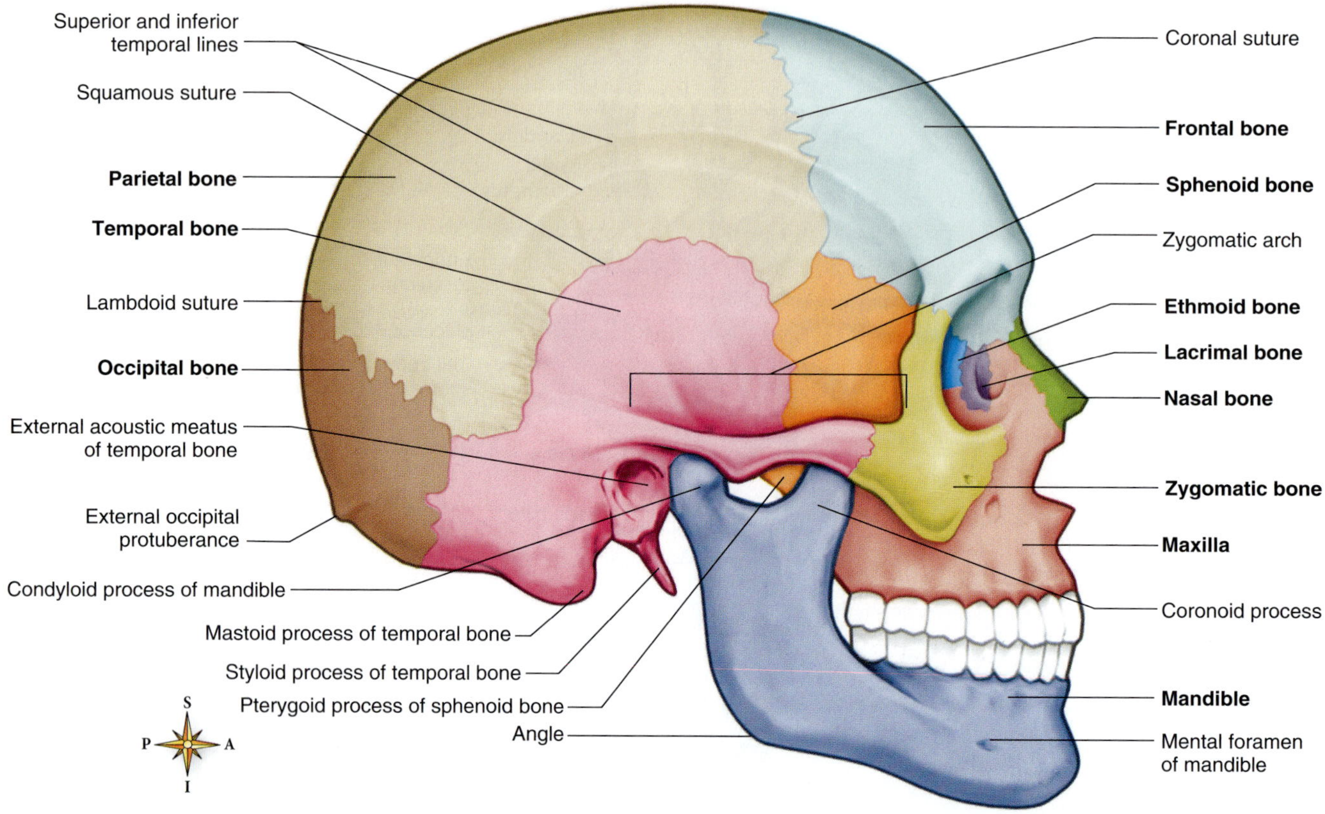

FIG. 34.2 Bones of the cranium. (From Vidic B, Suarez FR, eds. *Photographic Atlas of the Human Body.* St Louis: Mosby; 1984.)

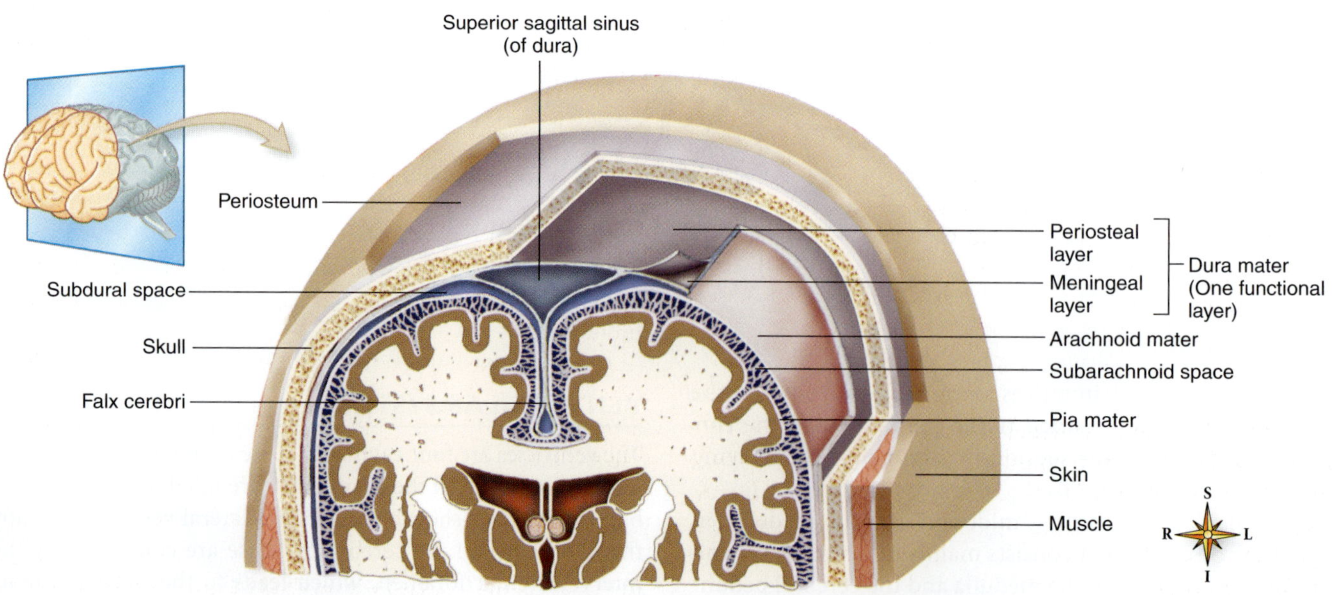

FIG. 34.3 Surgical layers of the scalp, galea, meninges, and brain. (From Abrahams P, Hutchings RT, Marks SC, eds. *McKinn's Color Atlas of Human Anatomy.* 4th ed. St Louis: Mosby; 1999.)

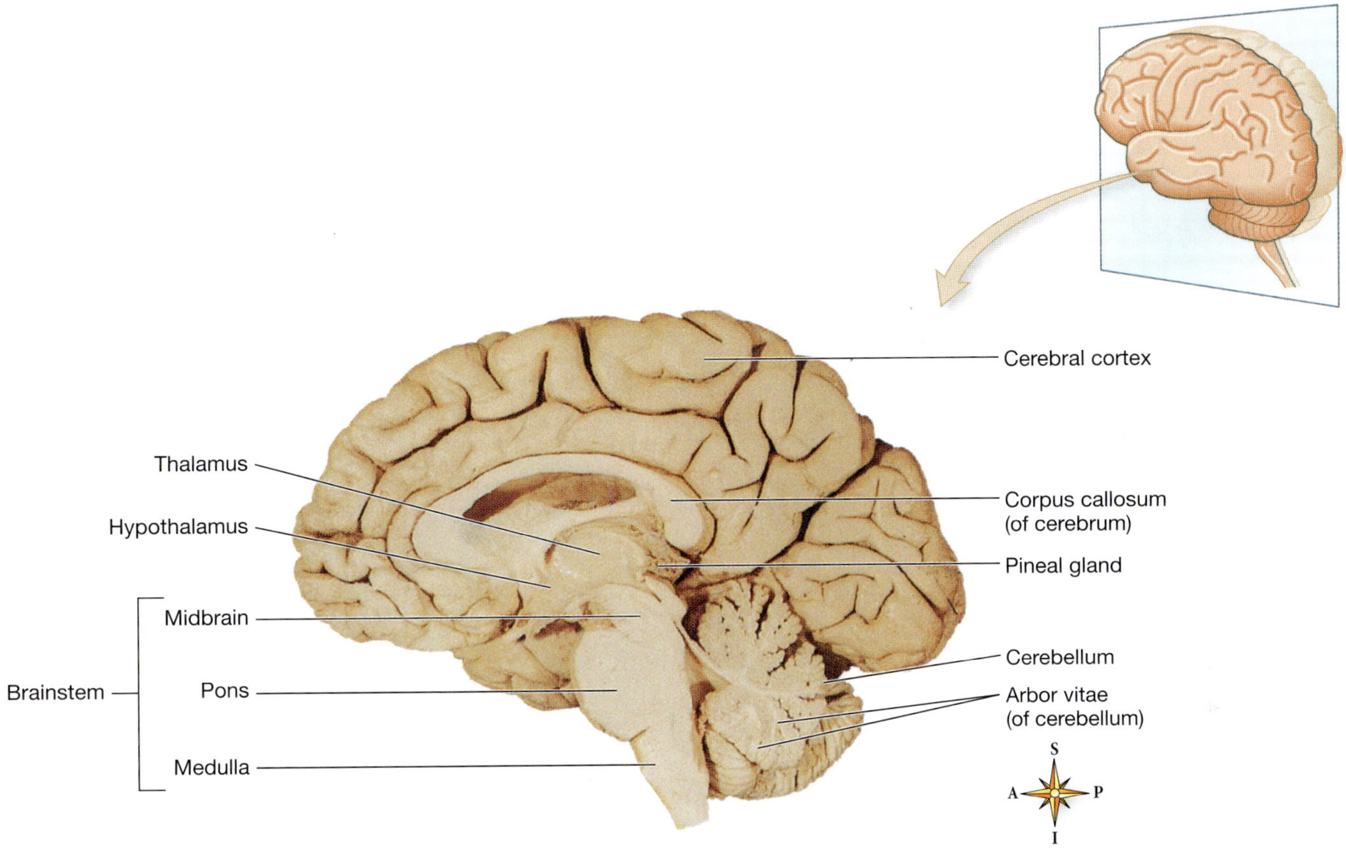

FIG. 34.4 Divisions of the brain. (From Applegate E. *The Anatomy and Physiology Learning System.* 2nd ed. St Louis: WB Saunders; 2000.)

near the base of the brain. The CSF leaves the fourth ventricle through three openings and then circulates around the brainstem and cord.

BLOOD SUPPLY TO THE BRAIN

To function adequately, the brain requires 20% more oxygen than the other organs in the body. It receives arterial blood from two systems, the internal carotid arteries and the vertebral arteries. These systems communicate through a structure called the *circle of Willis,* which is located at the base of the brain (Fig. 34.6). The circle of Willis gives rise to the other arteries that supply blood to the cerebral hemispheres and ensures continuity of the blood supply to the brain if any of the arteries are compromised. Blood is carried away from the brain by the cerebral veins that drain into the dural sinuses and internal jugular veins.

VERTEBRAL COLUMN

The vertebral column provides structure and protects the spinal cord. The vertebral column is composed of 24 bones, or vertebrae, in addition to the sacrum and coccyx, which are separate in childhood but become fused in adulthood (Fig. 34.7):

- 7 cervical vertebrae
- 12 thoracic vertebrae
- 5 lumbar vertebrae
- 5 sacral vertebrae (fused as one)
- 1 coccygeal vertebra, which also is a fused structure containing from 1 to 3 separate vertebrae

The vertebrae are referred to by a numerical designation preceded by the first letter of the region where they are located (e.g., the first cervical vertebra is C-1; the first thoracic vertebra is T-1).

The atlas, or first cervical vertebra (C-1), supports the skull and is fused with the second vertebra, the axis (C-2), to provide rotational movement of the neck. The remaining vertebrae are similar in structure and appearance. Each vertebra has a body with a circular opening through which the spinal cord passes. Two pedicles extend backward from the body and form the transverse processes, which project laterally and support the articulating surfaces, known as the *facets.* Each vertebra has openings (intervertebral foramina) for the passage of spinal nerves. Muscles and ligaments hold the vertebral column together.

The vertebrae are separated by cartilaginous cushions called *intervertebral discs.* The tough outer layer of the disc is the annulus fibrosis, and the jelly-like center layer is the nucleus pulposus (Fig. 34.8).

SPINAL CORD

The spinal cord is located within the vertebral canal and is continuous with the medulla oblongata of the hindbrain. The cord originates at the foramen magnum, a large opening at the base

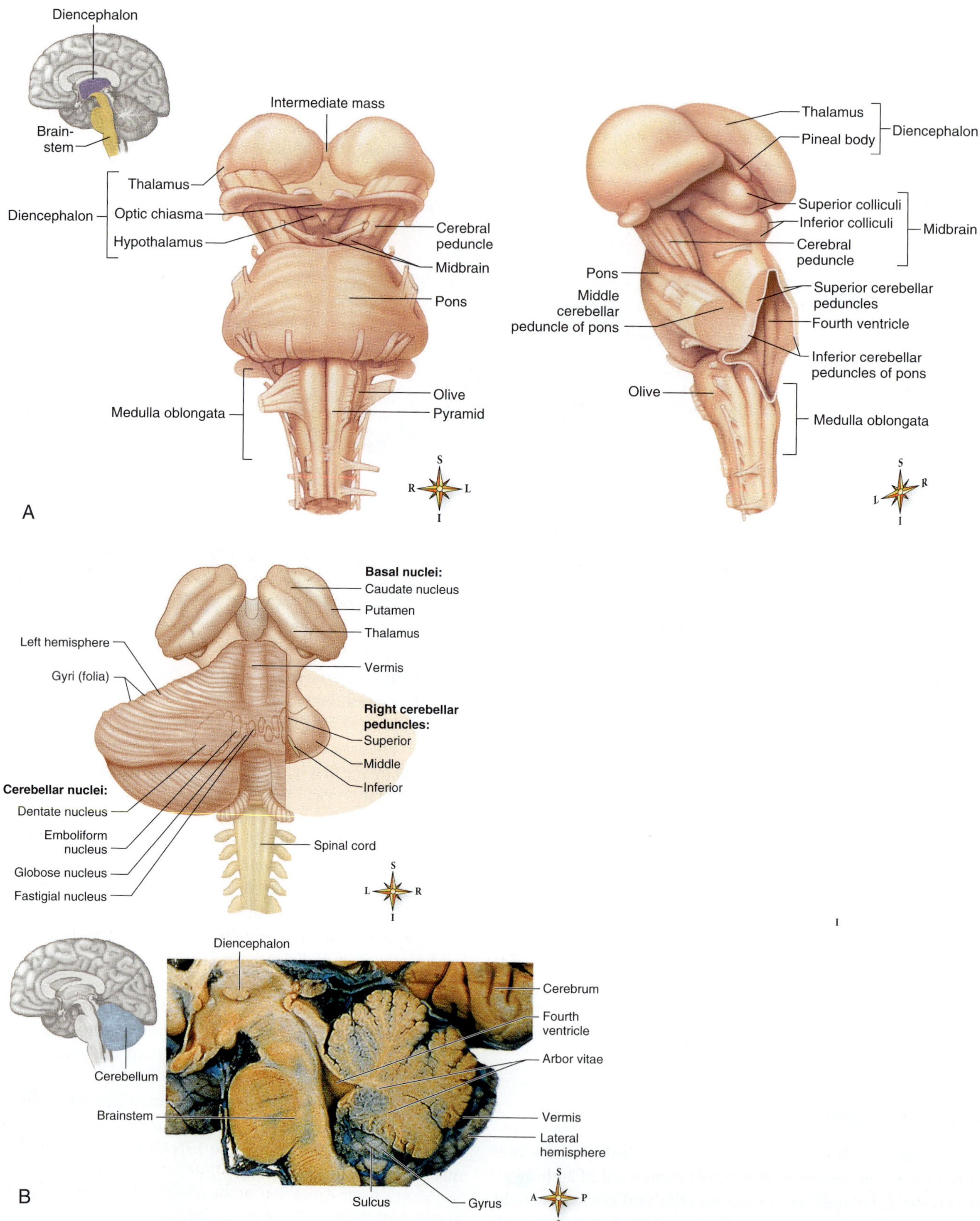

FIG. 34.5 (A) Cerebellum. (B) Brainstem. (From Abrahams P, Hutchings RT, Marks SC, eds. *McKinn's Color Atlas of Human Anatomy*. 4th ed. St Louis: Mosby; 1999.)

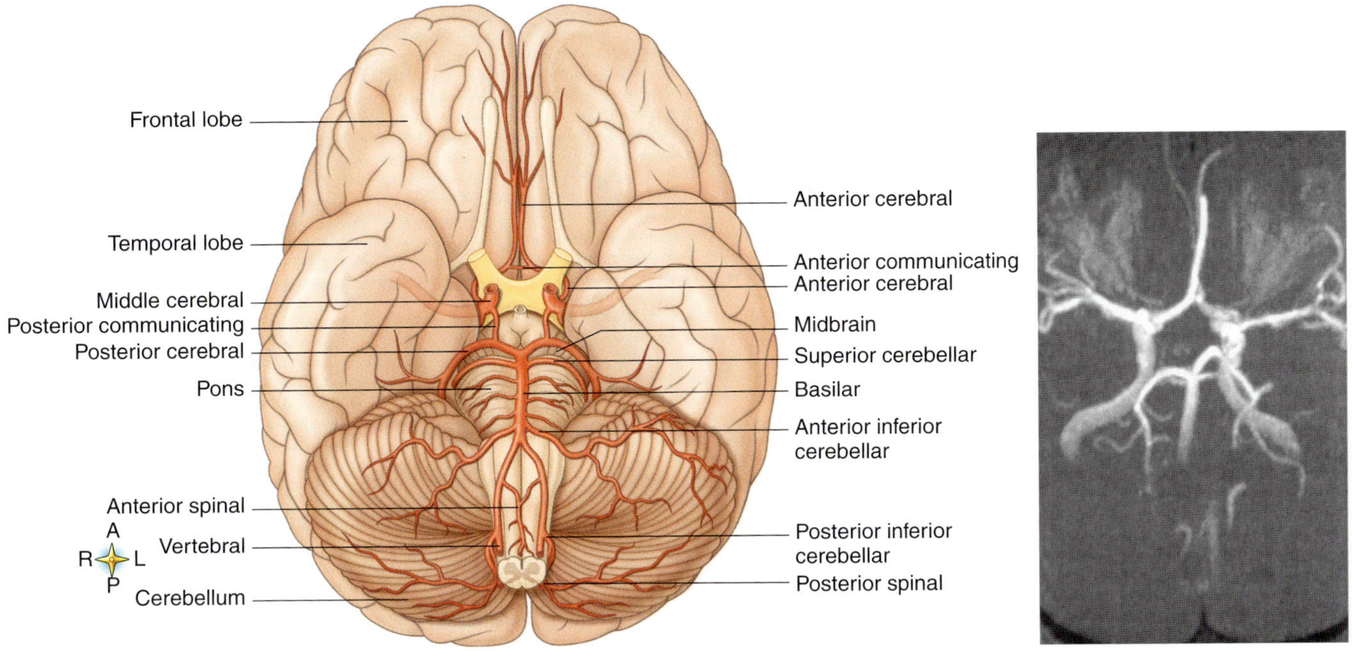

FIG. 34.6 Arteries of the brain. (From Drake R, Vogl AW, Mitchell AWM, eds. *Gray's Anatomy for Students*. Edinburgh: Elsevier; 2015; Abrahams P, Hutchings RT, Marks SC, eds. *McKinn's Color Atlas of Human Anatomy*. 5th ed. St Louis: Mosby; 2003.)

of the skull, and terminates in the cauda equina at the first and second lumbar vertebrae. The spinal cord has 31 segments: 8 cervical, 12 thoracic, 5 lumbar, 5 sacral, and 1 coccygeal.

Structurally, the spinal cord is somewhat flat on the dorsoventral side. It has an outer layer of white matter and an inner body of gray matter. A cross-section of the cord reveals that the gray matter forms a rough H shape. The two dorsal portions of the H are called the *dorsal horns* and the two ventral portions are called the *ventral horns*. The cross portion of the H is called the *gray commissure,* and this portion encompasses a canal that traverses the length of the cord. The cord is surrounded by the meninges—the outside dura mater, the arachnoid mater, and the inner pia mater. These are contiguous with the brainstem and continue beyond the spinal cord to the level of the second or third sacral vertebra.

Blood Supply to the Spinal Cord

Blood is supplied to the spinal cord via the branches of the vertebral artery, posterior spinal arteries, posterior inferior cerebral arteries, and various regions of the aorta. The anterior and posterior spinal veins are responsible for venous drainage from the cord.

CRANIAL NERVES

The cranial nerves are 12 pairs of nerves that originate in the brain and are responsible for the sensory and motor functions of the body. Each of the 12 pairs is designated by a Roman numeral, and each has a particular function:

- *I (olfactory):* Responsible for the sense of smell
- *II (optic):* Conveys impulses for sight
- *III (oculomotor):* Controls muscles that move the eye and iris
- *IV (trochlear):* Controls the oblique muscle of the eye
- *V (trigeminal):* A sensory nerve that controls the sensations of the face, forehead, mouth, nose, and top of the head
- *VI (abducens):* Controls lateral movement of the eye
- *VII (facial):* A motor nerve that controls the muscles in the face and scalp, as well as tears and salivation
- *VIII (vestibulocochlear [acoustic]):* Controls hearing and equilibrium
- *IX (glossopharyngeal):* Controls the sense of taste and pharyngeal movement, as well as the parotid gland and salivation
- *X (vagus):* Innervates the pharyngeal and laryngeal muscles, heart, pancreas, lungs, and digestive systems; also controls the sensory paths of the abdominal viscera, the pleura, and the thoracic viscera
- *XI (accessory):* Has two parts, a cranial portion and a spinal portion. The cranial portion joins the vagus nerve to help control the pharyngeal and laryngeal muscles. The spinal portion controls the trapezius and sternocleidomastoid muscles.
- *XII (hypoglossal):* Innervates the muscles of the tongue

SPINAL NERVES

The spinal nerves occur in pairs and originate from the spinal cord near their corresponding vertebrae. Each spinal nerve has two roots, a dorsal root and a ventral root. The dorsal root has an area of enlargement called the *dorsal root ganglion*. Each spinal nerve forms two branches, called *rami* (sing., ramus).

The cervical and thoracic nerves exit the spinal column through the vertebral foramina in a lateral direction. The lumbar, sacral, and coccygeal nerve roots exit from the distal spinal cord at the first lumbar vertebra. These particular

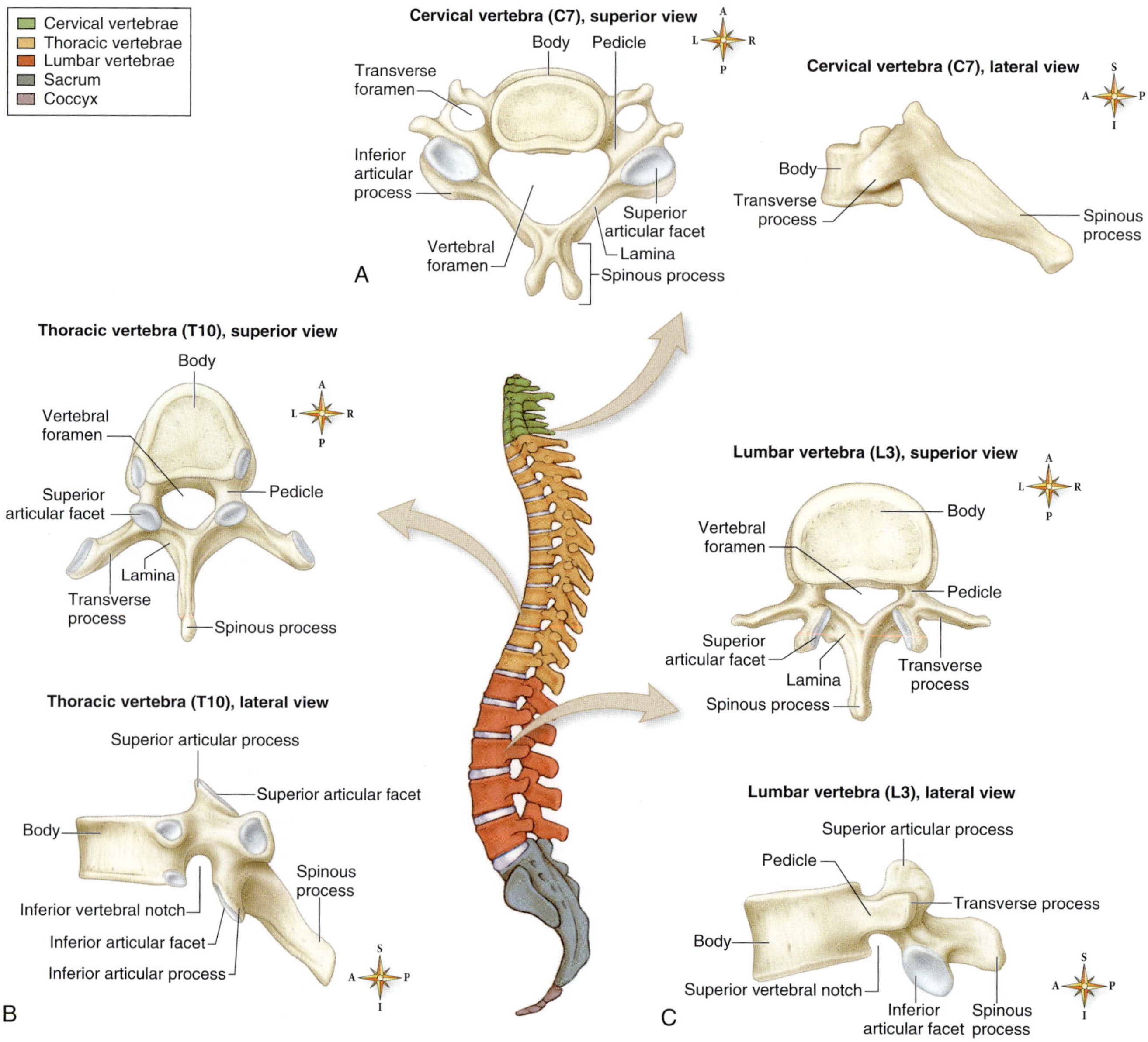

FIG. 34.7 Spinal column—comparison of the vertebrae. (A) Cervical vertebra (C7). (B) Thoracic vertebra (T10). (C) Lumbar vertebra (L3). (From Patton KT, Thibodeau GA, Douglas MM. *Essentials of Anatomy and Physiology—Text and Anatomy and Physiology Online Course.* St Louis: Elsevier-Mosby; 2012.)

nerve roots descend below the terminal point of the spinal cord and are referred to collectively as the *cauda equina* (horse's tail).

AUTONOMIC NERVOUS SYSTEM

The autonomic nervous system (ANS) is an involuntary system that transmits signals for vital functions such as the heart rate, respiration, and digestion. It connects the CNS to the visceral organs via the cranial and spinal nerves. The ANS can be further subdivided into complementary, sympathetic, and parasympathetic components. The sympathetic component is responsible for the "fight-or-flight" mechanism the body uses in response to a threat. The sympathetic response results in the diversion of blood (via vasoconstriction) from nonessential organs and systems (e.g., the gastrointestinal system and skin) to the brain, heart, lungs, and muscles. The parasympathetic component is responsible for the resting functions that promote energy conservation through the dilation of blood vessels and relaxation of muscle groups, as is seen with increased blood flow to the gastrointestinal tract to promote the digestion of food. The ANS and the CNS work together to maintain homeostasis.

SOMATIC NERVOUS SYSTEM

The somatic nervous system (SNS) connects the CNS to the skin and skeletal muscles via the cranial and spinal nerves. It is described as a voluntary system because many of its actions (e.g., blinking the eyelids) can be controlled. The SNS keeps the body in touch with its surroundings by processing sensory activity and controlling muscles.

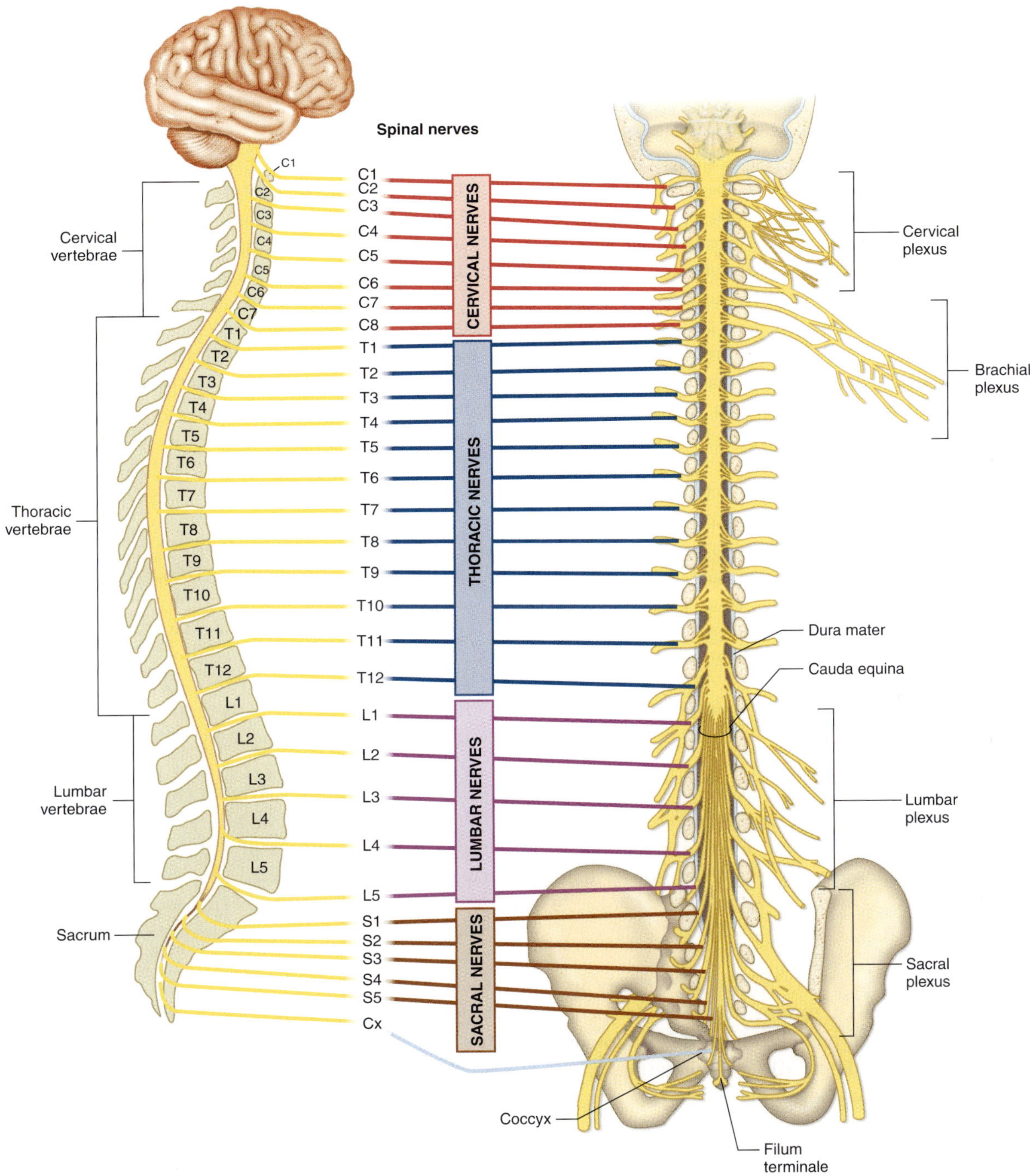

FIG. 34.8 Detail of the spine. The spinal nerves. Note that there are 31 pairs. Spinal cord injury involving the spinal nerves may affect the corresponding nerves and distal enervation. (From Patton KT, Thibodeau GA, Douglas MM. *Essentials of Anatomy and Physiology—Text and Anatomy and Physiology Online Course*. St Louis: Elsevier-Mosby; 2012.)

PERIPHERAL NERVES

Peripheral nerves are composed of small bundles of nerve fibers, called *fascicles,* which are surrounded by a sheath called the *endoneurium.* The perineurium, which is composed of fibers of connective tissue, extends within the spaces between the nerve fibers and binds them together. The nerve unit is bound together by the epineurium.

DIAGNOSTIC PROCEDURES

HISTORY AND PHYSICAL EXAMINATION

The patient's history is taken and a physical examination is performed to determine past and present symptoms, trauma, and neurological illness or pathological abnormalities. Many neurological problems are not visible; therefore specialized techniques are used during the physical examination to evaluate the CNS and PNS. In examining the patient, the neurosurgeon focuses on gait, speech, and mental status. Assessment of the patient's motor tone, strength, reflex response, and flexibility also is a critical element of the examination.

The patient's cerebellar function is evaluated by testing balance and coordination. Sensory function generally is evaluated during the cranial nerve examination.

IMAGING STUDIES

A variety of imaging studies may be performed before neurosurgery as part of the patient's diagnostic workup. Relevant studies must be available in the operating room or uploaded to the computer before the surgery begins.

Computed Tomography

Computed tomography (CT) is the gold standard for the evaluation of many cranial vascular disorders (e.g., **aneurysm**, acute hemorrhage). (Chapter 7 includes a discussion of the technical aspects of CT.)

Magnetic Resonance Imaging

Magnetic resonance imaging (MRI) is used extensively in neurosurgery for the diagnosis of tumors, abscesses, ligament damage, and disc herniation. It provides clear visualization of these structures. In some facilities, MRI is done intraoperatively, either with a portable unit or in a dedicated operating suite. (Chapter 6 includes a description of the technology used in MRI.)

Functional Magnetic Resonance Imaging

Functional MRI (fMRI) is used for preoperative brain mapping, which allows the neurosurgeon to localize areas of the brain responsible for certain motor skills, language, and sensory functions. Preoperative mapping also can determine the need for intraoperative mapping. Images of the brain are captured while the patient is asked to do certain tasks (e.g., recite a list of objects). These images are processed by the MRI computer software, which generates three-dimensional images showing the active areas of the brain.

Stereotactic Magnetic Resonance Imaging

Stereotactic MRI combines standard MRI technology with a head frame or magnetic markers, called *fiducials,* to pinpoint a particular location in the brain and provide precise coordinates for surgery. This procedure greatly enhances surgical precision for a variety of interventions.

Magnetic Resonance Angiography

Combined with MRI technology, magnetic resonance angiography (MRA) produces very detailed images of vascular structures. It is useful for visualizing the cerebral circulation.

Angiography (Arteriography)

In angiography, an arterial catheter is used to inject a contrast medium into the patient's arterial system. The contrast medium outlines the structure of the vessels. Angiography often is used in the diagnosis of cerebral aneurysms and **arteriovenous malformations (AVMs).** The principles of angiography are discussed in Chapter 30.

Digital Subtraction Angiography

Digital subtraction angiography (DSA) is an imaging technique used with standard angiography for the selective isolation of vascular structures. Images are obtained before and after injection of the contrast medium. The precontrast image is "subtracted" from the data, revealing the vascular structure only. This technology is used less routinely since the advent of three-dimensional CT angiography.

Three-Dimensional CT Angiography

In three-dimensional CT angiography, a contrast medium is used to provide images of the intracranial vasculature, which later are reconstructed in a three-dimensional view by the CT program software. This technology is less invasive than DSA.

Myelography

Although myelography has been largely replaced by MRI, some surgeons use x-rays to visualize the spinal cord. For these imaging studies, a contrast medium is injected into the subarachnoid space of the cervical or lumbar spine. Plain x-rays are then taken to record the images produced by the contrast medium.

Discography

Discography is an imaging technique used to evaluate the pathology of an intervertebral disc (e.g., herniation). In this procedure, a small amount of contrast dye is injected directly into the disc, and the patient's response is monitored in terms of the intensity and location of the pain resulting from the injection. Fluoroscopy is used for real-time assessment of the disc during the test. A CT scan may be performed afterward for a more detailed anatomical view of the disc.

Ultrasound

Ultrasound technology often is used before neurosurgery to assess the blood flow in the cerebral blood vessels. It is used intraoperatively for real-time imaging of cysts, tumors, and other structures in the brain or spinal cord.

Electroencephalogram

An electroencephalogram (EEG) measures the electrical activity of the brain. It typically is obtained to evaluate seizure disorders, head injuries, dementia, and metabolic conditions affecting the brain. In the perioperative setting, it can be used during a procedure to monitor the depth of anesthesia or to monitor brain activity in procedures that require occlusion of the carotid artery.

ELECTROMYOGRAPHY

Electromyography (EMG) measures the conduction rate of motor nerves. During this test, needle electrodes are placed in the muscle, and a low-voltage current is delivered. The period between stimulus and muscle contraction is measured. This test often is used to evaluate loss of nerve conduction caused by a herniated disc, **spondylosis** (narrowing of a bony tract or tunnel), or other types of impingement disorders.

SOMATOSENSORY EVOKED POTENTIALS

The somatosensory evoked potentials (SSEP) test measures sensory impulses from the body to the brain. This test may be performed preoperatively to assess nerve damage, or it may be performed intraoperatively to monitor changes in the nerves in spinal, carotid artery, or cerebral aneurysm surgery. Electrodes or fine needles are used to stimulate selected nerves, and function is determined by the elapsed time between stimulus and response.

CASE PLANNING

PSYCHOLOGICAL CONSIDERATIONS

All patients undergoing surgery arrive in the operating room with concerns about their safety and the surgical outcome. Because of the delicate nature of neurosurgery and the risk of impaired function after the surgery, neurosurgical patients often are very fearful or anxious. Patients facing cranial surgery may fear that they will not awaken after the surgery or that they will lose their sight, hearing, or mobility. The fear of losing cognitive ability is very strong in many patients.

Often patients who appear to be unaware or even unconscious are actually highly aware of their surroundings. Although voluntary movement may be impaired, their sensory perception may be fully intact. The perioperative team can provide important emotional and psychological support to the patient.

INSTRUMENTS

Neurosurgical instrumentation is often daunting to team members who are new to the specialty. Hundreds of different instruments are available, each having a particular shape and use. General surgery instruments are used for soft tissue access to neurological structures. Once exposure is achieved, specialty instruments are used to provide retraction and exposure, remove bone, extract disc fragments, and manipulate the delicate tissue of the brain and spinal cord.

Instrumentation specific to the neurosurgical procedure is discussed in the surgical techniques section. Commonly used instruments are shown in the Neurosurgical Instruments table.

Microsurgical instruments are used in cranial surgery, spinal surgery, and some peripheral nerve procedures. These instruments are delicate and must be handled with care. When the surgeon is using an instrument under the microscope, the surgical technologist must remember that the surgeon is working within a very limited visual field. The scrub must anticipate which instrument will be needed next and pass it in correct spatial orientation so that the surgeon does not have to look away from the field to receive it.

Decontamination and sterilization processing for neurosurgical instruments generally is identical to processing for other instruments. However, special processing is required for instruments used in known or suspected cases of Creutzfeldt-Jakob disease (CJD). CJD is a fatal disease of the nervous system that is caused by a prion, which cannot be destroyed by normal disinfection and sterilization methods. Although guidelines for decontamination vary by institution, recommendations include the use of disposable instruments, which are isolated and incinerated upon disposal. (A discussion of prion disease can be found in Chapter 10.)

NEUROSURGICAL INSTRUMENTS

Neurosurgical power instruments. (A) Hall perforator drill. (B) Burr guards. L-shaped guards prevent the drill tip from penetrating the cranial meninges. (C) Midas Rex drill and guards (Medtronic, Minneapolis, MN).

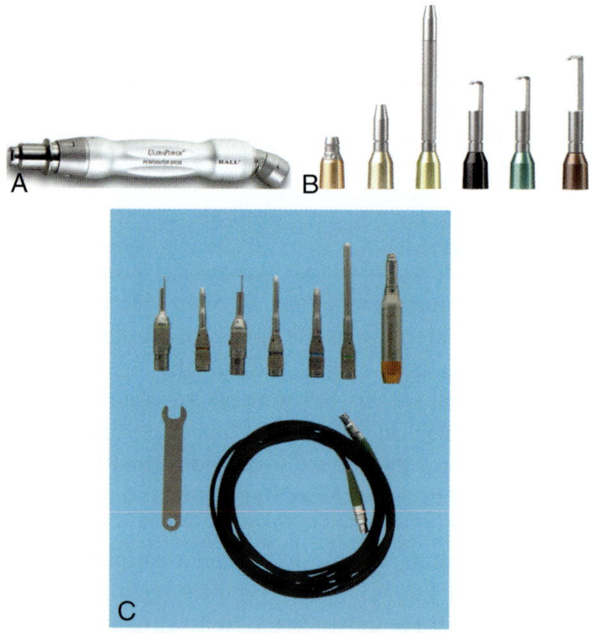

(From Tighe SM. *Instrumentation for the Operating Room*. 6th ed. St Louis: Mosby; 2003.)

STEVENSON ALLIGATOR SCIS 5⅜″

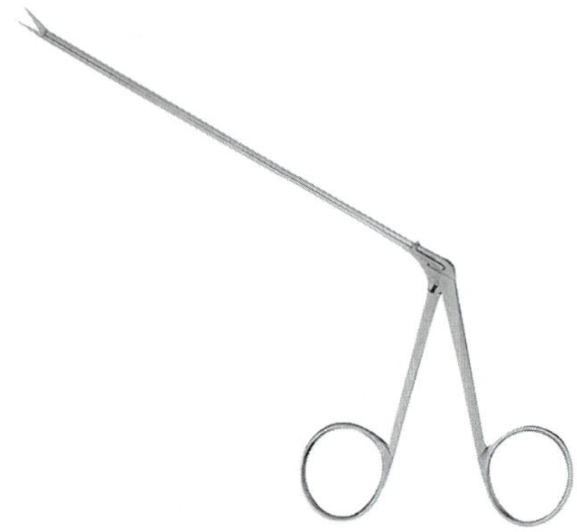

(Courtesy and copyright Becton, Dickson and Company.)

Yasargil MICRO SCIS 9″

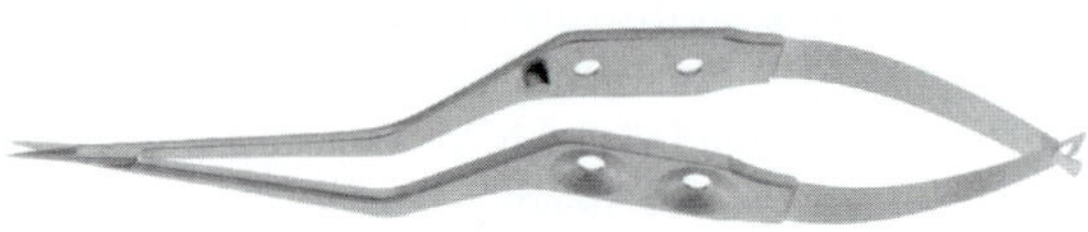

(Courtesy and copyright Becton, Dickson and Company.)

DANDY NEUROSURGICAL SCIS 6¾″

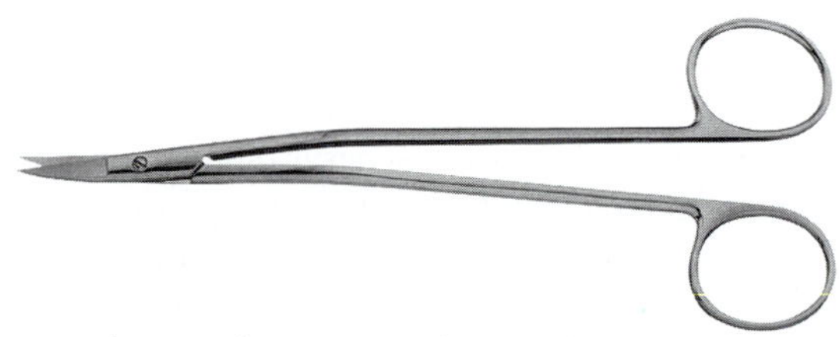

(Courtesy and copyright Becton, Dickson and Company.)

STRULLEY DISSECTING SCIS 8″

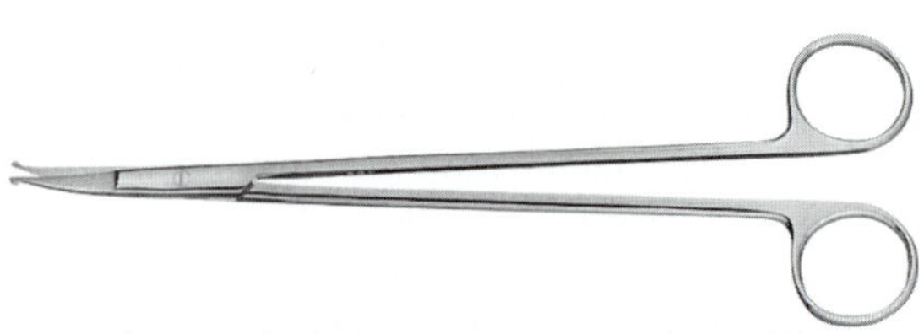

(Courtesy and copyright Becton, Dickson and Company.)

ADSON TISSUE FCPS 6″

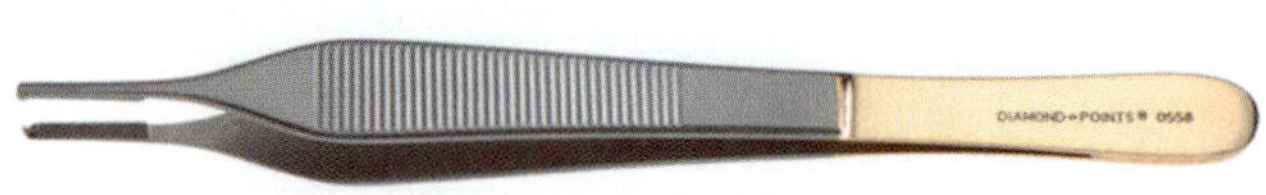

(Courtesy and copyright Becton, Dickson and Company.)

GERALD FCPS 1 × 2 TEETH 5½″

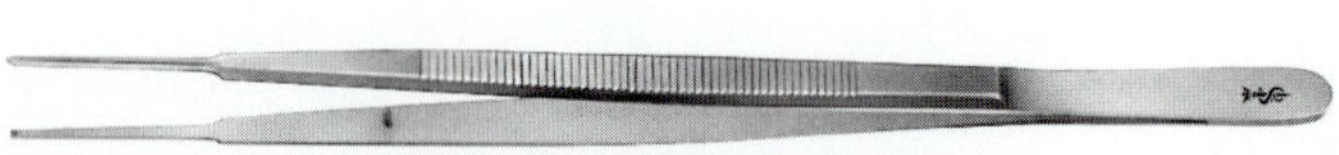

(Photo courtesy Aesculap, Inc., Center Valley, PA.)

CUSHING ANGLED TISSUE FCPS 7″

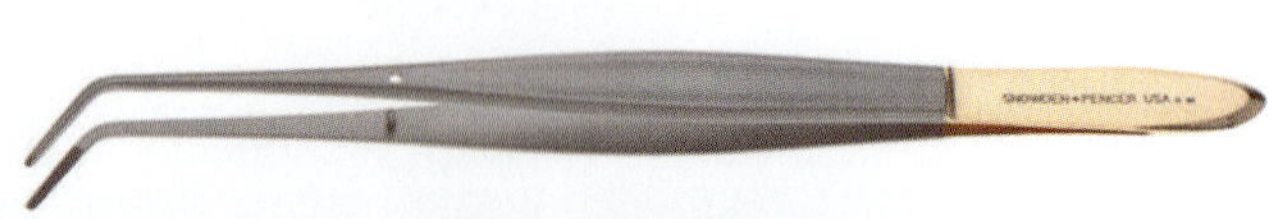

(Courtesy and copyright Becton, Dickson and Company.)

NEUROSURGICAL INSTRUMENTS—cont'd

CUSHING BAYONET FCPS 7″

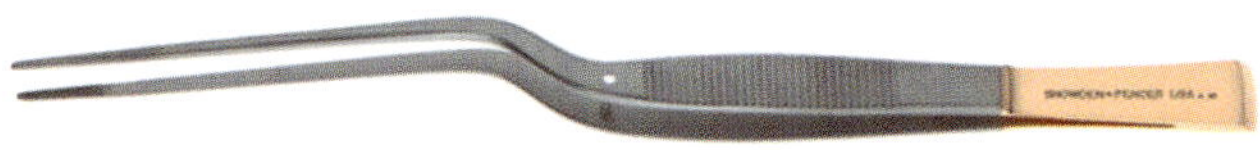

(Courtesy and copyright Becton, Dickson and Company.)

FRAZIER DURA HOOK 6″

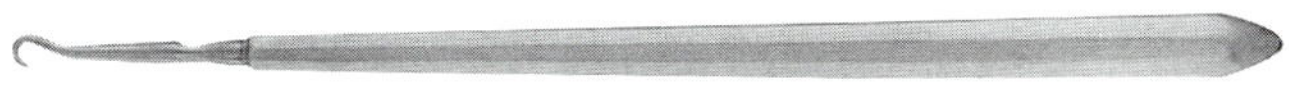

(Courtesy and copyright Becton, Dickson and Company.)

HORSLEY DURA SEPARATOR 6¾″

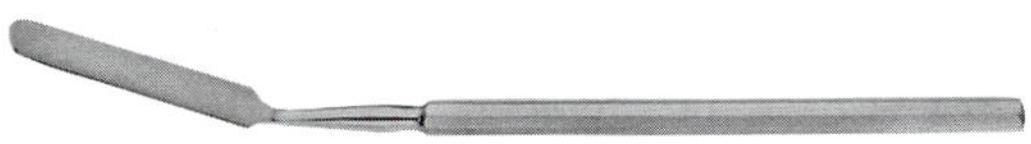

(Courtesy and copyright Becton, Dickson and Company.)

CUSHING PITUITARY SPOONS 9¼″

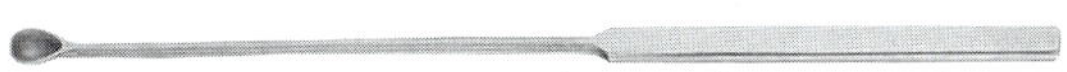

(Courtesy and copyright Becton, Dickson and Company.)

PENFIELD DISSECTOR #2 7½″

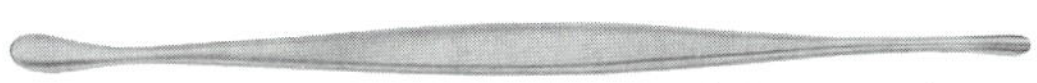

(Courtesy and copyright Becton, Dickson and Company.)

PENFIELD DISSECTOR #4 7½″

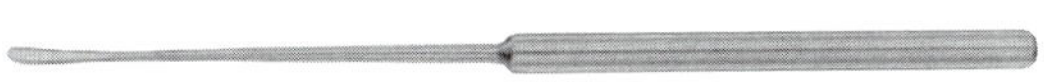

(Courtesy and copyright Becton, Dickson and Company.)

RANEY SCALP CLIP APPLICATION FRCP 6¼″

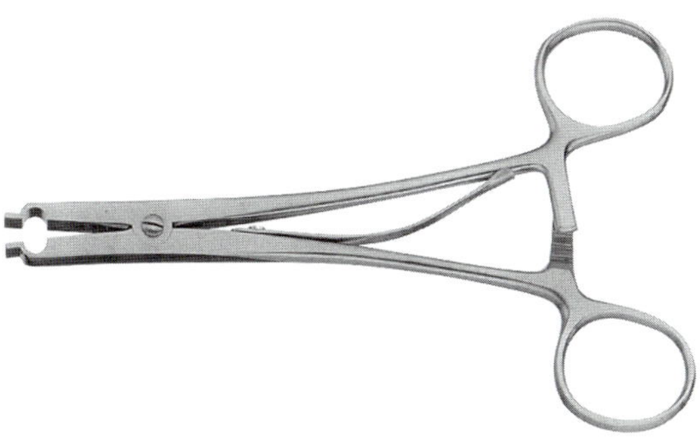

ADSON ANUERYSM NEEDLE 9″

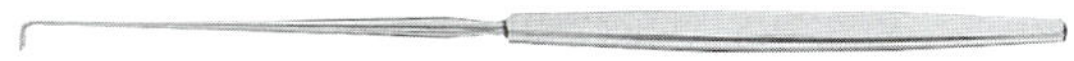

(Courtesy and copyright Becton, Dickson and Company.)

ADSON BLUNT DISSECTING HOOK 8¼″

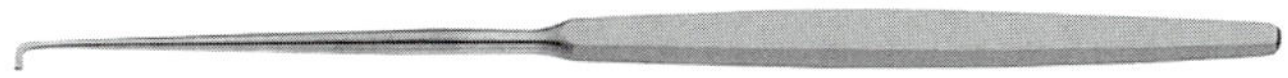

(Courtesy and copyright Becton, Dickson and Company.)

SACHS NERVE SEPARATOR 7¾″

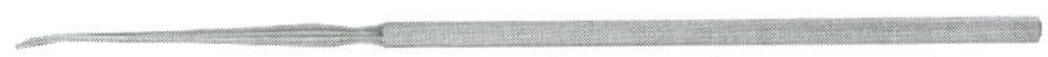

(Courtesy and copyright Becton, Dickson and Company.)

PENFIELD DISSECTOR #1 7½″

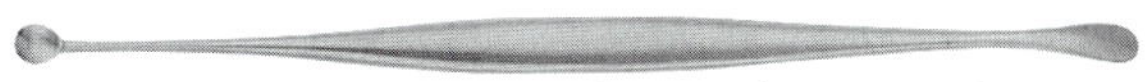

(Courtesy and copyright Becton, Dickson and Company.)

PENFIELD DISSECTOR #3 7½″

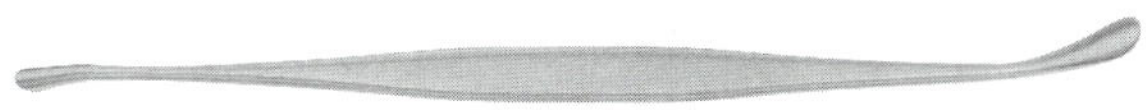

(Courtesy and copyright Becton, Dickson and Company.)

PENFIELD DISSECTOR #5 7½″

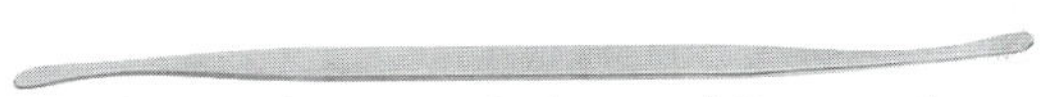

(Courtesy and copyright Becton, Dickson and Company.)

RANEY SCALP CLIP CARTRIDGE

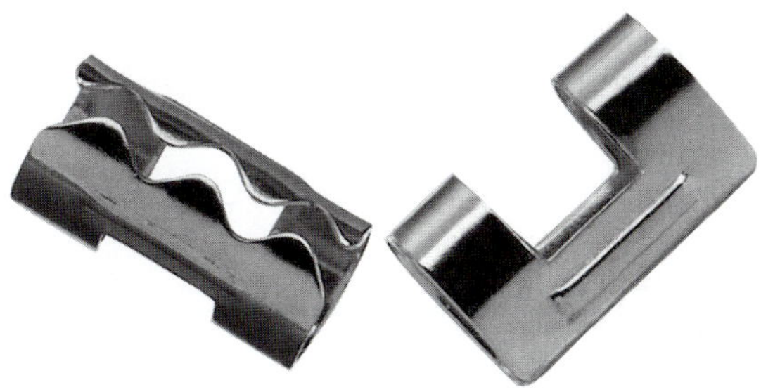

(Courtesy and copyright Becton, Dickson and Company.)

NEUROSURGICAL INSTRUMENTS—cont'd

YASARGIL ANEURYSM OCCLUDING CLIP

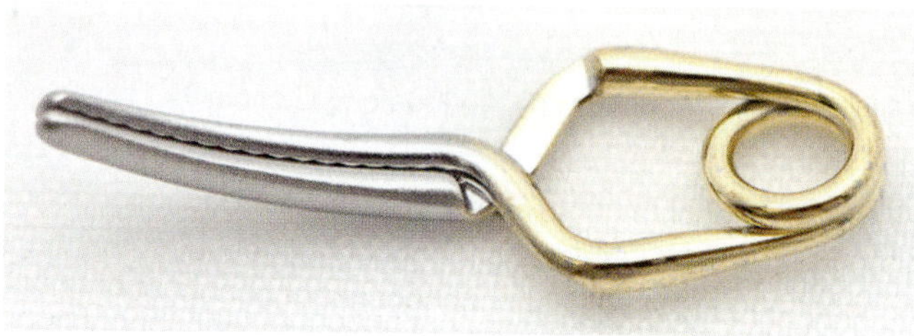

(Millennium Surgical Corp.)

FRAZIER SUCTION CANNULA 5″

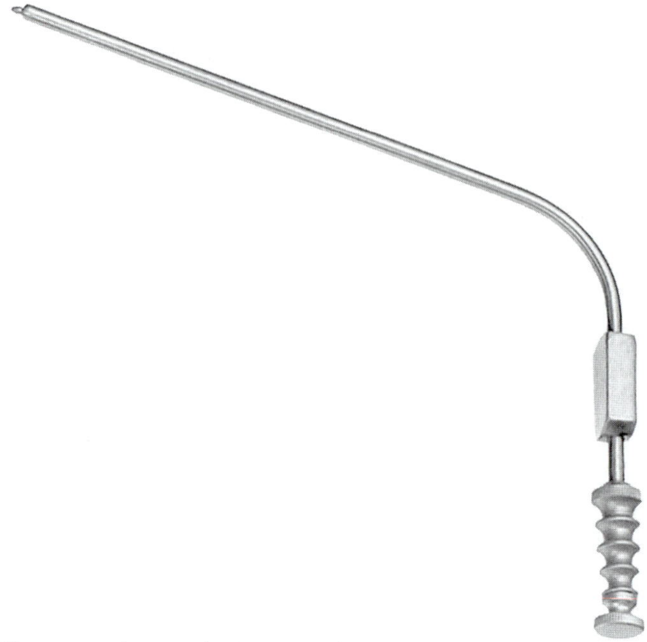

(Courtesy and copyright Becton, Dickson and Company.)

MURPHY BALL RETRACTOR 9″

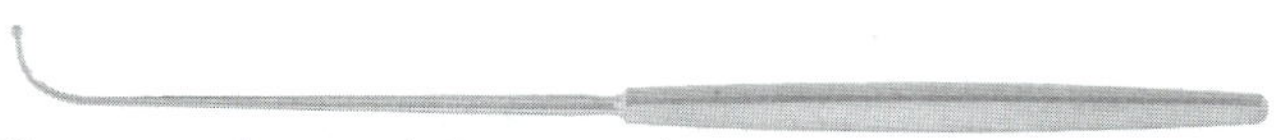

(Courtesy and copyright Becton, Dickson and Company.)

DAVIS BRAIN RETRACTOR 7½″

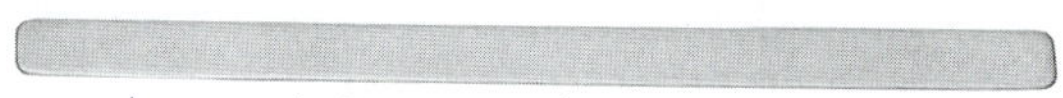

(Courtesy and copyright Becton, Dickson and Company.)

JANSON SCALP RETRACTOR 4⅝″

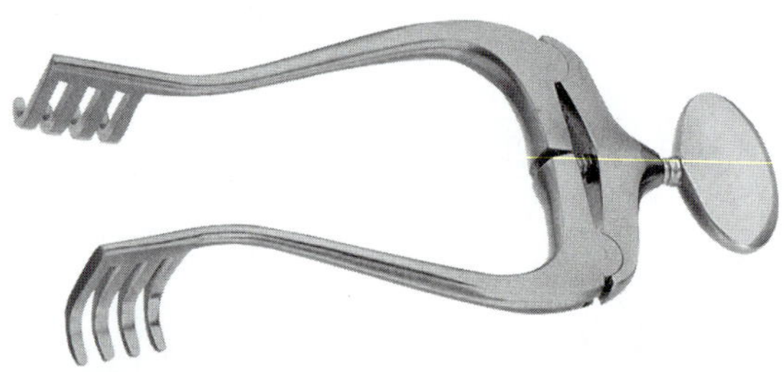

(Courtesy and copyright Becton, Dickson and Company.)

SPINAL INSTRUMENTS

BIPOLAR FORCEPS STRAIGHT 7″

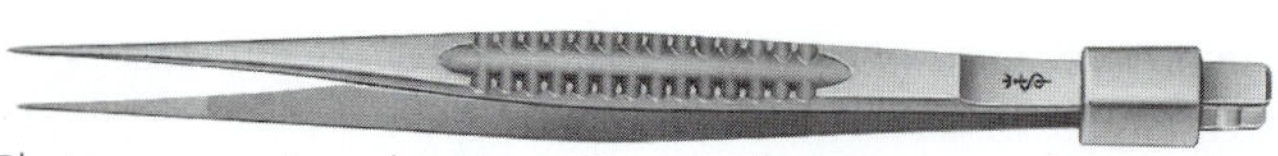

(Photo courtesy Aesculap, Inc., Center Valley, PA.)

BAYONET FORCEPS SMOOTH 7″

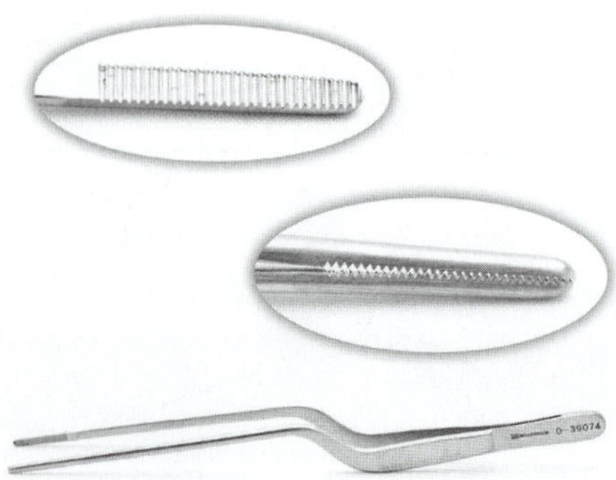

(Millennium Surgical Corp.)

NEUROSURGICAL INSTRUMENTS —cont'd

ADSON BAYONET FORCEPS 7″

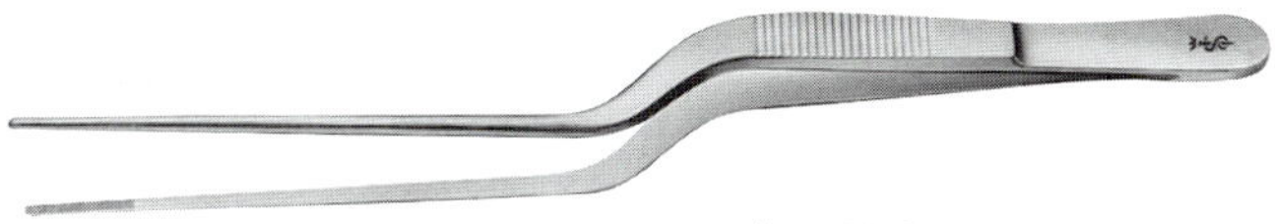

(Photo courtesy Aesculap, Inc., Center Valley, PA.)

SPINAL LIGAMENT FRCP 1 × 2 TEETH 7 ½″

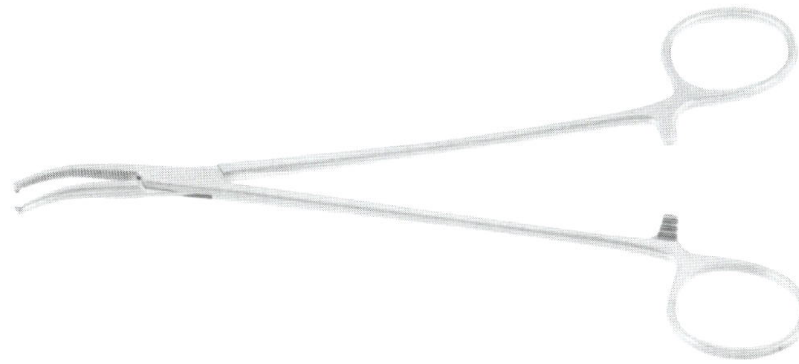

(Courtesy and copyright Becton, Dickson and Company)

CUSHING RONGEUR STRAIGHT 7″

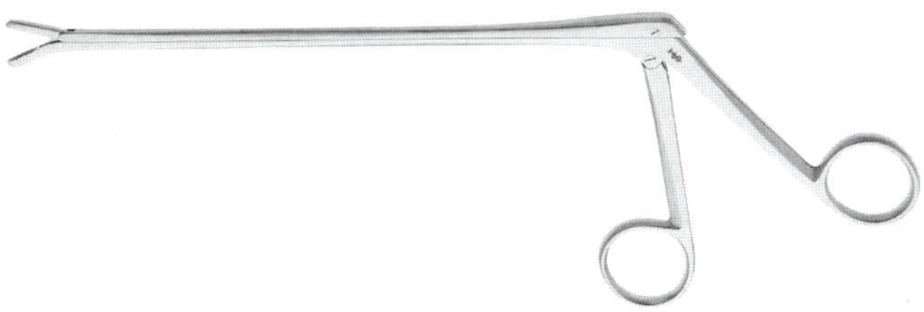

(Photo courtesy Aesculap, Inc., Center Valley, PA.)

CUSHING RONGEUR UP-BITE 7″

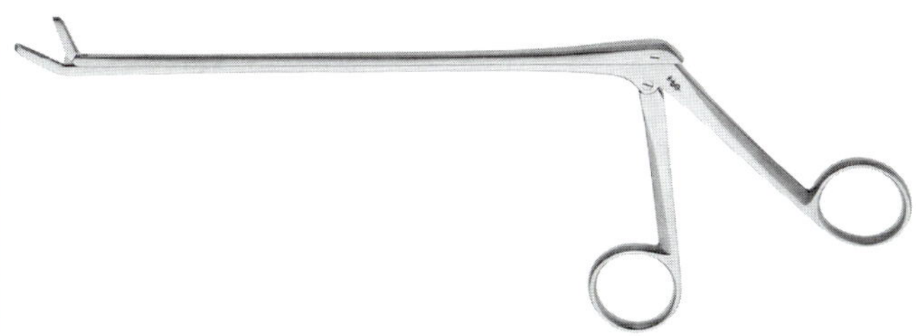

(Photo courtesy Aesculap, Inc., Center Valley, PA.)

KERRISON RONGEUR DOWN-BITE 7″

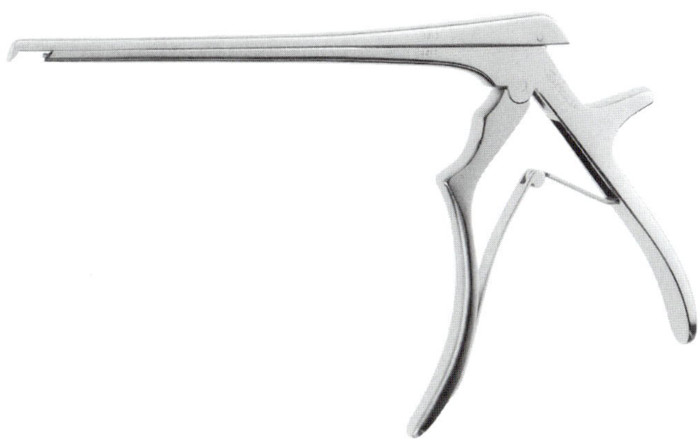

(Photo courtesy Aesculap, Inc., Center Valley, PA.)

KERRISON RONGEUR UP-BITE 7″

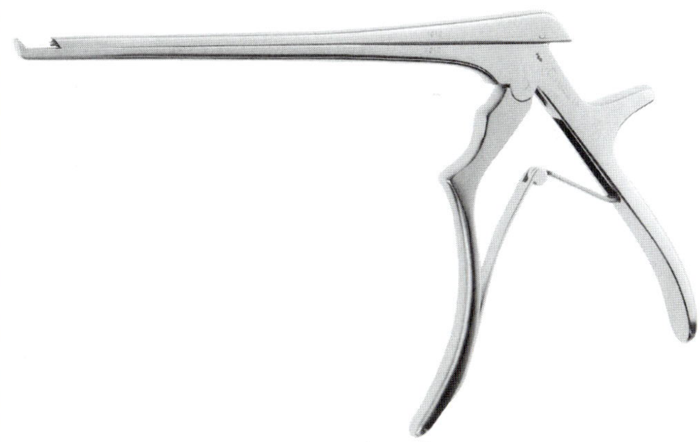

(Photo courtesy Aesculap, Inc., Center Valley, PA.)

PITUITARY RONGEUR 7″

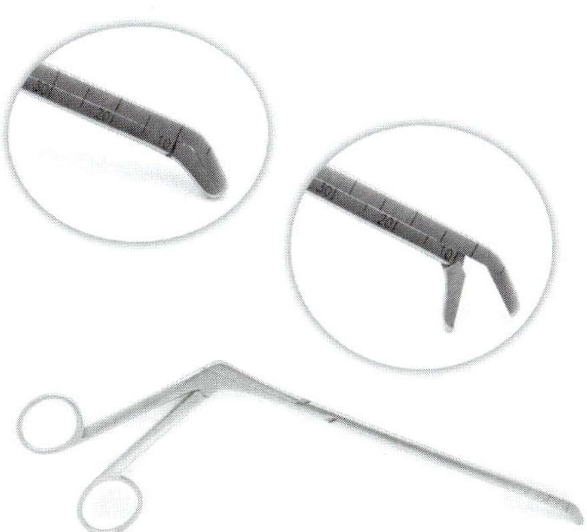

(Millennium Surgical Group.)

CASPER RONGEUR SERRATED 5½″

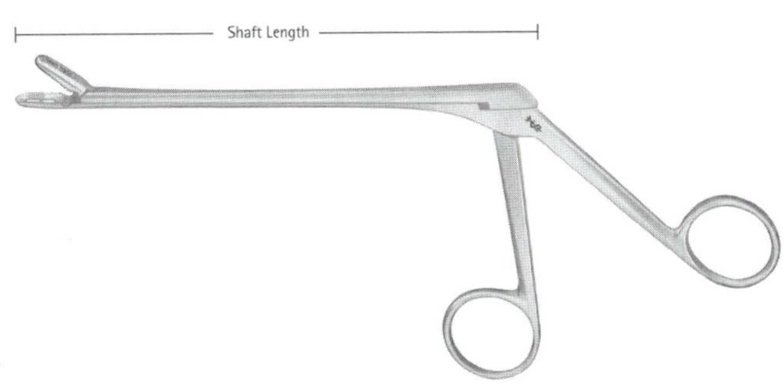

(Photo courtesy Aesculap, Inc., Center Valley, PA.)

NEUROSURGICAL INSTRUMENTS —cont'd

LEKSELL DOUBLE ACTION RONGEUR 9 ¾″

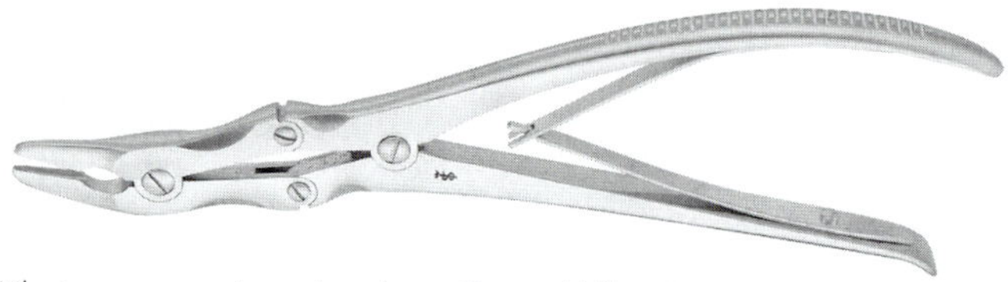

(Photo courtesy Aesculap, Inc., Center Valley, PA.)

CURETTE STRAIGHT AND ANGLED 7″

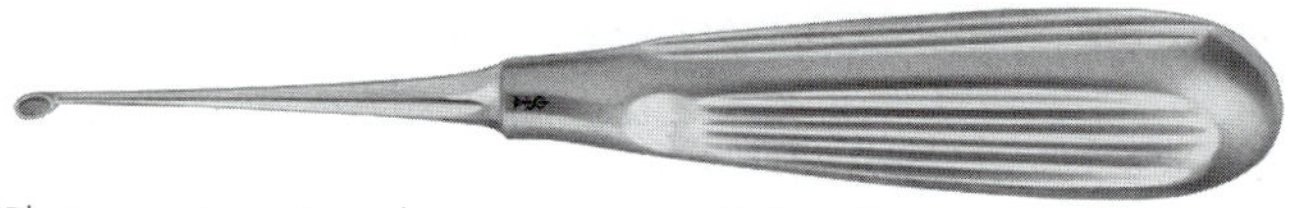

(Photo courtesy Aesculap, Inc., Center Valley, PA.)

CLOWARD LAMINA SPREADER 6″

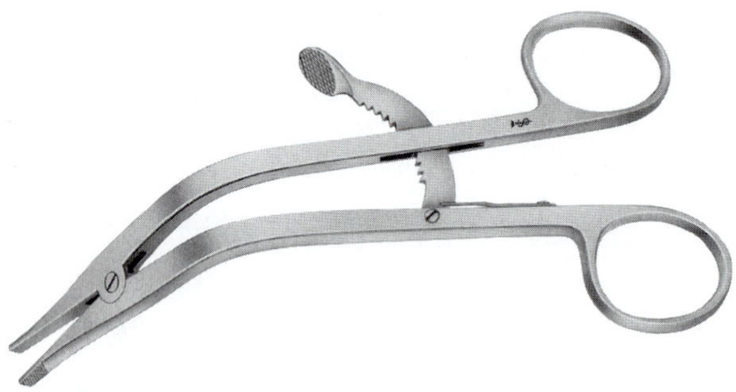

(Photo courtesy Aesculap, Inc., Center Valley, PA.)

SCOVILLE LAMINECTOMY RETRACTOR 7″

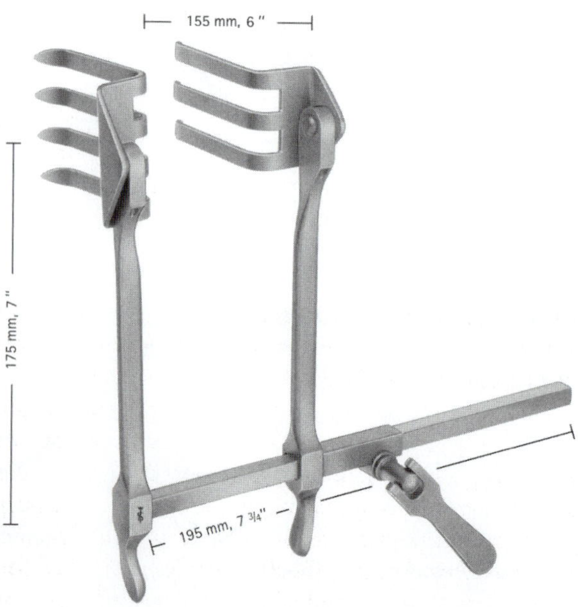

(Photo courtesy Aesculap, Inc., Center Valley, PA.)

COBB ELEVATOR 11″

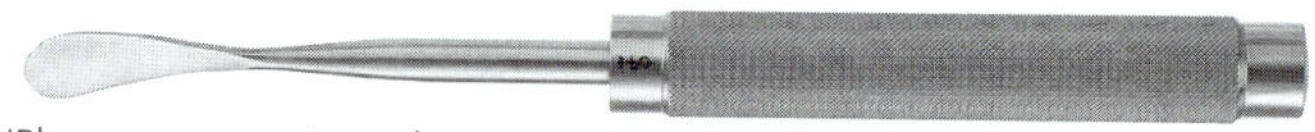

(Photo courtesy Aesculap, Inc., Center Valley, PA.)

ADSON (BECKMANN) RETRACTOR 12¾″

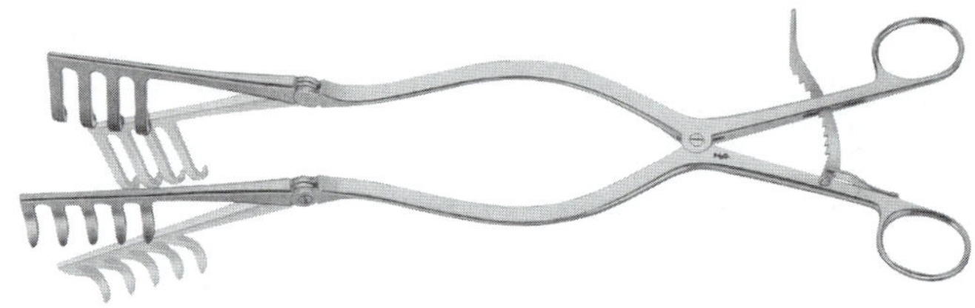

(Photo courtesy Aesculap, Inc., Center Valley, PA.)

MEYERDING RETRACTOR 10″

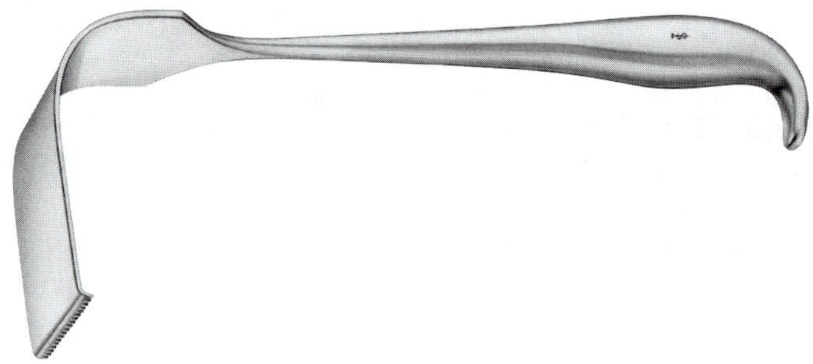

(Photo courtesy Aesculap, Inc., Center Valley, PA.)

TAYLOR SPINAL RETRACTOR 7¼″

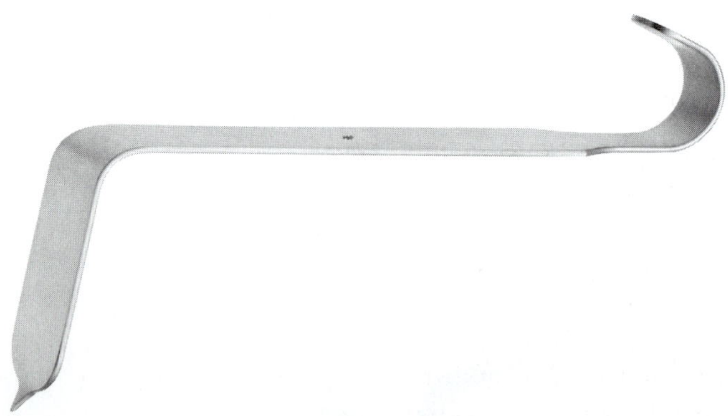

(Photo courtesy Aesculap, Inc., Center Valley, PA.)

POWER INSTRUMENTS

Power instruments are used to remove and shape bone. Power drills and saws are used for cutting and remodeling bone. Neurosurgical power equipment can be pneumatic (air-powered) or powered by battery or electricity. The surgical technologist is responsible for the safe handling of power instruments on the surgical field. Switches must always be in the safety position, except during use, to prevent injury in the event of inadvertent activation. The surgical technologist is also responsible for irrigating the tip of the drill when it is in use, to prevent overheating of tissue. Commonly used power systems are the Midas Rex system, the Hall perforator, and the Codman craniotome. A complete discussion of the care and use of power drills is provided in Chapter 30.

During a craniotomy, a perforator bit is used to drill holes in the cranial bones. The perforator is used with a power drill, called a *craniotome,* which is equipped with a safety clutch that stops the drill bit before it touches the dura.

IMPLANTS

Various implant materials, including bone, biosynthetics, plates, screws, rods, clips, shunts, coils, and chemotherapeutic wafers, are implanted in the course of many neurosurgical procedures. In general, surgical technologists must take care in handling any implantable device to ensure its sterility and integrity. The scrub must also document the manufacturer's serial and lot numbers and any other identifying features in the patient chart. When multiple devices are implanted, the scrub must communicate clearly with the circulator to ensure that the implant locations are noted in the patient record.

> Further information on isolation and sterilization measures is available on the website of the Centers for Disease Control and Prevention (CDC), at http://www.cdc.gov.

The U.S. Food and Drug Administration (FDA) regulates the tracking of certain implantable devices and requires that manufacturers have processes in place to locate devices in the event of a recall. The FDA regulations govern devices for which failure would result in serious, adverse health consequences, those that are intended to be left in the human body for at least 1 year, and any implantable device that is life sustaining or life supporting and is used outside of a health care facility. Facilities may develop policies and procedures for tracking any implantable device, but at minimum they must track the devices identified by the FDA. Typical information used in tracking includes the following:

- Device identification (e.g., lot number, serial number, model or batch number)
- Date of manufacture and shipping
- Name, address, telephone number, and Social Security number of the patient into whom the device was implanted
- Location where the device was implanted
- Name, address, and telephone number of the physician who implanted the device

On occasion, a previously implanted device is removed during a procedure. This process is known as *explantation.* Surgical technologists should be familiar with their facility's policies regarding explanted devices; all explanted devices are sent for pathological examination before their final disposition. Note that in the event of device failure, the device may be referred to the manufacturer according to policy.

WOUND MANAGEMENT

Sponges

Radiopaque 4 × 4 sponges are used in neurosurgical procedures to absorb blood and fluid and control bleeding. In addition to these, the neurosurgeon uses small, square, felted sponges made of cotton or rayon to control bleeding on neural and vascular tissue. These are commonly referred to as "patties" or "cottonoids." Radiopaque threads are sewn into the body of each sponge, which also has a strong string, colored green, for visibility in the wound. Patties are supplied in a variety of sizes. The felted consistency allows the surgeon to use the sponge as a filter when suction is applied to the neural tissue. Patties should be kept moist throughout the procedure and offered to the surgeon from a basin or a flat ribbon retractor. When used patties are discarded on the field, the scrub should immediately remove them. Used sponges may be dropped onto an extra draped Mayo stand or small table for counting purposes.

Small cotton balls with radiopaque markers and strings also are used in neurosurgery. These are soaked with saline or a vasoconstriction drug.

Drugs and Irrigation

Drugs that are managed by the scrub most commonly include the following:

1. Hemostatic agents
2. Irrigation fluids
3. Antibiotics in solution with injectable saline
4. Antispasmodic drugs

The temperature of the irrigation solution is very important. For tissue damage to be prevented, the temperature should be below 120°F (48.9°C). Fluid that is too cold may contribute to hypothermia in the patient. A piston syringe is used to irrigate the tissue. A catheter or needle-tip irrigator similar to that used in eye surgery may also be used during microsurgery or nerve repair.

Drains

Various drains are used in neurosurgery to evacuate blood and serum and to eliminate dead space in the surgical wound. A lumbar drain may be placed in the subarachnoid space before a surgical procedure to remove CSF from the spinal canal or brain; this decompresses the tissue. A lumbar drain can also be used to monitor **intracranial pressure (ICP).** As an alternative, a ventricular drain may be placed for the same purpose. Strict aseptic technique is maintained during the placement of this type of drain, because the drain acts as a direct conduit to the CNS, providing a portal of entry for infection. A separate surgical setup should be created for placement of the lumbar or ventricular drain.

Suture

Silk and nylon sutures are commonly used on neural tissue for dural retraction, closure, and repair. Peripheral nerve anastomosis is usually performed with fine nylon or polypropylene suture. Wire and mesh plates are used to secure the cranial bones after craniotomy. Staples are generally used for skin closure in the scalp and back.

Dressings

Wound dressings are applied at the end of a neurosurgical procedure to protect the incision and provide an environment for wound healing. Spinal incisions are dressed with nonadherent Telfa and absorbent gauze pads secured with tape. Cranial dressings tend to be more complex and more difficult to secure. A single nonadherent strip (Telfa or mesh) is placed over the incision. Square gauze and bulky fluff gauze are added, followed by soft rolled gauze, which is wrapped around the head to secure the dressings. If an external brace is required, it is applied over the dressing.

ANESTHESIA

Neurosurgery of the cranium and spine is usually performed with the patient under general anesthesia. Selected procedures, such as the placement of brain electrodes, can be performed with the patient awake or under light sedation. Depending on the patient's condition, an "awake" intubation may be required for safety in some procedures of the cervical spine.

Regional anesthesia can be used in peripheral nerve repair. The Bier block (see Chapter 13) is commonly used for nerve repair or transposition in the arm. The scalp incision site is routinely injected with a vasoconstrictive drug in a local anesthetic carrier (lidocaine) to maintain local vasoconstriction and a drier surgical field.

Extensive physiological monitoring is carried out during all cranial procedures.

Thermoregulation is an important consideration for neurosurgical patients undergoing general anesthesia because most procedures are lengthy. Hypothermia can interfere with clotting, alter the metabolism of drugs, and impair wound healing. The anesthesia provider implements a variety of measures to minimize the risk of intraoperative hyperthermia, such as warming the anesthetic gases and fluids and using warm blankets and forced-air warming blankets. Infants undergoing neurosurgical procedures are very vulnerable to the effects of hypothermia. An infrared light system is often used to keep the infant warm and reduce the risk.

Smooth emergence from anesthesia is extremely important to minimize the risk of laryngospasm and struggling. Often the surgical dressing is applied before the reversal agents are given to avoid overstimulating the patient, which may increase blood pressure.

PATIENT POSITIONING

Cranial procedures are often performed with the patient in the prone or supine position with the head extended over the operating table and secured with a fixation frame. Surgery of the spine is performed with the patient in the prone or lateral position.

Head Stabilization

During cranial surgery, various specialized positioning devices are used, including headrests and fixation devices that attach to the operating table. Many different types of headrests are available, some designed with pins that are inserted into the patient's cranium. The patient is first positioned with the headrest in place, and the pins are then reattached to the headrest to immobilize the head completely.

Two types of head stabilizers commonly used are the Mayfield headrest and the three-pin fixation stabilizer (Fig. 34.9). Skull tongs (e.g., Gardner-Wells tongs) may also be used to secure the patient's head in a particular position and as a means for attaching traction devices. The scrub establishes a small sterile field on a prep table for the neurosurgeon to use when inserting the fixation pins or tongs. The scrub may also assist the surgeon with insertion or removal of the device.

Operating Table

A specialty operating table is used in neurosurgery for spinal and some cranial procedures. These come with many accessories to optimize safe positioning. The Andrews bed and the Jackson spinal table are two examples of specialized operating tables, which allow for a wide variety of customized positions with clearance for C-arm fluoroscopy. An alternative to a dedicated spinal table is a laminectomy frame (e.g., the Wilson frame), which is positioned on the operating table and adjusted to elevate the patient's thorax (see Chapter 16).

Prepping and Draping

Once the patient has been positioned, the skin prep is performed. When necessary, hair removal should be done as close to the time of surgery as possible. Head hair is removed only when it would interfere with the surgery. If the surgeon has ordered hair clipping, it is performed outside the operating room. Generally, hair removal is limited to the amount necessary to facilitate the incision and ensure a clean surgical field; rarely is the entire head shaved. Instead the hair is held back with rubber bands and water-based gel. The patient's hair may be saved and returned to the patient as personal property. In preparation for procedures of the cervical spine, the surgeon may order the patient's nape to be shaved to the level of the ears. If the patient's hair is long, it should be secured to the top of the head with an elastic band. Neurosurgical procedures, such as those involving harvesting of a bone or fat graft, require a second surgical prep.

Drapes may be sewn directly to the scalp with silk sutures, adhesive drapes may be used, or surgical skin staple clips may be used. In any case involving the head, it is wise to have extra drapes available to secure a large sterile field. A specialized craniotomy drape with an attached fluid collection system is often used for cranial surgery.

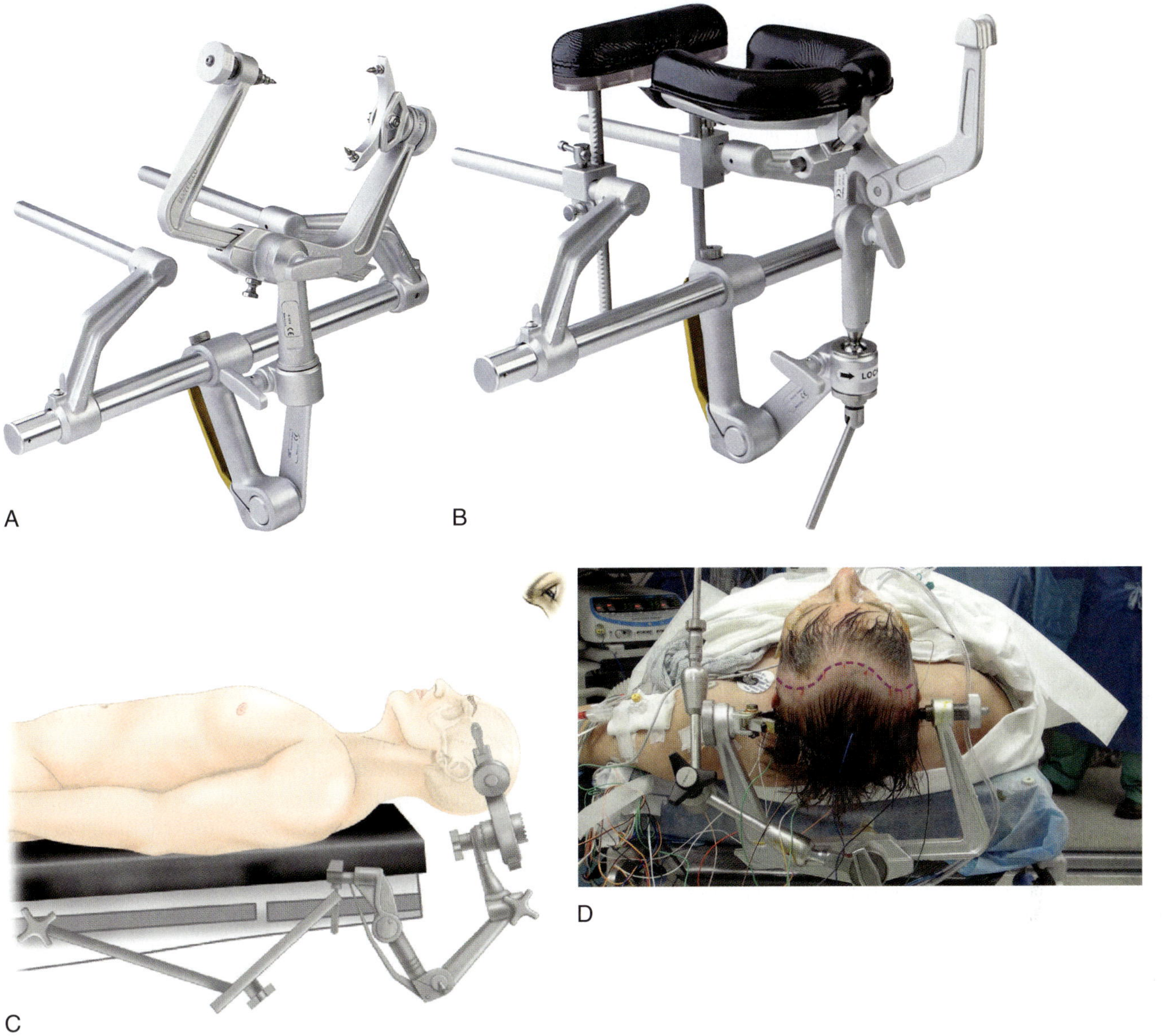

A B C D

FIG. 34.9 Mayfield and horse shoe head positioner. Cranial positioning system. (A) This system uses sterile pins that penetrate the cranium and stabilize the head during surgery. (B) Padded horse shoe positioner. (C) Patient in position using Mayfield positioner. Note that the head extends beyond the operating table edge, allowing the surgeons open access on all sides. (D) Patient in position showing skin incision. Note that the patient's hair has not been shaved. In this case a water-based gel can be used to part the hair and position it away from the incision. Elastic bands are often used to hold sections of hair. (From Quiñones-Hinojosa A, Rincon-Torroella J. *Video Atlas of Neurosurgery: Contemporary Tumor and Skull Base Surgery*. Edinburgh: Elsevier; 2017.)

CRANIAL PROCEDURES

CRANIOTOMY

Access to the brain requires surgical access through the superficial tissues of the scalp, bony cranium, and neural tissues. Generically, this is called a **craniotomy.** Open procedures of the brain start with this technique, which is described here. There will be some variations in the craniotomy depending on the pathology and the optimal location for approaching the anatomy.

Once the surgical technologist understands the anatomy and basic procedure for craniotomy, he or she can easily adapt to variations. A generic approach is presented here.

POSITION:	Supine; Fowler; prone
INCISION:	Depending on the pathology
PREP AND DRAPING:	Craniotomy
INSTRUMENTS:	Craniotomy set

Technical Points and Discussion

1. ***The patient is prepped and draped.***
Preparation of the patient includes positioning, skin marking, and infiltration of local anesthetic with epinephrine for hemostasis. The exact position depends on the pathology and selected access chosen by the surgeon. Many procedures are performed with the patient in the supine, Fowler, and prone positions. If complete stabilization of the head is necessary, a Mayfield or similar head frame is used. This requires the insertion of sharp pins that penetrate the skull and attach to the frame, which in turn is attached to the

operating table. During procedures in which the head must be repositioned during the surgery, the supine position with the head resting on a foam or gel doughnut can be used. In cases where access is temporal, the head is turned to the side and the opposite shoulder elevated slightly. A padded horseshoe headrest may also be used. This type of frame is attached to the head of the table and provides circumferential access to the patient's head and neck.

The surgeon marks the incision line, including the burr holes. This is followed by routine craniotomy draping. The craniotomy draping technique requires exposure of the operative site and full-body coverage. Plastic sterile drapes, including towel drapes and an incise drape over the incision area, may be used. A fluid pouch is attached to the top drape for drainage of blood and solutions away from the sterile field.

Before the incisions are made, the surgeon may inject the area with local anesthetic and epinephrine for hemostasis.

2. ***The scalp is incised and the pericranium elevated.***
To begin the procedure, the surgeon uses a #10 or #20 blade to make the skin incision following the skin marks. The incision is made through the full thickness of the scalp down to the bone. The scalp is highly vascular; the scrub should have the electrosurgical unit (ESU) and numerous sponges available. For hemostasis of the wound edge to be established and maintained, *Raney hemostatic clips* are applied over the full thickness of the scalp flap, including the drapes. The scalp flap is turned back and secured with sutures or a hook retractor. The tissue is covered with moist sponges.

After hemostasis is secured, a periosteal elevator is used to separate the pericranium from the bone.

3. ***A bone flap is created.***
The method used to raise the cranial flap involves drilling burr holes in the bone at suitable intervals. A saw is then used to cut the bone from one burr hole to the next. Burr holes are made with a *craniotome* and perforator bit. The tip has a dura protector that prevents penetration of soft tissue. While the burr holes are being made, the scrub must irrigate the perforator bit to prevent friction and thermal injury to the underlying tissue. Suction is applied adjacent to the irrigation stream to remove any bone particles from the field. The scrub should have bone wax prepared to control bleeding at the bone edges. The bipolar ESU is also used for hemostasis. The **bone flap** is removed from the field and placed in a secure location on the back table. The surgeon may require that the bone flap be maintained in an antibiotic solution or saline.

4. ***The dura is incised.***
In nonemergency situations, the surgeon uses a dura hook to elevate the dura and then incises it with a #15 blade. Metzenbaum or dural scissors are used to create a larger opening. The dura is retracted by means of fine sutures. The dura must be protected from drying and shrinkage during the procedure. This is commonly done by placing strips of moist Telfa over the exposed dura and tacking them with stay sutures. With the dura incised and retracted, the brain is exposed and a specific procedure carried out. The scrub is responsible for assisting in the management of the wound, as well as providing needed instruments during the procedure.

CRANIAL CLOSURE Cranial closure may vary with specific procedures. However, in general, closure consists of three or four layers. The dura is closed with a running suture of size 4-0 or 3-0 polypropylene or nylon. DuraSeal or fibrin glue may be applied to the suture line to make it watertight. The bone flap is secured with metal or resorbable plates, pins, mesh, or clamps. After the Raney clips are removed, the galea is closed with interrupted sutures of size 2-0 Vicryl or other synthetic absorbable material. Skin is closed with size 3-0 or 4-0 monofilament synthetic sutures or skin staples.

IMPORTANT TO KNOW *A* ***craniectomy*** *procedure is one in which the bone flap is not repositioned during closure. It may be replaced with an implant or the bone may be kept in sterile conditions and replaced weeks or months after surgery.*

Technical points of craniotomy are illustrated in Figs. 34.10 and 34.11.

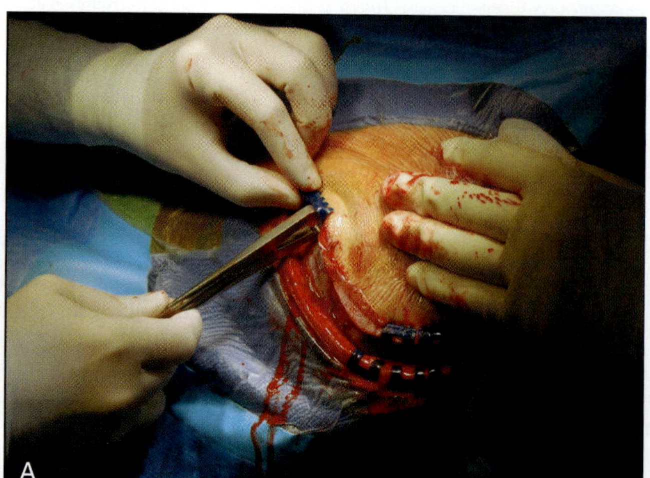

FIG. 34.10 Craniotomy. (A) Elevation of the skin flap and placement of Raney clips on the edges of the incision.

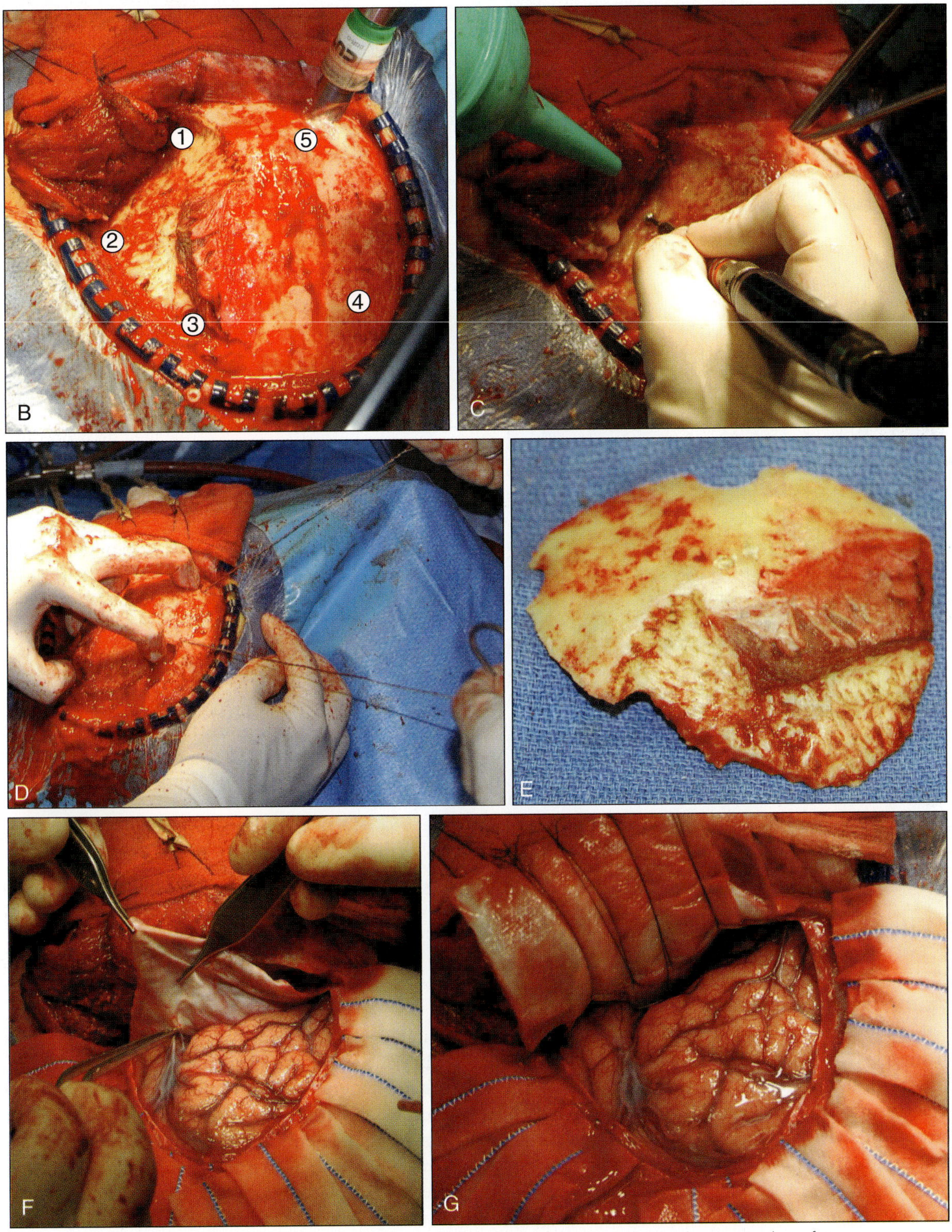

FIG. 34.10, cont'd (B and C) Drilling burr holes using a perforator with guard to protect the soft tissues underneath. (D) A Gigli saw, shown at the 4-o'clock position as a fine wire, is used to cut the bone between each bur hole. (E) The flap is released and placed on the back table in a protected area. (F) The dura is incised and folded back. (G) The cerebrum is exposed. Note the neurosurgical patties, which have been overlapped around the incision and dura. (From Jandial R, McCormick P, Black P, eds. *Core Techniques in Operative Neurosurgery.* Philadelphia: Elsevier; 2011.)

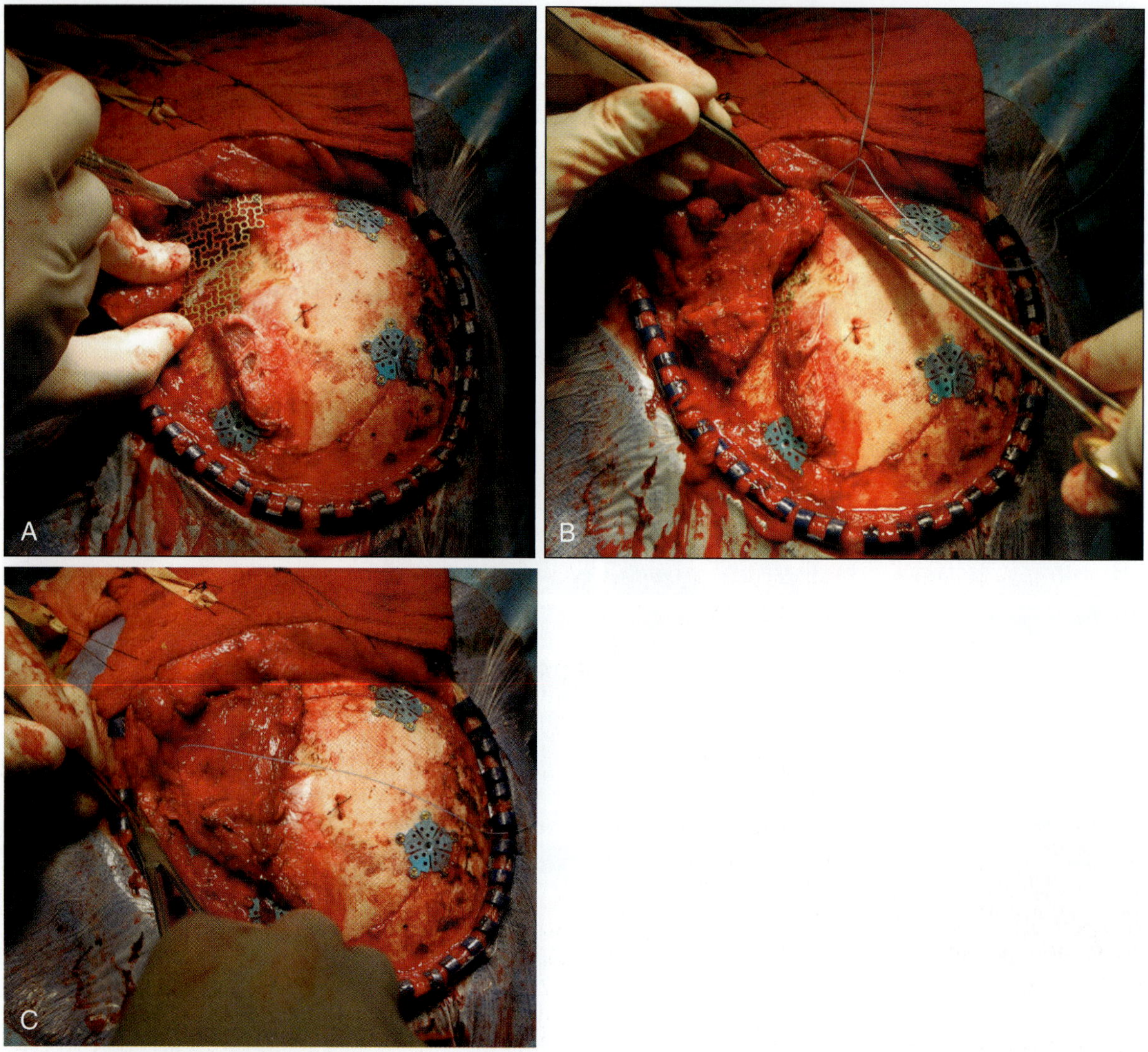

FIG. 34.11 Craniotomy closure. (A) The dura has been closed and the bone flap replaced. Titanium mesh and burr hole covers are used to hold the bone flap in place. (B) The muscle is sutured to the titanium mesh. (C) The scalp is realigned and sutured in two layers. (From Jandial R, McCormick P, Black P, eds. *Core Techniques in Operative Neurosurgery.* Philadelphia: Elsevier; 2011.)

CEREBRAL ANEURYSM SURGERY

Aneurysm surgery is performed to isolate and clip a cerebral aneurysm while preserving blood flow to the nearby vessels. Aneurysm clips are available from a variety of manufacturers but share common characteristics. The clip is composed of a body, a pivot point, and two blades. The blades of the clip come in different lengths and are configured in a variety of ways, including straight, curved, and angled up, down, or sideways, to allow for anatomical variation.

The scrub should be familiar with the basic aneurysm clips and clip appliers. Clips are supplied as permanent or temporary devices. Temporary clips have blades that open wider than permanent clips, and they also have lower closing force. They are used to occlude the arterial source to the aneurysm temporarily or to test-occlude the base of the aneurysm before the permanent clip is applied. Single-use clips are generally gold colored, for easy identification, and should be discarded after use. These are shown in the Neurosurgical Instruments table.

Permanent clips have a greater closing force and are designed to remain in place as a permanent implant. Fenestrated clips have an open blade. These clips may be used for indirect access to the aneurysm. A Sundt-type clip has a Teflon-lined lumen and is used to encircle the vessel completely when bleeding is encountered. Clip appliers may have a spring-loaded configuration, a pistol grip, or a hinged shaft to improve visualization. The scrub should have at least two clip appliers for each type of clip used. An anterior communicating aneurysm is described here.

PATHOLOGY

An intracranial aneurysm is a weakened and bulging artery within the cerebral circulation. Aneurysms can take many forms and shapes. A weakened arterial wall occurs as a congenital defect or as a result of trauma or infection. As blood flows through the vessel, the weakened aneurysm wall becomes thin. This creates a high risk of sudden rupture and hemorrhage, which can be quickly fatal. The anterior communicating artery aneurysm is the most common pathology of the circle of Willis arterial system.

POSITION:	Supine
INCISION:	Cranial
PREP AND DRAPING:	Cranial
INSTRUMENTS:	Craniotomy set; aneurysm set

Technical Points and Discussion

1. ***A lumbar drain may be placed before the patient is positioned.***
A lumbar drain, connected to a drainage bag with a stopcock, may be inserted by the surgeon before the patient is prepped or positioned. The drain is used to control the volume of CSF in the ventricles, if needed, during the procedure. The anesthesia provider opens the stopcock and releases CSF into the drainage bag to promote brain relaxation and reduce the ICP. The scrub should ensure that the lumbar drain is prepared and isolated in a separate sterile field. Drains are supplied in a prepackaged kit with all the necessary components for insertion. The scrub may be responsible for assisting the surgeon in the insertion of the drain.

2. ***The patient is prepped and draped.***
The patient is always placed in a three-point pin cranial fixation system to ensure absolute head stability and immobility. After the pins are placed and attached to the fixation device, the patient is positioned. The approach for most cerebral aneurysms is a frontal, bifrontal, or frontotemporal (i.e., pterional) craniotomy. The craniotomy is performed as previously described.

3. ***A self-retaining retractor system is put in place.***
A self-retaining brain retractor system is positioned after the dura is opened and tacked back from the surgical field. Moistened cottonoids or Gelfoam strips are placed beneath the retractor blades for cushioning and hydration. The retractors are essential for gentle, consistent retraction of the cerebral tissue. The system allows for the placement of retractors in almost any direction. Each system is configured differently, but all are designed to be secured to the patient's head, to the skull pin fixation device, or to a post and coupling attached to the operating bed. The surgeon may periodically adjust the retractor blades to ensure that the tissue beneath remains perfused and the brain is not bruised.

4. ***The arachnoid is opened.***
The draped operating microscope is brought to the field and positioned. At this point, the surgeon may request a draped sitting stool with an arm rest. The arachnoid is opened with microscissors, hooks, dissectors, and a microbipolar ESU. As the arachnoid is opened, CSF is released, which further relaxes the brain.

5. ***The arachnoid webs and other tissue are dissected away as necessary to allow for visualization of key intracranial structures.***
Dissection continues until the surgeon can see the aneurysm. Dissection must be meticulous to avoid undue manipulation of the aneurysm. The surgeon needs a large supply of moistened cottonoids and suction during this phase of the procedure. The microscopic suction tips can easily become occluded with blood and debris. The scrub should have several suction tips available on the field so that the tips can be changed out quickly with minimal interruption to the flow of the procedure.

6. ***One or more clips are applied to the base of the aneurysm.***
The aneurysm will be occluded at its base by means of an aneurysm clip. When handling aneurysm clips, the scrub should take care not to compress the clips or manipulate them in any way while loading them in the applier. The clip should be compressed only by the surgeon immediately before placement, because opening and closing the clip can weaken its grip, causing it to seat incorrectly.
The surgeon prepares the aneurysm for occlusion by continuing to isolate and identify the proximal and distal vasculature. This phase of the surgery requires careful handling of tissues because of the risk of rupture, which can occur at any time during the procedure but is more likely to happen during dissection. The scrub should always be prepared for the possibility of rupture by having a temporary clip loaded on a clip applier. If rupture occurs, suction and moistened cottonoids are needed immediately.
The surgeon places the clip across the neck of the aneurysm. Additional clips are used as necessary to ensure that the aneurysm and its feeder vessels are occluded.

7. ***The aneurysm sac is drained.***
Once the aneurysm is occluded, the surgeon requires a 30-gauge needle attached to the syringe to aspirate the aneurysm sac. This maneuver removes any blood in the aneurysm and allows the surgeon to establish that there is no filling of the aneurysm and the clip is secure. After clip placement, the surgeon may request a cottonoid moistened with papaverine to apply to the vessels surrounding the aneurysm to prevent vessel spasm. In cases of giant aneurysms, the surgeon may open the dome of the aneurysm (aneurysmectomy) after the clips are placed to evacuate blood, clots, or tissue debris. If a clip cannot be applied

to occlude the aneurysm, the surgeon may attempt to occlude it by wrapping or coating the vessel with a piece of the galea, methylmethacrylate, or cyanoacrylate.

8. ***The wound is closed.***
Wound closure follows as described for a craniotomy. The pin fixation device is removed before the patient emerges from anesthesia.

Technical points of the procedure are illustrated in Fig. 34.12.

ARTERIOVENOUS MALFORMATION RESECTION

AVM is an abnormal communication or fistula between the arteries and the veins. AVMs are commonly diagnosed in adults between 20 and 40 years of age. As the connection becomes larger under pressure, blood is diverted from surrounding brain tissue. When this occurs, multiple hemorrhages from the dilated blood vessels can cause seizures and subarachnoid hemorrhage.

Some AVMs may be very complex and involve many vessels, making surgical resection risky. A multidisciplinary approach often is used in treating these patients. An interventional radiologist may be involved in the patient's care before surgery to embolize the AVM and reduce its size. During **embolization,** platinum coils, glue, or microscopic plastic particles are placed in the vessels feeding the AVM. The materials close off the feeder vessels, reducing the vascularity of the AVM and hence the chance of rupture. Embolization may also be used after craniotomy for AVM resection, if required, to secure additional vessels not accessible during open surgery. Radiosurgery with the gamma knife is another option that may be used as an adjunct to surgery.

The procedure to resect an AVM is similar to that for clipping a cerebral aneurysm. A craniotomy approach is used, and the AVM is exposed by the same techniques described in the previous section. Because of the complexity of the vascular structure of most AVMs, microscopic dissection to identify the feeder vessels can be prolonged. A microtipped bipolar ESU is used extensively during this dissection. The scrub should have several microbipolar forceps available to allow for rapid exchange when the tips become coated with eschar. The scrub should observe the dissection on the video monitor to anticipate when the bipolar instrument will have to be exchanged, to make sure that the flow of instruments, sponges, and other materials is seamless, and to ensure that the surgeon does not have to look away from the microscope.

Once the AVM is exposed, the surgeon uses the bipolar ESU to occlude smaller vessels. Multiple aneurysm clips are placed on the larger feeder vessels. The AVM is then resected with the bipolar ESU. The scrub should be prepared with strips of Surgicel and Gelfoam to line the AVM cavity. The wound is closed as described for cerebral aneurysm clipping.

ENDOSCOPICALLY ASSISTED CORRECTION OF CRANIOSYNOSTOSIS

In simple craniosynostosis surgery, the infant's prematurely closed cranial suture lines are excised. This leaves a gap in the sutures which allows the brain to develop normally. The following discussion describes how a single strip of fused bone is removed. More complex surgery may require removal of large portions of connective tissue from the cranium with multiple repairs and remolding of the cranial bones. The surgery is performed with a 0-degree, 4-mm telescope so that visualization of the scissors can be maintained while the cranium is excised.

PATHOLOGY

In the newborn, the individual bones that make up the cranium are separated by flexible connective tissues. These are called *sutures.* These soft tissue boundaries allow the brain to expand rapidly in the first 3 months of life, after which the bone edges lose flexibility and the bones fuse. Craniosynostosis is a congenital deformity that results from premature closure of one or more of the cranial sutures of the skull, which can have different effects on the skull, generally causing growth restriction perpendicular to the suture. Growth restriction leads to increased cranial pressure and neurological changes. The surgery may be performed urgently.

POSITION:	Supine for anterior exposure; prone for posterior exposure
INCISION:	Cranial
PREP AND DRAPING:	Cranial
INSTRUMENTS:	Minor craniosynostosis set including #15 blade, Senn retractors, Penfield elevators, Cushing periosteal elevator, Adson forceps, bayonet forceps, straight and curved hemostats, Mayo scissors, Tessier bone-cutting scissors, bipolar ESU, Gelfoam
POSSIBLE EXTRAS:	Kerrison rongeurs

Technical Points and Discussion

1. ***The patient is prepped and draped.***
The infant is placed in the supine or prone position. If the prone position is necessary, the patient is first anesthetized and intubated and then turned to the prone position. The incision lines are marked and the cranium prepped. The incision sites are infiltrated with bupivacaine and epinephrine.

2. ***The incisions are made.***
To begin the procedure, the surgeon makes a small incision, which is carried through the skin and connective tissue. The incisions can be made with the monopolar ESU on very low setting or with the skin knife. The connective tissue is dissected using a periosteal elevator.

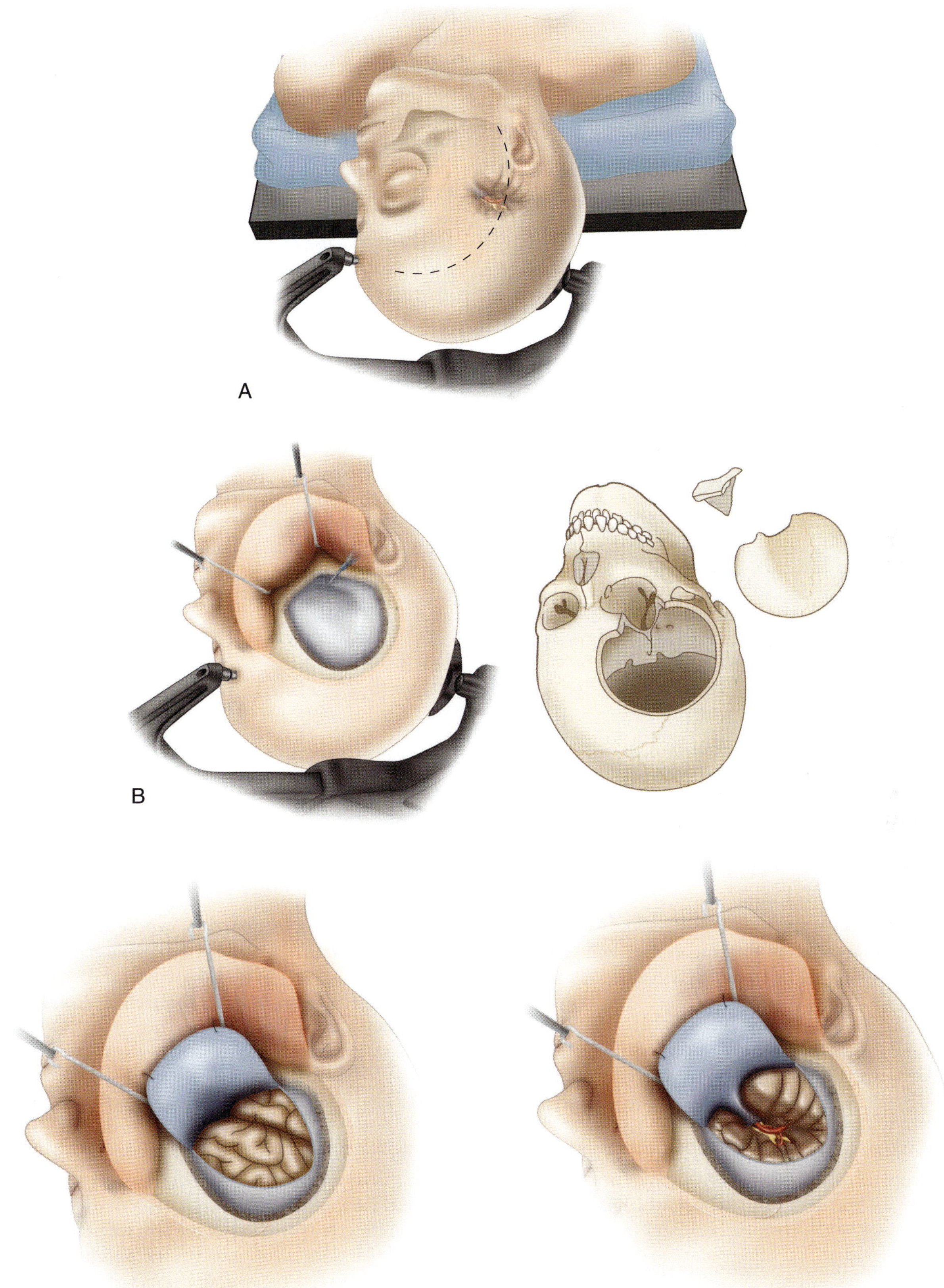

FIG. 34.12 Cerebral aneurysm. (A) Incision for pterional craniotomy. (B) The skin flap is raised to expose the dura and the bone flap is removed. (C) The dural incision is made, exposing the vasculature.

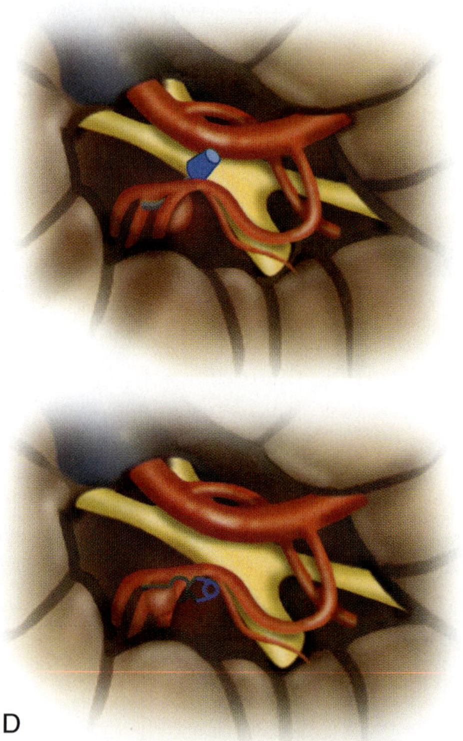

D

FIG. 34.12, cont'd (D) The aneurysm is clipped (shown at the 8 o'clock position). (From Jandial R, McCormick P, Black P, eds. *Core Techniques in Operative Neurosurgery.* Philadelphia: Elsevier; 2011.)

3. ***The dura is separated from the bone.***
   Blunt dissection is carried out between the cranium and dura. The fused suture is incised.
   Using curved Mayo scissors or rongeurs, the surgeon cuts the bone on each side of the fused suture. The strip of bone tissue is extracted.

4. ***Hemostasis is secured.***
   Hemostasis is secured by the bipolar ESU and Gelfoam soaked in thrombin. The wound is irrigated with antibiotic solution.

5. ***The wound is closed.***
   The galea is closed with size 4-0 Vicryl. The skin is closed with 4-0 rapid absorption polyglactin suture. The wound is dressed with nonadherent dressing. An abdominal pad is placed over the primary dressing and secured with netting.
   Recovery takes place in the PACU. Within a few days, the patient is fitted with a soft helmet, which is worn for 6 to 8 months while the cranium heals.

Technical points of the procedure are shown in Fig. 34.13.

CRANIOPLASTY

In a **cranioplasty,** a bone graft or prosthetic material is used to cover a missing portion of the cranium after trauma or disease. Many new technologies are available to restore continuity to the cranium. When native (patient's own) bone is secured, various metal and resorbable systems are used. If a prosthesis is required, there are several alternatives. Titanium mesh, calcium phosphate, or methylmethacrylate cement may be used. A more complex method is to use three-dimensional imaging and computer-aided design (CAD) to create a custom-made acrylic prosthesis that exactly fits the patient's cranial profile. Each of these systems is commercially sold with technical manuals on their use and method of implanting. Specific on-site training is also available from the manufacturer. A simple method used to create a flap with methylmethacrylate (MME) is presented here. An alternative use of MME cement is to use titanium mesh to cover the defect, with bone cement spread over the outer surface and edges of the mesh to provide a smooth surface.

PATHOLOGY

Deformities of the skull resulting from trauma or disease may leave a portion of the brain and dura mater exposed. If the cranial defect is clean (e.g., in closed trauma), the repair may be performed immediately. If the wound is contaminated (e.g., bone flap infection, open trauma), repair is delayed. The bone flap created by craniotomy may have been removed and stored under sterile conditions to allow the brain to expand and to reduce the ICP.

POSITION:	According to the location of the flap
INCISION:	Cranial to expose the bone
PREP AND DRAPING:	Cranial
INSTRUMENTS:	Cranioplasty set, including drill, methylmethacrylate cranioplasty set with closed vacuum mixing system

Technical Points and Discussion

1. ***The patient is positioned, prepped, and draped for access to a particular area of the cranium.***

2. ***An incision is made in the connective tissues, which are prepared as for a craniotomy.***
   The scalp is incised over the defect as for a craniotomy.

3. ***The edges of the defect are remodeled.***
   Depending on the nature of the previous injury or disease, remnants of bone may be present in the affected area. If bone fragments are present, the surgeon uses a rongeur to reduce them. If the affected area is completely devoid of bone, the surgeon trims the periphery of the area with rongeurs to form a saucer-like ledge. This prevents the prosthesis from slipping below the level of the skull and helps seat it in place. The scrub should retain all the bits of trimmed bone as specimens. The wound is irrigated with warm saline solution. An antibiotic irrigant also may be used at this time.

4. ***The methylmethacrylate is prepared and molded to fit the defect.***
   The scrub uses a commercially prepared cranioplasty kit containing a premeasured amount of powder and solvent

to form the methylmethacrylate prosthesis. Methylmethacrylate is flammable and must be mixed in a specifically designed closed vacuum system. While the cement is still doughy, the scrub places it in the plastic bag provided in the kit and passes it to the surgeon. The surgeon then flattens and molds the bag over the cranial defect to fit. The surgeon removes the molded cement from the defect to allow the cement to cure. While the cement is curing (usually 15 to 20 minutes), the surgeon may assess the wound for any small bleeders. During this time, the scrub should prepare a closure system to fix the prosthesis in place. After handling the uncured cement, team members should change gloves.

5. ***The prosthesis is secured to the edges of the defect.*** When the cement plate has hardened, rough spots are smoothed with a large burr attached to a power drill or craniotome. The surgeon then fits the cement plate into the defect and secures it using a closure system (e.g., plates, screws). The wound is irrigated and closed in routine fashion.

VENTRICULOPERITONEAL SHUNT

Ventricular shunting is used to divert the CSF away from the ventricles of the brain to another location in the body, such as the peritoneal cavity, where the CSF can be absorbed. This reduces ICP. Shunt systems vary by manufacturer, but common components include a ventricular catheter, a CSF reservoir, a valve, and a peritoneal catheter. Valves are designed for one-way flow and are supplied with a variety of pressure and flow settings. The scrub should read the manufacturer's specifications and instructions before the procedure is performed. As with all Silastic or other implant materials, the shunt should be handled as little as possible and protected from contamination by lint, dust, or glove powder. The shunt components are often soaked in antibiotic solution before they are implanted according to the surgeon's orders. The scrub is responsible for priming the assembly with saline and ensuring that no air is present in the system. Because ventricular shunting may be

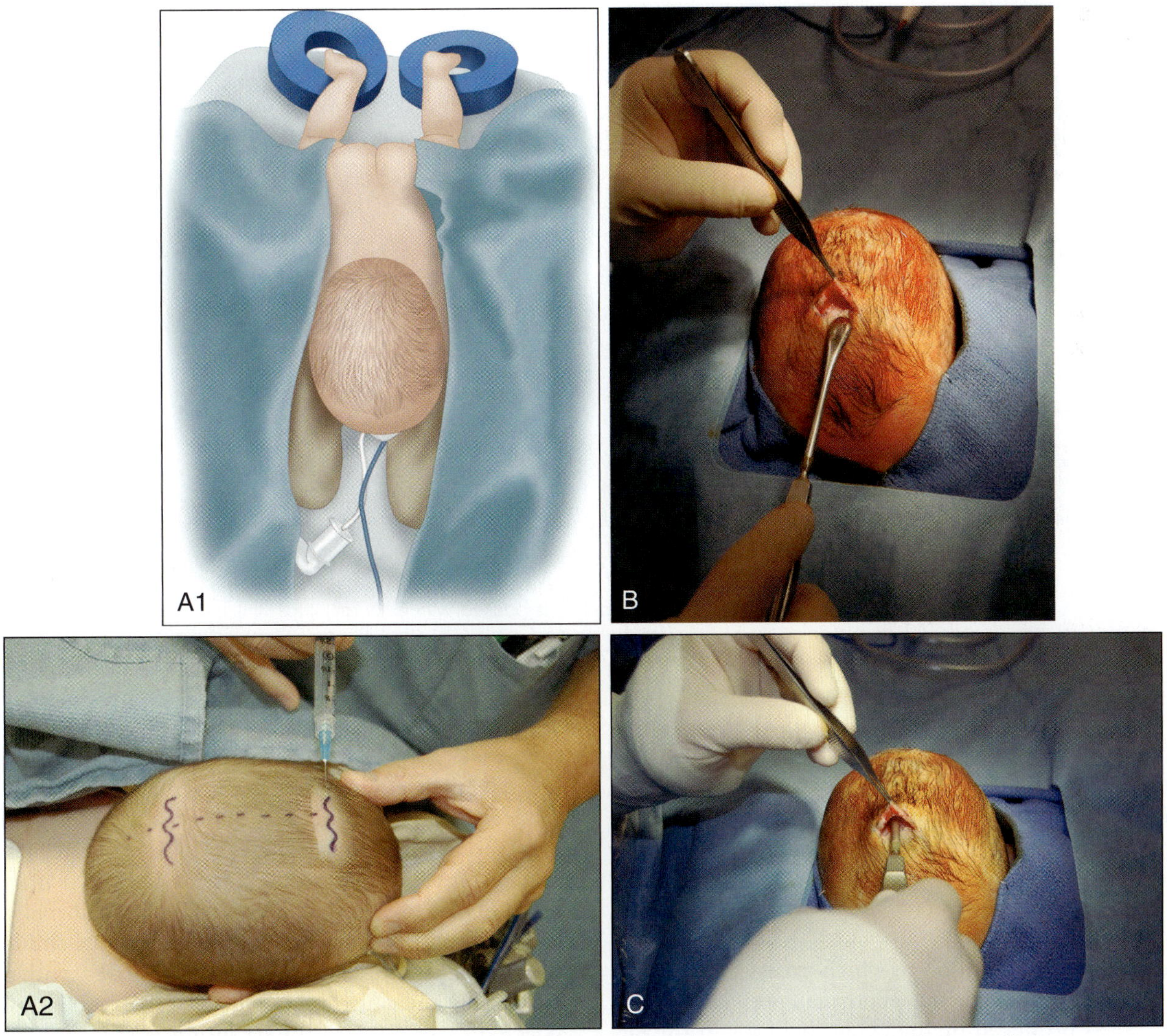

FIG. 34.13 Craniosynostosis. (A1) The patient is placed in the "sphinx" position. (A2) The scalp is infiltrated with bupivacaine and epinephrine for hemostasis. (B) The scalp is incised and lifted from the cranium by means of an elevator. (C) A dissection plane is created between the inner table of the fused sagittal suture and the dura.

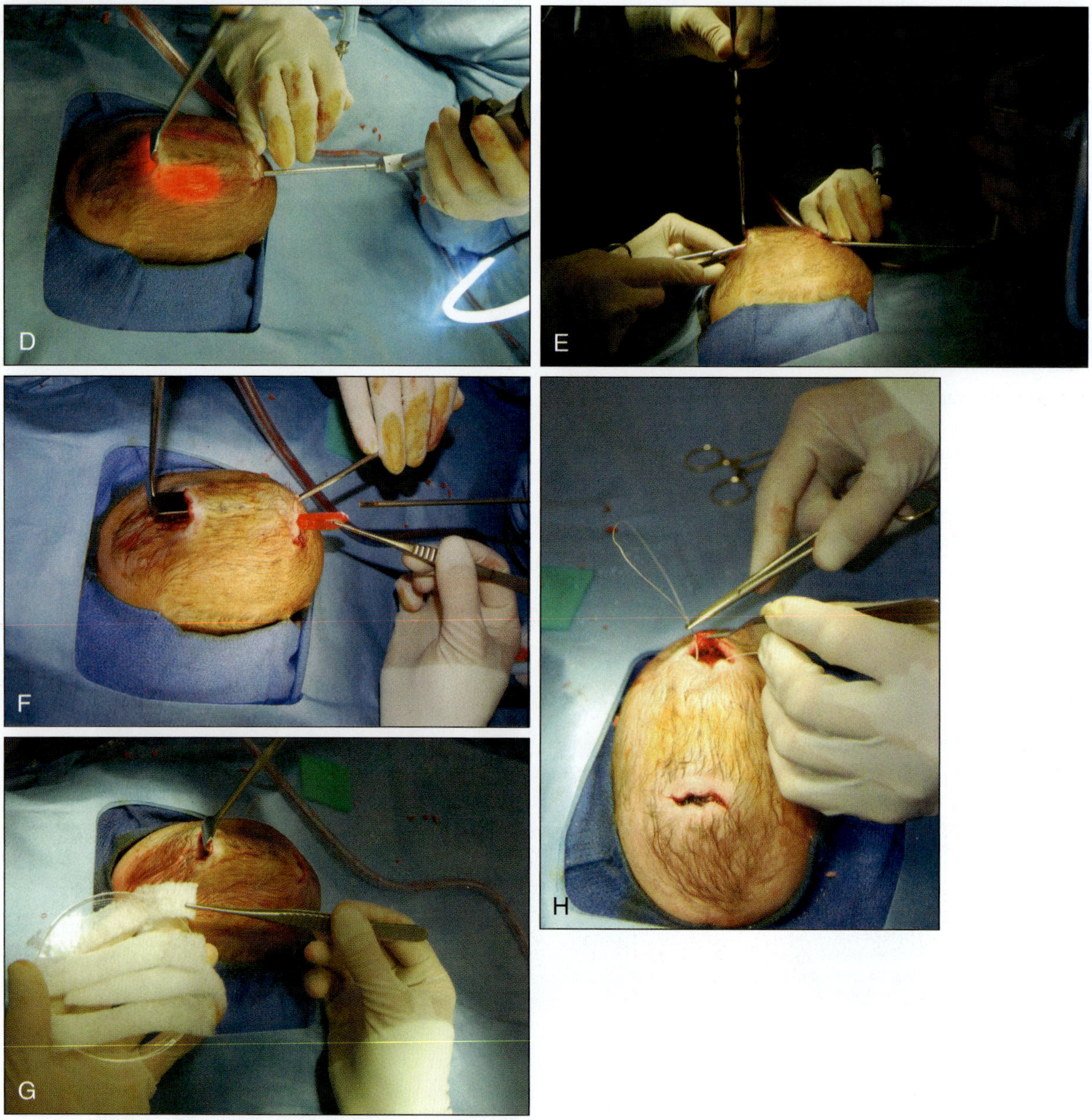

FIG. 34.13, cont'd (D) A lighted endoscope is positioned between the scalp and bone. (E) Mayo scissors are used to cut the fused suture on each side. A hook retractor can be seen at the 12 o'clock position. (F) The suture strip is removed. (G) The defect is packed with Gelfoam strips. (H) The wounds are closed. (A1 from Applegate E. From Jandial R, McCormick P, Black P, eds. *Core Techniques in Operative Neurosurgery*. Philadelphia: Elsevier; 2011.)

performed on adults or children, the scrub should ensure that the instruments and sutures selected are appropriate for the age and size of the patient.

PATHOLOGY

Hydrocephalus is a condition in which excess CSF is present in the ventricles, placing abnormal pressure on the tissues. CSF is produced by the epidermal cells in the lateral third and fourth ventricles. CSF circulates through the foramen of Monro into the third ventricle, through the cerebral aqueduct (aqueduct of Sylvius), and into the fourth ventricle. From the fourth ventricle, it flows through the cerebromedullar cistern down the spinal cord and over the cerebral hemispheres. Hydrocephalus can occur as a result of an overproduction of CSF, or it may be the result of a condition that interferes with the normal absorption of fluid. Hydrocephalus can develop in children and adults. Persistent hydrocephalus can interfere with cerebral blood flow and cause enlargement of the skull in infants. In selected cases, surgical intervention is aimed at removing the excess fluid to relieve pressure on the brain. A ventriculoperitoneal (VP) shunt is most often used to divert CSF when more conservative treatment has failed.

POSITION:	Supine
INCISION:	Cranial, abdomen
PREP AND DRAPING:	Two sites are prepped: cranium and abdomen
INSTRUMENTS:	Craniotomy, minor general surgery; laparotomy; VP shunt system

Technical Points and Discussion

1. ***The patient is positioned, prepped, and draped.***
The surgeon may choose a frontal, parietal, or occipital approach to place the ventricular catheter. The patient is positioned supine with the head slightly rotated away from the side of the shunt insertion. The shoulder on the operative side is elevated by means of a gel pad. The incision lines are marked.

2. ***An abdominal incision is made.***
The surgeon makes a 3- to 5-cm incision in the upper right quadrant using a #15 blade. Monopolar ESU with a needlepoint is used to deepen the incision. The scrub should have Senn retractors available. The muscles are bluntly separated. The abdominal peritoneum is elevated with two curved mosquito clamps and then divided with scissors or a #11 blade. When hemostasis is maintained, the incision is covered with a sterile towel while the cranial incision is made.

3. ***A craniotomy is performed.***
The surgeon makes a curved incision in the scalp using the needle ESU or a #15 blade. Suction should be immediately available. A small burr hole is made using a high-speed drill. Traction sutures are placed in the dura.

4. ***A subcutaneous tunnel is made.***
A passageway is made bluntly by means of a tunneler from the cranial opening, under the neck muscle and into the peritoneum at the level of the abdominal incision. A distal catheter is passed through the tunneler, which is then removed.

5. ***The valve assembly is introduced.***
A self-retaining retractor is placed in the cranial wound. An anti-siphon valve is attached to the proximal end of the distal catheter. The surgeon then makes a small hole in the dura using a dura hook and scissors. Intraoperative ultrasound may be used to confirm the location of the ventricle before catheter insertion is attempted. The scrub loads the ventricular catheter on an introducer, and the surgeon inserts it through the burr hole into the lateral ventricle. The introducer is removed and CSF flow through the catheter is confirmed. If no CSF flow is present, the catheter is removed, the introducer is replaced, and the procedure is attempted again. When CSF flow is confirmed, the reservoir and valve are attached to the ventricular catheter and secured with size 2-0 silk sutures. The surgeon tests the pump and secures the catheter to the peritoneum using size 3-0 Vicryl sutures.

6. ***The wounds are closed.***
The incisions are closed with absorbable synthetic suture. The scalp and abdominal skin incisions are closed with staples or with interrupted 4-0 nylon suture. The wounds are dressed with Telfa and flat gauze.

The most common complication after ventricular shunt placement is shunt malfunction as a result of blockage of the valve or catheter. This complication can occur shortly after placement or at any time after the shunt is in place. Overdrainage or underdrainage also can occur and can cause patients to exhibit a variety of symptoms ranging from headache to neurological deficits. Shunts placed in infants and children need to be replaced periodically to accommodate their growth.

This procedure is illustrated in Fig. 34.14.

TRANSNASAL TRANSSPHENOIDAL (TNTS) HYPOPHYSECTOMY

The goal of transnasal transsphenoidal (TNTS) hypophysectomy is to remove all or a part of the pituitary gland. This procedure may be performed to slow the growth and spread of an endocrine-dependent malignant tumor or to excise a pituitary tumor. The surgical approach is through the sphenoid.

An endoscopic approach is aided by the use of the microscope and C-arm fluoroscopy.

PATHOLOGY

The pituitary gland is responsible for the storage, release, and secretion of a variety of hormones. The gland is attached by a stalk to the hypothalamus and rests in the sella turcica. It is adjacent to critical structures such as the optic chiasma and cavernous sinuses, which contain several cranial nerves and the internal carotid arteries. Because the gland is uniquely located, symptoms from a tumor are often noticed as visual field anomalies or may be related to pressure on cranial nerves III through VI. Tumors may damage the adjacent brain tissue through mass effect by displacing structures, blocking CSF flow, or creating pressure.

POSITION:	Beach chair with the head in three-pin fixation. The neck is flexed toward the right shoulder
INCISION:	Transsphenoidal
PREP AND DRAPING:	The nose and face including intranasal mucosa; abdomen
INSTRUMENTS:	Transsphenoidal set; intranasal microinstruments; minor general surgery set; neurodissectors, scissors, probes, and elevators; bipolar ESU; sinuscope with 0-degree and 30-degree lenses

TECHNICAL POINTS AND DISCUSSION

Transsphenoidal hypophysectomy requires an interdisciplinary approach. An otorhinolaryngologist participates in the

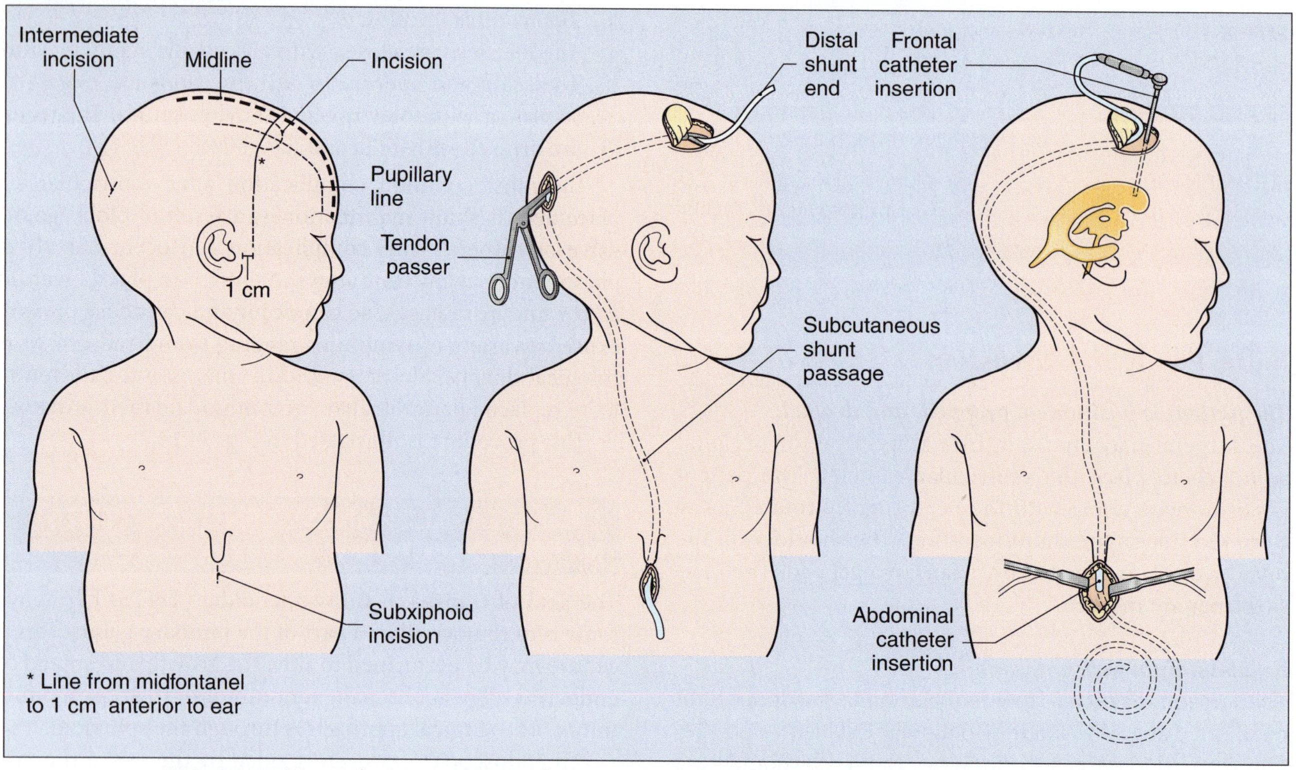

FIG. 34.14 Ventriculoperitoneal shunt. The patient is positioned and exact positions are marked. A subcutaneous tunnel is created for the shunt, and the catheter is inserted. (From Rengachary S, Ellenbogen R, eds. *Principles of Neurosurgery.* 2nd ed. St Louis: Mosby; 2005.)

surgery during access to the sella turcica. An open or endoscopic approach may be used. The scrub should have combined sinus instrumentation available. Specialized pituitary instrumentation, which includes self-retaining specula, long pituitary spoons and scoops, rongeurs, and curettes, should also be available. The operating microscope may be prepared and draped before the start of surgery.

Before the start of surgery, the scrub should prepare a side table that includes supplies needed for the injection and application of a local anesthetic. Supplies include nasal specula, cottonoids, syringes, and several 25-gauge needles. The circulating nurse dispenses topical cocaine and lidocaine with epinephrine to this nonsterile field. Before beginning the procedure, the surgeon injects the nasal and gingival mucosa to provide hemostasis.

The scrub is also responsible for preparing a *separate* sterile setup with a few basic instruments for obtaining a fat graft from the abdomen. The fat graft is harvested before the transsphe-noidal procedure begins, to maintain the flow from a clean to a contaminated area.

1. ***The patient is positioned, prepped, and draped.***
The patient is placed in the three-point pin fixation device and positioned in the beach chair position with the neck flexed toward the left and the head rotated to the right.

   The surgical approach is from the patient's right side. After the patient has been positioned, the C-arm is used to confirm that the positioning is accurate for access to the sella. Often the floor is marked with a piece of tape where the C-arm's wheels are placed so that it can be repositioned in the same location during the procedure. The face is draped with towels to exclude the upper face, followed by an adhesive barrier drape across the bridge of the nose to secure the towel drapes. The abdomen is draped for a small lower right abdominal incision. The thigh may also be used as a graft site. The face is prepped, including the nose and its submucosal tissues. An abdominal prep is also performed. Local anesthetic with epinephrine is instilled in the nasal mucosa.

2. ***The tissues are prepared with hemostatic drugs.***
To secure hemostasis before the incision and using the endoscope and a long handheld nasal speculum, the otorhinolaryngologist injects the nasal submucosa and gingival mucosa with lidocaine with epinephrine. The anesthesia provider may insert a throat pack so that any blood or fluid from the procedure does not enter the patient's stomach, which would cause postoperative nausea and vomiting.

   The scrub should note the number of cottonoids placed in the nose for reconciliation during the sponge count. Although a counted sponge is not typically used for the throat pack, the scrub should note its presence and ensure that it is removed at the end of the procedure.

3. ***A graft is harvested from the abdomen or thigh.***
The procedure begins with the harvesting of the fat graft from the abdomen. The surgeon makes a small incision below the belt line. A small amount of subcutaneous fat is removed with the monopolar ESU and Metzenbaum scissors. The fat may be harvested from any location in the abdomen, but the site is usually chosen for a cosmetic

result. Alternately, muscle may be removed from the patient's thigh. The scrub should keep the tissue graft in a basin filled with saline or wrapped in a moistened Telfa strip on the back table until it is needed. The surgeon uses 2-0 polyglactin suture to close the subcutaneous tissue. The skin can be closed with staples or running subcuticular stitches of 3-0 or 4-0 nylon or polypropylene suture. The scrub should protect the incision with a sterile towel for the remainder of the procedure.

4. ***The sphenoid is entered.***
   Before entering the sphenoid, the scrub drapes the C-arm, and the radiology technician moves it into place. Fluoroscopy is used at this stage to confirm exposure of the sphenoid sinus and the floor of the sella.
   Once exposure is confirmed, a diamond-tip high-speed drill and irrigator are used to enter the sphenoid. The opening is enlarged using a rongeur. The scrub should collect loose bone tissue as specimen.

5. ***The tumor is resected.***
   The dura is exposed as the sphenoid space is enlarged. Using a #11 blade, the surgeon incises the dura. A large tumor is usually seen as soon as the dura is opened. Smaller tumors require dissection through the pituitary using a blunt probe or dissector. Tumor tissue is removed piecemeal with ring curettes, enucleators, and microdissectors. The scrub must collect all tumor tissue for analysis. A frozen section may be performed early in the dissection.
   Occasionally the tumor may not be fully identified. In this case, a lumbar drain may be inserted into the bone cavity and preservative-free saline injected into the space. This increases the ICP. Another technique is to enlarge the bony space further with the use of rongeurs. A 30-degree endoscope may also be used.
   Bleeding is controlled with cottonoids soaked in epinephrine. Gelfoam packing may also be used.

6. ***A fat graft is placed in the sella.***
   Using the fat graft or muscle tissue obtained at the start of the procedure, the surgeon packs the floor of the sella to prevent or manage a CSF leak. In the case of very large macroadenomas, the anterior wall of the sella may require reconstruction with a bioabsorbable or titanium plate. Very small tumors often do not require a graft. Fibrin sealant may be used if needed. The nose is packed with Merocel.

7. ***The pin fixation is removed.***
   The patient is returned to a supine position, and the pin fixation device is removed before the patient emerges from anesthesia.

Technical points of the procedures are illustrated in Fig. 34.15.

Patients who have undergone transsphenoidal hypophysectomy are monitored in the intensive care unit postoperatively for changes in neurological status and CSF leakage. Because the pituitary gland has been manipulated or partly resected, patients may experience symptoms related to underproduction or overproduction of the various hormones controlled by the gland. These symptoms may be present immediately postoperatively or may manifest in the weeks or months after the procedure. Some patients require lifelong hormonal replacement after hypophysectomy.

ENDOSCOPIC THIRD VENTRICULOSCOPY

The third ventricle of the brain provides excellent access to the foramen of Monro (refer to the Surgical Anatomy section). Third-ventricle endoscopy has been continually developed to provide a safe means of relieving ventricular obstruction to restore CSF circulation. Stereotactic techniques may also be used to improve accuracy.

PATHOLOGY

Conditions that may be treated with endoscopic ventriculostomy include the following:
- Occlusive hydrocephalus
- Intraventricular tumors
- Colloid cyst
- Arachnoid cyst
- Pineal cyst
- Intraparenchymal cyst

Cysts may develop in the third ventricle and attach to the roof or floor. Various malignant or benign tumors may form in the third ventricle or may metastasize from other sites. The presence of a cyst or tumor may cause hydrocephalus, or hydrocephalus may be the result of other conditions.

Obstructive hydrocephalus is often treated by ventriculoscopy. There are two types of hydrocephalus. Obstructive hydrocephalus occurs when there is blockage in the CSF drainage system. This usually occurs at the cerebral aqueduct and is caused most often by congenital malformation or tumor. Communicating hydrocephalus occurs when the absorptive systems of the brain are disrupted. This can be caused by meningitis and subarachnoid hemorrhage. Ventriculoscopy can be effective in treating obstructive hydrocephalus by removing the source of the blockage.

VENTRICULOSCOPE

The ventriculoscope is available in rigid or flexible design. Like other endoscopes used for operative procedures, the rigid scope is favored in surgery because of the endoscope sheath, which contains ports for the insertion of instruments.

The rigid telescope is a standard Hopkins scope with 0-degree, 6-degree, and 30-degree lenses. The sheath is fitted to accept a blunt obturator.

Both rigid and flexible instruments are used with the rigid ventriculoscope, including grasping forceps, cup forceps, ventriculoscopy forceps, scissors, bipolar forceps, and bipolar rod.

A guillotine knife with footplate is used to cut tissue without risk of injury to nearby blood vessels.

A scope-holding system that attaches to the operating table is sometimes used to stabilize the ventriculoscope during surgery. This allows the surgeon to use both hands to perform the surgery in the absence of an assistant.

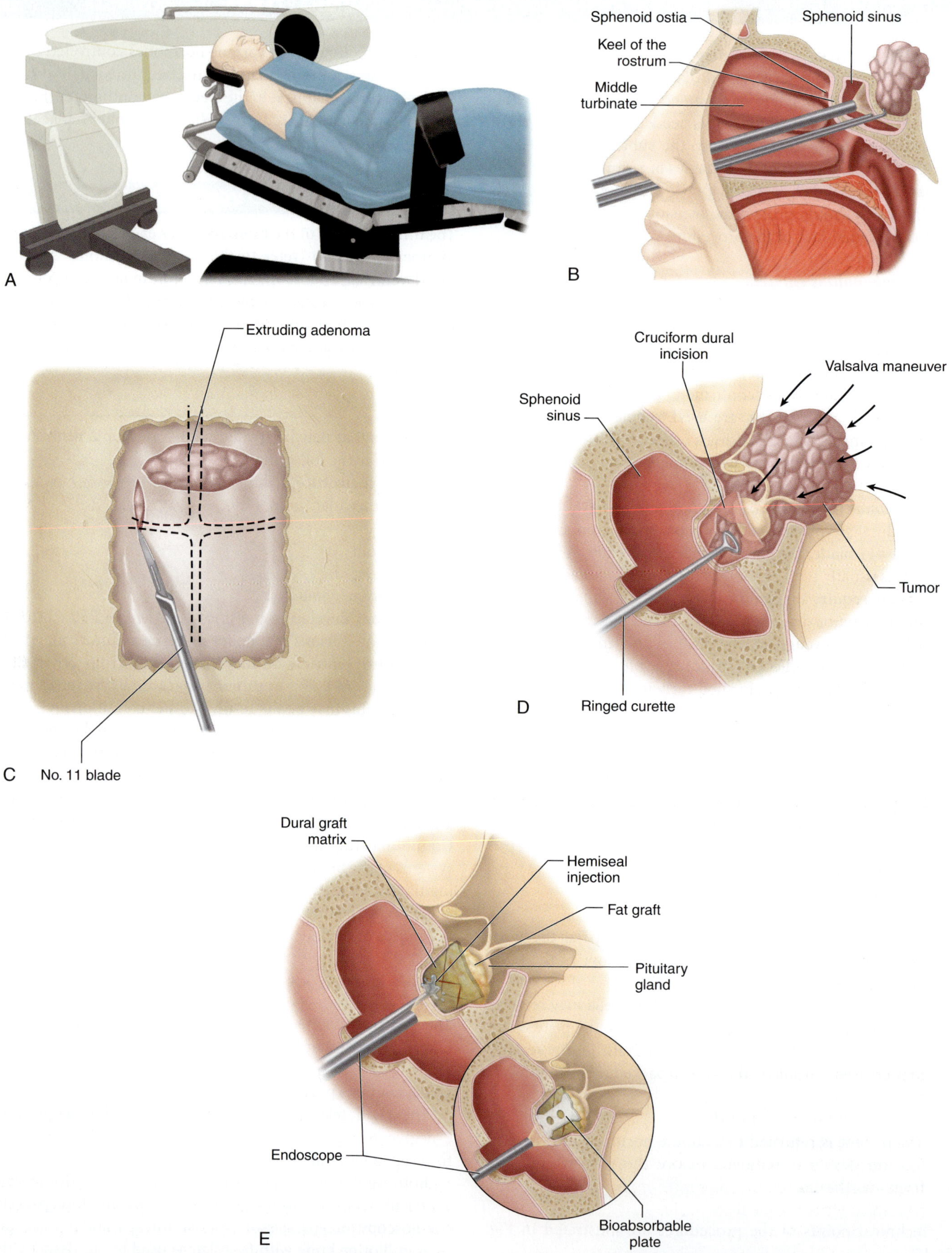

FIG. 34.15 Transsphenoidal hypophysectomy. (A) Patient position with reference to C-arm. (B) Orientation of the sagittal plane is verified with the C-arm. Note position of endoscope and forceps. (C) The sphenoid is entered with a high-speed drill and extended with rongeurs. The dura is incised with a #11 blade. (D) The tumor is removed with ring curettes. A Valsalva maneuver causes the tumor to be pushed into the bony opening. (E) When the tumor has been removed, the cavity is packed with Surgicel. A plate may be inserted if necessary, for support. (From Jandial R, McCormick P, Black P, eds. *Core Techniques in Operative Neurosurgery*. Philadelphia: Elsevier; 2011.)

POSITION:	Supine
INCISION:	Cranial
PREP AND DRAPING:	Cranial
INSTRUMENTS:	Ventriculoscope and its instruments; bipolar ESU; craniotomy set; craniotome and burrs; Fogarty catheter
POSSIBLE EXTRAS:	Stereotactic equipment

Technical Points and Discussion

1. ***The patient is positioned, prepped, and draped.***
   If stereotactic instrumentation is used for ventriculoscopy, the stereotactic system is applied as described, and the patient is placed under general anesthesia. Patients undergoing ventriculoscopy without stereotactic instrumentation are positioned supine, with the head resting on a soft headrest and elevated 30 degrees to promote venous drainage, minimize CSF loss, and reduce the likelihood of air entering the patient's vasculature.

2. ***An incision is made and a burr hole is placed.***
   After marking the incision and injecting it with lidocaine and epinephrine, the surgeon incises the skin and creates a burr hole over the right lateral ventricle. The dura is opened with scissors or a #11 blade, and the bipolar ESU is used for hemostasis.

3. ***The dura is opened and the operating sheath is placed.***
   The surgeon inserts the operating sheath with a trocar through the burr hole into the lateral ventricle. The trocar is removed once the sheath is in place. Some surgeons prefer to use a disposable catheter and sheath, which can be stapled to the drapes for stability.

   Sterile intravenous tubing is attached to the irrigation port and passed off the field to be attached to a bag of warmed Ringer lactate. A rigid endoscope is connected to the video camera and adjusted as necessary to ensure a clear image. The endoscope is passed through the cannula and the irrigation is started. The surgeon adjusts the flow of irrigation fluid as necessary, using the stopcock on the port to ensure that any bleeding is cleared from the field and the ventricles remain distended. The scrub should be prepared with suction to keep the surgical field clear of irrigation fluid.

4. ***The floor of the ventricle is opened.***
   The surgeon passes the endoscope into the lateral ventricle and navigates the scope through the foramen of Monro to visualize the floor of the third ventricle, which is opened with a blunt instrument, forceps, or blunt wire (Fig. 34.16). The hole is then widened using a Fogarty balloon catheter (arterial type), which is inserted into the endoscope sheath and opened slowly. The surgeon assesses the ventricle for any bleeding, which is controlled with the bipolar ESU.

5. ***The ventriculoscope is withdrawn.***
   The surgeon removes the endoscope and sheath and places Gelfoam in the burr hole for hemostasis. A ventricular drain may be placed before closure. Closure proceeds as described for the burr hole procedure.

STEREOTACTIC SURGERY

The term ***stereotactic*** is derived from Greek, meaning to *touch in space*. This technique combines images such as those produced during CT, MRI, and magnetic resonance to form a 3-D data map. This is called *image registration* and is the first stage of stereotaxis. The next stage is to attach a lightweight frame or imaging markers to the patient. These sophisticated devices create multiple reference points in relation to the 3-D map. The new image projects real-time reference points, including the surgical instruments for extremely fine orientation in areas of the brain that are difficult or too dangerous to enter by conventional means. As described earlier, there are two approaches used to create the reference point: *frame-based* and *frameless* surgery. It is important to have a basic understanding of each type.

FRAME-BASED SURGERY

The patient arrives several hours before surgery. With the patient under local anesthesia, the frame is fitted to the patient's head (for cranial surgery). With the frame in place, 3-D images are taken by CT, angiography, and MRI (unless contraindicated). Both the frame and the target pathology are included in the images, and accurate values for distance, height, and depth are captured in relation to the frame. During surgery, instruments can be attached to the frame and will be registered in real time during the procedure, guiding the surgeon through the optimal low-risk path to the target tissue.

FRAMELESS SURGERY

In the frameless technique, markers, called *fiducials*, are securely fixed to the patient's scalp before the brain is imaged. During the surgical procedure, the fiducials are captured (registered) with the 3-D images, providing reference points in relation to the target tissue. A digital camera senses the positions of the instruments and integrates their images along with the real-time 3-D view of the anatomy.

LEARNING THE TECHNOLOGY

Complex technology such as that used in stereotactic surgery requires advance study of the equipment, software, and instruments. The procedures take place in the operating room and in the interventional radiology department. The surgical technologist can take advantage of in-service training and opportunities to observe the procedures to become familiar with the terminology and techniques required. An outline of basic steps is provided here.

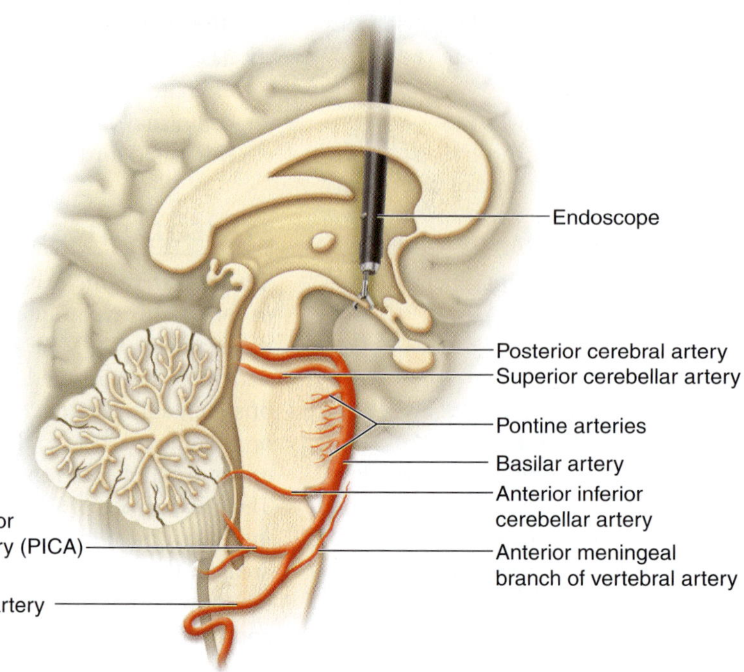

FIG. 34.16 Ventriculostomy for treatment of hydrocephalus. The endoscope is passed into the third ventricle and through the floor of the ventricle and into the space below. This creates drainage for the CSF. (From Jandial R, McCormick P, Black P, eds. *Core Techniques in Operative Neurosurgery.* Philadelphia: Elsevier; 2011.)

PATHOLOGY

The stereotactic approach may be used for tumor biopsy or removal, resection of AVMs, brain mapping, implantation of electrodes, catheter placement, ventriculostomy, and the treatment of movement disorders and intractable pain. It is used in conjunction with minimally invasive radiosurgical techniques to ablate tumors and AVMs and to treat functional disorders such as trigeminal neuralgia, Parkinson disease, and essential tremor.

POSITION:	According to the location of the pathology
INCISION:	According to the location of the pathology
PREP AND DRAPING:	Cranial
INSTRUMENTS:	Craniotomy set, stereotactic equipment and accessories

Technical Points and Discussion

1. ***The patient is fitted with a frame or fiducials and undergoes imaging.***
If a framed system is used, the patient's skin is infiltrated with local anesthetic at the skull pin insertion points. The patient undergoes a preoperative MRI or CT scan.
With the frame (or fiducials) in place, the patient is sent for CT or MRI, where predetermined anatomical landmarks are used as guides and the coordinates are determined. The computer determines the target trajectory.

2. ***A craniotomy is performed.***
The patient is transferred to the operating room with the frame or fiducials in place. General anesthesia is used if the procedure will be extensive. The surgeon places burr holes as previously described. After making the burr holes, the surgeon uses hollow cannulas, coagulating electrodes, cryosurgical probes, wire loops, and other biopsy instruments to access and treat target areas in the brain.
At the close of the procedure, the frame or fiducials are removed and the cranium is closed.

SPINAL PROCEDURES

ANTERIOR CERVICAL DISCECTOMY AND FUSION (OPEN)

The goal of an anterior cervical discectomy is to excise one or more herniated cervical discs. Spinal fusion restores continuity to the spine after the disc is removed.

Pathology

The most common indications for anterior cervical discectomy and fusion are a herniated cervical disc and stenosis. A patient with a herniated cervical disc has pain in the neck, shoulders, or arms, accompanied by numbness and weakness in the hands and arms. Depending on the level of herniation, the patient may experience more severe symptoms, such as difficulty walking.

Cervical spondylosis is a degenerative condition generally attributed to age-related changes in the cervical discs.

During the aging process, the discs lose fluid, fragment, and collapse. As the discs collapse, increased mechanical stress is placed on the bone, which may result in the formation of bony spurs along the spinal canal. Symptoms of cervical spondylosis include neck and shoulder pain, pain in the back of the head, and numbness and weakness in the arms. If spondylosis is severe, the spinal cord may be affected (myelopathy), and the patient may experience symptoms such as problems with walking and balance.

POSITION:	Supine; arms at the patient's sides; operative hip elevated
INCISION:	Anterior neck
PREP AND DRAPING:	Anterior neck
INSTRUMENTS:	Laminectomy set, bone graft set including Cloward instruments and Caspar retractor, osteotomes and chisels, high-speed drill with diamond burrs, small bone plates and screws

Technical Points and Discussion

1. ***The patient is positioned, prepped, and draped.***
The patient is placed in the supine position. Cervical traction may be applied with Gardner-Wells tongs. The right or left hip is elevated on a small bean bag or gel roll. This facilitates exposure of the iliac crest for removal of the bone graft. The surgeon marks both sites and infiltrates them with lidocaine with epinephrine. Both sites are prepped and draped in routine fashion.

2. ***A bone graft is obtained and placed in antibiotic solution.***
Two methods are used to take the bone graft. The Cloward method uses a special dowel cutter that creates a "plug" of bone from the iliac crest. Alternatively, an osteotome and a mallet can be used to shear the surface of the iliac crest and create short slivers of bone. Regardless of the method, the surgeon incises the iliac crest and deepens the incision with the monopolar ESU. When the bone has been exposed, a self-retaining retractor is placed in the wound. The surgeon uses a periosteal elevator to strip the crest of periosteum. The graft is then harvested and placed in antibiotic solution.
Bleeding vessels on the surface of the iliac crest are controlled with bone putty, and the surface is smoothed with a rasp or rongeur. The wound is irrigated and may or may not be closed at this time. Some surgeons pack the wound with sponges and delay closure until the fusion procedure is completed, in case an additional bone graft is needed. If the surgeon chooses to close the wound at this point, a sponge count is taken. After verification of the count, the surgeon closes the wound in layers with size 0 or 1-0 absorbable synthetic suture on a cutting needle and closes the skin with subcuticular stitches or staples. A drain may be placed before closure. The wound should be covered with a sterile towel for the duration of the procedure.

3. ***A transverse vertical incision is made in the neck.***
The surgeon makes a transverse incision in the skin crease of the neck at the level of the cricoid cartilage. The incision is extended through the platysma muscle with Metzenbaum scissors or the monopolar ESU. Using the scissors for both blunt and sharp dissection, the surgeon defines the medial edge of the sternocleidomastoid muscle. This plane of dissection is carried laterally between the carotid artery and medially between the esophagus and trachea. A small self-retaining retractor is placed in the wound. Hemostasis is maintained with the monopolar and bipolar ESUs.

4. ***The vertebrae are exposed.***
The surgeon incises the muscle fibers to expose the vertebrae. A layer of fascia overlying the vertebrae is incised with a #15 knife blade mounted on a #7 handle. A small handheld retractor may be needed by the assistant to help retract the muscle to expose the vertebrae. Next, the surgeon incises and removes the anterior longitudinal ligament.

5. ***The level is verified.***
With the disc then clearly visible, radiographs are taken to verify the diseased disc. The surgeon inserts one or two spinal needles into the disc body for identification of the disc level under C-arm fluoroscopy. Once the anatomy has been confirmed, the surgeon places a self-retaining retractor (e.g., a Cloward or Caspar retractor) in the wound. Care is taken in placing these retractors to avoid damaging the carotid artery and esophagus. Usually a combination of sharp and dull blades is used. The retractor systems allow for customization with a variety of blade curvatures, lengths, and retraction surfaces.

6. ***The disc is removed.***
With the retractors in place, the surgeon incises the disc with a #15 knife blade. The surgeon may use an intervertebral spreader to expose the disc. Pituitary rongeurs and fine curettes are used to remove the disc piece by piece. The scrub should remove the bits of disc from the rongeur or curette with a moistened 4 × 4 sponge. The surgeon usually presents the tip of the rongeur toward the scrub so that the tip can be wiped clean. The tissue is maintained as a specimen.

7. ***The interspace is enlarged.***
A small drill bit or burr may be used to expose the dura within the interspace. The dura then is elevated with a sharp nerve hook or dura hook and incised with a #15 knife blade. When the interspace has been adequately enlarged and the disc removed, the surgeon identifies the posterior longitudinal ligament, which may be removed with ligament forceps and a #15 blade. The surgeon uses a depth gauge and calipers to measure the defect. These measurements are used to size the bone graft.

8. ***The graft is prepared.***
While the bone graft is being prepared, the neck wound should be covered with a saline-soaked 4 × 4 sponge to prevent tissue drying and with a sterile towel to protect it

from contamination. The surgeon examines the graft and trims it to the appropriate size to fit into the intervertebral space. This is done with small bone rongeurs. Any extra bits of bone from the graft must be saved, because they may be used later to fill the interspace.

9. ***The graft is implanted into the interspace.***
The surgeon places the graft in the interspace and taps it with a mallet so that it fits snugly between the vertebrae. If the Cloward dowel cutter has been used, the Cloward impactor is used to place the graft.

10. ***A small plate is placed over the interspace.***
Plates and screws are used to secure the bone graft in place and provide stabilization during healing. In this instance, the surgeon drills pilot holes in the vertebrae on either side of the graft. The scrub should irrigate the burr while the holes are drilled. The surgeon places the plate in position and secures it with screws. Fluoroscopy is used to confirm the position of the bone graft, plate, and screws.

11. ***The wound is irrigated and closed.***
The wound is then irrigated with normal saline or antibiotic solution. Bleeding vessels are controlled with the monopolar and bipolar ESUs or a topical hemostatic agent. If it was not closed at the start of the procedure, the hip wound is closed at this time. The surgeon closes the cervical incision in layers with 3-0 polyglactin sutures and staples. Both wounds are dressed in routine fashion, and a rigid cervical collar is placed to help support the neck and maintain cervical alignment.

When the patient is moved from the operating table to the stretcher, particular care is taken to keep the head in alignment with the body to prevent dislodgment of the graft. Technical points of the procedure are illustrated in Fig. 34.17.

Postoperative hemorrhage, edema, and CSF leakage are possible after any surgery on the spine.

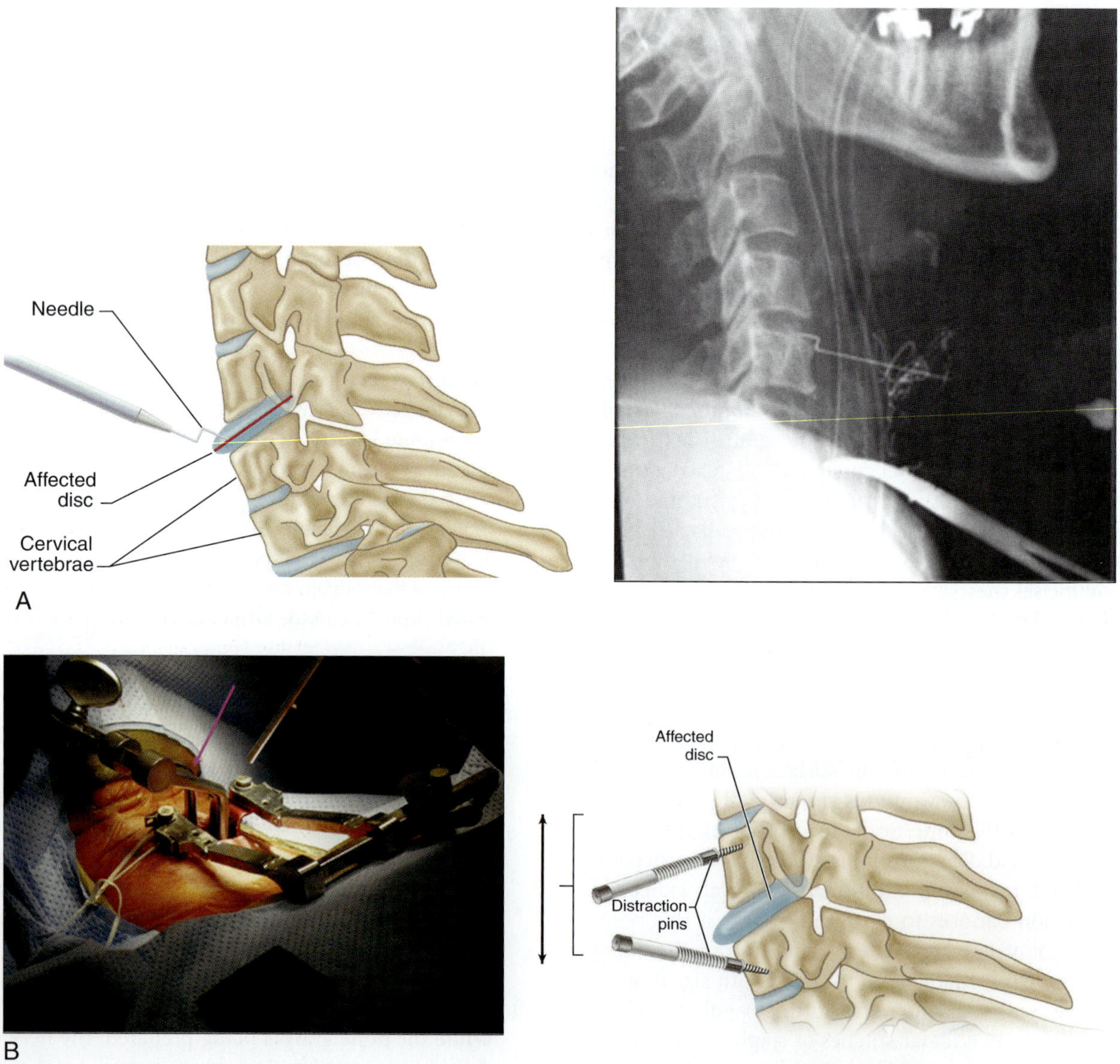

FIG. 34.17 Anterior cervical fusion. (A) A radiopaque marker (needle) is inserted at the affected disc so that the level can be verified on fluoroscopy. (B) Distraction pins (which work like a retractor) are inserted to separate the disc spaces above and below the affected disc to increase the working space.

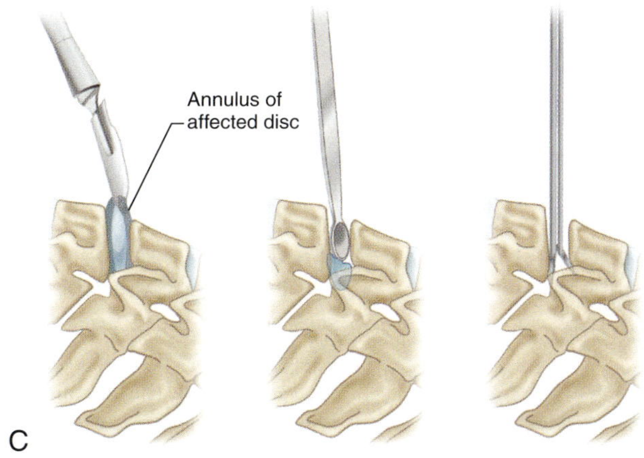

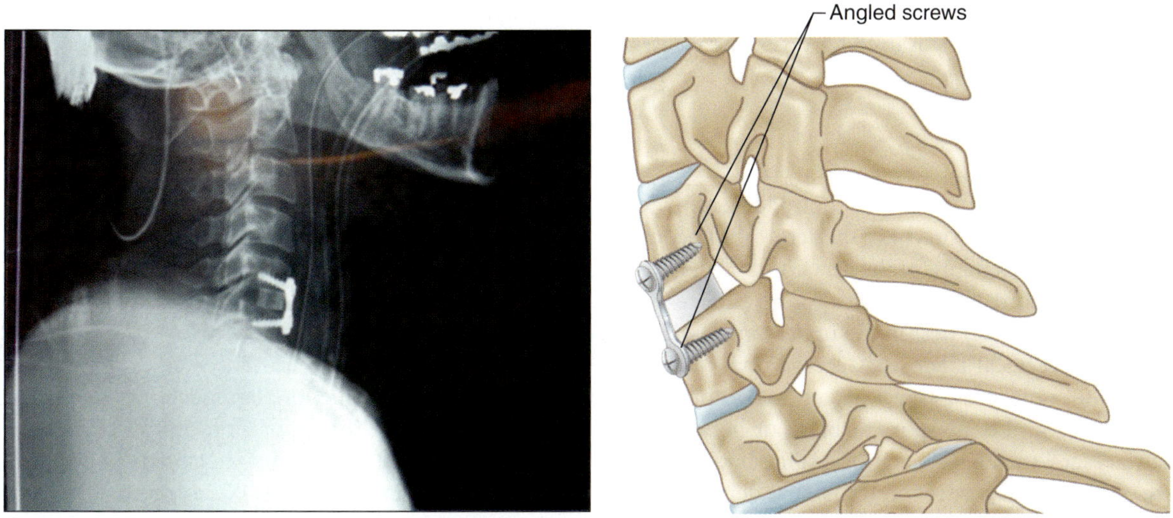

FIG. 34.17, cont'd (C) The annulus (fibrous covering on the disc) is incised. Curettes and pituitary rongeurs are used to remove the disc piecemeal. (D) A bone graft is inserted into the cleaned disc space. This is reinforced with a small plate and screws. (From Jandial R, McCormick P, Black P, eds. *Core Techniques in Operative Neurosurgery*. Philadelphia: Elsevier; 2011.)

ANTERIOR ENDOSCOPIC CERVICAL DECOMPRESSION OF DISC AND FORAMEN

In this procedure, a herniated intervertebral disc is removed and the foramen enlarged by the endoscopic surgery technique. During the procedure, EMG neurophysiological monitoring may be performed by the anesthesia provider.

PATHOLOGY

See Anterior Cervical Fusion (Open).

POSITION:	Supine
INCISION:	Lateral neck
PREP AND DRAPING:	Neck
INSTRUMENTS:	Cervical endoscope and discectomy set; 3.5-mm 6-degree cervical endoscope, endoscopic graspers and forceps, probe, knife, rasp, burr, endoscopic bipolar forceps, imaging system

Technical Points and Discussion

1. ***The patient is prepped and draped.***
The patient is placed in the supine position with the shoulders elevated on roll-positioning devices to hyperextend the neck slightly. The surgeon marks the incision point and anatomical landmarks and checks the level of the disc using an 18-gauge spinal needle inserted into the disc under fluoroscopy. The lower face, neck, and thorax are prepped and draped as for a thyroid procedure.

2. ***An incision is made and guidewire inserted.***
A 3-mm incision is made and a guidewire stylet inserted into the needle. The needle is then removed. A 2.5- or 3.5-mm combination cannula and dilator are introduced into the disc interspace.

3. ***The annulus is incised.***
The dilator is removed and a trephine is introduced. This is used to incise the annulus (tissue layer covering the disc) in a circular pattern.

4. ***The disc is removed.***
Disc tissue is now removed by means of curettes and forceps. A discectome is introduced through the cannula. This instrument contains a high-pressure irrigation and suction system with a guillotine cutting blade, curettes, knives, and grasping forceps. The disc is removed piecemeal under endoscopic and fluoroscopic guidance. Large bone spurs can be removed by means of a burr. When all traces of tissue have been removed, the cannula and instruments are withdrawn, and the wound is closed with Steri-Strips.

POSTERIOR CERVICAL LAMINECTOMY

Posterior cervical laminectomy is performed to access the cervical spinal cord and to remove a portion of the cervical lamina. A Jackson or Allen table is used for posterior access to the cervical spine.

PATHOLOGY

Posterior cervical laminectomy may be required to access neurological tumors. Tumors may occur in the cervical spinal cord or form in the vertebral elements of the cervical spine. Patients with cervical spinal cord tumors typically experience neck pain and numbness and weakness in the upper extremities.

In older adults, cervical stenosis is a common condition that may affect the spinal cord. Cervical stenosis occurs when the discs degenerate and bone spurs form on or between the vertebral surfaces, or the ligaments in the spine buckle, causing pressure on the spinal cord. Symptoms vary, depending on the amount of compression and the location of the stenosis. Most often, symptoms include pain and numbness that radiate down the patient's arm. Cervical stenosis, left untreated, can seriously damage the spinal cord.

Traumatic injury may result in fracture of the cervical spine and damage to the spinal cord, resulting in a variety of neurological deficits, depending on the level of injury. Decompression laminectomy may be necessary to remove bone fragments and fuse or fixate the spine to prevent ongoing damage to the cord.

POSITION:	Prone with Mayfield head brace
INCISION:	Anterior neck
PREP AND DRAPING:	Laminectomy
INSTRUMENTS:	Laminectomy; posterior cervical fusion set; standard bone set; high-speed drill and burrs; fixation plates and screws

Technical Points and Discussion

1. ***The patient is anesthetized and intubated on the gurney and turned into position on the operating table.***
For safe protection of the patient's airway, the patient is anesthetized and intubated on the transport gurney. The surgical team then turns the patient onto the operating table in the prone position. The anesthesia provider manages the patient's head, continuing to protect the airway. This procedure can be reviewed in Chapter 16.

2. ***A midline incision is made.***
The surgeon marks the incision site, which is then prepped and draped. After palpating the cervical spinous processes to determine the location of the incision, the surgeon makes a midline incision using a #10 blade.
The surgeon uses sharp dissection with Metzenbaum scissors and blunt finger dissection to separate the muscle layers. The incision is then carried to the spinous processes with the ESU. Fluoroscopy is used to confirm the level. A self-retaining retractor (e.g., Beckman-Adson retractor) is placed to help maintain exposure. Dissection continues until the spinous processes are visualized.

3. ***The periosteum is removed.***
The surgeon uses a variety of periosteal elevators (e.g., Cobb or Key elevator) to clean the periosteum off the bone and gain exposure. Moistened cottonoids and Gelfoam may be used to aid hemostasis.
Intraoperative fluoroscopy is used to verify the level of the lamina after exposure is completed. A spinal needle is inserted into the disc space and used as a marker.

4. ***Bone is removed.***
The surgeon begins the laminectomy with a Leksell rongeur to remove the spinous process and then uses Kerrison rongeurs in a variety of sizes to remove smaller pieces of bone. The scrub removes pieces of bone from the instruments with a moistened 4 × 4 sponge. Bone fragments should be kept as specimens. The surgeon may also use a high-speed drill (e.g., the Midas Rex) and 3-mm burr to create an opening in the lamina. The remaining bone is taken down with the use of Kerrison up- and down-biting rongeurs. The ligamentum flavum is removed with ligamentum forceps and a #15 blade. If necessary, the disc is removed with pituitary rongeurs and curettes, as described for an anterior discectomy. A bone plate may be inserted over the defect as for anterior discectomy.

5. ***The wound is closed.***
When the laminectomy and discectomy are completed, the surgeon irrigates the wound with antibiotic solution and secures hemostasis with the ESU. The wound is closed in layers with size 0 or 1-0 polyglactin suture on a cutting needle. The skin is usually closed with staples.
The wound is dressed with a simple gauze dressing. A rigid cervical collar is applied before the patient emerges from anesthesia. The collar provides stabilization while the laminectomy heals.

THORACIC CORPECTOMY

The corpora are the body of the spine. The goal of this procedure is to remove one or more vertebrae and their discs. This is followed by a bone graft and stabilization hardware attached to the existing bone structure. The procedure is performed through a lateral thoracotomy position, with the patient in the lateral decubitus position. Refer to Chapter 16 to review this position. Thoracotomy access is described in Chapter 31.

PATHOLOGY

Corpectomy is a complex procedure performed for spinal disease, including the following:

- Spinal fractures and compression of the cord
- Primary or metastatic tumor
- Herniated disc with migration and spinal cord impingement
- Infection—osteomyelitis or discitis

Technical Points and Discussion

1. ***The patient is prepped and draped.***
The patient is placed in the lateral decubitus position. Before the prep and drape, the operative level is verified by fluoroscopy or a standard x-ray. A marker is used for reference points. The incision will be made over the rib two vertebral levels above the diseased vertebra(e). The incision follows the anatomical boundary of the rib.
2. ***The incision is made.***
A skin incision is made over the selected rib and carried into subcutaneous tissue and muscle behind the pleura. The muscle is either divided or may be retracted by means of a large rake or Richardson retractors to expose the rib. The thoracic nerve is identified to avoid being injured. The level is again checked by means of an 18-gauge spinal needle and fluoroscopy. The rib is then resected by, first, removal of the periosteum with an elevator and then excision of the rib with a rib cutter. The scrub should maintain the rib in a moist condition on the back table. The lung is collapsed by the anesthesia provider, and a rib-spreading retractor is positioned. The incision is carried to the pleura.
3. ***The pleura is incised and retracted.***
The surgeon grasps the pleura using fine-toothed forceps and incises a section. The segmental vessels are identified, clamped, and ligated with size 2-0 silk.
4. ***The discs are removed and corpectomy performed.***
The two discs are removed using pituitary rongeurs and curettes. The corpectomy (removal of the vertebrae) is then performed with Kerrison rongeurs, osteotomes, and a high-speed drill. The scrub should collect the bone pieces and keep them moist on the back table for use as a graft later in the procedure.
5. ***The corpectomy defect is reconstructed.***
The defect left by the corpectomy is now repaired. If the bone cage system is used, the patient's bone tissue with an extender or synthetic demineralized bone matrix can be used to pack the bone cage cylinder (see Posterior Lumbar Interbody Fusion). If only an autograft is used, this is taken from the iliac crest autograft (described in Anterior Cervical Fusion and Discectomy, Open).
6. ***Metal fixation plates may be used to support the graft.***
Orthopedic screws and plates can be placed at this time. To place the screws, the surgeon identifies the entrance hole of the screw. The screw holes are then drilled and tapped. One or more plates are placed across the vertebra(e) and screws inserted for fixation.
7. ***The wound is irrigated and closed.***
Hemostasis is achieved with bone putty and ESU. The wound is then irrigated and closed in layers.

Technical points are illustrated in Fig. 34.18.

POSTERIOR LUMBAR INTERBODY FUSION (PLIF)

The posterior lumbar interbody fusion (PLIF) procedure involves removal of the lumbar lamina and diseased intervertebral disc, and implantation of a bone graft in the intervertebral space to restrict movement. An alternative approach to PLIF is the ALIF, the anterior approach through the abdomen. Intervertebral bone cages are used to create stability in the space. The cage is a titanium cylinder that allows the bone graft material to fuse with existing bone while providing stability during the healing process. Bone graft material is inserted into the cage, which is then placed in the intervertebral space. Biosynthetic bone graft material is gaining in popularity over traditional use of the iliac crest autograft, which is very painful postoperatively.

PATHOLOGY

Lumbar laminectomy as a stand-alone procedure most often is performed to decompress the spinal column in cases of spinal stenosis, to remove a diseased disc, or as a step in a more extensive surgery to correct a spinal deformity.

Discectomy is used to treat a herniation of the intervertebral disc. This is a tear in the outer ring (annulus fibrosis) that allows the softer middle portion of the disc (nucleus pulposus) to bulge out. Disc herniation occurs most frequently between the fourth and fifth lumbar vertebrae or between the fifth lumbar vertebra and the sacrum. Surgery is most often performed for degenerative disc disease (DDD).

POSITION:	Prone, supine position may be used to harvest the bone graft
INCISION:	Lower midline back, iliac crest for the bone graft
PREP AND DRAPING:	Back, abdomen
INSTRUMENTS:	Laminectomy set; osteotomes and chisels; minor general surgery set
POSSIBLE EXTRAS:	Cage system for bone graft; high-speed drill with cutting burrs

Technical Points and Discussion

1. ***The patient is anesthetized, prepped, and draped.***
After induction on the gurney and placement of an endotracheal tube, the patient is placed in the prone position on a laminectomy frame (e.g., Wilson or Jackson frame) or a specialized spinal operating table. Note that if an autograft is to be used, the patient is placed in the supine

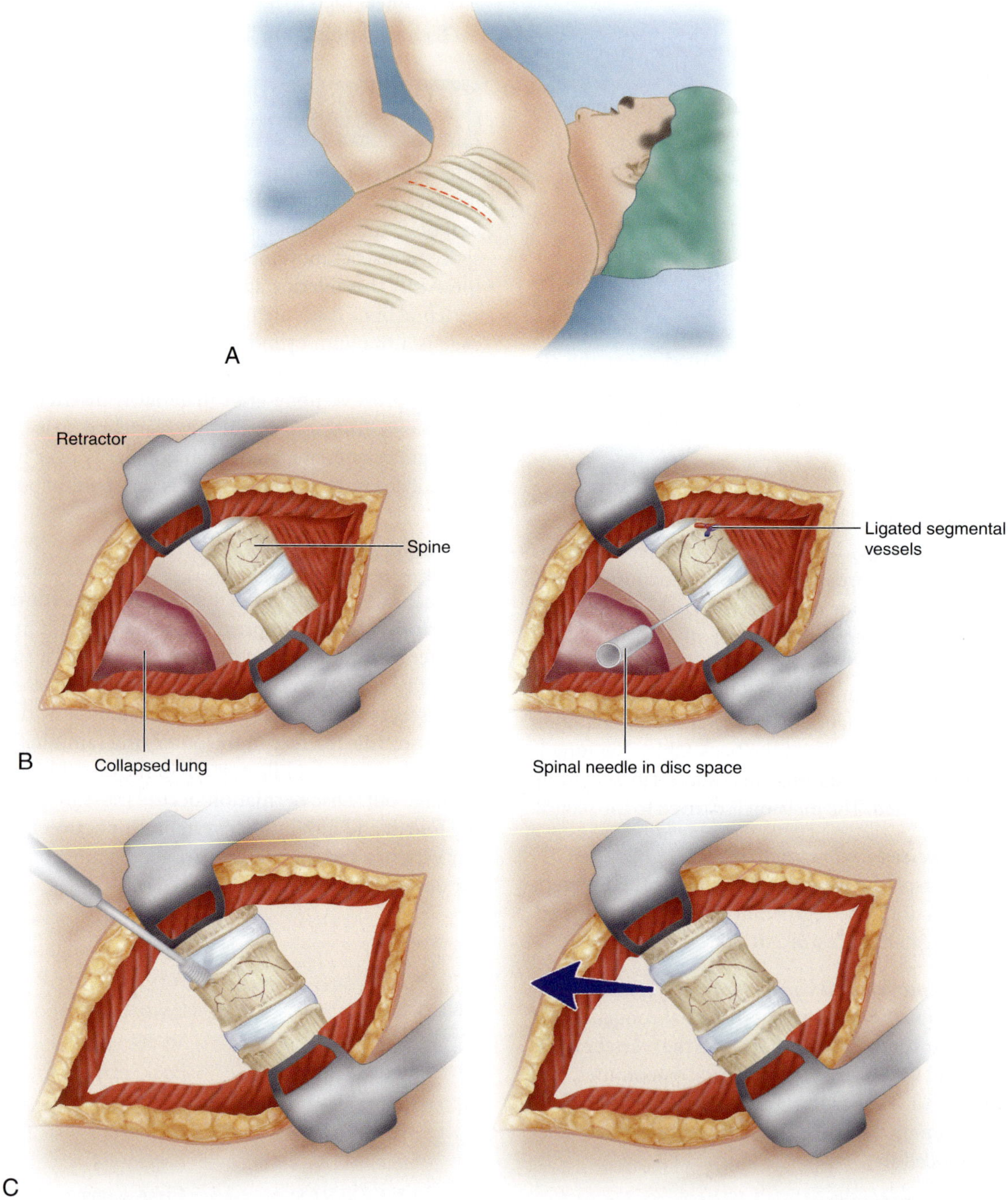

FIG. 34.18 Thoracic corpectomy. (A) A posterolateral incision is made. A rib may be removed for access to the spine. (B) The incision is carried across or behind the pleura. This exposes the spine. A needle is inserted into the affected disc to validate the level on fluoroscopy. (C) The pedicle (bony connection between the lamina and body of the vertebra) is taken down with a high-speed drill and Kerrison rongeur. This exposes the spinal canal.

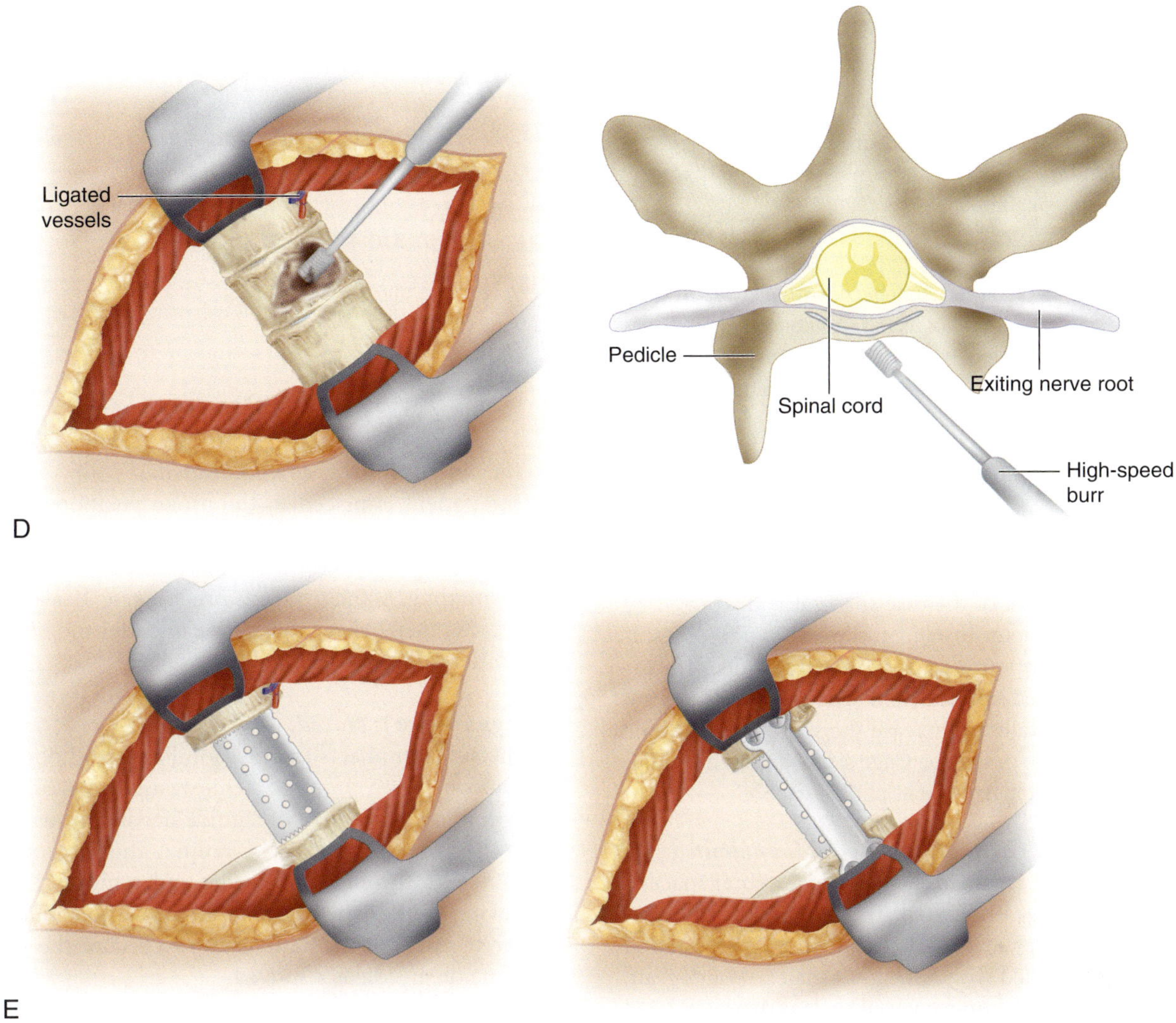

FIG. 34.18, cont'd (D) The corpectomy is performed with the high-speed drill and rongeurs, leaving some bone for support. (E) The corpectomy defect is supported with a bone cage packed with bone graft material. (From Jandial R, McCormick P, Black P, eds. *Core Techniques in Operative Neurosurgery.* Philadelphia: Elsevier; 2011.)

position for this part of the procedure and then turned to the prone position for the posterior procedure. (Refer to Anterior Cervical Discectomy and Fusion for a description of the bone graft harvesting procedure.)

2. ***The incision is made.***
To begin the anterior procedure, the surgeon may inject the incisional site with a small amount of local anesthetic with epinephrine to aid hemostasis. A midline vertical incision is made over the spine with a #20 knife blade. The surgeon deepens the wound with the knife or monopolar ESU to the level of the fascia. The fascia is dissected with toothed forceps and the monopolar ESU. Two angled Weitlaner or Beckman retractors are inserted into the wound for better exposure.

3. ***The wound is packed.***
The scrub should have a large number of unfolded 4 × 4 sponges available at this time. The surgeon packs the sponges along the vertebrae with periosteal elevators. This is done both to aid hemostasis and to expose the vertebrae by retracting the larger back muscles. Because the wound is now deep, the surgeon may replace the wound retractors with Meyerding or Taylor retractors. Fluoroscopy is used to verify the correct level. A spinal needle is inserted into the proposed space for identification.

4. ***The lamina is excised.***
The surgeon uses a large rongeur to remove small pieces of the spinous process and expose the lamina. Up- and down-biting Kerrison rongeurs then are used to excise the lamina and create access to the disc. As with all laminectomy procedures, the scrub may be required to clean the tip of the rongeur as it is presented after each bite of the rongeur.

The surgeon may also use a high-speed drill with a cutting burr to remove the bony facets. Any bone chips removed must be retained as specimens. After the lamina has been removed, cottonoid sponges are used instead of 4 × 4 sponges. To prevent the dura from tearing, the surgeon uses a nerve hook or Freer-type elevator to loosen any dura attached to the lamina. The scrub should have bone putty prepared to help control bleeding.

5. ***The ligamentum flavum is incised.***
The surgeon identifies the ligamentum flavum (one of the ligaments that connects each vertebra to the next) and incises it with a #15 knife blade mounted on a #7 handle. Down-biting Kerrison rongeurs are used to remove any ligament that obstructs the surgeon's view of the disc. The disc is now approachable.

6. ***The disc is removed.***
The assistant retracts the vertebral nerve with a Love retractor or similar nerve root retractor as the surgeon snips off pieces of the bulging disc with a Takahashi or pituitary rongeur. As the disc is removed, the surgeon may use a curette for further evacuation. These specimens should be kept separate from the bone fragments previously retrieved. The scrub must remain alert during this maneuver to keep the instrument tips clean, because the surgeon cannot turn away from the wound.

7. ***The disc space is distracted.***
For increased height of the disc space, it is distracted by means of the distractor instrument, which is part of a spinal fusion set. Distraction means to separate bone. The instrument is inserted into the joint space, and the jaws are opened incrementally to increase the space. This is done under fluoroscopic guidance. Cage sizers are then used to verify the correct measurement of the space.

8. ***A cage system with bone graft material is implanted.***
For stability to be regained in the intervertebral space, a device called a *cage* is inserted. This is a hollow titanium cylinder. The cages are inserted into the intervertebral space and are packed with bone graft material (autograft, cadaver, or synthetic bone material such as demineralized bone matrix). A cage system introducer is used to place the cage in the intervertebral space.

9. ***Fixation screws and plates may be inserted.***
Pedicle screws and plates may be used to provide further stability. A commercial system of spinal fusion instruments and plates is used according to the manufacturer's technical directions.

10. ***The wound is closed.***
After final fluoroscopic assessment of the repair has been made, the wound is irrigated and closed. The fascial layer is usually closed with size 0 absorbable synthetic sutures and a large cutting needle. Before closing the muscle layer, the surgeon may inject a long-acting local anesthetic to control postoperative pain. The muscle and subcutaneous layers are closed with 2-0 sutures. The skin is closed with staples or nonabsorbable synthetic sutures. The wound is dressed in routine fashion. Technical points are shown in Fig. 34.19.

MINIMALLY INVASIVE LUMBAR DISCECTOMY

During microdiscectomy, a small window is made in the lamina for access to an intervertebral disc. This is a minimally invasive approach to lumbar laminectomy and discectomy. Microdiscectomy may be performed with the patient under general anesthesia, local anesthesia, or local anesthesia with sedation.

PATHOLOGY

See Posterior Lumbar Interbody Fusion

POSITION:	Prone using Andrews table or spinal frame
INCISION:	Lumbar spine
PREP AND DRAPING:	Lumbar
INSTRUMENTS:	Spinal endoscopic set with instruments; minor set; bipolar ESU

Technical Points and Discussion

1. ***The patient is prepped and draped.***
The patient is placed in the prone position on a spinal frame or on an Andrews table. If general anesthesia is used, induction and intubation take place before patient positioning. Some surgeons prefer using local anesthesia, because they believe that they can better monitor the patient's responses to pain.

2. ***A guidewire is placed.***
The surgeon injects the incision line with lidocaine with epinephrine to promote hemostasis. The C-arm is used to confirm placement of a guide needle through the skin to the level of the affected lamina. The surgeon passes a guidewire through the needle and removes the needle, leaving the guidewire in place. The scrub should be prepared with a hemostatic clamp to secure the guidewire while the needle is removed.

3. ***A dilator is placed over the guidewire.***
A dilating tube is placed over the guidewire to separate the soft tissue and muscle. The surgeon removes the guidewire and leaves the dilating tube in place. A sequence of progressively larger tubes is placed over the existing tube to further dilate the space.

4. ***A cannula is placed over the dilating tubes and docked on the lamina.***
A cannula is placed over the dilating tubes and docked on the lamina. The retractor is secured to a post that clamps onto the operating bed for stability. The dilating tubes are removed, leaving the cannula in place. The operating microscope is positioned and adjusted. Alternately, an endoscope attached to a camera and monitoring system may be used.

5. ***Muscle and other soft tissue are removed from the lamina.***
The scrub places a long electrode on the monopolar ESU, and the surgeon uses it through the tubular retractor to remove any remaining muscle or soft tissue overlying the lamina. A small window of bone is removed through the retractor with a Kerrison or Leksell rongeur. Some surgeons prefer to use a high-speed power drill with a long cutting burr for removing the bone. The surgeon removes a window of bone, preserving the ligamentum flavum underneath to protect the dura.

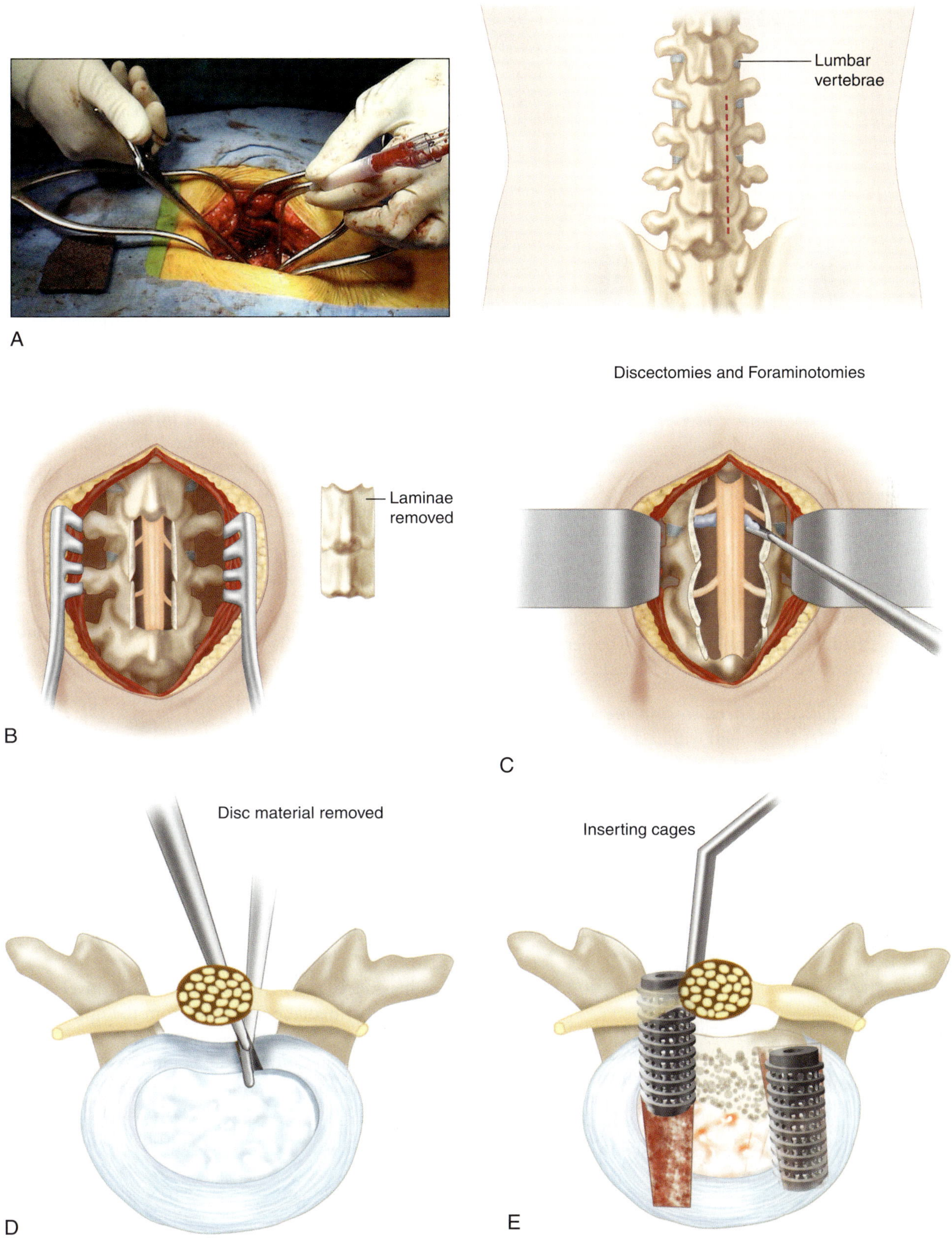

FIG. 34.19 Posterior lumbar interbody fusion (PLIF). (A) A midline spinal incision is made and carried to the spinal column. (B) A laminectomy is performed. Note Beckman retractor in place. (C) The foramen (spaces between vertebrae housing the spinal nerves) is opened up to create more space for the spinal nerves. The disc annulus is incised. (D) The disc is removed by means of pituitary rongeurs and curettes. (E) Bone grafts and cages are placed in the disc space.

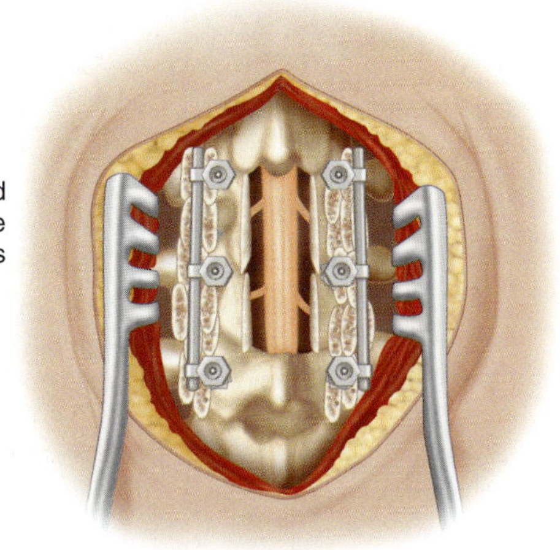

FIG. 34.19, cont'd (F) Plates and screws may be implanted for increased support. (From Jandial R, McCormick P, Black P, eds. *Core Techniques in Operative Neurosurgery.* Philadelphia: Elsevier; 2011.)

6. ***The disc is exposed and removed.***
A nerve root retractor is passed through the tubular retractor, and the nerve root is gently retracted. The epidural veins are coagulated with the bipolar ESU and dissected off the disc space. An endoscopic knife is used to incise the disc surface. The surgeon uses disc rongeurs to remove any extruded portions of the disc. The nerve root retractor is removed and the area is inspected.

7. ***The wound is irrigated and hemostasis achieved.***
The surgeon irrigates the wound with lactated Ringer solution to ensure that all debris is cleared and to visualize any areas of bleeding. Any necessary hemostasis is accomplished with the bipolar ESU and Gelfoam pledgets soaked in topical thrombin.

8. ***The wound is closed.***
The tubular retractor is removed. The wound edges are approximated with Steri-Strips or Dermabond glue.

RHIZOTOMY

This procedure is performed to relieve pain originating in the facet joints. Degenerative disease and bone spurs, which impinge on the nerves, may develop in the joints. In the procedure, the nerves are detached on both sides by bipolar ESU. The approach is through the skin, with a metal sheath and dilators used to make space for the bipolar ESU. The procedure is performed with the patient under local anesthetic.

POSITION:	Prone
INCISION:	Bilateral over the diseased facet joints
PREP AND DRAPING:	As for laminectomy
INSTRUMENTS:	Minimally invasive retractor and dilator system; monopolar ESU; rhizotomy set

Technical Points and Discussion

1. ***The facet joints are verified on fluoroscopy.***
The patient is placed in the prone position on the operating table. Using fluoroscopy, the surgeon uses a spinal needle to localize the facet joints. The levels and entry points are marked on the skin. The patient is then prepped and draped.

2. ***An incision is made over the entry point.***
The surgeon injects local anesthetic into the operative entry point. Using a #10 blade, the surgeon makes a small incision in the skin and subcutaneous tissue.

3. ***An introducer is placed in the tissue over the facet.***
The introducer acts as a probe, which tunnels through the soft tissue, leaving a tract for the next instruments. This is done under fluoroscopy for guidance.

4. ***Dilators are inserted over the introducer.***
Dilators are inserted over the introducer to widen the tract and provide retraction.

5. ***The nerve is visualized and removed.***
Using the bipolar ESU, the surgeon removes the nerve attachment from the facet joint.

6. ***The procedure is performed on the opposite side.***
The incisions are closed with fibrin adhesive and Steri-Strips.

PERIPHERAL NERVE PROCEDURES

ULNAR NERVE TRANSPOSITION

The surgical goal of an ulnar nerve transposition is to free the ulnar nerve from a groove on the medial epicondyle, thereby restoring function and eliminating desensitization of the affected arm. The surgery is performed with use of the pneumatic tourniquet. Local anesthesia may be used.

Pathology

The ulnar nerve is a peripheral nerve that travels through the groove of the medial epicondyle from the upper to the lower arm. The ulnar nerve can be injured by trauma, elbow fractures, dislocations, and repeated bending of the elbow as part of occupational or recreational activities. Symptoms generally include reduced sensation in the affected arm, hand atrophy, or, in severe cases, a clawhand deformity.

POSITION:	Supine with the arm on an operative arm board
INCISION:	Upper arm between the medial epicondyle and olecranon
PREP AND DRAPING:	Upper arm
INSTRUMENTS:	Basic general surgery set; nerve retractors; medium and small self-retaining retractors; bipolar ESU

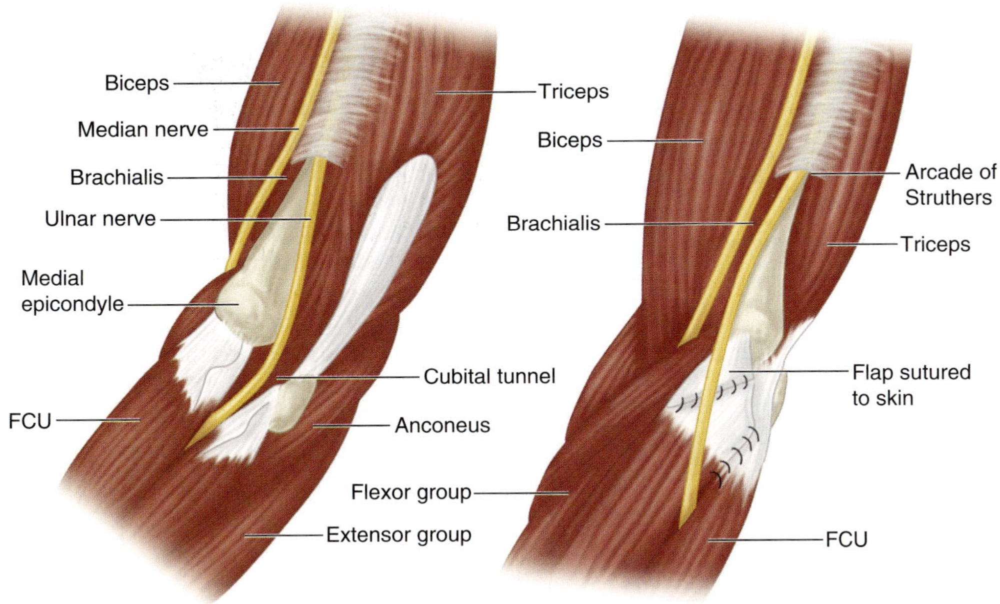

FIG. 34.20 Entrapment of the ulnar nerve and transposition. These two figures show the trapped nerve *(left)* and creation of a fascia sling, which prevents the nerve from re-entering the cubital tunnel *(right)*. (From Lee D, Neviaser R. *Operative Techniques: Shoulder and Elbow Surgery*. Philadelphia: Saunders Elsevier; 2011.)

Technical Points and Discussion

1. ***The patient is prepped and draped.***
The patient is placed in the supine position with the operative arm on an arm table, suspended over the patient, or laid across the patient's body, depending on the surgeon's preference. A pneumatic tourniquet is applied to the upper arm, and the procedure for exsanguination is performed.

2. ***The incision is made.***
The surgeon makes the skin incision over the median epicondyle. Using blunt and sharp dissection with Metzenbaum scissors, the surgeon mobilizes the ulnar nerve. Delicate scissors are used to free a section of the nerve, and moist umbilical tapes, vessel loops, or a Penrose drain is looped around the nerve to aid manipulation.

3. ***A fascia flap is developed.***
The surgeon continues the dissection around the nerve to free a portion extending from above the elbow to below the elbow. A flap of fascia over the medial epicondyle is created with scissors. The nerve then is transposed from the groove at the back of the medial epicondyle of the humerus to the front of the epicondyle and positioned under the fascial flap.

4. ***The flap is sutured.***
The fascial flap is loosely approximated with 2-0 Dexon sutures to protect the nerve. The tourniquet pressure is released, and the wound is checked for bleeders. The bipolar or monopolar ESU is used for hemostasis as needed.

5. ***The wound is closed.***
The wound is irrigated with sterile saline or an antibiotic solution, closed in layers with Dexon suture, and dressed with gauze. A splint or cast is applied to the arm.

Transposition of the ulnar nerve is illustrated in Fig. 34.20.

CARPAL TUNNEL RELEASE

The goal of surgical carpal tunnel release is to free an entrapped median volar nerve and restore function of the wrist. An open or a minimally invasive technique may be used. The procedure is performed under regional or general anesthesia. A pneumatic tourniquet is used to create a bloodless field. The open technique is described here.

PATHOLOGY

Carpal tunnel syndrome occurs when the median nerve in the carpal tunnel of the wrist is compressed. A variety of factors may contribute to nerve compression, including an anatomical decrease in the size of the carpal tunnel, wrist fracture, post-traumatic arthritis, and inflammatory disease, such as rheumatoid arthritis. External conditions, such as vibration, prolonged direct pressure, and repetitive movement, may contribute to or trigger the condition. Carpal tunnel syndrome occurs most often in adults from 30 to 60 years of age and is more common in women than in men. Patients experience numbness and tingling in the fingers and pain in the hand that often radiates up the forearm.

POSITION:	Supine with arm on a hand table
INCISION:	Palm of the hand
PREP AND DRAPING:	Hand
INSTRUMENTS:	Plastic surgery handset; bipolar ESU; vessel loops

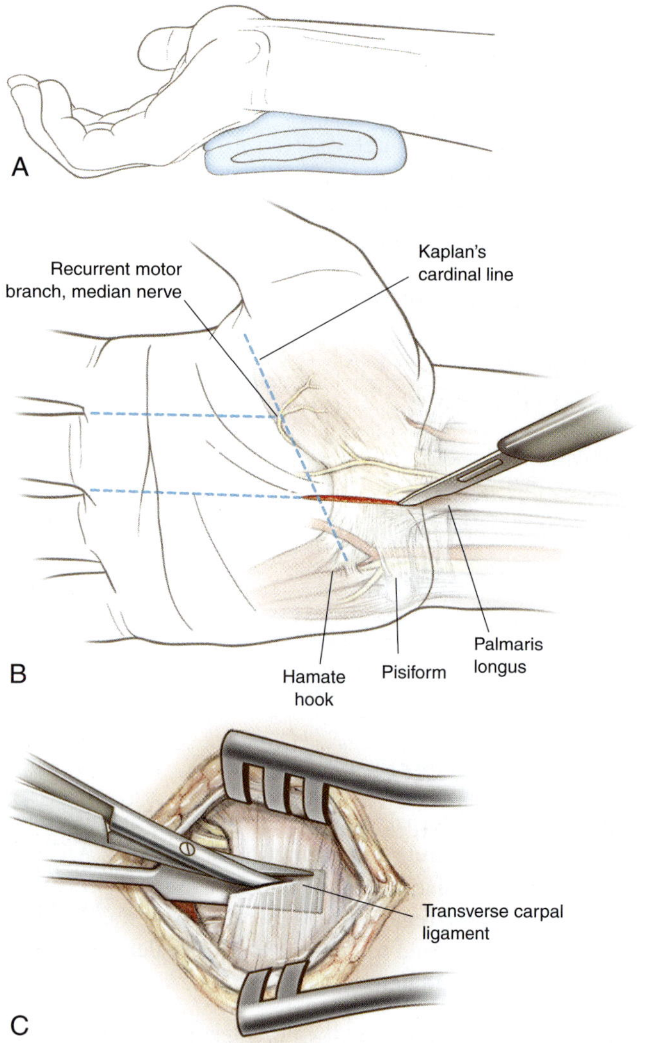

FIG. 34.21 Open carpal tunnel release. (A) Position of the hand for surgery. (B) Skin incision and anatomy. (C) Exposure of the median nerve with fine dissecting scissors. (From Miller MD, Chlabra AB, Hurwitz SR, Milhalko WM. *Orthopaedic Surgical Approaches*. Philadelphia: WB Saunders; 2008.)

Technical Points and Discussion

1. ***The patient is prepped and draped.***
The patient is positioned supine on the operating room table with the affected arm resting on a hand table.

2. ***A curvilinear or longitudinal incision is made in the palm and extended to the wrist.***
The surgeon uses a #15 blade to create a longitudinal or curvilinear incision in the skin (Fig. 34.21). Blunt dissection with small Metzenbaum scissors exposes the fascia, which is retracted with small Weitlaner retractors, skin hooks, or sharp Senn retractors. The flexor tendon is exposed and retracted. The surgeon identifies both the flexor tendon and the neurovascular bundle that lies close to the tendon.

3. ***The carpal ligament is retracted and divided.***
The transverse carpal ligament is then visualized, and the midsection is incised with a #15 blade. Tenotomy scissors are used to lengthen the incision to release the carpal ligament and median nerve. A small curved clamp may be passed under the tendon along its length to verify that all attachments have been released. The incision is irrigated with sterile saline.

4. ***The tourniquet is deflated and the wound is inspected for bleeding.***
The tourniquet pressure is released and the wound is checked for bleeders, which are controlled with the bipolar ESU.

5. ***The wound is closed.***
The surgeon may inject the incision with bupivacaine to control postoperative pain. The connective tissue is closed with size 3-0 Vicryl sutures. Skin is closed with an absorbable subcuticular suture or interrupted nylon size 3-0. A bulky compression dressing of gauze fluffs and a splint is applied.

Arthroscopic Technique

Carpal tunnel release may also be performed as minimally invasive surgery (MIS) with EndoWrist instruments. The anesthesia considerations, prepping, draping, and tourniquet use are as described for open carpal tunnel release. An advantage of the endoscopic approach is that it uses one or two small incisions over the palm of the hand instead of the extensive incision described for the open approach. The carpal ligament is directly below the incisions, in the distal area of the palm just below the wrist. The carpal ligament is incised longitudinally. This releases the pressure on the nerve as it passes through the ligament. Wound closure and dressing application are as described for the open technique.

Carpal tunnel release is most often performed in the outpatient setting, and the patient is discharged within hours of the procedure. Immediate and long-term postoperative complications are rare.

PERIPHERAL NERVE RESECTION AND REPAIR

In peripheral nerve repair, a severed nerve, usually in the hand or forearm, is anastomosed to restore function. The procedure to repair a severed peripheral nerve is usually performed as an emergency. If nerve repair is delayed, the risk of a poor outcome increases. Common methods of peripheral nerve repair are the funicular suture technique and the epineural suture technique. In the funicular technique, the funiculi (the fibers that make up the nerve) are joined individually. In the epineural technique, the epineurium (the component of connective tissue that surrounds the nerve) is anastomosed and the individual funiculi are not sutured together. An alternative to direct anastomosis of the severed ends or transplanted autograft is the use of a biograft *nerve conduit*. This is a commercially available biograft that can be used to bridge nerve gaps of less than 3 mm.

PATHOLOGY

Peripheral nerve injuries are commonly caused by industrial or home accidents involving tools or machinery. Successful repair depends on the patient's age, the extent of injury to adjacent tissue, and the type of injury to the nerve. An injury may be a clean-cut type (e.g., caused by a sharp object such as a knife or glass shard) or an injury that causes the nerve to shatter. If the nerve is severely damaged, it may be replaced with a nerve graft taken from another location in the body. The procedure described here is an upper extremity nerve repair. Note that the procedure may be performed using the operating microscope.

POSITION:	Supine with operative arm on hand table
INCISION:	Hand
PREP AND DRAPING:	Hand and arm
INSTRUMENTS:	Microinstruments; hand retraction system; bipolar ESU, balanced salt solution for irrigation; operating microscope; surgical loupes
POSSIBLE EXTRAS:	Nerve stimulator

Technical Points and Discussion

1. ***The patient is positioned supine with the arm resting on the hand table.***
The patient is positioned supine with the affected arm or hand resting on a hand table. A pneumatic tourniquet is used as previously described. If the limb has been extensively damaged, the surgeon may debride (excise any devitalized or ragged tissue) before beginning the nerve repair. Debridement usually takes place in conjunction with the skin prep or immediately after it. If the surgeon wants to perform the skin prep and debridement, the scrub or circulator should supply the surgeon with sterile saline solution, sponges, antiseptic soap, a fine scalpel, tissue forceps, and dissecting scissors.
When debridement has been completed, the limb is draped in routine fashion, and the tourniquet is inflated. Some surgeons drape the limb first and then perform the debridement.

2. ***The injured nerve is mobilized.***
The first step of the actual procedure is the mobilization of the injured nerve. The surgeon uses fine dissecting scissors and thumb forceps to gently free the severed nerve from its surrounding tissue.

3. ***The nerve is trimmed.***
Before the anastomosis is started, the jagged ends of the nerve must be severed. Two fine traction sutures are placed through each end of the nerve and are used to bring the nerve ends into approximation. The surgeon incises the ends of the nerve with a #15 blade to ensure that the damaged fibers are removed and clean edges are available for the anastomosis. A moistened wooden tongue blade or Silastic block may be used as a firm surface on which to place the nerve. The nerve ends are cut serially in 1-mm slices under the operating microscope until the ends appear satisfactory for anastomosis.

4. ***The nerve is repaired.***
In the epineural technique, the surgeon places several 6-0 or 7-0 nylon sutures, one through each quadrant of the nerve. For funicular repair, each individual funiculus is joined with interrupted sutures of 10-0 nylon. During the anastomosis, the scrub should irrigate the nerve frequently with balanced saline solution, to prevent the nerve from drying out.

5. ***The nerve graft is prepared and implanted.***
If a nerve conduit is used, the surgical technologist places the appropriately sized collagen graft in sterile saline for 5 minutes, or according to the manufacturer's instructions. After soaking, the graft will assume a hydrated appearance and is ready for use. Size 8-0 or 9-0 nylon sutures are used to attach the graft. The severed ends of the nerve are threaded inside the graft, and four mattress sutures are used to tack the graft in place at each end. The wound is then irrigated with normal saline or lactated Ringer solution before wound closure.

6. ***The wound is closed and dressed.***
After the repair, the tourniquet is released and the wound bed is inspected for bleeders. Hemostasis is maintained with the bipolar ESU, Gelfoam strips, and topical thrombin as necessary. The tissue layers are approximated with 3-0 and 4-0 polyglactin interrupted sutures. A dressing of cotton gauze and plaster splints or other casting material is used to immobilize the limb until healing is complete.

Fig. 34.22 illustrates the technique used in peripheral nerve repair.

KEY CONCEPTS

- Neurosurgery is a specialty encompassing procedures of the brain and cranium, spine, and peripheral nerves.
- In preparation for brain surgery, the patient's head is usually positioned over the edge of the operating table and secured by sharp tongs or metal pins that are inserted into the bone and attached to a head brace.
- The scalp is highly vascular, requiring special preparation for hemostasis. Scalp (Raney) clips are placed close together over the edges of the incision to prevent bleeding during surgery. These are removed before wound closure.
- Access to the brain for open procedures requires the creation of a bone flap. This is a plate of bone lifted at the beginning of the procedure and replaced at wound closure.
- A craniotome is a specialty drill used to create burr holes for cranial access. This drill is fitted with a special guard that prevents the drill from entering soft tissue (i.e., the dura).
- Methods of hemostasis used during neurosurgery include neurosponges (patties), cotton balls, bipolar and monopolar coagulation, topical thrombin, local filtration with anesthetic and epinephrine, and topical hemostatic agents such as Gelfoam, Avitene, and Surgicel.
- It is vital that the tissues exposed during neurosurgery be kept moist throughout the procedure. Common methods

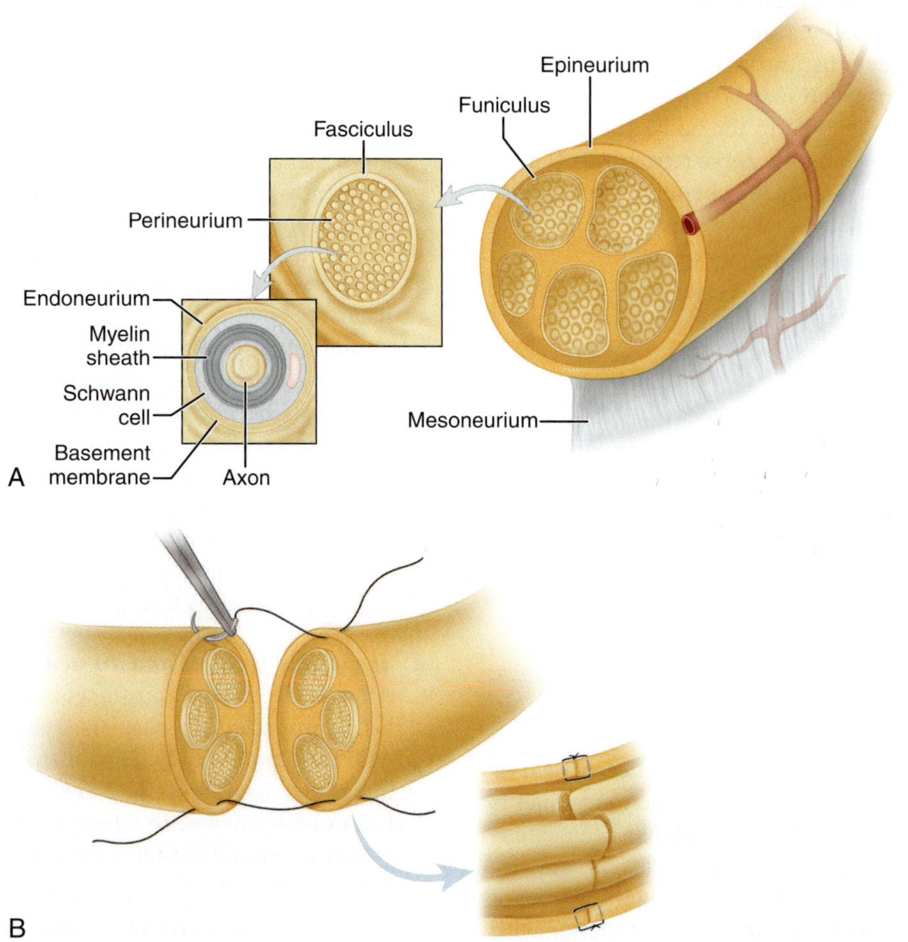

FIG. 34.22 Peripheral nerve repair. (A) Basic anatomy of a nerve. Note that individual nerve fibers called funiculi are bundled and covered by a protective layer (epineurium). (B) During repair, the epineurium alone can be joined by suture as shown. (From Canale S, Beaty J, eds. *Campbell's Operative Orthopaedics*. 12th ed. Philadelphia: Elsevier Mosby; 2013.)

are topical irrigation, application of wet Telfa strips, and moist surgical sponges.

- During cranioplasty, a section of the cranium is replaced with allograft bone, a metal plate, or synthetic cements in combination with mesh devices.
- Transsphenoidal surgery requires multidisciplinary techniques involving the nasal sinuses and bones and those of the floor of the cranial cavity.
- Impingement of the spinal cord or nerves can cause pain and may result in neurological symptoms such as numbness or paralysis.
- There are many different techniques used to stabilize the spine after removal of the pedicles, lamina, and disc. The most common technique is to replace the disc with an autograft from the hip or rib. This can be packed into the space as is, or contained in a metal mesh cage that provides strength while the transplanted bone fuses with the existing bone of the spine. Plates and screws are also used to support the vertebra(e).
- The goal of all nerve entrapment surgery is to release the bone or soft connective tissues causing the constriction.

REVIEW QUESTIONS

1. Why is hemostasis particularly important during cranial surgery?
2. How does the body normally shunt CSF out of the brain?
3. What precautions should be taken to prevent loss of or damage to the bone flap during craniotomy?
4. Why are burr holes required to remove a bone flap?
5. Name several specialty instrument sets that may be needed during neurosurgery.
6. Neurosurgical procedures can be lengthy. What safety and environmental precautions are particularly important to protect the patient from injury during a long procedure?
7. The Fowler position carries a high risk of embolism. Explain why.
8. Why is a subdural hematoma an emergency condition?
9. What methods of hemostasis are used during cranial surgery?
10. During laminectomy, small bits of bone are removed from the lamina in rapid succession. What is the role of the scrub during this part of the procedure?

11. In what cranial procedures might a fat graft be needed?
12. Describe the supplies that may be needed for debridement of a hand after an industrial accident.

BIBLIOGRAPHY

Asthagiri A, Pouratian N, Sherman J, et al. Advances in brain tumor surgery. *Neurol Clin*. 2007;25:975.

Brackmann DE, Green JD. Translabyrinth approach for acoustic tumor removal. *Neurosurg Clin North Am*. 2008;19:251.

Brown JA. Principles of pain management. In: Rengachary SS, Ellenbogen RG, eds. *Principles of Neurosurgery*. 2nd ed. St. Louis: Mosby; 2005.

Canale S, Beaty J, eds. *Campbell's Operative Orthopaedics*. 12th ed. Philadelphia: Elsevier Mosby; 2013.

Drake JM, Iantosca MR. Cerebrospinal fluid shunting and management of pediatric hydrocephalus. In: Schmidek HH, Roberts DW, eds. *Operative Neurosurgical Techniques: Indications, Methods and Results*. 5th ed. Philadelphia: WB Saunders; 2006.

Drummond JC, Patel PM. Neurosurgical anesthesia. In: Miller RD, ed. *Miller's Anesthesia*. 6th ed. Philadelphia: Churchill Livingstone; 2005.

Fanciullo GJ, Ball PA. Spinal cord stimulation and intraspinal infusions for pain. In: Schmidek HH, Roberts DW, eds. *Operative Neurosurgical Techniques: Indications, Methods and Results*. 5th ed. Philadelphia: WB Saunders; 2006.

Freeman BL. Scoliosis and kyphosis. In: Canale ST, Beaty JH, eds. *Campbell's Operative Orthopaedics*. 11th ed. Philadelphia: Mosby; 2008.

Jandial R, McCormick P, Black P, eds. *Core Techniques in Operative Neurosurgery*. Philadelphia: Elsevier; 2011.

Jobe MT, Martinez SF. Peripheral nerve injuries. In: Canale ST, Beaty JH, eds. *Campbell's Operative Orthopaedics*. 11th ed. Philadelphia: Mosby; 2008.

Kim D, Kim K, Kim Y, eds. *Minimally Invasive Percutaneous Spinal Techniques*. Philadelphia: Elsevier; 2011.

Lonser RR. Apfelbaum RI: Neurovascular decompression in surgical disorders of cranial nerves V, VII, IX, and X. In: Schmidek HH, Roberts DW, eds. *Operative Neurosurgical Techniques: Indications, Methods and Results*. 5th ed. Philadelphia: WB Saunders; 2006.

Polletti CE. Open cordotomy and medullary tractotomy. In: Schmidek HH, Roberts DW, eds. *Operative Neurosurgical Techniques: Indications, Methods and Results*. 5th ed. Philadelphia: WB Saunders; 2006.

Roberts GA, Dacey RG. General techniques of aneurysm surgery. In: LeRoux PD, Winn HR, Newell DW, eds. *Management of Cerebral Aneurysms*. Philadelphia: WB Saunders; 2004.

Schmidek HH, Roberts DW, eds. *Schmidek and Sweet's Operative Neurosurgical Techniques: Indications, Methods and Results*. 5th ed. Philadelphia: WB Saunders; 2006.

Seidel HM, Ball JW, Dains JE, Benedict GW, eds. *Mosby's Guide to Physical Examination*. 6th ed. St. Louis: Mosby; 2007.

Shen FH, Samartzis D, Khanna AJ, Anderson DG. Minimally invasive techniques for lumbar interbody fusions. *Orthoped Clin North Am*. 2007;38:373.

St-Arnaud D, Paquin M. Safe positioning for neurosurgical patients. *AORN J*. 2008;87:1156.

Sugarman RA. Structure and function of the neurologic system. In: McCance KL, Huether SE, eds. *Pathophysiology: The Biologic Basis for Disease in Adults and Children*. 5th ed. St. Louis: Mosby; 2006.

Sutton LN. Spinal dysraphism. In: Rengachary SS, Ellenbogen RG, eds. *Principles of Neurosurgery*. 2nd ed. St. Louis: Mosby; 2005.

Tarlov EC, Magge SN. Microsurgery of ruptured lumbar intervertebral disc. In: Schmidek HH, Roberts DW, eds. *Operative Neurosurgical Techniques: Indications, Methods and Results*. 5th ed. Philadelphia: WB Saunders; 2006.

U.S. Food and Drug Administration. *Medical Device Reporting*; 2016. https://www.fda.gov/medical-devices/medical-device-safety/medical-device-reporting-mdr-how-report-medical-device-problems. Accessed September 5, 2019.

Wang PP, Avellino AA. Hydrocephalus in children. In: Rengachary SS, Ellenbogen RG, eds. *Principles of Neurosurgery*. 2nd ed. St. Louis: Mosby; 2005.

Wright PE. Carpal tunnel, ulnar tunnel, and stenosing tenosynovitis. In: Canale ST, Beaty JH, eds. *Campbell's Operative Orthopaedics*. 11th ed. Philadelphia: Mosby; 2008.

Yaremchuk MJ. Surgical repair of major defects of the scalp and skull. In: Schmidek HH, Roberts DW, eds. *Operative Neurosurgical Techniques: Indications, Methods and Results*. 5th ed. Philadelphia: WB Saunders; 2006.

Yeung AT, Yeung CA. Minimally invasive techniques for the management of lumbar disc herniation. *Orthoped Clin Nor Am*. 2007;38:363.

35 EMERGENCY TRAUMA SURGERY

LEARNING OBJECTIVES

After studying this chapter, the reader will be able to:

1. Explain the trauma system used in the United States
2. Describe the lethal triangle of trauma physiology
3. Discuss compartment syndrome
4. Describe the principles of Advanced Trauma Life Support (ATLS) trauma management
5. Explain what is meant by *damage control surgery*
6. Discuss the elements of case planning for common trauma surgeries

TERMINOLOGY

Advanced Trauma Life Support (ATLS): A program established by the American College of Surgeons for protocols and training in trauma medicine.

Algorithms: Treatment pathways established to allow systematic and consistent methods of medical and surgical management.

Blunt injury: Trauma that results in deep tissue injury without rupture of the skin.

Cardiac rupture: Tearing of the atria or ventricles as a result of trauma.

Cardiac tamponade: Pressure on the heart, causing restriction and damage to the conduction system.

Coagulopathy: Condition in which the body's normal blood clotting mechanism ceases to function, characteristic in severe multi-trauma.

Compartment syndrome: Increased pressure in any compartment of the body such as the cranium, abdominal cavity, or a limb caused by trauma.

Contusions: Bruising.

Damage control surgery: Surgery whose objective is to stop hemorrhage and prevent sepsis without attempting reconstruction or anatomical continuity.

Definitive diagnosis: Evidence-based diagnosis of a medical problem using normal investigative procedures such as imaging studies.

Definitive procedure: A planned surgical procedure, usually with specific objectives for reconstruction or restoring function of anatomical structures.

Exsanguinating: Hemorrhage with the potential to deplete the patient's total blood volume.

Flail chest: Rib fracture in at least three adjacent ribs at both points of attachment. This condition requires immediate surgery.

Focused assessment with ultrasound for trauma (FAST): A protocol of ATLS in which ultrasound is used in a focused area to diagnose severe trauma.

Hemorrhagic shock: A type of shock characterized by vascular failure resulting from severe bleeding.

Hemothorax: Bleeding into the pleural space.

Metabolic acidosis: A potentially lethal physiological condition occurring in shock, characterized by abnormally low blood pH.

Occult injury: An injury that is not detected in normal assessment procedures.

Penetrating injury: Tissue damage that occurs when an object enters the body through the skin or the body is propelled against an object, breaking the skin.

Pneumothorax: Injury that results in air in the pleural space causing displacement or collapse of the respiratory structures.

Resuscitation: In trauma medicine, the process of restoring physiological balance after severe trauma.

Trauma is the leading cause of death among individuals between the age of 1 and 45 years and the third leading cause of death in all age groups. The World Health Organization predicts that injury will be the leading cause of death and disability in all age groups by 2020. Most civilian trauma patients arrive at the emergency department after normal working hours and on weekends, when fewer staff members are available. A systems approach is used to focus all available resources on lifesaving measures.

The current principles of trauma medicine and surgery have been heavily influenced by the work of US armed forces in Iraq and Afghanistan. As a result of these experiences, new trauma techniques have been developed, especially in the areas of resuscitation and staged surgical repair. At the same time, older procedures that were thought to be lifesaving in the civilian environment have been refined or discarded. For example, in the 1970s and 1980s, full-body pneumatic anti-shock garments were routinely used to control exsanguinating injuries. The device—a tubular pneumatic body suit—was placed on the victim and then inflated as a tamponade against severe hypotension in the trunk area. Although the results did raise the victim's blood pressure, many patients inevitably died as a result of blood loss related to hypertension caused by the device. Some blood-clotting products that were developed for battle situations caused severe burns, and some increased the hemorrhage on removal. These products, however, led to the development of more sophisticated resuscitation techniques and chemical hemostatics that are used in both civilian and military medicine.

This chapter is an introduction to the fundamentals of trauma surgery. The material in this discussion assumes that the surgical technologist has already acquired more than minimal training in all aspects of the nonemergency role and is ready to approach the more intense study of trauma surgery. The new vocabulary and concepts introduced here serve as a basis for increased learning by practice. Naturally, there will be variations on these practices and specific methodologies. However, the principles of trauma care are fairly constant.

Preparation of the surgical technologist in an emergency role involves several important domains of practice. Most of the skills acquired in routine surgical procedures contribute to advanced practice in emergency situations. Although some additional techniques are necessary, the focus is more on *how* these familiar skills are applied, and above all, *prioritization* of tasks.

During a true surgical emergency, more so than in any other scenario, teamwork is key to a successful outcome for the patient. In all types of emergencies, urgency and *timing* require that one person (the surgeon in this case) be the decision maker. In a true emergency, there is little or no time for discussion or dispute. A sudden change in the patient's condition can result in a swift reordering of priorities and actions. This may mean a change of instrumentation from one system to another, such as orthopedic to vascular instruments, or sudden need for autotransfusion equipment. The role of the surgical technologist is therefore critical to the pace and flow of a procedure.

Although the ability to respond quickly to the demands of the surgery is important, so is *accuracy*. Accuracy in emergency terms means "getting it right the first time." Rapid response is ineffective or harmful if the response is incorrect. An instrument or suture passed in the wrong position, passing an inappropriate type or size of retractor for the needed exposure, incorrectly identified medications, and garbled communication are examples of errors that cost time and increase patient risk.

Clear communication is the pivot point of team efforts in an emergency. There may be many people attending the patient at one time during the emergency. These can include several circulators, more than one scrub person and even a scrub team, surgical specialists (scrubbed or not), and other medical personnel present in the operating room during the setup and operative procedure. This is an opportunity for not only shared expertise but also miscommunication. The atmosphere may be distracting and noisy with multiple activities and requests to the circulators for medications, instruments, and assessment results. The surgical technologist must therefore be attentive not only to the tasks at hand but also to the responsibility of clear communication, which should be deliberate, clearly spoken, and precise. Timing in communication is also very important. During the procedure, the scrub is dependent on the circulator to distribute needed items on the sterile field. However, the scrub must also be sensitive to the fact that the circulator must meet the requirements of the whole team while maintaining communication with other professionals outside the department such as the laboratory, blood bank, and intensive care unit (ICU). The basic tasks of the surgical technologist in the assistant circulator role are listed in Box 35.1.

TRAUMA SYSTEMS

The current trauma system in the United States provides for a specific designation of the health care facilities that are capable of treating emergency trauma. Trauma centers are designated by a numerical system, levels I through V, with level I having the greatest capacity to handle all types of trauma. These designations are based on criteria established by the Committee on Trauma of the American College of Surgeons and by individual state laws. The criteria are extensive and include such things such as the number and type of trauma specialists (e.g., neurology, orthopedics, and pediatrics), equipment

BOX 35.1 Tasks of the Surgical Technologist in the Assistant Circulator Role in Trauma Surgery

1. Gather and distribute sterile supplies in a logical manner (first to be used, first opened).
2. Handle the patient meticulously during transport and positioning.
3. Ensure that adequate amounts of irrigation solutions are prewarmed.
4. Assistance in maintaining patient normothermia using warm air blankets as directed by the anesthesia care provider.
5. Participate in sponge management and counting.
6. Set up and monitor the use of nonsterile equipment and attachments.
7. Maintain a safe operative environment by managing blood and fluid spillage on floors and other nonsterile surfaces.
8. Participate in communication between the sterile team and others involved in the multidisciplinary care team outside the surgical department (e.g., laboratory, x-ray, blood bank, central supply).
9. Assist in arranging for immediate postoperative patient transport and destination (ICU, trauma ICU, pediatric ICU).
10. Obtain the results of imaging or other investigations performed in the preoperative period.
11. Maintain documentation in real time, as events occur, if possible.
12. Obtain whole blood or blood products from the blood bank, according to facility policy.

ICU, Intensive care unit.

available, and ability to transport victims quickly. Assessment capacity, community education in trauma prevention, and ability to perform a variety of specialty trauma procedures are also considered in the classification system. Communication between the field and facility is also of primary importance. Level I trauma centers must have state-of-the-art equipment that enables rescue and transport teams to communicate with facility trauma specialists in real time.

Physician certification in trauma care is achieved through the American College of Surgeons' **Advanced Trauma Life Support (ATLS)** course, which is globally recognized (see https://www.facs.org/quality-programs/trauma/atls). The course focuses on ATLS treatment guidelines and protocols for trauma management. Non-physician health personnel may audit the course in some regions, but certification is reserved for licensed physicians only.

TRAUMA INJURIES

Unintentional trauma, such as automobile accidents (including pedestrian versus automobile), falls, bicycle accidents, and industrial accidents, leading to serious and lethal injury, has yielded injury patterns that are somewhat predictable. Intentional injuries such as those caused by firearms and other weapons have also been studied extensively in the past decade. To become familiar with the type of surgical interventions that are used to treat injuries, it is helpful to classify injuries by type. In **blunt injury,** the skin is unbroken, and the injuries are internal. In civilian populations, blunt injuries occur most commonly from motor vehicle accidents, falls, and interpersonal violence. In **penetrating injury,** the object that causes the injury creates an open wound and deeper injuries. Penetrating injury is most commonly caused by gunshot and knife attack. All surgical procedures involving open traumatic injury are graded as *contaminated.* Recall however that all surgical procedures adhere to the same standards of sterile technique.

Table 35.1 shows blunt trauma mechanisms and their associated injuries.

TRAUMA PATHOPHYSIOLOGY

The decision to perform emergency trauma surgery and the extent of the surgery are based on a unique set of criteria. A complex chain of physiological events occurs in severe trauma cases, especially in multiple trauma patients. These events often require a deviation from medical and surgical **algorithms** (treatment pathways) that usually guide the surgeon and other attending consultants toward a course of action. The mechanisms are complex, and many are not completely understood, even by specialists. However, an understanding of very basic trauma physiology is important to appreciate the decisions that must be made during all phases of trauma management.

LETHAL TRIANGLE

Three physiological conditions are a primary focus of assessment and decision making in severely injured patients. Together, the three conditions are called the "triangle of death," lethal triangle, or lethal triad. The three conditions are as follows:

- *Hypothermia:* Subnormal core body temperature for an extended period of time
- *Metabolic acidosis:* Lower-than-normal blood pH
- *Coagulopathy:* Potentially lethal disorder of the normal blood-clotting system

Patients who survive the first hour after injury are at risk for these conditions, which are related to hemorrhage, shock, and the body's immune response to trauma.

Hemorrhagic Shock

In Chapter 13, it was stated that there are a number of different kinds of shock, caused by different pathologies. In this discussion, the focus is on **hemorrhagic shock.** This is vascular failure caused by prolonged, severe blood loss, the most common cause of mortality in trauma.

The body's compensatory mechanisms that are triggered by hemorrhage occur at the microcirculatory level. In the healthy body, blood delivers oxygen to the cells and also carries metabolic waste out of the cells. The microcirculatory pathway responsible for these functions is called the *nutrient pathway.* The *non-nutrient pathway* provides warmth to the entire body, from core to extremities, necessary to sustain life. During severe hemorrhage and a drop in blood pressure, vasoconstriction occurs in the peripheral circulation. This mechanism preserves blood flow to the heart, kidneys, and brain. However, the diversion of blood to these vital structures causes the extremities, abdominal organs, and muscles to become deprived of normal circulation. In response to the loss of peripheral circulation, the cells begin to take on interstitial fluid from the vascular system. This decreases blood pressure further. At the same time, certain inflammatory chemicals are released in the body, and these are ultimately toxic to the non-vital organs in the absence of a normal circulatory system. Inflammatory factors cause swelling in the peripheral tissues and organs, resulting in further ischemia and blood stasis, micro clotting, and tissue death.

Hypothermia

In the initial stages of hypovolemic shock, the blood vessels constrict, causing increased vascular resistance. If shock deepens, further compensation occurs in the body as described earlier. In a healthy individual, body heat is produced by the consumption of oxygen in the cells through aerobic metabolism. This is especially pronounced in the muscles and abdominal organs. During shock, these tissues are deprived of adequate blood flow, stalling the aerobic metabolism. This in turn causes life-threatening hypothermia. Nearly all critical trauma patients are hypothermic by the time medical care is available. The hypothermic state can be made more severe through skin exposure during the initial assessment when clothing is removed, as well as lack of warmth during transport to the medical facility and even during treatment. Therefore steps to restore and maintain the patient's core temperature are a critical component of patient care before, during, and after emergency surgery. Persistent hypothermia quickly leads to other life-threatening physiological changes, described next.

TABLE 35.1 Mechanisms of Blunt Injury

Mechanism of Injury	Additional Considerations	Potential Associated Injuries
MOTOR VEHICLE COLLISIONS		
Head-on collision		Facial injuries Lower extremity injuries and upper extremity Aortic injuries
Rear-end collision		Hyperextension injuries of cervical spine Cervical spine fractures Central cord syndrome
Lateral (T-bone) collision		Thoracic injuries Abdominal injuries—spleen, liver Pelvic injuries Clavicle, humerus, rib fractures
Rollover	Greater chance of ejection Significant mechanism of injury	Crush injuries Compression fractures of the spine
Ejection from vehicle	Likely unrestrained Significant mortality	Spinal and pelvic injuries
Windshield damage	Likely unrestrained	Closed head injuries, coup and contrecoup injuries Facial fractures Skull fractures Cervical spine fractures
Steering wheel damage	Likely unrestrained	Thoracic injuries Sternal and rib fractures, flail chest Cardiac contusion Aortic injuries Hemo-/pneumothorax
Dashboard and front panel damage		Pelvic and acetabular injuries Dislocated hip
RESTRAINT/SEAT BELT USE		
Proper three-point restraint	Decreased morbidity	Sternal and rib fractures, pulmonary contusions
Lap belt only		Chance fractures, abdominal injuries, head and facial injuries/fractures
Shoulder belt only		Cervical spine injuries/fractures, "submarine" out of restraint devices (possible ejection)
Airbag deployment	Front-end collisions Less severe head/upper torso injuries Not effective for lateral impacts More severe injuries in children (improper front seat placement)	Upper extremity soft tissue injuries/fractures Lower extremity injuries/fractures
PEDESTRIAN VERSUS AUTOMOBILE		
Low speed (braking automobile)		Tibia and fibula fractures, knee injuries
High speed		Waddle triad—tibia/fibula or femur fractures, truncal injuries, craniofacial injuries "Thrown" pedestrians at risk for multisystem injuries
BICYCLE AND MOTORCYCLE ACCIDENTS		
Automobile vs. bicycle		Closed head injuries "Handlebar" injuries Spleen/liver lacerations Additional intraabdominal injuries Consider penetrating injuries
Non–automobile-related		Extremity injuries "Handlebar" injuries
Falls from a great height		Mortality 50% at 36–60 feet

Continued

TABLE 35.1 Mechanisms of Blunt Injury—cont'd

Mechanism of Injury	Additional Considerations	Potential Associated Injuries
Vertical impact		Calcaneal and lower extremity fractures Pelvic fractures Closed head injuries Cervical spine fractures Renal and renal vascular injuries
Horizontal impact		Craniofacial fractures Hand and wrist fractures Abdominal and thoracic visceral injuries Aortic injuries

Modified from Martin R, Meredith J. Management of acute trauma. In Townsend CM Jr, Beauchamp RD, Evers BM, Mattox KL, eds. *Sabiston Textbook of Surgery*. 19th ed. Philadelphia: WB Saunders; 2012.

Coagulopathy

During hemorrhage, the autonomic nervous system triggers the release of angiotensin, vasopressin, antidiuretic hormone, glucagon, cortisol, epinephrine, and norepinephrine. In the *early* stages of hemorrhagic shock, these hormones and the biochemical changes they cause are beneficial. They increase cardiac output and peripheral vasoconstriction, protecting the heart and brain from oxygen starvation. It is even common for blood pressure to remain within normal limits during the early compensatory stage of shock, even in the presence of severe hemorrhage. However, in the next stage of shock, further constriction of capillaries results in cellular death of those tissues deprived of blood and oxygen.

One of the primary consequences of the mechanisms just described is **coagulopathy** (dysfunction of the normal blood clotting process). Continued hypothermia and capillary constriction lead to fluid shifts that dilute the circulating blood. Total platelet supply and coagulation factors necessary for clotting also become diluted or lost completely with the addition of intravenous crystalloid fluids given as a strategy of treatment. In compensation for blood loss, the body releases additional thrombin. However, at this stage, circulation is sluggish, and this causes thrombin to be withdrawn from the vascular system and deposited in organs, leading to thrombin depletion, cellular destruction, and eventual failure. This constellation of events is called *disseminated intravascular coagulation (DIC)*. Even if major hemorrhage is halted through surgery or other mechanical means, *microhemorrhage* remains unchecked in DIC because the circulating platelets, thrombin, and coagulation factors have been deposited in the viscera and are ineffectual. DIC may be prevented by replacing the lost coagulation factors *early* in the crisis. However, the spiral of events can occur very rapidly, and once past a certain point, the process is irreversible.

NOTE *DIC can occur in all forms of shock.*

Metabolic Acidosis

During shock, lack of oxygen supply to muscles and abdominal organs causes another phenomenon called **metabolic acidosis** (abnormally low blood pH). As tissue perfusion decreases during hemorrhage and shock, cells are not oxygenated. The shift from aerobic to anaerobic metabolism at the cellular level creates the waste product lactic acid. Without a circulatory system or other normal physiological process to rid the body of metabolic waste, serum lactate levels rise, resulting in life-threatening metabolic acidosis.

COMPARTMENT SYNDROME

The compensatory mechanisms in acute injury can lead to the condition called **compartment syndrome.** In simple terms, this is tissue swelling within a closed area such as muscle bundles (surrounded by sheets of fascia and encased by superficial tissues) or the abdomen. When the tissue swelling reaches a critical point, circulation to the area is blocked, and the oxygen-deprived tissues become necrotic. Acute compartment syndrome (ACS) requires emergency surgery to relieve the pressure. Compartment syndrome can occur anywhere in the body but is seen most commonly in the abdomen, in limbs, and in brain injury. Surgical management of ACS is discussed later in the chapter.

NOTE *Acute compartment syndrome, or ACS, which can affect any closed compartment of the body, unfortunately has the same acronym as abdominal compartment syndrome (ACS), which refers only to the abdominal cavity. Acute abdominal compartment syndrome (AACS) is another term that refers to abdominal compartment syndrome that arises suddenly.*

ATLS PRINCIPLES OF TRAUMA MANAGEMENT

Lifesaving trauma management under the ATLS guidelines is based on specific objectives:

- The clinical problem that is the most lethal (the greatest threat to life) is treated first.
- Treatment is initiated even when a **definitive diagnosis** (a diagnosis confirmed by assessment or investigation) is not established.
- Treatment may be initiated even when there is no detailed history.

ATLS trauma assessment is performed in two stages, the primary survey and the secondary survey.

PREHOSPITAL CARE AND THE GOLDEN HOUR

Prehospital care takes place before the patient arrives at the trauma center. First responders such as emergency medical technologists, trauma nurses, and rescue personnel arriving on the scene of the trauma are involved in prehospital care in the field and in transit. The principles of care in the first hour are based on a concept known as the *Golden Hour.* This refers to the first critical hour after injury. Trauma-related morbidity and mortality are partially related to the time elapsed between the trauma event and resuscitation attempts. About 50% of victims with injury to the aorta, heart, spinal cord, or brainstem die from their injuries within minutes of the trauma. A further 30% of victims die in the first few hours. Of these, half will have died from hemorrhage and the remaining from damage to the central nervous system. Overall, hemorrhage is the primary cause of death in traumatic injury.

Field Care: The Primary Survey

The primary survey is the initial patient assessment, performed by first responders. Elements of the survey follow the ABCDE sequence:

1. **Airway and cervical spine control:** The patient's own or an artificial airway is secured, and the cervical spine is stabilized with a rigid collar to prevent further injury and to maintain the airway.
2. **Breathing and oxygenation:** The patient is assessed for thoracic injury such as pneumothorax, flail chest, or hemothorax (discussed later) that may compromise breathing. In the case of an open thorax, immediate artificial ventilation is established. Broken ribs or a crushed sternum may also prevent adequate ventilation.
3. **Circulation and hemorrhage:** Blood loss resulting from hemorrhage must be controlled in the early phase of the emergency to prevent coagulopathy and eventual exsanguination. Multiple intravenous lines are established for blood testing and administration of fluids and drugs. **Occult injury** is undetected injury (such as hidden hemorrhage). It is a significant clinical problem in the prehospital and emergency department phases.
4. **Dysfunction and disability of the central nervous system:** Traumatic brain injury (TBI) may result in the cessation of vital functions, including respiration. A rapid neurological assessment is performed to ascertain whether TBI has occurred.
5. **Exposure of injuries and environmental control (thermoregulation):** Once vital functions are restored, the full extent of the victim's injuries is assessed. This requires removal of clothing and steps to prevent or treat hypothermia.

The primary survey may determine the need for immediate emergency surgery if the patient is stable enough; the secondary survey is started right away. Resuscitation begins immediately in the early assessment stages of trauma and continues as long as necessary.

Resuscitation

Resuscitation is the process of restoring physiological balance in injury. In the context of trauma, resuscitation refers to treatment for the effects of hemorrhagic shock, including establishing normal circulating blood volume (hemodynamics), tissue perfusion, and vascular tone. Resuscitation is initiated as soon as medical help is available and continues throughout the prehospital, emergency department, preoperative, surgical, and ICU phases of recovery.

The process of trauma resuscitation is not a straightforward case of replacing blood or restoring normal fluid balance. This is because increased intravascular fluids such as colloids and crystalloids can dilute the circulating blood, platelet, and coagulation factors and can result in decreased oxygen supply to vital organs. As blood pressure is increased, the rate of blood loss also increases. Increasing the blood pressure can also disrupt or dislodge clots that have already been formed. Resuscitation is therefore a critical part of trauma response that requires careful monitoring and reevaluation throughout the emergency. The primary objectives of resuscitation in hemorrhagic shock are to achieve and maintain normothermia and to maintain the patient's intravascular volume in a balanced state of sufficient oxygen-carrying capacity, adequate levels of coagulation factors, and fluid pressure without increasing hemorrhage. Resuscitation involves placing at least two large-bore venous cannulas for mechanical pump infusion of blood products, plasma, colloids, crystalloid, and washed salvaged blood. The pump maintains fluids between 38°C and 40°C.

Hospital Care: The Secondary Survey

The secondary survey is performed once the patient is stable enough to be moved. However, a patient requiring *immediate, lifesaving surgery* may be transported directly to the operating room after the primary assessment. The secondary assessment includes a head-to-toe examination to look for less obvious injuries that may also be critical. In this phase, the patient is able to undergo investigations including ultrasound, radiology, and magnetic resonance imaging (MRI). Further interventions such as placing additional intravenous lines, a urinary catheter, or a nasogastric tube are performed at this time. An important aspect of the secondary survey is the verbal history obtained from the patient or witnesses who can provide details of the trauma. This can assist with the diagnosis obtained through imaging studies and other tests. If time does not allow complex investigations, the attending physician attempts to find out about the patient's general health, allergies, and other information that may affect the treatment plan. This is done by interviewing the victim's family, if they are available.

NOTE *All multiple-trauma patients recover in the ICU for continued resuscitation and monitoring.*

DAMAGE CONTROL SURGERY

The decision to perform emergency surgery even in the absence of a definitive diagnosis is highly influenced by the physiological events described earlier. Once the decision is made, the extent of surgical repair may be limited to **damage control surgery.** This is a specific surgical strategy whose exact technique depends on the body systems involved and the likelihood of improving the prognosis using surgical intervention. The goal of damage control surgery is to focus solely on lifesaving maneuvers:

- Control of hemorrhage
- Control of fecal spillage (abdominal and pelvic injury)
- Packing a body cavity
- Delayed or phased closure of the wound
- Relief of compartment syndrome
- Splinting or external fixation to prevent extension of injuries

Damage control surgery is based on the concept that the severely wounded patient is physiologically unstable and may quickly succumb to exsanguinating hemorrhage leading to deepening shock, hypothermia, inadequate organ perfusion, and coagulopathy. A secondary but immediate concern is sepsis caused by wound contamination. Damage control surgery stops the immediate cause of potential harm without extensive or elaborate reconstruction to restore anatomical form or continuity of tissues. It focuses on the immediate dangers so that the patient can be quickly moved to the ICU for continued resuscitation. Damage control surgery can be performed on any area of the body. The most common types are thoracic, abdominal, retroperitoneal, cranial, and orthopedic. Each system requires slightly different surgical techniques and equipment. These are discussed later in the chapter. If the patient is stabilized in 12 to 48 hours, he or she can then be returned to surgery for a **definitive procedure** (surgical treatment using a planned method and techniques intended to provide a lasting repair). The procedure often involves extensive wound repair in one or multiple (staged) procedures. If during resuscitation the patient shows no improvement or there is evidence of continuing hemorrhage, damage control surgery can be repeated to find and correct the source of the bleeding. Staged or phased procedures after damage control surgery are therefore performed for more extensive reconstruction, as a lifesaving measure in the presence of further hemorrhage, or to treat compartment syndrome.

CASE PLANNING FOR TRAUMA SURGERY

Trauma surgery may not follow a step-by-step routine that is common to specific procedures with definitive objectives, such as those described in earlier chapters. The surgeon does rely on preoperative investigations for a diagnosis when they are available. However, emergency surgery, by nature, is often investigative. For this reason, case planning should be guided by the regional anatomy (e.g., abdominal, orthopedic, thoracic) involved when precise information is unavailable preoperatively.

All health care facility surgical departments prepare emergency case carts in preparation for specific emergencies likely to arrive for treatment. These include basic setups for craniotomy, cesarean section, and abdominal aneurysm. Emergency carts may be adapted for other types of emergencies, or a general emergency cart may be prepared and placed on standby. This contains linens, drapes, towels, Mayo covers, extra table drapes, and general surgery instruments and supplies. Even when emergency carts are prepared ahead of time, case planning according to the body system (e.g., orthopedic, cranial, abdominal, and thoracic) and anatomical location will help the surgical team to quickly assemble other equipment needed to start an emergency procedure.

INSTRUMENTS

Planning for instrumentation should start with basic instruments and be modified according to the systems involved, with specialty instruments distributed on the sterile field during the case setup or as needed. A multiple-injury patient may require multiple system instruments. To avoid having instrument sets opened but not used, specialty instruments can be placed unopened on a cart outside the operating room in the sterile core. In this way they are easily and quickly available without adding more equipment to the setup. On the other hand, if it is known that the patient has both thoracic and abdominal injuries, it is wise to have both sets open so that the scrub can prepare both as time allows.

SOLUTIONS AND DRUGS

Copious amounts of irrigation solution are often needed during trauma surgery. These are used to flush and clean the wound of tissue debris and foreign objects. If major debridement is required and has not been performed in the emergency department, additional warm fluids will be needed. The scrubbed surgical technologists should have two separate suction systems, including separate tubing, suction tips, and irrigation devices. All solutions must be distributed warm and maintained warm during the surgery to combat hypothermia, which is an important element of the lethal triangle described earlier. Antibiotic irrigation is likely to be used in open trauma cases and can be distributed as needed at the close of surgery. To track blood loss, the circulator may place empty solution bottles in a designated area of the room for counting when time permits.

SUTURE AND HEMOSTATIC DEVICES

Hemostasis is a priority in all trauma surgery. The choice of suture therefore depends on the systems involved. Suture ligatures and free ties should be available throughout the surgery. Initially, 2-0 and 3-0 nonabsorbent ligatures should be immediately available. A general rule to follow is that nonabsorbent suture material will be favored in open trauma or possible bowel contamination of the wound because of the risk of infection, which would quickly dissolve absorbent materials. Size 0 would be needed in the event of major blood vessel damage, whereas 2-0 and 3-0 are adequate for smaller branching and peripheral vessels. It is best to have two sizes of tapered curved needles available for suture ligatures because these can be used on blood vessels and also on vascular bundles that may be encountered in deep tissue layers. Two electrosurgical unit (ESU) systems (handpieces and power units) should be available. One can be held in reserve until called for by the surgeons.

Thrombin-based tissue sealants are used only if there is no coagulopathy present because *these depend on an intact coagulation response.* Dry hemostats such as gelatin, collagen, and oxidized cellulose may also be ineffective in the presence of coagulopathy. However, in the absence of this condition, the scrub should anticipate the need for topical hemostatic agents, including thrombin-based materials.

The choice of skin closure materials is usually deferred until the close of surgery. In the case of damage control surgery, the wound may be left open without sutures, or a single-layer closure in heavy nonabsorbent material may be used. The type of closure may not be known until the extent of the trauma is determined and the condition of the patient is assessed at the end of surgery. Wound drains will be secured using nonabsorbent suture, size 2-0 or 3-0, on a 3⁄8 cutting needle.

AUTOTRANSFUSION

Autotransfusion is the salvaging of blood at the operative or trauma site and reinfusion into the patient. Its primary use is during surgical cases in which large blood loss is anticipated, such as orthopedic procedures. Autotransfusion equipment is set up before or during surgery, and sterile connections are passed to the scrubbed team. A number of different companies, such as Medtronic and Haemonetics, manufacture and sell autotransfusion systems.

The equipment and specific technology may vary among manufacturers, but the concepts remain the same. Free blood is collected in the wound by suction and routed through blood tubing directly attached to the device, which rinses, anticoagulates, and filters the blood cells to remove unwanted components. Blood is then collected within the system and is immediately available for reinfusion. Autotransfusion is acceptable to some patients who, for religious, cultural, or other reasons, decline transfusion of blood donated from another individual. Advantages of autotransfusion are decreased risk of communicable disease transmission by banked blood, increased hematocrit ratio in the blood, and immediate availability of blood during surgery. Auto transfusion systems include the power unit and cell-washing system, blood tubing and bags, suction catheter, and filters. Equipment setup includes sterile and nonsterile components. Depending on the type and manufacturer, the setup is relatively straightforward. The surgical technologist may be trained on setup and use of a specific unit by the company representative or by a facility staff member who is familiar with the unit.

IMPORTANT TO KNOW *It may be safe to assume, for planning purposes, that autotransfusion may be used in cases of severe hemorrhage. The unit and accessories should be placed on standby but not opened during case preparation unless requested by the surgeon.*

DRAINS AND DRESSINGS

The physiological changes brought about by trauma cause severe edema in the regional tissues, including those not directly injured. Postoperative serosanguinous pooling is controlled with wound drains, whereas fluid and electrolyte imbalance is managed through systemic resuscitative measures. Thoracic wounds require a closed chest drainage system (Pleur-Evac type), which is discussed in Chapter 31. Abdominal, pelvic, and other soft tissue trauma may require suction drainage by one or more drain systems such as a Hemovac, Jackson-Pratt, or negative-pressure wound therapy (NPWT) system (e.g., Wound V.A.C.).

Dressings and packing used in trauma surgery vary according to the type of wound and its classification, the tissues involved, and whether the wound will be packed and left without any primary closure until the next stage of repair. The clinical information needed to make this decision is often not known until the full extent of the injuries has been assessed during the surgical procedure.

SPONGES

The nature of trauma surgery and the objectives of damage control procedures require all possible methods of hemostasis, including the use of many surgical sponges. A large surgical wound may require 100 or more laparotomy sponges, which must be immediately available on the sterile field, with many packs held in reserve for immediate distribution as needed. Whereas a normal abdominal or thoracic case may require 10 to 20 lap sponges to start the case, in trauma surgery at least 40 should be available as soon as the procedure begins. The 4 × 4 sponge mounted on sponge forceps is usually only required for deep swabbing in a relatively dry wound.

Tracking sponges during emergency trauma surgery can be problematic. An initial (baseline) count may not have been possible because of the urgency of the procedure, and additional sponges may be provided without a proper count. At a minimum, the number of sponge packs (groups of 5 or 10) can be recorded as they are distributed on the field. This does not guarantee a correct count but can serve as a basis for estimation. The scrub and circulator must use practical judgment about the need to count sponges during the procedure. As time allows, the circulator retrieves bloodied sponges discarded off the sterile field and places them in a sponge holder as usual, to be counted when an opportunity arises. Wound packing is a technique of damage control surgery and is described later in the chapter. Although it is not ideal, the surgeon may use laparotomy sponges for packing the abdominal cavity, and these remain in place until the next procedure (usually within 24 hours). Whenever possible, every effort to account for sponges is made. This is true whether placed in the emergency department or during surgery in the operating room.

Special closure and dressing techniques such as planned open abdominal wound require items that can be gathered toward the end of the procedure. These include plastic viscera bags, Velcro sheets, plastic draping sheets, and Silastic mesh.

MANAGEMENT OF FORENSIC EVIDENCE

Forensic medicine is a complex topic in which the methods and means of crimes, including interpersonal violence, are studied. The surgical technologist working in an urban trauma facility is likely to have some contact with forensic evidence. Although an extended discussion of forensics is beyond the scope of this textbook, the surgical technologist should be familiar with some aspects of evidence management.

The concepts of forensics were introduced in Chapter 3, and some guidelines for managing forensic evidence were presented in Chapter 19. However, it is worth reviewing these with regard to trauma surgery.

Death from firearms is the second leading cause of mortality in the United States, and approximately 115,000 cases of firearm injury are treated each year. The most common firearm used in personal violence is the handgun. However, other weapons are also used, and many of these are fire-jacketed or exploding bullets. The manner in which these weapons are handled on the surgical field may determine whether they can be used as legal evidence. Therefore it is very important for the surgical technologist to use technique that is consistent with maintaining specimens correctly:

- When passing any instrument that will come in contact with a bullet, fragment, shrapnel, or other ballistic item, also ensure that the tips of the instrument are protected with rubber shods or completely covered with a sponge. Markings on the fragment or bullet may not be visible without magnification but are nevertheless present on all weapons.
- Avoid any contact between the bullet or fragment and other metal, such as a metal container or other bullets retrieved. Do not toss a projectile into a basin. Pad the basin and set the projectile into it. Careless handling can easily scratch the item and obscure evidential marks.
- Place ballistic fragments or whole bullets in separate containers and label them according to the exact location, as identified by the surgeon.
- Use plastic containers to avoid damage to the projectile.
- Projectiles should be sent in a dry container unless directed otherwise by the laboratory. ***Do not wash the item before submitting it to pathology.***
- Fragments of cloth or other debris removed from a wound must be preserved as specimens, and the exact location must be documented.
- When labeling specimens, do not speculate on the type of projectile. It will be later identified by law enforcement officials.

PREOPERATIVE CARE OF THE PATIENT

MOVING AND HANDLING

Positioning the trauma patient requires precise coordination among members of the surgical team. The real potential for extending the patient's injuries exists during moving and handling. Although splints and spinal support may have been applied at the scene of the accident or in the emergency department, *occult injuries* (those not detected during the assessment) may exist. For example, fractured bone ends can easily tear through adjacent blood vessels, nerves, and other soft tissue. Sudden movement of the body may shift blood clots. Particular attention is given to maintaining stability of the spine. To minimize this risk, basic precautions are exercised:

- All moves are directed by one person—the anesthesia provider or surgeon. It is necessary to have a lead person in charge of coordinating the moves to avoid further injury to the patient.
- Patients often arrive in the operating room with stabilization devices in place. These include vacuum or rigid splints for extremities, torso splints, and the cervical collar for maintaining alignment of the cervical spine. No support devices are removed until the anesthesia provider and surgeon state that it is safe to do so.
- Sudden shifts in fluid balance can occur during moving and handling. Active bleeding and shock can cause shifts in fluid spacing, which can become more severe with sudden postural changes. Postural changes such as raising and lowering the lower extremities must be made slowly with physiological monitoring in place.
- When moving and handling the pregnant patient, care is taken to avoid the compression of the vena cava, which can compromise fetal circulation. The patient should always be maintained in left lateral position.

MAINTAINING PATIENT NORMOTHERMIA

Maintaining the patient's core temperature as close to normal as possible is a major goal of emergency treatment. This means that exposure is kept to an absolute minimum and that warmed blankets are available all times during preoperative preparations. A warm-air heating blanket can be used intermittently between investigations in different locations of the facility. All intravenous infusion and irrigation solutions are prewarmed. The room temperature is prewarmed no higher than 29.4°C (85°F) and maintained until active warming devices achieve normothermia.

AIRWAY

Maintaining the patient's airway is a priority of the anesthesia provider. An emergency airway such as a tracheostomy or cricothyroidotomy may have been performed in the emergency department. This may be converted to a different type when the patient arrives in the operating room. In this case, the anesthesia provider may require surgical assistance and instruments to perform the procedure.

CONTINUING PHYSIOLOGICAL EVALUATION

The unstable trauma patient is continually evaluated for physiological changes from the time he or she arrives at the health care facility. Baseline tests that are performed in the emergency department are repeated at regular intervals. These include tests for blood gases, electrolyte levels, oxygen saturation, platelet and other blood components, and renal function, as well as many others. Some of the tests are urgent, and the results are needed to detect life-threatening metabolic changes. In these cases, the laboratory is notified when the patient arrives so that time can be dedicated to the emergency.

A runner may be identified in the surgical department or among the circulating team to transport blood samples quickly and to communicate with the laboratory staff. In many facilities, reports can be read out over the communication system directly from departments within the hospital to the operating room where the patient is being treated.

Imaging procedures that were performed during the secondary assessment can be uploaded to the operating room's dedicated computer almost immediately. However, not all hospitals have such capabilities, and the physical output of any imaging studies will have to be retrieved from where they were taken back to the operating room.

EMOTIONAL SUPPORT

The conscious trauma patient may arrive at the emergency department disoriented and frightened. Powerful emotional reactions to trauma can affect the body's physiological mechanisms through the same chemicals that induce and prolong metabolic shock. Health care personnel can and should offer reassurance to the patient and provide orientation as to where the patient is and what is happening. In a severe emergency, all activity is focused on lifesaving measures. However, whenever possible, it is important to provide some measure of emotional comfort.

The family of the patient is likely to arrive during the most urgent phases of assessment. The operating room supervisor or person in a similar role is often responsible for seeing that family members have a quiet place to wait. This person also provides intermittent updates on the patient's condition.

RECORDS AND CONSENT

Consent for invasive procedures, including emergency surgery, is obtained from the patient if he or she is able, or from responsible individuals according to hospital policy. Documentation of all care is vital so that subsequent care providers have accurate information on what was done and when throughout the assessment and treatment plan. The collection of forensic evidence and related documentation is also mandatory. This normally takes place in the emergency department but may be continued in the operating room.

OPENING A CASE AND STERILE SETUP

Teams that work together on a regular basis are able to plan the amount of time needed to open a case for a particular procedure fairly accurately. However, emergency trauma surgery presents challenges that are not conducive to preplanning. Often the extent of the injuries is not known to the team until the patient arrives in the department. The patient's condition may fluctuate, requiring nursing personnel to divide their time between direct patient care and distributing sterile items to the sterile team. In many cases, there may be very little time between the patient's arrival in the operating room and the start of surgery. This means that the scrub may be donning gown and gloves at the same time the surgeons arrive. In this situation, assistant circulators can be very valuable to help get the case opened and underway.

In emergency circumstances, some of the usual routines are abbreviated. This includes sponge and instrument counts. Although this is not an ideal situation, the American College of Surgeons has stated that standardized counting procedures may be suspended in life-threatening situations. The Association of periOperative Registered Nurses (AORN) has also stated in their recommended practices that surgical counts may be waived in circumstances in which the time required presents an unacceptable delay in patient care.

During the setup for a complex emergency case there is a tendency to bring in many more instruments and supplies than will be needed. Although it is wise to have items immediately available, it is also important to consider which supplies and instruments are certainly needed and which can be held in reserve. Another consideration is not to overload the back table with so many instruments and supplies that they cannot be located quickly as needed. Professional judgment and experience determine which items should be immediately available and which should be held in reserve. If there is a high probability that extra instrument sets are needed, these can be opened onto smaller instrument tables at the periphery of the sterile field.

ORDER OF SETUP

A general rule that most surgical technologists follow when setting up for an emergency is to prepare items in order of their immediate use on the field. The term *up* means "up on the Mayo, ready to use." The following is a suggested order:

1. Gowns, gloves, drapes arranged in the order of use
2. Draping completed
3. ESU, suction up
4. Light handles in place
5. Knife mounted and up
6. Four laparotomy sponges on the field, four in warm saline for immediate use
7. Superficial and self-retaining retractors up
8. Hemostats up

Once the wound is opened, preparations are made for the evacuation of free blood and wound packing.

Trauma patients who arrive with an open thorax as a result of emergency department thoracotomy require a modification of the suggested sequence. Retraction and exposure may be the first surgical objective, followed by the rapid control of bleeding.

IMPORTANT TO KNOW *It is wise to keep in mind at all times during an emergency that if the problem cannot be visualized, it cannot be managed. This means that adequate retraction, lighting, and removal of blood and clots from the wound are extremely important.*

SKIN PREP AND DRAPING

The decision to modify the skin prep for emergency technique lies with the medical and nursing team. The area of the prep is usually not clearly delineated unless the patient workup (assessment, history, and diagnostic and assessment procedures) indicates that the patient is stable and normal protocols can be followed. However, damage control surgery is performed in many trauma cases, and by definition, these procedures may be carried out because of severe hemorrhage that precludes "normal" patient prep.

As with the surgical prep, draping may be performed with fewer drapes, possibly excluding all but the top drape. In any event, discussion on this should be avoided once the patient is in the room. The surgical technologist takes direction from the surgeon, who will normally relate this information while the patient is being transferred to the operating table. Sometimes it is necessary to provide a variety of drapes so that the surgeon can select the type she or he wants as the drapes are applied.

MANAGING THE STERILE FIELD IN EMERGENCY TRAUMA

Management of the sterile field during emergency trauma surgery requires a high degree of attention to the wound itself and the immediate needs for instruments and supplies. Unlike other types of surgery in which there are known steps and procedures, trauma surgery is performed according to a succession of priorities that can change rapidly. It can be helpful to remember that the surgical priorities are to control and prevent hemorrhage and minimize contamination (in the case of bowel spillage and large penetrating wounds that may contain fragments). ***These objectives are the basis of surgical management and apply to all types of trauma surgery.***

ROLE OF THE SCRUBBED SURGICAL TECHNOLOGIST

The role of the scrubbed surgical technologist is to provide the most efficient and safest means of expediting the procedure. This means carrying out most of the usual tasks of the scrub role while predicting immediate needs. For example, as stated earlier, retraction must precede hemostasis in most cases. However, if the bleeding is **exsanguinating** (capable of depleting the patient's total blood volume), the area is first packed to slow the flow. Hemostasis can be achieved using suture ligatures or anastomosis (of a lacerated blood vessel). The process of hemostasis is predictable even if the steps of the entire procedure are not clear at the start.

Infection Control

Infection is the second leading cause of mortality in trauma patients. Containment methods are used during surgery to limit tissue exposure to bowel contents or foreign objects. Bowel technique, which is described in Chapter 22, is used to the extent that is possible within the limits of time. Debridement, described later, and irrigation are other methods used to prevent sepsis. As with hemostasis, the techniques used to mitigate wound contamination are predictable, and the surgical technologist can plan for them ahead of time.

Rapid Procedural Changes

Elements of surgery that are not so predictable are sudden changes in the course of the surgery, such as those that occur when occult injury is discovered or the patient's physiological status suddenly deteriorates, requiring a change in surgical strategy. These examples demonstrate the need to watch the wound even while performing other tasks such as clearing away instruments from the top drape or preparing supplies.

LAPAROTOMY WITH STAGED CLOSURE

Abdominal injury is the leading cause of trauma morbidity and mortality in all age groups. Blunt trauma is caused by motor vehicle accidents, including motorcycles, pedestrian versus vehicle encounters, falls, and assault. Penetrating wounds are most commonly caused by knife or gunshot. Difficulty in rapid and accurate diagnosis may lead to a high rate of occult abdominal injuries to vital organs and vascular structures of the abdomen. Most commonly injured are the spleen, liver, pancreas, small bowel, and retroperitoneal structures, with accompanying injuries to the omentum and mesentery. Damage control laparotomy with staged closure is an exploratory process in which the sources of hemorrhage are found and controlled. No reconstruction is attempted unless absolutely necessary. The abdomen is packed using sponges, left open, and protected with transparent wound cover (see description following).

In the stable patient, diagnosis of abdominal injury is performed mainly by computed tomography (CT) or **focused assessment with ultrasound for trauma (FAST).** In some cases, diagnostic peritoneal lavage (DPL) may be performed using a peritoneal catheter set. This can be done in the emergency department or in surgery. Unstable patients may be taken to surgery before a definitive diagnosis is made. This means that the need to immediately address obvious exsanguinating hemorrhage outweighs the time required to pinpoint the exact location of the hemorrhage in the abdomen in the assessment phase. The surgical objective in all damage control surgery is to secure hemostasis and prevent sepsis as quickly as possible to return the patient to the ICU for complete resuscitation.

CASE PLANNING FOR ABDOMINAL TRAUMA

Following the general recommendations for case planning discussed earlier, the ST should have a general surgery or laparotomy instrument set. He or she should also be prepared for subphrenic, retroperitoneal, and pelvic exploration. In this case, extra-long instruments should be on hand for an adult patient. Vascular clamps should be available for all emergency laparotomies.

Good exposure is critical to the success of emergency abdominal surgery in the presence of hemorrhage. Self-retaining retractors (e.g., the Bookwalter or Omni) and handheld wide Deaver and Richardson retractors should be included in the instrument setup. They must be immediately available at the start of the procedure. Box 35.2 lists suggested instruments and materials to *supplement* a major laparotomy set for a total abdominal exploration. These may be opened immediately at the start of surgery or held in reserve for distribution to the field as needed.

A variety of ligating materials and linear staplers are normally required. Size 2-0 and 0 non-absorbable stick ties and free ties should be prepared.

ABDOMINAL COMPARTMENT SYNDROME

Abdominal compartment syndrome is a complication requiring emergency response. A combination of immune response to tissue trauma and resuscitative procedures leads to severe edema of any closed compartment of the body, including the abdomen. In the closed abdomen (one that has been primarily closed at surgery), the intraabdominal pressure is greater than what can be tolerated by the vascular system. This results in tissue death from ischemia and can also cause mechanical obstruction to breathing. Elevated central venous pressure also leads to increased intracranial pressure, rupture of the retinal capillaries, and decreased cardiac output resulting from tamponade.

The treatment for ACS is immediate surgical opening of the abdominal cavity. Temporary abdominal closure as described below is intended to prevent ACS while following the protocols for damage control surgery (Table 35.2).

BOX 35.2 Suggested Instruments and Materials for Emergency Damage Control Laparotomy

RETRACTORS
Omni self-retaining, with specialty blades
Deaver set, wide
Harrington and various sizes of Deavers

CLAMPS
Long right-angle (Mixter type), delicate tip
Kidney pedicle
Vascular clamps: Satinsky, DeBakey straight, curved, tangential occlusion

FORCEPS
Vascular forceps, standard and long, straight atraumatic
DeBakey type, single-tooth delicate

SUPPLIES AND MATERIALS
One or two bowel bags
Elastic vessel loops
Shods for hemostats

DAMAGE CONTROL TECHNIQUES: ABDOMEN

Damage control technique for abdominal trauma consists of the following steps:

1. *Pack the wound in a systematic manner.*
2. *Evaluate for active bleeding and repair.*
3. *Evaluate for bowel spillage and repair.*
4. *Perform minimal or no primary closure.*
5. *Apply abdominal coverings.*

As soon as the skin incision is made, the surgical technologist should have at least eight laparotomy sponges moistened with warm saline and wrung dry. Two suction systems and an ESU should also be immediately available. Once the incision has been extended with the knife and ESU, the abdomen is evacuated for blood, clots, and fluid. Packing may begin as soon as the abdomen has been evacuated, or it may be only partially packed during exploration. If possible, the scrub should take

TABLE 35.2 Techniques for Temporary Abdominal Closure

Technique	Description	Mechanism
Vacuum-assisted closure (VAC)	A perforated plastic sheet covers the viscera, and a sponge is placed between the fascial edges. The wound is covered by an airtight seal, which is pierced by a suction drain connected to a suction pump and fluid collection system.	The (active and adjustable) negative pressure supplied by the pump keeps constant tension on the fascial edges while it collects excess abdominal fluid and helps resolve edema.
Vacuum pack	A perforated plastic sheet covers the viscera, damp surgical towels are placed in the wound, and a surgical drain is placed on the towels. An airtight seal covers the wound, and negative pressure is applied through the drain.	The negative pressure keeps constant tension on the fascial edges, and excess fluid is collected.
Artificial burr (Wittmann patch)	Two opposite Velcro sheets (hooks and loops, one on each side) are sutured to the fascial edges. The Velcro sheets connect in the middle.	This technique allows for easy access and stepwise closure of the fascia.
Dynamic retention sutures	The viscera are covered with a sheet (e.g., ISODrape, Microtek [Microban], Huntersville, NC). Horizontal sutures are placed through a large-diameter catheter and through the entire abdominal wall on both sides.	The sutures keep tension on the fascia and may be tightened to allow staged closure of the fascia. This may be combined with a vacuum system.
Plastic silo (Bogota bag)	A sterile x-ray film cassette bag or sterile 3-L urology irrigation bag is sutured between the fascial edges or the skin and opened in the middle.	This is an easy technique that allows for easy access. The bag may be reduced in size to approximate the fascial edges.
Mesh, sheet	An absorbable or nonabsorbable mesh or sheet is sutured between the fascial edges. Examples are Dexon, Marlex, or Vicryl mesh. Examples of sheets are Silastic or silicone sheets.	The mesh or sheet may be reduced in size to allow closure. Non-absorbable mesh may be removed or left in place at the edges of the wound.

Modified from Diaz J, Duton W, Miller R. The difficult abdominal wall. In Townsend CM Jr, Beauchamp RD, Evers BM, Mattox KL, eds. *Sabiston Textbook of Surgery*. 19th ed. Philadelphia: WB Saunders; 2012.

note of how many sponges have been positioned in each quadrant. If the patient has an intact coagulation process, packing all four quadrants using laparotomy sponges absorbs free abdominal blood and fluid, slows the bleeding, and allows the surgeon to identify the origin of the hemorrhage. In contrast to nonemergency surgery, meticulous repair is avoided.

The most common abdominal injuries are to the liver, spleen, pancreas, small intestine, and mesentery. The injuries may extend into the pelvic cavity and also include these structures. Injury to the solid organs (such as liver or pancreatic injury) may require partial resection or total removal (such as splenectomy) to control hemorrhage. Refer to Chapter 22 for details on these procedures.

STAGED ABDOMINAL CLOSURE

Damage control surgery for abdominal injury is managed by leaving the abdomen open for at least the first 24 hours until the patient is stabilized. The methods used for protecting the abdominal contents vary according to the surgeon's training and experience with certain materials. Even though the abdomen is not closed surgically, the tissues must be covered to protect them. Before the wound is covered, the cavities are thoroughly irrigated and checked again for hemorrhage and a count performed.

METHODS OF ABDOMINAL PROTECTION

One method of covering the wound is to enclose the viscera in a plastic pouch or bag that is secured to the skin as shown in Fig. 35.1. This method provides good protection but is time consuming to implement.

The most commonly used method is to cover the abdomen with a series of plastic drapes. A Steri-drape 1010 is used for the first layer. Two Jackson-Pratt suction drainage tubes are placed at the fascia margins. An Ioban (iodophor-impregnated) plastic drape is placed over this (Fig. 35.2).

A third option is closed vacuum suction (wound VAC). In this technique, several layers of protection are used. First, a layer of wound VAC sponges is lapped over the viscera and stapled under the fascia edges. The fascia is then partially closed using no. PDS sutures placed 5 cm apart. A clear plastic VAC covering is placed over the sponges and peripheral skin; an opening is made in the plastic at the wound edges. Finally, a black VAC sponge is placed over the white sponges and plastic skin covering. This is fixed with an occlusive dressing and suction tubing. This system allows evacuation of the wound with an aseptic closure. The VAC dressings can be removed, and the fascia can be closed in stages between the re-application of the VAC dressings (Fig. 35.3).

ORTHOPEDIC TRAUMA

Among the indications for urgent damage control surgery of the skeletal system are near amputation, crushing injury, potentially septic trauma, and pelvic fracture. The objective of early intervention in these cases is to prevent further injury related to vascular and soft tissue damage, decrease the risk of sepsis, prevent or treat compartment syndrome, and decrease blood loss. Stabilization of the bones is therefore often the surgical priority for fractures. In selected cases, conversion to definitive intramedullary nailing of long bones may be attempted. In near amputation such as that shown in Fig. 35.4, repair of major vascular structures may require emergency reconstruction. However, the decision to proceed with a definitive vascular procedure is weighed against causing further immune system reaction by a prolonged surgical procedure. Complex pelvic fracture is associated with high mortality rate. This is related to instability of the pelvic ring and multiple injuries to the venous system that are difficult to access surgically. Repair of soft tissue in orthopedic trauma usually takes place over several days and includes phased debridement to assess tissue viability.

PREOPERATIVE CARE OF THE ORTHOPEDIC PATIENT

Potential complications in the multiple orthopedic trauma patient are as follows:

- *Life-threatening hemorrhage:* Hemorrhage may be addressed with direct pressure on the wound. Early stabilization is critical.
- *Infection from open fractures:* Antibiotic therapy is started early in treatment. Further contamination is avoided by keeping the wounds covered with sterile barriers (e.g.,

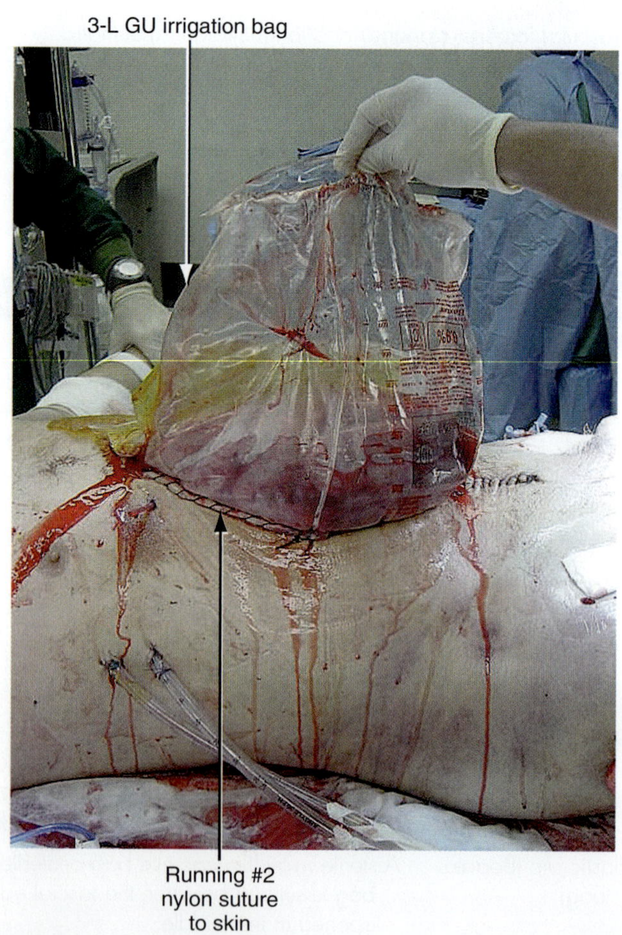

FIG. 35.1 A "Bogota bag" technique of damage control abdominal surgery. The viscera are contained within a plastic pouch (here, a genitourinary irrigation bag is used). The wound edges are secured to the bag to seal it. The viscera will be reduced into the abdomen in subsequent surgeries. (From Cioffi W, et al, eds. *Atlas of Trauma Emergency Surgical Techniques*. Philadelphia: Saunders; 2014.)

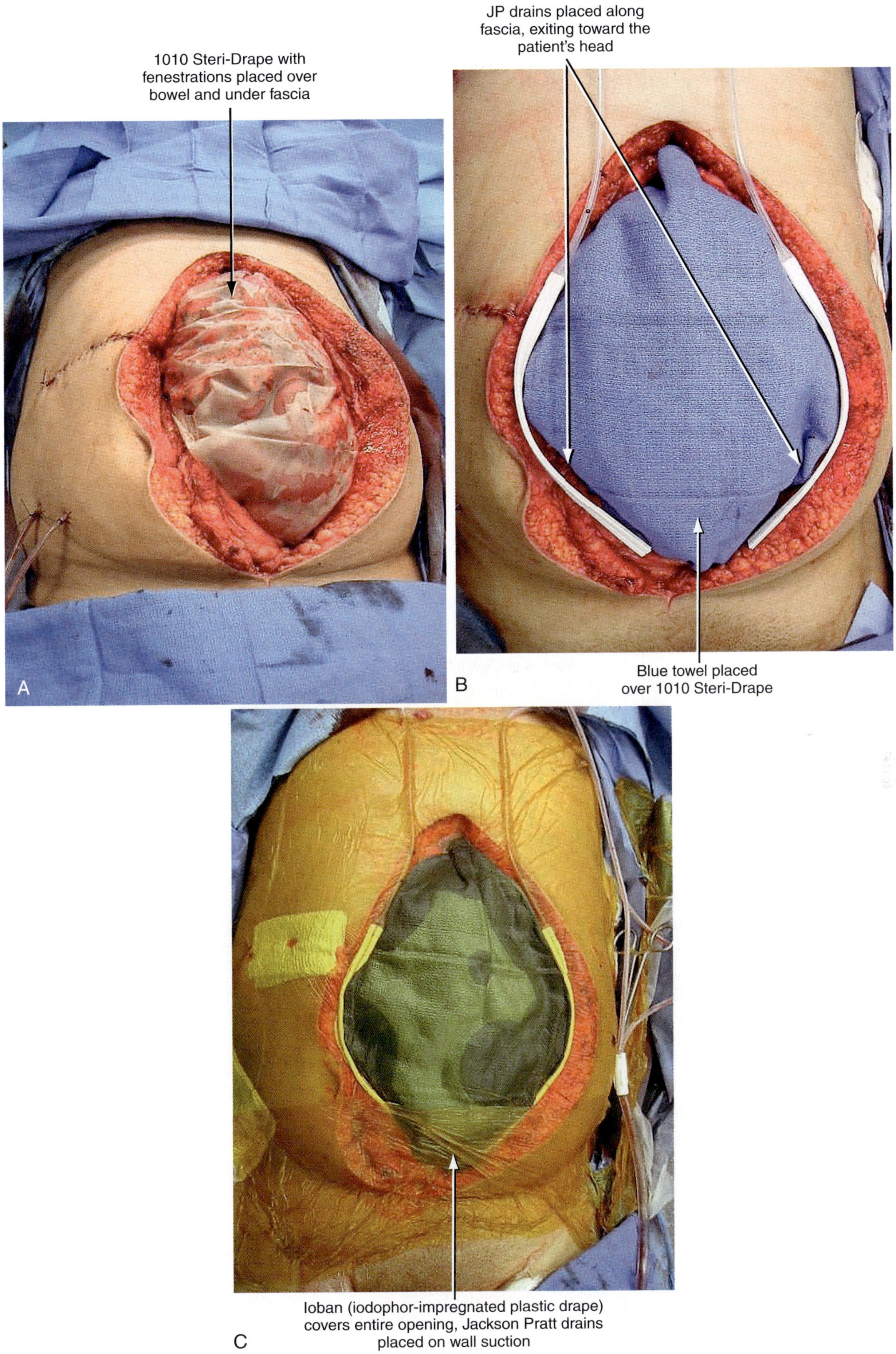

FIG. 35.2 Phased abdominal closure using multiple layers. (A) A Steri-drape 1010 is placed over the viscera and under the fascia. (B) Jackson-Pratt drains are placed on the fascia margins. A surgery towel may be used to cover the first layer of plastic. (C) An Ioban drape containing iodophor covers the towel. (From Cioffi W, et al, eds. *Atlas of Trauma Emergency Surgical Techniques*. Philadelphia: Saunders; 2014.)

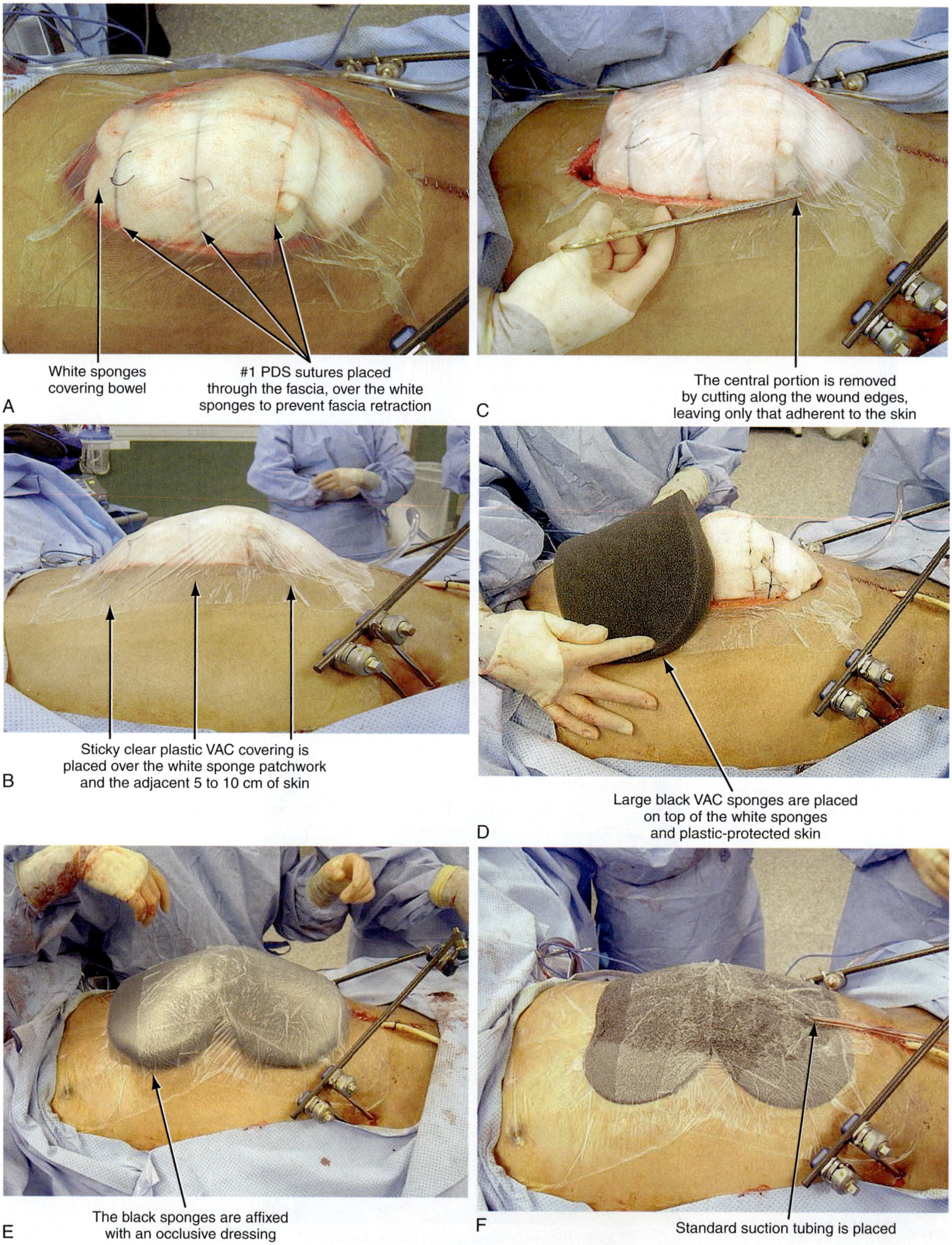

FIG. 35.3 Vacuum-assisted closure (VAC). (A) VAC sponges are used to cover the viscera. PDS sutures are placed through the fascia and over the sponges. (B) Clear plastic covers the sponges. (C) Central portion is removed. (D) VAC black sponge is placed over the white sponges. (E) An occlusive dressing is placed over the black sponge. (F) Suction is applied. (From Cioffi W, et al, eds. *Atlas of Trauma Emergency Surgical Techniques*. Philadelphia: Saunders; 2014.)

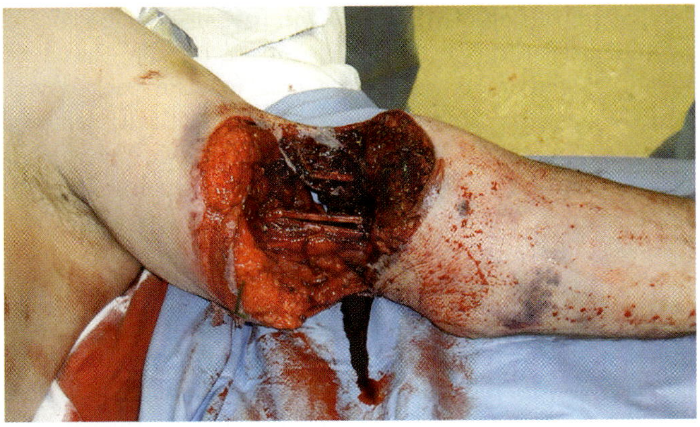

FIG. 35.4 Near amputation of the forearm. (From Canale S, Beaty J. *Campbell's Operative Orthopaedics*. 12th ed. Philadelphia: Mosby.)

loose dressings, drapes) and exposing tissues only when necessary in the preoperative period.

- *Neurological injury:* Care is taken during wound assessment to avoid causing or extending nerve damage.
- *Vascular damage, compartment syndrome, and limb loss:* Transporting, moving, and handling the patient can result in the extension of injuries including vascular damage. Compartment syndrome may occur early and must be treated quickly.
- *Loss of limb function:* Full debridement and identification of nerves, tendons, and blood vessels for reconstruction take place once the patient is stabilized. Debridement may be repeated within 24 hours.

Preoperative care of the patient is directed toward the prevention or treatment of these complications. The surgical technologist in an assistant circulator role may be directly or indirectly involved in presurgical care of the patient. Good communication is essential because there may be many people in the circulator role and the environment may be noisy.

Preoperative care of the patient may include debridement in the emergency department. If the primary assessment reveals exsanguinating hemorrhage, emergency surgery takes precedence over debridement. In this case, the patient may arrive in the operating room very quickly after transport to the health care facility. If there is a pelvic fracture, the patient may have a pelvic binder in place; this is released only with direction from the surgeon and anesthesia care provider. Limb traction may have been applied in the emergency department. If so, the anesthesia provider and surgeon direct all transfers to maintain traction. Anesthesia is started as soon as it is clinically safe, and the patient can be carefully positioned, prepped, and draped.

CASE PLANNING

Instruments and Equipment

Instrumentation required for orthopedic damage control surgery includes a major orthopedic set and general surgery instruments. Vascular instruments should be available on standby. Soft tissue repair may be delayed for phased procedures; however, one set of soft tissue instruments and equipment is needed for clean debridement and another for the

BOX 35.3 Suggested Equipment Used in Damage Control

- Low- and high-speed drills (low speed usually preferred) with extra drill bits
- Hand drill
- Kirschner wires
- Threaded Steinmann pins
- Heavy pin cutters
- Pin or clamp and frame fixation system (surgeon's preference) and olive wires
- Self-tapping screw fixation system
- Intramedullary nailing system, dynamic or static locking (surgeon's preference)

surgical repair. Open fracture of the long bones is most often stabilized with an external fixation system. If the method is preplanned before the patient arrives, naturally this equipment and hardware is included in the setup. However, if the stabilization methodology is not known, the surgical technologist should have certain equipment available to open on immediate request. A suggested list is shown in Box 35.3.

A high-impact pelvic fracture with open fracture of the leg is initially stabilized using a pin and frame external fixation system. This allows exploration of the wound. Severe pelvic fracture is associated with a high rate of tissue damage to the pelvic structures and severe hemorrhage arising from the venous system. Wound exploration requires right-angle clamps; fine long, curved hemostats; and narrow retractors, such as a Deaver set. If there is involvement of the lower intestinal or genitourinary tract, these instruments sets must also be available. An ample supply of Silastic vessel loops with bolsters and clamp shods should also be available.

Drapes

Emergency orthopedic surgery can require large amounts of irrigation solution for both debridement and normal surgical wound irrigation. Impermeable drapes, gowns, and cover sheets are therefore used whenever possible. Runoff from irrigation solutions must be controlled using pocket drapes. Sterile team members should have leggings available to prevent soaking through the scrub suit.

DAMAGE CONTROL ORTHOPEDIC SURGERY

The primary goals of damage control orthopedic surgery are the control of hemorrhage, stabilization of fractures, and prevention of sepsis.

The surgical technologist in the scrub role maintains a high level of wound management as described in detail in Chapter 19. Particular highlights of wound management in the multiple trauma orthopedic patient are as follows:

- Assist in maintaining hemostasis using all appropriate technologies available.
- Prepare and have ready appropriate-size instruments for the tissues.
- Clear the sterile field of all instruments not in use; maintain a clean, orderly field.

- Keep tissues moist.
- Protect the sterile field and maintain strict aseptic technique.

DEBRIDEMENT OF FRACTURES

Wound debridement is the removal of nonviable or dead tissue and debris from a traumatic or infected wound. Patients with open traumatic wounds, with or without fracture, are at high risk for infection; therefore debridement is a necessary part of treatment. The procedure may be performed in the emergency department before an emergent surgical procedure or as a part of the procedure. However, if immediate lifesaving surgery is required, debridement may be performed at the patient's bedside after both the patient and fracture are stabilized.

Open fractures are by definition contaminated and require some level of debridement, which may include excision of skin edges and deeper tissues that have been crushed or macerated in the trauma.

In preparation for debridement, the wound is draped with an extra-wide margin exposed beyond the periphery of the wound. The area is prepped as usual but extended to include a large anatomical region such as the entire limb. Debridement is performed using the surgical knife, Metzenbaum or fine scissors such as tenotomy or pediatric-size Metzenbaum, toothed tissue forceps, and the appropriate retractors for the tissue involved. Hemostasis is maintained as usual with ligation or ESU. The wound may be enlarged to encompass muscle, fascia, and in some cases devitalized medullary canal tissue. Tissue and debris may be collected in basins placed on the field. The surgeon will reduce or cut back the tissue margins until bleeding occurs; this signals that the tissue is viable. All tissue and non-tissue fragments are saved as specimens. Viable bone fragments recovered during debridement must be kept moistened with saline because they may be used during repair.

After surgical debridement, the wound must be copiously irrigated. Routine low-pressure irrigation using a bulb or Asepto syringe may be used, or the surgeon may use a pulsating lavage system. In either case, warm normal saline is used. Topical bacitracin may be used as an additive to the irrigation solution. Regardless of the mechanics of irrigation, the surgical technologist should prepare the surgical field for large quantities of fluid. Debridement may be repeated within 6 to 8 hours.

EMERGENCY TREATMENT OF FRACTURES

External fixation is currently the most common method of damage control orthopedic surgery. This strategy plays a significant role in stabilization to prevent further tissue damage, pain control, and maintaining limb length. All attempts will be made to resuscitate the multiple trauma patient to the point where damage control surgery can be attempted. This is because further insult to the body increases the immune responses, which lead to the deterioration of the patient's condition.

Control of hemorrhage takes priority in damage control orthopedic surgery. If the source of the bleeding has been identified and is accessible, the area may be packed with lap sponges, and the packs may be systematically removed to secure hemostasis. In the case of unstable pelvic fracture, abdominal, retroperitoneal, or pelvic structures may be severely injured. A focused assessment with ultrasound performed preoperatively aids in the identification of free blood. In the case of abdominal or pelvic bleeding, a laparotomy may be required to secure hemostasis. Bleeding in the retroperitoneal cavity is more difficult to identify and stop because it often arises from the venous plexus, which is difficult to access. Also, an unstable pelvic ring may extend the injuries. Because of these difficulties, a pelvic stabilizer may be applied at the start of surgery or in the emergency department. The C-clamp stabilizer is a temporary bar device held in place with pins. A pelvic binder is used in the preoperative and intraoperative stages to maintain stability (Fig. 35.5). A more complex external or internal fixation system replaces the C-clamp or binder during the first or later phased surgeries.

Long bone fractures are initially stabilized using an external fixation system such as the *Ilizarov system*, cage, or lateral fixator. These are held in place with pins or wires. Once the fractures are stabilized, the limb can be moved without any risk of further tissue damage (Fig. 35.6). Application of the device is straightforward. The scrub should have the surgeon's preferred system, including the bar and wire components and tools needed to assemble and adjust the framework.

THORACIC INJURY

Blunt thoracic injury accounts for at least 20% of all trauma mortality and contributes to 50% of all trauma mortality in the United States. The main cause of all thoracic injury is motor vehicle accidents. Life-threatening injuries to the thoracic structures and chest wall include those that cause mechanical impingement on respiratory and cardiac function, injury to the heart and great vessels, pulmonary injuries, and other soft tissue injuries such as esophageal and diaphragmatic trauma.

Open thoracotomy may be performed in the emergency department to evacuate a **cardiac tamponade** (hemorrhage into the pericardial sac sufficient to prevent the heart from contracting effectively) or to control hemorrhage of the heart, lung, or large vessels, including the aorta. Once the immediate emergency has been addressed, the patient is then transferred rapidly to the operating room for further surgery. Indications for immediate surgical intervention include tension pneumothorax, open pneumothorax, flail chest, massive hemothorax, and pericardial tamponade. These conditions are described later.

CASE PLANNING

Case planning for thoracic emergency should include instrumentation and supplies for three systems:

- Cardiovascular
- Respiratory
- Orthopedic

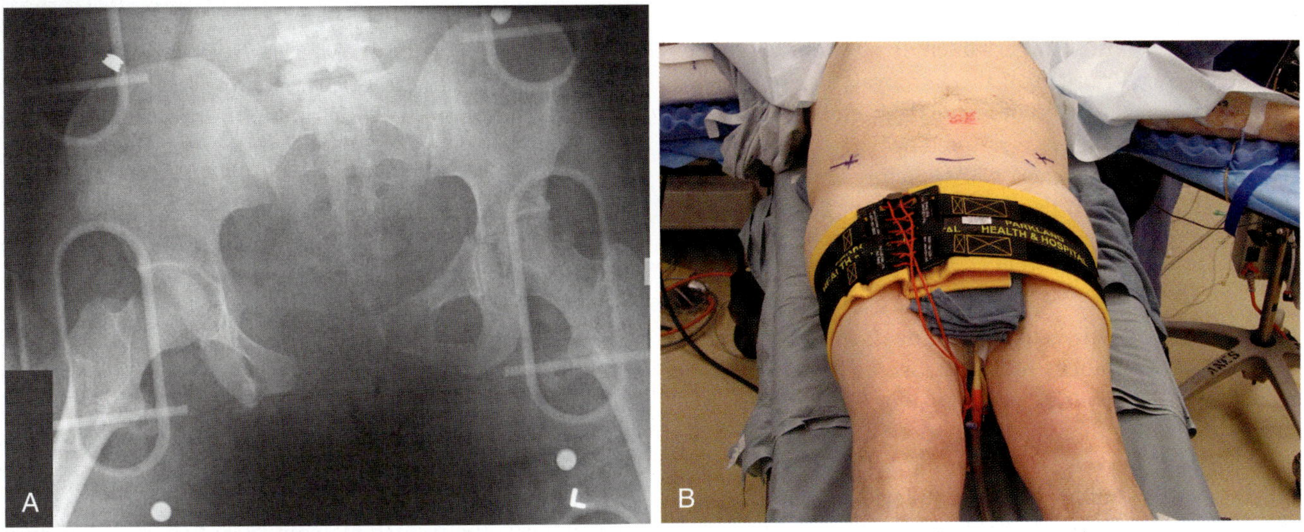

FIG. 35.5 Pelvic stabilizer. (A) Radiograph showing pelvic fracture. (B) External compression device used to provide stability to a pelvic fracture. (From Canale S, Beaty J, eds. *Campbell's Operative Orthopaedics*. 12th ed. Philadelphia: Mosby; 2013.)

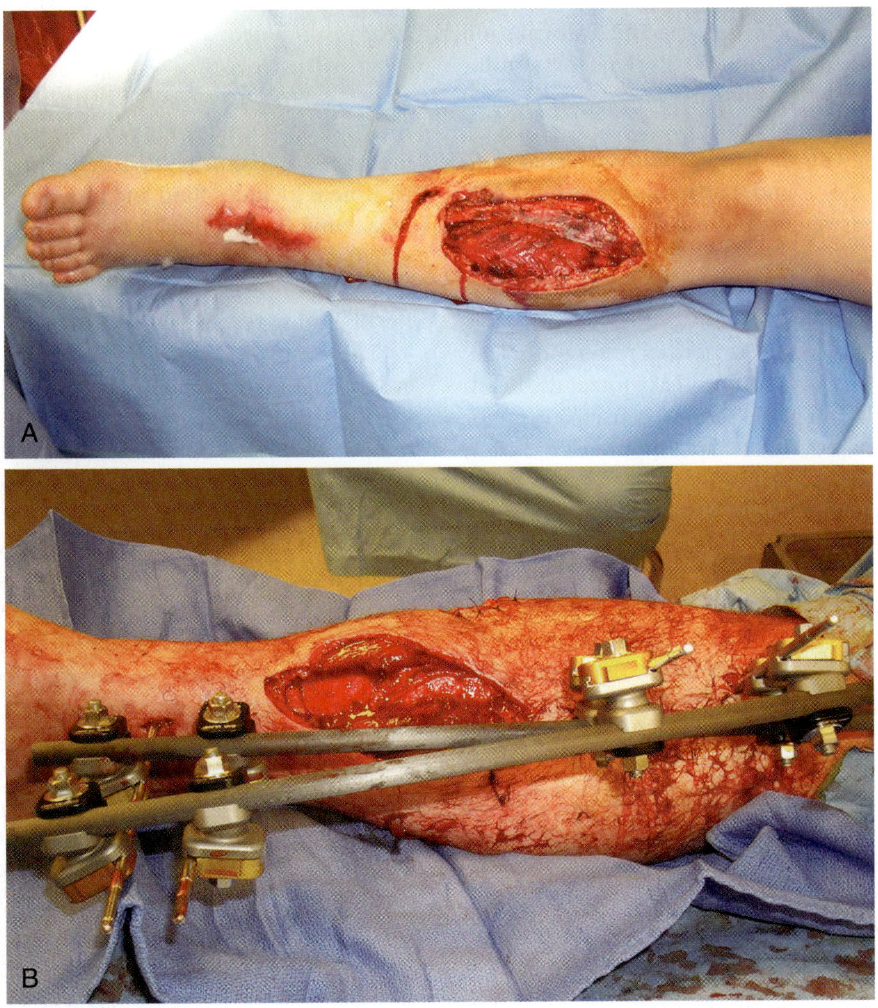

FIG. 35.6 Damage control surgery. External fixation using a unilateral pin and bar fixation device. (From Canale S, Beaty J, eds. *Campbell's Operative Orthopaedics*. 11th ed. Philadelphia: Mosby; 2009.)

The most urgent (lethal) injury is of course treated first, but total damage control surgery often involves at least two of the three systems. Priorities of the cardiovascular system are focused on the management of hemorrhage and cardiac function. The respiratory system is restored by repair of the injured structures including the chest wall. Fractures of the ribs can be life threatening when the fractured end punctures or lacerates vital soft tissues or in the case of multiple rib fracture that impinges on the lung (flail chest), described later in this section.

Rapid setup and delivery of instruments for damage control thoracotomy should be prioritized by the following:

1. ***Exposure of the injuries and source of hemorrhage.*** This translates to suction (at least two suction systems immediately available), sponges, and appropriate retractors. A Finochietto self-retaining and Deaver set should be available from the start of surgery.
2. ***Removal of free blood and clots.*** Prepare a large basin to receive clots. Have at least 10 to 15 lap sponges dipped in warm saline and wrung dry. Always have at least 30 sponges in reserve for immediate use.
3. ***Have cardiovascular sutures available according to the surgeon's preference card.* If the specific information is not available, have 2-0 and 3-0 Prolene or similar monofilament suture.** Fibrin glue may also be used to seal wounds in damage control surgery.
4. ***The strategy for chest wall closure is usually deferred until the end of the case.*** The wound may be closed in one layer. Chest tubes and underwater seal drainage are required.

INJURIES OF THE CHEST WALL

The chest wall must remain intact for normal respiration. Disruption in the rib and sternal structures that protect the heart, lungs, and great vessels can have serious consequences for the respiratory and cardiac systems. Open injury of the chest wall in which negative pressure is lost requires immediate lifesaving measures to restore respiratory function. This can be done in the field or in the emergency department. A common method for sealing the chest wall is the application of petrolatum gauze over the wound, which is an effective temporary sealant. Evacuation of air is performed using needle thoracostomy or immediate insertion of chest tubes. Extensive open chest wounds require mechanical ventilation.

CARDIOVASCULAR TRAUMA

Blunt Cardiac Rupture

Cardiac rupture is the tearing of the ventricles or atria, pericardium, chordae, valves, or other associated structures. It is among the most lethal of thoracic injuries and may include "explosive" rupture of the ascending aorta and shearing of the descending aorta, which occurs as the first rib and clavicle strike the vertebral column in high-speed, high-energy impact. Diagnosis is made by investigating the mechanism of the injury from witnesses and through echocardiogram. Cardiovascular trauma is usually accompanied by other serious injuries, including pulmonary, abdominal, and head injury. Diagnosis of these is generally based on focused sonogram and radiography, and survival is often based on an intact pericardium and ability to control hemorrhage from other sites. The most common cause of blunt cardiovascular trauma is a motor vehicle accident in which the driver impacts the steering wheel. Other causes are falls, blast injury, and crushing injury. Cardiac injury can be complicated by conduction disorder, dysrhythmia, and intraventricular thrombi. Treatment for cardiac rupture may be performed in the emergency department initially by pericardiocentesis, emergency thoracotomy, and pericardiotomy. The patient is then immediately transported to the operating room. The patient who has had thoracotomy in the emergency department may arrive with an inflated Foley catheter controlling a small hole in the heart or direct manual compression on larger wounds. Only about 10% require bypass for repair in the operating room. The surgical treatment is the immediate control of hemostasis and repair of the ruptured myocardium and other damaged structures. Damage control surgery of the heart includes packing the chest cavity and rapid repair of the structures using abbreviated traditional means and temporary closure of the thoracic cavity. A definitive procedure follows when the patient has been resuscitated.

Penetrating Cardiac Wound

Penetrating wounds of the heart caused by civilian gunshot or knife are now common in urban areas. Emergency department treatment includes fluid and blood resuscitation and tube thoracostomy (insertion of a chest tube) to treat pneumothorax, which usually occurs with penetrating wounds. Echocardiography is performed quickly, and the patient is transferred to the operating room.

The most lethal complications in penetrating cardiac injury are exsanguinating hemorrhage into the pleural cavity resulting in cardiac tamponade. The patient with increasing cardiac tamponade must be treated quickly, and this may require immediate emergency department thoracotomy.

Gunshot wounds to the thorax are associated with high mortality, especially with high-velocity bullets. Knife wounds result in the laceration of structures that can often be repaired, if the patient is treated quickly to avoid fatal hemorrhage. Other less frequent causes of penetrating wounds to the heart and vessels are various types of impalement injuries related to industrial and home accidents.

Surgical treatment includes the evacuation of free blood, restoring heart function, and repair of damaged tissues. This requires a complete cardiovascular setup with repair sutures or the surgeon's choice. The repair may be definitive but somewhat abbreviated. For example, suturing over pledgets may be too time consuming. Patch grafts are preferred over tube grafts.

Aortic Injury

Injury to the aorta is most often the result of a high-speed, head-on collision (unrestrained passenger or driver) or high-impact lateral blow to the chest. Car versus pedestrian accidents, a fall from a great height, and ejection from a motor vehicle also contribute to the incidence of aortic trauma. Mortality is high, especially with the complete rupture of the aorta.

Of patients with blunt aorta injury, 60% to 90% die at the scene of the accident or shortly after arrival in the trauma center. Diagnosis may be difficult, especially in the multiple-trauma patient. Echocardiography, FAST, and radiography are used in the assessment, along with the analysis of the mechanism of injury and presenting symptoms.

Surgical repair of the aorta is definitive and may require cardiopulmonary bypass to prevent postoperative paraplegia related to cross-clamping the aorta. Synthetic grafts or direct anastomosis are techniques used in repair. Although most procedures require open surgery for the assessment and repair of associated injuries, some cases of aortic trauma can be managed using endovascular stenting via the femoral or iliac artery.

PULMONARY TRAUMA

Pulmonary trauma occurs most frequently in motor vehicle accidents as described earlier for cardiovascular injury. An additional cause is a blast injury, which occurs in intentional violence and occasionally in industrial accidents. Pulmonary injury ranges from severe lung and bronchial tears to a variety of conditions in which respiration is compromised because of loss of the lungs' mechanical ability to expand; 35% to 75% of pulmonary **contusions** (bruising of the lung parenchyma leading to hemorrhage into the alveolar spaces) occur because of blunt chest trauma. It is the most common thoracic injury in children.

Any pulmonary injury that compromises ventilation and gas exchange must be treated emergently. Treatment begins in the emergency department with thoracostomy or possible thoracotomy and is continued in the operating room. Emergency surgery requires a basic emergency setup, including major thoracic and vascular instruments. An autotransfusion system should also be available.

Flail Chest

Flail chest a critical condition in which three or more *adjacent* ribs are separated from the chest wall. The segment of ribs then moves freely over the soft tissues of the thorax, where the cut edges of the ribs can lacerate soft tissues. The flail segment moves *paradoxically:* inward with inspiration and outward on expiration, resulting in the inability to contribute to lung expansion. In some cases, the flail extends into the sternum. The significance of a flail chest is the loss of respiratory mechanisms and probable injury to the lungs (Fig. 35.7).

The goal of treatment is to restore ventilation and treat underlying injuries. Intubation and assisted ventilation are performed in extreme cases so that surgery can be initiated on injuries to the internal structures, which are almost always present and account for 8% to 35% mortality with flail chest.

Pneumothorax

Pneumothorax is the presence of air in the potential space between the lung and pleura, which prevents full expansion of the lung. This condition is always found in penetrating pleural injury. Three types of pneumothorax include *simple, communicating,* and *tension.*

A *simple pneumothorax* is one in which there is no communication with atmospheric air and no thoracic structures are displaced (Fig. 35.8). This can be caused by a fractured rib end entering the pleural space on impact or from a gunshot or stab wound.

Communicating pneumothorax occurs when the pleural wound communicates with the outside atmosphere. This results in the collapse of the lung on the affected side with the complete loss of ventilation (Fig. 35.9). This type of pneumothorax is sometimes referred to as a "sucking" chest wound because of the sound made as air is forced in and out of the wound during attempted respiration.

Tension pneumothorax occurs when air in the pleural space increases to a point where the mediastinum, lung, and great vessels are pushed and eventually compressed into the opposite side of the chest cavity. This is a potentially lethal injury resulting in rapid hypoxia, shock, and acidosis.

Pneumothorax is detected using CT scan and FAST. Treatment can be initiated in the field or in the emergency department by needle thoracostomy or by the insertion of chest tube in the case of tension pneumothorax. The presence of underlying injuries may require rapid transfer to the operating room.

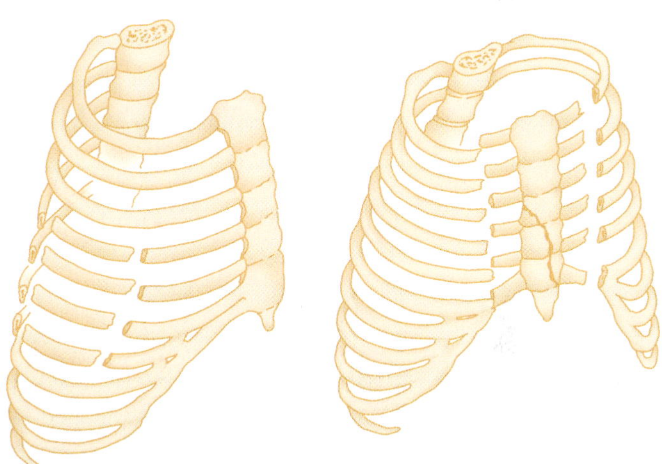

FIG. 35.7 Flail chest. Note that adjacent ribs are fractured in two sections, creating a lateral or central section that is free floating. Flail chest is an indication for immediate emergency surgery. (From Marx J, Hockberger R, Walls R, eds. *Rosen's Emergency Medicine: Concepts and Clinical Practice.* 7th ed. Philadelphia: WB Saunders; 2010.)

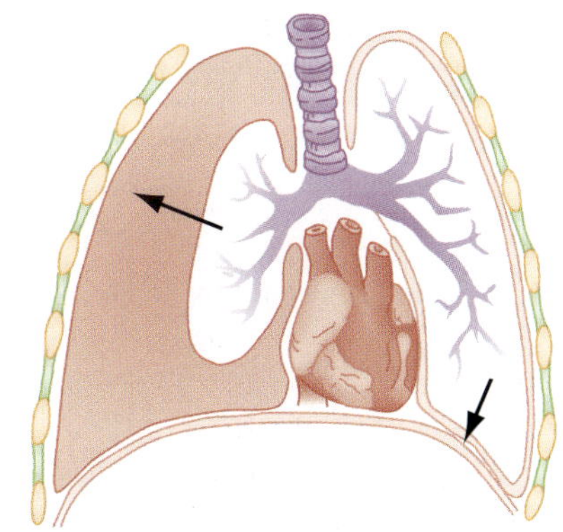

FIG. 35.8 Closed pneumothorax. This is a simple pneumothorax in the right lung with air in the pleural cavity and collapse of the lung. (From Marx J, Hockberger R, Walls R, eds. *Rosen's Emergency Medicine: Concepts and Clinical Practice.* 7th ed. Philadelphia: WB Saunders; 2010.)

Hemothorax

Hemothorax is free blood in the pleural cavity, which reduces lung capacity by the same mechanisms as pneumothorax. A common cause is the laceration of lung tissue, including the parenchyma (lung covering). Emergency thoracotomy is performed when blood reaches or exceeds 1500 mL. The patient can quickly become hypovolemic with complications related to failed gas exchange.

The surgical goal in this case is to repair the lacerations, restore respiratory function, and replace the blood loss. A thoracostomy is performed in the emergency department for initial treatment. In this case, a size 36- to 40-Fr chest tube is inserted under local anesthetic and connected to an underwater sealed drainage system. The patient is then transferred to the operating room.

Lacerated Lung

Pulmonary laceration or deep pulmonary laceration is associated with hemothorax and multiple rib fractures. A severe laceration can arise from the bronchi or from the lung tissue. In these cases, the patient may undergo emergency department thoracotomy to clamp the tissue and then may be moved quickly to the operating room for complete repair. Damage control surgery may include lobectomy in selected cases. However, initially the bleeding is controlled with rapid suturing. Some surgeons prefer to use staples for a temporary repair (Fig. 35.10).

Diaphragm Injury

Diaphragmatic injury occurs most frequently with motor vehicle accidents and falls from a great height. This injury involves the herniation of abdominal contents into the thoracic cavity through a defect in the diaphragm. This presents a risk of strangulation of abdominal structures that is made worse as the negative intrathoracic pressure pulls the organs into the thoracic cavity. Rupture of the diaphragm caused by blunt or penetrating trauma can be lethal and requires emergency surgery. Surgery can be performed laparoscopically, but full evaluation of all injuries often requires open surgery. The method of repair is definitive unless additional injuries indicate damage control laparotomy.

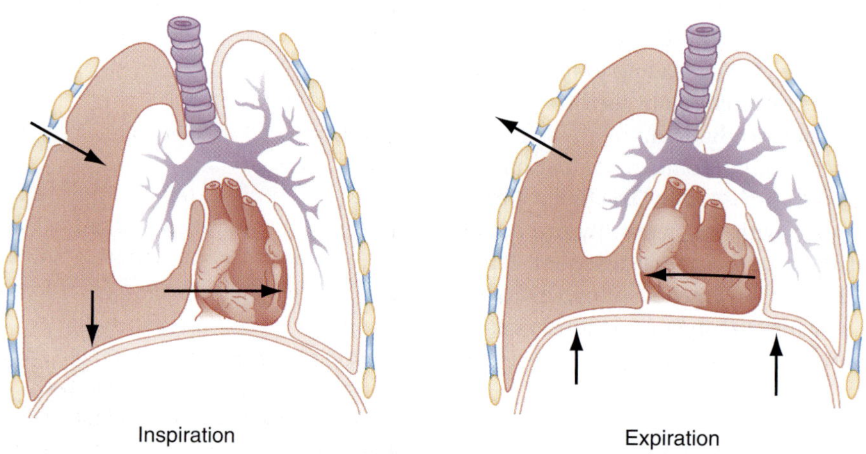

FIG. 35.9 Communicating pneumothorax. The right lung is collapsed, and there is a defect in the chest wall that communicates to the outside. (From Marx J, Hockberger R, Walls R, eds. *Rosen's Emergency Medicine: Concepts and Clinical Practice.* 7th ed. Philadelphia: WB Saunders; 2010.)

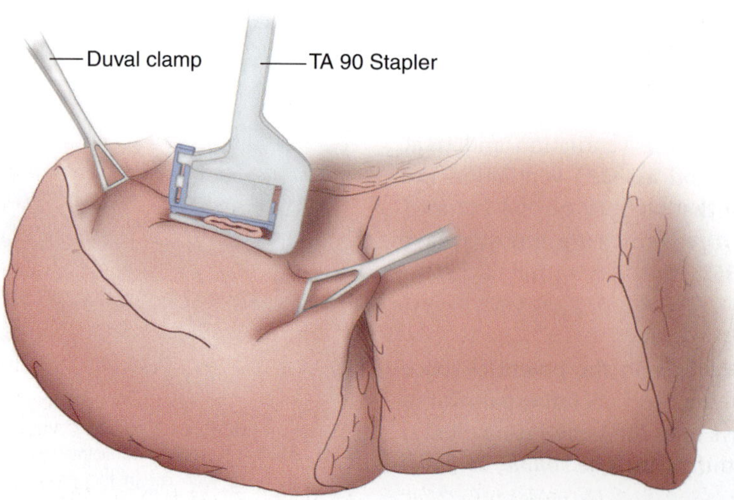

FIG. 35.10 Laceration of the lung closed with TA stapling device. (From Cioffi W, et al, eds. *Atlas of Trauma Emergency Surgical Techniques.* Philadelphia: Saunders; 2014.)

MAJOR PERIPHERAL VASCULAR TRAUMA

Trauma of the major arteries may threaten limb viability or vital structures and is therefore considered extremely urgent. In the United States, 70% to 90% of peripheral vascular injuries occur as a result of penetrating trauma related to violence. Gunshot wounds remain the leading cause of death in individuals from 15 to 34 years. Ninety percent of victims are males.

The method of assessment in vascular trauma depends on the severity of the wounds and the patient's condition at the time of arrival at the health care facility. Patients with severe, pulsating hemorrhage from an open wound and other obvious indications of limb-threatening injury are often taken directly to the operating room without preoperative diagnostic workup. Intraoperative angiography may be performed after bleeding is under control and the patient is hemodynamically stable. Other less serious but nonetheless urgent cases are diagnosed using color flow Doppler, CT scan, and MRI. The value of diagnostic procedures must be weighed against the time required to produce the results.

Specific areas of vascular injury are often associated with another trauma. For example, the most common vascular injury is to the femoral artery and vein caused by hip fracture. Trauma to the iliac artery is almost always accompanied by the involvement of the intestine, bladder, and pelvis. In this case, damage control laparotomy is performed. The most common arterial injury of the arm is the brachial artery, seen mostly with penetrating trauma, fracture of the humerus, and animal bites.

Vascular injury is divided into two major categories according to the cause—penetrating and blunt trauma.

PENETRATING TRAUMA

In civilian medicine, penetrating trauma to blood vessels is most frequently caused by gunshot and knife wounds. The trajectory, perimeters of wound damage, and path of bullets have been expertly studied in the field of ballistics. Data gathered by civilian, military, and human rights organizations have greatly benefited the surgeon's ability to predict the extent of trauma and therefore more effective exploratory surgery and treatment.

Ballistics

There is wide variation in penetrating ability, lateral tissue damage, and shape of bullet wounds, according to the type of weapon and bullet involved. Surgeons are challenged to learn about new or modified weapons that are introduced into the community and used for civilian interpersonal violence. All bullets produce a typically elongated track. Jacketed or semijacketed types also expand (explode) early in impact or late in the path. This means that tissue damage and vascular injury may occur distant from the entry wound. Shotgun or pellet wounds present a larger scope of impact that may result in the migration of fragments into distant tissues.

Knife Trauma

Knife trauma results in partial or total severing of vascular structures. Small wounds may be easily explored and treated, whereas larger, deeper penetrating wounds can be fatal and require emergency surgery.

BLUNT TRAUMA

Blunt vascular trauma occurs as a result of crushing injuries such as those that occur in motor vehicle or industrial accidents. A fractured long bone may also impinge on vascular bundles, causing occlusion and limb ischemia. Loss of blood supply to the lower limb forces the tissue into anaerobic metabolism, accumulation of lactic acid, and tissue death.

CASE PLANNING

Urgent vascular trauma surgery commonly includes other systems. A vascular setup and general surgery instruments should be prepared along with all supplies needed for a major vascular case including drugs, solutions, hemostatics, Silastic vessel loops, and other vascular supplies, such as Fogarty catheters for removing thrombi in damaged vessels. Orthopedic and amputation instruments should also be available for limb surgery.

Sutures and supplies should include basic peripheral vascular sutures such as Mersilene, Prolene, or Pronova on vascular needles. Grafting is usually not performed in emergency surgery. Instead, direct repair and anastomosis techniques are used. As soon as the technologist is able to identify (or is informed) of the vessels to be repaired, the appropriate-size sutures should be quickly prepared. It is better to have made an intelligent guess than to have no repair sutures available. Both single-arm and double-arm (for anastomosis) sutures should be immediately available. Unless the surgeon identifies which suture materials are needed for ties, silk, size 2-0 and 0, should be prepared on right-angle passers to start the case.

In cases in which the limb is in danger of ischemia and compartment syndrome, the anesthesia provider and surgeon may implement a forced cooling protocol to slow the metabolism in the limb. In this case, sterile ice slush and cold irrigation may be required on the field.

SURGICAL TREATMENT

Preoperative treatment in the emergency department includes resuscitative measures and attempts to stanch the hemorrhage, if the source can be accessed. A Foley catheter may be inserted at the wound site and used as a tamponade. In some cases, vascular repair may not take precedence over other life-threatening injuries, which are addressed first while arterial or venous injuries are treated by direct compression. The patient is transferred to the operating room as soon as possible in the presence of exsanguinating vascular trauma complicated with other injuries.

If the vascular injury involves a major neurovascular bundle or the limb has been severely mangled, amputation may be performed. A generalized list of priorities of the surgery will be as follows:

- Exposure to the site of injury
- Gaining access to the injured vessels by evacuation, retraction, and careful dissection
- Hemorrhage control by clamping or direct pressure followed by direct repair or temporary graft
- Blood and fluid replacement (continued resuscitation)
- Repair or removal of bone or foreign body fragments to prevent further injury

The type of repair performed on the vessels depends on the patient's condition. Damage control surgery for major injury favors direct repair of the vessel including anastomosis. However, a temporary synthetic graft may be implanted for a short period (usually no more than 24 hours) to perfuse a limb in an unstable patient.

INJURIES OF THE BRAIN AND SPINAL CORD

TBI accounts for approximately one-third of all deaths from trauma, representing about 52,000 deaths each year. The main causes of TBI are falls and motor vehicle accidents. TBI is the leading cause of death in patients younger than 25 years. Two-thirds of total deaths resulting from brain injury in the birth to 4-year-old group are the result of child abuse. The objective of emergency medical and surgical intervention is to avert secondary injuries related to increased cranial pressure and the physiological changes that occur with severe head trauma.

BLUNT TRAUMA

Because brain injury is irreversible, all attempts are made to prevent secondary events that accompany the initial trauma. These include the management of hemorrhage and intracranial pressure resulting from bleeding and cerebral edema. These can occur with blunt trauma to the head or when the head in motion (such as in a fast-moving vehicle) is suddenly stopped. This has two effects: the shearing injury of neural tissue and blood vessels and the physical impact of the brain against the cranium. These can result in the rupture of blood vessels, laceration of tissue, and *avulsion* (separation or tearing away of one tissue layer from another).

Assessment for head injury relies on laboratory findings and imaging studies using CT neuroimaging and MRI. The decision for emergency neurosurgery depends on the presence of other life-threatening injuries and the patient's hemodynamic status. Damage control surgery includes drilling burr holes in the cranium and ventriculostomy (placement of a drainage catheter in a ventricular space to relieve pressure). Definitive surgery to relieve intracranial pressure related to hemorrhage is craniotomy with the evacuation of blood and clots and securing hemostasis.

PENETRATING BRAIN INJURY

The most common cause of penetrating brain injury in the United States is gunshot. Gunshot wounds account for approximately 21,000 deaths per year. As with injury to other systems by gunshot, the type of weapon, speed and type of bullet, and exact path in the tissue determine the lethality of the injury. Patients who survive the initial impact are evaluated for the location of the injured tissue, extent of hemorrhage, and secondary effects—mainly hypoxia, ischemia, and hypotension. Emergency surgical management is usually craniotomy for the control of intracranial pressure.

CASE PLANNING

Planning for craniotomy is detailed and requires many specialty instruments and supplies. Therefore an emergency craniotomy cart is available on standby in health care facilities that receive trauma patients. The cart contains essential items including but not limited to standard linens, suction tubing, ESU equipment, hemostatic materials, scalp clips, surgical sponges, and neurosurgical instrument sets. Preparing for multiple-injury cases that include an emergency neurosurgical procedure plus additional setups can be difficult because of the amount of neurosurgical equipment required. A sequential setup may be possible if the surgeon knows ahead of time the priority of multiple repairs. Two or more setups can be confined to separate back tables that are brought forward in order of need. Damage control neurosurgery (see later discussion) requires few instruments, and the equipment can be quickly separated from the emergency cart. The scrub can then switch back tables as needed. An alternative strategy is that more than one scrubbed team operates simultaneously on different injuries. In this case, each team has a dedicated setup.

Positioning

Positioning the patient requires care to maintain the spine in a neutral position. Cervical spine injury is not ruled out until a conclusive (often time-consuming) assessment has been completed. The urgency of surgery may override full evaluation. The patient usually arrives with a stabilizing cervical collar, and transfer to the operating table requires log rolling with a lateral transfer device. The supine position can be used if cervical injury has been completely ruled out. In this case, the head is turned with the affected side up. A prone or beach chair position may also be used if it does not interfere with the surgery of other systems.

Draping

Draping for emergency craniotomy with multiple injury sites must accommodate these sites. In such cases, the top drape can be extended only as far as the periphery of the other site, and a second procedure drape is used to overlap the craniotomy drape. A penetrating brain injury is considered contaminated because the penetrating object is not sterile and scalp tissue, including hair, is often dragged into the wound.

EMERGENCY NEUROSURGICAL PROCEDURES

Depending on the location of the injury and source of hemorrhage, a number of different approaches are used in emergency neurosurgery. These are described here.

- **Subdural hematoma:** Hematoma between the dura and brain. These are often associated with acceleration-deceleration trauma.

- **Epidural hematoma:** Hematoma arising between the dura and deepest layer of the cranium. These are usually associated with fracture and can be rapidly fatal.
- **Traumatic subarachnoid hemorrhage:** This type of injury may be associated with the tearing of subarachnoid vessels.
- **Intracerebral hematoma:** A traumatic intracerebral hematoma occurs as a shearing injury that ruptures small arteries deep within the brain. They occur as a result of impact of the brain against the cranial vault rather than as a direct injury. Traumatic (direct) intracerebral injury carries a high mortality rate.

NOTE *The procedures for craniotomy and cranioplasty are detailed in Chapter 34.*

SPINAL TRAUMA

Approximately 50% of spinal injuries are caused by motor vehicle accidents in patients who were unrestrained at the time of the accident. Most of the remaining 50% are caused by falls, gunshot wounds, or sport injuries.

Spinal cord injury occurs when the supporting ligaments, intervertebral discs, and bony structures are disrupted, causing the spine to move in opposing directions. The protective structures that hold the spine in alignment occur as two separate columns. If one column remains intact, it acts as a brace against injury. However, if both the posterior and anterior columns are disrupted, the likelihood of spinal cord injury is greatly increased.

Primary injury to the spinal cord can worsen at any time during transport and treatment as long as the spinal column is unsupported. Therefore the stability of the spine is a primary consideration in emergency response. Emergency personnel in the field now apply cervical and full-body stabilization devices to accident victims, sometime before they are extricated from the accident debris. Stabilization devices are not removed until there is definitive evidence that no spinal injury exists.

Many different types of spinal fractures have been identified. Injury to the spinal cord depends on the direction of impact and penetration of the spinal cord by bone or other connective tissues, such as the ligaments that extend along the spinal column. Diagnostic imaging (CT, MRI) and laboratory tests are used to confirm a diagnosis.

These data are kept by the National Spinal Cord Injury Association: https://www.nscisc.uab.edu/Public_Pages/Database.

TYPES OF SPINAL CORD INJURIES

Spinal cord injuries are divided into two main types, primary and secondary. Primary injury occurs when blunt or penetrating trauma severs neural tissue in the spinal column. Primary injury also occurs when a dural hematoma impinges on the cord. Secondary injury occurs as a result of a cascade of physiological changes that occur with trauma, including the lethal triad discussed previously, and injury related to moving and handling the patient after admission to the health care facility.

A further classification of spinal cord lesions is the complete and incomplete lesion. *Complete* lesions cause complete loss of motor and sensory function distal to the injury. *Incomplete* lesions result in varying degrees of combined motor and sensory loss depending on the nature of the lesion, its location, and the extent of injury. Emergency surgery is usually not performed on patients with complete lesions. However, an incomplete lesion can benefit from exploratory surgery that includes removal of foreign bodies, bone fragments, or other tissue impinging on the spinal cord, removal of hematomas, and mechanical stabilization using a spinal orthopedic system or by application of a halo brace. These procedures are performed on stabilized patients.

NECK TRAUMA

Life-threatening neck trauma of the soft tissues may involve the airway, blood vessels, and laryngeal structures. Severe hemorrhage from any of the vital structures can result in shock or obstructed airway. Three classifications of neck trauma are blunt, penetrating, and strangulating (also called *near hanging*), and these account for up to 5% of all traumatic injuries. Blunt trauma is rare compared with other mechanisms of injury.

A penetrating injury is most commonly related to gunshot and knife wounds and shrapnel from explosives.

Emergency response for injuries of the neck depends on the structures suspected of injury. Diagnosis employs a combination of physical assessment for signs of hemorrhage, airway obstruction, and neurological damage, in addition to imaging studies—CT scan and MRI.

PREOPERATIVE CARE OF THE PATIENT

Cervical spine injury is not ruled out in the patient with severe neck trauma, and field response includes placement of a cervical collar. Intubation may be required, and in this case rapid sequence intubation (RSI) is performed. In this technique, a fast-acting, short-duration sedative is administered and orotracheal intubation is performed unless there is massive facial trauma. If RSI is not possible, a surgical airway such as cricothyrotomy is performed in the emergency department or in the field. Care of the patient in the immediate preoperative phase is the same as for all trauma patients, with attention to preventing hypothermia, spinal protection, and monitoring vital signs while in transit. Although many neck injuries can be treated conservatively, those involving major blood vessels or the airway may require immediate surgery. A gunshot wound may contain pellets that can migrate into an open blood vessel and into the heart or brain. Severe hemorrhage of the carotid, subclavian, or jugular vein may cause blockage to the airway.

CASE PLANNING

Case planning for neck trauma must include vascular instruments, sutures, and supplies such as those used in carotid surgery (refer to Chapter 30). Fine dissecting instruments should also be available for the exploration of the upper respiratory structures. This will require a variety of retractors, such as those used in thyroid procedures and for carotid endarterectomy. Drugs and hemostatic agents should be distributed as for carotid procedures.

Patients are normally positioned supine with prep and draping as for wide thyroidectomy. In the event of cervical fracture, stabilization devices will be managed by the anesthesia care provider, and positioning is carried out with care to maintain a neutral spine.

SURGICAL MANAGEMENT OF NECK INJURY

Surgical management of vascular injuries in the neck is usually definitive unless there are other, more urgent concurrent injuries that require immediate attention. Direct anastomosis or patch graft techniques are used to control vascular hemorrhage. Airway trauma may also be treated by direct repair with tracheostomy. Combined laryngotracheal trauma usually occurs in blunt trauma in motor vehicle accidents and also in near-hanging incidents. A fractured cricoid cartilage leads to airway obstruction. Immediate control of hemorrhage and removal of airway obstruction are the surgical objectives in these cases.

KEY CONCEPTS

- The Committee on Trauma of the American College of Surgeons has developed extensive criteria for the designation of trauma facilities. These facilities are graded according to their capacity to attend trauma patients and other criteria involving community trauma response.
- The physiological consequences of multiple or severe trauma can develop into an irreversible cascade of events initiated by the immune system. These are often called the "lethal triad" and include severe hypotension, metabolic acidosis, and coagulopathy.
- Treatment protocols for the lethal triad are initiated as soon as medical help is available to trauma victims. Actions taken in the first hour often determine whether the injuries are fatal.
- Compartment syndrome is the severe compression of tissues within a compartment of the body, including the cranium, abdomen, or limb. Unless relieved, compartment syndrome can lead to ischemia and necrosis of the tissue involved.
- ATLS trauma management defines specific protocols and objectives. The main objectives are to treat life-threatening clinical problems such as severe hemorrhage immediately and then transport the patient to the ICU for resuscitation. Phased surgical procedures then follow when the patient is stable.
- Damage control surgery is defined as surgery that only addresses hemorrhage and the threat of sepsis. Reconstructive and other types of prolonged procedures are delayed until the patient is stable.
- Case planning for emergency trauma surgery includes a multisystem approach based on possible surgical interventions. The surgical technologist can develop expertise in trauma surgery by building on the principles and techniques of nonemergency surgery.

REVIEW QUESTIONS

1. The trauma system used in the United States involves assigning numeric levels to health care facilities. Explain this system.
2. Explain what is meant by the "golden hour" as it applies to emergency trauma.
3. Explain compartment syndrome.
4. Define "lethal triangle" as it applies to emergency trauma. Briefly describe the elements of the triangle.
5. How does case planning for emergency trauma surgery differ from case planning of nonemergency cases?
6. Why is it no longer recommended to perform extensive repair and reconstruction surgery in the initial stages of emergency trauma?
7. Explain the *primary survey,* which is performed by first responders in the field.
8. Describe the appropriate care of forensic specimens during surgery and the rationale for using this protocol.
9. Why are displaced pelvic fractures life threatening?
10. Distinguish between flail chest, pneumothorax, and hemothorax.

BIBLIOGRAPHY

American College of Surgeons: *Statement on the prevention of retained foreign bodies after surgery*. Accessed November 2, 2016. http://bulletin.facs.org/2016/10/revised-statement-on-the-prevention-of-unintentionally-retained-surgical-items-after-surgery/.

AORN. *Recommended Practices for Prevention of Retained Surgical Items. Association of periOperative Registered Nurses: Guidelines for Perioperative Practice*. Denver: AORN; 2015.

Association of periOperative Registered Nurses (AORN). Unplanned perioperative hypothermia. In: *Standards, Recommended Practices and Guidelines*. Denver: AORN; 2011.

Borden Institute and the U.S. *Department of Defense: Emergency War Surgery, third United States Revision*. Washington, DC: U.S. Government Printing Office; 2004.

Canale S, Beaty J, eds. *Campbell's Operative Orthopedics*. 12th ed. Philadelphia: Mosby; 2013.

Cioffi W, et al., ed. *Atlas of Trauma Emergency Surgical Techniques*. Saunders; 2014.

Martin R, Meredith J. Management of acute trauma. In: Townsend Jr CM, Beauchamp RD, Evers BM, Mattox KL, eds. *Sabiston Textbook of Surgery*. 19th ed. Philadelphia: WB Saunders; 2012.

Marx J, Hockberger R, Walls R, eds. *Rosen's Emergency Medicine: Concepts and Clinical Practice*. 7th ed. Philadelphia: WB Saunders; 2010.

Miller R, Eriksson L, Fleisher L, Weiner-Kronish J, Young W, eds. *Miller's Anesthesia*. 7th ed. Philadelphia: Churchill Livingstone; 2009.

Roberts J, Hedges J, eds. *Clinical Procedures in Emergency Medicine*. 5th ed. Philadelphia: WB Saunders; 2010.

Townsend CM, Beauchamp DR, Evers M, Mattox KL, eds. *Sabiston Textbook of Surgery*. 19th ed. Philadelphia: WB Saunders; 2012.

36 DISASTER PREPAREDNESS AND RESPONSE

LEARNING OBJECTIVES

After studying this chapter, the reader will be able to:

1. Discuss different types of disasters
2. Discuss the common features of a disaster
3. Explain the role of government agencies during a disaster
4. Explain what is meant by an *all-hazards* approach to disaster planning
5. Define the four phases of the disaster cycle
6. Locate documents useful for making a home disaster plan
7. Describe the main components and strategy used by communities to prepare their local disaster plan
8. Define the incident command system and explain how it works
9. Describe basic human needs in a disaster
10. List the primary components of a health care facility disaster plan
11. Discuss ethical dilemmas that accompany disasters
12. Explain the possible roles of the surgical technologist during a disaster

TERMINOLOGY

Agency for Healthcare Research and Quality (AHRQ): Agency that provides disaster-related research, resources, training, and recommendations for health care facilities, communities, and individuals.

All-hazards approach: An integrated strategy for disaster management that focuses on the common features of all disasters, regardless of the cause or origin.

American Red Cross: National organization that provides humanitarian assistance and technical support during disasters and emergencies.

Bioterrorism: The intentional release of biological agents (e.g., bacteria, viruses, mycotoxins) to create illness and death in humans, animals, and the environment. Modes of transmission include air, water, and food.

Declared state of emergency: A status conferred on a disaster by the state governor or the president (for a federal declaration). An official declaration of emergency entitles the state in which the disaster occurs to receive federal aid through the Federal Emergency Management Agency (FEMA).

Disaster: A catastrophic event that affects a large portion of the population and poses significant risk to human life and property. A disaster overwhelms local resources and requires outside assistance.

Disaster recovery: A phase of the disaster cycle in which the community returns to a functional level after a disaster. Recovery has no defined interval and may take years.

Emergency: A more geographically isolated event than a disaster that can be handled by local emergency services, such as ambulances, the fire department, or paramedics.

Federal Emergency Management Agency (FEMA): Federal agency responsible for all aspects of coordination, management, and response for nationally declared disasters. It also provides extensive training programs in disaster preparedness management and response for professionals and members of the community.

Logistics supply chain: The event-related process of handling material goods from the point of procurement, to the point of delivery to the end user.

Mass casualty event (MCE): An emergency in which the number of victims overwhelms the human and material capacity of available health care services. An MCE is usually associated with a geographically isolated event (e.g., transportation accident, industrial accident).

Mitigation: A process or intervention intended to reduce the level of injury or harm. For example, mitigation against the effects of a hurricane includes early warning systems that may predict the strength and location of the storm.

National Fire Protection Association (NFPA): Organization that develops and distributes codes and standards that aim to lessen the threat of fire and hazards as well as their potential impact in the community.

Natural disaster: Widespread damage and risk of injury caused by forces of nature, such as a hurricane, a tornado, an earthquake, floods, and extreme heat or cold.

Pandemic: A public health emergency in which an infectious disease spreads throughout a large population, often across international boundaries.

TERMINOLOGY (CONT.)

Shelter-in-place: During a disaster, individuals may be required (or may choose) to shelter-in-place rather than evacuate the hazardous areas. This means that people remain where they are until the environment is safe or until rescue workers can reach the site.

Surge capacity: The number of patients a health care facility can manage in an emergency.

Vulnerability: Exposure to the risk of harm. In disaster management, vulnerable populations are those with a higher than normal risk. This may be related to their age, mobility, inaccessibility, or other condition that hinders or prevents aid.

In recent years, natural and human-made disasters have revealed a need for increased disaster preparedness among all sectors of the community, including health care. As a result, government, social, and professional groups have increased funding for research, training, and implementation of disaster programs designed to inform the public, create new systems, and train professionals in disaster preparedness. The World Health Organization (WHO), the Centers for Disease Control and Prevention (CDC), and many academic institutions and national health organizations now provide training at all levels of disaster management. Recognizing that different types of disasters require common response strategies, training for disaster is based on an **all-hazards approach,** in which communities and disaster specialists learn basic management and responses that can be applied with some modification to many different types of emergencies.

Disaster preparedness training is required for health care professionals, including those in allied health. The Commission on Accreditation of Allied Health Education Programs (CAAHEP) has added emergency preparedness to its accreditation standards. The organization has stated that allied health students "must have an understanding of their specific role in an emergency environment, both as citizens and health care professionals."

Disaster preparedness training and management is a broad interdisciplinary process that involves many agencies and individuals. This chapter is intended to introduce the surgical technologist to disaster terminology, core principles, and the disaster environment. It is not intended to train people in management or other roles specific to disasters. These roles depend on the emergency plan of the health care facility and may require more extensive training. Many courses are available on all-hazard preparedness, including those for health professionals. For a list of agencies that provide all-hazard courses, refer to the last section of this chapter, Resources for Students and Instructors.

ACRONYMS

Government and international institutions often use a variety of acronyms to define documents, agencies, and doctrines. These are usually familiar to those who work in those sectors but are confusing for others. Acronyms used in this chapter are necessary for studying federal government documents and processes. A list is provided here for reference:

AHRQ	Agency for Healthcare Research and Quality
CDC	Centers for Disease Control and Prevention
DHHS	Department of Health and Human Services
DHS	Department of Homeland Security
DHSES	Division of Homeland Security and Emergency Services
DMAT	Disaster Medical Assistance Team
EMA	Emergency management agency
EOC	Emergency operations center
FCC	Federal Communications Commission
FEMA	Federal Emergency Management Agency
HazMat	Hazardous materials
HICS	Hospital incident command system
HRSA	Health Resources and Services Administration
MCE	Mass casualty event
NDMS	National Disaster Medical System
NIMS	National Incident Management System
NRF	National Response Framework
NWS	National Weather Service
START	Simple triage and rapid treatment
WHO	World Health Organization

TRAINING

Although currently no standardized curriculum exists regarding disaster preparedness for health care professionals, the need for such a curriculum has been nationally recognized. Individual professional organizations are responding to this

BOX 36.1 Proposed Health Care Worker Competencies for Disaster Training

1. Recognize a potential critical event and implement initial actions.
2. Apply the principles of critical event management.
3. Demonstrate critical event safety principles.
4. Understand the institution's emergency operations plan.
5. Demonstrate effective critical event communications.
6. Understand the incident command system and the health care worker's role in it.
7. Demonstrate the knowledge and skills needed to fulfill the health care worker's role during a critical event.

From Hsu E, Thomas T, Bass E, et al. Health care worker competencies for disaster training. *BMC Med Educ.* 2006;6:19.

need by creating objectives and guidance statements. While this work is in progress, allied health and other professionals can increase their capacity to respond to disaster and mass casualty events by taking specific courses in disaster management. This chapter is an introduction to the disaster environment in accordance with the academic requirements of CAAHEP.

A number of government agencies and academic institutions offer excellent disaster preparedness courses (see resources at the end of this chapter), and many of them are free, available as podcasts or live broadcasts. A wealth of federal, state, and community disaster training is available at all levels, including advanced academic degrees for disaster managers. These are intended for students and instructors. Advanced courses are also available in specific topics, such as **bioterrorism,** public health, and infectious disease. Basic competencies for disaster training are shown in Box 36.1.

CLASSIFICATION AND DEFINITION OF DISASTERS

A **disaster** is a catastrophic event that poses a large-scale risk to human life and property. Most importantly, a disaster *overwhelms local resources and requires outside assistance.* Disasters are often associated with human tragedy and widespread environmental devastation.

It is important to distinguish between a disaster and an emergency. A disaster causes widespread disruption in the social order, as well as injury and loss of property. In other words, disasters have far-reaching *social* consequences. An **emergency** is a more geographically isolated event that can be handled by local emergency services, such as ambulances, the fire department, or paramedics. For example, a motor vehicle accident or house fire can have tragic implications for those directly involved; however, unlike a disaster, these emergencies do not threaten the entire community.

A **mass casualty event (MCE)** is a localized emergency, such as a transportation accident (e.g., major air crash), explosion, or structural collapse in which the number of victims overwhelms local health care services. A mass casualty event may overwhelm local health care services, but it does not usually constitute a large-scale disaster requiring federal assistance.

TYPES OF DISASTERS

Disasters and emergencies are classified by type and cause. The type of disaster can influence the response and may have implications for federal or state funding and reimbursement for property loss.

Traditionally, disasters were classified simply as "human-made" or "natural." However, today's global and regional disasters do not fit easily into these categories. Although we sometimes use these terms for broad discussion, root causes such as globalization, climate conditions, and widespread environmental degradation have blurred the categories. It is easy to see how the definitions lose meaning when we discuss whether a flood was caused by a torrential storm, loss of topsoil and vegetation related to farming practices, or poor engineering of levees on a flood plain. The current nomenclature for hazards used by the Federal Emergency Management Agency is *Natural, Technological/Accidental, Pandemic,* and *Terrorist.*

We then define the disaster specifically according to probable causes (Table 36.1). A classification of disasters indicates the level of response needed:

- Level I: Local emergency teams are able to manage the immediate consequences and aftermath of the event.
- Level II: Regional assistance from surrounding communities is required.
- Level III: Statewide and federal assistance is required because the effects of the disaster have overwhelmed local and regional resources.

Natural Disasters

A **natural disaster** is one that arises from a force of nature, such as a hurricane, a tornado, an earthquake, floods, and extreme heat or cold. Natural disasters are often complicated by other environmental factors, including those caused by populations. Overcrowding in communities, failure to meet building codes or lack of building codes, and even inequitable health care systems can place vulnerable populations at an even higher risk when a disaster occurs. The more we study the effects of population growth, land use, and other social and technological pressures, the more apparent it is that human presence and activities may be the root cause of many disasters described as "natural." For example, mud slides and flooding may be initiated by excessive rainfall, but the root cause often is deforestation and urbanization of natural flood plains, which alter the geography. The following are considered to be natural disasters:

- *Blizzard:* A winter storm characterized by high wind and blowing snow, resulting in low or no visibility. Blizzard conditions are often extremely cold. High winds can also pick up fallen snow, causing blizzard conditions.
- *Ice storm:* Freezing rain falls during an ice storm, covering all exposed areas with a thick, slippery, glass-like layer of ice. The weight of the ice causes the collapse of roofs, power lines, trees, and other solid structures. Transportation is halted because of dangerous road conditions, and power outages are widespread.

TABLE 36.1 Natural and Human-Made Disasters, Health Risks, and Mitigation

Type of Disaster	Health Risks/Effects	Mitigation/Response
CLIMATIC		
Flood	Drowning Overflow of sanitation collection sites Driving through or into water Contamination of drinking water	Early warning Environmental surveillance Structural preparation Land use planning and preparation
Hurricane	Drowning Injury from debris Massive property damage	Surveillance Early warning Evacuation
Tornado	Injury from debris Structural collapse Massive property damage	Surveillance Early warning Safety shelter Evacuation
Winter storm	Vehicle accidents Hypothermia Carbon monoxide poisoning Structural collapse from ice and snow Ice jams Flooding	Identification of shelters Establishment of shelter-in-place plan Adequate supplies of sand, salt, heavy equipment Distribution of weather radios Extra food stocks in communities
Extreme heat	Heat cramps Heat exhaustion Heat stroke Fatal hyperthermia	Identification of vulnerable groups Surveillance
Earthquake	Injury and death resulting from structural collapse Risk of tsunami	Strategies for rescue Building and retrofitting for structural soundness (to prevent structural collapse)
Wildfire	Smoke inhalation Carbon monoxide poisoning Burns Injury from falling structures Heat stress (especially for responders) Electrical hazard	Evacuation plan Management of hazardous fuel in wild lands and forests Community awareness and education Build backfires Create fire breaks
Tsunami	Drowning Injury from structural collapse and high-velocity debris	Earthquake surveillance and early warning systems Evacuation
Volcano	Asphyxiation from toxic gas and ash Inundation by mud and lava	Early warning Evacuation
Landslides, avalanches, and mudslides	Drowning, inundation by mud and debris Injury related to high-velocity debris and water Electrical risks Disrupted roadways/lack of access to health care	Land use and urban planning Environmental surveillance Early warning Community education
INFECTIOUS DISEASE		
Pandemic, emerging infectious diseases, epidemic	Flu viruses	Adequate stockpile of vaccine Adequate stockpile of medical supplies and drugs Community education Surveillance
UNINTENTIONAL AND TECHNICAL DISASTER		
Transportation accident (train, air disaster, motor vehicle, marine)	Traumatic injuries Burns Drowning	Response includes search and rescue. Federal agencies may become involved in investigations.
Explosion	Burns Head and other traumatic injury Ear injury	Following safety standards in the workplace Workplace training in safety and first aid

TABLE 36.1 Natural and Human-Made Disasters, Health Risks, and Mitigation—cont'd

Type of Disaster	Health Risks/Effects	Mitigation/Response
Hazardous material spill	Burns Lung injury Nerve damage Systemic poisoning	Early detection of the agent Early identification of the agent Protective measures according to type of agent Decontamination areas may be needed for victims and hazardous materials crews that work on the front line
Radiation	Nuclear accident	Protection from radioactive fallout Protection from contamination in the area Safe use of food and water Monitoring and treatment of victims of radiation exposure
INTENTIONAL VIOLENCE/TERRORISM		
Bioterrorism	Anthrax Botulism Plague Smallpox Tularemia Viral hemorrhagic fevers	Enhanced diagnosis capacity Surveillance Establishment of case definitions Training and education Preparation of health care facilities Establishment of safe areas
Chemical	Caustic agents Pulmonary Explosives Flammable gas and liquid Blistering agents Nerve agents Blood agents Dioxins Oxidizers Incapacitating agents Respiratory (pulmonary) agents Metals Vomiting agents Toxic alcohols	Early detection of the chemical Early identification of the agent Rapid surveillance and reporting systems Specific training for primary health workers Personal protective equipment (PPE) for workers and civilians Availability of specialists in rapid removal Provision of shelter-in-place Case definitions of adverse effects Preparatory training before an incident occurs
Radiation	Dirty bombs Nuclear blast Radiation poisoning	Protection from radioactive fallout Protection from contamination in the area Safe use of food and water Monitoring and treatment of victims of radiation exposure
Explosion or bombing	Blast injury Burns Injury from high-velocity debris	Community education about disaster plans Health care facilities prepared for mass casualty

- *Extreme heat:* Temperatures that exceed the body's ability to regulate itself result in death, unless the body can be externally cooled. During a heat wave, power grids may fail because of overload from urban use of air conditioners. People who do not have the means to cool the body are most vulnerable, including older adults, poor, and homeless. More people die as a result of heat waves in the United States than from any other weather-related disaster.
- *Drought:* A climate condition that features lack of rain (precipitation) is called a *drought.* Drought conditions result in failed crops and low water levels in reservoirs meant for human use. The most famous drought in recent history was during the 1930s in the central region of the country (the Dust Bowl). In severe drought conditions such as those that occurred during the Depression, thousands of families were forced to leave their land and homes to seek food and work.
- *Earthquake:* Movement of earth's tectonic plates that causes them to move past each other results in pressure on the boundary. When the pressure reaches a critical level, an earthquake occurs. Earthquake disaster can cause massive loss of life and property resulting from collapsed structures. Water and power lines are often affected, and logistic systems for bringing in aid may be crippled for weeks.
- *Flood:* Floods are usually related to both weather and land use. Poor drainage, lack of engineered waterways, and construction in flood plains with a known history of previous mass flooding contribute to loss of life and

property during a flood. The risks among populations are often related to inability or refusal to evacuate the flood area as warnings are issued.

- *Forest fire:* Forest fires occur every year in the United States as a result of lightning strikes and more commonly from human activity near large forest lands. As urban communities continue to encroach on wild forest lands, fires become increasingly common.
- *Hurricane:* A combination of conditions including warm oceans, moisture, light winds, and a weather disturbance can lead to a hurricane. Most hurricanes do not reach land but remain over the ocean. However, as the conditions build, the hurricane can move quickly, reaching coastal and urban communities very fast. Hurricane categories are based on the Saffir-Simpson scale. A Category 3 or higher is a major event with sustained winds of 74 mph or higher.

> The federal government's Agency for Toxic Substances and Disease Registry provides HazMat Emergency Preparedness Training and Tools for Responders, including a dictionary of hazardous materials, on their website: http://www.atsdr.cdc.gov/hazmat-emergency-preparedness.html or search for "ATSDR HazMat."

- *Tornado:* This is a narrow rotating column of air that forms during a thunderstorm. The column or "funnel" extends from the base of the thunderstorm to the ground, moving rapidly across the land while rotating extremely fast. Although the energy released during a tornado is very destructive, the actual footprint may be small (perhaps only 100 or 200 yards) in comparison to a hurricane.
- *Tsunami:* An earthquake or volcano generated on the ocean floor can create very long, powerful waves on the ocean surface. Such a wave is called a *tsunami* or *tidal wave.* On the open ocean, the wave can be very shallow. However, as it reaches shallow land near shore, the height of the wave increases. Waves of enormous speed and force can completely destroy structures in their path. Just before reaching the shore, water on the coastline retracts quickly, often below the lowest tidal point. Once on shore, the tsunami crosses the shoreline, going far inland, and then pulls back, taking with it most of the debris created by the wave.
- *Snow avalanche:* Snow avalanches are familiar to most people who ski or live in mountainous areas. Avalanches are large swaths of snow, ice, and rock that fall along slip planes weakened by warm weather or water. The avalanche may take along trees, boulders, and buildings in its path.
- *Mudslide:* Similar to an avalanche, a mudslide is the release of thousands of tons of mud from an incline. The cause is usually unstable slippage planes that may be natural (related to the type of soil) and made active by loss of topsoil and vegetation. Mudslides commonly occur in regions that have been cleared for forestry activity or urbanization. Particular types of soil are prone to slides, and houses or whole communities built in these areas are at high risk. A mudslide can be fast moving and very destructive, carrying debris, trees, buildings, and boulders in its path.

Technological Disasters

Technological or industrial disasters are *unintentional* events caused by human activity, compounded by error or negligence. They can be caused by the release and spread of toxic substances involved in manufacturing, transportation, building, and extraction of natural resources such as oil and minerals. In many of these disasters, specific methods are used to contain and neutralize toxic materials. Technological disaster can be particularly frightening for communities because many of the dangers are hidden and represent an unknown. The effects of these disasters are often experienced for decades, as we have seen in Chernobyl and in the 1984 Bhopal disaster in India. At Bhopal, an accident at the Union Carbide plant released a pesticide component into the air, immediately killing at least 4000 people and causing lifelong disability in an estimated 400,000 others. The following are technological disasters:

- *Explosion:* Large-scale explosions can occur where flammable materials are used in manufacturing or in large storage facilities, including oil refineries, chemical plants, and manufacturing facilities. Victims at the site of the disaster suffer severe injury from the blast and fire. Communities are affected if chemicals are released into the environment. This can have short-term or long-term health implications.
- *Hazardous material accident:* Hazardous material accidents occur in conditions similar to those for explosions, with greater risk in refineries and other locations where large amounts of hazardous materials are stored or manufactured. Disaster response in this type of situation depends on identification of the hazardous material and the ability to contain the material or to mitigate the effects. HazMat specialists are needed to manage and advise on the response.
- *Radiation accident:* Radiation accidents such as the Fukushima nuclear crisis and Chernobyl are uncommon but devastating to communities. The unpredictable outcome of a radiation disaster can create fear and anxiety for many decades after the event. During the disaster, containment of the leak and evacuation of the population are the two main features of community and technical responses. Specialists in radiation technology are needed on site to help manage the disaster and evacuate victims to appropriate treatment centers in the region.
- *Transportation accident:* Large-scale aviation, vehicle, and train accidents often result in mass casualty events. If the accident is caused by environmental conditions such as snow, fog, or ice storm, these can complicate rescue efforts and prevent emergency crews from reaching health care facilities. Air accidents that occur over urban areas multiply the effects many times. In all mass casualty situations, triage and treatment begin at the site of the accident unless it is unsafe to remain in the area.

Pandemic

A **pandemic** is a wide-scale, rapidly contagious infectious disease, whereas an epidemic is localized to a specific population. In recent years, human immunodeficiency virus/acquired immunodeficiency syndrome (HIV/AIDS), influenza, and coronavirus have been the major causes of worldwide pandemics. Community response to pandemics and epidemics includes prevention through public health practices such as immunization, health education, and testing. At the clinical level, containment of the infectious agent requires isolation, strict hand washing, disinfection, and sterilization of patient care items. Although clinics are often very busy with flu patients during the winter season, there are few occasions when all services are overwhelmed, and these are usually temporary.

Acts of Terrorism

Current community and public health attention to all-hazards approach began with the events of 9/11 and other terrorist threats that followed. Extensive education, planning, and preventive measures have been put in place to enable a response to a variety of terrorist threats and actual events.

- *Bioterrorism:* This is the intentional release of harmful biological agents (disease-causing bacteria or viruses) into the environment. A specific group of biological agents is associated with bioterrorism for their properties. They are easy to disseminate into the environment on a warhead or other means, they are rapidly fatal with high public health impact, and they require specific treatment and complex methods to mitigate their effects. The most common agents associated with bioterrorism are anthrax, botulism, plague, smallpox, tularemia, and viral hemorrhagic fevers. Some emerging infectious diseases such as hantavirus are also being considered as possible threats.
- *Chemical terrorism:* This is the use of chemical agents for intentional harm in the population. Chemicals include blistering and caustic agents that enter the respiratory system and the nerve gas groups that cause paralysis. Flammable chemicals such as napalm used during the Vietnam War are also in this group. Disaster planning for biological and biochemical terrorism is complex and highly technical. Special procedures for detection, analysis, and protection against individual chemicals and biotoxins are a specialty in disaster preparedness. HazMat training is provided by the CDC and other government agencies.
- *Bombing/direct attack:* A direct terrorist attack, as what occurred on 9/11 and in the Oklahoma City bombing, creates a mass casualty event in which all disaster preparedness systems for rescue, triage, evacuation, and national security are immediately put in place. In addition to the health emergency services, civil and national defense alerts are also activated. These may involve military presence at the site of the disaster. Chain of command may change according to the priority set by government agencies such as Homeland Security. State and national responders may be rapidly deployed to the area of the bombing.

DISASTER MANAGEMENT AND GOVERNMENT STRUCTURES

Disaster management is the strategy used in preparedness and response at different levels of government (federal, state, and local) and by communities themselves. A primary feature of disaster management is rapid, decisive, effective action. This requires a somewhat hierarchical management structure. Because all disaster plans involve government agencies, each level of governance (federal, regional or state, community) *flows from the one above it.* For example, the state disaster plan is based on the procedures and protocols of the federal agencies. Facility plans (including those for health care facilities) must be in accordance with state and federal systems such as those directed by the Occupational Safety and Health Administration (OSHA) and the Department of Health and Human Services (DHHS).

Disaster plans and protocols are consolidated at each government level through that level's emergency system following the *chain of command.* At the community and facility level, each has its own protocols for the disaster plan that are compatible with state and federal regulations. This means that doctors, nurses, or allied health professionals do not have to know the detailed points of the federal government disaster plan (discussed later), but they must understand and be able to practice the disaster plan for their community and for the health care facility and the department in which they work. On the other hand, *disaster managers* (specialists in the management aspects of disaster) must be familiar with all levels of the disaster plan.

FEDERAL LEVEL: AGENCIES AND ROLES

Governmental and nongovernmental agencies contribute to management and coordination during a disaster. The type of agency and the level of involvement depend on the nature of the disaster, the size of the affected population, and the location and extent of the affected area. The federal framework for disasters management is implemented by the Department of Homeland Security (DHS), which ensures that the disaster response is consistent with the country's doctrines and laws (especially constitutional law). This is especially important during a terrorist attack of any kind. The key policy document of the DHS is called the *National Response Framework (NRF).* The information and guidance of the framework contains the following sections:

- Roles and responsibilities (of disaster managers)
- Actions (policy and procedure)
- Organization (how the nation is organized in a disaster)
- Planning
- Resources

The *principles (doctrine)* of the framework are listed in Box 36.2.

FEDERAL EMERGENCY MANAGEMENT AGENCY

The **Federal Emergency Management Agency (FEMA)** is responsible for the coordination, management, and response for nationally *declared disasters.* It also conducts training programs in disaster preparedness, management, and response for professionals and nonprofessionals. FEMA assistance is only available in disasters that have been "declared" a **state of emergency** by the governor of the state where the disaster occurred. Once the governor has declared a disaster, a formal request is made to the federal government. This results in a

The NRF document can be accessed at https://www.fema.gov/media-library/assets/documents/117791 or by searching online for "FEMA National Response Framework."

federal declaration of the disaster that releases federal funding and other resources to help out with the disaster.

FEMA collaborates with many different partners, including community-based organizations, to implement disaster response. Its four federal partners are as follows:

1. Federal Communications Commission (FCC)
2. National Weather Service (NWS)
3. National Disaster Medical System (NDMS)
4. Department of Health and Human Services (DHHS)

NATIONAL INCIDENT MANAGEMENT SYSTEM

FEMA uses the *National Incident Management System (NIMS)* to implement its work. NIMS defines the management structure, objectives, chain of command, and procedures necessary for disaster coordination and response. NIMS is intended for use by all levels of government, nongovernmental organizations, and the private sector. There are five main components and many subsections in the system. The five components are as follows:

- Preparedness
- Communications and Information Management
- Resource Management
- Command and Management
- Ongoing Management and Maintenance

Training for NIMS is available through FEMA, which maintains a large database of resources and references. NIMS courses can be taken on site, and individuals can access online training (see later links) through the agency's Center for Domestic Preparedness and Emergency Management Institute.

HEALTH RESOURCES AND SERVICES ADMINISTRATION

Health Resources and Services Administration (HRSA), an agency of the Department of Health and Human Services, oversees two primary agencies that are involved in the medical (health) response to disaster management:

- **Agency for Healthcare Research and Quality (AHRQ).** This agency provides disaster-related research, resources, training, and recommendations for health care facilities, communities, and individuals.
- National Disaster Medical System (NDMS). This agency maintains a database of trained on-call medical, paramedical, and allied health personnel for emergency deployment during a disaster. It also trains first responders. NDMS response teams are established in each state, and trained professionals are recruited as needed to maintain a full team. Specialist teams include the following:
    - Disaster Medical Assistance Team (DMAT)
    - Disaster Mortuary Operations Response Team (DMORT)
    - National Veterinary Response Team (NVRT)
    - National Nurse Response Team (NNRT)
    - National Pharmacy Response Team (NPRT)

BOX 36.2 Key Principles of the National Response Framework

1. Engaged partnership
2. Tiered response
3. Scalable, flexible, and adaptable operational capabilities
4. Unity of effort through unified command
5. Readiness to act

Disaster Medical Assistance Team

DMAT is the on-call volunteer health assistance team for FEMA. Individuals on DMAT teams are deployed in their usual roles as health care professionals and perform associated tasks. Individuals on the DMAT teams must be available for rapid deployment and able to work in resource-poor disaster environments. Health professionals with specific skills such as radiation, chemical, or other types of trauma are needed in special circumstances. Health care professionals, including surgical technologists, who are interested in applying can make application to their state or local DMAT organization. For information on state DMAT teams, go to https://www.phe.gov/Preparedness/responders/ndms/ndms-teams/Pages/dmat.aspx. Community members may also join their local Community Emergency Response Team (CERT). See https://www.ready.gov/community-emergency-response-team. Additional opportunities for volunteering exist with the Emergency System for the Advance Registration of Volunteer Health Professionals (ESAR-VHP).

CENTERS FOR DISEASE CONTROL AND PREVENTION

Among its many programs and mandates, the CDC is a key information, training, and research organization for disasters and emergencies. Through local partners, it provides public health education to inform people about existing and emerging threats to the population. It provides research and strategic guidelines for all types of health problems, including those resulting from bioterrorism, environmental and technical disaster, infectious disease outbreak, and other public health issues. The CDC Coordinating Office for Terrorism Preparedness and Emergency Response (COTPER) is a federally supported agency that funds technical assistance and stockpiles the drugs, antidotes, vaccines, and medical supplies needed during a disaster. Its Emergency Operations Center monitors threats so that disaster response can be more efficiently and effectively coordinated. The agency also provides extensive disaster training for health care providers and the public.

STATE AND LOCAL LEVELS: AGENCIES AND ROLES

Disaster planning, management, and coordination at the state level are implemented through each state's emergency management agency or EMA (e.g., the Alabama Emergency Management Agency, the Colorado Office of Emergency Management, and the Florida Division of Emergency Management). State EMAs coordinate closely with FEMA and local emergency management agencies (LEMAs).

Governmental and nongovernmental agencies are involved in disaster coordination and response at the local level. Local governments are responsible for management, using protocols and guidelines established by the EMA and FEMA. Individual agencies provide services according to their capacity and expertise. Their local knowledge is particularly helpful in coordinating with state and federal disaster managers. The **American Red Cross** and other nongovernmental agencies provide humanitarian assistance and technical support during disasters and emergencies. Local chapters of the Red Cross also provide courses and training for health care professionals and the community. Individuals who wish to volunteer to help in community disaster response can register with the Red Cross through their state EMA. (Further information is available at the organization's website, https://www.redcross.org/volunteer/volunteer-opportunities/disaster-volunteer.html.) Local communities plan for disasters with the help of FEMA guidelines and disaster specialists.

DISASTER CYCLE

Up to this point, we have discussed types of disasters and the government structures that are involved in setting guidelines, structures, documents, and chain of command for a disaster. From here, we move to the community level, the facility, and the actual events of the disaster. The *disaster cycle* (Fig. 36.1) is a framework for action from the start of planning until communities are able to function again after a disaster. The disaster cycle is a convenient structure for planning and implementation. This framework is used in mainstream disaster planning at all levels and can be changed as needs arise. One or more of the phases may take place at different times or at the same time. The important fact to take away is that the disaster cycle provides grouping of the complex action points of all hazard preparedness.

I. PREPAREDNESS

The preparedness phase is the first step in planning for a disaster. It encompasses numerous complex activities that have a common goal. This is to ensure that individuals, communities, and government sectors are able to respond effectively to different types of disasters. Planning is carried out using the guidelines, procedures, and recommendations provided by governmental agencies (e.g., FEMA), health agencies (e.g., the CDC), and research and academic institutions experienced in disaster management. When a disaster occurs in a hospital, medical office, or stand-alone surgery center, an executable plan must be in place to prevent wasted resources, both human and material. Without adequate planning, the disaster environment can rapidly deteriorate, increasing loss of life and property.

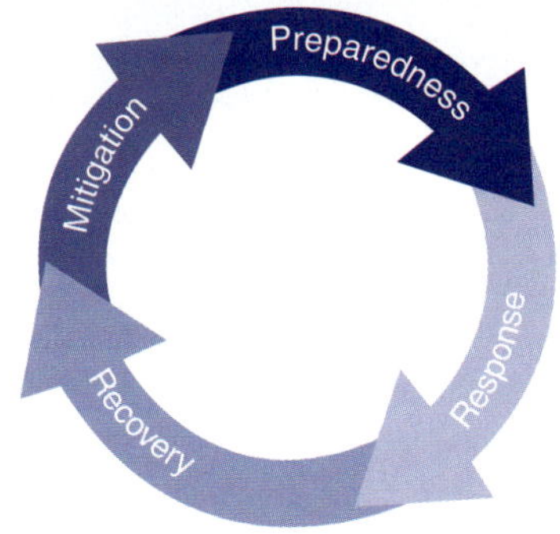

FIG. 36.1 The disaster cycle—planning and implementation model.

Local Team Building

Local team building for disaster planning is derived from the community. Experts from the community form the basis of the team, which has the capacity to discuss important issues and create a working plan. Representatives or lead coordinators from important sectors include the following:

- Law enforcement
- Fire service
- Public works, water, and sanitation
- Public health
- Emergency medical services
- Emergency paramedical services
- Search and rescue
- Ambulance service
- Social and children's services
- Mental health practitioners
- Public health specialists
- Water and sanitation engineers
- Veterinary service
- Structural specialists
- Health care facility management

Other groups such as utility companies, community service organizations, and transportation authorities can provide support input to the planning process.

Risk Analysis and Mitigation Strategy

Once the team is formed, a risk analysis is carried out to target the most likely hazards in that particular community. Even though the overall approach is "all hazards," there are certain mitigation activities that must be carried out according to areas of vulnerability. For example, an area may be near chemical, nuclear, or fuel plants that might create a community-wide disaster in the event of an accident. Natural risks such as flooding, hurricane, and tsunami may also be potential hazards. Each community considers its risks and plans accordingly within the all-hazard framework. Once the risk assessment has been completed, the risk reduction plan is designed. This is where specific technical recommendations are made to protect people and property.

Resource Assessment

No plan can be implemented without the resources to do it. At this point, communities must assess their capacity to fulfill the disaster plan. This includes available communication services, logistical capacity, and human resources.

TABLE 36.2 Primary Objectives of a Local Disaster Plan

Objective	Explanation
1. Activation of emergency response personnel	Based on which organizations have been identified in planning phase. The level of activation depends on the predetermined threshold or trigger.
2. Command post operations center	Responding personnel need a place to meet. This may correspond with the emergency operations center (EOC).
3. Public announcements, hazard and service information	People in the community need to receive updated information about the emergency. The plan must include methods for information dissemination.
4. Management of resources	During a disaster, resources can be depleted or used inefficiently. The plan includes a resource management team that coordinates private and government sources of all types of resources.
5. Restoration of vital services	Critical services such as power, fuel, sewer, and roadways are essential to aiding victims and preventing additional emergency situations. A strategy for restoration of vital services is addressed at the planning stage.

Response Plan

The response plan is developed with consideration of the assessment of resources, risk evaluation, and input from specific community interest and service groups. The plan addresses the process of activation, what will be done and how, who is involved, and the criteria for triggering the response. It includes the sequence of different responses, levels of action, and the actual organization of the response. There is no single plan that fits all communities. A list of general components for an emergency plan is shown in Table 36.2.

In addition to the main disaster preparedness plan, states require specific plans to meet health and safety codes. Examples of these are the following:

- Plan for Hazardous Materials Incident Response (HazMat Plan)
- Risk Management Plan for toxic flammable explosive substances, which includes management of oil spills and other chemicals released into the water or air
- Dam Failure Emergency Action Plan for mitigation and response to dam failure
- Crowd Control Plan used for mitigation of crowd disasters involving venues with a capacity of more than 5000 people
- Radiological Emergency Response Plan, specific to commercial nuclear power plants and hazards associated with nuclear disaster
- School Safety Plan developed to protect school children in event of disaster
- Hospital Disaster Plan, specific to health care facilities, employees, and patients
- Nursing Home Disaster plan to provide mitigation and response to patients and staff
- Adult Health Care Facility Disaster Emergency Plan for protection of residences and shelters of adults in the community
- Electric Utility Storm Plan designed to protect the population and restore power in an emergency or disaster
- Airport Emergency Plan to mitigate and plan for hazards associated with airports and their use in disaster

Local Incident Command System

The local incident command system (ICS) is the on-site (local) disaster management process used during all disasters. The system is designed during the preparation phase and implemented during the response. Many operational sectors in the community such as health care facilities, law enforcement, public works, and schools are integrated into the system in which one or several commanders take the lead, and various sector leaders work under the commanders' line management. Horizontal and vertical communication within the ICS promotes coordination, information gathering, appropriate response, and analysis during an ongoing disaster. This top-down approach is necessary so that decisions affecting people's lives and property can be made quickly by experienced disaster managers. Individual sectors within the ICS include planning, logistics, health, communications, operations, finance, and others.

The ICS is used to overcome coordination problems common to disasters and emergencies, such as the following:

- Competing goals or standards among agencies
- Many responders with no specific tasks or objectives
- Poor communication among responders and agencies
- Lack of clarity about what is to be done and how
- No clear chain of command
- No overall plan or the responders are unaware of the plan

The ICS may be implemented locally for a single facility, such as a hospital, or it may be strategically based to provide management for the entire community or state. A more complex command system may include *incident commanders,* who are heads of organizations involved in the disaster. This system is then called *incident command.* When implemented for an individual health facility such as a hospital, it is called an *HICS* (hospital incident command system). The ICS mandate must follow the NIMS structure and protocols for consistency and efficient use of resources during an emergency. The operational goals of an ICS are to accomplish the following:

- Meet the needs of the incident
- Provide a system under which different agencies can rapidly become operational
- Provide logistic and administrative support to operational staff
- Prevent duplication of efforts

Coordination

Coordination is the process by which the efforts and activities of groups and individuals are organized to make the most efficient use of resources. Disaster-planning coordination prevents duplication of efforts and gaps in service and takes place throughout the disaster cycle. The coordinating body may be a specially trained team or individuals who manage a particular sector, such as health, logistics, or administrative duties. Coordinators are responsible for meshing the activities of service providers or front-line responders and ensuring that they are in compliance with the disaster plan, standards, and recommendations. Uncoordinated groups actually may become a burden or a risk during the response phase. Coordination requires a clear, concise plan; a means of communication during the disaster; and trained individuals to oversee the coordination. Good coordination requires an overall plan that is both strategic and realistic. All health care facilities coordinate efforts to put their disaster plan in order. They coordinate with other local agencies and service providers and meet regularly to review their plan.

Logistics and Supply Chains

During a disaster, normal supply chains and locations of goods, including food, are often disrupted. Disaster preparedness therefore includes extensive logistical planning for emergency procurement, storage, and distribution of supplies and equipment. Categories of supplies and materials needed in a disaster include shelter materials, medical supplies, food and water, nonfood items (e.g., blankets, tarpaulins, soap), and communications equipment. The **logistics supply chain,** the stages of supply from procurement to end user, may require predisaster placement or stockpiling. Local disaster agencies ensure that all responders are familiar with the regional plan so that the supply chain can be activated quickly and smoothly. Points of distribution (PODs) of supplies are preplanned along with alternative sites. The federal government's *Strategic National Stockpile* of drugs and medical supplies, maintained by the CDC, is available in the event of terrorist attack, disease outbreak, or other public health emergency. Antibiotics, emergency medicines, airway equipment, intravenous fluids, and dressing materials are included in "push packs" for immediate distribution in an emergency.

Emergency Exercises

Exercises in which disaster responders do a "dry run" of a disaster are an essential part of disaster preparedness. Hospitals and other types of health care facilities are required by The Joint Commission to implement a facility exercise at least once a year. However, it is also important that local or regional agencies and responders perform emergency exercises that include all those who would be involved in the event of a disaster. Predisaster exercises are valuable for revealing gaps and weaknesses in overall plans, which can be resolved before a disaster occurs. Analysis of lessons learned from large emergencies or previous disasters is also important in strategic planning before a disaster or mass casualty event occurs.

Personal and Family Preparedness

National and state agencies encourage individuals and families to prepare for a disaster or local emergency in specific ways to mitigate the effects of the disaster on personal health, safety, and communication.

IMPORTANT TO KNOW *A model plan includes logistical problems that may arise, such as inability to access drinking water, failure of usual communication systems (phone, Internet), and evacuation. Methods of evacuation and designated meeting places for families are also included in the model plan. The plan may also include provisions for pet evacuation.*

Shelter in disasters is crucial for health and safety. Any plan for disaster or emergency includes a strategy for sheltering in place. This requires preplanning to maintain a supply of food, water, and other necessities at home or work site, including pet care. Prolonged sheltering may be necessary in emergencies in which it is impossible to move people or when a group of people have no alternative but to stay where they are. Examples of this are groups that have been moved to large sports stadiums or other public facilities until individual homes or shelters can be provided.

A model plan includes an evacuation kit containing a 3-day supply of personal and "survival" items. This type of simple "go bag" is also important for health care providers who may be called out to assist in an emergency. It should include your wallet, copies of personal identification cards or passport, and contact information.

II. MITIGATION

Mitigation, or risk reduction, is a process or activity that minimizes the impact of an event. In general, when a disaster cannot be averted or avoided, mitigation is used to reduce the disaster's effects on people, the infrastructure, property, and the environment. Mitigation is sometimes placed first on the disaster cycle or in association with preparedness. It may also occur as part of the response.

Many types and levels of mitigation can be used, depending on the type of disaster and the environment in which it occurs. For example, structural mitigation may involve changing planning and building codes or actually rebuilding structures so that they can withstand the forces of an earthquake. The engineering and construction of structures, such as dams, seawalls, and defensible spaces, are mitigation activities. Construction of an elaborate communications (i.e., with LEMA) and technological infrastructure, such as early warning and detection systems, is also a part of the mitigation process, as is isolating patients with contagious disease.

III. RESPONSE

The process of disaster response is complex and often very difficult. The environment is stressful and often disturbing, and the work is demanding. Even the best preparation and coordination plans can be quickly overwhelmed by the unpredictable events

For more information on this program, see http://www.cdc.gov/phpr/stockpile/index.htm.

Excellent resources for developing personal and family all-hazard preparedness plans are available from the Centers for Disease Control and from FEMA. Refer to https://www.redcross.org/get-help/how-to-prepare-for-emergencies/make-a-plan.html. An additional resource on animals in emergency can be accessed at https://www.redcross.org/about-us/news-and-events/news/Pet-First-Aid-Awareness-Month-Get-the-Red-Cross-App.html.

and conditions of a disaster. The work of preparation is over; now is the time to implement the plan. You hope for the best but understand that not every detail can be accounted for in the planning stage. Things can go wrong—but you do your best and remember your ethical mandates to do no harm. Remain cooperative and keep your head, even under great psychological pressure. Keep track of your own mental and physical health status.

Community Disaster Response

Although specific types of disasters create particular needs in a population, many scenarios are common, especially in natural disasters in which significant human needs and damage to the infrastructure occur. Some common scenarios are as follows:

- Loss of shelter (buildings or other means of escaping environmental hazards)
- Sudden requirement to shelter large numbers of people
- Disruption or alteration of communications, including access to electronic information
- Disruption, alteration, or destruction of the usual methods of transport
- Sudden need for large-scale health care services
- Sudden need for relocation of patients and newly injured
- Disproportionate effects on vulnerable sectors of society (older adults, impoverished, chronically ill, homeless, and others)
- Diversion of logistical support normally available for health needs
- Loss of infrastructure (systems and structures)
- Shortage of human resources
- Disruption, alteration, or destruction of power sources
- Disruption or destruction of water supply lines
- Possible contamination of drinking water
- Rapid depletion of medical supplies
- Scarcity of food
- Diversion of human resources and changes in roles

It is not possible to predict all the effects of all disasters. However, part of disaster planning and management is to assess the life-threatening effects of the disaster, prioritize needs, and analyze the best use of resources.

Human Needs in a Disaster

Many disaster response activities are implemented to provide basic, immediate human needs: shelter, sanitation, food and water, and medical assistance.

EVACUATION AND SHELTER Shelter protects people from environmental conditions, including extreme weather. It also offers an element of safety and a sense of security. Shelter may be a single building or a group of buildings away from the disaster area, or it may be temporary structures, such as tents. Shelter also offers protection from injury or further harm. In a disaster, shelter or protection may be the most immediate human need. Naturally, food and water are essential for life, but people's first instinct is to escape harm, and this often equates with shelter or evacuation. Evacuation is a way of moving people away from a disaster to protect them from catastrophic morbidity and mortality. Once an order has been made for evacuation, messages are sent out through local radio and other media that are still accessible. It is often part of the disaster scenario. People are assisted with transportation during an organized evacuation. Evacuation teams composed of community responders such as fire and other emergency personnel are identified in the predisaster planning stage. Vulnerable individuals in the population must be identified during the disaster planning phase. Some people cannot evacuate because of illness, physical incapacity, or lack of understanding of the risks. Others choose not to evacuate because they do not want to leave their home or pets. This may increase their risk of injury and often poses additional hazards for rescuers, who must come in to assist late in the disaster. Gaps in these services can create a separate type of humanitarian crisis in which people are left homeless and dependent on agencies for long periods.

The alternative to evacuation is **shelter-in-place,** in which people remain where they are, usually in a building or other structure, in a relatively safe location within the structure. A safe room or location sometimes can be fitted to resist debris impact or to prevent contamination by outside air. The decision to shelter-in-place is based on risk analysis and is usually communicated to the population through the media. An example of a disaster that may require shelter-in-place is a tornado or other extreme weather event in which people remain below ground until the disaster is declared over. A chemical disaster or bioterrorism is another type of event in which remaining inside to avoid toxic fumes or vapor may be the safest course of action.

MEDICAL AID Medical aid in a disaster is carried out in existing health care facilities or mobile clinics. During the planning phase of disaster management, all facilities that are equipped to take patients are involved in medical aid. Stand-alone offices and smaller facilities are assigned roles according to their capacity. The type of aid needed depends on the nature of the disaster. For example, earthquakes that cause buildings to collapse result in a high rate of orthopedic and other crush injuries. Chemical disasters result in toxicity and may include large numbers of burn victims. Transporting victims who need medical aid is a difficult problem when roads are blocked by collapsed structures or flooded with water.

INFECTION CONTROL Prevention of disease transmission is one of the primary objectives during a disaster. Infection control applies to evacuation facilities (shelters and camps), health care facilities, and community health. Important operational needs related to disease prevention in the disaster setting include, but are not limited to, the following:

- Control of infectious disease in evacuation centers
- Safe water
- Sanitation
- Health messages to the community
- Safe disposal of medical waste
- Collection and destruction of garbage
- Control of animal and insect pests in congested areas
- Shelter from harsh environments

Infection control procedures during a disaster must be followed as closely as possible. This includes wearing personal protective equipment (e.g., hand protection and masks) when handling body fluids and rigorous hand washing. When hand-washing facilities are not available, bottled water or an alcohol-based hand rub is used to prevent cross-infection. If the disaster itself is caused by an infectious agent, such as during a bioterrorism attack, community volunteers and HazMat teams will distribute appropriate protective clothing, respirators, and eye protection to those people closest to the focal point of the disaster. Decontamination procedures must be set up at a health care facility where appropriate equipment and supplies are available.

FOOD Food security often is threatened during a disaster because the normal means of procuring and transporting food are interrupted or destroyed. Food shortages also create panic in an unstable environment. Problems with the food pipeline sometimes emerge days, rather than hours, after the onset of a disaster because supply lines may be destroyed or the disaster environment prevents a sufficient flow of food into the logistics pipeline.

MENTAL HEALTH NEEDS Social and psychological assistance is needed in every disaster. People are best able to use their innate coping strategies when the social structure is maintained. Disaster response therefore includes measures to reunite families and maintain social cohesiveness. Although critical incident counseling during a disaster is controversial, immediate psychological aid can assist some individuals traumatized by the effects of a disaster. Mental health providers are among those who are needed in the immediate and short-term disaster response.

PROTECTION Protection from criminal threat may be necessary during a disaster or emergency, especially when resources are scarce and the usual protection measures are diminished or absent. In large disasters, local law enforcement agencies often divert personnel to lifesaving and rescue efforts. Curfews may be enforced during a disaster to help prevent violence and loss of property.

VULNERABLE POPULATIONS The term **vulnerability** (exposure to risk) often is discussed in association with disasters and emergencies. Vulnerable populations are those with a particularly high risk of injury or harm as a result of the disaster. People living in a floodplain, those living in substandard housing, people with learning and physical disabilities, and older adults are particularly vulnerable in disasters. They may not fully appreciate the danger of the situation or may not be able to respond to evacuation orders. Poorly constructed housing and physical isolation also contribute to vulnerability. Disaster planning at the community level includes the ability to locate and assist special needs populations and those living in difficult physical circumstances.

REUNIFICATION Often in disasters, family members are separated, and there may be no way for them to contact each other. The Red Cross has a mandate to assist families in reunification during disaster. There are different methods and means for providing reunification, which depends on collecting names and other information and funneling it through one or two sources. Electronic reunification is sometimes the best method of keeping a database, and local radio stations can assist in making announcements. It may be necessary for families to have more than one designated person to be the center point of communication in case that person loses contact with the others for some reason. The local Red Cross agency is almost always the best way to begin the process because they have many years of experience in reunification.

Health Care Facility Disaster Response

The following is a mass casualty disaster scenario with events as they may occur in a health care facility. Not all services are represented in this short scenario, but these examples may be helpful in understanding the disaster environment and for tabletop analysis.

Local community members and the media report that an explosion and fire have taken place at 2:00 a.m. in a large local furniture factory located in a semiurban area, in which there is also forestry activity. The fire is being fueled by the structure itself, its contents, and a large chemical warehouse where flammable materials are stored. The fire is spreading rapidly, and there are many injuries from the explosion and collapse of the building. The families living near the factory are low-income factory workers, and their houses are low-quality structures mainly made of chip wood. The community has one hospital with a helipad. The nearest large health care facility is 100 miles away.

1. Within minutes of the explosion, the first victims arrive at the 100-bed health care facility by private car from surrounding neighborhoods. News arrives that hundreds of severely wounded people will follow shortly.
2. The emergency department staff rushes to evacuate all existing nonurgent patients from the department.
3. The hospital incident command system has been activated, and hospital staff is called in according to the facility emergency plan. The command center is put in place at the security desk.
4. The hospital administrator contacts other county and state emergency managers to notify them of the disaster and possible need for assistance.
5. Department heads report to the command center and call as many of their employees as possible. All incoming staff report to the command center before going to their units. Job sheets are filled out for special assignments according to need and urgency.
6. ICU and nursing management begin to discharge patients who do not need essential medical care. Local taxi and

volunteer vehicles are found to take patients who are able to be discharged immediately to make room for emergency cases.

7. Emergency communication systems are in place, but there are not enough VHF radios. The mobile network system is overloaded. The primary communications system in the emergency department is used to make radio calls.
8. The emergency services—ambulance, fire, and other rescue vehicles—have all been deployed, and victims are being brought in by emergency crews. Triage has been performed by doctors and nurses in the emergency vehicles and near the hospital entrance. All patients are identified using numbered disaster tags.
9. A runner is sent to all departments to inform them of the type and approximate number of victims they can expect.
10. A triage area is established outside the emergency department, but people from the community arrive and enter the area looking for loved ones. There are two hospital security officers who recruit three other hospital staff to help with crowd control. A visitor control center is then set up in the lobby and manned by two social services staff. A third is on the way.
11. A temporary morgue has been set up, but it is far from the emergency department, requiring travel outside the building to avoid patients and the public.
12. The hospital administrator contacts the county emergency office to request RACES (Radio Amateur Civil Emergency Service) personnel to assist in providing radio communications.
13. Perioperative personnel have arrived and start setting up rooms for emergency surgery. The operating room supervisor contacts the central supply department to request extra supplies. A runner is assigned to transport the needed supplies.
14. Clinical staff has arrived and are already on duty in the treatment areas (e.g., surgery, radiology, blood bank). Technical staff are deployed to the operating room to help with instrument processing and transportation of patients.
15. Police and other law enforcement professionals arrive to help with crowd control and communications.
16. Members of the maintenance department lock all outside doors except those for employees, the emergency department, and the front lobby.
17. A headquarters for members of the media is set up in the hospital cafe.
18. Housekeeping staff bring additional beds from the supply room and create additional ward areas.
19. There are 35 burn victims who need airway care. They are triaged by two emergency department doctors. Eight of the victims need immediate intubation. The anesthesia technologist and two respiratory therapists are brought in to assist in intubation of the victims.
20. A phone line in the medical records department is designated for receiving outside calls and communication with relatives.
21. The incident command system, which includes bringing in regional actors to assist in the emergency, is partially effective. However, there are not enough managers to direct and coordinate the efforts.
22. Triage is notified when operating rooms and recovery areas are ready to take additional patients.
23. As the initial wave of victims is cared for at the hospital level, community organizations are setting up shelter accommodation in the town. Emergency vehicles arrive from other state regions to take victims to other facilities for care.
24. The hospital's helicopter is joined by an additional flight crew and helicopter to assist.
25. Emergency cases continue to be seen well into the next day, and evacuation of residents from the fire area is ongoing. The fire is still burning but is moving away from the town center. The emergency services will be working for another 6 days to care for victims and place people in temporary shelters.

In the fictional scene just described, we can see activation of many different types of emergency services that require preplanning.

However, even with the best planning, there is no way to predict exactly how the health care facility or community will cope with the needs of people during a specific disaster event. The health care needs of populations in disaster or emergency events vary widely according to the type of event, the location, and population density. Some disasters result in high morbidity, but low mortality, whereas in others such as earthquakes, fewer people are injured than killed. In the early days of a disaster, the focus is on survival and rescue. After the initial burden of victims has been handled, other needs emerge, including management of patients who were not urgent at the time of the disaster but who nevertheless need care. Chronic disease, reproductive, and mental health needs can become critical when patients do not have access to health care services.

OPERATIONAL CONSIDERATIONS DURING THE RESPONSE

Communication A disaster or large-scale emergency may result in loss of usual methods of communication, or existing networks may be overwhelmed as people try to connect with relatives, friends, and service providers. A major health care facility has the ability to communicate using satellite or high-frequency radio. Health and safety messages to the community are more difficult but can be achieved by radio transmission. Local radio stations are particularly effective in transferring health messages and providing links between individuals and families. Staff will be oriented to disaster communications during drills and training sessions. At least three different communication systems will be activated for backup. All hospital employees are normally oriented to emergency alert signals (fire and patient emergency codes) during the first week of employment. The usual emergency alert systems for the hospital may be suspended during a community disaster. Within the health care facility during disaster response, one area is converted to a communications room for internal and external use. Communication generated from the health care facility is limited to essential transmissions only. A media representative is also needed to work from the communications area. This is necessary because people's need for information may override accuracy in reporting, resulting in a worsening situation of public anxiety.

Medical Facility Evacuation Evacuation of a medical facility may sometimes be necessary because of structural hazards or immediate threat from fire, a chemical, or bioterrorism. The decision to evacuate patients is difficult because in the midst of a disaster, managers must evaluate the risks of moving people as compared to the dangers of staying in place. In general, a structural evaluation must be made by qualified personnel such as facility engineers. Medical personnel must ensure that care of the patients can be continued and that the evacuation destination is safer than the location being evacuated. Naturally, when there is an immediate undeniable threat, such as a structural fire that is out of control, the objective is to move people as quickly as possible away from harm. Planning before a disaster occurs can help set thresholds for threats that require evacuation. Evacuation may be partial (moving to another part of the building or outside) or complete (moving to another facility). The procedures and protocols for a facility evacuation can be located in the disaster guidelines for that facility. Patient evacuation is carried out by trained first responders.

Surge Capacity **Surge capacity** is the ability of a health care facility to quickly increase its capability to receive and treat patients. In disasters that have a high burden of injuries, this becomes a critical issue. A system for transferring patients from one facility to another may not be functional (e.g., flooded roads or building debris may block access). Health care facilities can determine the maximum number of casualties they can receive, but the environment of the disaster may not permit the movement of patients to other locations. Strategies to increase surge capacity include discharge of elective cases, not admitting nonemergency cases, and conversion of nonpatient areas into makeshift wards. Calling in staff from other health care facilities is often necessary to reach surge capacity, but space to work in, supplies, drugs, and medical equipment are also needed.

> A set of job action sheets for the California Emergency Services Authority can be accessed online at http://hicscenter.org/SitePages/Job%20Action%20Sheets%20(JASs).aspx, or search for "California Emergency Job Sheets." This website provides good examples of typical job sheets used in many different kinds of disasters.

Staff Assignments One of the first events to occur in health care facility disaster management is activation of the emergency plan, including the deployment of all facility staff. Disaster plans for all health care facilities include a protocol for callout of staff. In most cases, staff is called in by a member of the facility incident command system. Individuals report to their incident command station and then their usual duty area, or they may be assigned tasks at another location. Facility departments are assigned roles during development of the disaster response plan or by the incident commander at the time of the event. Roles are assigned using a *job action sheet* (JAS). This is a tool used to define a person's functional role during an emergency. The JAS is completed by the unit leader or section leader for that professional. The important data include the position (which may not be the person's usual role), whom to report to, the purpose of the role, and tasks to be completed and in what order. The disaster plan must designate the exact reporting or assembly area for staff and the names of those who are assigned. The role of the surgical technologist during disaster response is most likely his or her usual role in the operating room, which may include helping with instrument and equipment reprocessing.

IMPORTANT TO KNOW *The surgical technologist will never be required to perform tasks that are outside his or her legal and ethical scope of practice.*

Note that the ICS is enacted at the management level, not the operational level. The "hands-on" roles and responsibilities are delegated by the facility ICS manager according to the disaster plan for that facility.

Triage Triage is a process in which casualties are given emergency medical treatment according to the probability of their survival. The surgical technologist is expected to support the role of triage as needed. Triage is a necessary procedure when the number of people needing medical attention overwhelms the services available. The process requires rapid, clear, decisive thinking and action by medical personnel. No standard scoring system is used in triage. However, a common practice is to differentiate patients by the following parameters:

- Those not needing emergency care
- Those with the greatest chance of survival with medical care
- Those for whom medical intervention will aid survival
- Those whose chance of survival would not increase with medical intervention

Triage is performed at the disaster or mass casualty site, in transit to a health care facility by emergency vehicle, or in the health care facility itself. People with minor injuries and their families often crowd to a medical facility for reassurance during a disaster. However, an attempt must be made to triage each person to ensure that a seriously injured or ill person is not overlooked. Triaged individuals are assigned a category and tagged using a color or other code tags that can be identified by other health care workers (Fig. 36.2).

In very large disasters where there are mass casualties, such as 9/11, a rapid triage system is used by emergency medical personnel. The START (simple triage and rapid treatment) system is used when the number of casualties overwhelms the capacity to fully assess victims. The system uses basic metabolic signs: respiration, perfusion, and mental status. Training in the START system is available at health care facilities and as part of overall disaster training in the community.

Advanced first aid courses, including first responder techniques, are available for communities and through disaster training management groups. To access these courses, refer to the list of resources at the end of this chapter.

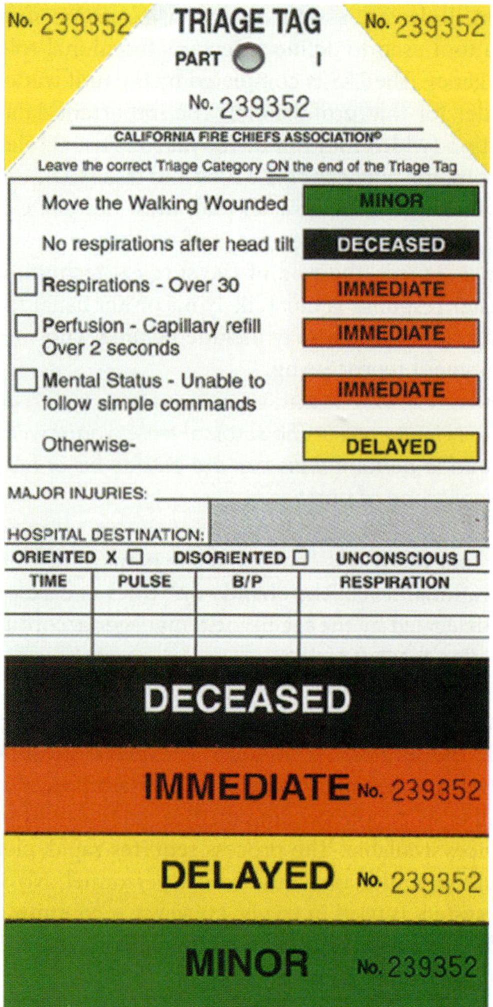

FIG. 36.2 Triage system tag used to identify victims according to survival chances. (From Marx J, ed. *Rosen's Emergency Medicine, Concepts and Clinical Practice*. 7th ed. St Louis: Mosby; 2010.)

Supplies and Drugs Supplies are managed during an emergency by the procurement officer and his or her staff. Accounting must be kept for all supplies, even if the system is streamlined for emergency purposes. This is necessary so that as supplies are depleted, an immediate rough inventory and request for a regional stockpile can be made. In some events, a request for medical supplies is made at the beginning of the disaster, with knowledge of what supplies are likely to run out.

Drugs are managed by the pharmacy department with runners actively assisting in distribution of drugs following orders. Orders must be recorded and dispensed in a way that allows tracking.

Items that require refrigeration can be kept cold using the facility's emergency generator or cold packs that are prepacked and ready for use in emergency.

Morgue A facility morgue is set up near the back of the hospital if overflow room is needed. The location should be selected to prevent casual or accidental viewing of bodies by visitors. The morgue is usually an assigned task of the pathology department. Someone from the department stays on duty at all times, and bodies are removed from the premises as soon as feasible. Disaster tags are necessary for all bodies, and all forms must be filled out at the time the body is delivered to the morgue area.

Protection of Facility Records Protection of medical records during disasters is a topic that is currently being debated by disaster managers and health care facilities. Unless the facility keeps electronic records off-site or in multiple sites, there is no easy way to solve the problem of lost or damaged records. In large disasters, patients may travel far from their usual health care facility for treatment or may be relocated for extended periods of time without their records, unless they keep updated documents with them. There are also questions about the security of all electronic medical records.

IV. RECOVERY

The recovery phase of a disaster is not defined by a particular event or activity. **Disaster recovery** is a complex process in which the risk of morbidity and mortality is reduced or mitigated to a level at which the community can cope. This does not mean that losses are reverted to predisaster levels. Complete "recovery" from a major disaster may take many years.

Recovery activities and objectives are targeted at all components of society. This includes not only repair and reconstruction of physical structures but also recovery from the economic, social, and psychological effects of the disaster. This means that disaster recovery is built into the planning and response phase. Available resources (human and material) are first targeted toward survival and then toward regaining an acceptable level of normality within the community.

Humanitarian Aid and Professionals

International aid workers are usually sent to an emergency or disaster by individual United Nations or nongovernmental organizations. International responders are professionals, specially trained in international humanitarian response. Most have at least a bachelor-level education in their profession, with additional training or experience in the international context. In the health sector, doctors, nurses, anesthesiologists, midwives, and nurse practitioners are needed to fulfill the roles and responsibilities created by complex emergencies such as conflict and disaster.

Surgical technologists may enter the field of international aid. Because few people are deployed for a given disaster, all aid professionals are required to have extensive experience, professional training, or both. One person may be required to do the job of three people, with cross-cutting responsibilities within the team. Top coordinators in the specific sectors (e.g., medical, logistics, shelter, nutrition) are usually master's level trained with additional certification in security, team management, and other sectors according to their role.

The minimum entry degree for health responders is the bachelor of nursing with certifications in tropical medicine and/or public health in disaster. Health professionals are managed by the agencies that contract with them for a disaster.

Further information on international relief resources and career opportunities is available at the website http://reliefweb.int. This is the designated website for the United Nations Office for Coordination of Humanitarian Affairs. A mirror site can be accessed by searching for "Relief web."

ETHICAL DILEMMAS IN DISASTER

We observe the best and worst in human behavior during a disaster. Communities all around the world pull together when there is a common threat. People are often surprised at the level of personal sacrifice and courage seen in emergency situations. In fact, it is very common for people to empathize with others and to offer comfort, shelter, and sustenance. But there is another side of disaster that reveals the tragedy of choice, perceived need, and perceived loss. Here are some examples of situations in which these issues become very real:

1. Marginalized populations such as those living in poverty, older adults, physically and mentally challenged, and chronically ill are often invisible during a disaster. Their needs have not been preplanned. They cannot advocate for themselves and rely on others to advocate for them. If the social and political will is not there, they may be forgotten in a crisis.
2. People who have immediate access to disaster assistance are helped first. If disaster assistance is unable to reach all the people who need aid, those who can travel are better able to travel to the assistance.
3. Individuals' perceived needs are often very different from each other. The perception of what is essential for survival or even comfort may be far above or below what the reality of the situation can provide or that agencies should provide.
4. Disaster assistance agencies and managers must make choices during mass disaster. Who should be rescued first? What criteria are used? What priority should be given to aiding animals?
5. Should people be compensated by the government for loss that occurred during a disaster?
6. In multiple disasters within a state or region, how can we decide where to place resources?

These questions and many more are often debated publicly by community leaders, emergency and disaster specialists, and ethicists. Students involved in disaster response should debate the legal and ethical implications of these issues to explore or provide clarity about one's personal convictions and to understand those of others.

RESOURCES FOR STUDENTS AND INSTRUCTORS

In appreciation of the need for resources on disaster plans and disaster management in the classroom, the following list is provided to assist surgical technologist students, instructors, and others who need quick access to essential, trustworthy information, including online training courses. In most cases, the title of the document describes the content. Where it is not clear, a brief explanation is provided. Each website has been assessed for relevance to the CAAHEP requirements:

- Division of Homeland Security and Emergency Services
  Provides federal and state planning documents, training, and other resources
- FEMA Emergency Management Institute
  Training courses online and on-site
- FEMA Introduction to the Incident Command System for Healthcare/Hospitals
  Training course online
- Institute for Disaster and Emergency Preparedness
  All-hazards courses online
- FEMA, Emergency Management Institute
  Independent Study Program
- Department of Homeland Security, National Response Framework, 2008
  The federal document for all disasters
- NOVA Institute for Disaster and Emergency Preparedness
  Provides courses, education, and training for groups. Works with all major disaster agencies
- FEMA, Incident Command System (ICS)
- The International Disaster Database, Centre for Research on the Epidemiology of Disasters (CRED)
  Epidemiology of past disasters, including disaster profiles, lists, and trends

KEY CONCEPTS

- Disasters overwhelm local resources and require outside assistance.
- An important factor that distinguishes a disaster from an emergency is that an emergency is a geographically isolated event that can be handled by local health and emergency services.
- A mass casualty event is a localized emergency, such as a transportation accident (e.g., major air crash), explosion, or structural collapse in which the number of victims overwhelms local health care services.
- The two main categories of disasters are natural disasters and human-made disasters.
- Natural disasters are caused by forces of nature, such as a hurricane, a tornado, an earthquake, floods, and extreme heat or cold.
- Human-made disasters are the result of intentional or unintentional human action, such as technical accidents (e.g., chemical or radiation disasters) and terrorist and conflict-related disasters.
- Although many different types of disasters can occur, they often have common characteristics because they affect individuals and the community in general.
- Vulnerable populations are those with a particularly high risk for injury or harm as a result of a disaster.
- Federal and local agencies are responsible for the management of a disaster. The Federal Emergency Management Agency is responsible for overall coordination and management of nationally declared disasters.

- Only a disaster that is a declared state of emergency by the governor of the state where the disaster occurred qualifies for FEMA assistance.
- The National Incident Management System is a set of guidelines that defines the management structure, objectives, and chain of command during a disaster.
- At the state level, disasters are managed by that state's emergency management agency.
- The all-hazards approach is a disaster management strategy that emphasizes the common elements of all types of disasters. It is defined by four phases: mitigation, preparedness, response, and recovery.
- Mitigation or risk reduction is a process or activity that minimizes the impact of a disaster.
- The preparation phase of a disaster includes numerous coordinated activities with the common goal of ensuring that individuals, communities, and government sectors can respond effectively to a variety of different types of disasters.
- The objective of disaster response is to prevent injuries and loss of life and to protect against property loss.
- Evacuation is a way of moving people away from a disaster to prevent catastrophic morbidity and mortality.
- The alternative to evacuation is shelter-in-place in which people remain where they are (usually in a building or other structure) in a relatively safe location within the structure.
- Currently, no national standard exists for training health care professionals in the all-hazards approach to disaster preparedness. Allied health and other professionals can increase their ability to respond to disaster and mass casualty events by taking specific courses in disaster management.
- Primary care and allied health professionals usually assist in a disaster by performing their normal role and occasionally by performing tasks that are outside their usual job description, but not outside their scope of practice.
- Surgical technologists are trained in a variety of professional skills that are needed during a disaster. The specific role of the surgical technologist may be determined at the time of the disaster.
- International disasters include all the elements of a disaster in developed countries, as well as other constraints and complexities, such as conflict, war, and an unstable or failed government.
- In the health sector, doctors, nurses, anesthesiologists, midwives, and nurse practitioners are needed to fulfill the roles and duties created by complex emergencies, such as conflict and natural disaster.

REVIEW QUESTIONS

1. What are some of the differences between a disaster and an emergency?
2. Differentiate between a natural disaster and a human-made disaster.
3. Define *state of emergency.* What government official declares a state of emergency, and why is this done?
4. What is the all-hazards approach to disaster preparedness and management?
5. Define *mitigation.* Give several examples of mitigation in natural disaster management.
6. What is an incident command system? Why is this used during a disaster?

CASE STUDIES

CASE 1

An earthquake has occurred; the epicenter is approximately 50 miles from your workplace. You hear on the radio that all primary health care and allied health care employees should be on standby for immediate duty. You receive a call to come into the facility and remain on duty there for an "indefinite period of time." You will be staying at the hospital until the first phase of the disaster has passed. How will you prepare yourself mentally for this assignment? Can you predict what coping mechanisms you will use to respond to the coming days of work, which will bring an unusual level of fatigue and stress?

CASE 2

One of the important issues to consider in disaster planning is "altered care." Currently, a debate is going on among disaster professionals and health care workers about the reality of health and care standards in the disaster environment. The Agency for Healthcare Research and Quality has stated that to save as many people as possible during a disaster, compromises in health care delivery are necessary; this is called "altered care." The AHRQ points out that this may mean restricting medical supplies to certain types of patients or using ventilators only for surgical patients. It also might mean compromise in normal isolation techniques. In some disasters, two or more surgical patients may be operated on side by side in the same operating room. If you were asked to discuss this topic among your peers, what would you add to the discussion? This is both an ethical and a technical discussion. What is your opinion about what surgical practices could be altered during a disaster?

CASE 3

Discuss the significance of having an incident command system structure during a disaster or mass casualty event. Top-down management has advantages and disadvantages. Discuss these in detail. Apply any previous experience you have had with management in analyzing a possible disaster scenario in which all major decisions come from one central location. What would happen if you overrode the system and ignored a few directives (even though you believe it to be in the best interest of the patients)?

CASE 4

You are employed by a busy medical center as a certified surgical technologist and team manager for orthopedics. Your supervisor notifies you that you must attend 2-day training on disaster preparedness. Your colleagues, who must also attend, do not want to "waste" the time and feel that the information is too far removed from day-to-day practice. What response in favor of disaster preparedness will you give them? How would you encourage others to become more engaged in the training?

BIBLIOGRAPHY

Agency for Health Care Research and Quality (AHRQ). *Mass Medical Care with Scarce Resources: A Community Planning Guide*. AHRQ Pub. No. 07-0001. http://www.ahrq.gov/. Accessed July 2016.

American Medical Association/American Public Health Association (AMA/APHA). *Improving Health System Preparedness for Terrorism and Mass Casualty Events*. https://stacks.cdc.gov/view/cdc/6891. Accessed September 3, 2019.

American Nurses Association. *Adapting Standards of Care Under Extreme Conditions: Guidance for Professionals During Disasters, Pandemics, and Other Extreme Emergencies, Columbia School of Nursing*. New York: American Nurses Association; 2008.

Association of periOperative Registered Nurses (AORN). AORN guidance statement: mass casualty, triage, and evacuation. *AORN J*. 2011;85:792–800.

Centers for Disease Control and Prevention. *Public Health Preparedness: Strengthening CDC's Emergency Response: A CDC Report on Terrorism Preparedness and Emergency Response (TPER)-Funded Activities*. http://www.cdc.gov/phpr/reportingonreadiness.htm. Accessed July 5, 2016.

Coppola D, ed. *Introduction to International Disaster Management*. Oxford: Butterworth-Heinemann; 2007.

Department of Homeland Security. *National Response Framework*; 2008. https://www.epa.gov/emergency-response/national-response-framework-nrf. Accessed September 3, 2019.

Health Systems Research. *Altered Standards of Care in Mass Casualty Events*. AHRQ Pub. No. 037-0043; 2005. https://asprtracie.hhs.gov/technical-resources/resource/491/altered-standards-of-care-in-mass-casualty-eventsf. Accessed September 3, 2019.

Hsu E, Thomas T, Bass E, et al. Health care worker competencies for disaster training. *BMC Med Edu*. 2006;6:19.

APPENDIX

A COMMON PATHOLOGY BY SYSTEM

Note: Infectious disease organisms are discussed in Chapter 8. Pathologies associated with surgical treatment are discussed by system in their respective chapters.

SKIN AND SUPERFICIAL TISSUES	
Basal cell carcinoma	Slow-growing neoplasm of the skin related to excessive exposure to ultraviolet light.
Cellulitis	Bacterial infection of superficial tissues, especially in immunocompromised patients.
Chemical injury	Burn caused by strong alkaline or acidic chemicals; results in tissue necrosis and liquefaction.
Cold thermal injury	Tissue necrosis related to prolonged exposure to freezing temperature.
Electrical injury	Trauma related to electrical systems, lightning, or electrical devices. May result in paralysis, cardiopulmonary arrest, and burns.
Keratosis	Horn-like skin lesion related to excessive exposure to ultraviolet light.
Melanoma	Rapidly growing, potentially metastatic neoplasm originating in the melanocyte of the skin.
Nevus	Circumscribed pigmented lesion of the skin or connective tissue, usually congenital. May be a cancerous precursor lesion.
Squamous cell carcinoma	Neoplasm of the squamous cells.
SKELETAL SYSTEM AND CONNECTIVE TISSUES	
Ankylosing spondylitis	Inflammatory arthritic condition associated with other inflammatory diseases, such as inflammatory bowel disease, psoriasis, and rheumatoid disease.
Avascular necrosis	Infarction of bone and marrow tissue resulting in ischemia and necrosis; may be idiopathic or related to trauma.
Bursitis	Inflammation of the joint capsule related to disease or injury.
Carpal tunnel syndrome	Inflammation of the medial tendon sheath related to overuse or repetitive use.
Cyst	Fluid-filled sac encapsulated by a membrane.
Degenerative disc	Condition in which fibrocartilage or softer nucleus of the intervertebral disc is damaged through the aging process, injury, or disease, resulting in degeneration of the tissues and instability of the spine.
Fibromyalgia	Condition of widespread pain located in "tender points" that can be elicited by digital compression.
Gout	A disease caused by deposition of monosodium urate in the tissue related to hyperuricemia. The disease results in arthritis and soft tissue inflammation.
Infectious arthritis	Acute bacterial infection of a joint space. Most commonly affects the knee; usually caused by *Staphylococcus aureus* infection.
Marfan syndrome	Inherited connective tissue disease that may affect numerous body systems. Manifestation depends on the system that is affected.
Muscular dystrophy	Genetic disorder resulting in progressive muscle weakness and degeneration.
Myasthenia gravis	Autoimmune disorder resulting in extreme muscle weakness. May affect any muscle of the body.
Osteomalacia	Extreme softening of the bones resulting in deformity. May be due to vitamin D deficiency or other disease process.
Paget disease	Inherited chronic disease of the axial skeleton that results in bone destruction and disorders of the osteoblast cells. The cause is unknown.
Pectus carinatum	Congenital deformity of the chest wall most commonly resulting in protrusion of the upper sternum and depression of the lower anterolateral chest wall.

Continued

Pectus excavatum	Congenital deformity of the chest wall resulting in depression of the sternum that may restrict breathing.
Radial dysplasia	Historical term for *radial longitudinal deficiency.* The condition results in a shortened forearm with radial deviation and is associated with other systemic diseases.
Rheumatoid arthritis	Inflammatory autoimmune disorder affecting the joints. The disease tends to be progressive and affects other body systems.
Rickets	Nutritional disease related to deficiency of calcium phosphate or vitamin D.
Talipes equinovarus	Congenital deformity involving the calcaneotalar–navicular complex of the foot.
NERVOUS SYSTEM	
Arteriovenous malformation	In the nervous system, it refers to an abnormal connection between arteries and veins without capillaries. The cause is unknown.
Astrocytoma	Tumor of the astrocyte cells occurring in the brain or spinal cord; may become rapidly malignant.
Cerebral palsy	Term used to describe a large group of disorders caused by disturbances in fetal development. May present as problems of development, orthopedic deformity, perception, and cognition.
Encephalitis	General term meaning inflammation of the brain.
Glioma	Tumor of the neuroglial cells arising from the brain or spinal cord.
Meningioma	Slow-growing tumor arising from the arachnoid cells of the arachnoid villi; most are benign.
Parkinson disease	Degenerative disease of the extrapyramidal dopaminergic system. The disease is characterized by four main signs: tremor, rigidity, akinesia (loss of muscle movement), and postural problems.
Seizure disorder (epilepsy)	Electrical disturbance in brain activity resulting in unprovoked seizures. There are many causes.
EAR, NOSE, AND THROAT	
Choanal atresia	Congenital stricture of the choana.
Infection	The most common infections are otitis externa (swimmer's ear) and atopic dermatitis. Other causes can be viruses and fungi.
Infection/inflammation	Infections of the nose may be caused by bacteria or fungi. The most common causes of inflammation of the nose are allergies and nasal polyps.
Laryngitis	Inflammation of the larynx; a symptom of many different diseases affecting the throat.
Mastoiditis	Infection of the mastoid cavity; may be associated with severe otitis media. With the introduction of modern antibiotics, the condition is rarely seen in developed countries.
Meniere disease	The cause of Meniere disease is unknown. It is characterized by recurrent vertigo (dizziness) that lasts several hours, sensorineural hearing loss at low frequency, and ringing in the ears (tinnitus).
Nonmalignant tumor	Nonmalignant tumors include juvenile nasal angiofibroma and inverting papilloma. Although these are not cancerous, they can cause nasal obstruction.
Otitis externa	Superficial infection of the outer ear.
Otitis media	Infection of the middle ear. May be acute or chronic. It is more common in childhood, especially when children are exposed to cigarette smoke and other air pollutants.
Polyp	Lobular growth on mucous membrane tissue of the same tissue origin.
Ruptured tympanic membrane	Tear or puncture of the tympanic membrane usually associated with infection of the middle ear.
Sinusitis	Inflammation or infection of the air cavities of the nose and face.
Tinnitus	Ringing or other sounds in the ear; may be idiopathic or symptomatic of a number of ear diseases.
Trauma	Injury to the external ear can result in avulsion of the ear or hematoma.
Vertigo	A sensation of dizziness.
EYE	
Cataract	Opacity of the lens of the eye usually related to aging process.
Conjunctivitis	Inflammation of the conjunctiva related to infection or allergy.
Glaucoma	A group of diseases related to increased intraocular pressure and damage to the optic nerve. Increased pressure may be due to blockage of aqueous humor circulation or drainage.
Macular degeneration	Age-related complex degeneration of the photoreceptors, retinal pigment epithelium, and choriocapillaris of the eye, leading to blindness.

CARDIOVASCULAR SYSTEM	
Aneurysm	Outpocketing or ballooning of an artery or heart chamber in an area weakened by disease or congenital defect. The aneurysm may continue to progress, growing larger until it ruptures.
Angina	Chest pain associated with blockage of the coronary artery, most commonly resulting from arteriosclerosis. Blockage results in ischemia of the heart muscle and pain. Occurs most commonly on exertion.
Arteriosclerosis	A group of vascular diseases characterized by hardening and stiffening of the arteries caused by calcium deposits and fatty substances in the arterial wall. The disease is related to age, smoking, diabetes, and hypertension.
Atelectasis	Condition in which the lung alveoli remain collapsed because of hypoxia related to trauma or because of disease.
Atherosclerosis	The most common form of arteriosclerosis; an obstructive disease of the arteries in which the vessels are infiltrated with calcium and fatty fibrous deposits, causing reduced elasticity, as well as obstruction and ischemia. Risk factors include smoking, a high-fat diet, obesity, and inactivity.
Cardiac fibrillation	Ineffective quivering or uncoordinated movement of the heart muscle rather than normal regular contraction of the atria and ventricles.
Congestive heart failure	Failure of the heart to pump related to cardiac tissue damage or disease. Right heart failure results in inability to pump blood into the pulmonary circulation, causing peripheral edema and congestion of the abdominal viscera. Left heart failure causes blood to back up into the pulmonary circulation with overload.
Coronary artery disease	Arteriosclerosis of the coronary arteries leading to cardiac ischemia.
Embolus	A moving vascular obstruction—usually a blood clot, but may also be a fat globule, plaque, air, or foreign body.
Endocarditis	Inflammation or infection of the endocardium lining the heart chambers.
Gangrene	Tissue necrosis as a result of ischemia and loss of oxygen to the tissue. Dry gangrene is not related to bacterial infection.
Heart block	Damage or disease of the conduction cells of the heart resulting in inability to initiate or sustain electrical activity necessary for contraction of the muscle. Heart block may be partial or complete.
Intermittent claudication	Not a disease, but a symptom—intermittent muscle pain on exertion related to arteriosclerosis. The pain is relieved with rest.
Mitral stenosis	Hardening and malfunction of the mitral valve.
Murmur	Not a disease, but a sign of valvular disorder that can be detected on auscultation.
Myocardial infarction	Necrosis of heart muscle resulting from ischemia (lack of blood supply and therefore oxygen); often associated with coronary artery disease.
Myocarditis	Inflammation or infection of the heart muscle.
Pericarditis	Inflammation or infection of the pericardium surrounding the heart.
Raynaud syndrome	Spasm of the blood vessels of the fingers and toes in a cold environment or during stress, resulting in blanching of the skin. The condition is often idiopathic (no known cause).
Rheumatic heart disease	An acute manifestation of the streptococcal disease rheumatic fever that becomes chronic over time. Rheumatic heart disease usually affects the heart valves, causing deformities and malfunction.
Thrombophlebitis	The presence of a thrombus in a superficial or deep vein with accompanying inflammation.
Thrombus	A stationary blood clot or other obstruction in the vascular system.
BLOOD AND LYMPH	
Anemia	Deficiency of red cells or hemoglobin related to excessive blood loss or destruction (hemolytic anemia).
Aplastic anemia	Bone marrow depression related to stem cell disease and loss of blood cells, white blood cells, and platelets.
Hodgkin disease	Malignant lymphoma; cancer of the lymph system and structures.
Leukemia	Cancer of the hematopoietic stem cells.
Polycythemia	Abnormally high total red blood cell mass with hematocrit greater than 55%.

Continued

RESPIRATORY SYSTEM	
Atelectasis	Collapse of entire or part of the lung.
Aspiration	Inhalation of an object, particle, or liquid into the airway.
Bronchitis	Inflammation of the bronchi.
Chronic obstructive pulmonary disease	Inflammatory disease of the respiratory system caused by exposure to cigarette smoke. The main features of the disease are airflow limitation, chronic airway irritation, mucus production, and airway scarring.
Cystic fibrosis	Genetic disorder affecting multiple systems, including dehydrated secretions in the pulmonary system, pancreas, liver, and intestinal tract requiring long-term care.
Empyema	Suppurative infection in the lung; lung abscess.
Pleuritis	Inflammation or infection of the pleural sac.
Pneumothorax	Positive pressure in the pleural cavity resulting from presence of air.
Pulmonary effusion	Not a disease but a symptom—accumulation of fluid in the pleural space. There are multiple causes related to disease or trauma.
Pulmonary embolus	An embolus that has entered the respiratory circulation with potential to cause death resulting from ischemia and necrosis of lung tissue.
GASTROINTESTINAL SYSTEM	
Celiac disease	Inflammatory condition of the small intestine, which is related to ingestion of wheat, rye, and barley and is associated with genetic factors.
Crohn disease	Inflammatory and ulcerative condition of the small intestine related to genetic predisposition.
Diverticular disease	Abnormal outpockets within the intestinal lining that trap material and become infected.
Esophageal atresia	Narrowing or stricture of the esophagus resulting from congenital defect or disease.
Esophageal varices	Engorged veins of the esophagus as a result of blood that has backed up from the hepatic circulation.
Fistula	A tract, usually congenital in origin, which penetrates the esophagus and emerges outside the organ.
Hiatal hernia	Herniation of a portion of the stomach at the juncture with the diaphragm, allowing the stomach to slide partially into the thoracic cavity.
Inflammatory bowel disease	Multiple inflammatory pathologies arising from the large and small intestines; many are related to autoimmunity.
Intussusception	Telescoping of bowel tissue, usually in a child, leading to obstruction. If undetected, can cause ischemia and necrosis.
Nutritional/psychiatric diseases	Anorexia and bulimia nervosa are two disorders found only in Western society in which the individual refuses food and purges the body of nutrition to the point of death.
Obstruction	Any condition of the bowel that creates a physical obstruction of bowel contents or causes bowel tissue to lose peristaltic tone.
Peptic ulcer disease	Ulceration of the stomach or duodenum is mainly caused by *Helicobacter pylori* bacteria and ingestion of noxious substances.
Pyloric stenosis	Congenital defect involving thickened bands of muscle tissue at the pyloric sphincter that prevent nutritional intake.
Salivary gland disorders	These include salivary gland stones, infection, and neoplasms of the glands.
Sjögren syndrome	Inflammatory disease that may affect the functioning of the salivary glands.
Volvulus	Twisted or looped section of bowel leading to obstruction and necrosis.
LIVER, PANCREAS, AND SPLEEN	
Cholecystitis	Inflammation or infection of the gallbladder.
Cholelithiasis	Presence of gallstones in the bile ducts or gallbladder.
Cirrhosis	Disease of the liver in which the tissue becomes sclerotic and inflamed and ceases to function normally.
Cirrhosis and portal hypertension	End-stage alcoholic liver disease characterized by fibrosis of the liver, which prevents the flow of blood and bile. Blood backs up into the portal vein, causing congestion and rupture of the esophageal venous plexus.

Diabetes type 1	Autoimmune disease resulting in destruction of insulin-producing cells in the pancreas and alterations in normal carbohydrate metabolism.
Diabetes type 2	Acquired disease in which there is relative resistance to insulin and dysfunction of the beta cells in the pancreas.
Pancreatitis	Inflammatory disease of the pancreas and peripancreatic fat that often results in tissue fibrosis and necrosis. Chronic pancreatitis is most commonly associated with alcohol abuse or biliary disease.
Portal hypertension	Impaired hepatic circulation due to sclerosis of the liver sinusoids, causing blood to back up into the digestive tract.
ENDOCRINE DISORDERS	
Hyperadrenalism (Cushing disease)	Disorder in which excessive glucocorticoid is produced; related to pituitary adenoma secreting adrenocorticotropic hormone.
Hypoadrenalism (Addison disease)	Disease of adrenal insufficiency as a result of bilateral destruction of the adrenal cortex, usually as a result of autoimmune causes.
Hyperparathyroidism	Abnormally high production of parathyroid hormone, which regulates calcium and phosphorus in the body.
Hyperthyroidism (Graves disease)	Autoimmune disease resulting in multinodular thyroid gland and excessive production of thyroid hormone.
Hypothyroidism (Hashimoto disease)	Hypothyroidism may be congenital or acquired. Thyroid hormone is essential for brain development in the fetus. In adults, hypothyroidism is caused by thyroidectomy or radiation of the thyroid for cancer treatment.
Thyroid nodule	Usually benign, may be related to iodine deficiency or cystic condition of the thyroid.
FEMALE REPRODUCTIVE SYSTEM	
Abnormal uterine bleeding	Uterine bleeding that occurs at irregular intervals. Note: The term *dysfunctional uterine bleeding* is no longer used.
Cystocele	Herniation of the bladder into the anterior vaginal wall, usually related to multiple childbirths and weakening of the vaginal tissue.
Endometriosis	Presence of endometrial tissue in locations of the body other than the uterine lining. The tissue remains under hormonal control and may bleed and become painful.
Fibrocystic disease	Usually refers to the breast, in which one or more cysts can develop within the connective tissue. Polycystic disease refers to ovarian cysts.
Leiomyoma	Benign tumor of the myometrium.
Menorrhagia	Regular menstrual bleeding but excessive flow.
Pelvic inflammatory disease	Refers to an infectious process. Usually related to *Chlamydia* but may also be caused by any other sexually transmitted disease.
Rectocele	Herniation of the rectal wall into the posterior vaginal wall, usually related to multiple childbirths and weakening of the vaginal tissue.
OBSTETRICAL COMPLICATIONS	
Abruptio placentae	Premature separation of the placenta from the uterine wall, often related to high blood pressure during pregnancy.
Breech presentation	Occurs when the baby's feet, knees, or buttocks are delivered ahead of the rest of the body.
Cephalopelvic disproportion	Occurs when the mother's birth canal is too small or the baby is too large for delivery.
Ectopic pregnancy	Implantation of the fertilized ovum occurring outside the uterus, usually in the fallopian tube.
Nuchal cord	Condition in which the umbilical cord is wrapped one or more times around the baby's neck, with risk of compression of the cord against the birth canal.
Preeclampsia	Hypertension during pregnancy that contributes to high risk for the woman and fetus.
Spontaneous abortion	Loss of pregnancy before the 20th week of gestation.
MALE REPRODUCTIVE SYSTEM	
Balanitis and balanoposthitis	Inflammation of the glans or foreskin; may be related to infection.
Benign prostatic hypertrophy	Enlargement of the prostate gland, usually with age. Although benign, may cause voiding problems.

Continued

Cryptorchidism	Undescended testicle in the child or adult usually related to congenital defect. May result in sterility if left untreated.
Epispadias	Rare congenital defect in which the anterior urethra is incompletely developed, resulting in a meatus located on the ventral side of the penis or in other locations depending on the extent of the defect.
Erectile dysfunction	Inability to achieve or maintain erectile function of the penis. It may be related to many different causes, including functional, medical, and emotional origins.
Hydrocele	Fluid-filled sac arising in the layers of the tunica vaginalis of the testicle, often related to inguinal hernia or other inguinal defect.
Hypospadias	Congenital defect in which the external urethral meatus is located on the ventral side of the penis; accompanied by stricture.
Orchitis	Inflammation or infection of the testicle.
Phimosis, paraphimosis	Tightness in the prepuce preventing retraction over the glans or return to its normal position. May be related to infection or scarring.
Prostatitis	Inflammation or infection of the prostate gland.
Spermatocele	Fluid-filled cyst at the spermatic cord.
Testicular torsion	Twisting of the testicle on itself, resulting in ischemia and necrosis. The condition usually occurs as a sports injury but may have underlying structural causes.
Varicocele	Abnormal dilation of the testicular blood vessels.
UROGENITAL SYSTEM	
Addison disease	Adrenal insufficiency. A rare disorder with many different causes, including autoimmune disease and certain tumors.
Calculi (stones)	Stones are formed by crystalline minerals and salts precipitated from filtrate produced in the kidney.
Cancer of the bladder	The most common form of urinary tract cancer; tumors are derived from the bladder lining.
Cancer of the kidney	Primary cancer of the kidney arises from the cortex and renal pelvis. The greatest risk factor is smoking.
Cushing syndrome	Overproduction of glucocorticoid, which is secreted by the adrenal glands; the condition can be related to several pathological conditions of the pituitary gland, an adrenal tumor, or other tumors.
Cystic kidney disease	Renal cysts originate in the nephron as a result of obstruction. Fluid-filled cysts impinge on vascular structures causing loss of kidney function. Cystic disease may be acquired or congenital. Polycystic disease is hereditary and has no treatment.
Cystitis	Infection of the urinary bladder.
End-stage renal disease	Renal failure that cannot be reversed. It has many causes, including diabetes, hypertension, systemic lupus erythematosus, nephrotic syndrome, and infection (ingestion of *Escherichia coli* is a common cause of renal failure).
Glomerulonephritis	Kidney infection and autoimmune disorders may affect any part of the nephron and glomerulus. Glomerulonephritis is a general term, rather than a specific disease.
Hydronephrosis	Distention and loss of function of the ureter or renal pelvis related to urinary reflux (backward movement of urine) caused by obstruction such as a stricture, stone, or tumor.
Neurogenic bladder disorder	A general term that refers to pathogenic loss of bladder function related to neurological damage. The common causes are spinal cord injury, cerebrovascular accident, brain lesion, peripheral nerve disease, and infection.
Polycystic disease	Inherited disease in which fluid-filled cysts replace normal kidney tissue.
Trauma to the bladder	Traumatic injury to the bladder occurs most often in motor vehicle accidents and is related to pelvic fracture.
Trauma to the kidney	Injury to the kidney is usually caused by a blow to the flank or back. Most commonly occurs during contact sports or as a result of intentional violence.
Urinary incontinence	The most common cause of urinary incontinence is loss of sphincter control at the bladder neck. This may be related to multiple childbirths or advancing age. Hypertrophy of the prostate also causes involuntary loss of urine.
Urinary reflux	Backward flow of urine or filtrate in the renal system.
Urinary retention	Retention of urine related to medical or psychological problem.

Urinary tract infection (UTI)	Infection of the lower urinary tract. It is commonly caused by *E. coli* contamination of the distal urethra or by a sexually transmitted disease. Chronic UTIs may result in scarring of the urethra that requires surgery.
Wilms tumor (nephroblastoma)	The most common tumor in children—arising in the kidney.
GENETIC DISORDERS	
Achondroplasia	Deficiency of growth hormone resulting in short stature but normal body proportions.
Albinism	Inherited condition of melanin production resulting in little or no pigment in the skin, eyes, or hair.
Developmental disorder	Any physical or mental condition that results in delay or arrest of normal physical, social, or mental development.
Down syndrome	Genetic condition in which a person has 47 rather than the normal 46 chromosomes. The condition is accompanied by many defects, including developmental delay, structural deformity, and delayed mental and social development.
Marfan syndrome	See Skeletal System and Connective Tissues.
Phenylketonuria	Inherited metabolic defect in which a baby is born without the ability to break down phenylalanine, an essential amino acid.
Sickle cell disorder	Inherited disorder of the blood cells in which healthy red blood cells are replaced with more fragile sickle-shaped cells, which carry less oxygen and may cause vessel blockages.
Tay-Sachs disease	A congenital defect of chromosome 15 that results in inability to produce hexosaminidase A, which helps break down gangliosides in nerve cells. The condition is usually fatal.

APPENDIX B

DRUGS AND SUBSTANCES ASSOCIATED WITH SURGERY

Common Surgical Medications

Category	Type	Examples
ANTIINFECTIVES		
Antibiotics	Aminoglycosides	Amikacin Gentamicin Neomycin Tobramycin
	Antiretrovirals	Didanosine Efavirenz Lamivudine Stavudine Zidovudine
	Cephalosporins	Cefotaxime Cefoxitin Ceftriaxone Cefuroxime
	Fluoroquinolones	Ciprofloxacin Gemifloxacin Levofloxacin
	Lincosamines, vancomycin, ketolides	Clindamycin Vancomycin Telithromycin
	Macrolides	Azithromycin Clarithromycin Erythromycin
	Penicillins	Amoxicillin Ampicillin Penicillin G Penicillin V Piperacillin Ticarcillin
	Sulfonamides	Sulfadiazine Sulfamethoxazole and trimethoprim Sulfisoxazole
	Tetracyclines	Doxycycline Minocycline Tetracycline Tigecycline
Antiviral	Antiretroviral	Didanosine Efavirenz Lamivudine Stavudine Zidovudine

Continued

Common Surgical Medications—cont'd

Category	Type	Examples
Antifungal	Systemic	Amphotericin Anidulafungin Caspofungin Micafungin
BLOOD		
Blood Derivatives	—	Whole blood Packed red cells Leukoreduced red blood cells Frozen-thawed red cells Platelet concentrate Fresh frozen plasma Cryoprecipitate Factor IX prothrombin concentrate Granulocyte concentrate
Anticoagulants	Heparins	Unfractionated heparin Low-molecular-weight heparin Warfarin (Coumadin)
	Thrombolytics	Recombinant tissue plasminogen activator Urokinase
Coagulants		Topical thrombin
CENTRAL NERVOUS SYSTEM AGENTS		
General Anesthetics	Inhalation	Nitrous oxide Isoflurane Sevoflurane Desflurane Enflurane
	Dissociative	Ketamine
Analgesics	Opiates	Morphine Codeine Hydromorphone Hydrocodone Oxycodone Oxymorphone
	Nonopiates	Ibuprofen (antiinflammatory) Diclofenac (antiinflammatory) Acetaminophen
Sedatives/Hypnotics	Intravenous	Propofol Etomidate Dexmedetomidine
	Barbiturates	Thiopental Methohexital
	Benzodiazepines	Midazolam Lorazepam Alprazolam Diazepam
Neuromuscular Blocking	Depolarizing	Succinylcholine
	Nondepolarizing	Atracurium Cisatracurium Pancuronium Rocuronium Vecuronium

Common Surgical Medications—cont'd

Category	Type	Examples
DIAGNOSTIC AGENTS		
Contrast Media	Iodinated	Diatrizoate Metrizoate
	Paramagnetic	Gadoxetate disodium Gadopentetate dimeglumine Gadobenate dimeglumine
ELECTROLYTE AND FLUID BALANCE		
Crystalloids	Normal saline—0.9% sodium chloride Lactated Ringer solution PlasmaLyte (balanced crystalloid) Dextrose 0.5% in water (D_5W)	
Electrolytes/Solutes	Sodium Potassium Calcium Magnesium Chloride Lactate Bicarbonate Gluconate	
Colloids	Albumin Hydroxyethyl starches Gelatins Dextran	
Diuretics	Acetazolamide Bumetanide Furosemide Hydrochlorothiazide Indapamide hemihydrate Amiloride HCl (potassium sparing) Spironolactone (potassium sparing)	
LOCAL ANESTHETICS		
Injectable	Procaine Chloroprocaine Lidocaine Mepivacaine Prilocaine Bupivacaine Ropivacaine	
Topical	Benzocaine Cocaine Dibucaine Lidocaine Tetracaine	
GASTROINTESTINAL DRUGS		
Histamine-2 Receptor	Cimetidine Famotidine Ranitidine	
Gastric Proton-Pump Inhibitors	Lansoprazole Omeprazole Rabeprazole Pantoprazole Esomeprazole	

Continued

Common Surgical Medications—cont'd

Category	Type	Examples
Antiemetics	Dolasetron Droperidol Granisetron Metoclopramide Ondansetron	
OBSTETRICAL DRUGS		
Oxytocics	Carboprost Dinoprostone Oxytocin Syntometrine Ergometrine	
CORTICOSTEROIDS		
Corticosteroids	Dexamethasone Prednisone Betamethasone	
CARDIAC DRUGS		
Antianginals	Amlodipine Atenolol Diltiazem Isosorbide Nifedipine Nitroglycerin Propranolol Verapamil	
Antiarrhythmics	Adenosine Amiodarone Atropine Digoxin Esmolol Isoproterenol Lidocaine Procainamide Quinidine Verapamil	
Antihypertensives	Amlodipine Candesartan Captopril Doxazosin Felodipine Lisinopril Losartan Nitroprusside	
Inotropics	Dobutamine Dopamine Digoxin Epinephrine Milrinone	
Vasodilators	Ambrisentan Bosentan Iloprost Nesiritide Nimodipine Sildenafil	
HEMOSTATIC DEVICES (HEMOSTASIS)		
Gelatin Sponge	Gelfoam Surgifoam	

Common Surgical Medications—cont'd

Category	Type	Examples
Collagen Powder	Avitene EndoAvitene Instat MCH	
Oxidized Cellulose	Surgicel gauze or sponge tuft	
Fibrin Combination Sealant	Tisseel FloSeal Surgiflo Crosseal Omnex CoSeal Dermabond	
Other	Platelet gel Ostene bone putty BioGlue	
DYES AND STAINS		
	Gentian violet Methylene blue Indigo carmine Lugol solution	
CHEMOTHERAPEUTIC AGENTS		
Intravesical	Doxorubicin Epirubicin Thiotepa Mitomycin Interferon Gemcitabine	

Medications Used During Ophthalmic Surgery

Drug/Brand Name	Description/Uses
MYDRIATICS (DRUGS THAT DILATE THE PUPIL BUT PERMIT FOCUSING)	
Phenylephrine (Neo-Synephrine, Mydfrin), 2.5%, 10%	Objective examination of the retina, testing of refraction, and easier removal of lenses; mydriatics may be used alone or with a cycloplegic drug.
CYCLOPLEGICS (DRUGS THAT PARALYZE ACCOMMODATION AND INHIBIT FOCUSING)	
Tropicamide (Mydriacyl), 1%	Anticholinergic, dilation of the pupil, examination of the fundus, and refraction.
Atropine, 1%	Dilates the pupil, inhibits focusing; potent anticholinergic, with a long duration of action (7–14 days).
Cyclopentolate (Cyclogyl), 1%, 2%	Anticholinergic; dilates the pupil, inhibits focusing.
Scopolamine hydrobromide (Isopto Hyoscine), 0.25%	Anticholinergic; dilates the pupil, inhibits focusing.
Homatropine hydrobromide (Isopto Homatropine), 2%, 5%	Anticholinergic; dilates the pupil, inhibits focusing.
Epinephrine (1:1,000) preservative free (PF)	Dilates the pupil; added to bottles of balanced salt solution (BSS) for irrigation to maintain pupil dilation during cataract surgery or vitrectomy.
MIOTICS	
Carbachol (Miostat), 0.01%	Potent cholinergic; constricts the pupil, used intraocularly during anterior segment surgery.
Carbachol (Isopto Carbachol), 0.75%, 1.5%, 2.25%, 3%	Potent cholinergic; constricts the pupil, used topically to reduce intraocular pressure (IOP) in glaucoma.
Acetylcholine chloride (Miochol-E), 1%	Cholinergic; rapidly constricts the pupil, used intraocularly during anterior segment surgery; reconstitute immediately before using.
Pilocarpine hydrochloride, 1%, 4%	Cholinergic; constricts the pupil, used topically to lower IOP in glaucoma.

Continued

Medications Used During Ophthalmic Surgery—cont'd

Drug/Brand Name	Description/Uses
TOPICAL ANESTHETICS	
Tetracaine hydrochloride (Pontocaine), 0.05%	*Onset:* 5–20 s *Duration of action:* 10–20 min
Proparacaine hydrochloride (Ophthaine), 0.05%	*Onset:* 5–20 s *Duration of action:* 10–20 min
INJECTABLE ANESTHETICS	
Lidocaine (Xylocaine), 1%, 2%, 4%	*Onset:* 4–6 min *Duration of action:* 40–60 min, 120 min with epinephrine
Methylparaben Free (MPF)	PF; adjunct to topical anesthetic.
Bupivacaine (Marcaine, Sensorcaine), 0.25%, 0.50%, 0.75%	*Onset:* 5–11 min *Duration of action:* 8–12 h with epinephrine; often used in 0.75% strength in combination with lidocaine for blocks.
Mepivacaine (Carbocaine), 1%, 2%	*Onset:* 3–5 min *Duration of action:* 2 h (longer with epinephrine)
Etidocaine (Duranest), 1%	*Onset:* 3 min *Duration of action:* 5–10 h
ADDITIVES TO LOCAL ANESTHETICS	
Epinephrine, 1:50,000–1:200,000	Combined with injectable local anesthetics to prolong anesthesia and reduce bleeding.
Hyaluronidase	Enzyme mixed with anesthetics (75 units per 10 mL) to increase diffusion of anesthetic through tissue, improving the effectiveness of the block; contraindicated if skin inflammation or malignancy is present.
VISCOELASTICS	
Sodium hyaluronate (Healon, Amvisc, Provisc, Vitrax) in a sterile syringe assembly with blunt-tip cannula	Lubricant and support; maintains separation between tissues to protect the endothelium and maintain the anterior chamber intraocularly; removed from anterior chamber to prevent postoperative increase in pressure; should be refrigerated (except Vitrax); allow 30 min to warm to room temperature.
Sodium chondroitin–sodium hyaluronate (Viscoat) in a sterile syringe assembly with blunt-tip cannula	Maintains a deep chamber for anterior segment procedures, protects epithelium of cornea, and improves visualization; may be used to coat intraocular lens before implantation; should be refrigerated.
DuoVisc	Packages of separate syringes of Provisc and Viscoat in the same box.
VISCOADHERENTS	
Hydroxypropyl methylcellulose 2% (OcuCoat) in a sterile syringe assembly with blunt-tip cannula	Maintains a deep chamber for anterior segment procedures, protects epithelium of cornea, and may be used to coat the intraocular lens before implantation; removed from the anterior chamber at the end of procedure; stored at room temperature.
Hydroxyethylcellulose (Gonioscopic Prism Solution)	Bonds gonioscopic prisms to the eye; stored at room temperature.
Hydroxypropyl methylcellulose 2.5% (Goniosol)	Bonds gonioscopic prisms to the eye; stored at room temperature.
IRRIGANTS	
BSS, Endosol	Used to keep the cornea moist during surgery; also used as an internal irrigant in the anterior or posterior segment.
BSS enriched with bicarbonate, dextrose, and glutathione (BSS Plus, Endosol Extra)	Used as an internal irrigant in the anterior or posterior segment; must be reconstituted immediately before use by adding part I to part II with the transfer device.
HYPEROSMOTIC AGENTS	
Mannitol (Osmitrol)	Intravenous (IV) osmotic diuretic; increases the osmolarity of the plasma, causing the osmotic pressure gradient to pull free fluid from the eye into the plasma, thereby reducing the IOP.
Glycerin (Osmoglyn, Glyrol)	Oral osmotic diuretic given in chilled juice or cola; increases the osmolarity of the plasma, causing the osmotic pressure gradient to pull free fluid from the eye into the plasma, thereby reducing the IOP.

Medications Used During Ophthalmic Surgery—cont'd

Drug/Brand Name	Description/Uses
ANTIINFLAMMATORY AGENTS	
Betamethasone sodium phosphate and betamethasone acetate suspension (Celestone)	Glucocorticoid; injected subconjunctivally after surgery for prophylaxis; also used to treat severe allergic and inflammatory conditions.
Dexamethasone (Decadron)	Adrenocorticosteroid; injected subconjunctivally after surgery for prophylaxis; also used to treat severe allergic and inflammatory conditions and intraocularly for endophthalmitis.
Methylprednisolone acetate suspension (Depo-Medrol)	Glucocorticoid; injected subconjunctivally after surgery for prophylaxis; also used to treat severe allergic and inflammatory conditions.
ANTIINFECTIVE DRUGS	
Polymyxin B/bacitracin (Polysporin ointment)	Topical treatment of superficial ocular infections of the conjunctiva or cornea; also used prophylactically after surgery.
Polymyxin B/neomycin/bacitracin (Neosporin ointment)	Topical treatment of superficial infections of the external eye; used prophylactically after surgery; hypersensitivity to neomycin is possible.
Neomycin and polymyxin B sulfates and dexamethasone (Maxitrol ointment or suspension)	Topical treatment of steroid-responsive inflammatory ocular conditions or bacterial infections of the external eye; hypersensitivity to neomycin is possible.
Tobramycin/dexamethasone (TobraDex)	Topical treatment or prevention of superficial infections of the external part of the eye; also has antiinflammatory properties.
Cefazolin (Ancef, Kefzol)	Injected subconjunctivally for prophylaxis after eye procedures; also used topically, intraocularly, and systematically for endophthalmitis.
Gentamicin sulfate (Garamycin)	Injected subconjunctivally for prophylaxis after eye procedures; also used topically, subconjunctivally, and intraocularly for endophthalmitis.
Ceftazidime (Fortaz, Tazicef, Tazidime)	Injected subconjunctivally and intraocularly for the treatment of endophthalmitis.
OTHER DRUGS	
Cocaine, 1%–4%	Used topically only, never injected; used on cornea to loosen epithelium before debridement and on nasal packing to reduce congestion of mucosa.
5-Fluorouracil (5-FU)	Antimetabolite used topically to inhibit scar formation in glaucoma-filtering procedures; handle and discard in compliance with the regulations of the Occupational Safety and Health Administration (OSHA) and health care facility's policies for safe use of antineoplastics.
Mitomycin (Mutamycin)	Antimetabolite used topically to inhibit scar formation in glaucoma-filtering procedures and pterygium excision; handle and discard in compliance with OSHA's and health care facility's policies for safe use of antineoplastics.
Tissue plasminogen activator (TPA) (Activase)	Thrombolytic agent; used for the treatment of fibrin formation in patients who have had vitrectomy and for the lysis of clots on the retina.
Fluorescein	*IV diagnostic aid:* Used in fluorescein angiography to diagnose retinal disorders. *Topical stain:* Fluorescein strip temporarily stains the cornea yellow-green in areas of denuded corneal epithelium.
Timolol maleate (Timoptic)	Beta-adrenergic receptor blocking agent; used in the treatment of elevated IOP in ocular hypertension or open-angle glaucoma.
Acetazolamide sodium (Diamox)	Carbonic anhydrase inhibitor; given IV to reduce the secretion of aqueous humor, resulting in a drop in IOP; also has a diuretic effect.
Dextrose, 50%	Added to BSS, Endosol, BSS Plus, or Endosol Extra for patients with diabetes during intraocular procedures.

From Rothrock JC. *Alexander's Care of the Patient in Surgery*. 13th ed. St Louis: Mosby; 2007.

APPENDIX

C MATH REVIEW

Fundamental skills in math are necessary for patient safety and documentation and are required of surgical technologists who participate in the medication process and in other roles requiring calculations. Practical use of math skills by surgical technologists includes the following:

- Drug calculations, including concentration, dosage, ratio, conversion, and amount delivered
- Reporting and documentation, including vital signs, weight, height, and age
- Measuring and reporting irrigation fluid used during surgery
- Calculation of time (duration) using the international system

These and many other tasks require the use of math. The basic tools necessary for computations are reviewed in this section. Students or graduates should never hesitate to ask for help or to consult with a colleague about a calculation or other math process because patient safety is the most important consideration in the completion of required tasks.

NOTE *This math review assumes that the reader can carry out very basic math skills in addition, subtraction, multiplication, and division of whole numbers, with or without using a calculator.*

FRACTIONS

A fraction is a number often written in the form a/b, where *a* represents the numerator (the value above the line) and *b* represents the denominator (the value below the line). When *a* is less than *b*, the fraction has a value less than 1 and is referred to as a **proper fraction.** When *a* is equal to *b*, the fraction has a value of 1. When *a* is greater than *b*, the fraction has a value greater than 1 and is called an **improper fraction.**

Examples:

⅔ has a value less than 1

$3/3$ has a value equal to 1

$5/3$ has a value greater than 1

A **mixed fraction** is one that contains a whole number *and* a fractional amount. For example, 3½ is a mixed fraction. It is sometimes necessary to convert the mixed fraction into an improper fraction to perform a calculation.

To convert 3½ into a fractional amount:

- Multiply the whole number by the denominator of the fraction, add the numerator, and place this value over the denominator:

$3 \times 2 = 6$

$6 + 1 = 7$

Answer: 7/2 = 3½

Convert 5¾ into a fraction.

$5 \times 4 = 20$

$20 + 3 = 23$

Answer: $23/4 = 5\frac{3}{4}$

COMMON DENOMINATORS

Fractions have common denominators when the denominators of the fractions are the same numbers.

$2/7$ and $6/7$ have common denominators of 7

$4/9$ and $7/6$ do not have common denominators

$8/3$ and $8/10$ do not have common denominators

EQUIVALENT FRACTIONS

Two fractions are **equivalent** if they represent the same *value.* Multiplying any number by 1 does not change the value of the original number. Therefore when a fraction is multiplied by a fraction that equals 1, the fraction will look different but will have the same value as the original fraction.

- Multiply the both the numerator and denominator of the fraction $5/6$ by 2.

$$\frac{5}{6} \times \frac{2}{2} = \frac{10}{12} \text{ Therefore, } \frac{5}{6} = \frac{10}{12}$$

$$\text{And } \frac{14}{3} \times \frac{3}{3} = \frac{42}{27} \text{ Therefore, } \frac{14}{9} = \frac{42}{27}$$

Keep this process in mind. We will use it later.

LIKE FRACTIONS

Fractions are considered like when they have the same denominator.

- ¾ and $7/4$ are like fractions because they have the same denominator. They have a **common denominator.**
- ¾ and $7/5$ are not like fractions because they do not have the same denominator.

SIMPLIFYING FRACTIONS

It is often necessary to reduce a fraction to its simplest terms. This is called **simplification.**

A fraction that has been reduced to its most simple terms is one whose numerator and denominator cannot be evenly divided by the same number greater than 1.

To simplify the fraction, the numerator and denominator are *divided* by the same number to get the smallest equivalent fraction.

- $7/12$ cannot be simplified because no whole number greater than 1 can divide into 7 and 12 evenly.
- $8/12$ can be simplified because 8 and 12 can both be divided evenly by 4.
- To simplify the fraction, we divide 8 by 4, which equals 2, and we divide 12 by 4, which equals 3. This fraction simplifies or reduces to $2/3$.
- $35/20$ can be simplified because 35 and 20 can both be evenly divided by 5. To simplify the fraction, divide 35 by 5 (which equals 7) and divide 20 by 5 (which equals 4). The fraction simplifies or reduces to $7/4$.

MULTIPLYING FRACTIONS

To multiply one fraction by another fraction, multiply the numerators of the two fractions to determine a new numerator and multiply the denominators of the two fractions to determine a new denominator:

$$\frac{3}{5}\times\frac{4}{7}=\frac{12}{35}$$

$$\frac{2}{3}\times\frac{5}{11}=\frac{10}{33}$$

To multiply a fraction by a whole number, convert the whole number to a fraction by making it the numerator with a denominator of 1.

- **Multiply** $4/5$ by 7: $\frac{4}{5}\times 7=$

$$\frac{4}{5}\times\frac{7}{1}=\frac{28}{5}$$

DIVIDING FRACTIONS

To divide a fraction by another fraction, we invert the second fraction (the inverted fraction is then called the **reciprocal**) and multiply the first fraction by that reciprocal:

$\frac{3}{5}+\frac{4}{7}$	We are given a fraction to divide by another fraction.
$\frac{3}{5}\times\frac{7}{4}$	We find the reciprocal of the second fraction and *multiply* the two fractions.
$\frac{3\times 7}{5\times 4}$	We multiply numerators by numerators and denominators by denominators.
$\frac{21}{20}$	Three-fifths divided by four-sevenths equals twenty-one twentieths.

Here is another example of division:

$\frac{2}{3}\div\frac{5}{11}$	Divide two-thirds by five-elevenths.
$\frac{2}{3}\times\frac{11}{5}$	Find the reciprocal (inversion) of the second fraction and multiply the two fractions.
$\frac{2\times 11}{3\times 5}$	We multiply the numerator of one fraction by the numerator of the other fraction and denominator of one fraction by the denominator of the other fraction.
$\frac{22}{15}$	Two-thirds divided by five-elevenths equals twenty-two fifteenths.

ADDING AND SUBTRACTING FRACTIONS

When adding or subtracting *like* fractions, add the numerators while keeping the common denominator.

$$\frac{3}{4}+\frac{4}{5}=\frac{7}{5}$$

However, when adding or subtracting *unlike* fractions, it is necessary to find the **lowest common denominator** or **LCD** (the smallest number that can divide into both denominators evenly).

$\frac{3}{2}+\frac{9}{8}=?$	The denominators are not the same, so we must determine the LCD. This is the smallest number that both denominators can divide into evenly. One way to do this is to multiply the first fraction by 1, which does not change its value but only its appearance.
$\frac{3}{2}\sum\frac{4}{4}+\frac{9}{8}=$	To convert the first fraction to an equivalent fraction that has 8 as a denominator, multiply the 2 by 4 to get our common denominator of 8. Since we multiplied the denominator by 4, we must also multiply the numerator by 4 to get a fraction equivalent to the original fraction. Remember that $4/4$ equals 1 and does not change the value of $3/2$.
$\frac{12}{8}+\frac{9}{8}=$	Now we have two fractions with the same (common) denominators.
$\frac{21}{8}$	Twelve-eighths added to nine-eighths equals twenty-one eighths.

DECIMALS

Decimal numbers are a way of writing any number in groups of 10, using the decimal point as a separator between *multiples* of 10 and *parts* or fractions of 10. The location of the number in relation to the decimal point tells us its value. Numbers to the right of the point are fractions of 10, and those to the left of the point are multiples of 10, as shown here:

Multiples of 10 mn Fractions of 10							
Thousands (1000s)	Hundreds (100s)	Tens (10s)	Ones (1s)	Σ	Tenths (1/10s)	Hundredths (1/100s)	Thousandths (1/1000s)
1000.	100.	10.	1.		.1	.01	.001

Note that the "ones" represent the number of single base units. This could be milligrams, liters, milliliters, degrees, or any other base unit.

The number 5.8 is read five and eight-tenths or *five point eight.* This means there are 5 whole base units plus $\frac{8}{10}$ of a base unit.

Ones	Σ	Tenths
5	Σ	8

The number 25.75 is read twenty-five and seventy-five hundredths *or twenty-five point seven five.*

It means 20 units of 10, plus 5 single units, plus 7 tenths of a unit, plus 5 one-hundredths of a unit. Notice how all the values to the right of the point are fractions, whereas those to the left are whole numbers. The point is just a separator and has no value itself.

Hundreds	Tens	Ones	Σ	Tenths	Hundredths
	2	5	Σ	7	5

The following number is *3619 point 475* or 3619.475.

Thousands	Hundreds	Tens	Ones	Σ	Tenths	Hundredths	Thousandths
3	6	1	9	Σ	4	7	5

ROUNDING DECIMAL NUMBERS

Sometimes when doing calculations, it is necessary to *round up* or *round down* a decimal value. For example: 1/3 = 0.33333333333 and so on to infinity.

In certain calculations, for example, we are told (or we know) that the result must be rounded to a certain place such as the nearest tenth, nearest thousandth, or nearest whole number. The procedure for rounding is as follows:

Rounding Decimal Numbers

1. Find the digit in the place you are asked to round to.
2. Look at the very next digit to the right.
3. If the digit immediately to the right is 5 or more, round up.
4. If the digit immediately to the right is 4 or less, do nothing.

Round *up* the following number to the nearest tenth:
Example: Round up 35.89.

The place we are asked to round to is the tenth. In this value, 8 is in the tenths place. The number immediately after the 8 is 9.

9 is greater than 5, so we *raise* the 8 by one.

35.87 rounded to the nearest tenth = 35.9.

But we do not round off numbers automatically! Only when doing calculations that require it. For example, if the patient's temperature is 37.5°, we do not report it as 38°. It remains 37.5°.

Example: Round down 0.428571 to the nearest tenth:

The 4 is in the tenths place and the 2 is immediately to its right. Because 2 is less than 5, the 4 in the tenths place remains 4 tenths.

ADDING AND SUBTRACTING DECIMALS

To add decimals, line up the numbers to be added so that the decimal points also line up. Then simply add as usual, keeping the decimal in position:

$$\frac{567.01 + 2.03}{569.04}$$

To subtract, line up the numbers with decimal points in line also:

$$\frac{423.04 - 10.92}{412.12}$$

MULTIPLYING DECIMALS

To multiply decimal values, set up and work the calculation as you would any multiplication problem—by calculator or by hand, without consideration of the decimal points. When you have calculated the result, count the total decimal point places represented by all factors to be multiplied. In the following problem, there are four places total: two for each factor. Place the decimal point that same number of places, in this case four, counting right to left:

$$\frac{2.25 \times 2.15}{4.8375}$$

DIVIDING DECIMALS

To divide a decimal value by a whole number using long division, first set up the problem as you would any other but be sure to keep the decimal point in place.

6.375
4)25.50
24
1.5
1.2
0.30
0.28
.20
.20
00

To correctly place the decimal point in the answer, simply move the decimal up to the result in line with the original point.

To divide a decimal value by *another decimal value,* set up the problem, keeping decimals in place at first.

To determine the correct position of the decimal under the division sign, move the divisor decimal over to the right so that it becomes a whole number. Count the number of places you moved it and adjust the dividend decimal the same number of places.

6.375
4)25.50
24
1.5
1.2
0.30
0.28
.20
.20
00

CONVERTING A DECIMAL TO A FRACTION

1. Count the number of decimal places.
2. Move the decimal point that many places to the right.
3. Write the answer all over a denominator with a 1 followed by that number of zeros.

Example: Convert the decimal 4.38 to a fraction:

4.38	There are **two** decimal places represented by the number.
438.	Move the decimal point **two** places to the right.
438/100	Write the result all over a denominator with 1 followed by **two**zeros.
4.38 = 438/100	Result

Example: Convert the decimal 67.3 to a fraction:

67.3	There is **one** decimal place represented by the number.
673.	Move the decimal point **one** place to the right.
673/10	Write the result all over 1 followed by **one** zero.
67.3 = 673/10	Result

CONVERTING FRACTIONS TO DECIMALS

If the denominator of the fraction is a power of 10, such as 1/1000, 1/100, 1/10, and 1/1, we can easily write a decimal of equivalent value.

$\frac{1}{1} = 1.0$	$\frac{1}{10} = 0.1$	$\frac{1}{100} = 0.01$	$\frac{1}{1000} = 0.001$
$\frac{8}{1} = 8.0$	$\frac{8}{10} = 0.8$	$\frac{8}{100} = 0.08$	$\frac{8}{1000} = 0.008$
$\frac{170}{1} = 170.0$	$\frac{170}{10} = 17$	$\frac{170}{100} = 1.7$	$\frac{170}{1000} = 0.17$
$\frac{2953}{1} = 2953.0$	$\frac{2953}{10} = 295.3$	$\frac{2953}{100} = 29.53$	$\frac{2953}{1000} = 2.953$

If the denominator is *not a power of 10,* we can use division to convert fractions to their decimal equivalent.

3/5 is the same as 3 is divided by 5 and can be written as

3 ÷ 5 or 5)3.0 = 0.6

This means that 3 ÷ 5 = 0.6.

We keep the 0 in the answer as a placeholder to represent the fact that there are zero ones.

NOTE *Recall that the "do not use" documentation protocol introduced in Chapter 3 and again in Chapter 13 states that in medicine we never use a trailing zero (such as 3.0 or 25.0) after a decimal amount. A place-holding zero is not a trailing zero.*

PERCENT

Percent (%) always means *for each one hundred* or *parts of one hundred.* Percent is used to compare quantities. For example, we may read that 98% of a certain population has been vaccinated for measles. This means that for each 100 people in the population, 98 have been vaccinated for measles. This can also be expressed as the fraction 98/100. A student may be required to solo scrub 75% of cases given to her in a year. This means that for every 100 cases assigned to her, she must scrub 75 alone, without assistance, or 75/100. Remember that when working with percents, we are working with comparisons. That is, we are always comparing a number to 100.

To perform any mathematical problems using percent, it is necessary to convert the percent into a decimal or fraction.

Working with percents, decimals, and fractions is not difficult. The following boxes show how.

Convert a percentage into a decimal value:
1. Replace the percent sign (%) with × 0.01 (times 0.01).
2. Perform the multiplication by moving the decimal point to the left two points.

- Convert 36% into a decimal value.

$$36 \times 0.01 = 0.36$$
$$36\% = 0.36$$

- Convert 25.5% into a decimal value.

$$25 \times 0.01 = 0.255$$
$$25.5\% = 0.255$$

Examples:
What percent does .25 represent?

$$25 \times 100 = 25\%$$

One-third (⅓) represents what percent of the whole?

$$1/3 \times 100 =$$
$$1/3 \times 100/1 =$$
$$100/3 = 33.333333$$
$$(\text{rounded to the nearest one}) = 33\%$$

UNITS OF MEASUREMENT

Measurement is a way of quantifying things in a way that is universally understood. **Units of measurement** represent distinct quantities that are expressed as numbers followed by the unit itself (e.g., 10 milliliters, 5 pounds, 100 kilograms). The most common measurements used in medicine are the following:

- *Weight*—the heaviness of something, caused by gravity; also called *mass*
- *Length*—the distance from one point and another
- *Volume*—the amount of space a liquid or solid takes up
- *Temperature*—a measurement of heat

There are, of course, many other types of measurement. However, these are only occasionally encountered in clinical medicine.

International Units were introduced in Chapter 13 of the text. Here we will work with unit calculations to have a more complete understanding of this concept. International Units are a system of measurement that represents *biological activity* or *potency* as a measure. Do not confuse the number of international units of a drug with metric system weights and measure. They are not the same. Three drugs presented in international units are insulin, heparin, and thrombin. Two of these drugs, heparin and thrombin, are commonly used in surgery.

SYSTEMS OF MEASUREMENT

Throughout history, people have developed different ways to quantify things. Having a system of measurement was particularly important for trading when everyone had to agree on amounts being bought or sold. Early civilizations and cultures each had their own systems of measurement, usually corresponding to objects found in the environment—a seed, bean, the length of a man's foot or hand, and so on. In modern times, the need for a system that could be used globally led to adaptation of the *metric system* for science and medicine. You will see other systems of measurement in textbooks. The apothecary system and household system are two that were used historically but are no longer considered safe for medical use. The apothecary system was originally developed for physicians and apothecaries (those who mixed and sold drugs) dating back to the 1600s. The system was officially banned in the United States in the early 1970s. The household system was used only for liquid measurement and is inaccurate and confusing. This system has also been replaced by the metric system. It is very unlikely that you will encounter the apothecary or household system in actual practice. However, you may occasionally see measurements in the American system.

All systems of measurement are expressed in distinct units of quantity called **base units.** Examples of base units in the American system are inch, foot, yard, ounce, pound, mile, and degree Fahrenheit. Base units of the metric system are the gram, liter, meter, and degree Celsius. Later in this discussion you will see how to use the metric system and how to convert common measurements from the American system to metric system.

THE METRIC SYSTEM

The metric system is based on units of 10. These are shown in the box below.

Base Units in the Metric System

Mass (Weight)	Length	Volume	Temperature
Gram (g)	Meter (m)	Liter (l)	Degrees Celsius/ centigrade (° C)

In the metric system, everything is expressed as *multiples* or *fractions* of 10.

To know whether the thing being measured is a *multiple* or *fraction* of 10, simply look at the prefix.

Multiples of 10 Prefixes

- **10** times the base unit has the prefix **deka-:**
  1 dekagram = 10 grams
  1 dekameter = 10 meters
  1 dekaliter = 10 liters
- **100** times the base unit has the prefix **hecto-:**
  1 hectogram = 100 grams
  1 hectometer = 100 meters
  1 hectoliter = 100 liters
- **1000** times the base unit has the prefix **kilo-:**
  1 kilogram = 1000 grams
  1 kilometer = 1000 meters
  1 kiloliter = 1000 liters

Fraction (Part) of 10 Unit Prefixes

- **One hundredth** (1/100) of the base unit has the prefix **centi-:**
  1 centigram = 1 hundredth (1/100) of a gram
  1 centimeter = 1 hundredth (1/100) of a meter
  1 centiliter = 1 hundredth (1/100) of a liter
- **One thousandth** (1/1000) of the base unit has the prefix **milli-:**
  1 milligram = 1 thousandth (1/1000) of a gram

1 milliliter = 1 thousandth (1/1000) of a liter
1 millimeter = 1 thousandth (1/1000) of a meter

- **One millionth** (1/1,000,000) of the base unit has the prefix **micro-:**
  1 microgram = 1 millionth (1/1,000,000) of a gram
- **One thousand millionth** (1/1,000,000,000) of a base unit has the prefix **nano-:**
  1 nanogram = 1 thousand millionth (1/1,000,000,000) of a gram

If we map the prefixes in a line, we can see that each position represents multiples or fractions of 1 unit. Those to the right of the unit mark are fractions, whereas those to the left are multiples.

Kilo	Hecto	Deka	[unit]	Deci	Centi	Milli
1000	100	10	1	1/10	1/100	1/1000

UNIT CONVERSION

UNIT CONVERSION WITHIN THE METRIC SYSTEM

Unit conversion within the metric system is not difficult because the system is based on units of 10. Try to work with whole numbers when calculating conversions. For example, instead of converting 0.252 milligrams, use its equivalent, which is 252 micrograms. Another reason to use whole numbers is that there is always the risk that a decimal can be put in the wrong place, resulting in very large errors.

To convert within the metric system, first keep in mind that each place along the line of units is based on multiples or fractions of 1 unit, as shown earlier.

One simple way to convert is to multiply or divide as necessary and move the decimal point to the right or left.

To move the decimal point, use the following rules:

- Each of the metric units 1 gram, 1 milligram, 1 microgram, and 1 nanogram (those used in medicine) differs from the next by a factor of 1000. That is, 1 kg = 1000 g; 1 g = 1000 mg; 1 mg = 1000 mcg; 1 mcg = 1000 ng.
- To convert from a larger unit to a smaller unit, *multiply* the larger unit by the conversion factor. Move the decimal point three places to the right. Use zeros to fill empty places as needed.
- To convert from a smaller unit to a larger unit, move the decimal point three places to the left. Use zeros to fill the empty places as needed.

Examples:

Convert 0.25 g to milligrams. This requires converting from the larger unit (gram) to the smaller unit (milligram), so we multiply times 1000.

$$1000 \times 0.25 = 250 \text{ mg}$$

The decimal point is moved three places to the *right* and a zero used to fill in the number of places.

Convert 5000 g to kilograms. This requires converting from the smaller unit to the larger, so we divide by 1000.

$$5000/1000 = 5 \text{ g}$$

The decimal point is moved three places to the *left*.

UNIT CONVERSION BETWEEN SYSTEMS

Whenever we perform calculations of any kind, all the units in the problem must be expressed in the same system. In medicine, all units must be converted to the metric system. Metric conversion charts have detailed formulas for many different types of measurements. Several common conversions are discussed next.

Celsius and Fahrenheit

- To convert a temperature **from Celsius to Fahrenheit,** use the conversion formula

$$F = \frac{9}{5}(C + 32)$$

- To convert a temperature **from Fahrenheit to Celsius,** use the conversion formula

$$C = \frac{5}{9}(F - 32)$$

The surgeon requires solutions for cystoscopic irrigation to be warmed no more than 98° Fahrenheit. The solution warmer is calibrated in degrees Celsius (centigrade). What is the appropriate temperature for the solutions in Celsius?

Worked Example

$C = \frac{5}{9}(F - 32)$	Set up the problem.
$C = \frac{5}{9}(98 - 32)$	Substitute the "F" with the 98° temperature in the formula.
$C = \frac{5}{9}(66)$	Simplify inside the parentheses.
$C = 36.6666$	Round up.
$C = 37$	The cystoscopic irrigation should be warmed to no more than 37° Celsius.

Kilograms and Pounds

- To convert **kilograms to pounds,** use the conversion formula **p = (kg)(2.205).**
- To convert **pounds to kilograms,** use the conversion formula **kg = (p)(0.4536).**

The patient's weight is written in the chart in *pounds.* You must calculate the weight in *kilograms* to determine whether the regular operating table or a bariatric table is required. *Convert the patient's weight at 380 pounds to kilograms.*

Worked Example

kg = (p)(0.4536)	Set up the problem.
kg = (380)(0.4536)	Substitute *p* with 380 pounds.
kg = 172.368	Round down.
kg = 172	The patient weighs approximately 172 kg.

Millimeters or Centimeters and Inches

- To convert centimeters to inches, use the conversion formula **i = (cm)(0.3937).**
- To convert inches to centimeters, use the conversion formula **cm = (i)(2.54).**

The orthopedic surgeon requests a malleolar countersink tap, size 4¾ inches. What is the metric size?

Worked Example

cm = (i)(2.54)	Set up the problem.
cm = (4.75)(2.54)	Substitute *i* for 4.75 inches (given).
cm = 12.065	Round down.
cm = 12.1	The malleolar countersink tape is size 12.1 to the nearest tenth of a centimeter.

RATIOS

Ratios are used frequently to express drug concentration. The surgical technologist must be able to interpret and work with ratios. Like percentage, ratio is a way of comparing values. A ratio can be expressed as a series of numbers separated by one or more colons, as a fraction, and as a percent. Some examples of ratios are shown here:

1. A class has 3 female students for every 5 male students. The ratio of female to male students is 1 to 3, also written as 1:3 or ⅓.
2. One can of frozen orange juice concentrate is mixed with 4 cans of water to make orange juice drink. The ratio of frozen orange juice concentrate to water is 1 to 4, also written as 1:4 or ¼. For every 1 can of concentrate, there are 4 cans of water in the orange juice drink.
3. The surgery supply room has 100 Foley catheters in stock. Of these, 25 are pediatric sizes and the rest are adult sizes. The ratio of pediatric-size catheters to adult-size catheters is 25 to 75, also written as 25:75 or 25/75, which reduces to ⅓.

The following discussion on drug concentration illustrates how ratio is used in perioperative pharmacology.

CONCENTRATION

Learning how to calculate drug concentration is one of the most important skills required of surgical technologists. All drugs are ordered by strength, which is the same as concentration. But what does this actually mean in terms of numbers? How can we determine concentration of a drug? There are three ways in which concentration is expressed, as shown in the following box.

How Is Concentration Expressed?

1. By mixing a solid substance in a liquid, called *percent of weight per volume* of a solution.
2. By diluting or mixing one solution with another, called *percent of volume per volume* of a solution.
3. By mixing a solid substance with another solid substance, known as *percent of weight per weight* of a substance.

PERCENT WEIGHT PER VOLUME (% W/V)

The concentration of a solution is expressed in weight per volume, and the abbreviation for this is % w/v. A solution is a liquid containing a *solute* or solid substance dissolved in a *solvent,* which is a liquid such as water. The base unit of *weight* in the metric system is the gram. The base unit of *volume* in the metric system is the liter. Therefore weight per volume is expressed as grams and liters. Weight per volume is the most common method of expressing drug concentration.

Sterile saline is an example of a solution used commonly in surgery. Saline solution is composed of sodium chloride (a solid) plus water. Consider the following partial label for sterile saline used as an irrigation fluid:

Sodium Chloride 0.9%—Contents 1 liter not for injection

How do we know exactly how many grams of sodium chloride is contained in the liter knowing that the concentration is 0.9%?

Answer: % weight per volume means number of grams per 100 mL.

Now let's look at the entire label for sodium chloride 9%:

Sodium Chloride 0.9%—Contents 1 liter not for injection. Each 100 mL of 0.9% Sodium Chloride Irrigation, USP contains: Sodium chloride 900 mg. Sodium Chloride, USP is chemically designated NaCl, a white crystalline powder, freely soluble in water. Water for injection is chemically designated H_2O.

Example: Calculate the amount of lidocaine in a solution of 2% lidocaine.

1. Convert 2% to a decimal value:
2. Replace the percent sign (%) with × 0.01 (times 0.01) just as you did earlier to convert a percentage to a decimal.
3. Perform the multiplication by moving the decimal point two points to the **left.**

Answer: 2 × 0.01 = .0001 g lidocaine.

PERCENT OF VOLUME PER VOLUME (%V/V)

Volume is a liquid measurement. In the metric system, the base unit for measuring liquids is the liter. Therefore volume per volume is measured as parts or fractions of a liter. This standard compares the amount of one liquid with another. Many drugs used in surgery must be calculated and measured in percent volume per volume. The drug order is often expressed as a ratio.

Example:

Prepare 50 mL of a solution containing 25% Hypaque and intravenous sodium chloride 0.9% *in a ratio of 1:2.*

First, let's break the problem down and see what we have and what we are asked to do. The drug Hypaque is available in different concentrations. In this case, we obtain 25% Hypaque, prepared by the manufacturer. We do not need to analyze the drug itself. We also have intravenous saline already available as a 0.9% solution.

Remember, we are not calculating the amount of actual drug in each solution; we are only asked to mix the two in a specific proportion.

Have:

- *Hypaque solution* 25% w/v (let's assume we obtain 50 mL of this solution from the circulator).
- *Sterile saline for intravenous use* 0.9% w/v (let's assume we obtain 100 mL from the circulator).

Need:

- 50 mL solution containing Hypaque 25% solution and sterile saline 0.9% solution in a ratio of 1 to 2.

Calculations:

- Which of these solutions should represent 1 part and which should represent 2 parts? *Answer:* The first solution mentioned is Hypaque, so it is the first number of the ratio: Hypaque 1 part, saline 2 parts.
- What amounts of each solution should we mix to arrive at the desired concentration? *Answer:* We can prepare any amount of final solution as long as the ratio of 1 to 2 remains the same. If we start with 25 mL Hypaque, we must add 50 mL saline. This gives us *75 mL of the final solution.* We can then draw up 50 mL of the final solution. We could just as easily start with 20 mL of Hypaque and add 40 mL of saline (1 part to 2 parts). This preserves the 1-to-2 ratio.

In Real Practice:

Remember that all drugs must be labeled, and any measuring device, such as a syringe, must be dedicated to that drug (used only with that drug) and also labeled. In the example just given, one container is used to hold saline and the other Hypaque. A third container is used to hold the mixed solution, which must also have a dedicated delivery device. This becomes extremely important when mixing high-alert drugs such as epinephrine and heparin. You will always have an opportunity to consult with a colleague (usually the circulator) to deliver the correct dose in the correct amount. Do not be embarrassed about this. It is common practice for nursing and allied health professionals to help each other achieve safe practice.

EXPRESSIONS CONTAINING "IN"

In surgery, we often see the word *in* to refer to the ratio of drug to solution. The most common reference using *in* or *to* is the concentration of epinephrine in lidocaine. For example, the surgeon may request local anesthetic as follows: **1% lidocaine with epinephrine 1 to 200,000.**

This order is the equivalent of **1% lidocaine with epinephrine 1:200,000,** which demonstrates the ratio of 1% lidocaine to epinephrine. Remember that the 1% refers only to the lidocaine, not the epinephrine.

The key here is to know that 1 to 200,000 or 1:200,000 means **1 gram (g) in 200,000 mL.**

Example:

How much epinephrine is contained in a 20-mL vial of the drug 1% lidocaine with epinephrine 1:200,000?

- We know that there is 1 gram for every 200,000 mL.
- Convert grams to milligrams: 1 gram = 1000 milligrams.
- There is 1000 mg/200,000 mL.

Answer: 1000/200,000 × 20 = 0.1 mg epinephrine in the vial.

PARTS PER MILLION

Parts per million is a method of expressing solutions that are very dilute. Dilution of disinfectants is often expressed in parts per million (ppm). We saw earlier that **percent** solution means parts per one hundred. Parts per million means equivalent to 1 gram in 1,000,000 mL, which is 1 mg per liter. In real practice, you will not be asked to calculate parts per million. However, you may see parts per millions expressed as a concentration for liquid disinfectant. The correct dilution factor for a given use (such as terminal disinfection of operating room furniture) for the antiseptic will be clearly stated on the container.

PROPORTIONS

A true proportion represents *two ratios* that are equal. This is similar to equivalent fractions, which were discussed earlier. A ratio of 2 to 5 is equivalent to a ratio of 6 to 15 and can therefore be written as follows:

2:5:6:15 or $\frac{2}{5} = \frac{6}{15}$ or
" 2 is in the same ratio to 5 as 6 in the ratio to 15" or
" 2 is to 5 as 6 is to 15" .

INTERNATIONAL TIME

Example: You are asked to calculate the number of hours you worked overtime in a week. Your normal work week is 40 hours per week. Here is the schedule you worked based on the 24-hour clock system:

Monday:	7:00 to 22:00
Tuesday	7:00 to 18:30
Wednesday:	7:00 to 15:00
Thursday:	7:00 to 16:00
Friday:	7:00 to 19:30
Saturday:	11:00 to 18:00
Sunday:	Off

How many overtime hours did you work?

Determine the number of hours you worked each day by subtracting the beginning time of each day from the ending time of each day. The 30 minutes after 18 hours on Tuesday and the 30 minutes after 19 hours on Friday represent ½ hour each.

Monday:	22 − 7 = 15 hours
Tuesday:	18½ − 7 = 11½ hours
Wednesday:	15 − 7 = 8 hours
Thursday:	16 − 7 = 9 hours
Friday:	19½ − 7 = 12½ hours
Saturday:	18 − 11 = 9 hours
Sunday:	Off

The total time worked is 15 + 11½ + 8 + 9 + 12½ + 9 = 65 hours worked, which indicates that you worked 25 hours of overtime.

GLOSSARY

Abandonment: A health care professional's failure to stay with a patient and provide care, especially when there is an implied contract to do so.
Abdominal peritoneum: The serous membrane lining the walls of the abdominal cavity. The retroperitoneum is the posterior aspect. In surgical discussions, "abdominal" usually refers to the anterior aspect.
Abduction: Movement of a joint or body part away from the body.
ABHES: Accrediting Bureau of Health Education Schools. An organization that offers accreditation to higher education institutions.
Ablate: To remove or destroy tissue.
Ablation: The complete destruction of tissue.
ABO blood group: Inherited antigens are found on the surface of an individual's red blood cells. These antigens identify the blood group (i.e., type A blood has type A antigens). Also known as *blood type.*
Absorbable suture: Suture material that is broken down and metabolized by the body.
Accommodation: A process in which the lens continually changes shape to maintain the focus of an image on the retina.
Accountability: Accepting responsibility for one's actions. In a professional context, this means that roles and actions accepted by an individual within the context of their occupation require the person to accept responsibility for the consequences of carrying them out.
Accreditation (of a health care facility): The process by which a hospital or other health care facility is evaluated by an independent organization. Accredited facilities are those that meet the standards of the accreditation agency.
ACS: American College of Surgeons. A professional organization that establishes educational and practice standards for surgeons and surgical residency programs.
Active electrode: In electrosurgery, the point of the electrosurgical instrument that delivers current to tissue.
Active electrode monitoring (AEM): A method of reducing the risk of patient burns during monopolar electrosurgery. AEM systems stop the electrical current whenever resistance is high anywhere in the circuit.
Activities of daily living (ADLs): Basic activities and tasks necessary for day-to-day self-care, such as dressing, bathing, toileting, and meal preparation.
Acute illness: Sudden onset of disease or trauma or disease of short duration, usually 3 weeks or less.
Adhesion: Scar formation of the abdominal viscera.
Administration: Individuals who manage an institution, plan its activities, and provide oversight for day-to-day operations and employees. The administration is also a liaison between the facility and the community, government, and media.
Administrative laws: Laws created by an agency or a department of the US government.
Adnexa: A collective term for the ovaries, fallopian tubes, and their connective and vascular attachments.
Advance directive: A document in which a person gives instructions about his or her medical care in the event that the individual cannot speak for himself or herself. Examples are a living will and a medical power of attorney.
Advance health care directive: A written document stating an individual's specific wishes regarding his or her health care to be enacted in the event the person is unable to make decisions.
Adverse reaction: An unexpected, harmful reaction to a drug.
Aerobes: Organisms that favor an environment with oxygen. Strict aerobes cannot live without oxygen.
Aerosol droplets: Droplets of moisture small enough to remain suspended in the air; such a droplet can carry microorganisms within it.
Aesthetic surgery: Surgery that is performed to improve appearance but not necessarily function; also called *cosmetic surgery.*
Aggression: The exertion of power over others through intimidation, sarcasm, or bullying.
Agonist: A drug that produces a response in the body by binding to a receptor.
Air exchange: The exchange of air between areas separated by a physical boundary. Standards for air exchange are regulated by health and safety organizations.
Airborne transmission precautions: Precautions that prevent airborne transfer of disease organisms in the environment.
Airway: The anatomical passageway or artificial tube through which the patient breathes.
Algorithms: Treatment pathways established to allow systematic and consistent methods of medical and surgical management
Allergy: Hypersensitivity to a substance; a response produced by the immune system.
Allied health profession: A profession that follows the principles of medicine and nursing but focuses on an expertise set apart from those practices.
Allograft: A tissue graft in which the donor and recipient are of the same species.
Alloy: A combination of several different kinds of metals. Alloys are used in the manufacturing of stainless steel.
AMA: American Medical Association. An association founded in 1847 comprising medical doctors whose mission is to promote healthy lifestyles across all patient populations.
Amniotic fluid: Fluid surrounding the fetus in the uterus.
Amniotic membranes: Two membranes that encase the fetus, amniotic fluid, and placenta during pregnancy.
Ampere: A unit measuring the amount of energy passing a given point in a stated period of time.
Amplification: In wave science, the phenomenon of increasing wave height by lining up the peaks and troughs of individual waves.
Amplitude: In electromagnetic wave energy, the height of a wave.

Anaerobes: Organisms that prefer an oxygen-poor environment. Strict anaerobes cannot survive in the presence of oxygen.
Analgesia: The absence of pain, produced by specific drugs.
Anastomosis: A surgical technique in which two hollow structures such as portions of the intestine or blood vessels are joined together by sutures or other means. End-to-end anastomosis is the joining of two end sections after a section has been removed. End-to-side anastomosis is the jointing of an end section to the side of another section.
Anesthesia: The absence of sensory awareness or medically induced unconsciousness.
Anesthesia machine: A biotechnical device used to deliver anesthetic and medical gases. The modern term is *anesthesia workstation.*
Anesthesia provider (AP): A professional who is licensed to administer anesthetic agents and manage the patient throughout the period of anesthesia.
Anesthesia technician: An allied health professional trained to assist the anesthesia provider.
Anesthesiologist: A physician specialist in anesthesia and pain management.
Anesthetic: A drug that reduces or blocks sensation or induces unconsciousness.
ANSI: American National Standards Institute. An organization that establishes business and health standards to serve as a baseline for assessment.
Antagonist: A drug or chemical that blocks a receptor-mediated response.
Antegrade: Toward the normal direction of flow (e.g., from the kidney to the bladder).
Anterograde amnesia: In anesthesia, the patient's inability to recall events that occur after the administration of specific drugs. After the drug is metabolized and cleared from the body, normal recall returns.
Antibiotics: Drugs that inhibit the growth of or kill bacteria.
Antiseptic: Chemical agent approved for use on the skin that inhibits the growth and reproduction of microorganisms.
Antiseptic: A chemical used to remove microbes from the skin.
Anxiolytic: A drug that reduces anxiety.
AORN: Association of periOperative Registered Nurses. The professional organization for surgical nurses; originally known as the *Association of Operating Room Nurses.*
APGAR score: Method of assessing neonates according to respiratory rate, color, reflex response, heart rate, and body tone.
Apnea: Absence of breathing.
Approximate: To bring tissues together by sutures or other means.
ARC/STSA: Accreditation Review Council on Education in Surgical Technology and Surgical Assisting. ARC/STSA establishes, maintains, and promotes quality standards for education programs in surgical technology and surgical first assisting.
Arch bars: Metal plates wired to the teeth to occlude the jaw during maxillofacial surgery or during healing. Arch bars maintain the patient's normal bite (occlusion).
Argon: An inert gas used in electrosurgery to direct and shroud the electrical current.
Arterial blood gases (ABGs): A blood test that measures the level of oxygen and carbon dioxide and the pH of the blood.
Arteriovenous fistula (or AV shunt): Surgically created vascular access for patients undergoing hemodialysis.
Arthroscopy: Endoscopic surgery of a joint.
Asepsis: The absence of pathogenic microorganisms on an animate surface or on body tissue. Literally, asepsis means "without infection," whereas sepsis literally means "with infection."
Aseptic technique: Methods or practices in health care that reduce or prevent the spread of infection.
Aspiration: Inhalation of fluid or solid matter into the lungs.
Assertiveness: Communicating one's personal and professional needs to others; protecting one's own rights while respecting those of others.
Assistant circulator: The surgical technologist in the nonsterile role of the surgical team responsible for monitoring the conditions in the operating room that are related to patient care, safety, documentation, distribution of sterile supplies, and counts. A registered perioperative nurse in this role would be considered a circulator and will have additional responsibilities.
AST: Association of Surgical Technologists. The professional association for surgical technologists that strives to uphold and support the standards of patient care and the profession.
Atom: A discrete unit made of matter consisting of charged and uncharged particles.
Auscultation: Listening to the lungs, heart, or abdomen through the stethoscope.
Autograft: The surgical transplantation of tissue from one part of the body to another in the same individual.
Autotransfusion: Also called *blood salvaging.* A method of retrieving blood lost at the operative site, reprocessing it, and infusing it back to the patient.
Auxiliary water channel: A channel in the flexible endoscope that conveys irrigation fluid to the tip.
Back table: A large stainless steel table on which most of the sterile surgical supplies and instruments are organized for use during surgery. Before surgery, the back table is covered with a sterile drape, and sterile instruments and other equipment are opened onto its surface.
Bactericidal: Able to kill bacteria.
Bacteriostatic: Chemical agent capable of inhibiting the growth of bacteria.
Benign: A term used to characterize a tumor that does not have the capability to spread to other parts of the body and is usually composed of tissue similar to its tissue of origin.
Bicortical screws: Screws that penetrate both cortical layers and the intervening spongy layer of the bone.
Bier block: Regional anesthesia in which the anesthetic agent is injected into a vein.
Billroth I procedure: A gastroduodenostomy, or surgical anastomosis, of the stomach and the duodenum.
Billroth II procedure: A gastrojejunostomy, or surgical anastomosis, of the stomach and the jejunum.
Bioavailability: The extent and rate at which a drug or its metabolites (products of breakdown) enter the systemic circulation and reach the site of action.
Bioburden: The number of contaminating microbes on an object or substance.
Biofilm: Dense colonies of bacteria that adhere tightly to surfaces.
Biological grafts: Grafts derived from live tissue, whether human or animal.
Biological indicator: A quality control mechanism used in the process of sterilization. It consists of a closed system containing harmless, spore-forming bacteria that can be rapidly cultured after the sterilization process.
Biomedical engineering technician: Professional who specializes in the maintenance, repair, and safe operation of devices used in patient care.
Biopsy: Removal of a sample of tissue for pathological analysis.
Biopsy channel: A channel that extends the full length of a flexible endoscope through which to retrieve biopsy tissue.

Biosynthetic: A type of graft or implant material made of synthetic absorbable material.

Bipolar circuit: An electrosurgical circuit in which current travels from the power unit through an instrument containing two opposite poles in contact with the tissue and then returns it directly to the energy source.

Birth canal: The maternal pelvis and soft structures through which the baby passes during birth.

Bispectral index system (BIS): A monitoring method used to determine the patient's level of consciousness and prevent intraoperative awareness.

Blended mode: In electrosurgery, a combination of intermediate frequency and intermediate wave intervals to produce a specific effect on tissue.

Blood-borne pathogens: Harmful microorganisms that may be present in and transmitted through human blood and body fluids.

Blowout fracture: A severe fracture of the orbital cavity in which a portion of the globe may extrude outside the cavity.

Blunt dissection: The technique of separating tissue layers by teasing them apart with a rough sponge dissector, blunt instrument, or manually.

Body image: In psychology, the way a person sees himself or herself through the eyes of others. A negative body image can severely affect a patient's sense of identity, as well as social and personal interactions.

Body language: Communication through facial expressions, posture, and gestures.

Boiling point: The temperature of a substance when its state changes from a liquid to a gas.

Bowel technique: A method of preventing cross-contamination between the bowel contents and nearby tissues.

Bowie–Dick Test: A test that identifies air leaks and ineffective air removal in the steam sterilization process.

Box lock: A ratchet mechanism that holds a surgical instrument in the closed position

Breathing bag: The reservoir breathing apparatus of the anesthesia machine. Gases are titrated and shunted into the breathing bag, which is connected to the patient's airway.

Breech presentation: Presentation of the baby during delivery in which the buttocks or feet deliver first.

Bridle suture: In ophthalmic surgery, a temporary traction suture placed through the sclera used to pull the globe laterally for exposure of the posterolateral surface. It is called a *bridle suture* because of its resemblance to the reins of a horse's bridle.

Bronchospasm: Partial or complete closure of the bronchial tubes as a result of spasm.

CAAHEP: Commission on Accreditation of Allied Health Education Programs. Accredits health science programs, including those for surgical technology.

Calculi: Stones caused by the precipitation of minerals, such as calcium, and other substances from the kidney filtrate.

Camera control unit (CCU): The main control source for the video camera. The unit captures video signals from the camera head and processes them for display on the monitor.

Cannula: In minimally invasive surgery, a cannula is a slender tube inserted through the body wall and used to receive and stabilize telescopic instruments.

Capacitative coupling: In minimally invasive surgery, the unintended transmission of electricity from the active electrode to an adjacent conductive pathway, sometimes resulting in a patient burn.

Capacitive coupling: A specific burn hazard of monopolar endoscopic surgery. It occurs when current passes unintentionally through instrument insulation and adjacent conductive material into tissue.

Capillary action: The ability of suture material to absorb fluid.

Carbon dioxide: An inert gas used in laser surgery and for sufflation of the abdomen during laparoscopy.

Case cart system: A method of preparing equipment and instruments for a surgical case. Equipment is prepared and assembled by the central services or supply department and sent to the operating room in a closed stainless steel cart.

Case planning: Systematic preparation for a surgical procedure.

Cataract: Clouding of vision caused by a disease in which the crystalline lens of the eye, its capsule, or both become opaque. This prevents light from focusing on the retina, resulting in visual distortion. Cataracts may develop as a result of the aging process, disease, or injury.

Cavitation: The mechanism of ultrasonic cleaning in which air bubbles implode (burst inward), releasing particles of soil or tissue debris.

Cavitron Ultrasonic Surgical Aspirator (CUSA): This instrument destroys tissue through the use of high-frequency sound waves (ultrasound).

Certified registered nurse anesthetist (CRNA): An advance trained and certified nurse licensed to provide anesthesia.

Central core: A restricted area of the operating room, where sterile supplies and immediate-use (flash) sterilizers may be located.

Central nervous system depression: This refers to a decrease in sensory awareness caused by drugs or a pathological condition.

Central processing unit (CPU): The component of a computer that contains the circuitry, memory, and power controls.

Cerclage: A procedure in which a suture ligature is placed around the cervix to prevent spontaneous abortion.

Certification: Acknowledgment by a private agency that a person has achieved a minimum level of knowledge and skill.

Cerumen: A substance produced by the cerumen glands of the ear (i.e., ear wax).

Chain of command: A hierarchy of personnel positions that establishes both vertical and horizontal relationships between positions.

Chemical barrier: The barrier formed by the residual action of a disinfectant or antiseptic; it not only reduces the number of microorganisms on a surface but also prevents recolonization (regrowth) for a limited period.

Chemical indicator: A method of testing a sterilization parameter. Chemical strips sensitive to physical conditions, such as temperature, are placed with the item being sterilized and change color when the parameter is reached; sometimes called a *chemical monitor.*

Chemical name: The name of a drug that reflects its molecular structure.

Chemical sterilization: A process that uses chemical agents to achieve sterilization.

Chisel: An orthopedic instrument used to shave bone; one side is straight and the other is beveled.

Cholesteatoma: A benign tumor of the middle ear caused by the shedding of keratin.

Chronic illness: An illness that has continued for months, weeks, or years.

-cidal: A suffix indicating death. For example, bactericidal means "able to kill bacteria."

Circuit: The path of free electrons as they move through conductive material. In a closed circuit, the electrons proceed unhindered and electrical energy is maintained; in an open circuit, the path of the electrons is interrupted, which stops the flow of current.

Cirrhosis: A disease of the liver in which the tissue hardens and the venous drainage becomes blocked.

Clean: The absence of visible soil on a surface.
Cleaning: A process that removes organic or inorganic soil or debris using friction, detergent, and water.
Coagulum: A sticky, semiliquid substance that forms when tissue is altered by electrical or ultrasonic energy.
Cobalt-60 radiation: A method of institutional bulk sterilization used by manufacturers to sterilize prepackaged equipment using ionizing radiation.
Coherent light waves: Light waves that are lined up so that the troughs and peaks are matched.
Coitus: Sexual intercourse.
Colposcopy: Microscopic examination of the cervix.
Coma: The deepest state of unconsciousness, in which most brain activity ceases.
Complete blood count (CBC): A blood test that measures specific components, including the hemoglobin, hematocrit, red blood cells, and white blood cells.
Composite graft: A biological graft composed of different types of tissues such as skin and muscle.
Compression injury: Tissue injury caused by continuous pressure over an area.
Computed tomography (CT): An imaging technique that allows physicians to obtain cross-sectional x-ray views of the patient. The result is a CT scan.
Concentration: A measure of the quantity of a substance per unit of volume or weight.
Conduction: The transfer of heat from one substance to another by the natural movement of molecules, which sets other molecules in motion.
Conductivity: The relative ability of a substance to transmit free electrons or electricity.
Consciousness: Neurological state in which a patient is able to sense environmental stimuli such as sight, sound, touch, pressure, pain, heat, and cold.
Consensus: Agreement among members of a group.
Containment and confinement: A foundation concept of aseptic technique in which sterile and nonsterile surfaces are separated by physical barriers or distance (space).
Contaminated: Rendered nonsterile and unacceptable for use in critical areas of the body.
Contaminated: Describes a sterile surface which has come in contact with a nonsterile surface.
Contamination: The consequence of physical contact between a sterile surface and a nonsterile surface. Contamination results in the potential or actual transfer of microbes to normally sterile tissue or an inanimate object.
Continuing education: More formally called *professional development.* It demonstrates an ongoing learning process in an individual's profession. Continuing education (CE) credits are provided by a professional organization. Credits are earned by attending lectures and in-service presentations or by study and examination. Usually, only peer-reviewed professional literature qualifies for CE credits.
Continuous-wave lasers: Lasers that emit the laser light continuously rather than in pulses.
Contracture: Scar tissue that lacks flexibility, causing constriction and pain.
Contraindications: Contraindications to a protocol, drug, or procedure are circumstances that make its use medically inadvisable because it increases the risk of injury or harm.
Contrast media: Radiopaque solutions (i.e., not penetrated by x-rays) that are introduced into body cavities and vessels to outline their inside surfaces.
Contrast medium: A fluid that is not penetrable by x-rays, used to determine the contours of a part of the body.
Control head: The proximal section of a flexible endoscope where the controls are located.
Controlled substances: Drugs that have the potential for abuse. Controlled substances are rated according to their risk potential; these ratings are called *schedules.*
Convection: The displacement of cool air by warm air. Convection usually creates currents as the warm air rises and the cool air falls.
Cord prolapse: Complication of pregnancy in which the umbilical cord emerges from the uterus during labor and may be compressed against the maternal pelvis or the vagina. This can obstruct blood supply to the fetus.
Coroner's case: A patient death that requires investigation by the coroner, as well as an autopsy on the deceased.
Count: A systematic method of accounting for items that may be retained in the patient during surgery.
Cryoablation: A method of tissue destruction in which a probe is inserted into a tumor or tissue mass. High-pressure argon gas is injected into the probe, causing the surrounding tissue to freeze and eventually slough.
Cryosurgery: The use of extremely low temperature to destroy diseased tissue.
Cryotherapy: A technique in which a cold probe is used to freeze tissue, such as the sclera, ciliary body (for glaucoma), or retinal layers, after detachment.
CST: Certified surgical technologist. A surgical technologist who has successfully passed the certification examination given by the National Board of Surgical Technology and Surgical Assisting.
CST–CFA: Certified surgical technologist–certified first assistant. A surgical technologist with advanced training who has successfully passed the certification examination for surgical first assistants and is credentialed by the National Board of Surgical Technology and Surgical Assisting.
Cultural competence: Knowledge of and ability to provide support and care to individuals of cultures and belief systems different from one's own.
Culture: The process of growing a microbe in a laboratory setting so that it can be studied and tested.
Curettage: The removal of tissue by scraping with a surgical curette.
Cutting mode: In electrosurgery, the use of high voltage and relatively low frequency to cut through tissue.
Cystocele: A herniation of the bladder into the vaginal wall.
Damages: Money awarded in a civil lawsuit to compensate the injured party.
Debridement: The removal of devitalized tissue, debris, and foreign objects from a wound. Debridement is performed on trauma injuries, burns, and infected wounds either before surgery or as part of the surgical procedure.
Decontamination: A process in which recently used and soiled medical devices, including instruments, are made safe for personnel to handle.
Decontamination area: A room or department in which soiled instruments and equipment are cleaned of gross matter and processed to remove microorganisms.
Defamation: A derogatory statement concerning another person's skill, character, or reputation.
Dehiscence: Separation of the edges of a surgical wound during healing.
Delegation: The assignment of one's duties to another person. In medicine, the person who delegates a duty retains accountability for the action of the person to whom it is delegated.

Delirium: A state of confusion and disorientation. In the past, delirium was defined as a distinct stage of induction and emergence from general anesthesia. However, this stage is rarely demonstrated in association with modern anesthetics.

Dentition: The number, type, and pattern of the teeth.

Dependent areas of the body: Areas of the body subject to pressure from gravity and weight. For example, the sacrum is a dependent area when a person is in the supine position.

Deposition: The testimony of a witness given under oath and transcribed by a court reporter during the pretrial phase of a civil lawsuit.

Dermatome: A medical device used for removing single-thickness skin grafts.

Dermoid cyst: A mass arising from the germ layers of the embryo that contains tissue remnants, including hair and teeth.

Detachable suture: A suture-needle combination in which the suture can be easily removed from the needle by pulling it sharply.

Detergent: A chemical that breaks down organic debris by emulsification (separation into small particles) to aid in cleaning.

Determination of death: A formal medical process to determine brain death.

Diagnostic endoscopy: A diagnostic procedure in which a long, flexible, fiberoptic tube is inserted into a body cavity for viewing and diagnosis.

Diastolic pressure: The pressure exerted on the walls of the blood vessels during the resting phase of cardiac contraction.

Diathermy: Low-power cautery used to mark the sclera over an area of retinal detachment.

Differential count: A test that determines the number of each type of white blood cell in a specimen of blood.

Diffusion: Uniform dispersal of particles in a solution or across a membrane.

Digital output recorder: During video-assisted surgery, digital signals are captured from the video camera and transmitted to an image system. The digital output recorder processes these signals.

Dilator: Graduated, smooth instrument that is used to increase the circumference of an orifice.

Dilemma: A situation or personal conflict that arises from a need to make a decision when none of the choices are acceptable.

Diluent: The liquid component of a drug that must be reconstituted from a powder to a solution for the purposes of administration.

Direct coupling: The transfer of electrical current from an active electrode to another conductive instrument by accident or as part of the electrosurgical process.

Direct current (DC): A type of low-voltage electrical current in which electrons flow in one direction to complete a circuit. Battery power uses direct current.

Direct inguinal hernia: A hernia caused by a weakness in the inguinal floor.

Direct transmission: The transfer of microbes by direct physical contact with the microbes.

Discharge against medical advice (AMA): Self-discharge by a patient who has not necessarily met discharge criteria.

Discharge criteria: Objective criteria used to determine whether a patient is safe for discharge from the health care facility.

Disinfection: Destruction of microorganisms by heat or chemical means.

Disinfection: A process that results in the destruction of microorganisms on an inanimate (nonliving) object or surface.

Dispersive electrode: A component of the electrosurgical circuit that spreads current at the point where it exits the body and thus prevents injury.

Dissecting sponge: A small compact sponge used to dissect soft tissue planes; also referred to as a *sponge dissector.* The dissecting sponge is always mounted on a clamp for use in the surgical wound.

DNAR: "Do not attempt resuscitation." Emphasizes the patient's desire to refuse intervention to resuscitate.

DNR: "Do not resuscitate." An official request to refrain from certain types of resuscitation, usually cardiopulmonary resuscitation.

Docking: In robotic surgery, the process of positioning the robotic arm in the exact location over the patient so that instruments can be safely attached to their ports in the body cavity.

Doppler effect: The effect perceived when the origin or receiver of sound waves moves. The perception is a change in the frequency of the waves and corresponding pitch.

Doppler studies: A technique that uses ultrasonic waves to measure blood flow in a vessel.

Doppler ultrasound: A medical device that uses the Doppler effect and ultrasonic waves to measure and record blood flow as well as tissue density and shape.

Dosage: The regulated administration of prescribed amounts of a drug. Dosage is expressed as a quantity of drug per unit of time.

Dose: The quantity of a drug to be taken at one time or the stated amount of drug per unit of distribution (e.g., 0.5 mg per milliliter of solution).

Double gloving: Wearing two pairs of gloves, one over the other, to reduce the risk of contamination as a result of glove failure or puncture.

Double-action rongeur: A bone-cutting instrument with two hinges in the middle. This increases the leverage and strength of the instrument.

Droplet nuclei: Dried remnants of previously moist secretions containing microorganisms. Droplet nuclei are an important source of disease transmission.

Drug: A chemical substance that, when taken into the body, has a physiological effect.

Drug administration: The giving of a drug to a person by any route.

Duty cycle: In electrosurgery, the duration of current flow sometimes is referred to as the duty cycle. The duty cycle can intermittently be applied to produce the desired effect on tissue.

Eclampsia: A seizure during pregnancy, usually as a result of pregnancy-induced hypertension.

Ectopic pregnancy: Implantation of the fertilized ovum outside the uterus.

Efficiency: The economic use of time and energy to prevent unnecessary expenditure of work, materials, and time.

Effusion: Fluid in the middle ear.

Electrocardiography: A noninvasive assessment of the heart's electrical activity displayed on a graph, the electrocardiogram. In the United States, electrocardiogram is abbreviated correctly as ECG. EKG is the European abbreviation.

Electrocution: Severe burns, cardiac disturbances, or death as a result of electrical current discharged into the body.

Electrolytic fluid: Fluids that contain electrolytes and therefore can transmit an electrical current.

Electromagnetic field: A three-dimensional pattern of force created by the attraction and repulsion of charged particles around a magnet.

Electromagnetic waves: The natural phenomenon of wave energy, such as electricity, light, and radio broadcasts. The type of energy is determined by the frequency of the waves.

Electron: A negatively charged particle that orbits the nucleus of an atom.

Electrostatic discharge: The sudden release of electrical energy from surfaces where charged particles have accumulated because of friction.

Electrosurgery: The direct use of electricity to cut and coagulate tissue.

Electrosurgical unit (ESU): The power generator and control source in the electrosurgical system.

Electrosurgical vessel sealing: A type of bipolar electrosurgery in which tissue is welded together using low-voltage, low-temperature, high-frequency current.

Element: A pure substance composed of atoms, each with the same number of protons (e.g., iron, copper, uranium).

Elevator: A straight instrument with a curved sharp or dull tip used to separate tissue layers such as periosteum from bone.

Elevator channel: A channel that extends the full length of a flexible endoscope and conveys biopsy forceps or other instruments.

Elimination: The physiological process of removing cellular and chemical waste products from the body.

Embolism: A clot of blood, air, organic material, or a foreign body that moves freely in the vascular system. An embolus travels from larger to smaller vessels until it cannot pass through a vessel. At that level, it interrupts the flow of blood and may cause severe disease or death.

Emergence: The stage in general anesthesia at which the anesthetic agent is withdrawn and the patient regains consciousness.

Emoticons: Small images or acronyms used to convey emotion in email and SMS (text message) communication.

End of life: A period within which death is expected, usually within days, weeks, or months.

Endocoupler: A device that connects the telescope to the camera.

Endoscopic procedures: Medical assessment of body cavities using a fiber-optic instrument (endoscope).

Endospore: The dormant stage of some bacteria that allows them to survive in extreme environmental conditions, including heat, cold, and exposure to chemicals. Endospores are commonly referred to as *spores.*

Endotracheal tube: An artificial airway (tube) that is inserted into the patient's trachea to maintain patency.

Entry site: In microbial transmission, the sites where microorganisms enter the body.

Enucleation: Surgical removal of the globe and accessory attachments.

Environmental cleaning: The process of cleaning the surfaces in patient care areas, including the operating room. This includes floors, cabinets, equipment, lights, and furniture.

Enzymatic cleaner: A specific chemical used in detergents and cleaners to penetrate and break down biological debris, such as blood.

Epidural: A type of anesthesia in which the anesthetic is delivered through a small catheter into the epidural space of the spinal cord.

Episiotomy: A perineal incision made during the second stage of labor to prevent the tearing of tissue.

Epistaxis: Bleeding arising from the nasal cavity.

Eschar: Burned tissue fragments that can accumulate on the electrosurgical tip during use; eschar can cause sparking and become a source of ignition.

Escharotomy: Excision of eschar to release stricture in surrounding tissues.

Esmarch bandage: A rolled bandage made of rubber or latex that is used to exsanguinate blood from a limb before inflating a pneumatic tourniquet.

Esophageal varices: Distended veins of the esophagus, caused by advanced liver disease. The condition occurs as a result of portal vein obstruction arising from fibrosis of the liver. Esophageal varices may bleed profusely.

Ethical dilemmas: Situations in which ethical choices involve conflicting values.

Ethical dilemma: A situation in which one must make a decision and none of the options are acceptable.

Ethics: Core values that define one's relationship with others or the environment.

Ethylene oxide (EO): A highly flammable gas that is capable of sterilizing an object.

Event related: An activity or process linked with an event.

Event-related sterility: A wrapped sterile item may become contaminated by environmental conditions or events, such as a puncture in the wrapper. Event-related sterility refers to sterility based on the absence of such events. The shelf life of a sterilized pack is event related, not time related.

Evert: To turn outward or inside out.

Evidence-based practice: Professional practices and their standards based on established scientific research rather than opinion or tradition.

Evisceration: The protrusion of abdominal viscera through a wound or surgical incision.

Excimer: A type of lasing energy that is created when electrons are removed from the lasing medium.

Excitation source: In laser technology, the energy that causes the atoms of a lasing medium (gas or solid) to vibrate.

Exenteration: Complete surgical removal of organs or tissue blocs.

Exploratory laparotomy: A laparotomy performed to examine the abdominal cavity when less invasive measures fail to confirm a diagnosis.

Exposure time: This is the amount of time goods are held in specific conditions during disinfection or the sterilization process. Exposure time varies with the size of the load, type of materials being sterilized, and the type of agent used. Exposure time is sometimes called the *hold time.*

Extracorporeal shock wave lithotripsy (ESWL): A procedure in which ultrasonic sound waves are used to pulverize kidney or gallbladder stones.

Extubation: Withdrawal of an artificial airway.

Facilitator: A group leader who coordinates the direction and flow of a group meeting without influencing the content of people's contributions. It is similar to an *enabling* position, in which people are encouraged to express ideas without fear of judgment.

Fasciotomy: Longitudinal incisions made in the fascia to release severe swelling or stricture, which can result in necrosis.

Feedback: The response to a message; a component of effective communication.

Fenestrated drape: A sterile sheet with a hole or "window" *(fenestration)* that exposes the incision site. The fenestrated drape is positioned after other drapes and towels have been placed in keeping with the procedure. Fenestrated drapes are differentiated by type (e.g., laparotomy, thyroid, kidney, eye, ear, and extremity drapes).

Fetal demise: Death of the fetus.

Fibroid: See Leiomyoma.

Fistula: An abnormal tract or passage leading from one organ to another or from an organ to the skin; usually caused by infection.

Flammable: Capable of burning.

Fluoroscopy: A radiological technique that provides real-time images of an anatomical region.

Focal point: The exact location where light rays converge after passing through a convex lens.
Foley catheter: A retention catheter with an expandable balloon at the distal end.
Fomite: An intermediate inanimate source in the process of disease transmission. An object, such as a contaminated surgical instrument or medical device, can become a fomite in disease transmission.
Fowler position: In this position the patient is recumbent in a sitting or modified sitting position for exposure to the head, posterior neck and cranium, anterior chest area, face, and shoulders.
Frequency: In physics, the number of waves that pass a point in 1 second. The unit of measurement for frequency is the hertz (Hz).
Friable: A descriptive term for tissue that means fragile and easily torn; friable tissue may bleed profusely. Some disease states produce friable tissue. The liver and spleen normally are friable.
Frozen section: A procedure in which a tissue specimen is flash frozen and sectioned for examination under the microscope. The procedure is used to verify suspected cancer during surgery.
Fulguration: A process of tissue surface destruction used in electrosurgery.
Full-thickness skin graft (FTSG): A skin graft composed of the epidermis and dermis.
Gain: In electronics, the intensity of the signal.
Gas plasma sterilization: A process that uses the form of matter known as plasma during the sterilization process.
Gas scavenging: The capture and safe removal of extraneous anesthetic gases from the anesthesia machine.
Gastrostomy: A surgical opening through the stomach wall connecting to the outside of the body or another hollow anatomical structure.
General anesthesia: Anesthesia associated with a state of unconsciousness. General anesthesia is not a fixed state of unconsciousness, but rather, ranges along a continuum from semi-responsiveness to profound unresponsiveness.
Generation: In pharmacology, refers to a drug group that was developed from a previous prototype (e.g., first-generation cephalosporin).
Generic drug: A drug that is manufactured and sold under its formulary name.
Generic name: The formulary name of a drug that is assigned by the U.S. Adopted Names Council.
Gestational age: The age of the fetus as measured in the number of weeks from conception.
Glasgow Coma Scale (GCS): A standardized method of measuring a patient's response to external stimuli and thus his or her level of consciousness.
Glaucoma: A group of diseases characterized by the elevation of intraocular pressure. Sustained pressure on the optic nerve and other structures may result in ischemia and blindness.
Glomerular filtration rate (GFR): An indication of kidney function in which serum creatinine (normally filtered by the kidney) is measured.
Gouge: A V- or U-shaped bone chisel.
Graft: An implant used to replace or augment existing tissue. A graft may be obtained from the patient, another person, an animal source, or synthetic or biosynthetic materials.
Gravity-displacement sterilizer: A type of steam sterilizer that removes air by gravity.
Gross contamination: Contamination of a large area of tissue by a highly infective source.
Grounding: A path for electrical current to flow unimpeded through a material and disperse back to the source or disperse into the ground.
Grounding pad: An alternate name for the *patient return electrode.*
Groupthink: In sociology and group behavior theory, the conformity of a group to one way of thinking and behaving. Groupthink creates two factions: those who agree (in-group) and those who disagree (out-group). This generates resentment and conflict in the workplace.
Half-life: The time required for one half of a drug to be cleared from the body.
Hand disinfection: The systematic application of antiseptic foam or gel on the hands and arms before gowning and gloving for a sterile procedure. Hand disinfection may be used as an alternative to the traditional hand scrub under certain conditions.
Hand washing: A specific technique used to remove soil, debris, and dead cells from the hands. Hand washing with an antiseptic also reduces the number of microorganisms on the skin.
Handover (hand-off): A verbal and written report from one nurse to another to provide updated patient information.
Haptic feedback: Tactile feedback, conveyed from tissue to the hand when a surgical instrument is used.
Harmonics: The quality of sound related to the frequency of the sound waves.
Heart-beating cadaver: A cadaver maintained on cardiopulmonary support to provide tissue perfusion. This is done to maintain viability of organs for donation.
Hematocrit (Hct): The ratio of red blood cells to plasma, measured as a percentage.
Hematoma: A blood-filled space in tissue, the result of a bleeding vessel.
Hemoglobin (Hgb): The oxygen-carrying molecule found in red blood cells. The amount of hemoglobin in the patient's blood is measured in grams per deciliter (g/dL).
Hemorrhage: Continuous bleeding from a pathological cause.
Hemostat: A surgical clamp most often used to occlude a blood vessel.
Hemostasis: Absence of bleeding.
Hemostatic agent: Substance applied to bleeding tissue to enhance clotting.
Hernia: A protrusion of tissue under the skin through a weakened area of the body wall.
High definition (HD): A type of video format. The clarity of the image is based on the number of signals (pixels) emitted by the camera. HD format has a 16:9 aspect ratio, which is seven times greater than standard definition.
High-efficiency particulate air (HEPA) filters: Filters installed in the operating room ventilation system that remove 99.97% of particles equal to or larger than 0.3 μm.
High-level disinfection (HLD): A process that reduces the bioburden to an absolute minimum.
High-vacuum sterilizer: A type of steam sterilizer that removes air in the chamber by vacuum and refills it with pressurized steam. Also known as a *prevacuum sterilizer.*
Holmium: YAG:A solid crystal lasing medium that penetrates a wide variety of substances, including renal and biliary stones and soft tissue.
Homeostasis: A state of balance in physiological functions.
Horizontal abuse: Verbal abuse or sabotage of people of equal job or professional ranking.
Hook wire: A device used to pinpoint the exact location of a mass detected during a mammogram (also referred to as a *hook needle*). A fine wire is inserted into the mass during the examination, and the tissue around the needle is removed for pathological examination and definitive diagnosis.
Hospital policy: Rules or regulations that hospital employees are required to follow. They are created to protect patients and employees from harm and to ensure smooth operation of the hospital.

Hot wire: In electrical circuits, the hot wire is the one that carries the electrical current.

Hydro dressing: A dressing impregnated with a water-based gel. This type of dressing prevents the wound from drying.

Hyperextension: Extension of a joint beyond its normal anatomical range.

Hyperflexion: Flexion of a joint beyond its normal anatomical range.

Hyperplasia: An excessive proliferation of tissue.

Hypersensitivity: Allergic immune response to a substance causing a range of symptoms from mild inflammation to anaphylactic shock and death.

Hypertrophic scar: A raised scar characterized by excess collagen.

Hypertrophy: Enlargement of an organ or tissue.

Hypothermia: Body temperature that is below normal.

Hypoxia: Lack of oxygen in the tissue.

Imaging studies: Diagnostic tests that produce a picture or image.

Imaging system: The combined components of the minimally invasive surgery system, which create the image captured in the focal view of the telescope.

Immediate-use steam sterilization (IUSS): Rapid sterilization of instruments to be used immediately. This process was previously called *flash sterilization.*

Impedance: The constriction of electrical current by a nonconductive material or an area of high density. This results in the transformation of electricity into heat.

Impervious: Waterproof.

Implant: A synthetic, natural, or biosynthetic substance used to fill in or replace an anatomical structure.

Implant: Defined by the U.S. Food and Drug Administration (FDA) as "a device that is placed into a surgically or naturally formed cavity of the human body if it is intended to remain there for a period of 30 days or more."

Implanted electronic device (IED): An electronic device that monitors and corrects physiological conditions. Electrosurgery may interfere with the function of such devices, which include pacemakers, internal defibrillators, deep brain stimulators, ventricular assist devices, and others.

Incarcerated hernia: Herniated tissue that is trapped in an abdominal wall defect. Incarcerated tissue requires emergency surgery to prevent ischemia and tissue necrosis.

Incident report: A written description of any event that caused harm or presented the risk of harm to a patient or staff in the course of normal health care.

Incise drape: A plastic adhesive drape that is positioned over the incision site after surgical skin prep. The incise drape creates a sterile surface over the skin.

Incisional hernia: The postoperative herniation of tissue into the tissue layers around an abdominal incision. This may occur in the immediate postoperative period or later, after the incision has healed.

Incomplete abortion: Expulsion of the fetus with retained placenta before 20 weeks' gestation.

Indirect inguinal hernia: A hernia that protrudes into the membranous sac of the spermatic cord. This condition usually is due to a congenital defect in the abdominal wall.

Induction: Initiation of general anesthesia with a drug that causes unconsciousness.

Indwelling catheter: A urethral or ureteral catheter that is left in place for continuous drainage.

Inert: Causing little or no reaction in tissue or with other materials.

Infection: The state or condition in which pathogenic microorganisms invade and colonize in the body or body tissues.

Inflammation: The body's nonspecific reaction to injury or infection that results in redness, heat, swelling, and pain.

Informed consent: A process or legal document that describes the patient's surgical procedure and the risks, consequences, and benefits of that procedure.

Insertion tube: The long, narrow portion of the flexible endoscope that is inserted into the body.

Instrument channel: A channel that extends the full length of a flexible endoscope and conveys instruments during flexible endoscopy.

Insufflation: In minimally invasive surgery, inflation of the abdominal or thoracic cavity with carbon dioxide gas.

Insulate: To cover or surround a conductive substance with nonconductive material.

Insulator: A substance that does not conduct electrical current and is used to prevent electricity from seeking an alternate path.

Insurance: A contract in which the insurance company agrees to defend the policy holder if that individual is sued for acts covered by the policy.

Integrated operating room: A type of structural and engineering design in which digital and computerized components such as cameras, monitors, and environmental controls can be controlled from a central location in the room.

Internal drives: Data storage devices that are an integral part of the computer.

Internet: A worldwide public network of computers that are connected by wires, fiberoptic cables, or satellite signals. Computers connected to this system can receive and transmit data to other computers in the system.

Interrupted sutures: A technique of bringing tissue together by placing individual sutures close together.

Intranet: A computer network within a facility or an organization that can be accessed only by those employed or affiliated with the organization.

Intraoperative awareness (IOA): A rare condition in which a patient undergoing general anesthesia is able to feel pain and other noxious stimuli but is unable to react.

Intraosseous: Refers to administration of a drug directly into the bone marrow.

Intrathecal: Refers to administration of a drug into the spinal canal.

Intravasation: The absorption of the fluid into the vascular system, leading to increased blood pressure and possible death related to fluid overload.

Intravascular volume: Fluid volume within the blood vessels.

Intubation: The process of inserting an invasive artificial airway.

Invasive procedure: A medical or surgical procedure in which the protective surfaces of the body such as skin or mucous membrane are penetrated.

Ischemia: Loss of blood supply to a body part either by compression or as a result of a blockage in blood vessels. Prolonged ischemia causes tissue death from lack of oxygen to the tissue.

Isolated circuit: An electrical circuit that has no ground reference or method of conducting current into the ground at the site of use. Current is directed from the energy source, through the patient, and back to the source.

Job description: A document that specifies the duties, responsibilities, location, pay, and management structure of a job.

Job title: The name of a job, such as "Certified Surgical Technologist" or "Chief of Surgery."

Keloid: Excess scar tissue occurring in dark-skinned individuals. The scar may become bulbous and usually does not reduce over time.

Keratoplasty: Surgery of the cornea. The term *penetrating keratoplasty* refers to corneal transplantation.

Kick bucket: A stainless steel bucket mounted in a frame on wheels used for soiled surgical sponges during the procedure.
Kraske position: Also called *jackknife position,* the patient lies prone with the middle section of the table flexed at a slight angle.
Kübler-Ross, Elisabeth: A Swiss psychiatrist who proposed a theory of developmental or psychological stages of the dying experience.
Labor: The process of regular contraction of the uterine muscle that results in birth.
Laminar air flow: An unidirectional ultraclean air delivery system that creates a "curtain" of super clean air around the sterile field.
Laminar airflow (LAF) system: A ventilation system that moves a contained volume of air in layers at a continuous velocity, with 800 to 900 air exchanges per hour.
Laparotomy: A procedure in which the abdominal cavity is surgically opened. The techniques used for laparotomy are used for all open surgical procedures of the abdomen.
Laryngeal mask airway (LMA): An airway consisting of a tube and small mask that fits internally over the patient's larynx.
Laryngoscope: A lighted instrument used during endotracheal intubation.
Laryngospasm: Muscular spasm of the larynx, which may result in obstruction.
Laser: Acronym for light amplification by stimulated emission of radiation.
Laser classifications: Industry and international system for grading laser energy according to its ability to cause injury.
Laser head: The component of the laser system that holds the lasing medium.
Laser medium: A solid or gas that is sensitive to atomic excitation by an energy source, which creates intense laser light and energy.
Lateral position: In this position the patient lies on his or her side for exposure to the opposite lateral chest and flank.
Lateral transfer: Transferring the patient from one horizontal surface to another, such as from a bed to a gurney.
Latex: A naturally occurring substance obtained from the sap of rubber trees and used in the manufacture of medical devices, supplies, and patient care items.
Laws: Standards of conduct that apply to all people in a given society.
Le Fort I fracture: A horizontal fracture of the maxilla that causes the hard palate and alveolar process to become separated from the rest of the maxilla. The fracture extends into the lower nasal septum, lateral maxillary sinus, and palatine bones.
Le Fort II fracture: A fracture that extends from the nasal bone to the frontal processes of the maxilla, lacrimal bones, and inferior orbital floor. It may extend into the orbital foramen. Inferiorly, it extends into the anterior maxillary sinus and the pterygoid plates.
Le Fort III fracture: This fracture involves separation of all the facial bones from their cranial base. It includes fracture of the zygoma, maxilla, and nasal bones.
LEEP: Loop electrode excision procedure. In this technique, an electrosurgical loop is used to remove a core of tissue from the cervical canal.
Leiomyoma: A fibrous, benign tumor of the uterus that usually arises from the myometrium.
Liable: Legally responsible and accountable.
Libel: Defamation of a person in writing.
Licensure: Professional status, granted by state government, which defines the limits (scope) of practice and regulates those who hold a license.
Ligate: To place a loop or tie around a blood vessel or duct.
Light cable: The fiber-optic light cable that transmits light from the source to the endoscopic instrument; sometimes called a *light guide.*
Light source: A device that controls and emits light for endoscopic procedures.
Linea alba: A strip of avascular tissue that follows the midline and extends from the pubis to the xiphoid process.
Lithotomy position: Used for exposure to the perineum for gynecological and urological procedures. In this position the patient's legs are elevated and placed in stirrups or leg crutches.
Living will: A legal document stating the patient's wishes regarding care in the event the patient is unable to speak for himself or herself.
Lobectomy: Surgical removal of one or more anatomical sections of the liver or lung.
Low-level disinfection: A method used to disinfect patient care items that contact only the skin.
Magnetic field: A three-dimensional force pattern created by the positive and negative charges of a polar magnet.
Magnetic resonance imaging (MRI): A diagnostic technique that uses radiofrequency signals and magnetic energy to produce images.
Malignant: A term used to characterize tissue that shows disorganized, uncontrolled growth (cancer). Malignant tissue has the potential to spread to distant areas of the body. It is then termed *metastatic.*
Malignant hyperthermia: A rare state of hypermetabolism that occurs in association with inhalation anesthetics and neuromuscular blocking agents. In extreme cases, the condition causes hyperpyrexia, seizures, and cardiac arrhythmia.
Malpractice: Negligence (as defined by the law) committed by a professional.
Maslow's hierarchy of human needs: A model of human achievement and self-actualization developed by psychologist Abraham Maslow.
Mastectomy: A procedure in which breast tissue, including the skin, areola, and nipple, is removed, but the lymph nodes are not removed (also called a *simple mastectomy*).
Master controllers: In robotic surgery, the nonsterile hand controls that manipulate surgical instruments.
Material Safety Data Sheet (MSDS): A government-mandated requirement for all chemicals used in the workplace. The MSDS describes the formulation, safe use, precautions, and emergency response.
Maxillomandibular fixation (MMF): See Arch bars.
Mayo stand: A small open-ended adjustable table used during surgery. Instruments and supplies to be required immediately are placed on the Mayo stand
McBurney incision: An incision in which the oblique right muscle is manually split to allow for removal of the appendix.
Mean arterial pressure (MAP): The average amount of pressure exerted throughout the cardiac cycle.
Meatotomy: A procedure in which a small incision is made in the urethral meatus to relieve a stricture.
Meconium: Fecal waste that accumulates while the fetus is in the uterus. It is passed within the first few days after birth.
Medical device: Any equipment, instrument, implant, material, or apparatus used in the diagnosis, treatment, or monitoring of patients.
Medical ethics: A branch of ethics concerned with the practice of medicine.
Medical power of attorney: A legal document that confers authority of an individual to make health care decisions for another person.
Menarche: The onset of menstruation, menses.

Menorrhagia: Excessive bleeding during menses.
Message: The idea, concept, thought, or feeling expressed during communication.
Metastasis: The spread of cancerous cells to a local or distant area of the body.
Missed abortion: An abortion in which the products of conception are no longer viable but are retained in the uterus.
Mobility: The ability of an organism to move. As a protective mechanism, mobility allows an organism to move away from harmful stimuli.
Moderate Sedation: Defined by the American Society of Anesthesiologists and the Joint Commission as sedation during a diagnostic or therapeutic procedure that goes no deeper than the moderate stage or lighter. Under moderate sedation, the patient must be able to control his or her own airway.
Modified radical mastectomy: A procedure in which the entire breast, nipple, and areolar region are removed. The lymph nodes also are usually removed.
Mohs surgery: A procedure in which a malignant tissue mass is removed and cut into sections before frozen section. These are used to map the tumor and determine the exact location of malignant margins.
Molecule: A specific substance made up of elements that are bonded together.
Monitored anesthesia care (MAC): Defined by the American Society of Anesthesiologists as sedation at a level appropriate for managing a patient's needs and includes close physiological monitoring. The anesthetist/anesthesiologist must be able to convert to general anesthesia as needed. See Moderate Sedation for differentiation.
Monopolar circuit: In electrosurgery, a continuous path of electricity that flows from the electrosurgical unit to the active electrode, through the patient and the return electrode, and then back to the electrosurgical unit.
Morbid obesity: A condition in which the patient's body mass index (BMI) is 40 or higher, and the individual is at least 100 pounds (45 kg) over the ideal weight.
Muscle recession: Surgery in which the eye muscle is reattached to reposition the globe.
Muscle resection: Surgical shortening of an eye muscle to pull the globe into correct position.
Nasogastric (NG) tube: A flexible tube inserted through the nose and advanced into the stomach. The NG tube is used to decompress the stomach or to provide a means of feeding the patient liquid nutrients and medication.
Nasolaryngoscope: A flexible endoscope that is passed through the nose for visualization of the larynx.
Nasopharyngeal airway: Artificial airway between the nostril and the nasopharynx; used in semiconscious patients or when an oral airway is not feasible.
National Certifying Examination for Surgical Technologists: A comprehensive written examination required for official certification by the Association of Surgical Technologists, developed by NBSTSA.
NBSTSA: National Board of Surgical Technology and Surgical Assisting. NBSTSA (formerly the Liaison Council on Certification for the Surgical Technologist) is responsible for all certification-related decisions, such as eligibility, renewal, and revocation, as well as developing the certification examination.
NCCT: National Center for Competency Testing. A nonprofit organization that provides a certification examination for nonaccredited programs, as well as on-the-job training for other trained surgical technologists whose programs are not recognized by the Association of Surgical Technologists.
Necrosis: Tissue death.
Negligence: Negligence as it applies to health professionals can occur in two ways: it can be a failure to do something that a reasonable person, guided by the ordinary professional considerations would do; or it can be the act of doing something that a reasonable and prudent person would not do.
Neodymium: YAG:A solid lasing medium known for its attraction to protein and deep penetration into tissue.
Neoplasm: A tumor, which may be benign or malignant.
Neuromuscular blocking agent: A drug that blocks nerve conduction in striated muscle tissue.
Neutral zone: An area of the sterile field designated for the exchange of sharps. A magnetic pad or basin can be used for sharps so that hand-to-hand exchange can be avoided.
Neuropathy: Permanent or temporary nerve injury that results in numbness or loss of function of a body part.
Neutron: A subatomic particle located in the nucleus of the atom. It has no electrical charge.
No-hands technique: A method of transferring sharp instruments on the surgical field without hand-to-hand contact. A neutral zone is identified, and sharps are exchanged in this zone.
No-touch technique: All sharp items used in surgery are handled with an instrument, not the hand to prevent injury and transmission of blood-borne disease.
Non-absorbable suture: Suture material that resists breakdown in the body.
Nonconductive: The quality of a substance that resists the transfer of electrons and therefore electrical current.
Nonelectrolyte: Solutions that do not contain electrolytes. These must be used for bladder distention or continuous irrigation whenever electrosurgery is performed.
Non–heart-beating cadaver: A cadaver in which perfusion at and after death was not possible. Only tissues that do not require perfusion may be procured for donation from a non-heart-beating cadaver.
Nonsterile: Applies to objects that have been processed by a sterilization method and shown to have been effective by chemical or biologic tests.
Nonsterile personnel: In surgery, team members who remain outside the boundary of the sterile field and do not come in direct contact with sterile equipment, sterile areas, or the surgical wound. The circulator, anesthesia care provider, and radiographic technician are examples of nonsterile team members.
Nonwoven: A fabric or material that is bonded together as opposed to a process of interweaving individual threads.
Normal spontaneous vaginal delivery (NSVD): A normal delivery of the fetus, without the need for medical intervention.
Norms: Behaviors that are accepted as part of the environment and culture of a group. Norms are usually established by custom and popular acceptance rather than by law, although the two may not be mutually exclusive.
Nosocomial infection: Another term for *hospital-acquired infection (HAI)* or *health care–acquired infection;* an infection acquired as a result of being in a health care facility.
Nuchal cord: A complication of pregnancy in which the umbilical cord is wrapped around the neck of the fetus. This may lead to obstructed blood flow to the fetus.
Nuclear medicine: Medical procedures that use radioactive particles to track and target tissues in the body.
Nucleus: The center of an atom.
Obturator: A blunt-nosed rod that is inserted through the sheath of a rigid endoscope or hysteroscope to protect the tissue as the instrument is advanced.

Occlusion: In maxillofacial surgery, this refers to the patient's bite pattern when the jaw is closed.

Occupational exposure: Exposure to hazards in the workplace; for example, exposure to hazardous chemicals or contact with potentially infected blood and body fluids.

Odontectomy: Tooth extraction.

Onset: The point at which a drug begins to exert a physiological effect in the body.

Operating room (OR): A designated room in the surgical suite that qualifies as a restricted area where surgery and other invasive procedures that require an aseptic field can be performed. The term *OR* is often used to refer to the entire surgical department or surgical suite.

Opportunistic infection: Infection in a weakened individual, or as a result of specific drugs, usually by colonization of a bacterium that does not usually cause disease. The host may be debilitated by another disease or their immune system may be compromised.

Optical angle: The angle at which light is transmitted at the distal end of an endoscope.

Optical resonant cavity: The component of a laser system in which the lasing medium is contained and light is transformed.

Oromaxillofacial surgery: Surgery involving the bones of the face, primarily for repair of fractures and reconstruction of congenital anomalies.

Oropharyngeal airway (OPA): Artificial airway that is inserted over the tongue into the larynx; used in patients in whom endotracheal intubation is difficult or contraindicated.

ORT: Operating room technician. Former name for surgical technologists (the name was changed to *surgical technologist* in the early 1970s).

Orthostatic (postural) blood pressure: Refers to a technique used to check the patient's blood pressure in the upright and recumbent positions.

Ossicles: The bones of the middle ear that conduct sound (i.e., the malleus, incus, and stapes).

-ostomy: A suffix that refers to an opening between two hollow organs—for example, gastroduodenostomy, a surgical procedure that joins the stomach and duodenum.

Ostomy: A technique in which a new opening is made between a tubular structure such as the intestine or ureter and the outside of the body.

Ototoxic: A substance that can injure the ear.

Oxidizers: Agents or substances capable of supporting fire.

Oxygen-enriched atmosphere (OEA): An environment that contains a high percentage of oxygen and therefore presents a high risk for fire.

Packing: A method of applying a dressing to a body cavity. In nasal procedures, ¼- or ½-inch (0.63- or 1.25-cm) gauze strips are inserted into the nasal cavity to absorb drainage, control bleeding, or expose the mucosa to topical medication. "Packing" a wound may refer to any dressing that is introduced into an anatomical space or cavity.

Palpating: Assessing a part of the body by feeling the outline, density, movement, or other attributes.

Papanicolaou (Pap) test: A diagnostic test in which epithelial cells are taken from the endocervical canal and examined for abnormalities that can lead to cervical cancer.

Papilloma: A benign epithelial tumor characterized by a branching or lobular tumor (also called a *papillary tumor*).

Paranasal sinuses: Air cells surrounding or on the periphery of the nasal cavities. These are the maxillary, ethmoid, sphenoid, and frontal sinuses.

Parenteral: Refers to administration of a drug by injection.

Paresis: Paralysis of a structure (e.g., vocal cord paresis).

Partial thromboplastin time (PTT): A test of blood coagulation used in patients receiving heparin to determine the correct level of anticoagulation.

Parturition: Birth.

Pathogen: A disease-causing (pathogenic) microorganism.

Patient return electrode (PRE): A critical component of the monopolar electrosurgical circuit, the PRE is a conductive pad that captures electricity and shunts it safely out of the body and back to the electrosurgical unit.

Patient-centered care: Therapeutic care, communication, and intervention provided according to the unique needs of the patient and centered on those needs.

Peak effect: The period of maximum effect of a drug.

Peracetic acid: A chemical used in the sterilization of critical items.

Percutaneous: A term for a procedure that is performed "through the skin." For example, in percutaneous nephroscopy, the nephroscope is inserted into the kidney through a skin incision.

Perforation: A defect in the tympanic membrane caused by trauma or infection.

Perfusion: Circulation of blood to specific tissue, organ, system, or the whole body. Perfusion is necessary to maintain cell life.

Perineum: The anatomical area between the posterior vestibule and the anus.

Periodic table: A standardized chart of all known elements.

Perjury: The crime of intentionally lying or falsifying information during court testimony after a person has sworn to tell the truth.

Personal protective equipment (PPE): Clothing or equipment that protects the wearer from direct contact with hazardous chemicals or potentially infectious body fluids.

Personnel policy: A policy that sets forth the health care facility's job descriptions, role delineations, requirements for employment, and rules of conduct for personnel.

Phacoemulsification: A process whereby high-frequency sound waves are used to emulsify tissue, such as a cataract.

Pharmacodynamics: The biochemical and physiological effects of drugs and their mechanisms of action in the body.

Pharmacokinetics: The movement of a drug through the tissues and cells of the body, including the processes of absorption, distribution, and localization in tissues; biotransformation; and excretion by mechanical and chemical means.

Pharmacology: The study of drugs and their action in the body.

Phonation: Vibration of the vocal cords during speaking or vocalization.

Photo damage: Damage to the skin caused by ultraviolet light.

Photon: In physics, the name given to a light particle.

Physical barrier: In surgery, a barrier that separates a sterile surface from a nonsterile surface. Examples are sterile surgical gloves, gowns, and drapes. A physical barrier, such as a clean surgical cap, prevents a bacteria-laden surface, such as the hair, from shedding microorganisms.

Physical monitor: A device that automatically provides output on the physical parameters of the sterilization process. Output includes printouts, gauges, and a digital display.

Physiological: Refers to the biochemical and metabolic processes of an organism.

Physiological monitoring: Assessment of the patient's vital metabolic functions.

PID: Pelvic inflammatory disease, caused by a sexually transmitted disease. It causes scarring of the fallopian tubes and adhesions in the abdominal and pelvic cavities.

Pixel: The smallest unit of color displayed as a computer image. The entire image is made up of many pixels.

Placenta: The organ that transfers selected nutrients to the fetus during pregnancy.

Placenta previa: A complication of pregnancy in which the placenta implants completely or partly over the cervical os. In this position, the placenta begins to bleed as it separates from the cervix during labor.

Placental abruption: Premature separation of the placenta from the uterine wall after 20 weeks' gestation and before the fetus is delivered.

Plasma: A gaseous state in which the atom's nucleus becomes separated from the electrons.

Plication: Folding of tissue and securing it in place surgically.

Pneumatic tourniquet: An air-filled tourniquet used to prevent blood flow to an extremity during surgery.

Pneumoperitoneum: Distension of the abdomen with carbon dioxide gas during laparoscopy. This is necessary to visualize the surgical anatomy.

Polyp: Excessive proliferation of the mucosal epithelium.

Porcine: Derived from pig tissue.

Port: In minimally invasive surgery, an opening in the body created by a sharp trocar or blunt obturator and maintained with a cannula that remains in place to receive MIS instruments during surgery.

Post-exposure prophylaxis (PEP): Voluntary procedures a person may undertake following potential exposure to blood-borne pathogens.

Positive air flow: The operating room environment is engineered for positive and negative pressure areas to maintain asepsis. A positive pressure system is maintained in areas where clean air is critically important. A high pressure gradient prevents air from less-clean areas from entering the critical area.

Positron emission tomography (PET): A type of medical imaging that measures specific metabolic activity in the target tissue.

Postanesthesia care unit (PACU): The critical care area where patients are taken after surgery for monitoring and evaluation as they emerge from anesthesia.

Postexposure prophylaxis (PEP): Recommended procedures to help prevent the development of blood-borne diseases after an exposure incident such as a needlestick injury.

Postmortem care: Physical care of the body to prepare it for viewing by the family and for mortuary procedures.

Potassium-titanyl-phosphate (KTP): A low-power lasing medium that produces a very small diameter beam well suited to microsurgery.

Practice acts: State laws that establish and regulate the conditions under which professionals may practice including licensure, registration, educational requirements, scope of duties, and functions.

Prenatal: The period of pregnancy before birth.

Preoperative medication: One or more drugs administered before surgery to prevent complications related to the surgical procedure or anesthesia.

Prescription: An order for a licensed drug written by an authorized health care provider.

Presentation: Refers to the part of the baby that descends into the birth canal first.

Primary intention: The wound-healing process after a clean surgical repair.

Prion: An infectious protein particle that is a unique pathogenic substance containing no nucleic acid. The prion is resistant to most forms of disinfection and sterilization normally used in the health care setting.

Procedure room: A treatment area for procedures that do not require an aseptic field but may be performed using sterile instruments and supplies. It may be located in the surgical department or in a separate area of the facility.

Process challenge monitoring: A sealed, harmless bacteria sample included in a load of goods to be sterilized. The sample is recovered after the sterilization process and cultured to test for viability.

Professional attributes: Positive behaviors and traits of a professional, highly regarded by the public and professional peers. They include traits such as honesty, reliability, tact, diplomacy, and commitment to the profession.

Professional ethics: Ethical behavior established by authoritative peers of a particular profession, such as medicine or law.

Prognosis: A prediction of the patient's medical outcome (e.g., poor prognosis, good prognosis).

Proprietary name: The patented name given to a drug by its manufacturer.

Proprietary school: Private, for-profit school.

Protective reflexes: Nervous system responses to harmful environmental stimuli, such as pain, obstruction of the airway, and extreme temperature. Coughing, blinking, shivering, and withdrawal (from painful stimuli) are protective reflexes.

Prothrombin time (PT): A measurement of the time required for blood to clot.

Pterygium: A triangular membrane that arises from the medial canthus; the tissue may extend over the cornea, causing blindness.

Ptosis: Drooping or sagging of any anatomical structure.

Pulmonary embolism (PE): An obstruction in a pulmonary vessel caused by a blood clot, air bubble, or foreign body. The embolism causes sudden pain and loss of oxygen to the tissues that are served by the obstructed vessel.

Pulse oximeter: A monitoring device that measures the patient's hemoglobin oxygen saturation by means of spectrometry.

Pulse pressure: A measurement of the difference between the systolic pressure and diastolic pressure. This can be a significant sign of metabolic disturbance.

Pulsed-wave lasers: Lasers that apply the laser light intermittently to the target tissue.

Punitive: Actions intended to punish a person who has violated the law.

Q-switched lasers: An alternate name for pulsed-wave lasers.

Radiant exposure: In laser technology, the combination of the concentration of laser energy and the length of time tissue is exposed to it.

Radioactive seeds: Small particles of radioactive material implanted in tissue for cancer treatment.

Radiofrequency: Electromagnetic energy in which the frequency is in the area of radio transmission. In electrosurgery, radiofrequency electromagnetic waves are used to produce the desired surgical effect.

Radionuclides or isotopes: In nuclear medicine, radioactive particles are directed at the nucleus of a selected element to create energy. These special elements are referred to as radionuclides or isotopes.

Radiopaque: A substance that is impenetrable by x-rays.

Range of motion: The normal anatomical movement of an extremity.

Raytec: A surgical sponge folded to 4 inches by 4 inches. The Raytec derives its name from one of the companies that manufactures surgical sponges.

Receiver: The person to whom a message is communicated by a sender.

Reduce: To manipulate herniated tissue back into its normal anatomical position.

Reflection: Communication with the patient that helps the individual connect his or her current feelings with events in the environment.

Reflux: Flow of a body fluid in the direction opposite its normal path. Urinary reflux is backward flow of urine into the ureter or kidney.

Refraction: A phenomenon of physics in which light rays are bent as they pass through a transparent medium that is denser than air. In the eye, refraction occurs as light enters the front of the eye and passes through the cornea, lens, aqueous humor, and vitreous.

Regional block: Anesthesia in a specific area of the body, achieved by injection of an anesthetic around a major nerve or group of nerves.

Regulations: Laws that are enforced by state and federal agencies.

Reprocessing: Activities or tasks that prepare contaminated medical devices for use on another patient.

Required request law: A law requiring medical personnel to request organ recovery from a deceased's family.

Resection: A surgical technique in which a section of an organ or tissue is usually removed because of disease or trauma. Resection requires closure or repair of the remaining tissue edges along the line of resection.

Resectoscope: A surgical endoscope used in morcellation or tissue fragmentation.

Resident flora: Microorganisms are normally present in specific tissues. Resident flora is necessary to the function of these tissues or structures—also called *normal flora.*

Resident microorganisms: The microorganisms that normally colonize certain tissues of the body, usually without harm to the host.

Residual activity: The antimicrobial action of an antiseptic or a disinfectant that continues after the solution has dried.

Resistance: In electricity, the measurement of a substance's ability to inhibit the flow of electricity.

Restricted area: A designated space within the operating room department where surgical and other invasive procedures are performed. Traffic in the restricted area is limited to authorized personnel and patients who may only enter the area through a semi-restricted area. Patients and personnel must wear surgical attire and cover the head and facial hair. Masks are required in the presence of open sterile supplies or where personnel are in the process of scrubbing or have completed the surgical scrub.

Restricted zone: An area of the operating room with the highest level asepsis. The main difference between semi-restricted and restricted is the requirement for surgical masks in restricted zones.

Retained foreign object: An item that is inadvertently left inside the patient during surgery.

Retention catheter: A type of urinary catheter that remains in place. Also called an *indwelling* or *Foley catheter.*

Retrograde pyelography: Imaging studies of the renal pelvis in which a contrast medium is instilled through a transurethral catheter. Retrograde refers to flow, which is opposite the normal direction.

Return electrode monitoring (REM): A safety system used in electrosurgery in which the PRE transmits continuous feedback on the quality of impedance in the electrode and stops the current when it becomes dangerously high.

Reusable: A designation used by manufacturers to indicate that a medical device can be reprocessed for use on more than one patient.

Reverse cutting needing: A suture needle containing a sharp edge along the inside curve.

Reverse Trendelenburg: A position in which the operating table is tilted downward feet first.

Rigor mortis: The natural stiffening of the body that starts approximately 15 minutes after death and lasts about 24 hours.

Ring stand: A stainless steel frame designed to hold sterile fluid basins during surgery.

Risk: The statistical probability of a given event on the basis of the number of such events that have already occurred in a defined population.

Risk management: The process of tracking, evaluating, and studying accidents and incidents to protect patients and employees.

Robot: A mechanical device that can be programmed to perform tasks.

Role confusion: Lack of clarity about one's job duties and responsibilities.

Roller board: A lateral transfer device composed of serial rollers covered in heavy plastic fabric.

Rongeur: A hinged instrument with sharp, cupped tips that is used to extract pieces of bone or other connective tissue.

Rule of nines: A method of estimating the percentage of burned tissue which relates to the patient's prognosis.

Rumor: Information with questionable validity.

Running suture: A method of suturing that uses one continuous suture strand for tissue approximation.

Safe Medical Device Act: A federal regulation that requires the reporting of any incident causing death or injury that is suspected to be the result of a medical device.

Scrub: Role and name commonly applied to the surgical technologist or licensed nurse in the sterile scrub role during surgery.

Scrubbed personnel: In surgery, members of the surgical team who have performed hand antisepsis, donned sterile attire, and move within the sterile field. Also called *sterile personnel.*

Sedation: A state of consciousness in which an individual is only partially aware of sensory stimuli. Depression of the central nervous system. Deep sedation results in loss of sensory awareness.

Sedative: A drug that induces a range of unconscious states. The effects are dose dependent. At low doses, sedatives cause some drowsiness. Increasing the dose causes central nervous system depression, ending in loss of consciousness.

Segmental resection: Surgical removal of tissue or an organ in segments defined by its blood supply.

Selective absorption: The absorption of a lasing medium into tissue being lased, according to its color and density.

Semi-restricted area: A designated area in the surgery department in which personnel must wear surgical attire and cover the head and facial hair.

Semi-restricted zone: An area of the operating room that has specific requirements for the use of surgical attire and access to other areas of the department.

Sender: The person who communicates a message to another.

Sensation: The ability to feel stimuli in the environment (e.g., pain, heat, touch, visual stimuli, sound).

Sensorineural hearing loss: Hearing impairment arising from the cochlea, auditory nerve, or central nervous system.

Sentinel event: An unexpected incident resulting in serious physical injury, psychological harm, or death. The near miss of injury or harm is also considered a sentinel event.

Sentinel lymph node biopsy (SLNB): A procedure in which one or more lymph nodes are removed to determine whether a tumor has metastasized. Other lymph nodes may be removed periodically to determine whether metastasis has occurred.

Serosa: The delicate outer tissue layer of most organs.

Serosanguineous fluid: Exudate or discharge containing serum and blood.
Sexual harassment: An extreme abuse of power in which an individual uses sexualized language, gestures, or unwanted touch to coerce or intimidate another person.
Shank: The area between the tip and the finger ring of an instrument.
Sharps: Any object that can penetrate the skin and has the potential to cause injury and infection. Sharps include but are not limited to needles, scalpels, broken glass, and exposed ends of dental wires.
Shear injury: Tissue injury or necrosis occurring when two tissue planes are forcefully pulled in opposite directions. Shearing usually occurs when the body is pulled or slides by gravity across a high-friction surface, such as a bed sheet.
Side effects: Anticipated effects of a drug other than those intended. Side effects may be uncomfortable for the patient or may have a positive outcome.
Single-action rongeur: A bone-cutting instrument that has one hinge.
Single-stage prep: Also called a *paint prep.* The skin prep is performed using only antiseptic solution, which is applied to the skin at the operative site.
Single-use items: Instruments and devices intended for one-time use on one patient only.
Skin flap: A flap that is created by an incision made in the skin, which is cut away from the underlying tissue to which it is attached. The flap can be increased in size or "raised" as it is enlarged by dissection.
Slander: Spoken defamation.
Smoke plume: Smoke created during the use of an electrosurgical unit (ESU) or laser. This smoke contains toxic chemicals, vapors, blood fragments, and viruses.
Solid: A state of matter in which the molecules are bonded very tightly. Characteristics of solids are hardness and the ability to break apart into other solid pieces.
Solution: Any liquid drug or chemical combined with water.
Spatula needle: A flat-tipped suture needle commonly used in ophthalmic surgery.
Spaulding system: A system used to determine the level of microbial destruction required for medical devices and supplies. Each level is based on the risk of infection associated with the area of the body where the device is used.
Specific gravity: The ratio of the density of a fluid compared to water. The specific gravity of urine is an important diagnostic tool.
Sphygmomanometer: An instrument used to measure blood pressure.
Split-thickness (or partial-thickness) skin graft (STSG): A skin graft that consists of the epidermis and a portion of the papillary dermis.
Sporicidal: Able to kill spores.
Spray coagulation: An alternate term for fulguration.
Squames: Dead flattened skin cells that are normally shed from the epidermis as new skin cells emerge. Squames can be laden with potentially pathogenic bacteria.
Squaring the incision: Refers to placing four towels in a square around the incision site.
Staghorn stone: A large, jagged kidney stone that forms in the renal pelvis.
Staging: An international method of classifying tissue to determine the level of metastasis in cancer.
Standard definition (SD): A type of video format. The clarity of an image is based on the number of signals (pixels) emitted by the camera. A standard definition format displays 640 × 480 pixels in a rectangular image.
Standard Precautions: Guidelines issued by the Centers for Disease Control and Prevention (CDC) to reduce the risk of disease transmitted by blood-borne and other pathogens.
Standards of conduct: A set of rules or guidelines an organization establishes for its members. The rules pertain to how people behave and are based on the principles that the organization values, such as professionalism and personal integrity.
States of matter: The physical forms of matter. The four states of matter are gas, liquid, solid, and plasma.
Static electricity: The buildup of charged particles on a surface.
Statutes: Laws passed by state legislative bodies.
Stent: A supportive catheter that is placed in a duct or tube to allow fluids to pass through.

Stereoscopic viewer:
Sterile: Completely free of all microorganisms.

In robotic surgery, the binocular lens system of the surgeon's console.

Sterile field: An area that includes the draped patient, all sterile tables, and sterile equipment in the immediate area of the patient. The surgical incision is the center of the sterile field.
Sterile item: Any item or medical device that has been exposed to a process that destroys all microbes, including spores.
Sterile team member: Members of the surgical team who have performed a surgical scrub or hand and arm antisepsis procedure. They don sterile gown and gloves and either perform the surgery or assist. Sterile personnel include the surgeon, assistant(s), and scrub.
Sterile setup: The process of organizing and arranging sterile supplies and equipment before surgery to create the sterile field.
Sterility: A state in which an inanimate surface or tissue harbors absolutely no viable microorganisms.
Sterilization: A process by which all microorganisms, including bacterial spores, are destroyed.
Stoma appliance: A two- or three-piece medical device used to collect drainage from a stoma. The appliance is attached to the patient's skin and completely covers the stoma. This allows for free drainage into a collection device or bag.
Stoma: An opening created in a hollow organ and sutured to the skin to drain the organ's contents (e.g., an intestinal or ureteral stoma). A stoma may be a temporary or permanent method of bypass.
STD: Sexually transmitted disease: Sexually transmitted diseaseThis acronym is used among *medical practitioners*. The term STI (sexually transmitted infection) is a more socially acceptable term, used more commonly in social contexts.
Strabismus: Inability to coordinate the extraocular muscles, which prevents binocular vision.
Straight catheter: A urinary catheter used to drain the bladder one time (sometimes called a *Robinson catheter*).
Strangulated hernia: A hernia in which abdominal tissue has become trapped between the layers of an abdominal wall defect. The strangulated tissue usually becomes swollen as a result of venous congestion. Lack of blood supply can lead to tissue necrosis.
Stricture: A narrowing in a lumen such as the esophagus or urethra, caused by disease or trauma.
Strike-through contamination: An event in which a sterile surface becomes contaminated by liquid or fluid wicked from a nonsterile surface.
Subcutaneous mastectomy: A procedure in which the breast is removed, but the skin, nipple, and areola are left intact (also called a *lumpectomy*).
Subpoena: A court order requiring its recipient to appear and testify at a trial or deposition. Medical records can also be the subject of subpoenas.

Suppurative: Having developed pus and fluid.

Surgeon's preference card: A database or card system listing the methods, materials, and techniques used by each surgeon for specific procedures.

Surgical conscience: In surgery, the ethical motivation to practice excellent aseptic technique to protect the patient from infection. Surgical conscience implies that the health care professional practices excellent technique, regardless of whether others are observing.

Surgical scrub: A specific technique for scrubbing the hands and arms before donning sterile surgical gown and gloves just before surgery. The scrub is performed with timed or counted strokes using detergent-based antiseptic.

Surgical site infection (SSI): Postoperative infection of the surgical wound. An SSI may be caused by contamination during surgery or acquired during the healing process.

Surgical wound: All the tissue layers of the surgical incision.

Swage: The area of an atraumatic suture where the suture strand is fused to the needle.

Synthetic grafts: Grafts derived from synthetic material compatible with body tissue. Synthetic grafts may be soft, semisolid, or liquid.

Systolic pressure: The pressure exerted by blood on the walls of vessels during the contraction phase of the cardiac cycle.

Tamponade: An instrument or other device that puts pressure on tissue to control bleeding.

Tapered needle: A suture needle that has a round body that tapers to a sharp point.

Technetium-99: A radioactive substance used to identify sentinel lymph nodes.

Tenaculum: A grasping instrument with sharp pointed tips, generally used to manipulate or grasp tissue.

Tensile strength: The amount of force or stress a suture can withstand before breaking.

Terminal cleaning: A daily process in which exposed surfaces of the operating room are cleaned and disinfected.

The Joint Commission: The accrediting organization for hospitals and other health care facilities in the United States.

Therapeutic communication: A purposeful method of communication in which the caregiver responds to the explicit or implicit needs of the patient.

Therapeutic touch: The purposeful touching of another person to convey empathy, care, and comfort.

Therapeutic window: Range of drug doses that are effective without causing toxicity.

Thermal conductivity: The ability of a substance to conduct heat. Different substances have different abilities to conduct or transmit heat.

Thermoregulation: A complex physiological process in which the body maintains a temperature that is optimal for survival.

Throw: A loop that forms a knot.

Tie on a passer: A strand of suture material attached to the tip of an instrument.

TIMEOUT: A procedure in which the surgical team affirms the identity of the patient, correct procedure, and location (side), verification of informed consent, and other documents necessary to proceed with the surgery—formally called the *Universal Protocol*. The procedure is mandated by The Joint Commission.

Tincture: Any chemical or substance combined with alcohol.

TM: The tympanic membrane.

TNM classification system: An international system for determining the extent of metastasis and the level of cell differentiation, two important factors in the treatment and prognosis of cancer.

Topical: Refers to the application of a drug to the skin or mucous membranes.

Topical anesthesia: Anesthesia of superficial nerves of the skin or mucous membranes.

Torsion: Twisting of an organ or a structure on itself. Torsion may cause local ischemia and necrosis.

Tort: Legal wrongdoing that results in injury to a person or property.

Traction injury: A nerve injury caused by stretching or compression of the nerve.

Trade name: The name given to a drug by the company that produces and sells it.

Traffic patterns: The movement of people and equipment into, out of, and within the surgical environment.

Transcervical: Literally, "through the cervix." In surgery, a transcervical approach means that surgery is performed by passing instruments through the cervix.

Transcutaneous: Literally "through the skin"; it refers to a procedure in which a needle or other medical device is inserted through the skin.

Transdermal: Refers to administration of a drug by absorption through the skin, such as with ointments or patches impregnated with the drug.

Transfer board: A plastic board that is used during a lateral transfer.

Transient flora: Microorganisms that do not normally colonize in tissue but are the result of contact with the environment.

Transitional area: An area in which surgical personnel or visitors prepare to enter the semi-restricted areas. Transitional areas include the locker rooms and changing rooms.

Transmission-based precautions: Guidelines to prevent the spread of infectious disease by patients known to be infected.

Transsphenoidal: Literally, "across or through the sphenoid bone." Surgery of the pituitary gland may be performed by approaching it through the sphenoid bone.

Transurethral: Surgical access through the urethral orifice. The term also may describe an instrument that enters the bladder through the urethral meatus.

Trendelenburg position: The position in which a prone or supine patient is tilted with the head down.

Tumor marker: An antigen present on the tumor cell, or a substance (protein, hormone, or other chemical) released by cancer cells into the blood.

Tunable dye laser: A type of laser formed by the combination of argon gas and specific dyes that alter tissue absorption of the lasing beam.

Turnover: Cleaning, disinfection, and preparation of the operating room between patients.

Two-stage prep: Preparation of the skin including washing with antiseptic soap followed by application of antiseptic tincture or solution.

U.S. Pharmacopeia (USP): An organization that establishes standards for drugs approved by the U.S. Food and Drug Administration (FDA) for their labeled use. All approved drugs have been tested for consumer safety, and written information is available about their pharmacological action, use, risks, and dosage.

Ultrasonic energy: High-frequency energy created by vibration or excitation of molecules. This type of energy destroys tissue by breaking molecular bonds.

Ultrasound: A technology that transforms high-frequency wave energy into visual images on a screen.

Unconsciousness: Neurological state characterized by complete inability to respond to external stimuli. Unconsciousness can be induced with drugs or may be caused by trauma or disease.

Undermine: A surgical technique in which a plane of tissue is created or an existing tissue plane is lifted.

Underwriters Laboratories (UL): A nonprofit agency that tests and certifies electrical equipment in the United States.

Universal Protocol: A procedure for verifying the patient's identity, correct surgical procedure, site, and side. The procedure is initiated as a TIMEOUT and takes place after the patient has been positioned, prepped, and draped but before the first incision.

Unrestricted area: An area of the surgical environment in which people dressed in street clothes may enter.

Unrestricted zone: An area of the operating room that is maintained at the lowest level of asepsis.

Unretrieved device fragment: A portion of a medical device that has broken off or come apart in the body and is not detected or removed. Examples are fragments of a broken surgical needle or a hinge pin of a surgical instrument.

Vector: A living intermediate carrier of microorganisms from one host to another.

Ventilation: The mechanical process of pulling air into the lungs during inhalation and the released of carbon dioxide during exhalation.

Ventral hernia: A weakness in the abdominal wall, usually resulting in protrusion of abdominal viscera against the peritoneum and abdominal fascia.

Verbal abuse: Deliberate attempts to devalue, intimidate, bully, or embarrass another person using loud, vulgar, sexualized, or intimidating language.

Vertical abuse: Bullying, attempts to devalue, intimidate, or embarrass an individual. This occurs between two people of different levels of hierarchy in an organization.

Virion: A complete virus particle.

Virulence: The degree to which a microorganism is capable of causing disease.

Viscera: The organs or tissue of the abdominal cavity.

Vital signs: Cardinal signs of well-being: pain, temperature, pulse, respiration, and blood pressure. These are measured to assess a patient's basic metabolic status.

Volatile: A substance with a low boiling point such as alcohol that converts to a vapor at low temperature.

Voltage: The electrical force in a circuit, measured as the amount of force that passes a given point over a stated period.

Washer–sterilizer/disinfector: Equipment that washes and decontaminates instruments so that they can be safely handled by personnel.

Wave: In physics, a naturally occurring phenomenon in which energy is transmitted in the form of peaks (high points) and troughs (low points).

Wavelength: The distance between peaks in a complete wave cycle.

White balance: A procedure for adjusting the light color of the video camera to other components of the system.

Win–lose solution: In conflict resolution, a solution that leaves one party satisfied but the other party dissatisfied.

Win–win solution: In conflict resolution, a solution that allows both parties in a conflict to gain.

Wire localization: A biopsy procedure in which a hook wire is inserted (under fluoroscopy) into tissue suspected of being cancerous to identify its location.

World Wide Web: In computer technology, a network of links to data via an Internet system. The Web uses a special computer language protocol and is only one of many types of systems for transmitting data through a computer network.

Woven wrappers: Also called *linen* or *cloth wrappers,* these are fabric cloths used to wrap clean, disinfected supplies in preparation for a sterilization process.

Xenograft: A graft made up of tissue taken from one species and grafted into another species (e.g., a porcine graft implanted into human tissue).

INDEX

Note: Page numbers followed by *f*, *t*, or *b* indicate figures, tables, or boxes, respectively.

D

E

N

O

P

Q

R

X

Y

Z

SURGICAL PROCEDURES

CHAPTER 22 General Surgery
Open Repair of an Indirect Inguinal Hernia
Laparoscopic Repair of a Direct Inguinal Hernia (TAPP Approach)
Robotic Repair of an Indirect Inguinal Hernia
Open Repair of Incisional Hernia
Incisional Hernia Repair (Laparoscopic)
Umbilical Hernia Repair (Open)
Repair of Umbilical Hernia (Laparoscopic)
Laparotomy
Gastrectomy, Billroth I and II (Open)
Laparoscopic Band Gastroplasty
Roux-En-Y Gastric Bypass (Laparoscopic)
Nissen Fundoplication (Laparoscopic)
Segmental Resection of the Small Intestine (Open)
End Ileostomy
Intestinal Stoma
Right Hemicolectomy (Open)
Robotic Assisted Low Anterior Resection (LAR)
Appendectomy (Laparoscopic)
Excisional Hemorrhoidectomy
Surgical Treatment for Anal Fistula
Cholecystectomy (Laparoscopic)
Cholecystectomy (Open)
Splenectomy
Splenectomy (Laparoscopic)
Pancreaticoduodenectomy (Whipple Procedure)
Segmental Resection of the Liver (Open)
Wire Localization and Breast Biopsy
Sentinel Lymph Node Biopsy
Breast-Conserving Surgery for a Mass (Lumpectomy, Segmental Mastectomy) with Axillary Dissection
Modified Radical Mastectomy
Minimally Invasive Video-Assisted Thyroidectomy (MIVAT)
Thyroidectomy (Open)

CHAPTER 23 Gynecological and Obstetrical Surgery
Hysteroscopic Endometrial Ablation
Myomectomy
Dilation and Curettage
Vaginal Hysterectomy
Repair of a Cystocele and Rectocele (Anterior-Posterior Repair)
Repair of a Vesicovaginal Fistula
Removal of a Bartholin Gland Cyst
Simple Vulvectomy
Removal of Condyloma Acuminata
Laparoscopic Management of and Ovarian Cyst
Tuboplasty
Diagnostic Laparoscopy
Laparoscopic Tubal Ligation
Laparoscopic Management of an Ovarian Mass
Laparoscopic-Assisted Vaginal Hysterectomy
Total Abdominal Hysterectomy with Bilateral Salpingo-oophorectomy
Robotic-Assisted Hysterectomy
Radical Hysterectomy with Lymphadenectomy
Pelvic Exenteration
Cesarean Delivery

CHAPTER 24 Genitourinary Surgery
Routine Diagnostic Cystoscopy
Transurethral Resection of a Bladder Tumor (TURBT)
Cystectomy with the Ileal Conduit
Percutaneous Nephrolithotomy (PCNL)
Simple Nephrectomy (Flank Incision)
Kidney Transplant
Transurethral Resection of the Prostate
Simple Prostatectomy (Suprapubic)
Perineal Prostatectomy (Open)
Robotic-Assisted Laparoscopic Prostatectomy (RALP)
Circumcision (Adult)
Partial Penectomy
Insertion of Penile Implant
Hydrocelectomy
Orchiectomy

CHAPTER 25 Ophthalmic Surgery
Excision of a Chalazion
Dacryocystorhinostomy
Muscle Resection and Recession
Penetrating Keratoplasty (Corneal Transplantation)
Extracapsular Cataract Extraction (Phacoemulsification)
Anterior Vitrectomy
Scleral Buckling Procedure for Detached Retina
Filtering Procedures and Trabeculectomy
Removal of the Eye
Repair of Entropion Lower Lid
Repair of Ectropion Lower Lid

CHAPTER 26 Surgery of the Ear, Nose, Pharynx, and Larynx
Endoscopic Tympanotomy
Myringotomy
Myringoplasty
Tympanoplasty
Mastoidectomy
Stapedectomy
Cochlear Implant
Endoscopic Sinus Surgery
Caldwell-Luc Procedure
Turbinectomy/Turbinate Reduction
Septoplasty
Open Rhinoplasty
Tonsillectomy
Adenoidectomy
Uvulopalatopharyngoplasty
Laryngoscopy
Tracheotomy/Tracheostomy
Parotidectomy
Modified Radical Neck Dissection
Glossectomy
Laryngectomy
Temporomandibular Joint Arthroplasty

CHAPTER 27 Oral and Maxillofacial Surgery
Open Reduction and Internal Fixation: Orbital Floor Fracture
Maxillomandibular Fixation (Application of Arch Bars)
Open Reduction/Internal Fixation: Midface Fracture
Open Reduction and Internal Fixation: Mandibular Fracture
Tooth Extraction

CHAPTER 28 Plastic and Reconstructive Surgery
Surgical Management of Burns
Debridement of Burns
Split-Thickness Skin Graft
Full-Thickness Skin Graft
Flap Graft
Mohs Micrographic Surgery